The Comparative
Guide to
American Hospitals

Volume 2

Second Edition

The Comparative Guide to American Hospitals

Volume 2: Southern Region

4,383 Hospitals with Key Personnel and
24 Quality Measures in Treating Heart Attack, Heart Failure,
Pneumonia, Pregnancy and Surgical Infection Prevention

A SEDGWICK PRESS Book

Grey House
Publishing

PUBLISHER . . . . Leslie Mackenzie
EDITOR. . . . . David Garoogian
EDITORIAL DIRECTOR. . . . . Laura Mars-Proietti
PRODUCTION MANAGER . . . . Karen Stevens
MARKETING DIRECTOR . . . . Jessica Moody

A Sedgewick Press Book
Grey House Publishing, Inc.
185 Millerton Road
Millerton, NY 12546
518.789.8700
FAX 518.789.0545
www.greyhouse.com
e-mail: books @greyhouse.com

10 9 8 7 6 5 4 3 2

Comparative guide to American hospitals. Vol. 1, Eastern region; [ed. David Garoogian]. -- 2nd ed. (2007)

   v. ; cm.

   Includes index.
   "4,383 hospitals with key personnel and 24 quality measures in treating heart attack, heart failure, pneumonia, pregnancy and surgical infection prevention."

1. Hospitals--United States--Directories. 2. Hospitals--United States--Periodicals. 3. Hospitals--Ratings--United States--Statistics--Periodicals. 4. Myocardial infarction--Hospitals--United States--Directories. 5. Heart failure--Hospitals--United States--Directories. 6. Pneumonia--Hospitals--United States--Directories. I. Garoogian, David.

RA977 .C66
610/.025

4-Volume Set	ISBN: 978-1-59237-182-2
Volume 1	ISBN: 978-1-59237-280-5
Volume 2	**ISBN: 978-1-59237-281-2**
Volume 3	ISBN: 978-1-59237-282-9
Volume 4	ISBN: 978-1-59237-283-6

Table of Contents

Introduction
User's Guide

Section One

Hospital Rankings and Profiles

Alabama. 1

Arkansas 40

Florida 68

Georgia 141

Louisiana 192

Mississippi. 234

Puerto Rico 265

South Carolina. 284

Texas 309

Section Two

State-by-State Statistical Summary. 433

Appendix A

Hospital Mortality. 457

Appendix B

Glossary of Terms. 463

Index

Hospital Profile Index. 467

Introduction

Welcome to the second edition of *The Comparative Guide to American Hospitals*. It reports on how 4,383 hospitals in America measure up when caring for patients with a number of specific conditions. The first edition reported on **Heart Attacks, Heart Failure** and **Pneumonia**. In this second edition, each hospital profile includes additional data on **Pregnancy Care** and **Surgical Infection Prevention**. Also new are two Appendixes - **30-Day Mortality Data** and **Glossary of Terms**.

The content of this work is based on a Federal study (Hospital Compare) in which short-term acute care and critical access hospitals around the country voluntarily reported on quality measures in order to receive an incentive payment established by the Medicare Prescription Drug, Improvement and Modernization Act of 2003. Each hospital is rated on 24 recognized quality measures - **Seven More Than Last Edition** -- and is compared to both state and national averages, and to the top hospitals in the country (best practices).

Due to the increased data, and the regional use of such data, this edition is comprised of four regional volumes - **Eastern, Southern, Central** and **Western**. In addition to comprehensive hospital profiles for all states in the region, each volume includes a **State-by-State Statistical Summary**.

Each hospital profile in *The Comparative Guide to American Hospitals* is comprised of data from Hospital Compare (the Medicare sponsored web site) and The Joint Commission plus value-added data from Grey House's *Directory of Hospital Personnel*. You will find **20,700 key contact names** managing the care at 4,383 hospitals - that's 5,509 more names at 180 more hospitals than last edition. In addition, each state chapter includes **State Rankings**.

Section One: Hospital Rankings & State Profiles

The first section of each regional volume of *The Comparative Guide to American Hospitals* is arranged alphabetically by state. Each state starts with a ranking section that rates hospitals in that state on how often they meet the accepted quality protocols. Following the ranking section, hospital profiles are listed first by city, then alpha within city. Profiles include name, address, phone, fax, web site and number of licensed beds. Further, each profile includes an average of 10 key medical contacts -- **Five More Than Last Edition** -- including hospital administration, patients, and those who provide products and services to the industry -- representing not only the facility's top administration but also the physicians specifically responsible for the care of heart, pneumonia, and pregnant patients, as well as surgical infection prevention.

The first section of *The Comparative Guide to American Hospitals*:

- **Evaluates 24 Quality Measures:** The quality measures rated in *The Comparative Guide to American Hospitals* are based on accepted, effective treatments supported by the Centers for Medicare & Medical Services of the US Department of Health & Human Services and the Hospital Quality Alliance (HQA) - a public/private collaboration established to promote on hospital quality of care. HQA represents consumers, hospitals, doctors, employers, accrediting organizations and Federal agencies.

- **Examines Critical Conditions: Heart Attack Care** measures include aspirin at arrival and discharge, beta blockers at arrival and discharge, use of ACE/ARB inhibitors, and PCI administration and fibrinolytic medication timing. **Heart Failure Care** measures include LVF assessment, use of ACE/ARB inhibitors, discharge instructions and smoking cessation advice. **Pneumonia Care** measures include use of initial antibiotics and pneumococcal vaccine, use of oxygenation and blood culture results, smoking cessation advice, and administration of influenza vaccine. **Surgical Infection Prevention** measures *(NEW)* include use of prophylactic antibiotics. **Pregnancy Care** measures *(NEW)* include inpatient neonatal mortality, and degree of vaginal lacerations.

Section Two: Statistical Summary, Appendixes & Index

The second section of *The Comparative Guide to American Hospitals includes:*

- **Regional State-by-State Statistical Summary Tables** show at a glance how hospitals in the same state score and compare with each other. They are arranged alphabetically by state in easy-to-read landscape format.

- **Appendix A: 30-Day Mortality Chart** *(NEW)* lists hospitals nationwide that are "better" or "worse" than the national average, plus a State Summary of Hospital Mortality.

- **Appendix B: Glossary of Terms** *(NEW)* provides a list of 60 medical terms to make the best use possible of the data in this edition.

- **Regional Hospital Profile Index** lists hospitals alphabetically, including city and state.

This completely revised second edition of *The Comparative Guide to American Hospitals,* **now in four regional volumes,** is a valuable guide for the entire medical community, with more hospitals, more criteria measures and more key executives than the first edition. It offers an indispensable snapshot of how hospitals measure up, not only to established "best practices," but also to each other.

We welcome your comments to this edition.

User's Guide

Shown below is a fictitious listing illustrating the kind of information that is or might be included in a Hospital Profile. Each numbered item of information is described in the paragraphs following the example.

❶ **Bowling Green Medical Center**
250 Park Street
Bowling Green, KY 42101
E-mail: SKWebb@mcbg.org
URL: www.mcbg.org
Ownership: Voluntary non-profit - Private
Emergency Services: Yes

Phone: 270-745-1255
Fax: 270-745-1253

Accredited: Yes
Licensed Beds: 330

❷ **Key Personnel:**
CEO/President . . . . Wayne Bush, MD
Emergency Room Director . . . . Pliois Prerost
Director Medical/Surgical Nursing . . . . Kathleen Riley, RN
Chief OB/GYN . . . . Joseph Gass, MD
Surgery Chair . . . . James Bergin, MD
Chief Radiology . . . . Ken Bartholomew, MD

	Measure	Cases	This Hospital	State Average	U.S. Average	Top Hospital
❸						
❹	**Heart Attack Care**					
	ACE Inhibitor or ARB for LVSD	63	73%	75%	82%	100%
	Aspirin at Arrival	191	95%	89%	92%	100%
	Aspirin at Discharge	243	96%	86%	90%	100%
	Beta Blocker at Arrival	140	91%	82%	87%	100%
	Beta Blocker at Discharge	274	97%	86%	90%	100%
	Fibrinolytic Medication Timing[1]	10	10%	31%	31%	100%
	PCI Within 90 Minutes of Arrival[1]	6	17%	44%	54%	95%
	Smoking Cessation Advice	147	100%	84%	88%	100%
❺	**Heart Failure Care**					
	ACE Inhibitor or ARB for LVSD	162	84%	78%	82%	100%
	Discharge Instructions	394	50%	59%	61%	93%
	Evaluation of LVS Function	466	90%	79%	83%	99%
	Smoking Cessation Advice	123	100%	82%	82%	100%
❻	**Pneumonia Care**					
	Appropriate Initial Antibiotic	277	84%	82%	83%	94%
	Blood Culture Timing	225	92%	89%	90%	100%
	Influenza Vaccine	87	84%	76%	70%	100%
	Initial Antibiotic Timing	382	69%	82%	80%	93%
	Oxygenation Assessment	483	100%	99%	99%	100%
	Pneumococcal Vaccine	284	87%	75%	69%	94%
	Smoking Cessation Advice	170	100%	84%	80%	100%
❼	**Surgical Infection Prevention**					
	Prophylactic Antibiotic Given[3]	427	89%	74%	77%	95%
	Prophylactic Antibiotic Selection	245	87%	85%	90%	100%
	Prophylactic Antibiotic Stopped[3]	424	91%	69%	72%	95%
❽	**Pregnancy Care**					
	Inpatient Neonatal Mortality	1,979	0.25%	-	-	-
	Third or Fourth Degree Laceration	1,283	4.36%	3.25%	3.63%	3.27%

❶ **Hospital Name and Record Header:** hospital name; alternate name (if applicable); street address; phone; fax; e-mail; URL; ownership; accredited (Yes/No); emergency services (Yes/No); and number of licensed beds. *Source: Directory of Hospital Personnel, 2007, Grey House Publishing; www.hospitalcompare.hhs.gov, Centers for Medicare & Medicaid Services (CMS), an agency of the U.S. Department of Health and Human Services (DHHS) along with the Hospital Quality Alliance (HQA).*

❷ **Key Personnel:** includes the names of key personnel primarily related to the five conditions covered in this publication. *Source: Directory of Hospital Personnel, 2007, Grey House Publishing*

❸ **Hospital Compare Data:** each table contains data covering the five conditions and twenty-four associated measures contained in the Hospital Compare database. There are six columns:

> **Measure:** the twenty-four quality measures reported.
>
> There are five possible footnotes:
>
> > 1. *The number of cases is too small (n<25) for purposes of reliably predicting hospital performance.*
> > For each measure, the rate is displayed as a percent of the number of patients for whom the measured treatment is appropriate. For hospitals with small numbers of patients for whom the measured treatment is appropriate during the reporting period (fewer than 25 patients), the calculated rate may not be predictive of the hospital's future performance. As the quality data base is expanded to a full rolling four quarters of data for each measure, the number of cases used to determine hospitals' rates will likely increase, thereby increasing the reliability and stability of the rates. Note: This footnote does not necessarily reflect hospital size or overall patient volume.
> >
> > 2. *Measure reflects the hospital's indication that its submission was based upon a sample of its relevant discharges.*
> > Rates are based on the cases reported by hospitals. A rate may be based upon the total number of cases treated by a hospital, or for a facility with a large caseload, a rate may be based on a random sample of the cases the hospital treated. This footnote indicates that a hospital chose to submit data for a sample of its total cases (following specific rules for how to the select the cases).
> >
> > 3. *Rate reflects fewer than the maximum possible quarters of data for the measure.*
> > Each rate reflects the care provided over a specific time period, up to a maximum of four quarters. The number of quarters of data available is determined by when hospitals first began to report data using a specific measure. For example, for the ten measures in the "Starter Set", the maximum number of quarters for which a hospital could have provided data is four quarters. For measures added more recently, the maximum will be fewer than four quarters. This footnote indicates that the hospital's rate was based on data from fewer than the maximum possible number of quarters that the measure was generally collected.
> >
> > 4. *Inaccurate information submitted and suppressed for one or more quarters.*
> > Hospitals are required to submit accurate, reportable data to the Centers for Medicare and Medicaid Services (CMS). The rates for these measures were calculated by excluding data that had been suppressed for one or more quarters because they were identified as inaccurate.
> >
> > 5. *No data is available from the hospital for this measure.*
> > Hospitals volunteer to provide data for reporting on Hospital Compare. This footnote is applied when the hospital did not submit any cases for a measure.
>
> **Cases:** the size of the data sample (number of patients) for each hospital and quality measure. In addition, the notation "0" is applied when a hospital provided care to patients with a condition, such as pneumonia, but the cases that the hospital submitted did not meet the specific criteria for being included in the calculation of the measure.
>
> **This Hospital:** the performance rate that the hospital achieved for each quality measure. This value is expressed as a percentage of the sample size that was measured.
>
> **State Average:** the average rate for all hospitals reporting data in the state the hospital is located in.
>
> **U.S. Average:** the average rate for all hospitals reporting nationwide.
>
> **Top Hospital:** the average rate for the 90th percentile (or top 10%) of hospitals reporting data.
>
> *Note:* A two-step process was used to calculate the national and state comparison group rates. The national and state comparison rates for each measure were calculated using all of the data submitted to the QIO Clinical Data Warehouse for hospitals with at least one case that met the measure's inclusion criteria (that is, for which the denominator was greater than zero).

First, the individual hospital performance rates were calculated using the method described above for all hospitals. Next, hospitals with "0 patients" were excluded from the calculation. For the determination of the 90th percentile (or top 10%) of hospitals on a national basis, the individual rates were then rank ordered and the top 10th percentile score identified. For the national and state averages, a simple average was constructed where the numerator was the sum of all non-excluded hospitals' scores and the denominator was the total number of hospitals, each calculated at either the national or individual state level.

❹ Heart Attack Care

Every year, about one million people suffer a heart attack (acute myocardial infarction or AMI). AMI is among the leading causes of hospital admission for Medicare beneficiaries, age 65 and older.

Scientific evidence indicates that the following process of care measures represent the best practices for the treatment of AMI. Higher scores are better.

- **ACE Inhibitor or ARB for LVSD** - AMI patients with left ventricular systolic dysfunction (LVSD) and without angiotensin converting enzyme inhibitor (ACE inhibitor) contraindications or angiotensin receptor blocker (ARB) contraindications who are prescribed an ACE inhibitor or an ARB at hospital discharge.

- **Aspirin at Arrival** - Acute myocardial infarction (AMI) patients without aspirin contraindications who received aspirin within 24 hours before or after hospital arrival.

- **Aspirin at Discharge** - AMI patients without aspirin contraindications who were prescribed aspirin at hospital discharge.

- **Beta Blocker at Arrival** - AMI patients without beta-blocker contraindications who received a beta-blocker within 24 hours after hospital arrival.

- **Beta Blocker at Discharge** - AMI patients without beta-blocker contraindications who were prescribed a beta-blocker at hospital discharge.

- **Fibrinolytic Medication Timing** - AMI patients receiving fibrinolytic therapy during the hospital stay and having a time from hospital arrival to fibrinolysis of 30 minutes or less.

- **PCI Within 90 Minutes of Arrival** - AMI patients receiving Percutaneous Coronary Intervention (PCI) during the hospital stay with a time from hospital arrival to PCI of 90 minutes or less.

- **Smoking Cessation Advice** - AMI patients with a history of smoking cigarettes, who are given smoking cessation advice or counseling during a hospital stay.

❺ Heart Failure Care

Heart failure is the most common hospital admission diagnosis in patients age 65 or older, accounting for more than 700,000 hospitalizations among Medicare beneficiaries every year. It is associated with severe functional impairments and high rates of mortality and morbidity.

Substantial scientific evidence indicates that the following process of care measures represent the best practices for the treatment of heart failure. Higher scores are better.

- **ACE Inhibitor or ARB for LVSD** - Heart failure patients with left ventricular systolic dysfunction (LVSD) and without angiotensin converting enzyme inhibitor (ACE inhibitor) contraindications or angiotensin receptor blocker (ARB) contraindications who are prescribed an ACE inhibitor or an ARB at hospital discharge.

- **Discharge Instructions** - Heart failure patients discharged home with written instructions or educational material given to patient or care giver at discharge or during the hospital stay addressing all of the following: activity level, diet, discharge medications, follow-up appointment, weight monitoring, and what to do if symptoms worsen.

- **Evaluation of LVS Function** - Heart failure patients with documentation in the hospital record that an evaluation of the left ventricular systolic (LVS) function was performed before arrival, during hospitalization, or is planned for after discharge.

- **Smoking Cessation Advice** - Heart failure patients with a history of smoking cigarettes, who are given smoking cessation advice or counseling during a hospital stay.

❻ Pneumonia Care

Community acquired pneumonia is a major contributor to illness and mortality in the United States, causing four million episodes of illness and nearly one million hospital admissions each year.

Scientific evidence indicates that the following process of care measures represent the best practices for the treatment of community-acquired pneumonia. Higher scores are better.

- **Appropriate Initial Antibiotic** - Immunocompetent patients with pneumonia who receive an initial antibiotic regimen that is consistent with current guidelines.

- **Blood Culture Timing** - Pneumonia patients whose initial emergency room blood culture specimen was collected prior to first hospital dose of antibiotics.

- **Influenza Vaccination** - Pneumonia patients age 50 years and older, hospitalized during October, November, December, January, or February who were screened for influenza vaccine status and were vaccinated prior to discharge, if indicated.

- **Initial Antibiotic Timing** - Pneumonia inpatients who receive antibiotics within 4 hours of hospital arrival. Evidence shows better outcomes for administration times less than four hours.

- **Oxygenation Assessment** - Pneumonia inpatients who receive an oxygenation assessment, arterial blood gas (ABG), or pulse oximetry within 24 hours of hospital arrival.

- **Pneumococcal Vaccination** - Pneumonia inpatients age 65 and older who were screened for pneumococcal vaccine status and were administered the vaccine prior to discharge, if indicated.

- **Smoking Cessation Advice** - Pneumonia patients with a history of smoking cigarettes, who are given smoking cessation advice or counseling during a hospital stay.

❼ Surgical Infection Prevention

Hospitals can reduce the risk of wound infection after surgery by providing the right medicines at the right time on the day of surgery. Studies show a strong association of reduced incidence of post-operative infection with administration of antibiotics within the one hour prior to surgery. After the incision is closed, however, studies show that prolonged administration of prophylaxis with antibiotics may increase the risk of certain other infections at no additional benefit to the surgical patient.

Scientific evidence indicates that the following process of care measures represent the best practices for the prevention of infections after selected surgeries (colon surgery, hip and knee arthroplasty, abdominal and vaginal hysterectomy, cardiac surgery (including coronary artery bypass grafts (CABG)) and vascular surgery). Higher scores are better.

- **Prophylactic Antibiotic Given** - Surgical patients who received prophylactic antibiotics within 1 hour prior to surgical incision.

- **Prophylactic Antibiotic Selection** - Surgical patients who received the recommended antibiotics for their particular type of surgery.

- **Prophylactic Antibiotic Stopped** - Surgical patients whose prophylactic antibiotics were discontinued within 24 hours after surgery end time.

❽ Pregnancy Care

- **Inpatient Neonatal Mortality** - This measure reports how often infants died before 28 days of birth; it is adjusted to reflect the fact that some babies are sicker than others at or shortly after birth.

- **Third or Fourth Degree Laceration** - This measure reports how often patients have significant tears between the vagina and anus while having a baby. These types of tears can lead to other medical complications.

Information about Hospital Performance

Hospital performance rates tell you the proportion of cases where a hospital provided the recommended process of care. Only patients meeting the inclusion criteria for a measure are included in the calculation of the rate for a measure. A rate of 88% means that the hospital provided the recommended process of care 88% of the time. For example, the rates for initial antibiotic timing tell you the percentage of patients who received their first dose of antibiotics within four hours of arrival to the hospital. The ultimate goal for all measures listed (except Pregnancy Care) is 100%. With the two measures under Pregnancy Care, lower numbers are preferable. Hospitals with effective quality improvement programs are continually working toward this goal.

Confidence Intervals

The table below enables the user to calculate confidence intervals for each reported measure.

Confidence intervals can be used to estimate the precision of the calculated rates for an individual hospital. A confidence interval is the range of values, within which an estimated value or rate is likely to fall. A confidence interval is a statistical determination of the degree of certainty associated with an estimated value. As can be seen in the table of estimated values (below), large differences between individual hospitals' rates may be significant, and small differences between hospitals are usually not significant.

The smaller the sample size, the greater the difference in rates must be order for that difference to be statistically meaningful. Also, as sample size varies between hospitals, it is difficult to precisely compare their rates, without considering the confidence intervals.

Over time, as the quality data base is expanded, a full four quarters of data will ultimately be available, so the number of cases used to determine hospitals' rates will likely increase, thereby increasing the reliability and stability of the rates.

Estimating Confidence Intervals for the Quality Measures: Estimated Values for Proportion Data

Sample Size	Observed Rate								
	10%	20%	30%	40%	50%	60%	70%	80%	90%
< 25	*	*	24.9	26.6	27.2	26.6	24.9	*	*
25 - 75	8.3	11.1	12.7	13.6	13.9	13.6	12.7	11.1	8.3
76 - 125	5.9	7.8	9.0	9.6	9.8	9.6	9.0	7.8	5.9
126 - 175	4.8	6.4	7.3	7.8	8.0	7.8	7.3	6.4	4.8
176 - 225	4.2	5.5	6.4	6.8	6.9	6.8	6.4	5.5	4.2
226 -275	3.7	5.0	5.7	6.1	6.2	6.1	5.7	5.0	3.7
276+	2.9	3.9	4.5	4.8	4.9	4.8	4.5	3.9	2.9

*Source: CMS/OCSQ/QIG. The values in the table are the approximate amount to add and subtract from the observed rate to estimate a 95 percent confidence interval for the given sample size. (Interpolation between the values in the table is appropriate.) * Estimates of an interval in these cells exceed the natural limits for proportions.*

Source of Data

The information in this book comes from the quality data submitted by hospitals to the QIO Clinical Data Warehouse for inpatient discharges. Heart Attack Care, Heart Failure Care, Pneumonia Care, Pregnancy Care and Surgical Infection Prevention data is from www.hospitalcompare.hhs.gov, a website tool developed by the Centers for Medicare & Medicaid Services (CMS). Data covers October 2005 through September 2006. Hospital Mortality data is also from www.hospitalcompare.hhs.gov. Data covers July 2005 through June 2006.

Pregnancy Care data is from www.qualitycheck.org, a service of The Joint Commission. The Joint Commission (formerly the Joint Commission on Accreditation of Healthcare Organizations (JCAHO)), is a US-based non-profit organization formed in 1951 with a mission to maintain and elevate the standards of healthcare delivery through evaluation and accreditation of healthcare organizations. Data covers January 2006 through December 2006.

Heart Attack Care

1. ACE Inhibitor or ARB for LVSD

Hospital Name	City	Rate	Cases
Flowers Hospital	Dothan	98%	56
Brookwood Medical Center	Birmingham	94%	50
Springhill Medical Center	Mobile	94%	32
University of South Alabama Medical Center	Mobile	94%	31
Eliza Coffee Memorial Hospital	Florence	92%	87
Medical Center East	Birmingham	92%	90
Trinity Medical Center	Birmingham	92%	114
East Alabama Medical Center	Opelika	91%	80
Southeast Alabama Medical Center	Dothan	90%	148
Thomas Hospital	Fairhope	90%	59
Huntsville Hospital	Huntsville	88%	260
Physicians Medical Center Carraway	Birmingham	88%	32
Princeton Baptist Medical Center	Birmingham	87%	131
Decatur General Hospital	Decatur	86%	44
Northeast Alabama Regional Medical Center	Anniston	82%	50
UAB Hospital	Birmingham	81%	88
Shelby Baptist Medical Center	Alabaster	80%	61
Providence Hospital	Mobile	79%	38
Baptist Medical Center	Montgomery	78%	64
DCH Regional Medical Center	Tuscaloosa	77%	60
Mobile Infirmary Medical Center	Mobile	74%	61
Vaughan Regional Med Ctr-Parkway Campus	Selma	74%	27
Gadsden Regional Medical Center	Gadsden	72%	39
Saint Vincent's Hospital	Birmingham	72%	60
Riverview Regional Medical Center	Gadsden	67%	52
Jackson Hospital and Clinic	Montgomery	62%	52

2. Aspirin at Arrival

Hospital Name	City	Rate	Cases
Cooper Green Mercy Hospital	Birmingham	100%	25
Physicians Medical Center Carraway	Birmingham	100%	105
South Baldwin Regional Medical Center	Foley	100%	54
Decatur General Hospital	Decatur	99%	142
Eliza Coffee Memorial Hospital	Florence	99%	213
Flowers Hospital	Dothan	99%	158
Saint Vincent's Hospital	Birmingham	99%	224
University of South Alabama Medical Center	Mobile	99%	68
DCH Regional Medical Center	Tuscaloosa	98%	161
Huntsville Hospital	Huntsville	98%	557
Mobile Infirmary Medical Center	Mobile	98%	168
Russell Medical Center	Alexander City	98%	52
Trinity Medical Center	Birmingham	98%	208
UAB Hospital	Birmingham	98%	177
Walker Baptist Medical Center	Jasper	98%	57
Baptist Medical Center East	Montgomery	97%	29
Brookwood Medical Center	Birmingham	97%	146
Coosa Valley Baptist Medical Center	Sylacauga	97%	32
Cullman Regional Medical Center	Cullman	97%	62
East Alabama Medical Center	Opelika	97%	233
Medical Center East	Birmingham	97%	274
Northeast Alabama Regional Medical Center	Anniston	97%	177
Princeton Baptist Medical Center	Birmingham	97%	299
Providence Hospital	Mobile	97%	181
Stringfellow Memorial Hospital	Anniston	97%	59
Southeast Alabama Medical Center	Dothan	96%	284
Thomas Hospital	Fairhope	96%	176
UAB Medical West	Bessemer	96%	56
Baptist Medical Center	Montgomery	95%	106
Springhill Medical Center	Mobile	92%	116
Helen Keller Memorial Hospital	Sheffield	91%	34
Shelby Baptist Medical Center	Alabaster	91%	171
Crestwood Medical Center	Huntsville	90%	84
Riverview Regional Medical Center	Gadsden	90%	169
Lawrence Medical Center	Moulton	89%	37
Gadsden Regional Medical Center	Gadsden	86%	120
Jackson Hospital and Clinic	Montgomery	86%	173
George H Lanier Memorial Hospital	Valley	84%	25
Vaughan Regional Med Ctr-Parkway Campus	Selma	84%	97
Marshall Medical Center South	Boaz	60%	30

3. Aspirin at Discharge

Hospital Name	City	Rate	Cases
Flowers Hospital	Dothan	100%	274
Thomas Hospital	Fairhope	100%	256
Trinity Medical Center	Birmingham	100%	418
Walker Baptist Medical Center	Jasper	100%	43
Eliza Coffee Memorial Hospital	Florence	99%	336
Saint Vincent's Hospital	Birmingham	99%	227
UAB Hospital	Birmingham	99%	325

Baptist Medical Center	Montgomery	98%	220
DCH Regional Medical Center	Tuscaloosa	98%	258
Southeast Alabama Medical Center	Dothan	98%	511
Decatur General Hospital	Decatur	97%	149
Huntsville Hospital	Huntsville	97%	985
Mobile Infirmary Medical Center	Mobile	97%	231
Princeton Baptist Medical Center	Birmingham	97%	409
Brookwood Medical Center	Birmingham	96%	182
East Alabama Medical Center	Opelika	96%	310
South Baldwin Regional Medical Center	Foley	96%	26
Stringfellow Memorial Hospital	Anniston	96%	53
Medical Center East	Birmingham	95%	298
Physicians Medical Center Carraway	Birmingham	95%	137
Providence Hospital	Mobile	95%	207
Springhill Medical Center	Mobile	95%	111
University of South Alabama Medical Center	Mobile	95%	97
Crestwood Medical Center	Huntsville	94%	79
Northeast Alabama Regional Medical Center	Anniston	94%	180
Shelby Baptist Medical Center	Alabaster	93%	180
Vaughan Regional Med Ctr-Parkway Campus	Selma	93%	56
Gadsden Regional Medical Center	Gadsden	92%	146
Jackson Hospital and Clinic	Montgomery	92%	235
Riverview Regional Medical Center	Gadsden	92%	171
Russell Medical Center	Alexander City	91%	46
UAB Medical West	Bessemer	90%	39
Cullman Regional Medical Center	Cullman	87%	31
Lawrence Medical Center	Moulton	71%	28

4. Beta Blocker at Arrival

Hospital Name	City	Rate	Cases
Baptist Medical Center East	Montgomery	100%	32
Flowers Hospital	Dothan	100%	121
Walker Baptist Medical Center	Jasper	100%	47
Physicians Medical Center Carraway	Birmingham	98%	99
Russell Medical Center	Alexander City	98%	52
Saint Vincent's Hospital	Birmingham	98%	174
University of South Alabama Medical Center	Mobile	98%	55
Brookwood Medical Center	Birmingham	97%	138
Trinity Medical Center	Birmingham	97%	190
Eliza Coffee Memorial Hospital	Florence	96%	191
Mobile Infirmary Medical Center	Mobile	96%	116
Princeton Baptist Medical Center	Birmingham	96%	239
Baptist Medical Center	Montgomery	95%	86
Huntsville Hospital	Huntsville	95%	468
Medical Center East	Birmingham	95%	249
Decatur General Hospital	Decatur	94%	131
UAB Hospital	Birmingham	94%	156
Southeast Alabama Medical Center	Dothan	93%	233
Cullman Regional Medical Center	Cullman	90%	49
East Alabama Medical Center	Opelika	90%	156
Northeast Alabama Regional Medical Center	Anniston	90%	108
Coosa Valley Baptist Medical Center	Sylacauga	89%	27
Thomas Hospital	Fairhope	89%	134
South Baldwin Regional Medical Center	Foley	88%	42
Springhill Medical Center	Mobile	88%	60
Providence Hospital	Mobile	87%	107
Riverview Regional Medical Center	Gadsden	87%	130
Crestwood Medical Center	Huntsville	86%	70
DCH Regional Medical Center	Tuscaloosa	86%	126
UAB Medical West	Bessemer	86%	59
Vaughan Regional Med Ctr-Parkway Campus	Selma	86%	87
Helen Keller Memorial Hospital	Sheffield	85%	26
Gadsden Regional Medical Center	Gadsden	78%	98
Shelby Baptist Medical Center	Alabaster	78%	128
Jackson Hospital and Clinic	Montgomery	76%	124
Lawrence Medical Center	Moulton	71%	34
Stringfellow Memorial Hospital	Anniston	70%	40
Marshall Medical Center South	Boaz	44%	25

5. Beta Blocker at Discharge

Hospital Name	City	Rate	Cases
Flowers Hospital	Dothan	100%	282
Princeton Baptist Medical Center	Birmingham	100%	381
Walker Baptist Medical Center	Jasper	100%	37
Brookwood Medical Center	Birmingham	99%	184
Trinity Medical Center	Birmingham	99%	416
Physicians Medical Center Carraway	Birmingham	98%	143
Russell Medical Center	Alexander City	98%	46
Springhill Medical Center	Mobile	98%	125
Baptist Medical Center	Montgomery	97%	251
East Alabama Medical Center	Opelika	97%	305
Huntsville Hospital	Huntsville	97%	946
Southeast Alabama Medical Center	Dothan	97%	505
Thomas Hospital	Fairhope	97%	242

NOTE: Hospital profiles are in alphabetical order by state, then city, then hospital within the city; Rankings are sorted by rate in descending order and exclude hospitals with less than 25 cases; (1) The number of cases is too small (n<25) for purposes of reliably predicting hospital performance; (2) Measure reflects the hospital's indication that its submission was based upon a sample of its relevant discharges; (3) Rate reflects fewer than the maximum possible quarters of data for the measure; (4) Inaccurate information submitted and suppressed for one or more quarters; (5) No data is available from the hospital for this measure; Please refer to the User's Guide for a full explanation of data

DCH Regional Medical Center	Tuscaloosa	96%	252
Mobile Infirmary Medical Center	Mobile	96%	246
South Baldwin Regional Medical Center	Foley	96%	28
Decatur General Hospital	Decatur	95%	153
Medical Center East	Birmingham	95%	315
UAB Hospital	Birmingham	95%	316
Providence Hospital	Mobile	94%	217
Shelby Baptist Medical Center	Alabaster	94%	170
Eliza Coffee Memorial Hospital	Florence	93%	330
UAB Medical West	Bessemer	93%	43
Saint Vincent's Hospital	Birmingham	92%	225
University of South Alabama Medical Center	Mobile	92%	95
Crestwood Medical Center	Huntsville	91%	77
Vaughan Regional Med Ctr-Parkway Campus	Selma	90%	59
Northeast Alabama Regional Medical Center	Anniston	89%	184
Cullman Regional Medical Center	Cullman	88%	32
Gadsden Regional Medical Center	Gadsden	88%	157
Riverview Regional Medical Center	Gadsden	88%	175
Jackson Hospital and Clinic	Montgomery	87%	239
Stringfellow Memorial Hospital	Anniston	79%	56
Lawrence Medical Center	Moulton	67%	30

6. Fibrinolytic Medication Timing

Hospital Name	City	Rate	Cases
Physicians Medical Center Carraway	Birmingham	50%	38

7. PCI Within 90 Minutes of Arrival

Hospital Name	City	Rate	Cases
Huntsville Hospital	Huntsville	88%	33

8. Smoking Cessation Advice

Hospital Name	City	Rate	Cases
Baptist Medical Center	Montgomery	100%	113
DCH Regional Medical Center	Tuscaloosa	100%	119
Flowers Hospital	Dothan	100%	123
Gadsden Regional Medical Center	Gadsden	100%	77
Medical Center East	Birmingham	100%	146
Northeast Alabama Regional Medical Center	Anniston	100%	95
Physicians Medical Center Carraway	Birmingham	100%	78
Riverview Regional Medical Center	Gadsden	100%	64
Stringfellow Memorial Hospital	Anniston	100%	31
University of South Alabama Medical Center	Mobile	100%	70
Walker Baptist Medical Center	Jasper	100%	26
East Alabama Medical Center	Opelika	99%	144
Princeton Baptist Medical Center	Birmingham	99%	168
Southeast Alabama Medical Center	Dothan	99%	218
Brookwood Medical Center	Birmingham	98%	65
Huntsville Hospital	Huntsville	98%	415
Providence Hospital	Mobile	98%	88
Eliza Coffee Memorial Hospital	Florence	97%	160
Saint Vincent's Hospital	Birmingham	97%	69
Thomas Hospital	Fairhope	96%	112
Mobile Infirmary Medical Center	Mobile	95%	104
Decatur General Hospital	Decatur	94%	54
Trinity Medical Center	Birmingham	94%	172
Springhill Medical Center	Mobile	93%	55
Crestwood Medical Center	Huntsville	87%	31
UAB Hospital	Birmingham	87%	127
Jackson Hospital and Clinic	Montgomery	81%	95
Shelby Baptist Medical Center	Alabaster	78%	83

Heart Failure Care

9. ACE Inhibitor or ARB for LVSD

Hospital Name	City	Rate	Cases
Cooper Green Mercy Hospital	Birmingham	100%	62
Flowers Hospital	Dothan	100%	109
Mizell Memorial Hospital	Opp	100%	29
Trinity Medical Center	Birmingham	99%	146
Walker Baptist Medical Center	Jasper	99%	91
East Alabama Medical Center	Opelika	97%	304
Springhill Medical Center	Mobile	97%	177
UAB Medical West	Bessemer	96%	75
Medical Center Enterprise	Enterprise	94%	32
Community Hospital	Tallassee	93%	43
George H Lanier Memorial Hospital	Valley	93%	87
Parkway Medical Center Hospital	Decatur	93%	30
Physicians Medical Center Carraway	Birmingham	93%	88
Cullman Regional Medical Center	Cullman	92%	89
University of South Alabama Medical Center	Mobile	92%	140
Prattville Baptist Hospital	Prattville	91%	33
Providence Hospital	Mobile	91%	149

Athens-Limestone Hospital	Athens	90%	51
Crestwood Medical Center	Huntsville	89%	87
Infirmary West	Mobile	89%	44
Northwest Medical Center	Winfield	89%	28
Medical Center East	Birmingham	88%	136
Decatur General Hospital	Decatur	87%	143
Southeast Alabama Medical Center	Dothan	87%	319
Brookwood Medical Center	Birmingham	84%	182
Huntsville Hospital	Huntsville	84%	591
DCH Regional Medical Center	Tuscaloosa	83%	116
DeKalb Regional Medical Center	Fort Payne	83%	60
Helen Keller Memorial Hospital	Sheffield	83%	64
UAB Hospital	Birmingham	83%	320
Monroe County Hospital	Monroeville	82%	45
Atmore Community Hospital	Atmore	81%	26
Eliza Coffee Memorial Hospital	Florence	81%	138
Princeton Baptist Medical Center	Birmingham	81%	238
Randolph Health Systems Medical Center	Roanoke	81%	26
Stringfellow Memorial Hospital	Anniston	81%	101
Vaughan Evergreen Medical Center	Evergreen	81%	42
Baptist Medical Center	Montgomery	80%	145
Vaughan Regional Med Ctr-Parkway Campus	Selma	80%	192
Coosa Valley Baptist Medical Center	Sylacauga	79%	57
Gadsden Regional Medical Center	Gadsden	79%	131
Marshall Medical Center South	Boaz	79%	66
Riverview Regional Medical Center	Gadsden	79%	130
Russell Medical Center	Alexander City	79%	28
Jackson Hospital and Clinic	Montgomery	78%	114
L V Stabler Memorial Hospital	Greenville	78%	36
Northeast Alabama Regional Medical Center	Anniston	78%	226
South Baldwin Regional Medical Center	Foley	78%	67
Baptist Medical Center East	Montgomery	77%	57
Cherokee Medical Center	Centre	77%	31
Saint Vincent's Hospital	Birmingham	77%	195
Thomas Hospital	Fairhope	76%	97
Northport Medical Center	Northport	75%	28
Citizens Baptist Medical Center	Talladega	73%	49
Woodland Medical Center	Cullman	72%	40
Mobile Infirmary Medical Center	Mobile	65%	130
Shelby Baptist Medical Center	Alabaster	62%	121
Saint Clair Regional Hospital	Pell City	61%	28
Andalusia Regional Hospital	Andalusia	59%	37

10. Discharge Instructions

Hospital Name	City	Rate	Cases
Parkway Medical Center Hospital	Decatur	100%	102
Walker Baptist Medical Center	Jasper	99%	165
Lawrence Medical Center	Moulton	98%	42
Russellville Hospital	Russellville	97%	65
Flowers Hospital	Dothan	94%	274
Georgiana Hospital	Georgiana	92%	52
Hartselle Medical Center	Hartselle	91%	70
Lakeland Community Hospital	Haleyville	91%	68
L V Stabler Memorial Hospital	Greenville	90%	79
Monroe County Hospital	Monroeville	90%	119
Northport Medical Center	Northport	89%	70
Cullman Regional Medical Center	Cullman	87%	172
Wiregrass Medical Center	Geneva	87%	67
Andalusia Regional Hospital	Andalusia	86%	149
Decatur General Hospital	Decatur	85%	304
Medical Center East	Birmingham	85%	271
Baptist Medical Center	Montgomery	84%	268
Woodland Medical Center	Cullman	82%	87
Marshall Medical Center South	Boaz	81%	116
Prattville Baptist Hospital	Prattville	81%	88
Shoals Hospital	Muscle Shoals	81%	59
University of South Alabama Medical Center	Mobile	80%	232
East Alabama Medical Center	Opelika	79%	583
DeKalb Regional Medical Center	Fort Payne	78%	95
Southeast Alabama Medical Center	Dothan	78%	696
Trinity Medical Center	Birmingham	78%	308
Jacksonville Medical Center	Jacksonville	76%	37
Marion Regional Wellness Center	Hamilton	76%	46
Medical Center Enterprise	Enterprise	76%	89
Huntsville Hospital	Huntsville	75%	1126
DCH Regional Medical Center	Tuscaloosa	73%	245
Brookwood Medical Center	Birmingham	72%	355
South Baldwin Regional Medical Center	Foley	72%	192
Cooper Green Mercy Hospital	Birmingham	71%	107
Northeast Alabama Regional Medical Center	Anniston	71%	430
Thomas Hospital	Fairhope	71%	201
Helen Keller Memorial Hospital	Sheffield	70%	181
Atmore Community Hospital	Atmore	69%	59
Saint Clair Regional Hospital	Pell City	69%	89

NOTE: Hospital profiles are in alphabetical order by state, then city, then hospital within the city; Rankings are sorted by rate in descending order and exclude hospitals with less than 25 cases; (1) The number of cases is too small (n<25) for purposes of reliably predicting hospital performance; (2) Measure reflects the hospital's indication that its submission was based upon a sample of its relevant discharges; (3) Rate reflects fewer than the maximum possible quarters of data for the measure; (4) Inaccurate information submitted and suppressed for one or more quarters; (5) No data is available from the hospital for this measure; Please refer to the User's Guide for a full explanation of data

Hospital Name	City	Rate	Cases
Crestwood Medical Center	Huntsville	68%	189
Princeton Baptist Medical Center	Birmingham	67%	383
Marshall Medical Center North	Guntersville	66%	71
Saint Vincent's Hospital	Birmingham	66%	422
Eliza Coffee Memorial Hospital	Florence	65%	346
Lakeview Community Hospital	Eufaula	65%	63
Providence Hospital	Mobile	65%	477
Physicians Medical Center Carraway	Birmingham	64%	191
Baptist Medical Center East	Montgomery	58%	186
Jackson Hospital and Clinic	Montgomery	58%	311
Mobile Infirmary Medical Center	Mobile	57%	262
Russell Medical Center	Alexander City	56%	62
UAB Medical West	Bessemer	55%	186
Community Hospital	Tallassee	52%	73
Coosa Valley Baptist Medical Center	Sylacauga	51%	84
Stringfellow Memorial Hospital	Anniston	51%	208
Highlands Medical Center	Scottsboro	50%	125
Cherokee Medical Center	Centre	49%	43
Northwest Medical Center	Winfield	47%	76
Riverview Regional Medical Center	Gadsden	47%	277
Springhill Medical Center	Mobile	45%	455
Citizens Baptist Medical Center	Talladega	44%	110
Fayette Medical Center	Fayette	44%	55
Gadsden Regional Medical Center	Gadsden	44%	260
D W McMillan Memorial Hospital	Brewton	42%	74
Vaughan Evergreen Medical Center	Evergreen	42%	144
UAB Hospital	Birmingham	41%	516
George H Lanier Memorial Hospital	Valley	38%	178
Medical Center Blount	Oneonta	35%	40
Troy Regional Medical Center	Troy	35%	48
Shelby Baptist Medical Center	Alabaster	32%	271
Infirmary West	Mobile	31%	59
Vaughan Regional Med Ctr-Parkway Campus	Selma	31%	364
Pickens County Medical Center	Carrollton	27%	48
Grove Hill Memorial Hospital	Grove Hill	24%	54
Dale Medical Center	Ozark	21%	56
Mizell Memorial Hospital	Opp	19%	77
Lake Martin Community Hospital	Dadeville	18%	33
Athens-Limestone Hospital	Athens	16%	115
Bullock County Hospital	Union Springs	12%	26
Randolph Health Systems Medical Center	Roanoke	8%	37
Jackson Medical Center	Jackson	6%	47
Wedowee Hospital	Wedowee	4%	55
Bryan W Whitfield Memorial Hospital	Demopolis	1%	93
Clay County Hospital	Ashland	1%	67
Crenshaw Baptist Hospital	Luverne	0%	26

11. Evaluation of LVS Function

Hospital Name	City	Rate	Cases
Community Hospital	Tallassee	100%	87
Flowers Hospital	Dothan	100%	304
Hartselle Medical Center	Hartselle	100%	86
Walker Baptist Medical Center	Jasper	100%	205
East Alabama Medical Center	Opelika	99%	648
Providence Hospital	Mobile	99%	527
UAB Medical West	Bessemer	99%	200
Marshall Medical Center South	Boaz	98%	168
Medical Center East	Birmingham	98%	316
Springhill Medical Center	Mobile	98%	496
Gadsden Regional Medical Center	Gadsden	97%	348
Medical Center Enterprise	Enterprise	97%	103
Parkway Medical Center Hospital	Decatur	97%	127
Princeton Baptist Medical Center	Birmingham	97%	443
DeKalb Regional Medical Center	Fort Payne	96%	119
George H Lanier Memorial Hospital	Valley	96%	187
Shoals Hospital	Muscle Shoals	96%	68
South Baldwin Regional Medical Center	Foley	96%	225
D W McMillan Memorial Hospital	Brewton	95%	78
Marshall Medical Center North	Guntersville	95%	94
Prattville Baptist Hospital	Prattville	95%	104
Russellville Hospital	Russellville	95%	80
Stringfellow Memorial Hospital	Anniston	95%	232
Trinity Medical Center	Birmingham	95%	372
UAB Hospital	Birmingham	95%	549
Jacksonville Medical Center	Jacksonville	94%	53
Mobile Infirmary Medical Center	Mobile	94%	309
Southeast Alabama Medical Center	Dothan	94%	773
University of South Alabama Medical Center	Mobile	94%	232
Cooper Green Mercy Hospital	Birmingham	93%	108
Huntsville Hospital	Huntsville	93%	1301
North Baldwin Infirmary	Bay Minette	93%	28
Physicians Medical Center Carraway	Birmingham	93%	224
Pickens County Medical Center	Carrollton	93%	55
Shelby Baptist Medical Center	Alabaster	93%	305
Baptist Medical Center East	Montgomery	92%	200
Brookwood Medical Center	Birmingham	92%	424
Crestwood Medical Center	Huntsville	92%	234
Eliza Coffee Memorial Hospital	Florence	92%	409
Infirmary West	Mobile	92%	63
L V Stabler Memorial Hospital	Greenville	92%	92
Russell Medical Center	Alexander City	92%	86
Thomas Hospital	Fairhope	92%	240
Decatur General Hospital	Decatur	91%	364
Marion Regional Wellness Center	Hamilton	90%	50
Atmore Community Hospital	Atmore	89%	70
Baptist Medical Center	Montgomery	89%	291
Lakeland Community Hospital	Haleyville	88%	90
Mizell Memorial Hospital	Opp	88%	92
Northeast Alabama Regional Medical Center	Anniston	88%	502
Citizens Baptist Medical Center	Talladega	87%	126
Cullman Regional Medical Center	Cullman	87%	193
Randolph Health Systems Medical Center	Roanoke	87%	55
Saint Vincent's Hospital	Birmingham	87%	468
Vaughan Regional Med Ctr-Parkway Campus	Selma	87%	412
Athens-Limestone Hospital	Athens	86%	154
DCH Regional Medical Center	Tuscaloosa	86%	288
Dale Medical Center	Ozark	86%	63
Florala Memorial Hospital	Florala	86%	28
Helen Keller Memorial Hospital	Sheffield	85%	215
Jackson Hospital and Clinic	Montgomery	85%	353
Medical Center Blount	Oneonta	85%	66
Monroe County Hospital	Monroeville	85%	132
Woodland Medical Center	Cullman	85%	140
Northwest Medical Center	Winfield	83%	103
Riverview Regional Medical Center	Gadsden	82%	366
Thomasville Infirmary	Thomasville	82%	89
Andalusia Regional Hospital	Andalusia	80%	183
Coosa Valley Baptist Medical Center	Sylacauga	80%	112
Fayette Medical Center	Fayette	80%	71
Troy Regional Medical Center	Troy	80%	64
Cherokee Medical Center	Centre	79%	67
Northport Medical Center	Northport	78%	79
Lawrence Medical Center	Moulton	76%	45
Vaughan Evergreen Medical Center	Evergreen	72%	158
Grove Hill Memorial Hospital	Grove Hill	71%	56
Saint Clair Regional Hospital	Pell City	70%	98
Jackson Medical Center	Jackson	60%	52
Lakeview Community Hospital	Eufaula	58%	89
Crenshaw Baptist Hospital	Luverne	56%	32
Wedowee Hospital	Wedowee	49%	59
Highlands Medical Center	Scottsboro	48%	157
Wiregrass Medical Center	Geneva	46%	76
Lake Martin Community Hospital	Dadeville	43%	49
Greene County Hospital	Eutaw	38%	47
Bryan W Whitfield Memorial Hospital	Demopolis	37%	105
Clay County Hospital	Ashland	37%	83
Georgiana Hospital	Georgiana	35%	54
Hale County Hospital	Greensboro	23%	39
Bullock County Hospital	Union Springs	13%	38

12. Smoking Cessation Advice

Hospital Name	City	Rate	Cases
Baptist Medical Center	Montgomery	100%	81
DCH Regional Medical Center	Tuscaloosa	100%	45
Decatur General Hospital	Decatur	100%	70
East Alabama Medical Center	Opelika	100%	143
Flowers Hospital	Dothan	100%	50
Helen Keller Memorial Hospital	Sheffield	100%	45
Monroe County Hospital	Monroeville	100%	35
Parkway Medical Center Hospital	Decatur	100%	27
Prattville Baptist Hospital	Prattville	100%	29
Princeton Baptist Medical Center	Birmingham	100%	86
Providence Hospital	Mobile	100%	96
Riverview Regional Medical Center	Gadsden	100%	66
Stringfellow Memorial Hospital	Anniston	100%	60
UAB Medical West	Bessemer	100%	52
University of South Alabama Medical Center	Mobile	100%	98
Walker Baptist Medical Center	Jasper	100%	45
Northeast Alabama Regional Medical Center	Anniston	99%	113
Medical Center East	Birmingham	98%	54
South Baldwin Regional Medical Center	Foley	98%	47
Gadsden Regional Medical Center	Gadsden	97%	60
Physicians Medical Center Carraway	Birmingham	97%	68
Huntsville Hospital	Huntsville	96%	254
Saint Vincent's Hospital	Birmingham	96%	69
Brookwood Medical Center	Birmingham	94%	69
Eliza Coffee Memorial Hospital	Florence	93%	61
Lakeview Community Hospital	Eufaula	93%	29

NOTE: Hospital profiles are in alphabetical order by state, then city, then hospital within the city; Rankings are sorted by rate in descending order and exclude hospitals with less than 25 cases; (1) The number of cases is too small (n<25) for purposes of reliably predicting hospital performance; (2) Measure reflects the hospital's indication that its submission was based upon a sample of its relevant discharges; (3) Rate reflects fewer than the maximum possible quarters of data for the measure; (4) Inaccurate information submitted and suppressed for one or more quarters; (5) No data is available from the hospital for this measure; Please refer to the User's Guide for a full explanation of data

Hospital Name	City	Rate	Cases
Athens-Limestone Hospital	Athens	92%	25
Cullman Regional Medical Center	Cullman	92%	37
Thomas Hospital	Fairhope	92%	40
Woodland Medical Center	Cullman	92%	25
George H Lanier Memorial Hospital	Valley	89%	47
Jackson Hospital and Clinic	Montgomery	89%	85
Vaughan Regional Med Ctr-Parkway Campus	Selma	89%	75
Crestwood Medical Center	Huntsville	87%	47
Mobile Infirmary Medical Center	Mobile	87%	84
Southeast Alabama Medical Center	Dothan	86%	152
Springhill Medical Center	Mobile	86%	76
Highlands Medical Center	Scottsboro	85%	34
Marshall Medical Center South	Boaz	85%	33
Cooper Green Mercy Hospital	Birmingham	82%	61
Citizens Baptist Medical Center	Talladega	78%	27
Trinity Medical Center	Birmingham	77%	66
Shelby Baptist Medical Center	Alabaster	66%	53
UAB Hospital	Birmingham	63%	134

Pneumonia Care

13. Appropriate Initial Antibiotic

Hospital Name	City	Rate	Cases
Hartselle Medical Center	Hartselle	95%	56
Walker Baptist Medical Center	Jasper	95%	269
Bibb Medical Center	Centreville	94%	36
Elba General Hospital & Nursing Home	Elba	94%	47
Flowers Hospital	Dothan	93%	134
Medical Center Enterprise	Enterprise	93%	118
D W McMillan Memorial Hospital	Brewton	92%	60
East Alabama Medical Center	Opelika	91%	108
Northwest Medical Center	Winfield	91%	114
Decatur General Hospital	Decatur	90%	193
Eliza Coffee Memorial Hospital	Florence	90%	316
Helen Keller Memorial Hospital	Sheffield	90%	90
Northport Medical Center	Northport	90%	68
Coosa Valley Baptist Medical Center	Sylacauga	89%	101
Gadsden Regional Medical Center	Gadsden	89%	194
Jackson Medical Center	Jackson	89%	76
Princeton Baptist Medical Center	Birmingham	89%	212
Infirmary West	Mobile	88%	57
Southeast Alabama Medical Center	Dothan	88%	209
Trinity Medical Center	Birmingham	88%	133
Woodland Medical Center	Cullman	87%	98
Pickens County Medical Center	Carrollton	86%	87
UAB Medical West	Bessemer	86%	172
Community Hospital	Tallassee	85%	52
Northeast Alabama Regional Medical Center	Anniston	85%	169
Riverview Regional Medical Center	Gadsden	85%	229
Highlands Medical Center	Scottsboro	84%	193
UAB Hospital	Birmingham	84%	88
Clay County Hospital	Ashland	83%	59
Grove Hill Memorial Hospital	Grove Hill	83%	41
Lawrence Medical Center	Moulton	83%	106
Marshall Medical Center North	Guntersville	83%	132
Physicians Medical Center Carraway	Birmingham	83%	140
Providence Hospital	Mobile	83%	270
Russellville Hospital	Russellville	83%	109
Stringfellow Memorial Hospital	Anniston	83%	156
Brookwood Medical Center	Birmingham	82%	292
Cherokee Medical Center	Centre	82%	44
Lakeland Community Hospital	Haleyville	82%	248
Medical Center East	Birmingham	82%	297
Shelby Baptist Medical Center	Alabaster	82%	176
Springhill Medical Center	Mobile	82%	121
Baptist Medical Center East	Montgomery	81%	106
Cullman Regional Medical Center	Cullman	81%	171
DeKalb Regional Medical Center	Fort Payne	81%	104
Fayette Medical Center	Fayette	81%	85
Huntsville Hospital	Huntsville	81%	525
Shoals Hospital	Muscle Shoals	81%	88
Citizens Baptist Medical Center	Talladega	80%	86
DCH Regional Medical Center	Tuscaloosa	80%	199
Lakeview Community Hospital	Eufaula	80%	76
North Baldwin Infirmary	Bay Minette	80%	40
Athens-Limestone Hospital	Athens	79%	167
Crenshaw Baptist Medical Center	Luverne	79%	38
Marion Regional Wellness Center	Hamilton	79%	94
Monroe County Hospital	Monroeville	79%	102
University of South Alabama Medical Center	Mobile	79%	72
Atmore Community Hospital	Atmore	78%	32
Chilton Medical Center	Clanton	78%	36
Crestwood Medical Center	Huntsville	78%	155
Medical Center Blount	Oneonta	78%	79
Parkway Medical Center Hospital	Decatur	78%	93
Prattville Baptist Hospital	Prattville	78%	120
Saint Clair Regional Hospital	Pell City	78%	130
Saint Vincent's Hospital	Birmingham	78%	395
Cooper Green Mercy Hospital	Birmingham	77%	70
George H Lanier Memorial Hospital	Valley	77%	70
Lake Martin Community Hospital	Dadeville	77%	26
South Baldwin Regional Medical Center	Foley	77%	108
Andalusia Regional Hospital	Andalusia	76%	95
Jacksonville Medical Center	Jacksonville	76%	80
Mizell Memorial Hospital	Opp	74%	87
Mobile Infirmary Medical Center	Mobile	74%	77
Vaughan Evergreen Medical Center	Evergreen	74%	47
Baptist Medical Center	Montgomery	73%	73
Marshall Medical Center South	Boaz	73%	172
Thomas Hospital	Fairhope	73%	103
L V Stabler Memorial Hospital	Greenville	70%	69
Vaughan Regional Med Ctr-Parkway Campus	Selma	70%	117
Jackson Hospital and Clinic	Montgomery	69%	91
Russell Medical Center	Alexander City	68%	53
Troy Regional Medical Center	Troy	63%	52
Dale Medical Center	Ozark	61%	74
Wiregrass Medical Center	Geneva	55%	131
Bryan W Whitfield Memorial Hospital	Demopolis	53%	58

14. Blood Culture Timing

Hospital Name	City	Rate	Cases
Elba General Hospital & Nursing Home	Elba	100%	26
Flowers Hospital	Dothan	100%	131
Hartselle Medical Center	Hartselle	100%	37
Parkway Medical Center Hospital	Decatur	98%	59
Wiregrass Medical Center	Geneva	98%	40
Walker Baptist Medical Center	Jasper	97%	287
D W McMillan Memorial Hospital	Brewton	96%	50
Northwest Medical Center	Winfield	96%	50
Prattville Baptist Hospital	Prattville	96%	122
Shoals Hospital	Muscle Shoals	96%	57
Trinity Medical Center	Birmingham	96%	135
Woodland Medical Center	Cullman	96%	75
Crestwood Medical Center	Huntsville	95%	101
Decatur General Hospital	Decatur	95%	136
Fayette Medical Center	Fayette	95%	62
Medical Center Enterprise	Enterprise	95%	97
Northeast Alabama Regional Medical Center	Anniston	95%	167
Community Hospital	Tallassee	94%	34
George H Lanier Memorial Hospital	Valley	94%	50
L V Stabler Memorial Hospital	Greenville	94%	33
Providence Hospital	Mobile	94%	152
Stringfellow Memorial Hospital	Anniston	94%	97
Thomas Hospital	Fairhope	94%	67
Troy Regional Medical Center	Troy	94%	31
Cullman Regional Medical Center	Cullman	93%	122
Eliza Coffee Memorial Hospital	Florence	93%	135
Monroe County Hospital	Monroeville	93%	54
Citizens Baptist Medical Center	Talladega	92%	61
Coosa Valley Baptist Medical Center	Sylacauga	92%	74
Helen Keller Memorial Hospital	Sheffield	92%	75
Marshall Medical Center South	Boaz	92%	136
Princeton Baptist Medical Center	Birmingham	92%	167
Lakeland Community Hospital	Haleyville	91%	58
UAB Medical West	Bessemer	91%	158
Highlands Medical Center	Scottsboro	90%	92
Northport Medical Center	Northport	90%	62
Marion Regional Wellness Center	Hamilton	89%	64
Marshall Medical Center North	Guntersville	89%	114
Pickens County Medical Center	Carrollton	89%	37
Shelby Baptist Medical Center	Alabaster	89%	96
Southeast Alabama Medical Center	Dothan	89%	116
Athens-Limestone Hospital	Athens	88%	85
DeKalb Regional Medical Center	Fort Payne	88%	65
Jacksonville Medical Center	Jacksonville	88%	50
Saint Clair Regional Hospital	Pell City	88%	50
Brookwood Medical Center	Birmingham	87%	212
Jackson Hospital and Clinic	Montgomery	87%	89
Vaughan Regional Med Ctr-Parkway Campus	Selma	87%	68
Gadsden Regional Medical Center	Gadsden	86%	206
Mobile Infirmary Medical Center	Mobile	86%	78
DCH Regional Medical Center	Tuscaloosa	85%	155
Dale Medical Center	Ozark	85%	53
Lawrence Medical Center	Moulton	85%	39
Russell Medical Center	Alexander City	85%	62
Baptist Medical Center	Montgomery	84%	81
South Baldwin Regional Medical Center	Foley	84%	75
University of South Alabama Medical Center	Mobile	84%	70

NOTE: Hospital profiles are in alphabetical order by state, then city, then hospital within the city; Rankings are sorted by rate in descending order and exclude hospitals with less than 25 cases; (1) The number of cases is too small (n<25) for purposes of reliably predicting hospital performance; (2) Measure reflects the hospital's indication that its submission was based upon a sample of its relevant discharges; (3) Rate reflects fewer than the maximum possible quarters of data for the measure; (4) Inaccurate information submitted and suppressed for one or more quarters; (5) No data is available from the hospital for this measure; Please refer to the User's Guide for a full explanation of data

Hospital Name	City	Rate	Cases
Infirmary West	Mobile	83%	52
Medical Center Blount	Oneonta	83%	58
East Alabama Medical Center	Opelika	82%	74
Mizell Memorial Hospital	Opp	82%	33
Andalusia Regional Hospital	Andalusia	81%	52
Baptist Medical Center East	Montgomery	81%	80
Huntsville Hospital	Huntsville	81%	458
Russellville Hospital	Russellville	80%	76
Medical Center East	Birmingham	79%	135
Lakeview Community Hospital	Eufaula	78%	51
Riverview Regional Medical Center	Gadsden	78%	134
Cherokee Medical Center	Centre	75%	28
Saint Vincent's Hospital	Birmingham	75%	231
UAB Hospital	Birmingham	74%	139
Physicians Medical Center Carraway	Birmingham	73%	105
Springhill Medical Center	Mobile	71%	45
Cooper Green Mercy Hospital	Birmingham	60%	43

15. Influenza Vaccine

Hospital Name	City	Rate	Cases
Marion Regional Wellness Center	Hamilton	97%	32
East Alabama Medical Center	Opelika	96%	27
Medical Center Enterprise	Enterprise	95%	42
Flowers Hospital	Dothan	94%	49
Decatur General Hospital	Decatur	91%	35
Prattville Baptist Hospital	Prattville	90%	29
Gadsden Regional Medical Center	Gadsden	89%	65
Marshall Medical Center North	Guntersville	89%	38
DCH Regional Medical Center	Tuscaloosa	88%	59
South Baldwin Regional Medical Center	Foley	88%	34
Stringfellow Memorial Hospital	Anniston	84%	37
Cullman Regional Medical Center	Cullman	78%	45
Lawrence Medical Center	Moulton	78%	27
Walker Baptist Medical Center	Jasper	78%	51
Huntsville Hospital	Huntsville	77%	159
Marshall Medical Center South	Boaz	77%	26
Southeast Alabama Medical Center	Dothan	77%	48
Baptist Medical Center East	Montgomery	74%	27
Crestwood Medical Center	Huntsville	74%	31
Thomas Hospital	Fairhope	74%	27
DeKalb Regional Medical Center	Fort Payne	69%	36
Fayette Medical Center	Fayette	69%	26
Jackson Hospital and Clinic	Montgomery	69%	26
Mobile Infirmary Medical Center	Mobile	64%	28
Saint Vincent's Hospital	Birmingham	63%	79
Physicians Medical Center Carraway	Birmingham	61%	49
Springhill Medical Center	Mobile	59%	29
Eliza Coffee Memorial Hospital	Florence	57%	94
Shelby Baptist Medical Center	Alabaster	54%	50
Highlands Medical Center	Scottsboro	50%	38
Wiregrass Medical Center	Geneva	50%	32
Medical Center East	Birmingham	48%	58
Northwest Medical Center	Winfield	48%	25
Riverview Regional Medical Center	Gadsden	47%	53
Andalusia Regional Hospital	Andalusia	45%	31
Princeton Baptist Medical Center	Birmingham	44%	70
Providence Hospital	Mobile	43%	83
UAB Medical West	Bessemer	33%	46
Lakeland Community Hospital	Haleyville	3%	71

16. Initial Antibiotic Timing

Hospital Name	City	Rate	Cases
D W McMillan Memorial Hospital	Brewton	97%	64
Elba General Hospital & Nursing Home	Elba	96%	48
Hartselle Medical Center	Hartselle	96%	75
Parkway Medical Center Hospital	Decatur	96%	106
Fayette Medical Center	Fayette	95%	109
L V Stabler Memorial Hospital	Greenville	93%	84
Marion Regional Wellness Center	Hamilton	93%	123
Eliza Coffee Memorial Hospital	Florence	92%	458
Medical Center Enterprise	Enterprise	92%	160
Brookwood Medical Center	Birmingham	91%	337
Flowers Hospital	Dothan	91%	170
Thomasville Infirmary	Thomasville	91%	35
Citizens Baptist Medical Center	Talladega	90%	99
Marshall Medical Center North	Guntersville	90%	178
Walker Baptist Medical Center	Jasper	90%	393
Atmore Community Hospital	Atmore	89%	37
Coosa Valley Baptist Medical Center	Sylacauga	89%	104
Lawrence Medical Center	Moulton	89%	91
Northwest Medical Center	Winfield	89%	130
Medical Center Blount	Oneonta	88%	121
Prattville Baptist Hospital	Prattville	88%	145
Princeton Baptist Medical Center	Birmingham	88%	281

Hospital Name	City	Rate	Cases
Georgiana Hospital	Georgiana	87%	38
Russellville Hospital	Russellville	87%	143
Cherokee Medical Center	Centre	86%	58
Florala Memorial Hospital	Florala	86%	63
Helen Keller Memorial Hospital	Sheffield	86%	125
Wiregrass Medical Center	Geneva	86%	120
Andalusia Regional Hospital	Andalusia	85%	106
Cullman Regional Medical Center	Cullman	85%	193
J Paul Jones Hospital	Camden	85%	27
Jackson Medical Center	Jackson	85%	78
Lakeland Community Hospital	Haleyville	85%	346
Lakeview Community Hospital	Eufaula	85%	88
Woodland Medical Center	Cullman	85%	124
Dale Medical Center	Ozark	84%	80
Marshall Medical Center South	Boaz	84%	221
Decatur General Hospital	Decatur	83%	235
East Alabama Medical Center	Opelika	83%	148
Grove Hill Memorial Hospital	Grove Hill	83%	29
Highlands Medical Center	Scottsboro	82%	232
Monroe County Hospital	Monroeville	82%	102
Saint Clair Regional Hospital	Pell City	82%	116
Troy Regional Medical Center	Troy	81%	75
UAB Medical West	Bessemer	81%	302
Baptist Medical Center East	Montgomery	80%	130
Chilton Medical Center	Clanton	80%	44
Springhill Medical Center	Mobile	80%	156
Thomas Hospital	Fairhope	80%	116
Clay County Hospital	Ashland	79%	71
Pickens County Medical Center	Carrollton	79%	104
Stringfellow Memorial Hospital	Anniston	79%	163
DeKalb Regional Medical Center	Fort Payne	78%	127
George H Lanier Memorial Hospital	Valley	78%	83
Russell Medical Center	Alexander City	78%	83
Shoals Hospital	Muscle Shoals	78%	98
Trinity Medical Center	Birmingham	78%	206
University of South Alabama Medical Center	Mobile	78%	101
North Baldwin Infirmary	Bay Minette	76%	58
Saint Vincent's Hospital	Birmingham	76%	404
Community Hospital	Tallassee	75%	60
Northport Medical Center	Northport	75%	100
Physicians Medical Center Carraway	Birmingham	75%	212
Southeast Alabama Medical Center	Dothan	75%	195
Jacksonville Medical Center	Jacksonville	74%	82
Lake Martin Community Hospital	Dadeville	74%	38
Medical Center East	Birmingham	74%	288
Infirmary West	Mobile	73%	81
Riverview Regional Medical Center	Gadsden	73%	246
Shelby Baptist Medical Center	Alabaster	73%	231
Gadsden Regional Medical Center	Gadsden	72%	318
Providence Hospital	Mobile	72%	297
Baptist Medical Center	Montgomery	70%	116
Bibb Medical Center	Centreville	69%	36
DCH Regional Medical Center	Tuscaloosa	69%	301
Northeast Alabama Regional Medical Center	Anniston	69%	286
South Baldwin Regional Medical Center	Foley	68%	137
Mobile Infirmary Medical Center	Mobile	67%	147
Vaughan Evergreen Medical Center	Evergreen	67%	42
Bryan W Whitfield Memorial Hospital	Demopolis	65%	80
Athens-Limestone Hospital	Athens	64%	171
Crestwood Medical Center	Huntsville	64%	173
UAB Hospital	Birmingham	64%	180
Huntsville Hospital	Huntsville	63%	784
Vaughan Regional Med Ctr-Parkway Campus	Selma	60%	139
Mizell Memorial Hospital	Opp	58%	85
Jackson Hospital and Clinic	Montgomery	55%	164
Cooper Green Mercy Hospital	Birmingham	46%	94
Crenshaw Baptist Hospital	Luverne	42%	55

17. Oxygenation Assessment

Hospital Name	City	Rate	Cases
Andalusia Regional Hospital	Andalusia	100%	134
Bibb Medical Center	Centreville	100%	49
Brookwood Medical Center	Birmingham	100%	426
Cherokee Medical Center	Centre	100%	66
Chilton Medical Center	Clanton	100%	46
Community Hospital	Tallassee	100%	74
Cullman Regional Medical Center	Cullman	100%	238
D W McMillan Memorial Hospital	Brewton	100%	80
Dale Medical Center	Ozark	100%	106
Elba General Hospital & Nursing Home	Elba	100%	70
Eliza Coffee Memorial Hospital	Florence	100%	470
Florala Memorial Hospital	Florala	100%	87
Flowers Hospital	Dothan	100%	230
Gadsden Regional Medical Center	Gadsden	100%	390

NOTE: Hospital profiles are in alphabetical order by state, then city, then hospital within the city; Rankings are sorted by rate in descending order and exclude hospitals with less than 25 cases; (1) The number of cases is too small (n<25) for purposes of reliably predicting hospital performance; (2) Measure reflects the hospital's indication that its submission was based upon a sample of its relevant discharges; (3) Rate reflects fewer than the maximum possible quarters of data for the measure; (4) Inaccurate information submitted and suppressed for one or more quarters; (5) No data is available from the hospital for this measure; Please refer to the User's Guide for a full explanation of data

Hospital Name	City	Rate	Cases
Grove Hill Memorial Hospital	Grove Hill	100%	48
Hartselle Medical Center	Hartselle	100%	86
Helen Keller Memorial Hospital	Sheffield	100%	147
Highlands Medical Center	Scottsboro	100%	272
Huntsville Hospital	Huntsville	100%	934
Infirmary West	Mobile	100%	92
J Paul Jones Hospital	Camden	100%	33
Jackson Medical Center	Jackson	100%	84
Jacksonville Medical Center	Jacksonville	100%	93
L V Stabler Memorial Hospital	Greenville	100%	89
Lake Martin Community Hospital	Dadeville	100%	54
Lawrence Medical Center	Moulton	100%	127
Marion Regional Wellness Center	Hamilton	100%	153
Marshall Medical Center North	Guntersville	100%	219
Marshall Medical Center South	Boaz	100%	263
Medical Center Enterprise	Enterprise	100%	192
Mobile Infirmary Medical Center	Mobile	100%	174
Monroe County Hospital	Monroeville	100%	134
North Baldwin Infirmary	Bay Minette	100%	63
Northeast Alabama Regional Medical Center	Anniston	100%	345
Northwest Medical Center	Winfield	100%	151
Parkway Medical Center Hospital	Decatur	100%	119
Princeton Baptist Medical Center	Birmingham	100%	341
Randolph Health Systems Medical Center	Roanoke	100%	29
Russell Medical Center	Alexander City	100%	122
Saint Vincent's Hospital	Birmingham	100%	508
Shelby Baptist Medical Center	Alabaster	100%	298
Thomas Hospital	Fairhope	100%	153
Thomasville Infirmary	Thomasville	100%	43
Trinity Medical Center	Birmingham	100%	281
UAB Hospital	Birmingham	100%	243
University of South Alabama Medical Center	Mobile	100%	106
Vaughan Evergreen Medical Center	Evergreen	100%	57
Vaughan Regional Med Ctr-Parkway Campus	Selma	100%	164
Walker Baptist Medical Center	Jasper	100%	459
Woodland Medical Center	Cullman	100%	145
Baptist Medical Center	Montgomery	99%	153
Baptist Medical Center East	Montgomery	99%	162
Cooper Green Mercy Hospital	Birmingham	99%	100
Crestwood Medical Center	Huntsville	99%	197
DCH Regional Medical Center	Tuscaloosa	99%	385
DeKalb Regional Medical Center	Fort Payne	99%	153
Decatur General Hospital	Decatur	99%	279
East Alabama Medical Center	Opelika	99%	178
Lakeland Community Hospital	Haleyville	99%	398
Medical Center Blount	Oneonta	99%	134
Northport Medical Center	Northport	99%	123
Prattville Baptist Hospital	Prattville	99%	177
Riverview Regional Medical Center	Gadsden	99%	315
Saint Clair Regional Hospital	Pell City	99%	146
South Baldwin Regional Medical Center	Foley	99%	153
Southeast Alabama Medical Center	Dothan	99%	270
UAB Medical West	Bessemer	99%	336
Atmore Community Hospital	Atmore	98%	46
Fayette Medical Center	Fayette	98%	119
George H Lanier Memorial Hospital	Valley	98%	95
Georgiana Hospital	Georgiana	98%	46
Medical Center East	Birmingham	98%	376
Physicians Medical Center Carraway	Birmingham	98%	246
Russellville Hospital	Russellville	98%	176
Springhill Medical Center	Mobile	98%	195
Bryan W Whitfield Memorial Hospital	Demopolis	97%	92
Citizens Baptist Medical Center	Talladega	97%	117
Clay County Hospital	Ashland	97%	86
Coosa Valley Baptist Medical Center	Sylacauga	97%	122
Providence Hospital	Mobile	97%	353
Shoals Hospital	Muscle Shoals	97%	115
Stringfellow Memorial Hospital	Anniston	97%	216
Wiregrass Medical Center	Geneva	97%	159
Athens-Limestone Hospital	Athens	96%	211
Lakeview Community Hospital	Eufaula	96%	114
Troy Regional Medical Center	Troy	96%	83
Crenshaw Baptist Hospital	Luverne	95%	62
Jackson Hospital and Clinic	Montgomery	95%	190
Mizell Memorial Hospital	Opp	95%	128
Pickens County Medical Center	Carrollton	94%	108
Medical Center Enterprise	Enterprise	97%	114
Decatur General Hospital	Decatur	94%	146
East Alabama Medical Center	Opelika	94%	96
Hartselle Medical Center	Hartselle	91%	58
Marshall Medical Center South	Boaz	90%	126
Walker Baptist Medical Center	Jasper	90%	242
L V Stabler Memorial Hospital	Greenville	89%	45
Lakeland Community Hospital	Haleyville	89%	222
Prattville Baptist Hospital	Prattville	89%	93
Brookwood Medical Center	Birmingham	87%	250
Helen Keller Memorial Hospital	Sheffield	87%	94
Stringfellow Memorial Hospital	Anniston	87%	110
Gadsden Regional Medical Center	Gadsden	85%	220
Cullman Regional Medical Center	Cullman	84%	156
Jacksonville Medical Center	Jacksonville	84%	55
Huntsville Hospital	Huntsville	83%	474
DCH Regional Medical Center	Tuscaloosa	82%	196
George H Lanier Memorial Hospital	Valley	82%	51
Marshall Medical Center North	Guntersville	82%	124
Russellville Hospital	Russellville	81%	93
Atmore Community Hospital	Atmore	79%	33
Eliza Coffee Memorial Hospital	Florence	79%	285
Baptist Medical Center East	Montgomery	78%	96
Mobile Infirmary Medical Center	Mobile	78%	81
D W McMillan Memorial Hospital	Brewton	77%	44
Shoals Hospital	Muscle Shoals	77%	77
Northwest Medical Center	Winfield	76%	76
South Baldwin Regional Medical Center	Foley	76%	95
Woodland Medical Center	Cullman	76%	87
Mizell Memorial Hospital	Opp	75%	80
Community Hospital	Tallassee	74%	34
Crestwood Medical Center	Huntsville	72%	109
Southeast Alabama Medical Center	Dothan	72%	169
Fayette Medical Center	Fayette	71%	72
Trinity Medical Center	Birmingham	71%	165
Baptist Medical Center	Montgomery	68%	72
Thomas Hospital	Fairhope	68%	95
Wiregrass Medical Center	Geneva	67%	83
Monroe County Hospital	Monroeville	66%	73
Jackson Hospital and Clinic	Montgomery	65%	113
UAB Medical West	Bessemer	65%	177
Physicians Medical Center Carraway	Birmingham	64%	144
Athens-Limestone Hospital	Athens	62%	95
DeKalb Regional Medical Center	Fort Payne	62%	85
Cherokee Medical Center	Centre	61%	38
Jackson Medical Center	Jackson	61%	33
Troy Regional Medical Center	Troy	61%	46
Pickens County Medical Center	Carrollton	60%	68
Medical Center Blount	Oneonta	58%	76
Saint Clair Regional Hospital	Pell City	58%	72
Shelby Baptist Medical Center	Alabaster	58%	168
Bibb Medical Center	Centreville	57%	28
Providence Hospital	Mobile	57%	214
Riverview Regional Medical Center	Gadsden	57%	183
Highlands Medical Center	Scottsboro	56%	156
Northeast Alabama Regional Medical Center	Anniston	56%	189
Citizens Baptist Medical Center	Talladega	55%	55
Lawrence Medical Center	Moulton	54%	48
Russell Medical Center	Alexander City	53%	70
Vaughan Regional Med Ctr-Parkway Campus	Selma	53%	89
Northport Medical Center	Northport	52%	54
Saint Vincent's Hospital	Birmingham	52%	307
Andalusia Regional Hospital	Andalusia	51%	73
Springhill Medical Center	Mobile	49%	112
Infirmary West	Mobile	48%	33
Vaughan Evergreen Medical Center	Evergreen	47%	30
Coosa Valley Baptist Medical Center	Sylacauga	44%	61
Dale Medical Center	Ozark	44%	57
Princeton Baptist Medical Center	Birmingham	44%	186
Lakeview Community Hospital	Eufaula	39%	75
Medical Center East	Birmingham	39%	221
Clay County Hospital	Ashland	38%	47
North Baldwin Infirmary	Bay Minette	34%	38
Crenshaw Baptist Hospital	Luverne	29%	38
UAB Hospital	Birmingham	28%	110
Lake Martin Community Hospital	Dadeville	24%	29
Bryan W Whitfield Memorial Hospital	Demopolis	16%	43

18. Pneumococcal Vaccine

Hospital Name	City	Rate	Cases
Elba General Hospital & Nursing Home	Elba	100%	42
Parkway Medical Center Hospital	Decatur	100%	55
Florala Memorial Hospital	Florala	98%	56
Marion Regional Wellness Center	Hamilton	98%	101
Flowers Hospital	Dothan	97%	153

19. Smoking Cessation Advice

Hospital Name	City	Rate	Cases
Baptist Medical Center	Montgomery	100%	50
East Alabama Medical Center	Opelika	100%	51
Flowers Hospital	Dothan	100%	58
Medical Center East	Birmingham	100%	89

NOTE: Hospital profiles are in alphabetical order by state, then city, then hospital within the city; Rankings are sorted by rate in descending order and exclude hospitals with less than 25 cases; (1) The number of cases is too small (n<25) for purposes of reliably predicting hospital performance; (2) Measure reflects the hospital's indication that its submission was based upon a sample of its relevant discharges; (3) Rate reflects fewer than the maximum possible quarters of data for the measure; (4) Inaccurate information submitted and suppressed for one or more quarters; (5) No data is available from the hospital for this measure; Please refer to the User's Guide for a full explanation of data

Hospital	City	Rate	Cases
Medical Center Enterprise	Enterprise	100%	42
Parkway Medical Center Hospital	Decatur	100%	32
Prattville Baptist Hospital	Prattville	100%	49
Riverview Regional Medical Center	Gadsden	100%	72
South Baldwin Regional Medical Center	Foley	100%	34
Stringfellow Memorial Hospital	Anniston	100%	77
UAB Medical West	Bessemer	100%	78
University of South Alabama Medical Center	Mobile	100%	52
Walker Baptist Medical Center	Jasper	100%	163
Wiregrass Medical Center	Geneva	100%	42
Lawrence Medical Center	Moulton	98%	43
Northeast Alabama Regional Medical Center	Anniston	98%	88
Princeton Baptist Medical Center	Birmingham	98%	102
Russellville Hospital	Russellville	98%	54
Helen Keller Memorial Hospital	Sheffield	97%	39
Lakeland Community Hospital	Haleyville	97%	102
DCH Regional Medical Center	Tuscaloosa	96%	90
Decatur General Hospital	Decatur	95%	86
Gadsden Regional Medical Center	Gadsden	95%	102
Highlands Medical Center	Scottsboro	95%	61
Baptist Medical Center East	Montgomery	94%	32
Cullman Regional Medical Center	Cullman	94%	68
Eliza Coffee Memorial Hospital	Florence	94%	89
Marshall Medical Center North	Guntersville	94%	50
Providence Hospital	Mobile	94%	78
Saint Vincent's Hospital	Birmingham	94%	82
Brookwood Medical Center	Birmingham	93%	70
Physicians Medical Center Carraway	Birmingham	92%	75
Southeast Alabama Medical Center	Dothan	92%	88
Marion Regional Wellness Center	Hamilton	91%	33
Jackson Hospital and Clinic	Montgomery	90%	40
Lakeview Community Hospital	Eufaula	90%	42
Vaughan Regional Med Ctr-Parkway Campus	Selma	90%	29
Northport Medical Center	Northport	88%	42
DeKalb Regional Medical Center	Fort Payne	86%	37
Fayette Medical Center	Fayette	85%	33
Andalusia Regional Hospital	Andalusia	84%	38
Marshall Medical Center South	Boaz	84%	69
Huntsville Hospital	Huntsville	83%	240
Infirmary West	Mobile	83%	36
Citizens Baptist Medical Center	Talladega	82%	33
Coosa Valley Baptist Medical Center	Sylacauga	82%	33
Crestwood Medical Center	Huntsville	81%	57
Northwest Medical Center	Winfield	81%	37
Woodland Medical Center	Cullman	81%	42
Athens-Limestone Hospital	Athens	80%	56
Springhill Medical Center	Mobile	79%	43
Dale Medical Center	Ozark	78%	32
Thomas Hospital	Fairhope	78%	27
Trinity Medical Center	Birmingham	78%	64
George H Lanier Memorial Hospital	Valley	77%	26
Mobile Infirmary Medical Center	Mobile	76%	41
Medical Center Blount	Oneonta	68%	28
Cooper Green Mercy Hospital	Birmingham	64%	59
Shelby Baptist Medical Center	Alabaster	59%	95
UAB Hospital	Birmingham	48%	64
Saint Clair Regional Hospital	Pell City	47%	38
Pickens County Medical Center	Carrollton	29%	28
Marshall Medical Center North	Guntersville	89%	151
Brookwood Medical Center	Birmingham	88%	1059
Medical Center East	Birmingham	88%	1249
UAB Medical West	Bessemer	87%	349
DCH Regional Medical Center	Tuscaloosa	86%	262
Russellville Hospital	Russellville	86%	86
L V Stabler Memorial Hospital	Greenville	85%	33
Russell Medical Center	Alexander City	84%	231
Crestwood Medical Center	Huntsville	83%	797
Trinity Medical Center	Birmingham	83%	760
University of South Alabama Medical Center	Mobile	82%	182
D W McMillan Memorial Hospital	Brewton	81%	26
Saint Vincent's Hospital	Birmingham	81%	358
Baptist Medical Center East	Montgomery	80%	87
Infirmary West	Mobile	80%	98
Jacksonville Medical Center	Jacksonville	80%	107
Thomas Hospital	Fairhope	79%	471
HealthSouth Medical Center	Birmingham	78%	27
Baptist Medical Center	Montgomery	77%	208
Northeast Alabama Regional Medical Center	Anniston	77%	415
Providence Hospital	Mobile	77%	235
Shelby Baptist Medical Center	Alabaster	76%	401
Woodland Medical Center	Cullman	75%	59
North Baldwin Infirmary	Bay Minette	74%	39
Andalusia Regional Hospital	Andalusia	73%	118
Coosa Valley Baptist Medical Center	Sylacauga	72%	87
UAB Hospital	Birmingham	72%	556
Citizens Baptist Medical Center	Talladega	68%	77
George H Lanier Memorial Hospital	Valley	65%	104
Stringfellow Memorial Hospital	Anniston	65%	75
Springhill Medical Center	Mobile	64%	859
DeKalb Regional Medical Center	Fort Payne	56%	171
Parkway Medical Center Hospital	Decatur	55%	143
Physicians Medical Center Carraway	Birmingham	53%	167
Troy Regional Medical Center	Troy	41%	41
Cooper Green Mercy Hospital	Birmingham	40%	65
Athens-Limestone Hospital	Athens	38%	183
Vaughan Regional Med Ctr-Parkway Campus	Selma	28%	157
South Baldwin Regional Medical Center	Foley	15%	151
Highlands Medical Center	Scottsboro	1%	73

21. Prophylactic Antibiotic Selection

Hospital Name	City	Rate	Cases
Athens-Limestone Hospital	Athens	100%	38
Coosa Valley Baptist Medical Center	Sylacauga	100%	27
Decatur General Hospital	Decatur	100%	88
HealthSouth Medical Center	Birmingham	100%	27
Medical Center Enterprise	Enterprise	100%	84
Southeast Alabama Medical Center	Dothan	100%	70
Walker Baptist Medical Center	Jasper	100%	90
Flowers Hospital	Dothan	99%	285
Princeton Baptist Medical Center	Birmingham	99%	80
Trinity Medical Center	Birmingham	99%	255
East Alabama Medical Center	Opelika	97%	253
Eliza Coffee Memorial Hospital	Florence	97%	196
Medical Center East	Birmingham	96%	318
Northport Medical Center	Northport	96%	110
Providence Hospital	Mobile	96%	78
Cullman Regional Medical Center	Cullman	95%	132
Helen Keller Memorial Hospital	Sheffield	95%	40
Mobile Infirmary Medical Center	Mobile	95%	93
Andalusia Regional Hospital	Andalusia	94%	51
Baptist Medical Center East	Montgomery	94%	31
Brookwood Medical Center	Birmingham	94%	145
Gadsden Regional Medical Center	Gadsden	94%	206
Jackson Hospital and Clinic	Montgomery	94%	103
Thomas Hospital	Fairhope	93%	72
Springhill Medical Center	Mobile	92%	283
Marshall Medical Center North	Guntersville	91%	54
Northeast Alabama Regional Medical Center	Anniston	91%	125
University of South Alabama Medical Center	Mobile	91%	44
Physicians Medical Center Carraway	Birmingham	90%	49
Russell Medical Center	Alexander City	90%	50
Crestwood Medical Center	Huntsville	89%	106
Saint Vincent's Hospital	Birmingham	89%	82
UAB Medical West	Bessemer	89%	91
DeKalb Regional Medical Center	Fort Payne	88%	48
Northwest Medical Center	Winfield	88%	26
Parkway Medical Center Hospital	Decatur	88%	40
Huntsville Hospital	Huntsville	87%	192
DCH Regional Medical Center	Tuscaloosa	86%	69
Citizens Baptist Medical Center	Talladega	85%	26
Baptist Medical Center	Montgomery	81%	69
Marshall Medical Center South	Boaz	80%	41

Surgical Infection Prevention

20. Prophylactic Antibiotic Given

Hospital Name	City	Rate	Cases
Flowers Hospital	Dothan	100%	1133
Cullman Regional Medical Center	Cullman	98%	440
Decatur General Hospital	Decatur	97%	246
East Alabama Medical Center	Opelika	96%	1021
Medical Center Enterprise	Enterprise	96%	341
Walker Baptist Medical Center	Jasper	96%	275
Princeton Baptist Medical Center	Birmingham	95%	319
Gadsden Regional Medical Center	Gadsden	94%	758
Monroe County Hospital	Monroeville	94%	51
Northport Medical Center	Northport	94%	468
Northwest Medical Center	Winfield	94%	111
Southeast Alabama Medical Center	Dothan	94%	212
Fayette Medical Center	Fayette	93%	29
Jackson Hospital and Clinic	Montgomery	93%	359
Mobile Infirmary Medical Center	Mobile	93%	361
Helen Keller Memorial Hospital	Sheffield	91%	121
Marshall Medical Center South	Boaz	91%	148
Shoals Hospital	Muscle Shoals	91%	44
Riverview Regional Medical Center	Gadsden	90%	360
Eliza Coffee Memorial Hospital	Florence	89%	678
Huntsville Hospital	Huntsville	89%	836

NOTE: Hospital profiles are in alphabetical order by state, then city, then hospital within the city; Rankings are sorted by rate in descending order and exclude hospitals with less than 25 cases; (1) The number of cases is too small (n<25) for purposes of reliably predicting hospital performance; (2) Measure reflects the hospital's indication that its submission was based upon a sample of its relevant discharges; (3) Rate reflects fewer than the maximum possible quarters of data for the measure; (4) Inaccurate information submitted and suppressed for one or more quarters; (5) No data is available from the hospital for this measure; Please refer to the User's Guide for a full explanation of data

Shelby Baptist Medical Center	Alabaster	79%	139
UAB Hospital	Birmingham	73%	85
Riverview Regional Medical Center	Gadsden	71%	68
Vaughan Regional Med Ctr-Parkway Campus	Selma	68%	40
Cooper Green Mercy Hospital	Birmingham	66%	29
South Baldwin Regional Medical Center	Foley	48%	40

22. Prophylactic Antibiotic Stopped

Hospital Name	City	Rate	Cases
Flowers Hospital	Dothan	99%	1097
Medical Center Enterprise	Enterprise	98%	328
Parkway Medical Center Hospital	Decatur	97%	134
Monroe County Hospital	Monroeville	92%	50
East Alabama Medical Center	Opelika	91%	961
Marshall Medical Center North	Guntersville	91%	152
Citizens Baptist Medical Center	Talladega	90%	72
Jacksonville Medical Center	Jacksonville	90%	104
Princeton Baptist Medical Center	Birmingham	90%	306
Decatur General Hospital	Decatur	89%	236
Highlands Medical Center	Scottsboro	88%	72
D W McMillan Memorial Hospital	Brewton	85%	26
Eliza Coffee Memorial Hospital	Florence	85%	650
L V Stabler Memorial Hospital	Greenville	85%	33
Marshall Medical Center South	Boaz	85%	142
Northport Medical Center	Northport	85%	445
Jackson Hospital and Clinic	Montgomery	84%	357
Cullman Regional Medical Center	Cullman	82%	423
Walker Baptist Medical Center	Jasper	81%	258
Baptist Medical Center East	Montgomery	80%	83
Russell Medical Center	Alexander City	79%	223
Huntsville Hospital	Huntsville	78%	830
George H Lanier Memorial Hospital	Valley	77%	98
Helen Keller Memorial Hospital	Sheffield	77%	119
Shoals Hospital	Muscle Shoals	77%	43
Thomas Hospital	Fairhope	76%	457
Troy Regional Medical Center	Troy	76%	41
Infirmary West	Mobile	75%	99
Southeast Alabama Medical Center	Dothan	75%	203
Trinity Medical Center	Birmingham	72%	738
DCH Regional Medical Center	Tuscaloosa	71%	241
Springhill Medical Center	Mobile	70%	798
Baptist Medical Center	Montgomery	69%	196
Brookwood Medical Center	Birmingham	69%	1001
Crestwood Medical Center	Huntsville	69%	764
North Baldwin Infirmary	Bay Minette	69%	35
Russellville Hospital	Russellville	69%	85
Shelby Baptist Medical Center	Alabaster	69%	384
Woodland Medical Center	Cullman	69%	58
Providence Hospital	Mobile	66%	230
Athens-Limestone Hospital	Athens	65%	179
Mobile Infirmary Medical Center	Mobile	65%	343
Cooper Green Mercy Hospital	Birmingham	62%	50
Northeast Alabama Regional Medical Center	Anniston	62%	382
Northwest Medical Center	Winfield	62%	110
Vaughan Regional Med Ctr-Parkway Campus	Selma	62%	115
UAB Medical West	Bessemer	58%	329
Medical Center East	Birmingham	57%	1222
Physicians Medical Center Carraway	Birmingham	56%	121
DeKalb Regional Medical Center	Fort Payne	55%	164
Stringfellow Memorial Hospital	Anniston	55%	66
UAB Hospital	Birmingham	54%	546
Andalusia Regional Hospital	Andalusia	52%	118
Saint Vincent's Hospital	Birmingham	51%	335
University of South Alabama Medical Center	Mobile	50%	173
Gadsden Regional Medical Center	Gadsden	48%	726
Riverview Regional Medical Center	Gadsden	42%	336
South Baldwin Regional Medical Center	Foley	38%	147
Fayette Medical Center	Fayette	31%	29
Coosa Valley Baptist Medical Center	Sylacauga	24%	83
HealthSouth Medical Center	Birmingham	23%	26

Pregnancy Care

23. Inpatient Neonatal Mortality

Hospital Name	City	Rate	Cases
Flowers Hospital	Dothan	0.00%	1190
Jacksonville Medical Center	Jacksonville	0.00%	242
East Alabama Medical Center	Opelika	0.12%	1658
Marshall Medical Center North	Guntersville	0.25%	403
Baptist Medical Center East	Montgomery	0.63%	638
Huntsville Hospital	Huntsville	0.71%	983
Baptist Medical Center	Montgomery	1.32%	303
UAB Hospital	Birmingham	1.93%	831

24. Third or Fourth Degree Laceration

Hospital Name	City	Rate	Cases
Jacksonville Medical Center	Jacksonville	0.50%	202
Baptist Medical Center	Montgomery	0.63%	158
East Alabama Medical Center	Opelika	2.02%	1140
UAB Hospital	Birmingham	2.52%	2774
Baptist Medical Center East	Montgomery	3.86%	2148
Huntsville Hospital	Huntsville	4.65%	581
Flowers Hospital	Dothan	6.51%	676
Marshall Medical Center North	Guntersville	9.44%	286

NOTE: Hospital profiles are in alphabetical order by state, then city, then hospital within the city; Rankings are sorted by rate in descending order and exclude hospitals with less than 25 cases; (1) The number of cases is too small (n<25) for purposes of reliably predicting hospital performance; (2) Measure reflects the hospital's indication that its submission was based upon a sample of its relevant discharges; (3) Rate reflects fewer than the maximum possible quarters of data for the measure; (4) Inaccurate information submitted and suppressed for one or more quarters; (5) No data is available from the hospital for this measure; Please refer to the User's Guide for a full explanation of data

Shelby Baptist Medical Center

1000 First Street North
Alabaster, AL 35007
E-mail: kay.sertell@bhsala.com
URL: www.baptistmedical.org
Ownership: Voluntary non-profit - Church
Emergency Services: Yes

Phone: 205-620-8100
Fax: 205-620-7187

Accredited: Yes
Licensed Beds: 210

Key Personnel:
Chief Medical Staff . . . . Ginger L Alred, MD
Emergency Room . . . . Debbie Ritchie, RN
Chief Radiology . . . . Charles M Mead, MD
Director Respiratory Therapy . . . . Gene Sanders

Measure	Cases	This Hospital	State Average	U.S. Average	Top Hospital
Heart Attack Care					
ACE Inhibitor or ARB for LVSD	61	80%	78%	82%	100%
Aspirin at Arrival	171	91%	87%	92%	100%
Aspirin at Discharge	180	93%	87%	90%	100%
Beta Blocker at Arrival	128	78%	81%	87%	100%
Beta Blocker at Discharge	170	94%	86%	90%	100%
Fibrinolytic Medication Timing	0	-	25%	31%	100%
PCI Within 90 Minutes of Arrival[1]	14	43%	61%	54%	95%
Smoking Cessation Advice	83	78%	85%	88%	100%
Heart Failure Care					
ACE Inhibitor or ARB for LVSD	121	62%	80%	82%	100%
Discharge Instructions	271	32%	54%	61%	93%
Evaluation of LVS Function	305	93%	79%	83%	99%
Smoking Cessation Advice	53	66%	78%	82%	100%
Pneumonia Care					
Appropriate Initial Antibiotic	176	82%	81%	83%	94%
Blood Culture Timing	96	89%	89%	90%	100%
Influenza Vaccine	50	54%	62%	70%	100%
Initial Antibiotic Timing	231	73%	79%	80%	93%
Oxygenation Assessment	298	100%	99%	99%	100%
Pneumococcal Vaccine	168	58%	61%	69%	94%
Smoking Cessation Advice	95	59%	77%	80%	100%
Surgical Infection Prevention					
Prophylactic Antibiotic Given[2]	401	76%	74%	77%	95%
Prophylactic Antibiotic Selection[2]	139	79%	88%	90%	100%
Prophylactic Antibiotic Stopped[2]	384	69%	70%	72%	95%
Pregnancy Care					
Inpatient Neonatal Mortality	-	-	-	-	-
Third or Fourth Degree Laceration	-	-	3.32%	3.63%	3.27%

Russell Medical Center

Alternate Name: Russell Hospital
3316 Highway 280
Alexander City, AL 35010
E-mail: skelley@russellmedcenter.com
URL: www.russellmedcenter.com
Ownership: Voluntary non-profit - Private
Emergency Services: Yes

Phone: 256-329-7100
Fax: 256-329-7186

Accredited: Yes
Licensed Beds: 75

Key Personnel:
President/CEO . . . . Frank W Harris
Catheterization Lab . . . . Ricky Browning
Emergency Room . . . . Edwina Segrest
Emergency Room . . . . Michelle Goldhagen, MD
ICU . . . . Sharon Davis
Medical/Surgical Nursing . . . . Shana Hobbs
Women's Health . . . . Tanya McKee
Respiratory Therapy . . . . Greg Studdard

Measure	Cases	This Hospital	State Average	U.S. Average	Top Hospital
Heart Attack Care					
ACE Inhibitor or ARB for LVSD[1]	12	75%	78%	82%	100%
Aspirin at Arrival	52	98%	87%	92%	100%
Aspirin at Discharge	46	91%	87%	90%	100%
Beta Blocker at Arrival	52	98%	81%	87%	100%
Beta Blocker at Discharge	46	98%	86%	90%	100%
Fibrinolytic Medication Timing[1]	2	0%	25%	31%	100%
PCI Within 90 Minutes of Arrival[1]	4	25%	61%	54%	95%
Smoking Cessation Advice[1]	23	74%	85%	88%	100%
Heart Failure Care					

Measure	Cases	This Hospital	State Average	U.S. Average	Top Hospital
ACE Inhibitor or ARB for LVSD	28	79%	80%	82%	100%
Discharge Instructions	62	56%	54%	61%	93%
Evaluation of LVS Function	86	92%	79%	83%	99%
Smoking Cessation Advice[1]	18	56%	78%	82%	100%
Pneumonia Care					
Appropriate Initial Antibiotic	53	68%	81%	83%	94%
Blood Culture Timing	62	85%	89%	90%	100%
Influenza Vaccine[1]	19	53%	62%	70%	100%
Initial Antibiotic Timing	83	78%	79%	80%	93%
Oxygenation Assessment	122	100%	99%	99%	100%
Pneumococcal Vaccine	70	53%	61%	69%	94%
Smoking Cessation Advice[1]	19	58%	77%	80%	100%
Surgical Infection Prevention					
Prophylactic Antibiotic Given	231	84%	74%	77%	95%
Prophylactic Antibiotic Selection	50	90%	88%	90%	100%
Prophylactic Antibiotic Stopped	223	79%	70%	72%	95%
Pregnancy Care					
Inpatient Neonatal Mortality	-	-	-	-	-
Third or Fourth Degree Laceration	-	-	3.32%	3.63%	3.27%

Andalusia Regional Hospital

Alternate Name: Community Hospital of Andalusia
849 S Three Notch Street
PO Box 760
Andalusia, AL 36420
URL: www.andalusiaregional.com
Ownership: Proprietary
Emergency Services: No

Phone: 334-222-8466
Fax: 334-427-0349

Accredited: Yes
Licensed Beds: 113

Key Personnel:
CEO . . . . Michael A Callahan
CNO . . . . Melissa Davis
Chief Medical Staff . . . . Tim Day, MD

Measure	Cases	This Hospital	State Average	U.S. Average	Top Hospital
Heart Attack Care					
ACE Inhibitor or ARB for LVSD	0	-	78%	82%	100%
Aspirin at Arrival[1]	2	50%	87%	92%	100%
Aspirin at Discharge[1]	3	67%	87%	90%	100%
Beta Blocker at Arrival[1]	3	100%	81%	87%	100%
Beta Blocker at Discharge[1]	4	100%	86%	90%	100%
Fibrinolytic Medication Timing	0	-	25%	31%	100%
PCI Within 90 Minutes of Arrival	0	-	61%	54%	95%
Smoking Cessation Advice	0	-	85%	88%	100%
Heart Failure Care					
ACE Inhibitor or ARB for LVSD	37	59%	80%	82%	100%
Discharge Instructions	149	86%	54%	61%	93%
Evaluation of LVS Function	183	80%	79%	83%	99%
Smoking Cessation Advice[1]	22	100%	78%	82%	100%
Pneumonia Care					
Appropriate Initial Antibiotic	95	76%	81%	83%	94%
Blood Culture Timing	52	81%	89%	90%	100%
Influenza Vaccine	31	45%	62%	70%	100%
Initial Antibiotic Timing	106	85%	79%	80%	93%
Oxygenation Assessment	134	100%	99%	99%	100%
Pneumococcal Vaccine	73	51%	61%	69%	94%
Smoking Cessation Advice	38	84%	77%	80%	100%
Surgical Infection Prevention					
Prophylactic Antibiotic Given[2,3]	118	73%	74%	77%	95%
Prophylactic Antibiotic Selection[2]	51	94%	88%	90%	100%
Prophylactic Antibiotic Stopped[2,3]	118	52%	70%	72%	95%
Pregnancy Care					
Inpatient Neonatal Mortality	-	-	-	-	-
Third or Fourth Degree Laceration	-	-	3.32%	3.63%	3.27%

Northeast Alabama Regional Medical Center

400 E 10th Street
PO Box 2208
Anniston, AL 36207
URL: www.rmccares.org
Ownership: Government - Local
Emergency Services: Yes

Phone: 256-235-5121
Fax: 256-235-5608

Accredited: Yes
Licensed Beds: 372

Key Personnel:
President/CEO . . . . Allen P Fletcher

NOTE: Hospital profiles are in alphabetical order by state, then city, then hospital within the city; Rankings are sorted by rate in descending order and exclude hospitals with less than 25 cases; (1) The number of cases is too small (n<25) for purposes of reliably predicting hospital performance; (2) Measure reflects the hospital's indication that its submission was based upon a sample of its relevant discharges; (3) Rate reflects fewer than the maximum possible quarters of data for the measure; (4) Inaccurate information submitted and suppressed for one or more quarters; (5) No data is available from the hospital for this measure; Please refer to the User's Guide for a full explanation of data

Chief Medical Staff. . . . . Jefferson Trupp, MD
Cardiac Lab . . . . Bess Tingle
Catheterization Lab . . . . Todd Geoff
Emergency Room . . . . Traci Gaither
Infection Control. . . . . Trish Samples
ICU. . . . . Carolyn Moncrief
Intensive/Coronary Care . . . . Wendy Davidson
Medical/Surgical Nursing . . . . Joy Webb
OB/GYN Womens Health. . . . . Elaine Davis
Respiratory/Cardiopulmonary. . . . . Danny Schneck

Measure	Cases	This Hospital	State Average	U.S. Average	Top Hospital
Heart Attack Care					
ACE Inhibitor or ARB for LVSD	50	82%	78%	82%	100%
Aspirin at Arrival	177	97%	87%	92%	100%
Aspirin at Discharge	180	94%	87%	90%	100%
Beta Blocker at Arrival	108	90%	81%	87%	100%
Beta Blocker at Discharge	184	89%	86%	90%	100%
Fibrinolytic Medication Timing[1]	1	0%	25%	31%	100%
PCI Within 90 Minutes of Arrival[1]	11	91%	61%	54%	95%
Smoking Cessation Advice	95	100%	85%	88%	100%
Heart Failure Care					
ACE Inhibitor or ARB for LVSD	226	78%	80%	82%	100%
Discharge Instructions	430	71%	54%	61%	93%
Evaluation of LVS Function	502	88%	79%	83%	99%
Smoking Cessation Advice	113	99%	78%	82%	100%
Pneumonia Care					
Appropriate Initial Antibiotic	169	85%	81%	83%	94%
Blood Culture Timing	167	95%	89%	90%	100%
Influenza Vaccine[4,5]	-	-	62%	70%	100%
Initial Antibiotic Timing	286	69%	79%	80%	93%
Oxygenation Assessment	345	100%	99%	99%	100%
Pneumococcal Vaccine	189	56%	61%	69%	94%
Smoking Cessation Advice	88	98%	77%	80%	100%
Surgical Infection Prevention					
Prophylactic Antibiotic Given[3]	415	77%	74%	77%	95%
Prophylactic Antibiotic Selection	125	91%	88%	90%	100%
Prophylactic Antibiotic Stopped[3]	382	62%	70%	72%	95%
Pregnancy Care					
Inpatient Neonatal Mortality	-	-	-	-	-
Third or Fourth Degree Laceration	-	-	3.32%	3.63%	3.27%

Stringfellow Memorial Hospital

301 E 18th Street   Phone: 256-235-8900
Anniston, AL 36207   Fax: 256-235-8751
E-mail: info@StringfellowHealth.com
URL: www.stringfellowhealth.com
Ownership: Proprietary   Accredited: Yes
Emergency Services: Yes   Licensed Beds: 125
Key Personnel:
CEO/Administrator. . . . . Rich Ellis
Chief Medical Staff. . . . . Wilfredo Granna, MD
Emergency Room . . . . Preston McDonald, MD
Director Medical/Surgical Nursing . . . . Jan Stowe
Director Respiratory Therapy . . . . Lynne Suggs

Measure	Cases	This Hospital	State Average	U.S. Average	Top Hospital
Heart Attack Care					
ACE Inhibitor or ARB for LVSD[1]	8	88%	78%	82%	100%
Aspirin at Arrival	59	97%	87%	92%	100%
Aspirin at Discharge	53	96%	87%	90%	100%
Beta Blocker at Arrival	40	70%	81%	87%	100%
Beta Blocker at Discharge	56	79%	86%	90%	100%
Fibrinolytic Medication Timing[1]	1	0%	25%	31%	100%
PCI Within 90 Minutes of Arrival[1]	6	17%	61%	54%	95%
Smoking Cessation Advice	31	100%	85%	88%	100%
Heart Failure Care					
ACE Inhibitor or ARB for LVSD	101	81%	80%	82%	100%
Discharge Instructions	208	51%	54%	61%	93%
Evaluation of LVS Function	232	95%	79%	83%	99%
Smoking Cessation Advice	60	100%	78%	82%	100%
Pneumonia Care					
Appropriate Initial Antibiotic	156	83%	81%	83%	94%

Measure	Cases	This Hospital	State Average	U.S. Average	Top Hospital
Blood Culture Timing	97	94%	89%	90%	100%
Influenza Vaccine	37	84%	62%	70%	100%
Initial Antibiotic Timing	163	79%	79%	80%	93%
Oxygenation Assessment	216	97%	99%	99%	100%
Pneumococcal Vaccine	110	87%	61%	69%	94%
Smoking Cessation Advice	77	100%	77%	80%	100%
Surgical Infection Prevention					
Prophylactic Antibiotic Given[2]	75	65%	74%	77%	95%
Prophylactic Antibiotic Selection[1,2]	12	58%	88%	90%	100%
Prophylactic Antibiotic Stopped[2]	66	55%	70%	72%	95%
Pregnancy Care					
Inpatient Neonatal Mortality	-	-	-	-	-
Third or Fourth Degree Laceration	-	-	3.32%	3.63%	3.27%

Clay County Hospital

Alternate Name: Clay County Hospital & Nursing Home
83825 Highway 9   Phone: 256-354-2131
PO Box 1270   Fax: 256-354-1230
Ashland, AL 36251
E-mail: kjackson@clayhosp.org
URL: www.claycountyhospital.com
Ownership: Govt - Hospital District or Authority   Accredited: No
Emergency Services: Yes   Licensed Beds: 53
Key Personnel:
Administrator . . . . Linda U Jordan
Chief Medical Staff. . . . . Dwain Rush, MD
Infection Control. . . . . Becky Macoy, RN
Director Medical/Surgical Nursing . . . . Ann Fisher, RN
Director Radiology . . . . Debbie Upchurch, RT
Director Respiratory Therapy . . . . Hal Harris

Measure	Cases	This Hospital	State Average	U.S. Average	Top Hospital
Heart Attack Care					
ACE Inhibitor or ARB for LVSD	0	-	78%	82%	100%
Aspirin at Arrival[1]	4	75%	87%	92%	100%
Aspirin at Discharge[1]	4	75%	87%	90%	100%
Beta Blocker at Arrival[1]	3	33%	81%	87%	100%
Beta Blocker at Discharge[1]	5	40%	86%	90%	100%
Fibrinolytic Medication Timing	0	-	25%	31%	100%
PCI Within 90 Minutes of Arrival	0	-	61%	54%	95%
Smoking Cessation Advice	0	-	85%	88%	100%
Heart Failure Care					
ACE Inhibitor or ARB for LVSD[1]	11	64%	80%	82%	100%
Discharge Instructions	67	1%	54%	61%	93%
Evaluation of LVS Function	83	37%	79%	83%	99%
Smoking Cessation Advice[1]	12	58%	78%	82%	100%
Pneumonia Care					
Appropriate Initial Antibiotic	59	83%	81%	83%	94%
Blood Culture Timing[1]	18	89%	89%	90%	100%
Influenza Vaccine[1]	15	60%	62%	70%	100%
Initial Antibiotic Timing	71	79%	79%	80%	93%
Oxygenation Assessment	86	97%	99%	99%	100%
Pneumococcal Vaccine	47	38%	61%	69%	94%
Smoking Cessation Advice[1]	19	63%	77%	80%	100%
Surgical Infection Prevention					
Prophylactic Antibiotic Given[5]	-	-	74%	77%	95%
Prophylactic Antibiotic Selection[5]	-	-	88%	90%	100%
Prophylactic Antibiotic Stopped[5]	-	-	70%	72%	95%
Pregnancy Care					
Inpatient Neonatal Mortality	-	-	-	-	-
Third or Fourth Degree Laceration	-	-	3.32%	3.63%	3.27%

Athens-Limestone Hospital

700 West Market Street   Phone: 256-233-9292
Athens, AL 35611   Fax: 256-233-9277
E-mail: info@athenslimestonehospital.com
URL: www.athenslimestonehospital.com
Ownership: Govt - Hospital District or Authority   Accredited: Yes
Emergency Services: Yes   Licensed Beds: 101
Key Personnel:
CEO. . . . . Cary Payne
Chief Medical Staff. . . . . Paul Noel, MD

NOTE: Hospital profiles are in alphabetical order by state, then city, then hospital within the city; Rankings are sorted by rate in descending order and exclude hospitals with less than 25 cases; (1) The number of cases is too small (n<25) for purposes of reliably predicting hospital performance; (2) Measure reflects the hospital's indication that its submission was based upon a sample of its relevant discharges; (3) Rate reflects fewer than the maximum possible quarters of data for the measure; (4) Inaccurate information submitted and suppressed for one or more quarters; (5) No data is available from the hospital for this measure; Please refer to the User's Guide for a full explanation of data

Measure	Cases	This Hospital	State Average	U.S. Average	Top Hospital
Heart Attack Care					
ACE Inhibitor or ARB for LVSD[1]	3	33%	78%	82%	100%
Aspirin at Arrival[1]	13	92%	87%	92%	100%
Aspirin at Discharge[1]	4	100%	87%	90%	100%
Beta Blocker at Arrival[1]	16	69%	81%	87%	100%
Beta Blocker at Discharge[1]	4	100%	86%	90%	100%
Fibrinolytic Medication Timing	0	-	25%	31%	100%
PCI Within 90 Minutes of Arrival	0	-	61%	54%	95%
Smoking Cessation Advice	0	-	85%	88%	100%
Heart Failure Care					
ACE Inhibitor or ARB for LVSD	51	90%	80%	82%	100%
Discharge Instructions	115	16%	54%	61%	93%
Evaluation of LVS Function	154	86%	79%	83%	99%
Smoking Cessation Advice	25	92%	78%	82%	100%
Pneumonia Care					
Appropriate Initial Antibiotic	167	79%	81%	83%	94%
Blood Culture Timing	85	88%	89%	90%	100%
Influenza Vaccine[4,5]	-	-	62%	70%	100%
Initial Antibiotic Timing	171	64%	79%	80%	93%
Oxygenation Assessment	211	96%	99%	99%	100%
Pneumococcal Vaccine	95	62%	61%	69%	94%
Smoking Cessation Advice	56	84%	77%	80%	100%
Surgical Infection Prevention					
Prophylactic Antibiotic Given	183	38%	74%	77%	95%
Prophylactic Antibiotic Selection	38	100%	88%	90%	100%
Prophylactic Antibiotic Stopped	179	65%	70%	72%	95%
Pregnancy Care					
Inpatient Neonatal Mortality	-	-	-	-	-
Third or Fourth Degree Laceration	-	-	3.32%	3.63%	3.27%

Atmore Community Hospital

Alternate Name: Greenlawn Hospital
401 Medical Park Drive
Atmore, AL 36502
URL: www.ebaptisthealthcare.org/AtmoreCommunityHospital
Ownership: Voluntary non-profit - Other
Emergency Services: Yes

Phone: 334-368-2500
Fax: 334-368-6362
Accredited: Yes
Licensed Beds: 51

Key Personnel:
CEO . . . . Bob Gowing
OB/GYN Womens Health . . . . Bob Wade

Measure	Cases	This Hospital	State Average	U.S. Average	Top Hospital
Heart Attack Care					
ACE Inhibitor or ARB for LVSD[1]	1	100%	78%	82%	100%
Aspirin at Arrival[1]	7	71%	87%	92%	100%
Aspirin at Discharge[1]	3	67%	87%	90%	100%
Beta Blocker at Arrival[1]	1	0%	81%	87%	100%
Beta Blocker at Discharge[1]	2	100%	86%	90%	100%
Fibrinolytic Medication Timing	0	-	25%	31%	100%
PCI Within 90 Minutes of Arrival	0	-	61%	54%	95%
Smoking Cessation Advice[1]	1	100%	85%	88%	100%
Heart Failure Care					
ACE Inhibitor or ARB for LVSD	26	81%	80%	82%	100%
Discharge Instructions	59	69%	54%	61%	93%
Evaluation of LVS Function	70	89%	79%	83%	99%
Smoking Cessation Advice[1]	21	95%	78%	82%	100%
Pneumonia Care					
Appropriate Initial Antibiotic	32	78%	81%	83%	94%
Blood Culture Timing[1]	18	94%	89%	90%	100%
Influenza Vaccine[1]	8	62%	62%	70%	100%
Initial Antibiotic Timing	37	89%	79%	80%	93%
Oxygenation Assessment	46	98%	99%	99%	100%
Pneumococcal Vaccine	33	79%	61%	69%	94%
Smoking Cessation Advice[1]	10	90%	77%	80%	100%
Surgical Infection Prevention					
Prophylactic Antibiotic Given[5]	-	-	74%	77%	95%
Prophylactic Antibiotic Selection[5]	-	-	88%	90%	100%
Prophylactic Antibiotic Stopped[5]	-	-	70%	72%	95%
Pregnancy Care					
Inpatient Neonatal Mortality	-	-	-	-	-

			3.32%	3.63%	3.27%
Third or Fourth Degree Laceration	-	-	3.32%	3.63%	3.27%

North Baldwin Infirmary

1815 Hand Avenue
PO Box 1409
Bay Minette, AL 36507
URL: www.northbaldwinhospital.com
Ownership: Voluntary non-profit - Private
Emergency Services: Yes

Phone: 251-937-5521
Fax: 251-937-1657

Accredited: No

Key Personnel:
Administrator . . . . William McLaughlin
Chief Medical Staff . . . . John Crowell
Emergency Room . . . . Margaret Roley, RN
Director Medical/Surgical Nursing . . . . Margaret Roley, RN
OB/GYN Womens Health . . . . Marla Gleson, MD
Chief Radiology . . . . Larry Arcement, MD
Director Respiratory Therapy . . . . Paul Hicks

Measure	Cases	This Hospital	State Average	U.S. Average	Top Hospital
Heart Attack Care					
ACE Inhibitor or ARB for LVSD[3]	0	-	78%	82%	100%
Aspirin at Arrival[1,3]	2	100%	87%	92%	100%
Aspirin at Discharge[1,3]	1	100%	87%	90%	100%
Beta Blocker at Arrival[1,3]	1	100%	81%	87%	100%
Beta Blocker at Discharge[1,3]	1	100%	86%	90%	100%
Fibrinolytic Medication Timing[3]	0	-	25%	31%	100%
PCI Within 90 Minutes of Arrival	0	-	61%	54%	95%
Smoking Cessation Advice[3]	0	-	85%	88%	100%
Heart Failure Care					
ACE Inhibitor or ARB for LVSD[1]	9	89%	80%	82%	100%
Discharge Instructions[1]	23	0%	54%	61%	93%
Evaluation of LVS Function	28	93%	79%	83%	99%
Smoking Cessation Advice[1]	8	62%	78%	82%	100%
Pneumonia Care					
Appropriate Initial Antibiotic	40	80%	81%	83%	94%
Blood Culture Timing[1]	23	87%	89%	90%	100%
Influenza Vaccine[1]	5	40%	62%	70%	100%
Initial Antibiotic Timing	58	76%	79%	80%	93%
Oxygenation Assessment	63	100%	99%	99%	100%
Pneumococcal Vaccine	38	34%	61%	69%	94%
Smoking Cessation Advice[1]	11	55%	77%	80%	100%
Surgical Infection Prevention					
Prophylactic Antibiotic Given	39	74%	74%	77%	95%
Prophylactic Antibiotic Selection[1]	12	92%	88%	90%	100%
Prophylactic Antibiotic Stopped	35	69%	70%	72%	95%
Pregnancy Care					
Inpatient Neonatal Mortality	-	-	-	-	-
Third or Fourth Degree Laceration	-	-	3.32%	3.63%	3.27%

UAB Medical West

995 9th Avenue Southwest
Bessemer, AL 35021
URL: www.uab.edu
Ownership: Voluntary non-profit - Other
Emergency Services: Yes

Phone: 205-481-7000
Fax: 205-481-7994

Accredited: Yes
Licensed Beds: 300

Key Personnel:
CEO . . . . Timothy J Thornton
Director Respiratory Therapy . . . . Lisa Montil

Measure	Cases	This Hospital	State Average	U.S. Average	Top Hospital
Heart Attack Care					
ACE Inhibitor or ARB for LVSD[1]	16	94%	78%	82%	100%
Aspirin at Arrival	56	96%	87%	92%	100%
Aspirin at Discharge	39	90%	87%	90%	100%
Beta Blocker at Arrival	59	86%	81%	87%	100%
Beta Blocker at Discharge	43	93%	86%	90%	100%
Fibrinolytic Medication Timing[1]	1	0%	25%	31%	100%
PCI Within 90 Minutes of Arrival	0	-	61%	54%	95%
Smoking Cessation Advice[1]	17	100%	85%	88%	100%
Heart Failure Care					
ACE Inhibitor or ARB for LVSD	75	96%	80%	82%	100%
Discharge Instructions	186	55%	54%	61%	93%
Evaluation of LVS Function	200	99%	79%	83%	99%

NOTE: Hospital profiles are in alphabetical order by state, then city, then hospital within the city; Rankings are sorted by rate in descending order and exclude hospitals with less than 25 cases; (1) The number of cases is too small (n<25) for purposes of reliably predicting hospital performance; (2) Measure reflects the hospital's indication that its submission was based upon a sample of its relevant discharges; (3) Rate reflects fewer than the maximum possible quarters of data for the measure; (4) Inaccurate information submitted and suppressed for one or more quarters; (5) No data is available from the hospital for this measure; Please refer to the User's Guide for a full explanation of data

Smoking Cessation Advice	52	100%	78%	82%	100%

Pneumonia Care

Appropriate Initial Antibiotic	172	86%	81%	83%	94%
Blood Culture Timing	158	91%	89%	90%	100%
Influenza Vaccine	46	33%	62%	70%	100%
Initial Antibiotic Timing	302	81%	79%	80%	93%
Oxygenation Assessment	336	99%	99%	99%	100%
Pneumococcal Vaccine	177	65%	61%	69%	94%
Smoking Cessation Advice	78	100%	77%	80%	100%

Surgical Infection Prevention

Prophylactic Antibiotic Given	349	87%	74%	77%	95%
Prophylactic Antibiotic Selection	91	89%	88%	90%	100%
Prophylactic Antibiotic Stopped	329	58%	70%	72%	95%

Pregnancy Care

Inpatient Neonatal Mortality	-	-	-	-	-
Third or Fourth Degree Laceration	-	-	3.32%	3.63%	3.27%

Brookwood Medical Center

2010 Brookwood Medical Center Drive   Phone: 205-877-1000
Birmingham, AL 35209   Fax: 205-877-2279
URL: www.bwmc.com
Ownership: Proprietary   Accredited: Yes
Emergency Services: Yes   Licensed Beds: 586
Key Personnel:
President/CEO..........................Garry Gause
Chief Medical Staff.....................Bradley Dennis, MD
Emergency Room ....Jackie Dillard
Infection Control.......................Cathy Sanders
ICU ....Linda Suther
Intensive/Coronary Care ....Linda Suther
OB/GYN Women's Health ....Jackie Martinek

Measure	Cases	This Hospital	State Average	U.S. Average	Top Hospital
Heart Attack Care					
ACE Inhibitor or ARB for LVSD	50	94%	78%	82%	100%
Aspirin at Arrival	146	97%	87%	92%	100%
Aspirin at Discharge	182	96%	87%	90%	100%
Beta Blocker at Arrival	138	97%	81%	87%	100%
Beta Blocker at Discharge	184	99%	86%	90%	100%
Fibrinolytic Medication Timing	0	-	25%	31%	100%
PCI Within 90 Minutes of Arrival[1]	14	71%	61%	54%	95%
Smoking Cessation Advice	65	98%	85%	88%	100%
Heart Failure Care					
ACE Inhibitor or ARB for LVSD	182	84%	80%	82%	100%
Discharge Instructions	355	72%	54%	61%	93%
Evaluation of LVS Function	424	92%	79%	83%	99%
Smoking Cessation Advice	69	94%	78%	82%	100%
Pneumonia Care					
Appropriate Initial Antibiotic	292	82%	81%	83%	94%
Blood Culture Timing	212	87%	89%	90%	100%
Influenza Vaccine[4,5]	-	-	62%	70%	100%
Initial Antibiotic Timing	337	91%	79%	80%	93%
Oxygenation Assessment	426	100%	99%	99%	100%
Pneumococcal Vaccine	250	87%	61%	69%	94%
Smoking Cessation Advice	70	93%	77%	80%	100%
Surgical Infection Prevention					
Prophylactic Antibiotic Given[2]	1,059	88%	74%	77%	95%
Prophylactic Antibiotic Selection[2]	145	94%	88%	90%	100%
Prophylactic Antibiotic Stopped[2]	1,001	69%	70%	72%	95%
Pregnancy Care					
Inpatient Neonatal Mortality	-	-	-	-	-
Third or Fourth Degree Laceration	-	-	3.32%	3.63%	3.27%

Callahan Eye Foundation Hospital

1720 University Boulevard   Phone: 205-325-8100
Birmingham, AL 35249   Fax: 205-325-8547
URL: www.health.vab.edu/eyes
Ownership: Voluntary non-profit - Private Accredited: Yes
Emergency Services: Yes   Licensed Beds: 106
Key Personnel:
Senior VP..............................Raymond Butler
CEO...................................David Hoidal
Chief Medical Staff.....................Robert Morris, MD

Emergency Room ....Judy Cocheanien, RN

Measure	Cases	This Hospital	State Average	U.S. Average	Top Hospital
Heart Attack Care					
ACE Inhibitor or ARB for LVSD[5]	-	-	78%	82%	100%
Aspirin at Arrival[5]	-	-	87%	92%	100%
Aspirin at Discharge[5]	-	-	87%	90%	100%
Beta Blocker at Arrival[5]	-	-	81%	87%	100%
Beta Blocker at Discharge[5]	-	-	86%	90%	100%
Fibrinolytic Medication Timing[5]	-	-	25%	31%	100%
PCI Within 90 Minutes of Arrival[5]	-	-	61%	54%	95%
Smoking Cessation Advice[5]	-	-	85%	88%	100%
Heart Failure Care					
ACE Inhibitor or ARB for LVSD[5]	-	-	80%	82%	100%
Discharge Instructions[5]	-	-	54%	61%	93%
Evaluation of LVS Function[5]	-	-	79%	83%	99%
Smoking Cessation Advice[5]	-	-	78%	82%	100%
Pneumonia Care					
Appropriate Initial Antibiotic[5]	-	-	81%	83%	94%
Blood Culture Timing[5]	-	-	89%	90%	100%
Influenza Vaccine[5]	-	-	62%	70%	100%
Initial Antibiotic Timing[5]	-	-	79%	80%	93%
Oxygenation Assessment[5]	-	-	99%	99%	100%
Pneumococcal Vaccine[5]	-	-	61%	69%	94%
Smoking Cessation Advice[5]	-	-	77%	80%	100%
Surgical Infection Prevention					
Prophylactic Antibiotic Given[5]	-	-	74%	77%	95%
Prophylactic Antibiotic Selection[5]	-	-	88%	90%	100%
Prophylactic Antibiotic Stopped[5]	-	-	70%	72%	95%
Pregnancy Care					
Inpatient Neonatal Mortality	-	-	-	-	-
Third or Fourth Degree Laceration	-	-	3.32%	3.63%	3.27%

Cooper Green Mercy Hospital

1515 6th Avenue S   Phone: 205-930-3200
Birmingham, AL 35233   Fax: 205-930-3497
URL: www.coopergreenmercyhospital.org
Ownership: Government - Local   Accredited: Yes
Emergency Services: Yes   Licensed Beds: 319
Key Personnel:
CEO/Medical Director ....Sandral Hullett
Chief Medical Staff.....................Rick Player, MD
Emergency Room ....Jacqueline Perry
Director Medical/Surgical Nursing ....Jackie Smith, RN
Chief OB/GYN ....Rowell Ashford, MD
Chief Radiology ....William Cason, MD
Director Respiratory Therapy..............Anthony Johnson

Measure	Cases	This Hospital	State Average	U.S. Average	Top Hospital
Heart Attack Care					
ACE Inhibitor or ARB for LVSD[1,2]	4	100%	78%	82%	100%
Aspirin at Arrival[2]	25	100%	87%	92%	100%
Aspirin at Discharge[1,2]	21	100%	87%	90%	100%
Beta Blocker at Arrival[1,2]	24	100%	81%	87%	100%
Beta Blocker at Discharge[1,2]	23	100%	86%	90%	100%
Fibrinolytic Medication Timing[2]	0	-	25%	31%	100%
PCI Within 90 Minutes of Arrival[2]	0	-	61%	54%	95%
Smoking Cessation Advice[1,2]	20	85%	85%	88%	100%
Heart Failure Care					
ACE Inhibitor or ARB for LVSD	62	100%	80%	82%	100%
Discharge Instructions	107	71%	54%	61%	93%
Evaluation of LVS Function	108	93%	79%	83%	99%
Smoking Cessation Advice	61	82%	78%	82%	100%
Pneumonia Care					
Appropriate Initial Antibiotic	70	77%	81%	83%	94%
Blood Culture Timing	43	60%	89%	90%	100%
Influenza Vaccine[1]	9	33%	62%	70%	100%
Initial Antibiotic Timing	94	46%	79%	80%	93%
Oxygenation Assessment	100	99%	99%	99%	100%
Pneumococcal Vaccine[1]	10	70%	61%	69%	94%
Smoking Cessation Advice	59	64%	77%	80%	100%
Surgical Infection Prevention					

NOTE: Hospital profiles are in alphabetical order by state, then city, then hospital within the city; Rankings are sorted by rate in descending order and exclude hospitals with less than 25 cases; (1) The number of cases is too small (n<25) for purposes of reliably predicting hospital performance; (2) Measure reflects the hospital's indication that its submission was based upon a sample of its relevant discharges; (3) Rate reflects fewer than the maximum possible quarters of data for the measure; (4) Inaccurate information submitted and suppressed for one or more quarters; (5) No data is available from the hospital for this measure; Please refer to the User's Guide for a full explanation of data

Prophylactic Antibiotic Given[3]	65	40%	74%	77%	95%
Prophylactic Antibiotic Selection	29	66%	88%	90%	100%
Prophylactic Antibiotic Stopped[3]	50	62%	70%	72%	95%
Pregnancy Care					
Inpatient Neonatal Mortality	-	-	-	-	-
Third or Fourth Degree Laceration	-	-	3.32%	3.63%	3.27%

HealthSouth Medical Center

1201 11th Avenue S
Birmingham, AL 35205
URL: www.healthsouth.com
Ownership: Govt - Hospital District or Authority
Emergency Services: Yes

Phone: 205-930-7000
Fax: 205-930-7141

Accredited: Yes
Licensed Beds: 219

Key Personnel:
President/CEO . . . . Jay Grinney
Catheterization Lab . . . . Anderson Morris, MD
Emergency Room Manager . . . . Tommy Roberts
Emergency Room . . . . Adam Robertson, MD
Infection Control Coordinator . . . . Meredith Lutz, RN
Director Surgical Services . . . . Betsy Karr
Respiratory Manager . . . . Bobby Crumpton

Measure	Cases	This Hospital	State Average	U.S. Average	Top Hospital
Heart Attack Care					
ACE Inhibitor or ARB for LVSD[3]	0	-	78%	82%	100%
Aspirin at Arrival[3]	0	-	87%	92%	100%
Aspirin at Discharge[3]	0	-	87%	90%	100%
Beta Blocker at Arrival[3]	0	-	81%	87%	100%
Beta Blocker at Discharge[3]	0	-	86%	90%	100%
Fibrinolytic Medication Timing[3]	0	-	25%	31%	100%
PCI Within 90 Minutes of Arrival	0	-	61%	54%	95%
Smoking Cessation Advice[3]	0	-	85%	88%	100%
Heart Failure Care					
ACE Inhibitor or ARB for LVSD[1,3]	2	0%	80%	82%	100%
Discharge Instructions[1,3]	3	33%	54%	61%	93%
Evaluation of LVS Function[1,3]	6	33%	79%	83%	99%
Smoking Cessation Advice[1,3]	1	100%	78%	82%	100%
Pneumonia Care					
Appropriate Initial Antibiotic[1,3]	5	100%	81%	83%	94%
Blood Culture Timing[1,3]	2	100%	89%	90%	100%
Influenza Vaccine[5]	-	-	62%	70%	100%
Initial Antibiotic Timing[1,3]	5	100%	79%	80%	93%
Oxygenation Assessment[1,3]	10	100%	99%	99%	100%
Pneumococcal Vaccine[1,3]	5	40%	61%	69%	94%
Smoking Cessation Advice[1,3]	1	0%	77%	80%	100%
Surgical Infection Prevention					
Prophylactic Antibiotic Given[3]	27	78%	74%	77%	95%
Prophylactic Antibiotic Selection	27	100%	88%	90%	100%
Prophylactic Antibiotic Stopped[3]	26	23%	70%	72%	95%
Pregnancy Care					
Inpatient Neonatal Mortality	-	-	-	-	-
Third or Fourth Degree Laceration	-	-	3.32%	3.63%	3.27%

Medical Center East

50 Medical Park E Drive
Birmingham, AL 35235
URL: www.ehs.org
Ownership: Voluntary non-profit - Private
Emergency Services: Yes

Phone: 205-838-3000
Fax: 205-838-3326

Accredited: Yes
Licensed Beds: 282

Key Personnel:
CEO . . . . George McGowen
Chief Medical Staff . . . . Adeeb Thomas, MD
OB/GYN Womens Health . . . . Andrew Lemons, MD
Director Radiology . . . . Billy Connely
Director Respiratory Therapy . . . . Doug Clements

Measure	Cases	This Hospital	State Average	U.S. Average	Top Hospital
Heart Attack Care					
ACE Inhibitor or ARB for LVSD	90	92%	78%	82%	100%
Aspirin at Arrival	274	97%	87%	92%	100%
Aspirin at Discharge	298	95%	87%	90%	100%
Beta Blocker at Arrival	249	95%	81%	87%	100%
Beta Blocker at Discharge	315	95%	86%	90%	100%

Fibrinolytic Medication Timing[1]	1	100%	25%	31%	100%
PCI Within 90 Minutes of Arrival[1]	19	84%	61%	54%	95%
Smoking Cessation Advice	146	100%	85%	88%	100%
Heart Failure Care					
ACE Inhibitor or ARB for LVSD	136	88%	80%	82%	100%
Discharge Instructions	271	85%	54%	61%	93%
Evaluation of LVS Function	316	98%	79%	83%	99%
Smoking Cessation Advice	54	98%	78%	82%	100%
Pneumonia Care					
Appropriate Initial Antibiotic	297	82%	81%	83%	94%
Blood Culture Timing	135	79%	89%	90%	100%
Influenza Vaccine	58	48%	62%	70%	100%
Initial Antibiotic Timing	288	74%	79%	80%	93%
Oxygenation Assessment	376	98%	99%	99%	100%
Pneumococcal Vaccine	221	39%	61%	69%	94%
Smoking Cessation Advice	89	100%	77%	80%	100%
Surgical Infection Prevention					
Prophylactic Antibiotic Given	1,249	88%	74%	77%	95%
Prophylactic Antibiotic Selection	318	96%	88%	90%	100%
Prophylactic Antibiotic Stopped	1,222	57%	70%	72%	95%
Pregnancy Care					
Inpatient Neonatal Mortality	-	-	-	-	-
Third or Fourth Degree Laceration	-	-	3.32%	3.63%	3.27%

Physicians Medical Center Carraway

1600 Carraway Boulevard
Birmingham, AL 35234

Toll-Free: 800-727-8218
Phone: 205-502-6000
Fax: 205-502-5720

E-mail: webmaster@carraway.com
URL: www.carraway.org
Ownership: Voluntary non-profit - Private
Emergency Services: Yes

Accredited: Yes
Licensed Beds: 617

Key Personnel:
CEO . . . . Martin Nowak, FACHE
Emergency Department Director . . . . Mike Skellie
Infection Control . . . . Louise Standridge, RN

Measure	Cases	This Hospital	State Average	U.S. Average	Top Hospital
Heart Attack Care					
ACE Inhibitor or ARB for LVSD	32	88%	78%	82%	100%
Aspirin at Arrival	105	100%	87%	92%	100%
Aspirin at Discharge	137	95%	87%	90%	100%
Beta Blocker at Arrival	99	98%	81%	87%	100%
Beta Blocker at Discharge	143	98%	86%	90%	100%
Fibrinolytic Medication Timing	38	50%	25%	31%	100%
PCI Within 90 Minutes of Arrival	0	-	61%	54%	95%
Smoking Cessation Advice	78	100%	85%	88%	100%
Heart Failure Care					
ACE Inhibitor or ARB for LVSD	88	93%	80%	82%	100%
Discharge Instructions	191	64%	54%	61%	93%
Evaluation of LVS Function	224	93%	79%	83%	99%
Smoking Cessation Advice	68	97%	78%	82%	100%
Pneumonia Care					
Appropriate Initial Antibiotic	140	83%	81%	83%	94%
Blood Culture Timing	105	73%	89%	90%	100%
Influenza Vaccine	49	61%	62%	70%	100%
Initial Antibiotic Timing	212	75%	79%	80%	93%
Oxygenation Assessment	246	98%	99%	99%	100%
Pneumococcal Vaccine	144	64%	61%	69%	94%
Smoking Cessation Advice	75	92%	77%	80%	100%
Surgical Infection Prevention					
Prophylactic Antibiotic Given[2,3]	167	53%	74%	77%	95%
Prophylactic Antibiotic Selection[2]	49	90%	88%	90%	100%
Prophylactic Antibiotic Stopped[2,3]	121	56%	70%	72%	95%
Pregnancy Care					
Inpatient Neonatal Mortality	-	-	-	-	-
Third or Fourth Degree Laceration	-	-	3.32%	3.63%	3.27%

NOTE: Hospital profiles are in alphabetical order by state, then city, then hospital within the city; Rankings are sorted by rate in descending order and exclude hospitals with less than 25 cases; (1) The number of cases is too small (n<25) for purposes of reliably predicting hospital performance; (2) Measure reflects the hospital's indication that its submission was based upon a sample of its relevant discharges; (3) Rate reflects fewer than the maximum possible quarters of data for the measure; (4) Inaccurate information submitted and suppressed for one or more quarters; (5) No data is available from the hospital for this measure; Please refer to the User's Guide for a full explanation of data

Princeton Baptist Medical Center

701 Princeton Avenue SW
Birmingham, AL 35211
Ownership: Voluntary non-profit - Church
Emergency Services: Yes

Phone: 205-783-3000
Fax: 205-783-7233
Accredited: Yes

Measure	Cases	This Hospital	State Average	U.S. Average	Top Hospital
Heart Attack Care					
ACE Inhibitor or ARB for LVSD	131	87%	78%	82%	100%
Aspirin at Arrival	299	97%	87%	92%	100%
Aspirin at Discharge	409	97%	87%	90%	100%
Beta Blocker at Arrival	239	96%	81%	87%	100%
Beta Blocker at Discharge	381	100%	86%	90%	100%
Fibrinolytic Medication Timing[1]	3	33%	25%	31%	100%
PCI Within 90 Minutes of Arrival[1]	6	33%	61%	54%	95%
Smoking Cessation Advice	168	99%	85%	88%	100%
Heart Failure Care					
ACE Inhibitor or ARB for LVSD	238	81%	80%	82%	100%
Discharge Instructions	383	67%	54%	61%	93%
Evaluation of LVS Function	443	97%	79%	83%	99%
Smoking Cessation Advice	86	100%	78%	82%	100%
Pneumonia Care					
Appropriate Initial Antibiotic[2]	212	89%	81%	83%	94%
Blood Culture Timing[2]	167	92%	89%	90%	100%
Influenza Vaccine[2]	70	44%	62%	70%	100%
Initial Antibiotic Timing[2]	281	88%	79%	80%	93%
Oxygenation Assessment[2]	341	100%	99%	99%	100%
Pneumococcal Vaccine[2]	186	44%	61%	69%	94%
Smoking Cessation Advice[2]	102	98%	77%	80%	100%
Surgical Infection Prevention					
Prophylactic Antibiotic Given[2]	319	95%	74%	77%	95%
Prophylactic Antibiotic Selection[2]	80	99%	88%	90%	100%
Prophylactic Antibiotic Stopped[2]	306	90%	70%	72%	95%
Pregnancy Care					
Inpatient Neonatal Mortality	-	-	-	-	-
Third or Fourth Degree Laceration	-	-	3.32%	3.63%	3.27%

Saint Vincent's Hospital

810 Saint Vincent's Drive
Birmingham, AL 35205
URL: www.stv.org
Ownership: Voluntary non-profit - Other
Emergency Services: Yes
Key Personnel:
CEO. . . . . Vincent Capone
Chief Medical Staff. . . . . Ralph Yarbrough, MD
Chief Radiology . . . . John Mussleman, MD
Director Respiratory Therapy . . . . Richard Crocker

Phone: 205-939-7000
Fax: 205-930-2157

Accredited: Yes
Licensed Beds: 338

Measure	Cases	This Hospital	State Average	U.S. Average	Top Hospital
Heart Attack Care					
ACE Inhibitor or ARB for LVSD	60	72%	78%	82%	100%
Aspirin at Arrival	224	99%	87%	92%	100%
Aspirin at Discharge	227	99%	87%	90%	100%
Beta Blocker at Arrival	174	98%	81%	87%	100%
Beta Blocker at Discharge	225	92%	86%	90%	100%
Fibrinolytic Medication Timing	0	-	25%	31%	100%
PCI Within 90 Minutes of Arrival[1]	8	75%	61%	54%	95%
Smoking Cessation Advice	69	97%	85%	88%	100%
Heart Failure Care					
ACE Inhibitor or ARB for LVSD	195	77%	80%	82%	100%
Discharge Instructions	422	66%	54%	61%	93%
Evaluation of LVS Function	468	87%	79%	83%	99%
Smoking Cessation Advice	69	96%	78%	82%	100%
Pneumonia Care					
Appropriate Initial Antibiotic	395	78%	81%	83%	94%
Blood Culture Timing	231	75%	89%	90%	100%
Influenza Vaccine	79	63%	62%	70%	100%
Initial Antibiotic Timing	404	76%	79%	80%	93%
Oxygenation Assessment	508	100%	99%	99%	100%
Pneumococcal Vaccine	307	52%	61%	69%	94%
Smoking Cessation Advice	82	94%	77%	80%	100%

Measure	Cases	This Hospital	State Average	U.S. Average	Top Hospital
Surgical Infection Prevention					
Prophylactic Antibiotic Given[2]	358	81%	74%	77%	95%
Prophylactic Antibiotic Selection[2]	82	89%	88%	90%	100%
Prophylactic Antibiotic Stopped[2]	335	51%	70%	72%	95%
Pregnancy Care					
Inpatient Neonatal Mortality	-	-	-	-	-
Third or Fourth Degree Laceration	-	-	3.32%	3.63%	3.27%

Trinity Medical Center

800 Montclair Road
Birmingham, AL 35213

Toll-Free: 877-227-8478
Phone: 205-592-1000
Fax: 205-599-4958

URL: www.trinitymedicalonline.com
Ownership: Proprietary
Emergency Services: Yes
Key Personnel:

Accredited: Yes
Licensed Beds: 560

CEO. . . . . Vicki Briggs
Chief of Medical Staff. . . . . J.T. Eagan, Jr, MD
Hospital Advisory Council/Chief Surgery . . . . . . Lynda McLean
Catheterization Lab . . . . Bonnie Payne
Emergency Room . . . . Karen Faircloth
Infection Control. . . . . Ginger Smith
Intensive/Coronary Care . . . . Linda Suther
Medical/Surgical Nursing . . . . Nina Norflect Jamie Hacker
OB/GYN Womens Health. . . . . Nancy Holland
Respiratory/Cardiopulmonary. . . . . Melvin Grindberg

Measure	Cases	This Hospital	State Average	U.S. Average	Top Hospital
Heart Attack Care					
ACE Inhibitor or ARB for LVSD	114	92%	78%	82%	100%
Aspirin at Arrival	208	98%	87%	92%	100%
Aspirin at Discharge	418	100%	87%	90%	100%
Beta Blocker at Arrival	190	97%	81%	87%	100%
Beta Blocker at Discharge	416	99%	86%	90%	100%
Fibrinolytic Medication Timing[1]	6	50%	25%	31%	100%
PCI Within 90 Minutes of Arrival[1]	3	67%	61%	54%	95%
Smoking Cessation Advice	172	94%	85%	88%	100%
Heart Failure Care					
ACE Inhibitor or ARB for LVSD	146	99%	80%	82%	100%
Discharge Instructions	308	78%	54%	61%	93%
Evaluation of LVS Function	372	95%	79%	83%	99%
Smoking Cessation Advice	66	77%	78%	82%	100%
Pneumonia Care					
Appropriate Initial Antibiotic	133	88%	81%	83%	94%
Blood Culture Timing	135	96%	89%	90%	100%
Influenza Vaccine[4,5]	-	-	62%	70%	100%
Initial Antibiotic Timing	206	78%	79%	80%	93%
Oxygenation Assessment	281	100%	99%	99%	100%
Pneumococcal Vaccine	165	71%	61%	69%	94%
Smoking Cessation Advice	64	78%	77%	80%	100%
Surgical Infection Prevention					
Prophylactic Antibiotic Given[2,3]	760	83%	74%	77%	95%
Prophylactic Antibiotic Selection[2]	255	99%	88%	90%	100%
Prophylactic Antibiotic Stopped[2,3]	738	72%	70%	72%	95%
Pregnancy Care					
Inpatient Neonatal Mortality	-	-	-	-	-
Third or Fourth Degree Laceration	-	-	3.32%	3.63%	3.27%

UAB Hospital

Alternate Name: University of Alabama Hospital
619 19th Street South
Birmingham, AL 35249
URL: www.health.uab.edu
Ownership: Government - State
Emergency Services: Yes
Key Personnel:

Phone: 205-934-4011
Fax: 205-934-1273

Accredited: Yes
Licensed Beds: 908

CEO. . . . . David Hoidal
Chief Medical Staff. . . . . Scott Buchalter, MD
Emergency Room . . . . Mary Ellen Sharp
Infection Control. . . . . William Dismukes, MD
Medical/Surgical Nursing . . . . Dana Ellis
OB/GYN Womens Health. . . . . Robert Goldenberg, MD
Technical Director Respiratory Therapy . . . . . . Herman Meyers

NOTE: Hospital profiles are in alphabetical order by state, then city, then hospital within the city; Rankings are sorted by rate in descending order and exclude hospitals with less than 25 cases; (1) The number of cases is too small (n<25) for purposes of reliably predicting hospital performance; (2) Measure reflects the hospital's indication that its submission was based upon a sample of its relevant discharges; (3) Rate reflects fewer than the maximum possible quarters of data for the measure; (4) Inaccurate information submitted and suppressed for one or more quarters; (5) No data is available from the hospital for this measure; Please refer to the User's Guide for a full explanation of data

Measure	Cases	This Hospital	State Average	U.S. Average	Top Hospital
Heart Attack Care					
ACE Inhibitor or ARB for LVSD	88	81%	78%	82%	100%
Aspirin at Arrival	177	98%	87%	92%	100%
Aspirin at Discharge	325	99%	87%	90%	100%
Beta Blocker at Arrival	156	94%	81%	87%	100%
Beta Blocker at Discharge	316	95%	86%	90%	100%
Fibrinolytic Medication Timing	0	-	25%	31%	100%
PCI Within 90 Minutes of Arrival[1]	7	71%	61%	54%	95%
Smoking Cessation Advice	127	87%	85%	88%	100%
Heart Failure Care					
ACE Inhibitor or ARB for LVSD[2]	320	83%	80%	82%	100%
Discharge Instructions[2]	516	41%	54%	61%	93%
Evaluation of LVS Function[2]	549	95%	79%	83%	99%
Smoking Cessation Advice[2]	134	63%	78%	82%	100%
Pneumonia Care					
Appropriate Initial Antibiotic[2]	88	84%	81%	83%	94%
Blood Culture Timing[2]	139	74%	89%	90%	100%
Influenza Vaccine[1,2]	19	58%	62%	70%	100%
Initial Antibiotic Timing[2]	180	64%	79%	80%	93%
Oxygenation Assessment[2]	243	100%	99%	99%	100%
Pneumococcal Vaccine[2]	110	28%	61%	69%	94%
Smoking Cessation Advice[2]	64	48%	77%	80%	100%
Surgical Infection Prevention					
Prophylactic Antibiotic Given[2]	556	72%	74%	77%	95%
Prophylactic Antibiotic Selection[2]	85	73%	88%	90%	100%
Prophylactic Antibiotic Stopped[2]	546	54%	70%	72%	95%
Pregnancy Care					
Inpatient Neonatal Mortality[2]	831	1.93%	-	-	-
Third or Fourth Degree Laceration	2,774	2.52%	3.32%	3.63%	3.27%

Marshall Medical Center South

Alternate Name: Boaz-Albertville Medical Center
US Highway 431 N   Phone: 256-593-8310
Boaz, AL 35957   Fax: 256-840-3636
URL: www.mmcenters.com/mmcsouth.php
Ownership: Govt - Hospital District or Authority   Accredited: Yes
Emergency Services: Yes   Licensed Beds: 150
Key Personnel:
Chief Medical Staff . . . . Linda Smith
Director Infection/Disease Control . . . . Ann Thorne
CCU Spvg. Nurse . . . . Kerry Quinn, RN
Director Medical/Surgical Nursing . . . . Margaret Cheek, RN
Director Respiratory Therapy . . . . Angela Meadows

Measure	Cases	This Hospital	State Average	U.S. Average	Top Hospital
Heart Attack Care					
ACE Inhibitor or ARB for LVSD[1]	8	62%	78%	82%	100%
Aspirin at Arrival	30	60%	87%	92%	100%
Aspirin at Discharge[1]	11	82%	87%	90%	100%
Beta Blocker at Arrival	25	44%	81%	87%	100%
Beta Blocker at Discharge[1]	10	70%	86%	90%	100%
Fibrinolytic Medication Timing	0	-	25%	31%	100%
PCI Within 90 Minutes of Arrival	0	-	61%	54%	95%
Smoking Cessation Advice[1]	1	100%	85%	88%	100%
Heart Failure Care					
ACE Inhibitor or ARB for LVSD	66	79%	80%	82%	100%
Discharge Instructions	116	81%	54%	61%	93%
Evaluation of LVS Function	168	98%	79%	83%	99%
Smoking Cessation Advice	33	85%	78%	82%	100%
Pneumonia Care					
Appropriate Initial Antibiotic	172	73%	81%	83%	94%
Blood Culture Timing	136	92%	89%	90%	100%
Influenza Vaccine	26	77%	62%	70%	100%
Initial Antibiotic Timing	221	84%	79%	80%	93%
Oxygenation Assessment	263	100%	99%	99%	100%
Pneumococcal Vaccine	126	90%	61%	69%	94%
Smoking Cessation Advice	69	84%	77%	80%	100%
Surgical Infection Prevention					
Prophylactic Antibiotic Given[2]	148	91%	74%	77%	95%
Prophylactic Antibiotic Selection[2]	41	80%	88%	90%	100%
Prophylactic Antibiotic Stopped[2]	142	85%	70%	72%	95%

Measure	Cases	This Hospital	State Average	U.S. Average	Top Hospital
Pregnancy Care					
Inpatient Neonatal Mortality	-	-	-	-	-
Third or Fourth Degree Laceration	-	-	3.32%	3.63%	3.27%

D W McMillan Memorial Hospital

1301 Belleville Avenue   Phone: 251-867-8061
Brewton, AL 36426   Fax: 251-809-8486
URL: www.ebaptisthealthcare.org/DWMcMillanMemorialHospital
Ownership: Govt - Hospital District or Authority   Accredited: Yes
Emergency Services: Yes   Licensed Beds: 91
Key Personnel:
CEO . . . . Phillip L Parker

Measure	Cases	This Hospital	State Average	U.S. Average	Top Hospital
Heart Attack Care					
ACE Inhibitor or ARB for LVSD[1]	1	100%	78%	82%	100%
Aspirin at Arrival[1]	3	100%	87%	92%	100%
Aspirin at Discharge[1]	2	50%	87%	90%	100%
Beta Blocker at Arrival[1]	2	100%	81%	87%	100%
Beta Blocker at Discharge[1]	2	50%	86%	90%	100%
Fibrinolytic Medication Timing[1]	1	100%	25%	31%	100%
PCI Within 90 Minutes of Arrival	0	-	61%	54%	95%
Smoking Cessation Advice	0	-	85%	88%	100%
Heart Failure Care					
ACE Inhibitor or ARB for LVSD[1]	19	63%	80%	82%	100%
Discharge Instructions	74	42%	54%	61%	93%
Evaluation of LVS Function	78	95%	79%	83%	99%
Smoking Cessation Advice[1]	19	84%	78%	82%	100%
Pneumonia Care					
Appropriate Initial Antibiotic	60	92%	81%	83%	94%
Blood Culture Timing	50	96%	89%	90%	100%
Influenza Vaccine[1]	12	92%	62%	70%	100%
Initial Antibiotic Timing	64	97%	79%	80%	93%
Oxygenation Assessment	80	100%	99%	99%	100%
Pneumococcal Vaccine	44	77%	61%	69%	94%
Smoking Cessation Advice[1]	22	91%	77%	80%	100%
Surgical Infection Prevention					
Prophylactic Antibiotic Given[3]	26	81%	74%	77%	95%
Prophylactic Antibiotic Selection[1]	14	93%	88%	90%	100%
Prophylactic Antibiotic Stopped[3]	26	85%	70%	72%	95%
Pregnancy Care					
Inpatient Neonatal Mortality	-	-	-	-	-
Third or Fourth Degree Laceration	-	-	3.32%	3.63%	3.27%

J Paul Jones Hospital

317 McWilliams Avenue   Phone: 334-682-4131
Camden, AL 36726   Fax: 334-682-4131
Ownership: Government - Local   Accredited: No
Emergency Services: Yes   Licensed Beds: 32
Key Personnel:
CEO . . . . Elizabeth Kennedy
Chief Medical Staff . . . . Willie White, MD
Emergency Room . . . . Sheila Roe, RN
Infection Control . . . . Gladys Luker, RN
Respiratory/Cardiopulmonary . . . . Sheila Roe, RN

Measure	Cases	This Hospital	State Average	U.S. Average	Top Hospital
Heart Attack Care					
ACE Inhibitor or ARB for LVSD	0	-	78%	82%	100%
Aspirin at Arrival[1]	5	80%	87%	92%	100%
Aspirin at Discharge[1]	4	100%	87%	90%	100%
Beta Blocker at Arrival[1]	4	75%	81%	87%	100%
Beta Blocker at Discharge[1]	3	100%	86%	90%	100%
Fibrinolytic Medication Timing[3]	0	-	25%	31%	100%
PCI Within 90 Minutes of Arrival	0	-	61%	54%	95%
Smoking Cessation Advice[3]	0	-	85%	88%	100%
Heart Failure Care					
ACE Inhibitor or ARB for LVSD	0	-	80%	82%	100%
Discharge Instructions[1,3]	2	0%	54%	61%	93%
Evaluation of LVS Function[1]	12	0%	79%	83%	99%
Smoking Cessation Advice[1,3]	1	0%	78%	82%	100%
Pneumonia Care					

NOTE: Hospital profiles are in alphabetical order by state, then city, then hospital within the city; Rankings are sorted by rate in descending order and exclude hospitals with less than 25 cases; (1) The number of cases is too small (n<25) for purposes of reliably predicting hospital performance; (2) Measure reflects the hospital's indication that its submission was based upon a sample of its relevant discharges; (3) Rate reflects fewer than the maximum possible quarters of data for the measure; (4) Inaccurate information submitted and suppressed for one or more quarters; (5) No data is available from the hospital for this measure; Please refer to the User's Guide for a full explanation of data

Measure	Cases	This Hospital	State Average	U.S. Average	Top Hospital
Appropriate Initial Antibiotic[1,2,3]	3	100%	81%	83%	94%
Blood Culture Timing[2,3]	0	-	89%	90%	100%
Influenza Vaccine[4,5]	-	-	62%	70%	100%
Initial Antibiotic Timing[2]	27	85%	79%	80%	93%
Oxygenation Assessment[2]	33	100%	99%	99%	100%
Pneumococcal Vaccine[1,2]	22	0%	61%	69%	94%
Smoking Cessation Advice[2,3]	0	-	77%	80%	100%
Surgical Infection Prevention					
Prophylactic Antibiotic Given[5]	-	-	74%	77%	95%
Prophylactic Antibiotic Selection[5]	-	-	88%	90%	100%
Prophylactic Antibiotic Stopped[5]	-	-	70%	72%	95%
Pregnancy Care					
Inpatient Neonatal Mortality	-	-	-	-	-
Third or Fourth Degree Laceration	-	-	3.32%	3.63%	3.27%

Pickens County Medical Center

PO Box 478
Carrollton, AL 35447
URL: www.dchsystem.com
Ownership: Voluntary non-profit - Other
Emergency Services: Yes

Phone: 205-367-8111
Fax: 205-367-2121

Accredited: No
Licensed Beds: 56

Key Personnel:
President/CEO . . . . H Wayne McElroy
Chief Medical Staff . . . . James L Parker, MD
Emergency Room . . . . William R Brooke, MD
Medical/Surgical Coordinator . . . . Teresa Cochran, RN
Director Radiology . . . . Anita Sullivan
Director Cardiopulmonary Services . . . . Sharon Crawford

Measure	Cases	This Hospital	State Average	U.S. Average	Top Hospital
Heart Attack Care					
ACE Inhibitor or ARB for LVSD[1]	2	100%	78%	82%	100%
Aspirin at Arrival[1]	7	43%	87%	92%	100%
Aspirin at Discharge[1]	4	100%	87%	90%	100%
Beta Blocker at Arrival[1]	7	29%	81%	87%	100%
Beta Blocker at Discharge[1]	3	67%	86%	90%	100%
Fibrinolytic Medication Timing	0	-	25%	31%	100%
PCI Within 90 Minutes of Arrival	0	-	61%	54%	95%
Smoking Cessation Advice[1]	1	0%	85%	88%	100%
Heart Failure Care					
ACE Inhibitor or ARB for LVSD[1]	17	94%	80%	82%	100%
Discharge Instructions	48	27%	54%	61%	93%
Evaluation of LVS Function	55	93%	79%	83%	99%
Smoking Cessation Advice[1]	2	0%	78%	82%	100%
Pneumonia Care					
Appropriate Initial Antibiotic	87	86%	81%	83%	94%
Blood Culture Timing	37	89%	89%	90%	100%
Influenza Vaccine[1]	24	50%	62%	70%	100%
Initial Antibiotic Timing	104	79%	79%	80%	93%
Oxygenation Assessment	108	94%	99%	99%	100%
Pneumococcal Vaccine	68	60%	61%	69%	94%
Smoking Cessation Advice	28	29%	77%	80%	100%
Surgical Infection Prevention					
Prophylactic Antibiotic Given[1,3]	13	77%	74%	77%	95%
Prophylactic Antibiotic Selection[1]	2	100%	88%	90%	100%
Prophylactic Antibiotic Stopped[1,3]	13	100%	70%	72%	95%
Pregnancy Care					
Inpatient Neonatal Mortality	-	-	-	-	-
Third or Fourth Degree Laceration	-	-	3.32%	3.63%	3.27%

Cherokee Medical Center

400 Northwood Drive
Centre, AL 35960
URL: www.cherokeemedicalcenter.com
Ownership: Voluntary non-profit - Private
Emergency Services: Yes

Phone: 256-927-5531
Fax: 256-927-1304

Accredited: Yes
Licensed Beds: 60

Key Personnel:
CEO . . . . Peter Salman
Emergency Room . . . . Becky Smith, RN

Measure	Cases	This Hospital	State Average	U.S. Average	Top Hospital
Heart Attack Care					

Measure	Cases	This Hospital	State Average	U.S. Average	Top Hospital
ACE Inhibitor or ARB for LVSD[1]	2	50%	78%	82%	100%
Aspirin at Arrival[1]	7	43%	87%	92%	100%
Aspirin at Discharge[1]	2	100%	87%	90%	100%
Beta Blocker at Arrival[1]	3	67%	81%	87%	100%
Beta Blocker at Discharge[1]	2	100%	86%	90%	100%
Fibrinolytic Medication Timing[1]	2	50%	25%	31%	100%
PCI Within 90 Minutes of Arrival	0	-	61%	54%	95%
Smoking Cessation Advice	0	-	85%	88%	100%
Heart Failure Care					
ACE Inhibitor or ARB for LVSD	31	77%	80%	82%	100%
Discharge Instructions	43	49%	54%	61%	93%
Evaluation of LVS Function	67	79%	79%	83%	99%
Smoking Cessation Advice[1]	12	83%	78%	82%	100%
Pneumonia Care					
Appropriate Initial Antibiotic	44	82%	81%	83%	94%
Blood Culture Timing	28	75%	89%	90%	100%
Influenza Vaccine[1]	11	45%	62%	70%	100%
Initial Antibiotic Timing	58	86%	79%	80%	93%
Oxygenation Assessment	66	100%	99%	99%	100%
Pneumococcal Vaccine	38	61%	61%	69%	94%
Smoking Cessation Advice[1]	16	75%	77%	80%	100%
Surgical Infection Prevention					
Prophylactic Antibiotic Given[2,3]	0	-	74%	77%	95%
Prophylactic Antibiotic Selection[2]	0	-	88%	90%	100%
Prophylactic Antibiotic Stopped[2,3]	0	-	70%	72%	95%
Pregnancy Care					
Inpatient Neonatal Mortality	-	-	-	-	-
Third or Fourth Degree Laceration	-	-	3.32%	3.63%	3.27%

Bibb Medical Center

208 Pierson Ave
Centreville, AL 35042
Ownership: Government - Local
Emergency Services: Yes

Phone: 205-926-4881

Accredited: No

Measure	Cases	This Hospital	State Average	U.S. Average	Top Hospital
Heart Attack Care					
ACE Inhibitor or ARB for LVSD[5]	-	-	78%	82%	100%
Aspirin at Arrival[5]	-	-	87%	92%	100%
Aspirin at Discharge[5]	-	-	87%	90%	100%
Beta Blocker at Arrival[5]	-	-	81%	87%	100%
Beta Blocker at Discharge[5]	-	-	86%	90%	100%
Fibrinolytic Medication Timing[5]	-	-	25%	31%	100%
PCI Within 90 Minutes of Arrival[5]	-	-	61%	54%	95%
Smoking Cessation Advice[5]	-	-	85%	88%	100%
Heart Failure Care					
ACE Inhibitor or ARB for LVSD[1]	3	100%	80%	82%	100%
Discharge Instructions[1]	14	7%	54%	61%	93%
Evaluation of LVS Function[1]	16	19%	79%	83%	99%
Smoking Cessation Advice[1]	3	67%	78%	82%	100%
Pneumonia Care					
Appropriate Initial Antibiotic	36	94%	81%	83%	94%
Blood Culture Timing[1]	8	75%	89%	90%	100%
Influenza Vaccine[1]	11	27%	62%	70%	100%
Initial Antibiotic Timing	36	69%	79%	80%	93%
Oxygenation Assessment	49	100%	99%	99%	100%
Pneumococcal Vaccine	28	57%	61%	69%	94%
Smoking Cessation Advice[1]	7	71%	77%	80%	100%
Surgical Infection Prevention					
Prophylactic Antibiotic Given[5]	-	-	74%	77%	95%
Prophylactic Antibiotic Selection[5]	-	-	88%	90%	100%
Prophylactic Antibiotic Stopped[5]	-	-	70%	72%	95%
Pregnancy Care					
Inpatient Neonatal Mortality	-	-	-	-	-
Third or Fourth Degree Laceration	-	-	3.32%	3.63%	3.27%

Washington County Hospital

Alternate Name: Washington County Hospital & Nursing Home

NOTE: Hospital profiles are in alphabetical order by state, then city, then hospital within the city; Rankings are sorted by rate in descending order and exclude hospitals with less than 25 cases; (1) The number of cases is too small (n<25) for purposes of reliably predicting hospital performance; (2) Measure reflects the hospital's indication that its submission was based upon a sample of its relevant discharges; (3) Rate reflects fewer than the maximum possible quarters of data for the measure; (4) Inaccurate information submitted and suppressed for one or more quarters; (5) No data is available from the hospital for this measure; Please refer to the User's Guide for a full explanation of data

14600 St Stephens Avenue
PO Box 1299
Chatom, AL 36518
URL: www.wchnh.org
Ownership: Government - Local
Emergency Services: Yes

Phone: 251-847-2223
Fax: 251-847-3808

Accredited: Yes
Licensed Beds: 25

Key Personnel:
CEO. . . . . Douglas Tanner
Chief Medical Staff. . . . . James Hassell

Measure	Cases	This Hospital	State Average	U.S. Average	Top Hospital
Heart Attack Care					
ACE Inhibitor or ARB for LVSD[5]	-	-	78%	82%	100%
Aspirin at Arrival[5]	-	-	87%	92%	100%
Aspirin at Discharge[5]	-	-	87%	90%	100%
Beta Blocker at Arrival[5]	-	-	81%	87%	100%
Beta Blocker at Discharge[5]	-	-	86%	90%	100%
Fibrinolytic Medication Timing[5]	-	-	25%	31%	100%
PCI Within 90 Minutes of Arrival[5]	-	-	61%	54%	95%
Smoking Cessation Advice[5]	-	-	85%	88%	100%
Heart Failure Care					
ACE Inhibitor or ARB for LVSD[1]	3	33%	80%	82%	100%
Discharge Instructions[1]	10	0%	54%	61%	93%
Evaluation of LVS Function[1]	13	38%	79%	83%	99%
Smoking Cessation Advice[1]	2	0%	78%	82%	100%
Pneumonia Care					
Appropriate Initial Antibiotic[1]	8	100%	81%	83%	94%
Blood Culture Timing[1]	2	100%	89%	90%	100%
Influenza Vaccine	0	-	62%	70%	100%
Initial Antibiotic Timing[1]	10	100%	79%	80%	93%
Oxygenation Assessment[1]	11	100%	99%	99%	100%
Pneumococcal Vaccine[1]	5	20%	61%	69%	94%
Smoking Cessation Advice	0	-	77%	80%	100%
Surgical Infection Prevention					
Prophylactic Antibiotic Given[5]	-	-	74%	77%	95%
Prophylactic Antibiotic Selection[5]	-	-	88%	90%	100%
Prophylactic Antibiotic Stopped[5]	-	-	70%	72%	95%
Pregnancy Care					
Inpatient Neonatal Mortality	-	-	-	-	-
Third or Fourth Degree Laceration	-	-	3.32%	3.63%	3.27%

Chilton Medical Center

1010 Lay Dam Road
Clanton, AL 35045
URL: www.sunlinkhealth.com
Ownership: Voluntary non-profit - Private
Emergency Services: Yes

Phone: 205-755-2500
Fax: 205-280-3569

Accredited: Yes
Licensed Beds: 60

Key Personnel:
CEO. . . . . Robert M Thornton Jr
Cardiac Lab . . . . Dollie Carroll
Emergency Room . . . . Cheryl Ellison
Infection Control. . . . . Joyce Shanks
Medical/Surgical Nursing . . . . Corley Clecker
Respiratory/Cardiopulmonary. . . . . Shawn Bright

Measure	Cases	This Hospital	State Average	U.S. Average	Top Hospital
Heart Attack Care					
ACE Inhibitor or ARB for LVSD[3]	0	-	78%	82%	100%
Aspirin at Arrival[1,3]	2	0%	87%	92%	100%
Aspirin at Discharge[1,3]	1	0%	87%	90%	100%
Beta Blocker at Arrival[1,3]	2	0%	81%	87%	100%
Beta Blocker at Discharge[1,3]	1	0%	86%	90%	100%
Fibrinolytic Medication Timing[3]	0	-	25%	31%	100%
PCI Within 90 Minutes of Arrival[5]	-	-	61%	54%	95%
Smoking Cessation Advice[1,3]	1	100%	85%	88%	100%
Heart Failure Care					
ACE Inhibitor or ARB for LVSD[1]	3	67%	80%	82%	100%
Discharge Instructions[1]	12	58%	54%	61%	93%
Evaluation of LVS Function[1]	15	93%	79%	83%	99%
Smoking Cessation Advice	0	-	78%	82%	100%
Pneumonia Care					
Appropriate Initial Antibiotic	36	78%	81%	83%	94%
Blood Culture Timing[1]	19	74%	89%	90%	100%

Influenza Vaccine[1]	7	71%	62%	70%	100%
Initial Antibiotic Timing	44	80%	79%	80%	93%
Oxygenation Assessment	46	100%	99%	99%	100%
Pneumococcal Vaccine[1]	24	67%	61%	69%	94%
Smoking Cessation Advice[1]	7	100%	77%	80%	100%
Surgical Infection Prevention					
Prophylactic Antibiotic Given[5]	-	-	74%	77%	95%
Prophylactic Antibiotic Selection[5]	-	-	88%	90%	100%
Prophylactic Antibiotic Stopped[5]	-	-	70%	72%	95%
Pregnancy Care					
Inpatient Neonatal Mortality	-	-	-	-	-
Third or Fourth Degree Laceration	-	-	3.32%	3.63%	3.27%

Cullman Regional Medical Center

1912 Alabama Highway 157
Cullman, AL 35058
Ownership: Govt - Hospital District or Authority   Accredited: Yes
Emergency Services: Yes

Phone: 256-737-2000

Measure	Cases	This Hospital	State Average	U.S. Average	Top Hospital
Heart Attack Care					
ACE Inhibitor or ARB for LVSD[1]	7	86%	78%	82%	100%
Aspirin at Arrival	62	97%	87%	92%	100%
Aspirin at Discharge	31	87%	87%	90%	100%
Beta Blocker at Arrival	49	90%	81%	87%	100%
Beta Blocker at Discharge	32	88%	86%	90%	100%
Fibrinolytic Medication Timing[1]	1	0%	25%	31%	100%
PCI Within 90 Minutes of Arrival	0	-	61%	54%	95%
Smoking Cessation Advice[1]	7	100%	85%	88%	100%
Heart Failure Care					
ACE Inhibitor or ARB for LVSD	89	92%	80%	82%	100%
Discharge Instructions	172	87%	54%	61%	93%
Evaluation of LVS Function	193	87%	79%	83%	99%
Smoking Cessation Advice	37	92%	78%	82%	100%
Pneumonia Care					
Appropriate Initial Antibiotic	171	81%	81%	83%	94%
Blood Culture Timing	122	93%	89%	90%	100%
Influenza Vaccine	45	78%	62%	70%	100%
Initial Antibiotic Timing	193	85%	79%	80%	93%
Oxygenation Assessment	238	100%	99%	99%	100%
Pneumococcal Vaccine	156	84%	61%	69%	94%
Smoking Cessation Advice	68	94%	77%	80%	100%
Surgical Infection Prevention					
Prophylactic Antibiotic Given	440	98%	74%	77%	95%
Prophylactic Antibiotic Selection	132	95%	88%	90%	100%
Prophylactic Antibiotic Stopped	423	82%	70%	72%	95%
Pregnancy Care					
Inpatient Neonatal Mortality	-	-	-	-	-
Third or Fourth Degree Laceration	-	-	3.32%	3.63%	3.27%

Woodland Medical Center

Alternate Name: Woodland Community Hospital
1910 Cherokee Avenue SW
Cullman, AL 35055
URL: www.woodlandmedicalcenter.com
Ownership: Proprietary
Emergency Services: Yes

Phone: 256-739-3500
Fax: 256-736-1093

Accredited: Yes
Licensed Beds: 100

Key Personnel:
CEO. . . . . Mary Irons
Chief Medical Staff. . . . . Michael Schendel, MD
Director Medical/Surgical Nursing . . . . Sherri Jackson, RN
OB/GYN Womens Health. . . . . Christopher L Baldwin, MD
Chief Radiology . . . . Levon Jimmerson
Director Respiratory Therapy . . . . Matthew Johnson

Measure	Cases	This Hospital	State Average	U.S. Average	Top Hospital
Heart Attack Care					
ACE Inhibitor or ARB for LVSD[1]	4	75%	78%	82%	100%
Aspirin at Arrival[1]	16	81%	87%	92%	100%
Aspirin at Discharge[1]	9	44%	87%	90%	100%
Beta Blocker at Arrival[1]	18	78%	81%	87%	100%
Beta Blocker at Discharge[1]	11	82%	86%	90%	100%

NOTE: Hospital profiles are in alphabetical order by state, then city, then hospital within the city; Rankings are sorted by rate in descending order and exclude hospitals with less than 25 cases; (1) The number of cases is too small (n<25) for purposes of reliably predicting hospital performance; (2) Measure reflects the hospital's indication that its submission was based upon a sample of its relevant discharges; (3) Rate reflects fewer than the maximum possible quarters of data for the measure; (4) Inaccurate information submitted and suppressed for one or more quarters; (5) No data is available from the hospital for this measure; Please refer to the User's Guide for a full explanation of data

Fibrinolytic Medication Timing	0	-	25%	31%	100%
PCI Within 90 Minutes of Arrival	0	-	61%	54%	95%
Smoking Cessation Advice[1]	3	100%	85%	88%	100%
Heart Failure Care					
ACE Inhibitor or ARB for LVSD	40	72%	80%	82%	100%
Discharge Instructions	87	82%	54%	61%	93%
Evaluation of LVS Function	140	85%	79%	83%	99%
Smoking Cessation Advice	25	92%	78%	82%	100%
Pneumonia Care					
Appropriate Initial Antibiotic	98	87%	81%	83%	94%
Blood Culture Timing	75	96%	89%	90%	100%
Influenza Vaccine[1]	17	71%	62%	70%	100%
Initial Antibiotic Timing	124	85%	79%	80%	93%
Oxygenation Assessment	145	100%	99%	99%	100%
Pneumococcal Vaccine	87	76%	61%	69%	94%
Smoking Cessation Advice	42	81%	77%	80%	100%
Surgical Infection Prevention					
Prophylactic Antibiotic Given[2,3]	59	75%	74%	77%	95%
Prophylactic Antibiotic Selection[1,2]	18	83%	88%	90%	100%
Prophylactic Antibiotic Stopped[2,3]	58	69%	70%	72%	95%
Pregnancy Care					
Inpatient Neonatal Mortality	-	-	-	-	-
Third or Fourth Degree Laceration	-	-	3.32%	3.63%	3.27%

Lake Martin Community Hospital

201 Mariarden Road   Phone: 256-825-7821
Dadeville, AL 36853
Ownership: Government - Federal   Accredited: No
Emergency Services: Yes

Measure	Cases	This Hospital	State Average	U.S. Average	Top Hospital
Heart Attack Care					
ACE Inhibitor or ARB for LVSD[1]	2	0%	78%	82%	100%
Aspirin at Arrival[1]	10	60%	87%	92%	100%
Aspirin at Discharge[1]	8	25%	87%	90%	100%
Beta Blocker at Arrival[1]	10	80%	81%	87%	100%
Beta Blocker at Discharge[1]	7	57%	86%	90%	100%
Fibrinolytic Medication Timing	0	-	25%	31%	100%
PCI Within 90 Minutes of Arrival	0	-	61%	54%	95%
Smoking Cessation Advice[1]	1	0%	85%	88%	100%
Heart Failure Care					
ACE Inhibitor or ARB for LVSD[1]	1	0%	80%	82%	100%
Discharge Instructions	33	18%	54%	61%	93%
Evaluation of LVS Function	49	43%	79%	83%	99%
Smoking Cessation Advice[1]	9	22%	78%	82%	100%
Pneumonia Care					
Appropriate Initial Antibiotic	26	77%	81%	83%	94%
Blood Culture Timing[1]	14	93%	89%	90%	100%
Influenza Vaccine[1]	7	57%	62%	70%	100%
Initial Antibiotic Timing	38	74%	79%	80%	93%
Oxygenation Assessment	54	100%	99%	99%	100%
Pneumococcal Vaccine	29	24%	61%	69%	94%
Smoking Cessation Advice[1]	19	32%	77%	80%	100%
Surgical Infection Prevention					
Prophylactic Antibiotic Given[5]	-	-	74%	77%	95%
Prophylactic Antibiotic Selection[5]	-	-	88%	90%	100%
Prophylactic Antibiotic Stopped[5]	-	-	70%	72%	95%
Pregnancy Care					
Inpatient Neonatal Mortality	-	-	-	-	-
Third or Fourth Degree Laceration	-	-	3.32%	3.63%	3.27%

Decatur General Hospital

1201 7th Street SE   Phone: 256-341-2000
Decatur, AL 35609   Fax: 256-306-1645
URL: www.decaturgeneral.org
Ownership: Govt - Hospital District or Authority   Accredited: Yes
Emergency Services: Yes   Licensed Beds: 273
Key Personnel:
President/CEO. . . . . James W Hahn
Medical Staff President . . . . Stephen Suggs, MD

Measure	Cases	This Hospital	State Average	U.S. Average	Top Hospital

---

Heart Attack Care					
ACE Inhibitor or ARB for LVSD	44	86%	78%	82%	100%
Aspirin at Arrival	142	99%	87%	92%	100%
Aspirin at Discharge	149	97%	87%	90%	100%
Beta Blocker at Arrival	131	94%	81%	87%	100%
Beta Blocker at Discharge	153	95%	86%	90%	100%
Fibrinolytic Medication Timing[1]	3	67%	25%	31%	100%
PCI Within 90 Minutes of Arrival[1]	1	100%	61%	54%	95%
Smoking Cessation Advice	54	94%	85%	88%	100%
Heart Failure Care					
ACE Inhibitor or ARB for LVSD	143	87%	80%	82%	100%
Discharge Instructions	304	85%	54%	61%	93%
Evaluation of LVS Function	364	91%	79%	83%	99%
Smoking Cessation Advice	70	100%	78%	82%	100%
Pneumonia Care					
Appropriate Initial Antibiotic[2]	193	90%	81%	83%	94%
Blood Culture Timing[2]	136	95%	89%	90%	100%
Influenza Vaccine	35	91%	62%	70%	100%
Initial Antibiotic Timing[2]	235	83%	79%	80%	93%
Oxygenation Assessment[2]	279	99%	99%	99%	100%
Pneumococcal Vaccine[2]	146	94%	61%	69%	94%
Smoking Cessation Advice[2]	86	95%	77%	80%	100%
Surgical Infection Prevention					
Prophylactic Antibiotic Given[2]	246	97%	74%	77%	95%
Prophylactic Antibiotic Selection[2]	88	100%	88%	90%	100%
Prophylactic Antibiotic Stopped[2]	236	89%	70%	72%	95%
Pregnancy Care					
Inpatient Neonatal Mortality	-	-	-	-	-
Third or Fourth Degree Laceration	-	-	3.32%	3.63%	3.27%

Parkway Medical Center Hospital

1874 Beltline Road SW   Phone: 256-350-2211
Decatur, AL 35601   Fax: 256-350-8415
URL: www.parkwaymedicalcenter.com
Ownership: Proprietary   Accredited: Yes
Emergency Services: Yes   Licensed Beds: 120
Key Personnel:
CEO. . . . . Phillip Mazzuca
Chief Medical Staff. . . . . David Francis, MD
Emergency Room . . . . Ann Harrison
Director Medical/Surgical Nursing . . . . Ann Harrison
Chief Radiology . . . . Vernon Hurst, MD
Director Respiratory Therapy . . . . Martha Nelson

Measure	Cases	This Hospital	State Average	U.S. Average	Top Hospital
Heart Attack Care					
ACE Inhibitor or ARB for LVSD[1]	2	100%	78%	82%	100%
Aspirin at Arrival[1]	14	79%	87%	92%	100%
Aspirin at Discharge[1]	4	75%	87%	90%	100%
Beta Blocker at Arrival[1]	17	82%	81%	87%	100%
Beta Blocker at Discharge[1]	5	80%	86%	90%	100%
Fibrinolytic Medication Timing	0	-	25%	31%	100%
PCI Within 90 Minutes of Arrival	0	-	61%	54%	95%
Smoking Cessation Advice[1]	1	100%	85%	88%	100%
Heart Failure Care					
ACE Inhibitor or ARB for LVSD	30	93%	80%	82%	100%
Discharge Instructions	102	100%	54%	61%	93%
Evaluation of LVS Function	127	97%	79%	83%	99%
Smoking Cessation Advice	27	100%	78%	82%	100%
Pneumonia Care					
Appropriate Initial Antibiotic	93	78%	81%	83%	94%
Blood Culture Timing	59	98%	89%	90%	100%
Influenza Vaccine[1]	21	100%	62%	70%	100%
Initial Antibiotic Timing	106	96%	79%	80%	93%
Oxygenation Assessment	119	100%	99%	99%	100%
Pneumococcal Vaccine	55	100%	61%	69%	94%
Smoking Cessation Advice	32	100%	77%	80%	100%
Surgical Infection Prevention					
Prophylactic Antibiotic Given[2,3]	143	55%	74%	77%	95%
Prophylactic Antibiotic Selection[2]	40	88%	88%	90%	100%
Prophylactic Antibiotic Stopped[2,3]	134	97%	70%	72%	95%
Pregnancy Care					

NOTE: Hospital profiles are in alphabetical order by state, then city, then hospital within the city; Rankings are sorted by rate in descending order and exclude hospitals with less than 25 cases; (1) The number of cases is too small (n<25) for purposes of reliably predicting hospital performance; (2) Measure reflects the hospital's indication that its submission was based upon a sample of its relevant discharges; (3) Rate reflects fewer than the maximum possible quarters of data for the measure; (4) Inaccurate information submitted and suppressed for one or more quarters; (5) No data is available from the hospital for this measure; Please refer to the User's Guide for a full explanation of data

Inpatient Neonatal Mortality	-	-	-	-	-
Third or Fourth Degree Laceration	-	-	3.32%	3.63%	3.27%

Bryan W Whitfield Memorial Hospital

105 US W Highway 80 E   Phone: 334-289-4000
PO Box 890   Fax: 334-287-2594
Demopolis, AL 36732
E-mail: info@bwwmh.com
URL: www.bwwmh.com
Ownership: Govt - Hospital District or Authority   Accredited: Yes
Emergency Services: Yes   Licensed Beds: 99
Key Personnel:
Administrator/CEO . . . . Michael D Marshall
Chief Medical Staff . . . . Reese M Holifield, MD
Nurse Manager Med/Surg Services . . . . Vanessa Mills
Nurse Manager Maternal/Infant Department . . . Natasha Horne
Nurse Manager of Surgical Services . . . . Betty Johnson
Director od Respiratory Services . . . . Kayla Hasty

Measure	Cases	This Hospital	State Average	U.S. Average	Top Hospital
Heart Attack Care					
ACE Inhibitor or ARB for LVSD[1]	1	100%	78%	82%	100%
Aspirin at Arrival[1]	18	56%	87%	92%	100%
Aspirin at Discharge[1]	12	92%	87%	90%	100%
Beta Blocker at Arrival[1]	19	47%	81%	87%	100%
Beta Blocker at Discharge[1]	12	58%	86%	90%	100%
Fibrinolytic Medication Timing	0	-	25%	31%	100%
PCI Within 90 Minutes of Arrival	0	-	61%	54%	95%
Smoking Cessation Advice[1]	1	0%	85%	88%	100%
Heart Failure Care					
ACE Inhibitor or ARB for LVSD[1]	7	100%	80%	82%	100%
Discharge Instructions	93	1%	54%	61%	93%
Evaluation of LVS Function	105	37%	79%	83%	99%
Smoking Cessation Advice[1]	18	22%	78%	82%	100%
Pneumonia Care					
Appropriate Initial Antibiotic	58	53%	81%	83%	94%
Blood Culture Timing[1]	7	86%	89%	90%	100%
Influenza Vaccine[1]	13	0%	62%	70%	100%
Initial Antibiotic Timing	80	65%	79%	80%	93%
Oxygenation Assessment	92	97%	99%	99%	100%
Pneumococcal Vaccine	43	16%	61%	69%	94%
Smoking Cessation Advice[1]	22	50%	77%	80%	100%
Surgical Infection Prevention					
Prophylactic Antibiotic Given[1,3]	23	61%	74%	77%	95%
Prophylactic Antibiotic Selection[1]	8	88%	88%	90%	100%
Prophylactic Antibiotic Stopped[1,3]	23	83%	70%	72%	95%
Pregnancy Care					
Inpatient Neonatal Mortality	-	-	-	-	-
Third or Fourth Degree Laceration	-	-	3.32%	3.63%	3.27%

Flowers Hospital

4370 West Main Street   Phone: 334-793-5000
Dothan, AL 36305   Fax: 334-793-4613
URL: www.flowershospital.com
Ownership: Proprietary   Accredited: Yes
Emergency Services: Yes   Licensed Beds: 235
Key Personnel:
President/CEO . . . . L Keith Granger

Measure	Cases	This Hospital	State Average	U.S. Average	Top Hospital
Heart Attack Care					
ACE Inhibitor or ARB for LVSD	56	98%	78%	82%	100%
Aspirin at Arrival	158	99%	87%	92%	100%
Aspirin at Discharge	274	100%	87%	90%	100%
Beta Blocker at Arrival	121	100%	81%	87%	100%
Beta Blocker at Discharge	282	100%	86%	90%	100%
Fibrinolytic Medication Timing[1]	2	0%	25%	31%	100%
PCI Within 90 Minutes of Arrival[1]	9	78%	61%	54%	95%
Smoking Cessation Advice	123	100%	85%	88%	100%
Heart Failure Care					
ACE Inhibitor or ARB for LVSD	109	100%	80%	82%	100%
Discharge Instructions	274	94%	54%	61%	93%

Evaluation of LVS Function	304	100%	79%	83%	99%
Smoking Cessation Advice	50	100%	78%	82%	100%
Pneumonia Care					
Appropriate Initial Antibiotic	134	93%	81%	83%	94%
Blood Culture Timing	131	100%	89%	90%	100%
Influenza Vaccine	49	94%	62%	70%	100%
Initial Antibiotic Timing	170	91%	79%	80%	93%
Oxygenation Assessment	230	100%	99%	99%	100%
Pneumococcal Vaccine	153	97%	61%	69%	94%
Smoking Cessation Advice	58	100%	77%	80%	100%
Surgical Infection Prevention					
Prophylactic Antibiotic Given	1,133	100%	74%	77%	95%
Prophylactic Antibiotic Selection	285	99%	88%	90%	100%
Prophylactic Antibiotic Stopped	1,097	99%	70%	72%	95%
Pregnancy Care					
Inpatient Neonatal Mortality	1,190	0.00%	-	-	-
Third or Fourth Degree Laceration	676	6.51%	3.32%	3.63%	3.27%

Southeast Alabama Medical Center

1108 Ross Clark Circle   Phone: 334-793-8111
Dothan, AL 36301   Fax: 334-793-8751
URL: www.samc.org
Ownership: Govt - Hospital District or Authority   Accredited: Yes
Emergency Services: Yes   Licensed Beds: 400
Key Personnel:
CEO . . . . Ronald S Owen
Administrator/COO . . . . Charlie Brannen
Chief Medical Staff . . . . Ralph Filmore, MD
Emergency Room . . . . Jim Jones, DO
OB/GYN Womens Health . . . . Terance Bubreuil, MD
Chief Radiology . . . . Chirstopher Ahmed, MD
Director Pulmonary Medicine . . . . Sue Tillis

Measure	Cases	This Hospital	State Average	U.S. Average	Top Hospital
Heart Attack Care					
ACE Inhibitor or ARB for LVSD	148	90%	78%	82%	100%
Aspirin at Arrival	284	96%	87%	92%	100%
Aspirin at Discharge	511	98%	87%	90%	100%
Beta Blocker at Arrival	233	93%	81%	87%	100%
Beta Blocker at Discharge	505	97%	86%	90%	100%
Fibrinolytic Medication Timing	0	-	25%	31%	100%
PCI Within 90 Minutes of Arrival[1]	15	60%	61%	54%	95%
Smoking Cessation Advice	218	99%	85%	88%	100%
Heart Failure Care					
ACE Inhibitor or ARB for LVSD	319	87%	80%	82%	100%
Discharge Instructions	696	78%	54%	61%	93%
Evaluation of LVS Function	773	94%	79%	83%	99%
Smoking Cessation Advice	152	86%	78%	82%	100%
Pneumonia Care					
Appropriate Initial Antibiotic	209	88%	81%	83%	94%
Blood Culture Timing	116	89%	89%	90%	100%
Influenza Vaccine	48	77%	62%	70%	100%
Initial Antibiotic Timing	195	75%	79%	80%	93%
Oxygenation Assessment	270	99%	99%	99%	100%
Pneumococcal Vaccine	169	72%	61%	69%	94%
Smoking Cessation Advice	88	92%	77%	80%	100%
Surgical Infection Prevention					
Prophylactic Antibiotic Given[2,3]	212	94%	74%	77%	95%
Prophylactic Antibiotic Selection[2]	70	100%	88%	90%	100%
Prophylactic Antibiotic Stopped[2,3]	203	75%	70%	72%	95%
Pregnancy Care					
Inpatient Neonatal Mortality	-	-	-	-	-
Third or Fourth Degree Laceration	-	-	3.32%	3.63%	3.27%

Elba General Hospital & Nursing Home

987 Drayton Street   Phone: 334-897-2257
Elba, AL 36323   Fax: 334-897-6549
Ownership: Govt - Hospital District or Authority   Accredited: No
Emergency Services: Yes   Licensed Beds: 125
Key Personnel:
CEO . . . . Ellen C Briley
Chief Medical Staff . . . . Lance K Dyess, MD
Emergency Room . . . . Jan Wicker

NOTE: Hospital profiles are in alphabetical order by state, then city, then hospital within the city; Rankings are sorted by rate in descending order and exclude hospitals with less than 25 cases; (1) The number of cases is too small (n<25) for purposes of reliably predicting hospital performance; (2) Measure reflects the hospital's indication that its submission was based upon a sample of its relevant discharges; (3) Rate reflects fewer than the maximum possible quarters of data for the measure; (4) Inaccurate information submitted and suppressed for one or more quarters; (5) No data is available from the hospital for this measure; Please refer to the User's Guide for a full explanation of data

Director Medical/Surgical Nursing . . . . Jan Wicker, RN
Chief Radiology . . . . Dudley Terrell, MD
Director Respiratory Therapy . . . . June McIlwain

Measure	Cases	This Hospital	State Average	U.S. Average	Top Hospital
Heart Attack Care					
ACE Inhibitor or ARB for LVSD[3]	0	-	78%	82%	100%
Aspirin at Arrival[1,3]	2	100%	87%	92%	100%
Aspirin at Discharge[1,3]	2	100%	87%	90%	100%
Beta Blocker at Arrival[1,3]	2	100%	81%	87%	100%
Beta Blocker at Discharge[1,3]	2	100%	86%	90%	100%
Fibrinolytic Medication Timing[3]	0	-	25%	31%	100%
PCI Within 90 Minutes of Arrival	0	-	61%	54%	95%
Smoking Cessation Advice[3]	0	-	85%	88%	100%
Heart Failure Care					
ACE Inhibitor or ARB for LVSD[1]	1	100%	80%	82%	100%
Discharge Instructions[1]	16	100%	54%	61%	93%
Evaluation of LVS Function[1]	17	100%	79%	83%	99%
Smoking Cessation Advice[1]	2	100%	78%	82%	100%
Pneumonia Care					
Appropriate Initial Antibiotic	47	94%	81%	83%	94%
Blood Culture Timing	26	100%	89%	90%	100%
Influenza Vaccine[4,5]	-	-	62%	70%	100%
Initial Antibiotic Timing	48	96%	79%	80%	93%
Oxygenation Assessment	70	100%	99%	99%	100%
Pneumococcal Vaccine	42	100%	61%	69%	94%
Smoking Cessation Advice[1]	12	100%	77%	80%	100%
Surgical Infection Prevention					
Prophylactic Antibiotic Given[5]	-	-	74%	77%	95%
Prophylactic Antibiotic Selection[5]	-	-	88%	90%	100%
Prophylactic Antibiotic Stopped[5]	-	-	70%	72%	95%
Pregnancy Care					
Inpatient Neonatal Mortality	-	-	-	-	-
Third or Fourth Degree Laceration	-	-	3.32%	3.63%	3.27%

Medical Center Enterprise

400 N Edwards Street
Enterprise, AL 36330   Phone: 334-347-0584
Ownership: Proprietary
Emergency Services: Yes   Accredited: Yes

Measure	Cases	This Hospital	State Average	U.S. Average	Top Hospital
Heart Attack Care					
ACE Inhibitor or ARB for LVSD[1]	2	100%	78%	82%	100%
Aspirin at Arrival[1]	10	90%	87%	92%	100%
Aspirin at Discharge[1]	7	71%	87%	90%	100%
Beta Blocker at Arrival[1]	7	71%	81%	87%	100%
Beta Blocker at Discharge[1]	6	83%	86%	90%	100%
Fibrinolytic Medication Timing[1]	1	0%	25%	31%	100%
PCI Within 90 Minutes of Arrival	0	-	61%	54%	95%
Smoking Cessation Advice[1]	1	100%	85%	88%	100%
Heart Failure Care					
ACE Inhibitor or ARB for LVSD	32	94%	80%	82%	100%
Discharge Instructions	89	76%	54%	61%	93%
Evaluation of LVS Function	103	97%	79%	83%	99%
Smoking Cessation Advice[1]	15	100%	78%	82%	100%
Pneumonia Care					
Appropriate Initial Antibiotic	118	93%	81%	83%	94%
Blood Culture Timing	97	95%	89%	90%	100%
Influenza Vaccine	42	95%	62%	70%	100%
Initial Antibiotic Timing	160	92%	79%	80%	93%
Oxygenation Assessment	192	100%	99%	99%	100%
Pneumococcal Vaccine	114	97%	61%	69%	94%
Smoking Cessation Advice	42	100%	77%	80%	100%
Surgical Infection Prevention					
Prophylactic Antibiotic Given	341	96%	74%	77%	95%
Prophylactic Antibiotic Selection	84	100%	88%	90%	100%
Prophylactic Antibiotic Stopped	328	98%	70%	72%	95%
Pregnancy Care					
Inpatient Neonatal Mortality	-	-	-	-	-
Third or Fourth Degree Laceration	-	-	3.32%	3.63%	3.27%

Lakeview Community Hospital

820 W Washington Street
Eufaula, AL 36027   Phone: 334-688-7000
URL: www.chs.net   Fax: 334-687-0028
Ownership: Proprietary
Emergency Services: Yes   Accredited: Yes
Key Personnel: Licensed Beds: 74
CEO. . . . . Steve Honeycutt
Chief Medical Staff. . . . . William King, MD
OB/GYN Women's Health . . . . AH Savel
Respiratory Care . . . . Junior Williams

Measure	Cases	This Hospital	State Average	U.S. Average	Top Hospital
Heart Attack Care					
ACE Inhibitor or ARB for LVSD[3]	0	-	78%	82%	100%
Aspirin at Arrival[1,3]	4	100%	87%	92%	100%
Aspirin at Discharge[1,3]	2	50%	87%	90%	100%
Beta Blocker at Arrival[1,3]	2	50%	81%	87%	100%
Beta Blocker at Discharge[1,3]	2	50%	86%	90%	100%
Fibrinolytic Medication Timing[1,3]	1	0%	25%	31%	100%
PCI Within 90 Minutes of Arrival	0	-	61%	54%	95%
Smoking Cessation Advice[3]	0	-	85%	88%	100%
Heart Failure Care					
ACE Inhibitor or ARB for LVSD[1]	23	74%	80%	82%	100%
Discharge Instructions	63	65%	54%	61%	93%
Evaluation of LVS Function	89	58%	79%	83%	99%
Smoking Cessation Advice	29	93%	78%	82%	100%
Pneumonia Care					
Appropriate Initial Antibiotic	76	80%	81%	83%	94%
Blood Culture Timing	51	78%	89%	90%	100%
Influenza Vaccine[1]	19	53%	62%	70%	100%
Initial Antibiotic Timing	88	85%	79%	80%	93%
Oxygenation Assessment	114	96%	99%	99%	100%
Pneumococcal Vaccine	75	39%	61%	69%	94%
Smoking Cessation Advice	42	90%	77%	80%	100%
Surgical Infection Prevention					
Prophylactic Antibiotic Given[1,3]	6	67%	74%	77%	95%
Prophylactic Antibiotic Selection[1]	2	0%	88%	90%	100%
Prophylactic Antibiotic Stopped[1,3]	4	50%	70%	72%	95%
Pregnancy Care					
Inpatient Neonatal Mortality	-	-	-	-	-
Third or Fourth Degree Laceration	-	-	3.32%	3.63%	3.27%

Greene County Hospital

509 Wilson Avenue
Eutaw, AL 35462   Phone: 205-372-3388
Ownership: Voluntary non-profit - Other   Fax: 205-372-2716
Emergency Services: Yes   Accredited: No
Key Personnel: Licensed Beds: 20
CEO. . . . . Robert J Coker, Jr
Chief Medical Staff. . . . . S Faroogai
Emergency Room . . . . Myra Marzette

Measure	Cases	This Hospital	State Average	U.S. Average	Top Hospital
Heart Attack Care					
ACE Inhibitor or ARB for LVSD[5]	-	-	78%	82%	100%
Aspirin at Arrival[5]	-	-	87%	92%	100%
Aspirin at Discharge[5]	-	-	87%	90%	100%
Beta Blocker at Arrival[5]	-	-	81%	87%	100%
Beta Blocker at Discharge[5]	-	-	86%	90%	100%
Fibrinolytic Medication Timing[5]	-	-	25%	31%	100%
PCI Within 90 Minutes of Arrival[5]	-	-	61%	54%	95%
Smoking Cessation Advice[5]	-	-	85%	88%	100%
Heart Failure Care					
ACE Inhibitor or ARB for LVSD	0	-	80%	82%	100%
Discharge Instructions[1,3]	9	22%	54%	61%	93%
Evaluation of LVS Function	47	38%	79%	83%	99%
Smoking Cessation Advice[1,3]	2	0%	78%	82%	100%
Pneumonia Care					
Appropriate Initial Antibiotic[1,3]	3	100%	81%	83%	94%
Blood Culture Timing[1,3]	1	100%	89%	90%	100%
Influenza Vaccine[5]	-	-	62%	70%	100%

NOTE: Hospital profiles are in alphabetical order by state, then city, then hospital within the city; Rankings are sorted by rate in descending order and exclude hospitals with less than 25 cases; (1) The number of cases is too small (n<25) for purposes of reliably predicting hospital performance; (2) Measure reflects the hospital's indication that its submission was based upon a sample of its relevant discharges; (3) Rate reflects fewer than the maximum possible quarters of data for the measure; (4) Inaccurate information submitted and suppressed for one or more quarters; (5) No data is available from the hospital for this measure; Please refer to the User's Guide for a full explanation of data

	Cases	This Hospital	State Average	U.S. Average	Top Hospital
Initial Antibiotic Timing[1,3]	9	44%	79%	80%	93%
Oxygenation Assessment[1]	15	100%	99%	99%	100%
Pneumococcal Vaccine[1,3]	6	0%	61%	69%	94%
Smoking Cessation Advice[3]	0	-	77%	80%	100%
Surgical Infection Prevention					
Prophylactic Antibiotic Given[5]	-	-	74%	77%	95%
Prophylactic Antibiotic Selection[5]	-	-	88%	90%	100%
Prophylactic Antibiotic Stopped[5]	-	-	70%	72%	95%
Pregnancy Care					
Inpatient Neonatal Mortality	-	-	-	-	-
Third or Fourth Degree Laceration	-	-	3.32%	3.63%	3.27%

Vaughan Evergreen Medical Center

Alternate Name: Evergreen Medical Center

101 Crestview Avenue
Evergreen, AL 36401
Ownership: Proprietary
Emergency Services: Yes

Phone: 334-418-4100
Fax: 334-875-5223
Accredited: No
Licensed Beds: 44

Key Personnel:
CEO. . . . . Steve Mahan
Chief Medical Staff. . . . . William Deacor
Emergency Room Director. . . . . Anita Elliison
Director Respiratory Therapy . . . . Jackie Moulcire

Measure	Cases	This Hospital	State Average	U.S. Average	Top Hospital
Heart Attack Care					
ACE Inhibitor or ARB for LVSD	0	-	78%	82%	100%
Aspirin at Arrival[1]	5	100%	87%	92%	100%
Aspirin at Discharge[1]	2	100%	87%	90%	100%
Beta Blocker at Arrival[1]	6	83%	81%	87%	100%
Beta Blocker at Discharge[1]	2	100%	86%	90%	100%
Fibrinolytic Medication Timing	0	-	25%	31%	100%
PCI Within 90 Minutes of Arrival	0	-	61%	54%	95%
Smoking Cessation Advice	0	-	85%	88%	100%
Heart Failure Care					
ACE Inhibitor or ARB for LVSD	42	81%	80%	82%	100%
Discharge Instructions	144	42%	54%	61%	93%
Evaluation of LVS Function	158	72%	79%	83%	99%
Smoking Cessation Advice[1]	21	86%	78%	82%	100%
Pneumonia Care					
Appropriate Initial Antibiotic	47	74%	81%	83%	94%
Blood Culture Timing[1]	11	91%	89%	90%	100%
Influenza Vaccine[1]	9	56%	62%	70%	100%
Initial Antibiotic Timing	42	67%	79%	80%	93%
Oxygenation Assessment	57	100%	99%	99%	100%
Pneumococcal Vaccine	30	47%	61%	69%	94%
Smoking Cessation Advice[1]	10	90%	77%	80%	100%
Surgical Infection Prevention					
Prophylactic Antibiotic Given[5]	-	-	74%	77%	95%
Prophylactic Antibiotic Selection[5]	-	-	88%	90%	100%
Prophylactic Antibiotic Stopped[5]	-	-	70%	72%	95%
Pregnancy Care					
Inpatient Neonatal Mortality	-	-	-	-	-
Third or Fourth Degree Laceration	-	-	3.32%	3.63%	3.27%

Thomas Hospital

750 Morphy Avenue
PO Box 929
Fairhope, AL 36532
E-mail: info@thomashospital.com
URL: www.thomashospital.com
Ownership: Govt - Hospital District or Authority
Emergency Services: No

Phone: 251-928-2375
Fax: 251-928-8028

Accredited: Yes
Licensed Beds: 150

Key Personnel:
President/CEO. . . . . Owen Bailey
Chief Medical Staff. Gary Nelson, MD
Cardiac Lab . . . . Ernie Livingston
Catheterization Lab . . . . Ernie Livingston
Emergency Room . . . . Carrie Sullivan
Infection Control. . . . . Patti Thames, RN
ICU . . . . Donna Ingraham
Intensive Coronary Unit . . . . Kim Devilbiss, RN
Medical Surgical Nursing . . . . Tina Blair, RN

Director Medical/Surgical Affairs . . . . Dr Michael McBrearty
OB/GYN/Women's Health . . . . Vicky Whitman, RN
Director Respiratory Therapy . . . . Lisa Scott

Measure	Cases	This Hospital	State Average	U.S. Average	Top Hospital
Heart Attack Care					
ACE Inhibitor or ARB for LVSD	59	90%	78%	82%	100%
Aspirin at Arrival	176	96%	87%	92%	100%
Aspirin at Discharge	256	100%	87%	90%	100%
Beta Blocker at Arrival	134	89%	81%	87%	100%
Beta Blocker at Discharge	242	97%	86%	90%	100%
Fibrinolytic Medication Timing	0	-	25%	31%	100%
PCI Within 90 Minutes of Arrival[1]	16	75%	61%	54%	95%
Smoking Cessation Advice	112	96%	85%	88%	100%
Heart Failure Care					
ACE Inhibitor or ARB for LVSD	97	76%	80%	82%	100%
Discharge Instructions	201	71%	54%	61%	93%
Evaluation of LVS Function	240	92%	79%	83%	99%
Smoking Cessation Advice	40	92%	78%	82%	100%
Pneumonia Care					
Appropriate Initial Antibiotic	103	73%	81%	83%	94%
Blood Culture Timing	67	94%	89%	90%	100%
Influenza Vaccine	27	74%	62%	70%	100%
Initial Antibiotic Timing	116	80%	79%	80%	93%
Oxygenation Assessment	153	100%	99%	99%	100%
Pneumococcal Vaccine	95	68%	61%	69%	94%
Smoking Cessation Advice	27	78%	77%	80%	100%
Surgical Infection Prevention					
Prophylactic Antibiotic Given[2,3]	471	79%	74%	77%	95%
Prophylactic Antibiotic Selection[2]	72	93%	88%	90%	100%
Prophylactic Antibiotic Stopped[2,3]	457	76%	70%	72%	95%
Pregnancy Care					
Inpatient Neonatal Mortality	-	-	-	-	-
Third or Fourth Degree Laceration	-	-	3.32%	3.63%	3.27%

Fayette Medical Center

1653 Temple Avenue
PO Drawer 710
Fayette, AL 35555
URL: www.dchsystem.com
Ownership: Voluntary non-profit - Other
Emergency Services: Yes

Phone: 205-932-5966
Fax: 205-932-1260

Accredited: Yes
Licensed Beds: 61

Key Personnel:
Administrator . . . . Harold Reed
Director Respiratory Therapy . . . . Kim Jordan

Measure	Cases	This Hospital	State Average	U.S. Average	Top Hospital
Heart Attack Care					
ACE Inhibitor or ARB for LVSD[1]	2	0%	78%	82%	100%
Aspirin at Arrival[1]	12	67%	87%	92%	100%
Aspirin at Discharge[1]	6	67%	87%	90%	100%
Beta Blocker at Arrival[1]	11	64%	81%	87%	100%
Beta Blocker at Discharge[1]	5	80%	86%	90%	100%
Fibrinolytic Medication Timing	0	-	25%	31%	100%
PCI Within 90 Minutes of Arrival	0	-	61%	54%	95%
Smoking Cessation Advice	0	-	85%	88%	100%
Heart Failure Care					
ACE Inhibitor or ARB for LVSD[1]	19	58%	80%	82%	100%
Discharge Instructions	55	44%	54%	61%	93%
Evaluation of LVS Function	71	80%	79%	83%	99%
Smoking Cessation Advice[1]	10	80%	78%	82%	100%
Pneumonia Care					
Appropriate Initial Antibiotic	85	81%	81%	83%	94%
Blood Culture Timing	62	95%	89%	90%	100%
Influenza Vaccine	26	69%	62%	70%	100%
Initial Antibiotic Timing	109	95%	79%	80%	93%
Oxygenation Assessment	119	98%	99%	99%	100%
Pneumococcal Vaccine	72	71%	61%	69%	94%
Smoking Cessation Advice	33	85%	77%	80%	100%
Surgical Infection Prevention					
Prophylactic Antibiotic Given	29	93%	74%	77%	95%
Prophylactic Antibiotic Selection[1]	9	100%	88%	90%	100%

NOTE: Hospital profiles are in alphabetical order by state, then city, then hospital within the city; Rankings are sorted by rate in descending order and exclude hospitals with less than 25 cases; (1) The number of cases is too small (n<25) for purposes of reliably predicting hospital performance; (2) Measure reflects the hospital's indication that its submission was based upon a sample of its relevant discharges; (3) Rate reflects fewer than the maximum possible quarters of data for the measure; (4) Inaccurate information submitted and suppressed for one or more quarters; (5) No data is available from the hospital for this measure; Please refer to the User's Guide for a full explanation of data

Prophylactic Antibiotic Stopped	29	31%	70%	72%	95%
Pregnancy Care					
Inpatient Neonatal Mortality	-	-	-	-	-
Third or Fourth Degree Laceration	-	-	3.32%	3.63%	3.27%

Florala Memorial Hospital

24273 5th Avenue   Phone: 334-858-3287
Florala, AL 36442   Fax: 334-858-3287
Ownership: Voluntary non-profit - Private   Accredited: No
Emergency Services: Yes   Licensed Beds: 23

Key Personnel:
Chairman/CEO. . . . . Blair Henson
Chief Medical Staff. . . . . S Vishwanath, MD

Measure	Cases	This Hospital	State Average	U.S. Average	Top Hospital
Heart Attack Care					
ACE Inhibitor or ARB for LVSD[3]	0	-	78%	82%	100%
Aspirin at Arrival[1,3]	2	100%	87%	92%	100%
Aspirin at Discharge[1,3]	2	100%	87%	90%	100%
Beta Blocker at Arrival[3]	0	-	81%	87%	100%
Beta Blocker at Discharge[3]	0	-	86%	90%	100%
Fibrinolytic Medication Timing[5]	-	-	25%	31%	100%
PCI Within 90 Minutes of Arrival[5]	-	-	61%	54%	95%
Smoking Cessation Advice[5]	-	-	85%	88%	100%
Heart Failure Care					
ACE Inhibitor or ARB for LVSD[1]	3	100%	80%	82%	100%
Discharge Instructions[1,3]	8	100%	54%	61%	93%
Evaluation of LVS Function	28	86%	79%	83%	99%
Smoking Cessation Advice[3]	0	-	78%	82%	100%
Pneumonia Care					
Appropriate Initial Antibiotic[1,3]	10	80%	81%	83%	94%
Blood Culture Timing[1,3]	2	100%	89%	90%	100%
Influenza Vaccine[5]	-	-	62%	70%	100%
Initial Antibiotic Timing	63	86%	79%	80%	93%
Oxygenation Assessment	87	100%	99%	99%	100%
Pneumococcal Vaccine	56	98%	61%	69%	94%
Smoking Cessation Advice[1,3]	3	100%	77%	80%	100%
Surgical Infection Prevention					
Prophylactic Antibiotic Given[5]	-	-	74%	77%	95%
Prophylactic Antibiotic Selection[5]	-	-	88%	90%	100%
Prophylactic Antibiotic Stopped[5]	-	-	70%	72%	95%
Pregnancy Care					
Inpatient Neonatal Mortality	-	-	-	-	-
Third or Fourth Degree Laceration	-	-	3.32%	3.63%	3.27%

Eliza Coffee Memorial Hospital

205 Marengo Street   Phone: 256-768-9191
Florence, AL 35630   Fax: 256-768-9420
URL: chgroup.org
Ownership: Govt - Hospital District or Authority   Accredited: Yes
Emergency Services: Yes

Key Personnel:
President/CEO. . . . . Carl Bailey
Catheterization Lab . . . . Rick Williams
Director Emergency Room. . . . . Jan Hannah
Infection Control. . . . . Pam Floyd
ICU . . . . Patrice Crosby
Intensive/Coronary Care . . . . Patrice Crosby
OB/GYN Womens Health. . . . . Beth Bevis
Respiratory/Cardiopulmonary. . . . . David Bowling

Measure	Cases	This Hospital	State Average	U.S. Average	Top Hospital
Heart Attack Care					
ACE Inhibitor or ARB for LVSD	87	92%	78%	82%	100%
Aspirin at Arrival	213	99%	87%	92%	100%
Aspirin at Discharge	336	99%	87%	90%	100%
Beta Blocker at Arrival	191	96%	81%	87%	100%
Beta Blocker at Discharge	330	93%	86%	90%	100%
Fibrinolytic Medication Timing	0	-	25%	31%	100%
PCI Within 90 Minutes of Arrival[1]	22	82%	61%	54%	95%
Smoking Cessation Advice	160	97%	85%	88%	100%
Heart Failure Care					

Measure	Cases	This Hospital	State Average	U.S. Average	Top Hospital
ACE Inhibitor or ARB for LVSD	138	81%	80%	82%	100%
Discharge Instructions	346	65%	54%	61%	93%
Evaluation of LVS Function	409	92%	79%	83%	99%
Smoking Cessation Advice	61	93%	78%	82%	100%
Pneumonia Care					
Appropriate Initial Antibiotic	316	90%	81%	83%	94%
Blood Culture Timing	135	93%	89%	90%	100%
Influenza Vaccine	94	57%	62%	70%	100%
Initial Antibiotic Timing	458	92%	79%	80%	93%
Oxygenation Assessment	470	100%	99%	99%	100%
Pneumococcal Vaccine	285	79%	61%	69%	94%
Smoking Cessation Advice	89	94%	77%	80%	100%
Surgical Infection Prevention					
Prophylactic Antibiotic Given[3]	678	89%	74%	77%	95%
Prophylactic Antibiotic Selection	196	97%	88%	90%	100%
Prophylactic Antibiotic Stopped[3]	650	85%	70%	72%	95%
Pregnancy Care					
Inpatient Neonatal Mortality	-	-	-	-	-
Third or Fourth Degree Laceration	-	-	3.32%	3.63%	3.27%

South Baldwin Regional Medical Center

Alternate Name: South Baldwin Hospital
1613 N McKenzie Street   Phone: 251-949-3400
Foley, AL 36535   Fax: 251-949-3404
URL: www.southbaldwinrmc.com
Ownership: Proprietary   Accredited: Yes
Emergency Services: Yes   Licensed Beds: 82

Key Personnel:
President/CEO. . . . . Stephen Penninoton
Chief Medical Staff. Dennis McNulty, DO
Catheterization Lab . . . . David Godfrey
Emergency Room . . . . Will McDaniel
Infection Control. . . . . Vicki Coyle
ICU . . . . Sharon Dunkin
Intensive Coronary. Sharon Dunkin
Director Medical/Surgical Nursing . . . . Mike Brantly, RN
Chief Radiology . . . . Henry Koehler
Director Respiratory Therapy . . . . Alex Belmont

Measure	Cases	This Hospital	State Average	U.S. Average	Top Hospital
Heart Attack Care					
ACE Inhibitor or ARB for LVSD[1]	6	83%	78%	82%	100%
Aspirin at Arrival	54	100%	87%	92%	100%
Aspirin at Discharge	26	96%	87%	90%	100%
Beta Blocker at Arrival	42	88%	81%	87%	100%
Beta Blocker at Discharge	28	96%	86%	90%	100%
Fibrinolytic Medication Timing	0	-	25%	31%	100%
PCI Within 90 Minutes of Arrival	0	-	61%	54%	95%
Smoking Cessation Advice[1]	5	100%	85%	88%	100%
Heart Failure Care					
ACE Inhibitor or ARB for LVSD	67	78%	80%	82%	100%
Discharge Instructions	192	72%	54%	61%	93%
Evaluation of LVS Function	225	96%	79%	83%	99%
Smoking Cessation Advice	47	98%	78%	82%	100%
Pneumonia Care					
Appropriate Initial Antibiotic	108	77%	81%	83%	94%
Blood Culture Timing	75	84%	89%	90%	100%
Influenza Vaccine	34	88%	62%	70%	100%
Initial Antibiotic Timing	137	68%	79%	80%	93%
Oxygenation Assessment	153	99%	99%	99%	100%
Pneumococcal Vaccine	95	76%	61%	69%	94%
Smoking Cessation Advice	34	100%	77%	80%	100%
Surgical Infection Prevention					
Prophylactic Antibiotic Given[2,3]	151	15%	74%	77%	95%
Prophylactic Antibiotic Selection[2]	40	48%	88%	90%	100%
Prophylactic Antibiotic Stopped[2,3]	147	38%	70%	72%	95%
Pregnancy Care					
Inpatient Neonatal Mortality	-	-	-	-	-
Third or Fourth Degree Laceration	-	-	3.32%	3.63%	3.27%

NOTE: Hospital profiles are in alphabetical order by state, then city, then hospital within the city; Rankings are sorted by rate in descending order and exclude hospitals with less than 25 cases; (1) The number of cases is too small (n<25) for purposes of reliably predicting hospital performance; (2) Measure reflects the hospital's indication that its submission was based upon a sample of its relevant discharges; (3) Rate reflects fewer than the maximum possible quarters of data for the measure; (4) Inaccurate information submitted and suppressed for one or more quarters; (5) No data is available from the hospital for this measure; Please refer to the User's Guide for a full explanation of data

DeKalb Regional Medical Center

200 Medical Center Drive
Fort Payne, AL 35968
URL: www.dekalbregional.com
Ownership: Voluntary non-profit - Church
Emergency Services: Yes

Phone: 256-845-3150
Fax: 256-997-2512

Accredited: Yes
Licensed Beds: 134

Key Personnel:
President/CEO . . . . Mary Elizabeth O'Brien
Chief Medical Staff . . . . Daniel M Mince, MD
Director Emergency Services . . . . Betty Miller, RN
Director OB/GYN/Women's Health . . . . Donna Etheredge, RNC BSN
Director Radiology . . . . Gaye Roberts
Director Cardiopulmonary Services . . . . Vicki Kay

Measure	Cases	This Hospital	State Average	U.S. Average	Top Hospital
Heart Attack Care					
ACE Inhibitor or ARB for LVSD[1]	5	80%	78%	82%	100%
Aspirin at Arrival[1]	24	92%	87%	92%	100%
Aspirin at Discharge[1]	12	83%	87%	90%	100%
Beta Blocker at Arrival[1]	19	95%	81%	87%	100%
Beta Blocker at Discharge[1]	12	92%	86%	90%	100%
Fibrinolytic Medication Timing	0	-	25%	31%	100%
PCI Within 90 Minutes of Arrival	0	-	61%	54%	95%
Smoking Cessation Advice[1]	5	60%	85%	88%	100%
Heart Failure Care					
ACE Inhibitor or ARB for LVSD	60	83%	80%	82%	100%
Discharge Instructions	95	78%	54%	61%	93%
Evaluation of LVS Function	119	96%	79%	83%	99%
Smoking Cessation Advice[1]	20	100%	78%	82%	100%
Pneumonia Care					
Appropriate Initial Antibiotic	104	81%	81%	83%	94%
Blood Culture Timing	65	88%	89%	90%	100%
Influenza Vaccine	36	69%	62%	70%	100%
Initial Antibiotic Timing	127	78%	79%	80%	93%
Oxygenation Assessment	153	99%	99%	99%	100%
Pneumococcal Vaccine	85	62%	61%	69%	94%
Smoking Cessation Advice	37	86%	77%	80%	100%
Surgical Infection Prevention					
Prophylactic Antibiotic Given[2,3]	171	56%	74%	77%	95%
Prophylactic Antibiotic Selection[2]	48	88%	88%	90%	100%
Prophylactic Antibiotic Stopped[2,3]	164	55%	70%	72%	95%
Pregnancy Care					
Inpatient Neonatal Mortality	-	-	-	-	-
Third or Fourth Degree Laceration	-	-	3.32%	3.63%	3.27%

Gadsden Regional Medical Center

Alternate Name: Baptist Hospital of Gadsden
1007 Goodyear Avenue
Gadsden, AL 35903
E-mail: grmcphysicianservices@gadsdenregional.com
URL: www.gadsdenregional.com
Ownership: Proprietary
Emergency Services: Yes

Phone: 256-494-4000
Fax: 256-494-4474

Accredited: Yes
Licensed Beds: 346

Key Personnel:
CEO . . . . Doug DeGraaf
Chief Medical Staff . . . . Bruce Head, MD
Cardiac Lab . . . . Carol Davis
Catheterization Lab Director . . . . Carol Davis
Emergency Room Director . . . . Pam Rosson
Director Infection/Disease Control . . . . Teresa Fox, RN
ICU . . . . Delite Cruit
Medical Surgical Nursing Director . . . . Amy Ragsdale
Director Women & Children Center . . . . Judy Swafford
Director Radiology . . . . Bill Ross
Director Respiratory/Cardiology . . . . David Bearden

Measure	Cases	This Hospital	State Average	U.S. Average	Top Hospital
Heart Attack Care					
ACE Inhibitor or ARB for LVSD	39	72%	78%	82%	100%
Aspirin at Arrival	120	86%	87%	92%	100%
Aspirin at Discharge	146	92%	87%	90%	100%
Beta Blocker at Arrival	98	78%	81%	87%	100%
Beta Blocker at Discharge	157	88%	86%	90%	100%

Measure	Cases	This Hospital	State Average	U.S. Average	Top Hospital
Fibrinolytic Medication Timing[1]	17	24%	25%	31%	100%
PCI Within 90 Minutes of Arrival[1]	10	50%	61%	54%	95%
Smoking Cessation Advice	77	100%	85%	88%	100%
Heart Failure Care					
ACE Inhibitor or ARB for LVSD	131	79%	80%	82%	100%
Discharge Instructions	260	44%	54%	61%	93%
Evaluation of LVS Function	348	97%	79%	83%	99%
Smoking Cessation Advice	60	97%	78%	82%	100%
Pneumonia Care					
Appropriate Initial Antibiotic	194	89%	81%	83%	94%
Blood Culture Timing	206	86%	89%	90%	100%
Influenza Vaccine	65	89%	62%	70%	100%
Initial Antibiotic Timing	318	72%	79%	80%	93%
Oxygenation Assessment	390	100%	99%	99%	100%
Pneumococcal Vaccine	220	85%	61%	69%	94%
Smoking Cessation Advice	102	95%	77%	80%	100%
Surgical Infection Prevention					
Prophylactic Antibiotic Given	758	94%	74%	77%	95%
Prophylactic Antibiotic Selection	206	94%	88%	90%	100%
Prophylactic Antibiotic Stopped	726	48%	70%	72%	95%
Pregnancy Care					
Inpatient Neonatal Mortality	-	-	-	-	-
Third or Fourth Degree Laceration	-	-	3.32%	3.63%	3.27%

Riverview Regional Medical Center

Alternate Name: Holy Name of Jesus Medical Center
600 South 3rd Street
Gadsden, AL 35901
Ownership: Proprietary
Emergency Services: Yes

Phone: 256-543-5200
Fax: 256-543-5888
Accredited: Yes
Licensed Beds: 281

Key Personnel:
President/CEO . . . . J Matt Hayes
Chief Medical Staff . . . . Richael Wells
Chief Catheterization Laboratory . . . . Ricky Browning
Emergency Room . . . . Crystal Robertson
Infection Control . . . . Donna Pruin, RN
ICU . . . . Betty Fortenberry
Director Medical Surgical Nursing . . . . Marye Elliott, RN
OB/GYN/Women's Health . . . . Cathy Gilbert, RN
Respiratory/Cardiopulmonary . . . . Christy Hood

Measure	Cases	This Hospital	State Average	U.S. Average	Top Hospital
Heart Attack Care					
ACE Inhibitor or ARB for LVSD	52	67%	78%	82%	100%
Aspirin at Arrival	169	90%	87%	92%	100%
Aspirin at Discharge	171	92%	87%	90%	100%
Beta Blocker at Arrival	130	87%	81%	87%	100%
Beta Blocker at Discharge	175	88%	86%	90%	100%
Fibrinolytic Medication Timing[1]	4	50%	25%	31%	100%
PCI Within 90 Minutes of Arrival[1]	5	40%	61%	54%	95%
Smoking Cessation Advice	64	100%	85%	88%	100%
Heart Failure Care					
ACE Inhibitor or ARB for LVSD	130	79%	80%	82%	100%
Discharge Instructions	277	47%	54%	61%	93%
Evaluation of LVS Function	366	82%	79%	83%	99%
Smoking Cessation Advice	66	100%	78%	82%	100%
Pneumonia Care					
Appropriate Initial Antibiotic	229	85%	81%	83%	94%
Blood Culture Timing	134	78%	89%	90%	100%
Influenza Vaccine	53	47%	62%	70%	100%
Initial Antibiotic Timing	246	73%	79%	80%	93%
Oxygenation Assessment	315	99%	99%	99%	100%
Pneumococcal Vaccine	183	57%	61%	69%	94%
Smoking Cessation Advice	72	100%	77%	80%	100%
Surgical Infection Prevention					
Prophylactic Antibiotic Given[2]	360	90%	74%	77%	95%
Prophylactic Antibiotic Selection[2]	68	71%	88%	90%	100%
Prophylactic Antibiotic Stopped[2]	336	42%	70%	72%	95%
Pregnancy Care					
Inpatient Neonatal Mortality	-	-	-	-	-
Third or Fourth Degree Laceration	-	-	3.32%	3.63%	3.27%

NOTE: Hospital profiles are in alphabetical order by state, then city, then hospital within the city; Rankings are sorted by rate in descending order and exclude hospitals with less than 25 cases; (1) The number of cases is too small (n<25) for purposes of reliably predicting hospital performance; (2) Measure reflects the hospital's indication that its submission was based upon a sample of its relevant discharges; (3) Rate reflects fewer than the maximum possible quarters of data for the measure; (4) Inaccurate information submitted and suppressed for one or more quarters; (5) No data is available from the hospital for this measure; Please refer to the User's Guide for a full explanation of data

Wiregrass Medical Center

1200 W Maple Avenue
Geneva, AL 36340
URL: www.wiregrassmedicalcenter.org
Ownership: Govt - Hospital District or Authority
Emergency Services: Yes

Phone: 334-684-3655
Fax: 334-684-0299

Accredited: Yes
Licensed Beds: 83

Key Personnel:
Interim CEO . . . . Greg Dykes
ER Director . . . . Mirilyn Boyd
Director of Infection Control . . . . Judy Brown
ICU Director . . . . Shan Wood
Surgery Supervisor . . . . Norma Hughes
Chief Radiology . . . . John Tomberlin
Director Respiratory Therapy . . . . OD Mitchum

Measure	Cases	This Hospital	State Average	U.S. Average	Top Hospital
Heart Attack Care					
ACE Inhibitor or ARB for LVSD	0	-	78%	82%	100%
Aspirin at Arrival[1]	9	100%	87%	92%	100%
Aspirin at Discharge[1]	5	60%	87%	90%	100%
Beta Blocker at Arrival[1]	9	56%	81%	87%	100%
Beta Blocker at Discharge[1]	5	80%	86%	90%	100%
Fibrinolytic Medication Timing	0	-	25%	31%	100%
PCI Within 90 Minutes of Arrival	0	-	61%	54%	95%
Smoking Cessation Advice	0	-	85%	88%	100%
Heart Failure Care					
ACE Inhibitor or ARB for LVSD[1]	9	22%	80%	82%	100%
Discharge Instructions	67	87%	54%	61%	93%
Evaluation of LVS Function	76	46%	79%	83%	99%
Smoking Cessation Advice[1]	21	100%	78%	82%	100%
Pneumonia Care					
Appropriate Initial Antibiotic	131	55%	81%	83%	94%
Blood Culture Timing	40	98%	89%	90%	100%
Influenza Vaccine	32	50%	62%	70%	100%
Initial Antibiotic Timing	120	86%	79%	80%	93%
Oxygenation Assessment	159	97%	99%	99%	100%
Pneumococcal Vaccine	83	67%	61%	69%	94%
Smoking Cessation Advice	42	100%	77%	80%	100%
Surgical Infection Prevention					
Prophylactic Antibiotic Given[1,3]	15	47%	74%	77%	95%
Prophylactic Antibiotic Selection[1]	7	14%	88%	90%	100%
Prophylactic Antibiotic Stopped[1,3]	15	27%	70%	72%	95%
Pregnancy Care					
Inpatient Neonatal Mortality	-	-	-	-	-
Third or Fourth Degree Laceration	-	-	3.32%	3.63%	3.27%

Georgiana Hospital

Alternate Name: Georgiana Doctors Community Hospital
515 Miranda Street
Georgiana, AL 36033
Ownership: Proprietary
Emergency Services: Yes

Phone: 334-376-2205
Fax: 334-376-9080

Accredited: No
Licensed Beds: 22

Key Personnel:
CEO . . . . Harry Cole
Chief of Medical Staff . . . . Geoffery Vorts
Emergency Room . . . . Cathy Cates

Measure	Cases	This Hospital	State Average	U.S. Average	Top Hospital
Heart Attack Care					
ACE Inhibitor or ARB for LVSD[1]	1	100%	78%	82%	100%
Aspirin at Arrival[1]	18	61%	87%	92%	100%
Aspirin at Discharge[1]	14	71%	87%	90%	100%
Beta Blocker at Arrival[1]	18	50%	81%	87%	100%
Beta Blocker at Discharge[1]	15	60%	86%	90%	100%
Fibrinolytic Medication Timing[1]	4	0%	25%	31%	100%
PCI Within 90 Minutes of Arrival	0	-	61%	54%	95%
Smoking Cessation Advice[1]	2	100%	85%	88%	100%
Heart Failure Care					
ACE Inhibitor or ARB for LVSD[1]	16	31%	80%	82%	100%
Discharge Instructions	52	92%	54%	61%	93%
Evaluation of LVS Function	54	35%	79%	83%	99%
Smoking Cessation Advice[1]	12	100%	78%	82%	100%
Pneumonia Care					

Measure	Cases	This Hospital	State Average	U.S. Average	Top Hospital
Appropriate Initial Antibiotic[1]	19	74%	81%	83%	94%
Blood Culture Timing	0	-	89%	90%	100%
Influenza Vaccine[1]	8	75%	62%	70%	100%
Initial Antibiotic Timing	38	87%	79%	80%	93%
Oxygenation Assessment	46	98%	99%	99%	100%
Pneumococcal Vaccine[1]	24	67%	61%	69%	94%
Smoking Cessation Advice[1]	10	100%	77%	80%	100%
Surgical Infection Prevention					
Prophylactic Antibiotic Given[5]	-	-	74%	77%	95%
Prophylactic Antibiotic Selection[5]	-	-	88%	90%	100%
Prophylactic Antibiotic Stopped[5]	-	-	70%	72%	95%
Pregnancy Care					
Inpatient Neonatal Mortality	-	-	-	-	-
Third or Fourth Degree Laceration	-	-	3.32%	3.63%	3.27%

Hale County Hospital

508 Green Street
Greensboro, AL 36744
Ownership: Government - Local
Emergency Services: Yes

Phone: 334-624-3024
Fax: 334-624-3800

Accredited: No
Licensed Beds: 39

Key Personnel:
CEO . . . . Richard McGill
Chief of Medical Staff . . . . Izzeddin Kamalmaz
Director Medical Surgical Nursing . . . . Shay Whaley
Chief Radiology . . . . Delbert Honn, MD

Measure	Cases	This Hospital	State Average	U.S. Average	Top Hospital
Heart Attack Care					
ACE Inhibitor or ARB for LVSD[5]	-	-	78%	82%	100%
Aspirin at Arrival[5]	-	-	87%	92%	100%
Aspirin at Discharge[5]	-	-	87%	90%	100%
Beta Blocker at Arrival[5]	-	-	81%	87%	100%
Beta Blocker at Discharge[5]	-	-	86%	90%	100%
Fibrinolytic Medication Timing[5]	-	-	25%	31%	100%
PCI Within 90 Minutes of Arrival[5]	-	-	61%	54%	95%
Smoking Cessation Advice[5]	-	-	85%	88%	100%
Heart Failure Care					
ACE Inhibitor or ARB for LVSD	0	-	80%	82%	100%
Discharge Instructions[1,3]	13	92%	54%	61%	93%
Evaluation of LVS Function	39	23%	79%	83%	99%
Smoking Cessation Advice[1,3]	3	100%	78%	82%	100%
Pneumonia Care					
Appropriate Initial Antibiotic[1,3]	2	100%	81%	83%	94%
Blood Culture Timing[3]	0	-	89%	90%	100%
Influenza Vaccine[5]	-	-	62%	70%	100%
Initial Antibiotic Timing[1]	5	80%	79%	80%	93%
Oxygenation Assessment[1]	14	100%	99%	99%	100%
Pneumococcal Vaccine[1]	8	0%	61%	69%	94%
Smoking Cessation Advice[3]	0	-	77%	80%	100%
Surgical Infection Prevention					
Prophylactic Antibiotic Given[5]	-	-	74%	77%	95%
Prophylactic Antibiotic Selection[5]	-	-	88%	90%	100%
Prophylactic Antibiotic Stopped[5]	-	-	70%	72%	95%
Pregnancy Care					
Inpatient Neonatal Mortality	-	-	-	-	-
Third or Fourth Degree Laceration	-	-	3.32%	3.63%	3.27%

L V Stabler Memorial Hospital

29 LV Stabler Drive
Greenville, AL 36037
URL: www.lvstabler.com
Ownership: Proprietary
Emergency Services: Yes

Phone: 334-383-2317
Fax: 334-382-0305

Accredited: Yes
Licensed Beds: 72

Key Personnel:
CEO . . . . Bobby Ginn
Cardiac Lab . . . . Terri Bagents
Emergency Room . . . . Ginger Salter
Infection Control . . . . Chris Killebrew
ICU . . . . Kimberli Weaver
Intensive/Coronary Care . . . . Kimberli Weaver
Medical Surgical Nursing . . . . Kimberli Weaver
OB/GYN Women's Health . . . . William Thomas, MD
Respiratory/Cardiopulmonary . . . . Terri Bagents

NOTE: Hospital profiles are in alphabetical order by state, then city, then hospital within the city; Rankings are sorted by rate in descending order and exclude hospitals with less than 25 cases; (1) The number of cases is too small (n<25) for purposes of reliably predicting hospital performance; (2) Measure reflects the hospital's indication that its submission was based upon a sample of its relevant discharges; (3) Rate reflects fewer than the maximum possible quarters of data for the measure; (4) Inaccurate information submitted and suppressed for one or more quarters; (5) No data is available from the hospital for this measure; Please refer to the User's Guide for a full explanation of data

Measure	Cases	This Hospital	State Average	U.S. Average	Top Hospital
Heart Attack Care					
ACE Inhibitor or ARB for LVSD	0	-	78%	82%	100%
Aspirin at Arrival[1]	11	82%	87%	92%	100%
Aspirin at Discharge[1]	7	86%	87%	90%	100%
Beta Blocker at Arrival[1]	11	82%	81%	87%	100%
Beta Blocker at Discharge[1]	7	86%	86%	90%	100%
Fibrinolytic Medication Timing	0	-	25%	31%	100%
PCI Within 90 Minutes of Arrival	0	-	61%	54%	95%
Smoking Cessation Advice[1]	1	0%	85%	88%	100%
Heart Failure Care					
ACE Inhibitor or ARB for LVSD	36	78%	80%	82%	100%
Discharge Instructions	79	90%	54%	61%	93%
Evaluation of LVS Function	92	92%	79%	83%	99%
Smoking Cessation Advice[1]	19	95%	78%	82%	100%
Pneumonia Care					
Appropriate Initial Antibiotic	69	70%	81%	83%	94%
Blood Culture Timing	33	94%	89%	90%	100%
Influenza Vaccine[1]	14	93%	62%	70%	100%
Initial Antibiotic Timing	84	93%	79%	80%	93%
Oxygenation Assessment	89	100%	99%	99%	100%
Pneumococcal Vaccine	45	89%	61%	69%	94%
Smoking Cessation Advice[1]	16	88%	77%	80%	100%
Surgical Infection Prevention					
Prophylactic Antibiotic Given[2,3]	33	85%	74%	77%	95%
Prophylactic Antibiotic Selection[1,2]	12	92%	88%	90%	100%
Prophylactic Antibiotic Stopped[2,3]	33	85%	70%	72%	95%
Pregnancy Care					
Inpatient Neonatal Mortality	-	-	-	-	-
Third or Fourth Degree Laceration	-	-	3.32%	3.63%	3.27%

Grove Hill Memorial Hospital

295 S Jackson Street
Grove Hill, AL 36451
Ownership: Government - Local
Emergency Services: No

Phone: 251-275-3191
Fax: 251-275-4281
Accredited: No
Licensed Beds: 50

Key Personnel:

CEO . . . . Doug Sewell
Chief of Medical Staff . . . . Raff Neal
Chief Radiology . . . . Himath Singh, MD
Chief of Respiratory . . . . Calton Barmer

Measure	Cases	This Hospital	State Average	U.S. Average	Top Hospital
Heart Attack Care					
ACE Inhibitor or ARB for LVSD[1]	1	0%	78%	82%	100%
Aspirin at Arrival[1]	8	62%	87%	92%	100%
Aspirin at Discharge[1]	2	100%	87%	90%	100%
Beta Blocker at Arrival[1]	7	57%	81%	87%	100%
Beta Blocker at Discharge[1]	2	100%	86%	90%	100%
Fibrinolytic Medication Timing	0	-	25%	31%	100%
PCI Within 90 Minutes of Arrival	0	-	61%	54%	95%
Smoking Cessation Advice	0	-	85%	88%	100%
Heart Failure Care					
ACE Inhibitor or ARB for LVSD[1]	11	64%	80%	82%	100%
Discharge Instructions	54	24%	54%	61%	93%
Evaluation of LVS Function	56	71%	79%	83%	99%
Smoking Cessation Advice[1]	5	20%	78%	82%	100%
Pneumonia Care					
Appropriate Initial Antibiotic	41	83%	81%	83%	94%
Blood Culture Timing[1]	11	91%	89%	90%	100%
Influenza Vaccine[1]	9	56%	62%	70%	100%
Initial Antibiotic Timing	29	83%	79%	80%	93%
Oxygenation Assessment	48	100%	99%	99%	100%
Pneumococcal Vaccine[1]	22	55%	61%	69%	94%
Smoking Cessation Advice[1]	7	0%	77%	80%	100%
Surgical Infection Prevention					
Prophylactic Antibiotic Given[1,3]	1	0%	74%	77%	95%
Prophylactic Antibiotic Selection[5]	-	-	88%	90%	100%
Prophylactic Antibiotic Stopped[3]	0	-	70%	72%	95%
Pregnancy Care					
Inpatient Neonatal Mortality	-	-	-	-	-

Third or Fourth Degree Laceration	-	-	3.32%	3.63%	3.27%

Marshall Medical Center North

Alternate Name: Guntersville-Arab Medical Center
8000 Alabama Highway 69
Guntersville, AL 35976
E-mail: jwillmon@mmcnorth.com
URL: www.mmcenters.com/mmcnorth.php
Ownership: Govt - Hospital District or Authority
Emergency Services: Yes

Phone: 256-753-8000
Fax: 256-753-8007

Accredited: Yes
Licensed Beds: 90

Key Personnel:

President/CEO . . . . Gary R Gore
Chief Medical Staff . . . . John Packard, MD
Emergency Room . . . . Wanda Stone, RN
Infection Control . . . . Nilda Strickun, RN
ICU . . . . Wanda Stone, RN
Medical/Surgical Nursing . . . . Kathy Woodruff, RN
OB/GYN Womens Health . . . . Kathy Woodruff, RN
Respiratory/Cardiopulmonary . . . . Greg Allred

Measure	Cases	This Hospital	State Average	U.S. Average	Top Hospital
Heart Attack Care					
ACE Inhibitor or ARB for LVSD[3]	0	-	78%	82%	100%
Aspirin at Arrival[1,3]	4	75%	87%	92%	100%
Aspirin at Discharge[1,3]	1	100%	87%	90%	100%
Beta Blocker at Arrival[1,3]	6	83%	81%	87%	100%
Beta Blocker at Discharge[1,3]	3	100%	86%	90%	100%
Fibrinolytic Medication Timing[3]	0	-	25%	31%	100%
PCI Within 90 Minutes of Arrival	0	-	61%	54%	95%
Smoking Cessation Advice[3]	0	-	85%	88%	100%
Heart Failure Care					
ACE Inhibitor or ARB for LVSD[1]	21	95%	80%	82%	100%
Discharge Instructions	71	66%	54%	61%	93%
Evaluation of LVS Function	94	95%	79%	83%	99%
Smoking Cessation Advice[1]	9	100%	78%	82%	100%
Pneumonia Care					
Appropriate Initial Antibiotic	132	83%	81%	83%	94%
Blood Culture Timing	114	89%	89%	90%	100%
Influenza Vaccine	38	89%	62%	70%	100%
Initial Antibiotic Timing	178	90%	79%	80%	93%
Oxygenation Assessment	219	100%	99%	99%	100%
Pneumococcal Vaccine	124	82%	61%	69%	94%
Smoking Cessation Advice	50	94%	77%	80%	100%
Surgical Infection Prevention					
Prophylactic Antibiotic Given	151	89%	74%	77%	95%
Prophylactic Antibiotic Selection	54	91%	88%	90%	100%
Prophylactic Antibiotic Stopped	152	91%	70%	72%	95%
Pregnancy Care					
Inpatient Neonatal Mortality	403	0.25%	-	-	-
Third or Fourth Degree Laceration	286	9.44%	3.32%	3.63%	3.27%

Lakeland Community Hospital

42024 Highway 195 E
Haleyville, AL 35565
Ownership: Voluntary non-profit - Church
Emergency Services: Yes

Phone: 205-485-7117

Accredited: Yes

Measure	Cases	This Hospital	State Average	U.S. Average	Top Hospital
Heart Attack Care					
ACE Inhibitor or ARB for LVSD	0	-	78%	82%	100%
Aspirin at Arrival[1]	11	91%	87%	92%	100%
Aspirin at Discharge[1]	7	100%	87%	90%	100%
Beta Blocker at Arrival[1]	13	85%	81%	87%	100%
Beta Blocker at Discharge[1]	8	100%	86%	90%	100%
Fibrinolytic Medication Timing	0	-	25%	31%	100%
PCI Within 90 Minutes of Arrival	0	-	61%	54%	95%
Smoking Cessation Advice[1]	1	100%	85%	88%	100%
Heart Failure Care					
ACE Inhibitor or ARB for LVSD[1]	15	87%	80%	82%	100%
Discharge Instructions	68	91%	54%	61%	93%
Evaluation of LVS Function	90	88%	79%	83%	99%
Smoking Cessation Advice[1]	18	94%	78%	82%	100%

NOTE: Hospital profiles are in alphabetical order by state, then city, then hospital within the city; Rankings are sorted by rate in descending order and exclude hospitals with less than 25 cases; (1) The number of cases is too small (n<25) for purposes of reliably predicting hospital performance; (2) Measure reflects the hospital's indication that its submission was based upon a sample of its relevant discharges; (3) Rate reflects fewer than the maximum possible quarters of data for the measure; (4) Inaccurate information submitted and suppressed for one or more quarters; (5) No data is available from the hospital for this measure; Please refer to the User's Guide for a full explanation of data

Pneumonia Care					
Appropriate Initial Antibiotic	248	82%	81%	83%	94%
Blood Culture Timing	58	91%	89%	90%	100%
Influenza Vaccine	71	3%	62%	70%	100%
Initial Antibiotic Timing	346	85%	79%	80%	93%
Oxygenation Assessment	398	99%	99%	99%	100%
Pneumococcal Vaccine	222	89%	61%	69%	94%
Smoking Cessation Advice	102	97%	77%	80%	100%
Surgical Infection Prevention					
Prophylactic Antibiotic Given[1,2,3]	4	25%	74%	77%	95%
Prophylactic Antibiotic Selection[1,2]	1	100%	88%	90%	100%
Prophylactic Antibiotic Stopped[1,2,3]	4	25%	70%	72%	95%
Pregnancy Care					
Inpatient Neonatal Mortality	-	-	-	-	-
Third or Fourth Degree Laceration	-	-	3.32%	3.63%	3.27%

Marion Regional Wellness Center

Alternate Name: NMMC-Hamilton
1256 Military Street S
Hamilton, AL 35570   Phone: 205-921-6200
E-mail: mbmc@scnet.net
URL: www.nmhs.net
Ownership: Voluntary non-profit - Private   Accredited: Yes
Emergency Services: Yes   Licensed Beds: 57
Key Personnel:
President/CEO . . . . John Heer
Administrator . . . . Donald Jones
Director Respiratory Therapy . . . . Stephen Proctor

Measure	Cases	This Hospital	State Average	U.S. Average	Top Hospital
Heart Attack Care					
ACE Inhibitor or ARB for LVSD[1,3]	1	100%	78%	82%	100%
Aspirin at Arrival[1,3]	3	100%	87%	92%	100%
Aspirin at Discharge[1,3]	2	100%	87%	90%	100%
Beta Blocker at Arrival[1,3]	2	100%	81%	87%	100%
Beta Blocker at Discharge[1,3]	3	100%	86%	90%	100%
Fibrinolytic Medication Timing[3]	0	-	25%	31%	100%
PCI Within 90 Minutes of Arrival[5]	-	-	61%	54%	95%
Smoking Cessation Advice[3]	0	-	85%	88%	100%
Heart Failure Care					
ACE Inhibitor or ARB for LVSD[1]	17	82%	80%	82%	100%
Discharge Instructions	46	76%	54%	61%	93%
Evaluation of LVS Function	50	90%	79%	83%	99%
Smoking Cessation Advice[1]	6	100%	78%	82%	100%
Pneumonia Care					
Appropriate Initial Antibiotic	94	79%	81%	83%	94%
Blood Culture Timing	64	89%	89%	90%	100%
Influenza Vaccine	32	97%	62%	70%	100%
Initial Antibiotic Timing	123	93%	79%	80%	93%
Oxygenation Assessment	153	100%	99%	99%	100%
Pneumococcal Vaccine	101	98%	61%	69%	94%
Smoking Cessation Advice	33	91%	77%	80%	100%
Surgical Infection Prevention					
Prophylactic Antibiotic Given[1,3]	2	100%	74%	77%	95%
Prophylactic Antibiotic Selection[1]	2	100%	88%	90%	100%
Prophylactic Antibiotic Stopped[1,3]	2	100%	70%	72%	95%
Pregnancy Care					
Inpatient Neonatal Mortality	-	-	-	-	-
Third or Fourth Degree Laceration	-	-	3.32%	3.63%	3.27%

Hartselle Medical Center

201 Pine Street NW   Phone: 256-773-6511
PO Box 969   Fax: 256-773-4010
Hartselle, AL 35640
URL: www.hartsellemedicalcenter.com
Ownership: Proprietary   Accredited: Yes
Emergency Services: Yes   Licensed Beds: 150
Key Personnel:
CEO. . . . . Jeff Rains
Chief of Medical Staff . . . . Amit Bohra, MD
Director of Cardiology/Cardiac Lab. . . . . Paddy Lawn
Emergency Room . . . . June Davis
Director Medical/Surgical Nursing . . . . Mitzie Pouncey

Chief Radiology . . . . Lee Creel, DDS
Director Respiratory Therapy . . . . Sherry Taylor

Measure	Cases	This Hospital	State Average	U.S. Average	Top Hospital
Heart Attack Care					
ACE Inhibitor or ARB for LVSD	0	-	78%	82%	100%
Aspirin at Arrival[1]	3	100%	87%	92%	100%
Aspirin at Discharge[1]	1	100%	87%	90%	100%
Beta Blocker at Arrival[1]	2	100%	81%	87%	100%
Beta Blocker at Discharge[1]	4	100%	86%	90%	100%
Fibrinolytic Medication Timing	0	-	25%	31%	100%
PCI Within 90 Minutes of Arrival	0	-	61%	54%	95%
Smoking Cessation Advice	0	-	85%	88%	100%
Heart Failure Care					
ACE Inhibitor or ARB for LVSD[1]	18	100%	80%	82%	100%
Discharge Instructions	70	91%	54%	61%	93%
Evaluation of LVS Function	86	100%	79%	83%	99%
Smoking Cessation Advice[1]	8	100%	78%	82%	100%
Pneumonia Care					
Appropriate Initial Antibiotic	56	95%	81%	83%	94%
Blood Culture Timing	37	100%	89%	90%	100%
Influenza Vaccine[1]	15	100%	62%	70%	100%
Initial Antibiotic Timing	75	96%	79%	80%	93%
Oxygenation Assessment	86	100%	99%	99%	100%
Pneumococcal Vaccine	58	91%	61%	69%	94%
Smoking Cessation Advice[1]	18	100%	77%	80%	100%
Surgical Infection Prevention					
Prophylactic Antibiotic Given[1,2,3]	5	60%	74%	77%	95%
Prophylactic Antibiotic Selection[1,2]	4	100%	88%	90%	100%
Prophylactic Antibiotic Stopped[1,2,3]	5	20%	70%	72%	95%
Pregnancy Care					
Inpatient Neonatal Mortality	-	-	-	-	-
Third or Fourth Degree Laceration	-	-	3.32%	3.63%	3.27%

Crestwood Medical Center

One Hospital Drive   Phone: 256-882-3100
Huntsville, AL 35801   Fax: 256-880-4246
URL: www.crestwoodmedcenter.com
Ownership: Proprietary   Accredited: Yes
Emergency Services: Yes   Licensed Beds: 150
Key Personnel:
CEO. . . . . Bradley E Jones
Chief Medical Staff . . . . James A Flatt, MD
ER Director . . . . Bob Phillips
Infection Control. . . . . Mae Mason
ICU . . . . Lora Porter
Medical & Surgical Nursing . . . . Nancy Walker
Chief of OB/GYN . . . . Edith Aguaye

Measure	Cases	This Hospital	State Average	U.S. Average	Top Hospital
Heart Attack Care					
ACE Inhibitor or ARB for LVSD[1]	15	87%	78%	82%	100%
Aspirin at Arrival	84	90%	87%	92%	100%
Aspirin at Discharge	79	94%	87%	90%	100%
Beta Blocker at Arrival	70	86%	81%	87%	100%
Beta Blocker at Discharge	77	91%	86%	90%	100%
Fibrinolytic Medication Timing[1]	1	0%	25%	31%	100%
PCI Within 90 Minutes of Arrival[1]	4	100%	61%	54%	95%
Smoking Cessation Advice	31	87%	85%	88%	100%
Heart Failure Care					
ACE Inhibitor or ARB for LVSD	87	89%	80%	82%	100%
Discharge Instructions	189	68%	54%	61%	93%
Evaluation of LVS Function	234	92%	79%	83%	99%
Smoking Cessation Advice	47	87%	78%	82%	100%
Pneumonia Care					
Appropriate Initial Antibiotic	155	78%	81%	83%	94%
Blood Culture Timing	101	95%	89%	90%	100%
Influenza Vaccine	31	74%	62%	70%	100%
Initial Antibiotic Timing	173	64%	79%	80%	93%
Oxygenation Assessment	197	99%	99%	99%	100%
Pneumococcal Vaccine	109	72%	61%	69%	94%
Smoking Cessation Advice	57	81%	77%	80%	100%

NOTE: Hospital profiles are in alphabetical order by state, then city, then hospital within the city; Rankings are sorted by rate in descending order and exclude hospitals with less than 25 cases; (1) The number of cases is too small (n<25) for purposes of reliably predicting hospital performance; (2) Measure reflects the hospital's indication that its submission was based upon a sample of its relevant discharges; (3) Rate reflects fewer than the maximum possible quarters of data for the measure; (4) Inaccurate information submitted and suppressed for one or more quarters; (5) No data is available from the hospital for this measure; Please refer to the User's Guide for a full explanation of data

Surgical Infection Prevention					
Prophylactic Antibiotic Given[2]	797	83%	74%	77%	95%
Prophylactic Antibiotic Selection[2]	106	89%	88%	90%	100%
Prophylactic Antibiotic Stopped[2]	764	69%	70%	72%	95%
Pregnancy Care					
Inpatient Neonatal Mortality	-	-	-	-	-
Third or Fourth Degree Laceration	-	-	3.32%	3.63%	3.27%

Huntsville Hospital

101 Sivley Road
Huntsville, AL 35801
URL: www.huntsvillehospitalal.org
Ownership: Govt - Hospital District or Authority
Emergency Services: Yes

Phone: 256-265-1000
Fax: 256-517-8484

Accredited: Yes
Licensed Beds: 901

Key Personnel:
Administrator/CEO . . . . Joe Austin
Chief Medical Staff. . . . . Sherrie Squyres, MD
Cardiac Lab . . . . Mike Carter
Catheterization Lab . . . . Mike Carter
Emergency Room . . . . Barbara Pierce
Director Infection/Disease Control . . . . Cindy Mize
OB/GYN Womens Health. . . . . Paula Woodfin

Measure	Cases	This Hospital	State Average	U.S. Average	Top Hospital
Heart Attack Care					
ACE Inhibitor or ARB for LVSD	260	88%	78%	82%	100%
Aspirin at Arrival	557	98%	87%	92%	100%
Aspirin at Discharge	985	97%	87%	90%	100%
Beta Blocker at Arrival	468	95%	81%	87%	100%
Beta Blocker at Discharge	946	97%	86%	90%	100%
Fibrinolytic Medication Timing[1]	4	25%	25%	31%	100%
PCI Within 90 Minutes of Arrival	33	88%	61%	54%	95%
Smoking Cessation Advice	415	98%	85%	88%	100%
Heart Failure Care					
ACE Inhibitor or ARB for LVSD	591	84%	80%	82%	100%
Discharge Instructions	1,126	75%	54%	61%	93%
Evaluation of LVS Function	1,301	93%	79%	83%	99%
Smoking Cessation Advice	254	96%	78%	82%	100%
Pneumonia Care					
Appropriate Initial Antibiotic	525	81%	81%	83%	94%
Blood Culture Timing	458	81%	89%	90%	100%
Influenza Vaccine	159	77%	62%	70%	100%
Initial Antibiotic Timing	784	63%	79%	80%	93%
Oxygenation Assessment	934	100%	99%	99%	100%
Pneumococcal Vaccine	474	83%	61%	69%	94%
Smoking Cessation Advice	240	83%	77%	80%	100%
Surgical Infection Prevention					
Prophylactic Antibiotic Given[2]	836	89%	74%	77%	95%
Prophylactic Antibiotic Selection[2]	192	87%	88%	90%	100%
Prophylactic Antibiotic Stopped[2]	830	78%	70%	72%	95%
Pregnancy Care					
Inpatient Neonatal Mortality[2]	983	0.71%	-	-	-
Third or Fourth Degree Laceration[2]	581	4.65%	3.32%	3.63%	3.27%

Jackson Medical Center

Alternate Name: Vaughan Jackson Medical Center
220 Hospital Drive
Jackson, AL 36545
URL: www.jacksonmedicalcenter.com
Ownership: Proprietary
Emergency Services: Yes

Phone: 251-246-9021
Fax: 251-246-1108

Accredited: No
Licensed Beds: 35

Key Personnel:
CEO. . . . . Teresa F Grimes
Chief Medical Staff. . . . . Jared Ellis, MD

Measure	Cases	This Hospital	State Average	U.S. Average	Top Hospital
Heart Attack Care					
ACE Inhibitor or ARB for LVSD	0	-	78%	82%	100%
Aspirin at Arrival[1]	1	100%	87%	92%	100%
Aspirin at Discharge	0	-	87%	90%	100%
Beta Blocker at Arrival	0	-	81%	87%	100%
Beta Blocker at Discharge	0	-	86%	90%	100%

			25%	31%	100%
Fibrinolytic Medication Timing	0	-	25%	31%	100%
PCI Within 90 Minutes of Arrival	0	-	61%	54%	95%
Smoking Cessation Advice	0	-	85%	88%	100%
Heart Failure Care					
ACE Inhibitor or ARB for LVSD[1]	5	60%	80%	82%	100%
Discharge Instructions	47	6%	54%	61%	93%
Evaluation of LVS Function	52	60%	79%	83%	99%
Smoking Cessation Advice[1]	7	43%	78%	82%	100%
Pneumonia Care					
Appropriate Initial Antibiotic	76	89%	81%	83%	94%
Blood Culture Timing[1]	16	94%	89%	90%	100%
Influenza Vaccine[1]	17	47%	62%	70%	100%
Initial Antibiotic Timing	78	85%	79%	80%	93%
Oxygenation Assessment	84	100%	99%	99%	100%
Pneumococcal Vaccine	33	61%	61%	69%	94%
Smoking Cessation Advice[1]	19	47%	77%	80%	100%
Surgical Infection Prevention					
Prophylactic Antibiotic Given[5]	-	-	74%	77%	95%
Prophylactic Antibiotic Selection[5]	-	-	88%	90%	100%
Prophylactic Antibiotic Stopped[5]	-	-	70%	72%	95%
Pregnancy Care					
Inpatient Neonatal Mortality	-	-	-	-	-
Third or Fourth Degree Laceration	-	-	3.32%	3.63%	3.27%

Jacksonville Medical Center

1701 Pelham Road S
Jacksonville, AL 36265
E-mail: webmaster@jmchealth.com
URL: www.jmchealth.com
Ownership: Proprietary
Emergency Services: Yes

Phone: 256-435-4970
Fax: 256-435-8116

Accredited: Yes
Licensed Beds: 89

Key Personnel:
CEO . . . . Roger Collins
Director Cardiopulmonary . . . . Jeff Green
Director Emergency Medicine . . . . William Tyndall, MD
Director Emergency . . . . Rebecca Pierce
Director Medical/Surgical Unit . . . . Sharon Abernathy
OB/GYN Womens Health. . . . . Shan Young, MD
Director Radiology . . . . Jeff Green

Measure	Cases	This Hospital	State Average	U.S. Average	Top Hospital
Heart Attack Care					
ACE Inhibitor or ARB for LVSD[1]	1	100%	78%	82%	100%
Aspirin at Arrival[1]	8	100%	87%	92%	100%
Aspirin at Discharge[1]	2	100%	87%	90%	100%
Beta Blocker at Arrival[1]	6	83%	81%	87%	100%
Beta Blocker at Discharge[1]	4	75%	86%	90%	100%
Fibrinolytic Medication Timing	0	-	25%	31%	100%
PCI Within 90 Minutes of Arrival	0	-	61%	54%	95%
Smoking Cessation Advice	0	-	85%	88%	100%
Heart Failure Care					
ACE Inhibitor or ARB for LVSD[1]	9	100%	80%	82%	100%
Discharge Instructions	37	76%	54%	61%	93%
Evaluation of LVS Function	53	94%	79%	83%	99%
Smoking Cessation Advice[1]	7	100%	78%	82%	100%
Pneumonia Care					
Appropriate Initial Antibiotic	80	76%	81%	83%	94%
Blood Culture Timing	50	88%	89%	90%	100%
Influenza Vaccine[1]	10	90%	62%	70%	100%
Initial Antibiotic Timing	82	74%	79%	80%	93%
Oxygenation Assessment	93	100%	99%	99%	100%
Pneumococcal Vaccine	55	84%	61%	69%	94%
Smoking Cessation Advice[1]	23	100%	77%	80%	100%
Surgical Infection Prevention					
Prophylactic Antibiotic Given	107	80%	74%	77%	95%
Prophylactic Antibiotic Selection[1]	19	68%	88%	90%	100%
Prophylactic Antibiotic Stopped	104	90%	70%	72%	95%
Pregnancy Care					
Inpatient Neonatal Mortality	242	0.00%	-	-	-
Third or Fourth Degree Laceration	202	0.50%	3.32%	3.63%	3.27%

NOTE: Hospital profiles are in alphabetical order by state, then city, then hospital within the city; Rankings are sorted by rate in descending order and exclude hospitals with less than 25 cases; (1) The number of cases is too small (n<25) for purposes of reliably predicting hospital performance; (2) Measure reflects the hospital's indication that its submission was based upon a sample of its relevant discharges; (3) Rate reflects fewer than the maximum possible quarters of data for the measure; (4) Inaccurate information submitted and suppressed for one or more quarters; (5) No data is available from the hospital for this measure; Please refer to the User's Guide for a full explanation of data

Walker Baptist Medical Center

3400 Highway 78 E
Jasper, AL 35501
URL: www.bhsala.com/walker
Ownership: Govt - Hospital District or Authority
Emergency Services: Yes

Phone: 205-387-4000
Fax: 205-387-4011

Accredited: Yes
Licensed Beds: 197

Key Personnel:
President . . . . Joel W Tate
Chief Medical Staff . . . . Harvey McCulloch, MD
OB/GYN Womens Health . . . . Carolyn Waldrep
Chief Radiology . . . . James Bradley, MD
Director Respiratory Therapy . . . . Deborah Channell

Measure	Cases	This Hospital	State Average	U.S. Average	Top Hospital
Heart Attack Care					
ACE Inhibitor or ARB for LVSD[1]	9	100%	78%	82%	100%
Aspirin at Arrival	57	98%	87%	92%	100%
Aspirin at Discharge	43	100%	87%	90%	100%
Beta Blocker at Arrival	47	100%	81%	87%	100%
Beta Blocker at Discharge	37	100%	86%	90%	100%
Fibrinolytic Medication Timing[1]	5	40%	25%	31%	100%
PCI Within 90 Minutes of Arrival	0	-	61%	54%	95%
Smoking Cessation Advice	26	100%	85%	88%	100%
Heart Failure Care					
ACE Inhibitor or ARB for LVSD[2]	91	99%	80%	82%	100%
Discharge Instructions[2]	165	99%	54%	61%	93%
Evaluation of LVS Function[2]	205	100%	79%	83%	99%
Smoking Cessation Advice[2]	45	100%	78%	82%	100%
Pneumonia Care					
Appropriate Initial Antibiotic	269	95%	81%	83%	94%
Blood Culture Timing	287	97%	89%	90%	100%
Influenza Vaccine	51	78%	62%	70%	100%
Initial Antibiotic Timing	393	90%	79%	80%	93%
Oxygenation Assessment	459	100%	99%	99%	100%
Pneumococcal Vaccine	242	90%	61%	69%	94%
Smoking Cessation Advice	163	100%	77%	80%	100%
Surgical Infection Prevention					
Prophylactic Antibiotic Given[2]	275	96%	74%	77%	95%
Prophylactic Antibiotic Selection[2]	90	100%	88%	90%	100%
Prophylactic Antibiotic Stopped[2]	258	81%	70%	72%	95%
Pregnancy Care					
Inpatient Neonatal Mortality	-	-	-	-	-
Third or Fourth Degree Laceration	-	-	3.32%	3.63%	3.27%

Crenshaw Baptist Hospital

101 Hospital Circle
Luverne, AL 36049
E-mail: mplowden@baptistfirst.org
Ownership: Voluntary non-profit - Church
Emergency Services: Yes

Phone: 334-335-3374
Fax: 334-335-5636

Accredited: No
Licensed Beds: 65

Key Personnel:
Hospital Administrator . . . . Moultrie D Plowden
Emergency Room . . . . Jeanie Colquitt
Infection Control . . . . Cynthia Butts
Medical/Surgical Nursing . . . . MaryAnn King, RN
OB/GYN Womens Health . . . . Carol Dillon
Chief Radiology . . . . Ken Lyons, ART
Respiratory/Cardiopulmonary . . . . Melanie Foster

Measure	Cases	This Hospital	State Average	U.S. Average	Top Hospital
Heart Attack Care					
ACE Inhibitor or ARB for LVSD[1]	1	100%	78%	82%	100%
Aspirin at Arrival[1]	4	75%	87%	92%	100%
Aspirin at Discharge[1]	3	100%	87%	90%	100%
Beta Blocker at Arrival[1]	4	75%	81%	87%	100%
Beta Blocker at Discharge[1]	3	100%	86%	90%	100%
Fibrinolytic Medication Timing	0	-	25%	31%	100%
PCI Within 90 Minutes of Arrival	0	-	61%	54%	95%
Smoking Cessation Advice	0	-	85%	88%	100%
Heart Failure Care					
ACE Inhibitor or ARB for LVSD[1]	11	55%	80%	82%	100%
Discharge Instructions	26	0%	54%	61%	93%
Evaluation of LVS Function	32	56%	79%	83%	99%

Smoking Cessation Advice[1]	6	17%	78%	82%	100%
Pneumonia Care					
Appropriate Initial Antibiotic	38	79%	81%	83%	94%
Blood Culture Timing[1]	21	100%	89%	90%	100%
Influenza Vaccine[1]	8	88%	62%	70%	100%
Initial Antibiotic Timing	55	42%	79%	80%	93%
Oxygenation Assessment	62	95%	99%	99%	100%
Pneumococcal Vaccine	38	29%	61%	69%	94%
Smoking Cessation Advice[1]	15	13%	77%	80%	100%
Surgical Infection Prevention					
Prophylactic Antibiotic Given[3]	0	-	74%	77%	95%
Prophylactic Antibiotic Selection	0	-	88%	90%	100%
Prophylactic Antibiotic Stopped[3]	0	-	70%	72%	95%
Pregnancy Care					
Inpatient Neonatal Mortality	-	-	-	-	-
Third or Fourth Degree Laceration	-	-	3.32%	3.63%	3.27%

Infirmary West

5600 Girby Rd
Mobile, AL 36693
Ownership: Government - State
Emergency Services: No

Phone: 251-660-5236

Accredited: Yes

Measure	Cases	This Hospital	State Average	U.S. Average	Top Hospital
Heart Attack Care					
ACE Inhibitor or ARB for LVSD[1]	2	50%	78%	82%	100%
Aspirin at Arrival[1]	20	85%	87%	92%	100%
Aspirin at Discharge[1]	8	88%	87%	90%	100%
Beta Blocker at Arrival[1]	15	80%	81%	87%	100%
Beta Blocker at Discharge[1]	9	89%	86%	90%	100%
Fibrinolytic Medication Timing	0	-	25%	31%	100%
PCI Within 90 Minutes of Arrival	0	-	61%	54%	95%
Smoking Cessation Advice[1]	2	100%	85%	88%	100%
Heart Failure Care					
ACE Inhibitor or ARB for LVSD	44	89%	80%	82%	100%
Discharge Instructions	59	31%	54%	61%	93%
Evaluation of LVS Function	63	92%	79%	83%	99%
Smoking Cessation Advice[1]	16	88%	78%	82%	100%
Pneumonia Care					
Appropriate Initial Antibiotic	57	88%	81%	83%	94%
Blood Culture Timing	52	83%	89%	90%	100%
Influenza Vaccine[1]	14	57%	62%	70%	100%
Initial Antibiotic Timing	81	73%	79%	80%	93%
Oxygenation Assessment	92	100%	99%	99%	100%
Pneumococcal Vaccine	33	48%	61%	69%	94%
Smoking Cessation Advice	36	83%	77%	80%	100%
Surgical Infection Prevention					
Prophylactic Antibiotic Given[2]	98	80%	74%	77%	95%
Prophylactic Antibiotic Selection[1,2]	16	69%	88%	90%	100%
Prophylactic Antibiotic Stopped[2]	99	75%	70%	72%	95%
Pregnancy Care					
Inpatient Neonatal Mortality	-	-	-	-	-
Third or Fourth Degree Laceration	-	-	3.32%	3.63%	3.27%

Mobile Infirmary Medical Center

5 Mobile Infirmary Circle
Mobile, AL 36607
URL: www.mimc.com
Ownership: Voluntary non-profit - Private
Emergency Services: Yes

Phone: 251-435-2400
Fax: 251-435-3920

Accredited: Yes
Licensed Beds: 704

Key Personnel:
President/CEO . . . . E Chandler Bramlett
Chief Medical Staff . . . . William Schulte, MD
Emergency Room . . . . William E Admire Jr
CCU Spvg. Nurse . . . . Cindy Buhring, RN
Director Medical/Surgical Nursing . . . . Pamela Gilbert, RN
Chief Radiology . . . . Douglas Hungerford, MD
Director Respiratory Therapy . . . . Barry Jones

Measure	Cases	This Hospital	State Average	U.S. Average	Top Hospital
Heart Attack Care					
ACE Inhibitor or ARB for LVSD[2]	61	74%	78%	82%	100%

NOTE: Hospital profiles are in alphabetical order by state, then city, then hospital within the city; Rankings are sorted by rate in descending order and exclude hospitals with less than 25 cases; (1) The number of cases is too small (n<25) for purposes of reliably predicting hospital performance; (2) Measure reflects the hospital's indication that its submission was based upon a sample of its relevant discharges; (3) Rate reflects fewer than the maximum possible quarters of data for the measure; (4) Inaccurate information submitted and suppressed for one or more quarters; (5) No data is available from the hospital for this measure; Please refer to the User's Guide for a full explanation of data

Measure	Cases	This Hospital	State Average	U.S. Average	Top Hospital
Aspirin at Arrival[2]	168	98%	87%	92%	100%
Aspirin at Discharge[2]	231	97%	87%	90%	100%
Beta Blocker at Arrival[2]	116	96%	81%	87%	100%
Beta Blocker at Discharge[2]	246	96%	86%	90%	100%
Fibrinolytic Medication Timing[1,2]	1	0%	25%	31%	100%
PCI Within 90 Minutes of Arrival[1,2]	10	50%	61%	54%	95%
Smoking Cessation Advice[2]	104	95%	85%	88%	100%
Heart Failure Care					
ACE Inhibitor or ARB for LVSD[2]	130	65%	80%	82%	100%
Discharge Instructions[2]	262	57%	54%	61%	93%
Evaluation of LVS Function[2]	309	94%	79%	83%	99%
Smoking Cessation Advice[2]	84	87%	78%	82%	100%
Pneumonia Care					
Appropriate Initial Antibiotic[2]	77	74%	81%	83%	94%
Blood Culture Timing[2]	78	86%	89%	90%	100%
Influenza Vaccine[2]	28	64%	62%	70%	100%
Initial Antibiotic Timing[2]	147	67%	79%	80%	93%
Oxygenation Assessment[2]	174	100%	99%	99%	100%
Pneumococcal Vaccine[2]	81	78%	61%	69%	94%
Smoking Cessation Advice[2]	41	76%	77%	80%	100%
Surgical Infection Prevention					
Prophylactic Antibiotic Given[2]	361	93%	74%	77%	95%
Prophylactic Antibiotic Selection[2]	93	95%	88%	90%	100%
Prophylactic Antibiotic Stopped[2]	343	65%	70%	72%	95%
Pregnancy Care					
Inpatient Neonatal Mortality	-	-	-	-	-
Third or Fourth Degree Laceration	-	-	3.32%	3.63%	3.27%

Providence Hospital

6801 Airport Boulevard
PO Box 850429
Mobile, AL 36608
URL: www.providencehospital.org
Ownership: Voluntary non-profit - Church
Emergency Services: Yes

Phone: 251-633-1000
Fax: 251-633-1411

Accredited: Yes
Licensed Beds: 349

Key Personnel:
President/CEO . . . . Clark P Christianson
Chief Medical Staff . . . . James Simpson
Director Catheterization Laboratory . . . . Donna Padgett
Acting Director Catheterization Lab . . . . John Host
Director Infection/Disease Control . . . . Anne Doss
CCU Spvg. Nurse . . . . Carolyn Anderson, RN
Director Medical/Surgical Nursing . . . . Valorie Dearmon, RN
Chief OB/GYN . . . . Kirby Plessala, MD
Chief Radiology . . . . Allen Oaks, MD
Director Pulmonary Medicine . . . . Dan Scarcliff

Measure	Cases	This Hospital	State Average	U.S. Average	Top Hospital
Heart Attack Care					
ACE Inhibitor or ARB for LVSD	38	79%	78%	82%	100%
Aspirin at Arrival	181	97%	87%	92%	100%
Aspirin at Discharge	207	95%	87%	90%	100%
Beta Blocker at Arrival	107	87%	81%	87%	100%
Beta Blocker at Discharge	217	94%	86%	90%	100%
Fibrinolytic Medication Timing	0	-	25%	31%	100%
PCI Within 90 Minutes of Arrival[1]	13	54%	61%	54%	95%
Smoking Cessation Advice	88	98%	85%	88%	100%
Heart Failure Care					
ACE Inhibitor or ARB for LVSD	149	91%	80%	82%	100%
Discharge Instructions	477	65%	54%	61%	93%
Evaluation of LVS Function	527	99%	79%	83%	99%
Smoking Cessation Advice	96	100%	78%	82%	100%
Pneumonia Care					
Appropriate Initial Antibiotic	270	83%	81%	83%	94%
Blood Culture Timing	152	94%	89%	90%	100%
Influenza Vaccine	83	43%	62%	70%	100%
Initial Antibiotic Timing	297	72%	79%	80%	93%
Oxygenation Assessment	353	97%	99%	99%	100%
Pneumococcal Vaccine	214	57%	61%	69%	94%
Smoking Cessation Advice	78	94%	77%	80%	100%
Surgical Infection Prevention					
Prophylactic Antibiotic Given[2]	235	77%	74%	77%	95%
Prophylactic Antibiotic Selection[2]	78	96%	88%	90%	100%

Measure	Cases	This Hospital	State Average	U.S. Average	Top Hospital
Prophylactic Antibiotic Stopped[2]	230	66%	70%	72%	95%
Pregnancy Care					
Inpatient Neonatal Mortality	-	-	-	-	-
Third or Fourth Degree Laceration	-	-	3.32%	3.63%	3.27%

Springhill Medical Center

Alternate Name: Springhill Memorial Hospital
3719 Dauphin Street
Mobile, AL 36608
E-mail: dsweeney@springhill.org
URL: www.springhillmedicalcenter.com
Ownership: Proprietary
Emergency Services: Yes

Phone: 251-344-9630
Fax: 251-460-5248

Accredited: Yes
Licensed Beds: 252

Key Personnel:
CEO . . . . Bill A Mason
Chief Medical Staff . . . . John Sands, MD
Catheterization Lab . . . . Don Williams, RN
Emergency Room . . . . Jeff Triboulet, RN
Infection Control . . . . Dan McRae, RN
Director Respiratory Therapy . . . . Joe Woulard

Measure	Cases	This Hospital	State Average	U.S. Average	Top Hospital
Heart Attack Care					
ACE Inhibitor or ARB for LVSD	32	94%	78%	82%	100%
Aspirin at Arrival	116	92%	87%	92%	100%
Aspirin at Discharge	111	95%	87%	90%	100%
Beta Blocker at Arrival	60	88%	81%	87%	100%
Beta Blocker at Discharge	125	98%	86%	90%	100%
Fibrinolytic Medication Timing	0	-	25%	31%	100%
PCI Within 90 Minutes of Arrival[1]	3	33%	61%	54%	95%
Smoking Cessation Advice	55	93%	85%	88%	100%
Heart Failure Care					
ACE Inhibitor or ARB for LVSD	177	97%	80%	82%	100%
Discharge Instructions	455	45%	54%	61%	93%
Evaluation of LVS Function	496	98%	79%	83%	99%
Smoking Cessation Advice	76	86%	78%	82%	100%
Pneumonia Care					
Appropriate Initial Antibiotic	121	82%	81%	83%	94%
Blood Culture Timing	45	71%	89%	90%	100%
Influenza Vaccine	29	59%	62%	70%	100%
Initial Antibiotic Timing	156	80%	79%	80%	93%
Oxygenation Assessment	195	98%	99%	99%	100%
Pneumococcal Vaccine	112	49%	61%	69%	94%
Smoking Cessation Advice	43	79%	77%	80%	100%
Surgical Infection Prevention					
Prophylactic Antibiotic Given	859	64%	74%	77%	95%
Prophylactic Antibiotic Selection	283	92%	88%	90%	100%
Prophylactic Antibiotic Stopped	798	70%	70%	72%	95%
Pregnancy Care					
Inpatient Neonatal Mortality	-	-	-	-	-
Third or Fourth Degree Laceration	-	-	3.32%	3.63%	3.27%

University of South Alabama Medical Center

2451 Fillingim Street
Mobile, AL 36617
URL: www.southalabama.edu/usamc
Ownership: Government - State
Emergency Services: Yes

Phone: 251-471-7000
Fax: 251-470-1672

Accredited: Yes
Licensed Beds: 406

Key Personnel:
Administrator . . . . Beth Anderson
Director of Cardiology/Cardiac Lab . . . . Frank Petty John
Chief Catheterization Laboratory . . . . Martin A Alpert, MD
Emergency Room . . . . Frank Pettyjohn, MD
Director Infection/Disease Control . . . . Keith Ramsey
Director Medical/Surgical Nursing . . . . Sandee Leonard
Chief Radiology . . . . Stephen Teplick
Director Respiratory Therapy . . . . Jimmy Norwood

Measure	Cases	This Hospital	State Average	U.S. Average	Top Hospital
Heart Attack Care					
ACE Inhibitor or ARB for LVSD	31	94%	78%	82%	100%
Aspirin at Arrival	68	99%	87%	92%	100%
Aspirin at Discharge	97	95%	87%	90%	100%

NOTE: Hospital profiles are in alphabetical order by state, then city, then hospital within the city; Rankings are sorted by rate in descending order and exclude hospitals with less than 25 cases; (1) The number of cases is too small (n<25) for purposes of reliably predicting hospital performance; (2) Measure reflects the hospital's indication that its submission was based upon a sample of its relevant discharges; (3) Rate reflects fewer than the maximum possible quarters of data for the measure; (4) Inaccurate information submitted and suppressed for one or more quarters; (5) No data is available from the hospital for this measure; Please refer to the User's Guide for a full explanation of data

Measure	Cases	This Hospital	State Average	U.S. Average	Top Hospital
Beta Blocker at Arrival	55	98%	81%	87%	100%
Beta Blocker at Discharge	95	92%	86%	90%	100%
Fibrinolytic Medication Timing	0	-	25%	31%	100%
PCI Within 90 Minutes of Arrival[1]	3	67%	61%	54%	95%
Smoking Cessation Advice	70	100%	85%	88%	100%
Heart Failure Care					
ACE Inhibitor or ARB for LVSD	140	92%	80%	82%	100%
Discharge Instructions	232	80%	54%	61%	93%
Evaluation of LVS Function	232	94%	79%	83%	99%
Smoking Cessation Advice	98	100%	78%	82%	100%
Pneumonia Care					
Appropriate Initial Antibiotic	72	79%	81%	83%	94%
Blood Culture Timing	70	84%	89%	90%	100%
Influenza Vaccine[1]	8	50%	62%	70%	100%
Initial Antibiotic Timing	101	78%	79%	80%	93%
Oxygenation Assessment	106	100%	99%	99%	100%
Pneumococcal Vaccine[1]	13	23%	61%	69%	94%
Smoking Cessation Advice	52	100%	77%	80%	100%
Surgical Infection Prevention					
Prophylactic Antibiotic Given[2]	182	82%	74%	77%	95%
Prophylactic Antibiotic Selection[2]	44	91%	88%	90%	100%
Prophylactic Antibiotic Stopped[2]	173	50%	70%	72%	95%
Pregnancy Care					
Inpatient Neonatal Mortality	-	-	-	-	-
Third or Fourth Degree Laceration	-	-	3.32%	3.63%	3.27%

Monroe County Hospital

2016 South Alabama Avenue
Monroeville, AL 36461
Ownership: Government - Local
Emergency Services: Yes

Phone: 251-575-3111

Accredited: Yes

Measure	Cases	This Hospital	State Average	U.S. Average	Top Hospital
Heart Attack Care					
ACE Inhibitor or ARB for LVSD[1]	1	100%	78%	82%	100%
Aspirin at Arrival[1]	10	100%	87%	92%	100%
Aspirin at Discharge[1]	6	83%	87%	90%	100%
Beta Blocker at Arrival[1]	11	91%	81%	87%	100%
Beta Blocker at Discharge[1]	7	100%	86%	90%	100%
Fibrinolytic Medication Timing	0	-	25%	31%	100%
PCI Within 90 Minutes of Arrival	0	-	61%	54%	95%
Smoking Cessation Advice	0	-	85%	88%	100%
Heart Failure Care					
ACE Inhibitor or ARB for LVSD	45	82%	80%	82%	100%
Discharge Instructions	119	90%	54%	61%	93%
Evaluation of LVS Function	132	85%	79%	83%	99%
Smoking Cessation Advice	35	100%	78%	82%	100%
Pneumonia Care					
Appropriate Initial Antibiotic	102	79%	81%	83%	94%
Blood Culture Timing	54	93%	89%	90%	100%
Influenza Vaccine[1]	17	65%	62%	70%	100%
Initial Antibiotic Timing	102	82%	79%	80%	93%
Oxygenation Assessment	134	100%	99%	99%	100%
Pneumococcal Vaccine	73	66%	61%	69%	94%
Smoking Cessation Advice[1]	21	100%	77%	80%	100%
Surgical Infection Prevention					
Prophylactic Antibiotic Given	51	94%	74%	77%	95%
Prophylactic Antibiotic Selection[1]	10	100%	88%	90%	100%
Prophylactic Antibiotic Stopped	50	92%	70%	72%	95%
Pregnancy Care					
Inpatient Neonatal Mortality	-	-	-	-	-
Third or Fourth Degree Laceration	-	-	3.32%	3.63%	3.27%

Baptist Medical Center

2105 E S Boulevard
Montgomery, AL 36116
Ownership: Voluntary non-profit - Church
Emergency Services: Yes
Key Personnel:
President/CEO . . . . Victor D Butler
Chief Medical Staff . . . . Bill Boyel
Chief Catheterization Laboratory . . . . John Finklea, MD

Phone: 334-288-2100
Fax: 334-273-4204
Accredited: Yes
Licensed Beds: 454

Emergency Room . . . . John Moorehouse, MD
Director Medical/Surgical Nursing . . . . Peggy Bunson
OB/GYN Womens Health . . . . F Kim Whittington, MD
Chief Radiology . . . . William McGuffin
Director Respiratory Therapy . . . . Julie Hall

Measure	Cases	This Hospital	State Average	U.S. Average	Top Hospital
Heart Attack Care					
ACE Inhibitor or ARB for LVSD	64	78%	78%	82%	100%
Aspirin at Arrival	106	95%	87%	92%	100%
Aspirin at Discharge	220	98%	87%	90%	100%
Beta Blocker at Arrival	86	95%	81%	87%	100%
Beta Blocker at Discharge	251	97%	86%	90%	100%
Fibrinolytic Medication Timing[1]	1	0%	25%	31%	100%
PCI Within 90 Minutes of Arrival[1]	5	20%	61%	54%	95%
Smoking Cessation Advice	113	100%	85%	88%	100%
Heart Failure Care					
ACE Inhibitor or ARB for LVSD	145	80%	80%	82%	100%
Discharge Instructions	268	84%	54%	61%	93%
Evaluation of LVS Function	291	89%	79%	83%	99%
Smoking Cessation Advice	81	100%	78%	82%	100%
Pneumonia Care					
Appropriate Initial Antibiotic	73	73%	81%	83%	94%
Blood Culture Timing	81	84%	89%	90%	100%
Influenza Vaccine[1]	16	62%	62%	70%	100%
Initial Antibiotic Timing	116	70%	79%	80%	93%
Oxygenation Assessment	153	99%	99%	99%	100%
Pneumococcal Vaccine	72	68%	61%	69%	94%
Smoking Cessation Advice	50	100%	77%	80%	100%
Surgical Infection Prevention					
Prophylactic Antibiotic Given[3]	208	77%	74%	77%	95%
Prophylactic Antibiotic Selection	69	81%	88%	90%	100%
Prophylactic Antibiotic Stopped[3]	196	69%	70%	72%	95%
Pregnancy Care					
Inpatient Neonatal Mortality[2]	303	1.32%	-	-	-
Third or Fourth Degree Laceration[2]	158	0.63%	3.32%	3.63%	3.27%

Baptist Medical Center East

400 Taylor Road
Montgomery, AL 36117
URL: www.baptistfirst.org
Ownership: Voluntary non-profit - Private
Emergency Services: Yes
Key Personnel:
CEO . . . . Russ Tyner
Administrator . . . . Mindy Burdick
Chief of Medical Staff . . . . Kathy Lindsey
Director of Emergency Room . . . . Kemmy Farmer

Phone: 334-244-8500
Fax: 334-244-8300

Accredited: Yes
Licensed Beds: 150

Measure	Cases	This Hospital	State Average	U.S. Average	Top Hospital
Heart Attack Care					
ACE Inhibitor or ARB for LVSD[1]	3	67%	78%	82%	100%
Aspirin at Arrival	29	97%	87%	92%	100%
Aspirin at Discharge[1]	16	88%	87%	90%	100%
Beta Blocker at Arrival	32	100%	81%	87%	100%
Beta Blocker at Discharge[1]	21	95%	86%	90%	100%
Fibrinolytic Medication Timing	0	-	25%	31%	100%
PCI Within 90 Minutes of Arrival	0	-	61%	54%	95%
Smoking Cessation Advice[1]	5	100%	85%	88%	100%
Heart Failure Care					
ACE Inhibitor or ARB for LVSD	57	77%	80%	82%	100%
Discharge Instructions	186	58%	54%	61%	93%
Evaluation of LVS Function	200	92%	79%	83%	99%
Smoking Cessation Advice[1]	24	83%	78%	82%	100%
Pneumonia Care					
Appropriate Initial Antibiotic	106	81%	81%	83%	94%
Blood Culture Timing	80	81%	89%	90%	100%
Influenza Vaccine	27	74%	62%	70%	100%
Initial Antibiotic Timing	130	80%	79%	80%	93%
Oxygenation Assessment	162	99%	99%	99%	100%
Pneumococcal Vaccine	96	78%	61%	69%	94%

NOTE: Hospital profiles are in alphabetical order by state, then city, then hospital within the city; Rankings are sorted by rate in descending order and exclude hospitals with less than 25 cases; (1) The number of cases is too small (n<25) for purposes of reliably predicting hospital performance; (2) Measure reflects the hospital's indication that its submission was based upon a sample of its relevant discharges; (3) Rate reflects fewer than the maximum possible quarters of data for the measure; (4) Inaccurate information submitted and suppressed for one or more quarters; (5) No data is available from the hospital for this measure; Please refer to the User's Guide for a full explanation of data

Measure	Cases	This Hospital	State Average	U.S. Average	Top Hospital
Smoking Cessation Advice	32	94%	77%	80%	100%
Surgical Infection Prevention					
Prophylactic Antibiotic Given[3]	87	80%	74%	77%	95%
Prophylactic Antibiotic Selection	31	94%	88%	90%	100%
Prophylactic Antibiotic Stopped[3]	83	80%	70%	72%	95%
Pregnancy Care					
Inpatient Neonatal Mortality[2]	638	0.63%	-	-	-
Third or Fourth Degree Laceration	2,148	3.86%	3.32%	3.63%	3.27%

Jackson Hospital and Clinic

1725 Pine Street
Montgomery, AL 36106
URL: www.jackson.org
Ownership: Voluntary non-profit - Private
Emergency Services: Yes

Phone: 334-293-8000
Fax: 334-293-8972

Accredited: Yes
Licensed Beds: 281

Key Personnel:
President/CEO. . . . . Donald M Ball
President Medical Staff . . . . Patrick Ryan, MD
Catheterization Lab . . . . Teresa Bigbie
Infection Control. . . . . Janice Smith

Measure	Cases	This Hospital	State Average	U.S. Average	Top Hospital
Heart Attack Care					
ACE Inhibitor or ARB for LVSD[2]	52	62%	78%	82%	100%
Aspirin at Arrival[2]	173	86%	87%	92%	100%
Aspirin at Discharge[2]	235	92%	87%	90%	100%
Beta Blocker at Arrival[2]	124	76%	81%	87%	100%
Beta Blocker at Discharge[2]	239	87%	86%	90%	100%
Fibrinolytic Medication Timing[2]	0	-	25%	31%	100%
PCI Within 90 Minutes of Arrival[1,2]	9	33%	61%	54%	95%
Smoking Cessation Advice[2]	95	81%	85%	88%	100%
Heart Failure Care					
ACE Inhibitor or ARB for LVSD[2]	114	78%	80%	82%	100%
Discharge Instructions[2]	311	58%	54%	61%	93%
Evaluation of LVS Function[2]	353	85%	79%	83%	99%
Smoking Cessation Advice[2]	85	89%	78%	82%	100%
Pneumonia Care					
Appropriate Initial Antibiotic[2]	91	69%	81%	83%	94%
Blood Culture Timing[2]	89	87%	89%	90%	100%
Influenza Vaccine[2]	26	69%	62%	70%	100%
Initial Antibiotic Timing[2]	164	55%	79%	80%	93%
Oxygenation Assessment[2]	190	95%	99%	99%	100%
Pneumococcal Vaccine[2]	113	65%	61%	69%	94%
Smoking Cessation Advice[2]	40	90%	77%	80%	100%
Surgical Infection Prevention					
Prophylactic Antibiotic Given[2]	359	93%	74%	77%	95%
Prophylactic Antibiotic Selection[2]	103	94%	88%	90%	100%
Prophylactic Antibiotic Stopped[2]	357	84%	70%	72%	95%
Pregnancy Care					
Inpatient Neonatal Mortality[2]	-	-	-	-	-
Third or Fourth Degree Laceration	-	-	3.32%	3.63%	3.27%

Lawrence Medical Center

Alternate Name: Lawrence County Hospital
202 Hospital Street
Moulton, AL 35650
Ownership: Proprietary
Emergency Services: Yes

Phone: 256-974-2200
Fax: 256-974-2299
Accredited: Yes
Licensed Beds: 98

Key Personnel:
CEO. . . . . Thomas Dunning
Chief Medical Staff. . . . . Charles Coffey
ER Director . . . . Anita Lacy
Infection Control. . . . . Melody Farley
ICU Director. . . . . Anita Lacy
Intensive/Coronary Care . . . . Anita Lacy
Medical/Surgical Nursing . . . . Cynthia Pressley
Director Radiology. . . . . Dean White
Respiratory Coordinator. . . . . Debbie Moss

Measure	Cases	This Hospital	State Average	U.S. Average	Top Hospital
Heart Attack Care					
ACE Inhibitor or ARB for LVSD[1]	5	80%	78%	82%	100%
Aspirin at Arrival	37	89%	87%	92%	100%

Measure	Cases	This Hospital	State Average	U.S. Average	Top Hospital
Aspirin at Discharge	28	71%	87%	90%	100%
Beta Blocker at Arrival	34	71%	81%	87%	100%
Beta Blocker at Discharge	30	67%	86%	90%	100%
Fibrinolytic Medication Timing	0	-	25%	31%	100%
PCI Within 90 Minutes of Arrival	0	-	61%	54%	95%
Smoking Cessation Advice[1]	8	100%	85%	88%	100%
Heart Failure Care					
ACE Inhibitor or ARB for LVSD[1]	11	91%	80%	82%	100%
Discharge Instructions	42	98%	54%	61%	93%
Evaluation of LVS Function	45	76%	79%	83%	99%
Smoking Cessation Advice[1]	9	89%	78%	82%	100%
Pneumonia Care					
Appropriate Initial Antibiotic	106	83%	81%	83%	94%
Blood Culture Timing	39	85%	89%	90%	100%
Influenza Vaccine	27	78%	62%	70%	100%
Initial Antibiotic Timing	91	89%	79%	80%	93%
Oxygenation Assessment	127	100%	99%	99%	100%
Pneumococcal Vaccine	48	54%	61%	69%	94%
Smoking Cessation Advice	43	98%	77%	80%	100%
Surgical Infection Prevention					
Prophylactic Antibiotic Given[5]	-	-	74%	77%	95%
Prophylactic Antibiotic Selection[5]	-	-	88%	90%	100%
Prophylactic Antibiotic Stopped[5]	-	-	70%	72%	95%
Pregnancy Care					
Inpatient Neonatal Mortality	-	-	-	-	-
Third or Fourth Degree Laceration	-	-	3.32%	3.63%	3.27%

Shoals Hospital

Alternate Name: Medical Center Shoals
201 Avalon Avenue
PO Box 3359
Muscle Shoals, AL 35662
URL: www.chgroup.org
Ownership: Govt - Hospital District or Authority
Emergency Services: Yes

Phone: 256-386-1600
Fax: 256-386-1115

Accredited: Yes
Licensed Beds: 144

Key Personnel:
Administrator . . . . Jody Pigg
Chief Medical Staff. . . . . Dr. Brad McAnalley
Catheterization Lab . . . . Ricky Williams
Emergency Room . . . . Sheila Felton

Measure	Cases	This Hospital	State Average	U.S. Average	Top Hospital
Heart Attack Care					
ACE Inhibitor or ARB for LVSD[1]	1	100%	78%	82%	100%
Aspirin at Arrival[1]	12	83%	87%	92%	100%
Aspirin at Discharge[1]	3	100%	87%	90%	100%
Beta Blocker at Arrival[1]	13	100%	81%	87%	100%
Beta Blocker at Discharge[1]	4	100%	86%	90%	100%
Fibrinolytic Medication Timing[1]	1	0%	25%	31%	100%
PCI Within 90 Minutes of Arrival	0	-	61%	54%	95%
Smoking Cessation Advice[1]	2	50%	85%	88%	100%
Heart Failure Care					
ACE Inhibitor or ARB for LVSD[1]	14	86%	80%	82%	100%
Discharge Instructions	59	81%	54%	61%	93%
Evaluation of LVS Function	68	96%	79%	83%	99%
Smoking Cessation Advice[1]	9	78%	78%	82%	100%
Pneumonia Care					
Appropriate Initial Antibiotic	88	81%	81%	83%	94%
Blood Culture Timing	57	96%	89%	90%	100%
Influenza Vaccine[4,5]	-	-	62%	70%	100%
Initial Antibiotic Timing	98	78%	79%	80%	93%
Oxygenation Assessment	115	97%	99%	99%	100%
Pneumococcal Vaccine	77	77%	61%	69%	94%
Smoking Cessation Advice[1]	16	62%	77%	80%	100%
Surgical Infection Prevention					
Prophylactic Antibiotic Given	44	91%	74%	77%	95%
Prophylactic Antibiotic Selection[1]	8	100%	88%	90%	100%
Prophylactic Antibiotic Stopped	43	77%	70%	72%	95%
Pregnancy Care					
Inpatient Neonatal Mortality	-	-	-	-	-
Third or Fourth Degree Laceration	-	-	3.32%	3.63%	3.27%

NOTE: Hospital profiles are in alphabetical order by state, then city, then hospital within the city; Rankings are sorted by rate in descending order and exclude hospitals with less than 25 cases; (1) The number of cases is too small (n<25) for purposes of reliably predicting hospital performance; (2) Measure reflects the hospital's indication that its submission was based upon a sample of its relevant discharges; (3) Rate reflects fewer than the maximum possible quarters of data for the measure; (4) Inaccurate information submitted and suppressed for one or more quarters; (5) No data is available from the hospital for this measure; Please refer to the User's Guide for a full explanation of data

Northport Medical Center

Alternate Name: Northport Hospital-DCH
2700 Hospital Drive
Northport, AL 35476   Phone: 205-333-4500
                          Fax: 205-333-4588
URL: www.dchsystem.com
Ownership: Govt - Hospital District or Authority   Accredited: Yes
Emergency Services: Yes   Licensed Beds: 204
Key Personnel:
President/CEO . . . . Charles L Stewart
Chief Medical Staff . . . . Dr. Jerry Palmer
Emergency Room . . . . Janice Neill
Emergency Room . . . . Rhonda Turnipseed
Infection Control . . . . Ellen Cockrell
ICU . . . . Rhonda Turnnepseed, RN
CCU Spvg. Nurse . . . . Rhonda Turnipseed, RN
Medical/Surgical Nursing . . . . Barbara Lesson
OB/GYN Womens Health. . . . . Carolyn Hawkins
Manager Respiratory Therapy . . . . Paul Abel

Measure	Cases	This Hospital	State Average	U.S. Average	Top Hospital
Heart Attack Care					
ACE Inhibitor or ARB for LVSD[1]	1	100%	78%	82%	100%
Aspirin at Arrival[1]	5	100%	87%	92%	100%
Aspirin at Discharge[1]	3	100%	87%	90%	100%
Beta Blocker at Arrival[1]	6	100%	81%	87%	100%
Beta Blocker at Discharge[1]	5	100%	86%	90%	100%
Fibrinolytic Medication Timing	0	-	25%	31%	100%
PCI Within 90 Minutes of Arrival	0	-	61%	54%	95%
Smoking Cessation Advice[1]	1	100%	85%	88%	100%
Heart Failure Care					
ACE Inhibitor or ARB for LVSD	28	75%	80%	82%	100%
Discharge Instructions	70	89%	54%	61%	93%
Evaluation of LVS Function	79	78%	79%	83%	99%
Smoking Cessation Advice[1]	11	100%	78%	82%	100%
Pneumonia Care					
Appropriate Initial Antibiotic	68	90%	81%	83%	94%
Blood Culture Timing	62	90%	89%	90%	100%
Influenza Vaccine[4,5]	-	-	62%	70%	100%
Initial Antibiotic Timing	100	75%	79%	80%	93%
Oxygenation Assessment	123	99%	99%	99%	100%
Pneumococcal Vaccine	54	52%	61%	69%	94%
Smoking Cessation Advice	42	88%	77%	80%	100%
Surgical Infection Prevention					
Prophylactic Antibiotic Given	468	94%	74%	77%	95%
Prophylactic Antibiotic Selection	110	96%	88%	90%	100%
Prophylactic Antibiotic Stopped	445	85%	70%	72%	95%
Pregnancy Care					
Inpatient Neonatal Mortality	-	-	-	-	-
Third or Fourth Degree Laceration	-	-	3.32%	3.63%	3.27%

Medical Center Blount

Alternate Name: Blount Memorial Hospital
150 Gilbreath Drive
Oneonta, AL 35121   Phone: 205-274-3000
                          Fax: 205-274-3056
E-mail: smbusenlehner@ehs-inc.com
URL: www.medicalcenterblount.com
Ownership: Voluntary non-profit - Private   Accredited: No
Emergency Services: Yes   Licensed Beds: 101
Key Personnel:
CEO . . . . Jacki Jennings
Chief Medical Staff . . . . John Smith, MD
Emergency Room . . . . Stephen Avram, MD
Chief Radiology . . . . Constantine Morros, MD
Director Respiratory Therapy . . . . Jim Doty

Measure	Cases	This Hospital	State Average	U.S. Average	Top Hospital
Heart Attack Care					
ACE Inhibitor or ARB for LVSD[1]	1	0%	78%	82%	100%
Aspirin at Arrival[1]	7	86%	87%	92%	100%
Aspirin at Discharge[1]	5	80%	87%	90%	100%
Beta Blocker at Arrival[1]	7	100%	81%	87%	100%
Beta Blocker at Discharge[1]	5	100%	86%	90%	100%
Fibrinolytic Medication Timing[1]	2	0%	25%	31%	100%

Measure	Cases	This Hospital	State Average	U.S. Average	Top Hospital
PCI Within 90 Minutes of Arrival	0	-	61%	54%	95%
Smoking Cessation Advice[1]	1	0%	85%	88%	100%
Heart Failure Care					
ACE Inhibitor or ARB for LVSD[1]	17	76%	80%	82%	100%
Discharge Instructions	40	35%	54%	61%	93%
Evaluation of LVS Function	66	85%	79%	83%	99%
Smoking Cessation Advice[1]	14	71%	78%	82%	100%
Pneumonia Care					
Appropriate Initial Antibiotic	79	78%	81%	83%	94%
Blood Culture Timing	58	83%	89%	90%	100%
Influenza Vaccine[1]	19	47%	62%	70%	100%
Initial Antibiotic Timing	121	88%	79%	80%	93%
Oxygenation Assessment	134	99%	99%	99%	100%
Pneumococcal Vaccine	76	58%	61%	69%	94%
Smoking Cessation Advice	28	68%	77%	80%	100%
Surgical Infection Prevention					
Prophylactic Antibiotic Given[1]	8	62%	74%	77%	95%
Prophylactic Antibiotic Selection[1]	1	100%	88%	90%	100%
Prophylactic Antibiotic Stopped[1]	7	100%	70%	72%	95%
Pregnancy Care					
Inpatient Neonatal Mortality	-	-	-	-	-
Third or Fourth Degree Laceration	-	-	3.32%	3.63%	3.27%

East Alabama Medical Center

2000 Pepperell Parkway
Opelika, AL 36801   Phone: 334-749-3411
                          Fax: 334-528-1764
URL: www.eamc.org
Ownership: Govt - Hospital District or Authority   Accredited: Yes
Emergency Services: Yes   Licensed Beds: 348
Key Personnel:
CEO . . . . Terry Andrus
Chief Medical Staff . . . . Michael Gunter, MD
Emergency Room . . . . Melissa Rogers, RN
Director Medical/Surgical Nursing . . . . Lexie Butler, RN
OB/GYN Womens Health. . . . . Steven Litsey, MD
Chief Radiology . . . . David Montiel, MD
Director Respiratory Therapy . . . . Nancy Strickland

Measure	Cases	This Hospital	State Average	U.S. Average	Top Hospital
Heart Attack Care					
ACE Inhibitor or ARB for LVSD	80	91%	78%	82%	100%
Aspirin at Arrival	233	97%	87%	92%	100%
Aspirin at Discharge	310	96%	87%	90%	100%
Beta Blocker at Arrival	156	90%	81%	87%	100%
Beta Blocker at Discharge	305	97%	86%	90%	100%
Fibrinolytic Medication Timing	0	-	25%	31%	100%
PCI Within 90 Minutes of Arrival[1]	8	75%	61%	54%	95%
Smoking Cessation Advice	144	99%	85%	88%	100%
Heart Failure Care					
ACE Inhibitor or ARB for LVSD	304	97%	80%	82%	100%
Discharge Instructions	583	79%	54%	61%	93%
Evaluation of LVS Function	648	99%	79%	83%	99%
Smoking Cessation Advice	143	100%	78%	82%	100%
Pneumonia Care					
Appropriate Initial Antibiotic	108	91%	81%	83%	94%
Blood Culture Timing	74	82%	89%	90%	100%
Influenza Vaccine	27	96%	62%	70%	100%
Initial Antibiotic Timing	148	83%	79%	80%	93%
Oxygenation Assessment	178	99%	99%	99%	100%
Pneumococcal Vaccine	96	94%	61%	69%	94%
Smoking Cessation Advice	51	100%	77%	80%	100%
Surgical Infection Prevention					
Prophylactic Antibiotic Given	1,021	96%	74%	77%	95%
Prophylactic Antibiotic Selection	253	97%	88%	90%	100%
Prophylactic Antibiotic Stopped	961	91%	70%	72%	95%
Pregnancy Care					
Inpatient Neonatal Mortality	1,658	0.12%	-	-	-
Third or Fourth Degree Laceration	1,140	2.02%	3.32%	3.63%	3.27%

NOTE: Hospital profiles are in alphabetical order by state, then city, then hospital within the city; Rankings are sorted by rate in descending order and exclude hospitals with less than 25 cases; (1) The number of cases is too small (n<25) for purposes of reliably predicting hospital performance; (2) Measure reflects the hospital's indication that its submission was based upon a sample of its relevant discharges; (3) Rate reflects fewer than the maximum possible quarters of data for the measure; (4) Inaccurate information submitted and suppressed for one or more quarters; (5) No data is available from the hospital for this measure; Please refer to the User's Guide for a full explanation of data

Mizell Memorial Hospital

702 Main Street
Opp, AL 36467
E-mail: rlemaire@mizellmh.com
URL: www.mizellmh.com
Ownership: Voluntary non-profit - Private
Emergency Services: Yes

Phone: 334-493-3541
Fax: 334-493-9664

Accredited: No
Licensed Beds: 99

Key Personnel:

CEO . . . . Allen Foster
ER Director . . . . Dr Steve Davis
ICU . . . . Patricia Hill, CRNP
Medical/Surgical Nursing . . . . Patricia Hill, CRNP
Surgical Services Director . . . . Fay Bedsole
Director Respiratory Therapy . . . . James Anderson

Measure	Cases	This Hospital	State Average	U.S. Average	Top Hospital
Heart Attack Care					
ACE Inhibitor or ARB for LVSD[1,3]	1	100%	78%	82%	100%
Aspirin at Arrival[1,3]	5	100%	87%	92%	100%
Aspirin at Discharge[1,3]	4	100%	87%	90%	100%
Beta Blocker at Arrival[1,3]	8	100%	81%	87%	100%
Beta Blocker at Discharge[1,3]	6	100%	86%	90%	100%
Fibrinolytic Medication Timing[1,3]	2	50%	25%	31%	100%
PCI Within 90 Minutes of Arrival[5]	-	-	61%	54%	95%
Smoking Cessation Advice[1,3]	1	100%	85%	88%	100%
Heart Failure Care					
ACE Inhibitor or ARB for LVSD[2]	29	100%	80%	82%	100%
Discharge Instructions[2]	77	19%	54%	61%	93%
Evaluation of LVS Function[2]	92	88%	79%	83%	99%
Smoking Cessation Advice[1,2]	12	83%	78%	82%	100%
Pneumonia Care					
Appropriate Initial Antibiotic	87	74%	81%	83%	94%
Blood Culture Timing	33	82%	89%	90%	100%
Influenza Vaccine[1]	15	7%	62%	70%	100%
Initial Antibiotic Timing	85	58%	79%	80%	93%
Oxygenation Assessment	128	95%	99%	99%	100%
Pneumococcal Vaccine	80	75%	61%	69%	94%
Smoking Cessation Advice[1]	24	83%	77%	80%	100%
Surgical Infection Prevention					
Prophylactic Antibiotic Given[1]	11	73%	74%	77%	95%
Prophylactic Antibiotic Selection[1]	5	80%	88%	90%	100%
Prophylactic Antibiotic Stopped[1]	10	90%	70%	72%	95%
Pregnancy Care					
Inpatient Neonatal Mortality	-	-	-	-	-
Third or Fourth Degree Laceration	-	-	3.32%	3.63%	3.27%

Dale Medical Center

Alternate Name: Dale County Hospital
126 Hospital Avenue
Ozark, AL 36360
URL: www.dalemedical.org
Ownership: Govt - Hospital District or Authority
Emergency Services: No

Phone: 334-774-2601
Fax: 334-774-0258

Accredited: No
Licensed Beds: 89

Key Personnel:

CEO . . . . Vernon Johnson
Emergency Room . . . . Lisa Sanders
Infection Control . . . . Jan Hamm

Measure	Cases	This Hospital	State Average	U.S. Average	Top Hospital
Heart Attack Care					
ACE Inhibitor or ARB for LVSD[1]	1	0%	78%	82%	100%
Aspirin at Arrival[1]	19	84%	87%	92%	100%
Aspirin at Discharge[1]	5	80%	87%	90%	100%
Beta Blocker at Arrival[1]	14	79%	81%	87%	100%
Beta Blocker at Discharge[1]	6	67%	86%	90%	100%
Fibrinolytic Medication Timing[1]	1	100%	25%	31%	100%
PCI Within 90 Minutes of Arrival	0	-	61%	54%	95%
Smoking Cessation Advice[1]	1	100%	85%	88%	100%
Heart Failure Care					
ACE Inhibitor or ARB for LVSD[1]	9	89%	80%	82%	100%
Discharge Instructions	56	21%	54%	61%	93%
Evaluation of LVS Function	63	86%	79%	83%	99%
Smoking Cessation Advice[1]	16	69%	78%	82%	100%

Measure	Cases	This Hospital	State Average	U.S. Average	Top Hospital
Pneumonia Care					
Appropriate Initial Antibiotic	74	61%	81%	83%	94%
Blood Culture Timing	53	85%	89%	90%	100%
Influenza Vaccine[1]	8	100%	62%	70%	100%
Initial Antibiotic Timing	80	84%	79%	80%	93%
Oxygenation Assessment	106	100%	99%	99%	100%
Pneumococcal Vaccine	57	44%	61%	69%	94%
Smoking Cessation Advice	32	78%	77%	80%	100%
Surgical Infection Prevention					
Prophylactic Antibiotic Given[1,3]	11	27%	74%	77%	95%
Prophylactic Antibiotic Selection[1]	8	100%	88%	90%	100%
Prophylactic Antibiotic Stopped[1,3]	11	73%	70%	72%	95%
Pregnancy Care					
Inpatient Neonatal Mortality	-	-	-	-	-
Third or Fourth Degree Laceration	-	-	3.32%	3.63%	3.27%

Saint Clair Regional Hospital

2805 Hospital Drive
Pell City, AL 35125
URL: www.stclairregional.com
Ownership: Government - Local
Emergency Services: Yes

Phone: 205-338-3301
Fax: 205-814-2145

Accredited: No
Licensed Beds: 82

Key Personnel:

CEO . . . . Douglas H Beverly
Director Medical/Surgical Nursing . . . . Elaine Staples, RN
OB/GYN Womens Health . . . . A Williamson Huff, MD
Chief Radiology . . . . Darrell Lovell
Director Respiratory Therapy . . . . Gloria Layton

Measure	Cases	This Hospital	State Average	U.S. Average	Top Hospital
Heart Attack Care					
ACE Inhibitor or ARB for LVSD	0	-	78%	82%	100%
Aspirin at Arrival[1]	7	86%	87%	92%	100%
Aspirin at Discharge[1]	3	67%	87%	90%	100%
Beta Blocker at Arrival[1]	7	43%	81%	87%	100%
Beta Blocker at Discharge[1]	3	33%	86%	90%	100%
Fibrinolytic Medication Timing[1]	3	33%	25%	31%	100%
PCI Within 90 Minutes of Arrival	0	-	61%	54%	95%
Smoking Cessation Advice[1]	1	100%	85%	88%	100%
Heart Failure Care					
ACE Inhibitor or ARB for LVSD	28	61%	80%	82%	100%
Discharge Instructions	89	69%	54%	61%	93%
Evaluation of LVS Function	98	70%	79%	83%	99%
Smoking Cessation Advice[1]	23	35%	78%	82%	100%
Pneumonia Care					
Appropriate Initial Antibiotic[2]	130	78%	81%	83%	94%
Blood Culture Timing[2]	50	88%	89%	90%	100%
Influenza Vaccine[1]	24	79%	62%	70%	100%
Initial Antibiotic Timing[2]	116	82%	79%	80%	93%
Oxygenation Assessment[2]	146	99%	99%	99%	100%
Pneumococcal Vaccine[2]	72	58%	61%	69%	94%
Smoking Cessation Advice[2]	38	47%	77%	80%	100%
Surgical Infection Prevention					
Prophylactic Antibiotic Given[1,3]	1	0%	74%	77%	95%
Prophylactic Antibiotic Selection[1]	1	100%	88%	90%	100%
Prophylactic Antibiotic Stopped[1,3]	1	100%	70%	72%	95%
Pregnancy Care					
Inpatient Neonatal Mortality	-	-	-	-	-
Third or Fourth Degree Laceration	-	-	3.32%	3.63%	3.27%

Summit Hospital

4401 River Chase Drive
Phenix City, AL 36867
Ownership: Government - State
Emergency Services: Yes

Phone: 334-732-3456

Accredited: Yes

Measure	Cases	This Hospital	State Average	U.S. Average	Top Hospital
Heart Attack Care					
ACE Inhibitor or ARB for LVSD[3]	0	-	78%	82%	100%
Aspirin at Arrival[1,3]	2	50%	87%	92%	100%
Aspirin at Discharge[1,3]	1	100%	87%	90%	100%
Beta Blocker at Arrival[1,3]	2	100%	81%	87%	100%

NOTE: Hospital profiles are in alphabetical order by state, then city, then hospital within the city; Rankings are sorted by rate in descending order and exclude hospitals with less than 25 cases; (1) The number of cases is too small (n<25) for purposes of reliably predicting hospital performance; (2) Measure reflects the hospital's indication that its submission was based upon a sample of its relevant discharges; (3) Rate reflects fewer than the maximum possible quarters of data for the measure; (4) Inaccurate information submitted and suppressed for one or more quarters; (5) No data is available from the hospital for this measure; Please refer to the User's Guide for a full explanation of data

Beta Blocker at Discharge[1,3]	1	0%	86%	90%	100%
Fibrinolytic Medication Timing[3]	0	-	25%	31%	100%
PCI Within 90 Minutes of Arrival	0	-	61%	54%	95%
Smoking Cessation Advice[3]	0	-	85%	88%	100%
Heart Failure Care					
ACE Inhibitor or ARB for LVSD[1,3]	2	100%	80%	82%	100%
Discharge Instructions[1,3]	5	0%	54%	61%	93%
Evaluation of LVS Function[1,3]	5	60%	79%	83%	99%
Smoking Cessation Advice[3]	0	-	78%	82%	100%
Pneumonia Care					
Appropriate Initial Antibiotic[1,3]	2	100%	81%	83%	94%
Blood Culture Timing[1,3]	1	100%	89%	90%	100%
Influenza Vaccine[5]	-	-	62%	70%	100%
Initial Antibiotic Timing[1,3]	3	67%	79%	80%	93%
Oxygenation Assessment[1,3]	3	100%	99%	99%	100%
Pneumococcal Vaccine[1,3]	1	0%	61%	69%	94%
Smoking Cessation Advice[1,3]	2	50%	77%	80%	100%
Surgical Infection Prevention					
Prophylactic Antibiotic Given[1,3]	1	100%	74%	77%	95%
Prophylactic Antibiotic Selection[1]	1	100%	88%	90%	100%
Prophylactic Antibiotic Stopped[1,3]	1	100%	70%	72%	95%
Pregnancy Care					
Inpatient Neonatal Mortality	-	-	-	-	-
Third or Fourth Degree Laceration	-	-	3.32%	3.63%	3.27%

Prattville Baptist Hospital

Alternate Name: Northridge Medical Center
124 South Memorial Drive
Prattville, AL 36067
URL: www.baptistfirst.org/facilities/prattville.htm
Ownership: Voluntary non-profit - Private
Emergency Services: Yes

Phone: 334-365-0651
Fax: 334-361-3131

Accredited: Yes
Licensed Beds: 85

Key Personnel:
Administrator . . . . Ginger Irsik
Chief of Medical Staff . . . . Ed Foxhall
Emergency Room . . . . Danny Perry
Medical/Surgical Nursing . . . . Lisa Hudson, RN
Respiratory/Cardiopulmonary . . . . Kim Quinney

Measure	Cases	This Hospital	State Average	U.S. Average	Top Hospital
Heart Attack Care					
ACE Inhibitor or ARB for LVSD[1]	2	50%	78%	82%	100%
Aspirin at Arrival[1]	17	82%	87%	92%	100%
Aspirin at Discharge[1]	5	80%	87%	90%	100%
Beta Blocker at Arrival[1]	15	87%	81%	87%	100%
Beta Blocker at Discharge[1]	6	83%	86%	90%	100%
Fibrinolytic Medication Timing	0	-	25%	31%	100%
PCI Within 90 Minutes of Arrival	0	-	61%	54%	95%
Smoking Cessation Advice[1]	1	100%	85%	88%	100%
Heart Failure Care					
ACE Inhibitor or ARB for LVSD	33	91%	80%	82%	100%
Discharge Instructions	88	81%	54%	61%	93%
Evaluation of LVS Function	104	95%	79%	83%	99%
Smoking Cessation Advice	29	100%	78%	82%	100%
Pneumonia Care					
Appropriate Initial Antibiotic	120	78%	81%	83%	94%
Blood Culture Timing	122	96%	89%	90%	100%
Influenza Vaccine	29	90%	62%	70%	100%
Initial Antibiotic Timing	145	88%	79%	80%	93%
Oxygenation Assessment	177	99%	99%	99%	100%
Pneumococcal Vaccine	93	89%	61%	69%	94%
Smoking Cessation Advice	49	100%	77%	80%	100%
Surgical Infection Prevention					
Prophylactic Antibiotic Given[1,3]	13	85%	74%	77%	95%
Prophylactic Antibiotic Selection[1]	7	71%	88%	90%	100%
Prophylactic Antibiotic Stopped[1,3]	15	80%	70%	72%	95%
Pregnancy Care					
Inpatient Neonatal Mortality	-	-	-	-	-
Third or Fourth Degree Laceration	-	-	3.32%	3.63%	3.27%

Red Bay Hospital

211 Hospital Road
Red Bay, AL 35582
URL: www.redbayhospital.com
Ownership: Voluntary non-profit - Other
Emergency Services: Yes

Phone: 256-356-9532
Fax: 256-356-2809

Accredited: Yes
Licensed Beds: 33

Key Personnel:
Director Infection/Disease Control . . . . K Paten

Measure	Cases	This Hospital	State Average	U.S. Average	Top Hospital
Heart Attack Care					
ACE Inhibitor or ARB for LVSD[5]	-	-	78%	82%	100%
Aspirin at Arrival[5]	-	-	87%	92%	100%
Aspirin at Discharge[5]	-	-	87%	90%	100%
Beta Blocker at Arrival[5]	-	-	81%	87%	100%
Beta Blocker at Discharge[5]	-	-	86%	90%	100%
Fibrinolytic Medication Timing[5]	-	-	25%	31%	100%
PCI Within 90 Minutes of Arrival[5]	-	-	61%	54%	95%
Smoking Cessation Advice[5]	-	-	85%	88%	100%
Heart Failure Care					
ACE Inhibitor or ARB for LVSD[3]	0	-	80%	82%	100%
Discharge Instructions[1,3]	3	0%	54%	61%	93%
Evaluation of LVS Function[1,3]	5	20%	79%	83%	99%
Smoking Cessation Advice[1,3]	1	0%	78%	82%	100%
Pneumonia Care					
Appropriate Initial Antibiotic[1,3]	3	67%	81%	83%	94%
Blood Culture Timing[1,3]	1	100%	89%	90%	100%
Influenza Vaccine[5]	-	-	62%	70%	100%
Initial Antibiotic Timing[1,3]	3	67%	79%	80%	93%
Oxygenation Assessment[1,3]	5	60%	99%	99%	100%
Pneumococcal Vaccine[1,3]	3	67%	61%	69%	94%
Smoking Cessation Advice[1,3]	1	0%	77%	80%	100%
Surgical Infection Prevention					
Prophylactic Antibiotic Given[5]	-	-	74%	77%	95%
Prophylactic Antibiotic Selection[5]	-	-	88%	90%	100%
Prophylactic Antibiotic Stopped[5]	-	-	70%	72%	95%
Pregnancy Care					
Inpatient Neonatal Mortality	-	-	-	-	-
Third or Fourth Degree Laceration	-	-	3.32%	3.63%	3.27%

Randolph Health Systems Medical Center

59928 Highway 22
PO Box 670
Roanoke, AL 36274
URL: www.randolphmedicalcenter.org
Ownership: Govt - Hospital District or Authority
Emergency Services: Yes

Phone: 334-863-4111
Fax: 334-863-8663

Accredited: No
Licensed Beds: 40

Key Personnel:
President . . . . Gil McKenzie
CEO . . . . Tim Harlin
Emergency Room . . . . Van Wheeles, RN
Infection Control . . . . Frnaces Williamson, RN
Director Radiology . . . . Kay Turner
Respiratory Care . . . . Linda Ross

Measure	Cases	This Hospital	State Average	U.S. Average	Top Hospital
Heart Attack Care					
ACE Inhibitor or ARB for LVSD[3]	0	-	78%	82%	100%
Aspirin at Arrival[1,3]	2	100%	87%	92%	100%
Aspirin at Discharge[3]	0	-	87%	90%	100%
Beta Blocker at Arrival[3]	0	-	81%	87%	100%
Beta Blocker at Discharge[3]	0	-	86%	90%	100%
Fibrinolytic Medication Timing[3]	0	-	25%	31%	100%
PCI Within 90 Minutes of Arrival[5]	-	-	61%	54%	95%
Smoking Cessation Advice[3]	0	-	85%	88%	100%
Heart Failure Care					
ACE Inhibitor or ARB for LVSD	26	81%	80%	82%	100%
Discharge Instructions	37	8%	54%	61%	93%
Evaluation of LVS Function	55	87%	79%	83%	99%
Smoking Cessation Advice[1]	8	25%	78%	82%	100%
Pneumonia Care					
Appropriate Initial Antibiotic[1]	17	100%	81%	83%	94%
Blood Culture Timing[1]	10	80%	89%	90%	100%

NOTE: Hospital profiles are in alphabetical order by state, then city, then hospital within the city; Rankings are sorted by rate in descending order and exclude hospitals with less than 25 cases; (1) The number of cases is too small (n<25) for purposes of reliably predicting hospital performance; (2) Measure reflects the hospital's indication that its submission was based upon a sample of its relevant discharges; (3) Rate reflects fewer than the maximum possible quarters of data for the measure; (4) Inaccurate information submitted and suppressed for one or more quarters; (5) No data is available from the hospital for this measure; Please refer to the User's Guide for a full explanation of data

Influenza Vaccine[1]	4	0%	62%	70%	100%
Initial Antibiotic Timing[1]	21	67%	79%	80%	93%
Oxygenation Assessment	29	100%	99%	99%	100%
Pneumococcal Vaccine[1]	15	7%	61%	69%	94%
Smoking Cessation Advice[1]	7	14%	77%	80%	100%
Surgical Infection Prevention					
Prophylactic Antibiotic Given[5]	-	-	74%	77%	95%
Prophylactic Antibiotic Selection[5]	-	-	88%	90%	100%
Prophylactic Antibiotic Stopped[5]	-	-	70%	72%	95%
Pregnancy Care					
Inpatient Neonatal Mortality	-	-	-	-	-
Third or Fourth Degree Laceration	-	-	3.32%	3.63%	3.27%

Russellville Hospital

15155 Highway 43
Russellville, AL 35653
Ownership: Proprietary
Emergency Services: Yes

Phone: 256-331-3889
Fax: 256-331-3897
Accredited: Yes

Measure	Cases	This Hospital	State Average	U.S. Average	Top Hospital
Heart Attack Care					
ACE Inhibitor or ARB for LVSD[1]	1	100%	78%	82%	100%
Aspirin at Arrival[1]	21	100%	87%	92%	100%
Aspirin at Discharge[1]	14	86%	87%	90%	100%
Beta Blocker at Arrival[1]	17	88%	81%	87%	100%
Beta Blocker at Discharge[1]	14	93%	86%	90%	100%
Fibrinolytic Medication Timing	0	-	25%	31%	100%
PCI Within 90 Minutes of Arrival	0	-	61%	54%	95%
Smoking Cessation Advice[1]	1	100%	85%	88%	100%
Heart Failure Care					
ACE Inhibitor or ARB for LVSD[1]	19	89%	80%	82%	100%
Discharge Instructions	65	97%	54%	61%	93%
Evaluation of LVS Function	80	95%	79%	83%	99%
Smoking Cessation Advice[1]	16	94%	78%	82%	100%
Pneumonia Care					
Appropriate Initial Antibiotic	109	83%	81%	83%	94%
Blood Culture Timing	76	80%	89%	90%	100%
Influenza Vaccine[1]	23	65%	62%	70%	100%
Initial Antibiotic Timing	143	87%	79%	80%	93%
Oxygenation Assessment	176	98%	99%	99%	100%
Pneumococcal Vaccine	93	81%	61%	69%	94%
Smoking Cessation Advice	54	98%	77%	80%	100%
Surgical Infection Prevention					
Prophylactic Antibiotic Given[2,3]	86	86%	74%	77%	95%
Prophylactic Antibiotic Selection[1,2]	24	83%	88%	90%	100%
Prophylactic Antibiotic Stopped[2,3]	85	69%	70%	72%	95%
Pregnancy Care					
Inpatient Neonatal Mortality	-	-	-	-	-
Third or Fourth Degree Laceration	-	-	3.32%	3.63%	3.27%

Highlands Medical Center

380 Woods Cove Road
Scottsboro, AL 35768
URL: www.highlandsmedcenter.com
Ownership: Govt - Hospital District or Authority   Accredited: Yes
Emergency Services: Yes
Key Personnel:
CEO. . . . . Thomas O'Lackey

Phone: 256-259-4444
Fax: 256-218-3656

Measure	Cases	This Hospital	State Average	U.S. Average	Top Hospital
Heart Attack Care					
ACE Inhibitor or ARB for LVSD[1]	2	50%	78%	82%	100%
Aspirin at Arrival[1]	19	68%	87%	92%	100%
Aspirin at Discharge[1]	15	60%	87%	90%	100%
Beta Blocker at Arrival[1]	21	52%	81%	87%	100%
Beta Blocker at Discharge[1]	15	53%	86%	90%	100%
Fibrinolytic Medication Timing[1]	1	0%	25%	31%	100%
PCI Within 90 Minutes of Arrival	0	-	61%	54%	95%
Smoking Cessation Advice[1]	3	67%	85%	88%	100%
Heart Failure Care					
ACE Inhibitor or ARB for LVSD[1]	19	63%	80%	82%	100%
Discharge Instructions	125	50%	54%	61%	93%

Evaluation of LVS Function	157	48%	79%	83%	99%
Smoking Cessation Advice	34	85%	78%	82%	100%
Pneumonia Care					
Appropriate Initial Antibiotic	193	84%	81%	83%	94%
Blood Culture Timing	92	90%	89%	90%	100%
Influenza Vaccine	38	50%	62%	70%	100%
Initial Antibiotic Timing	232	82%	79%	80%	93%
Oxygenation Assessment	272	100%	99%	99%	100%
Pneumococcal Vaccine	156	56%	61%	69%	94%
Smoking Cessation Advice	61	95%	77%	80%	100%
Surgical Infection Prevention					
Prophylactic Antibiotic Given[3]	73	1%	74%	77%	95%
Prophylactic Antibiotic Selection[1]	23	91%	88%	90%	100%
Prophylactic Antibiotic Stopped[3]	72	88%	70%	72%	95%
Pregnancy Care					
Inpatient Neonatal Mortality	-	-	-	-	-
Third or Fourth Degree Laceration	-	-	3.32%	3.63%	3.27%

Vaughan Regional Med Ctr-Parkway Campus

1015 Medical Center Parkway
Selma, AL 36701
Ownership: Proprietary
Emergency Services: Yes

Phone: 334-418-4100

Accredited: Yes

Measure	Cases	This Hospital	State Average	U.S. Average	Top Hospital
Heart Attack Care					
ACE Inhibitor or ARB for LVSD	27	74%	78%	82%	100%
Aspirin at Arrival	97	84%	87%	92%	100%
Aspirin at Discharge	56	93%	87%	90%	100%
Beta Blocker at Arrival	87	86%	81%	87%	100%
Beta Blocker at Discharge	59	90%	86%	90%	100%
Fibrinolytic Medication Timing[1]	7	43%	25%	31%	100%
PCI Within 90 Minutes of Arrival	0	-	61%	54%	95%
Smoking Cessation Advice[1]	8	100%	85%	88%	100%
Heart Failure Care					
ACE Inhibitor or ARB for LVSD	192	80%	80%	82%	100%
Discharge Instructions	364	31%	54%	61%	93%
Evaluation of LVS Function	412	87%	79%	83%	99%
Smoking Cessation Advice	75	89%	78%	82%	100%
Pneumonia Care					
Appropriate Initial Antibiotic	117	70%	81%	83%	94%
Blood Culture Timing	68	87%	89%	90%	100%
Influenza Vaccine[1]	23	48%	62%	70%	100%
Initial Antibiotic Timing	139	60%	79%	80%	93%
Oxygenation Assessment	164	100%	99%	99%	100%
Pneumococcal Vaccine	89	53%	61%	69%	94%
Smoking Cessation Advice	29	90%	77%	80%	100%
Surgical Infection Prevention					
Prophylactic Antibiotic Given[3]	157	28%	74%	77%	95%
Prophylactic Antibiotic Selection	40	68%	88%	90%	100%
Prophylactic Antibiotic Stopped[3]	115	62%	70%	72%	95%
Pregnancy Care					
Inpatient Neonatal Mortality	-	-	-	-	-
Third or Fourth Degree Laceration	-	-	3.32%	3.63%	3.27%

Helen Keller Memorial Hospital

1300 S Montgomery Avenue
PO Box 610
Sheffield, AL 35660
E-mail: info@helenkeller.com
URL: www.helenkeller.com
Ownership: Govt - Hospital District or Authority   Accredited: Yes
Emergency Services: Yes   Licensed Beds: 185
Key Personnel:
President/CEO. . . . . William H Anderson, FACHE
Chief Medical Staff. Richard Deal
Emergency Room . . . . David Gardner
OB/GYN Womens Health. . . . . Larry Stutts, MD
Chief Radiology . . . . Brent Fritts
Director Respiratory Therapy . . . . Ronda Hood

Phone: 256-386-4154
Fax: 256-386-4469

Measure	Cases	This Hospital	State Average	U.S. Average	Top Hospital

NOTE: Hospital profiles are in alphabetical order by state, then city, then hospital within the city; Rankings are sorted by rate in descending order and exclude hospitals with less than 25 cases; (1) The number of cases is too small (n<25) for purposes of reliably predicting hospital performance; (2) Measure reflects the hospital's indication that its submission was based upon a sample of its relevant discharges; (3) Rate reflects fewer than the maximum possible quarters of data for the measure; (4) Inaccurate information submitted and suppressed for one or more quarters; (5) No data is available from the hospital for this measure; Please refer to the User's Guide for a full explanation of data

Heart Attack Care					
ACE Inhibitor or ARB for LVSD[1]	6	50%	78%	82%	100%
Aspirin at Arrival	34	91%	87%	92%	100%
Aspirin at Discharge[1]	19	84%	87%	90%	100%
Beta Blocker at Arrival	26	85%	81%	87%	100%
Beta Blocker at Discharge[1]	19	79%	86%	90%	100%
Fibrinolytic Medication Timing	0	-	25%	31%	100%
PCI Within 90 Minutes of Arrival	0	-	61%	54%	95%
Smoking Cessation Advice[1]	7	86%	85%	88%	100%
Heart Failure Care					
ACE Inhibitor or ARB for LVSD	64	83%	80%	82%	100%
Discharge Instructions	181	70%	54%	61%	93%
Evaluation of LVS Function	215	85%	79%	83%	99%
Smoking Cessation Advice	45	100%	78%	82%	100%
Pneumonia Care					
Appropriate Initial Antibiotic	90	90%	81%	83%	94%
Blood Culture Timing	75	92%	89%	90%	100%
Influenza Vaccine[1]	20	100%	62%	70%	100%
Initial Antibiotic Timing	125	86%	79%	80%	93%
Oxygenation Assessment	147	100%	99%	99%	100%
Pneumococcal Vaccine	94	87%	61%	69%	94%
Smoking Cessation Advice	39	97%	77%	80%	100%
Surgical Infection Prevention					
Prophylactic Antibiotic Given[2,3]	121	91%	74%	77%	95%
Prophylactic Antibiotic Selection[2]	40	95%	88%	90%	100%
Prophylactic Antibiotic Stopped[2,3]	119	77%	70%	72%	95%
Pregnancy Care					
Inpatient Neonatal Mortality	-	-	-	-	-
Third or Fourth Degree Laceration	-	-	3.32%	3.63%	3.27%

Coosa Valley Baptist Medical Center

Alternate Name: Coosa Valley Medical Center
315 W Hickory Street
Sylacauga, AL 35150   Phone: 256-249-5000
URL: www.cvhealth.net   Fax: 256-249-5622
Ownership: Voluntary non-profit - Other
Emergency Services: Yes   Accredited: Yes
                                  Licensed Beds: 223
Key Personnel:
CEO . . . . Glenn C Sisk
Chief Medical Staff . . . . Stephen Bowen, MD
Emergency Room . . . . Tina Brooks, RN
Director Medical/Surgical Nursing . . . . Lynn Vaughn
Obstetrics/Gyneology . . . . Patricia Sanders, MD
Chief Radiology . . . . Oswald C Carr, MD
Director Respiratory Therapy . . . . Carolyn Gregor

Measure	Cases	This Hospital	State Average	U.S. Average	Top Hospital
Heart Attack Care					
ACE Inhibitor or ARB for LVSD[1]	6	67%	78%	82%	100%
Aspirin at Arrival	32	97%	87%	92%	100%
Aspirin at Discharge[1]	14	93%	87%	90%	100%
Beta Blocker at Arrival	27	89%	81%	87%	100%
Beta Blocker at Discharge[1]	15	93%	86%	90%	100%
Fibrinolytic Medication Timing	0	-	25%	31%	100%
PCI Within 90 Minutes of Arrival	0	-	61%	54%	95%
Smoking Cessation Advice[1]	3	67%	85%	88%	100%
Heart Failure Care					
ACE Inhibitor or ARB for LVSD[2]	57	79%	80%	82%	100%
Discharge Instructions[2]	84	51%	54%	61%	93%
Evaluation of LVS Function[2]	112	80%	79%	83%	99%
Smoking Cessation Advice[1,2]	21	86%	78%	82%	100%
Pneumonia Care					
Appropriate Initial Antibiotic	101	89%	81%	83%	94%
Blood Culture Timing	74	92%	89%	90%	100%
Influenza Vaccine[1]	20	60%	62%	70%	100%
Initial Antibiotic Timing	104	89%	79%	80%	93%
Oxygenation Assessment	122	97%	99%	99%	100%
Pneumococcal Vaccine	61	44%	61%	69%	94%
Smoking Cessation Advice	33	82%	77%	80%	100%
Surgical Infection Prevention					
Prophylactic Antibiotic Given[3]	87	72%	74%	77%	95%
Prophylactic Antibiotic Selection	27	100%	88%	90%	100%
Prophylactic Antibiotic Stopped[3]	83	24%	70%	72%	95%

Pregnancy Care					
Inpatient Neonatal Mortality	-	-	-	-	-
Third or Fourth Degree Laceration	-	-	3.32%	3.63%	3.27%

Citizens Baptist Medical Center

Alternate Name: Citizens Hospital
604 Stone Avenue
PO Drawer 978   Toll-Free: 877-222-7847
Talladega, AL 35161   Phone: 256-362-8111
E-mail: info@bhsala.com   Fax: 256-761-4658
URL: www.bhsala.com
Ownership: Voluntary non-profit - Private   Accredited: Yes
Emergency Services: Yes   Licensed Beds: 122
Key Personnel:
President/CEO . . . . Steven L Gautney
Chief Staff . . . . Leigh Murphy, MD
Emergency Room Department Manager . . . . . . Deborah Rutledge
Director Radiology . . . . Byron Patterson
Director Respiratory Therapy . . . . William Howard

Measure	Cases	This Hospital	State Average	U.S. Average	Top Hospital
Heart Attack Care					
ACE Inhibitor or ARB for LVSD[1]	4	100%	78%	82%	100%
Aspirin at Arrival[1]	24	88%	87%	92%	100%
Aspirin at Discharge[1]	16	94%	87%	90%	100%
Beta Blocker at Arrival[1]	11	64%	81%	87%	100%
Beta Blocker at Discharge[1]	16	94%	86%	90%	100%
Fibrinolytic Medication Timing	0	-	25%	31%	100%
PCI Within 90 Minutes of Arrival	0	-	61%	54%	95%
Smoking Cessation Advice[1]	1	100%	85%	88%	100%
Heart Failure Care					
ACE Inhibitor or ARB for LVSD	49	73%	80%	82%	100%
Discharge Instructions	110	44%	54%	61%	93%
Evaluation of LVS Function	126	87%	79%	83%	99%
Smoking Cessation Advice	27	78%	78%	82%	100%
Pneumonia Care					
Appropriate Initial Antibiotic	86	80%	81%	83%	94%
Blood Culture Timing	61	92%	89%	90%	100%
Influenza Vaccine[1]	24	50%	62%	70%	100%
Initial Antibiotic Timing	99	90%	79%	80%	93%
Oxygenation Assessment	117	97%	99%	99%	100%
Pneumococcal Vaccine	55	55%	61%	69%	94%
Smoking Cessation Advice	33	82%	77%	80%	100%
Surgical Infection Prevention					
Prophylactic Antibiotic Given[3]	77	68%	74%	77%	95%
Prophylactic Antibiotic Selection	26	85%	88%	90%	100%
Prophylactic Antibiotic Stopped[3]	72	90%	70%	72%	95%
Pregnancy Care					
Inpatient Neonatal Mortality	-	-	-	-	-
Third or Fourth Degree Laceration	-	-	3.32%	3.63%	3.27%

Community Hospital

805 Friendship Road
PO Box 780700   Phone: 334-283-6541
Tallassee, AL 36078   Fax: 334-283-3758
E-mail: kmonroe@communityhospitalal.org
URL: www.chal.org
Ownership: Voluntary non-profit - Private   Accredited: No
Emergency Services: No   Licensed Beds: 69
Key Personnel:
Administrator/CEO . . . . Jennie Rhinehart
Chief Medical Staff . . . . Mike Wells
ER Coordinator . . . . Rebecca Carroll, RN
Infection Control . . . . Heather Brawner
Medical/Surgical Nursing . . . . Vicki Wadkins
Director Respiratory Therapy . . . . Terry Adair

Measure	Cases	This Hospital	State Average	U.S. Average	Top Hospital
Heart Attack Care					
ACE Inhibitor or ARB for LVSD	0	-	78%	82%	100%
Aspirin at Arrival[1]	7	86%	87%	92%	100%
Aspirin at Discharge[1]	6	67%	87%	90%	100%
Beta Blocker at Arrival[1]	7	100%	81%	87%	100%

Measure	Cases	This Hospital	State Average	U.S. Average	Top Hospital
Beta Blocker at Discharge[1]	6	83%	86%	90%	100%
Fibrinolytic Medication Timing	0	-	25%	31%	100%
PCI Within 90 Minutes of Arrival	0	-	61%	54%	95%
Smoking Cessation Advice	0	-	85%	88%	100%
Heart Failure Care					
ACE Inhibitor or ARB for LVSD	43	93%	80%	82%	100%
Discharge Instructions	73	52%	54%	61%	93%
Evaluation of LVS Function	87	100%	79%	83%	99%
Smoking Cessation Advice[1]	19	53%	78%	82%	100%
Pneumonia Care					
Appropriate Initial Antibiotic	52	85%	81%	83%	94%
Blood Culture Timing	34	94%	89%	90%	100%
Influenza Vaccine[1]	12	75%	62%	70%	100%
Initial Antibiotic Timing	60	75%	79%	80%	93%
Oxygenation Assessment	74	100%	99%	99%	100%
Pneumococcal Vaccine	34	74%	61%	69%	94%
Smoking Cessation Advice[1]	17	82%	77%	80%	100%
Surgical Infection Prevention					
Prophylactic Antibiotic Given[1]	12	83%	74%	77%	95%
Prophylactic Antibiotic Selection[1]	3	100%	88%	90%	100%
Prophylactic Antibiotic Stopped[1]	12	92%	70%	72%	95%
Pregnancy Care					
Inpatient Neonatal Mortality	-	-	-	-	-
Third or Fourth Degree Laceration	-	-	3.32%	3.63%	3.27%

Thomasville Infirmary

33700 Highway 43
Thomasville, AL 36784
Ownership: Proprietary
Emergency Services: Yes

Phone: 334-636-4431
Fax: 334-636-6212
Accredited: No
Licensed Beds: 49

Key Personnel:
Interim CEO . . . . Mickey Rabuka
Chief Medical Staff . . . . T B Darji, MD
Director Respiratory Therapy . . . . Curtis Chapman

Measure	Cases	This Hospital	State Average	U.S. Average	Top Hospital
Heart Attack Care					
ACE Inhibitor or ARB for LVSD[1]	1	100%	78%	82%	100%
Aspirin at Arrival[1]	8	75%	87%	92%	100%
Aspirin at Discharge[1]	2	100%	87%	90%	100%
Beta Blocker at Arrival[1]	6	50%	81%	87%	100%
Beta Blocker at Discharge[1]	2	100%	86%	90%	100%
Fibrinolytic Medication Timing[3]	0	-	25%	31%	100%
PCI Within 90 Minutes of Arrival	0	-	61%	54%	95%
Smoking Cessation Advice[3]	0	-	85%	88%	100%
Heart Failure Care					
ACE Inhibitor or ARB for LVSD[1]	21	90%	80%	82%	100%
Discharge Instructions[1,3]	17	6%	54%	61%	93%
Evaluation of LVS Function	89	82%	79%	83%	99%
Smoking Cessation Advice[1,3]	2	0%	78%	82%	100%
Pneumonia Care					
Appropriate Initial Antibiotic[1,3]	3	100%	81%	83%	94%
Blood Culture Timing[1,3]	3	100%	89%	90%	100%
Influenza Vaccine[5]	-	-	62%	70%	100%
Initial Antibiotic Timing	35	91%	79%	80%	93%
Oxygenation Assessment	43	100%	99%	99%	100%
Pneumococcal Vaccine[1]	22	91%	61%	69%	94%
Smoking Cessation Advice[1,3]	1	0%	77%	80%	100%
Surgical Infection Prevention					
Prophylactic Antibiotic Given[1,3]	17	94%	74%	77%	95%
Prophylactic Antibiotic Selection[5]	-	-	88%	90%	100%
Prophylactic Antibiotic Stopped[1,3]	17	12%	70%	72%	95%
Pregnancy Care					
Inpatient Neonatal Mortality	-	-	-	-	-
Third or Fourth Degree Laceration	-	-	3.32%	3.63%	3.27%

Troy Regional Medical Center

1330 Highway 231 S
Troy, AL 36081
URL: www.attentushealthcare.com/troyregional
Ownership: Proprietary
Emergency Services: No

Phone: 334-670-5000
Fax: 334-566-7490

Accredited: Yes
Licensed Beds: 97

Key Personnel:
OB/GYN Womens Health . . . . Cheryl Gospel
Chief Radiology . . . . Terry Hughes
Director Respiratory Therapy . . . . Terry Hughes

Measure	Cases	This Hospital	State Average	U.S. Average	Top Hospital
Heart Attack Care					
ACE Inhibitor or ARB for LVSD[1]	2	100%	78%	82%	100%
Aspirin at Arrival[1]	11	73%	87%	92%	100%
Aspirin at Discharge[1]	8	75%	87%	90%	100%
Beta Blocker at Arrival[1]	8	75%	81%	87%	100%
Beta Blocker at Discharge[1]	7	71%	86%	90%	100%
Fibrinolytic Medication Timing	0	-	25%	31%	100%
PCI Within 90 Minutes of Arrival	0	-	61%	54%	95%
Smoking Cessation Advice[1]	2	0%	85%	88%	100%
Heart Failure Care					
ACE Inhibitor or ARB for LVSD[1]	17	59%	80%	82%	100%
Discharge Instructions	48	35%	54%	61%	93%
Evaluation of LVS Function	64	80%	79%	83%	99%
Smoking Cessation Advice[1]	15	80%	78%	82%	100%
Pneumonia Care					
Appropriate Initial Antibiotic	52	63%	81%	83%	94%
Blood Culture Timing	31	94%	89%	90%	100%
Influenza Vaccine[1]	21	62%	62%	70%	100%
Initial Antibiotic Timing	75	81%	79%	80%	93%
Oxygenation Assessment	83	96%	99%	99%	100%
Pneumococcal Vaccine	46	61%	61%	69%	94%
Smoking Cessation Advice[1]	18	78%	77%	80%	100%
Surgical Infection Prevention					
Prophylactic Antibiotic Given[3]	41	41%	74%	77%	95%
Prophylactic Antibiotic Selection[1]	20	85%	88%	90%	100%
Prophylactic Antibiotic Stopped[3]	41	76%	70%	72%	95%
Pregnancy Care					
Inpatient Neonatal Mortality	-	-	-	-	-
Third or Fourth Degree Laceration	-	-	3.32%	3.63%	3.27%

DCH Regional Medical Center

809 University Boulevard East
Tuscaloosa, AL 35401
URL: www.dchsystem.com
Ownership: Govt - Hospital District or Authority
Emergency Services: Yes

Phone: 205-759-7111
Fax: 205-759-6984

Accredited: Yes
Licensed Beds: 583

Key Personnel:
President/CEO . . . . Brian Kindred
Chief Medical Staff . . . . David Rice, MD
Emergency Room . . . . Perry Lovely, MD
Infection Control . . . . Royce Roby
ICU . . . . Sheila Bresnahan, RN
Respiratory/Cardiopulmonary . . . . Byron Truelove

Measure	Cases	This Hospital	State Average	U.S. Average	Top Hospital
Heart Attack Care					
ACE Inhibitor or ARB for LVSD	60	77%	78%	82%	100%
Aspirin at Arrival	161	98%	87%	92%	100%
Aspirin at Discharge	258	98%	87%	90%	100%
Beta Blocker at Arrival	126	86%	81%	87%	100%
Beta Blocker at Discharge	252	96%	86%	90%	100%
Fibrinolytic Medication Timing[1]	1	0%	25%	31%	100%
PCI Within 90 Minutes of Arrival[1]	9	78%	61%	54%	95%
Smoking Cessation Advice	119	100%	85%	88%	100%
Heart Failure Care					
ACE Inhibitor or ARB for LVSD	116	83%	80%	82%	100%
Discharge Instructions	245	73%	54%	61%	93%
Evaluation of LVS Function	288	86%	79%	83%	99%
Smoking Cessation Advice	45	100%	78%	82%	100%
Pneumonia Care					
Appropriate Initial Antibiotic	199	80%	81%	83%	94%

NOTE: Hospital profiles are in alphabetical order by state, then city, then hospital within the city; Rankings are sorted by rate in descending order and exclude hospitals with less than 25 cases; (1) The number of cases is too small (n<25) for purposes of reliably predicting hospital performance; (2) Measure reflects the hospital's indication that its submission was based upon a sample of its relevant discharges; (3) Rate reflects fewer than the maximum possible quarters of data for the measure; (4) Inaccurate information submitted and suppressed for one or more quarters; (5) No data is available from the hospital for this measure; Please refer to the User's Guide for a full explanation of data

	155	85%	89%	90%	100%
Blood Culture Timing	155	85%	89%	90%	100%
Influenza Vaccine	59	88%	62%	70%	100%
Initial Antibiotic Timing	301	69%	79%	80%	93%
Oxygenation Assessment	385	99%	99%	99%	100%
Pneumococcal Vaccine	196	82%	61%	69%	94%
Smoking Cessation Advice	90	96%	77%	80%	100%
Surgical Infection Prevention					
Prophylactic Antibiotic Given	262	86%	74%	77%	95%
Prophylactic Antibiotic Selection	69	86%	88%	90%	100%
Prophylactic Antibiotic Stopped	241	71%	70%	72%	95%
Pregnancy Care					
Inpatient Neonatal Mortality	-	-	-	-	-
Third or Fourth Degree Laceration	-	-	3.32%	3.63%	3.27%

Bullock County Hospital

102 W Conecuh Avenue
Union Springs, AL 36089
E-mail: bullockcountyhospital@hotmail.com
Ownership: Govt - Hospital District or Authority
Emergency Services: Yes

Phone: 334-738-2140
Fax: 334-738-2146

Accredited: No
Licensed Beds: 30

Key Personnel:
Administrator . . . . Daniel Hall
Chief Medical Staff . . . . Tahir Siddiq, MD
Emergency Room . . . . Tahir Siddig, MD
Infection Control . . . . Concetta Braughton, DON
Medical Surgical Nursing . . . . Concetta Braughton, DON

Measure	Cases	This Hospital	State Average	U.S. Average	Top Hospital
Heart Attack Care					
ACE Inhibitor or ARB for LVSD[3]	0	-	78%	82%	100%
Aspirin at Arrival[3]	0	-	87%	92%	100%
Aspirin at Discharge[3]	0	-	87%	90%	100%
Beta Blocker at Arrival[1,3]	1	100%	81%	87%	100%
Beta Blocker at Discharge[1,3]	1	100%	86%	90%	100%
Fibrinolytic Medication Timing[3]	0	-	25%	31%	100%
PCI Within 90 Minutes of Arrival[5]	-	-	61%	54%	95%
Smoking Cessation Advice[3]	0	-	85%	88%	100%
Heart Failure Care					
ACE Inhibitor or ARB for LVSD[1]	1	100%	80%	82%	100%
Discharge Instructions	26	12%	54%	61%	93%
Evaluation of LVS Function	38	13%	79%	83%	99%
Smoking Cessation Advice[1]	2	50%	78%	82%	100%
Pneumonia Care					
Appropriate Initial Antibiotic[1]	12	83%	81%	83%	94%
Blood Culture Timing[1]	7	86%	89%	90%	100%
Influenza Vaccine[1]	8	25%	62%	70%	100%
Initial Antibiotic Timing[1]	18	83%	79%	80%	93%
Oxygenation Assessment[1]	20	100%	99%	99%	100%
Pneumococcal Vaccine[1]	9	44%	61%	69%	94%
Smoking Cessation Advice[1]	2	0%	77%	80%	100%
Surgical Infection Prevention					
Prophylactic Antibiotic Given[5]	-	-	74%	77%	95%
Prophylactic Antibiotic Selection[5]	-	-	88%	90%	100%
Prophylactic Antibiotic Stopped[5]	-	-	70%	72%	95%
Pregnancy Care					
Inpatient Neonatal Mortality	-	-	-	-	-
Third or Fourth Degree Laceration	-	-	3.32%	3.63%	3.27%

George H Lanier Memorial Hospital

4800 48th Street
Valley, AL 36854
URL: www.lanierhospital.com
Ownership: Voluntary non-profit - Other
Emergency Services: Yes

Phone: 334-756-9180
Fax: 334-756-6698

Accredited: Yes
Licensed Beds: 210

Key Personnel:
CEO . . . . Robert J Humphrey
Chief Medical Staff . . . . Eric Hemberg
Emergency Room . . . . Lance Strength, RN
OB/GYN Womens Health . . . . Arthur F Perkins, MD
Chief Radiology . . . . Eugene R Long, MD
Director Respiratory Therapy . . . . Dorothea Penn

Measure	Cases	This Hospital	State Average	U.S. Average	Top Hospital

Heart Attack Care					
ACE Inhibitor or ARB for LVSD[1]	3	33%	78%	82%	100%
Aspirin at Arrival	25	84%	87%	92%	100%
Aspirin at Discharge[1]	9	78%	87%	90%	100%
Beta Blocker at Arrival[1]	23	91%	81%	87%	100%
Beta Blocker at Discharge[1]	10	70%	86%	90%	100%
Fibrinolytic Medication Timing[1]	1	0%	25%	31%	100%
PCI Within 90 Minutes of Arrival	0	-	61%	54%	95%
Smoking Cessation Advice	0	-	85%	88%	100%
Heart Failure Care					
ACE Inhibitor or ARB for LVSD	87	93%	80%	82%	100%
Discharge Instructions	178	38%	54%	61%	93%
Evaluation of LVS Function	187	96%	79%	83%	99%
Smoking Cessation Advice	47	89%	78%	82%	100%
Pneumonia Care					
Appropriate Initial Antibiotic	70	77%	81%	83%	94%
Blood Culture Timing	50	94%	89%	90%	100%
Influenza Vaccine[1]	19	63%	62%	70%	100%
Initial Antibiotic Timing	83	78%	79%	80%	93%
Oxygenation Assessment	95	98%	99%	99%	100%
Pneumococcal Vaccine	51	82%	61%	69%	94%
Smoking Cessation Advice	26	77%	77%	80%	100%
Surgical Infection Prevention					
Prophylactic Antibiotic Given	104	65%	74%	77%	95%
Prophylactic Antibiotic Selection	0	-	88%	90%	100%
Prophylactic Antibiotic Stopped	98	77%	70%	72%	95%
Pregnancy Care					
Inpatient Neonatal Mortality	-	-	-	-	-
Third or Fourth Degree Laceration	-	-	3.32%	3.63%	3.27%

Wedowee Hospital

209 N Main Street
PO Box 307
Wedowee, AL 36278
Ownership: Govt - Hospital District or Authority
Emergency Services: Yes

Phone: 256-357-2111
Fax: 256-357-2165

Accredited: No
Licensed Beds: 34

Key Personnel:
CEO . . . . John L Robertson
CEO . . . . Ferrel Turner
Director Infection/Disease Control . . . . Ruth Bailey
Director Respiratory Therapy . . . . Becky Prince

Measure	Cases	This Hospital	State Average	U.S. Average	Top Hospital
Heart Attack Care					
ACE Inhibitor or ARB for LVSD	0	-	78%	82%	100%
Aspirin at Arrival	0	-	87%	92%	100%
Aspirin at Discharge	0	-	87%	90%	100%
Beta Blocker at Arrival	0	-	81%	87%	100%
Beta Blocker at Discharge	0	-	86%	90%	100%
Fibrinolytic Medication Timing	0	-	25%	31%	100%
PCI Within 90 Minutes of Arrival	0	-	61%	54%	95%
Smoking Cessation Advice	0	-	85%	88%	100%
Heart Failure Care					
ACE Inhibitor or ARB for LVSD[1]	10	80%	80%	82%	100%
Discharge Instructions	55	4%	54%	61%	93%
Evaluation of LVS Function	59	49%	79%	83%	99%
Smoking Cessation Advice[1]	9	22%	78%	82%	100%
Pneumonia Care					
Appropriate Initial Antibiotic[1]	21	81%	81%	83%	94%
Blood Culture Timing[1]	3	100%	89%	90%	100%
Influenza Vaccine[1]	7	0%	62%	70%	100%
Initial Antibiotic Timing[1]	22	82%	79%	80%	93%
Oxygenation Assessment[1]	24	88%	99%	99%	100%
Pneumococcal Vaccine[1]	14	14%	61%	69%	94%
Smoking Cessation Advice[1]	2	50%	77%	80%	100%
Surgical Infection Prevention					
Prophylactic Antibiotic Given[5]	-	-	74%	77%	95%
Prophylactic Antibiotic Selection[5]	-	-	88%	90%	100%
Prophylactic Antibiotic Stopped[5]	-	-	70%	72%	95%
Pregnancy Care					
Inpatient Neonatal Mortality	-	-	-	-	-
Third or Fourth Degree Laceration	-	-	3.32%	3.63%	3.27%

NOTE: Hospital profiles are in alphabetical order by state, then city, then hospital within the city; Rankings are sorted by rate in descending order and exclude hospitals with less than 25 cases; (1) The number of cases is too small (n<25) for purposes of reliably predicting hospital performance; (2) Measure reflects the hospital's indication that its submission was based upon a sample of its relevant discharges; (3) Rate reflects fewer than the maximum possible quarters of data for the measure; (4) Inaccurate information submitted and suppressed for one or more quarters; (5) No data is available from the hospital for this measure; Please refer to the User's Guide for a full explanation of data

Elmore Community Hospital

Alternate Name: Central Alabama Medical Center
500 Hospital Drive
Wetumpka, AL 36092
Ownership: Proprietary
Emergency Services: Yes

Phone: 334-567-4311
Fax: 334-567-5919
Accredited: No
Licensed Beds: 69

Key Personnel:

Administrator . . . . Gordon Faulk
Chief Medical Staff. . . . . Spencer Coleman, MD
Emergency Room . . . . Becky Turner, RN
Director Medical/Surgical Nursing . . . . Emily Mann, RN
Chief Radiology . . . . Stanley Winslow, MD
Director Respiratory Therapy . . . . Richard Johns

Measure	Cases	This Hospital	State Average	U.S. Average	Top Hospital
Heart Attack Care					
ACE Inhibitor or ARB for LVSD[5]	-	-	78%	82%	100%
Aspirin at Arrival[5]	-	-	87%	92%	100%
Aspirin at Discharge[5]	-	-	87%	90%	100%
Beta Blocker at Arrival[5]	-	-	81%	87%	100%
Beta Blocker at Discharge[5]	-	-	86%	90%	100%
Fibrinolytic Medication Timing[5]	-	-	25%	31%	100%
PCI Within 90 Minutes of Arrival[5]	-	-	61%	54%	95%
Smoking Cessation Advice[5]	-	-	85%	88%	100%
Heart Failure Care					
ACE Inhibitor or ARB for LVSD[1,3]	4	50%	80%	82%	100%
Discharge Instructions[1,3]	6	0%	54%	61%	93%
Evaluation of LVS Function[1,3]	23	48%	79%	83%	99%
Smoking Cessation Advice[1,3]	3	0%	78%	82%	100%
Pneumonia Care					
Appropriate Initial Antibiotic[1,3]	3	67%	81%	83%	94%
Blood Culture Timing[1,3]	5	100%	89%	90%	100%
Influenza Vaccine[5]	-	-	62%	70%	100%
Initial Antibiotic Timing[1,3]	13	85%	79%	80%	93%
Oxygenation Assessment[1,3]	16	94%	99%	99%	100%
Pneumococcal Vaccine[1,3]	11	0%	61%	69%	94%
Smoking Cessation Advice[1,3]	3	33%	77%	80%	100%
Surgical Infection Prevention					
Prophylactic Antibiotic Given[5]	-	-	74%	77%	95%
Prophylactic Antibiotic Selection[5]	-	-	88%	90%	100%
Prophylactic Antibiotic Stopped[5]	-	-	70%	72%	95%
Pregnancy Care					
Inpatient Neonatal Mortality	-	-	-	-	-
Third or Fourth Degree Laceration	-	-	3.32%	3.63%	3.27%

Northwest Medical Center

Alternate Name: Winfield Carraway Hospital
1530 US Highway 43
Winfield, AL 35594
URL: www.northwestmedcenter.com
Ownership: Proprietary
Emergency Services: Yes

Phone: 205-487-7000
Fax: 205-487-7891

Accredited: Yes
Licensed Beds: 71

Key Personnel:

President/CEO. . . . . William F Carpenter, III
Chief Medical Staff. . . . . Dan Avery, MD
Cardiac Lab . . . . Rhonda Taylor, RN
Emergency Room . . . . Lisa Chaffin, RN
Emergency Room . . . . Tim Jordan, MD
Infection Control. . . . . Sherri White, RN
ICU . . . . Lisa Chaffin, RN
Medical/Surgical Nursing . . . . Robin Wise, RN
OB/GYN Womens Health. . . . . Will Lenanan
Chief Radiology . . . . Scott Loveless, MD
Director Respiratory Therapy . . . . Lesa Hamm

Measure	Cases	This Hospital	State Average	U.S. Average	Top Hospital
Heart Attack Care					
ACE Inhibitor or ARB for LVSD[1]	1	100%	78%	82%	100%
Aspirin at Arrival[1]	8	88%	87%	92%	100%
Aspirin at Discharge[1]	4	100%	87%	90%	100%
Beta Blocker at Arrival[1]	12	92%	81%	87%	100%
Beta Blocker at Discharge[1]	8	88%	86%	90%	100%
Fibrinolytic Medication Timing[1]	1	0%	25%	31%	100%

Measure	Cases	This Hospital	State Average	U.S. Average	Top Hospital
PCI Within 90 Minutes of Arrival	0	-	61%	54%	95%
Smoking Cessation Advice	0	-	85%	88%	100%
Heart Failure Care					
ACE Inhibitor or ARB for LVSD	28	89%	80%	82%	100%
Discharge Instructions	76	47%	54%	61%	93%
Evaluation of LVS Function	103	83%	79%	83%	99%
Smoking Cessation Advice[1]	22	86%	78%	82%	100%
Pneumonia Care					
Appropriate Initial Antibiotic	114	91%	81%	83%	94%
Blood Culture Timing	50	96%	89%	90%	100%
Influenza Vaccine	25	48%	62%	70%	100%
Initial Antibiotic Timing	130	89%	79%	80%	93%
Oxygenation Assessment	151	100%	99%	99%	100%
Pneumococcal Vaccine	76	76%	61%	69%	94%
Smoking Cessation Advice	37	81%	77%	80%	100%
Surgical Infection Prevention					
Prophylactic Antibiotic Given	111	94%	74%	77%	95%
Prophylactic Antibiotic Selection	26	88%	88%	90%	100%
Prophylactic Antibiotic Stopped	110	62%	70%	72%	95%
Pregnancy Care					
Inpatient Neonatal Mortality	-	-	-	-	-
Third or Fourth Degree Laceration	-	-	3.32%	3.63%	3.27%

Hill Hospital of Sumter County

Alternate Name: Hill Hospital of York
751 Derby Drive
York, AL 36925
E-mail: hillhospital@yahoo.com
URL: www.hillhospitalhomestead.com/hillhospitalhomepage.html
Ownership: Voluntary non-profit - Other
Emergency Services: Yes

Phone: 205-392-5263
Fax: 205-392-9974

Accredited: No
Licensed Beds: 33

Key Personnel:

Chief Medical Staff. . . . . Gary Walson, DO
Infection Control. . . . . Cynthia Brown, RN

Measure	Cases	This Hospital	State Average	U.S. Average	Top Hospital
Heart Attack Care					
ACE Inhibitor or ARB for LVSD[5]	-	-	78%	82%	100%
Aspirin at Arrival[5]	-	-	87%	92%	100%
Aspirin at Discharge[5]	-	-	87%	90%	100%
Beta Blocker at Arrival[5]	-	-	81%	87%	100%
Beta Blocker at Discharge[5]	-	-	86%	90%	100%
Fibrinolytic Medication Timing[5]	-	-	25%	31%	100%
PCI Within 90 Minutes of Arrival[5]	-	-	61%	54%	95%
Smoking Cessation Advice[5]	-	-	85%	88%	100%
Heart Failure Care					
ACE Inhibitor or ARB for LVSD	0	-	80%	82%	100%
Discharge Instructions[1]	2	0%	54%	61%	93%
Evaluation of LVS Function[1]	5	20%	79%	83%	99%
Smoking Cessation Advice	0	-	78%	82%	100%
Pneumonia Care					
Appropriate Initial Antibiotic[1,2]	1	0%	81%	83%	94%
Blood Culture Timing[1,2]	1	100%	89%	90%	100%
Influenza Vaccine[1]	1	0%	62%	70%	100%
Initial Antibiotic Timing[1,2]	4	75%	79%	80%	93%
Oxygenation Assessment[1,2]	5	100%	99%	99%	100%
Pneumococcal Vaccine[1,2]	3	0%	61%	69%	94%
Smoking Cessation Advice[1,2]	2	0%	77%	80%	100%
Surgical Infection Prevention					
Prophylactic Antibiotic Given[5]	-	-	74%	77%	95%
Prophylactic Antibiotic Selection[5]	-	-	88%	90%	100%
Prophylactic Antibiotic Stopped[5]	-	-	70%	72%	95%
Pregnancy Care					
Inpatient Neonatal Mortality	-	-	-	-	-
Third or Fourth Degree Laceration	-	-	3.32%	3.63%	3.27%

NOTE: Hospital profiles are in alphabetical order by state, then city, then hospital within the city; Rankings are sorted by rate in descending order and exclude hospitals with less than 25 cases; (1) The number of cases is too small (n<25) for purposes of reliably predicting hospital performance; (2) Measure reflects the hospital's indication that its submission was based upon a sample of its relevant discharges; (3) Rate reflects fewer than the maximum possible quarters of data for the measure; (4) Inaccurate information submitted and suppressed for one or more quarters; (5) No data is available from the hospital for this measure; Please refer to the User's Guide for a full explanation of data

Heart Attack Care

1. ACE Inhibitor or ARB for LVSD

Hospital Name	City	Rate	Cases
White River Medical Center	Batesville	96%	54
NW Medical Center Benton County	Bentonville	94%	51
Saint Mary-Rogers Memorial Hospital	Rogers	92%	26
Baptist Health Medical Center	Little Rock	90%	88
Saint Bernard's Medical Center	Jonesboro	90%	100
Saint Edward Mercy Medical Center	Fort Smith	90%	91
Washington Regional Medical Center	Fayetteville	88%	64
Jefferson Regional Medical Center	Pine Bluff	87%	75
Baxter Regional Medical Center	Mountain Home	84%	88
Saint Joseph's Mercy Health Center	Hot Spgs Natl Pk	83%	53
UAMS Medical Center	Little Rock	82%	33
Sparks Regional Medical Center	Fort Smith	78%	46
Northwest Medical Center	Springdale	77%	35
Arkansas Heart Hospital	Little Rock	75%	126
White County Medical Center	Searcy	75%	36
Baptist Health Med Ctr-North Little Rock	North Little Rock	74%	43
Conway Regional Medical Center	Conway	73%	37
Saint Vincent Infirmary Medical Center	Little Rock	68%	63

2. Aspirin at Arrival

Hospital Name	City	Rate	Cases
Arkansas Heart Hospital	Little Rock	99%	87
Baptist Health Medical Center	Little Rock	99%	163
NW Medical Center Benton County	Bentonville	99%	143
Saint Joseph's Mercy Health Center	Hot Spgs Natl Pk	99%	181
Saint Mary-Rogers Memorial Hospital	Rogers	99%	120
White River Medical Center	Batesville	99%	136
Baptist Health Med Ctr-North Little Rock	North Little Rock	98%	171
National Park Medical Center	Hot Springs	98%	59
Northwest Medical Center	Springdale	98%	165
NEA Medical Center	Jonesboro	97%	92
North Arkansas Regional Medical Center	Harrison	97%	33
Rebsamen Medical Center	Jacksonville	97%	30
Saint Bernard's Medical Center	Jonesboro	97%	215
Conway Regional Medical Center	Conway	96%	123
Saint Edward Mercy Medical Center	Fort Smith	96%	157
Saint Vincent Infirmary Medical Center	Little Rock	96%	145
UAMS Medical Center	Little Rock	96%	97
Saint Mary's Regional Medical Center	Russellville	95%	41
Baxter Regional Medical Center	Mountain Home	94%	270
Jefferson Regional Medical Center	Pine Bluff	94%	163
Washington Regional Medical Center	Fayetteville	94%	183
White County Medical Center	Searcy	94%	102
Saline Memorial Hospital	Benton	93%	43
Sparks Regional Medical Center	Fort Smith	93%	188
Arkansas Methodist Hospital	Paragould	92%	98
Summit Medical Center	Van Buren	90%	29
Medical Center of South Arkansas	El Dorado	89%	27
Great River Medical Center	Blytheville	74%	31

3. Aspirin at Discharge

Hospital Name	City	Rate	Cases
Saint Joseph's Mercy Health Center	Hot Spgs Natl Pk	100%	209
Saint Mary-Rogers Memorial Hospital	Rogers	100%	132
Baptist Health Medical Center	Little Rock	98%	327
Jefferson Regional Medical Center	Pine Bluff	98%	232
NEA Medical Center	Jonesboro	98%	173
Northwest Medical Center	Springdale	98%	199
NW Medical Center Benton County	Bentonville	97%	126
Saint Edward Mercy Medical Center	Fort Smith	97%	253
Washington Regional Medical Center	Fayetteville	97%	267
White County Medical Center	Searcy	97%	99
Saint Bernard's Medical Center	Jonesboro	96%	368
Saint Vincent Infirmary Medical Center	Little Rock	96%	244
White River Medical Center	Batesville	96%	132
Baptist Health Med Ctr-North Little Rock	North Little Rock	95%	213
UAMS Medical Center	Little Rock	95%	88
Sparks Regional Medical Center	Fort Smith	94%	220
National Park Medical Center	Hot Springs	92%	60
Arkansas Heart Hospital	Little Rock	91%	435
Arkansas Methodist Hospital	Paragould	91%	82
Baxter Regional Medical Center	Mountain Home	89%	300
Conway Regional Medical Center	Conway	87%	140

4. Beta Blocker at Arrival

Hospital Name	City	Rate	Cases
White River Medical Center	Batesville	100%	119
Baptist Health Medical Center	Little Rock	99%	131

Saint Mary-Rogers Memorial Hospital	Rogers	98%	93
Saint Edward Mercy Medical Center	Fort Smith	97%	118
NW Medical Center Benton County	Bentonville	94%	104
Saint Mary's Regional Medical Center	Russellville	94%	32
Sparks Regional Medical Center	Fort Smith	94%	186
Baxter Regional Medical Center	Mountain Home	93%	256
Jefferson Regional Medical Center	Pine Bluff	93%	144
Saint Joseph's Mercy Health Center	Hot Spgs Natl Pk	91%	145
Saint Vincent Infirmary Medical Center	Little Rock	91%	104
Baptist Health Med Ctr-North Little Rock	North Little Rock	90%	126
Medical Center of South Arkansas	El Dorado	90%	30
NEA Medical Center	Jonesboro	90%	68
Arkansas Methodist Hospital	Paragould	89%	76
Rebsamen Medical Center	Jacksonville	89%	27
Saint Bernard's Medical Center	Jonesboro	89%	140
Arkansas Heart Hospital	Little Rock	88%	80
National Park Medical Center	Hot Springs	88%	52
Washington Regional Medical Center	Fayetteville	88%	161
Summit Medical Center	Van Buren	86%	28
UAMS Medical Center	Little Rock	85%	67
White County Medical Center	Searcy	83%	88
Conway Regional Medical Center	Conway	82%	119
Northwest Medical Center	Springdale	81%	127
Great River Medical Center	Blytheville	73%	30
Saline Memorial Hospital	Benton	73%	33

5. Beta Blocker at Discharge

Hospital Name	City	Rate	Cases
Saint Mary-Rogers Memorial Hospital	Rogers	99%	142
Baptist Health Medical Center	Little Rock	98%	340
NW Medical Center Benton County	Bentonville	98%	133
Baptist Health Med Ctr-North Little Rock	North Little Rock	97%	211
Saint Edward Mercy Medical Center	Fort Smith	97%	257
UAMS Medical Center	Little Rock	96%	102
White River Medical Center	Batesville	96%	144
Saint Bernard's Medical Center	Jonesboro	95%	368
Saint Vincent Infirmary Medical Center	Little Rock	95%	243
Sparks Regional Medical Center	Fort Smith	95%	224
White County Medical Center	Searcy	95%	110
Baxter Regional Medical Center	Mountain Home	94%	297
Saint Joseph's Mercy Health Center	Hot Spgs Natl Pk	94%	156
Jefferson Regional Medical Center	Pine Bluff	93%	232
Northwest Medical Center	Springdale	92%	207
Arkansas Methodist Hospital	Paragould	91%	78
Medical Center of South Arkansas	El Dorado	90%	29
Washington Regional Medical Center	Fayetteville	90%	267
Arkansas Heart Hospital	Little Rock	89%	414
NEA Medical Center	Jonesboro	89%	141
National Park Medical Center	Hot Springs	89%	54
Conway Regional Medical Center	Conway	80%	141

8. Smoking Cessation Advice

Hospital Name	City	Rate	Cases
Arkansas Methodist Hospital	Paragould	100%	29
Baxter Regional Medical Center	Mountain Home	100%	109
Saint Edward Mercy Medical Center	Fort Smith	100%	137
Saint Joseph's Mercy Health Center	Hot Spgs Natl Pk	100%	93
Saint Vincent Infirmary Medical Center	Little Rock	100%	111
UAMS Medical Center	Little Rock	100%	57
Arkansas Heart Hospital	Little Rock	99%	195
Baptist Health Med Ctr-North Little Rock	North Little Rock	99%	97
NEA Medical Center	Jonesboro	99%	78
Saint Bernard's Medical Center	Jonesboro	99%	192
White County Medical Center	Searcy	98%	51
White River Medical Center	Batesville	98%	52
Baptist Health Medical Center	Little Rock	97%	153
National Park Medical Center	Hot Springs	97%	30
Saint Mary-Rogers Memorial Hospital	Rogers	96%	53
Jefferson Regional Medical Center	Pine Bluff	95%	98
NW Medical Center Benton County	Bentonville	95%	57
Northwest Medical Center	Springdale	95%	81
Conway Regional Medical Center	Conway	89%	55
Washington Regional Medical Center	Fayetteville	86%	101
Sparks Regional Medical Center	Fort Smith	84%	85

Heart Failure Care

9. ACE Inhibitor or ARB for LVSD

Hospital Name	City	Rate	Cases
Baptist Memorial Hospital-Forrest City	Forrest City	100%	34
Chicot Memorial Hospital	Lake Village	97%	38
Arkansas Methodist Hospital	Paragould	96%	49
Ouachita Medical Center	Camden	96%	28

NOTE: Hospital profiles are in alphabetical order by state, then city, then hospital within the city; Rankings are sorted by rate in descending order and exclude hospitals with less than 25 cases; (1) The number of cases is too small (n<25) for purposes of reliably predicting hospital performance; (2) Measure reflects the hospital's indication that its submission was based upon a sample of its relevant discharges; (3) Rate reflects fewer than the maximum possible quarters of data for the measure; (4) Inaccurate information submitted and suppressed for one or more quarters; (5) No data is available from the hospital for this measure; Please refer to the User's Guide for a full explanation of data

Saint Joseph's Mercy Health Center	Hot Spgs Natl Pk	96%	135
Saint Mary-Rogers Memorial Hospital	Rogers	96%	78
White River Medical Center	Batesville	95%	125
Crittenden Memorial Hospital	West Memphis	94%	72
NEA Medical Center	Jonesboro	93%	102
Medical Park Hospital	Hope	90%	42
Baptist Health Medical Center	Little Rock	89%	362
National Park Medical Center	Hot Springs	88%	43
Northwest Medical Center	Springdale	88%	92
Stuttgart Regional Medical Center	Stuttgart	88%	32
Saint Vincent Infirmary Medical Center	Little Rock	86%	228
Magnolia Hospital	Magnolia	85%	41
Saint Bernard's Medical Center	Jonesboro	85%	317
Washington Regional Medical Center	Fayetteville	85%	148
Saint Edward Mercy Medical Center	Fort Smith	84%	103
Baptist Health Med Ctr-North Little Rock	North Little Rock	83%	133
Medical Center of South Arkansas	El Dorado	82%	66
NW Medical Center Benton County	Bentonville	82%	38
Summit Medical Center	Van Buren	81%	26
Saint Mary's Regional Medical Center	Russellville	79%	53
Sparks Regional Medical Center	Fort Smith	79%	151
UAMS Medical Center	Little Rock	79%	192
Jefferson Regional Medical Center	Pine Bluff	78%	232
White County Medical Center	Searcy	77%	91
North Arkansas Regional Medical Center	Harrison	74%	38
Great River Medical Center	Blytheville	73%	30
Rebsamen Medical Center	Jacksonville	72%	29
Arkansas Heart Hospital	Little Rock	69%	327
Baxter Regional Medical Center	Mountain Home	68%	169
Helena Regional Medical Center	Helena	67%	61
Hot Springs County Medical Center	Malvern	67%	36
Conway Regional Medical Center	Conway	66%	73
Saline Memorial Hospital	Benton	50%	52

10. Discharge Instructions

Hospital Name	City	Rate	Cases
Baptist Memorial Hospital-Forrest City	Forrest City	100%	88
Crittenden Memorial Hospital	West Memphis	95%	209
Medical Park Hospital	Hope	94%	66
Washington Regional Medical Center	Fayetteville	91%	258
Arkansas Methodist Hospital	Paragould	89%	146
Baptist Health Medical Center	Arkadelphia	85%	33
NEA Medical Center	Jonesboro	82%	196
White River Medical Center	Batesville	82%	253
NW Medical Center Benton County	Bentonville	80%	75
Saint Joseph's Mercy Health Center	Hot Spgs Natl Pk	80%	282
Magnolia Hospital	Magnolia	78%	90
Arkansas Heart Hospital	Little Rock	77%	461
Bradley County Medical Center	Warren	77%	53
White County Medical Center	Searcy	76%	202
Ashley County Medical Center	Crossett	75%	32
Conway Regional Medical Center	Conway	75%	134
Northwest Medical Center	Springdale	75%	152
South Mississippi County Regional Med Ctr	Osceola	75%	48
Saint Mary-Rogers Memorial Hospital	Rogers	74%	165
Chicot Memorial Hospital	Lake Village	72%	141
Saint Mary's Regional Medical Center	Russellville	72%	116
Baxter Regional Medical Center	Mountain Home	71%	279
UAMS Medical Center	Little Rock	71%	263
Sparks Regional Medical Center	Fort Smith	69%	323
North Arkansas Regional Medical Center	Harrison	68%	109
CrossRidge Community Hospital	Wynne	67%	36
Stuttgart Regional Medical Center	Stuttgart	67%	96
Baptist Health Medical Center	Little Rock	65%	649
Ozark Health Medical Center	Clinton	65%	26
Jefferson Regional Medical Center	Pine Bluff	62%	343
Ouachita Medical Center	Camden	62%	87
Harris Hospital and Clinic	Newport	60%	67
Saint Edward Mercy Medical Center	Fort Smith	60%	229
Saint Vincent Medical Center North	Sherwood	60%	53
Saint Bernard's Medical Center	Jonesboro	59%	506
Helena Regional Medical Center	Helena	58%	167
Medical Center of South Arkansas	El Dorado	58%	128
Drew Memorial Hospital	Monticello	57%	42
Johnson Regional Medical Center	Clarksville	55%	71
Baptist Health Med Ctr-North Little Rock	North Little Rock	54%	247
Summit Medical Center	Van Buren	54%	80
Mena Medical Center	Mena	53%	59
National Park Medical Center	Hot Springs	52%	89
Great River Medical Center	Blytheville	48%	62
Saint Vincent Infirmary Medical Center	Little Rock	44%	423
Saline Memorial Hospital	Benton	42%	90
Hot Springs County Medical Center	Malvern	33%	111
Saint John's Hospital-Berryville	Berryville	29%	41

Siloam Springs Memorial Hospital	Siloam Springs	25%	71
Randolph County Medical Center	Pocahontas	20%	25

11. Evaluation of LVS Function

Hospital Name	City	Rate	Cases
Baptist Health Medical Center	Heber Springs	100%	26
Saint Mary-Rogers Memorial Hospital	Rogers	100%	211
White River Medical Center	Batesville	100%	333
Medical Center of South Arkansas	El Dorado	99%	173
Medical Park Hospital	Hope	99%	122
Saint Bernard's Medical Center	Jonesboro	99%	613
Saint Edward Mercy Medical Center	Fort Smith	99%	286
Baptist Health Med Ctr-North Little Rock	North Little Rock	98%	285
NEA Medical Center	Jonesboro	98%	222
Jefferson Regional Medical Center	Pine Bluff	97%	440
North Arkansas Regional Medical Center	Harrison	97%	142
Piggott Community Hospital	Piggott	97%	39
Saint Anthony's Healthcare Center	Morrilton	97%	38
Saint Joseph's Mercy Health Center	Hot Spgs Natl Pk	97%	345
UAMS Medical Center	Little Rock	97%	288
Washington Regional Medical Center	Fayetteville	97%	292
Baptist Health Medical Center	Little Rock	96%	762
Baptist Memorial Hospital-Forrest City	Forrest City	96%	98
National Park Medical Center	Hot Springs	95%	106
Stuttgart Regional Medical Center	Stuttgart	95%	127
Arkansas Methodist Hospital	Paragould	94%	214
Baxter Regional Medical Center	Mountain Home	94%	357
Chicot Memorial Hospital	Lake Village	94%	172
White County Medical Center	Searcy	93%	254
Northwest Medical Center	Springdale	92%	198
Saint Mary's Regional Medical Center	Russellville	92%	153
Saline Memorial Hospital	Benton	92%	116
Crittenden Memorial Hospital	West Memphis	91%	236
Saint Vincent Infirmary Medical Center	Little Rock	91%	508
Stone County Medical Center	Mountain View	91%	33
Harris Hospital and Clinic	Newport	90%	127
NW Medical Center Benton County	Bentonville	90%	93
Rebsamen Medical Center	Jacksonville	90%	91
Lawrence Memorial Hospital	Walnut Ridge	89%	47
Sparks Regional Medical Center	Fort Smith	89%	430
Arkansas Heart Hospital	Little Rock	88%	512
Great River Medical Center	Blytheville	87%	76
Saint Vincent Medical Center North	Sherwood	87%	68
Johnson Regional Medical Center	Clarksville	83%	84
CrossRidge Community Hospital	Wynne	82%	50
South Mississippi County Regional Med Ctr	Osceola	82%	65
Summit Medical Center	Van Buren	82%	122
Baptist Health Medical Center	Arkadelphia	78%	46
Helena Regional Medical Center	Helena	76%	254
Magnolia Hospital	Magnolia	76%	103
Drew Memorial Hospital	Monticello	75%	52
Hot Springs County Medical Center	Malvern	71%	135
Southwest Regional Medical Centre	Little Rock	71%	31
Conway Regional Medical Center	Conway	69%	156
De Queen Regional Medical Center	De Queen	69%	36
Howard Memorial Hospital	Nashville	68%	25
Ouachita Medical Center	Camden	67%	105
Ozark Health Medical Center	Clinton	67%	46
Siloam Springs Memorial Hospital	Siloam Springs	67%	85
Booneville Community Hospital	Booneville	65%	34
Mena Medical Center	Mena	62%	74
Ashley County Medical Center	Crossett	59%	39
Saint John's Hospital-Berryville	Berryville	55%	49
Randolph County Medical Center	Pocahontas	54%	39
McGehee-Desha County Hospital	McGehee	53%	30
De Witt Hospital & Nursing Home	De Witt	15%	26
Bradley County Medical Center	Warren	13%	62
Chambers Memorial Hospital	Danville	6%	140

12. Smoking Cessation Advice

Hospital Name	City	Rate	Cases
Crittenden Memorial Hospital	West Memphis	100%	57
Medical Center of South Arkansas	El Dorado	100%	53
Medical Park Hospital	Hope	100%	29
NEA Medical Center	Jonesboro	100%	41
UAMS Medical Center	Little Rock	100%	98
Arkansas Heart Hospital	Little Rock	99%	75
Baptist Health Medical Center	Little Rock	99%	110
Saint Bernard's Medical Center	Jonesboro	99%	151
Saint Vincent Infirmary Medical Center	Little Rock	99%	100
Washington Regional Medical Center	Fayetteville	99%	67
Baptist Health Med Ctr-North Little Rock	North Little Rock	98%	59
Saint Joseph's Mercy Health Center	Hot Spgs Natl Pk	98%	87
Conway Regional Medical Center	Conway	97%	32

NOTE: Hospital profiles are in alphabetical order by state, then city, then hospital within the city; Rankings are sorted by rate in descending order and exclude hospitals with less than 25 cases; (1) The number of cases is too small (n<25) for purposes of reliably predicting hospital performance; (2) Measure reflects the hospital's indication that its submission was based upon a sample of its relevant discharges; (3) Rate reflects fewer than the maximum possible quarters of data for the measure; (4) Inaccurate information submitted and suppressed for one or more quarters; (5) No data is available from the hospital for this measure; Please refer to the User's Guide for a full explanation of data

Northwest Medical Center	Springdale	97%	30
Saint Edward Mercy Medical Center	Fort Smith	97%	59
Baxter Regional Medical Center	Mountain Home	96%	52
Saint Mary-Rogers Memorial Hospital	Rogers	96%	25
Arkansas Methodist Hospital	Paragould	93%	41
Helena Regional Medical Center	Helena	93%	55
White River Medical Center	Batesville	93%	54
Jefferson Regional Medical Center	Pine Bluff	92%	107
White County Medical Center	Searcy	91%	35
Saint Mary's Regional Medical Center	Russellville	86%	29
North Arkansas Regional Medical Center	Harrison	84%	25
Great River Medical Center	Blytheville	83%	30
Sparks Regional Medical Center	Fort Smith	65%	60
Chambers Memorial Hospital	Danville	53%	34

Pneumonia Care

13. Appropriate Initial Antibiotic

Hospital Name	City	Rate	Cases
Baptist Health Medical Center	Heber Springs	98%	63
Lawrence Memorial Hospital	Walnut Ridge	97%	35
Ozark Health Medical Center	Clinton	96%	73
CrossRidge Community Hospital	Wynne	93%	69
Johnson Regional Medical Center	Clarksville	92%	105
Mena Medical Center	Mena	91%	57
White River Medical Center	Batesville	91%	132
Stuttgart Regional Medical Center	Stuttgart	89%	53
White County Medical Center	Searcy	89%	141
Bradley County Medical Center	Warren	88%	48
Saint Bernard's Medical Center	Jonesboro	88%	266
Saint John's Hospital-Berryville	Berryville	88%	95
Saint Mary's Regional Medical Center	Russellville	88%	178
Saint Mary-Rogers Memorial Hospital	Rogers	88%	154
Hot Springs County Medical Center	Malvern	87%	109
McGehee-Desha County Hospital	McGehee	87%	31
Medical Center of South Arkansas	El Dorado	87%	94
UAMS Medical Center	Little Rock	87%	119
Chicot Memorial Hospital	Lake Village	85%	61
Great River Medical Center	Blytheville	85%	54
Saint Joseph's Mercy Health Center	Hot Spgs Natl Pk	85%	253
Baptist Memorial Hospital-Forrest City	Forrest City	84%	62
NEA Medical Center	Jonesboro	84%	141
Ouachita Medical Center	Camden	84%	91
Stone County Medical Center	Mountain View	84%	98
Harris Hospital and Clinic	Newport	83%	84
Jefferson Regional Medical Center	Pine Bluff	82%	197
NW Medical Center Benton County	Bentonville	82%	71
Saint Edward Mercy Medical Center	Fort Smith	82%	101
South Mississippi County Regional Med Ctr	Osceola	82%	34
Sparks Regional Medical Center	Fort Smith	82%	212
Conway Regional Medical Center	Conway	81%	160
Saint Vincent Infirmary Medical Center	Little Rock	81%	187
Saline Memorial Hospital	Benton	81%	117
Siloam Springs Memorial Hospital	Siloam Springs	81%	91
Magnolia Hospital	Magnolia	80%	59
Medical Park Hospital	Hope	80%	70
North Arkansas Regional Medical Center	Harrison	80%	191
Northwest Medical Center	Springdale	80%	110
Randolph County Medical Center	Pocahontas	80%	65
Baptist Health Med Ctr-North Little Rock	North Little Rock	79%	118
Baxter Regional Medical Center	Mountain Home	79%	207
Delta Memorial Hospital	Dumas	79%	28
Washington Regional Medical Center	Fayetteville	79%	103
Arkansas Methodist Hospital	Paragould	78%	232
National Park Medical Center	Hot Springs	76%	101
Saint Anthony's Healthcare Center	Morrilton	76%	50
Saint Vincent Medical Center North	Sherwood	75%	71
Crittenden Memorial Hospital	West Memphis	74%	72
Drew Memorial Hospital	Monticello	74%	70
Summit Medical Center	Van Buren	74%	117
Baptist Health Medical Center	Little Rock	73%	251
De Witt Hospital & Nursing Home	De Witt	73%	26
Booneville Community Hospital	Booneville	70%	37
Helena Regional Medical Center	Helena	69%	108
Arkansas Heart Hospital	Little Rock	41%	29

14. Blood Culture Timing

Hospital Name	City	Rate	Cases
Randolph County Medical Center	Pocahontas	100%	30
Siloam Springs Memorial Hospital	Siloam Springs	100%	53
Medical Center of South Arkansas	El Dorado	99%	68
Saint Mary-Rogers Memorial Hospital	Rogers	99%	133
Ozark Health Medical Center	Clinton	98%	64
Conway Regional Medical Center	Conway	97%	106

Hospital Name	City	Rate	Cases
Saint Vincent Medical Center North	Sherwood	97%	30
Howard Memorial Hospital	Nashville	96%	27
Magnolia Hospital	Magnolia	96%	53
NEA Medical Center	Jonesboro	96%	93
Baptist Health Med Ctr-North Little Rock	North Little Rock	95%	60
Lawrence Memorial Hospital	Walnut Ridge	95%	43
National Park Medical Center	Hot Springs	95%	81
Saline Memorial Hospital	Benton	95%	106
Sparks Regional Medical Center	Fort Smith	95%	194
Baptist Health Medical Center	Heber Springs	94%	34
Stuttgart Regional Medical Center	Stuttgart	94%	49
Washington Regional Medical Center	Fayetteville	94%	72
Baxter Regional Medical Center	Mountain Home	93%	172
Crittenden Memorial Hospital	West Memphis	93%	61
Hot Springs County Medical Center	Malvern	93%	76
North Arkansas Regional Medical Center	Harrison	93%	130
Saint Bernard's Medical Center	Jonesboro	93%	210
Saint Joseph's Mercy Health Center	Hot Spgs Natl Pk	93%	233
White County Medical Center	Searcy	93%	138
White River Medical Center	Batesville	93%	132
Baptist Memorial Hospital-Forrest City	Forrest City	92%	65
Harris Hospital and Clinic	Newport	92%	36
Medical Park Hospital	Hope	92%	51
Saint Vincent Infirmary Medical Center	Little Rock	92%	166
Stone County Medical Center	Mountain View	92%	52
Great River Medical Center	Blytheville	91%	33
Northwest Medical Center	Springdale	91%	94
Saint John's Hospital-Berryville	Berryville	91%	44
Summit Medical Center	Van Buren	91%	87
Baptist Health Medical Center	Little Rock	90%	192
Helena Regional Medical Center	Helena	90%	62
Saint Edward Mercy Medical Center	Fort Smith	90%	92
Arkansas Methodist Hospital	Paragould	88%	161
Mena Medical Center	Mena	88%	34
Saint Mary's Regional Medical Center	Russellville	87%	129
UAMS Medical Center	Little Rock	86%	176
Jefferson Regional Medical Center	Pine Bluff	85%	134
Ouachita Medical Center	Camden	84%	73
Johnson Regional Medical Center	Clarksville	83%	71
NW Medical Center Benton County	Bentonville	78%	72

15. Influenza Vaccine

Hospital Name	City	Rate	Cases
Saint Edward Mercy Medical Center	Fort Smith	100%	26
White River Medical Center	Batesville	98%	59
Medical Park Hospital	Hope	96%	28
Saint Mary-Rogers Memorial Hospital	Rogers	94%	51
Summit Medical Center	Van Buren	94%	31
Saint Joseph's Mercy Health Center	Hot Spgs Natl Pk	89%	72
Saint Mary's Regional Medical Center	Russellville	88%	42
NW Medical Center Benton County	Bentonville	86%	35
North Arkansas Regional Medical Center	Harrison	83%	54
Ouachita Medical Center	Camden	76%	33
Stone County Medical Center	Mountain View	76%	25
Baptist Health Medical Center	Little Rock	75%	56
Medical Center of South Arkansas	El Dorado	75%	28
NEA Medical Center	Jonesboro	75%	44
Saint Bernard's Medical Center	Jonesboro	75%	76
Sparks Regional Medical Center	Fort Smith	75%	60
Helena Regional Medical Center	Helena	73%	33
Saint Vincent Infirmary Medical Center	Little Rock	71%	72
Northwest Medical Center	Springdale	64%	28
Washington Regional Medical Center	Fayetteville	58%	26
Jefferson Regional Medical Center	Pine Bluff	56%	52
Baxter Regional Medical Center	Mountain Home	51%	75
UAMS Medical Center	Little Rock	49%	51
Saline Memorial Hospital	Benton	38%	39
Conway Regional Medical Center	Conway	32%	38

16. Initial Antibiotic Timing

Hospital Name	City	Rate	Cases
De Witt Hospital & Nursing Home	De Witt	94%	31
Piggott Community Hospital	Piggott	94%	36
Booneville Community Hospital	Booneville	93%	45
Hot Springs County Medical Center	Malvern	93%	176
Baptist Health Medical Center	Arkadelphia	92%	53
Medical Park Hospital	Hope	92%	132
Saint John's Hospital-Berryville	Berryville	92%	97
Saint Mary-Rogers Memorial Hospital	Rogers	92%	200
Baxter Regional Medical Center	Mountain Home	91%	291
Chambers Memorial Hospital	Danville	91%	79
Helena Regional Medical Center	Helena	91%	151
Saint Mary's Regional Medical Center	Russellville	91%	195
Ashley County Medical Center	Crossett	90%	18

NOTE: Hospital profiles are in alphabetical order by state, then city, then hospital within the city; Rankings are sorted by rate in descending order and exclude hospitals with less than 25 cases; (1) The number of cases is too small (n<25) for purposes of reliably predicting hospital performance; (2) Measure reflects the hospital's indication that its submission was based upon a sample of its relevant discharges; (3) Rate reflects fewer than the maximum possible quarters of data for the measure; (4) Inaccurate information submitted and suppressed for one or more quarters; (5) No data is available from the hospital for this measure; Please refer to the User's Guide for a full explanation of data

Hospital Name	City	Rate	Cases
Lawrence Memorial Hospital	Walnut Ridge	90%	63
CrossRidge Community Hospital	Wynne	89%	92
Medical Center of South Arkansas	El Dorado	89%	112
North Arkansas Regional Medical Center	Harrison	89%	218
Stuttgart Regional Medical Center	Stuttgart	89%	91
NEA Medical Center	Jonesboro	88%	174
National Park Medical Center	Hot Springs	88%	129
Ozark Health Medical Center	Clinton	88%	98
Stone County Medical Center	Mountain View	88%	82
Randolph County Medical Center	Pocahontas	87%	69
Arkansas Heart Hospital	Little Rock	86%	29
Johnson Regional Medical Center	Clarksville	86%	143
Ouachita Medical Center	Camden	86%	142
Saline Memorial Hospital	Benton	86%	169
White County Medical Center	Searcy	86%	195
Baptist Health Medical Center	Heber Springs	85%	72
Conway Regional Medical Center	Conway	85%	189
Magnolia Hospital	Magnolia	85%	88
Summit Medical Center	Van Buren	85%	131
Howard Memorial Hospital	Nashville	84%	45
McGehee-Desha County Hospital	McGehee	84%	49
Rebsamen Medical Center	Jacksonville	84%	116
Saint Joseph's Mercy Health Center	Hot Spgs Natl Pk	84%	344
Baptist Memorial Hospital-Forrest City	Forrest City	83%	89
Chicot Memorial Hospital	Lake Village	83%	65
Harris Hospital and Clinic	Newport	83%	104
Arkansas Methodist Hospital	Paragould	82%	272
Baptist Health Med Ctr-North Little Rock	North Little Rock	82%	173
Siloam Springs Memorial Hospital	Siloam Springs	82%	127
NW Medical Center Benton County	Bentonville	81%	100
Bradley County Medical Center	Warren	80%	56
Saint Vincent Infirmary Medical Center	Little Rock	80%	264
Mena Medical Center	Mena	79%	81
Crittenden Memorial Hospital	West Memphis	78%	88
Saint Anthony's Healthcare Center	Morrilton	78%	45
Delta Memorial Hospital	Dumas	77%	31
White River Medical Center	Batesville	77%	184
Jefferson Regional Medical Center	Pine Bluff	76%	267
Saint Bernard's Medical Center	Jonesboro	76%	372
Drew Memorial Hospital	Monticello	75%	85
Southwest Regional Medical Centre	Little Rock	75%	48
Great River Medical Center	Blytheville	72%	68
Northwest Medical Center	Springdale	67%	158
Saint Vincent Medical Center North	Sherwood	67%	81
Sparks Regional Medical Center	Fort Smith	67%	317
Saint Edward Mercy Medical Center	Fort Smith	66%	140
Washington Regional Medical Center	Fayetteville	64%	138
South Mississippi County Regional Med Ctr	Osceola	63%	51
Baptist Health Medical Center	Little Rock	60%	345
UAMS Medical Center	Little Rock	55%	228

17. Oxygenation Assessment

Hospital Name	City	Rate	Cases
Arkansas Heart Hospital	Little Rock	100%	35
Arkansas Methodist Hospital	Paragould	100%	320
Ashley County Medical Center	Crossett	100%	31
Baptist Health Medical Center	Heber Springs	100%	88
Baptist Health Medical Center	Little Rock	100%	413
Baptist Health Med Ctr-North Little Rock	North Little Rock	100%	193
Baptist Memorial Hospital-Forrest City	Forrest City	100%	108
Baxter Regional Medical Center	Mountain Home	100%	341
Booneville Community Hospital	Booneville	100%	60
Chambers Memorial Hospital	Danville	100%	94
Conway Regional Medical Center	Conway	100%	238
CrossRidge Community Hospital	Wynne	100%	102
De Queen Regional Medical Center	De Queen	100%	29
Delta Memorial Hospital	Dumas	100%	37
Drew Memorial Hospital	Monticello	100%	108
Harris Hospital and Clinic	Newport	100%	107
Howard Memorial Hospital	Nashville	100%	49
Johnson Regional Medical Center	Clarksville	100%	165
Lawrence Memorial Hospital	Walnut Ridge	100%	77
McGehee-Desha County Hospital	McGehee	100%	59
Medical Center of South Arkansas	El Dorado	100%	130
Medical Park Hospital	Hope	100%	157
NEA Medical Center	Jonesboro	100%	212
NW Medical Center Benton County	Bentonville	100%	127
National Park Medical Center	Hot Springs	100%	144
North Arkansas Regional Medical Center	Harrison	100%	285
Northwest Medical Center	Springdale	100%	189
Ozark Health Medical Center	Clinton	100%	119
Piggott Community Hospital	Piggott	100%	45
Randolph County Medical Center	Pocahontas	100%	85
Rebsamen Medical Center	Jacksonville	100%	149

Hospital Name	City	Rate	Cases
Saint Anthony's Healthcare Center	Morrilton	100%	72
Saint Edward Mercy Medical Center	Fort Smith	100%	178
Saint John's Hospital-Berryville	Berryville	100%	122
Saint Joseph's Mercy Health Center	Hot Spgs Natl Pk	100%	433
Saint Mary's Regional Medical Center	Russellville	100%	253
Saint Mary-Rogers Memorial Hospital	Rogers	100%	251
Saint Vincent Infirmary Medical Center	Little Rock	100%	317
Saint Vincent Medical Center North	Sherwood	100%	87
Saline Memorial Hospital	Benton	100%	211
Southwest Regional Medical Centre	Little Rock	100%	61
Stone County Medical Center	Mountain View	100%	116
UAMS Medical Center	Little Rock	100%	335
Washington Regional Medical Center	Fayetteville	100%	169
White River Medical Center	Batesville	100%	229
Helena Regional Medical Center	Helena	99%	161
Magnolia Hospital	Magnolia	99%	103
Mena Medical Center	Mena	99%	95
Ouachita Medical Center	Camden	99%	167
Saint Bernard's Medical Center	Jonesboro	99%	448
Siloam Springs Memorial Hospital	Siloam Springs	99%	147
Sparks Regional Medical Center	Fort Smith	99%	390
Stuttgart Regional Medical Center	Stuttgart	99%	103
Summit Medical Center	Van Buren	99%	154
Baptist Health Medical Center	Arkadelphia	98%	59
Hot Springs County Medical Center	Malvern	98%	180
Jefferson Regional Medical Center	Pine Bluff	98%	298
Chicot Memorial Hospital	Lake Village	97%	71
South Mississippi County Regional Med Ctr	Osceola	97%	65
Great River Medical Center	Blytheville	96%	80
De Witt Hospital & Nursing Home	De Witt	94%	34
White County Medical Center	Searcy	94%	236
Crittenden Memorial Hospital	West Memphis	93%	105
Bradley County Medical Center	Warren	86%	66

18. Pneumococcal Vaccine

Hospital Name	City	Rate	Cases
Piggott Community Hospital	Piggott	100%	35
Baptist Memorial Hospital-Forrest City	Forrest City	97%	61
Summit Medical Center	Van Buren	95%	77
NEA Medical Center	Jonesboro	94%	131
Saint Joseph's Mercy Health Center	Hot Spgs Natl Pk	92%	282
Baptist Health Medical Center	Heber Springs	91%	56
Baxter Regional Medical Center	Mountain Home	91%	229
Medical Park Hospital	Hope	91%	101
Baptist Health Medical Center	Arkadelphia	90%	40
NW Medical Center Benton County	Bentonville	90%	94
Howard Memorial Hospital	Nashville	89%	35
Lawrence Memorial Hospital	Walnut Ridge	89%	54
Baptist Health Med Ctr-North Little Rock	North Little Rock	88%	113
Saint Mary's Regional Medical Center	Russellville	88%	135
Saint Mary-Rogers Memorial Hospital	Rogers	88%	170
Harris Hospital and Clinic	Newport	87%	54
Ozark Health Medical Center	Clinton	86%	80
South Mississippi County Regional Med Ctr	Osceola	86%	35
CrossRidge Community Hospital	Wynne	85%	79
White River Medical Center	Batesville	85%	144
Stuttgart Regional Medical Center	Stuttgart	84%	61
Arkansas Methodist Hospital	Paragould	83%	168
Medical Center of South Arkansas	El Dorado	81%	68
Saint Bernard's Medical Center	Jonesboro	81%	262
Saint Edward Mercy Medical Center	Fort Smith	81%	95
North Arkansas Regional Medical Center	Harrison	79%	192
National Park Medical Center	Hot Springs	78%	78
Baptist Health Medical Center	Little Rock	76%	229
Stone County Medical Center	Mountain View	75%	76
Saint Anthony's Healthcare Center	Morrilton	73%	48
Saint John's Hospital-Berryville	Berryville	73%	79
Saint Vincent Infirmary Medical Center	Little Rock	72%	191
Johnson Regional Medical Center	Clarksville	70%	99
Magnolia Hospital	Magnolia	70%	61
White County Medical Center	Searcy	70%	163
Chicot Memorial Hospital	Lake Village	68%	40
Northwest Medical Center	Springdale	68%	116
Jefferson Regional Medical Center	Pine Bluff	66%	155
Sparks Regional Medical Center	Fort Smith	66%	212
Washington Regional Medical Center	Fayetteville	64%	98
McGehee-Desha County Hospital	McGehee	62%	34
Randolph County Medical Center	Pocahontas	62%	61
Helena Regional Medical Center	Helena	59%	95
Ouachita Medical Center	Camden	59%	104
Booneville Community Hospital	Booneville	55%	38
Crittenden Memorial Hospital	West Memphis	52%	46
Siloam Springs Memorial Hospital	Siloam Springs	51%	75
Hot Springs County Medical Center	Malvern	50%	98

NOTE: Hospital profiles are in alphabetical order by state, then city, then hospital within the city; Rankings are sorted by rate in descending order and exclude hospitals with less than 25 cases; (1) The number of cases is too small (n<25) for purposes of reliably predicting hospital performance; (2) Measure reflects the hospital's indication that its submission was based upon a sample of its relevant discharges; (3) Rate reflects fewer than the maximum possible quarters of data for the measure; (4) Inaccurate information submitted and suppressed for one or more quarters; (5) No data is available from the hospital for this measure; Please refer to the User's Guide for a full explanation of data

Mena Medical Center	Mena	49%	67
Saint Vincent Medical Center North	Sherwood	49%	49
Conway Regional Medical Center	Conway	47%	142
Rebsamen Medical Center	Jacksonville	44%	95
Saline Memorial Hospital	Benton	39%	111
Southwest Regional Medical Centre	Little Rock	39%	28
UAMS Medical Center	Little Rock	36%	118
Drew Memorial Hospital	Monticello	35%	52
Chambers Memorial Hospital	Danville	34%	56
Arkansas Heart Hospital	Little Rock	31%	26
Great River Medical Center	Blytheville	27%	33
Bradley County Medical Center	Warren	21%	39

19. Smoking Cessation Advice

Hospital Name	City	Rate	Cases
Baptist Memorial Hospital-Forrest City	Forrest City	100%	28
Drew Memorial Hospital	Monticello	100%	30
Medical Center of South Arkansas	El Dorado	100%	40
Medical Park Hospital	Hope	100%	38
Baxter Regional Medical Center	Mountain Home	99%	96
UAMS Medical Center	Little Rock	99%	106
NEA Medical Center	Jonesboro	98%	65
Saint Vincent Infirmary Medical Center	Little Rock	98%	93
Arkansas Methodist Hospital	Paragould	96%	112
Baptist Health Medical Center	Little Rock	96%	76
Saint Joseph's Mercy Health Center	Hot Spgs Natl Pk	96%	118
Baptist Health Med Ctr-North Little Rock	North Little Rock	95%	39
Saint Mary-Rogers Memorial Hospital	Rogers	95%	61
Saint Bernard's Medical Center	Jonesboro	94%	172
Conway Regional Medical Center	Conway	93%	54
National Park Medical Center	Hot Springs	93%	58
White County Medical Center	Searcy	93%	54
Saint Edward Mercy Medical Center	Fort Smith	92%	49
North Arkansas Regional Medical Center	Harrison	89%	61
Stuttgart Regional Medical Center	Stuttgart	89%	28
Harris Hospital and Clinic	Newport	88%	33
Helena Regional Medical Center	Helena	88%	41
White River Medical Center	Batesville	84%	50
Saint Mary's Regional Medical Center	Russellville	83%	65
Hot Springs County Medical Center	Malvern	82%	49
Northwest Medical Center	Springdale	81%	52
Washington Regional Medical Center	Fayetteville	80%	45
Jefferson Regional Medical Center	Pine Bluff	79%	73
Sparks Regional Medical Center	Fort Smith	79%	86
NW Medical Center Benton County	Bentonville	78%	27
Summit Medical Center	Van Buren	72%	60
Ozark Health Medical Center	Clinton	71%	28
Siloam Springs Memorial Hospital	Siloam Springs	69%	35
Johnson Regional Medical Center	Clarksville	67%	51
Saline Memorial Hospital	Benton	63%	38

Surgical Infection Prevention

20. Prophylactic Antibiotic Given

Hospital Name	City	Rate	Cases
NEA Medical Center	Jonesboro	97%	379
Medical Center of South Arkansas	El Dorado	96%	535
North Arkansas Regional Medical Center	Harrison	96%	185
Saint Joseph's Mercy Health Center	Hot Spgs Natl Pk	95%	587
Saint Bernard's Medical Center	Jonesboro	94%	728
White River Medical Center	Batesville	94%	354
Baptist Memorial Hospital-Forrest City	Forrest City	93%	55
Healthpark Hospital	Hot Springs	93%	214
Saint Mary's Regional Medical Center	Russellville	93%	376
Arkansas Methodist Hospital	Paragould	92%	117
Baptist Health Med Ctr-North Little Rock	North Little Rock	92%	747
Arkansas Heart Hospital	Little Rock	91%	605
Rebsamen Medical Center	Jacksonville	89%	36
Saint Edward Mercy Medical Center	Fort Smith	89%	227
National Park Medical Center	Hot Springs	88%	213
Baptist Health Medical Center	Little Rock	85%	486
Saint Vincent Infirmary Medical Center	Little Rock	83%	221
NW Medical Center Benton County	Bentonville	82%	254
Northwest Medical Center	Springdale	81%	420
Arkansas Surgical Hospital	North Little Rock	80%	586
Mena Medical Center	Mena	80%	30
Summit Medical Center	Van Buren	80%	82
Saint Mary-Rogers Memorial Hospital	Rogers	79%	224
Baxter Regional Medical Center	Mountain Home	78%	713
White County Medical Center	Searcy	78%	331
Conway Regional Medical Center	Conway	76%	617
Jefferson Regional Medical Center	Pine Bluff	74%	933
Surgical Hospital of Jonesboro	Jonesboro	74%	192
UAMS Medical Center	Little Rock	74%	303

21. Prophylactic Antibiotic Selection

Hospital Name	City	Rate	Cases
Arkansas Heart Hospital	Little Rock	100%	186
Arkansas Surgical Hospital	North Little Rock	100%	185
Summit Medical Center	Van Buren	100%	26
Baptist Health Med Ctr-North Little Rock	North Little Rock	99%	192
Medical Center of South Arkansas	El Dorado	99%	150
NEA Medical Center	Jonesboro	99%	105
Saint Vincent Infirmary Medical Center	Little Rock	99%	74
White County Medical Center	Searcy	99%	149
North Arkansas Regional Medical Center	Harrison	97%	35
Northwest Medical Center	Springdale	97%	118
Saint Bernard's Medical Center	Jonesboro	97%	144
Saint Joseph's Mercy Health Center	Hot Spgs Natl Pk	97%	58
Saint Mary's Regional Medical Center	Russellville	97%	101
Sparks Regional Medical Center	Fort Smith	96%	98
Saint Edward Mercy Medical Center	Fort Smith	95%	65
Saint Mary-Rogers Memorial Hospital	Rogers	95%	62
Healthpark Hospital	Hot Springs	94%	34
NW Medical Center Benton County	Bentonville	94%	62
Washington Regional Medical Center	Fayetteville	94%	79
White River Medical Center	Batesville	94%	132
Crittenden Memorial Hospital	West Memphis	93%	30
Jefferson Regional Medical Center	Pine Bluff	91%	237
Arkansas Methodist Hospital	Paragould	90%	29
National Park Medical Center	Hot Springs	90%	42
Baptist Health Medical Center	Little Rock	88%	158
Saline Memorial Hospital	Benton	88%	51
Baxter Regional Medical Center	Mountain Home	86%	170
Conway Regional Medical Center	Conway	81%	146
UAMS Medical Center	Little Rock	56%	73

22. Prophylactic Antibiotic Stopped

Hospital Name	City	Rate	Cases
Saint Vincent Medical Center North	Sherwood	99%	84
Arkansas Methodist Hospital	Paragould	94%	113
Medical Center of South Arkansas	El Dorado	93%	520
Mena Medical Center	Mena	93%	27
Rebsamen Medical Center	Jacksonville	93%	29
Surgical Hospital of Jonesboro	Jonesboro	92%	190
Saint Mary-Rogers Memorial Hospital	Rogers	90%	212
White County Medical Center	Searcy	90%	300
Bradley County Medical Center	Warren	89%	27
North Arkansas Regional Medical Center	Harrison	89%	174
UAMS Medical Center	Little Rock	88%	292
Saint Bernard's Medical Center	Jonesboro	87%	698
Baptist Health Med Ctr-North Little Rock	North Little Rock	86%	720
National Park Medical Center	Hot Springs	86%	200
Ouachita Medical Center	Camden	84%	62
White River Medical Center	Batesville	82%	342
Arkansas Heart Hospital	Little Rock	81%	595
Baptist Health Medical Center	Little Rock	80%	475
Saint Joseph's Mercy Health Center	Hot Spgs Natl Pk	79%	540
Jefferson Regional Medical Center	Pine Bluff	77%	892
Saint Vincent Infirmary Medical Center	Little Rock	77%	216
Baptist Memorial Hospital-Forrest City	Forrest City	76%	54
Saint Edward Mercy Medical Center	Fort Smith	76%	221
Sparks Regional Medical Center	Fort Smith	76%	287
Arkansas Surgical Hospital	North Little Rock	72%	584
NEA Medical Center	Jonesboro	71%	375
Saint Mary's Regional Medical Center	Russellville	71%	369
Baxter Regional Medical Center	Mountain Home	70%	681
Crittenden Memorial Hospital	West Memphis	70%	84
Great River Medical Center	Blytheville	68%	47
Conway Regional Medical Center	Conway	67%	601
Washington Regional Medical Center	Fayetteville	64%	189
Southwest Regional Medical Centre	Little Rock	57%	83
Northwest Medical Center	Springdale	56%	409
Harris Hospital and Clinic	Newport	52%	64
NW Medical Center Benton County	Bentonville	50%	242
Randolph County Medical Center	Pocahontas	44%	32
Saline Memorial Hospital	Benton	36%	225

NOTE: Hospital profiles are in alphabetical order by state, then city, then hospital within the city; Rankings are sorted by rate in descending order and exclude hospitals with less than 25 cases; (1) The number of cases is too small (n<25) for purposes of reliably predicting hospital performance; (2) Measure reflects the hospital's indication that its submission was based upon a sample of its relevant discharges; (3) Rate reflects fewer than the maximum possible quarters of data for the measure; (4) Inaccurate information submitted and suppressed for one or more quarters; (5) No data is available from the hospital for this measure; Please refer to the User's Guide for a full explanation of data

Healthpark Hospital	Hot Springs	28%	191
Summit Medical Center	Van Buren	27%	82
Johnson Regional Medical Center	Clarksville	17%	63

Pregnancy Care

23. Inpatient Neonatal Mortality

Hospital Name	City	Rate	Cases
Rebsamen Medical Center	Jacksonville	0.00%	466
Saline Memorial Hospital	Benton	0.00%	492
Sparks Regional Medical Center	Fort Smith	0.00%	1135
Saint Bernard's Medical Center	Jonesboro	0.07%	1412
Northwest Medical Center	Springdale	0.38%	3661
Saint Vincent Infirmary Medical Center	Little Rock	0.54%	2042
Baptist Health Medical Center	Little Rock	0.60%	2853
Crittenden Memorial Hospital	West Memphis	1.00%	799
UAMS Medical Center	Little Rock	1.97%	2029

24. Third or Fourth Degree Laceration

Hospital Name	City	Rate	Cases
Crittenden Memorial Hospital	West Memphis	1.05%	569
Rebsamen Medical Center	Jacksonville	1.57%	318
Baptist Health Medical Center	Little Rock	2.96%	1553
Northwest Medical Center	Springdale	3.31%	2511
Sparks Regional Medical Center	Fort Smith	3.84%	730
Saint Bernard's Medical Center	Jonesboro	4.00%	925
Saline Memorial Hospital	Benton	4.68%	342
Saint Vincent Infirmary Medical Center	Little Rock	5.88%	1446
UAMS Medical Center	Little Rock	6.37%	1224

NOTE: Hospital profiles are in alphabetical order by state, then city, then hospital within the city; Rankings are sorted by rate in descending order and exclude hospitals with less than 25 cases; (1) The number of cases is too small (n<25) for purposes of reliably predicting hospital performance; (2) Measure reflects the hospital's indication that its submission was based upon a sample of its relevant discharges; (3) Rate reflects fewer than the maximum possible quarters of data for the measure; (4) Inaccurate information submitted and suppressed for one or more quarters; (5) No data is available from the hospital for this measure; Please refer to the User's Guide for a full explanation of data

Baptist Health Medical Center

3050 Twin Rivers Drive
Arkadelphia, AR 71923
URL: www.baptist-health.org
Ownership: Voluntary non-profit - Other
Emergency Services: Yes

Phone: 870-245-2622
Fax: 870-245-1198

Accredited: Yes
Licensed Beds: 57

Key Personnel:
Emergency Room Director . . . . Tom Tobin
Respiratory . . . . Phyllis Morris

Measure	Cases	This Hospital	State Average	U.S. Average	Top Hospital
Heart Attack Care					
ACE Inhibitor or ARB for LVSD[3]	0	-	82%	82%	100%
Aspirin at Arrival[1,3]	2	50%	88%	92%	100%
Aspirin at Discharge[1,3]	2	50%	87%	90%	100%
Beta Blocker at Arrival[1,3]	2	100%	82%	87%	100%
Beta Blocker at Discharge[1,3]	2	100%	86%	90%	100%
Fibrinolytic Medication Timing[3]	0	-	41%	31%	100%
PCI Within 90 Minutes of Arrival	0	-	46%	54%	95%
Smoking Cessation Advice[3]	0	-	91%	88%	100%
Heart Failure Care					
ACE Inhibitor or ARB for LVSD[1]	8	50%	78%	82%	100%
Discharge Instructions	33	85%	65%	61%	93%
Evaluation of LVS Function	46	78%	81%	83%	99%
Smoking Cessation Advice[1]	3	100%	86%	82%	100%
Pneumonia Care					
Appropriate Initial Antibiotic[1]	23	83%	83%	83%	94%
Blood Culture Timing[1]	19	100%	93%	90%	100%
Influenza Vaccine[1]	11	100%	70%	70%	100%
Initial Antibiotic Timing	53	92%	82%	80%	93%
Oxygenation Assessment	59	98%	99%	99%	100%
Pneumococcal Vaccine	40	90%	68%	69%	94%
Smoking Cessation Advice[1]	7	86%	83%	80%	100%
Surgical Infection Prevention					
Prophylactic Antibiotic Given[1,3]	15	100%	73%	77%	95%
Prophylactic Antibiotic Selection[1]	15	100%	90%	90%	100%
Prophylactic Antibiotic Stopped[1,3]	15	67%	74%	72%	95%
Pregnancy Care					
Inpatient Neonatal Mortality	-	-	-	-	-
Third or Fourth Degree Laceration	-	-	3.82%	3.63%	3.27%

White River Medical Center

1710 Harrison Street
PO Box 2197
Batesville, AR 72501
E-mail: smace@mail.wrmc.com
URL: www.wrmc.com
Ownership: Voluntary non-profit - Private
Emergency Services: Yes

Phone: 870-262-1200
Fax: 870-612-6094

Accredited: No
Licensed Beds: 167

Key Personnel:
CEO. . . . . Gary L Bebow
Chief of Medical Staff. Neaville Germ, MD
Director of Cardiology/Cardiac Lab. . . . . Robert Wright
Emergency Room . . . . Sisy Ford
Emergency Room . . . . Jeff Mares, RN
Director Medical/Surgical Nursing . . . . Gwenda Dobbs, RN
Director Respiratory Therapy . . . . Jay Williams

Measure	Cases	This Hospital	State Average	U.S. Average	Top Hospital
Heart Attack Care					
ACE Inhibitor or ARB for LVSD	54	96%	82%	82%	100%
Aspirin at Arrival	136	99%	88%	92%	100%
Aspirin at Discharge	132	96%	87%	90%	100%
Beta Blocker at Arrival	119	100%	82%	87%	100%
Beta Blocker at Discharge	144	96%	86%	90%	100%
Fibrinolytic Medication Timing[1]	12	50%	41%	31%	100%
PCI Within 90 Minutes of Arrival[1]	4	75%	46%	54%	95%
Smoking Cessation Advice	52	98%	91%	88%	100%
Heart Failure Care					
ACE Inhibitor or ARB for LVSD	125	95%	78%	82%	100%
Discharge Instructions	253	82%	65%	61%	93%
Evaluation of LVS Function	333	100%	81%	83%	99%
Smoking Cessation Advice	54	93%	86%	82%	100%

Measure	Cases	This Hospital	State Average	U.S. Average	Top Hospital
Pneumonia Care					
Appropriate Initial Antibiotic	132	91%	83%	83%	94%
Blood Culture Timing	132	93%	93%	90%	100%
Influenza Vaccine	59	98%	70%	70%	100%
Initial Antibiotic Timing	184	77%	82%	80%	93%
Oxygenation Assessment	229	100%	99%	99%	100%
Pneumococcal Vaccine	144	85%	68%	69%	94%
Smoking Cessation Advice	50	84%	83%	80%	100%
Surgical Infection Prevention					
Prophylactic Antibiotic Given[3]	354	94%	73%	77%	95%
Prophylactic Antibiotic Selection	132	94%	90%	90%	100%
Prophylactic Antibiotic Stopped[3]	342	82%	74%	72%	95%
Pregnancy Care					
Inpatient Neonatal Mortality	-	-	-	-	-
Third or Fourth Degree Laceration	-	-	3.82%	3.63%	3.27%

Saline Memorial Hospital

1 Medical Park Drive
Benton, AR 72015
E-mail: ContactUs@salinememorial.org
URL: www.salinememorial.org
Ownership: Voluntary non-profit - Private
Emergency Services: Yes

Phone: 501-776-6000
Fax: 501-776-6768

Accredited: Yes
Licensed Beds: 153

Key Personnel:
CEO. . . . . James Richardson
Chief of Medical Staff. . . . . Daniel Scartaya
Emergency Room Head. . . . . Melissa Dockery

Measure	Cases	This Hospital	State Average	U.S. Average	Top Hospital
Heart Attack Care					
ACE Inhibitor or ARB for LVSD[1]	4	50%	82%	82%	100%
Aspirin at Arrival	43	93%	88%	92%	100%
Aspirin at Discharge[1]	13	54%	87%	90%	100%
Beta Blocker at Arrival	33	73%	82%	87%	100%
Beta Blocker at Discharge[1]	12	83%	86%	90%	100%
Fibrinolytic Medication Timing[1]	7	57%	41%	31%	100%
PCI Within 90 Minutes of Arrival	0	-	46%	54%	95%
Smoking Cessation Advice[1]	4	75%	91%	88%	100%
Heart Failure Care					
ACE Inhibitor or ARB for LVSD	52	50%	78%	82%	100%
Discharge Instructions	90	42%	65%	61%	93%
Evaluation of LVS Function	116	92%	81%	83%	99%
Smoking Cessation Advice[1]	15	93%	86%	82%	100%
Pneumonia Care					
Appropriate Initial Antibiotic	117	81%	83%	83%	94%
Blood Culture Timing	106	95%	93%	90%	100%
Influenza Vaccine	39	38%	70%	70%	100%
Initial Antibiotic Timing	169	86%	82%	80%	93%
Oxygenation Assessment	211	100%	99%	99%	100%
Pneumococcal Vaccine	111	39%	68%	69%	94%
Smoking Cessation Advice	38	63%	83%	80%	100%
Surgical Infection Prevention					
Prophylactic Antibiotic Given	224	60%	73%	77%	95%
Prophylactic Antibiotic Selection	51	88%	90%	90%	100%
Prophylactic Antibiotic Stopped	225	36%	74%	72%	95%
Pregnancy Care					
Inpatient Neonatal Mortality	492	0.00%	-	-	-
Third or Fourth Degree Laceration	342	4.68%	3.82%	3.63%	3.27%

NW Medical Center Benton County

3000 Medical Center Parkway
Bentonville, AR 72712
URL: www.northwesthealth.com
Ownership: Proprietary
Emergency Services: Yes

Phone: 479-553-1000
Fax: 479-553-1900

Accredited: Yes
Licensed Beds: 73

Key Personnel:
CEO. . . . . Gary Looper

Measure	Cases	This Hospital	State Average	U.S. Average	Top Hospital
Heart Attack Care					
ACE Inhibitor or ARB for LVSD	51	94%	82%	82%	100%
Aspirin at Arrival	143	99%	88%	92%	100%

NOTE: Hospital profiles are in alphabetical order by state, then city, then hospital within the city; Rankings are sorted by rate in descending order and exclude hospitals with less than 25 cases; (1) The number of cases is too small (n<25) for purposes of reliably predicting hospital performance; (2) Measure reflects the hospital's indication that its submission was based upon a sample of its relevant discharges; (3) Rate reflects fewer than the maximum possible quarters of data for the measure; (4) Inaccurate information submitted and suppressed for one or more quarters; (5) No data is available from the hospital for this measure; Please refer to the User's Guide for a full explanation of data

Aspirin at Discharge	126	97%	87%	90%	100%
Beta Blocker at Arrival	104	94%	82%	87%	100%
Beta Blocker at Discharge	133	98%	86%	90%	100%
Fibrinolytic Medication Timing[1]	2	0%	41%	31%	100%
PCI Within 90 Minutes of Arrival[1]	5	0%	46%	54%	95%
Smoking Cessation Advice	57	95%	91%	88%	100%
Heart Failure Care					
ACE Inhibitor or ARB for LVSD	38	82%	78%	82%	100%
Discharge Instructions	75	80%	65%	61%	93%
Evaluation of LVS Function	93	90%	81%	83%	99%
Smoking Cessation Advice[1]	24	88%	86%	82%	100%
Pneumonia Care					
Appropriate Initial Antibiotic	71	82%	83%	83%	94%
Blood Culture Timing	72	78%	93%	90%	100%
Influenza Vaccine	35	86%	70%	70%	100%
Initial Antibiotic Timing	100	81%	82%	80%	93%
Oxygenation Assessment	127	100%	99%	99%	100%
Pneumococcal Vaccine	94	90%	68%	69%	94%
Smoking Cessation Advice	27	78%	83%	80%	100%
Surgical Infection Prevention					
Prophylactic Antibiotic Given	254	82%	73%	77%	95%
Prophylactic Antibiotic Selection	62	94%	90%	90%	100%
Prophylactic Antibiotic Stopped	242	50%	74%	72%	95%
Pregnancy Care					
Inpatient Neonatal Mortality	-	-	-	-	-
Third or Fourth Degree Laceration	-	-	3.82%	3.63%	3.27%

Saint John's Hospital-Berryville

214 Carter Street
Berryville, AR 72616

Toll-Free: 800-827-3355
Phone: 870-423-3355
Fax: 870-423-5233

E-mail: info@stjohnsberryville.com
URL: www.stjohnsberryville.com
Ownership: Voluntary non-profit - Church
Emergency Services: No

Accredited: Yes
Licensed Beds: 50

Key Personnel:
CEO . . . . Rudy Darling
Chief Medical Staff. Richard Taylor, MD
Emergency Room . . . . Larry Ginn
Director Medical/Surgical Nursing . . . . Wendy Turner
OB/GYN Womens Health. . . . . Eric Spann, MD
Director Radiology . . . . Gary Jordan
Director Respiratory Therapy . . . . Brian Harp

Measure	Cases	This Hospital	State Average	U.S. Average	Top Hospital
Heart Attack Care					
ACE Inhibitor or ARB for LVSD[1]	2	100%	82%	82%	100%
Aspirin at Arrival[1]	13	85%	88%	92%	100%
Aspirin at Discharge[1]	12	92%	87%	90%	100%
Beta Blocker at Arrival[1]	16	75%	82%	87%	100%
Beta Blocker at Discharge[1]	10	100%	86%	90%	100%
Fibrinolytic Medication Timing	0	-	41%	31%	100%
PCI Within 90 Minutes of Arrival	0	-	46%	54%	95%
Smoking Cessation Advice[1]	3	100%	91%	88%	100%
Heart Failure Care					
ACE Inhibitor or ARB for LVSD[1]	6	100%	78%	82%	100%
Discharge Instructions	41	29%	65%	61%	93%
Evaluation of LVS Function	49	55%	81%	83%	99%
Smoking Cessation Advice[1]	7	43%	86%	82%	100%
Pneumonia Care					
Appropriate Initial Antibiotic	95	88%	83%	83%	94%
Blood Culture Timing	44	91%	93%	90%	100%
Influenza Vaccine[1]	22	73%	70%	70%	100%
Initial Antibiotic Timing	97	92%	82%	80%	93%
Oxygenation Assessment	122	100%	99%	99%	100%
Pneumococcal Vaccine	79	73%	68%	69%	94%
Smoking Cessation Advice[1]	23	61%	83%	80%	100%
Surgical Infection Prevention					
Prophylactic Antibiotic Given[5]	-	-	73%	77%	95%
Prophylactic Antibiotic Selection[5]	-	-	90%	90%	100%
Prophylactic Antibiotic Stopped[5]	-	-	74%	72%	95%
Pregnancy Care					
Inpatient Neonatal Mortality	-	-	-	-	-

Third or Fourth Degree Laceration			-	-	3.82%	3.63%	3.27%

Great River Medical Center

1520 N Division Street
Blytheville, AR 72315
E-mail: info@greatrivermc.com
URL: www.greatrivermc.com
Ownership: Voluntary non-profit - Other
Emergency Services: Yes

Phone: 870-838-7300
Fax: 870-838-7493

Accredited: Yes
Licensed Beds: 168

Key Personnel:
Administrator . . . . Ian Watson
Chief Staff . . . . Karen Hester, MD
Emergency Room . . . . Lisa Alsup
Infection Control. . . . . Willa Warren
ICU . . . . Creseana Gist
Respiratory/Cardiopulmonary. . . . . Jim Wages

Measure	Cases	This Hospital	State Average	U.S. Average	Top Hospital
Heart Attack Care					
ACE Inhibitor or ARB for LVSD[1]	1	100%	82%	82%	100%
Aspirin at Arrival	31	74%	88%	92%	100%
Aspirin at Discharge[1]	17	82%	87%	90%	100%
Beta Blocker at Arrival	30	73%	82%	87%	100%
Beta Blocker at Discharge[1]	17	88%	86%	90%	100%
Fibrinolytic Medication Timing	0	-	41%	31%	100%
PCI Within 90 Minutes of Arrival	0	-	46%	54%	95%
Smoking Cessation Advice[1]	6	100%	91%	88%	100%
Heart Failure Care					
ACE Inhibitor or ARB for LVSD	30	73%	78%	82%	100%
Discharge Instructions	62	48%	65%	61%	93%
Evaluation of LVS Function	76	87%	81%	83%	99%
Smoking Cessation Advice	30	83%	86%	82%	100%
Pneumonia Care					
Appropriate Initial Antibiotic	54	85%	83%	83%	94%
Blood Culture Timing	33	91%	93%	90%	100%
Influenza Vaccine[1]	14	36%	70%	70%	100%
Initial Antibiotic Timing	68	72%	82%	80%	93%
Oxygenation Assessment	80	96%	99%	99%	100%
Pneumococcal Vaccine	33	27%	68%	69%	94%
Smoking Cessation Advice[1]	18	89%	83%	80%	100%
Surgical Infection Prevention					
Prophylactic Antibiotic Given[2]	49	27%	73%	77%	95%
Prophylactic Antibiotic Selection[1,2]	11	91%	90%	90%	100%
Prophylactic Antibiotic Stopped[2]	47	68%	74%	72%	95%
Pregnancy Care					
Inpatient Neonatal Mortality[5]	0	0.00%	-	-	-
Third or Fourth Degree Laceration[5]	0	0.00%	3.82%	3.63%	3.27%

Booneville Community Hospital

880 W Main Street
PO Box 290
Booneville, AR 72927
E-mail: gldelforge@hotmail.com
URL: www.boonevillehospital.com
Ownership: Government - Local
Emergency Services: Yes

Phone: 479-675-2800
Fax: 479-675-4842

Accredited: No
Licensed Beds: 25

Key Personnel:
CEO . . . . Gary DelForge
Chief Medical Staff. William Daniel, MD
Emergency Room . . . . Erum Akhter, MD
Emergency Room . . . . LeAnn Box
Director Infection/Disease Control . . . . Nikki Parker
Medical/Surgical Nursing . . . . LeAnn Box, RN
Chief Radiology . . . . Karyn Johnson
Respiratory/Therapy Director . . . . Mara Cree

Measure	Cases	This Hospital	State Average	U.S. Average	Top Hospital
Heart Attack Care					
ACE Inhibitor or ARB for LVSD[3]	0	-	82%	82%	100%
Aspirin at Arrival[1,3]	2	50%	88%	92%	100%
Aspirin at Discharge[1,3]	1	100%	87%	90%	100%
Beta Blocker at Arrival[1,3]	1	0%	82%	87%	100%

NOTE: Hospital profiles are in alphabetical order by state, then city, then hospital within the city; Rankings are sorted by rate in descending order and exclude hospitals with less than 25 cases; (1) The number of cases is too small (n<25) for purposes of reliably predicting hospital performance; (2) Measure reflects the hospital's indication that its submission was based upon a sample of its relevant discharges; (3) Rate reflects fewer than the maximum possible quarters of data for the measure; (4) Inaccurate information submitted and suppressed for one or more quarters; (5) No data is available from the hospital for this measure; Please refer to the User's Guide for a full explanation of data

Beta Blocker at Discharge[1,3]	1	100%	86%	90%	100%
Fibrinolytic Medication Timing[3]	0	-	41%	31%	100%
PCI Within 90 Minutes of Arrival	0	-	46%	54%	95%
Smoking Cessation Advice[3]	0	-	91%	88%	100%
Heart Failure Care					
ACE Inhibitor or ARB for LVSD[1]	5	60%	78%	82%	100%
Discharge Instructions[1]	19	63%	65%	61%	93%
Evaluation of LVS Function	34	65%	81%	83%	99%
Smoking Cessation Advice[1]	6	83%	86%	82%	100%
Pneumonia Care					
Appropriate Initial Antibiotic	37	70%	83%	83%	94%
Blood Culture Timing[1]	5	100%	93%	90%	100%
Influenza Vaccine[1]	10	30%	70%	70%	100%
Initial Antibiotic Timing	45	93%	82%	80%	93%
Oxygenation Assessment	60	100%	99%	99%	100%
Pneumococcal Vaccine	38	55%	68%	69%	94%
Smoking Cessation Advice[1]	16	69%	83%	80%	100%
Surgical Infection Prevention					
Prophylactic Antibiotic Given[5]	-	-	73%	77%	95%
Prophylactic Antibiotic Selection[5]	-	-	90%	90%	100%
Prophylactic Antibiotic Stopped[5]	-	-	74%	72%	95%
Pregnancy Care					
Inpatient Neonatal Mortality	-	-	-	-	-
Third or Fourth Degree Laceration	-	-	3.82%	3.63%	3.27%

Ouachita Medical Center

638 California Street
Camden, AR 71701
E-mail: ocmc@ipa.net
URL: www.ouachitamedcenter.com
Ownership: Voluntary non-profit - Private
Emergency Services: Yes

Phone: 870-836-1000
Fax: 870-836-1358

Accredited: Yes
Licensed Beds: 98

Key Personnel:
Chairman/CEO. . . . . CC McAllister
Chief Medical Staff. . . . . Milton Brinson
Director Respiratory Therapy . . . . Debra Radford

Measure	Cases	This Hospital	State Average	U.S. Average	Top Hospital
Heart Attack Care					
ACE Inhibitor or ARB for LVSD[1]	4	75%	82%	82%	100%
Aspirin at Arrival[1]	23	83%	88%	92%	100%
Aspirin at Discharge[1]	10	90%	87%	90%	100%
Beta Blocker at Arrival[1]	23	91%	82%	87%	100%
Beta Blocker at Discharge[1]	14	86%	86%	90%	100%
Fibrinolytic Medication Timing[1]	4	75%	41%	31%	100%
PCI Within 90 Minutes of Arrival	0	-	46%	54%	95%
Smoking Cessation Advice[1]	1	100%	91%	88%	100%
Heart Failure Care					
ACE Inhibitor or ARB for LVSD	28	96%	78%	82%	100%
Discharge Instructions	87	62%	65%	61%	93%
Evaluation of LVS Function	105	67%	81%	83%	99%
Smoking Cessation Advice[1]	19	89%	86%	82%	100%
Pneumonia Care					
Appropriate Initial Antibiotic	91	84%	83%	83%	94%
Blood Culture Timing	73	84%	93%	90%	100%
Influenza Vaccine	33	76%	70%	70%	100%
Initial Antibiotic Timing	142	86%	82%	80%	93%
Oxygenation Assessment	167	99%	99%	99%	100%
Pneumococcal Vaccine	104	59%	68%	69%	94%
Smoking Cessation Advice[1]	24	100%	83%	80%	100%
Surgical Infection Prevention					
Prophylactic Antibiotic Given[1,3]	15	20%	73%	77%	95%
Prophylactic Antibiotic Selection[1]	16	100%	90%	90%	100%
Prophylactic Antibiotic Stopped[3]	62	84%	74%	72%	95%
Pregnancy Care					
Inpatient Neonatal Mortality	-	-	-	-	-
Third or Fourth Degree Laceration	-	-	3.82%	3.63%	3.27%

Johnson Regional Medical Center

Alternate Name: Johnson County Regional Hospital

1100 Poplar Street
Clarksville, AR 72830
URL: www.jrmc.com
Ownership: Voluntary non-profit - Private
Emergency Services: Yes

Phone: 479-754-5454
Fax: 501-754-4019

Accredited: No
Licensed Beds: 68

Key Personnel:
Administrator/CEO . . . . Ken Wood
Chief Medical Staff. . . . . Scott Kuykendall
Emergency Room . . . . Milton Teal
Infection Control. . . . . Renay Storms
ICU . . . . Liza Gerot
OB/GYN Womens Health. . . . . Linda Tate
Respiratory/Cardiopulmonary. . . . . Deanna Yates

Measure	Cases	This Hospital	State Average	U.S. Average	Top Hospital
Heart Attack Care					
ACE Inhibitor or ARB for LVSD[1]	4	75%	82%	82%	100%
Aspirin at Arrival[1]	24	83%	88%	92%	100%
Aspirin at Discharge[1]	17	82%	87%	90%	100%
Beta Blocker at Arrival[1]	19	84%	82%	87%	100%
Beta Blocker at Discharge[1]	11	100%	86%	90%	100%
Fibrinolytic Medication Timing[1]	2	100%	41%	31%	100%
PCI Within 90 Minutes of Arrival	0	-	46%	54%	95%
Smoking Cessation Advice[1]	3	67%	91%	88%	100%
Heart Failure Care					
ACE Inhibitor or ARB for LVSD[1]	16	81%	78%	82%	100%
Discharge Instructions	71	55%	65%	61%	93%
Evaluation of LVS Function	84	83%	81%	83%	99%
Smoking Cessation Advice[1]	13	62%	86%	82%	100%
Pneumonia Care					
Appropriate Initial Antibiotic	105	92%	83%	83%	94%
Blood Culture Timing	71	83%	93%	90%	100%
Influenza Vaccine[4,5]	-	-	70%	70%	100%
Initial Antibiotic Timing	143	86%	82%	80%	93%
Oxygenation Assessment	165	100%	99%	99%	100%
Pneumococcal Vaccine	99	70%	68%	69%	94%
Smoking Cessation Advice	51	67%	83%	80%	100%
Surgical Infection Prevention					
Prophylactic Antibiotic Given	65	20%	73%	77%	95%
Prophylactic Antibiotic Selection[1]	11	91%	90%	90%	100%
Prophylactic Antibiotic Stopped	63	17%	74%	72%	95%
Pregnancy Care					
Inpatient Neonatal Mortality	-	-	-	-	-
Third or Fourth Degree Laceration	-	-	3.82%	3.63%	3.27%

Ozark Health Medical Center

Alternate Name: Van Buren County Memorial Hospital
Highway 65 S
Clinton, AR 72031
E-mail: ozark@artelco.com
Ownership: Voluntary non-profit - Private
Emergency Services: Yes

Phone: 501-745-7000
Fax: 501-745-2472

Accredited: No

Key Personnel:
CEO. . . . . Kirk Reamey
Chief of Medical Staff. . . . . Harry Starns
Emergency Room . . . . Lef Sessions
Emergency Room . . . . Jose Abiseid, MD
Director Medical/Surgical Nursing . . . . Harriet Gugelimo, RN
Chief Radiology . . . . Keith Beil, MD
Director Respiratory Therapy . . . . Denise Huggins

Measure	Cases	This Hospital	State Average	U.S. Average	Top Hospital
Heart Attack Care					
ACE Inhibitor or ARB for LVSD[5]	-	-	82%	82%	100%
Aspirin at Arrival[5]	-	-	88%	92%	100%
Aspirin at Discharge[5]	-	-	87%	90%	100%
Beta Blocker at Arrival[5]	-	-	82%	87%	100%
Beta Blocker at Discharge[5]	-	-	86%	90%	100%
Fibrinolytic Medication Timing[5]	-	-	41%	31%	100%
PCI Within 90 Minutes of Arrival[5]	-	-	46%	54%	95%
Smoking Cessation Advice[5]	-	-	91%	88%	100%
Heart Failure Care					
ACE Inhibitor or ARB for LVSD[5]	-	-	78%	82%	100%

NOTE: Hospital profiles are in alphabetical order by state, then city, then hospital within the city; Rankings are sorted by rate in descending order and exclude hospitals with less than 25 cases; (1) The number of cases is too small (n<25) for purposes of reliably predicting hospital performance; (2) Measure reflects the hospital's indication that its submission is based upon a sample of its relevant discharges; (3) Rate reflects fewer than the maximum possible quarters of data for the measure; (4) Inaccurate information submitted and suppressed for one or more quarters; (5) No data is available from the hospital for this measure; Please refer to the User's Guide for a full explanation of data

Discharge Instructions	26	65%	65%	61%	93%
Evaluation of LVS Function	46	67%	81%	83%	99%
Smoking Cessation Advice[5]	-	-	86%	82%	100%
Pneumonia Care					
Appropriate Initial Antibiotic	73	96%	83%	83%	94%
Blood Culture Timing	64	98%	93%	90%	100%
Influenza Vaccine[1]	14	100%	70%	70%	100%
Initial Antibiotic Timing	98	88%	82%	80%	93%
Oxygenation Assessment	119	100%	99%	99%	100%
Pneumococcal Vaccine	80	86%	68%	69%	94%
Smoking Cessation Advice	28	71%	83%	80%	100%
Surgical Infection Prevention					
Prophylactic Antibiotic Given[5]	-	-	73%	77%	95%
Prophylactic Antibiotic Selection[5]	-	-	90%	90%	100%
Prophylactic Antibiotic Stopped[5]	-	-	74%	72%	95%
Pregnancy Care					
Inpatient Neonatal Mortality	-	-	-	-	-
Third or Fourth Degree Laceration	-	-	3.82%	3.63%	3.27%

Conway Regional Medical Center

2302 College Avenue
Conway, AR 72032
E-mail: info@conwayregional.org
URL: www.conwayregional.org
Ownership: Voluntary non-profit - Private
Emergency Services: Yes

Phone: 501-329-3831
Fax: 501-450-2283

Accredited: Yes
Licensed Beds: 116

Key Personnel:
CEO . . . . James Summersett
Chief Medical Staff . . . . Paul McChristian
Director Respiratory Therapy . . . . Kenneth Rains

Measure	Cases	This Hospital	State Average	U.S. Average	Top Hospital
Heart Attack Care					
ACE Inhibitor or ARB for LVSD	37	73%	82%	82%	100%
Aspirin at Arrival	123	96%	88%	92%	100%
Aspirin at Discharge	140	87%	87%	90%	100%
Beta Blocker at Arrival	119	82%	82%	87%	100%
Beta Blocker at Discharge	141	80%	86%	90%	100%
Fibrinolytic Medication Timing[1]	3	67%	41%	31%	100%
PCI Within 90 Minutes of Arrival[1]	9	56%	46%	54%	95%
Smoking Cessation Advice	55	89%	91%	88%	100%
Heart Failure Care					
ACE Inhibitor or ARB for LVSD	73	66%	78%	82%	100%
Discharge Instructions	134	75%	65%	61%	93%
Evaluation of LVS Function	156	69%	81%	83%	99%
Smoking Cessation Advice	32	97%	86%	82%	100%
Pneumonia Care					
Appropriate Initial Antibiotic	160	81%	83%	83%	94%
Blood Culture Timing	106	97%	93%	90%	100%
Influenza Vaccine	38	32%	70%	70%	100%
Initial Antibiotic Timing	189	85%	82%	80%	93%
Oxygenation Assessment	238	100%	99%	99%	100%
Pneumococcal Vaccine	142	47%	68%	69%	94%
Smoking Cessation Advice	54	93%	83%	80%	100%
Surgical Infection Prevention					
Prophylactic Antibiotic Given	617	76%	73%	77%	95%
Prophylactic Antibiotic Selection	146	81%	90%	90%	100%
Prophylactic Antibiotic Stopped	601	67%	74%	72%	95%
Pregnancy Care					
Inpatient Neonatal Mortality	-	-	-	-	-
Third or Fourth Degree Laceration	-	-	3.82%	3.63%	3.27%

Ashley County Medical Center

Alternate Name: Ashley Memorial Hospital
1015 Unity Road
Crossett, AR 71635
URL: www.acmonline.org
Ownership: Voluntary non-profit - Private
Emergency Services: Yes

Phone: 870-364-4111
Fax: 870-364-1245

Accredited: No
Licensed Beds: 46

Key Personnel:
CEO . . . . Russ D Sword
Chief Medical Staff . . . . Phillip Rindt, MD
Emergency Room . . . . William Lynn, MD

Infection Control . . . . Myrna Bryan
ICU . . . . Nicki Miller
Director Radiology . . . . Ronnie Dillion, MD
Director Respiratory Therapy . . . . Kathy Childs

Measure	Cases	This Hospital	State Average	U.S. Average	Top Hospital
Heart Attack Care					
ACE Inhibitor or ARB for LVSD	0	-	82%	82%	100%
Aspirin at Arrival[1]	13	69%	88%	92%	100%
Aspirin at Discharge[1]	4	25%	87%	90%	100%
Beta Blocker at Arrival[1]	15	60%	82%	87%	100%
Beta Blocker at Discharge[1]	2	50%	86%	90%	100%
Fibrinolytic Medication Timing[1]	1	0%	41%	31%	100%
PCI Within 90 Minutes of Arrival	0	-	46%	54%	95%
Smoking Cessation Advice	0	-	91%	88%	100%
Heart Failure Care					
ACE Inhibitor or ARB for LVSD[1]	8	50%	78%	82%	100%
Discharge Instructions	32	75%	65%	61%	93%
Evaluation of LVS Function	39	59%	81%	83%	99%
Smoking Cessation Advice[1]	3	100%	86%	82%	100%
Pneumonia Care					
Appropriate Initial Antibiotic[1]	16	88%	83%	83%	94%
Blood Culture Timing[1]	9	100%	93%	90%	100%
Influenza Vaccine[1]	5	60%	70%	70%	100%
Initial Antibiotic Timing	29	90%	82%	80%	93%
Oxygenation Assessment	31	100%	99%	99%	100%
Pneumococcal Vaccine[1]	18	83%	68%	69%	94%
Smoking Cessation Advice[1]	9	100%	83%	80%	100%
Surgical Infection Prevention					
Prophylactic Antibiotic Given[5]	-	-	73%	77%	95%
Prophylactic Antibiotic Selection[5]	-	-	90%	90%	100%
Prophylactic Antibiotic Stopped[5]	-	-	74%	72%	95%
Pregnancy Care					
Inpatient Neonatal Mortality	-	-	-	-	-
Third or Fourth Degree Laceration	-	-	3.82%	3.63%	3.27%

Chambers Memorial Hospital

Highway 10 at Detroit
Danville, AR 72833
Ownership: Voluntary non-profit - Other
Emergency Services: Yes

Phone: 479-495-2241
Fax: 479-495-6290
Accredited: No
Licensed Beds: 41

Key Personnel:
CEO . . . . Scott Peek
Chief Medical Staff . . . . Philip Tippin, MD
OB/GYN Womens Health . . . . Philip Tippin, MD
Chief Radiology . . . . Don Riley
Director Respiratory Therapy . . . . Paula Dick

Measure	Cases	This Hospital	State Average	U.S. Average	Top Hospital
Heart Attack Care					
ACE Inhibitor or ARB for LVSD[1]	1	100%	82%	82%	100%
Aspirin at Arrival[1]	18	94%	88%	92%	100%
Aspirin at Discharge[1]	16	56%	87%	90%	100%
Beta Blocker at Arrival[1]	8	62%	82%	87%	100%
Beta Blocker at Discharge[1]	15	60%	86%	90%	100%
Fibrinolytic Medication Timing[3]	0	-	41%	31%	100%
PCI Within 90 Minutes of Arrival	0	-	46%	54%	95%
Smoking Cessation Advice	0	-	91%	88%	100%
Heart Failure Care					
ACE Inhibitor or ARB for LVSD[1]	7	57%	78%	82%	100%
Discharge Instructions[1,3]	17	12%	65%	61%	93%
Evaluation of LVS Function	140	6%	81%	83%	99%
Smoking Cessation Advice	34	53%	86%	82%	100%
Pneumonia Care					
Appropriate Initial Antibiotic[1,3]	11	82%	83%	83%	94%
Blood Culture Timing[3]	0	-	93%	90%	100%
Influenza Vaccine[5]	-	-	70%	70%	100%
Initial Antibiotic Timing	79	91%	82%	80%	93%
Oxygenation Assessment	94	100%	99%	99%	100%
Pneumococcal Vaccine	56	34%	68%	69%	94%
Smoking Cessation Advice[1]	20	55%	83%	80%	100%
Surgical Infection Prevention					

Measure	Cases	This Hospital	State Average	U.S. Average	Top Hospital
Prophylactic Antibiotic Given[1,3]	8	50%	73%	77%	95%
Prophylactic Antibiotic Selection[1]	8	38%	90%	90%	100%
Prophylactic Antibiotic Stopped[1,3]	8	88%	74%	72%	95%
Pregnancy Care					
Inpatient Neonatal Mortality	-	-	-	-	-
Third or Fourth Degree Laceration	-	-	3.82%	3.63%	3.27%

De Queen Regional Medical Center

Alternate Name: Columbia De Queen Regional Medical Center
1306 West Collin Raye Drive   Phone: 870-584-4111
De Queen, AR 71832   Fax: 870-584-4100
URL: www.dequeenmedicalcenter.com
Ownership: Voluntary non-profit - Private   Accredited: No
Emergency Services: Yes   Licensed Beds: 122
Key Personnel:
CEO . . . . Charles H Long
Chief Medical Staff . . . . Richard S Ridlon, MD
Director Medical/Surgical Nursing . . . . Ulonda Jamison, RN
OB/GYN Womens Health . . . . Gopal V Naik, MD
Chief Radiology . . . . Jerry Everett, MD
Director Respiratory Therapy . . . . Rex Jones

Measure	Cases	This Hospital	State Average	U.S. Average	Top Hospital
Heart Attack Care					
ACE Inhibitor or ARB for LVSD[3]	0	-	82%	82%	100%
Aspirin at Arrival[1,3]	1	100%	88%	92%	100%
Aspirin at Discharge[3]	0	-	87%	90%	100%
Beta Blocker at Arrival[1,3]	2	100%	82%	87%	100%
Beta Blocker at Discharge[1,3]	1	100%	86%	90%	100%
Fibrinolytic Medication Timing[3]	0	-	41%	31%	100%
PCI Within 90 Minutes of Arrival[5]	-	-	46%	54%	95%
Smoking Cessation Advice[3]	0	-	91%	88%	100%
Heart Failure Care					
ACE Inhibitor or ARB for LVSD[1,3]	15	47%	78%	82%	100%
Discharge Instructions[1,3]	15	53%	65%	61%	93%
Evaluation of LVS Function[3]	36	69%	81%	83%	99%
Smoking Cessation Advice[1,3]	4	25%	86%	82%	100%
Pneumonia Care					
Appropriate Initial Antibiotic[1,3]	18	89%	83%	83%	94%
Blood Culture Timing[1]	16	88%	93%	90%	100%
Influenza Vaccine[1]	10	50%	70%	70%	100%
Initial Antibiotic Timing[1,3]	20	55%	82%	80%	93%
Oxygenation Assessment[3]	29	100%	99%	99%	100%
Pneumococcal Vaccine[1,3]	20	65%	68%	69%	94%
Smoking Cessation Advice[1,3]	8	12%	83%	80%	100%
Surgical Infection Prevention					
Prophylactic Antibiotic Given[5]	-	-	73%	77%	95%
Prophylactic Antibiotic Selection[5]	-	-	90%	90%	100%
Prophylactic Antibiotic Stopped[5]	-	-	74%	72%	95%
Pregnancy Care					
Inpatient Neonatal Mortality	-	-	-	-	-
Third or Fourth Degree Laceration	-	-	3.82%	3.63%	3.27%

De Witt Hospital & Nursing Home

1641 S Whitehead Drive   Phone: 870-946-3571
De Witt, AR 72042   Fax: 870-946-4377
Ownership: Voluntary non-profit - Private   Accredited: No
Emergency Services: No   Licensed Beds: 25
Key Personnel:
CEO . . . . Darren Caldwell
Chief Medical Staff . . . . Stan Purleson
Emergency Room Director . . . . Karen Campbell, RN
Director Respiratory Therapy . . . . Tony Poole

Measure	Cases	This Hospital	State Average	U.S. Average	Top Hospital
Heart Attack Care					
ACE Inhibitor or ARB for LVSD[5]	-	-	82%	82%	100%
Aspirin at Arrival[5]	-	-	88%	92%	100%
Aspirin at Discharge[5]	-	-	87%	90%	100%
Beta Blocker at Arrival[5]	-	-	82%	87%	100%
Beta Blocker at Discharge[5]	-	-	86%	90%	100%
Fibrinolytic Medication Timing[5]	-	-	41%	31%	100%

Measure	Cases	This Hospital	State Average	U.S. Average	Top Hospital
PCI Within 90 Minutes of Arrival[5]	-	-	46%	54%	95%
Smoking Cessation Advice[5]	-	-	91%	88%	100%
Heart Failure Care					
ACE Inhibitor or ARB for LVSD[1]	1	0%	78%	82%	100%
Discharge Instructions[1]	19	100%	65%	61%	93%
Evaluation of LVS Function[1]	26	15%	81%	83%	99%
Smoking Cessation Advice[1]	1	100%	86%	82%	100%
Pneumonia Care					
Appropriate Initial Antibiotic	26	73%	83%	83%	94%
Blood Culture Timing[1]	3	100%	93%	90%	100%
Influenza Vaccine[1]	8	38%	70%	70%	100%
Initial Antibiotic Timing	31	94%	82%	80%	93%
Oxygenation Assessment	34	94%	99%	99%	100%
Pneumococcal Vaccine[1]	19	11%	68%	69%	94%
Smoking Cessation Advice[1]	3	67%	83%	80%	100%
Surgical Infection Prevention					
Prophylactic Antibiotic Given[5]	-	-	73%	77%	95%
Prophylactic Antibiotic Selection[5]	-	-	90%	90%	100%
Prophylactic Antibiotic Stopped[5]	-	-	74%	72%	95%
Pregnancy Care					
Inpatient Neonatal Mortality	-	-	-	-	-
Third or Fourth Degree Laceration	-	-	3.82%	3.63%	3.27%

Delta Memorial Hospital

300 E Pickens Street   Phone: 870-382-4303
Dumas, AR 71639   Fax: 870-382-6555
E-mail: xray@deltamem.org
URL: www.dumasar.org
Ownership: Voluntary non-profit - Private   Accredited: No
Emergency Services: Yes   Licensed Beds: 50
Key Personnel:
CEO . . . . Mark Deal
Director Respiratory Therapy . . . . Ashley Riley

Measure	Cases	This Hospital	State Average	U.S. Average	Top Hospital
Heart Attack Care					
ACE Inhibitor or ARB for LVSD[3]	0	-	82%	82%	100%
Aspirin at Arrival[1,3]	2	0%	88%	92%	100%
Aspirin at Discharge[1,3]	1	100%	87%	90%	100%
Beta Blocker at Arrival[1,3]	2	100%	82%	87%	100%
Beta Blocker at Discharge[1,3]	2	100%	86%	90%	100%
Fibrinolytic Medication Timing[3]	0	-	41%	31%	100%
PCI Within 90 Minutes of Arrival[5]	-	-	46%	54%	95%
Smoking Cessation Advice[3]	0	-	91%	88%	100%
Heart Failure Care					
ACE Inhibitor or ARB for LVSD[1]	3	100%	78%	82%	100%
Discharge Instructions[1]	17	59%	65%	61%	93%
Evaluation of LVS Function[1]	21	67%	81%	83%	99%
Smoking Cessation Advice[1]	5	80%	86%	82%	100%
Pneumonia Care					
Appropriate Initial Antibiotic	28	79%	83%	83%	94%
Blood Culture Timing[1]	16	94%	93%	90%	100%
Influenza Vaccine[4,5]	-	-	70%	70%	100%
Initial Antibiotic Timing	31	77%	82%	80%	93%
Oxygenation Assessment	37	100%	99%	99%	100%
Pneumococcal Vaccine[1]	15	67%	68%	69%	94%
Smoking Cessation Advice[1]	7	86%	83%	80%	100%
Surgical Infection Prevention					
Prophylactic Antibiotic Given[5]	-	-	73%	77%	95%
Prophylactic Antibiotic Selection[5]	-	-	90%	90%	100%
Prophylactic Antibiotic Stopped[5]	-	-	74%	72%	95%
Pregnancy Care					
Inpatient Neonatal Mortality	-	-	-	-	-
Third or Fourth Degree Laceration	-	-	3.82%	3.63%	3.27%

Medical Center of South Arkansas

700 W Grove Street   Phone: 870-863-2000
El Dorado, AR 71731   Fax: 870-863-2500
URL: www.themedcenter.net
Ownership: Proprietary   Accredited: Yes
Emergency Services: Yes   Licensed Beds: 360
Key Personnel:
CEO . . . . Luther Lewis

Chief Medical Staff . . . . Cheryl Barenberg
Emergency Room . . . . Marie Owens
Director Infection/Disease Control . . . . Bob Cook, RN
CCU Spvg. Nurse . . . . Becky Parnell
Director Respiratory Therapy . . . . Debbie Raper

Measure	Cases	This Hospital	State Average	U.S. Average	Top Hospital
Heart Attack Care					
ACE Inhibitor or ARB for LVSD[1]	5	100%	82%	82%	100%
Aspirin at Arrival	27	89%	88%	92%	100%
Aspirin at Discharge[1]	23	91%	87%	90%	100%
Beta Blocker at Arrival	30	90%	82%	87%	100%
Beta Blocker at Discharge	29	90%	86%	90%	100%
Fibrinolytic Medication Timing[1]	8	75%	41%	31%	100%
PCI Within 90 Minutes of Arrival[1]	1	0%	46%	54%	95%
Smoking Cessation Advice[1]	10	100%	91%	88%	100%
Heart Failure Care					
ACE Inhibitor or ARB for LVSD	66	82%	78%	82%	100%
Discharge Instructions	128	58%	65%	61%	93%
Evaluation of LVS Function	173	99%	81%	83%	99%
Smoking Cessation Advice	53	100%	86%	82%	100%
Pneumonia Care					
Appropriate Initial Antibiotic	94	87%	83%	83%	94%
Blood Culture Timing	68	99%	93%	90%	100%
Influenza Vaccine	28	75%	70%	70%	100%
Initial Antibiotic Timing	112	89%	82%	80%	93%
Oxygenation Assessment	130	100%	99%	99%	100%
Pneumococcal Vaccine	68	81%	68%	69%	94%
Smoking Cessation Advice	40	100%	83%	80%	100%
Surgical Infection Prevention					
Prophylactic Antibiotic Given	535	96%	73%	77%	95%
Prophylactic Antibiotic Selection	150	99%	90%	90%	100%
Prophylactic Antibiotic Stopped	520	93%	74%	72%	95%
Pregnancy Care					
Inpatient Neonatal Mortality	-	-	-	-	-
Third or Fourth Degree Laceration	-	-	3.82%	3.63%	3.27%

Washington Regional Medical Center

3215 N North Hills Blvd
Fayetteville, AR 72703
URL: www.wregional.com
Ownership: Voluntary non-profit - Private
Emergency Services: Yes

Phone: 479-713-1000
Fax: 479-713-1296

Accredited: Yes
Licensed Beds: 294

Key Personnel:
CEO . . . . Bill Bradley
Chief of Medical Staff . . . . David Ratcliffe
OB/GYN Womens Health . . . . Mark Pickhart, MD
Chief Radiology . . . . Kevin Pope, MD
Director Respiratory Therapy . . . . Nancy Bowen

Measure	Cases	This Hospital	State Average	U.S. Average	Top Hospital
Heart Attack Care					
ACE Inhibitor or ARB for LVSD	64	88%	82%	82%	100%
Aspirin at Arrival	183	94%	88%	92%	100%
Aspirin at Discharge	267	97%	87%	90%	100%
Beta Blocker at Arrival	161	88%	82%	87%	100%
Beta Blocker at Discharge	267	90%	86%	90%	100%
Fibrinolytic Medication Timing	0	-	41%	31%	100%
PCI Within 90 Minutes of Arrival[1]	6	67%	46%	54%	95%
Smoking Cessation Advice	101	86%	91%	88%	100%
Heart Failure Care					
ACE Inhibitor or ARB for LVSD	148	85%	78%	82%	100%
Discharge Instructions	258	91%	65%	61%	93%
Evaluation of LVS Function	292	97%	81%	83%	99%
Smoking Cessation Advice	67	99%	86%	82%	100%
Pneumonia Care					
Appropriate Initial Antibiotic	103	79%	83%	83%	94%
Blood Culture Timing	72	94%	93%	90%	100%
Influenza Vaccine	26	58%	70%	70%	100%
Initial Antibiotic Timing	138	64%	82%	80%	93%
Oxygenation Assessment	169	100%	99%	99%	100%
Pneumococcal Vaccine	98	64%	68%	69%	94%

Smoking Cessation Advice	45	80%	83%	80%	100%
Surgical Infection Prevention					
Prophylactic Antibiotic Given[3]	80	31%	73%	77%	95%
Prophylactic Antibiotic Selection	79	94%	90%	90%	100%
Prophylactic Antibiotic Stopped[3]	189	64%	74%	72%	95%
Pregnancy Care					
Inpatient Neonatal Mortality	-	-	-	-	-
Third or Fourth Degree Laceration	-	-	3.82%	3.63%	3.27%

Baptist Memorial Hospital-Forrest City

1601 Newcastle Road
Forrest City, AR 72335
URL: www.bmhcc.org
Ownership: Voluntary non-profit - Church
Emergency Services: Yes

Phone: 870-261-0000
Fax: 970-277-3516

Accredited: Yes
Licensed Beds: 118

Key Personnel:
Chief Medical Staff . . . . Frank Schwartz, MD
Director Infection/Disease Control . . . . Jerre Fisher, RN
CCU Spvg. Nurse . . . . Mary Baker, RN
Director Medical/Surgical Nursing . . . . Darlene Mansel
Chief OB/GYN . . . . Cem Sarinoglu, MD
Director Respiratory Therapy . . . . Nadine Stanley

Measure	Cases	This Hospital	State Average	U.S. Average	Top Hospital
Heart Attack Care					
ACE Inhibitor or ARB for LVSD[1,3]	2	50%	82%	82%	100%
Aspirin at Arrival[1,3]	10	70%	88%	92%	100%
Aspirin at Discharge[1,3]	7	86%	87%	90%	100%
Beta Blocker at Arrival[1,3]	7	100%	82%	87%	100%
Beta Blocker at Discharge[1,3]	8	88%	86%	90%	100%
Fibrinolytic Medication Timing[3]	0	-	41%	31%	100%
PCI Within 90 Minutes of Arrival	0	-	46%	54%	95%
Smoking Cessation Advice[3]	0	-	91%	88%	100%
Heart Failure Care					
ACE Inhibitor or ARB for LVSD	34	100%	78%	82%	100%
Discharge Instructions	88	100%	65%	61%	93%
Evaluation of LVS Function	98	96%	81%	83%	99%
Smoking Cessation Advice[1]	23	100%	86%	82%	100%
Pneumonia Care					
Appropriate Initial Antibiotic	62	84%	83%	83%	94%
Blood Culture Timing	65	92%	93%	90%	100%
Influenza Vaccine[1]	24	96%	70%	70%	100%
Initial Antibiotic Timing	89	83%	82%	80%	93%
Oxygenation Assessment	108	100%	99%	99%	100%
Pneumococcal Vaccine	61	97%	68%	69%	94%
Smoking Cessation Advice	28	100%	83%	80%	100%
Surgical Infection Prevention					
Prophylactic Antibiotic Given[2]	55	93%	73%	77%	95%
Prophylactic Antibiotic Selection[1,2]	17	94%	90%	90%	100%
Prophylactic Antibiotic Stopped[2]	54	76%	74%	72%	95%
Pregnancy Care					
Inpatient Neonatal Mortality	-	-	-	-	-
Third or Fourth Degree Laceration	-	-	3.82%	3.63%	3.27%

Saint Edward Mercy Medical Center

7301 Rogers Avenue
Fort Smith, AR 72903
URL: www.stedwardmercy.com
Ownership: Voluntary non-profit - Church
Emergency Services: Yes

Phone: 479-484-6000
Fax: 479-314-1770

Accredited: Yes
Licensed Beds: 349

Key Personnel:
CEO . . . . Jerry Stevenson
Chief Medical Staff . . . . Chrisca Van Asche, MD
Director of Cardiology/Cardiac Lab . . . . Timothy Waack
Emergency Room . . . . Jackie Wallace, RN
Director Medical/Surgical Nursing . . . . Dolly Shoemake, RN
Director Medical/Surgical Nursing . . . . Charlotte Hatwig, RN
Director Respiratory Therapy . . . . John McKinney, Jr

Measure	Cases	This Hospital	State Average	U.S. Average	Top Hospital
Heart Attack Care					
ACE Inhibitor or ARB for LVSD[2]	91	90%	82%	82%	100%
Aspirin at Arrival[2]	157	96%	88%	92%	100%

NOTE: Hospital profiles are in alphabetical order by state, then city, then hospital within the city; Rankings are sorted by rate in descending order and exclude hospitals with less than 25 cases; (1) The number of cases is too small (n<25) for purposes of reliably predicting hospital performance; (2) Measure reflects the hospital's indication that its submission was based upon a sample of its relevant discharges; (3) Rate reflects fewer than the maximum possible quarters of data for the measure; (4) Inaccurate information submitted and suppressed for one or more quarters; (5) No data is available from the hospital for this measure; Please refer to the User's Guide for a full explanation of data

Aspirin at Discharge[2]	253	97%	87%	90%	100%
Beta Blocker at Arrival[2]	118	97%	82%	87%	100%
Beta Blocker at Discharge[2]	257	97%	86%	90%	100%
Fibrinolytic Medication Timing[1,2]	9	11%	41%	31%	100%
PCI Within 90 Minutes of Arrival[1,2]	5	40%	46%	54%	95%
Smoking Cessation Advice[2]	137	100%	91%	88%	100%
Heart Failure Care					
ACE Inhibitor or ARB for LVSD[2]	103	84%	78%	82%	100%
Discharge Instructions[2]	229	60%	65%	61%	93%
Evaluation of LVS Function[2]	286	99%	81%	83%	99%
Smoking Cessation Advice[2]	59	97%	86%	82%	100%
Pneumonia Care					
Appropriate Initial Antibiotic[2]	101	82%	83%	83%	94%
Blood Culture Timing[2]	92	90%	93%	90%	100%
Influenza Vaccine[2]	26	100%	70%	70%	100%
Initial Antibiotic Timing[2]	140	66%	82%	80%	93%
Oxygenation Assessment[2]	178	100%	99%	99%	100%
Pneumococcal Vaccine[2]	95	81%	68%	69%	94%
Smoking Cessation Advice[2]	49	92%	83%	80%	100%
Surgical Infection Prevention					
Prophylactic Antibiotic Given[2]	227	89%	73%	77%	95%
Prophylactic Antibiotic Selection[2]	65	95%	90%	90%	100%
Prophylactic Antibiotic Stopped[2]	221	76%	74%	72%	95%
Pregnancy Care					
Inpatient Neonatal Mortality	-	-	-	-	-
Third or Fourth Degree Laceration	-	-	3.82%	3.63%	3.27%

Sparks Regional Medical Center

1311 S I Street
Fort Smith, AR 72901
URL: www.sparks.org
Ownership: Voluntary non-profit - Private
Emergency Services: Yes

Phone: 479-441-4000
Fax: 479-441-5462

Accredited: Yes
Licensed Beds: 510

Key Personnel:
CEO . . . . John Guest
Head Emergency Room . . . . Lee Johnson
Director Respiratory Therapy . . . . Paul Reano

Measure	Cases	This Hospital	State Average	U.S. Average	Top Hospital
Heart Attack Care					
ACE Inhibitor or ARB for LVSD	46	78%	82%	82%	100%
Aspirin at Arrival	188	93%	88%	92%	100%
Aspirin at Discharge	220	94%	87%	90%	100%
Beta Blocker at Arrival	186	94%	82%	87%	100%
Beta Blocker at Discharge	224	95%	86%	90%	100%
Fibrinolytic Medication Timing[1]	24	21%	41%	31%	100%
PCI Within 90 Minutes of Arrival[1]	7	14%	46%	54%	95%
Smoking Cessation Advice	85	84%	91%	88%	100%
Heart Failure Care					
ACE Inhibitor or ARB for LVSD	151	79%	78%	82%	100%
Discharge Instructions	323	69%	65%	61%	93%
Evaluation of LVS Function	430	89%	81%	83%	99%
Smoking Cessation Advice	60	65%	86%	82%	100%
Pneumonia Care					
Appropriate Initial Antibiotic	212	82%	83%	83%	94%
Blood Culture Timing	194	95%	93%	90%	100%
Influenza Vaccine	60	75%	70%	70%	100%
Initial Antibiotic Timing	317	67%	82%	80%	93%
Oxygenation Assessment	390	99%	99%	99%	100%
Pneumococcal Vaccine	212	66%	68%	69%	94%
Smoking Cessation Advice	86	79%	83%	80%	100%
Surgical Infection Prevention					
Prophylactic Antibiotic Given[2]	299	66%	73%	77%	95%
Prophylactic Antibiotic Selection[2]	98	96%	90%	90%	100%
Prophylactic Antibiotic Stopped[2]	287	76%	74%	72%	95%
Pregnancy Care					
Inpatient Neonatal Mortality	1,135	0.00%	-	-	-
Third or Fourth Degree Laceration	730	3.84%	3.82%	3.63%	3.27%

North Arkansas Regional Medical Center

620 N Willow Street
Harrison, AR 72601
URL: www.narmc.com
Ownership: Voluntary non-profit - Private
Emergency Services: Yes

Phone: 870-365-2000
Fax: 870-365-2430

Accredited: Yes
Licensed Beds: 174

Key Personnel:
President/CEO . . . . Timothy E Hill
Emergency Room Manager . . . . Cary Foley
Infection Control . . . . Kalen Youngs
Surgery Services Manager . . . . Carole Lichti
Respiratory Therapy Manager . . . . James Lawrence

Measure	Cases	This Hospital	State Average	U.S. Average	Top Hospital
Heart Attack Care					
ACE Inhibitor or ARB for LVSD[1]	12	75%	82%	82%	100%
Aspirin at Arrival	33	97%	88%	92%	100%
Aspirin at Discharge[1]	21	100%	87%	90%	100%
Beta Blocker at Arrival[1]	24	79%	82%	87%	100%
Beta Blocker at Discharge[1]	18	94%	86%	90%	100%
Fibrinolytic Medication Timing	0	-	41%	31%	100%
PCI Within 90 Minutes of Arrival	0	-	46%	54%	95%
Smoking Cessation Advice[1]	1	100%	91%	88%	100%
Heart Failure Care					
ACE Inhibitor or ARB for LVSD	38	74%	78%	82%	100%
Discharge Instructions	109	68%	65%	61%	93%
Evaluation of LVS Function	142	97%	81%	83%	99%
Smoking Cessation Advice	25	84%	86%	82%	100%
Pneumonia Care					
Appropriate Initial Antibiotic	191	80%	83%	83%	94%
Blood Culture Timing	130	93%	93%	90%	100%
Influenza Vaccine	54	83%	70%	70%	100%
Initial Antibiotic Timing	218	89%	82%	80%	93%
Oxygenation Assessment	285	100%	99%	99%	100%
Pneumococcal Vaccine	192	79%	68%	69%	94%
Smoking Cessation Advice	61	89%	83%	80%	100%
Surgical Infection Prevention					
Prophylactic Antibiotic Given	185	96%	73%	77%	95%
Prophylactic Antibiotic Selection	35	97%	90%	90%	100%
Prophylactic Antibiotic Stopped	174	89%	74%	72%	95%
Pregnancy Care					
Inpatient Neonatal Mortality	-	-	-	-	-
Third or Fourth Degree Laceration	-	-	3.82%	3.63%	3.27%

Baptist Health Medical Center

2319 Highway 110 W
Heber Springs, AR 72543
URL: www.baptist-health.org
Ownership: Voluntary non-profit - Church
Emergency Services: Yes

Phone: 501-206-3000
Fax: 501-206-3390

Accredited: Yes
Licensed Beds: 49

Key Personnel:
CEO . . . . Edward Lacy
Chief Medical Staff . . . . Tonya Little, MD
Emergency Room . . . . Crystal Sumpter, RN
Infection Control . . . . Tamara Wright
Director Respiratory Therapy . . . . Cathy Alexander

Measure	Cases	This Hospital	State Average	U.S. Average	Top Hospital
Heart Attack Care					
ACE Inhibitor or ARB for LVSD[1,3]	1	100%	82%	82%	100%
Aspirin at Arrival[3]	0	-	88%	92%	100%
Aspirin at Discharge[3]	0	-	87%	90%	100%
Beta Blocker at Arrival[3]	0	-	82%	87%	100%
Beta Blocker at Discharge[3]	0	-	86%	90%	100%
Fibrinolytic Medication Timing[3]	0	-	41%	31%	100%
PCI Within 90 Minutes of Arrival	0	-	46%	54%	95%
Smoking Cessation Advice[3]	0	-	91%	88%	100%
Heart Failure Care					
ACE Inhibitor or ARB for LVSD[1]	2	100%	78%	82%	100%
Discharge Instructions[1]	19	79%	65%	61%	93%
Evaluation of LVS Function	26	100%	81%	83%	99%
Smoking Cessation Advice[1]	6	100%	86%	82%	100%
Pneumonia Care					

NOTE: Hospital profiles are in alphabetical order by state, then city, then hospital within the city; Rankings are sorted by rate in descending order and exclude hospitals with less than 25 cases; (1) The number of cases is too small (n<25) for purposes of reliably predicting hospital performance; (2) Measure reflects the hospital's indication that its submission was based upon a sample of its relevant discharges; (3) Rate reflects fewer than the maximum possible quarters of data for the measure; (4) Inaccurate information submitted and suppressed for one or more quarters; (5) No data is available from the hospital for this measure; Please refer to the User's Guide for a full explanation of data

Measure	Cases	This Hospital	State Average	U.S. Average	Top Hospital
Appropriate Initial Antibiotic	63	98%	83%	83%	94%
Blood Culture Timing	34	94%	93%	90%	100%
Influenza Vaccine[1]	16	94%	70%	70%	100%
Initial Antibiotic Timing	72	85%	82%	80%	93%
Oxygenation Assessment	88	100%	99%	99%	100%
Pneumococcal Vaccine	56	91%	68%	69%	94%
Smoking Cessation Advice[1]	14	100%	83%	80%	100%
Surgical Infection Prevention					
Prophylactic Antibiotic Given[5]	-	-	73%	77%	95%
Prophylactic Antibiotic Selection[5]	-	-	90%	90%	100%
Prophylactic Antibiotic Stopped[5]	-	-	74%	72%	95%
Pregnancy Care					
Inpatient Neonatal Mortality	-	-	-	-	-
Third or Fourth Degree Laceration	-	-	3.82%	3.63%	3.27%

Helena Regional Medical Center

1801 Martin Luther King Drive
PO Box 788
Helena, AR 72342
URL: www.helenaregionalmedicalcenter.com
Ownership: Proprietary
Emergency Services: Yes

Phone: 870-338-5800
Fax: 870-816-3944

Accredited: Yes
Licensed Beds: 155

Key Personnel:
CEO. . . . . Tom Kinnebrew
Infection Control. . . . . Jamie Pryor
ICU . . . . Mattie Littlejohn, MD
Med/Surg Nursing . . . . Pam Johnston
OB/GYN Womens Health. . . . . Ruby Scottl

Measure	Cases	This Hospital	State Average	U.S. Average	Top Hospital
Heart Attack Care					
ACE Inhibitor or ARB for LVSD[1]	1	100%	82%	82%	100%
Aspirin at Arrival[1]	9	78%	88%	92%	100%
Aspirin at Discharge[1]	6	67%	87%	90%	100%
Beta Blocker at Arrival[1]	11	73%	82%	87%	100%
Beta Blocker at Discharge[1]	5	60%	86%	90%	100%
Fibrinolytic Medication Timing[1]	1	0%	41%	31%	100%
PCI Within 90 Minutes of Arrival	0	-	46%	54%	95%
Smoking Cessation Advice[1]	3	67%	91%	88%	100%
Heart Failure Care					
ACE Inhibitor or ARB for LVSD	61	67%	78%	82%	100%
Discharge Instructions	167	58%	65%	61%	93%
Evaluation of LVS Function	254	76%	81%	83%	99%
Smoking Cessation Advice	55	93%	86%	82%	100%
Pneumonia Care					
Appropriate Initial Antibiotic	108	69%	83%	83%	94%
Blood Culture Timing	62	90%	93%	90%	100%
Influenza Vaccine	33	73%	70%	70%	100%
Initial Antibiotic Timing	151	91%	82%	80%	93%
Oxygenation Assessment	161	99%	99%	99%	100%
Pneumococcal Vaccine	95	59%	68%	69%	94%
Smoking Cessation Advice	41	88%	83%	80%	100%
Surgical Infection Prevention					
Prophylactic Antibiotic Given[1,2,3]	19	26%	73%	77%	95%
Prophylactic Antibiotic Selection[1,2]	6	67%	90%	90%	100%
Prophylactic Antibiotic Stopped[1,2,3]	18	78%	74%	72%	95%
Pregnancy Care					
Inpatient Neonatal Mortality	-	-	-	-	-
Third or Fourth Degree Laceration	-	-	3.82%	3.63%	3.27%

Medical Park Hospital

Alternate Name: Medical Park Hospital
2001 S Main Street
Hope, AR 71801
URL: www.medicalparkhospitals.com
Ownership: Proprietary
Emergency Services: Yes

Phone: 870-777-2323
Fax: 870-722-7158

Accredited: Yes
Licensed Beds: 91

Key Personnel:
President/CEO. . . . . Jimmy Leopard
Chief Medical Staff. . . . . Matthew Walter, MD
Emergency Room . . . . Faye Hughes
Medical/Surgical Nursing . . . . Pennie Bobo
OB/GYN Womens Health. . . . . Stewart Rushton, MD

Chief Radiology . . . . Lawrence Bigongiari, MD
Director Respiratory Therapy . . . . Sandra Byrd

Measure	Cases	This Hospital	State Average	U.S. Average	Top Hospital
Heart Attack Care					
ACE Inhibitor or ARB for LVSD[1]	2	100%	82%	82%	100%
Aspirin at Arrival[1]	20	95%	88%	92%	100%
Aspirin at Discharge[1]	12	100%	87%	90%	100%
Beta Blocker at Arrival[1]	15	100%	82%	87%	100%
Beta Blocker at Discharge[1]	10	100%	86%	90%	100%
Fibrinolytic Medication Timing	0	-	41%	31%	100%
PCI Within 90 Minutes of Arrival	0	-	46%	54%	95%
Smoking Cessation Advice[1]	2	100%	91%	88%	100%
Heart Failure Care					
ACE Inhibitor or ARB for LVSD	42	90%	78%	82%	100%
Discharge Instructions	66	94%	65%	61%	93%
Evaluation of LVS Function	122	99%	81%	83%	99%
Smoking Cessation Advice	29	100%	86%	82%	100%
Pneumonia Care					
Appropriate Initial Antibiotic	70	80%	83%	83%	94%
Blood Culture Timing	51	92%	93%	90%	100%
Influenza Vaccine	28	96%	70%	70%	100%
Initial Antibiotic Timing	132	92%	82%	80%	93%
Oxygenation Assessment	157	100%	99%	99%	100%
Pneumococcal Vaccine	101	91%	68%	69%	94%
Smoking Cessation Advice	38	100%	83%	80%	100%
Surgical Infection Prevention					
Prophylactic Antibiotic Given[1]	23	83%	73%	77%	95%
Prophylactic Antibiotic Selection[1]	5	100%	90%	90%	100%
Prophylactic Antibiotic Stopped[1]	23	70%	74%	72%	95%
Pregnancy Care					
Inpatient Neonatal Mortality	-	-	-	-	-
Third or Fourth Degree Laceration	-	-	3.82%	3.63%	3.27%

Healthpark Hospital

1636 Higdon Ferry Road
Hot Springs, AR 71913
Ownership: Proprietary
Emergency Services: Yes

Phone: 501-520-2000

Accredited: No

Measure	Cases	This Hospital	State Average	U.S. Average	Top Hospital
Heart Attack Care					
ACE Inhibitor or ARB for LVSD[5]	-	-	82%	82%	100%
Aspirin at Arrival[5]	-	-	88%	92%	100%
Aspirin at Discharge[5]	-	-	87%	90%	100%
Beta Blocker at Arrival[5]	-	-	82%	87%	100%
Beta Blocker at Discharge[5]	-	-	86%	90%	100%
Fibrinolytic Medication Timing[5]	-	-	41%	31%	100%
PCI Within 90 Minutes of Arrival[5]	-	-	46%	54%	95%
Smoking Cessation Advice[5]	-	-	91%	88%	100%
Heart Failure Care					
ACE Inhibitor or ARB for LVSD[1]	1	100%	78%	82%	100%
Discharge Instructions[1]	7	57%	65%	61%	93%
Evaluation of LVS Function[1]	8	100%	81%	83%	99%
Smoking Cessation Advice[1]	2	100%	86%	82%	100%
Pneumonia Care					
Appropriate Initial Antibiotic[1]	15	87%	83%	83%	94%
Blood Culture Timing[1]	4	100%	93%	90%	100%
Influenza Vaccine[1]	6	50%	70%	70%	100%
Initial Antibiotic Timing[1]	18	83%	82%	80%	93%
Oxygenation Assessment[1]	21	100%	99%	99%	100%
Pneumococcal Vaccine[1]	19	63%	68%	69%	94%
Smoking Cessation Advice	0	-	83%	80%	100%
Surgical Infection Prevention					
Prophylactic Antibiotic Given[2]	214	93%	73%	77%	95%
Prophylactic Antibiotic Selection[2]	34	94%	90%	90%	100%
Prophylactic Antibiotic Stopped[2]	191	28%	74%	72%	95%
Pregnancy Care					
Inpatient Neonatal Mortality	-	-	-	-	-
Third or Fourth Degree Laceration	-	-	3.82%	3.63%	3.27%

NOTE: Hospital profiles are in alphabetical order by state, then city, then hospital within the city; Rankings are sorted by rate in descending order and exclude hospitals with less than 25 cases; (1) The number of cases is too small (n<25) for purposes of reliably predicting hospital performance; (2) Measure reflects the hospital's indication that its submission was based upon a sample of its relevant discharges; (3) Rate reflects fewer than the maximum possible quarters of data for the measure; (4) Inaccurate information submitted and suppressed for one or more quarters; (5) No data is available from the hospital for this measure; Please refer to the User's Guide for a full explanation of data

Levi Hospital

300 Prospect Avenue
Hot Springs Natl Pk, AR 71901
E-mail: bholsomback@levihospital.com
URL: www.levihospital.com
Ownership: Voluntary non-profit - Private
Emergency Services: Yes

Phone: 501-624-1281
Fax: 501-622-3500

Accredited: Yes
Licensed Beds: 89

Key Personnel:
President/CEO . . . . Patrick G McCabe, Jr
Chief Medical Staff . . . . Michael Goldman
Chief Radiology . . . . Erma Wimsett

Measure	Cases	This Hospital	State Average	U.S. Average	Top Hospital
Heart Attack Care					
ACE Inhibitor or ARB for LVSD[5]	-	-	82%	82%	100%
Aspirin at Arrival[5]	-	-	88%	92%	100%
Aspirin at Discharge[5]	-	-	87%	90%	100%
Beta Blocker at Arrival[5]	-	-	82%	87%	100%
Beta Blocker at Discharge[5]	-	-	86%	90%	100%
Fibrinolytic Medication Timing[5]	-	-	41%	31%	100%
PCI Within 90 Minutes of Arrival[5]	-	-	46%	54%	95%
Smoking Cessation Advice[5]	-	-	91%	88%	100%
Heart Failure Care					
ACE Inhibitor or ARB for LVSD[5]	-	-	78%	82%	100%
Discharge Instructions[5]	-	-	65%	61%	93%
Evaluation of LVS Function[5]	-	-	81%	83%	99%
Smoking Cessation Advice[5]	-	-	86%	82%	100%
Pneumonia Care					
Appropriate Initial Antibiotic[5]	-	-	83%	83%	94%
Blood Culture Timing[5]	-	-	93%	90%	100%
Influenza Vaccine[5]	-	-	70%	70%	100%
Initial Antibiotic Timing[5]	-	-	82%	80%	93%
Oxygenation Assessment[5]	-	-	99%	99%	100%
Pneumococcal Vaccine[5]	-	-	68%	69%	94%
Smoking Cessation Advice[5]	-	-	83%	80%	100%
Surgical Infection Prevention					
Prophylactic Antibiotic Given[5]	-	-	73%	77%	95%
Prophylactic Antibiotic Selection[5]	-	-	90%	90%	100%
Prophylactic Antibiotic Stopped[5]	-	-	74%	72%	95%
Pregnancy Care					
Inpatient Neonatal Mortality	-	-	-	-	-
Third or Fourth Degree Laceration	-	-	3.82%	3.63%	3.27%

National Park Medical Center

Alternate Name: AMI National Park Medical Center
1910 Malvern Avenue
Hot Springs, AR 71901
URL: www.nationalparkmedical.com
Ownership: Proprietary
Emergency Services: Yes

Phone: 501-321-1000
Fax: 501-321-2922

Accredited: Yes
Licensed Beds: 166

Key Personnel:
CEO . . . . Jerry D Mabry

Measure	Cases	This Hospital	State Average	U.S. Average	Top Hospital
Heart Attack Care					
ACE Inhibitor or ARB for LVSD[1]	14	57%	82%	82%	100%
Aspirin at Arrival	59	98%	88%	92%	100%
Aspirin at Discharge	60	92%	87%	90%	100%
Beta Blocker at Arrival	52	88%	82%	87%	100%
Beta Blocker at Discharge	54	89%	86%	90%	100%
Fibrinolytic Medication Timing[1]	4	100%	41%	31%	100%
PCI Within 90 Minutes of Arrival	0	-	46%	54%	95%
Smoking Cessation Advice	30	97%	91%	88%	100%
Heart Failure Care					
ACE Inhibitor or ARB for LVSD	43	88%	78%	82%	100%
Discharge Instructions	89	52%	65%	61%	93%
Evaluation of LVS Function	106	95%	81%	83%	99%
Smoking Cessation Advice[1]	16	94%	86%	82%	100%
Pneumonia Care					
Appropriate Initial Antibiotic	101	76%	83%	83%	94%
Blood Culture Timing	81	95%	93%	90%	100%
Influenza Vaccine[1]	19	68%	70%	70%	100%
Initial Antibiotic Timing	129	88%	82%	80%	93%

Measure	Cases	This Hospital	State Average	U.S. Average	Top Hospital
Oxygenation Assessment	144	100%	99%	99%	100%
Pneumococcal Vaccine	78	78%	68%	69%	94%
Smoking Cessation Advice	58	93%	83%	80%	100%
Surgical Infection Prevention					
Prophylactic Antibiotic Given	213	88%	73%	77%	95%
Prophylactic Antibiotic Selection	42	90%	90%	90%	100%
Prophylactic Antibiotic Stopped	200	86%	74%	72%	95%
Pregnancy Care					
Inpatient Neonatal Mortality	-	-	-	-	-
Third or Fourth Degree Laceration	-	-	3.82%	3.63%	3.27%

Saint Joseph's Mercy Health Center

300 Werner Street
PO Box 29001
Hot Springs Natl Pk, AR 71903
URL: www.saintjosephs.com
Ownership: Voluntary non-profit - Church
Emergency Services: Yes

Phone: 501-622-1000
Fax: 501-622-1199

Accredited: Yes
Licensed Beds: 309

Key Personnel:
President/CEO . . . . Randy Fale
Director Respiratory Therapy . . . . John Campbell

Measure	Cases	This Hospital	State Average	U.S. Average	Top Hospital
Heart Attack Care					
ACE Inhibitor or ARB for LVSD	53	83%	82%	82%	100%
Aspirin at Arrival	181	99%	88%	92%	100%
Aspirin at Discharge	209	100%	87%	90%	100%
Beta Blocker at Arrival	145	91%	82%	87%	100%
Beta Blocker at Discharge	156	94%	86%	90%	100%
Fibrinolytic Medication Timing[1]	20	60%	41%	31%	100%
PCI Within 90 Minutes of Arrival[1]	2	50%	46%	54%	95%
Smoking Cessation Advice	93	100%	91%	88%	100%
Heart Failure Care					
ACE Inhibitor or ARB for LVSD	135	96%	78%	82%	100%
Discharge Instructions	282	80%	65%	61%	93%
Evaluation of LVS Function	345	97%	81%	83%	99%
Smoking Cessation Advice	87	98%	86%	82%	100%
Pneumonia Care					
Appropriate Initial Antibiotic	253	85%	83%	83%	94%
Blood Culture Timing	233	93%	93%	90%	100%
Influenza Vaccine	72	89%	70%	70%	100%
Initial Antibiotic Timing	344	84%	82%	80%	93%
Oxygenation Assessment	433	100%	99%	99%	100%
Pneumococcal Vaccine	282	92%	68%	69%	94%
Smoking Cessation Advice	118	96%	83%	80%	100%
Surgical Infection Prevention					
Prophylactic Antibiotic Given[2]	587	95%	73%	77%	95%
Prophylactic Antibiotic Selection[2]	58	97%	90%	90%	100%
Prophylactic Antibiotic Stopped[2]	540	79%	74%	72%	95%
Pregnancy Care					
Inpatient Neonatal Mortality	-	-	-	-	-
Third or Fourth Degree Laceration	-	-	3.82%	3.63%	3.27%

Rebsamen Medical Center

1400 Braden Street
Jacksonville, AR 72076
Ownership: Voluntary non-profit - Other
Emergency Services: Yes

Phone: 501-985-7000
Fax: 501-982-3055

Accredited: Yes

Key Personnel:
CEO . . . . Kurt Meyer
Head of Catheterization . . . . David Johnson
Director Medical/Surgical Nursing . . . . Alice Jenson
Director Medical/Surgical Nursing . . . . Carolyn Webb
Chief Radiology . . . . Mike Miller
Director of Respiratory . . . . Cindy Stafford

Measure	Cases	This Hospital	State Average	U.S. Average	Top Hospital
Heart Attack Care					
ACE Inhibitor or ARB for LVSD[1]	6	50%	82%	82%	100%
Aspirin at Arrival	30	97%	88%	92%	100%
Aspirin at Discharge[1]	14	64%	87%	90%	100%
Beta Blocker at Arrival	27	89%	82%	87%	100%

NOTE: Hospital profiles are in alphabetical order by state, then city, then hospital within the city; Rankings are sorted by rate in descending order and exclude hospitals with less than 25 cases; (1) The number of cases is too small (n<25) for purposes of reliably predicting hospital performance; (2) Measure reflects the hospital's indication that its submission was based upon a sample of its relevant discharges; (3) Rate reflects fewer than the maximum possible quarters of data for the measure; (4) Inaccurate information submitted and suppressed for one or more quarters; (5) No data is available from the hospital for this measure; Please refer to the User's Guide for a full explanation of data

Measure	Cases	This Hospital	State Average	U.S. Average	Top Hospital
Beta Blocker at Discharge[1]	16	81%	86%	90%	100%
Fibrinolytic Medication Timing[3]	0	-	41%	31%	100%
PCI Within 90 Minutes of Arrival	0	-	46%	54%	95%
Smoking Cessation Advice[1,3]	2	100%	91%	88%	100%
Heart Failure Care					
ACE Inhibitor or ARB for LVSD	29	72%	78%	82%	100%
Discharge Instructions[1,3]	15	13%	65%	61%	93%
Evaluation of LVS Function	91	90%	81%	83%	99%
Smoking Cessation Advice[1,3]	3	67%	86%	82%	100%
Pneumonia Care					
Appropriate Initial Antibiotic[1,3]	18	83%	83%	83%	94%
Blood Culture Timing[1,3]	18	89%	93%	90%	100%
Influenza Vaccine[5]	-	-	70%	70%	100%
Initial Antibiotic Timing	116	84%	82%	80%	93%
Oxygenation Assessment	149	100%	99%	99%	100%
Pneumococcal Vaccine	95	44%	68%	69%	94%
Smoking Cessation Advice[1,3]	6	67%	83%	80%	100%
Surgical Infection Prevention					
Prophylactic Antibiotic Given[2,3]	36	89%	73%	77%	95%
Prophylactic Antibiotic Selection[5]	-	-	90%	90%	100%
Prophylactic Antibiotic Stopped[2,3]	29	93%	74%	72%	95%
Pregnancy Care					
Inpatient Neonatal Mortality	466	0.00%	-	-	-
Third or Fourth Degree Laceration	318	1.57%	3.82%	3.63%	3.27%

NEA Medical Center

3024 Stadium Boulevard
Jonesboro, AR 72401
URL: www.rmcnea.com
Ownership: Proprietary
Emergency Services: Yes

Phone: 870-972-7000
Fax: 870-972-7051

Accredited: Yes
Licensed Beds: 104

Key Personnel:
CEO . . . . William Lievense
Emergency Room . . . . Rick Cole

Measure	Cases	This Hospital	State Average	U.S. Average	Top Hospital
Heart Attack Care					
ACE Inhibitor or ARB for LVSD[1]	20	95%	82%	82%	100%
Aspirin at Arrival	92	97%	88%	92%	100%
Aspirin at Discharge	173	98%	87%	90%	100%
Beta Blocker at Arrival	68	90%	82%	87%	100%
Beta Blocker at Discharge	141	89%	86%	90%	100%
Fibrinolytic Medication Timing	0	-	41%	31%	100%
PCI Within 90 Minutes of Arrival[1]	4	75%	46%	54%	95%
Smoking Cessation Advice	78	99%	91%	88%	100%
Heart Failure Care					
ACE Inhibitor or ARB for LVSD	102	93%	78%	82%	100%
Discharge Instructions	196	82%	65%	61%	93%
Evaluation of LVS Function	222	98%	81%	83%	99%
Smoking Cessation Advice	41	100%	86%	82%	100%
Pneumonia Care					
Appropriate Initial Antibiotic	141	84%	83%	83%	94%
Blood Culture Timing	93	96%	93%	90%	100%
Influenza Vaccine	44	75%	70%	70%	100%
Initial Antibiotic Timing	174	88%	82%	80%	93%
Oxygenation Assessment	212	100%	99%	99%	100%
Pneumococcal Vaccine	131	94%	68%	69%	94%
Smoking Cessation Advice	65	98%	83%	80%	100%
Surgical Infection Prevention					
Prophylactic Antibiotic Given	379	97%	73%	77%	95%
Prophylactic Antibiotic Selection	105	99%	90%	90%	100%
Prophylactic Antibiotic Stopped	375	71%	74%	72%	95%
Pregnancy Care					
Inpatient Neonatal Mortality	-	-	-	-	-
Third or Fourth Degree Laceration	-	-	3.82%	3.63%	3.27%

Saint Bernard's Medical Center

225 E Jackson
Jonesboro, AR 72401

Toll-Free: 888-782-4555
Phone: 870-972-4100
Fax: 870-974-5112

URL: www.sbrmc.com
Ownership: Voluntary non-profit - Church
Emergency Services: Yes

Accredited: Yes
Licensed Beds: 375

Key Personnel:
President/CEO . . . . Ben E Owens
Administrator . . . . Scott Street
Chief Medical Staff . . . . BJ Cranfill, MD
Cardiac Lab . . . . Jo Yawn
Catheterization Lab . . . . Vonda Curtis
Emergency Room . . . . Katheryn Blackman
Infection Control . . . . Debbi Ledbetter, RN
Director Surgery . . . . Dorothy Byford, RN

Measure	Cases	This Hospital	State Average	U.S. Average	Top Hospital
Heart Attack Care					
ACE Inhibitor or ARB for LVSD	100	90%	82%	82%	100%
Aspirin at Arrival	215	97%	88%	92%	100%
Aspirin at Discharge	368	96%	87%	90%	100%
Beta Blocker at Arrival	140	89%	82%	87%	100%
Beta Blocker at Discharge	368	95%	86%	90%	100%
Fibrinolytic Medication Timing	0	-	41%	31%	100%
PCI Within 90 Minutes of Arrival[1]	7	100%	46%	54%	95%
Smoking Cessation Advice	192	99%	91%	88%	100%
Heart Failure Care					
ACE Inhibitor or ARB for LVSD	317	85%	78%	82%	100%
Discharge Instructions	506	59%	65%	61%	93%
Evaluation of LVS Function	613	99%	81%	83%	99%
Smoking Cessation Advice	151	99%	86%	82%	100%
Pneumonia Care					
Appropriate Initial Antibiotic	266	88%	83%	83%	94%
Blood Culture Timing	210	93%	93%	90%	100%
Influenza Vaccine	76	75%	70%	70%	100%
Initial Antibiotic Timing	372	76%	82%	80%	93%
Oxygenation Assessment	448	99%	99%	99%	100%
Pneumococcal Vaccine	262	81%	68%	69%	94%
Smoking Cessation Advice	172	94%	83%	80%	100%
Surgical Infection Prevention					
Prophylactic Antibiotic Given	728	94%	73%	77%	95%
Prophylactic Antibiotic Selection	144	97%	90%	90%	100%
Prophylactic Antibiotic Stopped	698	87%	74%	72%	95%
Pregnancy Care					
Inpatient Neonatal Mortality	1,412	0.07%	-	-	-
Third or Fourth Degree Laceration	925	4.00%	3.82%	3.63%	3.27%

Surgical Hospital of Jonesboro

909 Enterprise Drive
Jonesboro, AR 72401
Ownership: Proprietary
Emergency Services: Yes

Phone: 870-336-1100

Accredited: No

Measure	Cases	This Hospital	State Average	U.S. Average	Top Hospital
Heart Attack Care					
ACE Inhibitor or ARB for LVSD[5]	-	-	82%	82%	100%
Aspirin at Arrival[5]	-	-	88%	92%	100%
Aspirin at Discharge[5]	-	-	87%	90%	100%
Beta Blocker at Arrival[5]	-	-	82%	87%	100%
Beta Blocker at Discharge[5]	-	-	86%	90%	100%
Fibrinolytic Medication Timing[5]	-	-	41%	31%	100%
PCI Within 90 Minutes of Arrival[5]	-	-	46%	54%	95%
Smoking Cessation Advice[5]	-	-	91%	88%	100%
Heart Failure Care					
ACE Inhibitor or ARB for LVSD[5]	-	-	78%	82%	100%
Discharge Instructions[5]	-	-	65%	61%	93%
Evaluation of LVS Function[5]	-	-	81%	83%	99%
Smoking Cessation Advice[5]	-	-	86%	82%	100%
Pneumonia Care					
Appropriate Initial Antibiotic[5]	-	-	83%	83%	94%
Blood Culture Timing[5]	-	-	93%	90%	100%
Influenza Vaccine[5]	-	-	70%	70%	100%

NOTE: Hospital profiles are in alphabetical order by state, then city, then hospital within the city; Rankings are sorted by rate in descending order and exclude hospitals with less than 25 cases; (1) The number of cases is too small (n<25) for purposes of reliably predicting hospital performance; (2) Measure reflects the hospital's indication that its submission was based upon a sample of its relevant discharges; (3) Rate reflects fewer than the maximum possible quarters of data for the measure; (4) Inaccurate information submitted and suppressed for one or more quarters; (5) No data is available from the hospital for this measure; Please refer to the User's Guide for a full explanation of data

		This Hospital	State Average	U.S. Average	Top Hospital
Initial Antibiotic Timing[5]	-	-	82%	80%	93%
Oxygenation Assessment[5]	-	-	99%	99%	100%
Pneumococcal Vaccine[5]	-	-	68%	69%	94%
Smoking Cessation Advice[5]	-	-	83%	80%	100%
Surgical Infection Prevention					
Prophylactic Antibiotic Given[2]	192	74%	73%	77%	95%
Prophylactic Antibiotic Selection[1,2]	19	100%	90%	90%	100%
Prophylactic Antibiotic Stopped[2]	190	92%	74%	72%	95%
Pregnancy Care					
Inpatient Neonatal Mortality	-	-	-	-	-
Third or Fourth Degree Laceration	-	-	3.82%	3.63%	3.27%

Chicot Memorial Hospital

2729 Highway 65 & 82 South
Lake Village, AR 71653
Ownership: Government - Local
Emergency Services: Yes

Phone: 870-265-5351
Fax: 870-265-2091
Accredited: No
Licensed Beds: 25

Key Personnel:
Administrator/CEO . . . . Bruce A Bennett
Chief Medical Staff . . . . John R Russell, MD
Chief Radiology . . . . T Tuangsith, MD
Director Respiratory Therapy . . . . Clarence Johnson, CRRT

Measure	Cases	This Hospital	State Average	U.S. Average	Top Hospital
Heart Attack Care					
ACE Inhibitor or ARB for LVSD	0	-	82%	82%	100%
Aspirin at Arrival[1]	6	50%	88%	92%	100%
Aspirin at Discharge[1]	2	50%	87%	90%	100%
Beta Blocker at Arrival[1]	5	100%	82%	87%	100%
Beta Blocker at Discharge[1]	2	50%	86%	90%	100%
Fibrinolytic Medication Timing	0	-	41%	31%	100%
PCI Within 90 Minutes of Arrival	0	-	46%	54%	95%
Smoking Cessation Advice	0	-	91%	88%	100%
Heart Failure Care					
ACE Inhibitor or ARB for LVSD	38	97%	78%	82%	100%
Discharge Instructions	141	72%	65%	61%	93%
Evaluation of LVS Function	172	94%	81%	83%	99%
Smoking Cessation Advice[1]	24	75%	86%	82%	100%
Pneumonia Care					
Appropriate Initial Antibiotic	61	85%	83%	83%	94%
Blood Culture Timing[1]	14	100%	93%	90%	100%
Influenza Vaccine[4,5]	-	-	70%	70%	100%
Initial Antibiotic Timing	65	83%	82%	80%	93%
Oxygenation Assessment	71	97%	99%	99%	100%
Pneumococcal Vaccine	40	68%	68%	69%	94%
Smoking Cessation Advice[1]	16	88%	83%	80%	100%
Surgical Infection Prevention					
Prophylactic Antibiotic Given[1]	15	80%	73%	77%	95%
Prophylactic Antibiotic Selection[1]	3	100%	90%	90%	100%
Prophylactic Antibiotic Stopped[1]	15	100%	74%	72%	95%
Pregnancy Care					
Inpatient Neonatal Mortality	-	-	-	-	-
Third or Fourth Degree Laceration	-	-	3.82%	3.63%	3.27%

Arkansas Heart Hospital

1701 South Shackleford Road
Little Rock, AR 72211
URL: www.arheart.com
Ownership: Proprietary
Emergency Services: Yes

Phone: 501-219-7000
Fax: 501-219-7402

Accredited: Yes
Licensed Beds: 84

Key Personnel:
President/CEO . . . . Charlie Smith
Surgical Director . . . . C O Williams

Measure	Cases	This Hospital	State Average	U.S. Average	Top Hospital
Heart Attack Care					
ACE Inhibitor or ARB for LVSD	126	75%	82%	82%	100%
Aspirin at Arrival	87	99%	88%	92%	100%
Aspirin at Discharge	435	91%	87%	90%	100%
Beta Blocker at Arrival	80	88%	82%	87%	100%
Beta Blocker at Discharge	414	89%	86%	90%	100%
Fibrinolytic Medication Timing	0	-	41%	31%	100%

Measure	Cases	This Hospital	State Average	U.S. Average	Top Hospital
PCI Within 90 Minutes of Arrival	0	-	46%	54%	95%
Smoking Cessation Advice	195	99%	91%	88%	100%
Heart Failure Care					
ACE Inhibitor or ARB for LVSD	327	69%	78%	82%	100%
Discharge Instructions	461	77%	65%	61%	93%
Evaluation of LVS Function	512	88%	81%	83%	99%
Smoking Cessation Advice	75	99%	86%	82%	100%
Pneumonia Care					
Appropriate Initial Antibiotic	29	41%	83%	83%	94%
Blood Culture Timing[1]	15	80%	93%	90%	100%
Influenza Vaccine[1]	4	0%	70%	70%	100%
Initial Antibiotic Timing	29	86%	82%	80%	93%
Oxygenation Assessment	35	100%	99%	99%	100%
Pneumococcal Vaccine	26	31%	68%	69%	94%
Smoking Cessation Advice[1]	11	91%	83%	80%	100%
Surgical Infection Prevention					
Prophylactic Antibiotic Given[3]	605	91%	73%	77%	95%
Prophylactic Antibiotic Selection	186	100%	90%	90%	100%
Prophylactic Antibiotic Stopped[3]	595	81%	74%	72%	95%
Pregnancy Care					
Inpatient Neonatal Mortality	-	-	-	-	-
Third or Fourth Degree Laceration	-	-	3.82%	3.63%	3.27%

Baptist Health Medical Center

Alternate Name: Baptist Medical Center
9601 Interstate 630
Exit 7
Little Rock, AR 72205
URL: www.baptist-health.com
Ownership: Voluntary non-profit - Private
Emergency Services: Yes

Phone: 501-202-2000
Fax: 501-202-1280

Accredited: Yes
Licensed Beds: 787

Key Personnel:
President/CEO . . . . Russel D Harrington Jr
Chief Medical Staff . . . . Neal Beaton, MD
Emergency Room . . . . Marvin Leibovich, MD
Director Infection/Disease Control . . . . John Schultz, MD
OB/GYN Womens Health . . . . Rick Wyatt, MD
Director Radiology . . . . Cecile Shoptan, MD
Director Respiratory Therapy . . . . Marsha Lewis

Measure	Cases	This Hospital	State Average	U.S. Average	Top Hospital
Heart Attack Care					
ACE Inhibitor or ARB for LVSD	88	90%	82%	82%	100%
Aspirin at Arrival	163	99%	88%	92%	100%
Aspirin at Discharge	327	98%	87%	90%	100%
Beta Blocker at Arrival	131	99%	82%	87%	100%
Beta Blocker at Discharge	340	98%	86%	90%	100%
Fibrinolytic Medication Timing	0	-	41%	31%	100%
PCI Within 90 Minutes of Arrival[1]	13	31%	46%	54%	95%
Smoking Cessation Advice	153	97%	91%	88%	100%
Heart Failure Care					
ACE Inhibitor or ARB for LVSD	362	89%	78%	82%	100%
Discharge Instructions	649	65%	65%	61%	93%
Evaluation of LVS Function	762	96%	81%	83%	99%
Smoking Cessation Advice	110	99%	86%	82%	100%
Pneumonia Care					
Appropriate Initial Antibiotic	251	73%	83%	83%	94%
Blood Culture Timing	192	90%	93%	90%	100%
Influenza Vaccine	56	75%	70%	70%	100%
Initial Antibiotic Timing	345	60%	82%	80%	93%
Oxygenation Assessment	413	100%	99%	99%	100%
Pneumococcal Vaccine	229	76%	68%	69%	94%
Smoking Cessation Advice	76	96%	83%	80%	100%
Surgical Infection Prevention					
Prophylactic Antibiotic Given[3]	486	85%	73%	77%	95%
Prophylactic Antibiotic Selection	158	88%	90%	90%	100%
Prophylactic Antibiotic Stopped[3]	475	80%	74%	72%	95%
Pregnancy Care					
Inpatient Neonatal Mortality	2,853	0.60%	-	-	-
Third or Fourth Degree Laceration	1,553	2.96%	3.82%	3.63%	3.27%

NOTE: Hospital profiles are in alphabetical order by state, then city, then hospital within the city; Rankings are sorted by rate in descending order and exclude hospitals with less than 25 cases; (1) The number of cases is too small (n<25) for purposes of reliably predicting hospital performance; (2) Measure reflects the hospital's indication that its submission was based upon a sample of its relevant discharges; (3) Rate reflects fewer than the maximum possible quarters of data for the measure; (4) Inaccurate information submitted and suppressed for one or more quarters; (5) No data is available from the hospital for this measure; Please refer to the User's Guide for a full explanation of data

Saint Vincent Infirmary Medical Center

2 Saint Vincent Circle   Phone: 501-552-3000
Little Rock, AR 72205   Fax: 501-552-4510
URL: www.stvincenthealth.org
Ownership: Voluntary non-profit - Church   Accredited: Yes
Emergency Services: Yes   Licensed Beds: 611

Key Personnel:
President/CEO . . . . Diana T Hueter
Chief Medical Staff . . . . Gail A McCracken, MD
Emergency Room . . . . Leslie H Sessions, MD
Director Infection/Disease Control . . . . Kenny Kemp
Director Medical/Surgical Nursing . . . . Georgia Berry
OB/GYN Womens Health . . . . DB Allen, MD
Chief Radiology . . . . David Tamas, MD
Director Respiratory Therapy . . . . Duane Clausen

Measure	Cases	This Hospital	State Average	U.S. Average	Top Hospital
Heart Attack Care					
ACE Inhibitor or ARB for LVSD	63	68%	82%	82%	100%
Aspirin at Arrival	145	96%	88%	92%	100%
Aspirin at Discharge	244	96%	87%	90%	100%
Beta Blocker at Arrival	104	91%	82%	87%	100%
Beta Blocker at Discharge	243	95%	86%	90%	100%
Fibrinolytic Medication Timing	0	-	41%	31%	100%
PCI Within 90 Minutes of Arrival[1]	5	20%	46%	54%	95%
Smoking Cessation Advice	111	100%	91%	88%	100%
Heart Failure Care					
ACE Inhibitor or ARB for LVSD	228	86%	78%	82%	100%
Discharge Instructions	423	44%	65%	61%	93%
Evaluation of LVS Function	508	91%	81%	83%	99%
Smoking Cessation Advice	100	99%	86%	82%	100%
Pneumonia Care					
Appropriate Initial Antibiotic	187	81%	83%	83%	94%
Blood Culture Timing	166	92%	93%	90%	100%
Influenza Vaccine	72	71%	70%	70%	100%
Initial Antibiotic Timing	264	80%	82%	80%	93%
Oxygenation Assessment	317	100%	99%	99%	100%
Pneumococcal Vaccine	191	72%	68%	69%	94%
Smoking Cessation Advice	93	98%	83%	80%	100%
Surgical Infection Prevention					
Prophylactic Antibiotic Given[3]	221	83%	73%	77%	95%
Prophylactic Antibiotic Selection	74	99%	90%	90%	100%
Prophylactic Antibiotic Stopped[3]	216	77%	74%	72%	95%
Pregnancy Care					
Inpatient Neonatal Mortality	2,042	0.54%	-	-	-
Third or Fourth Degree Laceration	1,446	5.88%	3.82%	3.63%	3.27%

Southwest Regional Medical Centre

11401 Interstate 30   Phone: 501-455-7100
Little Rock, AR 72209   Fax: 501-455-7399
Ownership: Proprietary   Accredited: Yes
Emergency Services: Yes   Licensed Beds: 125

Key Personnel:
CEO/CFO . . . . Nancy Fodi
Emergency Room . . . . Shelly Goldthrope
Director of Respiratory . . . . Randy Freed

Measure	Cases	This Hospital	State Average	U.S. Average	Top Hospital
Heart Attack Care					
ACE Inhibitor or ARB for LVSD[1]	9	89%	82%	82%	100%
Aspirin at Arrival[1]	15	93%	88%	92%	100%
Aspirin at Discharge[1]	16	100%	87%	90%	100%
Beta Blocker at Arrival[1]	17	88%	82%	87%	100%
Beta Blocker at Discharge[1]	17	88%	86%	90%	100%
Fibrinolytic Medication Timing[3]	0	-	41%	31%	100%
PCI Within 90 Minutes of Arrival	0	-	46%	54%	95%
Smoking Cessation Advice[3]	0	-	91%	88%	100%
Heart Failure Care					
ACE Inhibitor or ARB for LVSD[1]	15	80%	78%	82%	100%
Discharge Instructions[1,3]	3	67%	65%	61%	93%
Evaluation of LVS Function	31	71%	81%	83%	99%
Smoking Cessation Advice[1,3]	1	0%	86%	82%	100%
Pneumonia Care					

Appropriate Initial Antibiotic[1,3]	4	75%	83%	83%	94%
Blood Culture Timing[1,3]	8	75%	93%	90%	100%
Influenza Vaccine[5]	-	-	70%	70%	100%
Initial Antibiotic Timing	48	75%	82%	80%	93%
Oxygenation Assessment	61	100%	99%	99%	100%
Pneumococcal Vaccine	28	39%	68%	69%	94%
Smoking Cessation Advice[1,3]	1	0%	83%	80%	100%
Surgical Infection Prevention					
Prophylactic Antibiotic Given[3]	89	73%	73%	77%	95%
Prophylactic Antibiotic Selection[5]	-	-	90%	90%	100%
Prophylactic Antibiotic Stopped[3]	83	57%	74%	72%	95%
Pregnancy Care					
Inpatient Neonatal Mortality	-	-	-	-	-
Third or Fourth Degree Laceration	-	-	3.82%	3.63%	3.27%

UAMS Medical Center

4301 W Markham Street   Phone: 501-686-7000
Little Rock, AR 72205   Fax: 501-686-5554
URL: www.uams.edu/medcenter
Ownership: Government - State   Accredited: Yes
Emergency Services: Yes   Licensed Beds: 400

Key Personnel:
CEO/Executive Director . . . . Richard A Pierson
Chief Catheterization Laboratory . . . . Jon Lindemann, MD
Emergency Room . . . . Gail Ray, MD
Director Infection/Disease Control . . . . Robert W Bradsher, MD
CCU Spvg. Nurse . . . . Mary Helen Forrest, RN
Director Medical/Surgical Nursing . . . . Carol Murry, RN
OB/GYN Womens Health . . . . J Gerald Quirk, MD
Chief Radiology . . . . Ernest Ferris, MD

Measure	Cases	This Hospital	State Average	U.S. Average	Top Hospital
Heart Attack Care					
ACE Inhibitor or ARB for LVSD	33	82%	82%	82%	100%
Aspirin at Arrival	97	96%	88%	92%	100%
Aspirin at Discharge	88	95%	87%	90%	100%
Beta Blocker at Arrival	67	85%	82%	87%	100%
Beta Blocker at Discharge	102	96%	86%	90%	100%
Fibrinolytic Medication Timing[1]	1	0%	41%	31%	100%
PCI Within 90 Minutes of Arrival[1]	4	50%	46%	54%	95%
Smoking Cessation Advice	57	100%	91%	88%	100%
Heart Failure Care					
ACE Inhibitor or ARB for LVSD	192	79%	78%	82%	100%
Discharge Instructions	263	71%	65%	61%	93%
Evaluation of LVS Function	288	97%	81%	83%	99%
Smoking Cessation Advice	98	100%	86%	82%	100%
Pneumonia Care					
Appropriate Initial Antibiotic	119	87%	83%	83%	94%
Blood Culture Timing	176	86%	93%	90%	100%
Influenza Vaccine	51	49%	70%	70%	100%
Initial Antibiotic Timing	228	55%	82%	80%	93%
Oxygenation Assessment	335	100%	99%	99%	100%
Pneumococcal Vaccine	118	36%	68%	69%	94%
Smoking Cessation Advice	106	99%	83%	80%	100%
Surgical Infection Prevention					
Prophylactic Antibiotic Given[2,3]	303	74%	73%	77%	95%
Prophylactic Antibiotic Selection[2]	73	56%	90%	90%	100%
Prophylactic Antibiotic Stopped[2,3]	292	88%	74%	72%	95%
Pregnancy Care					
Inpatient Neonatal Mortality	2,029	1.97%	-	-	-
Third or Fourth Degree Laceration	1,224	6.37%	3.82%	3.63%	3.27%

Magnolia Hospital

101 Hospital Drive   Phone: 870-235-3000
Magnolia, AR 71753   Fax: 870-235-3557
E-mail: nwarren@magnolia-net.com
URL: www.magnolia-net.com
Ownership: Government - Local   Accredited: Yes
Emergency Services: Yes   Licensed Beds: 70

Key Personnel:
Chief Medical Staff . . . . Fred Murphy, MD
Director Infection/Disease Control . . . . Robin Proctor, B.S.N.
Chief CCU . . . . Fred Murphy, MD

NOTE: Hospital profiles are in alphabetical order by state, then city, then hospital within the city; Rankings are sorted by rate in descending order and exclude hospitals with less than 25 cases; (1) The number of cases is too small (n<25) for purposes of reliably predicting hospital performance; (2) Measure reflects the hospital's indication that its submission was based upon a sample of its relevant discharges; (3) Rate reflects fewer than the maximum possible quarters of data for the measure; (4) Inaccurate information submitted and suppressed for one or more quarters; (5) No data is available from the hospital for this measure; Please refer to the User's Guide for a full explanation of data

Chief OB/GYN . . . . Frank Roberts, MD
Chief Radiology . . . . Robert Parkman, MD
Director Respiratory Therapy . . . . Paul Linder

Measure	Cases	This Hospital	State Average	U.S. Average	Top Hospital
Heart Attack Care					
ACE Inhibitor or ARB for LVSD[1]	1	100%	82%	82%	100%
Aspirin at Arrival[1]	13	92%	88%	92%	100%
Aspirin at Discharge[1]	4	75%	87%	90%	100%
Beta Blocker at Arrival[1]	6	100%	82%	87%	100%
Beta Blocker at Discharge[1]	3	100%	86%	90%	100%
Fibrinolytic Medication Timing[1]	7	57%	41%	31%	100%
PCI Within 90 Minutes of Arrival	0	-	46%	54%	95%
Smoking Cessation Advice[1]	1	100%	91%	88%	100%
Heart Failure Care					
ACE Inhibitor or ARB for LVSD	41	85%	78%	82%	100%
Discharge Instructions	90	78%	65%	61%	93%
Evaluation of LVS Function	103	76%	81%	83%	99%
Smoking Cessation Advice[1]	15	100%	86%	82%	100%
Pneumonia Care					
Appropriate Initial Antibiotic	59	80%	83%	83%	94%
Blood Culture Timing	53	96%	93%	90%	100%
Influenza Vaccine[1]	14	71%	70%	70%	100%
Initial Antibiotic Timing	88	85%	82%	80%	93%
Oxygenation Assessment	103	99%	99%	99%	100%
Pneumococcal Vaccine	61	70%	68%	69%	94%
Smoking Cessation Advice[1]	16	81%	83%	80%	100%
Surgical Infection Prevention					
Prophylactic Antibiotic Given[1,3]	13	46%	73%	77%	95%
Prophylactic Antibiotic Selection[1]	7	71%	90%	90%	100%
Prophylactic Antibiotic Stopped[1,3]	11	100%	74%	72%	95%
Pregnancy Care					
Inpatient Neonatal Mortality	-	-	-	-	-
Third or Fourth Degree Laceration	-	-	3.82%	3.63%	3.27%

Hot Springs County Medical Center

1001 Schneider Drive
Malvern, AR 72104
E-mail: Info@hscmc.org
URL: www.hscmc.org
Ownership: Voluntary non-profit - Private
Emergency Services: Yes

Phone: 501-332-1000
Fax: 501-332-7395

Accredited: No
Licensed Beds: 92

Key Personnel:
CEO. . . . . Phillip K Gilmore
Chief Medical Staff. . . . . Shane Higginbotham, MD
Emergency Room . . . . Robert Brown
Cardiology . . . . Charles Clogston
Director Respiratory Care. . . . . Lisa Goarl

Measure	Cases	This Hospital	State Average	U.S. Average	Top Hospital
Heart Attack Care					
ACE Inhibitor or ARB for LVSD[1]	1	100%	82%	82%	100%
Aspirin at Arrival[1]	9	89%	88%	92%	100%
Aspirin at Discharge[1]	5	80%	87%	90%	100%
Beta Blocker at Arrival[1]	6	50%	82%	87%	100%
Beta Blocker at Discharge[1]	7	86%	86%	90%	100%
Fibrinolytic Medication Timing	0	-	41%	31%	100%
PCI Within 90 Minutes of Arrival	0	-	46%	54%	95%
Smoking Cessation Advice	0	-	91%	88%	100%
Heart Failure Care					
ACE Inhibitor or ARB for LVSD	36	67%	78%	82%	100%
Discharge Instructions	111	33%	65%	61%	93%
Evaluation of LVS Function	135	71%	81%	83%	99%
Smoking Cessation Advice[1]	23	65%	86%	82%	100%
Pneumonia Care					
Appropriate Initial Antibiotic	109	87%	83%	83%	94%
Blood Culture Timing	76	93%	93%	90%	100%
Influenza Vaccine[4,5]	-	-	70%	70%	100%
Initial Antibiotic Timing	176	93%	82%	80%	93%
Oxygenation Assessment	180	98%	99%	99%	100%
Pneumococcal Vaccine	98	50%	68%	69%	94%
Smoking Cessation Advice	49	82%	83%	80%	100%

Measure	Cases	This Hospital	State Average	U.S. Average	Top Hospital
Surgical Infection Prevention					
Prophylactic Antibiotic Given[1,3]	14	71%	73%	77%	95%
Prophylactic Antibiotic Selection[1]	4	100%	90%	90%	100%
Prophylactic Antibiotic Stopped[1,3]	15	93%	74%	72%	95%
Pregnancy Care					
Inpatient Neonatal Mortality	-	-	-	-	-
Third or Fourth Degree Laceration	-	-	3.82%	3.63%	3.27%

McGehee-Desha County Hospital

900 S 3rd Street
McGehee, AR 71654
Ownership: Government - Local
Emergency Services: No

Phone: 870-222-5600
Fax: 870-222-4253
Accredited: No
Licensed Beds: 34

Key Personnel:
CEO. . . . . John Heard

Measure	Cases	This Hospital	State Average	U.S. Average	Top Hospital
Heart Attack Care					
ACE Inhibitor or ARB for LVSD[3]	0	-	82%	82%	100%
Aspirin at Arrival[1,3]	3	33%	88%	92%	100%
Aspirin at Discharge[1,3]	3	67%	87%	90%	100%
Beta Blocker at Arrival[1,3]	3	33%	82%	87%	100%
Beta Blocker at Discharge[1,3]	3	67%	86%	90%	100%
Fibrinolytic Medication Timing[3]	0	-	41%	31%	100%
PCI Within 90 Minutes of Arrival	0	-	46%	54%	95%
Smoking Cessation Advice[3]	0	-	91%	88%	100%
Heart Failure Care					
ACE Inhibitor or ARB for LVSD[1]	2	100%	78%	82%	100%
Discharge Instructions[1]	22	82%	65%	61%	93%
Evaluation of LVS Function	30	53%	81%	83%	99%
Smoking Cessation Advice[1]	4	100%	86%	82%	100%
Pneumonia Care					
Appropriate Initial Antibiotic	31	87%	83%	83%	94%
Blood Culture Timing[1]	15	93%	93%	90%	100%
Influenza Vaccine[1]	8	50%	70%	70%	100%
Initial Antibiotic Timing	49	84%	82%	80%	93%
Oxygenation Assessment	59	100%	99%	99%	100%
Pneumococcal Vaccine	34	62%	68%	69%	94%
Smoking Cessation Advice[1]	9	100%	83%	80%	100%
Surgical Infection Prevention					
Prophylactic Antibiotic Given[5]	-	-	73%	77%	95%
Prophylactic Antibiotic Selection[5]	-	-	90%	90%	100%
Prophylactic Antibiotic Stopped[5]	-	-	74%	72%	95%
Pregnancy Care					
Inpatient Neonatal Mortality	-	-	-	-	-
Third or Fourth Degree Laceration	-	-	3.82%	3.63%	3.27%

Mena Medical Center

311 N Morrow Street
Mena, AR 71953
Ownership: Government - Local
Emergency Services: No

Phone: 479-394-6100
Fax: 501-394-4577
Accredited: No
Licensed Beds: 65

Key Personnel:
President/CEO. . . . . Vincent D DiFranco
Emergency Room . . . . Andrew David, MD
Infection Control. . . . . Pam Posey, RN
ICU . . . . Darlene Hesterlee
OB/GYN Womens Health. . . . . Tara Milham
Respiratory/Cardiopulmonary. . . . . Russell Lockhart

Measure	Cases	This Hospital	State Average	U.S. Average	Top Hospital
Heart Attack Care					
ACE Inhibitor or ARB for LVSD[1]	2	100%	82%	82%	100%
Aspirin at Arrival[1]	9	100%	88%	92%	100%
Aspirin at Discharge[1]	9	89%	87%	90%	100%
Beta Blocker at Arrival[1]	6	33%	82%	87%	100%
Beta Blocker at Discharge[1]	8	50%	86%	90%	100%
Fibrinolytic Medication Timing	0	-	41%	31%	100%
PCI Within 90 Minutes of Arrival	0	-	46%	54%	95%
Smoking Cessation Advice[1]	1	100%	91%	88%	100%
Heart Failure Care					
ACE Inhibitor or ARB for LVSD[1]	14	43%	78%	82%	100%

NOTE: Hospital profiles are in alphabetical order by state, then city, then hospital within the city; Rankings are sorted by rate in descending order and exclude hospitals with less than 25 cases; (1) The number of cases is too small (n<25) for purposes of reliably predicting hospital performance; (2) Measure reflects the hospital's indication that its submission was based upon a sample of its relevant discharges; (3) Rate reflects fewer than the maximum possible quarters of data for the measure; (4) Inaccurate information submitted and suppressed for one or more quarters; (5) No data is available from the hospital for this measure; Please refer to the User's Guide for a full explanation of data

Discharge Instructions	59	53%	65%	61%	93%
Evaluation of LVS Function	74	62%	81%	83%	99%
Smoking Cessation Advice[1]	9	100%	86%	82%	100%
Pneumonia Care					
Appropriate Initial Antibiotic	57	91%	83%	83%	94%
Blood Culture Timing	34	88%	93%	90%	100%
Influenza Vaccine[1]	9	33%	70%	70%	100%
Initial Antibiotic Timing	81	79%	82%	80%	93%
Oxygenation Assessment	95	99%	99%	99%	100%
Pneumococcal Vaccine	67	49%	68%	69%	94%
Smoking Cessation Advice[1]	22	77%	83%	80%	100%
Surgical Infection Prevention					
Prophylactic Antibiotic Given[2,3]	30	80%	73%	77%	95%
Prophylactic Antibiotic Selection[1,2]	11	82%	90%	90%	100%
Prophylactic Antibiotic Stopped[2,3]	27	93%	74%	72%	95%
Pregnancy Care					
Inpatient Neonatal Mortality	-	-	-	-	-
Third or Fourth Degree Laceration	-	-	3.82%	3.63%	3.27%

Drew Memorial Hospital

778 Scogin Drive   Phone: 870-460-3539
Monticello, AR 71655   Fax: 870-460-3562
E-mail: sweast@drewmemorial.org
URL: www.drewmemorial.org
Ownership: Government - Local   Accredited: No
Emergency Services: No   Licensed Beds: 49
Key Personnel:
President/CEO. . . . . Richard L Goddard, MA
Emergency Room . . . . Bill Williams, MD
Infection Control. . . . . Barbara Barnes, RN
ICU . . . . Zelda Pryor, RN
Intensive/Coronary Care . . . . Zelda Pryor, RN
Medical/Surgical Manager . . . . Donna Sledge, RN
Director Surgery. . . . . Ginger Jeffers, RN
Director Radiology . . . . David Gossman, BSRT
Respiratory/Cardiopulmonary Director . . . . Cherie Brown, RRT

Measure	Cases	This Hospital	State Average	U.S. Average	Top Hospital
Heart Attack Care					
ACE Inhibitor or ARB for LVSD[3]	0	-	82%	82%	100%
Aspirin at Arrival[3]	0	-	88%	92%	100%
Aspirin at Discharge[3]	0	-	87%	90%	100%
Beta Blocker at Arrival[3]	0	-	82%	87%	100%
Beta Blocker at Discharge[3]	0	-	86%	90%	100%
Fibrinolytic Medication Timing[3]	0	-	41%	31%	100%
PCI Within 90 Minutes of Arrival	0	-	46%	54%	95%
Smoking Cessation Advice[3]	0	-	91%	88%	100%
Heart Failure Care					
ACE Inhibitor or ARB for LVSD[1]	15	73%	78%	82%	100%
Discharge Instructions	42	57%	65%	61%	93%
Evaluation of LVS Function	52	75%	81%	83%	99%
Smoking Cessation Advice[1]	17	94%	86%	82%	100%
Pneumonia Care					
Appropriate Initial Antibiotic	70	74%	83%	83%	94%
Blood Culture Timing[1]	22	100%	93%	90%	100%
Influenza Vaccine[1]	16	62%	70%	70%	100%
Initial Antibiotic Timing	85	75%	82%	80%	93%
Oxygenation Assessment	108	100%	99%	99%	100%
Pneumococcal Vaccine	52	35%	68%	69%	94%
Smoking Cessation Advice	30	100%	83%	80%	100%
Surgical Infection Prevention					
Prophylactic Antibiotic Given[1]	13	62%	73%	77%	95%
Prophylactic Antibiotic Selection[1]	7	100%	90%	90%	100%
Prophylactic Antibiotic Stopped[1]	13	85%	74%	72%	95%
Pregnancy Care					
Inpatient Neonatal Mortality	-	-	-	-	-
Third or Fourth Degree Laceration	-	-	3.82%	3.63%	3.27%

Saint Anthony's Healthcare Center
Alternate Name: Saint Anthony's Hospital

4 Hospital Drive   Phone: 501-977-2300
Morrilton, AR 72110   Fax: 501-977-2400
URL: stvincenthealth.com
Ownership: Voluntary non-profit - Church   Accredited: No
Emergency Services: Yes   Licensed Beds: 49
Key Personnel:
CEO. . . . . Jonathan Davis
Chief of Medical Staff. . . . . Jack Lyon, MD
Director/Emergency Room. . . . . Daphne Brown
Director/Infectious Control . . . . Holly Campbell
Director/Surgical Nursing . . . . Sharlene Mourot
Director/Respiratory . . . . Brian Dopson

Measure	Cases	This Hospital	State Average	U.S. Average	Top Hospital
Heart Attack Care					
ACE Inhibitor or ARB for LVSD	0	-	82%	82%	100%
Aspirin at Arrival[1]	2	100%	88%	92%	100%
Aspirin at Discharge[1]	2	100%	87%	90%	100%
Beta Blocker at Arrival[1]	4	100%	82%	87%	100%
Beta Blocker at Discharge[1]	3	100%	86%	90%	100%
Fibrinolytic Medication Timing	0	-	41%	31%	100%
PCI Within 90 Minutes of Arrival	0	-	46%	54%	95%
Smoking Cessation Advice	0	-	91%	88%	100%
Heart Failure Care					
ACE Inhibitor or ARB for LVSD[1]	18	89%	78%	82%	100%
Discharge Instructions[1]	24	71%	65%	61%	93%
Evaluation of LVS Function	38	97%	81%	83%	99%
Smoking Cessation Advice[1]	8	88%	86%	82%	100%
Pneumonia Care					
Appropriate Initial Antibiotic	50	76%	83%	83%	94%
Blood Culture Timing[1]	18	94%	93%	90%	100%
Influenza Vaccine[1]	9	100%	70%	70%	100%
Initial Antibiotic Timing	45	78%	82%	80%	93%
Oxygenation Assessment	72	100%	99%	99%	100%
Pneumococcal Vaccine	48	73%	68%	69%	94%
Smoking Cessation Advice[1]	20	80%	83%	80%	100%
Surgical Infection Prevention					
Prophylactic Antibiotic Given[5]	-	-	73%	77%	95%
Prophylactic Antibiotic Selection[5]	-	-	90%	90%	100%
Prophylactic Antibiotic Stopped[5]	-	-	74%	72%	95%
Pregnancy Care					
Inpatient Neonatal Mortality	-	-	-	-	-
Third or Fourth Degree Laceration	-	-	3.82%	3.63%	3.27%

Baxter Regional Medical Center

624 Hospital Drive   Phone: 870-508-1000
Mountain Home, AR 72653   Fax: 870-424-1650
URL: www.baxterregional.org
Ownership: Voluntary non-profit - Other   Accredited: No
Emergency Services: Yes   Licensed Beds: 268
Key Personnel:
CEO. . . . . Stephen M Erixon
Chief Medical Staff. Dr. Ed White
Cardiac Laboratory. Michele Pierski
Catheterization Laboratory. . . . . Michele Pierski
Director Emergency Room. . . . . Don Hunt
Emergency Room . . . . Don Huntk
Infection Control. . . . . Sherry McGoldrick
VP Med/Surg Nursing . . . . Shannon Morris
Director Womens Health . . . . Caron Alexander, MD
Director Radiology . . . . Randy Gontens, MD
Director Cardiopulmonary . . . . Cindy Hawthorne

Measure	Cases	This Hospital	State Average	U.S. Average	Top Hospital
Heart Attack Care					
ACE Inhibitor or ARB for LVSD	88	84%	82%	82%	100%
Aspirin at Arrival	270	94%	88%	92%	100%
Aspirin at Discharge	300	89%	87%	90%	100%
Beta Blocker at Arrival	256	93%	82%	87%	100%
Beta Blocker at Discharge	297	94%	86%	90%	100%
Fibrinolytic Medication Timing	0	-	41%	31%	100%
PCI Within 90 Minutes of Arrival[1]	19	32%	46%	54%	95%
Smoking Cessation Advice	109	100%	91%	88%	100%

Heart Failure Care				
ACE Inhibitor or ARB for LVSD	169	68%	78%	82%	100%
Discharge Instructions	279	71%	65%	61%	93%
Evaluation of LVS Function	357	94%	81%	83%	99%
Smoking Cessation Advice	52	96%	86%	82%	100%

Pneumonia Care				
Appropriate Initial Antibiotic	207	79%	83%	83%	94%
Blood Culture Timing	172	93%	93%	90%	100%
Influenza Vaccine	75	51%	70%	70%	100%
Initial Antibiotic Timing	291	91%	82%	80%	93%
Oxygenation Assessment	341	100%	99%	99%	100%
Pneumococcal Vaccine	229	91%	68%	69%	94%
Smoking Cessation Advice	96	99%	83%	80%	100%

Surgical Infection Prevention				
Prophylactic Antibiotic Given	713	78%	73%	77%	95%
Prophylactic Antibiotic Selection	170	86%	90%	90%	100%
Prophylactic Antibiotic Stopped	681	70%	74%	72%	95%

Pregnancy Care				
Inpatient Neonatal Mortality	-	-	-	-	-
Third or Fourth Degree Laceration	-	-	3.82%	3.63%	3.27%

Stone County Medical Center

2106 East Main Street
Mountain View, AR 72560
Ownership: Voluntary non-profit - Other
Emergency Services: Yes

Phone: 870-269-4361
Fax: 870-269-6593
Accredited: No
Licensed Beds: 25

Key Personnel:
Administrator/COO........................ Karen Craft

Measure	Cases	This Hospital	State Average	U.S. Average	Top Hospital
Heart Attack Care					
ACE Inhibitor or ARB for LVSD[1,3]	2	100%	82%	82%	100%
Aspirin at Arrival[1,3]	3	100%	88%	92%	100%
Aspirin at Discharge[1,3]	2	100%	87%	90%	100%
Beta Blocker at Arrival[1,3]	2	100%	82%	87%	100%
Beta Blocker at Discharge[1,3]	1	100%	86%	90%	100%
Fibrinolytic Medication Timing[3]	0	-	41%	31%	100%
PCI Within 90 Minutes of Arrival	0	-	46%	54%	95%
Smoking Cessation Advice[3]	0	-	91%	88%	100%
Heart Failure Care					
ACE Inhibitor or ARB for LVSD[1]	13	100%	78%	82%	100%
Discharge Instructions[1]	22	64%	65%	61%	93%
Evaluation of LVS Function	33	91%	81%	83%	99%
Smoking Cessation Advice[1]	3	33%	86%	82%	100%
Pneumonia Care					
Appropriate Initial Antibiotic	98	84%	83%	83%	94%
Blood Culture Timing	52	92%	93%	90%	100%
Influenza Vaccine	25	76%	70%	70%	100%
Initial Antibiotic Timing	82	88%	82%	80%	93%
Oxygenation Assessment	116	100%	99%	99%	100%
Pneumococcal Vaccine	76	75%	68%	69%	94%
Smoking Cessation Advice[1]	18	83%	83%	80%	100%
Surgical Infection Prevention					
Prophylactic Antibiotic Given[5]	-	-	73%	77%	95%
Prophylactic Antibiotic Selection[5]	-	-	90%	90%	100%
Prophylactic Antibiotic Stopped[5]	-	-	74%	72%	95%
Pregnancy Care					
Inpatient Neonatal Mortality	-	-	-	-	-
Third or Fourth Degree Laceration	-	-	3.82%	3.63%	3.27%

Pike County Memorial Hospital

315 E 13th Street
Murfreesboro, AR 71958
Ownership: Government - Local
Emergency Services: No

Phone: 870-285-3182
Fax: 870-285-3305
Accredited: No
Licensed Beds: 32

Key Personnel:
Administrator.............................. D Fritts
Director Infection/Disease Control .... Louise Marron, RN
Chief Radiology........................... Jim O'Neal

Measure	Cases	This Hospital	State Average	U.S. Average	Top Hospital
Heart Attack Care					

ACE Inhibitor or ARB for LVSD	0	-	82%	82%	100%
Aspirin at Arrival[1]	3	100%	88%	92%	100%
Aspirin at Discharge[1]	1	100%	87%	90%	100%
Beta Blocker at Arrival[1]	5	20%	82%	87%	100%
Beta Blocker at Discharge[1]	2	50%	86%	90%	100%
Fibrinolytic Medication Timing[1]	8	12%	41%	31%	100%
PCI Within 90 Minutes of Arrival	0	-	46%	54%	95%
Smoking Cessation Advice	0	-	91%	88%	100%

Heart Failure Care				
ACE Inhibitor or ARB for LVSD	0	-	78%	82%	100%
Discharge Instructions[1]	14	64%	65%	61%	93%
Evaluation of LVS Function[1]	14	7%	81%	83%	99%
Smoking Cessation Advice[1]	4	75%	86%	82%	100%

Pneumonia Care				
Appropriate Initial Antibiotic[1]	12	92%	83%	83%	94%
Blood Culture Timing	0	-	93%	90%	100%
Influenza Vaccine	0	-	70%	70%	100%
Initial Antibiotic Timing[1]	16	94%	82%	80%	93%
Oxygenation Assessment[1]	22	100%	99%	99%	100%
Pneumococcal Vaccine[1]	10	30%	68%	69%	94%
Smoking Cessation Advice[1]	5	60%	83%	80%	100%

Surgical Infection Prevention				
Prophylactic Antibiotic Given[5]	-	-	73%	77%	95%
Prophylactic Antibiotic Selection[5]	-	-	90%	90%	100%
Prophylactic Antibiotic Stopped[5]	-	-	74%	72%	95%

Pregnancy Care				
Inpatient Neonatal Mortality	-	-	-	-	-
Third or Fourth Degree Laceration	-	-	3.82%	3.63%	3.27%

Howard Memorial Hospital

800 West Leslie Street
Nashville, AR 71852
E-mail: hmh@cswnet.com
Ownership: Voluntary non-profit - Other
Emergency Services: No

Phone: 870-845-4400
Fax: 870-845-4178

Accredited: No
Licensed Beds: 25

Key Personnel:
President/CEO......................... Brian Thomas
Emergency Room .... Eddie Beene, RN
Emergency Room .... TJ Humphreys, MD
Infection Control...................... Jan Marshall
ICU .... Eddie Beene, RN
Medical/Surgical Nursing .... Tammy Penka
Respiratory/Cardiopulmonary.............. Gayla Beaird

Measure	Cases	This Hospital	State Average	U.S. Average	Top Hospital
Heart Attack Care					
ACE Inhibitor or ARB for LVSD[3]	0	-	82%	82%	100%
Aspirin at Arrival[1,3]	4	100%	88%	92%	100%
Aspirin at Discharge[1,3]	2	100%	87%	90%	100%
Beta Blocker at Arrival[1,3]	4	75%	82%	87%	100%
Beta Blocker at Discharge[1,3]	2	50%	86%	90%	100%
Fibrinolytic Medication Timing[3]	0	-	41%	31%	100%
PCI Within 90 Minutes of Arrival	0	-	46%	54%	95%
Smoking Cessation Advice[3]	0	-	91%	88%	100%
Heart Failure Care					
ACE Inhibitor or ARB for LVSD[1]	9	67%	78%	82%	100%
Discharge Instructions[1]	18	22%	65%	61%	93%
Evaluation of LVS Function	25	68%	81%	83%	99%
Smoking Cessation Advice[1]	6	83%	86%	82%	100%
Pneumonia Care					
Appropriate Initial Antibiotic[1]	20	85%	83%	83%	94%
Blood Culture Timing	27	96%	93%	90%	100%
Influenza Vaccine[1]	10	70%	70%	70%	100%
Initial Antibiotic Timing	45	84%	82%	80%	93%
Oxygenation Assessment	49	100%	99%	99%	100%
Pneumococcal Vaccine	35	89%	68%	69%	94%
Smoking Cessation Advice[1]	5	80%	83%	80%	100%
Surgical Infection Prevention					
Prophylactic Antibiotic Given[1,3]	8	88%	73%	77%	95%
Prophylactic Antibiotic Selection[1]	1	0%	90%	90%	100%
Prophylactic Antibiotic Stopped[1,3]	8	12%	74%	72%	95%
Pregnancy Care					

NOTE: Hospital profiles are in alphabetical order by state, then city, then hospital within the city; Rankings are sorted by rate in descending order and exclude hospitals with less than 25 cases; (1) The number of cases is too small (n<25) for purposes of reliably predicting hospital performance; (2) Measure reflects the hospital's indication that its submission was based upon a sample of its relevant discharges; (3) Rate reflects fewer than the maximum possible quarters of data for the measure; (4) Inaccurate information submitted and suppressed for one or more quarters; (5) No data is available from the hospital for this measure; Please refer to the User's Guide for a full explanation of data

Inpatient Neonatal Mortality	-	-	-	-	-
Third or Fourth Degree Laceration	-	-	3.82%	3.63%	3.27%

Harris Hospital and Clinic

1205 McCain Street
Newport, AR 72112
URL: www.harrishospital.com
Ownership: Proprietary
Emergency Services: Yes

Phone: 870-523-8911
Fax: 870-523-4437

Accredited: Yes
Licensed Beds: 133

Key Personnel:

CEO . . . . Butch Naylor
Chief Medical Staff. . . . . Hon Poon, MD
Emergency Room . . . . Andrea Winemiller
Emergency Room . . . . Sharon Rodgers, RN
OB/GYN Womens Health. . . . . Jabez Jackson, MD
Chief Radiology . . . . Mufiz Chauhan, MD
Director Respiratory Therapy . . . . Ed Joseph

Measure	Cases	This Hospital	State Average	U.S. Average	Top Hospital
Heart Attack Care					
ACE Inhibitor or ARB for LVSD[1]	4	100%	82%	82%	100%
Aspirin at Arrival[1]	11	91%	88%	92%	100%
Aspirin at Discharge[1]	5	100%	87%	90%	100%
Beta Blocker at Arrival[1]	8	100%	82%	87%	100%
Beta Blocker at Discharge[1]	5	100%	86%	90%	100%
Fibrinolytic Medication Timing	0	-	41%	31%	100%
PCI Within 90 Minutes of Arrival	0	-	46%	54%	95%
Smoking Cessation Advice	0	-	91%	88%	100%
Heart Failure Care					
ACE Inhibitor or ARB for LVSD[1]	21	90%	78%	82%	100%
Discharge Instructions	67	60%	65%	61%	93%
Evaluation of LVS Function	127	90%	81%	83%	99%
Smoking Cessation Advice[1]	19	89%	86%	82%	100%
Pneumonia Care					
Appropriate Initial Antibiotic	84	83%	83%	83%	94%
Blood Culture Timing	36	92%	93%	90%	100%
Influenza Vaccine[1]	16	100%	70%	70%	100%
Initial Antibiotic Timing	104	83%	82%	80%	93%
Oxygenation Assessment	107	100%	99%	99%	100%
Pneumococcal Vaccine	54	87%	68%	69%	94%
Smoking Cessation Advice	33	88%	83%	80%	100%
Surgical Infection Prevention					
Prophylactic Antibiotic Given[2,3]	73	30%	73%	77%	95%
Prophylactic Antibiotic Selection[1,2]	20	80%	90%	90%	100%
Prophylactic Antibiotic Stopped[2,3]	64	52%	74%	72%	95%
Pregnancy Care					
Inpatient Neonatal Mortality	-	-	-	-	-
Third or Fourth Degree Laceration	-	-	3.82%	3.63%	3.27%

Arkansas Surgical Hospital

5201 North Shore Drive
North Little Rock, AR 72118
Ownership: Voluntary non-profit - Private
Emergency Services: Yes

Phone: 501-748-8000

Accredited: Yes

Measure	Cases	This Hospital	State Average	U.S. Average	Top Hospital
Heart Attack Care					
ACE Inhibitor or ARB for LVSD[5]	-	-	82%	82%	100%
Aspirin at Arrival[5]	-	-	88%	92%	100%
Aspirin at Discharge[5]	-	-	87%	90%	100%
Beta Blocker at Arrival[5]	-	-	82%	87%	100%
Beta Blocker at Discharge[5]	-	-	86%	90%	100%
Fibrinolytic Medication Timing[5]	-	-	41%	31%	100%
PCI Within 90 Minutes of Arrival[5]	-	-	46%	54%	95%
Smoking Cessation Advice[5]	-	-	91%	88%	100%
Heart Failure Care					
ACE Inhibitor or ARB for LVSD[5]	-	-	78%	82%	100%
Discharge Instructions[5]	-	-	65%	61%	93%
Evaluation of LVS Function[5]	-	-	81%	83%	99%
Smoking Cessation Advice[5]	-	-	86%	82%	100%
Pneumonia Care					
Appropriate Initial Antibiotic[5]	-	-	83%	83%	94%

Measure	Cases	This Hospital	State Average	U.S. Average	Top Hospital
Blood Culture Timing[5]	-	-	93%	90%	100%
Influenza Vaccine[5]	-	-	70%	70%	100%
Initial Antibiotic Timing[5]	-	-	82%	80%	93%
Oxygenation Assessment[5]	-	-	99%	99%	100%
Pneumococcal Vaccine[5]	-	-	68%	69%	94%
Smoking Cessation Advice[5]	-	-	83%	80%	100%
Surgical Infection Prevention					
Prophylactic Antibiotic Given[2]	586	80%	73%	77%	95%
Prophylactic Antibiotic Selection[2]	185	100%	90%	90%	100%
Prophylactic Antibiotic Stopped[2]	584	72%	74%	72%	95%
Pregnancy Care					
Inpatient Neonatal Mortality	-	-	-	-	-
Third or Fourth Degree Laceration	-	-	3.82%	3.63%	3.27%

Baptist Health Med Ctr-North Little Rock

3333 Springhill Drive
North Little Rock, AR 72116
E-mail: roxannel@baptist-health.org
URL: www.baptist-health.org
Ownership: Voluntary non-profit - Other
Emergency Services: Yes

Phone: 501-202-3000
Fax: 501-202-3813

Accredited: Yes
Licensed Beds: 248

Key Personnel:

President/CEO. . . . . Russell D Harrington
Chief Medical Staff. . . . . Valerie McNee
Cardiac Lab . . . . Jim Proctor
Catheterization Lab . . . . Jim Proctor
Emergency Room . . . . Ricki Meimann
Emergency Room . . . . Pam Hicks
Infection Control. . . . . Becky Hawley
ICU . . . . Marisue Rowe
Intensive/Coronary Care . . . . Faye Nipps
Medical/Surgical Nursing . . . . Darlene Wallen
OB/GYN Womens Health. . . . . Naomi Wallis
Respiratory/Cardiopulmonary. . . . . James Lisenbey

Measure	Cases	This Hospital	State Average	U.S. Average	Top Hospital
Heart Attack Care					
ACE Inhibitor or ARB for LVSD[2]	43	74%	82%	82%	100%
Aspirin at Arrival	171	98%	88%	92%	100%
Aspirin at Discharge	213	95%	87%	90%	100%
Beta Blocker at Arrival	126	90%	82%	87%	100%
Beta Blocker at Discharge	211	97%	86%	90%	100%
Fibrinolytic Medication Timing	0	-	41%	31%	100%
PCI Within 90 Minutes of Arrival[1]	9	44%	46%	54%	95%
Smoking Cessation Advice	97	99%	91%	88%	100%
Heart Failure Care					
ACE Inhibitor or ARB for LVSD	133	83%	78%	82%	100%
Discharge Instructions	247	54%	65%	61%	93%
Evaluation of LVS Function	285	98%	81%	83%	99%
Smoking Cessation Advice	59	98%	86%	82%	100%
Pneumonia Care					
Appropriate Initial Antibiotic	118	79%	83%	83%	94%
Blood Culture Timing	60	95%	93%	90%	100%
Influenza Vaccine[1]	21	76%	70%	70%	100%
Initial Antibiotic Timing	173	82%	82%	80%	93%
Oxygenation Assessment	193	100%	99%	99%	100%
Pneumococcal Vaccine	113	88%	68%	69%	94%
Smoking Cessation Advice	39	95%	83%	80%	100%
Surgical Infection Prevention					
Prophylactic Antibiotic Given	747	92%	73%	77%	95%
Prophylactic Antibiotic Selection	192	99%	90%	90%	100%
Prophylactic Antibiotic Stopped	720	86%	74%	72%	95%
Pregnancy Care					
Inpatient Neonatal Mortality	-	-	-	-	-
Third or Fourth Degree Laceration	-	-	3.82%	3.63%	3.27%

South Mississippi County Regional Med Ctr

Alternate Name: SMC Regional Medical Center

NOTE: Hospital profiles are in alphabetical order by state, then city, then hospital within the city; Rankings are sorted by rate in descending order and exclude hospitals with less than 25 cases; (1) The number of cases is too small (n<25) for purposes of reliably predicting hospital performance; (2) Measure reflects the hospital's indication that its submission was based upon a sample of its relevant discharges; (3) Rate reflects fewer than the maximum possible quarters of data for the measure; (4) Inaccurate information submitted and suppressed for one or more quarters; (5) No data is available from the hospital for this measure; Please refer to the User's Guide for a full explanation of data

611 W Lee Avenue
Osceola, AR 72370
Ownership: Voluntary non-profit - Church
Emergency Services: Yes

Phone: 870-563-7000
Fax: 615-327-0898
Accredited: Yes
Licensed Beds: 25

Key Personnel:
CEO. . . . . Keith Broach
Chief Medical Staff. . . . . James Hudson, MD
Emergency Room . . . . Karen Lindley
Infection Control. . . . . Willa Warren
ICU . . . . Renee Debald
Intensive/Coronary Care . . . . Tammy Fleming
Medical/Surgical Nursing . . . . Holly Kirk
OB/GYN Womens Health. . . . . Millie Newell

Measure	Cases	This Hospital	State Average	U.S. Average	Top Hospital
Heart Attack Care					
ACE Inhibitor or ARB for LVSD[3]	0	-	82%	82%	100%
Aspirin at Arrival[1,3]	2	50%	88%	92%	100%
Aspirin at Discharge[1,3]	1	0%	87%	90%	100%
Beta Blocker at Arrival[1,3]	2	100%	82%	87%	100%
Beta Blocker at Discharge[1,3]	1	100%	86%	90%	100%
Fibrinolytic Medication Timing[3]	0	-	41%	31%	100%
PCI Within 90 Minutes of Arrival	0	-	46%	54%	95%
Smoking Cessation Advice[1,3]	1	0%	91%	88%	100%
Heart Failure Care					
ACE Inhibitor or ARB for LVSD[1]	7	14%	78%	82%	100%
Discharge Instructions	48	75%	65%	61%	93%
Evaluation of LVS Function	65	82%	81%	83%	99%
Smoking Cessation Advice[1]	15	80%	86%	82%	100%
Pneumonia Care					
Appropriate Initial Antibiotic	34	82%	83%	83%	94%
Blood Culture Timing[1]	14	100%	93%	90%	100%
Influenza Vaccine[1]	12	83%	70%	70%	100%
Initial Antibiotic Timing	51	63%	82%	80%	93%
Oxygenation Assessment	65	97%	99%	99%	100%
Pneumococcal Vaccine	35	86%	68%	69%	94%
Smoking Cessation Advice[1]	16	62%	83%	80%	100%
Surgical Infection Prevention					
Prophylactic Antibiotic Given[5]	-	-	73%	77%	95%
Prophylactic Antibiotic Selection[5]	-	-	90%	90%	100%
Prophylactic Antibiotic Stopped[5]	-	-	74%	72%	95%
Pregnancy Care					
Inpatient Neonatal Mortality	-	-	-	-	-
Third or Fourth Degree Laceration	-	-	3.82%	3.63%	3.27%

Arkansas Methodist Hospital

900 West Kingshighway
Paragould, AR 72450
URL: www.amhparagould.com
Ownership: Voluntary non-profit - Other
Emergency Services: Yes

Phone: 870-239-7000
Fax: 870-239-7400

Accredited: Yes
Licensed Beds: 129

Key Personnel:
President . . . . Ronald K Rooney
Chief Medical Staff. . . . . Dwight Williams, MD
Emergency Room . . . . Pat Ray, RN
OB/GYN Womens Health. . . . . Norman Smith, MD
Chief Radiology . . . . Edwin Bird, MD
Director Respiratory Therapy . . . . Renae Gardner

Measure	Cases	This Hospital	State Average	U.S. Average	Top Hospital
Heart Attack Care					
ACE Inhibitor or ARB for LVSD[1]	6	100%	82%	82%	100%
Aspirin at Arrival	98	92%	88%	92%	100%
Aspirin at Discharge	82	91%	87%	90%	100%
Beta Blocker at Arrival	76	89%	82%	87%	100%
Beta Blocker at Discharge	78	91%	86%	90%	100%
Fibrinolytic Medication Timing	0	-	41%	31%	100%
PCI Within 90 Minutes of Arrival	0	-	46%	54%	95%
Smoking Cessation Advice	29	100%	91%	88%	100%
Heart Failure Care					
ACE Inhibitor or ARB for LVSD	49	96%	78%	82%	100%
Discharge Instructions	146	89%	65%	61%	93%
Evaluation of LVS Function	214	94%	81%	83%	99%

Smoking Cessation Advice	41	93%	86%	82%	100%
Pneumonia Care					
Appropriate Initial Antibiotic	232	78%	83%	83%	94%
Blood Culture Timing	161	88%	93%	90%	100%
Influenza Vaccine[4,5]	-	-	70%	70%	100%
Initial Antibiotic Timing	272	82%	82%	80%	93%
Oxygenation Assessment	320	100%	99%	99%	100%
Pneumococcal Vaccine	168	83%	68%	69%	94%
Smoking Cessation Advice	112	96%	83%	80%	100%
Surgical Infection Prevention					
Prophylactic Antibiotic Given[3]	117	92%	73%	77%	95%
Prophylactic Antibiotic Selection	29	90%	90%	90%	100%
Prophylactic Antibiotic Stopped[3]	113	94%	74%	72%	95%
Pregnancy Care					
Inpatient Neonatal Mortality	-	-	-	-	-
Third or Fourth Degree Laceration	-	-	3.82%	3.63%	3.27%

Piggott Community Hospital

1206 Gordon Duckworth Drive
Piggott, AR 72454
Ownership: Government - Local
Emergency Services: Yes

Phone: 870-598-3881
Fax: 870-598-2437
Accredited: No
Licensed Beds: 35

Key Personnel:
CEO. . . . . James Magee
Chief Radiology . . . . James G Sheridan, MD
Director of Pulmonary/Respiratory Care. . . . . . . Dennis Blake

Measure	Cases	This Hospital	State Average	U.S. Average	Top Hospital
Heart Attack Care					
ACE Inhibitor or ARB for LVSD[1,3]	5	80%	82%	82%	100%
Aspirin at Arrival[1,3]	11	100%	88%	92%	100%
Aspirin at Discharge[1,3]	10	80%	87%	90%	100%
Beta Blocker at Arrival[1,3]	10	80%	82%	87%	100%
Beta Blocker at Discharge[1,3]	8	50%	86%	90%	100%
Fibrinolytic Medication Timing[3]	0	-	41%	31%	100%
PCI Within 90 Minutes of Arrival	0	-	46%	54%	95%
Smoking Cessation Advice[1,3]	3	100%	91%	88%	100%
Heart Failure Care					
ACE Inhibitor or ARB for LVSD[1,3]	15	80%	78%	82%	100%
Discharge Instructions[1,3]	16	94%	65%	61%	93%
Evaluation of LVS Function[3]	39	97%	81%	83%	99%
Smoking Cessation Advice[1,3]	5	80%	86%	82%	100%
Pneumonia Care					
Appropriate Initial Antibiotic[1,3]	24	92%	83%	83%	94%
Blood Culture Timing[5]	-	-	93%	90%	100%
Influenza Vaccine[1]	13	100%	70%	70%	100%
Initial Antibiotic Timing[3]	36	94%	82%	80%	93%
Oxygenation Assessment[3]	45	100%	99%	99%	100%
Pneumococcal Vaccine[3]	35	100%	68%	69%	94%
Smoking Cessation Advice[1,3]	8	100%	83%	80%	100%
Surgical Infection Prevention					
Prophylactic Antibiotic Given[5]	-	-	73%	77%	95%
Prophylactic Antibiotic Selection[5]	-	-	90%	90%	100%
Prophylactic Antibiotic Stopped[5]	-	-	74%	72%	95%
Pregnancy Care					
Inpatient Neonatal Mortality	-	-	-	-	-
Third or Fourth Degree Laceration	-	-	3.82%	3.63%	3.27%

Jefferson Regional Medical Center

1600 W 40th Avenue
Pine Bluff, AR 71603
URL: www.jrmc.org
Ownership: Voluntary non-profit - Other
Emergency Services: Yes

Phone: 870-541-7100
Fax: 870-541-7204

Accredited: Yes
Licensed Beds: 471

Key Personnel:
President/CEO. . . . . Robert P Atkinson
Cardiac Lab . . . . Bill Bledsoe
Catheterization Lab . . . . Malcolm Pearce, MD
Emergency Room . . . . John Skowronski, MD
Director Infection/Disease Control . . . . Michaelle Roberts
CCU Spvg. Nurse . . . . Shirley Atkinson, RN
Medical/Surgical Nursing . . . . Nancy Brown
OB/GYN Womens Health. . . . . Robert L Ross, MD

NOTE: Hospital profiles are in alphabetical order by state, then city, then hospital within the city; Rankings are sorted by rate in descending order and exclude hospitals with less than 25 cases; (1) The number of cases is too small (n<25) for purposes of reliably predicting hospital performance; (2) Measure reflects the hospital's indication that its submission was based upon a sample of its relevant discharges; (3) Rate reflects fewer than the maximum possible quarters of data for the measure; (4) Inaccurate information submitted and suppressed for one or more quarters; (5) No data is available from the hospital for this measure; Please refer to the User's Guide for a full explanation of data

Respiratory/Cardiopulmonary. . . . . John Lindsey

Measure	Cases	This Hospital	State Average	U.S. Average	Top Hospital
Heart Attack Care					
ACE Inhibitor or ARB for LVSD	75	87%	82%	82%	100%
Aspirin at Arrival	163	94%	88%	92%	100%
Aspirin at Discharge	232	98%	87%	90%	100%
Beta Blocker at Arrival	144	93%	82%	87%	100%
Beta Blocker at Discharge	232	93%	86%	90%	100%
Fibrinolytic Medication Timing[1]	9	22%	41%	31%	100%
PCI Within 90 Minutes of Arrival[1]	3	0%	46%	54%	95%
Smoking Cessation Advice	98	95%	91%	88%	100%
Heart Failure Care					
ACE Inhibitor or ARB for LVSD	232	78%	78%	82%	100%
Discharge Instructions	343	62%	65%	61%	93%
Evaluation of LVS Function	440	97%	81%	83%	99%
Smoking Cessation Advice	107	92%	86%	82%	100%
Pneumonia Care					
Appropriate Initial Antibiotic	197	82%	83%	83%	94%
Blood Culture Timing	134	85%	93%	90%	100%
Influenza Vaccine	52	56%	70%	70%	100%
Initial Antibiotic Timing	267	76%	82%	80%	93%
Oxygenation Assessment	298	98%	99%	99%	100%
Pneumococcal Vaccine	155	66%	68%	69%	94%
Smoking Cessation Advice	73	79%	83%	80%	100%
Surgical Infection Prevention					
Prophylactic Antibiotic Given	933	74%	73%	77%	95%
Prophylactic Antibiotic Selection	237	91%	90%	90%	100%
Prophylactic Antibiotic Stopped	892	77%	74%	72%	95%
Pregnancy Care					
Inpatient Neonatal Mortality	-	-	-	-	-
Third or Fourth Degree Laceration	-	-	3.82%	3.63%	3.27%

Randolph County Medical Center

2801 Medical Center Drive   Phone: 870-892-6000
Pocahontas, AR 72455   Fax: 870-892-8100
URL: www.chc.net
Ownership: Proprietary   Accredited: No
Emergency Services: Yes   Licensed Beds: 50
Key Personnel:
CEO. . . . . Terry G Whittington
Emergency Room . . . . Mandy Dollins, RN
Infection Control. Judy Downs, RN
ICU . . . . Linda Leach, RN
Medical/Surgical Nurse . . . . Becky Wilson, RN
CNO. . . . . Judy Haney, RN
Respiratory/Cardiopulmonary. . . . . Susan Hawkins

Measure	Cases	This Hospital	State Average	U.S. Average	Top Hospital
Heart Attack Care					
ACE Inhibitor or ARB for LVSD[1,3]	1	100%	82%	82%	100%
Aspirin at Arrival[1,3]	6	83%	88%	92%	100%
Aspirin at Discharge[1,3]	4	75%	87%	90%	100%
Beta Blocker at Arrival[1,3]	6	83%	82%	87%	100%
Beta Blocker at Discharge[1,3]	3	67%	86%	90%	100%
Fibrinolytic Medication Timing[3]	0	-	41%	31%	100%
PCI Within 90 Minutes of Arrival[5]	-	-	46%	54%	95%
Smoking Cessation Advice[3]	0	-	91%	88%	100%
Heart Failure Care					
ACE Inhibitor or ARB for LVSD[1]	8	88%	78%	82%	100%
Discharge Instructions	25	20%	65%	61%	93%
Evaluation of LVS Function	39	54%	81%	83%	99%
Smoking Cessation Advice[1]	6	100%	86%	82%	100%
Pneumonia Care					
Appropriate Initial Antibiotic	65	80%	83%	83%	94%
Blood Culture Timing	30	100%	93%	90%	100%
Influenza Vaccine[1]	22	41%	70%	70%	100%
Initial Antibiotic Timing	69	87%	82%	80%	93%
Oxygenation Assessment	85	100%	99%	99%	100%
Pneumococcal Vaccine	61	62%	68%	69%	94%
Smoking Cessation Advice[1]	12	100%	83%	80%	100%
Surgical Infection Prevention					

Measure	Cases	This Hospital	State Average	U.S. Average	Top Hospital
Prophylactic Antibiotic Given[3]	40	62%	73%	77%	95%
Prophylactic Antibiotic Selection[1]	22	95%	90%	90%	100%
Prophylactic Antibiotic Stopped[3]	32	44%	74%	72%	95%
Pregnancy Care					
Inpatient Neonatal Mortality	-	-	-	-	-
Third or Fourth Degree Laceration	-	-	3.82%	3.63%	3.27%

Saint Mary-Rogers Memorial Hospital

1200 W Walnut Street   Phone: 479-636-0200
Rogers, AR 72756   Fax: 501-636-2906
URL: www.mercyhealthnwa.smhs.com
Ownership: Voluntary non-profit - Church   Accredited: Yes
Emergency Services: Yes   Licensed Beds: 165
Key Personnel:
CEO. . . . . Susan Barrett
Chief Medical Staff. . . . . R Black
Emergency Room . . . . Carolyn Fries
OB/GYN Womens Health. . . . . Karen Lanier, MD
Surgery Service . . . . Forrest Parks
Chief Radiology . . . . Michael McAdams
Director of Pulmonary/Respiratory Care. . . . . . . David Jordan

Measure	Cases	This Hospital	State Average	U.S. Average	Top Hospital
Heart Attack Care					
ACE Inhibitor or ARB for LVSD	26	92%	82%	82%	100%
Aspirin at Arrival	120	99%	88%	92%	100%
Aspirin at Discharge	132	100%	87%	90%	100%
Beta Blocker at Arrival	93	98%	82%	87%	100%
Beta Blocker at Discharge	142	99%	86%	90%	100%
Fibrinolytic Medication Timing	0	-	41%	31%	100%
PCI Within 90 Minutes of Arrival[1]	7	100%	46%	54%	95%
Smoking Cessation Advice	53	96%	91%	88%	100%
Heart Failure Care					
ACE Inhibitor or ARB for LVSD	78	96%	78%	82%	100%
Discharge Instructions	165	74%	65%	61%	93%
Evaluation of LVS Function	211	100%	81%	83%	99%
Smoking Cessation Advice	25	96%	86%	82%	100%
Pneumonia Care					
Appropriate Initial Antibiotic	154	88%	83%	83%	94%
Blood Culture Timing	133	99%	93%	90%	100%
Influenza Vaccine	51	94%	70%	70%	100%
Initial Antibiotic Timing	200	92%	82%	80%	93%
Oxygenation Assessment	251	100%	99%	99%	100%
Pneumococcal Vaccine	170	88%	68%	69%	94%
Smoking Cessation Advice	61	95%	83%	80%	100%
Surgical Infection Prevention					
Prophylactic Antibiotic Given[2]	224	79%	73%	77%	95%
Prophylactic Antibiotic Selection[2]	62	95%	90%	90%	100%
Prophylactic Antibiotic Stopped[2]	212	90%	74%	72%	95%
Pregnancy Care					
Inpatient Neonatal Mortality	-	-	-	-	-
Third or Fourth Degree Laceration	-	-	3.82%	3.63%	3.27%

Saint Mary's Regional Medical Center

1808 W Main Street   Phone: 479-968-284I
Russellville, AR 72801   Fax: 479-964-9287
URL: www.saintmarysregional.com
Ownership: Proprietary   Accredited: Yes
Emergency Services: Yes   Licensed Beds: 170
Key Personnel:
CEO. . . . . Mike MacCoy
Chief Medical Staff. . . . . Anthony Harden, MD
Emergency Room . . . . Todd Carter, MD

Measure	Cases	This Hospital	State Average	U.S. Average	Top Hospital
Heart Attack Care					
ACE Inhibitor or ARB for LVSD[1]	8	88%	82%	82%	100%
Aspirin at Arrival	41	95%	88%	92%	100%
Aspirin at Discharge[1]	17	94%	87%	90%	100%
Beta Blocker at Arrival	32	94%	82%	87%	100%
Beta Blocker at Discharge[1]	15	93%	86%	90%	100%
Fibrinolytic Medication Timing[1]	9	56%	41%	31%	100%

NOTE: Hospital profiles are in alphabetical order by state, then city, then hospital within the city; Rankings are sorted by rate in descending order and exclude hospitals with less than 25 cases; (1) The number of cases is too small (n<25) for purposes of reliably predicting hospital performance; (2) Measure reflects the hospital's indication that its submission was based upon a sample of its relevant discharges; (3) Rate reflects fewer than the maximum possible quarters of data for the measure; (4) Inaccurate information submitted and suppressed for one or more quarters; (5) No data is available from the hospital for this measure; Please refer to the User's Guide for a full explanation of data

PCI Within 90 Minutes of Arrival	0	-	46%	54%	95%
Smoking Cessation Advice[1]	2	100%	91%	88%	100%
Heart Failure Care					
ACE Inhibitor or ARB for LVSD	53	79%	78%	82%	100%
Discharge Instructions	116	72%	65%	61%	93%
Evaluation of LVS Function	153	92%	81%	83%	99%
Smoking Cessation Advice	29	86%	86%	82%	100%
Pneumonia Care					
Appropriate Initial Antibiotic	178	88%	83%	83%	94%
Blood Culture Timing	129	87%	93%	90%	100%
Influenza Vaccine	42	88%	70%	70%	100%
Initial Antibiotic Timing	195	91%	82%	80%	93%
Oxygenation Assessment	253	100%	99%	99%	100%
Pneumococcal Vaccine	135	88%	68%	69%	94%
Smoking Cessation Advice	65	83%	83%	80%	100%
Surgical Infection Prevention					
Prophylactic Antibiotic Given	376	93%	73%	77%	95%
Prophylactic Antibiotic Selection	101	97%	90%	90%	100%
Prophylactic Antibiotic Stopped	369	71%	74%	72%	95%
Pregnancy Care					
Inpatient Neonatal Mortality	-	-	-	-	-
Third or Fourth Degree Laceration	-	-	3.82%	3.63%	3.27%

White County Medical Center

3214 E Race Ave
Searcy, AR 72143
URL: www.wcmc.org
Ownership: Proprietary   Phone: 501-268-6121
Emergency Services: Yes   Accredited: Yes
    Licensed Beds: 245
Key Personnel:
CEO. . . . . Ben Frank
Chief of Medical Staff. . . . . Shelly Tobey
OB/GYN Womens Health. . . . . Melissa Eats
Chief Radiology . . . . Jack Riddle
Director Respiratory Therapy . . . . Cindy Western

Measure	Cases	This Hospital	State Average	U.S. Average	Top Hospital
Heart Attack Care					
ACE Inhibitor or ARB for LVSD[3]	36	75%	82%	82%	100%
Aspirin at Arrival[3]	102	94%	88%	92%	100%
Aspirin at Discharge[3]	99	97%	87%	90%	100%
Beta Blocker at Arrival[3]	88	83%	82%	87%	100%
Beta Blocker at Discharge[3]	110	95%	86%	90%	100%
Fibrinolytic Medication Timing[1,3]	6	50%	41%	31%	100%
PCI Within 90 Minutes of Arrival[1]	11	36%	46%	54%	95%
Smoking Cessation Advice[3]	51	98%	91%	88%	100%
Heart Failure Care					
ACE Inhibitor or ARB for LVSD[3]	91	77%	78%	82%	100%
Discharge Instructions[3]	202	76%	65%	61%	93%
Evaluation of LVS Function[3]	254	93%	81%	83%	99%
Smoking Cessation Advice[3]	35	91%	86%	82%	100%
Pneumonia Care					
Appropriate Initial Antibiotic[3]	141	89%	83%	83%	94%
Blood Culture Timing[3]	138	93%	93%	90%	100%
Influenza Vaccine[5]	-	-	70%	70%	100%
Initial Antibiotic Timing[3]	195	86%	82%	80%	93%
Oxygenation Assessment[3]	236	94%	99%	99%	100%
Pneumococcal Vaccine[3]	163	70%	68%	69%	94%
Smoking Cessation Advice[3]	54	93%	83%	80%	100%
Surgical Infection Prevention					
Prophylactic Antibiotic Given[3]	331	78%	73%	77%	95%
Prophylactic Antibiotic Selection	149	99%	90%	90%	100%
Prophylactic Antibiotic Stopped[3]	300	90%	74%	72%	95%
Pregnancy Care					
Inpatient Neonatal Mortality	-	-	-	-	-
Third or Fourth Degree Laceration	-	-	3.82%	3.63%	3.27%

Saint Vincent Medical Center North

2215 Wildwood Avenue   Phone: 501-552-7100
Sherwood, AR 72120
Ownership: Voluntary non-profit - Church   Accredited: No
Emergency Services: No

Measure	Cases	This Hospital	State Average	U.S. Average	Top Hospital
Heart Attack Care					
ACE Inhibitor or ARB for LVSD[1]	2	50%	82%	82%	100%
Aspirin at Arrival[1]	18	94%	88%	92%	100%
Aspirin at Discharge[1]	8	100%	87%	90%	100%
Beta Blocker at Arrival[1]	18	83%	82%	87%	100%
Beta Blocker at Discharge[1]	8	100%	86%	90%	100%
Fibrinolytic Medication Timing	0	-	41%	31%	100%
PCI Within 90 Minutes of Arrival	0	-	46%	54%	95%
Smoking Cessation Advice[1]	1	100%	91%	88%	100%
Heart Failure Care					
ACE Inhibitor or ARB for LVSD[1]	20	85%	78%	82%	100%
Discharge Instructions	53	60%	65%	61%	93%
Evaluation of LVS Function	68	87%	81%	83%	99%
Smoking Cessation Advice[1]	15	100%	86%	82%	100%
Pneumonia Care					
Appropriate Initial Antibiotic	71	75%	83%	83%	94%
Blood Culture Timing	30	97%	93%	90%	100%
Influenza Vaccine[1]	17	71%	70%	70%	100%
Initial Antibiotic Timing	81	67%	82%	80%	93%
Oxygenation Assessment	87	100%	99%	99%	100%
Pneumococcal Vaccine	49	49%	68%	69%	94%
Smoking Cessation Advice[1]	20	100%	83%	80%	100%
Surgical Infection Prevention					
Prophylactic Antibiotic Given	89	58%	73%	77%	95%
Prophylactic Antibiotic Selection[1]	14	93%	90%	90%	100%
Prophylactic Antibiotic Stopped	84	99%	74%	72%	95%
Pregnancy Care					
Inpatient Neonatal Mortality	-	-	-	-	-
Third or Fourth Degree Laceration	-	-	3.82%	3.63%	3.27%

Siloam Springs Memorial Hospital

Alternate Name: Memorial Hospital
205 E Jefferson Street   Phone: 479-549-2478
Siloam Springs, AR 72761   Fax: 501-549-2486
Ownership: Government - Local   Accredited: Yes
Emergency Services: Yes   Licensed Beds: 73
Key Personnel:
CEO/President . . . . Tinny Mclean
Chief Medical Staff. . . . . Angela Sanmeier
Emergency Room . . . . Robin McAlister
Director Medical/Surgical Nursing . . . . Brenda Lea, RN
Director Respiratory Therapy . . . . Geoff Copeland

Measure	Cases	This Hospital	State Average	U.S. Average	Top Hospital
Heart Attack Care					
ACE Inhibitor or ARB for LVSD[1]	1	0%	82%	82%	100%
Aspirin at Arrival[1]	11	91%	88%	92%	100%
Aspirin at Discharge[1]	6	100%	87%	90%	100%
Beta Blocker at Arrival[1]	12	67%	82%	87%	100%
Beta Blocker at Discharge[1]	7	86%	86%	90%	100%
Fibrinolytic Medication Timing	0	-	41%	31%	100%
PCI Within 90 Minutes of Arrival	0	-	46%	54%	95%
Smoking Cessation Advice[1]	1	0%	91%	88%	100%
Heart Failure Care					
ACE Inhibitor or ARB for LVSD[1]	14	93%	78%	82%	100%
Discharge Instructions	71	25%	65%	61%	93%
Evaluation of LVS Function	85	67%	81%	83%	99%
Smoking Cessation Advice[1]	18	56%	86%	82%	100%
Pneumonia Care					
Appropriate Initial Antibiotic	91	81%	83%	83%	94%
Blood Culture Timing	53	100%	93%	90%	100%
Influenza Vaccine[1]	24	62%	70%	70%	100%
Initial Antibiotic Timing	127	82%	82%	80%	93%
Oxygenation Assessment	147	99%	99%	99%	100%
Pneumococcal Vaccine	75	51%	68%	69%	94%

NOTE: Hospital profiles are in alphabetical order by state, then city, then hospital within the city; Rankings are sorted by rate in descending order and exclude hospitals with less than 25 cases; (1) The number of cases is too small (n<25) for purposes of reliably predicting hospital performance; (2) Measure reflects the hospital's indication that its submission was based upon a sample of its relevant discharges; (3) Rate reflects fewer than the maximum possible quarters of data for the measure; (4) Inaccurate information submitted and suppressed for one or more quarters; (5) No data is available from the hospital for this measure; Please refer to the User's Guide for a full explanation of data

Smoking Cessation Advice	35	69%	83%	80%	100%
Surgical Infection Prevention					
Prophylactic Antibiotic Given[1,2,3]	23	30%	73%	77%	95%
Prophylactic Antibiotic Selection[1,2]	6	83%	90%	90%	100%
Prophylactic Antibiotic Stopped[1,2,3]	16	69%	74%	72%	95%
Pregnancy Care					
Inpatient Neonatal Mortality	-	-	-	-	-
Third or Fourth Degree Laceration	-	-	3.82%	3.63%	3.27%

Northwest Medical Center

Alternate Name: Springdale Memorial Hospital
609 W Maple Avenue
Springdale, AR 72764
URL: www.northwesthealth.org
Ownership: Proprietary
Emergency Services: Yes

Phone: 479-751-5711
Fax: 479-757-2928

Accredited: Yes
Licensed Beds: 222

Key Personnel:
CEO . . . . Bill Bradley
Chief Medical Staff . . . . Sanjay Patel, MD
Emergency Room . . . . Gail Bergland
Emergency Room . . . . Dana Bell, MD
Infection Control . . . . Sharon Jorde
ICU . . . . Carol Tulobaski
Director Medical/Surgical Nursing . . . . Faith Moore
Director Medical/Surgical Nursing . . . . Beverly Bowman, RN
OBGYN . . . . Juho Krepp
Chief Radiology . . . . Tom Picquet
Director Respiratory Therapy . . . . Kevin Wahl

Measure	Cases	This Hospital	State Average	U.S. Average	Top Hospital
Heart Attack Care					
ACE Inhibitor or ARB for LVSD	35	77%	82%	82%	100%
Aspirin at Arrival	165	98%	88%	92%	100%
Aspirin at Discharge	199	98%	87%	90%	100%
Beta Blocker at Arrival	127	81%	82%	87%	100%
Beta Blocker at Discharge	207	92%	86%	90%	100%
Fibrinolytic Medication Timing	0	-	41%	31%	100%
PCI Within 90 Minutes of Arrival[1]	10	80%	46%	54%	95%
Smoking Cessation Advice	81	95%	91%	88%	100%
Heart Failure Care					
ACE Inhibitor or ARB for LVSD	92	88%	78%	82%	100%
Discharge Instructions	152	75%	65%	61%	93%
Evaluation of LVS Function	198	92%	81%	83%	99%
Smoking Cessation Advice	30	97%	86%	82%	100%
Pneumonia Care					
Appropriate Initial Antibiotic	110	80%	83%	83%	94%
Blood Culture Timing	94	91%	93%	90%	100%
Influenza Vaccine	28	64%	70%	70%	100%
Initial Antibiotic Timing	158	67%	82%	80%	93%
Oxygenation Assessment	189	100%	99%	99%	100%
Pneumococcal Vaccine	116	68%	68%	69%	94%
Smoking Cessation Advice	52	81%	83%	80%	100%
Surgical Infection Prevention					
Prophylactic Antibiotic Given	420	81%	73%	77%	95%
Prophylactic Antibiotic Selection	118	97%	90%	90%	100%
Prophylactic Antibiotic Stopped	409	56%	74%	72%	95%
Pregnancy Care					
Inpatient Neonatal Mortality	3,661	0.38%	-	-	-
Third or Fourth Degree Laceration	2,511	3.31%	3.82%	3.63%	3.27%

Stuttgart Regional Medical Center

1703 N Buerkle Road
Stuttgart, AR 72160
E-mail: aholstead@stuttgart-medical.org
URL: www.stuttgart-medical.org
Ownership: Voluntary non-profit - Other
Emergency Services: Yes

Phone: 870-673-3511
Fax: 870-672-6869

Accredited: No
Licensed Beds: 49

Key Personnel:
Administrator/CEO . . . . John C Neal
Emergency Room . . . . Don Warner, RN
Infection Control . . . . Rachelle McCarthy, RN
ICU . . . . Janice York
Intensive/Coronary Care . . . . Janice York
OB/GYN Womens Health . . . . Frederick Hanson, MD

Respiratory/Cardiopulmonary . . . . Gary Davis

Measure	Cases	This Hospital	State Average	U.S. Average	Top Hospital
Heart Attack Care					
ACE Inhibitor or ARB for LVSD	0	-	82%	82%	100%
Aspirin at Arrival[1]	8	88%	88%	92%	100%
Aspirin at Discharge[1]	4	100%	87%	90%	100%
Beta Blocker at Arrival[1]	8	88%	82%	87%	100%
Beta Blocker at Discharge[1]	5	100%	86%	90%	100%
Fibrinolytic Medication Timing	0	-	41%	31%	100%
PCI Within 90 Minutes of Arrival	0	-	46%	54%	95%
Smoking Cessation Advice	0	-	91%	88%	100%
Heart Failure Care					
ACE Inhibitor or ARB for LVSD	32	88%	78%	82%	100%
Discharge Instructions	96	67%	65%	61%	93%
Evaluation of LVS Function	127	95%	81%	83%	99%
Smoking Cessation Advice[1]	15	93%	86%	82%	100%
Pneumonia Care					
Appropriate Initial Antibiotic	53	89%	83%	83%	94%
Blood Culture Timing	49	94%	93%	90%	100%
Influenza Vaccine[1]	19	95%	70%	70%	100%
Initial Antibiotic Timing	91	89%	82%	80%	93%
Oxygenation Assessment	103	99%	99%	99%	100%
Pneumococcal Vaccine	61	84%	68%	69%	94%
Smoking Cessation Advice	28	89%	83%	80%	100%
Surgical Infection Prevention					
Prophylactic Antibiotic Given[1]	22	100%	73%	77%	95%
Prophylactic Antibiotic Selection[1]	2	100%	90%	90%	100%
Prophylactic Antibiotic Stopped[1]	20	95%	74%	72%	95%
Pregnancy Care					
Inpatient Neonatal Mortality	-	-	-	-	-
Third or Fourth Degree Laceration	-	-	3.82%	3.63%	3.27%

Summit Medical Center

E Main & S 20th Streets
Van Buren, AR 72956
URL: www.summitmc.net
Ownership: Proprietary
Emergency Services: Yes

Phone: 479-474-3401
Fax: 501-474-4458

Accredited: Yes
Licensed Beds: 103

Key Personnel:
CEO . . . . Kevin Clement
Chief Medical Staff . . . . Brett Whatcott, DO
Director, Infection Control . . . . Beth Puckett, RN
ICU . . . . Landon Horton, RN
Medical/Surgical Nursing Director . . . . Landon Horton, RN
Respiratory/Cardiopulmonary Director . . . . Rhonda Dillon

Measure	Cases	This Hospital	State Average	U.S. Average	Top Hospital
Heart Attack Care					
ACE Inhibitor or ARB for LVSD[1]	3	67%	82%	82%	100%
Aspirin at Arrival	29	90%	88%	92%	100%
Aspirin at Discharge[1]	14	64%	87%	90%	100%
Beta Blocker at Arrival	28	86%	82%	87%	100%
Beta Blocker at Discharge[1]	14	93%	86%	90%	100%
Fibrinolytic Medication Timing[1]	2	0%	41%	31%	100%
PCI Within 90 Minutes of Arrival	0	-	46%	54%	95%
Smoking Cessation Advice[1]	1	100%	91%	88%	100%
Heart Failure Care					
ACE Inhibitor or ARB for LVSD	26	81%	78%	82%	100%
Discharge Instructions	80	54%	65%	61%	93%
Evaluation of LVS Function	122	82%	81%	83%	99%
Smoking Cessation Advice[1]	14	79%	86%	82%	100%
Pneumonia Care					
Appropriate Initial Antibiotic	117	74%	83%	83%	94%
Blood Culture Timing	87	91%	93%	90%	100%
Influenza Vaccine	31	94%	70%	70%	100%
Initial Antibiotic Timing	131	85%	82%	80%	93%
Oxygenation Assessment	154	99%	99%	99%	100%
Pneumococcal Vaccine	77	95%	68%	69%	94%
Smoking Cessation Advice	60	72%	83%	80%	100%
Surgical Infection Prevention					
Prophylactic Antibiotic Given	82	80%	73%	77%	95%

Prophylactic Antibiotic Selection	26	100%	90%	90%	100%
Prophylactic Antibiotic Stopped	82	27%	74%	72%	95%
Pregnancy Care					
Inpatient Neonatal Mortality	-	-	-	-	-
Third or Fourth Degree Laceration	-	-	3.82%	3.63%	3.27%

Lawrence Memorial Hospital

1309 W Main Street
PO Box 839
Walnut Ridge, AR 72476
E-mail: beagan@lawrencehealth.net
URL: www.lawrencehealth.net
Ownership: Government - Local
Emergency Services: Yes

Phone: 870-886-1200
Fax: 870-886-5340

Accredited: Yes
Licensed Beds: 195

Key Personnel:
President . . . . Leah Osbahr
Chief Medical Staff . . . . Paul Vellozo
Emergency Room . . . . Dennise Chadwick
Director Infection/Disease Control . . . . Teresa Milam
Director Medical/Surgical Nursing . . . . Linda Howell
Director Respiratory Therapy . . . . Roger Parker

Measure	Cases	This Hospital	State Average	U.S. Average	Top Hospital
Heart Attack Care					
ACE Inhibitor or ARB for LVSD[3]	0	-	82%	82%	100%
Aspirin at Arrival[1,3]	1	100%	88%	92%	100%
Aspirin at Discharge[3]	0	-	87%	90%	100%
Beta Blocker at Arrival[1,3]	1	0%	82%	87%	100%
Beta Blocker at Discharge[3]	0	-	86%	90%	100%
Fibrinolytic Medication Timing[3]	0	-	41%	31%	100%
PCI Within 90 Minutes of Arrival[5]	-	-	46%	54%	95%
Smoking Cessation Advice[3]	0	-	91%	88%	100%
Heart Failure Care					
ACE Inhibitor or ARB for LVSD[1]	18	78%	78%	82%	100%
Discharge Instructions[1]	16	88%	65%	61%	93%
Evaluation of LVS Function	47	89%	81%	83%	99%
Smoking Cessation Advice[1]	3	100%	86%	82%	100%
Pneumonia Care					
Appropriate Initial Antibiotic	35	97%	83%	83%	94%
Blood Culture Timing	43	95%	93%	90%	100%
Influenza Vaccine[1]	15	80%	70%	70%	100%
Initial Antibiotic Timing	63	90%	82%	80%	93%
Oxygenation Assessment	77	100%	99%	99%	100%
Pneumococcal Vaccine	54	89%	68%	69%	94%
Smoking Cessation Advice[1]	12	92%	83%	80%	100%
Surgical Infection Prevention					
Prophylactic Antibiotic Given[5]	-	-	73%	77%	95%
Prophylactic Antibiotic Selection[5]	-	-	90%	90%	100%
Prophylactic Antibiotic Stopped[5]	-	-	74%	72%	95%
Pregnancy Care					
Inpatient Neonatal Mortality	-	-	-	-	-
Third or Fourth Degree Laceration	-	-	3.82%	3.63%	3.27%

Bradley County Medical Center

404 S Bradley Street
Warren, AR 71671
Ownership: Voluntary non-profit - Private
Emergency Services: Yes

Phone: 870-226-3731
Fax: 870-226-7049
Accredited: No
Licensed Beds: 49

Key Personnel:
Chairman/CEO . . . . Harry Stevens
Chief Medical Staff . . . . James W Marsh, MD
Emergency Room . . . . Paullete Tolefree
Chief Radiology . . . . Beverly Weeks
Director Respiratory Therapy . . . . Judy Taylor, RRT

Measure	Cases	This Hospital	State Average	U.S. Average	Top Hospital
Heart Attack Care					
ACE Inhibitor or ARB for LVSD[3]	0	-	82%	82%	100%
Aspirin at Arrival[1,3]	2	100%	88%	92%	100%
Aspirin at Discharge[1,3]	1	100%	87%	90%	100%
Beta Blocker at Arrival[3]	0	-	82%	87%	100%
Beta Blocker at Discharge[1,3]	1	0%	86%	90%	100%
Fibrinolytic Medication Timing[3]	0	-	41%	31%	100%

PCI Within 90 Minutes of Arrival[5]	-	-	46%	54%	95%
Smoking Cessation Advice[3]	0	-	91%	88%	100%
Heart Failure Care					
ACE Inhibitor or ARB for LVSD[1]	3	67%	78%	82%	100%
Discharge Instructions	53	77%	65%	61%	93%
Evaluation of LVS Function	62	13%	81%	83%	99%
Smoking Cessation Advice[1]	4	100%	86%	82%	100%
Pneumonia Care					
Appropriate Initial Antibiotic	48	88%	83%	83%	94%
Blood Culture Timing[1]	10	90%	93%	90%	100%
Influenza Vaccine[1]	14	36%	70%	70%	100%
Initial Antibiotic Timing	56	80%	82%	80%	93%
Oxygenation Assessment	66	86%	99%	99%	100%
Pneumococcal Vaccine	39	21%	68%	69%	94%
Smoking Cessation Advice[1]	6	50%	83%	80%	100%
Surgical Infection Prevention					
Prophylactic Antibiotic Given[3]	37	51%	73%	77%	95%
Prophylactic Antibiotic Selection[5]	-	-	90%	90%	100%
Prophylactic Antibiotic Stopped[3]	27	89%	74%	72%	95%
Pregnancy Care					
Inpatient Neonatal Mortality	-	-	-	-	-
Third or Fourth Degree Laceration	-	-	3.82%	3.63%	3.27%

Crittenden Memorial Hospital

200 Tyler Avenue
West Memphis, AR 72301
URL: www.crittendenmemorial.org
Ownership: Voluntary non-profit - Other
Emergency Services: Yes

Phone: 870-735-1500
Fax: 870-732-7710

Accredited: Yes
Licensed Beds: 152

Key Personnel:
President/CEO . . . . Ross Hooper
Chief Medical Staff . . . . Paul J Huffstutter, MD
Cardiac Laboratory . . . . Frank Martin, MD
Emergency Room . . . . Lance Herrell
Director Infection/Disease Control . . . . Laura Staveley
ICU . . . . Donna Lanier
Medical Surgical Nursing . . . . Steve Earnshaw, RN
OB/GYN Womens Health . . . . James DeRoss, MD
Director Respiratory Therapy . . . . Robin Weaver

Measure	Cases	This Hospital	State Average	U.S. Average	Top Hospital
Heart Attack Care					
ACE Inhibitor or ARB for LVSD[1]	4	75%	82%	82%	100%
Aspirin at Arrival[1]	20	100%	88%	92%	100%
Aspirin at Discharge[1]	10	100%	87%	90%	100%
Beta Blocker at Arrival[1]	19	100%	82%	87%	100%
Beta Blocker at Discharge[1]	11	82%	86%	90%	100%
Fibrinolytic Medication Timing	0	-	41%	31%	100%
PCI Within 90 Minutes of Arrival	0	-	46%	54%	95%
Smoking Cessation Advice[1]	3	100%	91%	88%	100%
Heart Failure Care					
ACE Inhibitor or ARB for LVSD	72	94%	78%	82%	100%
Discharge Instructions	209	95%	65%	61%	93%
Evaluation of LVS Function	236	91%	81%	83%	99%
Smoking Cessation Advice	57	100%	86%	82%	100%
Pneumonia Care					
Appropriate Initial Antibiotic	72	74%	83%	83%	94%
Blood Culture Timing	61	93%	93%	90%	100%
Influenza Vaccine[1]	23	61%	70%	70%	100%
Initial Antibiotic Timing	88	78%	82%	80%	93%
Oxygenation Assessment	105	93%	99%	99%	100%
Pneumococcal Vaccine	46	52%	68%	69%	94%
Smoking Cessation Advice[1]	24	100%	83%	80%	100%
Surgical Infection Prevention					
Prophylactic Antibiotic Given[2,3]	83	60%	73%	77%	95%
Prophylactic Antibiotic Selection[2]	30	93%	90%	90%	100%
Prophylactic Antibiotic Stopped[2,3]	84	70%	74%	72%	95%
Pregnancy Care					
Inpatient Neonatal Mortality	799	1.00%	-	-	-
Third or Fourth Degree Laceration	569	1.05%	3.82%	3.63%	3.27%

NOTE: Hospital profiles are in alphabetical order by state, then city, then hospital within the city; Rankings are sorted by rate in descending order and exclude hospitals with less than 25 cases; (1) The number of cases is too small (n<25) for purposes of reliably predicting hospital performance; (2) Measure reflects the hospital's indication that its submission was based upon a sample of its relevant discharges; (3) Rate reflects fewer than the maximum possible quarters of data for the measure; (4) Inaccurate information submitted and suppressed for one or more quarters; (5) No data is available from the hospital for this measure; Please refer to the User's Guide for a full explanation of data

CrossRidge Community Hospital

310 S Falls Boulevard
Wynne, AR 72396
Ownership: Voluntary non-profit - Church
Emergency Services: Yes

Phone: 870-238-3300
Fax: 870-238-7432
Accredited: Yes
Licensed Beds: 25

Key Personnel:
Administrator . . . . Gary Sparks
Director Respiratory Therapy . . . . Carol Sparks

Measure	Cases	This Hospital	State Average	U.S. Average	Top Hospital
Heart Attack Care					
ACE Inhibitor or ARB for LVSD[3]	0	-	82%	82%	100%
Aspirin at Arrival[1,3]	1	100%	88%	92%	100%
Aspirin at Discharge[1,3]	1	100%	87%	90%	100%
Beta Blocker at Arrival[1,3]	1	100%	82%	87%	100%
Beta Blocker at Discharge[1,3]	1	100%	86%	90%	100%
Fibrinolytic Medication Timing[3]	0	-	41%	31%	100%
PCI Within 90 Minutes of Arrival[5]	-	-	46%	54%	95%
Smoking Cessation Advice[3]	0	-	91%	88%	100%
Heart Failure Care					
ACE Inhibitor or ARB for LVSD[1]	15	73%	78%	82%	100%
Discharge Instructions	36	67%	65%	61%	93%
Evaluation of LVS Function	50	82%	81%	83%	99%
Smoking Cessation Advice[1]	5	80%	86%	82%	100%
Pneumonia Care					
Appropriate Initial Antibiotic	69	93%	83%	83%	94%
Blood Culture Timing[1]	12	100%	93%	90%	100%
Influenza Vaccine[1]	21	95%	70%	70%	100%
Initial Antibiotic Timing	92	89%	82%	80%	93%
Oxygenation Assessment	102	100%	99%	99%	100%
Pneumococcal Vaccine	79	85%	68%	69%	94%
Smoking Cessation Advice[1]	15	87%	83%	80%	100%
Surgical Infection Prevention					
Prophylactic Antibiotic Given[5]	-	-	73%	77%	95%
Prophylactic Antibiotic Selection[5]	-	-	90%	90%	100%
Prophylactic Antibiotic Stopped[5]	-	-	74%	72%	95%
Pregnancy Care					
Inpatient Neonatal Mortality	-	-	-	-	-
Third or Fourth Degree Laceration	-	-	3.82%	3.63%	3.27%

NOTE: Hospital profiles are in alphabetical order by state, then city, then hospital within the city; Rankings are sorted by rate in descending order and exclude hospitals with less than 25 cases; (1) The number of cases is too small (n<25) for purposes of reliably predicting hospital performance; (2) Measure reflects the hospital's indication that its submission was based upon a sample of its relevant discharges; (3) Rate reflects fewer than the maximum possible quarters of data for the measure; (4) Inaccurate information submitted and suppressed for one or more quarters; (5) No data is available from the hospital for this measure; Please refer to the User's Guide for a full explanation of data

	Miami	63%	180
Kendall Medical Center	Miami	63%	180
North Florida Regional Medical Center	Gainesville	62%	98

Heart Attack Care

1. ACE Inhibitor or ARB for LVSD

Hospital Name	City	Rate	Cases
Cleveland Clinic Florida	Weston	100%	41
Fort Walton Beach Medical Center	Fort Walton Beach	100%	54
South Miami Hospital	Miami	100%	84
Venice Regional Medical Center	Venice	100%	74
Wuesthoff Health Systems	Rockledge	100%	68
Delray Medical Center	Delray Beach	99%	118
Lawnwood Regional Med Ctr & Heart Inst	Fort Pierce	99%	115
Westside Regional Medical Center	Plantation	99%	68
Holy Cross Hospital	Fort Lauderdale	98%	45
Aventura Hospital and Medical Center	Aventura	97%	79
Parrish Medical Center	Titusville	97%	38
Sacred Heart Health System	Pensacola	97%	74
Morton Plant Hospital	Clearwater	96%	155
North Ridge Medical Center	Fort Lauderdale	96%	54
Northside Hospital	Saint Petersburg	95%	37
Shands Jacksonville	Jacksonville	95%	65
Baptist Hospital	Miami	94%	127
Memorial Hospital West	Pembroke Pines	94%	36
Mercy Hospital	Miami	94%	79
Saint Luke's Hospital	Jacksonville	94%	32
Halifax Medical Center	Daytona Beach	93%	68
Saint Joseph's Hospital	Tampa	93%	178
Memorial Regional Hospital	Hollywood	92%	150
Hialeah Hospital	Miami	91%	35
Jackson Memorial Hospital	Miami	91%	66
NCH Downtown Naples Hospital	Naples	91%	120
Tallahassee Memorial Health Care Foundation	Tallahassee	91%	121
Florida Hospital Heartland Medical Center	Sebring	90%	31
Largo Medical Center	Largo	90%	48
Florida Medical Center	Lauderdale Lakes	89%	127
Northwest Medical Center	Margate	89%	27
Orlando Regional Healthcare	Orlando	89%	196
North Broward Medical Center	Deerfield Beach	88%	33
Florida Hospital Orlando	Orlando	87%	253
Helen Ellis Memorial Hospital	Tarpon Springs	87%	31
JFK Medical Center	Atlantis	87%	245
Oak Hill Hospital	Brooksville	87%	39
Saint Vincent's Medical Center	Jacksonville	87%	69
Sarasota Memorial Health Care Systems	Sarasota	87%	141
West Florida Regional Medical Center	Pensacola	87%	46
Baptist Medical Center	Jacksonville	86%	63
Ocala Regional Medical Center	Ocala	86%	106
Blake Medical Center	Bradenton	85%	67
Columbia Memorial Hospital of Jacksonville	Jacksonville	85%	65
Florida Hospital DeLand	Deland	85%	26
Holmes Regional Medical Center	Melbourne	85%	298
Regional Medical Center Bayonet Point	Hudson	85%	163
Saint Lucie Medical Center	Port Saint Lucie	85%	26
Bert Fish Medical Center	New Smyrna Beach	82%	28
Florida Hospital Waterman	Tavares	82%	28
Lakeland Regional Medical Center	Lakeland	82%	67
Leesburg Regional Medical Center	Leesburg	82%	114
Munroe Regional Medical Center	Ocala	82%	170
Osceola Regional Medical Center	Kissimmee	82%	66
Shands at the University of Florida	Gainesville	82%	128
Baptist Hospital	Pensacola	81%	54
Mount Sinai Medical Center	Miami	81%	99
Charlotte Regional Medical Center	Punta Gorda	80%	85
Lee Memorial Health System	Fort Myers	80%	59
Winter Haven Hospital	Winter Haven	80%	85
Capital Regional Medical Center	Tallahassee	79%	39
Tampa General Healthcare	Tampa	79%	102
Broward General Medical Center	Fort Lauderdale	78%	81
Martin Memorial Medical Center	Stuart	78%	36
Bayfront Medical Center	Saint Petersburg	77%	26
Central Florida Regional Hospital	Sanford	77%	48
Community Hospital	New Port Richey	76%	38
North Shore Medical Center	Miami	76%	41
Manatee Memorial Hospital	Bradenton	75%	93
Bay Medical Center	Panama City	74%	126
Flagler Hospital	Saint Augustine	74%	27
Citrus Memorial Hospital	Inverness	73%	55
Florida Hospital-Ormond Memorial	Ormond Beach	73%	96
Southwest Florida Regional Medical Center	Fort Myers	72%	86
Florida Hospital Fish Memorial	Orange City	71%	31
Brandon Regional Hospital	Brandon	70%	107
Florida Hospital Zephyrhills	Zephyrhills	69%	55
University Community Hospital	Tampa	69%	77
Cedars Medical Center	Miami	66%	118
Palm Beach Grdns Medical Center	Palm Beach Grdns	64%	198

2. Aspirin at Arrival

Hospital Name	City	Rate	Cases
Cleveland Clinic Florida	Weston	100%	87
Delray Medical Center	Delray Beach	100%	506
Holy Cross Hospital	Fort Lauderdale	100%	188
Homestead Hospital	Homestead	100%	88
Mariners Hospital	Tavernier	100%	32
Memorial Hospital Miramar	Miramar	100%	39
NCH Downtown Naples Hospital	Naples	100%	577
Palms of Pasadena Hospital	Saint Petersburg	100%	44
Saint Luke's Hospital	Jacksonville	100%	146
South Florida Baptist Hospital	Plant City	100%	33
South Miami Hospital	Miami	100%	185
Venice Regional Medical Center	Venice	100%	311
Charlotte Regional Medical Center	Punta Gorda	99%	151
Fort Walton Beach Medical Center	Fort Walton Beach	99%	164
Lawnwood Regional Med Ctr & Heart Inst	Fort Pierce	99%	189
Memorial Regional Hospital	Hollywood	99%	412
Mercy Hospital	Miami	99%	251
Saint Joseph's Hospital	Tampa	99%	494
Shands Jacksonville	Jacksonville	99%	208
Westside Regional Medical Center	Plantation	99%	328
Aventura Hospital and Medical Center	Aventura	98%	284
Baptist Hospital	Miami	98%	439
Baptist Medical Center Beaches	Jacksonville Bch	98%	105
Bayfront Medical Center	Saint Petersburg	98%	143
Memorial Hospital Pembroke	Pembroke Pines	98%	103
North Florida Regional Medical Center	Gainesville	98%	194
Pasco Regional Medical Center	Dade City	98%	44
Peace River Regional Medical Center	Port Charlotte	98%	54
Sacred Heart Health System	Pensacola	98%	226
Sebastian River Medical Center	Sebastian	98%	63
Seven Rivers Regional Medical Center	Crystal River	98%	112
Wuesthoff Health Systems	Rockledge	98%	205
Bay Medical Center	Panama City	97%	312
Cape Canaveral Hospital	Cocoa Beach	97%	90
Coral Gables Hospital	Miami	97%	119
Edward White Hospital	Saint Petersburg	97%	30
Florida Medical Center	Lauderdale Lakes	97%	323
Gulf Breeze Hospital	Gulf Breeze	97%	29
Halifax Medical Center	Daytona Beach	97%	367
HealthSouth Doctors' Hospital	Miami	97%	62
Hialeah Hospital	Miami	97%	216
Jackson Hospital	Marianna	97%	30
Lakeland Regional Medical Center	Lakeland	97%	284
Largo Medical Center	Largo	97%	267
Larkin Community Hospital	South Miami	97%	31
Leesburg Regional Medical Center	Leesburg	97%	262
Mease Hospital-Countryside	Safety Harbor	97%	158
Memorial Hospital West	Pembroke Pines	97%	264
Morton Plant Hospital	Clearwater	97%	415
Palm Springs General Hospital	Miami	97%	139
Palmetto General Hospital	Hialeah	97%	189
Pan American Hospital	Miami	97%	116
Saint Vincent's Medical Center	Jacksonville	97%	140
Shands at the University of Florida	Gainesville	97%	280
Sun Coast Hospital	Largo	97%	39
West Boca Medical Center	Boca Raton	97%	119
Winter Haven Hospital	Winter Haven	97%	299
Baptist Hospital	Pensacola	96%	145
Baptist Medical Center	Jacksonville	96%	152
Central Florida Regional Hospital	Sanford	96%	160
Citrus Memorial Hospital	Inverness	96%	282
Coral Springs Medical Center	Coral Springs	96%	93
Florida Hospital DeLand	Deland	96%	138
Florida Hospital Orlando	Orlando	96%	598
Good Samaritan Medical Center	West Palm Beach	96%	51
Indian River Memorial Hospital	Vero Beach	96%	134
JFK Medical Center	Atlantis	96%	729
Jackson Memorial Hospital	Miami	96%	223
Mount Sinai Medical Center	Miami	96%	184
Saint Mary's Medical Center	West Palm Beach	96%	46
Santa Rosa Medical Center	Milton	96%	52
Sarasota Memorial Health Care Systems	Sarasota	96%	420
Southwest Florida Regional Medical Center	Fort Myers	96%	226
Tallahassee Memorial Health Care Foundation	Tallahassee	96%	314
Wellington Regional Medical Center	Wellington	96%	51
Bert Fish Medical Center	New Smyrna Beach	95%	146
Blake Medical Center	Bradenton	95%	312
Brandon Regional Hospital	Brandon	95%	361
Florida Hospital-Ormond Memorial	Ormond Beach	95%	280

NOTE: Hospital profiles are in alphabetical order by state, then city, then hospital within the city; Rankings are sorted by rate in descending order and exclude hospitals with less than 25 cases; (1) The number of cases is too small (n<25) for purposes of reliably predicting hospital performance; (2) Measure reflects the hospital's indication that its submission was based upon a sample of its relevant discharges; (3) Rate reflects fewer than the maximum possible quarters of data for the measure; (4) Inaccurate information submitted and suppressed for one or more quarters; (5) No data is available from the hospital for this measure; Please refer to the User's Guide for a full explanation of data

Hospital Name	City	Rate	Cases
Manatee Memorial Hospital	Bradenton	95%	414
Martin Memorial Medical Center	Stuart	95%	149
Mease Hospital-Dunedin	Dunedin	95%	60
North Ridge Medical Center	Fort Lauderdale	95%	148
Northside Hospital	Saint Petersburg	95%	210
Palm Beach Grdns Medical Center	Palm Beach Grdns	95%	364
University Community Hospital	Tampa	95%	287
West Florida Regional Medical Center	Pensacola	95%	146
Broward General Medical Center	Fort Lauderdale	94%	155
Cape Coral Hospital	Cape Coral	94%	93
Community Hospital	New Port Richey	94%	219
Holmes Regional Medical Center	Melbourne	94%	426
Kendall Medical Center	Miami	94%	455
Munroe Regional Medical Center	Ocala	94%	319
Ocala Regional Medical Center	Ocala	94%	220
Parrish Medical Center	Titusville	94%	143
Tampa General Healthcare	Tampa	94%	252
Town and Country Hospital	Tampa	94%	33
Villages Regional Hospital	The Villages	94%	64
Englewood Community Hospital	Englewood	93%	116
Lee Memorial Health System	Fort Myers	93%	161
North Bay Medical Center	New Port Richey	93%	73
Orange Park Medical Center	Orange Park	93%	84
Orlando Regional Healthcare	Orlando	93%	388
Saint Anthony's Hospital	Saint Petersburg	93%	104
Columbia Memorial Hospital of Jacksonville	Jacksonville	92%	245
Florida Hospital Fish Memorial	Orange City	92%	206
Florida Hospital Flagler	Palm Coast	92%	177
Florida Hospital Zephyrhills	Zephyrhills	92%	226
Helen Ellis Memorial Hospital	Tarpon Springs	92%	134
Putnam Community Medical Center	Palatka	92%	86
Regional Medical Center Bayonet Point	Hudson	92%	344
Saint Lucie Medical Center	Port Saint Lucie	92%	200
South Lake Hospital	Clermont	92%	71
Highlands Regional Medical Center	Sebring	91%	44
North Broward Medical Center	Deerfield Beach	91%	164
Osceola Regional Medical Center	Kissimmee	91%	221
Bethesda Memorial Hospital	Boynton Beach	90%	125
Boca Raton Community Hospital	Boca Raton	90%	126
Cedars Medical Center	Miami	90%	242
Wuesthoff Medical Center-Melbourne	Melbourne	90%	30
DeSoto Memorial Hospital	Arcadia	89%	28
Doctors Hospital of Sarasota	Sarasota	89%	65
Flagler Hospital	Saint Augustine	89%	289
Florida Hospital Waterman	Tavares	89%	158
North Okaloosa Medical Center	Crestview	89%	46
Capital Regional Medical Center	Tallahassee	88%	89
Northwest Medical Center	Margate	88%	165
Raulerson Hospital	Okeechobee	88%	49
Saint Petersburg General Hospital	Saint Petersburg	88%	60
Brooksville Regional Hospital	Brooksville	87%	164
Florida Hospital Heartland Medical Center	Sebring	87%	119
Lehigh Regional Medical Center	Lehigh Acres	87%	52
Oak Hill Hospital	Brooksville	87%	223
University Hospital & Medical Center	Tamarac	87%	109
Jupiter Medical Center	Jupiter	86%	70
Shands at Lake Shore	Lake City	86%	81
Health Central	Ocoee	85%	94
North Shore Medical Center	Miami	84%	171
South Bay Hospital	Sun City Center	84%	95
Lakewood Ranch Medical Center	Bradenton	83%	46
Palms West Hospital	Loxahatchee	83%	52
Fawcett Memorial Hospital	Port Charlotte	82%	85
Columbia Hospital	West Palm Beach	80%	65
Heart of Florida Regional Medical Center	Davenport	79%	106
Imperial Point Medical Center	Fort Lauderdale	79%	33
Lake City Medical Center	Lake City	79%	48

3. Aspirin at Discharge

Hospital Name	City	Rate	Cases
Cleveland Clinic Florida	Weston	100%	140
Delray Medical Center	Delray Beach	100%	548
Venice Regional Medical Center	Venice	100%	260
Aventura Hospital and Medical Center	Aventura	99%	277
Baptist Hospital	Miami	99%	490
Fort Walton Beach Medical Center	Fort Walton Beach	99%	282
Halifax Medical Center	Daytona Beach	99%	364
Holy Cross Hospital	Fort Lauderdale	99%	266
Memorial Regional Hospital	Hollywood	99%	652
Mercy Hospital	Miami	99%	355
NCH Downtown Naples Hospital	Naples	99%	700
North Ridge Medical Center	Fort Lauderdale	99%	251
South Miami Hospital	Miami	99%	277
Tallahassee Memorial Health Care Foundation	Tallahassee	99%	399
West Florida Regional Medical Center	Pensacola	99%	201
Westside Regional Medical Center	Plantation	99%	333
Wuesthoff Health Systems	Rockledge	99%	223
Baptist Medical Center	Jacksonville	98%	402
Holmes Regional Medical Center	Melbourne	98%	744
Lawnwood Regional Med Ctr & Heart Inst	Fort Pierce	98%	369
Morton Plant Hospital	Clearwater	98%	601
Blake Medical Center	Bradenton	97%	282
Florida Hospital DeLand	Deland	97%	72
Lakeland Regional Medical Center	Lakeland	97%	309
Leesburg Regional Medical Center	Leesburg	97%	355
North Florida Regional Medical Center	Gainesville	97%	314
Northside Hospital	Saint Petersburg	97%	257
Orange Park Medical Center	Orange Park	97%	33
Saint Luke's Hospital	Jacksonville	97%	143
Sarasota Memorial Health Care Systems	Sarasota	97%	528
Shands Jacksonville	Jacksonville	97%	276
Shands at the University of Florida	Gainesville	97%	401
Tampa General Healthcare	Tampa	97%	329
Baptist Hospital	Pensacola	96%	206
Cape Coral Hospital	Cape Coral	96%	49
Central Florida Regional Hospital	Sanford	96%	224
Citrus Memorial Hospital	Inverness	96%	272
Jackson Memorial Hospital	Miami	96%	212
Largo Medical Center	Largo	96%	255
Lee Memorial Health System	Fort Myers	96%	199
Peace River Regional Medical Center	Port Charlotte	96%	28
Sacred Heart Health System	Pensacola	96%	312
Saint Joseph's Hospital	Tampa	96%	517
Sebastian River Medical Center	Sebastian	96%	25
Seven Rivers Regional Medical Center	Crystal River	96%	45
Southwest Florida Regional Medical Center	Fort Myers	96%	274
Charlotte Regional Medical Center	Punta Gorda	95%	311
Columbia Memorial Hospital of Jacksonville	Jacksonville	95%	335
Hialeah Hospital	Miami	95%	87
JFK Medical Center	Atlantis	95%	944
Memorial Hospital West	Pembroke Pines	95%	160
Munroe Regional Medical Center	Ocala	95%	345
Ocala Regional Medical Center	Ocala	95%	219
Orlando Regional Healthcare	Orlando	95%	607
Saint Vincent's Medical Center	Jacksonville	95%	283
University Community Hospital	Tampa	95%	372
West Boca Medical Center	Boca Raton	95%	57
Bay Medical Center	Panama City	94%	359
Florida Hospital Orlando	Orlando	94%	982
Florida Hospital-Ormond Memorial	Ormond Beach	94%	413
Florida Medical Center	Lauderdale Lakes	94%	420
Memorial Hospital Pembroke	Pembroke Pines	94%	32
North Broward Medical Center	Deerfield Beach	94%	64
Putnam Community Medical Center	Palatka	94%	33
Regional Medical Center Bayonet Point	Hudson	94%	625
Bethesda Memorial Hospital	Boynton Beach	93%	69
Broward General Medical Center	Fort Lauderdale	93%	208
Kendall Medical Center	Miami	93%	409
Pan American Hospital	Miami	93%	44
Saint Anthony's Hospital	Saint Petersburg	93%	73
Baptist Medical Center Beaches	Jacksonville Bch	92%	49
Florida Hospital Heartland Medical Center	Sebring	92%	59
Florida Hospital Zephyrhills	Zephyrhills	92%	185
Palm Beach Grdns Medical Center	Palm Beach Grdns	92%	782
Sun Coast Hospital	Largo	92%	25
Winter Haven Hospital	Winter Haven	92%	324
Bayfront Medical Center	Saint Petersburg	91%	168
Cape Canaveral Hospital	Cocoa Beach	91%	56
Doctors Hospital of Sarasota	Sarasota	91%	35
Flagler Hospital	Saint Augustine	91%	257
Manatee Memorial Hospital	Bradenton	91%	410
Martin Memorial Medical Center	Stuart	91%	91
Northwest Medical Center	Margate	90%	72
Palmetto General Hospital	Hialeah	90%	40
Indian River Memorial Hospital	Vero Beach	89%	62
Capital Regional Medical Center	Tallahassee	88%	86
Columbia Hospital	West Palm Beach	88%	32
Health Central	Ocoee	88%	48
Mease Hospital-Countryside	Safety Harbor	88%	57
Mease Hospital-Dunedin	Dunedin	88%	25
North Shore Medical Center	Miami	88%	82
Brandon Regional Hospital	Brandon	87%	350
Florida Hospital Fish Memorial	Orange City	87%	112
Jupiter Medical Center	Jupiter	87%	30
Boca Raton Community Hospital	Boca Raton	86%	42
Florida Hospital Flagler	Palm Coast	86%	86
Florida Hospital Waterman	Tavares	86%	86
Mount Sinai Medical Center	Miami	86%	313
North Bay Medical Center	New Port Richey	86%	28

NOTE: Hospital profiles are in alphabetical order by state, then city, then hospital within the city; Rankings are sorted by rate in descending order and exclude hospitals with less than 25 cases; (1) The number of cases is too small (n<25) for purposes of reliably predicting hospital performance; (2) Measure reflects the hospital's indication that its submission was based upon a sample of its relevant discharges; (3) Rate reflects fewer than the maximum possible quarters of data for the measure; (4) Inaccurate information submitted and suppressed for one or more quarters; (5) No data is available from the hospital for this measure; Please refer to the User's Guide for a full explanation of data

Hospital Name	City	Rate	Cases
University Hospital & Medical Center	Tamarac	84%	32
Osceola Regional Medical Center	Kissimmee	83%	245
Palm Springs General Hospital	Miami	83%	46
Community Hospital	New Port Richey	82%	89
Fawcett Memorial Hospital	Port Charlotte	82%	50
Saint Lucie Medical Center	Port Saint Lucie	82%	68
Coral Gables Hospital	Miami	81%	59
Cedars Medical Center	Miami	80%	286
Parrish Medical Center	Titusville	80%	60
South Bay Hospital	Sun City Center	79%	42
Bert Fish Medical Center	New Smyrna Beach	78%	65
Englewood Community Hospital	Englewood	78%	63
Brooksville Regional Hospital	Brooksville	76%	59
Oak Hill Hospital	Brooksville	73%	158
North Okaloosa Medical Center	Crestview	71%	28
Shands at Lake Shore	Lake City	71%	51
Coral Springs Medical Center	Coral Springs	69%	36
Heart of Florida Regional Medical Center	Davenport	69%	54
Helen Ellis Memorial Hospital	Tarpon Springs	68%	87
Palms West Hospital	Loxahatchee	57%	28

4. Beta Blocker at Arrival

Hospital Name	City	Rate	Cases
Cleveland Clinic Florida	Weston	100%	86
Fort Walton Beach Medical Center	Fort Walton Beach	100%	130
Homestead Hospital	Homestead	100%	77
Seven Rivers Regional Medical Center	Crystal River	100%	113
South Florida Baptist Hospital	Plant City	100%	33
Coral Gables Hospital	Miami	99%	108
Delray Medical Center	Delray Beach	99%	474
Holy Cross Hospital	Fort Lauderdale	99%	172
Memorial Hospital Pembroke	Pembroke Pines	99%	85
Mercy Hospital	Miami	99%	250
Palmetto General Hospital	Hialeah	99%	177
Saint Joseph's Hospital	Tampa	99%	379
Venice Regional Medical Center	Venice	99%	269
Baptist Medical Center Beaches	Jacksonville Bch	98%	95
Good Samaritan Medical Center	West Palm Beach	98%	46
Halifax Medical Center	Daytona Beach	98%	301
HealthSouth Doctors' Hospital	Miami	98%	57
Memorial Hospital West	Pembroke Pines	98%	167
NCH Downtown Naples Hospital	Naples	98%	507
Palms of Pasadena Hospital	Saint Petersburg	98%	44
Sacred Heart Health System	Pensacola	98%	221
Saint Mary's Medical Center	West Palm Beach	98%	45
West Boca Medical Center	Boca Raton	98%	118
Westside Regional Medical Center	Plantation	98%	307
Aventura Hospital and Medical Center	Aventura	97%	204
Broward General Medical Center	Fort Lauderdale	97%	112
Lawnwood Regional Med Ctr & Heart Inst	Fort Pierce	97%	163
Memorial Regional Hospital	Hollywood	97%	357
Pasco Regional Medical Center	Dade City	97%	34
Saint Luke's Hospital	Jacksonville	97%	118
Saint Petersburg General Hospital	Saint Petersburg	97%	33
Shands Jacksonville	Jacksonville	97%	181
South Miami Hospital	Miami	97%	146
Parrish Medical Center	Titusville	96%	118
Saint Vincent's Medical Center	Jacksonville	96%	139
Tallahassee Memorial Health Care Foundation	Tallahassee	96%	229
Baptist Hospital	Miami	95%	343
Bert Fish Medical Center	New Smyrna Beach	95%	133
Cape Canaveral Hospital	Cocoa Beach	95%	100
Highlands Regional Medical Center	Sebring	95%	39
North Ridge Medical Center	Fort Lauderdale	95%	142
Sarasota Memorial Health Care Systems	Sarasota	95%	389
Sebastian River Medical Center	Sebastian	95%	59
Wuesthoff Health Systems	Rockledge	95%	154
Baptist Medical Center	Jacksonville	94%	147
Coral Springs Medical Center	Coral Springs	94%	67
Florida Medical Center	Lauderdale Lakes	94%	325
Jackson Memorial Hospital	Miami	94%	180
Largo Medical Center	Largo	94%	170
Mease Hospital-Dunedin	Dunedin	94%	32
Morton Plant Hospital	Clearwater	94%	245
Orange Park Medical Center	Orange Park	94%	65
Putnam Community Medical Center	Palatka	94%	78
Bay Medical Center	Panama City	93%	290
Blake Medical Center	Bradenton	93%	228
Charlotte Regional Medical Center	Punta Gorda	93%	146
Hialeah Hospital	Miami	93%	170
JFK Medical Center	Atlantis	93%	517
Larkin Community Hospital	South Miami	93%	27
Northside Hospital	Saint Petersburg	93%	150
Saint Anthony's Hospital	Saint Petersburg	93%	85
Sun Coast Hospital	Largo	93%	42
Holmes Regional Medical Center	Melbourne	92%	383
Lakeland Regional Medical Center	Lakeland	92%	261
Lee Memorial Health System	Fort Myers	92%	119
Memorial Hospital Miramar	Miramar	92%	39
University Community Hospital	Tampa	92%	245
Baptist Hospital	Pensacola	91%	116
Florida Hospital Flagler	Palm Coast	91%	165
Mount Sinai Medical Center	Miami	91%	163
North Bay Medical Center	New Port Richey	91%	33
North Broward Medical Center	Deerfield Beach	91%	112
Palm Beach Grdns Medical Center	Palm Beach Grdns	91%	333
Southwest Florida Regional Medical Center	Fort Myers	91%	207
Florida Hospital DeLand	Deland	90%	112
Florida Hospital Fish Memorial	Orange City	90%	145
Helen Ellis Memorial Hospital	Tarpon Springs	90%	126
Indian River Memorial Hospital	Vero Beach	90%	144
Leesburg Regional Medical Center	Leesburg	90%	170
Martin Memorial Medical Center	Stuart	90%	106
Saint Lucie Medical Center	Port Saint Lucie	90%	185
Santa Rosa Medical Center	Milton	90%	50
Shands at the University of Florida	Gainesville	90%	246
Brooksville Regional Hospital	Brooksville	89%	157
Cape Coral Hospital	Cape Coral	89%	73
Central Florida Regional Hospital	Sanford	89%	113
Community Hospital	New Port Richey	89%	122
Jupiter Medical Center	Jupiter	89%	72
Lake City Medical Center	Lake City	89%	47
Manatee Memorial Hospital	Bradenton	89%	364
North Okaloosa Medical Center	Crestview	89%	45
Northwest Medical Center	Margate	89%	102
Palm Springs General Hospital	Miami	89%	123
Pan American Hospital	Miami	89%	119
Raulerson Hospital	Okeechobee	89%	44
Tampa General Healthcare	Tampa	89%	198
Winter Haven Hospital	Winter Haven	89%	265
Columbia Memorial Hospital of Jacksonville	Jacksonville	88%	184
Florida Hospital Orlando	Orlando	88%	520
Gulf Breeze Hospital	Gulf Breeze	88%	25
Mease Hospital-Countryside	Safety Harbor	88%	75
North Shore Medical Center	Miami	88%	145
Bayfront Medical Center	Saint Petersburg	87%	124
Boca Raton Community Hospital	Boca Raton	87%	127
Brandon Regional Hospital	Brandon	87%	230
North Florida Regional Medical Center	Gainesville	87%	143
Capital Regional Medical Center	Tallahassee	86%	69
Florida Hospital Heartland Medical Center	Sebring	86%	90
Jackson Hospital	Marianna	86%	29
Munroe Regional Medical Center	Ocala	86%	213
Orlando Regional Healthcare	Orlando	86%	266
Peace River Regional Medical Center	Port Charlotte	86%	37
Town and Country Hospital	Tampa	86%	37
University Hospital & Medical Center	Tamarac	86%	66
Citrus Memorial Hospital	Inverness	85%	260
Florida Hospital Zephyrhills	Zephyrhills	85%	206
Regional Medical Center Bayonet Point	Hudson	85%	324
Wellington Regional Medical Center	Wellington	85%	40
West Florida Regional Medical Center	Pensacola	85%	98
South Lake Hospital	Clermont	84%	43
Villages Regional Hospital	The Villages	84%	64
Florida Hospital Waterman	Tavares	83%	145
Florida Hospital-Ormond Memorial	Ormond Beach	83%	232
Kendall Medical Center	Miami	83%	322
Oak Hill Hospital	Brooksville	83%	189
Cedars Medical Center	Miami	82%	239
Shands at Lake Shore	Lake City	82%	82
Fawcett Memorial Hospital	Port Charlotte	81%	75
Englewood Community Hospital	Englewood	80%	118
Flagler Hospital	Saint Augustine	80%	224
Osceola Regional Medical Center	Kissimmee	80%	196
Bethesda Memorial Hospital	Boynton Beach	79%	77
Doctors Hospital of Sarasota	Sarasota	79%	29
Lakewood Ranch Medical Center	Bradenton	79%	47
Ocala Regional Medical Center	Ocala	79%	112
Health Central	Ocoee	76%	96
Lehigh Regional Medical Center	Lehigh Acres	75%	48
Columbia Hospital	West Palm Beach	72%	47
South Bay Hospital	Sun City Center	71%	62
Heart of Florida Regional Medical Center	Davenport	68%	102

5. Beta Blocker at Discharge

Hospital Name	City	Rate	Cases
Baptist Hospital	Miami	100%	510
Cleveland Clinic Florida	Weston	100%	142

NOTE: Hospital profiles are in alphabetical order by state, then city, then hospital within the city; Rankings are sorted by rate in descending order and exclude hospitals with less than 25 cases; (1) The number of cases is too small (n<25) for purposes of reliably predicting hospital performance; (2) Measure reflects the hospital's indication that its submission was based upon a sample of its relevant discharges; (3) Rate reflects fewer than the maximum possible quarters of data for the measure; (4) Inaccurate information submitted and suppressed for one or more quarters; (5) No data is available from the hospital for this measure; Please refer to the User's Guide for a full explanation of data

Hospital Name	City	Rate	Cases
Good Samaritan Medical Center	West Palm Beach	100%	30
Memorial Hospital Pembroke	Pembroke Pines	100%	32
Orange Park Medical Center	Orange Park	100%	46
Peace River Regional Medical Center	Port Charlotte	100%	33
Putnam Community Medical Center	Palatka	100%	43
Venice Regional Medical Center	Venice	100%	320
Delray Medical Center	Delray Beach	99%	541
Florida Hospital Heartland Medical Center	Sebring	99%	77
Fort Walton Beach Medical Center	Fort Walton Beach	99%	262
Holy Cross Hospital	Fort Lauderdale	99%	271
Memorial Hospital West	Pembroke Pines	99%	171
Morton Plant Hospital	Clearwater	99%	695
Northwest Medical Center	Margate	99%	93
South Miami Hospital	Miami	99%	297
Westside Regional Medical Center	Plantation	99%	334
Aventura Hospital and Medical Center	Aventura	98%	314
Lawnwood Regional Med Ctr & Heart Inst	Fort Pierce	98%	398
Lee Memorial Health System	Fort Myers	98%	220
Mease Hospital-Dunedin	Dunedin	98%	46
Memorial Regional Hospital	Hollywood	98%	652
NCH Downtown Naples Hospital	Naples	98%	666
Wuesthoff Health Systems	Rockledge	98%	255
Baptist Hospital	Pensacola	97%	204
Baptist Medical Center	Jacksonville	97%	404
Blake Medical Center	Bradenton	97%	249
Cape Canaveral Hospital	Cocoa Beach	97%	71
Halifax Medical Center	Daytona Beach	97%	378
Leesburg Regional Medical Center	Leesburg	97%	401
Mease Hospital-Countryside	Safety Harbor	97%	88
Mercy Hospital	Miami	97%	374
North Ridge Medical Center	Fort Lauderdale	97%	260
Ocala Regional Medical Center	Ocala	97%	260
Shands Jacksonville	Jacksonville	97%	271
Southwest Florida Regional Medical Center	Fort Myers	97%	286
Tallahassee Memorial Health Care Foundation	Tallahassee	97%	436
Bethesda Memorial Hospital	Boynton Beach	96%	92
Florida Hospital DeLand	Deland	96%	77
Florida Hospital Fish Memorial	Orange City	96%	109
Jackson Memorial Hospital	Miami	96%	231
Largo Medical Center	Largo	96%	278
Munroe Regional Medical Center	Ocala	96%	397
North Shore Medical Center	Miami	96%	101
Northside Hospital	Saint Petersburg	96%	270
Orlando Regional Healthcare	Orlando	96%	671
Parrish Medical Center	Titusville	96%	76
Sacred Heart Health System	Pensacola	96%	310
Seven Rivers Regional Medical Center	Crystal River	96%	50
Shands at the University of Florida	Gainesville	96%	403
University Community Hospital	Tampa	96%	394
West Florida Regional Medical Center	Pensacola	96%	210
Bert Fish Medical Center	New Smyrna Beach	95%	65
Brandon Regional Hospital	Brandon	95%	434
Cape Coral Hospital	Cape Coral	95%	62
Coral Gables Hospital	Miami	95%	64
Florida Hospital Orlando	Orlando	95%	1021
Florida Medical Center	Lauderdale Lakes	95%	434
Holmes Regional Medical Center	Melbourne	95%	762
JFK Medical Center	Atlantis	95%	946
Lakeland Regional Medical Center	Lakeland	95%	303
Saint Joseph's Hospital	Tampa	95%	529
Saint Luke's Hospital	Jacksonville	95%	181
Saint Vincent's Medical Center	Jacksonville	95%	293
Bay Medical Center	Panama City	94%	367
Boca Raton Community Hospital	Boca Raton	94%	53
Central Florida Regional Hospital	Sanford	94%	240
Columbia Memorial Hospital of Jacksonville	Jacksonville	94%	349
Doctors Hospital of Sarasota	Sarasota	94%	34
Hialeah Hospital	Miami	94%	94
Regional Medical Center Bayonet Point	Hudson	94%	640
Sarasota Memorial Health Care Systems	Sarasota	94%	548
Tampa General Healthcare	Tampa	94%	339
Winter Haven Hospital	Winter Haven	94%	328
Broward General Medical Center	Fort Lauderdale	93%	215
Citrus Memorial Hospital	Inverness	93%	278
North Broward Medical Center	Deerfield Beach	93%	91
Palm Beach Grdns Medical Center	Palm Beach Grdns	93%	815
Sun Coast Hospital	Largo	93%	30
West Boca Medical Center	Boca Raton	93%	61
Florida Hospital Waterman	Tavares	92%	89
Palmetto General Hospital	Hialeah	92%	51
Saint Anthony's Hospital	Saint Petersburg	92%	75
South Bay Hospital	Sun City Center	92%	53
Brooksville Regional Hospital	Brooksville	91%	75
Florida Hospital Flagler	Palm Coast	91%	79
Health Central	Ocoee	91%	53

Hospital Name	City	Rate	Cases
Jupiter Medical Center	Jupiter	91%	32
Fawcett Memorial Hospital	Port Charlotte	90%	61
Indian River Memorial Hospital	Vero Beach	90%	72
Kendall Medical Center	Miami	90%	494
Martin Memorial Medical Center	Stuart	90%	109
North Florida Regional Medical Center	Gainesville	90%	316
South Lake Hospital	Clermont	90%	30
Baptist Medical Center Beaches	Jacksonville Bch	89%	56
Charlotte Regional Medical Center	Punta Gorda	89%	332
Florida Hospital Zephyrhills	Zephyrhills	89%	184
Florida Hospital-Ormond Memorial	Ormond Beach	89%	419
Mount Sinai Medical Center	Miami	89%	339
Bayfront Medical Center	Saint Petersburg	88%	168
Helen Ellis Memorial Hospital	Tarpon Springs	88%	96
Manatee Memorial Hospital	Bradenton	87%	422
Palm Springs General Hospital	Miami	87%	52
Pan American Hospital	Miami	87%	46
Saint Lucie Medical Center	Port Saint Lucie	87%	79
Community Hospital	New Port Richey	86%	127
Coral Springs Medical Center	Coral Springs	86%	36
Flagler Hospital	Saint Augustine	86%	245
University Hospital & Medical Center	Tamarac	86%	50
Oak Hill Hospital	Brooksville	85%	176
Wellington Regional Medical Center	Wellington	84%	25
Capital Regional Medical Center	Tallahassee	83%	95
North Bay Medical Center	New Port Richey	83%	36
Osceola Regional Medical Center	Kissimmee	81%	254
Cedars Medical Center	Miami	79%	299
Englewood Community Hospital	Englewood	78%	76
Palms West Hospital	Loxahatchee	76%	25
Santa Rosa Medical Center	Milton	76%	29
Shands at Lake Shore	Lake City	75%	53
Heart of Florida Regional Medical Center	Davenport	73%	59
North Okaloosa Medical Center	Crestview	73%	26
Columbia Hospital	West Palm Beach	69%	32

6. Fibrinolytic Medication Timing

Hospital Name	City	Rate	Cases
Bert Fish Medical Center	New Smyrna Beach	62%	32
Saint Lucie Medical Center	Port Saint Lucie	42%	33
Florida Hospital Fish Memorial	Orange City	24%	25
Cedars Medical Center	Miami	18%	28

7. PCI Within 90 Minutes of Arrival

Hospital Name	City	Rate	Cases
Memorial Regional Hospital	Hollywood	87%	30
JFK Medical Center	Atlantis	47%	34

8. Smoking Cessation Advice

Hospital Name	City	Rate	Cases
Aventura Hospital and Medical Center	Aventura	100%	70
Baptist Hospital	Miami	100%	168
Cleveland Clinic Florida	Weston	100%	44
Community Hospital	New Port Richey	100%	28
Delray Medical Center	Delray Beach	100%	73
Florida Hospital Orlando	Orlando	100%	355
Florida Medical Center	Lauderdale Lakes	100%	101
Halifax Medical Center	Daytona Beach	100%	160
Holy Cross Hospital	Fort Lauderdale	100%	71
Lakeland Regional Medical Center	Lakeland	100%	115
Lawnwood Regional Med Ctr & Heart Inst	Fort Pierce	100%	147
Memorial Hospital West	Pembroke Pines	100%	56
Mercy Hospital	Miami	100%	64
North Ridge Medical Center	Fort Lauderdale	100%	68
Palm Beach Grdns Medical Center	Palm Beach Grdns	100%	219
Parrish Medical Center	Titusville	100%	25
Saint Anthony's Hospital	Saint Petersburg	100%	30
Saint Joseph's Hospital	Tampa	100%	197
Saint Luke's Hospital	Jacksonville	100%	59
Venice Regional Medical Center	Venice	100%	81
Wuesthoff Health Systems	Rockledge	100%	115
Baptist Medical Center	Jacksonville	99%	170
Bayfront Medical Center	Saint Petersburg	99%	69
Columbia Memorial Hospital of Jacksonville	Jacksonville	99%	177
Fort Walton Beach Medical Center	Fort Walton Beach	99%	110
JFK Medical Center	Atlantis	99%	272
Kendall Medical Center	Miami	99%	139
Lee Memorial Health System	Fort Myers	99%	87
Memorial Regional Hospital	Hollywood	99%	222
NCH Downtown Naples Hospital	Naples	99%	158
Ocala Regional Medical Center	Ocala	99%	90
Osceola Regional Medical Center	Kissimmee	99%	81
South Miami Hospital	Miami	99%	100

NOTE: Hospital profiles are in alphabetical order by state, then city, then hospital within the city; Rankings are sorted by rate in descending order and exclude hospitals with less than 25 cases; (1) The number of cases is too small (n<25) for purposes of reliably predicting hospital performance; (2) Measure reflects the hospital's indication that its submission was based upon a sample of its relevant discharges; (3) Rate reflects fewer than the maximum possible quarters of data for the measure; (4) Inaccurate information submitted and suppressed for one or more quarters; (5) No data is available from the hospital for this measure; Please refer to the User's Guide for a full explanation of data

Hospital Name	City	Rate	Cases
Southwest Florida Regional Medical Center	Fort Myers	99%	89
West Florida Regional Medical Center	Pensacola	99%	101
Winter Haven Hospital	Winter Haven	99%	108
Brandon Regional Hospital	Brandon	98%	180
Broward General Medical Center	Fort Lauderdale	98%	96
Florida Hospital-Ormond Memorial	Ormond Beach	98%	133
Largo Medical Center	Largo	98%	98
Leesburg Regional Medical Center	Leesburg	98%	114
North Florida Regional Medical Center	Gainesville	98%	115
Oak Hill Hospital	Brooksville	98%	48
Tallahassee Memorial Health Care Foundation	Tallahassee	98%	168
University Community Hospital	Tampa	98%	138
Bay Medical Center	Panama City	97%	145
Blake Medical Center	Bradenton	97%	73
Capital Regional Medical Center	Tallahassee	97%	33
Central Florida Regional Hospital	Sanford	97%	89
Holmes Regional Medical Center	Melbourne	97%	256
Morton Plant Hospital	Clearwater	97%	232
Northside Hospital	Saint Petersburg	97%	120
Baptist Hospital	Pensacola	96%	93
Charlotte Regional Medical Center	Punta Gorda	96%	103
Orlando Regional Healthcare	Orlando	96%	246
Shands Jacksonville	Jacksonville	96%	144
Shands at the University of Florida	Gainesville	96%	161
Tampa General Healthcare	Tampa	96%	137
Jackson Memorial Hospital	Miami	95%	96
Manatee Memorial Hospital	Bradenton	95%	154
Regional Medical Center Bayonet Point	Hudson	95%	208
Sacred Heart Health System	Pensacola	95%	128
Westside Regional Medical Center	Plantation	95%	64
Citrus Memorial Hospital	Inverness	94%	103
Flagler Hospital	Saint Augustine	94%	78
Munroe Regional Medical Center	Ocala	93%	143
Mount Sinai Medical Center	Miami	91%	97
Sarasota Memorial Health Care Systems	Sarasota	91%	142
Saint Vincent's Medical Center	Jacksonville	86%	104
Helen Ellis Memorial Hospital	Tarpon Springs	82%	28
Cedars Medical Center	Miami	80%	94
Florida Hospital Zephyrhills	Zephyrhills	75%	56

Heart Failure Care

9. ACE Inhibitor or ARB for LVSD

Hospital Name	City	Rate	Cases
Cleveland Clinic Florida	Weston	100%	97
Fort Walton Beach Medical Center	Fort Walton Beach	100%	74
Memorial Hospital Pembroke	Pembroke Pines	100%	73
Seven Rivers Regional Medical Center	Crystal River	100%	126
Venice Regional Medical Center	Venice	100%	140
Holy Cross Hospital	Fort Lauderdale	99%	191
Wuesthoff Health Systems	Rockledge	99%	180
Homestead Hospital	Homestead	98%	126
Memorial Hospital of Tampa	Tampa	98%	44
South Miami Hospital	Miami	98%	144
Delray Medical Center	Delray Beach	97%	178
Pasco Regional Medical Center	Dade City	97%	70
Peace River Regional Medical Center	Port Charlotte	97%	66
HealthSouth Doctors' Hospital	Miami	96%	45
Hialeah Hospital	Miami	96%	163
Putnam Community Medical Center	Palatka	96%	77
West Boca Medical Center	Boca Raton	96%	52
Lawnwood Regional Med Ctr & Heart Inst	Fort Pierce	95%	261
Mercy Hospital	Miami	95%	298
Sacred Heart Health System	Pensacola	95%	188
Halifax Medical Center	Daytona Beach	94%	311
South Florida Baptist Hospital	Plant City	94%	63
Mariners Hospital	Tavernier	93%	27
Memorial Regional Hospital	Hollywood	93%	486
Palms of Pasadena Hospital	Saint Petersburg	93%	42
Parrish Medical Center	Titusville	93%	104
Winter Haven Hospital	Winter Haven	93%	300
Aventura Hospital and Medical Center	Aventura	92%	173
Baptist Hospital	Miami	92%	319
Jackson Hospital	Marianna	92%	50
Sebastian River Medical Center	Sebastian	92%	96
Largo Medical Center	Largo	91%	110
Mease Hospital-Countryside	Safety Harbor	91%	150
Saint Joseph's Hospital	Tampa	91%	422
Shands Jacksonville	Jacksonville	91%	176
Sun Coast Hospital	Largo	91%	54
Bayfront Medical Center	Saint Petersburg	90%	134
Broward General Medical Center	Fort Lauderdale	90%	177
Coral Gables Hospital	Miami	90%	90
Memorial Hospital West	Pembroke Pines	90%	178
Morton Plant Hospital	Clearwater	90%	240
North Ridge Medical Center	Fort Lauderdale	90%	94
Sacred Heart Hospital on the Emerald Coast	Destin	90%	29
Saint Luke's Hospital	Jacksonville	90%	115
Town and Country Hospital	Tampa	90%	39
Westside Regional Medical Center	Plantation	90%	117
Cape Canaveral Hospital	Cocoa Beach	89%	95
Leesburg Regional Medical Center	Leesburg	89%	178
North Bay Medical Center	New Port Richey	89%	71
Raulerson Hospital	Okeechobee	89%	54
Saint Anthony's Hospital	Saint Petersburg	89%	98
Santa Rosa Medical Center	Milton	89%	45
Glades General Hospital	Belle Glade	88%	51
Gulf Breeze Hospital	Gulf Breeze	88%	25
Lehigh Regional Medical Center	Lehigh Acres	88%	66
Saint Cloud Regional Medical Center	Saint Cloud	88%	25
Mease Hospital-Dunedin	Dunedin	87%	90
Northwest Medical Center	Margate	87%	95
Bartow Regional Medical Center	Bartow	86%	37
Good Samaritan Medical Center	West Palm Beach	86%	77
Orange Park Medical Center	Orange Park	86%	122
Saint Mary's Medical Center	West Palm Beach	86%	81
Shands at the University of Florida	Gainesville	86%	324
Doctors Hospital of Sarasota	Sarasota	85%	65
JFK Medical Center	Atlantis	85%	493
North Shore Medical Center	Miami	85%	271
Tampa General Healthcare	Tampa	85%	336
Blake Medical Center	Bradenton	84%	130
Cape Coral Hospital	Cape Coral	84%	49
Florida Hospital Orlando	Orlando	84%	776
Jackson Memorial Hospital	Miami	84%	275
Lakeland Regional Medical Center	Lakeland	84%	157
Martin Memorial Medical Center	Stuart	84%	101
Munroe Regional Medical Center	Ocala	84%	229
Orlando Regional Healthcare	Orlando	84%	743
Saint Lucie Medical Center	Port Saint Lucie	84%	185
Sarasota Memorial Health Care Systems	Sarasota	84%	233
Florida Hospital Flagler	Palm Coast	83%	69
Manatee Memorial Hospital	Bradenton	83%	233
North Broward Medical Center	Deerfield Beach	83%	115
Northside Hospital	Saint Petersburg	83%	98
Saint Vincent's Medical Center	Jacksonville	83%	125
Southwest Florida Regional Medical Center	Fort Myers	83%	219
Baptist Hospital	Pensacola	82%	136
Baptist Medical Center	Jacksonville	82%	251
Baptist Medical Center Beaches	Jacksonville Bch	82%	85
Brooksville Regional Hospital	Brooksville	82%	141
Edward White Hospital	Saint Petersburg	82%	33
Flagler Hospital	Saint Augustine	82%	144
Florida Hospital Zephyrhills	Zephyrhills	82%	110
Imperial Point Medical Center	Fort Lauderdale	82%	50
Tallahassee Memorial Health Care Foundation	Tallahassee	82%	209
Wellington Regional Medical Center	Wellington	82%	62
Bay Medical Center	Panama City	81%	376
Charlotte Regional Medical Center	Punta Gorda	81%	253
Heart of Florida Regional Medical Center	Davenport	81%	160
Lee Memorial Health System	Fort Myers	81%	100
Lower Keys Medical Center	Key West	81%	31
Mount Sinai Medical Center	Miami	80%	173
NCH Downtown Naples Hospital	Naples	80%	456
Ocala Regional Medical Center	Ocala	80%	204
Palmetto General Hospital	Hialeah	80%	177
Pan American Hospital	Miami	80%	127
Regional Medical Center Bayonet Point	Hudson	80%	304
Coral Springs Medical Center	Coral Springs	79%	72
Helen Ellis Memorial Hospital	Tarpon Springs	79%	122
Community Hospital	New Port Richey	78%	156
Florida Hospital DeLand	Deland	78%	120
Health Central	Ocoee	78%	110
Palm Springs General Hospital	Miami	78%	160
University Community Hospital	Tampa	78%	176
Bethesda Memorial Hospital	Boynton Beach	77%	78
Columbia Memorial Hospital of Jacksonville	Jacksonville	77%	239
Saint Petersburg General Hospital	Saint Petersburg	77%	39
Wuesthoff Medical Center-Melbourne	Melbourne	77%	71
Bert Fish Medical Center	New Smyrna Beach	76%	70
Englewood Community Hospital	Englewood	76%	59
Fawcett Memorial Hospital	Port Charlotte	76%	103
Florida Hospital Fish Memorial	Orange City	76%	123
Florida Hospital Waterman	Tavares	76%	234
Florida Medical Center	Lauderdale Lakes	76%	203
Indian River Memorial Hospital	Vero Beach	76%	142
South Lake Hospital	Clermont	76%	75
West Florida Regional Medical Center	Pensacola	76%	127
Central Florida Regional Hospital	Sanford	75%	118

NOTE: Hospital profiles are in alphabetical order by state, then city, then hospital within the city; Rankings are sorted by rate in descending order and exclude hospitals with less than 25 cases; (1) The number of cases is too small (n<25) for purposes of reliably predicting hospital performance; (2) Measure reflects the hospital's indication that its submission was based upon a sample of its relevant discharges; (3) Rate reflects fewer than the maximum possible quarters of data for the measure; (4) Inaccurate information submitted and suppressed for one or more quarters; (5) No data is available from the hospital for this measure; Please refer to the User's Guide for a full explanation of data

Palm Beach Grdns Medical Center	Palm Beach Grdns	75%	351
Villages Regional Hospital	The Villages	75%	93
Citrus Memorial Hospital	Inverness	74%	112
Gulf Coast Medical Center	Panama City	74%	43
Holmes Regional Medical Center	Melbourne	74%	412
Lake Wales Medical Center	Lake Wales	74%	68
North Okaloosa Medical Center	Crestview	73%	52
Osceola Regional Medical Center	Kissimmee	73%	211
Boca Raton Community Hospital	Boca Raton	72%	206
Florida Hospital-Ormond Memorial	Ormond Beach	72%	211
Jupiter Medical Center	Jupiter	72%	81
University Hospital & Medical Center	Tamarac	72%	97
Florida Hospital Heartland Medical Center	Sebring	71%	206
Oak Hill Hospital	Brooksville	71%	108
Plantation General Hospital	Plantation	71%	76
Capital Regional Medical Center	Tallahassee	70%	158
Doctors Memorial Hospital	Perry	68%	28
Highlands Regional Medical Center	Sebring	66%	58
Cedars Medical Center	Miami	65%	371
Kendall Medical Center	Miami	65%	342
Palms West Hospital	Loxahatchee	65%	83
North Florida Regional Medical Center	Gainesville	64%	220
University Community Hospital of Carrollwood	Tampa	64%	42
Baptist Medical Center Nassau	Fernandina Bch	63%	27
Columbia Hospital	West Palm Beach	63%	67
Brandon Regional Hospital	Brandon	60%	179
South Bay Hospital	Sun City Center	59%	102
Lake City Medical Center	Lake City	54%	56
Shands at Lake Shore	Lake City	52%	33

10. Discharge Instructions

Hospital Name	City	Rate	Cases
Delray Medical Center	Delray Beach	100%	497
Holy Cross Hospital	Fort Lauderdale	100%	446
Mariners Hospital	Tavernier	100%	39
Hialeah Hospital	Miami	99%	368
Seven Rivers Regional Medical Center	Crystal River	99%	216
Larkin Community Hospital	South Miami	98%	41
Hendry Regional Medical Center	Clewiston	97%	29
North Ridge Medical Center	Fort Lauderdale	97%	176
Halifax Medical Center	Daytona Beach	96%	641
Jay Hospital	Jay	96%	46
Memorial Hospital Pembroke	Pembroke Pines	96%	237
Mercy Hospital	Miami	96%	496
Broward General Medical Center	Fort Lauderdale	95%	263
Fort Walton Beach Medical Center	Fort Walton Beach	95%	219
Osceola Regional Medical Center	Kissimmee	95%	401
Pan American Hospital	Miami	95%	240
Coral Gables Hospital	Miami	94%	223
Homestead Hospital	Homestead	94%	291
Memorial Hospital of Tampa	Tampa	94%	107
Cleveland Clinic Florida	Weston	93%	207
Coral Springs Medical Center	Coral Springs	93%	175
Shands at Starke	Starke	93%	43
Venice Regional Medical Center	Venice	93%	254
Aventura Hospital and Medical Center	Aventura	92%	425
Cape Canaveral Hospital	Cocoa Beach	92%	197
North Shore Medical Center	Miami	92%	494
Parrish Medical Center	Titusville	92%	182
Saint Mary's Medical Center	West Palm Beach	92%	168
Doctors Memorial Hospital	Bonifay	90%	48
Lawnwood Regional Med Ctr & Heart Inst	Fort Pierce	90%	493
Glades General Hospital	Belle Glade	89%	122
Winter Haven Hospital	Winter Haven	89%	436
Boca Raton Community Hospital	Boca Raton	88%	460
Memorial Hospital Miramar	Miramar	88%	122
Northwest Medical Center	Margate	88%	260
HealthSouth Doctors' Hospital	Miami	87%	153
South Miami Hospital	Miami	87%	311
Saint Lucie Medical Center	Port Saint Lucie	86%	369
Memorial Regional Hospital	Hollywood	85%	869
Palm Beach Grdns Medical Center	Palm Beach Grdns	85%	567
Lakeland Regional Medical Center	Lakeland	84%	280
Manatee Memorial Hospital	Bradenton	84%	475
Memorial Hospital West	Pembroke Pines	84%	463
Tallahassee Memorial Health Care Foundation	Tallahassee	84%	355
Lower Keys Medical Center	Key West	83%	90
Saint Anthony's Hospital	Saint Petersburg	83%	217
Wuesthoff Health Systems	Rockledge	83%	413
Baptist Hospital	Miami	82%	660
JFK Medical Center	Atlantis	82%	1037
North Broward Medical Center	Deerfield Beach	82%	214
South Lake Hospital	Clermont	82%	208
Palmetto General Hospital	Hialeah	81%	395
Putnam Community Medical Center	Palatka	81%	236
West Boca Medical Center	Boca Raton	81%	168
Palm Springs General Hospital	Miami	80%	316
Sacred Heart Health System	Pensacola	80%	342
Raulerson Hospital	Okeechobee	79%	234
Saint Vincent's Medical Center	Jacksonville	79%	244
Fawcett Memorial Hospital	Port Charlotte	77%	246
Englewood Community Hospital	Englewood	76%	131
Baptist Medical Center Beaches	Jacksonville Bch	75%	162
Florida Hospital Orlando	Orlando	75%	1762
Florida Hospital Waterman	Tavares	75%	403
Sacred Heart Hospital on the Emerald Coast	Destin	74%	74
Twin Cities Hospital	Niceville	74%	46
Holmes Regional Medical Center	Melbourne	73%	661
Kendall Medical Center	Miami	72%	679
Blake Medical Center	Bradenton	71%	408
Imperial Point Medical Center	Fort Lauderdale	71%	119
South Florida Baptist Hospital	Plant City	71%	119
Tampa General Healthcare	Tampa	71%	556
Westside Regional Medical Center	Plantation	71%	325
Florida Hospital-Ormond Memorial	Ormond Beach	70%	372
Mease Hospital-Dunedin	Dunedin	70%	159
Palms of Pasadena Hospital	Saint Petersburg	70%	132
University Community Hospital of Carrollwood	Tampa	70%	97
University Hospital & Medical Center	Tamarac	70%	244
Leesburg Regional Medical Center	Leesburg	69%	343
Mease Hospital-Countryside	Safety Harbor	68%	337
Shands Jacksonville	Jacksonville	68%	257
Charlotte Regional Medical Center	Punta Gorda	67%	407
Good Samaritan Medical Center	West Palm Beach	67%	206
Morton Plant Hospital	Clearwater	67%	523
Orange Park Medical Center	Orange Park	67%	257
Central Florida Regional Hospital	Sanford	66%	283
Doctors Hospital of Sarasota	Sarasota	66%	129
Santa Rosa Medical Center	Milton	66%	122
Indian River Memorial Hospital	Vero Beach	65%	63
Plantation General Hospital	Plantation	64%	131
Bethesda Memorial Hospital	Boynton Beach	63%	204
Community Hospital	New Port Richey	63%	346
Villages Regional Hospital	The Villages	63%	247
Lakewood Ranch Medical Center	Bradenton	62%	66
Saint Joseph's Hospital	Tampa	62%	811
Sebastian River Medical Center	Sebastian	62%	175
Shands Live Oak	Live Oak	62%	47
Wuesthoff Medical Center-Melbourne	Melbourne	60%	121
Saint Luke's Hospital	Jacksonville	59%	245
Florida Hospital Heartland Medical Center	Sebring	58%	382
Bayfront Medical Center	Saint Petersburg	57%	247
Florida Medical Center	Lauderdale Lakes	57%	393
Gulf Breeze Hospital	Gulf Breeze	57%	92
Baptist Hospital	Pensacola	56%	351
Wellington Regional Medical Center	Wellington	56%	208
Citrus Memorial Hospital	Inverness	54%	241
Northside Hospital	Saint Petersburg	54%	252
Pasco Regional Medical Center	Dade City	54%	166
Columbia Hospital	West Palm Beach	53%	186
Florida Hospital Zephyrhills	Zephyrhills	53%	294
North Bay Medical Center	New Port Richey	53%	152
Jupiter Medical Center	Jupiter	52%	178
Southwest Florida Regional Medical Center	Fort Myers	52%	460
Regional Medical Center Bayonet Point	Hudson	51%	549
University Community Hospital	Tampa	51%	351
Mount Sinai Medical Center	Miami	50%	305
Ocala Regional Medical Center	Ocala	49%	343
South Bay Hospital	Sun City Center	49%	253
Bay Medical Center	Panama City	48%	876
Palms West Hospital	Loxahatchee	47%	215
Lake City Medical Center	Lake City	46%	160
Lee Memorial Health System	Fort Myers	46%	195
West Florida Regional Medical Center	Pensacola	46%	240
NCH Downtown Naples Hospital	Naples	45%	887
Peace River Regional Medical Center	Port Charlotte	45%	175
Cape Coral Hospital	Cape Coral	44%	117
North Florida Regional Medical Center	Gainesville	44%	470
Columbia Memorial Hospital of Jacksonville	Jacksonville	43%	498
Munroe Regional Medical Center	Ocala	43%	364
Martin Memorial Medical Center	Stuart	42%	208
Saint Petersburg General Hospital	Saint Petersburg	42%	85
Florida Hospital Fish Memorial	Orange City	41%	342
Jackson Memorial Hospital	Miami	41%	509
Largo Medical Center	Largo	41%	332
Gulf Coast Medical Center	Panama City	40%	98
Health Central	Ocoee	39%	200
Florida Hospital DeLand	Deland	38%	242
Cedars Medical Center	Miami	37%	663

NOTE: Hospital profiles are in alphabetical order by state, then city, then hospital within the city; Rankings are sorted by rate in descending order and exclude hospitals with less than 25 cases; (1) The number of cases is too small (n<25) for purposes of reliably predicting hospital performance; (2) Measure reflects the hospital's indication that its submission was based upon a sample of its relevant discharges; (3) Rate reflects fewer than the maximum possible quarters of data for the measure; (4) Inaccurate information submitted and suppressed for one or more quarters; (5) No data is available from the hospital for this measure; Please refer to the User's Guide for a full explanation of data

Orlando Regional Healthcare	Orlando	37%	1408
Baptist Medical Center	Jacksonville	36%	502
Flagler Hospital	Saint Augustine	35%	366
Sarasota Memorial Health Care Systems	Sarasota	35%	423
Bert Fish Medical Center	New Smyrna Beach	34%	156
Brandon Regional Hospital	Brandon	34%	350
Brooksville Regional Hospital	Brooksville	32%	336
Shands at the University of Florida	Gainesville	32%	548
Town and Country Hospital	Tampa	32%	112
North Okaloosa Medical Center	Crestview	31%	135
Westchester General Hospital	Miami	30%	27
Highlands Regional Medical Center	Sebring	29%	160
Lehigh Regional Medical Center	Lehigh Acres	28%	164
Northwest Florida Community Hospital	Chipley	26%	35
Trinity Community Hospital	Jasper	26%	43
Bartow Regional Medical Center	Bartow	25%	139
Florida Hospital Flagler	Palm Coast	25%	191
Oak Hill Hospital	Brooksville	25%	357
Jackson Hospital	Marianna	24%	125
Edward White Hospital	Saint Petersburg	23%	93
Lake Wales Medical Center	Lake Wales	22%	180
Sun Coast Hospital	Largo	21%	111
Heart of Florida Regional Medical Center	Davenport	20%	398
DeSoto Memorial Hospital	Arcadia	18%	78
Capital Regional Medical Center	Tallahassee	17%	307
Helen Ellis Memorial Hospital	Tarpon Springs	12%	235
Shands at Lake Shore	Lake City	11%	141
Baptist Medical Center Nassau	Fernandina Bch	8%	65

11. Evaluation of LVS Function

Hospital Name	City	Rate	Cases
Cleveland Clinic Florida	Weston	100%	220
HealthSouth Doctors' Hospital	Miami	100%	177
Hialeah Hospital	Miami	100%	446
Holy Cross Hospital	Fort Lauderdale	100%	544
Homestead Hospital	Homestead	100%	323
Mariners Hospital	Tavernier	100%	46
Memorial Hospital Pembroke	Pembroke Pines	100%	270
Memorial Hospital West	Pembroke Pines	100%	523
Putnam Community Medical Center	Palatka	100%	275
South Miami Hospital	Miami	100%	360
Venice Regional Medical Center	Venice	100%	323
Aventura Hospital and Medical Center	Aventura	99%	552
Baptist Hospital	Miami	99%	760
Baptist Medical Center Nassau	Fernandina Bch	99%	76
Delray Medical Center	Delray Beach	99%	688
Glades General Hospital	Belle Glade	99%	128
Halifax Medical Center	Daytona Beach	99%	786
Leesburg Regional Medical Center	Leesburg	99%	426
Memorial Hospital of Tampa	Tampa	99%	144
Memorial Regional Hospital	Hollywood	99%	992
Mercy Hospital	Miami	99%	551
Orlando Regional Healthcare	Orlando	99%	1651
Peace River Regional Medical Center	Port Charlotte	99%	222
South Florida Baptist Hospital	Plant City	99%	146
Westside Regional Medical Center	Plantation	99%	394
Bayfront Medical Center	Saint Petersburg	98%	291
Flagler Hospital	Saint Augustine	98%	458
Florida Hospital DeLand	Deland	98%	351
Lawnwood Regional Med Ctr & Heart Inst	Fort Pierce	98%	586
Memorial Hospital Miramar	Miramar	98%	133
Northside Hospital	Saint Petersburg	98%	321
Orange Park Medical Center	Orange Park	98%	371
Osceola Regional Medical Center	Kissimmee	98%	458
Physicians Regional Medical Center	Naples	98%	60
Sacred Heart Health System	Pensacola	98%	389
Twin Cities Hospital	Niceville	98%	53
Wuesthoff Health Systems	Rockledge	98%	486
Baptist Medical Center	Jacksonville	97%	622
Broward General Medical Center	Fort Lauderdale	97%	282
Fort Walton Beach Medical Center	Fort Walton Beach	97%	283
Jackson Memorial Hospital	Miami	97%	569
Kendall Medical Center	Miami	97%	777
Largo Medical Center	Largo	97%	429
North Shore Medical Center	Miami	97%	571
Shands Jacksonville	Jacksonville	97%	298
Tallahassee Memorial Health Care Foundation	Tallahassee	97%	432
Cape Canaveral Hospital	Cocoa Beach	96%	239
Capital Regional Medical Center	Tallahassee	96%	395
Coral Gables Hospital	Miami	96%	295
Doctors Hospital of Sarasota	Sarasota	96%	194
Pan American Hospital	Miami	96%	323
Pasco Regional Medical Center	Dade City	96%	205
Sacred Heart Hospital on the Emerald Coast	Destin	96%	90
Saint Luke's Hospital	Jacksonville	96%	306
Shands at the University of Florida	Gainesville	96%	617
West Florida Regional Medical Center	Pensacola	96%	272
Winter Haven Hospital	Winter Haven	96%	532
Bethesda Memorial Hospital	Boynton Beach	95%	263
Brandon Regional Hospital	Brandon	95%	445
Good Samaritan Medical Center	West Palm Beach	95%	263
Lehigh Regional Medical Center	Lehigh Acres	95%	174
North Okaloosa Medical Center	Crestview	95%	165
Palmetto General Hospital	Hialeah	95%	462
Saint Joseph's Hospital	Tampa	95%	975
Saint Mary's Medical Center	West Palm Beach	95%	209
Seven Rivers Regional Medical Center	Crystal River	95%	280
Florida Hospital Heartland Medical Center	Sebring	94%	476
Florida Hospital Orlando	Orlando	94%	2113
Florida Hospital Waterman	Tavares	94%	485
Florida Hospital-Ormond Memorial	Ormond Beach	94%	503
Lower Keys Medical Center	Key West	94%	104
Manatee Memorial Hospital	Bradenton	94%	630
Martin Memorial Medical Center	Stuart	94%	270
Mount Sinai Medical Center	Miami	94%	373
Parrish Medical Center	Titusville	94%	234
Regional Medical Center Bayonet Point	Hudson	94%	674
Saint Petersburg General Hospital	Saint Petersburg	94%	134
Saint Vincent's Medical Center	Jacksonville	94%	310
South Lake Hospital	Clermont	94%	240
Town and Country Hospital	Tampa	94%	154
University Community Hospital	Tampa	94%	461
Charlotte Regional Medical Center	Punta Gorda	93%	464
Columbia Memorial Hospital of Jacksonville	Jacksonville	93%	615
Health Central	Ocoee	93%	268
JFK Medical Center	Atlantis	93%	1223
Mease Hospital-Countryside	Safety Harbor	93%	434
Morton Plant Hospital	Clearwater	93%	701
Northwest Medical Center	Margate	93%	333
Ocala Regional Medical Center	Ocala	93%	440
Palms West Hospital	Loxahatchee	93%	245
Sarasota Memorial Health Care Systems	Sarasota	93%	580
Shands at Starke	Starke	93%	58
South Bay Hospital	Sun City Center	93%	338
Tampa General Healthcare	Tampa	93%	605
West Boca Medical Center	Boca Raton	93%	223
Wuesthoff Medical Center-Melbourne	Melbourne	93%	149
Baptist Medical Center Beaches	Jacksonville Bch	92%	222
Brooksville Regional Hospital	Brooksville	92%	396
Cedars Medical Center	Miami	92%	777
Florida Hospital Fish Memorial	Orange City	92%	437
Blake Medical Center	Bradenton	91%	514
Central Florida Regional Hospital	Sanford	91%	356
Helen Ellis Memorial Hospital	Tarpon Springs	91%	308
Lake City Medical Center	Lake City	91%	214
Lakeland Regional Medical Center	Lakeland	91%	322
Lakewood Ranch Medical Center	Bradenton	91%	78
Lee Memorial Health System	Fort Myers	91%	238
Mease Hospital-Dunedin	Dunedin	91%	199
Munroe Regional Medical Center	Ocala	91%	454
North Bay Medical Center	New Port Richey	91%	196
Palm Beach Grdns Medical Center	Palm Beach Grdns	91%	672
Palm Springs General Hospital	Miami	91%	380
Saint Lucie Medical Center	Port Saint Lucie	91%	503
Santa Rosa Medical Center	Milton	91%	142
Sun Coast Hospital	Largo	91%	150
Cape Coral Hospital	Cape Coral	90%	143
Florida Hospital Flagler	Palm Coast	90%	241
Jay Hospital	Jay	90%	58
Jupiter Medical Center	Jupiter	90%	219
North Ridge Medical Center	Fort Lauderdale	90%	221
Coral Springs Medical Center	Coral Springs	89%	195
Holmes Regional Medical Center	Melbourne	89%	818
Larkin Community Hospital	South Miami	89%	73
NCH Downtown Naples Hospital	Naples	89%	1121
North Broward Medical Center	Deerfield Beach	89%	257
University Hospital & Medical Center	Tamarac	89%	318
Gulf Breeze Hospital	Gulf Breeze	88%	110
Lake Wales Medical Center	Lake Wales	88%	214
North Florida Regional Medical Center	Gainesville	88%	573
Saint Cloud Regional Medical Center	Saint Cloud	88%	80
Shands at Lake Shore	Lake City	88%	166
Villages Regional Hospital	The Villages	88%	279
Boca Raton Community Hospital	Boca Raton	87%	614
Florida Medical Center	Lauderdale Lakes	87%	528
Jackson Hospital	Marianna	87%	167
Saint Anthony's Hospital	Saint Petersburg	87%	281
Southwest Florida Regional Medical Center	Fort Myers	87%	531
University Community Hospital of Carrollwood	Tampa	87%	120

NOTE: Hospital profiles are in alphabetical order by state, then city, then hospital within the city; Rankings are sorted by rate in descending order and exclude hospitals with less than 25 cases; (1) The number of cases is too small (n<25) for purposes of reliably predicting hospital performance; (2) Measure reflects the hospital's indication that its submission was based upon a sample of its relevant discharges; (3) Rate reflects fewer than the maximum possible quarters of data for the measure; (4) Inaccurate information submitted and suppressed for one or more quarters; (5) No data is available from the hospital for this measure; Please refer to the User's Guide for a full explanation of data

Hospital Name	City	Rate	Cases
Baptist Hospital	Pensacola	86%	400
Bay Medical Center	Panama City	86%	1003
Citrus Memorial Hospital	Inverness	86%	297
Edward White Hospital	Saint Petersburg	86%	148
Imperial Point Medical Center	Fort Lauderdale	86%	139
Palms of Pasadena Hospital	Saint Petersburg	86%	176
Plantation General Hospital	Plantation	86%	153
Florida Hospital Zephyrhills	Zephyrhills	85%	349
Community Hospital	New Port Richey	84%	494
Fawcett Memorial Hospital	Port Charlotte	84%	312
Gulf Coast Medical Center	Panama City	84%	132
Highlands Regional Medical Center	Sebring	83%	208
Bert Fish Medical Center	New Smyrna Beach	82%	181
Heart of Florida Regional Medical Center	Davenport	82%	439
Wellington Regional Medical Center	Wellington	81%	200
Englewood Community Hospital	Englewood	80%	169
Indian River Memorial Hospital	Vero Beach	80%	458
Oak Hill Hospital	Brooksville	80%	418
Nature Coast Regional Hospital	Williston	78%	41
Columbia Hospital	West Palm Beach	75%	275
Westchester General Hospital	Miami	72%	47
Hendry Regional Medical Center	Clewiston	70%	30
Bartow Regional Medical Center	Bartow	69%	159
Raulerson Hospital	Okeechobee	67%	258
Doctors Memorial Hospital	Perry	66%	74
Gulf Coast Hospital	Fort Meyers	60%	25
Northwest Florida Community Hospital	Chipley	60%	40
Shands Live Oak	Live Oak	59%	61
DeSoto Memorial Hospital	Arcadia	56%	89
Sebastian River Medical Center	Sebastian	47%	153
Healthmark Regional Medical Center	Defuniak Springs	33%	30
Trinity Community Hospital	Jasper	30%	44
Doctors Memorial Hospital	Bonifay	22%	74

12. Smoking Cessation Advice

Hospital Name	City	Rate	Cases
Aventura Hospital and Medical Center	Aventura	100%	42
Coral Gables Hospital	Miami	100%	27
Florida Hospital DeLand	Deland	100%	59
Florida Medical Center	Lauderdale Lakes	100%	35
Fort Walton Beach Medical Center	Fort Walton Beach	100%	55
Good Samaritan Medical Center	West Palm Beach	100%	27
Halifax Medical Center	Daytona Beach	100%	201
Hialeah Hospital	Miami	100%	66
Holy Cross Hospital	Fort Lauderdale	100%	57
Homestead Hospital	Homestead	100%	84
Imperial Point Medical Center	Fort Lauderdale	100%	38
Kendall Medical Center	Miami	100%	65
Largo Medical Center	Largo	100%	59
Martin Memorial Medical Center	Stuart	100%	34
Mease Hospital-Dunedin	Dunedin	100%	25
Memorial Hospital Pembroke	Pembroke Pines	100%	46
Memorial Hospital West	Pembroke Pines	100%	52
Memorial Regional Hospital	Hollywood	100%	208
Mercy Hospital	Miami	100%	75
Morton Plant Hospital	Clearwater	100%	93
North Broward Medical Center	Deerfield Beach	100%	45
North Shore Medical Center	Miami	100%	124
Northwest Medical Center	Margate	100%	37
Osceola Regional Medical Center	Kissimmee	100%	44
Palmetto General Hospital	Hialeah	100%	71
Parrish Medical Center	Titusville	100%	39
Putnam Community Medical Center	Palatka	100%	66
Raulerson Hospital	Okeechobee	100%	58
Saint Anthony's Hospital	Saint Petersburg	100%	69
Saint Joseph's Hospital	Tampa	100%	171
Saint Luke's Hospital	Jacksonville	100%	42
Saint Vincent's Medical Center	Jacksonville	100%	42
Seven Rivers Regional Medical Center	Crystal River	100%	53
South Florida Baptist Hospital	Plant City	100%	43
Tallahassee Memorial Health Care Foundation	Tallahassee	100%	88
University Community Hospital	Tampa	100%	68
Venice Regional Medical Center	Venice	100%	43
Wuesthoff Health Systems	Rockledge	100%	108
Wuesthoff Medical Center-Melbourne	Melbourne	100%	25
Baptist Hospital	Miami	99%	85
Brooksville Regional Hospital	Brooksville	99%	86
Broward General Medical Center	Fort Lauderdale	99%	76
Charlotte Regional Medical Center	Punta Gorda	99%	70
Community Hospital	New Port Richey	99%	72
Florida Hospital Orlando	Orlando	99%	342
JFK Medical Center	Atlantis	99%	170
Lawnwood Regional Med Ctr & Heart Inst	Fort Pierce	99%	135
Leesburg Regional Medical Center	Leesburg	99%	73

Hospital Name	City	Rate	Cases
Palm Beach Grdns Medical Center	Palm Beach Grdns	99%	90
Saint Lucie Medical Center	Port Saint Lucie	99%	68
Tampa General Healthcare	Tampa	99%	154
Blake Medical Center	Bradenton	98%	47
Cape Canaveral Hospital	Cocoa Beach	98%	45
Mease Hospital-Countryside	Safety Harbor	98%	47
North Florida Regional Medical Center	Gainesville	98%	82
Sacred Heart Health System	Pensacola	98%	102
South Miami Hospital	Miami	98%	41
Westside Regional Medical Center	Plantation	98%	48
Columbia Memorial Hospital of Jacksonville	Jacksonville	97%	128
Fawcett Memorial Hospital	Port Charlotte	97%	38
Florida Hospital Flagler	Palm Coast	97%	36
Florida Hospital-Ormond Memorial	Ormond Beach	97%	77
NCH Downtown Naples Hospital	Naples	97%	122
Northside Hospital	Saint Petersburg	97%	60
Southwest Florida Regional Medical Center	Fort Myers	97%	87
Winter Haven Hospital	Winter Haven	97%	72
Doctors Hospital of Sarasota	Sarasota	96%	25
Glades General Hospital	Belle Glade	96%	26
Pan American Hospital	Miami	96%	28
Saint Mary's Medical Center	West Palm Beach	96%	46
Shands Jacksonville	Jacksonville	96%	83
University Hospital & Medical Center	Tamarac	96%	26
West Florida Regional Medical Center	Pensacola	96%	54
Lee Memorial Health System	Fort Myers	95%	42
Pasco Regional Medical Center	Dade City	95%	37
South Bay Hospital	Sun City Center	95%	41
Bayfront Medical Center	Saint Petersburg	94%	94
Jackson Hospital	Marianna	94%	31
Lake City Medical Center	Lake City	94%	32
Manatee Memorial Hospital	Bradenton	94%	144
Santa Rosa Medical Center	Milton	94%	48
Sarasota Memorial Health Care Systems	Sarasota	94%	68
South Lake Hospital	Clermont	94%	34
Baptist Hospital	Pensacola	93%	108
Brandon Regional Hospital	Brandon	93%	71
Florida Hospital Fish Memorial	Orange City	93%	58
Holmes Regional Medical Center	Melbourne	93%	132
North Bay Medical Center	New Port Richey	93%	30
Oak Hill Hospital	Brooksville	93%	61
Ocala Regional Medical Center	Ocala	93%	85
Orange Park Medical Center	Orange Park	93%	75
Central Florida Regional Hospital	Sanford	92%	97
Orlando Regional Healthcare	Orlando	92%	334
Bay Medical Center	Panama City	91%	238
Florida Hospital Heartland Medical Center	Sebring	91%	87
Mount Sinai Medical Center	Miami	91%	35
Regional Medical Center Bayonet Point	Hudson	91%	115
Sebastian River Medical Center	Sebastian	91%	32
Citrus Memorial Hospital	Inverness	90%	41
Baptist Medical Center Beaches	Jacksonville Bch	89%	27
North Okaloosa Medical Center	Crestview	89%	35
Plantation General Hospital	Plantation	89%	37
Florida Hospital Waterman	Tavares	87%	67
Shands at the University of Florida	Gainesville	87%	122
Capital Regional Medical Center	Tallahassee	86%	73
Flagler Hospital	Saint Augustine	86%	78
Lakeland Regional Medical Center	Lakeland	86%	49
Saint Petersburg General Hospital	Saint Petersburg	86%	28
Villages Regional Hospital	The Villages	86%	35
Boca Raton Community Hospital	Boca Raton	85%	26
Cedars Medical Center	Miami	85%	199
Health Central	Ocoee	85%	53
Palm Springs General Hospital	Miami	85%	26
Wellington Regional Medical Center	Wellington	85%	33
Heart of Florida Regional Medical Center	Davenport	84%	56
Munroe Regional Medical Center	Ocala	82%	73
Palms West Hospital	Loxahatchee	82%	34
Baptist Medical Center	Jacksonville	81%	149
Bartow Regional Medical Center	Bartow	77%	35
Shands at Lake Shore	Lake City	74%	35
Jackson Memorial Hospital	Miami	73%	137
Columbia Hospital	West Palm Beach	71%	42
Helen Ellis Memorial Hospital	Tarpon Springs	63%	43
Florida Hospital Zephyrhills	Zephyrhills	49%	53
Lehigh Regional Medical Center	Lehigh Acres	48%	33
Lake Wales Medical Center	Lake Wales	23%	35

Pneumonia Care

13. Appropriate Initial Antibiotic

Hospital Name	City	Rate	Cases
Homestead Hospital	Homestead	98%	241

NOTE: Hospital profiles are in alphabetical order by state, then city, then hospital within the city; Rankings are sorted by rate in descending order and exclude hospitals with less than 25 cases; (1) The number of cases is too small (n<25) for purposes of reliably predicting hospital performance; (2) Measure reflects the hospital's indication that its submission was based upon a sample of its relevant discharges; (3) Rate reflects fewer than the maximum possible quarters of data for the measure; (4) Inaccurate information submitted and suppressed for one or more quarters; (5) No data is available from the hospital for this measure; Please refer to the User's Guide for a full explanation of data

Hospital Name	City	Rate	Cases
Memorial Regional Hospital	Hollywood	97%	305
Baptist Hospital	Miami	95%	421
Bayfront Medical Center	Saint Petersburg	95%	166
Cleveland Clinic Florida	Weston	95%	83
Memorial Hospital West	Pembroke Pines	95%	320
Mercy Hospital	Miami	95%	202
Jackson Memorial Hospital	Miami	94%	200
North Shore Medical Center	Miami	94%	187
South Miami Hospital	Miami	94%	288
Delray Medical Center	Delray Beach	93%	257
Saint Mary's Medical Center	West Palm Beach	93%	165
DeSoto Memorial Hospital	Arcadia	92%	61
Florida Hospital DeLand	Deland	92%	225
Gulf Breeze Hospital	Gulf Breeze	92%	114
Kendall Medical Center	Miami	91%	464
North Florida Regional Medical Center	Gainesville	91%	204
South Lake Hospital	Clermont	91%	92
Venice Regional Medical Center	Venice	91%	164
Community Hospital	New Port Richey	90%	167
Florida Hospital Heartland Medical Center	Sebring	90%	193
Florida Hospital Orlando	Orlando	90%	929
Florida Hospital-Ormond Memorial	Ormond Beach	90%	154
Halifax Medical Center	Daytona Beach	90%	381
Lawnwood Regional Med Ctr & Heart Inst	Fort Pierce	90%	219
Mariners Hospital	Tavernier	90%	60
Memorial Hospital Pembroke	Pembroke Pines	90%	263
Morton Plant Hospital	Clearwater	90%	262
Mount Sinai Medical Center	Miami	90%	128
North Ridge Medical Center	Fort Lauderdale	90%	50
Ocala Regional Medical Center	Ocala	90%	294
Orange Park Medical Center	Orange Park	90%	303
Putnam Community Medical Center	Palatka	90%	185
Saint Luke's Hospital	Jacksonville	90%	87
Wellington Regional Medical Center	Wellington	90%	124
Baptist Hospital	Pensacola	89%	238
Baptist Medical Center Nassau	Fernandina Bch	89%	97
Cape Canaveral Hospital	Cocoa Beach	89%	192
Good Samaritan Medical Center	West Palm Beach	89%	217
Leesburg Regional Medical Center	Leesburg	89%	210
Memorial Hospital Miramar	Miramar	89%	134
Orlando Regional Healthcare	Orlando	89%	664
University Community Hospital of Carrollwood	Tampa	89%	146
University Hospital & Medical Center	Tamarac	89%	143
Bethesda Memorial Hospital	Boynton Beach	88%	139
Boca Raton Community Hospital	Boca Raton	88%	289
Broward General Medical Center	Fort Lauderdale	88%	113
Columbia Memorial Hospital of Jacksonville	Jacksonville	88%	301
Edward White Hospital	Saint Petersburg	88%	92
Florida Hospital Fish Memorial	Orange City	88%	262
Lakeland Regional Medical Center	Lakeland	88%	163
Memorial Hospital of Tampa	Tampa	88%	139
NCH Downtown Naples Hospital	Naples	88%	496
Northwest Medical Center	Margate	88%	194
Saint Anthony's Hospital	Saint Petersburg	88%	188
Southwest Florida Regional Medical Center	Fort Myers	88%	262
Villages Regional Hospital	The Villages	88%	202
West Boca Medical Center	Boca Raton	88%	192
Blake Medical Center	Bradenton	87%	217
Central Florida Regional Hospital	Sanford	87%	149
Coral Gables Hospital	Miami	87%	223
Doctors Hospital of Sarasota	Sarasota	87%	122
HealthSouth Doctors' Hospital	Miami	87%	167
Martin Memorial Medical Center	Stuart	87%	82
Palm Beach Grdns Medical Center	Palm Beach Grdns	87%	143
Palmetto General Hospital	Hialeah	87%	244
Palms of Pasadena Hospital	Saint Petersburg	87%	136
Parrish Medical Center	Titusville	87%	130
Saint Joseph's Hospital	Tampa	87%	252
Shands Live Oak	Live Oak	87%	39
Tallahassee Memorial Health Care Foundation	Tallahassee	87%	173
Florida Hospital Zephyrhills	Zephyrhills	86%	176
Munroe Regional Medical Center	Ocala	86%	176
North Broward Medical Center	Deerfield Beach	86%	123
North Okaloosa Medical Center	Crestview	86%	110
Plantation General Hospital	Plantation	86%	84
Regional Medical Center Bayonet Point	Hudson	86%	125
Saint Lucie Medical Center	Port Saint Lucie	86%	243
South Florida Baptist Hospital	Plant City	86%	132
Tampa General Healthcare	Tampa	86%	145
University Community Hospital	Tampa	86%	180
Winter Haven Hospital	Winter Haven	86%	367
Brooksville Regional Hospital	Brooksville	85%	227
Charlotte Regional Medical Center	Punta Gorda	85%	127
Heart of Florida Regional Medical Center	Davenport	85%	173
Holmes Regional Medical Center	Melbourne	85%	388
Holy Cross Hospital	Fort Lauderdale	85%	172
Imperial Point Medical Center	Fort Lauderdale	85%	94
Jupiter Medical Center	Jupiter	85%	116
Manatee Memorial Hospital	Bradenton	85%	215
Mease Hospital-Countryside	Safety Harbor	85%	265
Mease Hospital-Dunedin	Dunedin	85%	107
Northwest Florida Community Hospital	Chipley	85%	33
Sun Coast Hospital	Largo	85%	116
Baptist Medical Center Beaches	Jacksonville Bch	84%	202
Helen Ellis Memorial Hospital	Tarpon Springs	84%	108
Hialeah Hospital	Miami	84%	279
Lakewood Ranch Medical Center	Bradenton	84%	93
Saint Petersburg General Hospital	Saint Petersburg	84%	136
West Florida Regional Medical Center	Pensacola	84%	146
Wuesthoff Health Systems	Rockledge	84%	185
Cape Coral Hospital	Cape Coral	83%	92
Citrus Memorial Hospital	Inverness	83%	139
Coral Springs Medical Center	Coral Springs	83%	116
Florida Medical Center	Lauderdale Lakes	83%	90
Westside Regional Medical Center	Plantation	83%	186
Cedars Medical Center	Miami	82%	170
Columbia Hospital	West Palm Beach	82%	62
Glades General Hospital	Belle Glade	82%	50
Health Central	Ocoee	82%	114
Lake Wales Medical Center	Lake Wales	82%	94
Largo Medical Center	Largo	82%	211
Lee Memorial Health System	Fort Myers	82%	105
Sarasota Memorial Health Care Systems	Sarasota	82%	221
Seven Rivers Regional Medical Center	Crystal River	82%	154
Shands at Starke	Starke	82%	39
Westchester General Hospital	Miami	82%	65
Aventura Hospital and Medical Center	Aventura	81%	225
Bay Medical Center	Panama City	81%	344
Flagler Hospital	Saint Augustine	81%	160
North Bay Medical Center	New Port Richey	81%	99
Northside Hospital	Saint Petersburg	81%	275
Palms West Hospital	Loxahatchee	81%	137
Shands at the University of Florida	Gainesville	81%	160
Twin Cities Hospital	Niceville	81%	58
Baptist Medical Center	Jacksonville	80%	301
Bert Fish Medical Center	New Smyrna Beach	80%	127
Brandon Regional Hospital	Brandon	80%	319
Capital Regional Medical Center	Tallahassee	80%	86
Fawcett Memorial Hospital	Port Charlotte	80%	121
JFK Medical Center	Atlantis	80%	351
Lehigh Regional Medical Center	Lehigh Acres	80%	172
Sacred Heart Hospital on the Emerald Coast	Destin	80%	55
Town and Country Hospital	Tampa	80%	112
Fishermen's Hospital	Marathon	79%	28
Fort Walton Beach Medical Center	Fort Walton Beach	79%	156
Indian River Memorial Hospital	Vero Beach	79%	42
Oak Hill Hospital	Brooksville	79%	237
Osceola Regional Medical Center	Kissimmee	79%	298
Peace River Regional Medical Center	Port Charlotte	79%	160
Saint Vincent's Medical Center	Jacksonville	79%	117
Shands Jacksonville	Jacksonville	79%	96
South Bay Hospital	Sun City Center	79%	174
Gulf Coast Medical Center	Panama City	78%	181
Florida Hospital Waterman	Tavares	77%	180
Santa Rosa Medical Center	Milton	77%	137
Sebastian River Medical Center	Sebastian	77%	187
Pasco Regional Medical Center	Dade City	76%	131
Larkin Community Hospital	South Miami	75%	65
Florida Hospital Flagler	Palm Coast	74%	92
Jackson Hospital	Marianna	74%	91
Wuesthoff Medical Center-Melbourne	Melbourne	74%	85
Gulf Coast Hospital	Fort Myers	73%	59
Raulerson Hospital	Okeechobee	72%	149
Englewood Community Hospital	Englewood	71%	92
Highlands Regional Medical Center	Sebring	71%	150
Shands at Lake Shore	Lake City	70%	97
Lake City Medical Center	Lake City	69%	177
Doctors Memorial Hospital	Bonifay	67%	60
Palm Springs General Hospital	Miami	67%	247
Pan American Hospital	Miami	65%	223
Sacred Heart Health System	Pensacola	64%	219
Jay Hospital	Jay	61%	49
Bartow Regional Medical Center	Bartow	58%	108
Lower Keys Medical Center	Key West	50%	98

14. Blood Culture Timing

Hospital Name	City	Rate	Cases
Delray Medical Center	Delray Beach	100%	211
Seven Rivers Regional Medical Center	Crystal River	100%	115

NOTE: Hospital profiles are in alphabetical order by state, then city, then hospital within the city; Rankings are sorted by rate in descending order and exclude hospitals with less than 25 cases; (1) The number of cases is too small (n<25) for purposes of reliably predicting hospital performance; (2) Measure reflects the hospital's indication that its submission was based upon a sample of its relevant discharges; (3) Rate reflects fewer than the maximum possible quarters of data for the measure; (4) Inaccurate information submitted and suppressed for one or more quarters; (5) No data is available from the hospital for this measure; Please refer to the User's Guide for a full explanation of data

Memorial Hospital Miramar	Miramar	98%	125		Florida Hospital Waterman	Tavares	88%	206
Memorial Hospital Pembroke	Pembroke Pines	98%	286		Largo Medical Center	Largo	88%	171
South Miami Hospital	Miami	98%	341		Raulerson Hospital	Okeechobee	88%	102
Lake Wales Medical Center	Lake Wales	97%	77		Bethesda Memorial Hospital	Boynton Beach	87%	134
Lakeland Regional Medical Center	Lakeland	97%	169		Doctors Hospital of Sarasota	Sarasota	87%	103
Santa Rosa Medical Center	Milton	97%	131		Florida Hospital Heartland Medical Center	Sebring	87%	137
West Florida Regional Medical Center	Pensacola	97%	139		Holy Cross Hospital	Fort Lauderdale	87%	182
Cleveland Clinic Florida	Weston	96%	90		Indian River Memorial Hospital	Vero Beach	87%	38
Jay Hospital	Jay	96%	28		Jupiter Medical Center	Jupiter	87%	103
Pan American Hospital	Miami	96%	162		Sacred Heart Hospital on the Emerald Coast	Destin	87%	38
Cape Canaveral Hospital	Cocoa Beach	95%	203		Saint Luke's Hospital	Jacksonville	87%	106
Charlotte Regional Medical Center	Punta Gorda	95%	137		Sarasota Memorial Health Care Systems	Sarasota	87%	222
Columbia Hospital	West Palm Beach	95%	80		Shands at the University of Florida	Gainesville	87%	166
Florida Hospital DeLand	Deland	95%	251		South Lake Hospital	Clermont	87%	92
Good Samaritan Medical Center	West Palm Beach	95%	221		Wellington Regional Medical Center	Wellington	87%	143
Homestead Hospital	Homestead	95%	249		Aventura Hospital and Medical Center	Aventura	86%	290
Mease Hospital-Countryside	Safety Harbor	95%	286		Bayfront Medical Center	Saint Petersburg	86%	162
Mease Hospital-Dunedin	Dunedin	95%	109		Boca Raton Community Hospital	Boca Raton	86%	239
Memorial Regional Hospital	Hollywood	95%	359		Flagler Hospital	Saint Augustine	86%	115
Morton Plant Hospital	Clearwater	95%	239		Imperial Point Medical Center	Fort Lauderdale	86%	97
Palm Springs General Hospital	Miami	95%	189		Jackson Hospital	Marianna	86%	56
Saint Mary's Medical Center	West Palm Beach	95%	207		Oak Hill Hospital	Brooksville	86%	149
Hialeah Hospital	Miami	94%	281		Southwest Florida Regional Medical Center	Fort Myers	86%	285
Kendall Medical Center	Miami	94%	424		Sun Coast Hospital	Largo	86%	118
Lawnwood Regional Med Ctr & Heart Inst	Fort Pierce	94%	288		University Hospital & Medical Center	Tamarac	86%	137
Mariners Hospital	Tavernier	94%	47		Baptist Medical Center	Jacksonville	85%	324
Memorial Hospital of Tampa	Tampa	94%	144		Bartow Regional Medical Center	Bartow	85%	73
Mercy Hospital	Miami	94%	234		Florida Hospital Orlando	Orlando	85%	951
Northside Hospital	Saint Petersburg	94%	222		Glades General Hospital	Belle Glade	85%	55
Pasco Regional Medical Center	Dade City	94%	125		Lakewood Ranch Medical Center	Bradenton	85%	82
Putnam Community Medical Center	Palatka	94%	141		Manatee Memorial Hospital	Bradenton	85%	153
Sacred Heart Health System	Pensacola	94%	131		Martin Memorial Medical Center	Stuart	85%	105
South Florida Baptist Hospital	Plant City	94%	178		Mount Sinai Medical Center	Miami	85%	153
Brooksville Regional Hospital	Brooksville	93%	185		NCH Downtown Naples Hospital	Naples	85%	384
Highlands Regional Medical Center	Sebring	93%	123		Orlando Regional Healthcare	Orlando	85%	564
Holmes Regional Medical Center	Melbourne	93%	403		Shands Live Oak	Live Oak	85%	26
Lee Memorial Health System	Fort Myers	93%	116		Capital Regional Medical Center	Tallahassee	84%	86
Venice Regional Medical Center	Venice	93%	176		Florida Hospital Flagler	Palm Coast	84%	85
Winter Haven Hospital	Winter Haven	93%	379		Health Central	Ocoee	84%	101
Wuesthoff Medical Center-Melbourne	Melbourne	93%	58		Heart of Florida Regional Medical Center	Davenport	84%	105
Baptist Medical Center Beaches	Jacksonville Bch	92%	170		Leesburg Regional Medical Center	Leesburg	84%	251
Baptist Medical Center Nassau	Fernandina Bch	92%	105		North Shore Medical Center	Miami	84%	211
Coral Gables Hospital	Miami	92%	197		Tallahassee Memorial Health Care Foundation	Tallahassee	84%	152
Lake City Medical Center	Lake City	92%	80		University Community Hospital	Tampa	84%	150
Lehigh Regional Medical Center	Lehigh Acres	92%	74		Villages Regional Hospital	The Villages	84%	180
North Bay Medical Center	New Port Richey	92%	92		Englewood Community Hospital	Englewood	83%	58
Orange Park Medical Center	Orange Park	92%	447		Plantation General Hospital	Plantation	83%	102
Saint Anthony's Hospital	Saint Petersburg	92%	200		Saint Petersburg General Hospital	Saint Petersburg	83%	149
West Boca Medical Center	Boca Raton	92%	171		Baptist Hospital	Pensacola	82%	217
Wuesthoff Health Systems	Rockledge	92%	189		Ocala Regional Medical Center	Ocala	82%	211
Baptist Hospital	Miami	91%	459		Palms West Hospital	Loxahatchee	82%	80
DeSoto Memorial Hospital	Arcadia	91%	45		Bert Fish Medical Center	New Smyrna Beach	80%	86
Edward White Hospital	Saint Petersburg	91%	112		Central Florida Regional Hospital	Sanford	80%	104
Fawcett Memorial Hospital	Port Charlotte	91%	105		Community Hospital	New Port Richey	80%	117
Florida Hospital-Ormond Memorial	Ormond Beach	91%	138		Osceola Regional Medical Center	Kissimmee	80%	202
Florida Medical Center	Lauderdale Lakes	91%	89		Florida Hospital Zephyrhills	Zephyrhills	79%	101
Gulf Breeze Hospital	Gulf Breeze	91%	76		Sebastian River Medical Center	Sebastian	79%	121
Lower Keys Medical Center	Key West	91%	93		University Community Hospital of Carrollwood	Tampa	79%	99
Memorial Hospital West	Pembroke Pines	91%	341		Bay Medical Center	Panama City	78%	294
North Ridge Medical Center	Fort Lauderdale	91%	44		Brandon Regional Hospital	Brandon	78%	161
Peace River Regional Medical Center	Port Charlotte	91%	129		JFK Medical Center	Atlantis	78%	379
South Bay Hospital	Sun City Center	91%	170		Palmetto General Hospital	Hialeah	77%	213
Twin Cities Hospital	Niceville	91%	34		North Florida Regional Medical Center	Gainesville	76%	203
Blake Medical Center	Bradenton	90%	159		Cedars Medical Center	Miami	75%	195
Cape Coral Hospital	Cape Coral	90%	97		Gulf Coast Medical Center	Panama City	73%	83
Citrus Memorial Hospital	Inverness	90%	123		Shands Jacksonville	Jacksonville	71%	113
Columbia Memorial Hospital of Jacksonville	Jacksonville	90%	346		Westchester General Hospital	Miami	71%	41
Gulf Coast Hospital	Fort Meyers	90%	49		North Okaloosa Medical Center	Crestview	70%	64
HealthSouth Doctors' Hospital	Miami	90%	165		Saint Joseph's Hospital	Tampa	70%	290
Larkin Community Hospital	South Miami	90%	83		Town and Country Hospital	Tampa	70%	88
North Broward Medical Center	Deerfield Beach	90%	96		Palms of Pasadena Hospital	Saint Petersburg	69%	150
Northwest Medical Center	Margate	90%	156		Halifax Medical Center	Daytona Beach	68%	285
Palm Beach Grdns Medical Center	Palm Beach Grdns	90%	126		Jackson Memorial Hospital	Miami	68%	182
Parrish Medical Center	Titusville	90%	132		Regional Medical Center Bayonet Point	Hudson	68%	84
Saint Vincent's Medical Center	Jacksonville	90%	117					
Westside Regional Medical Center	Plantation	90%	166					

15. Influenza Vaccine

Hospital Name	City	Rate	Cases
Broward General Medical Center	Fort Lauderdale	89%	133
Coral Springs Medical Center	Coral Springs	89%	115
Florida Hospital Fish Memorial	Orange City	89%	228
Fort Walton Beach Medical Center	Fort Walton Beach	89%	132
Helen Ellis Memorial Hospital	Tarpon Springs	89%	73
Munroe Regional Medical Center	Ocala	89%	135
Saint Lucie Medical Center	Port Saint Lucie	89%	206
Shands at Lake Shore	Lake City	89%	47
Tampa General Healthcare	Tampa	89%	181

Hospital Name	City	Rate	Cases
Holy Cross Hospital	Fort Lauderdale	100%	55
Memorial Hospital Miramar	Miramar	100%	26
South Miami Hospital	Miami	100%	106
Good Samaritan Medical Center	West Palm Beach	98%	63
Cape Canaveral Hospital	Cocoa Beach	96%	57
Cleveland Clinic Florida	Weston	96%	28
HealthSouth Doctors' Hospital	Miami	96%	57

NOTE: Hospital profiles are in alphabetical order by state, then city, then hospital within the city; Rankings are sorted by rate in descending order and exclude hospitals with less than 25 cases; (1) The number of cases is too small (n<25) for purposes of reliably predicting hospital performance; (2) Measure reflects the hospital's indication that its submission was based upon a sample of its relevant discharges; (3) Rate reflects fewer than the maximum possible quarters of data for the measure; (4) Inaccurate information submitted and suppressed for one or more quarters; (5) No data is available from the hospital for this measure; Please refer to the User's Guide for a full explanation of data

Hospital Name	City	Rate	Cases
Memorial Hospital Pembroke	Pembroke Pines	96%	73
Hialeah Hospital	Miami	95%	77
Lawnwood Regional Med Ctr & Heart Inst	Fort Pierce	95%	80
Memorial Regional Hospital	Hollywood	95%	65
Memorial Hospital West	Pembroke Pines	94%	81
Wuesthoff Health Systems	Rockledge	94%	52
Putnam Community Medical Center	Palatka	92%	60
Saint Mary's Medical Center	West Palm Beach	92%	40
Peace River Regional Medical Center	Port Charlotte	90%	41
Pan American Hospital	Miami	89%	44
North Shore Medical Center	Miami	86%	36
Baptist Hospital	Miami	85%	120
Bethesda Memorial Hospital	Boynton Beach	85%	41
Pasco Regional Medical Center	Dade City	85%	55
Santa Rosa Medical Center	Milton	85%	46
Munroe Regional Medical Center	Ocala	84%	55
Ocala Regional Medical Center	Ocala	84%	92
Venice Regional Medical Center	Venice	84%	75
Homestead Hospital	Homestead	83%	52
Lee Memorial Health System	Fort Myers	81%	31
Coral Springs Medical Center	Coral Springs	80%	25
Tallahassee Memorial Health Care Foundation	Tallahassee	80%	46
West Boca Medical Center	Boca Raton	80%	44
Brooksville Regional Hospital	Brooksville	79%	66
Florida Hospital Waterman	Tavares	79%	66
Villages Regional Hospital	The Villages	79%	71
Winter Haven Hospital	Winter Haven	79%	141
Palm Beach Grdns Medical Center	Palm Beach Grdns	78%	40
West Florida Regional Medical Center	Pensacola	78%	46
Saint Luke's Hospital	Jacksonville	77%	26
Larkin Community Hospital	South Miami	76%	29
Saint Joseph's Hospital	Tampa	76%	95
Memorial Hospital of Tampa	Tampa	75%	32
Orlando Regional Healthcare	Orlando	75%	224
Sebastian River Medical Center	Sebastian	75%	60
Florida Hospital Heartland Medical Center	Sebring	74%	57
Mease Hospital-Countryside	Safety Harbor	74%	91
Florida Medical Center	Lauderdale Lakes	73%	30
Morton Plant Hospital	Clearwater	73%	89
Raulerson Hospital	Okeechobee	73%	49
Baptist Medical Center Nassau	Fernandina Bch	72%	25
Baptist Hospital	Pensacola	71%	73
Doctors Hospital of Sarasota	Sarasota	70%	53
Northwest Medical Center	Margate	70%	53
University Hospital & Medical Center	Tamarac	70%	50
Seven Rivers Regional Medical Center	Crystal River	69%	42
Bert Fish Medical Center	New Smyrna Beach	68%	34
Lakeland Regional Medical Center	Lakeland	68%	41
Sarasota Memorial Health Care Systems	Sarasota	67%	57
Westside Regional Medical Center	Plantation	67%	49
Heart of Florida Regional Medical Center	Davenport	66%	47
Sacred Heart Health System	Pensacola	66%	41
Fort Walton Beach Medical Center	Fort Walton Beach	65%	40
JFK Medical Center	Atlantis	65%	129
Palmetto General Hospital	Hialeah	65%	40
Manatee Memorial Hospital	Bradenton	64%	50
North Florida Regional Medical Center	Gainesville	64%	76
Palms West Hospital	Loxahatchee	62%	32
Saint Anthony's Hospital	Saint Petersburg	62%	58
South Florida Baptist Hospital	Plant City	62%	45
Wellington Regional Medical Center	Wellington	62%	37
Largo Medical Center	Largo	61%	82
South Bay Hospital	Sun City Center	60%	70
Tampa General Healthcare	Tampa	60%	55
Baptist Medical Center	Jacksonville	59%	99
Orange Park Medical Center	Orange Park	59%	118
Charlotte Regional Medical Center	Punta Gorda	58%	48
Saint Vincent's Medical Center	Jacksonville	58%	33
Holmes Regional Medical Center	Melbourne	57%	96
Parrish Medical Center	Titusville	57%	42
Blake Medical Center	Bradenton	56%	75
Englewood Community Hospital	Englewood	56%	27
Lake City Medical Center	Lake City	56%	52
Gulf Coast Medical Center	Panama City	55%	44
Saint Lucie Medical Center	Port Saint Lucie	55%	53
Fawcett Memorial Hospital	Port Charlotte	53%	38
Florida Hospital Fish Memorial	Orange City	53%	77
Lower Keys Medical Center	Key West	52%	25
Mease Hospital-Dunedin	Dunedin	52%	42
Baptist Medical Center Beaches	Jacksonville Bch	51%	55
Regional Medical Center Bayonet Point	Hudson	51%	47
Southwest Florida Regional Medical Center	Fort Myers	51%	110
Central Florida Regional Hospital	Sanford	49%	45
Osceola Regional Medical Center	Kissimmee	49%	79
Edward White Hospital	Saint Petersburg	47%	38
Highlands Regional Medical Center	Sebring	46%	56
Brandon Regional Hospital	Brandon	44%	61
Columbia Memorial Hospital of Jacksonville	Jacksonville	43%	74
Oak Hill Hospital	Brooksville	43%	68
Jupiter Medical Center	Jupiter	42%	31
Boca Raton Community Hospital	Boca Raton	41%	85
Jackson Memorial Hospital	Miami	41%	46
Kendall Medical Center	Miami	41%	116
Northside Hospital	Saint Petersburg	41%	73
Aventura Hospital and Medical Center	Aventura	40%	73
Mount Sinai Medical Center	Miami	40%	25
North Bay Medical Center	New Port Richey	40%	25
Saint Petersburg General Hospital	Saint Petersburg	40%	45
University Community Hospital	Tampa	36%	25
Shands at the University of Florida	Gainesville	34%	50
Community Hospital	New Port Richey	33%	61
Jackson Hospital	Marianna	32%	25
Florida Hospital Zephyrhills	Zephyrhills	29%	59
NCH Downtown Naples Hospital	Naples	28%	143
Cedars Medical Center	Miami	25%	59

16. Initial Antibiotic Timing

Hospital Name	City	Rate	Cases
Delray Medical Center	Delray Beach	95%	257
Sacred Heart Hospital on the Emerald Coast	Destin	94%	48
Mariners Hospital	Tavernier	93%	60
Memorial Hospital Miramar	Miramar	93%	150
Edward White Hospital	Saint Petersburg	92%	154
Memorial Hospital Pembroke	Pembroke Pines	92%	266
Venice Regional Medical Center	Venice	91%	263
North Ridge Medical Center	Fort Lauderdale	90%	71
South Miami Hospital	Miami	90%	372
West Boca Medical Center	Boca Raton	90%	234
Bayfront Medical Center	Saint Petersburg	89%	218
HealthSouth Doctors' Hospital	Miami	89%	174
Mercy Hospital	Miami	89%	295
Halifax Medical Center	Daytona Beach	88%	471
Mease Hospital-Dunedin	Dunedin	88%	115
Florida Hospital DeLand	Deland	87%	342
Memorial Hospital West	Pembroke Pines	87%	436
Bert Fish Medical Center	New Smyrna Beach	86%	170
Cleveland Clinic Florida	Weston	86%	84
Florida Hospital Flagler	Palm Coast	86%	113
Hialeah Hospital	Miami	86%	390
Holmes Regional Medical Center	Melbourne	86%	517
Imperial Point Medical Center	Fort Lauderdale	86%	125
Memorial Regional Hospital	Hollywood	85%	403
Sun Coast Hospital	Largo	85%	156
Good Samaritan Medical Center	West Palm Beach	84%	298
Pan American Hospital	Miami	84%	207
Physicians Regional Medical Center	Naples	84%	49
Saint Luke's Hospital	Jacksonville	84%	147
South Florida Baptist Hospital	Plant City	84%	166
Cape Coral Hospital	Cape Coral	83%	121
Columbia Hospital	West Palm Beach	83%	103
Florida Hospital Wauchula	Wauchula	83%	30
Florida Medical Center	Lauderdale Lakes	83%	125
Shands at Starke	Starke	83%	52
Wellington Regional Medical Center	Wellington	83%	163
Bethesda Memorial Hospital	Boynton Beach	82%	237
Coral Gables Hospital	Miami	82%	251
Glades General Hospital	Belle Glade	82%	55
Jay Hospital	Jay	82%	50
South Lake Hospital	Clermont	82%	110
Gulf Breeze Hospital	Gulf Breeze	81%	127
Holy Cross Hospital	Fort Lauderdale	81%	211
Lakewood Ranch Medical Center	Bradenton	81%	100
Lawnwood Regional Med Ctr & Heart Inst	Fort Pierce	81%	356
Pasco Regional Medical Center	Dade City	81%	141
Fawcett Memorial Hospital	Port Charlotte	80%	173
Homestead Hospital	Homestead	80%	298
Miami Jewish Home & Hosp for the Aged	Miami	80%	46
Northwest Florida Community Hospital	Chipley	80%	41
Shands Live Oak	Live Oak	80%	59
Baptist Medical Center Nassau	Fernandina Bch	79%	125
Boca Raton Community Hospital	Boca Raton	79%	304
Cape Canaveral Hospital	Cocoa Beach	79%	247
Doctors Memorial Hospital	Bonifay	79%	61
Doctors Memorial Hospital	Perry	79%	58
Fishermen's Hospital	Marathon	79%	29
Memorial Hospital of Tampa	Tampa	79%	203
Putnam Community Medical Center	Palatka	79%	275
Raulerson Hospital	Okeechobee	79%	189
Sarasota Memorial Health Care Systems	Sarasota	79%	320

NOTE: Hospital profiles are in alphabetical order by state, then city, then hospital within the city; Rankings are sorted by rate in descending order and exclude hospitals with less than 25 cases; (1) The number of cases is too small (n<25) for purposes of reliably predicting hospital performance; (2) Measure reflects the hospital's indication that its submission was based upon a sample of its relevant discharges; (3) Rate reflects fewer than the maximum possible quarters of data for the measure; (4) Inaccurate information submitted and suppressed for one or more quarters; (5) No data is available from the hospital for this measure; Please refer to the User's Guide for a full explanation of data

Hospital Name	City	Rate	Cases
Jackson Hospital	Marianna	78%	101
Martin Memorial Medical Center	Stuart	78%	153
Mease Hospital-Countryside	Safety Harbor	78%	281
North Bay Medical Center	New Port Richey	78%	103
Saint Mary's Medical Center	West Palm Beach	78%	287
Santa Rosa Medical Center	Milton	78%	151
Westside Regional Medical Center	Plantation	78%	249
Brooksville Regional Hospital	Brooksville	77%	284
Charlotte Regional Medical Center	Punta Gorda	77%	177
Florida Hospital Waterman	Tavares	77%	255
Jupiter Medical Center	Jupiter	77%	155
Palm Beach Grdns Medical Center	Palm Beach Grdns	77%	166
Saint Joseph's Hospital	Tampa	77%	391
Saint Petersburg General Hospital	Saint Petersburg	77%	228
Winter Haven Hospital	Winter Haven	77%	532
Community Hospital	New Port Richey	76%	245
Doctors Hospital of Sarasota	Sarasota	76%	193
Florida Hospital Orlando	Orlando	76%	1482
Florida Hospital-Ormond Memorial	Ormond Beach	76%	218
Kendall Medical Center	Miami	76%	619
University Hospital & Medical Center	Tamarac	76%	202
Citrus Memorial Hospital	Inverness	75%	178
Columbia Memorial Hospital of Jacksonville	Jacksonville	75%	416
Florida Hospital Zephyrhills	Zephyrhills	75%	174
Larkin Community Hospital	South Miami	75%	120
Lehigh Regional Medical Center	Lehigh Acres	75%	171
Orange Park Medical Center	Orange Park	75%	501
Palmetto General Hospital	Hialeah	75%	263
Saint Anthony's Hospital	Saint Petersburg	75%	219
Baptist Hospital	Pensacola	74%	318
Englewood Community Hospital	Englewood	74%	104
Lake Wales Medical Center	Lake Wales	74%	137
Parrish Medical Center	Titusville	74%	194
Seven Rivers Regional Medical Center	Crystal River	74%	149
Twin Cities Hospital	Niceville	74%	85
Bartow Regional Medical Center	Bartow	73%	122
Helen Ellis Memorial Hospital	Tarpon Springs	73%	139
Lee Memorial Health System	Fort Myers	73%	155
North Broward Medical Center	Deerfield Beach	73%	152
North Florida Regional Medical Center	Gainesville	73%	309
Palm Springs General Hospital	Miami	73%	292
Palms of Pasadena Hospital	Saint Petersburg	73%	199
Sebastian River Medical Center	Sebastian	73%	188
South Bay Hospital	Sun City Center	73%	238
Southwest Florida Regional Medical Center	Fort Myers	73%	437
Indian River Memorial Hospital	Vero Beach	72%	270
Lakeland Regional Medical Center	Lakeland	72%	240
NCH Downtown Naples Hospital	Naples	72%	527
North Okaloosa Medical Center	Crestview	72%	142
Bay Medical Center	Panama City	71%	475
Coral Springs Medical Center	Coral Springs	71%	133
Largo Medical Center	Largo	71%	303
Nature Coast Regional Hospital	Williston	71%	41
Saint Cloud Regional Medical Center	Saint Cloud	71%	84
Villages Regional Hospital	The Villages	71%	235
Wuesthoff Health Systems	Rockledge	71%	241
Baptist Medical Center Beaches	Jacksonville Bch	70%	261
DeSoto Memorial Hospital	Arcadia	70%	63
Lower Keys Medical Center	Key West	70%	105
Manatee Memorial Hospital	Bradenton	70%	264
Northwest Medical Center	Margate	70%	225
Town and Country Hospital	Tampa	70%	145
Broward General Medical Center	Fort Lauderdale	69%	183
Florida Hospital Heartland Medical Center	Sebring	69%	257
Fort Walton Beach Medical Center	Fort Walton Beach	69%	218
Ocala Regional Medical Center	Ocala	69%	401
Capital Regional Medical Center	Tallahassee	68%	139
Gulf Coast Hospital	Fort Meyers	68%	79
Plantation General Hospital	Plantation	68%	148
Flagler Hospital	Saint Augustine	67%	216
Peace River Regional Medical Center	Port Charlotte	67%	214
University Community Hospital of Carrollwood	Tampa	67%	172
Gulf Coast Medical Center	Panama City	66%	269
Saint Lucie Medical Center	Port Saint Lucie	66%	307
Wuesthoff Medical Center-Melbourne	Melbourne	66%	91
Morton Plant Hospital	Clearwater	65%	289
Mount Sinai Medical Center	Miami	65%	193
Northside Hospital	Saint Petersburg	65%	373
Orlando Regional Healthcare	Orlando	65%	956
West Florida Regional Medical Center	Pensacola	65%	202
Blake Medical Center	Bradenton	64%	272
Leesburg Regional Medical Center	Leesburg	64%	344
North Shore Medical Center	Miami	63%	262
Oak Hill Hospital	Brooksville	63%	321
Baptist Hospital	Miami	62%	535

Hospital Name	City	Rate	Cases
Lake City Medical Center	Lake City	62%	227
Regional Medical Center Bayonet Point	Hudson	62%	185
Tallahassee Memorial Health Care Foundation	Tallahassee	62%	226
Westchester General Hospital	Miami	62%	71
Baptist Medical Center	Jacksonville	61%	468
Shands at Lake Shore	Lake City	61%	102
University Community Hospital	Tampa	61%	236
Healthmark Regional Medical Center	Defuniak Springs	60%	40
Highlands Regional Medical Center	Sebring	60%	183
Heart of Florida Regional Medical Center	Davenport	59%	211
Munroe Regional Medical Center	Ocala	59%	245
Florida Hospital Fish Memorial	Orange City	58%	349
Sacred Heart Health System	Pensacola	58%	228
Saint Vincent's Medical Center	Jacksonville	57%	175
Central Florida Regional Hospital	Sanford	56%	217
JFK Medical Center	Atlantis	56%	547
Shands at the University of Florida	Gainesville	55%	238
Cedars Medical Center	Miami	54%	314
Health Central	Ocoee	53%	187
Osceola Regional Medical Center	Kissimmee	53%	342
Shands Jacksonville	Jacksonville	52%	162
Jackson Memorial Hospital	Miami	51%	326
Brandon Regional Hospital	Brandon	49%	388
Aventura Hospital and Medical Center	Aventura	48%	370
Tampa General Healthcare	Tampa	48%	255
Palms West Hospital	Loxahatchee	46%	140

17. Oxygenation Assessment

Hospital Name	City	Rate	Cases
Baptist Hospital	Miami	100%	695
Baptist Hospital	Pensacola	100%	350
Baptist Medical Center Beaches	Jacksonville Bch	100%	284
Bartow Regional Medical Center	Bartow	100%	152
Bay Medical Center	Panama City	100%	571
Bayfront Medical Center	Saint Petersburg	100%	244
Bert Fish Medical Center	New Smyrna Bch	100%	193
Bethesda Memorial Hospital	Boynton Beach	100%	263
Blake Medical Center	Bradenton	100%	322
Brooksville Regional Hospital	Brooksville	100%	347
Broward General Medical Center	Fort Lauderdale	100%	210
Cape Canaveral Hospital	Cocoa Beach	100%	286
Cape Coral Hospital	Cape Coral	100%	140
Capital Regional Medical Center	Tallahassee	100%	152
Citrus Memorial Hospital	Inverness	100%	231
Cleveland Clinic Florida	Weston	100%	120
Columbia Hospital	West Palm Beach	100%	132
Coral Springs Medical Center	Coral Springs	100%	174
Delray Medical Center	Delray Beach	100%	305
Doctors Hospital of Sarasota	Sarasota	100%	229
Englewood Community Hospital	Englewood	100%	116
Fawcett Memorial Hospital	Port Charlotte	100%	220
Fishermen's Hospital	Marathon	100%	36
Flagler Hospital	Saint Augustine	100%	265
Florida Hospital Fish Memorial	Orange City	100%	372
Florida Hospital Heartland Medical Center	Sebring	100%	287
Florida Hospital Orlando	Orlando	100%	1744
Florida Hospital Waterman	Tavares	100%	323
Florida Hospital Wauchula	Wauchula	100%	35
Florida Medical Center	Lauderdale Lakes	100%	147
Fort Walton Beach Medical Center	Fort Walton Beach	100%	245
Glades General Hospital	Belle Glade	100%	66
Good Samaritan Medical Center	West Palm Beach	100%	349
Gulf Breeze Hospital	Gulf Breeze	100%	153
Gulf Coast Hospital	Fort Meyers	100%	92
Halifax Medical Center	Daytona Beach	100%	576
Health Central	Ocoee	100%	202
HealthSouth Doctors' Hospital	Miami	100%	250
Heart of Florida Regional Medical Center	Davenport	100%	231
Hialeah Hospital	Miami	100%	438
Highlands Regional Medical Center	Sebring	100%	206
Holmes Regional Medical Center	Melbourne	100%	602
Holy Cross Hospital	Fort Lauderdale	100%	266
Homestead Hospital	Homestead	100%	344
Imperial Point Medical Center	Fort Lauderdale	100%	135
Indian River Memorial Hospital	Vero Beach	100%	350
JFK Medical Center	Atlantis	100%	668
Jackson Hospital	Marianna	100%	128
Jupiter Medical Center	Jupiter	100%	192
Kendall Medical Center	Miami	100%	660
Lake Wales Medical Center	Lake Wales	100%	151
Lakeland Regional Medical Center	Lakeland	100%	291
Lakewood Ranch Medical Center	Bradenton	100%	127
Largo Medical Center	Largo	100%	333

NOTE: Hospital profiles are in alphabetical order by state, then city, then hospital within the city; Rankings are sorted by rate in descending order and exclude hospitals with less than 25 cases; (1) The number of cases is too small (n<25) for purposes of reliably predicting hospital performance; (2) Measure reflects the hospital's indication that its submission was based upon a sample of its relevant discharges; (3) Rate reflects fewer than the maximum possible quarters of data for the measure; (4) Inaccurate information submitted and suppressed for one or more quarters; (5) No data is available from the hospital for this measure; Please refer to the User's Guide for a full explanation of data

Larkin Community Hospital	South Miami	100%	135
Lee Memorial Health System	Fort Myers	100%	193
Leesburg Regional Medical Center	Leesburg	100%	362
Lehigh Regional Medical Center	Lehigh Acres	100%	202
Lower Keys Medical Center	Key West	100%	140
Mariners Hospital	Tavernier	100%	73
Martin Memorial Medical Center	Stuart	100%	179
Mease Hospital-Countryside	Safety Harbor	100%	445
Mease Hospital-Dunedin	Dunedin	100%	208
Memorial Hospital Miramar	Miramar	100%	174
Memorial Hospital Pembroke	Pembroke Pines	100%	376
Memorial Hospital West	Pembroke Pines	100%	502
Memorial Hospital of Tampa	Tampa	100%	208
Memorial Regional Hospital	Hollywood	100%	506
Mercy Hospital	Miami	100%	354
Miami Jewish Home & Hosp for the Aged	Miami	100%	64
Morton Plant Hospital	Clearwater	100%	463
Munroe Regional Medical Center	Ocala	100%	306
NCH Downtown Naples Hospital	Naples	100%	654
Nature Coast Regional Hospital	Williston	100%	49
North Bay Medical Center	New Port Richey	100%	157
North Broward Medical Center	Deerfield Beach	100%	175
North Okaloosa Medical Center	Crestview	100%	158
North Shore Medical Center	Miami	100%	314
Northside Hospital	Saint Petersburg	100%	411
Northwest Florida Community Hospital	Chipley	100%	46
Northwest Medical Center	Margate	100%	274
Ocala Regional Medical Center	Ocala	100%	482
Orange Park Medical Center	Orange Park	100%	669
Orlando Regional Healthcare	Orlando	100%	1188
Osceola Regional Medical Center	Kissimmee	100%	396
Palmetto General Hospital	Hialeah	100%	311
Pan American Hospital	Miami	100%	236
Parrish Medical Center	Titusville	100%	243
Pasco Regional Medical Center	Dade City	100%	204
Physicians Regional Medical Center	Naples	100%	63
Raulerson Hospital	Okeechobee	100%	226
Regional Medical Center Bayonet Point	Hudson	100%	233
Sacred Heart Health System	Pensacola	100%	299
Sacred Heart Hospital on the Emerald Coast	Destin	100%	93
Saint Anthony's Hospital	Saint Petersburg	100%	372
Saint Cloud Regional Medical Center	Saint Cloud	100%	102
Saint Joseph's Hospital	Tampa	100%	648
Saint Lucie Medical Center	Port Saint Lucie	100%	383
Saint Mary's Medical Center	West Palm Beach	100%	301
Saint Vincent's Medical Center	Jacksonville	100%	241
Santa Rosa Medical Center	Milton	100%	193
Sarasota Memorial Health Care Systems	Sarasota	100%	421
Seven Rivers Regional Medical Center	Crystal River	100%	202
Shands Live Oak	Live Oak	100%	60
Shands at Starke	Starke	100%	64
Shands at the University of Florida	Gainesville	100%	319
South Florida Baptist Hospital	Plant City	100%	261
South Lake Hospital	Clermont	100%	144
South Miami Hospital	Miami	100%	475
Southwest Florida Regional Medical Center	Fort Myers	100%	509
Sun Coast Hospital	Largo	100%	210
Tallahassee Memorial Health Care Foundation	Tallahassee	100%	270
Twin Cities Hospital	Niceville	100%	108
Venice Regional Medical Center	Venice	100%	306
Wellington Regional Medical Center	Wellington	100%	205
West Florida Regional Medical Center	Pensacola	100%	247
Wuesthoff Health Systems	Rockledge	100%	294
Wuesthoff Medical Center-Melbourne	Melbourne	100%	115
Brandon Regional Hospital	Brandon	99%	466
Charlotte Regional Medical Center	Punta Gorda	99%	232
Columbia Memorial Hospital of Jacksonville	Jacksonville	99%	530
Community Hospital	New Port Richey	99%	296
DeSoto Memorial Hospital	Arcadia	99%	67
Edward White Hospital	Saint Petersburg	99%	182
Florida Hospital DeLand	Deland	99%	387
Florida Hospital Flagler	Palm Coast	99%	145
Gulf Coast Medical Center	Panama City	99%	304
Helen Ellis Memorial Hospital	Tarpon Springs	99%	155
Jackson Memorial Hospital	Miami	99%	352
Lawnwood Regional Med Ctr & Heart Inst	Fort Pierce	99%	411
Manatee Memorial Hospital	Bradenton	99%	312
North Ridge Medical Center	Fort Lauderdale	99%	81
Palm Beach Grdns Medical Center	Palm Beach Grdns	99%	203
Palms West Hospital	Loxahatchee	99%	165
Peace River Regional Medical Center	Port Charlotte	99%	266
Plantation General Hospital	Plantation	99%	162
Putnam Community Medical Center	Palatka	99%	302
Saint Luke's Hospital	Jacksonville	99%	209
Saint Petersburg General Hospital	Saint Petersburg	99%	278

Sebastian River Medical Center	Sebastian	99%	239
Shands Jacksonville	Jacksonville	99%	201
Shands at Lake Shore	Lake City	99%	118
Tampa General Healthcare	Tampa	99%	328
Town and Country Hospital	Tampa	99%	160
University Community Hospital	Tampa	99%	296
University Community Hospital of Carrollwood	Tampa	99%	193
Villages Regional Hospital	The Villages	99%	303
West Boca Medical Center	Boca Raton	99%	268
Westside Regional Medical Center	Plantation	99%	264
Winter Haven Hospital	Winter Haven	99%	605
Baptist Medical Center	Jacksonville	98%	576
Boca Raton Community Hospital	Boca Raton	98%	421
Cedars Medical Center	Miami	98%	343
Central Florida Regional Hospital	Sanford	98%	244
Coral Gables Hospital	Miami	98%	283
Florida Hospital-Ormond Memorial	Ormond Beach	98%	259
Lake City Medical Center	Lake City	98%	256
Oak Hill Hospital	Brooksville	98%	360
Palms of Pasadena Hospital	Saint Petersburg	98%	247
South Bay Hospital	Sun City Center	98%	286
Aventura Hospital and Medical Center	Aventura	97%	464
Baptist Medical Center Nassau	Fernandina Bch	97%	143
Doctors Memorial Hospital	Perry	97%	75
North Florida Regional Medical Center	Gainesville	97%	384
University Hospital & Medical Center	Tamarac	97%	226
Westchester General Hospital	Miami	97%	74
Florida Hospital Zephyrhills	Zephyrhills	96%	233
Jay Hospital	Jay	96%	73
Palm Springs General Hospital	Miami	96%	341
Mount Sinai Medical Center	Miami	95%	219
Healthmark Regional Medical Center	Defuniak Springs	90%	48
Doctors Memorial Hospital	Bonifay	88%	82

18. Pneumococcal Vaccine

Hospital Name	City	Rate	Cases
Holy Cross Hospital	Fort Lauderdale	100%	170
Memorial Hospital Miramar	Miramar	100%	92
South Miami Hospital	Miami	99%	310
Memorial Hospital West	Pembroke Pines	98%	264
Memorial Hospital Pembroke	Pembroke Pines	97%	196
Pan American Hospital	Miami	97%	155
Cleveland Clinic Florida	Weston	96%	71
Memorial Regional Hospital	Hollywood	96%	236
Homestead Hospital	Homestead	95%	160
Good Samaritan Medical Center	West Palm Beach	94%	210
HealthSouth Doctors' Hospital	Miami	94%	161
Peace River Regional Medical Center	Port Charlotte	94%	168
Delray Medical Center	Delray Beach	93%	216
Mariners Hospital	Tavernier	93%	44
Cape Canaveral Hospital	Cocoa Beach	92%	192
Hialeah Hospital	Miami	92%	299
Lawnwood Regional Med Ctr & Heart Inst	Fort Pierce	92%	240
Putnam Community Medical Center	Palatka	92%	182
Tallahassee Memorial Health Care Foundation	Tallahassee	92%	149
Florida Hospital Orlando	Orlando	90%	894
Saint Mary's Medical Center	West Palm Beach	90%	94
Baptist Hospital	Miami	89%	388
Pasco Regional Medical Center	Dade City	87%	135
Shands Live Oak	Live Oak	87%	31
Venice Regional Medical Center	Venice	87%	241
Bethesda Memorial Hospital	Boynton Beach	86%	162
Halifax Medical Center	Daytona Beach	86%	286
Larkin Community Hospital	South Miami	86%	77
Sacred Heart Hospital on the Emerald Coast	Destin	86%	63
Sarasota Memorial Health Care Systems	Sarasota	86%	282
Glades General Hospital	Belle Glade	85%	26
Saint Luke's Hospital	Jacksonville	85%	153
Brooksville Regional Hospital	Brooksville	84%	191
Community Hospital	New Port Richey	84%	193
Mercy Hospital	Miami	84%	261
Seven Rivers Regional Medical Center	Crystal River	84%	142
South Lake Hospital	Clermont	84%	89
Coral Springs Medical Center	Coral Springs	83%	86
Shands at Starke	Starke	83%	30
South Florida Baptist Hospital	Plant City	83%	148
Munroe Regional Medical Center	Ocala	82%	225
Santa Rosa Medical Center	Milton	82%	98
Cape Coral Hospital	Cape Coral	81%	95
Citrus Memorial Hospital	Inverness	81%	167
Wuesthoff Health Systems	Rockledge	81%	171
Coral Gables Hospital	Miami	80%	203
Florida Medical Center	Lauderdale Lakes	80%	103
Ocala Regional Medical Center	Ocala	80%	296

NOTE: Hospital profiles are in alphabetical order by state, then city, then hospital within the city; Rankings are sorted by rate in descending order and exclude hospitals with less than 25 cases; (1) The number of cases is too small (n<25) for purposes of reliably predicting hospital performance; (2) Measure reflects the hospital's indication that its submission was based upon a sample of its relevant discharges; (3) Rate reflects fewer than the maximum possible quarters of data for the measure; (4) Inaccurate information submitted and suppressed for one or more quarters; (5) No data is available from the hospital for this measure; Please refer to the User's Guide for a full explanation of data

Hospital Name	City	Rate	Cases
Doctors Memorial Hospital	Bonifay	79%	39
Manatee Memorial Hospital	Bradenton	79%	181
Twin Cities Hospital	Niceville	79%	66
Bert Fish Medical Center	New Smyrna Beach	78%	125
Florida Hospital Heartland Medical Center	Sebring	78%	210
Sebastian River Medical Center	Sebastian	78%	198
West Boca Medical Center	Boca Raton	78%	160
Winter Haven Hospital	Winter Haven	78%	386
Baptist Medical Center Beaches	Jacksonville Bch	77%	169
Baptist Medical Center Nassau	Fernandina Bch	77%	73
Bayfront Medical Center	Saint Petersburg	77%	115
Florida Hospital Waterman	Tavares	77%	205
Lee Memorial Health System	Fort Myers	77%	118
Florida Hospital-Ormond Memorial	Ormond Beach	76%	171
Gulf Breeze Hospital	Gulf Breeze	76%	95
Orlando Regional Healthcare	Orlando	76%	581
West Florida Regional Medical Center	Pensacola	76%	155
Wuesthoff Medical Center-Melbourne	Melbourne	76%	70
Leesburg Regional Medical Center	Leesburg	75%	233
Mease Hospital-Countryside	Safety Harbor	75%	296
North Shore Medical Center	Miami	75%	145
Parrish Medical Center	Titusville	74%	133
Villages Regional Hospital	The Villages	74%	223
Northwest Medical Center	Margate	73%	175
Palmetto General Hospital	Hialeah	73%	174
Saint Joseph's Hospital	Tampa	73%	274
Town and Country Hospital	Tampa	73%	84
Fawcett Memorial Hospital	Port Charlotte	72%	160
Morton Plant Hospital	Clearwater	72%	312
Aventura Hospital and Medical Center	Aventura	71%	307
Physicians Regional Medical Center	Naples	71%	35
Jay Hospital	Jay	70%	37
Lakewood Ranch Medical Center	Bradenton	70%	77
Orange Park Medical Center	Orange Park	70%	409
Palm Beach Grdns Medical Center	Palm Beach Grdns	70%	132
Saint Cloud Regional Medical Center	Saint Cloud	70%	61
Baptist Hospital	Pensacola	69%	194
Florida Hospital Flagler	Palm Coast	69%	77
Health Central	Ocoee	69%	108
Palms West Hospital	Loxahatchee	69%	89
Raulerson Hospital	Okeechobee	69%	143
Capital Regional Medical Center	Tallahassee	68%	77
Memorial Hospital of Tampa	Tampa	68%	120
Charlotte Regional Medical Center	Punta Gorda	67%	164
Doctors Hospital of Sarasota	Sarasota	67%	171
Fort Walton Beach Medical Center	Fort Walton Beach	67%	138
North Ridge Medical Center	Fort Lauderdale	67%	61
Westchester General Hospital	Miami	67%	54
Westside Regional Medical Center	Plantation	66%	146
Bay Medical Center	Panama City	65%	344
Flagler Hospital	Saint Augustine	65%	142
Tampa General Healthcare	Tampa	65%	110
Baptist Medical Center	Jacksonville	64%	252
Florida Hospital DeLand	Deland	64%	228
Highlands Regional Medical Center	Sebring	64%	149
JFK Medical Center	Atlantis	64%	434
Lake Wales Medical Center	Lake Wales	64%	86
Lakeland Regional Medical Center	Lakeland	64%	170
Saint Anthony's Hospital	Saint Petersburg	64%	183
Largo Medical Center	Largo	63%	226
Palms of Pasadena Hospital	Saint Petersburg	63%	188
Saint Lucie Medical Center	Port Saint Lucie	63%	241
Holmes Regional Medical Center	Melbourne	62%	377
North Bay Medical Center	New Port Richey	62%	80
Sacred Heart Health System	Pensacola	62%	176
University Hospital & Medical Center	Tamarac	62%	162
Blake Medical Center	Bradenton	60%	231
Saint Vincent's Medical Center	Jacksonville	60%	139
Lake City Medical Center	Lake City	58%	170
North Okaloosa Medical Center	Crestview	58%	96
Lehigh Regional Medical Center	Lehigh Acres	57%	119
Martin Memorial Medical Center	Stuart	57%	127
Mease Hospital-Dunedin	Dunedin	57%	137
Healthmark Regional Medical Center	Defuniak Springs	56%	32
Heart of Florida Regional Medical Center	Davenport	56%	131
Sun Coast Hospital	Largo	56%	109
Wellington Regional Medical Center	Wellington	56%	126
North Broward Medical Center	Deerfield Beach	55%	78
Imperial Point Medical Center	Fort Lauderdale	54%	72
Regional Medical Center Bayonet Point	Hudson	54%	158
Southwest Florida Regional Medical Center	Fort Myers	54%	336
Boca Raton Community Hospital	Boca Raton	53%	309
Edward White Hospital	Saint Petersburg	53%	115
Mount Sinai Medical Center	Miami	53%	138
Palm Springs General Hospital	Miami	53%	248
Florida Hospital Fish Memorial	Orange City	52%	226
Gulf Coast Hospital	Fort Meyers	52%	54
Jupiter Medical Center	Jupiter	52%	129
Kendall Medical Center	Miami	52%	444
Lower Keys Medical Center	Key West	52%	77
Doctors Memorial Hospital	Perry	51%	37
North Florida Regional Medical Center	Gainesville	51%	241
Oak Hill Hospital	Brooksville	49%	249
Shands Jacksonville	Jacksonville	49%	78
Englewood Community Hospital	Englewood	48%	79
Central Florida Regional Hospital	Sanford	47%	124
Columbia Hospital	West Palm Beach	47%	66
DeSoto Memorial Hospital	Arcadia	47%	38
Florida Hospital Zephyrhills	Zephyrhills	47%	143
Plantation General Hospital	Plantation	47%	43
South Bay Hospital	Sun City Center	47%	206
Miami Jewish Home & Hosp for the Aged	Miami	46%	52
Gulf Coast Medical Center	Panama City	45%	179
Jackson Memorial Hospital	Miami	45%	139
Brandon Regional Hospital	Brandon	44%	264
NCH Downtown Naples Hospital	Naples	44%	482
Columbia Memorial Hospital of Jacksonville	Jacksonville	42%	294
Shands at the University of Florida	Gainesville	42%	146
University Community Hospital	Tampa	42%	160
University Community Hospital of Carrollwood	Tampa	42%	95
Northside Hospital	Saint Petersburg	41%	253
Saint Petersburg General Hospital	Saint Petersburg	39%	162
Shands at Lake Shore	Lake City	39%	56
Indian River Memorial Hospital	Vero Beach	37%	247
Helen Ellis Memorial Hospital	Tarpon Springs	35%	97
Osceola Regional Medical Center	Kissimmee	34%	243
Cedars Medical Center	Miami	33%	203
Jackson Hospital	Marianna	26%	70
Bartow Regional Medical Center	Bartow	24%	82
Broward General Medical Center	Fort Lauderdale	19%	67

19. Smoking Cessation Advice

Hospital Name	City	Rate	Cases
Aventura Hospital and Medical Center	Aventura	100%	62
Baptist Hospital	Miami	100%	117
Baptist Hospital	Pensacola	100%	98
Brooksville Regional Hospital	Brooksville	100%	92
Community Hospital	New Port Richey	100%	87
Florida Hospital DeLand	Deland	100%	87
Florida Hospital Flagler	Palm Coast	100%	37
Florida Medical Center	Lauderdale Lakes	100%	25
Good Samaritan Medical Center	West Palm Beach	100%	61
Gulf Breeze Hospital	Gulf Breeze	100%	35
HealthSouth Doctors' Hospital	Miami	100%	51
Hialeah Hospital	Miami	100%	53
Holy Cross Hospital	Fort Lauderdale	100%	29
Homestead Hospital	Homestead	100%	103
Imperial Point Medical Center	Fort Lauderdale	100%	35
Largo Medical Center	Largo	100%	75
Larkin Community Hospital	South Miami	100%	49
Martin Memorial Medical Center	Stuart	100%	29
Mease Hospital-Dunedin	Dunedin	100%	48
Memorial Hospital Miramar	Miramar	100%	26
Memorial Hospital Pembroke	Pembroke Pines	100%	68
Memorial Hospital West	Pembroke Pines	100%	80
Memorial Hospital of Tampa	Tampa	100%	39
Memorial Regional Hospital	Hollywood	100%	118
Mercy Hospital	Miami	100%	44
North Shore Medical Center	Miami	100%	54
Palm Springs General Hospital	Miami	100%	26
Palmetto General Hospital	Hialeah	100%	46
Pan American Hospital	Miami	100%	25
Parrish Medical Center	Titusville	100%	49
Putnam Community Medical Center	Palatka	100%	77
Raulerson Hospital	Okeechobee	100%	53
Saint Luke's Hospital	Jacksonville	100%	39
Saint Mary's Medical Center	West Palm Beach	100%	95
South Bay Hospital	Sun City Center	100%	60
South Miami Hospital	Miami	100%	63
University Community Hospital of Carrollwood	Tampa	100%	40
University Hospital & Medical Center	Tamarac	100%	35
Venice Regional Medical Center	Venice	100%	47
West Boca Medical Center	Boca Raton	100%	32
Westside Regional Medical Center	Plantation	100%	45
Florida Hospital Orlando	Orlando	99%	405
Halifax Medical Center	Daytona Beach	99%	144
Santa Rosa Medical Center	Milton	99%	67
Wuesthoff Health Systems	Rockledge	99%	91
Bay Medical Center	Panama City	98%	163

NOTE: Hospital profiles are in alphabetical order by state, then city, then hospital within the city; Rankings are sorted by rate in descending order and exclude hospitals with less than 25 cases; The number of cases is too small (n<25) for purposes of reliably predicting hospital performance; (2) Measure reflects the hospital's indication that its submission was based upon a sample of its relevant discharges; (3) Rate reflects fewer than the maximum possible quarters of data for the measure; (4) Inaccurate information submitted and suppressed for one or more quarters; (5) No data is available from the hospital for this measure; Please refer to the User's Guide for a full explanation of data

Hospital Name	City	Rate	Cases
Bethesda Memorial Hospital	Boynton Beach	98%	48
Brandon Regional Hospital	Brandon	98%	116
Broward General Medical Center	Fort Lauderdale	98%	62
Charlotte Regional Medical Center	Punta Gorda	98%	52
Mease Hospital-Countryside	Safety Harbor	98%	85
North Florida Regional Medical Center	Gainesville	98%	90
Saint Anthony's Hospital	Saint Petersburg	98%	112
Saint Lucie Medical Center	Port Saint Lucie	98%	58
South Florida Baptist Hospital	Plant City	98%	66
West Florida Regional Medical Center	Pensacola	98%	45
Gulf Coast Medical Center	Panama City	97%	69
JFK Medical Center	Atlantis	97%	118
Jackson Hospital	Marianna	97%	36
Lawnwood Regional Med Ctr & Heart Inst	Fort Pierce	97%	106
Lower Keys Medical Center	Key West	97%	35
Oak Hill Hospital	Brooksville	97%	72
Peace River Regional Medical Center	Port Charlotte	97%	68
Saint Joseph's Hospital	Tampa	97%	162
Saint Vincent's Medical Center	Jacksonville	97%	29
Tallahassee Memorial Health Care Foundation	Tallahassee	97%	66
Blake Medical Center	Bradenton	96%	45
Cape Canaveral Hospital	Cocoa Beach	96%	56
Columbia Memorial Hospital of Jacksonville	Jacksonville	96%	147
Coral Gables Hospital	Miami	96%	27
Coral Springs Medical Center	Coral Springs	96%	46
Lake City Medical Center	Lake City	96%	52
Northwest Medical Center	Margate	96%	52
Osceola Regional Medical Center	Kissimmee	96%	56
Palm Beach Grdns Medical Center	Palm Beach Grdns	96%	28
Shands at the University of Florida	Gainesville	96%	99
Tampa General Healthcare	Tampa	96%	101
Wellington Regional Medical Center	Wellington	96%	46
Fort Walton Beach Medical Center	Fort Walton Beach	95%	76
North Bay Medical Center	New Port Richey	95%	43
Regional Medical Center Bayonet Point	Hudson	95%	43
Shands Jacksonville	Jacksonville	95%	57
Baptist Medical Center Beaches	Jacksonville Bch	94%	50
Bayfront Medical Center	Saint Petersburg	94%	63
Citrus Memorial Hospital	Inverness	94%	36
Mount Sinai Medical Center	Miami	94%	32
Cape Coral Hospital	Cape Coral	93%	30
Fawcett Memorial Hospital	Port Charlotte	93%	44
Kendall Medical Center	Miami	93%	86
Ocala Regional Medical Center	Ocala	93%	144
Plantation General Hospital	Plantation	93%	45
Flagler Hospital	Saint Augustine	92%	71
Leesburg Regional Medical Center	Leesburg	92%	61
Northside Hospital	Saint Petersburg	92%	105
Southwest Florida Regional Medical Center	Fort Myers	92%	102
Florida Hospital Fish Memorial	Orange City	91%	80
Florida Hospital Waterman	Tavares	91%	64
Morton Plant Hospital	Clearwater	91%	102
Palms West Hospital	Loxahatchee	91%	34
Capital Regional Medical Center	Tallahassee	90%	40
Doctors Hospital of Sarasota	Sarasota	90%	59
Heart of Florida Regional Medical Center	Davenport	90%	59
Lee Memorial Health System	Fort Myers	90%	39
Manatee Memorial Hospital	Bradenton	90%	77
Villages Regional Hospital	The Villages	90%	41
Winter Haven Hospital	Winter Haven	90%	114
Munroe Regional Medical Center	Ocala	89%	90
Orlando Regional Healthcare	Orlando	89%	330
Pasco Regional Medical Center	Dade City	89%	55
Saint Petersburg General Hospital	Saint Petersburg	89%	66
Florida Hospital Heartland Medical Center	Sebring	88%	50
Health Central	Ocoee	88%	40
Holmes Regional Medical Center	Melbourne	88%	121
North Broward Medical Center	Deerfield Beach	88%	40
University Community Hospital	Tampa	88%	56
Central Florida Regional Hospital	Sanford	87%	68
Florida Hospital-Ormond Memorial	Ormond Beach	87%	71
Lakeland Regional Medical Center	Lakeland	87%	91
Orange Park Medical Center	Orange Park	87%	134
North Okaloosa Medical Center	Crestview	86%	44
Sebastian River Medical Center	Sebastian	86%	57
Cedars Medical Center	Miami	85%	67
Town and Country Hospital	Tampa	85%	27
Edward White Hospital	Saint Petersburg	84%	45
Sarasota Memorial Health Care Systems	Sarasota	82%	78
Boca Raton Community Hospital	Boca Raton	80%	35
Highlands Regional Medical Center	Sebring	79%	28
Baptist Medical Center	Jacksonville	77%	151
Palms of Pasadena Hospital	Saint Petersburg	77%	39
Jupiter Medical Center	Jupiter	76%	25
NCH Downtown Naples Hospital	Naples	76%	124
Bartow Regional Medical Center	Bartow	75%	40
Florida Hospital Zephyrhills	Zephyrhills	75%	57
Sacred Heart Health System	Pensacola	75%	60
Bert Fish Medical Center	New Smyrna Beach	74%	43
Seven Rivers Regional Medical Center	Crystal River	74%	39
Baptist Medical Center Nassau	Fernandina Bch	73%	33
Jackson Memorial Hospital	Miami	70%	86
Shands at Lake Shore	Lake City	66%	38
Helen Ellis Memorial Hospital	Tarpon Springs	64%	39
South Lake Hospital	Clermont	62%	32
Sun Coast Hospital	Largo	56%	55
Lehigh Regional Medical Center	Lehigh Acres	47%	57
Lake Wales Medical Center	Lake Wales	36%	33

Surgical Infection Prevention

20. Prophylactic Antibiotic Given

Hospital Name	City	Rate	Cases
HealthSouth Doctors' Hospital	Miami	99%	546
Bethesda Memorial Hospital	Boynton Beach	97%	206
Cleveland Clinic Florida	Weston	97%	320
Memorial Hospital Pembroke	Pembroke Pines	97%	169
Baptist Hospital	Miami	96%	296
Cape Canaveral Hospital	Cocoa Beach	96%	437
Cedars Medical Center	Miami	96%	468
Delray Medical Center	Delray Beach	96%	1176
Mercy Hospital	Miami	96%	1252
Westside Regional Medical Center	Plantation	96%	540
Bay Medical Center	Panama City	95%	799
Coral Gables Hospital	Miami	95%	145
Hialeah Hospital	Miami	95%	123
Largo Medical Center	Largo	95%	279
North Shore Medical Center	Miami	95%	79
Palm Beach Grdns Medical Center	Palm Beach Grdns	95%	599
Venice Regional Medical Center	Venice	95%	449
Wuesthoff Health Systems	Rockledge	95%	664
Leesburg Regional Medical Center	Leesburg	94%	467
Plantation General Hospital	Plantation	94%	146
Sebastian River Medical Center	Sebastian	94%	204
Memorial Regional Hospital	Hollywood	93%	1000
North Ridge Medical Center	Fort Lauderdale	93%	580
Ocala Regional Medical Center	Ocala	93%	983
Orlando Regional Healthcare	Orlando	93%	3356
Seven Rivers Regional Medical Center	Crystal River	93%	497
Shands Jacksonville	Jacksonville	93%	270
South Miami Hospital	Miami	93%	245
Wuesthoff Medical Center-Melbourne	Melbourne	93%	290
Doctors Hospital of Sarasota	Sarasota	92%	226
Indian River Memorial Hospital	Vero Beach	92%	59
Palms of Pasadena Hospital	Saint Petersburg	92%	336
Tallahassee Memorial Health Care Foundation	Tallahassee	92%	713
Town and Country Hospital	Tampa	92%	136
Twin Cities Hospital	Niceville	92%	99
Winter Haven Hospital	Winter Haven	92%	738
Fawcett Memorial Hospital	Port Charlotte	91%	425
Florida Hospital DeLand	Deland	91%	410
Halifax Medical Center	Daytona Beach	91%	794
Helen Ellis Memorial Hospital	Tarpon Springs	91%	47
Holmes Regional Medical Center	Melbourne	91%	947
Martin Memorial Medical Center	Stuart	91%	241
Memorial Hospital West	Pembroke Pines	91%	583
Saint Petersburg General Hospital	Saint Petersburg	91%	225
Cape Coral Hospital	Cape Coral	90%	105
Munroe Regional Medical Center	Ocala	90%	673
Orange Park Medical Center	Orange Park	90%	519
Parrish Medical Center	Titusville	90%	231
Saint Lucie Medical Center	Port Saint Lucie	90%	472
South Lake Hospital	Clermont	90%	329
University Hospital & Medical Center	Tamarac	90%	178
West Boca Medical Center	Boca Raton	90%	163
Baptist Medical Center Beaches	Jacksonville Bch	89%	356
Brooksville Regional Hospital	Brooksville	89%	387
Edward White Hospital	Saint Petersburg	89%	126
Florida Medical Center	Lauderdale Lakes	89%	460
Heart of Florida Regional Medical Center	Davenport	89%	748
Memorial Hospital Miramar	Miramar	89%	213
Community Hospital	New Port Richey	88%	273
Englewood Community Hospital	Englewood	88%	168
Florida Hospital Heartland Medical Center	Sebring	88%	434
Lee Memorial Health System	Fort Myers	88%	339
NCH Downtown Naples Hospital	Naples	88%	2605
Palmetto General Hospital	Hialeah	88%	179
Santa Rosa Medical Center	Milton	88%	156
Capital Regional Medical Center	Tallahassee	87%	321

NOTE: Hospital profiles are in alphabetical order by state, then city, then hospital within the city; Rankings are sorted by rate in descending order and exclude hospitals with less than 25 cases; (1) The number of cases is too small (n<25) for purposes of reliably predicting hospital performance; (2) Measure reflects the hospital's indication that its submission was based upon a sample of its relevant discharges; (3) Rate reflects fewer than the maximum possible quarters of data for the measure; (4) Inaccurate information submitted and suppressed for one or more quarters; (5) No data is available from the hospital for this measure; Please refer to the User's Guide for a full explanation of data

Hospital Name	City	Rate	Cases
Florida Hospital Fish Memorial	Orange City	87%	432
Fort Walton Beach Medical Center	Fort Walton Beach	87%	246
JFK Medical Center	Atlantis	87%	905
Jackson Hospital	Marianna	87%	86
Oak Hill Hospital	Brooksville	87%	435
South Bay Hospital	Sun City Center	87%	227
Baptist Medical Center Nassau	Fernandina Bch	86%	109
Blake Medical Center	Bradenton	86%	895
Citrus Memorial Hospital	Inverness	86%	529
Florida Hospital Orlando	Orlando	86%	1434
Homestead Hospital	Homestead	86%	73
Kendall Medical Center	Miami	86%	330
Lawnwood Regional Med Ctr & Heart Inst	Fort Pierce	86%	428
North Florida Regional Medical Center	Gainesville	86%	315
Northwest Medical Center	Margate	86%	318
Shands at the University of Florida	Gainesville	86%	589
Sun Coast Hospital	Largo	86%	198
Northside Hospital	Saint Petersburg	85%	228
Health Central	Ocoee	84%	170
Saint Anthony's Hospital	Saint Petersburg	84%	149
Saint Mary's Medical Center	West Palm Beach	84%	192
Westchester General Hospital	Miami	84%	45
Central Florida Regional Hospital	Sanford	83%	390
Columbia Memorial Hospital of Jacksonville	Jacksonville	83%	314
Gulf Coast Hospital	Fort Meyers	83%	354
Lakeland Regional Medical Center	Lakeland	83%	534
Pan American Hospital	Miami	83%	242
Pasco Regional Medical Center	Dade City	83%	280
Sarasota Memorial Health Care Systems	Sarasota	83%	771
Boca Raton Community Hospital	Boca Raton	82%	1075
Peace River Regional Medical Center	Port Charlotte	82%	401
Raulerson Hospital	Okeechobee	82%	67
University Community Hospital of Carrollwood	Tampa	82%	76
Aventura Hospital and Medical Center	Aventura	81%	234
Lakewood Ranch Medical Center	Bradenton	81%	155
Mease Hospital-Dunedin	Dunedin	81%	103
Memorial Hospital of Tampa	Tampa	81%	129
South Florida Baptist Hospital	Plant City	81%	114
Tampa General Healthcare	Tampa	81%	1985
Manatee Memorial Hospital	Bradenton	80%	468
Osceola Regional Medical Center	Kissimmee	80%	528
Sacred Heart Hospital on the Emerald Coast	Destin	80%	183
Saint Joseph's Hospital	Tampa	80%	225
Villages Regional Hospital	The Villages	80%	123
Florida Hospital Zephyrhills	Zephyrhills	79%	328
Florida Hospital-Ormond Memorial	Ormond Beach	79%	866
Mount Sinai Medical Center	Miami	79%	547
Wellington Regional Medical Center	Wellington	79%	547
Fishermen's Hospital	Marathon	78%	69
Saint Luke's Hospital	Jacksonville	78%	282
Baptist Hospital	Pensacola	77%	741
Bert Fish Medical Center	New Smyrna Beach	77%	173
Brandon Regional Hospital	Brandon	77%	299
Broward General Medical Center	Fort Lauderdale	77%	245
Southwest Florida Regional Medical Center	Fort Myers	77%	345
Baptist Medical Center	Jacksonville	76%	1325
Gulf Breeze Hospital	Gulf Breeze	76%	419
Florida Hospital Flagler	Palm Coast	75%	371
Imperial Point Medical Center	Fort Lauderdale	75%	138
Morton Plant Hospital	Clearwater	75%	224
Palm Springs General Hospital	Miami	75%	123
Holy Cross Hospital	Fort Lauderdale	74%	292
Palms West Hospital	Loxahatchee	74%	307
Physicians Regional Medical Center	Naples	74%	77
Columbia Hospital	West Palm Beach	73%	219
Mease Hospital-Countryside	Safety Harbor	73%	168
Florida Hospital Waterman	Tavares	72%	579
Putnam Community Medical Center	Palatka	72%	141
Good Samaritan Medical Center	West Palm Beach	70%	227
Gulf Coast Medical Center	Panama City	70%	416
Jupiter Medical Center	Jupiter	70%	178
Bayfront Medical Center	Saint Petersburg	69%	586
Coral Springs Medical Center	Coral Springs	69%	170
North Broward Medical Center	Deerfield Beach	69%	186
University Community Hospital	Tampa	69%	323
North Bay Medical Center	New Port Richey	68%	111
Charlotte Regional Medical Center	Punta Gorda	65%	464
North Okaloosa Medical Center	Crestview	65%	227
West Florida Regional Medical Center	Pensacola	64%	288
Regional Medical Center Bayonet Point	Hudson	62%	566
Saint Vincent's Medical Center	Jacksonville	62%	321
Jackson Memorial Hospital	Miami	60%	298
Flagler Hospital	Saint Augustine	59%	259
Lower Keys Medical Center	Key West	57%	120
Shands at Lake Shore	Lake City	57%	101
Lehigh Regional Medical Center	Lehigh Acres	54%	140
Sacred Heart Health System	Pensacola	54%	349
Highlands Regional Medical Center	Sebring	53%	135
Lake Wales Medical Center	Lake Wales	50%	52
Bartow Regional Medical Center	Bartow	44%	36
Saint Cloud Regional Medical Center	Saint Cloud	44%	32

21. Prophylactic Antibiotic Selection

Hospital Name	City	Rate	Cases
Baptist Hospital	Miami	100%	73
Coral Gables Hospital	Miami	100%	31
Jackson Hospital	Marianna	100%	29
Seven Rivers Regional Medical Center	Crystal River	100%	57
Villages Regional Hospital	The Villages	100%	32
Leesburg Regional Medical Center	Leesburg	99%	124
Bert Fish Medical Center	New Smyrna Beach	98%	48
Bethesda Memorial Hospital	Boynton Beach	98%	41
Columbia Hospital	West Palm Beach	98%	47
Florida Hospital DeLand	Deland	98%	90
Gulf Coast Hospital	Fort Meyers	98%	85
Palm Beach Grdns Medical Center	Palm Beach Grdns	98%	129
Pasco Regional Medical Center	Dade City	98%	51
Aventura Hospital and Medical Center	Aventura	97%	67
Baptist Medical Center Beaches	Jacksonville Bch	97%	33
Citrus Memorial Hospital	Inverness	97%	150
Cleveland Clinic Florida	Weston	97%	76
Doctors Hospital of Sarasota	Sarasota	97%	72
Florida Hospital Heartland Medical Center	Sebring	97%	94
Good Samaritan Medical Center	West Palm Beach	97%	62
Gulf Breeze Hospital	Gulf Breeze	97%	93
Imperial Point Medical Center	Fort Lauderdale	97%	33
JFK Medical Center	Atlantis	97%	274
Kendall Medical Center	Miami	97%	134
Lakeland Regional Medical Center	Lakeland	97%	127
Largo Medical Center	Largo	97%	103
Mease Hospital-Dunedin	Dunedin	97%	30
Memorial Hospital Pembroke	Pembroke Pines	97%	39
Mercy Hospital	Miami	97%	316
North Bay Medical Center	New Port Richey	97%	34
South Florida Baptist Hospital	Plant City	97%	30
South Lake Hospital	Clermont	97%	73
Wellington Regional Medical Center	Wellington	97%	137
Winter Haven Hospital	Winter Haven	97%	198
Delray Medical Center	Delray Beach	96%	252
HealthSouth Doctors' Hospital	Miami	96%	137
Jupiter Medical Center	Jupiter	96%	45
North Broward Medical Center	Deerfield Beach	96%	47
North Ridge Medical Center	Fort Lauderdale	96%	150
Oak Hill Hospital	Brooksville	96%	126
Orlando Regional Healthcare	Orlando	96%	847
Plantation General Hospital	Plantation	96%	46
Saint Joseph's Hospital	Tampa	96%	69
Sarasota Memorial Health Care Systems	Sarasota	96%	192
Bay Medical Center	Panama City	95%	203
Blake Medical Center	Bradenton	95%	96
Fawcett Memorial Hospital	Port Charlotte	95%	87
Memorial Hospital West	Pembroke Pines	95%	41
Memorial Regional Hospital	Hollywood	95%	63
Northside Hospital	Saint Petersburg	95%	74
Regional Medical Center Bayonet Point	Hudson	95%	155
Shands at the University of Florida	Gainesville	95%	133
South Miami Hospital	Miami	95%	62
Bayfront Medical Center	Saint Petersburg	94%	64
Charlotte Regional Medical Center	Punta Gorda	94%	70
Edward White Hospital	Saint Petersburg	94%	33
Florida Hospital Orlando	Orlando	94%	363
Florida Medical Center	Lauderdale Lakes	94%	82
Holmes Regional Medical Center	Melbourne	94%	241
Holy Cross Hospital	Fort Lauderdale	94%	77
Martin Memorial Medical Center	Stuart	94%	71
Munroe Regional Medical Center	Ocala	94%	173
NCH Downtown Naples Hospital	Naples	94%	593
Ocala Regional Medical Center	Ocala	94%	242
Osceola Regional Medical Center	Kissimmee	94%	144
Southwest Florida Regional Medical Center	Fort Myers	94%	234
Sun Coast Hospital	Largo	94%	51
Tallahassee Memorial Health Care Foundation	Tallahassee	94%	180
West Florida Regional Medical Center	Pensacola	94%	114
Westside Regional Medical Center	Plantation	94%	133
Brooksville Regional Hospital	Brooksville	93%	55
Florida Hospital-Ormond Memorial	Ormond Beach	93%	195
Lehigh Regional Medical Center	Lehigh Acres	93%	29
Mease Hospital-Countryside	Safety Harbor	93%	61
Palmetto General Hospital	Hialeah	93%	44

NOTE: Hospital profiles are in alphabetical order by state, then city, then hospital within the city; Rankings are sorted by rate in descending order and exclude hospitals with less than 25 cases; (1) The number of cases is too small (n<25) for purposes of reliably predicting hospital performance; (2) Measure reflects the hospital's indication that its submission was based upon a sample of its relevant discharges; (3) Rate reflects fewer than the maximum possible quarters of data for the measure; (4) Inaccurate information submitted and suppressed for one or more quarters; (5) No data is available from the hospital for this measure; Please refer to the User's Guide for a full explanation of data

Hospital Name	City	Rate	Cases
Sacred Heart Health System	Pensacola	93%	86
Saint Petersburg General Hospital	Saint Petersburg	93%	67
Sebastian River Medical Center	Sebastian	93%	46
Cape Canaveral Hospital	Cocoa Beach	92%	95
Central Florida Regional Hospital	Sanford	92%	100
Palms West Hospital	Loxahatchee	92%	79
Parrish Medical Center	Titusville	92%	59
Putnam Community Medical Center	Palatka	92%	40
Raulerson Hospital	Okeechobee	92%	25
Saint Luke's Hospital	Jacksonville	92%	75
South Bay Hospital	Sun City Center	92%	66
Florida Hospital Flagler	Palm Coast	91%	96
Fort Walton Beach Medical Center	Fort Walton Beach	91%	110
Halifax Medical Center	Daytona Beach	91%	385
Health Central	Ocoee	91%	44
Lawnwood Regional Med Ctr & Heart Inst	Fort Pierce	91%	119
Lee Memorial Health System	Fort Myers	91%	86
Palms of Pasadena Hospital	Saint Petersburg	91%	80
Shands Jacksonville	Jacksonville	91%	70
Baptist Hospital	Pensacola	90%	157
Cape Coral Hospital	Cape Coral	90%	41
Englewood Community Hospital	Englewood	90%	51
Florida Hospital Waterman	Tavares	90%	134
Manatee Memorial Hospital	Bradenton	90%	126
North Florida Regional Medical Center	Gainesville	90%	136
Sacred Heart Hospital on the Emerald Coast	Destin	90%	51
University Hospital & Medical Center	Tamarac	90%	50
Wuesthoff Health Systems	Rockledge	90%	151
Cedars Medical Center	Miami	89%	101
Hialeah Hospital	Miami	89%	28
Memorial Hospital of Tampa	Tampa	89%	36
Orange Park Medical Center	Orange Park	89%	120
Saint Mary's Medical Center	West Palm Beach	89%	37
Santa Rosa Medical Center	Milton	89%	35
Tampa General Healthcare	Tampa	89%	517
University Community Hospital of Carrollwood	Tampa	89%	37
Venice Regional Medical Center	Venice	89%	93
Columbia Memorial Hospital of Jacksonville	Jacksonville	88%	137
Florida Hospital Zephyrhills	Zephyrhills	88%	67
Lakewood Ranch Medical Center	Bradenton	88%	26
Peace River Regional Medical Center	Port Charlotte	88%	68
West Boca Medical Center	Boca Raton	88%	42
Wuesthoff Medical Center-Melbourne	Melbourne	88%	76
Community Hospital	New Port Richey	87%	79
Flagler Hospital	Saint Augustine	87%	75
Morton Plant Hospital	Clearwater	87%	67
Pan American Hospital	Miami	87%	75
Town and Country Hospital	Tampa	86%	28
Heart of Florida Regional Medical Center	Davenport	85%	72
Mount Sinai Medical Center	Miami	84%	316
Saint Anthony's Hospital	Saint Petersburg	84%	49
Saint Vincent's Medical Center	Jacksonville	83%	83
Brandon Regional Hospital	Brandon	82%	99
Coral Springs Medical Center	Coral Springs	82%	40
Florida Hospital Fish Memorial	Orange City	82%	118
Jackson Memorial Hospital	Miami	82%	60
North Okaloosa Medical Center	Crestview	82%	40
Northwest Medical Center	Margate	82%	110
Helen Ellis Memorial Hospital	Tarpon Springs	81%	47
Palm Springs General Hospital	Miami	80%	41
Broward General Medical Center	Fort Lauderdale	79%	66
Boca Raton Community Hospital	Boca Raton	78%	210
Baptist Medical Center	Jacksonville	74%	78
University Community Hospital	Tampa	74%	90
Capital Regional Medical Center	Tallahassee	73%	26
Saint Lucie Medical Center	Port Saint Lucie	71%	100
Twin Cities Hospital	Niceville	68%	40
Gulf Coast Medical Center	Panama City	66%	82
Lower Keys Medical Center	Key West	58%	31
Saint Vincent's Medical Center	Jacksonville	91%	316
Baptist Medical Center Nassau	Fernandina Bch	90%	105
Citrus Memorial Hospital	Inverness	89%	483
Florida Hospital DeLand	Deland	89%	398
Largo Medical Center	Largo	89%	241
Pan American Hospital	Miami	89%	240
Westchester General Hospital	Miami	89%	44
Homestead Hospital	Homestead	87%	62
Venice Regional Medical Center	Venice	87%	433
Winter Haven Hospital	Winter Haven	87%	693
Cape Canaveral Hospital	Cocoa Beach	86%	414
Englewood Community Hospital	Englewood	86%	161
Jackson Hospital	Marianna	86%	84
Memorial Hospital Miramar	Miramar	86%	210
Orlando Regional Healthcare	Orlando	86%	3065
Saint Joseph's Hospital	Tampa	86%	198
Memorial Regional Hospital	Hollywood	85%	971
Twin Cities Hospital	Niceville	85%	99
Mease Hospital-Dunedin	Dunedin	84%	87
Mercy Hospital	Miami	84%	1229
Orange Park Medical Center	Orange Park	84%	498
Memorial Hospital West	Pembroke Pines	83%	553
Osceola Regional Medical Center	Kissimmee	83%	484
Delray Medical Center	Delray Beach	81%	1134
Gulf Coast Hospital	Fort Meyers	81%	351
Munroe Regional Medical Center	Ocala	81%	628
Bay Medical Center	Panama City	80%	769
Health Central	Ocoee	80%	167
Lee Memorial Health System	Fort Myers	80%	328
NCH Downtown Naples Hospital	Naples	80%	2452
Parrish Medical Center	Titusville	80%	225
Santa Rosa Medical Center	Milton	80%	153
Northwest Medical Center	Margate	79%	312
Shands Jacksonville	Jacksonville	79%	263
Westside Regional Medical Center	Plantation	79%	526
Charlotte Regional Medical Center	Punta Gorda	78%	450
Florida Hospital Zephyrhills	Zephyrhills	78%	308
Good Samaritan Medical Center	West Palm Beach	78%	219
Mease Hospital-Countryside	Safety Harbor	78%	145
Seven Rivers Regional Medical Center	Crystal River	78%	469
Halifax Medical Center	Daytona Beach	77%	779
North Okaloosa Medical Center	Crestview	77%	221
Plantation General Hospital	Plantation	77%	146
Saint Luke's Hospital	Jacksonville	77%	278
Bert Fish Medical Center	New Smyrna Beach	76%	162
Florida Hospital Fish Memorial	Orange City	76%	415
Peace River Regional Medical Center	Port Charlotte	76%	377
University Community Hospital	Tampa	76%	312
Bartow Regional Medical Center	Bartow	75%	36
Central Florida Regional Hospital	Sanford	75%	364
Florida Hospital Orlando	Orlando	75%	1383
Kendall Medical Center	Miami	75%	310
Lawnwood Regional Med Ctr & Heart Inst	Fort Pierce	75%	415
Tallahassee Memorial Health Care Foundation	Tallahassee	75%	690
Mount Sinai Medical Center	Miami	74%	538
North Bay Medical Center	New Port Richey	74%	89
Saint Mary's Medical Center	West Palm Beach	74%	185
Wuesthoff Health Systems	Rockledge	74%	635
Baptist Medical Center	Jacksonville	73%	1224
Doctors Hospital of Sarasota	Sarasota	73%	219
Palm Springs General Hospital	Miami	73%	121
Sacred Heart Hospital on the Emerald Coast	Destin	73%	177
Sarasota Memorial Health Care Systems	Sarasota	73%	754
South Florida Baptist Hospital	Plant City	73%	92
Lakeland Regional Medical Center	Lakeland	72%	510
Martin Memorial Medical Center	Stuart	72%	221
Shands at the University of Florida	Gainesville	72%	570
Tampa General Healthcare	Tampa	72%	1823
Boca Raton Community Hospital	Boca Raton	71%	1036
Cape Coral Hospital	Cape Coral	71%	100
Florida Hospital Heartland Medical Center	Sebring	71%	418
Saint Petersburg General Hospital	Saint Petersburg	71%	221
University Hospital & Medical Center	Tamarac	71%	167
Aventura Hospital and Medical Center	Aventura	70%	213
West Boca Medical Center	Boca Raton	70%	162
Brooksville Regional Hospital	Brooksville	69%	372
Edward White Hospital	Saint Petersburg	69%	118
Villages Regional Hospital	The Villages	69%	118
Jackson Memorial Hospital	Miami	68%	280
Cleveland Clinic Florida	Weston	67%	312
Hialeah Hospital	Miami	67%	96
Jupiter Medical Center	Jupiter	67%	174
Lehigh Regional Medical Center	Lehigh Acres	67%	133
Wuesthoff Medical Center-Melbourne	Melbourne	67%	283
Bayfront Medical Center	Saint Petersburg	66%	559

22. Prophylactic Antibiotic Stopped

Hospital Name	City	Rate	Cases
Lake Wales Medical Center	Lake Wales	96%	50
Memorial Hospital Pembroke	Pembroke Pines	96%	155
Physicians Regional Medical Center	Naples	95%	77
South Miami Hospital	Miami	95%	237
HealthSouth Doctors' Hospital	Miami	94%	525
Baptist Hospital	Miami	93%	286
Leesburg Regional Medical Center	Leesburg	93%	460
Sebastian River Medical Center	Sebastian	93%	195
Morton Plant Hospital	Clearwater	92%	200
Ocala Regional Medical Center	Ocala	92%	902
South Lake Hospital	Clermont	92%	326
North Shore Medical Center	Miami	91%	76

NOTE: Hospital profiles are in alphabetical order by state, then city, then hospital within the city; Rankings are sorted by rate in descending order and exclude hospitals with less than 25 cases; (1) The number of cases is too small (n<25) for purposes of reliably predicting hospital performance; (2) Measure reflects the hospital's indication that its submission was based upon a sample of its relevant discharges; (3) Rate reflects fewer than the maximum possible quarters of data for the measure; (4) Inaccurate information submitted and suppressed for one or more quarters; (5) No data is available from the hospital for this measure; Please refer to the User's Guide for a full explanation of data

Community Hospital	New Port Richey	66%	265
Town and Country Hospital	Tampa	66%	128
Wellington Regional Medical Center	Wellington	66%	542
Florida Hospital Flagler	Palm Coast	65%	365
Gulf Coast Medical Center	Panama City	65%	395
Holmes Regional Medical Center	Melbourne	65%	920
North Florida Regional Medical Center	Gainesville	65%	313
Florida Hospital Waterman	Tavares	64%	541
Memorial Hospital of Tampa	Tampa	64%	127
Baptist Hospital	Pensacola	63%	699
Brandon Regional Hospital	Brandon	63%	283
Palmetto General Hospital	Hialeah	63%	180
Pasco Regional Medical Center	Dade City	63%	252
Bethesda Memorial Hospital	Boynton Beach	62%	193
Cedars Medical Center	Miami	62%	462
Highlands Regional Medical Center	Sebring	62%	126
Manatee Memorial Hospital	Bradenton	62%	452
North Ridge Medical Center	Fort Lauderdale	62%	570
Southwest Florida Regional Medical Center	Fort Myers	62%	341
Capital Regional Medical Center	Tallahassee	61%	312
Fawcett Memorial Hospital	Port Charlotte	61%	409
Heart of Florida Regional Medical Center	Davenport	61%	740
Holy Cross Hospital	Fort Lauderdale	61%	279
Lakewood Ranch Medical Center	Bradenton	61%	145
South Bay Hospital	Sun City Center	61%	219
Columbia Memorial Hospital of Jacksonville	Jacksonville	60%	290
Gulf Breeze Hospital	Gulf Breeze	60%	394
Indian River Memorial Hospital	Vero Beach	60%	58
JFK Medical Center	Atlantis	60%	881
Regional Medical Center Bayonet Point	Hudson	60%	542
Northside Hospital	Saint Petersburg	59%	211
Florida Hospital-Ormond Memorial	Ormond Beach	58%	845
Sun Coast Hospital	Largo	58%	188
Oak Hill Hospital	Brooksville	57%	414
Sacred Heart Health System	Pensacola	57%	336
Saint Anthony's Hospital	Saint Petersburg	57%	136
Broward General Medical Center	Fort Lauderdale	56%	233
Helen Ellis Memorial Hospital	Tarpon Springs	55%	47
Columbia Hospital	West Palm Beach	54%	213
Palms West Hospital	Loxahatchee	54%	298
University Community Hospital of Carrollwood	Tampa	54%	72
Florida Medical Center	Lauderdale Lakes	53%	454
Fort Walton Beach Medical Center	Fort Walton Beach	53%	230
Raulerson Hospital	Okeechobee	52%	67
West Florida Regional Medical Center	Pensacola	51%	281
Baptist Medical Center Beaches	Jacksonville Bch	49%	333
Lower Keys Medical Center	Key West	48%	94
Putnam Community Medical Center	Palatka	48%	135
Saint Lucie Medical Center	Port Saint Lucie	45%	464
Coral Springs Medical Center	Coral Springs	44%	164
Flagler Hospital	Saint Augustine	44%	254
Palm Beach Grdns Medical Center	Palm Beach Grdns	42%	566
Palms of Pasadena Hospital	Saint Petersburg	42%	313
Blake Medical Center	Bradenton	39%	878
Coral Gables Hospital	Miami	37%	145
North Broward Medical Center	Deerfield Beach	33%	180
Shands at Lake Shore	Lake City	32%	91
Imperial Point Medical Center	Fort Lauderdale	26%	131
Fishermen's Hospital	Marathon	16%	68
Saint Cloud Regional Medical Center	Saint Cloud	16%	31

Pregnancy Care

23. Inpatient Neonatal Mortality

Hospital Name	City	Rate	Cases
Boca Raton Community Hospital	Boca Raton	0.00%	413
Wellington Regional Medical Center	Wellington	0.04%	2652
Saint Petersburg General Hospital	Saint Petersburg	0.06%	1587
Baptist Medical Center Beaches	Jacksonville Bch	0.13%	791
Florida Hospital Zephyrhills	Zephyrhills	0.14%	705
Mount Sinai Medical Center	Miami	0.19%	2158
Bethesda Memorial Hospital	Boynton Beach	0.26%	766
Baptist Medical Center Nassau	Fernandina Bch	0.38%	261
Capital Regional Medical Center	Tallahassee	0.41%	972
Sacred Heart Health System	Pensacola	0.43%	691
Plantation General Hospital	Plantation	0.63%	3780
Broward General Medical Center	Fort Lauderdale	0.65%	3524
Tampa General Healthcare	Tampa	0.65%	5567
Lakeland Regional Medical Center	Lakeland	0.67%	896
Shands at Lake Shore	Lake City	0.84%	238
Florida Hospital Heartland Medical Center	Sebring	0.94%	1069
Shands Jacksonville	Jacksonville	1.09%	733
Shands at the University of Florida	Gainesville	1.66%	1807

24. Third or Fourth Degree Laceration

Hospital Name	City	Rate	Cases
Baptist Medical Center Nassau	Fernandina Bch	0.44%	228
Florida Hospital Heartland Medical Center	Sebring	1.24%	726
Sacred Heart Health System	Pensacola	1.34%	373
Florida Hospital Zephyrhills	Zephyrhills	1.54%	456
Mount Sinai Medical Center	Miami	1.70%	1115
Shands at Lake Shore	Lake City	1.70%	176
Saint Petersburg General Hospital	Saint Petersburg	1.87%	1125
Broward General Medical Center	Fort Lauderdale	2.00%	2101
Shands at the University of Florida	Gainesville	2.03%	1032
Lakeland Regional Medical Center	Lakeland	2.13%	657
Shands Jacksonville	Jacksonville	2.19%	548
Plantation General Hospital	Plantation	2.43%	2060
Bethesda Memorial Hospital	Boynton Beach	2.57%	544
Capital Regional Medical Center	Tallahassee	3.24%	617
Tampa General Healthcare	Tampa	3.43%	3699
Wellington Regional Medical Center	Wellington	3.78%	1665
Boca Raton Community Hospital	Boca Raton	4.20%	1144
Baptist Medical Center Beaches	Jacksonville Bch	4.60%	695

NOTE: Hospital profiles are in alphabetical order by state, then city, then hospital within the city; Rankings are sorted by rate in descending order and exclude hospitals with less than 25 cases; (1) The number of cases is too small (n<25) for purposes of reliably predicting hospital performance; (2) Measure reflects the hospital's indication that its submission was based upon a sample of its relevant discharges; (3) Rate reflects fewer than the maximum possible quarters of data for the measure; (4) Inaccurate information submitted and suppressed for one or more quarters; (5) No data is available from the hospital for this measure; Please refer to the User's Guide for a full explanation of data

DeSoto Memorial Hospital

900 North Robert Avenue
Arcadia, FL 34266
E-mail: hr@dmh.org
URL: www.dmh.org
Ownership: Voluntary non-profit - Private
Emergency Services: Yes

Phone: 863-494-3535
Fax: 863-494-8400

Accredited: Yes
Licensed Beds: 49

Key Personnel:
CEO. . . . . Vince Sica
Chief Medical Staff. . . . . Wael Alokeh
Cardiopulmonary . . . . Patrica Collins
Emergency Department . . . . Lori Prescott
Infection Control. . . . . Yvonne Hunt
ICU . . . . Lori Prescott
Director Medical/Surgical Nursing . . . . Brenda Sabatta
Director Medical/Surgical Nursing . . . . Lisa Snelling
OB/GYN Womens Health. . . . . Kayum Mohammadbhoy, MD
Director Respiratory Therapy . . . . Dian Cox

Measure	Cases	This Hospital	State Average	U.S. Average	Top Hospital
Heart Attack Care					
ACE Inhibitor or ARB for LVSD[1]	1	0%	83%	82%	100%
Aspirin at Arrival	28	89%	93%	92%	100%
Aspirin at Discharge[1]	7	43%	88%	90%	100%
Beta Blocker at Arrival[1]	24	75%	89%	87%	100%
Beta Blocker at Discharge[1]	7	86%	92%	90%	100%
Fibrinolytic Medication Timing	0	-	33%	31%	100%
PCI Within 90 Minutes of Arrival	0	-	52%	54%	95%
Smoking Cessation Advice[1]	2	0%	92%	88%	100%
Heart Failure Care					
ACE Inhibitor or ARB for LVSD[1]	22	59%	82%	82%	100%
Discharge Instructions	78	18%	61%	61%	93%
Evaluation of LVS Function	89	56%	90%	83%	99%
Smoking Cessation Advice[1]	9	22%	91%	82%	100%
Pneumonia Care					
Appropriate Initial Antibiotic	61	92%	84%	83%	94%
Blood Culture Timing	45	91%	88%	90%	100%
Influenza Vaccine[1]	15	67%	64%	70%	100%
Initial Antibiotic Timing	63	70%	74%	80%	93%
Oxygenation Assessment	67	99%	99%	99%	100%
Pneumococcal Vaccine	38	47%	67%	69%	94%
Smoking Cessation Advice[1]	14	21%	90%	80%	100%
Surgical Infection Prevention					
Prophylactic Antibiotic Given[1]	3	100%	83%	77%	95%
Prophylactic Antibiotic Selection[1]	1	0%	90%	90%	100%
Prophylactic Antibiotic Stopped[1]	3	33%	70%	72%	95%
Pregnancy Care					
Inpatient Neonatal Mortality	-	-	-	-	-
Third or Fourth Degree Laceration	-	-	2.71%	3.63%	3.27%

JFK Medical Center

5301 S Congress Avenue
Atlantis, FL 33462
URL: www.jfkmc.com
Ownership: Voluntary non-profit - Private
Emergency Services: Yes

Phone: 561-965-7300
Fax: 561-642-3684

Accredited: Yes
Licensed Beds: 424

Key Personnel:
CEO. . . . . Phillip D Robinson
Chief Medical Staff. . . . . Jose F Arrascue, MD
Emergency Room . . . . Randall Wolff, MD
Director Infection/Disease Control . . . . Ellen Minden
Director Medical/Surgical Nursing . . . . Kathy Dassler
Chief Radiology . . . . Ann Regueiro
Director Respiratory Therapy . . . . Don Mofield

Measure	Cases	This Hospital	State Average	U.S. Average	Top Hospital
Heart Attack Care					
ACE Inhibitor or ARB for LVSD	245	87%	83%	82%	100%
Aspirin at Arrival	729	96%	93%	92%	100%
Aspirin at Discharge	944	95%	88%	90%	100%
Beta Blocker at Arrival	517	93%	89%	87%	100%
Beta Blocker at Discharge	946	95%	92%	90%	100%
Fibrinolytic Medication Timing[1]	1	100%	33%	31%	100%

Measure	Cases	This Hospital	State Average	U.S. Average	Top Hospital
PCI Within 90 Minutes of Arrival	34	47%	52%	54%	95%
Smoking Cessation Advice	272	99%	92%	88%	100%
Heart Failure Care					
ACE Inhibitor or ARB for LVSD	493	85%	82%	82%	100%
Discharge Instructions	1,037	82%	61%	61%	93%
Evaluation of LVS Function	1,223	93%	90%	83%	99%
Smoking Cessation Advice	170	99%	91%	82%	100%
Pneumonia Care					
Appropriate Initial Antibiotic	351	80%	84%	83%	94%
Blood Culture Timing	379	78%	88%	90%	100%
Influenza Vaccine	129	65%	64%	70%	100%
Initial Antibiotic Timing	547	56%	74%	80%	93%
Oxygenation Assessment	668	100%	99%	99%	100%
Pneumococcal Vaccine	434	64%	67%	69%	94%
Smoking Cessation Advice	118	97%	90%	80%	100%
Surgical Infection Prevention					
Prophylactic Antibiotic Given[3]	905	87%	83%	77%	95%
Prophylactic Antibiotic Selection	274	97%	90%	90%	100%
Prophylactic Antibiotic Stopped[3]	881	60%	70%	72%	95%
Pregnancy Care					
Inpatient Neonatal Mortality	-	-	-	-	-
Third or Fourth Degree Laceration	-	-	2.71%	3.63%	3.27%

Aventura Hospital and Medical Center

Alternate Name: Columbia Aventura Hospital and Medical Center
20900 Biscayne Boulevard
Aventura, FL 33180
URL: www.aventurahospital.com
Ownership: Voluntary non-profit - Private
Emergency Services: Yes

Phone: 305-682-7000
Fax: 305-682-7105

Accredited: Yes
Licensed Beds: 407

Key Personnel:
President/CEO. . . . . Davide Carbone
Chief Medical Staff. . . . . Mark Firestone, MD
Director Catheterization Lab. . . . . Dan Louther
Emergency Room . . . . James Provo, MD
Director Emergency Room. . . . . Linda Fitzpatrick, RM
Infection Control. . . . . Linda Kusek
ICU . . . . Florida Ong Santus
OB/GYN Womens Health. . . . . B Mitchell Grabois, MD
Respiratory/Cardiopulmonary. . . . . Frank Gomez

Measure	Cases	This Hospital	State Average	U.S. Average	Top Hospital
Heart Attack Care					
ACE Inhibitor or ARB for LVSD[2]	79	97%	83%	82%	100%
Aspirin at Arrival[2]	284	98%	93%	92%	100%
Aspirin at Discharge[2]	277	99%	88%	90%	100%
Beta Blocker at Arrival[2]	204	97%	89%	87%	100%
Beta Blocker at Discharge[2]	314	98%	92%	90%	100%
Fibrinolytic Medication Timing[1,2]	2	50%	33%	31%	100%
PCI Within 90 Minutes of Arrival[1,2]	4	50%	52%	54%	95%
Smoking Cessation Advice[2]	70	100%	92%	88%	100%
Heart Failure Care					
ACE Inhibitor or ARB for LVSD[2]	173	92%	82%	82%	100%
Discharge Instructions[2]	425	92%	61%	61%	93%
Evaluation of LVS Function[2]	552	99%	90%	83%	99%
Smoking Cessation Advice[2]	42	100%	91%	82%	100%
Pneumonia Care					
Appropriate Initial Antibiotic	225	81%	84%	83%	94%
Blood Culture Timing	290	86%	88%	90%	100%
Influenza Vaccine	73	40%	64%	70%	100%
Initial Antibiotic Timing	370	48%	74%	80%	93%
Oxygenation Assessment	464	97%	99%	99%	100%
Pneumococcal Vaccine	307	71%	67%	69%	94%
Smoking Cessation Advice	62	100%	90%	80%	100%
Surgical Infection Prevention					
Prophylactic Antibiotic Given[2,3]	234	81%	83%	77%	95%
Prophylactic Antibiotic Selection[2]	67	97%	90%	90%	100%
Prophylactic Antibiotic Stopped[2,3]	213	70%	70%	72%	95%
Pregnancy Care					
Inpatient Neonatal Mortality	-	-	-	-	-
Third or Fourth Degree Laceration	-	-	2.71%	3.63%	3.27%

NOTE: Hospital profiles are in alphabetical order by state, then city, then hospital within the city; Rankings are sorted by rate in descending order and exclude hospitals with less than 25 cases; (1) The number of cases is too small (n<25) for purposes of reliably predicting hospital performance; (2) Measure reflects the hospital's indication that its submission was based upon a sample of its relevant discharges; (3) Rate reflects fewer than the maximum possible quarters of data for the measure; (4) Inaccurate information submitted and suppressed for one or more quarters; (5) No data is available from the hospital for this measure; Please refer to the User's Guide for a full explanation of data

Bartow Regional Medical Center

Alternate Name: Columbia Bartow Memorial Hospital
2200 Osprey Boulevard   Phone: 863-533-8111
Bartow, FL 33830   Fax: 863-519-1420
URL: www.bartowregional.com
Ownership: Voluntary non-profit - Private   Accredited: Yes
Emergency Services: Yes   Licensed Beds: 56

Key Personnel:

CEO . . . . Justin M Davis
Chief Medical Staff . . . . Luis Farilli, MD
Emergency Room . . . . Catherine Crichlow, RN
Director Medical/Surgical Nursing . . . . Brenda Powers, RN
OB/GYN Womens Health . . . . Myrna Monreal, MD
Chief Radiology . . . . Raymond Larue, MD
Director Respiratory Therapy . . . . Kimberly Peterson

Measure	Cases	This Hospital	State Average	U.S. Average	Top Hospital
Heart Attack Care					
ACE Inhibitor or ARB for LVSD[1]	2	100%	83%	82%	100%
Aspirin at Arrival[1]	13	62%	93%	92%	100%
Aspirin at Discharge[1]	4	50%	88%	90%	100%
Beta Blocker at Arrival[1]	12	83%	89%	87%	100%
Beta Blocker at Discharge[1]	7	71%	92%	90%	100%
Fibrinolytic Medication Timing	0	-	33%	31%	100%
PCI Within 90 Minutes of Arrival	0	-	52%	54%	95%
Smoking Cessation Advice	0	-	92%	88%	100%
Heart Failure Care					
ACE Inhibitor or ARB for LVSD	37	86%	82%	82%	100%
Discharge Instructions	139	25%	61%	61%	93%
Evaluation of LVS Function	159	69%	90%	83%	99%
Smoking Cessation Advice	35	77%	91%	82%	100%
Pneumonia Care					
Appropriate Initial Antibiotic	108	58%	84%	83%	94%
Blood Culture Timing	73	85%	88%	90%	100%
Influenza Vaccine[1]	24	25%	64%	70%	100%
Initial Antibiotic Timing	122	73%	74%	80%	93%
Oxygenation Assessment	152	100%	99%	99%	100%
Pneumococcal Vaccine	82	24%	67%	69%	94%
Smoking Cessation Advice	40	75%	90%	80%	100%
Surgical Infection Prevention					
Prophylactic Antibiotic Given[2]	36	44%	83%	77%	95%
Prophylactic Antibiotic Selection[1,2]	5	40%	90%	90%	100%
Prophylactic Antibiotic Stopped[2]	36	75%	70%	72%	95%
Pregnancy Care					
Inpatient Neonatal Mortality	-	-	-	-	-
Third or Fourth Degree Laceration	-	-	2.71%	3.63%	3.27%

Glades General Hospital

1201 South Main Street   Phone: 561-996-6571
Belle Glade, FL 33430   Fax: 561-996-2898
URL: www.gladesgeneral.org
Ownership: Government - Local
Emergency Services: Yes   Accredited: Yes
    Licensed Beds: 73

Key Personnel:

CEO . . . . Ruth McDaniel
Chief Medical Staff . . . . Antonio Mendez, MD
Emergency Room Director . . . . Sharon Jones
Infection Control . . . . Nancy O'Neal
Respiratory/Cardiopulmonary Director . . . . Richard Young

Measure	Cases	This Hospital	State Average	U.S. Average	Top Hospital
Heart Attack Care					
ACE Inhibitor or ARB for LVSD[3]	0	-	83%	82%	100%
Aspirin at Arrival[1,3]	8	100%	93%	92%	100%
Aspirin at Discharge[1,3]	2	100%	88%	90%	100%
Beta Blocker at Arrival[1,3]	6	100%	89%	87%	100%
Beta Blocker at Discharge[1,3]	2	100%	92%	90%	100%
Fibrinolytic Medication Timing[3]	0	-	33%	31%	100%
PCI Within 90 Minutes of Arrival	0	-	52%	54%	95%
Smoking Cessation Advice[1,3]	1	0%	92%	88%	100%
Heart Failure Care					
ACE Inhibitor or ARB for LVSD[3]	51	88%	82%	82%	100%
Discharge Instructions[3]	122	89%	61%	61%	93%

Measure	Cases	This Hospital	State Average	U.S. Average	Top Hospital
Evaluation of LVS Function[3]	128	99%	90%	83%	99%
Smoking Cessation Advice[3]	26	96%	91%	82%	100%
Pneumonia Care					
Appropriate Initial Antibiotic[3]	50	82%	84%	83%	94%
Blood Culture Timing	55	85%	88%	90%	100%
Influenza Vaccine[4,5]	-	-	64%	70%	100%
Initial Antibiotic Timing[3]	55	82%	74%	80%	93%
Oxygenation Assessment[3]	66	100%	99%	99%	100%
Pneumococcal Vaccine[3]	26	85%	67%	69%	94%
Smoking Cessation Advice[1,3]	12	83%	90%	80%	100%
Surgical Infection Prevention					
Prophylactic Antibiotic Given[1,3]	24	96%	83%	77%	95%
Prophylactic Antibiotic Selection[1]	8	100%	90%	90%	100%
Prophylactic Antibiotic Stopped[1,3]	23	91%	70%	72%	95%
Pregnancy Care					
Inpatient Neonatal Mortality	-	-	-	-	-
Third or Fourth Degree Laceration	-	-	2.71%	3.63%	3.27%

Boca Raton Community Hospital

800 Meadows Rd   Phone: 561-362-5002
Boca Raton, FL 33486
Ownership: Voluntary non-profit - Private   Accredited: Yes
Emergency Services: Yes

Measure	Cases	This Hospital	State Average	U.S. Average	Top Hospital
Heart Attack Care					
ACE Inhibitor or ARB for LVSD[1]	17	82%	83%	82%	100%
Aspirin at Arrival	126	90%	93%	92%	100%
Aspirin at Discharge	42	86%	88%	90%	100%
Beta Blocker at Arrival	127	87%	89%	87%	100%
Beta Blocker at Discharge	53	94%	92%	90%	100%
Fibrinolytic Medication Timing[1]	2	0%	33%	31%	100%
PCI Within 90 Minutes of Arrival	0	-	52%	54%	95%
Smoking Cessation Advice[1]	8	62%	92%	88%	100%
Heart Failure Care					
ACE Inhibitor or ARB for LVSD	206	72%	82%	82%	100%
Discharge Instructions	460	88%	61%	61%	93%
Evaluation of LVS Function	614	87%	90%	83%	99%
Smoking Cessation Advice	26	85%	91%	82%	100%
Pneumonia Care					
Appropriate Initial Antibiotic	289	88%	84%	83%	94%
Blood Culture Timing	239	86%	88%	90%	100%
Influenza Vaccine	85	41%	64%	70%	100%
Initial Antibiotic Timing	304	79%	74%	80%	93%
Oxygenation Assessment	421	98%	99%	99%	100%
Pneumococcal Vaccine	309	53%	67%	69%	94%
Smoking Cessation Advice	35	80%	90%	80%	100%
Surgical Infection Prevention					
Prophylactic Antibiotic Given	1,075	82%	83%	77%	95%
Prophylactic Antibiotic Selection	210	78%	90%	90%	100%
Prophylactic Antibiotic Stopped	1,036	71%	70%	72%	95%
Pregnancy Care					
Inpatient Neonatal Mortality[2]	413	0.00%	-	-	-
Third or Fourth Degree Laceration	1,144	4.20%	2.71%	3.63%	3.27%

West Boca Medical Center

21644 State Road 7   Phone: 561-488-8000
Boca Raton, FL 33428   Fax: 561-488-8105
URL: www.westbocamedctr.com
Ownership: Proprietary   Accredited: Yes
Emergency Services: Yes   Licensed Beds: 185

Key Personnel:

CEO . . . . Walt Mickens
Chief Medical Officer . . . . Dr Jennifer Daley
Director Medical/Surgical Nursing . . . . Candace Carracher
Chief Radiology . . . . Lee Katims, MD
Director Respiratory Therapy . . . . Mike Davis

Measure	Cases	This Hospital	State Average	U.S. Average	Top Hospital
Heart Attack Care					
ACE Inhibitor or ARB for LVSD[1]	12	92%	83%	82%	100%
Aspirin at Arrival	119	97%	93%	92%	100%

NOTE: Hospital profiles are in alphabetical order by state, then city, then hospital within the city; Rankings are sorted by rate in descending order and exclude hospitals with less than 25 cases; (1) The number of cases is too small (n<25) for purposes of reliably predicting hospital performance; (2) Measure reflects the hospital's indication that its submission was based upon a sample of its relevant discharges; (3) Rate reflects fewer than the maximum possible quarters of data for the measure; (4) Inaccurate information submitted and suppressed for one or more quarters; (5) No data is available from the hospital for this measure; Please refer to the User's Guide for a full explanation of data

Aspirin at Discharge	57	95%	88%	90%	100%
Beta Blocker at Arrival	118	98%	89%	87%	100%
Beta Blocker at Discharge	61	93%	92%	90%	100%
Fibrinolytic Medication Timing[1]	4	75%	33%	31%	100%
PCI Within 90 Minutes of Arrival	0	-	52%	54%	95%
Smoking Cessation Advice[1]	2	100%	92%	88%	100%
Heart Failure Care					
ACE Inhibitor or ARB for LVSD	52	96%	82%	82%	100%
Discharge Instructions	168	81%	61%	61%	93%
Evaluation of LVS Function	223	93%	90%	83%	99%
Smoking Cessation Advice[1]	14	100%	91%	82%	100%
Pneumonia Care					
Appropriate Initial Antibiotic	192	88%	84%	83%	94%
Blood Culture Timing	171	92%	88%	90%	100%
Influenza Vaccine	44	80%	64%	70%	100%
Initial Antibiotic Timing	234	90%	74%	80%	93%
Oxygenation Assessment	268	99%	99%	99%	100%
Pneumococcal Vaccine	160	78%	67%	69%	94%
Smoking Cessation Advice	32	100%	90%	80%	100%
Surgical Infection Prevention					
Prophylactic Antibiotic Given[2]	163	90%	83%	77%	95%
Prophylactic Antibiotic Selection[2]	42	88%	90%	90%	100%
Prophylactic Antibiotic Stopped[2]	162	70%	70%	72%	95%
Pregnancy Care					
Inpatient Neonatal Mortality	-	-	-	-	-
Third or Fourth Degree Laceration	-	-	2.71%	3.63%	3.27%

Doctors Memorial Hospital

401 E Byrd Ave
Bonifay, FL 32425
URL: www.doctorsmemorialhospital.com
Ownership: Govt - Hospital District or Authority
Emergency Services: Yes

Phone: 850-547-1120
Fax: 850-547-4413

Accredited: Yes
Licensed Beds: 34

Key Personnel:
CEO. . . . . Robert Winkler
Chief Medical Staff. Mohammad Yunus
Emergency Room . . . . Joanne Royalty
Infection Control. . . . . Marta Peck

Measure	Cases	This Hospital	State Average	U.S. Average	Top Hospital
Heart Attack Care					
ACE Inhibitor or ARB for LVSD[5]	-	-	83%	82%	100%
Aspirin at Arrival[5]	-	-	93%	92%	100%
Aspirin at Discharge[5]	-	-	88%	90%	100%
Beta Blocker at Arrival[5]	-	-	89%	87%	100%
Beta Blocker at Discharge[5]	-	-	92%	90%	100%
Fibrinolytic Medication Timing[5]	-	-	33%	31%	100%
PCI Within 90 Minutes of Arrival[5]	-	-	52%	54%	95%
Smoking Cessation Advice[5]	-	-	92%	88%	100%
Heart Failure Care					
ACE Inhibitor or ARB for LVSD[1]	8	38%	82%	82%	100%
Discharge Instructions	48	90%	61%	61%	93%
Evaluation of LVS Function	74	22%	90%	83%	99%
Smoking Cessation Advice[1]	17	94%	91%	82%	100%
Pneumonia Care					
Appropriate Initial Antibiotic	60	67%	84%	83%	94%
Blood Culture Timing[1]	7	86%	88%	90%	100%
Influenza Vaccine[1]	15	87%	64%	70%	100%
Initial Antibiotic Timing	61	79%	74%	80%	93%
Oxygenation Assessment	82	88%	99%	99%	100%
Pneumococcal Vaccine	39	79%	67%	69%	94%
Smoking Cessation Advice[1]	19	89%	90%	80%	100%
Surgical Infection Prevention					
Prophylactic Antibiotic Given[5]	-	-	83%	77%	95%
Prophylactic Antibiotic Selection[5]	-	-	90%	90%	100%
Prophylactic Antibiotic Stopped[5]	-	-	70%	72%	95%
Pregnancy Care					
Inpatient Neonatal Mortality	-	-	-	-	-
Third or Fourth Degree Laceration	-	-	2.71%	3.63%	3.27%

Bethesda Memorial Hospital

2815 South Seacrest Boulevard
Boynton Beach, FL 33435
URL: www.bethesdahealthcare.com
Ownership: Voluntary non-profit - Private
Emergency Services: Yes

Phone: 561-737-7733
Fax: 561-737-4534

Accredited: Yes
Licensed Beds: 362

Key Personnel:
President/CEO. . . . . Robert B Hill
Medical Director Emergency Department. . . . . . Christopher Schirmer, MD

Measure	Cases	This Hospital	State Average	U.S. Average	Top Hospital
Heart Attack Care					
ACE Inhibitor or ARB for LVSD[1]	18	89%	83%	82%	100%
Aspirin at Arrival	125	90%	93%	92%	100%
Aspirin at Discharge	69	93%	88%	90%	100%
Beta Blocker at Arrival	77	79%	89%	87%	100%
Beta Blocker at Discharge	92	96%	92%	90%	100%
Fibrinolytic Medication Timing	0	-	33%	31%	100%
PCI Within 90 Minutes of Arrival	0	-	52%	54%	95%
Smoking Cessation Advice[1]	11	100%	92%	88%	100%
Heart Failure Care					
ACE Inhibitor or ARB for LVSD	78	77%	82%	82%	100%
Discharge Instructions	204	63%	61%	61%	93%
Evaluation of LVS Function	263	95%	90%	83%	99%
Smoking Cessation Advice[1]	21	100%	91%	82%	100%
Pneumonia Care					
Appropriate Initial Antibiotic	139	88%	84%	83%	94%
Blood Culture Timing	134	87%	88%	90%	100%
Influenza Vaccine	41	85%	64%	70%	100%
Initial Antibiotic Timing	237	82%	74%	80%	93%
Oxygenation Assessment	263	100%	99%	99%	100%
Pneumococcal Vaccine	162	86%	67%	69%	94%
Smoking Cessation Advice	48	98%	90%	80%	100%
Surgical Infection Prevention					
Prophylactic Antibiotic Given	206	97%	83%	77%	95%
Prophylactic Antibiotic Selection	41	98%	90%	90%	100%
Prophylactic Antibiotic Stopped	193	62%	70%	72%	95%
Pregnancy Care					
Inpatient Neonatal Mortality[2]	766	0.26%	-	-	-
Third or Fourth Degree Laceration[2]	544	2.57%	2.71%	3.63%	3.27%

Blake Medical Center

2020 59th Street W
Bradenton, FL 34209
URL: www.blakemedicalcenter.com
Ownership: Proprietary
Emergency Services: Yes

Phone: 941-792-6611

Accredited: Yes
Licensed Beds: 383

Key Personnel:
CEO. . . . . Daniel J Friedrich III
Chief Medical Staff. Janine Mylett, MD

Measure	Cases	This Hospital	State Average	U.S. Average	Top Hospital
Heart Attack Care					
ACE Inhibitor or ARB for LVSD	67	85%	83%	82%	100%
Aspirin at Arrival	312	95%	93%	92%	100%
Aspirin at Discharge	282	97%	88%	90%	100%
Beta Blocker at Arrival	228	93%	89%	87%	100%
Beta Blocker at Discharge	249	97%	92%	90%	100%
Fibrinolytic Medication Timing[1]	3	33%	33%	31%	100%
PCI Within 90 Minutes of Arrival[1]	4	50%	52%	54%	95%
Smoking Cessation Advice	73	97%	92%	88%	100%
Heart Failure Care					
ACE Inhibitor or ARB for LVSD	130	84%	82%	82%	100%
Discharge Instructions	408	71%	61%	61%	93%
Evaluation of LVS Function	514	91%	90%	83%	99%
Smoking Cessation Advice	47	98%	91%	82%	100%
Pneumonia Care					
Appropriate Initial Antibiotic	217	87%	84%	83%	94%
Blood Culture Timing	159	90%	88%	90%	100%
Influenza Vaccine	75	56%	64%	70%	100%
Initial Antibiotic Timing	272	64%	74%	80%	93%
Oxygenation Assessment	322	100%	99%	99%	100%

NOTE: Hospital profiles are in alphabetical order by state, then city, then hospital within the city; Rankings are sorted by rate in descending order and exclude hospitals with less than 25 cases; (1) The number of cases is too small (n<25) for purposes of reliably predicting hospital performance; (2) Measure reflects the hospital's indication that its submission was based upon a sample of its relevant discharges; (3) Rate reflects fewer than the maximum possible quarters of data for the measure; (4) Inaccurate information submitted and suppressed for one or more quarters; (5) No data is available from the hospital for this measure; Please refer to the User's Guide for a full explanation of data

Pneumococcal Vaccine	231	60%	67%	69%	94%
Smoking Cessation Advice	45	96%	90%	80%	100%

Surgical Infection Prevention					
Prophylactic Antibiotic Given[2]	895	86%	83%	77%	95%
Prophylactic Antibiotic Selection[2]	96	95%	90%	90%	100%
Prophylactic Antibiotic Stopped[2]	878	39%	70%	72%	95%

Pregnancy Care					
Inpatient Neonatal Mortality	-	-	-	-	-
Third or Fourth Degree Laceration	-	-	2.71%	3.63%	3.27%

Lakewood Ranch Medical Center

8330 Lakewood Ranch Boulevard
Bradenton, FL 34202
URL: www.lakewoodranchmedicalcenter.com
Ownership: Proprietary
Emergency Services: Yes

Phone: 941-782-2100
Fax: 941-782-2575

Accredited: Yes
Licensed Beds: 120

Key Personnel:
CEO. . . . . Lynn M Mergen
Chief OB/Pediatrics . . . . Jorge Alvarez, MD
Chief Surgery. . . . . Allesandro Golino, MD

Measure	Cases	This Hospital	State Average	U.S. Average	Top Hospital
Heart Attack Care					
ACE Inhibitor or ARB for LVSD[1]	7	86%	83%	82%	100%
Aspirin at Arrival	46	83%	93%	92%	100%
Aspirin at Discharge[1]	23	74%	88%	90%	100%
Beta Blocker at Arrival	47	79%	89%	87%	100%
Beta Blocker at Discharge[1]	23	83%	92%	90%	100%
Fibrinolytic Medication Timing[1]	3	33%	33%	31%	100%
PCI Within 90 Minutes of Arrival	0	-	52%	54%	95%
Smoking Cessation Advice[1]	3	33%	92%	88%	100%
Heart Failure Care					
ACE Inhibitor or ARB for LVSD[1]	19	79%	82%	82%	100%
Discharge Instructions	66	62%	61%	61%	93%
Evaluation of LVS Function	78	91%	90%	83%	99%
Smoking Cessation Advice[1]	6	100%	91%	82%	100%
Pneumonia Care					
Appropriate Initial Antibiotic	93	84%	84%	83%	94%
Blood Culture Timing	82	85%	88%	90%	100%
Influenza Vaccine[1]	16	69%	64%	70%	100%
Initial Antibiotic Timing	100	81%	74%	80%	93%
Oxygenation Assessment	127	100%	99%	99%	100%
Pneumococcal Vaccine	77	70%	67%	69%	94%
Smoking Cessation Advice[1]	23	65%	90%	80%	100%
Surgical Infection Prevention					
Prophylactic Antibiotic Given	155	81%	83%	77%	95%
Prophylactic Antibiotic Selection	26	88%	90%	90%	100%
Prophylactic Antibiotic Stopped	145	61%	70%	72%	95%
Pregnancy Care					
Inpatient Neonatal Mortality	-	-	-	-	-
Third or Fourth Degree Laceration	-	-	2.71%	3.63%	3.27%

Manatee Memorial Hospital

206 2nd Street E
Bradenton, FL 34208
E-mail: betty.chambliss@mmhhs.com
URL: www.manateememorial.com
Ownership: Voluntary non-profit - Private
Emergency Services: Yes

Phone: 941-745-6862
Fax: 941-745-6826

Accredited: Yes
Licensed Beds: 319

Key Personnel:
CEO. . . . . Moody L Chisholm
Catheterization Lab . . . . Paula Jefferson
Emergency Room Director. . . . . Linda Antes
Director-Surgery. . . . . Dan Magnusson
Respiratory/Cardiopulmonary Director . . . . Tom Andrews

Measure	Cases	This Hospital	State Average	U.S. Average	Top Hospital
Heart Attack Care					
ACE Inhibitor or ARB for LVSD	93	75%	83%	82%	100%
Aspirin at Arrival	414	95%	93%	92%	100%
Aspirin at Discharge	410	91%	88%	90%	100%
Beta Blocker at Arrival	364	89%	89%	87%	100%

Beta Blocker at Discharge	422	87%	92%	90%	100%
Fibrinolytic Medication Timing[1]	11	45%	33%	31%	100%
PCI Within 90 Minutes of Arrival[1]	14	64%	52%	54%	95%
Smoking Cessation Advice	154	95%	92%	88%	100%
Heart Failure Care					
ACE Inhibitor or ARB for LVSD	233	83%	82%	82%	100%
Discharge Instructions	475	84%	61%	61%	93%
Evaluation of LVS Function	630	94%	90%	83%	99%
Smoking Cessation Advice	144	94%	91%	82%	100%
Pneumonia Care					
Appropriate Initial Antibiotic	215	85%	84%	83%	94%
Blood Culture Timing	153	85%	88%	90%	100%
Influenza Vaccine	50	64%	64%	70%	100%
Initial Antibiotic Timing	264	70%	74%	80%	93%
Oxygenation Assessment	312	99%	99%	99%	100%
Pneumococcal Vaccine	181	79%	67%	69%	94%
Smoking Cessation Advice	77	90%	90%	80%	100%
Surgical Infection Prevention					
Prophylactic Antibiotic Given[3]	468	80%	83%	77%	95%
Prophylactic Antibiotic Selection	126	90%	90%	90%	100%
Prophylactic Antibiotic Stopped[3]	452	62%	70%	72%	95%
Pregnancy Care					
Inpatient Neonatal Mortality	-	-	-	-	-
Third or Fourth Degree Laceration	-	-	2.71%	3.63%	3.27%

Brandon Regional Hospital

Alternate Name: Humana Hospital-Brandon
119 Oakfield Drive
Brandon, FL 33511
URL: www.brandonhospital.com
Ownership: Proprietary
Emergency Services: Yes

Phone: 813-681-5551
Fax: 813-654-7203

Accredited: Yes
Licensed Beds: 277

Key Personnel:
CEO. . . . . Michael M Fencel
Cardiac Lab . . . . Leela Beers
Emergency Room . . . . Kathy Haddix-Hill
Intensive Coronary. . . . . Jim Milhollen
Chief Radiology . . . . Steve Rueter, MD
Director Respiratory Therapy . . . . Dave Mattson

Measure	Cases	This Hospital	State Average	U.S. Average	Top Hospital
Heart Attack Care					
ACE Inhibitor or ARB for LVSD	107	70%	83%	82%	100%
Aspirin at Arrival	361	95%	93%	92%	100%
Aspirin at Discharge	350	87%	88%	90%	100%
Beta Blocker at Arrival	230	87%	89%	87%	100%
Beta Blocker at Discharge	434	95%	92%	90%	100%
Fibrinolytic Medication Timing	0	-	33%	31%	100%
PCI Within 90 Minutes of Arrival[1]	20	60%	52%	54%	95%
Smoking Cessation Advice	180	98%	92%	88%	100%
Heart Failure Care					
ACE Inhibitor or ARB for LVSD	179	60%	82%	82%	100%
Discharge Instructions	350	34%	61%	61%	93%
Evaluation of LVS Function	445	95%	90%	83%	99%
Smoking Cessation Advice	71	93%	91%	82%	100%
Pneumonia Care					
Appropriate Initial Antibiotic	319	80%	84%	83%	94%
Blood Culture Timing	161	78%	88%	90%	100%
Influenza Vaccine	61	44%	64%	70%	100%
Initial Antibiotic Timing	388	49%	74%	80%	93%
Oxygenation Assessment	466	99%	99%	99%	100%
Pneumococcal Vaccine	264	44%	67%	69%	94%
Smoking Cessation Advice	116	98%	90%	80%	100%
Surgical Infection Prevention					
Prophylactic Antibiotic Given[2]	299	77%	83%	77%	95%
Prophylactic Antibiotic Selection[2]	99	82%	90%	90%	100%
Prophylactic Antibiotic Stopped[2]	283	63%	70%	72%	95%
Pregnancy Care					
Inpatient Neonatal Mortality	-	-	-	-	-
Third or Fourth Degree Laceration	-	-	2.71%	3.63%	3.27%

NOTE: Hospital profiles are in alphabetical order by state, then city, then hospital within the city; Rankings are sorted by rate in descending order and exclude hospitals with less than 25 cases; (1) The number of cases is too small (n<25) for purposes of reliably predicting hospital performance; (2) Measure reflects the hospital's indication that its submission was based upon a sample of its relevant discharges; (3) Rate reflects fewer than the maximum possible quarters of data for the measure; (4) Inaccurate information submitted and suppressed for one or more quarters; (5) No data is available from the hospital for this measure; Please refer to the User's Guide for a full explanation of data

Brooksville Regional Hospital

17240 Cortez Blvd
Brooksville, FL 34601
E-mail: elaine.rothen@brh.hma-corp.com
URL: www.brooksvilleregionalhospital.org
Ownership: Proprietary
Emergency Services: Yes

Phone: 352-796-5111
Fax: 352-544-5711

Accredited: Yes
Licensed Beds: 120

Key Personnel:
President/CEO.......................... Thomas D Barb
Chief Medical Staff...................... R.L. Rao, MD
Catheterization Lab .... Sheryl Clemente
Emergency Room .... Tracey Dellea, RN
Infection Control........................ Susan Napoleon
ICU .... Gina Swaggerty, RN
Medical Surgical Nursing .... Donna Carlsen
Respiratory/Cardiopulmonary............. Michael Alford

Measure	Cases	This Hospital	State Average	U.S. Average	Top Hospital
Heart Attack Care					
ACE Inhibitor or ARB for LVSD[1]	22	73%	83%	82%	100%
Aspirin at Arrival	164	87%	93%	92%	100%
Aspirin at Discharge	59	76%	88%	90%	100%
Beta Blocker at Arrival	157	89%	89%	87%	100%
Beta Blocker at Discharge	75	91%	92%	90%	100%
Fibrinolytic Medication Timing[1]	13	69%	33%	31%	100%
PCI Within 90 Minutes of Arrival	0	-	52%	54%	95%
Smoking Cessation Advice[1]	17	100%	92%	88%	100%
Heart Failure Care					
ACE Inhibitor or ARB for LVSD	141	82%	82%	82%	100%
Discharge Instructions	336	32%	61%	61%	93%
Evaluation of LVS Function	396	92%	90%	83%	99%
Smoking Cessation Advice	86	99%	91%	82%	100%
Pneumonia Care					
Appropriate Initial Antibiotic	227	85%	84%	83%	94%
Blood Culture Timing	185	93%	88%	90%	100%
Influenza Vaccine	66	79%	64%	70%	100%
Initial Antibiotic Timing	284	77%	74%	80%	93%
Oxygenation Assessment	347	100%	99%	99%	100%
Pneumococcal Vaccine	191	84%	67%	69%	94%
Smoking Cessation Advice	92	100%	90%	80%	100%
Surgical Infection Prevention					
Prophylactic Antibiotic Given[2]	387	89%	83%	77%	95%
Prophylactic Antibiotic Selection[2]	55	93%	90%	90%	100%
Prophylactic Antibiotic Stopped[2]	372	69%	70%	72%	95%
Pregnancy Care					
Inpatient Neonatal Mortality	-	-	-	-	-
Third or Fourth Degree Laceration	-	-	2.71%	3.63%	3.27%

Oak Hill Hospital

11375 Cortez Boulevard
Brooksville, FL 34613
URL: www.oakhillhospital.com
Ownership: Proprietary
Emergency Services: Yes

Phone: 352-596-6632
Fax: 352-597-3024

Accredited: Yes
Licensed Beds: 204

Key Personnel:
CEO.................................. Mickey Smith
Chief of Medical Staff................... Mahmoud Nimer, MD
CNO.................................. Walt Pannong, PhD

Measure	Cases	This Hospital	State Average	U.S. Average	Top Hospital
Heart Attack Care					
ACE Inhibitor or ARB for LVSD	39	87%	83%	82%	100%
Aspirin at Arrival	223	87%	93%	92%	100%
Aspirin at Discharge	158	73%	88%	90%	100%
Beta Blocker at Arrival	189	83%	89%	87%	100%
Beta Blocker at Discharge	176	85%	92%	90%	100%
Fibrinolytic Medication Timing[1]	3	100%	33%	31%	100%
PCI Within 90 Minutes of Arrival[1]	10	60%	52%	54%	95%
Smoking Cessation Advice	48	98%	92%	88%	100%
Heart Failure Care					
ACE Inhibitor or ARB for LVSD	108	71%	82%	82%	100%
Discharge Instructions	357	25%	61%	61%	93%
Evaluation of LVS Function	418	80%	90%	83%	99%

Measure	Cases	This Hospital	State Average	U.S. Average	Top Hospital
Smoking Cessation Advice	61	93%	91%	82%	100%
Pneumonia Care					
Appropriate Initial Antibiotic	237	79%	84%	83%	94%
Blood Culture Timing	149	86%	88%	90%	100%
Influenza Vaccine	68	43%	64%	70%	100%
Initial Antibiotic Timing	321	63%	74%	80%	93%
Oxygenation Assessment	360	98%	99%	99%	100%
Pneumococcal Vaccine	249	49%	67%	69%	94%
Smoking Cessation Advice	72	97%	90%	80%	100%
Surgical Infection Prevention					
Prophylactic Antibiotic Given[3]	435	87%	83%	77%	95%
Prophylactic Antibiotic Selection	126	96%	90%	90%	100%
Prophylactic Antibiotic Stopped[3]	414	57%	70%	72%	95%
Pregnancy Care					
Inpatient Neonatal Mortality	-	-	-	-	-
Third or Fourth Degree Laceration	-	-	2.71%	3.63%	3.27%

Cape Coral Hospital

636 Del Prado Blvd
Cape Coral, FL 33990
Ownership: Voluntary non-profit - Private
Emergency Services: Yes

Phone: 239-574-2323

Accredited: Yes

Measure	Cases	This Hospital	State Average	U.S. Average	Top Hospital
Heart Attack Care					
ACE Inhibitor or ARB for LVSD[1]	15	80%	83%	82%	100%
Aspirin at Arrival	93	94%	93%	92%	100%
Aspirin at Discharge	49	96%	88%	90%	100%
Beta Blocker at Arrival	73	89%	89%	87%	100%
Beta Blocker at Discharge	62	95%	92%	90%	100%
Fibrinolytic Medication Timing	0	-	33%	31%	100%
PCI Within 90 Minutes of Arrival	0	-	52%	54%	95%
Smoking Cessation Advice[1]	9	89%	92%	88%	100%
Heart Failure Care					
ACE Inhibitor or ARB for LVSD	49	84%	82%	82%	100%
Discharge Instructions	117	44%	61%	61%	93%
Evaluation of LVS Function	143	90%	90%	83%	99%
Smoking Cessation Advice[1]	23	96%	91%	82%	100%
Pneumonia Care					
Appropriate Initial Antibiotic[2]	92	83%	84%	83%	94%
Blood Culture Timing[2]	97	90%	88%	90%	100%
Influenza Vaccine[1]	21	71%	64%	70%	100%
Initial Antibiotic Timing[2]	121	83%	74%	80%	93%
Oxygenation Assessment[2]	140	100%	99%	99%	100%
Pneumococcal Vaccine[2]	95	81%	67%	69%	94%
Smoking Cessation Advice[2]	30	93%	90%	80%	100%
Surgical Infection Prevention					
Prophylactic Antibiotic Given	105	90%	83%	77%	95%
Prophylactic Antibiotic Selection	41	90%	90%	90%	100%
Prophylactic Antibiotic Stopped	100	71%	70%	72%	95%
Pregnancy Care					
Inpatient Neonatal Mortality	-	-	-	-	-
Third or Fourth Degree Laceration	-	-	2.71%	3.63%	3.27%

Northwest Florida Community Hospital

1360 Brickyard Road
Chipley, FL 32428
E-mail: marketing@nfch.org
URL: www.nfch.org
Ownership: Govt - Hospital District or Authority
Emergency Services: Yes

Phone: 850-638-1610
Fax: 850-638-6106

Accredited: Yes
Licensed Beds: 59

Key Personnel:
President .... Patrick A Schlenker
Chief Medical Staff...................... Samuel E Ward, MD
Director Infection/Disease Control .... Michelle W Fuller, RN
CCU Spvg. Nurse .... Anita Dowd, RN
Director Radiology .... Kim Hardy
Director Respiratory Therapy .... Larry Smith

Measure	Cases	This Hospital	State Average	U.S. Average	Top Hospital
Heart Attack Care					
ACE Inhibitor or ARB for LVSD[3]	0	-	83%	82%	100%

NOTE: Hospital profiles are in alphabetical order by state, then city, then hospital within the city; Rankings are sorted by rate in descending order and exclude hospitals with less than 25 cases; (1) The number of cases is too small (n<25) for purposes of reliably predicting hospital performance; (2) Measure reflects the hospital's indication that its submission was based upon a sample of its relevant discharges; (3) Rate reflects fewer than the maximum possible quarters of data for the measure; (4) Inaccurate information submitted and suppressed for one or more quarters; (5) No data is available from the hospital for this measure; Please refer to the User's Guide for a full explanation of data

Measure	Cases	This Hospital	State Average	U.S. Average	Top Hospital
Aspirin at Arrival[3]	0	-	93%	92%	100%
Aspirin at Discharge[3]	0	-	88%	90%	100%
Beta Blocker at Arrival[3]	0	-	89%	87%	100%
Beta Blocker at Discharge[3]	0	-	92%	90%	100%
Fibrinolytic Medication Timing[3]	0	-	33%	31%	100%
PCI Within 90 Minutes of Arrival[5]	-	-	52%	54%	95%
Smoking Cessation Advice[3]	0	-	92%	88%	100%
Heart Failure Care					
ACE Inhibitor or ARB for LVSD[1]	13	100%	82%	82%	100%
Discharge Instructions	35	26%	61%	61%	93%
Evaluation of LVS Function	40	60%	90%	83%	99%
Smoking Cessation Advice[1]	7	100%	91%	82%	100%
Pneumonia Care					
Appropriate Initial Antibiotic	33	85%	84%	83%	94%
Blood Culture Timing[1]	20	95%	88%	90%	100%
Influenza Vaccine[1]	7	100%	64%	70%	100%
Initial Antibiotic Timing	41	80%	74%	80%	93%
Oxygenation Assessment	46	100%	99%	99%	100%
Pneumococcal Vaccine[1]	16	62%	67%	69%	94%
Smoking Cessation Advice[1]	14	79%	90%	80%	100%
Surgical Infection Prevention					
Prophylactic Antibiotic Given[5]	-	-	83%	77%	95%
Prophylactic Antibiotic Selection[5]	-	-	90%	90%	100%
Prophylactic Antibiotic Stopped[5]	-	-	70%	72%	95%
Pregnancy Care					
Inpatient Neonatal Mortality	-	-	-	-	-
Third or Fourth Degree Laceration	-	-	2.71%	3.63%	3.27%

Morton Plant Hospital

300 Pinellas Street
Clearwater, FL 33756
URL: www.mortonplant.com
Ownership: Voluntary non-profit - Private
Emergency Services: Yes

Phone: 727-462-7000
Fax: 727-461-8101

Accredited: Yes
Licensed Beds: 687

Key Personnel:
President/CEO. . . . . Philip K Beauchamp, FACHE
Chief Medical Staff. . . . . John Babka, MD
Emergency Room . . . . Cheryl Young, RN
Director Infection/Disease Control . . . . Rebecca Carlson
CCU Spvg. Nurse . . . . Jackie Munroe
Director Medical/Surgical Nursing . . . . Pat Donnelly
Director Radiology . . . . Paul Amberg
Director Respiratory Therapy . . . . Terry Beard

Measure	Cases	This Hospital	State Average	U.S. Average	Top Hospital
Heart Attack Care					
ACE Inhibitor or ARB for LVSD	155	96%	83%	82%	100%
Aspirin at Arrival	415	97%	93%	92%	100%
Aspirin at Discharge	601	98%	88%	90%	100%
Beta Blocker at Arrival	245	94%	89%	87%	100%
Beta Blocker at Discharge	695	99%	92%	90%	100%
Fibrinolytic Medication Timing	0	-	33%	31%	100%
PCI Within 90 Minutes of Arrival	0	-	52%	54%	95%
Smoking Cessation Advice	232	97%	92%	88%	100%
Heart Failure Care					
ACE Inhibitor or ARB for LVSD	240	90%	82%	82%	100%
Discharge Instructions	523	67%	61%	61%	93%
Evaluation of LVS Function	701	93%	90%	83%	99%
Smoking Cessation Advice	93	100%	91%	82%	100%
Pneumonia Care					
Appropriate Initial Antibiotic	262	90%	84%	83%	94%
Blood Culture Timing	239	95%	88%	90%	100%
Influenza Vaccine	89	73%	64%	70%	100%
Initial Antibiotic Timing	289	65%	74%	80%	93%
Oxygenation Assessment	463	100%	99%	99%	100%
Pneumococcal Vaccine	312	72%	67%	69%	94%
Smoking Cessation Advice	102	91%	90%	80%	100%
Surgical Infection Prevention					
Prophylactic Antibiotic Given[2]	224	75%	83%	77%	95%
Prophylactic Antibiotic Selection[2]	67	87%	90%	90%	100%
Prophylactic Antibiotic Stopped[2]	200	92%	70%	72%	95%
Pregnancy Care					
Inpatient Neonatal Mortality	-	-	-	-	-

Measure	Cases	This Hospital	State Average	U.S. Average	Top Hospital
Third or Fourth Degree Laceration	-	-	2.71%	3.63%	3.27%

South Lake Hospital

1099 Citrus Tower Boulevard
Clermont, FL 34711
URL: www.southlakehospital.com
Ownership: Govt - Hospital District or Authority
Emergency Services: Yes

Phone: 352-394-4071
Fax: 352-241-7121

Accredited: Yes
Licensed Beds: 80

Key Personnel:
Executive Director/CEO. . . . . Leslie Longacre

Measure	Cases	This Hospital	State Average	U.S. Average	Top Hospital
Heart Attack Care					
ACE Inhibitor or ARB for LVSD[1]	9	56%	83%	82%	100%
Aspirin at Arrival	71	92%	93%	92%	100%
Aspirin at Discharge[1]	20	85%	88%	90%	100%
Beta Blocker at Arrival	43	84%	89%	87%	100%
Beta Blocker at Discharge	30	90%	92%	90%	100%
Fibrinolytic Medication Timing	0	-	33%	31%	100%
PCI Within 90 Minutes of Arrival	0	-	52%	54%	95%
Smoking Cessation Advice[1]	4	75%	92%	88%	100%
Heart Failure Care					
ACE Inhibitor or ARB for LVSD	75	76%	82%	82%	100%
Discharge Instructions	208	82%	61%	61%	93%
Evaluation of LVS Function	240	94%	90%	83%	99%
Smoking Cessation Advice	34	94%	91%	82%	100%
Pneumonia Care					
Appropriate Initial Antibiotic	92	91%	84%	83%	94%
Blood Culture Timing	92	87%	88%	90%	100%
Influenza Vaccine[4,5]	-	-	64%	70%	100%
Initial Antibiotic Timing	110	82%	74%	80%	93%
Oxygenation Assessment	144	100%	99%	99%	100%
Pneumococcal Vaccine	89	84%	67%	69%	94%
Smoking Cessation Advice	32	62%	90%	80%	100%
Surgical Infection Prevention					
Prophylactic Antibiotic Given	329	90%	83%	77%	95%
Prophylactic Antibiotic Selection	73	97%	90%	90%	100%
Prophylactic Antibiotic Stopped	326	92%	70%	72%	95%
Pregnancy Care					
Inpatient Neonatal Mortality	-	-	-	-	-
Third or Fourth Degree Laceration	-	-	2.71%	3.63%	3.27%

Hendry Regional Medical Center

Alternate Name: Hendry General Hospital
524 W Sagamore Ave
Clewiston, FL 33440
URL: www.HendryRegional.org
Ownership: Govt - Hospital District or Authority
Emergency Services: No

Phone: 863-983-9121
Fax: 863-983-0805

Accredited: Yes
Licensed Beds: 66

Key Personnel:
CEO. . . . . Craig R Cudworth
Chief Medical Staff. . . . . Adrian Fedele, MD
Emergency Room . . . . Tony Miracle
Director Infection/Disease Control . . . . Linda Reecer, RN
ICU . . . . Harriett Adams, RN
Director Medical/Surgical Nursing . . . . Alina Miracle, RN
Director Respiratory Therapy . . . . Ken Lazere

Measure	Cases	This Hospital	State Average	U.S. Average	Top Hospital
Heart Attack Care					
ACE Inhibitor or ARB for LVSD[1,3]	1	100%	83%	82%	100%
Aspirin at Arrival[1,3]	5	100%	93%	92%	100%
Aspirin at Discharge[1,3]	2	50%	88%	90%	100%
Beta Blocker at Arrival[1,3]	3	100%	89%	87%	100%
Beta Blocker at Discharge[1,3]	1	100%	92%	90%	100%
Fibrinolytic Medication Timing[1,3]	1	100%	33%	31%	100%
PCI Within 90 Minutes of Arrival	0	-	52%	54%	95%
Smoking Cessation Advice[1,3]	2	100%	92%	88%	100%
Heart Failure Care					
ACE Inhibitor or ARB for LVSD[1,3]	8	50%	82%	82%	100%
Discharge Instructions[3]	29	97%	61%	61%	93%
Evaluation of LVS Function[3]	30	70%	90%	83%	99%

NOTE: Hospital profiles are in alphabetical order by state, then city, then hospital within the city; Rankings are sorted by rate in descending order and exclude hospitals with less than 25 cases; (1) The number of cases is too small (n<25) for purposes of reliably predicting hospital performance; (2) Measure reflects the hospital's indication that its submission was based upon a sample of its relevant discharges; (3) Rate reflects fewer than the maximum possible quarters of data for the measure; (4) Inaccurate information submitted and suppressed for one or more quarters; (5) No data is available from the hospital for this measure; Please refer to the User's Guide for a full explanation of data

Measure	Cases	This Hospital	State Average	U.S. Average	Top Hospital
Smoking Cessation Advice[1,3]	6	100%	91%	82%	100%
Pneumonia Care					
Appropriate Initial Antibiotic[1,3]	12	92%	84%	83%	94%
Blood Culture Timing[1]	13	92%	88%	90%	100%
Influenza Vaccine[1]	1	0%	64%	70%	100%
Initial Antibiotic Timing[1,3]	9	56%	74%	80%	93%
Oxygenation Assessment[1,3]	15	100%	99%	99%	100%
Pneumococcal Vaccine[1,3]	7	86%	67%	69%	94%
Smoking Cessation Advice[1,3]	7	100%	90%	80%	100%
Surgical Infection Prevention					
Prophylactic Antibiotic Given[1,3]	3	100%	83%	77%	95%
Prophylactic Antibiotic Selection[5]	-	-	90%	90%	100%
Prophylactic Antibiotic Stopped[1,3]	3	100%	70%	72%	95%
Pregnancy Care					
Inpatient Neonatal Mortality	-	-	-	-	-
Third or Fourth Degree Laceration	-	-	2.71%	3.63%	3.27%

Cape Canaveral Hospital

Alternate Name: Cape Canaveral Hospital
701 W Cocoa Beach Causeway
Cocoa Beach, FL 32931
URL: www.health-first.org
Ownership: Voluntary non-profit - Private
Emergency Services: Yes

Phone: 321-799-7111
Fax: 321-799-8477

Accredited: Yes
Licensed Beds: 150

Key Personnel:
Chief Medical Staff. . . . . Thomas Garell
Director Infection/Disease Control . . . . Marilyn Zabin, RN
Chief Radiology . . . . Jeffrey Araj, MD

Measure	Cases	This Hospital	State Average	U.S. Average	Top Hospital
Heart Attack Care					
ACE Inhibitor or ARB for LVSD[1]	14	100%	83%	82%	100%
Aspirin at Arrival	90	97%	93%	92%	100%
Aspirin at Discharge	56	91%	88%	90%	100%
Beta Blocker at Arrival	100	95%	89%	87%	100%
Beta Blocker at Discharge	71	97%	92%	90%	100%
Fibrinolytic Medication Timing[1]	1	0%	33%	31%	100%
PCI Within 90 Minutes of Arrival	0	-	52%	54%	95%
Smoking Cessation Advice[1]	11	100%	92%	88%	100%
Heart Failure Care					
ACE Inhibitor or ARB for LVSD	95	89%	82%	82%	100%
Discharge Instructions	197	92%	61%	61%	93%
Evaluation of LVS Function	239	96%	90%	83%	99%
Smoking Cessation Advice	45	98%	91%	82%	100%
Pneumonia Care					
Appropriate Initial Antibiotic	192	89%	84%	83%	94%
Blood Culture Timing	203	95%	88%	90%	100%
Influenza Vaccine	57	96%	64%	70%	100%
Initial Antibiotic Timing	247	79%	74%	80%	93%
Oxygenation Assessment	286	100%	99%	99%	100%
Pneumococcal Vaccine	192	92%	67%	69%	94%
Smoking Cessation Advice	56	96%	90%	80%	100%
Surgical Infection Prevention					
Prophylactic Antibiotic Given[2]	437	96%	83%	77%	95%
Prophylactic Antibiotic Selection[2]	95	92%	90%	90%	100%
Prophylactic Antibiotic Stopped[2]	414	86%	70%	72%	95%
Pregnancy Care					
Inpatient Neonatal Mortality	-	-	-	-	-
Third or Fourth Degree Laceration	-	-	2.71%	3.63%	3.27%

Coral Gables Hospital

3100 Douglas Road
Miami, FL 33134
URL: www.coralgableshospital.com
Ownership: Proprietary
Emergency Services: Yes

Phone: 305-445-8461
Fax: 305-441-6879

Accredited: Yes
Licensed Beds: 273

Key Personnel:
CEO. . . . . Martha Garcia, RN
Emergency Room . . . . Donna Stevens, RN
Director Medical/Surgical Nursing . . . . Nelly Mercado, RN
OB/GYN Womens Health. . . . . Hernan Dominguez, MD
Chief Radiology . . . . Morton Blumberg, MD
Director Respiratory Therapy . . . . Donna Stevens, RN

Measure	Cases	This Hospital	State Average	U.S. Average	Top Hospital
Heart Attack Care					
ACE Inhibitor or ARB for LVSD[1]	12	83%	83%	82%	100%
Aspirin at Arrival	119	97%	93%	92%	100%
Aspirin at Discharge	59	81%	88%	90%	100%
Beta Blocker at Arrival	108	99%	89%	87%	100%
Beta Blocker at Discharge	64	95%	92%	90%	100%
Fibrinolytic Medication Timing[1]	8	50%	33%	31%	100%
PCI Within 90 Minutes of Arrival	0	-	52%	54%	95%
Smoking Cessation Advice[1]	6	100%	92%	88%	100%
Heart Failure Care					
ACE Inhibitor or ARB for LVSD	90	90%	82%	82%	100%
Discharge Instructions	223	94%	61%	61%	93%
Evaluation of LVS Function	295	96%	90%	83%	99%
Smoking Cessation Advice	27	100%	91%	82%	100%
Pneumonia Care					
Appropriate Initial Antibiotic	223	87%	84%	83%	94%
Blood Culture Timing	197	92%	88%	90%	100%
Influenza Vaccine[4,5]	-	-	64%	70%	100%
Initial Antibiotic Timing	251	82%	74%	80%	93%
Oxygenation Assessment	283	98%	99%	99%	100%
Pneumococcal Vaccine	203	80%	67%	69%	94%
Smoking Cessation Advice	27	96%	90%	80%	100%
Surgical Infection Prevention					
Prophylactic Antibiotic Given[2]	145	95%	83%	77%	95%
Prophylactic Antibiotic Selection[2]	31	100%	90%	90%	100%
Prophylactic Antibiotic Stopped[2]	145	37%	70%	72%	95%
Pregnancy Care					
Inpatient Neonatal Mortality	-	-	-	-	-
Third or Fourth Degree Laceration	-	-	2.71%	3.63%	3.27%

HealthSouth Doctors' Hospital

5000 University Drive
Miami, FL 33146
URL: www.healthsouth.com
Ownership: Voluntary non-profit - Other
Emergency Services: Yes

Phone: 706-308-3000
Fax: 786-308-3201

Accredited: Yes
Licensed Beds: 285

Key Personnel:
CEO. . . . . Lincoln Mendez
Chief Medical Staff. . . . . Richard Whittington, MD

Measure	Cases	This Hospital	State Average	U.S. Average	Top Hospital
Heart Attack Care					
ACE Inhibitor or ARB for LVSD[1]	3	100%	83%	82%	100%
Aspirin at Arrival	62	97%	93%	92%	100%
Aspirin at Discharge[1]	10	100%	88%	90%	100%
Beta Blocker at Arrival	57	98%	89%	87%	100%
Beta Blocker at Discharge[1]	17	100%	92%	90%	100%
Fibrinolytic Medication Timing[1]	3	100%	33%	31%	100%
PCI Within 90 Minutes of Arrival	0	-	52%	54%	95%
Smoking Cessation Advice[1]	1	100%	92%	88%	100%
Heart Failure Care					
ACE Inhibitor or ARB for LVSD	45	96%	82%	82%	100%
Discharge Instructions	153	87%	61%	61%	93%
Evaluation of LVS Function	177	100%	90%	83%	99%
Smoking Cessation Advice[1]	15	100%	91%	82%	100%
Pneumonia Care					
Appropriate Initial Antibiotic	167	87%	84%	83%	94%
Blood Culture Timing	165	90%	88%	90%	100%
Influenza Vaccine	57	96%	64%	70%	100%
Initial Antibiotic Timing	174	89%	74%	80%	93%
Oxygenation Assessment	250	100%	99%	99%	100%
Pneumococcal Vaccine	161	94%	67%	69%	94%
Smoking Cessation Advice	51	100%	90%	80%	100%
Surgical Infection Prevention					
Prophylactic Antibiotic Given	546	99%	83%	77%	95%
Prophylactic Antibiotic Selection	137	96%	90%	90%	100%
Prophylactic Antibiotic Stopped	525	94%	70%	72%	95%
Pregnancy Care					
Inpatient Neonatal Mortality	-	-	-	-	-
Third or Fourth Degree Laceration	-	-	2.71%	3.63%	3.27%

NOTE: Hospital profiles are in alphabetical order by state, then city, then hospital within the city; Rankings are sorted by rate in descending order and exclude hospitals with less than 25 cases; (1) The number of cases is too small (n<25) for purposes of reliably predicting hospital performance; (2) Measure reflects the hospital's indication that its submission was based upon a sample of its relevant discharges; (3) Rate reflects fewer than the maximum possible quarters of data for the measure; (4) Inaccurate information submitted and suppressed for one or more quarters; (5) No data is available from the hospital for this measure; Please refer to the User's Guide for a full explanation of data

Coral Springs Medical Center

3000 Coral Hills Drive
Coral Springs, FL 33065
URL: www.coralspringsmedicalcenter.org
Ownership: Govt - Hospital District or Authority
Emergency Services: Yes

Phone: 954-344-3000
Fax: 954-344-3146

Accredited: Yes
Licensed Beds: 200

Key Personnel:

CEO . . . . Deborah Mulvihill, RN/MSN
Chief Medical Staff . . . . Thomas Goldschmidt
Emergency Room . . . . Rachelle Zahniser
Director Infection/Disease Control . . . . Ava Dobin

Measure	Cases	This Hospital	State Average	U.S. Average	Top Hospital
Heart Attack Care					
ACE Inhibitor or ARB for LVSD[1]	11	82%	83%	82%	100%
Aspirin at Arrival	93	96%	93%	92%	100%
Aspirin at Discharge	36	69%	88%	90%	100%
Beta Blocker at Arrival	67	94%	89%	87%	100%
Beta Blocker at Discharge	36	86%	92%	90%	100%
Fibrinolytic Medication Timing[1]	8	38%	33%	31%	100%
PCI Within 90 Minutes of Arrival	0	-	52%	54%	95%
Smoking Cessation Advice[1]	5	100%	92%	88%	100%
Heart Failure Care					
ACE Inhibitor or ARB for LVSD	72	79%	82%	82%	100%
Discharge Instructions	175	93%	61%	61%	93%
Evaluation of LVS Function	195	89%	90%	83%	99%
Smoking Cessation Advice[1]	20	100%	91%	82%	100%
Pneumonia Care					
Appropriate Initial Antibiotic	116	83%	84%	83%	94%
Blood Culture Timing	115	89%	88%	90%	100%
Influenza Vaccine	25	80%	64%	70%	100%
Initial Antibiotic Timing	133	71%	74%	80%	93%
Oxygenation Assessment	174	100%	99%	99%	100%
Pneumococcal Vaccine	86	83%	67%	69%	94%
Smoking Cessation Advice	46	96%	90%	80%	100%
Surgical Infection Prevention					
Prophylactic Antibiotic Given	170	69%	83%	77%	95%
Prophylactic Antibiotic Selection	40	82%	90%	90%	100%
Prophylactic Antibiotic Stopped	164	44%	70%	72%	95%
Pregnancy Care					
Inpatient Neonatal Mortality	-	-	-	-	-
Third or Fourth Degree Laceration	-	-	2.71%	3.63%	3.27%

North Okaloosa Medical Center

151 Redstone Avenue SE
Crestview, FL 32539
Ownership: Voluntary non-profit - Private
Emergency Services: Yes

Phone: 850-689-8100
Fax: 850-689-8484
Accredited: Yes
Licensed Beds: 110

Key Personnel:

CEO . . . . Doug Sills
Emergency Room . . . . Russall Lewis
Nurse Manager OB/GYN/Women's Health . . . . . Bernice Toner

Measure	Cases	This Hospital	State Average	U.S. Average	Top Hospital
Heart Attack Care					
ACE Inhibitor or ARB for LVSD[1]	8	88%	83%	82%	100%
Aspirin at Arrival	46	89%	93%	92%	100%
Aspirin at Discharge	28	71%	88%	90%	100%
Beta Blocker at Arrival	45	89%	89%	87%	100%
Beta Blocker at Discharge	26	73%	92%	90%	100%
Fibrinolytic Medication Timing	0	-	33%	31%	100%
PCI Within 90 Minutes of Arrival	0	-	52%	54%	95%
Smoking Cessation Advice[1]	5	100%	92%	88%	100%
Heart Failure Care					
ACE Inhibitor or ARB for LVSD	52	73%	82%	82%	100%
Discharge Instructions	135	31%	61%	61%	93%
Evaluation of LVS Function	165	95%	90%	83%	99%
Smoking Cessation Advice	35	89%	91%	82%	100%
Pneumonia Care					
Appropriate Initial Antibiotic[2]	110	86%	84%	83%	94%
Blood Culture Timing[2]	64	70%	88%	90%	100%
Influenza Vaccine[1,2]	20	40%	64%	70%	100%

Measure	Cases	This Hospital	State Average	U.S. Average	Top Hospital
Initial Antibiotic Timing[2]	142	72%	74%	80%	93%
Oxygenation Assessment[2]	158	100%	99%	99%	100%
Pneumococcal Vaccine[2]	96	58%	67%	69%	94%
Smoking Cessation Advice[2]	44	86%	90%	80%	100%
Surgical Infection Prevention					
Prophylactic Antibiotic Given[2,3]	227	65%	83%	77%	95%
Prophylactic Antibiotic Selection[2]	40	82%	90%	90%	100%
Prophylactic Antibiotic Stopped[2,3]	221	77%	70%	72%	95%
Pregnancy Care					
Inpatient Neonatal Mortality	-	-	-	-	-
Third or Fourth Degree Laceration	-	-	2.71%	3.63%	3.27%

Seven Rivers Regional Medical Center

6201 N Suncoast Boulevard
Crystal River, FL 34428
E-mail: info@srrmc.hma-corp.com
URL: www.srrmc.com
Ownership: Proprietary
Emergency Services: Yes

Phone: 352-795-6560
Fax: 352-795-8369

Accredited: Yes
Licensed Beds: 128

Key Personnel:

CEO . . . . Joyce Brancato
Catheterization Lab Director . . . . Kay Burke
Emergency Room Director . . . . Lynne West, RN
Infection Control Coordinator . . . . Teresa Wright, RN
ICU Director . . . . Deanna Beverly, RN
Intensive/Coronary Director . . . . Deanna Beverly, RN
Medical Surgical Nursing Director . . . . Patricia Dourn, RN
CNO . . . . Cynthia Heitzman, RN
Respiratory Manager . . . . Al Barcena

Measure	Cases	This Hospital	State Average	U.S. Average	Top Hospital
Heart Attack Care					
ACE Inhibitor or ARB for LVSD[1]	24	100%	83%	82%	100%
Aspirin at Arrival	112	98%	93%	92%	100%
Aspirin at Discharge	45	96%	88%	90%	100%
Beta Blocker at Arrival	113	100%	89%	87%	100%
Beta Blocker at Discharge	50	96%	92%	90%	100%
Fibrinolytic Medication Timing	0	-	33%	31%	100%
PCI Within 90 Minutes of Arrival	0	-	52%	54%	95%
Smoking Cessation Advice[1]	12	100%	92%	88%	100%
Heart Failure Care					
ACE Inhibitor or ARB for LVSD	126	100%	82%	82%	100%
Discharge Instructions	216	99%	61%	61%	93%
Evaluation of LVS Function	280	95%	90%	83%	99%
Smoking Cessation Advice	53	100%	91%	82%	100%
Pneumonia Care					
Appropriate Initial Antibiotic	154	82%	84%	83%	94%
Blood Culture Timing	115	100%	88%	90%	100%
Influenza Vaccine	42	69%	64%	70%	100%
Initial Antibiotic Timing	149	74%	74%	80%	93%
Oxygenation Assessment	202	100%	99%	99%	100%
Pneumococcal Vaccine	142	84%	67%	69%	94%
Smoking Cessation Advice	39	74%	90%	80%	100%
Surgical Infection Prevention					
Prophylactic Antibiotic Given[2]	497	93%	83%	77%	95%
Prophylactic Antibiotic Selection[2]	57	100%	90%	90%	100%
Prophylactic Antibiotic Stopped[2]	469	78%	70%	72%	95%
Pregnancy Care					
Inpatient Neonatal Mortality	-	-	-	-	-
Third or Fourth Degree Laceration	-	-	2.71%	3.63%	3.27%

Pasco Regional Medical Center

Alternate Name: Humana Hospital Pasco
13100 Fort King Road
Dade City, FL 33525
URL: www.pascoregionalmc.com
Ownership: Proprietary
Emergency Services: Yes

Phone: 352-521-1100
Fax: 352-521-1196

Accredited: Yes
Licensed Beds: 120

Key Personnel:

President/CEO . . . . Michael J Arnd
Chief Medical Staff . . . . Joseph Hubaykah, MD
Emergency Room . . . . Sam Walton
Infection Control . . . . Rita Clark

NOTE: Hospital profiles are in alphabetical order by state, then city, then hospital within the city; Rankings are sorted by rate in descending order and exclude hospitals with less than 25 cases; (1) The number of cases is too small (n<25) for purposes of reliably predicting hospital performance; (2) Measure reflects the hospital's indication that its submission was based upon a sample of its relevant discharges; (3) Rate reflects fewer than the maximum possible quarters of data for the measure; (4) Inaccurate information submitted and suppressed for one or more quarters; (5) No data is available from the hospital for this measure; Please refer to the User's Guide for a full explanation of data

ICU . . . . Tina Nelson
Medical/Surgical Nursing . . . . Mia Buttleman

Measure	Cases	This Hospital	State Average	U.S. Average	Top Hospital
Heart Attack Care					
ACE Inhibitor or ARB for LVSD[1]	4	100%	83%	82%	100%
Aspirin at Arrival	44	98%	93%	92%	100%
Aspirin at Discharge[1]	14	100%	88%	90%	100%
Beta Blocker at Arrival	34	97%	89%	87%	100%
Beta Blocker at Discharge[1]	19	95%	92%	90%	100%
Fibrinolytic Medication Timing[1]	16	50%	33%	31%	100%
PCI Within 90 Minutes of Arrival	0	-	52%	54%	95%
Smoking Cessation Advice[1]	6	83%	92%	88%	100%
Heart Failure Care					
ACE Inhibitor or ARB for LVSD	70	97%	82%	82%	100%
Discharge Instructions	166	54%	61%	61%	93%
Evaluation of LVS Function	205	96%	90%	83%	99%
Smoking Cessation Advice	37	95%	91%	82%	100%
Pneumonia Care					
Appropriate Initial Antibiotic	131	76%	84%	83%	94%
Blood Culture Timing	125	94%	88%	90%	100%
Influenza Vaccine	55	85%	64%	70%	100%
Initial Antibiotic Timing	141	81%	74%	80%	93%
Oxygenation Assessment	204	100%	99%	99%	100%
Pneumococcal Vaccine	135	87%	67%	69%	94%
Smoking Cessation Advice	55	89%	90%	80%	100%
Surgical Infection Prevention					
Prophylactic Antibiotic Given[2]	280	83%	83%	77%	95%
Prophylactic Antibiotic Selection[2]	51	98%	90%	90%	100%
Prophylactic Antibiotic Stopped[2]	252	63%	70%	72%	95%
Pregnancy Care					
Inpatient Neonatal Mortality	-	-	-	-	-
Third or Fourth Degree Laceration	-	-	2.71%	3.63%	3.27%

Heart of Florida Regional Medical Center

40100 US Highway 27   Phone: 863-422-4971
Davenport, FL 33837   Fax: 863-419-2465
E-mail: hofrmc@gte.net
URL: www.heartofflorida.com
Ownership: Proprietary   Accredited: Yes
Emergency Services: Yes   Licensed Beds: 142
Key Personnel:
CEO. . . . . Ann Barnhart
Chief Medical Staff. . . . . Devendra Kahlon, MD
Infection Control. . . . . Nancy Draves
OB/GYN Women's Health . . . . Mark Alkass, MD
Manager Respiratory Therapy . . . . Tim Carlen

Measure	Cases	This Hospital	State Average	U.S. Average	Top Hospital
Heart Attack Care					
ACE Inhibitor or ARB for LVSD[1]	19	68%	83%	82%	100%
Aspirin at Arrival	106	79%	93%	92%	100%
Aspirin at Discharge	54	69%	88%	90%	100%
Beta Blocker at Arrival	102	68%	89%	87%	100%
Beta Blocker at Discharge	59	73%	92%	90%	100%
Fibrinolytic Medication Timing	0	-	33%	31%	100%
PCI Within 90 Minutes of Arrival	0	-	52%	54%	95%
Smoking Cessation Advice[1]	12	83%	92%	88%	100%
Heart Failure Care					
ACE Inhibitor or ARB for LVSD	160	81%	82%	82%	100%
Discharge Instructions	398	20%	61%	61%	93%
Evaluation of LVS Function	439	82%	90%	83%	99%
Smoking Cessation Advice	56	84%	91%	82%	100%
Pneumonia Care					
Appropriate Initial Antibiotic	173	85%	84%	83%	94%
Blood Culture Timing	105	84%	88%	90%	100%
Influenza Vaccine	47	66%	64%	70%	100%
Initial Antibiotic Timing	211	59%	74%	80%	93%
Oxygenation Assessment	231	100%	99%	99%	100%
Pneumococcal Vaccine	131	56%	67%	69%	94%
Smoking Cessation Advice	59	90%	90%	80%	100%
Surgical Infection Prevention					

| Prophylactic Antibiotic Given[2] | 748 | 89% | 83% | 77% | 95% |
| Prophylactic Antibiotic Selection[2] | 72 | 85% | 90% | 90% | 100% |
Prophylactic Antibiotic Stopped[2]	740	61%	70%	72%	95%
Pregnancy Care					
Inpatient Neonatal Mortality	-	-	-	-	-
Third or Fourth Degree Laceration	-	-	2.71%	3.63%	3.27%

Halifax Medical Center

303 N Clyde Morris Boulevard   Phone: 386-254-4000
Daytona Beach, FL 32114   Fax: 386-258-4860
URL: www.hfch.org/hmc
Ownership: Govt - Hospital District or Authority   Accredited: Yes
Emergency Services: Yes   Licensed Beds: 764
Key Personnel:
CEO. . . . . Jeff Feasel
Chief Medical Staff. . . . . Frank Herrero, MD
Catheterization Lab . . . . Donald Stoner, MD
Emergency Room . . . . Julie Woisard, RN
Emergency Room . . . . William Meek, MD
Infection Control. . . . . Richard Duma, MD
ICU . . . . Karen Locke, RN
Intensive Coronary Care . . . . Lori Myers, RN
OB/GYN Womens Health. . . . . John White, MD
Respiratory/Cardiopulmonary. . . . . Lyda Stelnicki

Measure	Cases	This Hospital	State Average	U.S. Average	Top Hospital
Heart Attack Care					
ACE Inhibitor or ARB for LVSD	68	93%	83%	82%	100%
Aspirin at Arrival	367	97%	93%	92%	100%
Aspirin at Discharge	364	99%	88%	90%	100%
Beta Blocker at Arrival	301	98%	89%	87%	100%
Beta Blocker at Discharge	378	97%	92%	90%	100%
Fibrinolytic Medication Timing[1]	8	12%	33%	31%	100%
PCI Within 90 Minutes of Arrival[1]	4	25%	52%	54%	95%
Smoking Cessation Advice	160	100%	92%	88%	100%
Heart Failure Care					
ACE Inhibitor or ARB for LVSD	311	94%	82%	82%	100%
Discharge Instructions	641	96%	61%	61%	93%
Evaluation of LVS Function	786	99%	90%	83%	99%
Smoking Cessation Advice	201	100%	91%	82%	100%
Pneumonia Care					
Appropriate Initial Antibiotic	381	90%	84%	83%	94%
Blood Culture Timing	285	68%	88%	90%	100%
Influenza Vaccine[4,5]	-	-	64%	70%	100%
Initial Antibiotic Timing	471	88%	74%	80%	93%
Oxygenation Assessment	576	100%	99%	99%	100%
Pneumococcal Vaccine	286	86%	67%	69%	94%
Smoking Cessation Advice	144	99%	90%	80%	100%
Surgical Infection Prevention					
Prophylactic Antibiotic Given	794	91%	83%	77%	95%
Prophylactic Antibiotic Selection	385	91%	90%	90%	100%
Prophylactic Antibiotic Stopped	779	77%	70%	72%	95%
Pregnancy Care					
Inpatient Neonatal Mortality	-	-	-	-	-
Third or Fourth Degree Laceration	-	-	2.71%	3.63%	3.27%

North Broward Medical Center

201 E Sample Road   Phone: 954-941-8300
Deerfield Beach, FL 33064   Fax: 954-781-4224
URL: www.browardhealth.org
Ownership: Govt - Hospital District or Authority   Accredited: Yes
Emergency Services: Yes   Licensed Beds: 409
Key Personnel:
President/CEO. . . . . Pauline Grant
Chief Medical Staff. . . . . Steven Shapiro, MD
Catheterization Lab . . . . Herold Altschuer, MD
Emergency Room . . . . Jerry Brooks, MD
Infection Control. . . . . Mel Koham, MD

Measure	Cases	This Hospital	State Average	U.S. Average	Top Hospital
Heart Attack Care					
ACE Inhibitor or ARB for LVSD	33	88%	83%	82%	100%
Aspirin at Arrival	164	91%	93%	92%	100%

NOTE: Hospital profiles are in alphabetical order by state, then city, then hospital within the city; Rankings are sorted by rate in descending order and exclude hospitals with less than 25 cases; (1) The number of cases is too small (n<25) for purposes of reliably predicting hospital performance; (2) Measure reflects the hospital's indication that its submission was based upon a sample of its relevant discharges; (3) Rate reflects fewer than the maximum possible quarters of data for the measure; (4) Inaccurate information submitted and suppressed for one or more quarters; (5) No data is available from the hospital for this measure; Please refer to the User's Guide for a full explanation of data

Aspirin at Discharge	64	94%	88%	90%	100%
Beta Blocker at Arrival	112	91%	89%	87%	100%
Beta Blocker at Discharge	91	93%	92%	90%	100%
Fibrinolytic Medication Timing[1]	5	40%	33%	31%	100%
PCI Within 90 Minutes of Arrival	0	-	52%	54%	95%
Smoking Cessation Advice[1]	10	100%	92%	88%	100%
Heart Failure Care					
ACE Inhibitor or ARB for LVSD[2]	115	83%	82%	82%	100%
Discharge Instructions[2]	214	82%	61%	61%	93%
Evaluation of LVS Function[2]	257	89%	90%	83%	99%
Smoking Cessation Advice[2]	45	100%	91%	82%	100%
Pneumonia Care					
Appropriate Initial Antibiotic[2]	123	86%	84%	83%	94%
Blood Culture Timing[2]	96	90%	88%	90%	100%
Influenza Vaccine[4,5]	-	-	64%	70%	100%
Initial Antibiotic Timing[2]	152	73%	74%	80%	93%
Oxygenation Assessment[2]	175	100%	99%	99%	100%
Pneumococcal Vaccine[2]	78	55%	67%	69%	94%
Smoking Cessation Advice[2]	40	88%	90%	80%	100%
Surgical Infection Prevention					
Prophylactic Antibiotic Given	186	69%	83%	77%	95%
Prophylactic Antibiotic Selection	47	96%	90%	90%	100%
Prophylactic Antibiotic Stopped	180	33%	70%	72%	95%
Pregnancy Care					
Inpatient Neonatal Mortality	-	-	-	-	-
Third or Fourth Degree Laceration	-	-	2.71%	3.63%	3.27%

Healthmark Regional Medical Center

4413 Us Hwy 331 S
Defuniak Springs, FL 32435
Ownership: Voluntary non-profit - Private
Emergency Services: Yes

Phone: 850-951-4500

Accredited: No

Measure	Cases	This Hospital	State Average	U.S. Average	Top Hospital
Heart Attack Care					
ACE Inhibitor or ARB for LVSD	0	-	83%	82%	100%
Aspirin at Arrival[1]	5	80%	93%	92%	100%
Aspirin at Discharge[1]	1	0%	88%	90%	100%
Beta Blocker at Arrival[1]	5	60%	89%	87%	100%
Beta Blocker at Discharge[1]	1	0%	92%	90%	100%
Fibrinolytic Medication Timing[3]	0	-	33%	31%	100%
PCI Within 90 Minutes of Arrival	0	-	52%	54%	95%
Smoking Cessation Advice[3]	0	-	92%	88%	100%
Heart Failure Care					
ACE Inhibitor or ARB for LVSD[1,2]	3	67%	82%	82%	100%
Discharge Instructions[1,2,3]	8	38%	61%	61%	93%
Evaluation of LVS Function[2]	30	33%	90%	83%	99%
Smoking Cessation Advice[1,2,3]	3	67%	91%	82%	100%
Pneumonia Care					
Appropriate Initial Antibiotic[1,2,3]	14	43%	84%	83%	94%
Blood Culture Timing[2,3]	0	-	88%	90%	100%
Influenza Vaccine[5]	-	-	64%	70%	100%
Initial Antibiotic Timing[2]	40	60%	74%	80%	93%
Oxygenation Assessment[2]	48	90%	99%	99%	100%
Pneumococcal Vaccine[2]	32	56%	67%	69%	94%
Smoking Cessation Advice[1,2,3]	8	38%	90%	80%	100%
Surgical Infection Prevention					
Prophylactic Antibiotic Given[3]	0	-	83%	77%	95%
Prophylactic Antibiotic Selection[5]	-	-	90%	90%	100%
Prophylactic Antibiotic Stopped[3]	0	-	70%	72%	95%
Pregnancy Care					
Inpatient Neonatal Mortality	-	-	-	-	-
Third or Fourth Degree Laceration	-	-	2.71%	3.63%	3.27%

Florida Hospital DeLand

701 West Plymouth
Deland, FL 32720
URL: www.fhdeland.org
Ownership: Voluntary non-profit - Private
Emergency Services: Yes
Key Personnel:
President/CEO . . . . Daryl Tol

Phone: 386-943-4522
Fax: 386-943-3674

Accredited: Yes
Licensed Beds: 156

Administrator . . . . Steve Otto
Chief Medical Staff. Hendrik Dinkla, MD
Director Surgical Services . . . . Penny Branch
Cardiopulmonary/Rehabilitative Services . . . . . . Jennifer Lyons
Director Cardiopulmonary . . . . Jennifer Lyons
Surgical Services Director . . . . Penny Branch
Infection Control . . . . Chrissie Kotwica
Director CCU/ICU . . . . Elisha Voigt
Birthcare Center Director . . . . Patricia Jamasen

Measure	Cases	This Hospital	State Average	U.S. Average	Top Hospital
Heart Attack Care					
ACE Inhibitor or ARB for LVSD	26	85%	83%	82%	100%
Aspirin at Arrival	138	96%	93%	92%	100%
Aspirin at Discharge	72	97%	88%	90%	100%
Beta Blocker at Arrival	112	90%	89%	87%	100%
Beta Blocker at Discharge	77	96%	92%	90%	100%
Fibrinolytic Medication Timing[1]	19	37%	33%	31%	100%
PCI Within 90 Minutes of Arrival	0	-	52%	54%	95%
Smoking Cessation Advice[1]	18	100%	92%	88%	100%
Heart Failure Care					
ACE Inhibitor or ARB for LVSD	120	78%	82%	82%	100%
Discharge Instructions	242	38%	61%	61%	93%
Evaluation of LVS Function	351	98%	90%	83%	99%
Smoking Cessation Advice	59	100%	91%	82%	100%
Pneumonia Care					
Appropriate Initial Antibiotic	225	92%	84%	83%	94%
Blood Culture Timing	251	95%	88%	90%	100%
Influenza Vaccine[4,5]	-	-	64%	70%	100%
Initial Antibiotic Timing	342	87%	74%	80%	93%
Oxygenation Assessment	387	99%	99%	99%	100%
Pneumococcal Vaccine	228	64%	67%	69%	94%
Smoking Cessation Advice	87	100%	90%	80%	100%
Surgical Infection Prevention					
Prophylactic Antibiotic Given	410	91%	83%	77%	95%
Prophylactic Antibiotic Selection	90	98%	90%	90%	100%
Prophylactic Antibiotic Stopped	398	89%	70%	72%	95%
Pregnancy Care					
Inpatient Neonatal Mortality	-	-	-	-	-
Third or Fourth Degree Laceration	-	-	2.71%	3.63%	3.27%

Delray Medical Center

Alternate Name: Delray Community Hospital
5352 Linton Boulevard
Delray Beach, FL 33484
URL: www.delraymedicalctr.com
Ownership: Proprietary
Emergency Services: Yes
Key Personnel:
CEO. . . . . Mitch Feldman
Chief Medical Staff. Bruce Barton, MD
Emergency Department . . . . Audrey Gregory
Director Respiratory Therapy . . . . Madeline Nava

Phone: 561-498-4440
Fax: 561-495-3103

Accredited: Yes
Licensed Beds: 343

Measure	Cases	This Hospital	State Average	U.S. Average	Top Hospital
Heart Attack Care					
ACE Inhibitor or ARB for LVSD	118	99%	83%	82%	100%
Aspirin at Arrival	506	100%	93%	92%	100%
Aspirin at Discharge	548	100%	88%	90%	100%
Beta Blocker at Arrival	474	99%	89%	87%	100%
Beta Blocker at Discharge	541	99%	92%	90%	100%
Fibrinolytic Medication Timing[1]	21	14%	33%	31%	100%
PCI Within 90 Minutes of Arrival[1]	19	95%	52%	54%	95%
Smoking Cessation Advice	73	100%	92%	88%	100%
Heart Failure Care					
ACE Inhibitor or ARB for LVSD	178	97%	82%	82%	100%
Discharge Instructions	497	100%	61%	61%	93%
Evaluation of LVS Function	688	99%	90%	83%	99%
Smoking Cessation Advice[1]	21	100%	91%	82%	100%
Pneumonia Care					
Appropriate Initial Antibiotic	257	93%	84%	83%	94%
Blood Culture Timing	211	100%	88%	90%	100%

NOTE: Hospital profiles are in alphabetical order by state, then city, then hospital within the city; Rankings are sorted by rate in descending order and exclude hospitals with less than 25 cases; (1) The number of cases is too small (n<25) for purposes of reliably predicting hospital performance; (2) Measure reflects the hospital's indication that its submission was based upon a sample of its relevant discharges; (3) Rate reflects fewer than the maximum possible quarters of data for the measure; (4) Inaccurate information submitted and suppressed for one or more quarters; (5) No data is available from the hospital for this measure; Please refer to the User's Guide for a full explanation of data

Influenza Vaccine[4,5]	-	-	64%	70%	100%
Initial Antibiotic Timing	257	95%	74%	80%	93%
Oxygenation Assessment	305	100%	99%	99%	100%
Pneumococcal Vaccine	216	93%	67%	69%	94%
Smoking Cessation Advice[1]	22	100%	90%	80%	100%
Surgical Infection Prevention					
Prophylactic Antibiotic Given[2]	1,176	96%	83%	77%	95%
Prophylactic Antibiotic Selection[2]	252	96%	90%	90%	100%
Prophylactic Antibiotic Stopped[2]	1,134	81%	70%	72%	95%
Pregnancy Care					
Inpatient Neonatal Mortality	-	-	-	-	-
Third or Fourth Degree Laceration	-	-	2.71%	3.63%	3.27%

Sacred Heart Hospital on the Emerald Coast

7800 US Highway 90 West   Toll-Free: 877-416-1600
Destin, FL 32550   Phone: 850-278-3000
                                            Fax: 850-278-3010

URL: www.sacredheartemerald.org
Ownership: Voluntary non-profit - Other   Accredited: Yes
Emergency Services: Yes

Measure	Cases	This Hospital	State Average	U.S. Average	Top Hospital
Heart Attack Care					
ACE Inhibitor or ARB for LVSD[1,2]	1	100%	83%	82%	100%
Aspirin at Arrival[1,2]	15	100%	93%	92%	100%
Aspirin at Discharge[1,2]	5	100%	88%	90%	100%
Beta Blocker at Arrival[1,2]	8	88%	89%	87%	100%
Beta Blocker at Discharge[1,2]	5	80%	92%	90%	100%
Fibrinolytic Medication Timing[2]	0	-	33%	31%	100%
PCI Within 90 Minutes of Arrival[2]	0	-	52%	54%	95%
Smoking Cessation Advice[1,2]	2	100%	92%	88%	100%
Heart Failure Care					
ACE Inhibitor or ARB for LVSD[2]	29	90%	82%	82%	100%
Discharge Instructions[2]	74	74%	61%	61%	93%
Evaluation of LVS Function[2]	90	96%	90%	83%	99%
Smoking Cessation Advice[1,2]	7	86%	91%	82%	100%
Pneumonia Care					
Appropriate Initial Antibiotic[2]	55	80%	84%	83%	94%
Blood Culture Timing[2]	38	87%	88%	90%	100%
Influenza Vaccine[1,2]	23	70%	64%	70%	100%
Initial Antibiotic Timing[2]	48	94%	74%	80%	93%
Oxygenation Assessment[2]	93	100%	99%	99%	100%
Pneumococcal Vaccine[2]	63	86%	67%	69%	94%
Smoking Cessation Advice[1,2]	23	91%	90%	80%	100%
Surgical Infection Prevention					
Prophylactic Antibiotic Given[2,3]	183	80%	83%	77%	95%
Prophylactic Antibiotic Selection[2]	51	90%	90%	90%	100%
Prophylactic Antibiotic Stopped[2,3]	177	73%	70%	72%	95%
Pregnancy Care					
Inpatient Neonatal Mortality	-	-	-	-	-
Third or Fourth Degree Laceration	-	-	2.71%	3.63%	3.27%

Mease Hospital-Dunedin

601 Main Street   Phone: 727-733-1111
Dunedin, FL 34698
Ownership: Government - Local   Accredited: Yes
Emergency Services: Yes

Measure	Cases	This Hospital	State Average	U.S. Average	Top Hospital
Heart Attack Care					
ACE Inhibitor or ARB for LVSD[1]	15	100%	83%	82%	100%
Aspirin at Arrival	60	95%	93%	92%	100%
Aspirin at Discharge	25	88%	88%	90%	100%
Beta Blocker at Arrival	32	94%	89%	87%	100%
Beta Blocker at Discharge	46	98%	92%	90%	100%
Fibrinolytic Medication Timing	0	-	33%	31%	100%
PCI Within 90 Minutes of Arrival	0	-	52%	54%	95%
Smoking Cessation Advice[1]	10	100%	92%	88%	100%
Heart Failure Care					
ACE Inhibitor or ARB for LVSD	90	87%	82%	82%	100%
Discharge Instructions	159	70%	61%	61%	93%
Evaluation of LVS Function	199	91%	90%	83%	99%

Smoking Cessation Advice	25	100%	91%	82%	100%
Pneumonia Care					
Appropriate Initial Antibiotic	107	85%	84%	83%	94%
Blood Culture Timing	109	95%	88%	90%	100%
Influenza Vaccine	42	52%	64%	70%	100%
Initial Antibiotic Timing	115	88%	74%	80%	93%
Oxygenation Assessment	208	100%	99%	99%	100%
Pneumococcal Vaccine	137	57%	67%	69%	94%
Smoking Cessation Advice	48	100%	90%	80%	100%
Surgical Infection Prevention					
Prophylactic Antibiotic Given[2]	103	81%	83%	77%	95%
Prophylactic Antibiotic Selection[2]	30	97%	90%	90%	100%
Prophylactic Antibiotic Stopped[2]	87	84%	70%	72%	95%
Pregnancy Care					
Inpatient Neonatal Mortality	-	-	-	-	-
Third or Fourth Degree Laceration	-	-	2.71%	3.63%	3.27%

Englewood Community Hospital

700 Medical Boulevard   Phone: 941-475-6571
Englewood, FL 34223   Fax: 941-473-7259
URL: www.englewoodcommunityhospital.com
Ownership: Proprietary   Accredited: Yes
Emergency Services: Yes   Licensed Beds: 100
Key Personnel:
CEO. . . . . Robert Meade
Chief Medical Staff. . . . . Raul Verde, MD

Measure	Cases	This Hospital	State Average	U.S. Average	Top Hospital
Heart Attack Care					
ACE Inhibitor or ARB for LVSD[1]	24	79%	83%	82%	100%
Aspirin at Arrival	116	93%	93%	92%	100%
Aspirin at Discharge	63	78%	88%	90%	100%
Beta Blocker at Arrival	118	80%	89%	87%	100%
Beta Blocker at Discharge	76	78%	92%	90%	100%
Fibrinolytic Medication Timing[1]	6	0%	33%	31%	100%
PCI Within 90 Minutes of Arrival	0	-	52%	54%	95%
Smoking Cessation Advice[1]	11	91%	92%	88%	100%
Heart Failure Care					
ACE Inhibitor or ARB for LVSD	59	76%	82%	82%	100%
Discharge Instructions	131	76%	61%	61%	93%
Evaluation of LVS Function	169	80%	90%	83%	99%
Smoking Cessation Advice[1]	13	77%	91%	82%	100%
Pneumonia Care					
Appropriate Initial Antibiotic	92	71%	84%	83%	94%
Blood Culture Timing	58	83%	88%	90%	100%
Influenza Vaccine	27	56%	64%	70%	100%
Initial Antibiotic Timing	104	74%	74%	80%	93%
Oxygenation Assessment	116	100%	99%	99%	100%
Pneumococcal Vaccine	79	48%	67%	69%	94%
Smoking Cessation Advice[1]	18	94%	90%	80%	100%
Surgical Infection Prevention					
Prophylactic Antibiotic Given[3]	168	88%	83%	77%	95%
Prophylactic Antibiotic Selection	51	90%	90%	90%	100%
Prophylactic Antibiotic Stopped[3]	161	86%	70%	72%	95%
Pregnancy Care					
Inpatient Neonatal Mortality	-	-	-	-	-
Third or Fourth Degree Laceration	-	-	2.71%	3.63%	3.27%

Baptist Medical Center Nassau

1250 South 18th Street   Phone: 904-321-3500
Fernandina Bch, FL 32034   Fax: 904-321-3511
URL: www.e-baptisthealth.com
Ownership: Government - Local   Accredited: Yes
Emergency Services: Yes   Licensed Beds: 54
Key Personnel:
President . . . . Jim Mayo
Chief Medical Staff. . . . . David Murray, MD
Emergency Room . . . . David Pietrasuik, MD
Infection Control. . . . . Ted Jones, RN
Intensive/Coronary Care . . . . Debbie Dunman
Medical/Surgical Nursing . . . . Wanda Linton, RN
Respiratory/Cardiopulmonary. . . . . Dale Wilcox, RT

NOTE: Hospital profiles are in alphabetical order by state, then city, then hospital within the city; Rankings are sorted by rate in descending order and exclude hospitals with less than 25 cases; (1) The number of cases is too small (n<25) for purposes of reliably predicting hospital performance; (2) Measure reflects the hospital's indication that its submission was based upon a sample of its relevant discharges; (3) Rate reflects fewer than the maximum possible quarters of data for the measure; (4) Inaccurate information submitted and suppressed for one or more quarters; (5) No data is available from the hospital for this measure; Please refer to the User's Guide for a full explanation of data

Measure	Cases	This Hospital	State Average	U.S. Average	Top Hospital
Heart Attack Care					
ACE Inhibitor or ARB for LVSD	0	-	83%	82%	100%
Aspirin at Arrival[1]	8	88%	93%	92%	100%
Aspirin at Discharge[1]	5	60%	88%	90%	100%
Beta Blocker at Arrival[1]	8	88%	89%	87%	100%
Beta Blocker at Discharge[1]	5	80%	92%	90%	100%
Fibrinolytic Medication Timing	0	-	33%	31%	100%
PCI Within 90 Minutes of Arrival	0	-	52%	54%	95%
Smoking Cessation Advice	0	-	92%	88%	100%
Heart Failure Care					
ACE Inhibitor or ARB for LVSD	27	63%	82%	82%	100%
Discharge Instructions	65	8%	61%	61%	93%
Evaluation of LVS Function	76	99%	90%	83%	99%
Smoking Cessation Advice[1]	10	70%	91%	82%	100%
Pneumonia Care					
Appropriate Initial Antibiotic	97	89%	84%	83%	94%
Blood Culture Timing	105	92%	88%	90%	100%
Influenza Vaccine	25	72%	64%	70%	100%
Initial Antibiotic Timing	125	79%	74%	80%	93%
Oxygenation Assessment	143	97%	99%	99%	100%
Pneumococcal Vaccine	73	77%	67%	69%	94%
Smoking Cessation Advice	33	73%	90%	80%	100%
Surgical Infection Prevention					
Prophylactic Antibiotic Given[2]	109	86%	83%	77%	95%
Prophylactic Antibiotic Selection[1,2]	21	86%	90%	90%	100%
Prophylactic Antibiotic Stopped[2]	105	90%	70%	72%	95%
Pregnancy Care					
Inpatient Neonatal Mortality	261	0.38%	-	-	-
Third or Fourth Degree Laceration	228	0.44%	2.71%	3.63%	3.27%

Broward General Medical Center

1600 South Andrews Avenue
Fort Lauderdale, FL 33316

Toll-Free: 800-528-4888
Phone: 954-355-4400
Fax: 954-468-8046

URL: www.browardhealth.org
Ownership: Govt - Hospital District or Authority
Emergency Services: Yes
Accredited: Yes
Licensed Beds: 744
Key Personnel:
President/CEO . . . . Joseph Scott
Chief Medical Staff . . . . Dr Callari
Cardiac Lab . . . . Michael Chizner, MD
Catheterization Lab . . . . Michael Chinzer, MD
Emergency Room . . . . Nabil ElSanadi, MD
Emergency Room . . . . Sue Zembal, RN
Infection Control . . . . Stephen Bowen, MD
Intensive/Coronary Care . . . . Kevin Hall
OB/Gyn/Women's Health . . . . Thomas Lowe, MD
OB/GYN Womens Health . . . . Christine Rosill, RN
Respiratory/Cardiopulmonary . . . . Yvette Noe

Measure	Cases	This Hospital	State Average	U.S. Average	Top Hospital
Heart Attack Care					
ACE Inhibitor or ARB for LVSD	81	78%	83%	82%	100%
Aspirin at Arrival	155	94%	93%	92%	100%
Aspirin at Discharge	208	93%	88%	90%	100%
Beta Blocker at Arrival	112	97%	89%	87%	100%
Beta Blocker at Discharge	215	93%	92%	90%	100%
Fibrinolytic Medication Timing[1]	1	0%	33%	31%	100%
PCI Within 90 Minutes of Arrival[1]	8	50%	52%	54%	95%
Smoking Cessation Advice	96	98%	92%	88%	100%
Heart Failure Care					
ACE Inhibitor or ARB for LVSD[2]	177	90%	82%	82%	100%
Discharge Instructions[2]	263	95%	61%	61%	93%
Evaluation of LVS Function[2]	282	97%	90%	83%	99%
Smoking Cessation Advice[2]	76	99%	91%	82%	100%
Pneumonia Care					
Appropriate Initial Antibiotic[2]	113	88%	84%	83%	94%
Blood Culture Timing[2]	133	89%	88%	90%	100%
Influenza Vaccine[1]	22	14%	64%	70%	100%
Initial Antibiotic Timing[2]	183	69%	74%	80%	93%
Oxygenation Assessment[2]	210	100%	99%	99%	100%

Measure	Cases	This Hospital	State Average	U.S. Average	Top Hospital
Pneumococcal Vaccine[2]	67	19%	67%	69%	94%
Smoking Cessation Advice[2]	62	98%	90%	80%	100%
Surgical Infection Prevention					
Prophylactic Antibiotic Given	245	77%	83%	77%	95%
Prophylactic Antibiotic Selection	66	79%	90%	90%	100%
Prophylactic Antibiotic Stopped	233	56%	70%	72%	95%
Pregnancy Care					
Inpatient Neonatal Mortality[2]	3,524	0.65%	-	-	-
Third or Fourth Degree Laceration[2]	2,101	2.00%	2.71%	3.63%	3.27%

Holy Cross Hospital

4725 N Federal Highway
Fort Lauderdale, FL 33308
E-mail: luisa.gutman@holy-cross.com
URL: www.holy-cross.com
Ownership: Voluntary non-profit - Church
Emergency Services: Yes

Phone: 954-771-8000
Fax: 954-267-6896

Accredited: Yes
Licensed Beds: 597

Key Personnel:
CEO . . . . John Johnson
Cardiac Lab . . . . Frank Schambeck
Catheterization Lab . . . . Joan Steele
Emergency Room . . . . Marilyn Staniford
Emergency Room . . . . Michael Neam
Infection Control . . . . Elisa Fabian
ICU . . . . Steve Seeley
Intensive/Coronary Care . . . . Steve Seeley
Medical/Surgical Nursing . . . . Steve Seeley
OB/GYN/Women's Health . . . . Joanne MacLean
Respiratory/Cardiopulmonary . . . . Frank Schambeck

Measure	Cases	This Hospital	State Average	U.S. Average	Top Hospital
Heart Attack Care					
ACE Inhibitor or ARB for LVSD	45	98%	83%	82%	100%
Aspirin at Arrival	188	100%	93%	92%	100%
Aspirin at Discharge	266	99%	88%	90%	100%
Beta Blocker at Arrival	172	99%	89%	87%	100%
Beta Blocker at Discharge	271	99%	92%	90%	100%
Fibrinolytic Medication Timing[1]	5	20%	33%	31%	100%
PCI Within 90 Minutes of Arrival[1]	4	25%	52%	54%	95%
Smoking Cessation Advice	71	100%	92%	88%	100%
Heart Failure Care					
ACE Inhibitor or ARB for LVSD	191	99%	82%	82%	100%
Discharge Instructions	446	100%	61%	61%	93%
Evaluation of LVS Function	544	100%	90%	83%	99%
Smoking Cessation Advice	57	100%	91%	82%	100%
Pneumonia Care					
Appropriate Initial Antibiotic	172	85%	84%	83%	94%
Blood Culture Timing	182	87%	88%	90%	100%
Influenza Vaccine	55	100%	64%	70%	100%
Initial Antibiotic Timing	211	81%	74%	80%	93%
Oxygenation Assessment	266	100%	99%	99%	100%
Pneumococcal Vaccine	170	100%	67%	69%	94%
Smoking Cessation Advice	29	100%	90%	80%	100%
Surgical Infection Prevention					
Prophylactic Antibiotic Given[2]	292	74%	83%	77%	95%
Prophylactic Antibiotic Selection[2]	77	94%	90%	90%	100%
Prophylactic Antibiotic Stopped[2]	279	61%	70%	72%	95%
Pregnancy Care					
Inpatient Neonatal Mortality	-	-	-	-	-
Third or Fourth Degree Laceration	-	-	2.71%	3.63%	3.27%

Imperial Point Medical Center

6401 N Federal Highway
Fort Lauderdale, FL 33308
URL: www.nbhd.org
Ownership: Govt - Hospital District or Authority
Emergency Services: Yes

Phone: 954-776-8500
Fax: 954-776-8520

Accredited: Yes
Licensed Beds: 204

Key Personnel:
President/CEO . . . . Alan Levine
Chief Medical Staff . . . . William Jensen, MD
Catheterization Lab . . . . Scott Carroll
Emergency Room . . . . Ellen McAuley, RN
Emergency Room . . . . Scott Meyer, MD

NOTE: Hospital profiles are in alphabetical order by state, then city, then hospital within the city; Rankings are sorted by rate in descending order and exclude hospitals with less than 25 cases; (1) The number of cases is too small (n<25) for purposes of reliably predicting hospital performance; (2) Measure reflects the hospital's indication that its submission was based upon a sample of its relevant discharges; (3) Rate reflects fewer than the maximum possible quarters of data for the measure; (4) Inaccurate information submitted and suppressed for one or more quarters; (5) No data is available from the hospital for this measure; Please refer to the User's Guide for a full explanation of data

Infection Control Director . . . . Carolyn Adams
ICU . . . . Barbara Donnelly
Respiratory/Cardiopulmonary . . . . Scott Carroll

Measure	Cases	This Hospital	State Average	U.S. Average	Top Hospital
Heart Attack Care					
ACE Inhibitor or ARB for LVSD[1]	3	67%	83%	82%	100%
Aspirin at Arrival	33	79%	93%	92%	100%
Aspirin at Discharge[1]	11	82%	88%	90%	100%
Beta Blocker at Arrival[1]	20	85%	89%	87%	100%
Beta Blocker at Discharge[1]	11	82%	92%	90%	100%
Fibrinolytic Medication Timing[1]	1	100%	33%	31%	100%
PCI Within 90 Minutes of Arrival	0	-	52%	54%	95%
Smoking Cessation Advice[1]	3	100%	92%	88%	100%
Heart Failure Care					
ACE Inhibitor or ARB for LVSD	50	82%	82%	82%	100%
Discharge Instructions	119	71%	61%	61%	93%
Evaluation of LVS Function	139	86%	90%	83%	99%
Smoking Cessation Advice	38	100%	91%	82%	100%
Pneumonia Care					
Appropriate Initial Antibiotic	94	85%	84%	83%	94%
Blood Culture Timing	97	86%	88%	90%	100%
Influenza Vaccine[4,5]	-	-	64%	70%	100%
Initial Antibiotic Timing	125	86%	74%	80%	93%
Oxygenation Assessment	135	100%	99%	99%	100%
Pneumococcal Vaccine	72	54%	67%	69%	94%
Smoking Cessation Advice	35	100%	90%	80%	100%
Surgical Infection Prevention					
Prophylactic Antibiotic Given	138	75%	83%	77%	95%
Prophylactic Antibiotic Selection	33	97%	90%	90%	100%
Prophylactic Antibiotic Stopped	131	26%	70%	72%	95%
Pregnancy Care					
Inpatient Neonatal Mortality	-	-	-	-	-
Third or Fourth Degree Laceration	-	-	2.71%	3.63%	3.27%

North Ridge Medical Center

5757 N Dixie Highway
Fort Lauderdale, FL 33334
URL: www.northridgemedical.com
Ownership: Proprietary
Emergency Services: Yes

Phone: 954-776-6000
Fax: 954-938-3229

Accredited: Yes
Licensed Beds: 332

Key Personnel:
Administrator/CEO . . . . Cliff Bauer
Chief Medical Staff . . . . Anthony Aberico
Director Infection/Disease Control . . . . Maria Wiener
ICU Supervising Nurse . . . . Carol Korbar
Director Respiratory Therapy . . . . Mark Rohrsted

Measure	Cases	This Hospital	State Average	U.S. Average	Top Hospital
Heart Attack Care					
ACE Inhibitor or ARB for LVSD	54	96%	83%	82%	100%
Aspirin at Arrival	148	95%	93%	92%	100%
Aspirin at Discharge	251	99%	88%	90%	100%
Beta Blocker at Arrival	142	95%	89%	87%	100%
Beta Blocker at Discharge	260	97%	92%	90%	100%
Fibrinolytic Medication Timing[1]	2	0%	33%	31%	100%
PCI Within 90 Minutes of Arrival[1]	15	40%	52%	54%	95%
Smoking Cessation Advice	68	100%	92%	88%	100%
Heart Failure Care					
ACE Inhibitor or ARB for LVSD	94	90%	82%	82%	100%
Discharge Instructions	176	97%	61%	61%	93%
Evaluation of LVS Function	221	90%	90%	83%	99%
Smoking Cessation Advice[1]	24	100%	91%	82%	100%
Pneumonia Care					
Appropriate Initial Antibiotic	50	90%	84%	83%	94%
Blood Culture Timing	44	91%	88%	90%	100%
Influenza Vaccine[1]	11	73%	64%	70%	100%
Initial Antibiotic Timing	71	90%	74%	80%	93%
Oxygenation Assessment	81	99%	99%	99%	100%
Pneumococcal Vaccine	61	67%	67%	69%	94%
Smoking Cessation Advice[1]	12	92%	90%	80%	100%
Surgical Infection Prevention					

	580	93%	83%	77%	95%
Prophylactic Antibiotic Given[2]	580	93%	83%	77%	95%
Prophylactic Antibiotic Selection[2]	150	96%	90%	90%	100%
Prophylactic Antibiotic Stopped[2]	570	62%	70%	72%	95%
Pregnancy Care					
Inpatient Neonatal Mortality	-	-	-	-	-
Third or Fourth Degree Laceration	-	-	2.71%	3.63%	3.27%

Gulf Coast Hospital

13681 Doctors Way
Fort Meyers, FL 33912
URL: www.gulfcoasthospital.com
Ownership: Proprietary
Emergency Services: Yes

Phone: 239-768-5000
Fax: 239-768-8379

Accredited: Yes
Licensed Beds: 107

Key Personnel:
CEO . . . . Mark F Weber
Chief Medical Staff . . . . David Reardin
Emergency Room . . . . Karen Reed

Measure	Cases	This Hospital	State Average	U.S. Average	Top Hospital
Heart Attack Care					
ACE Inhibitor or ARB for LVSD	0	-	83%	82%	100%
Aspirin at Arrival[1]	14	79%	93%	92%	100%
Aspirin at Discharge[1]	4	50%	88%	90%	100%
Beta Blocker at Arrival[1]	13	77%	89%	87%	100%
Beta Blocker at Discharge[1]	6	83%	92%	90%	100%
Fibrinolytic Medication Timing	0	-	33%	31%	100%
PCI Within 90 Minutes of Arrival	0	-	52%	54%	95%
Smoking Cessation Advice	0	-	92%	88%	100%
Heart Failure Care					
ACE Inhibitor or ARB for LVSD[1]	7	86%	82%	82%	100%
Discharge Instructions[1]	23	4%	61%	61%	93%
Evaluation of LVS Function	25	60%	90%	83%	99%
Smoking Cessation Advice[1]	1	100%	91%	82%	100%
Pneumonia Care					
Appropriate Initial Antibiotic	59	73%	84%	83%	94%
Blood Culture Timing	49	90%	88%	90%	100%
Influenza Vaccine[1]	15	67%	64%	70%	100%
Initial Antibiotic Timing	79	68%	74%	80%	93%
Oxygenation Assessment	92	100%	99%	99%	100%
Pneumococcal Vaccine	54	52%	67%	69%	94%
Smoking Cessation Advice[1]	20	100%	90%	80%	100%
Surgical Infection Prevention					
Prophylactic Antibiotic Given[2]	354	83%	83%	77%	95%
Prophylactic Antibiotic Selection[2]	85	98%	90%	90%	100%
Prophylactic Antibiotic Stopped[2]	351	81%	70%	72%	95%
Pregnancy Care					
Inpatient Neonatal Mortality	-	-	-	-	-
Third or Fourth Degree Laceration	-	-	2.71%	3.63%	3.27%

Lee Memorial Health System

2776 Cleveland Avenue
Fort Myers, FL 33901
URL: www.leememorial.org
Ownership: Govt - Hospital District or Authority
Emergency Services: Yes

Phone: 941-332-1111
Fax: 239-772-6565

Accredited: Yes
Licensed Beds: 948

Key Personnel:
Administrator/CEO . . . . James R Nathan
Chief Medical Staff . . . . Chuck Krivenko, MD

Measure	Cases	This Hospital	State Average	U.S. Average	Top Hospital
Heart Attack Care					
ACE Inhibitor or ARB for LVSD	59	80%	83%	82%	100%
Aspirin at Arrival	161	93%	93%	92%	100%
Aspirin at Discharge	199	96%	88%	90%	100%
Beta Blocker at Arrival	119	92%	89%	87%	100%
Beta Blocker at Discharge	220	98%	92%	90%	100%
Fibrinolytic Medication Timing[1]	1	0%	33%	31%	100%
PCI Within 90 Minutes of Arrival[1]	12	33%	52%	54%	95%
Smoking Cessation Advice	87	99%	92%	88%	100%
Heart Failure Care					
ACE Inhibitor or ARB for LVSD	100	81%	82%	82%	100%
Discharge Instructions	195	46%	61%	61%	93%

NOTE: Hospital profiles are in alphabetical order by state, then city, then hospital within the city; Rankings are sorted by rate in descending order and exclude hospitals with less than 25 cases; (1) The number of cases is too small (n<25) for purposes of reliably predicting hospital performance; (2) Measure reflects the hospital's indication that its submission was based upon a sample of its relevant discharges; (3) Rate reflects fewer than the maximum possible quarters of data for the measure; (4) Inaccurate information submitted and suppressed for one or more quarters; (5) No data is available from the hospital for this measure; Please refer to the User's Guide for a full explanation of data

		This	State	U.S.	Top
Evaluation of LVS Function	238	91%	90%	83%	99%
Smoking Cessation Advice	42	95%	91%	82%	100%
Pneumonia Care					
Appropriate Initial Antibiotic	105	82%	84%	83%	94%
Blood Culture Timing	116	93%	88%	90%	100%
Influenza Vaccine	31	81%	64%	70%	100%
Initial Antibiotic Timing	155	73%	74%	80%	93%
Oxygenation Assessment	193	100%	99%	99%	100%
Pneumococcal Vaccine	118	77%	67%	69%	94%
Smoking Cessation Advice	39	90%	90%	80%	100%
Surgical Infection Prevention					
Prophylactic Antibiotic Given	339	88%	83%	77%	95%
Prophylactic Antibiotic Selection	86	91%	90%	90%	100%
Prophylactic Antibiotic Stopped	328	80%	70%	72%	95%
Pregnancy Care					
Inpatient Neonatal Mortality	-	-	-	-	-
Third or Fourth Degree Laceration	-	-	2.71%	3.63%	3.27%

Southwest Florida Regional Medical Center

2727 Winkler Avenue
Fort Myers, FL 33901
URL: www.swfrmc.com
Ownership: Proprietary
Emergency Services: Yes

Phone: 239-939-1147
Fax: 239-939-8260

Accredited: Yes
Licensed Beds: 400

Key Personnel:
President/CEO . . . . Steve Royal
Chief Medical Staff . . . . Abraham Sadighi, MD
Director Catheterization Lab . . . . Paula Stafford, RN
Emergency Room . . . . Wanda Ruben
Director Infection/Disease Control . . . . Zelda Nottingham
Director Medical/Surgical Nursing . . . . Chris DeRose
Director Radiology . . . . Marcell Sizemore
Director Cardiopulmonary Services . . . . Mike MacDonald

Measure	Cases	This Hospital	State Average	U.S. Average	Top Hospital
Heart Attack Care					
ACE Inhibitor or ARB for LVSD	86	72%	83%	82%	100%
Aspirin at Arrival	226	96%	93%	92%	100%
Aspirin at Discharge	274	96%	88%	90%	100%
Beta Blocker at Arrival	207	91%	89%	87%	100%
Beta Blocker at Discharge	286	97%	92%	90%	100%
Fibrinolytic Medication Timing[1]	1	0%	33%	31%	100%
PCI Within 90 Minutes of Arrival[1]	12	42%	52%	54%	95%
Smoking Cessation Advice	89	99%	92%	88%	100%
Heart Failure Care					
ACE Inhibitor or ARB for LVSD	219	83%	82%	82%	100%
Discharge Instructions	460	52%	61%	61%	93%
Evaluation of LVS Function	531	87%	90%	83%	99%
Smoking Cessation Advice	87	97%	91%	82%	100%
Pneumonia Care					
Appropriate Initial Antibiotic	262	88%	84%	83%	94%
Blood Culture Timing	285	86%	88%	90%	100%
Influenza Vaccine	110	51%	64%	70%	100%
Initial Antibiotic Timing	437	73%	74%	80%	93%
Oxygenation Assessment	509	100%	99%	99%	100%
Pneumococcal Vaccine	336	54%	67%	69%	94%
Smoking Cessation Advice	102	92%	90%	80%	100%
Surgical Infection Prevention					
Prophylactic Antibiotic Given[2,3]	345	77%	83%	77%	95%
Prophylactic Antibiotic Selection[2]	234	94%	90%	90%	100%
Prophylactic Antibiotic Stopped[2,3]	341	62%	70%	72%	95%
Pregnancy Care					
Inpatient Neonatal Mortality	-	-	-	-	-
Third or Fourth Degree Laceration	-	-	2.71%	3.63%	3.27%

Lawnwood Regional Med Ctr & Heart Inst

1700 South 23rd Street
Fort Pierce, FL 34950
URL: www.lawnwoodmed.com
Ownership: Proprietary
Emergency Services: Yes

Phone: 772-461-4000
Fax: 877-567-8583

Accredited: Yes
Licensed Beds: 36

Measure	Cases	This Hospital	State Average	U.S. Average	Top Hospital
Heart Attack Care					
ACE Inhibitor or ARB for LVSD	115	99%	83%	82%	100%
Aspirin at Arrival	189	99%	93%	92%	100%
Aspirin at Discharge	369	98%	88%	90%	100%
Beta Blocker at Arrival	163	97%	89%	87%	100%
Beta Blocker at Discharge	398	98%	92%	90%	100%
Fibrinolytic Medication Timing[1]	8	38%	33%	31%	100%
PCI Within 90 Minutes of Arrival[1]	8	12%	52%	54%	95%
Smoking Cessation Advice	147	100%	92%	88%	100%
Heart Failure Care					
ACE Inhibitor or ARB for LVSD	261	95%	82%	82%	100%
Discharge Instructions	493	90%	61%	61%	93%
Evaluation of LVS Function	586	98%	90%	83%	99%
Smoking Cessation Advice	135	99%	91%	82%	100%
Pneumonia Care					
Appropriate Initial Antibiotic	219	90%	84%	83%	94%
Blood Culture Timing	288	94%	88%	90%	100%
Influenza Vaccine	80	95%	64%	70%	100%
Initial Antibiotic Timing	356	81%	74%	80%	93%
Oxygenation Assessment	411	99%	99%	99%	100%
Pneumococcal Vaccine	240	92%	67%	69%	94%
Smoking Cessation Advice	106	97%	90%	80%	100%
Surgical Infection Prevention					
Prophylactic Antibiotic Given[3]	428	86%	83%	77%	95%
Prophylactic Antibiotic Selection	119	91%	90%	90%	100%
Prophylactic Antibiotic Stopped[3]	415	75%	70%	72%	95%
Pregnancy Care					
Inpatient Neonatal Mortality	-	-	-	-	-
Third or Fourth Degree Laceration	-	-	2.71%	3.63%	3.27%

Fort Walton Beach Medical Center

Alternate Name: Humana Hospital-Fort Walton Beach
1000 Mar-Walt Drive
Fort Walton Beach, FL 32547
URL: www.fwbmc.com
Ownership: Proprietary
Emergency Services: Yes

Phone: 850-862-1111
Fax: 850-862-9149

Accredited: Yes
Licensed Beds: 247

Key Personnel:
CEO . . . . Wayne Campbell
Chief Medical Staff . . . . Thomas Holt
Cardiac Lab . . . . Stan Clark
Catheterization Lab . . . . Stan Clark
Emergency Room . . . . Cathy McIntyre
ICU . . . . Linda Davis
Intensive Coronary . . . . Linda Davis
Director Medical Surgical Nursing . . . . Marion Bach
OB/GYN/Women's Health . . . . Marian Bach
Director Respiratory Therapy . . . . Mark Herrington

Measure	Cases	This Hospital	State Average	U.S. Average	Top Hospital
Heart Attack Care					
ACE Inhibitor or ARB for LVSD	54	100%	83%	82%	100%
Aspirin at Arrival	164	99%	93%	92%	100%
Aspirin at Discharge	282	99%	88%	90%	100%
Beta Blocker at Arrival	130	100%	89%	87%	100%
Beta Blocker at Discharge	262	99%	92%	90%	100%
Fibrinolytic Medication Timing	0	-	33%	31%	100%
PCI Within 90 Minutes of Arrival[1]	12	42%	52%	54%	95%
Smoking Cessation Advice	110	99%	92%	88%	100%
Heart Failure Care					
ACE Inhibitor or ARB for LVSD	74	100%	82%	82%	100%
Discharge Instructions	219	95%	61%	61%	93%
Evaluation of LVS Function	283	97%	90%	83%	99%
Smoking Cessation Advice	55	100%	91%	82%	100%
Pneumonia Care					

NOTE: Hospital profiles are in alphabetical order by state, then city, then hospital within the city; Rankings are sorted by rate in descending order and exclude hospitals with less than 25 cases; (1) The number of cases is too small (n<25) for purposes of reliably predicting hospital performance; (2) Measure reflects the hospital's indication that its submission was based upon a sample of its relevant discharges; (3) Rate reflects fewer than the maximum possible quarters of data for the measure; (4) Inaccurate information submitted and suppressed for one or more quarters; (5) No data is available from the hospital for this measure; Please refer to the User's Guide for a full explanation of data

Measure	Cases	This Hospital	State Average	U.S. Average	Top Hospital
Appropriate Initial Antibiotic	156	79%	84%	83%	94%
Blood Culture Timing	132	89%	88%	90%	100%
Influenza Vaccine	40	65%	64%	70%	100%
Initial Antibiotic Timing	218	69%	74%	80%	93%
Oxygenation Assessment	245	100%	99%	99%	100%
Pneumococcal Vaccine	138	67%	67%	69%	94%
Smoking Cessation Advice	76	95%	90%	80%	100%
Surgical Infection Prevention					
Prophylactic Antibiotic Given[2]	246	87%	83%	77%	95%
Prophylactic Antibiotic Selection[2]	110	91%	90%	90%	100%
Prophylactic Antibiotic Stopped[2]	230	53%	70%	72%	95%
Pregnancy Care					
Inpatient Neonatal Mortality	-	-	-	-	-
Third or Fourth Degree Laceration	-	-	2.71%	3.63%	3.27%

North Florida Regional Medical Center

6500 Newberry Road   Phone: 352-333-4000
Gainesville, FL 32605   Fax: 352-333-4800
URL: www.nfrmc.com
Ownership: Proprietary   Accredited: Yes
Emergency Services: Yes   Licensed Beds: 278
Key Personnel:
CEO. . . . . Brian Robinson
Chief Radiology . . . . Robert Stouffer
Director Respiratory Therapy . . . . Dick Hahn

Measure	Cases	This Hospital	State Average	U.S. Average	Top Hospital
Heart Attack Care					
ACE Inhibitor or ARB for LVSD[2]	98	62%	83%	82%	100%
Aspirin at Arrival[2]	194	98%	93%	92%	100%
Aspirin at Discharge[2]	314	97%	88%	90%	100%
Beta Blocker at Arrival[2]	143	87%	89%	87%	100%
Beta Blocker at Discharge[2]	316	90%	92%	90%	100%
Fibrinolytic Medication Timing[2]	0	-	33%	31%	100%
PCI Within 90 Minutes of Arrival[1,2]	12	58%	52%	54%	95%
Smoking Cessation Advice[2]	115	98%	92%	88%	100%
Heart Failure Care					
ACE Inhibitor or ARB for LVSD[2]	220	64%	82%	82%	100%
Discharge Instructions[2]	470	44%	61%	61%	93%
Evaluation of LVS Function[2]	573	88%	90%	83%	99%
Smoking Cessation Advice[2]	82	98%	91%	82%	100%
Pneumonia Care					
Appropriate Initial Antibiotic[2]	204	91%	84%	83%	94%
Blood Culture Timing[2]	203	76%	88%	90%	100%
Influenza Vaccine	76	64%	64%	70%	100%
Initial Antibiotic Timing[2]	309	73%	74%	80%	93%
Oxygenation Assessment[2]	384	97%	99%	99%	100%
Pneumococcal Vaccine[2]	241	51%	67%	69%	94%
Smoking Cessation Advice[2]	90	98%	90%	80%	100%
Surgical Infection Prevention					
Prophylactic Antibiotic Given[2,3]	315	86%	83%	77%	95%
Prophylactic Antibiotic Selection[2]	136	90%	90%	90%	100%
Prophylactic Antibiotic Stopped[2,3]	313	65%	70%	72%	95%
Pregnancy Care					
Inpatient Neonatal Mortality	-	-	-	-	-
Third or Fourth Degree Laceration	-	-	2.71%	3.63%	3.27%

Shands at the University of Florida

Alternate Name: Shands Hospital at the University of Florida
1600 SW Archer Road   Toll-Free: 800-749-7424
Gainesville, FL 32608   Phone: 352-265-8000
                                       Fax: 352-265-7948
E-mail: consult@shands.ufl.edu
URL: www.shands.org
Ownership: Voluntary non-profit - Private   Accredited: Yes
Emergency Services: Yes   Licensed Beds: 1,953
Key Personnel:
President/CEO. . . . . Timothy M Goldfarb
Chief Medical Staff. . . . . Nikolaus Cassisi, MD
Emergency Room . . . . A Joseph Layon, MD
Director Infection/Disease Control . . . . Loretta L Fauerbach
CCU Spvg. Nurse . . . . Rose Rivers, RN
Director Medical/Surgical Nursing . . . . Rose Rivers, RN

OB/GYN Womens Health. . . . . I Keith Stone, MD
Director Respiratory Therapy . . . . Timothy J Coons, RRT

Measure	Cases	This Hospital	State Average	U.S. Average	Top Hospital
Heart Attack Care					
ACE Inhibitor or ARB for LVSD	128	82%	83%	82%	100%
Aspirin at Arrival	280	97%	93%	92%	100%
Aspirin at Discharge	401	97%	88%	90%	100%
Beta Blocker at Arrival	246	90%	89%	87%	100%
Beta Blocker at Discharge	403	96%	92%	90%	100%
Fibrinolytic Medication Timing[1]	1	0%	33%	31%	100%
PCI Within 90 Minutes of Arrival[1]	8	62%	52%	54%	95%
Smoking Cessation Advice	161	96%	92%	88%	100%
Heart Failure Care					
ACE Inhibitor or ARB for LVSD	324	86%	82%	82%	100%
Discharge Instructions	548	32%	61%	61%	93%
Evaluation of LVS Function	617	96%	90%	83%	99%
Smoking Cessation Advice	122	87%	91%	82%	100%
Pneumonia Care					
Appropriate Initial Antibiotic	160	81%	84%	83%	94%
Blood Culture Timing	166	87%	88%	90%	100%
Influenza Vaccine	50	34%	64%	70%	100%
Initial Antibiotic Timing	238	55%	74%	80%	93%
Oxygenation Assessment	319	100%	99%	99%	100%
Pneumococcal Vaccine	146	42%	67%	69%	94%
Smoking Cessation Advice	99	96%	90%	80%	100%
Surgical Infection Prevention					
Prophylactic Antibiotic Given	589	86%	83%	77%	95%
Prophylactic Antibiotic Selection	133	95%	90%	90%	100%
Prophylactic Antibiotic Stopped	570	72%	70%	72%	95%
Pregnancy Care					
Inpatient Neonatal Mortality[2]	1,807	1.66%	-	-	-
Third or Fourth Degree Laceration[2]	1,032	2.03%	2.71%	3.63%	3.27%

Campbellton Graceville Hospital

5429 College Drive   Phone: 850-263-7201
Graceville, FL 32440
Ownership: Govt - Hospital District or Authority   Accredited: No
Emergency Services: Yes

Measure	Cases	This Hospital	State Average	U.S. Average	Top Hospital
Heart Attack Care					
ACE Inhibitor or ARB for LVSD[5]	-	-	83%	82%	100%
Aspirin at Arrival[5]	-	-	93%	92%	100%
Aspirin at Discharge[5]	-	-	88%	90%	100%
Beta Blocker at Arrival[5]	-	-	89%	87%	100%
Beta Blocker at Discharge[5]	-	-	92%	90%	100%
Fibrinolytic Medication Timing[5]	-	-	33%	31%	100%
PCI Within 90 Minutes of Arrival[5]	-	-	52%	54%	95%
Smoking Cessation Advice[5]	-	-	92%	88%	100%
Heart Failure Care					
ACE Inhibitor or ARB for LVSD[1,3]	4	25%	82%	82%	100%
Discharge Instructions[1,3]	4	0%	61%	61%	93%
Evaluation of LVS Function[1,3]	8	50%	90%	83%	99%
Smoking Cessation Advice[3]	0	-	91%	82%	100%
Pneumonia Care					
Appropriate Initial Antibiotic[1,3]	2	100%	84%	83%	94%
Blood Culture Timing[3]	0	-	88%	90%	100%
Influenza Vaccine[5]	-	-	64%	70%	100%
Initial Antibiotic Timing[1,3]	3	100%	74%	80%	93%
Oxygenation Assessment[1,3]	3	100%	99%	99%	100%
Pneumococcal Vaccine[1,3]	3	0%	67%	69%	94%
Smoking Cessation Advice[3]	0	-	90%	80%	100%
Surgical Infection Prevention					
Prophylactic Antibiotic Given[5]	-	-	83%	77%	95%
Prophylactic Antibiotic Selection[5]	-	-	90%	90%	100%
Prophylactic Antibiotic Stopped[5]	-	-	70%	72%	95%
Pregnancy Care					
Inpatient Neonatal Mortality	-	-	-	-	-
Third or Fourth Degree Laceration	-	-	2.71%	3.63%	3.27%

NOTE: Hospital profiles are in alphabetical order by state, then city, then hospital within the city; Rankings are sorted by rate in descending order and exclude hospitals with less than 25 cases; (1) The number of cases is too small (n<25) for purposes of reliably predicting hospital performance; (2) Measure reflects the hospital's indication that its submission was based upon a sample of its relevant discharges; (3) Rate reflects fewer than the maximum possible quarters of data for the measure; (4) Inaccurate information submitted and suppressed for one or more quarters; (5) No data is available from the hospital for this measure; Please refer to the User's Guide for a full explanation of data

Gulf Breeze Hospital

1110 Gulf Breeze Parkway
Gulf Breeze, FL 32562
URL: www.ebaptisthealthcare.org/GulfBreezeHospital/Default
Ownership: Voluntary non-profit - Private
Emergency Services: Yes
Key Personnel:
Director Infection/Disease Control . . . . Carolynn Kindall

Phone: 850-934-2000
Fax: 850-934-2069
Accredited: Yes
Licensed Beds: 60

Measure	Cases	This Hospital	State Average	U.S. Average	Top Hospital
Heart Attack Care					
ACE Inhibitor or ARB for LVSD[1]	5	80%	83%	82%	100%
Aspirin at Arrival	29	97%	93%	92%	100%
Aspirin at Discharge[1]	20	100%	88%	90%	100%
Beta Blocker at Arrival	25	88%	89%	87%	100%
Beta Blocker at Discharge[1]	19	95%	92%	90%	100%
Fibrinolytic Medication Timing	0	-	33%	31%	100%
PCI Within 90 Minutes of Arrival	0	-	52%	54%	95%
Smoking Cessation Advice[1]	9	100%	92%	88%	100%
Heart Failure Care					
ACE Inhibitor or ARB for LVSD	25	88%	82%	82%	100%
Discharge Instructions	92	57%	61%	61%	93%
Evaluation of LVS Function	110	88%	90%	83%	99%
Smoking Cessation Advice[1]	15	93%	91%	82%	100%
Pneumonia Care					
Appropriate Initial Antibiotic	114	92%	84%	83%	94%
Blood Culture Timing	76	91%	88%	90%	100%
Influenza Vaccine[1]	22	73%	64%	70%	100%
Initial Antibiotic Timing	127	81%	74%	80%	93%
Oxygenation Assessment	153	100%	99%	99%	100%
Pneumococcal Vaccine	95	76%	67%	69%	94%
Smoking Cessation Advice	35	100%	90%	80%	100%
Surgical Infection Prevention					
Prophylactic Antibiotic Given	419	76%	83%	77%	95%
Prophylactic Antibiotic Selection	93	97%	90%	90%	100%
Prophylactic Antibiotic Stopped	394	60%	70%	72%	95%
Pregnancy Care					
Inpatient Neonatal Mortality	-	-	-	-	-
Third or Fourth Degree Laceration	-	-	2.71%	3.63%	3.27%

Hialeah Hospital

651 E 25th Street
Miami, FL 33013
URL: www.hialeahhosp.com
Ownership: Proprietary
Emergency Services: Yes
Key Personnel:
CEO. . . . . Clifford J Bauer
Chief Medical Staff. Jose Nunez, MD
Emergency Room . . . . Romon Vidal, MD
Director Infection/Disease Control . . . . Maggie Kane
Supervisor Medical/Surgical. . . . . Arletta Jackson
OB/GYN Womens Health. . . . . Laida Casandra, MD
Chief Radiology . . . . Mark Fasbinder, MD
Director Respiratory Therapy . . . . Jesus Rojas

Phone: 305-693-6100
Fax: 305-835-4252

Accredited: No
Licensed Beds: 378

Measure	Cases	This Hospital	State Average	U.S. Average	Top Hospital
Heart Attack Care					
ACE Inhibitor or ARB for LVSD	35	91%	83%	82%	100%
Aspirin at Arrival	216	97%	93%	92%	100%
Aspirin at Discharge	87	95%	88%	90%	100%
Beta Blocker at Arrival	170	93%	89%	87%	100%
Beta Blocker at Discharge	94	94%	92%	90%	100%
Fibrinolytic Medication Timing[1]	15	87%	33%	31%	100%
PCI Within 90 Minutes of Arrival	0	-	52%	54%	95%
Smoking Cessation Advice[1]	11	100%	92%	88%	100%
Heart Failure Care					
ACE Inhibitor or ARB for LVSD	163	96%	82%	82%	100%
Discharge Instructions	368	99%	61%	61%	93%
Evaluation of LVS Function	446	100%	90%	83%	99%
Smoking Cessation Advice	66	100%	91%	82%	100%
Pneumonia Care					
Appropriate Initial Antibiotic	279	84%	84%	83%	94%

Measure	Cases	This Hospital	State Average	U.S. Average	Top Hospital
Blood Culture Timing	281	94%	88%	90%	100%
Influenza Vaccine	77	95%	64%	70%	100%
Initial Antibiotic Timing	390	86%	74%	80%	93%
Oxygenation Assessment	438	100%	99%	99%	100%
Pneumococcal Vaccine	299	92%	67%	69%	94%
Smoking Cessation Advice	53	100%	90%	80%	100%
Surgical Infection Prevention					
Prophylactic Antibiotic Given[2]	123	95%	83%	77%	95%
Prophylactic Antibiotic Selection[2]	28	89%	90%	90%	100%
Prophylactic Antibiotic Stopped[2]	96	67%	70%	72%	95%
Pregnancy Care					
Inpatient Neonatal Mortality	-	-	-	-	-
Third or Fourth Degree Laceration	-	-	2.71%	3.63%	3.27%

Palm Springs General Hospital

1475 W 49th Street
Miami, FL 33012
Ownership: Voluntary non-profit - Private
Emergency Services: Yes
Key Personnel:
CEO. . . . . Carlos Milanes
Chief Medical Staff. Roberto Fernandez, MD
Emergency Room . . . . Theresa Bernanrd, RN
Director Medical/Surgical Nursing . . . . Karon Kurty, RN
Chief Radiology . . . . Stephen Kaul, MD
Director Respiratory Therapy . . . . Roger Depaz

Phone: 305-558-2500
Fax: 305-558-8679
Accredited: Yes
Licensed Beds: 247

Measure	Cases	This Hospital	State Average	U.S. Average	Top Hospital
Heart Attack Care					
ACE Inhibitor or ARB for LVSD[1]	23	83%	83%	82%	100%
Aspirin at Arrival	139	97%	93%	92%	100%
Aspirin at Discharge	46	83%	88%	90%	100%
Beta Blocker at Arrival	123	89%	89%	87%	100%
Beta Blocker at Discharge	52	87%	92%	90%	100%
Fibrinolytic Medication Timing[1]	15	40%	33%	31%	100%
PCI Within 90 Minutes of Arrival	0	-	52%	54%	95%
Smoking Cessation Advice	0	-	92%	88%	100%
Heart Failure Care					
ACE Inhibitor or ARB for LVSD	160	78%	82%	82%	100%
Discharge Instructions	316	80%	61%	61%	93%
Evaluation of LVS Function	380	91%	90%	83%	99%
Smoking Cessation Advice	26	85%	91%	82%	100%
Pneumonia Care					
Appropriate Initial Antibiotic	247	67%	84%	83%	94%
Blood Culture Timing	189	95%	88%	90%	100%
Influenza Vaccine[4,5]	-	-	64%	70%	100%
Initial Antibiotic Timing	292	73%	74%	80%	93%
Oxygenation Assessment	341	96%	99%	99%	100%
Pneumococcal Vaccine	248	53%	67%	69%	94%
Smoking Cessation Advice	26	100%	90%	80%	100%
Surgical Infection Prevention					
Prophylactic Antibiotic Given[3]	123	75%	83%	77%	95%
Prophylactic Antibiotic Selection	41	80%	90%	90%	100%
Prophylactic Antibiotic Stopped[3]	121	73%	70%	72%	95%
Pregnancy Care					
Inpatient Neonatal Mortality	-	-	-	-	-
Third or Fourth Degree Laceration	-	-	2.71%	3.63%	3.27%

Palmetto General Hospital

2001 W 68th Street
Hialeah, FL 33016
URL: www.palmettogeneral.com
Ownership: Proprietary
Emergency Services: Yes
Key Personnel:
President/CEO. . . . . Ana Mederos
Chief Medical Staff. Jose Gamez, MD
Director Cardiac Lab . . . . Gonzalo Arcentales
Director Catheterization Lab. . . . . Gonzalo Archentales
Director Emergency Room. . . . . Gene Letourneau
Emergency Room . . . . Richard Spirer, MD
Coordinator Infection Control . . . . Jose Luis Ruiz
Director Intensive/Coronary Care. . . . . Judy Martin

Phone: 305-823-5000
Fax: 305-364-2173

Accredited: Yes
Licensed Beds: 360

NOTE: Hospital profiles are in alphabetical order by state, then city, then hospital within the city; Rankings are sorted by rate in descending order and exclude hospitals with less than 25 cases; (1) The number of cases is too small (n<25) for purposes of reliably predicting hospital performance; (2) Measure reflects the hospital's indication that its submission was based upon a sample of its relevant discharges; (3) Rate reflects fewer than the maximum possible quarters of data for the measure; (4) Inaccurate information submitted and suppressed for one or more quarters; (5) No data is available from the hospital for this measure; Please refer to the User's Guide for a full explanation of data

Director Medical Surgical Nursing . . . . Brenda Wilson
Director OB/GYN/Women's Health. . . . . Beth Kelley
Director Radiology . . . . Cindy Siegel
Director Respiratory/Cardiopulmonary . . . . Justo Ruiz

Measure	Cases	This Hospital	State Average	U.S. Average	Top Hospital
Heart Attack Care					
ACE Inhibitor or ARB for LVSD[1]	16	88%	83%	82%	100%
Aspirin at Arrival	189	97%	93%	92%	100%
Aspirin at Discharge	40	90%	88%	90%	100%
Beta Blocker at Arrival	177	99%	89%	87%	100%
Beta Blocker at Discharge	51	92%	92%	90%	100%
Fibrinolytic Medication Timing[1]	3	0%	33%	31%	100%
PCI Within 90 Minutes of Arrival	0	-	52%	54%	95%
Smoking Cessation Advice[1]	12	100%	92%	88%	100%
Heart Failure Care					
ACE Inhibitor or ARB for LVSD	177	80%	82%	82%	100%
Discharge Instructions	395	81%	61%	61%	93%
Evaluation of LVS Function	462	95%	90%	83%	99%
Smoking Cessation Advice	71	100%	91%	82%	100%
Pneumonia Care					
Appropriate Initial Antibiotic	244	87%	84%	83%	94%
Blood Culture Timing	213	77%	88%	90%	100%
Influenza Vaccine	40	65%	64%	70%	100%
Initial Antibiotic Timing	263	75%	74%	80%	93%
Oxygenation Assessment	311	100%	99%	99%	100%
Pneumococcal Vaccine	174	73%	67%	69%	94%
Smoking Cessation Advice	46	100%	90%	80%	100%
Surgical Infection Prevention					
Prophylactic Antibiotic Given[2]	179	88%	83%	77%	95%
Prophylactic Antibiotic Selection[2]	44	93%	90%	90%	100%
Prophylactic Antibiotic Stopped[2]	180	63%	70%	72%	95%
Pregnancy Care					
Inpatient Neonatal Mortality	-	-	-	-	-
Third or Fourth Degree Laceration	-	-	2.71%	3.63%	3.27%

Memorial Regional Hospital

3501 Johnson Street
Hollywood, FL 33021
URL: www.mhs.net
Ownership: Govt - Hospital District or Authority
Emergency Services: Yes
Key Personnel:
Administrator . . . . JE Piriz
Chief Medical Staff. Kenneth Gelman, MD
Director Nursing/Emergency Services . . . . Rose Mary Bossman
OB/GYN Womens Health. . . . . Robert Siudmak, MD
Chief Radiology . . . . Robert Appelbaum, MD

Phone: 954-987-2000
Fax: 954-985-3453

Accredited: Yes
Licensed Beds: 684

Measure	Cases	This Hospital	State Average	U.S. Average	Top Hospital
Heart Attack Care					
ACE Inhibitor or ARB for LVSD	150	92%	83%	82%	100%
Aspirin at Arrival	412	99%	93%	92%	100%
Aspirin at Discharge	652	99%	88%	90%	100%
Beta Blocker at Arrival	357	97%	89%	87%	100%
Beta Blocker at Discharge	652	98%	92%	90%	100%
Fibrinolytic Medication Timing	0	-	33%	31%	100%
PCI Within 90 Minutes of Arrival	30	87%	52%	54%	95%
Smoking Cessation Advice	222	99%	92%	88%	100%
Heart Failure Care					
ACE Inhibitor or ARB for LVSD	486	93%	82%	82%	100%
Discharge Instructions	869	85%	61%	61%	93%
Evaluation of LVS Function	992	99%	90%	83%	99%
Smoking Cessation Advice	208	100%	91%	82%	100%
Pneumonia Care					
Appropriate Initial Antibiotic	305	97%	84%	83%	94%
Blood Culture Timing	359	95%	88%	90%	100%
Influenza Vaccine	65	95%	64%	70%	100%
Initial Antibiotic Timing	403	85%	74%	80%	93%
Oxygenation Assessment	506	100%	99%	99%	100%
Pneumococcal Vaccine	236	96%	67%	69%	94%
Smoking Cessation Advice	118	100%	90%	80%	100%

Measure	Cases	This Hospital	State Average	U.S. Average	Top Hospital
Surgical Infection Prevention					
Prophylactic Antibiotic Given[2]	1,000	93%	83%	77%	95%
Prophylactic Antibiotic Selection[2]	63	95%	90%	90%	100%
Prophylactic Antibiotic Stopped[2]	971	85%	70%	72%	95%
Pregnancy Care					
Inpatient Neonatal Mortality	-	-	-	-	-
Third or Fourth Degree Laceration	-	-	2.71%	3.63%	3.27%

Homestead Hospital

160 Northwest 13th Street
Homestead, FL 33030
URL: www.baptisthealth.net
Ownership: Voluntary non-profit - Private
Emergency Services: Yes
Key Personnel:
President/CEO. . . . . Brian Keeley
CEO. . . . . Bo Boulenger
Emergency Room . . . . Lloyd Tucker
Director Respiratory Therapy . . . . Karen Mella

Phone: 786-243-8000
Fax: 305-242-3557

Accredited: Yes
Licensed Beds: 120

Measure	Cases	This Hospital	State Average	U.S. Average	Top Hospital
Heart Attack Care					
ACE Inhibitor or ARB for LVSD[1]	8	100%	83%	82%	100%
Aspirin at Arrival	88	100%	93%	92%	100%
Aspirin at Discharge[1]	18	100%	88%	90%	100%
Beta Blocker at Arrival	77	100%	89%	87%	100%
Beta Blocker at Discharge[1]	20	100%	92%	90%	100%
Fibrinolytic Medication Timing[1]	2	0%	33%	31%	100%
PCI Within 90 Minutes of Arrival	0	-	52%	54%	95%
Smoking Cessation Advice[1]	5	100%	92%	88%	100%
Heart Failure Care					
ACE Inhibitor or ARB for LVSD	126	98%	82%	82%	100%
Discharge Instructions	291	94%	61%	61%	93%
Evaluation of LVS Function	323	100%	90%	83%	99%
Smoking Cessation Advice	84	100%	91%	82%	100%
Pneumonia Care					
Appropriate Initial Antibiotic	241	98%	84%	83%	94%
Blood Culture Timing	249	95%	88%	90%	100%
Influenza Vaccine	52	83%	64%	70%	100%
Initial Antibiotic Timing	298	80%	74%	80%	93%
Oxygenation Assessment	344	100%	99%	99%	100%
Pneumococcal Vaccine	160	95%	67%	69%	94%
Smoking Cessation Advice	103	100%	90%	80%	100%
Surgical Infection Prevention					
Prophylactic Antibiotic Given	73	86%	83%	77%	95%
Prophylactic Antibiotic Selection[1]	20	95%	90%	90%	100%
Prophylactic Antibiotic Stopped	62	87%	70%	72%	95%
Pregnancy Care					
Inpatient Neonatal Mortality	-	-	-	-	-
Third or Fourth Degree Laceration	-	-	2.71%	3.63%	3.27%

Regional Medical Center Bayonet Point

Alternate Name: HCA Bayonet/Hudson Point Medical Center
14000 Fivay Road
Hudson, FL 34667

URL: www.mchealth.com
Ownership: Proprietary
Emergency Services: Yes
Key Personnel:
CEO. . . . . Steve Rector
Chief Medical Staff. Marshall DeSantis, MD
Director Catheterization Lab. . . . . Julie Lauallani
Director Emergency Room. . . . . Pam Schlicher
Emergency Room . . . . Andrea O'Lenick
Infection Control. . . . . Barbara Haner
Director CCU . . . . Cavoy Foelders
Director Radiology . . . . Carol Corder
Director Respiratory Therapy . . . . Melanie White

Toll-Free: 800-432-7811
Phone: 727-819-2929
Fax: 727-868-6431

Accredited: Yes
Licensed Beds: 290

Measure	Cases	This Hospital	State Average	U.S. Average	Top Hospital
Heart Attack Care					
ACE Inhibitor or ARB for LVSD	163	85%	83%	82%	100%

NOTE: Hospital profiles are in alphabetical order by state, then city, then hospital within the city; Rankings are sorted by rate in descending order and exclude hospitals with less than 25 cases; (1) The number of cases is too small (n<25) for purposes of reliably predicting hospital performance; (2) Measure reflects the hospital's indication that its submission was based upon a sample of its relevant discharges; (3) Rate reflects fewer than the maximum possible quarters of data for the measure; (4) Inaccurate information submitted and suppressed for one or more quarters; (5) No data is available from the hospital for this measure; Please refer to the User's Guide for a full explanation of data

Measure	Cases	This Hospital	State Average	U.S. Average	Top Hospital
Aspirin at Arrival	344	92%	93%	92%	100%
Aspirin at Discharge	625	94%	88%	90%	100%
Beta Blocker at Arrival	324	85%	89%	87%	100%
Beta Blocker at Discharge	640	94%	92%	90%	100%
Fibrinolytic Medication Timing[1]	10	30%	33%	31%	100%
PCI Within 90 Minutes of Arrival[1]	3	33%	52%	54%	95%
Smoking Cessation Advice	208	95%	92%	88%	100%
Heart Failure Care					
ACE Inhibitor or ARB for LVSD	304	80%	82%	82%	100%
Discharge Instructions	549	51%	61%	61%	93%
Evaluation of LVS Function	674	94%	90%	83%	99%
Smoking Cessation Advice	115	91%	91%	82%	100%
Pneumonia Care					
Appropriate Initial Antibiotic	125	86%	84%	83%	94%
Blood Culture Timing	84	68%	88%	90%	100%
Influenza Vaccine	47	51%	64%	70%	100%
Initial Antibiotic Timing	185	62%	74%	80%	93%
Oxygenation Assessment	233	100%	99%	99%	100%
Pneumococcal Vaccine	158	54%	67%	69%	94%
Smoking Cessation Advice	43	95%	90%	80%	100%
Surgical Infection Prevention					
Prophylactic Antibiotic Given[3]	566	62%	83%	77%	95%
Prophylactic Antibiotic Selection	155	95%	90%	90%	100%
Prophylactic Antibiotic Stopped[3]	542	60%	70%	72%	95%
Pregnancy Care					
Inpatient Neonatal Mortality	-	-	-	-	-
Third or Fourth Degree Laceration	-	-	2.71%	3.63%	3.27%

Citrus Memorial Hospital

502 West Highland Boulevard
Inverness, FL 34452
E-mail: lringquist@citrusmh.org
URL: www.citrusmh.com
Ownership: Govt - Hospital District or Authority
Emergency Services: Yes

Phone: 352-344-6588
Fax: 352-341-0136

Accredited: Yes
Licensed Beds: 171

Key Personnel:
President/CEO . . . . Ryan Beaty
Chief Medical Staff . . . . Rama Nathan
Catheterization Laboratory Manager . . . . Eric Shifter
Manager Emergency Room . . . . Deborah Hamilton Ford, RN
Manager ICU/CCU . . . . Maggie Brest, RN
Manager Intensive/Coronary Care . . . . Maggie Brest, RN
Manager Medical Surgical Nursing . . . . Brenda Hilton
Manager Obstetrics . . . . Margie Leturno
Manager Respiratory/Cardiopulmonary . . . . David Batcheller

Measure	Cases	This Hospital	State Average	U.S. Average	Top Hospital
Heart Attack Care					
ACE Inhibitor or ARB for LVSD	55	73%	83%	82%	100%
Aspirin at Arrival	282	96%	93%	92%	100%
Aspirin at Discharge	272	96%	88%	90%	100%
Beta Blocker at Arrival	260	85%	89%	87%	100%
Beta Blocker at Discharge	278	93%	92%	90%	100%
Fibrinolytic Medication Timing[1]	1	100%	33%	31%	100%
PCI Within 90 Minutes of Arrival[1]	13	62%	52%	54%	95%
Smoking Cessation Advice	103	94%	92%	88%	100%
Heart Failure Care					
ACE Inhibitor or ARB for LVSD	112	74%	82%	82%	100%
Discharge Instructions	241	54%	61%	61%	93%
Evaluation of LVS Function	297	86%	90%	83%	99%
Smoking Cessation Advice	41	90%	91%	82%	100%
Pneumonia Care					
Appropriate Initial Antibiotic	139	83%	84%	83%	94%
Blood Culture Timing	123	90%	88%	90%	100%
Influenza Vaccine[4,5]	-	-	64%	70%	100%
Initial Antibiotic Timing	178	75%	74%	80%	93%
Oxygenation Assessment	231	100%	99%	99%	100%
Pneumococcal Vaccine	167	81%	67%	69%	94%
Smoking Cessation Advice	36	94%	90%	80%	100%
Surgical Infection Prevention					
Prophylactic Antibiotic Given	529	86%	83%	77%	95%
Prophylactic Antibiotic Selection	150	97%	90%	90%	100%
Prophylactic Antibiotic Stopped	483	89%	70%	72%	95%

Measure					
Pregnancy Care					
Inpatient Neonatal Mortality	-	-	-	-	-
Third or Fourth Degree Laceration	-	-	2.71%	3.63%	3.27%

Baptist Medical Center

800 Prudential Drive
Jacksonville, FL 32207
URL: www.e-baptisthealth.com
Ownership: Voluntary non-profit - Private
Emergency Services: Yes

Phone: 904-202-2000
Fax: 904-202-3134

Accredited: Yes
Licensed Beds: 601

Key Personnel:
Administrator . . . . Joe Mitrick, FACHE
President/CEO . . . . William C Mason
Administrator . . . . John Wilbankes
Chief Medical Staff . . . . William Z McLear, MD
Emergency Room . . . . Richard Stomberg, MD
Director Infection/Disease Control . . . . Edna Javis
OB/GYN Womens Health . . . . Cynthia Flanders
Director Pulmonary Services . . . . Carolyn Ivy

Measure	Cases	This Hospital	State Average	U.S. Average	Top Hospital
Heart Attack Care					
ACE Inhibitor or ARB for LVSD[2]	63	86%	83%	82%	100%
Aspirin at Arrival[2]	152	96%	93%	92%	100%
Aspirin at Discharge[2]	402	98%	88%	90%	100%
Beta Blocker at Arrival[2]	147	94%	89%	87%	100%
Beta Blocker at Discharge[2]	404	97%	92%	90%	100%
Fibrinolytic Medication Timing[1,2]	3	33%	33%	31%	100%
PCI Within 90 Minutes of Arrival[1,2]	7	14%	52%	54%	95%
Smoking Cessation Advice[2]	170	99%	92%	88%	100%
Heart Failure Care					
ACE Inhibitor or ARB for LVSD[2]	251	82%	82%	82%	100%
Discharge Instructions[2]	502	36%	61%	61%	93%
Evaluation of LVS Function[2]	622	97%	90%	83%	99%
Smoking Cessation Advice[2]	149	81%	91%	82%	100%
Pneumonia Care					
Appropriate Initial Antibiotic[2]	301	80%	84%	83%	94%
Blood Culture Timing[2]	324	85%	88%	90%	100%
Influenza Vaccine	99	59%	64%	70%	100%
Initial Antibiotic Timing[2]	468	61%	74%	80%	93%
Oxygenation Assessment[2]	576	98%	99%	99%	100%
Pneumococcal Vaccine[2]	252	64%	67%	69%	94%
Smoking Cessation Advice[2]	151	77%	90%	80%	100%
Surgical Infection Prevention					
Prophylactic Antibiotic Given[2]	1,325	76%	83%	77%	95%
Prophylactic Antibiotic Selection[2]	78	74%	90%	90%	100%
Prophylactic Antibiotic Stopped[2]	1,224	73%	70%	72%	95%
Pregnancy Care					
Inpatient Neonatal Mortality	-	-	-	-	-
Third or Fourth Degree Laceration	-	-	2.71%	3.63%	3.27%

Columbia Memorial Hospital of Jacksonville

Alternate Name: Memorial Medical Center of Jacksonville
3625 University Boulevard S
Jacksonville, FL 32216
URL: www.memorialhospitaljax.com
Ownership: Voluntary non-profit - Private
Emergency Services: Yes

Phone: 904-399-6111
Fax: 904-399-6817

Accredited: Yes
Licensed Beds: 353

Key Personnel:
Administrator/President . . . . Rex Etheredge
Chief Medical Staff . . . . Gary Decker, MD
Emergency Room . . . . Jorge Perez, MD
Director Infection/Disease Control . . . . Mary Lutz, RN
CCU Spvg. Nurse . . . . Barbara Johnston, RN
Director Medical/Surgical Nursing . . . . Jane Nieter-Clark
OB/GYN Womens Health . . . . Hormoz Khosravi, MD
Chief Radiology . . . . Patrick Gordon, MD
Director Respiratory Therapy . . . . Mary Pierce

Measure	Cases	This Hospital	State Average	U.S. Average	Top Hospital
Heart Attack Care					
ACE Inhibitor or ARB for LVSD	65	85%	83%	82%	100%
Aspirin at Arrival	245	92%	93%	92%	100%

NOTE: Hospital profiles are in alphabetical order by state, then city, then hospital within the city; Rankings are sorted by rate in descending order and exclude hospitals with less than 25 cases; (1) The number of cases is too small (n<25) for purposes of reliably predicting hospital performance; (2) Measure reflects the hospital's indication that its submission was based upon a sample of its relevant discharges; (3) Rate reflects fewer than the maximum possible quarters of data for the measure; (4) Inaccurate information submitted and suppressed for one or more quarters; (5) No data is available from the hospital for this measure; Please refer to the User's Guide for a full explanation of data

Measure	Cases	This Hospital	State Average	U.S. Average	Top Hospital
Aspirin at Discharge	335	95%	88%	90%	100%
Beta Blocker at Arrival	184	88%	89%	87%	100%
Beta Blocker at Discharge	349	94%	92%	90%	100%
Fibrinolytic Medication Timing[1]	4	50%	33%	31%	100%
PCI Within 90 Minutes of Arrival[1]	13	31%	52%	54%	95%
Smoking Cessation Advice	177	99%	92%	88%	100%
Heart Failure Care					
ACE Inhibitor or ARB for LVSD	239	77%	82%	82%	100%
Discharge Instructions	498	43%	61%	61%	93%
Evaluation of LVS Function	615	93%	90%	83%	99%
Smoking Cessation Advice	128	97%	91%	82%	100%
Pneumonia Care					
Appropriate Initial Antibiotic	301	88%	84%	83%	94%
Blood Culture Timing	346	90%	88%	90%	100%
Influenza Vaccine	74	43%	64%	70%	100%
Initial Antibiotic Timing	416	75%	74%	80%	93%
Oxygenation Assessment	530	99%	99%	99%	100%
Pneumococcal Vaccine	294	42%	67%	69%	94%
Smoking Cessation Advice	147	96%	90%	80%	100%
Surgical Infection Prevention					
Prophylactic Antibiotic Given[2,3]	314	83%	83%	77%	95%
Prophylactic Antibiotic Selection[2]	137	88%	90%	90%	100%
Prophylactic Antibiotic Stopped[2,3]	290	60%	70%	72%	95%
Pregnancy Care					
Inpatient Neonatal Mortality	-	-	-	-	-
Third or Fourth Degree Laceration	-	-	2.71%	3.63%	3.27%

Saint Luke's Hospital

4201 Belfort Road
Jacksonville, FL 32216
URL: www.mayoclinic.org/stlukes-jax
Ownership: Voluntary non-profit - Private
Emergency Services: Yes

Phone: 904-296-3700
Fax: 904-296-4698

Accredited: Yes
Licensed Beds: 289

Key Personnel:
CEO . . . . Terry Harvey
Emergency Room . . . . Kathy Coley, RN
Director Radiology . . . . Neal Wilson

Measure	Cases	This Hospital	State Average	U.S. Average	Top Hospital
Heart Attack Care					
ACE Inhibitor or ARB for LVSD	32	94%	83%	82%	100%
Aspirin at Arrival	146	100%	93%	92%	100%
Aspirin at Discharge	143	97%	88%	90%	100%
Beta Blocker at Arrival	118	97%	89%	87%	100%
Beta Blocker at Discharge	181	95%	92%	90%	100%
Fibrinolytic Medication Timing[1]	1	100%	33%	31%	100%
PCI Within 90 Minutes of Arrival[1]	9	78%	52%	54%	95%
Smoking Cessation Advice	59	100%	92%	88%	100%
Heart Failure Care					
ACE Inhibitor or ARB for LVSD	115	90%	82%	82%	100%
Discharge Instructions	245	59%	61%	61%	93%
Evaluation of LVS Function	306	96%	90%	83%	99%
Smoking Cessation Advice	42	100%	91%	82%	100%
Pneumonia Care					
Appropriate Initial Antibiotic	87	90%	84%	83%	94%
Blood Culture Timing	106	87%	88%	90%	100%
Influenza Vaccine	26	77%	64%	70%	100%
Initial Antibiotic Timing	147	84%	74%	80%	93%
Oxygenation Assessment	209	99%	99%	99%	100%
Pneumococcal Vaccine	153	85%	67%	69%	94%
Smoking Cessation Advice	39	100%	90%	80%	100%
Surgical Infection Prevention					
Prophylactic Antibiotic Given	282	78%	83%	77%	95%
Prophylactic Antibiotic Selection	75	92%	90%	90%	100%
Prophylactic Antibiotic Stopped	278	77%	70%	72%	95%
Pregnancy Care					
Inpatient Neonatal Mortality	-	-	-	-	-
Third or Fourth Degree Laceration	-	-	2.71%	3.63%	3.27%

Saint Vincent's Medical Center

1800 Barrs Street
Jacksonville, FL 32204
URL: www.stvincentshealth.com
Ownership: Voluntary non-profit - Church
Emergency Services: Yes

Phone: 904-308-7300
Fax: 904-308-7941

Accredited: Yes
Licensed Beds: 528

Key Personnel:
President/CEO . . . . John J Maher
Chief Medical Staff . . . . David E Pirrung, MD
Cardiac Lab . . . . Patti Stephenson
Catheterization Lab . . . . Patti Stephenson
Emergency Room . . . . Ralph Badanowski, MD
Emergency Room . . . . Lorraine Keith, RN
Infection Control . . . . Bonnie Viergutz
ICU . . . . Lorraine Keith, RN
Intensive/Coronary Care . . . . Lorraine Keith, RN
Medical/Surgical Nursing . . . . Joyce Bruffy, RN
OB/GYN Womens Health . . . . Pat Pataki, RN
Respiratory/Cardiopulmonary . . . . Bob Cook

Measure	Cases	This Hospital	State Average	U.S. Average	Top Hospital
Heart Attack Care					
ACE Inhibitor or ARB for LVSD[2]	69	87%	83%	82%	100%
Aspirin at Arrival[2]	140	97%	93%	92%	100%
Aspirin at Discharge[2]	283	95%	88%	90%	100%
Beta Blocker at Arrival[2]	139	96%	89%	87%	100%
Beta Blocker at Discharge[2]	293	95%	92%	90%	100%
Fibrinolytic Medication Timing[1,2]	1	0%	33%	31%	100%
PCI Within 90 Minutes of Arrival[1,2]	3	0%	52%	54%	95%
Smoking Cessation Advice[2]	104	86%	92%	88%	100%
Heart Failure Care					
ACE Inhibitor or ARB for LVSD[2]	125	83%	82%	82%	100%
Discharge Instructions[2]	244	79%	61%	61%	93%
Evaluation of LVS Function[2]	310	94%	90%	83%	99%
Smoking Cessation Advice[2]	42	100%	91%	82%	100%
Pneumonia Care					
Appropriate Initial Antibiotic[2,3]	117	79%	84%	83%	94%
Blood Culture Timing[2]	117	90%	88%	90%	100%
Influenza Vaccine[2]	33	58%	64%	70%	100%
Initial Antibiotic Timing[2]	175	57%	74%	80%	93%
Oxygenation Assessment[2]	241	100%	99%	99%	100%
Pneumococcal Vaccine[2]	139	60%	67%	69%	94%
Smoking Cessation Advice[2,3]	29	97%	90%	80%	100%
Surgical Infection Prevention					
Prophylactic Antibiotic Given[2]	321	62%	83%	77%	95%
Prophylactic Antibiotic Selection[2]	83	83%	90%	90%	100%
Prophylactic Antibiotic Stopped[2]	316	91%	70%	72%	95%
Pregnancy Care					
Inpatient Neonatal Mortality	-	-	-	-	-
Third or Fourth Degree Laceration	-	-	2.71%	3.63%	3.27%

Shands Jacksonville

Alternate Name: University Medical Center
655 W Eighth Street
Jacksonville, FL 32209
URL: www.shandsjacksonville.org
Ownership: Voluntary non-profit - Private
Emergency Services: Yes

Phone: 904-244-0411
Fax: 904-244-9668

Accredited: Yes
Licensed Beds: 696

Key Personnel:
President/Administrator . . . . Jim Burkhart
Senior Director Cardiovascular Services . . . . . . Monica Floyd Barrett
Catheterization Laboratory Supervisor . . . . Deanna Rewis
ICU . . . . Ginger Campbell, CNO
Intensive Coronary . . . . Ginger Campbell, CNO
Medical Surgical Nursing . . . . Ginger Campbell, CNO
OB/GYN/Women's Health . . . . Ginger Campbell

Measure	Cases	This Hospital	State Average	U.S. Average	Top Hospital
Heart Attack Care					
ACE Inhibitor or ARB for LVSD	65	95%	83%	82%	100%
Aspirin at Arrival	208	99%	93%	92%	100%
Aspirin at Discharge	276	97%	88%	90%	100%
Beta Blocker at Arrival	181	97%	89%	87%	100%

NOTE: Hospital profiles are in alphabetical order by state, then city, then hospital within the city; Rankings are sorted by rate in descending order and exclude hospitals with less than 25 cases; (1) The number of cases is too small (n<25) for purposes of reliably predicting hospital performance; (2) Measure reflects the hospital's indication that its submission was based upon a sample of its relevant discharges; (3) Rate reflects fewer than the maximum possible quarters of data for the measure; (4) Inaccurate information submitted and suppressed for one or more quarters; (5) No data is available from the hospital for this measure; Please refer to the User's Guide for a full explanation of data

Measure	Cases	This Hospital	State Average	U.S. Average	Top Hospital
Beta Blocker at Discharge	271	97%	92%	90%	100%
Fibrinolytic Medication Timing[1]	1	100%	33%	31%	100%
PCI Within 90 Minutes of Arrival[1]	6	67%	52%	54%	95%
Smoking Cessation Advice	144	96%	92%	88%	100%
Heart Failure Care					
ACE Inhibitor or ARB for LVSD	176	91%	82%	82%	100%
Discharge Instructions	257	68%	61%	61%	93%
Evaluation of LVS Function	298	97%	90%	83%	99%
Smoking Cessation Advice	83	96%	91%	82%	100%
Pneumonia Care					
Appropriate Initial Antibiotic	96	79%	84%	83%	94%
Blood Culture Timing	113	71%	88%	90%	100%
Influenza Vaccine[4,5]	-	-	64%	70%	100%
Initial Antibiotic Timing	162	52%	74%	80%	93%
Oxygenation Assessment	201	99%	99%	99%	100%
Pneumococcal Vaccine	78	49%	67%	69%	94%
Smoking Cessation Advice	57	95%	90%	80%	100%
Surgical Infection Prevention					
Prophylactic Antibiotic Given	270	93%	83%	77%	95%
Prophylactic Antibiotic Selection	70	91%	90%	90%	100%
Prophylactic Antibiotic Stopped	263	79%	70%	72%	95%
Pregnancy Care					
Inpatient Neonatal Mortality[2]	733	1.09%	-	-	-
Third or Fourth Degree Laceration[2]	548	2.19%	2.71%	3.63%	3.27%

Baptist Medical Center Beaches

1350 13th Avenue S
Jacksonville Bch, FL 32250
URL: e-baptisthealth.com
Ownership: Voluntary non-profit - Other
Emergency Services: Yes

Phone: 904-627-2900
Fax: 904-627-2975

Accredited: Yes
Licensed Beds: 146

Key Personnel:
Administrator . . . . Mark Slyter
CEO. . . . . Hugh Greene
Chief Medical Staff. . . . . Steve Shirley, MD
Director Medical/Surgical Nursing . . . . Martha Fletcher
Medical Staff Services . . . . Jeannette Brown
OB/GYN Womens Health. . . . . Sam Christian, MD

Measure	Cases	This Hospital	State Average	U.S. Average	Top Hospital
Heart Attack Care					
ACE Inhibitor or ARB for LVSD[1]	12	75%	83%	82%	100%
Aspirin at Arrival	105	98%	93%	92%	100%
Aspirin at Discharge	49	92%	88%	90%	100%
Beta Blocker at Arrival	95	98%	89%	87%	100%
Beta Blocker at Discharge	56	89%	92%	90%	100%
Fibrinolytic Medication Timing	0	-	33%	31%	100%
PCI Within 90 Minutes of Arrival	0	-	52%	54%	95%
Smoking Cessation Advice[1]	7	71%	92%	88%	100%
Heart Failure Care					
ACE Inhibitor or ARB for LVSD	85	82%	82%	82%	100%
Discharge Instructions	162	75%	61%	61%	93%
Evaluation of LVS Function	222	92%	90%	83%	99%
Smoking Cessation Advice	27	89%	91%	82%	100%
Pneumonia Care					
Appropriate Initial Antibiotic[2]	202	84%	84%	83%	94%
Blood Culture Timing[2]	170	92%	88%	90%	100%
Influenza Vaccine	55	51%	64%	70%	100%
Initial Antibiotic Timing[2]	261	70%	74%	80%	93%
Oxygenation Assessment[2]	284	100%	99%	99%	100%
Pneumococcal Vaccine[2]	169	77%	67%	69%	94%
Smoking Cessation Advice[2]	50	94%	90%	80%	100%
Surgical Infection Prevention					
Prophylactic Antibiotic Given[2]	356	89%	83%	77%	95%
Prophylactic Antibiotic Selection[2]	33	97%	90%	90%	100%
Prophylactic Antibiotic Stopped[2]	333	49%	70%	72%	95%
Pregnancy Care					
Inpatient Neonatal Mortality	791	0.13%	-	-	-
Third or Fourth Degree Laceration	695	4.60%	2.71%	3.63%	3.27%

Trinity Community Hospital

Alternate Name: Hamilton Memorial Hospital
506 NW 4th Street
Jasper, FL 32052
Ownership: Voluntary non-profit - Private
Emergency Services: Yes

Phone: 386-792-7200
Fax: 386-792-2084
Accredited: No
Licensed Beds: 42

Key Personnel:
Emergency Room . . . . Wayne A Rahming, MD
Supervisor ER . . . . Debbie Bourie
Infection Control. . . . . Lynn Burnham, LPN

Measure	Cases	This Hospital	State Average	U.S. Average	Top Hospital
Heart Attack Care					
ACE Inhibitor or ARB for LVSD[3]	0	-	83%	82%	100%
Aspirin at Arrival[3]	0	-	93%	92%	100%
Aspirin at Discharge[3]	0	-	88%	90%	100%
Beta Blocker at Arrival[3]	0	-	89%	87%	100%
Beta Blocker at Discharge[3]	0	-	92%	90%	100%
Fibrinolytic Medication Timing[1,3]	1	0%	33%	31%	100%
PCI Within 90 Minutes of Arrival	0	-	52%	54%	95%
Smoking Cessation Advice[3]	0	-	92%	88%	100%
Heart Failure Care					
ACE Inhibitor or ARB for LVSD	0	-	82%	82%	100%
Discharge Instructions	43	26%	61%	61%	93%
Evaluation of LVS Function	44	30%	90%	83%	99%
Smoking Cessation Advice[1]	4	0%	91%	82%	100%
Pneumonia Care					
Appropriate Initial Antibiotic[1]	5	80%	84%	83%	94%
Blood Culture Timing	0	-	88%	90%	100%
Influenza Vaccine[1]	1	0%	64%	70%	100%
Initial Antibiotic Timing[1]	7	43%	74%	80%	93%
Oxygenation Assessment[1]	7	100%	99%	99%	100%
Pneumococcal Vaccine[1]	6	17%	67%	69%	94%
Smoking Cessation Advice[1]	1	100%	90%	80%	100%
Surgical Infection Prevention					
Prophylactic Antibiotic Given[5]	-	-	83%	77%	95%
Prophylactic Antibiotic Selection[5]	-	-	90%	90%	100%
Prophylactic Antibiotic Stopped[5]	-	-	70%	72%	95%
Pregnancy Care					
Inpatient Neonatal Mortality	-	-	-	-	-
Third or Fourth Degree Laceration	-	-	2.71%	3.63%	3.27%

Jay Hospital

14114 Alabama Street
Jay, FL 32565
Ownership: Voluntary non-profit - Private
Emergency Services: Yes

Phone: 850-675-8000
Fax: 850-675-8070
Accredited: No
Licensed Beds: 55

Key Personnel:
CEO. . . . . Mark Faulkner
Emergency Room . . . . Kaprena Kelley, RN
Director Medical/Surgical Nursing . . . . Anita Caraway
Chief Radiology . . . . Arthur Parker, MD
Director Respiratory Therapy . . . . Karen Godwin

Measure	Cases	This Hospital	State Average	U.S. Average	Top Hospital
Heart Attack Care					
ACE Inhibitor or ARB for LVSD[1]	1	100%	83%	82%	100%
Aspirin at Arrival[1]	7	86%	93%	92%	100%
Aspirin at Discharge[1]	4	75%	88%	90%	100%
Beta Blocker at Arrival[1]	6	83%	89%	87%	100%
Beta Blocker at Discharge[1]	2	100%	92%	90%	100%
Fibrinolytic Medication Timing[1,3]	1	100%	33%	31%	100%
PCI Within 90 Minutes of Arrival	0	-	52%	54%	95%
Smoking Cessation Advice[1]	1	100%	92%	88%	100%
Heart Failure Care					
ACE Inhibitor or ARB for LVSD[1]	18	89%	82%	82%	100%
Discharge Instructions	46	96%	61%	61%	93%
Evaluation of LVS Function	58	90%	90%	83%	99%
Smoking Cessation Advice[1]	7	57%	91%	82%	100%
Pneumonia Care					
Appropriate Initial Antibiotic	49	61%	84%	83%	94%
Blood Culture Timing	28	96%	88%	90%	100%
Influenza Vaccine[1]	9	44%	64%	70%	100%

NOTE: Hospital profiles are in alphabetical order by state, then city, then hospital within the city; Rankings are sorted by rate in descending order and exclude hospitals with less than 25 cases; (1) The number of cases is too small (n<25) for purposes of reliably predicting hospital performance; (2) Measure reflects the hospital's indication that its submission was based upon a sample of its relevant discharges; (3) Rate reflects fewer than the maximum possible quarters of data for the measure; (4) Inaccurate information submitted and suppressed for one or more quarters; (5) No data is available from the hospital for this measure; Please refer to the User's Guide for a full explanation of data

Initial Antibiotic Timing	50	82%	74%	80%	93%
Oxygenation Assessment	73	96%	99%	99%	100%
Pneumococcal Vaccine	37	70%	67%	69%	94%
Smoking Cessation Advice[1]	20	60%	90%	80%	100%
Surgical Infection Prevention					
Prophylactic Antibiotic Given[5]	-	-	83%	77%	95%
Prophylactic Antibiotic Selection[5]	-	-	90%	90%	100%
Prophylactic Antibiotic Stopped[5]	-	-	70%	72%	95%
Pregnancy Care					
Inpatient Neonatal Mortality	-	-	-	-	-
Third or Fourth Degree Laceration	-	-	2.71%	3.63%	3.27%

Jupiter Medical Center

1210 S Old Dixie Highway
Jupiter, FL 33458
E-mail: ljones@jupitermed.com
URL: www.jupitermed.com
Ownership: Voluntary non-profit - Other
Emergency Services: Yes

Phone: 561-747-2234
Fax: 561-743-5042

Accredited: Yes
Licensed Beds: 156

Key Personnel:
CEO...R Michael Barry
Chief Medical Staff.......................Thomas Rowe, MD
Emergency Room.........................Michael Collins, MD
Director Medical/Surgical Nursing..........Alison Coleman
Chief Radiology...........................David Mullin
Director Respiratory Therapy..............Levi Weaver

Measure	Cases	This Hospital	State Average	U.S. Average	Top Hospital
Heart Attack Care					
ACE Inhibitor or ARB for LVSD[1,2]	8	75%	83%	82%	100%
Aspirin at Arrival[2]	70	86%	93%	92%	100%
Aspirin at Discharge[2]	30	87%	88%	90%	100%
Beta Blocker at Arrival[2]	72	89%	89%	87%	100%
Beta Blocker at Discharge[2]	32	91%	92%	90%	100%
Fibrinolytic Medication Timing[1,2]	2	50%	33%	31%	100%
PCI Within 90 Minutes of Arrival[2]	0	-	52%	54%	95%
Smoking Cessation Advice[1,2]	1	100%	92%	88%	100%
Heart Failure Care					
ACE Inhibitor or ARB for LVSD	81	72%	82%	82%	100%
Discharge Instructions	178	52%	61%	61%	93%
Evaluation of LVS Function	219	90%	90%	83%	99%
Smoking Cessation Advice[1]	14	71%	91%	82%	100%
Pneumonia Care					
Appropriate Initial Antibiotic[2]	116	85%	84%	83%	94%
Blood Culture Timing[2]	103	87%	88%	90%	100%
Influenza Vaccine[2]	31	42%	64%	70%	100%
Initial Antibiotic Timing[2]	155	77%	74%	80%	93%
Oxygenation Assessment[2]	192	100%	99%	99%	100%
Pneumococcal Vaccine[2]	129	52%	67%	69%	94%
Smoking Cessation Advice[2]	25	76%	90%	80%	100%
Surgical Infection Prevention					
Prophylactic Antibiotic Given[2]	178	70%	83%	77%	95%
Prophylactic Antibiotic Selection[2]	45	96%	90%	90%	100%
Prophylactic Antibiotic Stopped[2]	174	67%	70%	72%	95%
Pregnancy Care					
Inpatient Neonatal Mortality	-	-	-	-	-
Third or Fourth Degree Laceration	-	-	2.71%	3.63%	3.27%

Lower Keys Medical Center

Alternate Name: Lower Florida Keys Health System
5900 College Road
Key West, FL 33041
Ownership: Proprietary
Emergency Services: Yes

Phone: 305-294-5531
Fax: 305-296-2520
Accredited: Yes
Licensed Beds: 169

Key Personnel:
CEO.......................................Nicki Will
Chief of Medical Staff....................Jerome Covington, MD
Cardiology................................Dan Courtney
Director Emergency Room.................Sandy Rodeerica
Infection Control.........................Alice Brady
Director of Pulmonary...................Dan Courtney

Measure	Cases	This Hospital	State Average	U.S. Average	Top Hospital

Heart Attack Care					
ACE Inhibitor or ARB for LVSD[1]	2	100%	83%	82%	100%
Aspirin at Arrival[1]	22	91%	93%	92%	100%
Aspirin at Discharge[1]	7	86%	88%	90%	100%
Beta Blocker at Arrival[1]	18	89%	89%	87%	100%
Beta Blocker at Discharge[1]	7	100%	92%	90%	100%
Fibrinolytic Medication Timing[1]	1	0%	33%	31%	100%
PCI Within 90 Minutes of Arrival	0	-	52%	54%	95%
Smoking Cessation Advice[1]	2	50%	92%	88%	100%
Heart Failure Care					
ACE Inhibitor or ARB for LVSD	31	81%	82%	82%	100%
Discharge Instructions	90	83%	61%	61%	93%
Evaluation of LVS Function	104	94%	90%	83%	99%
Smoking Cessation Advice[1]	21	100%	91%	82%	100%
Pneumonia Care					
Appropriate Initial Antibiotic	98	50%	84%	83%	94%
Blood Culture Timing	93	91%	88%	90%	100%
Influenza Vaccine	25	52%	64%	70%	100%
Initial Antibiotic Timing	105	70%	74%	80%	93%
Oxygenation Assessment	140	100%	99%	99%	100%
Pneumococcal Vaccine	77	52%	67%	69%	94%
Smoking Cessation Advice	35	97%	90%	80%	100%
Surgical Infection Prevention					
Prophylactic Antibiotic Given[2]	120	57%	83%	77%	95%
Prophylactic Antibiotic Selection[2]	31	58%	90%	90%	100%
Prophylactic Antibiotic Stopped[2]	94	48%	70%	72%	95%
Pregnancy Care					
Inpatient Neonatal Mortality	-	-	-	-	-
Third or Fourth Degree Laceration	-	-	2.71%	3.63%	3.27%

Osceola Regional Medical Center

700 W Oak Street
Kissimmee, FL 34741
URL: www.osceolaregional.com
Ownership: Proprietary
Emergency Services: Yes

Phone: 407-846-2266
Fax: 407-518-3616

Accredited: Yes
Licensed Beds: 231

Key Personnel:
CEO.......................................E Timothy Cook
Chief Medical Staff.......................Dr. Raphael Jimenez
Associate Administrator...................Louis Caputo
Director Emergency.......................Joe Pimentel
Director Medical Surgical Nursing..........Jeanette Williams
Director OB/GYN Womens Health..........Ruth Reichard, MD
Chief Radiology...........................E Hampton Sessions, MD
Director Respiratory Therapy..............Lisa Livingston

Measure	Cases	This Hospital	State Average	U.S. Average	Top Hospital
Heart Attack Care					
ACE Inhibitor or ARB for LVSD	66	82%	83%	82%	100%
Aspirin at Arrival	221	91%	93%	92%	100%
Aspirin at Discharge	245	83%	88%	90%	100%
Beta Blocker at Arrival	196	80%	89%	87%	100%
Beta Blocker at Discharge	254	81%	92%	90%	100%
Fibrinolytic Medication Timing	0	-	33%	31%	100%
PCI Within 90 Minutes of Arrival[1]	13	31%	52%	54%	95%
Smoking Cessation Advice	81	99%	92%	88%	100%
Heart Failure Care					
ACE Inhibitor or ARB for LVSD	211	73%	82%	82%	100%
Discharge Instructions	401	95%	61%	61%	93%
Evaluation of LVS Function	458	98%	90%	83%	99%
Smoking Cessation Advice	44	100%	91%	82%	100%
Pneumonia Care					
Appropriate Initial Antibiotic	298	79%	84%	83%	94%
Blood Culture Timing	202	80%	88%	90%	100%
Influenza Vaccine	79	49%	64%	70%	100%
Initial Antibiotic Timing	342	53%	74%	80%	93%
Oxygenation Assessment	396	100%	99%	99%	100%
Pneumococcal Vaccine	243	34%	67%	69%	94%
Smoking Cessation Advice	56	96%	90%	80%	100%
Surgical Infection Prevention					
Prophylactic Antibiotic Given[3]	528	80%	83%	77%	95%
Prophylactic Antibiotic Selection	144	94%	90%	90%	100%
Prophylactic Antibiotic Stopped[3]	484	83%	70%	72%	95%

NOTE: Hospital profiles are in alphabetical order by state, then city, then hospital within the city; Rankings are sorted by rate in descending order and exclude hospitals with less than 25 cases; (1) The number of cases is too small (n<25) for purposes of reliably predicting hospital performance; (2) Measure reflects the hospital's indication that its submission was based upon a sample of its relevant discharges; (3) Rate reflects fewer than the maximum possible quarters of data for the measure; (4) Inaccurate information submitted and suppressed for one or more quarters; (5) No data is available from the hospital for this measure; Please refer to the User's Guide for a full explanation of data

Pregnancy Care					
Inpatient Neonatal Mortality	-	-	-	-	-
Third or Fourth Degree Laceration	-	-	2.71%	3.63%	3.27%

Lake City Medical Center

340 NW Commerce Drive   Phone: 386-719-9000
Lake City, FL 32055   Fax: 386-719-7787
URL: www.lakecitymedical.com
Ownership: Proprietary   Accredited: Yes
Emergency Services: Yes   Licensed Beds: 75
Key Personnel:
President/CEO..........................Gary Karsner
Chief Medical Staff......................Eric Ordinario, DO
Emergency Room ....Debbie Wingate, RN
Infection Control........................Mary Fuller
ICU ....Mark Fontaine
Respiratory/Cardiopulmonary...............Christine Goolsby

Measure	Cases	This Hospital	State Average	U.S. Average	Top Hospital
Heart Attack Care					
ACE Inhibitor or ARB for LVSD[1]	10	70%	83%	82%	100%
Aspirin at Arrival	48	79%	93%	92%	100%
Aspirin at Discharge[1]	19	53%	88%	90%	100%
Beta Blocker at Arrival	47	89%	89%	87%	100%
Beta Blocker at Discharge[1]	20	65%	92%	90%	100%
Fibrinolytic Medication Timing[1]	2	0%	33%	31%	100%
PCI Within 90 Minutes of Arrival	0	-	52%	54%	95%
Smoking Cessation Advice[1]	5	100%	92%	88%	100%
Heart Failure Care					
ACE Inhibitor or ARB for LVSD	56	54%	82%	82%	100%
Discharge Instructions	160	46%	61%	61%	93%
Evaluation of LVS Function	214	91%	90%	83%	99%
Smoking Cessation Advice	32	94%	91%	82%	100%
Pneumonia Care					
Appropriate Initial Antibiotic	177	69%	84%	83%	94%
Blood Culture Timing	80	92%	88%	90%	100%
Influenza Vaccine	52	56%	64%	70%	100%
Initial Antibiotic Timing	227	62%	74%	80%	93%
Oxygenation Assessment	256	98%	99%	99%	100%
Pneumococcal Vaccine	170	58%	67%	69%	94%
Smoking Cessation Advice	52	96%	90%	80%	100%
Surgical Infection Prevention					
Prophylactic Antibiotic Given[1,3]	19	26%	83%	77%	95%
Prophylactic Antibiotic Selection[1]	5	0%	90%	90%	100%
Prophylactic Antibiotic Stopped[1,3]	10	100%	70%	72%	95%
Pregnancy Care					
Inpatient Neonatal Mortality	-	-	-	-	-
Third or Fourth Degree Laceration	-	-	2.71%	3.63%	3.27%

Shands at Lake Shore

Alternate Name: Lake Shore Hospital
360 NE Franklin Street   Phone: 386-754-8000
Lake City, FL 32055   Fax: 386-754-8121
URL: www.shands.org
Ownership: Voluntary non-profit - Private   Accredited: Yes
Emergency Services: Yes   Licensed Beds: 99
Key Personnel:
CEO.................................Neil Whipkey
Chief Medical Staff......................Waseem Aziz, MD
Emergency Room ....Lowell Green
ICU ....Donna Reagan
OB/GYN...............................Shirley Lick
Surgery...............................Dee McRae
Director Respiratory Therapy..............Robert Flinn

Measure	Cases	This Hospital	State Average	U.S. Average	Top Hospital
Heart Attack Care					
ACE Inhibitor or ARB for LVSD[1]	9	56%	83%	82%	100%
Aspirin at Arrival	81	86%	93%	92%	100%
Aspirin at Discharge	51	71%	88%	90%	100%
Beta Blocker at Arrival	82	82%	89%	87%	100%
Beta Blocker at Discharge	53	75%	92%	90%	100%
Fibrinolytic Medication Timing	0	-	33%	31%	100%

Measure	Cases	This Hospital	State Average	U.S. Average	Top Hospital
PCI Within 90 Minutes of Arrival	0	-	52%	54%	95%
Smoking Cessation Advice[1]	12	58%	92%	88%	100%
Heart Failure Care					
ACE Inhibitor or ARB for LVSD	33	52%	82%	82%	100%
Discharge Instructions	141	11%	61%	61%	93%
Evaluation of LVS Function	166	88%	90%	83%	99%
Smoking Cessation Advice	35	74%	91%	82%	100%
Pneumonia Care					
Appropriate Initial Antibiotic	97	70%	84%	83%	94%
Blood Culture Timing	47	89%	88%	90%	100%
Influenza Vaccine[1]	22	45%	64%	70%	100%
Initial Antibiotic Timing	102	61%	74%	80%	93%
Oxygenation Assessment	118	99%	99%	99%	100%
Pneumococcal Vaccine	56	39%	67%	69%	94%
Smoking Cessation Advice	38	66%	90%	80%	100%
Surgical Infection Prevention					
Prophylactic Antibiotic Given	101	57%	83%	77%	95%
Prophylactic Antibiotic Selection[1]	18	100%	90%	90%	100%
Prophylactic Antibiotic Stopped	91	32%	70%	72%	95%
Pregnancy Care					
Inpatient Neonatal Mortality[2]	238	0.84%	-	-	-
Third or Fourth Degree Laceration[2]	176	1.70%	2.71%	3.63%	3.27%

Lake Wales Medical Center

410 South 11th Street   Phone: 863-676-1433
Lake Wales, FL 33853   Fax: 863-676-9323
URL: www.lakewalesmedicalcenter.com
Ownership: Proprietary   Accredited: Yes
Emergency Services: Yes   Licensed Beds: 154
Key Personnel:
CEO.................................Michael J Yungmann
Chief of Medical Staff...................Caroline Honculada, MD
Emergency Room ....Dave Seekins
Infection Control........................Marvette Isom, RN
ICU ....Flora Wilson, RN
Medical Surgical Nursing ....Julie Travis, RN
Respiratory Therapy.....................Chris Jessee

Measure	Cases	This Hospital	State Average	U.S. Average	Top Hospital
Heart Attack Care					
ACE Inhibitor or ARB for LVSD[1]	6	67%	83%	82%	100%
Aspirin at Arrival[1]	23	78%	93%	92%	100%
Aspirin at Discharge[1]	12	50%	88%	90%	100%
Beta Blocker at Arrival[1]	17	76%	89%	87%	100%
Beta Blocker at Discharge[1]	14	71%	92%	90%	100%
Fibrinolytic Medication Timing	0	-	33%	31%	100%
PCI Within 90 Minutes of Arrival	0	-	52%	54%	95%
Smoking Cessation Advice[1]	4	75%	92%	88%	100%
Heart Failure Care					
ACE Inhibitor or ARB for LVSD	68	74%	82%	82%	100%
Discharge Instructions	180	22%	61%	61%	93%
Evaluation of LVS Function	214	88%	90%	83%	99%
Smoking Cessation Advice	35	23%	91%	82%	100%
Pneumonia Care					
Appropriate Initial Antibiotic[2]	94	82%	84%	83%	94%
Blood Culture Timing[2]	77	97%	88%	90%	100%
Influenza Vaccine[1,2]	20	30%	64%	70%	100%
Initial Antibiotic Timing[2]	137	74%	74%	80%	93%
Oxygenation Assessment[2]	151	100%	99%	99%	100%
Pneumococcal Vaccine[2]	86	64%	67%	69%	94%
Smoking Cessation Advice[2]	33	36%	90%	80%	100%
Surgical Infection Prevention					
Prophylactic Antibiotic Given[2,3]	52	50%	83%	77%	95%
Prophylactic Antibiotic Selection[1,2]	12	92%	90%	90%	100%
Prophylactic Antibiotic Stopped[2,3]	50	96%	70%	72%	95%
Pregnancy Care					
Inpatient Neonatal Mortality	-	-	-	-	-
Third or Fourth Degree Laceration	-	-	2.71%	3.63%	3.27%

NOTE: Hospital profiles are in alphabetical order by state, then city, then hospital within the city; Rankings are sorted by rate in descending order and exclude hospitals with less than 25 cases; (1) The number of cases is too small (n<25) for purposes of reliably predicting hospital performance; (2) Measure reflects the hospital's indication that its submission was based upon a sample of its relevant discharges; (3) Rate reflects fewer than the maximum possible quarters of data for the measure; (4) Inaccurate information submitted and suppressed for one or more quarters; (5) No data is available from the hospital for this measure; Please refer to the User's Guide for a full explanation of data

Lakeland Regional Medical Center

1324 Lakeland Hills Boulevard
Lakeland, FL 33805
URL: www.lrmc.com
Ownership: Voluntary non-profit - Other
Emergency Services: Yes

Phone: 863-687-1100
Fax: 863-284-1979

Accredited: Yes
Licensed Beds: 851

Key Personnel:
CEO. . . . . Jack Stevens
Chief Medical Staff. . . . . Edwind Sammer
Emergency Room . . . . Marge Keck
Director Infection/Disease Control . . . . . . Julia Moody
OB/GYN Womens Health. . . . . Bindy Hankins
Chief Radiology . . . . Janet Fansler
Respiratory . . . . Conni Farmer

Measure	Cases	This Hospital	State Average	U.S. Average	Top Hospital
Heart Attack Care					
ACE Inhibitor or ARB for LVSD	67	82%	83%	82%	100%
Aspirin at Arrival	284	97%	93%	92%	100%
Aspirin at Discharge	309	97%	88%	90%	100%
Beta Blocker at Arrival	261	92%	89%	87%	100%
Beta Blocker at Discharge	303	95%	92%	90%	100%
Fibrinolytic Medication Timing[1]	3	0%	33%	31%	100%
PCI Within 90 Minutes of Arrival[1]	8	38%	52%	54%	95%
Smoking Cessation Advice	115	100%	92%	88%	100%
Heart Failure Care					
ACE Inhibitor or ARB for LVSD	157	84%	82%	82%	100%
Discharge Instructions	280	84%	61%	61%	93%
Evaluation of LVS Function	322	91%	90%	83%	99%
Smoking Cessation Advice	49	86%	91%	82%	100%
Pneumonia Care					
Appropriate Initial Antibiotic	163	88%	84%	83%	94%
Blood Culture Timing	169	97%	88%	90%	100%
Influenza Vaccine	41	68%	64%	70%	100%
Initial Antibiotic Timing	240	72%	74%	80%	93%
Oxygenation Assessment	291	100%	99%	99%	100%
Pneumococcal Vaccine	170	64%	67%	69%	94%
Smoking Cessation Advice	91	87%	90%	80%	100%
Surgical Infection Prevention					
Prophylactic Antibiotic Given	534	83%	83%	77%	95%
Prophylactic Antibiotic Selection	127	97%	90%	90%	100%
Prophylactic Antibiotic Stopped	510	72%	70%	72%	95%
Pregnancy Care					
Inpatient Neonatal Mortality[2]	896	0.67%	-	-	-
Third or Fourth Degree Laceration[2]	657	2.13%	2.71%	3.63%	3.27%

Largo Medical Center

201 14th Street SW
Largo, FL 33770
URL: www.largomedical.com
Ownership: Proprietary
Emergency Services: Yes

Phone: 727-588-5200
Fax: 727-588-5906

Accredited: Yes
Licensed Beds: 256

Key Personnel:
President/CEO. . . . . Thomas L Herron, FACHE
Administrator/COO. . . . . Lawrence W Kaufman
Chief of Cath Lab. . . . . Federico Lenz, MD
Catheterization Lab . . . . Steve Barber
Infection Control. . . . . Paula Bates
Intensive Coronary. Susan Finch
OB/GYN Womens Health. . . . . Ruth DePalantino
Vice Chief of Surgery . . . . Ricardo Requena, DO
Chief of Radiology . . . . Gregg Baran, MD

Measure	Cases	This Hospital	State Average	U.S. Average	Top Hospital
Heart Attack Care					
ACE Inhibitor or ARB for LVSD	48	90%	83%	82%	100%
Aspirin at Arrival	267	97%	93%	92%	100%
Aspirin at Discharge	255	96%	88%	90%	100%
Beta Blocker at Arrival	170	94%	89%	87%	100%
Beta Blocker at Discharge	278	96%	92%	90%	100%
Fibrinolytic Medication Timing[1]	3	33%	33%	31%	100%
PCI Within 90 Minutes of Arrival[1]	12	25%	52%	54%	95%

Measure	Cases	This Hospital	State Average	U.S. Average	Top Hospital
Smoking Cessation Advice	98	98%	92%	88%	100%
Heart Failure Care					
ACE Inhibitor or ARB for LVSD	110	91%	82%	82%	100%
Discharge Instructions	332	41%	61%	61%	93%
Evaluation of LVS Function	429	97%	90%	83%	99%
Smoking Cessation Advice	59	100%	91%	82%	100%
Pneumonia Care					
Appropriate Initial Antibiotic	211	82%	84%	83%	94%
Blood Culture Timing	171	88%	88%	90%	100%
Influenza Vaccine	82	61%	64%	70%	100%
Initial Antibiotic Timing	303	71%	74%	80%	93%
Oxygenation Assessment	333	100%	99%	99%	100%
Pneumococcal Vaccine	226	63%	67%	69%	94%
Smoking Cessation Advice	75	100%	90%	80%	100%
Surgical Infection Prevention					
Prophylactic Antibiotic Given[2,3]	279	95%	83%	77%	95%
Prophylactic Antibiotic Selection[2]	103	97%	90%	90%	100%
Prophylactic Antibiotic Stopped[2,3]	241	89%	70%	72%	95%
Pregnancy Care					
Inpatient Neonatal Mortality	-	-	-	-	-
Third or Fourth Degree Laceration	-	-	2.71%	3.63%	3.27%

Sun Coast Hospital

2025 Indian Rocks Road S
Largo, FL 33774
URL: www.suncoasthealthcare.com
Ownership: Voluntary non-profit - Private
Emergency Services: Yes

Phone: 727-581-9474
Fax: 727-587-7627

Accredited: Yes
Licensed Beds: 200

Key Personnel:
CEO. . . . . Larry Archbell
Chief Medical Staff. Ronald Walsh, DO
Emergency Room . . . . Peggy Dobbins, RN
OB/GYN Womens Health. . . . . Jennifer Hayes, DO
Chief Radiology . . . . J Eric Taylor, Jr, MD
Director Cardio-Pulmonary Services . . . . Carla Burton

Measure	Cases	This Hospital	State Average	U.S. Average	Top Hospital
Heart Attack Care					
ACE Inhibitor or ARB for LVSD[1]	11	55%	83%	82%	100%
Aspirin at Arrival	39	97%	93%	92%	100%
Aspirin at Discharge	25	92%	88%	90%	100%
Beta Blocker at Arrival	42	93%	89%	87%	100%
Beta Blocker at Discharge	30	93%	92%	90%	100%
Fibrinolytic Medication Timing	0	-	33%	31%	100%
PCI Within 90 Minutes of Arrival	0	-	52%	54%	95%
Smoking Cessation Advice[1]	6	33%	92%	88%	100%
Heart Failure Care					
ACE Inhibitor or ARB for LVSD	54	91%	82%	82%	100%
Discharge Instructions	111	21%	61%	61%	93%
Evaluation of LVS Function	150	91%	90%	83%	99%
Smoking Cessation Advice[1]	19	84%	91%	82%	100%
Pneumonia Care					
Appropriate Initial Antibiotic	116	85%	84%	83%	94%
Blood Culture Timing	118	86%	88%	90%	100%
Influenza Vaccine[4,5]	-	-	64%	70%	100%
Initial Antibiotic Timing	156	85%	74%	80%	93%
Oxygenation Assessment	210	100%	99%	99%	100%
Pneumococcal Vaccine	109	56%	67%	69%	94%
Smoking Cessation Advice	55	56%	90%	80%	100%
Surgical Infection Prevention					
Prophylactic Antibiotic Given	198	86%	83%	77%	95%
Prophylactic Antibiotic Selection	51	94%	90%	90%	100%
Prophylactic Antibiotic Stopped	188	58%	70%	72%	95%
Pregnancy Care					
Inpatient Neonatal Mortality	-	-	-	-	-
Third or Fourth Degree Laceration	-	-	2.71%	3.63%	3.27%

NOTE: Hospital profiles are in alphabetical order by state, then city, then hospital within the city; Rankings are sorted by rate in descending order and exclude hospitals with less than 25 cases; (1) The number of cases is too small (n<25) for purposes of reliably predicting hospital performance; (2) Measure reflects the hospital's indication that its submission was based upon a sample of its relevant discharges; (3) Rate reflects fewer than the maximum possible quarters of data for the measure; (4) Inaccurate information submitted and suppressed for one or more quarters; (5) No data is available from the hospital for this measure; Please refer to the User's Guide for a full explanation of data

Florida Medical Center

5000 West Oakland Park Boulevard
Lauderdale Lakes, FL 33313

Toll-Free: 800-222-9355
Phone: 954-735-6000
Fax: 954-677-2603

E-mail: sue.baron@tenethealth.com
URL: www.floridamedicalctr.com
Ownership: Proprietary   Accredited: Yes
Emergency Services: Yes   Licensed Beds: 459

Key Personnel:
CEO . . . . Aurelio M Fernandez
Chief Medical Staff . . . . Dr Robert Green, MD
Catheterization Lab . . . . Robert Dzwonkowski
Emergency Room . . . . Mary Jane Damavandi
Medical Director Emergency Room . . . . Louis Isaacson, DO
Director Infection Control . . . . Catherine Soumerai, RN
Director Surgical Services . . . . Mary Grimes, RN
Chief Radiology . . . . Edward Daver, MD
Director Cardiopulmonary . . . . Robert Dzwonkowski

Measure	Cases	This Hospital	State Average	U.S. Average	Top Hospital
Heart Attack Care					
ACE Inhibitor or ARB for LVSD	127	89%	83%	82%	100%
Aspirin at Arrival	323	97%	93%	92%	100%
Aspirin at Discharge	420	94%	88%	90%	100%
Beta Blocker at Arrival	325	94%	89%	87%	100%
Beta Blocker at Discharge	434	95%	92%	90%	100%
Fibrinolytic Medication Timing[1]	3	33%	33%	31%	100%
PCI Within 90 Minutes of Arrival[1]	18	56%	52%	54%	95%
Smoking Cessation Advice	101	100%	92%	88%	100%
Heart Failure Care					
ACE Inhibitor or ARB for LVSD	203	76%	82%	82%	100%
Discharge Instructions	393	57%	61%	61%	93%
Evaluation of LVS Function	528	87%	90%	83%	99%
Smoking Cessation Advice	35	100%	91%	82%	100%
Pneumonia Care					
Appropriate Initial Antibiotic	90	83%	84%	83%	94%
Blood Culture Timing	89	91%	88%	90%	100%
Influenza Vaccine	30	73%	64%	70%	100%
Initial Antibiotic Timing	125	83%	74%	80%	93%
Oxygenation Assessment	147	100%	99%	99%	100%
Pneumococcal Vaccine	103	80%	67%	69%	94%
Smoking Cessation Advice	25	100%	90%	80%	100%
Surgical Infection Prevention					
Prophylactic Antibiotic Given[2]	460	89%	83%	77%	95%
Prophylactic Antibiotic Selection[2]	82	94%	90%	90%	100%
Prophylactic Antibiotic Stopped[2]	454	53%	70%	72%	95%
Pregnancy Care					
Inpatient Neonatal Mortality	-	-	-	-	-
Third or Fourth Degree Laceration	-	-	2.71%	3.63%	3.27%

Leesburg Regional Medical Center

Alternate Name: LRMC
600 E Dixie Avenue
Leesburg, FL 34748

Toll-Free: 800-889-3755
Phone: 352-323-5762
Fax: 352-323-5009

URL: www.leesburgregional.org
Ownership: Voluntary non-profit - Private   Accredited: Yes
Emergency Services: Yes   Licensed Beds: 294

Key Personnel:
CEO . . . . Louis Bremer
Emergency Room . . . . Sharon Garbaravage
OB/GYN Womens Health . . . . Kathy Perfume, RN

Measure	Cases	This Hospital	State Average	U.S. Average	Top Hospital
Heart Attack Care					
ACE Inhibitor or ARB for LVSD	114	82%	83%	82%	100%
Aspirin at Arrival	262	97%	93%	92%	100%
Aspirin at Discharge	355	97%	88%	90%	100%
Beta Blocker at Arrival	170	90%	89%	87%	100%
Beta Blocker at Discharge	401	97%	92%	90%	100%
Fibrinolytic Medication Timing	0	-	33%	31%	100%
PCI Within 90 Minutes of Arrival[1]	20	30%	52%	54%	95%
Smoking Cessation Advice	114	98%	92%	88%	100%

Measure	Cases	This Hospital	State Average	U.S. Average	Top Hospital
Heart Failure Care					
ACE Inhibitor or ARB for LVSD	178	89%	82%	82%	100%
Discharge Instructions	343	69%	61%	61%	93%
Evaluation of LVS Function	426	99%	90%	83%	99%
Smoking Cessation Advice	73	99%	91%	82%	100%
Pneumonia Care					
Appropriate Initial Antibiotic	210	89%	84%	83%	94%
Blood Culture Timing	251	84%	88%	90%	100%
Influenza Vaccine[4,5]	-	-	64%	70%	100%
Initial Antibiotic Timing	344	64%	74%	80%	93%
Oxygenation Assessment	362	100%	99%	99%	100%
Pneumococcal Vaccine	233	75%	67%	69%	94%
Smoking Cessation Advice	61	92%	90%	80%	100%
Surgical Infection Prevention					
Prophylactic Antibiotic Given	467	94%	83%	77%	95%
Prophylactic Antibiotic Selection	124	99%	90%	90%	100%
Prophylactic Antibiotic Stopped	460	93%	70%	72%	95%
Pregnancy Care					
Inpatient Neonatal Mortality	-	-	-	-	-
Third or Fourth Degree Laceration	-	-	2.71%	3.63%	3.27%

Lehigh Regional Medical Center

1500 Lee Boulevard
Lehigh Acres, FL 33936

Phone: 239-369-2101
Fax: 239-368-4510

URL: www.lehighregional.com
Ownership: Proprietary   Accredited: Yes
Emergency Services: Yes   Licensed Beds: 88

Key Personnel:
CEO . . . . Randy Carson
Director Medical/Surgical Nursing . . . . Nancy Kaplan
OB/GYN Womens Health . . . . Robert Strathman
Chief Radiology . . . . Arthur Miller
Director Respiratory Therapy . . . . Kevin Suckerk

Measure	Cases	This Hospital	State Average	U.S. Average	Top Hospital
Heart Attack Care					
ACE Inhibitor or ARB for LVSD[1]	10	70%	83%	82%	100%
Aspirin at Arrival	52	87%	93%	92%	100%
Aspirin at Discharge[1]	21	57%	88%	90%	100%
Beta Blocker at Arrival	48	75%	89%	87%	100%
Beta Blocker at Discharge[1]	20	65%	92%	90%	100%
Fibrinolytic Medication Timing	0	-	33%	31%	100%
PCI Within 90 Minutes of Arrival	0	-	52%	54%	95%
Smoking Cessation Advice[1]	3	33%	92%	88%	100%
Heart Failure Care					
ACE Inhibitor or ARB for LVSD	66	88%	82%	82%	100%
Discharge Instructions	164	28%	61%	61%	93%
Evaluation of LVS Function	174	95%	90%	83%	99%
Smoking Cessation Advice	33	48%	91%	82%	100%
Pneumonia Care					
Appropriate Initial Antibiotic	172	80%	84%	83%	94%
Blood Culture Timing	74	92%	88%	90%	100%
Influenza Vaccine[4,5]	-	-	64%	70%	100%
Initial Antibiotic Timing	171	75%	74%	80%	93%
Oxygenation Assessment	202	100%	99%	99%	100%
Pneumococcal Vaccine	119	57%	67%	69%	94%
Smoking Cessation Advice	57	47%	90%	80%	100%
Surgical Infection Prevention					
Prophylactic Antibiotic Given[2]	140	54%	83%	77%	95%
Prophylactic Antibiotic Selection[2]	29	93%	90%	90%	100%
Prophylactic Antibiotic Stopped[2]	133	67%	70%	72%	95%
Pregnancy Care					
Inpatient Neonatal Mortality	-	-	-	-	-
Third or Fourth Degree Laceration	-	-	2.71%	3.63%	3.27%

Shands Live Oak

Alternate Name: Suwannee County Hospital

NOTE: Hospital profiles are in alphabetical order by state, then city, then hospital within the city; Rankings are sorted by rate in descending order and exclude hospitals with less than 25 cases; (1) The number of cases is too small (n<25) for purposes of reliably predicting hospital performance; (2) Measure reflects the hospital's indication that its submission was based upon a sample of its relevant discharges; (3) Rate reflects fewer than the maximum possible quarters of data for the measure; (4) Inaccurate information submitted and suppressed for one or more quarters; (5) No data is available from the hospital for this measure; Please refer to the User's Guide for a full explanation of data

1100 SW 11th Street
Live Oak, FL 32064
URL: www.shands.org
Ownership: Voluntary non-profit - Private
Emergency Services: Yes

Phone: 386-362-0800
Fax: 386-362-0841

Accredited: Yes
Licensed Beds: 30

Key Personnel:
Administrator . . . . Rhonda Sherrod, RN
Chief Medical Staff. . . . . Andrew Baff, MD
Emergency Room . . . . Robert Ftindell
Chief Radiology . . . . BS Hegde, MD
Director Respiratory Therapy . . . . Mark Hamilton

Measure	Cases	This Hospital	State Average	U.S. Average	Top Hospital
Heart Attack Care					
ACE Inhibitor or ARB for LVSD[3]	0	-	83%	82%	100%
Aspirin at Arrival[1,3]	3	100%	93%	92%	100%
Aspirin at Discharge[3]	0	-	88%	90%	100%
Beta Blocker at Arrival[1,3]	3	67%	89%	87%	100%
Beta Blocker at Discharge[3]	0	-	92%	90%	100%
Fibrinolytic Medication Timing[3]	0	-	33%	31%	100%
PCI Within 90 Minutes of Arrival[3]	0	-	52%	54%	95%
Smoking Cessation Advice[3]	0	-	92%	88%	100%
Heart Failure Care					
ACE Inhibitor or ARB for LVSD[1]	16	56%	82%	82%	100%
Discharge Instructions	47	62%	61%	61%	93%
Evaluation of LVS Function	61	59%	90%	83%	99%
Smoking Cessation Advice[1]	9	100%	91%	82%	100%
Pneumonia Care					
Appropriate Initial Antibiotic	39	87%	84%	83%	94%
Blood Culture Timing	26	85%	88%	90%	100%
Influenza Vaccine[1]	10	60%	64%	70%	100%
Initial Antibiotic Timing	59	80%	74%	80%	93%
Oxygenation Assessment	60	100%	99%	99%	100%
Pneumococcal Vaccine	31	87%	67%	69%	94%
Smoking Cessation Advice[1]	16	94%	90%	80%	100%
Surgical Infection Prevention					
Prophylactic Antibiotic Given[5]	-	-	83%	77%	95%
Prophylactic Antibiotic Selection[5]	-	-	90%	90%	100%
Prophylactic Antibiotic Stopped[5]	-	-	70%	72%	95%
Pregnancy Care					
Inpatient Neonatal Mortality	-	-	-	-	-
Third or Fourth Degree Laceration	-	-	2.71%	3.63%	3.27%

Palms West Hospital

Alternate Name: Palms West Hospital
13001 Southern Boulevard
Loxahatchee, FL 33470
URL: www.palmswesthospital.com
Ownership: Proprietary
Emergency Services: No

Phone: 561-798-3300
Fax: 561-791-8108

Accredited: Yes
Licensed Beds: 175

Key Personnel:
CEO. . . . . Heather Rohan
Emergency Room . . . . Judy Charriez, RN
Director Medical/Surgical Nursing . . . . Deborah Ford, RN
OB/GYN Womens Health. . . . . Moises Virelles, MD
Chief Radiology . . . . Donald Dewar, MD
Director Respiratory Therapy . . . . Elizabeth Howell

Measure	Cases	This Hospital	State Average	U.S. Average	Top Hospital
Heart Attack Care					
ACE Inhibitor or ARB for LVSD[1]	9	56%	83%	82%	100%
Aspirin at Arrival	52	83%	93%	92%	100%
Aspirin at Discharge	28	57%	88%	90%	100%
Beta Blocker at Arrival[1]	22	95%	89%	87%	100%
Beta Blocker at Discharge	25	76%	92%	90%	100%
Fibrinolytic Medication Timing	0	-	33%	31%	100%
PCI Within 90 Minutes of Arrival	0	-	52%	54%	95%
Smoking Cessation Advice[1]	9	100%	92%	88%	100%
Heart Failure Care					
ACE Inhibitor or ARB for LVSD	83	65%	82%	82%	100%
Discharge Instructions	215	47%	61%	61%	93%
Evaluation of LVS Function	245	93%	90%	83%	99%
Smoking Cessation Advice	34	82%	91%	82%	100%

Measure	Cases	This Hospital	State Average	U.S. Average	Top Hospital
Pneumonia Care					
Appropriate Initial Antibiotic	137	81%	84%	83%	94%
Blood Culture Timing	80	82%	88%	90%	100%
Influenza Vaccine	32	62%	64%	70%	100%
Initial Antibiotic Timing	140	46%	74%	80%	93%
Oxygenation Assessment	165	99%	99%	99%	100%
Pneumococcal Vaccine	89	69%	67%	69%	94%
Smoking Cessation Advice	34	91%	90%	80%	100%
Surgical Infection Prevention					
Prophylactic Antibiotic Given[3]	307	74%	83%	77%	95%
Prophylactic Antibiotic Selection	79	92%	90%	90%	100%
Prophylactic Antibiotic Stopped[3]	298	54%	70%	72%	95%
Pregnancy Care					
Inpatient Neonatal Mortality	-	-	-	-	-
Third or Fourth Degree Laceration	-	-	2.71%	3.63%	3.27%

Fishermen's Hospital

3301 Overseas Highway
Marathon, FL 33050
URL: www.fishermenshospital.com
Ownership: Proprietary
Emergency Services: Yes

Phone: 305-743-5533
Fax: 305-743-3962

Accredited: Yes
Licensed Beds: 58

Key Personnel:
CEO. . . . . Al Aboud
Emergency Room . . . . Sherryl Perry, RN
Director Medical/Surgical Nursing . . . . Stella Hork, RN
Chief Radiology . . . . Wayne Moccia, MD
Director Respiratory Therapy . . . . Kathy Huntt

Measure	Cases	This Hospital	State Average	U.S. Average	Top Hospital
Heart Attack Care					
ACE Inhibitor or ARB for LVSD[3]	0	-	83%	82%	100%
Aspirin at Arrival[1,3]	3	100%	93%	92%	100%
Aspirin at Discharge[3]	0	-	88%	90%	100%
Beta Blocker at Arrival[1,3]	3	100%	89%	87%	100%
Beta Blocker at Discharge[1,3]	1	100%	92%	90%	100%
Fibrinolytic Medication Timing[3]	0	-	33%	31%	100%
PCI Within 90 Minutes of Arrival	0	-	52%	54%	95%
Smoking Cessation Advice[3]	0	-	92%	88%	100%
Heart Failure Care					
ACE Inhibitor or ARB for LVSD[1]	9	100%	82%	82%	100%
Discharge Instructions[1]	20	25%	61%	61%	93%
Evaluation of LVS Function[1]	22	82%	90%	83%	99%
Smoking Cessation Advice[1]	4	100%	91%	82%	100%
Pneumonia Care					
Appropriate Initial Antibiotic	28	79%	84%	83%	94%
Blood Culture Timing[1]	14	93%	88%	90%	100%
Influenza Vaccine[1]	8	88%	64%	70%	100%
Initial Antibiotic Timing	29	79%	74%	80%	93%
Oxygenation Assessment	36	100%	99%	99%	100%
Pneumococcal Vaccine[1]	23	70%	67%	69%	94%
Smoking Cessation Advice[1]	10	90%	90%	80%	100%
Surgical Infection Prevention					
Prophylactic Antibiotic Given[2]	69	78%	83%	77%	95%
Prophylactic Antibiotic Selection[1,2]	15	87%	90%	90%	100%
Prophylactic Antibiotic Stopped[2]	68	16%	70%	72%	95%
Pregnancy Care					
Inpatient Neonatal Mortality	-	-	-	-	-
Third or Fourth Degree Laceration	-	-	2.71%	3.63%	3.27%

Northwest Medical Center

2801 North State Road 7
Margate, FL 33063
URL: www.northwestmed.com
Ownership: Proprietary
Emergency Services: Yes

Phone: 954-978-4000
Fax: 954-978-4183

Accredited: Yes
Licensed Beds: 215

Key Personnel:
CEO. . . . . Gina Melby
Chief Medical Staff. . . . . Steve Foster, MD
Catheterization Lab . . . . Laurie Siggins, RN
Emergency Room . . . . Adam Jhau, MD
Emergency Room . . . . Nadiney Giudice, RN
Infection Control. . . . . Jeannette Callaway

NOTE: Hospital profiles are in alphabetical order by state, then city, then hospital within the city; Rankings are sorted by rate in descending order and exclude hospitals with less than 25 cases; (1) The number of cases is too small (n<25) for purposes of reliably predicting hospital performance; (2) Measure reflects the hospital's indication that its submission was based upon a sample of its relevant discharges; (3) Rate reflects fewer than the maximum possible quarters of data for the measure; (4) Inaccurate information submitted and suppressed for one or more quarters; (5) No data is available from the hospital for this measure; Please refer to the User's Guide for a full explanation of data

ICU . . . . Carol Rhorstad, RN
Medical Surgical Nursing . . . . Beth Cooper, RN
OB/GYN/Women's Health . . . . Deb Block, RN
Respiratory/Cardiopulmonary. . . . . Olivene Gardner

Measure	Cases	This Hospital	State Average	U.S. Average	Top Hospital
Heart Attack Care					
ACE Inhibitor or ARB for LVSD	27	89%	83%	82%	100%
Aspirin at Arrival	165	88%	93%	92%	100%
Aspirin at Discharge	72	90%	88%	90%	100%
Beta Blocker at Arrival	102	89%	89%	87%	100%
Beta Blocker at Discharge	93	99%	92%	90%	100%
Fibrinolytic Medication Timing[1]	8	25%	33%	31%	100%
PCI Within 90 Minutes of Arrival	0	-	52%	54%	95%
Smoking Cessation Advice[1]	10	90%	92%	88%	100%
Heart Failure Care					
ACE Inhibitor or ARB for LVSD	95	87%	82%	82%	100%
Discharge Instructions	260	88%	61%	61%	93%
Evaluation of LVS Function	333	93%	90%	83%	99%
Smoking Cessation Advice	37	100%	91%	82%	100%
Pneumonia Care					
Appropriate Initial Antibiotic	194	88%	84%	83%	94%
Blood Culture Timing	156	90%	88%	90%	100%
Influenza Vaccine	53	70%	64%	70%	100%
Initial Antibiotic Timing	225	70%	74%	80%	93%
Oxygenation Assessment	274	100%	99%	99%	100%
Pneumococcal Vaccine	175	73%	67%	69%	94%
Smoking Cessation Advice	52	96%	90%	80%	100%
Surgical Infection Prevention					
Prophylactic Antibiotic Given[3]	318	86%	83%	77%	95%
Prophylactic Antibiotic Selection	110	82%	90%	90%	100%
Prophylactic Antibiotic Stopped[3]	312	79%	70%	72%	95%
Pregnancy Care					
Inpatient Neonatal Mortality	-	-	-	-	-
Third or Fourth Degree Laceration	-	-	2.71%	3.63%	3.27%

Jackson Hospital

4250 Hospital Drive
PO Box 1608
Marianna, FL 32446
E-mail: webmaster@JacksonHosp.com
URL: www.jacksonhosp.com
Ownership: Govt - Hospital District or Authority
Emergency Services: Yes
Key Personnel:

Phone: 850-526-2200
Fax: 850-482-6374

Accredited: Yes
Licensed Beds: 100

CEO . . . . John West
Chief Medical Staff. . . . . Gonzalo Oria, MD
Director Medical/Surgical Nursing . . . . Linda Henderson
Director Respiratory Therapy . . . . Scott Owen

Measure	Cases	This Hospital	State Average	U.S. Average	Top Hospital
Heart Attack Care					
ACE Inhibitor or ARB for LVSD[1]	10	90%	83%	82%	100%
Aspirin at Arrival	30	97%	93%	92%	100%
Aspirin at Discharge[1]	16	100%	88%	90%	100%
Beta Blocker at Arrival	29	86%	89%	87%	100%
Beta Blocker at Discharge[1]	19	95%	92%	90%	100%
Fibrinolytic Medication Timing	0	-	33%	31%	100%
PCI Within 90 Minutes of Arrival	0	-	52%	54%	95%
Smoking Cessation Advice[1]	5	100%	92%	88%	100%
Heart Failure Care					
ACE Inhibitor or ARB for LVSD	50	92%	82%	82%	100%
Discharge Instructions	125	24%	61%	61%	93%
Evaluation of LVS Function	167	87%	90%	83%	99%
Smoking Cessation Advice	31	94%	91%	82%	100%
Pneumonia Care					
Appropriate Initial Antibiotic	91	74%	84%	83%	94%
Blood Culture Timing	56	86%	88%	90%	100%
Influenza Vaccine	25	32%	64%	70%	100%
Initial Antibiotic Timing	101	78%	74%	80%	93%
Oxygenation Assessment	128	100%	99%	99%	100%
Pneumococcal Vaccine	70	26%	67%	69%	94%

Measure	Cases	This Hospital	State Average	U.S. Average	Top Hospital
Smoking Cessation Advice	36	97%	90%	80%	100%
Surgical Infection Prevention					
Prophylactic Antibiotic Given[3]	86	87%	83%	77%	95%
Prophylactic Antibiotic Selection	29	100%	90%	90%	100%
Prophylactic Antibiotic Stopped[3]	84	86%	70%	72%	95%
Pregnancy Care					
Inpatient Neonatal Mortality	-	-	-	-	-
Third or Fourth Degree Laceration	-	-	2.71%	3.63%	3.27%

Holmes Regional Medical Center

1350 S Hickory Street
Melbourne, FL 32901
URL: www.healthfirst.org
Ownership: Voluntary non-profit - Private
Emergency Services: Yes
Key Personnel:

Phone: 321-434-7000
Fax: 321-434-8587

Accredited: Yes
Licensed Beds: 468

President/CEO. . . . . Steve Bunker
Chief Medical Staff. . . . . Craig Badolato, MD
Director Emergency Services . . . . Barbara Ozmar, RN/MS
Emergency Room . . . . Scott Gettings, MD
Director Infection/Disease Control . . . . Stacy Westphal
CCU Spvg. Nurse . . . . Rose Mazanec-Freeman, RN
Director Medical/Surgical Nursing . . . . Joan Shinkus-Clark, RN
OB/GYN Womens Health. . . . . Rebecca Wagaman
Chief Radiology . . . . Martin Stern, MD
Director Respiratory Therapy . . . . Randy McGrath

Measure	Cases	This Hospital	State Average	U.S. Average	Top Hospital
Heart Attack Care					
ACE Inhibitor or ARB for LVSD[2]	298	85%	83%	82%	100%
Aspirin at Arrival[2]	426	94%	93%	92%	100%
Aspirin at Discharge[2]	744	98%	88%	90%	100%
Beta Blocker at Arrival[2]	383	92%	89%	87%	100%
Beta Blocker at Discharge[2]	762	95%	92%	90%	100%
Fibrinolytic Medication Timing[1,2]	4	25%	33%	31%	100%
PCI Within 90 Minutes of Arrival[1,2]	20	35%	52%	54%	95%
Smoking Cessation Advice[2]	256	97%	92%	88%	100%
Heart Failure Care					
ACE Inhibitor or ARB for LVSD[2]	412	74%	82%	82%	100%
Discharge Instructions[2]	661	73%	61%	61%	93%
Evaluation of LVS Function[2]	818	89%	90%	83%	99%
Smoking Cessation Advice[2]	132	93%	91%	82%	100%
Pneumonia Care					
Appropriate Initial Antibiotic[2]	388	85%	84%	83%	94%
Blood Culture Timing[2]	403	93%	88%	90%	100%
Influenza Vaccine[2]	96	57%	64%	70%	100%
Initial Antibiotic Timing[2]	517	86%	74%	80%	93%
Oxygenation Assessment[2]	602	100%	99%	99%	100%
Pneumococcal Vaccine[2]	377	62%	67%	69%	94%
Smoking Cessation Advice[2]	121	88%	90%	80%	100%
Surgical Infection Prevention					
Prophylactic Antibiotic Given[2]	947	91%	83%	77%	95%
Prophylactic Antibiotic Selection[2]	241	94%	90%	90%	100%
Prophylactic Antibiotic Stopped[2]	920	65%	70%	72%	95%
Pregnancy Care					
Inpatient Neonatal Mortality	-	-	-	-	-
Third or Fourth Degree Laceration	-	-	2.71%	3.63%	3.27%

Wuesthoff Medical Center-Melbourne

250 North Wickham Road
Melbourne, FL 32904
URL: www.wuesthoff.org
Ownership: Voluntary non-profit - Private
Emergency Services: Yes
Key Personnel:
President/CEO. . . . . Emil P Miller

Phone: 321-752-1200
Fax: 321-752-1698

Accredited: Yes
Licensed Beds: 65

Measure	Cases	This Hospital	State Average	U.S. Average	Top Hospital
Heart Attack Care					
ACE Inhibitor or ARB for LVSD[1]	7	100%	83%	82%	100%
Aspirin at Arrival	30	90%	93%	92%	100%
Aspirin at Discharge[1]	14	100%	88%	90%	100%
Beta Blocker at Arrival[1]	15	87%	89%	87%	100%

NOTE: Hospital profiles are in alphabetical order by state, then city, then hospital within the city; Rankings are sorted by rate in descending order and exclude hospitals with less than 25 cases; (1) The number of cases is too small (n<25) for purposes of reliably predicting hospital performance; (2) Measure reflects the hospital's indication that its submission was based upon a sample of its relevant discharges; (3) Rate reflects fewer than the maximum possible quarters of data for the measure; (4) Inaccurate information submitted and suppressed for one or more quarters; (5) No data is available from the hospital for this measure; Please refer to the User's Guide for a full explanation of data

Beta Blocker at Discharge[1]	18	100%	92%	90%	100%
Fibrinolytic Medication Timing	0	-	33%	31%	100%
PCI Within 90 Minutes of Arrival	0	-	52%	54%	95%
Smoking Cessation Advice[1]	2	100%	92%	88%	100%
Heart Failure Care					
ACE Inhibitor or ARB for LVSD	71	77%	82%	82%	100%
Discharge Instructions	121	60%	61%	61%	93%
Evaluation of LVS Function	149	93%	90%	83%	99%
Smoking Cessation Advice	25	100%	91%	82%	100%
Pneumonia Care					
Appropriate Initial Antibiotic	85	74%	84%	83%	94%
Blood Culture Timing	58	93%	88%	90%	100%
Influenza Vaccine[1]	22	73%	64%	70%	100%
Initial Antibiotic Timing	91	66%	74%	80%	93%
Oxygenation Assessment	115	100%	99%	99%	100%
Pneumococcal Vaccine	70	76%	67%	69%	94%
Smoking Cessation Advice[1]	23	100%	90%	80%	100%
Surgical Infection Prevention					
Prophylactic Antibiotic Given[2]	290	93%	83%	77%	95%
Prophylactic Antibiotic Selection[2]	76	88%	90%	90%	100%
Prophylactic Antibiotic Stopped[2]	283	67%	70%	72%	95%
Pregnancy Care					
Inpatient Neonatal Mortality	-	-	-	-	-
Third or Fourth Degree Laceration	-	-	2.71%	3.63%	3.27%

Baptist Hospital

Alternate Name: Baptist Hospital of Miami
8900 N Kendall Drive
Miami, FL 33176
URL: www.baptisthealth.net
Ownership: Voluntary non-profit - Private
Emergency Services: Yes

Phone: 786-596-1960
Fax: 786-596-2428

Accredited: Yes
Licensed Beds: 577

Key Personnel:
President/CEO. . . . . Bo Boulenger
Chief Medical Staff. . . . . Eugene Eisher, MD
Emergency Room . . . . David Nateman, MD
Emergency Room . . . . Becky Montesino, RN
Infection Control Director . . . . Barbara Russell, RN
ICU Director. . . . . Hal Augsburger
Respiratory/Cardiopulmonary Director . . . . John Bayer

Measure	Cases	This Hospital	State Average	U.S. Average	Top Hospital
Heart Attack Care					
ACE Inhibitor or ARB for LVSD	127	94%	83%	82%	100%
Aspirin at Arrival	439	98%	93%	92%	100%
Aspirin at Discharge	490	99%	88%	90%	100%
Beta Blocker at Arrival	343	95%	89%	87%	100%
Beta Blocker at Discharge	510	100%	92%	90%	100%
Fibrinolytic Medication Timing[1]	2	50%	33%	31%	100%
PCI Within 90 Minutes of Arrival[1]	14	100%	52%	54%	95%
Smoking Cessation Advice	168	100%	92%	88%	100%
Heart Failure Care					
ACE Inhibitor or ARB for LVSD	319	92%	82%	82%	100%
Discharge Instructions	660	82%	61%	61%	93%
Evaluation of LVS Function	760	99%	90%	83%	99%
Smoking Cessation Advice	85	99%	91%	82%	100%
Pneumonia Care					
Appropriate Initial Antibiotic	421	95%	84%	83%	94%
Blood Culture Timing	459	91%	88%	90%	100%
Influenza Vaccine	120	85%	64%	70%	100%
Initial Antibiotic Timing	535	62%	74%	80%	93%
Oxygenation Assessment	695	100%	99%	99%	100%
Pneumococcal Vaccine	388	89%	67%	69%	94%
Smoking Cessation Advice	117	100%	90%	80%	100%
Surgical Infection Prevention					
Prophylactic Antibiotic Given[2]	296	96%	83%	77%	95%
Prophylactic Antibiotic Selection[2]	73	100%	90%	90%	100%
Prophylactic Antibiotic Stopped[2]	286	93%	70%	72%	95%
Pregnancy Care					
Inpatient Neonatal Mortality	-	-	-	-	-
Third or Fourth Degree Laceration	-	-	2.71%	3.63%	3.27%

Bascom Palmer Eye Institute

900 NW 17th Street
Miami, FL 33136

Toll-Free: 800-329-7000
Phone: 305-326-6000
Fax: 305-326-6199

URL: www.bpei.med.miami.edu
Ownership: Voluntary non-profit - Other
Emergency Services: Yes

Accredited: Yes
Licensed Beds: 100

Key Personnel:
CEO. . . . . Dale Guffey
Chief Medical Staff. . . . . Paul Mendez, MD

Measure	Cases	This Hospital	State Average	U.S. Average	Top Hospital
Heart Attack Care					
ACE Inhibitor or ARB for LVSD[5]	-	-	83%	82%	100%
Aspirin at Arrival[5]	-	-	93%	92%	100%
Aspirin at Discharge[5]	-	-	88%	90%	100%
Beta Blocker at Arrival[5]	-	-	89%	87%	100%
Beta Blocker at Discharge[5]	-	-	92%	90%	100%
Fibrinolytic Medication Timing[5]	-	-	33%	31%	100%
PCI Within 90 Minutes of Arrival[5]	-	-	52%	54%	95%
Smoking Cessation Advice[5]	-	-	92%	88%	100%
Heart Failure Care					
ACE Inhibitor or ARB for LVSD[5]	-	-	82%	82%	100%
Discharge Instructions[5]	-	-	61%	61%	93%
Evaluation of LVS Function[5]	-	-	90%	83%	99%
Smoking Cessation Advice[5]	-	-	91%	82%	100%
Pneumonia Care					
Appropriate Initial Antibiotic[5]	-	-	84%	83%	94%
Blood Culture Timing[5]	-	-	88%	90%	100%
Influenza Vaccine[5]	-	-	64%	70%	100%
Initial Antibiotic Timing[5]	-	-	74%	80%	93%
Oxygenation Assessment[5]	-	-	99%	99%	100%
Pneumococcal Vaccine[5]	-	-	67%	69%	94%
Smoking Cessation Advice[5]	-	-	90%	80%	100%
Surgical Infection Prevention					
Prophylactic Antibiotic Given[5]	-	-	83%	77%	95%
Prophylactic Antibiotic Selection[5]	-	-	90%	90%	100%
Prophylactic Antibiotic Stopped[5]	-	-	70%	72%	95%
Pregnancy Care					
Inpatient Neonatal Mortality	-	-	-	-	-
Third or Fourth Degree Laceration	-	-	2.71%	3.63%	3.27%

Cedars Medical Center

Alternate Name: HCA, Cedars Medical Center
1400 NW 12th Avenue
Miami, FL 33136
URL: www.cedarsmedicalcenter.com
Ownership: Proprietary
Emergency Services: No

Phone: 305-325-5511
Fax: 305-325-4673

Accredited: Yes
Licensed Beds: 560

Key Personnel:
President/CEO. . . . . Anthony Degina
Chief Medical Staff. . . . . Jolly Varki, MD
Cardiology . . . . Anne Lee, RN
Respiratory Therapist. . . . . Dan Kinkade

Measure	Cases	This Hospital	State Average	U.S. Average	Top Hospital
Heart Attack Care					
ACE Inhibitor or ARB for LVSD	118	66%	83%	82%	100%
Aspirin at Arrival	242	90%	93%	92%	100%
Aspirin at Discharge	286	80%	88%	90%	100%
Beta Blocker at Arrival	239	82%	89%	87%	100%
Beta Blocker at Discharge	299	79%	92%	90%	100%
Fibrinolytic Medication Timing	28	18%	33%	31%	100%
PCI Within 90 Minutes of Arrival	0	-	52%	54%	95%
Smoking Cessation Advice	94	80%	92%	88%	100%
Heart Failure Care					
ACE Inhibitor or ARB for LVSD[2]	371	65%	82%	82%	100%
Discharge Instructions[2]	663	37%	61%	61%	93%
Evaluation of LVS Function[2]	777	92%	90%	83%	99%
Smoking Cessation Advice[2]	199	85%	91%	82%	100%
Pneumonia Care					
Appropriate Initial Antibiotic[2]	170	82%	84%	83%	94%
Blood Culture Timing[2]	195	75%	88%	90%	100%

NOTE: Hospital profiles are in alphabetical order by state, then city, then hospital within the city; Rankings are sorted by rate in descending order and exclude hospitals with less than 25 cases; (1) The number of cases is too small (n<25) for purposes of reliably predicting hospital performance; (2) Measure reflects the hospital's indication that its submission was based upon a sample of its relevant discharges; (3) Rate reflects fewer than the maximum possible quarters of data for the measure; (4) Inaccurate information submitted and suppressed for one or more quarters; (5) No data is available from the hospital for this measure; Please refer to the User's Guide for a full explanation of data

Measure	Cases	This Hospital	State Average	U.S. Average	Top Hospital
Influenza Vaccine	59	25%	64%	70%	100%
Initial Antibiotic Timing[2]	314	54%	74%	80%	93%
Oxygenation Assessment[2]	343	98%	99%	99%	100%
Pneumococcal Vaccine[2]	203	33%	67%	69%	94%
Smoking Cessation Advice[2]	67	85%	90%	80%	100%
Surgical Infection Prevention					
Prophylactic Antibiotic Given[2,3]	468	96%	83%	77%	95%
Prophylactic Antibiotic Selection[2]	101	89%	90%	90%	100%
Prophylactic Antibiotic Stopped[2,3]	462	62%	70%	72%	95%
Pregnancy Care					
Inpatient Neonatal Mortality	-	-	-	-	-
Third or Fourth Degree Laceration	-	-	2.71%	3.63%	3.27%

Jackson Memorial Hospital

1611 NW 12th Avenue
Miami, FL 33136
URL: www.jhsmiami.org
Ownership: Govt - Hospital District or Authority
Emergency Services: Yes

Phone: 305-585-1111
Fax: 305-326-8630

Accredited: Yes
Licensed Beds: 1,498

Key Personnel:
President/CEO . . . . Marvin O'Quinn
EVP/Chief Medical Officer . . . . Gerard A Kaiser, MD
SVP CAO Medical/Surgical Hosptial Center. . . . Eugene Bassett

Measure	Cases	This Hospital	State Average	U.S. Average	Top Hospital
Heart Attack Care					
ACE Inhibitor or ARB for LVSD[2]	66	91%	83%	82%	100%
Aspirin at Arrival[2]	223	96%	93%	92%	100%
Aspirin at Discharge[2]	212	96%	88%	90%	100%
Beta Blocker at Arrival[2]	180	94%	89%	87%	100%
Beta Blocker at Discharge[2]	231	96%	92%	90%	100%
Fibrinolytic Medication Timing[1,2]	18	33%	33%	31%	100%
PCI Within 90 Minutes of Arrival[1,2]	4	0%	52%	54%	95%
Smoking Cessation Advice[2]	96	95%	92%	88%	100%
Heart Failure Care					
ACE Inhibitor or ARB for LVSD[2]	275	84%	82%	82%	100%
Discharge Instructions[2]	509	41%	61%	61%	93%
Evaluation of LVS Function[2]	569	97%	90%	83%	99%
Smoking Cessation Advice[2]	137	73%	91%	82%	100%
Pneumonia Care					
Appropriate Initial Antibiotic[2]	200	94%	84%	83%	94%
Blood Culture Timing[2]	182	68%	88%	90%	100%
Influenza Vaccine[2]	46	41%	64%	70%	100%
Initial Antibiotic Timing[2]	326	51%	74%	80%	93%
Oxygenation Assessment[2]	352	99%	99%	99%	100%
Pneumococcal Vaccine[2]	139	45%	67%	69%	94%
Smoking Cessation Advice[2]	86	70%	90%	80%	100%
Surgical Infection Prevention					
Prophylactic Antibiotic Given[2]	298	60%	83%	77%	95%
Prophylactic Antibiotic Selection[2]	60	82%	90%	90%	100%
Prophylactic Antibiotic Stopped[2]	280	68%	70%	72%	95%
Pregnancy Care					
Inpatient Neonatal Mortality	-	-	-	-	-
Third or Fourth Degree Laceration	-	-	2.71%	3.63%	3.27%

Kendall Medical Center

11750 Bird Road
Miami, FL 33175
URL: www.kendalmed.com
Ownership: Proprietary
Emergency Services: Yes

Phone: 305-223-3000
Fax: 305-227-5503

Accredited: Yes
Licensed Beds: 412

Key Personnel:
President/CEO . . . . Victor Maya
Chief Medical Staff . . . . Fuad Ashkar, MD
Chief Catheterization Laboratory . . . . Mimi Gonzalez
Emergency Room . . . . Juan J Remos, MD
Director Infection/Disease Control . . . . Alberto Alea, MD
CCU Spvg. Nurse . . . . Vangie Bustos, RN
Director Medical/Surgical Nursing . . . . Ellen Uptak
Chief Radiology . . . . Roberto Calderon, MD
Director Respiratory Therapy . . . . Joe Miro

Measure	Cases	This Hospital	State Average	U.S. Average	Top Hospital

Measure	Cases	This Hospital	State Average	U.S. Average	Top Hospital
Heart Attack Care					
ACE Inhibitor or ARB for LVSD	180	63%	83%	82%	100%
Aspirin at Arrival	455	94%	93%	92%	100%
Aspirin at Discharge	409	93%	88%	90%	100%
Beta Blocker at Arrival	322	83%	89%	87%	100%
Beta Blocker at Discharge	494	90%	92%	90%	100%
Fibrinolytic Medication Timing[1]	7	14%	33%	31%	100%
PCI Within 90 Minutes of Arrival[1]	20	60%	52%	54%	95%
Smoking Cessation Advice	139	99%	92%	88%	100%
Heart Failure Care					
ACE Inhibitor or ARB for LVSD	342	65%	82%	82%	100%
Discharge Instructions	679	72%	61%	61%	93%
Evaluation of LVS Function	777	97%	90%	83%	99%
Smoking Cessation Advice	65	100%	91%	82%	100%
Pneumonia Care					
Appropriate Initial Antibiotic	464	91%	84%	83%	94%
Blood Culture Timing	424	94%	88%	90%	100%
Influenza Vaccine	116	41%	64%	70%	100%
Initial Antibiotic Timing	619	76%	74%	80%	93%
Oxygenation Assessment	660	100%	99%	99%	100%
Pneumococcal Vaccine	444	52%	67%	69%	94%
Smoking Cessation Advice	86	93%	90%	80%	100%
Surgical Infection Prevention					
Prophylactic Antibiotic Given[3]	330	86%	83%	77%	95%
Prophylactic Antibiotic Selection	134	97%	90%	90%	100%
Prophylactic Antibiotic Stopped[3]	310	75%	70%	72%	95%
Pregnancy Care					
Inpatient Neonatal Mortality	-	-	-	-	-
Third or Fourth Degree Laceration	-	-	2.71%	3.63%	3.27%

Mercy Hospital

3663 S Miami Avenue
Miami, FL 33133
URL: www.mercymiami.com
Ownership: Voluntary non-profit - Church
Emergency Services: Yes

Phone: 305-854-4400
Fax: 305-860-4723

Accredited: Yes
Licensed Beds: 483

Key Personnel:
President/CEO . . . . John E Matuska
Director Cardiac Lab . . . . Laura Dominguez
Emergency Room . . . . Cinara Navarro
Director Medical/Surgical Services. . . . . Nancy McCarthy, RN
Director Surgery/Women's Services. . . . . Frank Lago, RN
Director Radiology . . . . Kevin Gregory
Director Respiratory Therapy . . . . Reginald Severe

Measure	Cases	This Hospital	State Average	U.S. Average	Top Hospital
Heart Attack Care					
ACE Inhibitor or ARB for LVSD	79	94%	83%	82%	100%
Aspirin at Arrival	251	99%	93%	92%	100%
Aspirin at Discharge	355	99%	88%	90%	100%
Beta Blocker at Arrival	250	99%	89%	87%	100%
Beta Blocker at Discharge	374	97%	92%	90%	100%
Fibrinolytic Medication Timing[1]	1	0%	33%	31%	100%
PCI Within 90 Minutes of Arrival[1]	4	75%	52%	54%	95%
Smoking Cessation Advice	64	100%	92%	88%	100%
Heart Failure Care					
ACE Inhibitor or ARB for LVSD	298	95%	82%	82%	100%
Discharge Instructions	496	96%	61%	61%	93%
Evaluation of LVS Function	551	99%	90%	83%	99%
Smoking Cessation Advice	75	100%	91%	82%	100%
Pneumonia Care					
Appropriate Initial Antibiotic	202	95%	84%	83%	94%
Blood Culture Timing	234	94%	88%	90%	100%
Influenza Vaccine[4,5]	-	-	64%	70%	100%
Initial Antibiotic Timing	295	89%	74%	80%	93%
Oxygenation Assessment	354	100%	99%	99%	100%
Pneumococcal Vaccine	261	84%	67%	69%	94%
Smoking Cessation Advice	44	100%	90%	80%	100%
Surgical Infection Prevention					
Prophylactic Antibiotic Given	1,252	96%	83%	77%	95%
Prophylactic Antibiotic Selection	316	97%	90%	90%	100%
Prophylactic Antibiotic Stopped	1,229	84%	70%	72%	95%
Pregnancy Care					

NOTE: Hospital profiles are in alphabetical order by state, then city, then hospital within the city; Rankings are sorted by rate in descending order and exclude hospitals with less than 25 cases; (1) The number of cases is too small (n<25) for purposes of reliably predicting hospital performance; (2) Measure reflects the hospital's indication that its submission was based upon a sample of its relevant discharges; (3) Rate reflects fewer than the maximum possible quarters of data for the measure; (4) Inaccurate information submitted and suppressed for one or more quarters; (5) No data is available from the hospital for this measure; Please refer to the User's Guide for a full explanation of data

Measure	Cases	This Hospital	State Average	U.S. Average	Top Hospital
Inpatient Neonatal Mortality	-	-	-	-	-
Third or Fourth Degree Laceration	-	-	2.71%	3.63%	3.27%

Miami Jewish Home & Hosp for the Aged

5200 NE 2nd Avenue   Phone: 305-751-8626
Miami, FL 33137   Fax: 305-754-4530
E-mail: info@mjhha.org
URL: www.mjhha.org
Ownership: Voluntary non-profit - Private
Emergency Services: No   Accredited: Yes
       Licensed Beds: 494
Key Personnel:
President/CEO . . . . Harold Beck
Chief Medical Staff. Michael Silverman
Director Infection/Disease Control . . . . Erna Zemel
Director Respiratory Therapy . . . . Tim Brooks

Measure	Cases	This Hospital	State Average	U.S. Average	Top Hospital
Heart Attack Care					
ACE Inhibitor or ARB for LVSD[3]	0	-	83%	82%	100%
Aspirin at Arrival[1,3]	2	50%	93%	92%	100%
Aspirin at Discharge[1,3]	2	50%	88%	90%	100%
Beta Blocker at Arrival[1,3]	2	50%	89%	87%	100%
Beta Blocker at Discharge[1,3]	2	100%	92%	90%	100%
Fibrinolytic Medication Timing[3]	0	-	33%	31%	100%
PCI Within 90 Minutes of Arrival	0	-	52%	54%	95%
Smoking Cessation Advice[3]	0	-	92%	88%	100%
Heart Failure Care					
ACE Inhibitor or ARB for LVSD	0	-	82%	82%	100%
Discharge Instructions[1,3]	5	0%	61%	61%	93%
Evaluation of LVS Function[1]	16	75%	90%	83%	99%
Smoking Cessation Advice[3]	0	-	91%	82%	100%
Pneumonia Care					
Appropriate Initial Antibiotic[1]	5	40%	84%	83%	94%
Blood Culture Timing[1]	14	100%	88%	90%	100%
Influenza Vaccine[1]	12	58%	64%	70%	100%
Initial Antibiotic Timing	46	80%	74%	80%	93%
Oxygenation Assessment	64	100%	99%	99%	100%
Pneumococcal Vaccine	52	46%	67%	69%	94%
Smoking Cessation Advice[1]	1	0%	90%	80%	100%
Surgical Infection Prevention					
Prophylactic Antibiotic Given[3]	0	-	83%	77%	95%
Prophylactic Antibiotic Selection	0	-	90%	90%	100%
Prophylactic Antibiotic Stopped[3]	0	-	70%	72%	95%
Pregnancy Care					
Inpatient Neonatal Mortality	-	-	-	-	-
Third or Fourth Degree Laceration	-	-	2.71%	3.63%	3.27%

North Shore Medical Center

1100 NW 95th Street   Phone: 305-835-6000
Miami, FL 33150   Fax: 305-835-6163
URL: www.northshoremedical.com
Ownership: Voluntary non-profit - Private
Emergency Services: Yes   Accredited: Yes
       Licensed Beds: 357
Key Personnel:
President/CEO. . . . . Ana Mederos
Chief Medical Staff. Constantine Kitsos, MD
Cardiac Lab . . . . Dennis Reese
Emergency Room . . . . Vera Burke
Infection Control. . . . . Veronica Torres
ICU . . . . Edwina Crum, RN
Intensive/Coronary Care . . . . Edwina Crum
Medical Surgery Nurse. . . . . Sylvan Trepenier
OB/GYN Womens Health. . . . . Hortense Martin
Respiratory/Cardiopulmonary. . . . . Dennis Reese

Measure	Cases	This Hospital	State Average	U.S. Average	Top Hospital
Heart Attack Care					
ACE Inhibitor or ARB for LVSD	41	76%	83%	82%	100%
Aspirin at Arrival	171	84%	93%	92%	100%
Aspirin at Discharge	82	88%	88%	90%	100%
Beta Blocker at Arrival	145	88%	89%	87%	100%
Beta Blocker at Discharge	101	96%	92%	90%	100%
Fibrinolytic Medication Timing[1]	8	50%	33%	31%	100%

Measure	Cases	This Hospital	State Average	U.S. Average	Top Hospital
PCI Within 90 Minutes of Arrival	0	-	52%	54%	95%
Smoking Cessation Advice[1]	16	100%	92%	88%	100%
Heart Failure Care					
ACE Inhibitor or ARB for LVSD	271	85%	82%	82%	100%
Discharge Instructions	494	92%	61%	61%	93%
Evaluation of LVS Function	571	97%	90%	83%	99%
Smoking Cessation Advice	124	100%	91%	82%	100%
Pneumonia Care					
Appropriate Initial Antibiotic	187	94%	84%	83%	94%
Blood Culture Timing	211	84%	88%	90%	100%
Influenza Vaccine	36	86%	64%	70%	100%
Initial Antibiotic Timing	262	63%	74%	80%	93%
Oxygenation Assessment	314	100%	99%	99%	100%
Pneumococcal Vaccine	145	75%	67%	69%	94%
Smoking Cessation Advice	54	100%	90%	80%	100%
Surgical Infection Prevention					
Prophylactic Antibiotic Given[2]	79	95%	83%	77%	95%
Prophylactic Antibiotic Selection[1,2]	19	100%	90%	90%	100%
Prophylactic Antibiotic Stopped[2]	76	91%	70%	72%	95%
Pregnancy Care					
Inpatient Neonatal Mortality	-	-	-	-	-
Third or Fourth Degree Laceration	-	-	2.71%	3.63%	3.27%

Pan American Hospital

5959 NW 7th Street   Phone: 305-264-1000
Miami, FL 33126   Fax: 305-265-6504
E-mail: hospital@pahnet.org
URL: www.pahnet.org
Ownership: Voluntary non-profit - Private
Emergency Services: Yes   Accredited: Yes
       Licensed Beds: 146
Key Personnel:
Executive Director . . . . Vincente Sanchez

Measure	Cases	This Hospital	State Average	U.S. Average	Top Hospital
Heart Attack Care					
ACE Inhibitor or ARB for LVSD[1]	18	83%	83%	82%	100%
Aspirin at Arrival	116	97%	93%	92%	100%
Aspirin at Discharge	44	93%	88%	90%	100%
Beta Blocker at Arrival	119	89%	89%	87%	100%
Beta Blocker at Discharge	46	87%	92%	90%	100%
Fibrinolytic Medication Timing	0	-	33%	31%	100%
PCI Within 90 Minutes of Arrival	0	-	52%	54%	95%
Smoking Cessation Advice[1]	4	100%	92%	88%	100%
Heart Failure Care					
ACE Inhibitor or ARB for LVSD	127	80%	82%	82%	100%
Discharge Instructions	240	95%	61%	61%	93%
Evaluation of LVS Function	323	96%	90%	83%	99%
Smoking Cessation Advice	28	96%	91%	82%	100%
Pneumonia Care					
Appropriate Initial Antibiotic	223	65%	84%	83%	94%
Blood Culture Timing	162	96%	88%	90%	100%
Influenza Vaccine	44	89%	64%	70%	100%
Initial Antibiotic Timing	207	84%	74%	80%	93%
Oxygenation Assessment	236	100%	99%	99%	100%
Pneumococcal Vaccine	155	97%	67%	69%	94%
Smoking Cessation Advice	25	100%	90%	80%	100%
Surgical Infection Prevention					
Prophylactic Antibiotic Given	242	83%	83%	77%	95%
Prophylactic Antibiotic Selection	75	87%	90%	90%	100%
Prophylactic Antibiotic Stopped	240	89%	70%	72%	95%
Pregnancy Care					
Inpatient Neonatal Mortality	-	-	-	-	-
Third or Fourth Degree Laceration	-	-	2.71%	3.63%	3.27%

South Miami Hospital

6200 SW 73rd Street   Phone: 305-661-4611
Miami, FL 33143   Fax: 305-662-2759
E-mail: corporatepr@baptisthealth.net
URL: www.baptisthealth.net
Ownership: Voluntary non-profit - Private
Emergency Services: Yes   Accredited: Yes
       Licensed Beds: 336
Key Personnel:
President/CEO. . . . . D Wayne Brackin

NOTE: Hospital profiles are in alphabetical order by state, then city, then hospital within the city; Rankings are sorted by rate in descending order and exclude hospitals with less than 25 cases; (1) The number of cases is too small (n<25) for purposes of reliably predicting hospital performance; (2) Measure reflects the hospital's indication that its submission was based upon a sample of its relevant discharges; (3) Rate reflects fewer than the maximum possible quarters of data for the measure; (4) Inaccurate information submitted and suppressed for one or more quarters; (5) No data is available from the hospital for this measure; Please refer to the User's Guide for a full explanation of data

Chief Medical Staff. . . . . Juan Mella, MD
Director Catheterization Laboratory . . . . Daniel Crauthamer
Emergency Room . . . . Richard Walbert, MD
Director Infection/Disease Control . . . . Vicki Heitzer
CCU Spvg. Nurse . . . . Carol Biggs
Director Medical/Surgical Nursing . . . . Carol Biggs
OB/GYN Womens Health. . . . . James Esserman, MD
Chief Radiology . . . . Steven Olfzewski, MD
Director Respiratory Therapy . . . . Gale Jackson

Measure	Cases	This Hospital	State Average	U.S. Average	Top Hospital
Heart Attack Care					
ACE Inhibitor or ARB for LVSD	84	100%	83%	82%	100%
Aspirin at Arrival	185	100%	93%	92%	100%
Aspirin at Discharge	277	99%	88%	90%	100%
Beta Blocker at Arrival	146	97%	89%	87%	100%
Beta Blocker at Discharge	297	99%	92%	90%	100%
Fibrinolytic Medication Timing[1]	1	100%	33%	31%	100%
PCI Within 90 Minutes of Arrival[1]	9	78%	52%	54%	95%
Smoking Cessation Advice	100	99%	92%	88%	100%
Heart Failure Care					
ACE Inhibitor or ARB for LVSD	144	98%	82%	82%	100%
Discharge Instructions	311	87%	61%	61%	93%
Evaluation of LVS Function	360	100%	90%	83%	99%
Smoking Cessation Advice	41	98%	91%	82%	100%
Pneumonia Care					
Appropriate Initial Antibiotic	288	94%	84%	83%	94%
Blood Culture Timing	341	98%	88%	90%	100%
Influenza Vaccine	106	100%	64%	70%	100%
Initial Antibiotic Timing	372	90%	74%	80%	93%
Oxygenation Assessment	475	100%	99%	99%	100%
Pneumococcal Vaccine	310	99%	67%	69%	94%
Smoking Cessation Advice	63	100%	90%	80%	100%
Surgical Infection Prevention					
Prophylactic Antibiotic Given[2]	245	93%	83%	77%	95%
Prophylactic Antibiotic Selection[2]	62	95%	90%	90%	100%
Prophylactic Antibiotic Stopped[2]	237	95%	70%	72%	95%
Pregnancy Care					
Inpatient Neonatal Mortality	-	-	-	-	-
Third or Fourth Degree Laceration	-	-	2.71%	3.63%	3.27%

Westchester General Hospital

2500 SW 75th Avenue   Phone: 305-264-5252
Miami, FL 33155   Fax: 305-267-6920
Ownership: Proprietary   Accredited: Yes
Emergency Services: Yes   Licensed Beds: 160
Key Personnel:
CEO. . . . . Gilda Baldwin
Chief Medical Staff. . . . . Alisha Lond
Emergency Room . . . . Lorata Ziegler
Director Pulmonary Therapy . . . . M Leon

Measure	Cases	This Hospital	State Average	U.S. Average	Top Hospital
Heart Attack Care					
ACE Inhibitor or ARB for LVSD[1]	4	50%	83%	82%	100%
Aspirin at Arrival[1]	14	93%	93%	92%	100%
Aspirin at Discharge[1]	11	64%	88%	90%	100%
Beta Blocker at Arrival[1]	14	86%	89%	87%	100%
Beta Blocker at Discharge[1]	11	100%	92%	90%	100%
Fibrinolytic Medication Timing[1]	1	0%	33%	31%	100%
PCI Within 90 Minutes of Arrival	0	-	52%	54%	95%
Smoking Cessation Advice[1]	2	100%	92%	88%	100%
Heart Failure Care					
ACE Inhibitor or ARB for LVSD[1]	12	50%	82%	82%	100%
Discharge Instructions	27	30%	61%	61%	93%
Evaluation of LVS Function	47	72%	90%	83%	99%
Smoking Cessation Advice[1]	5	80%	91%	82%	100%
Pneumonia Care					
Appropriate Initial Antibiotic	65	82%	84%	83%	94%
Blood Culture Timing	41	71%	88%	90%	100%
Influenza Vaccine[1]	13	38%	64%	70%	100%
Initial Antibiotic Timing	71	62%	74%	80%	93%

Measure	Cases	This Hospital	State Average	U.S. Average	Top Hospital
Oxygenation Assessment	74	97%	99%	99%	100%
Pneumococcal Vaccine	54	67%	67%	69%	94%
Smoking Cessation Advice[1]	9	56%	90%	80%	100%
Surgical Infection Prevention					
Prophylactic Antibiotic Given	45	84%	83%	77%	95%
Prophylactic Antibiotic Selection[1]	14	93%	90%	90%	100%
Prophylactic Antibiotic Stopped	44	89%	70%	72%	95%
Pregnancy Care					
Inpatient Neonatal Mortality	-	-	-	-	-
Third or Fourth Degree Laceration	-	-	2.71%	3.63%	3.27%

Mount Sinai Medical Center

4300 Alton Road   Phone: 305-674-2121
Miami, FL 33140   Fax: 305-674-2334
E-mail: webmaster@msmc.com
URL: www.msmc.com
Ownership: Voluntary non-profit - Private   Accredited: Yes
Emergency Services: Yes   Licensed Beds: 701
Key Personnel:
President/CEO. . . . . Steven D Sonenreich
Chief Medical Staff. . . . . Kenneth Ratzan, MD
Director Cardiac Surgery . . . . Donald Williams, MD
Chief Catheterization Laboratory . . . . Paul Vignola, MD
Emergency Room . . . . Art Diskin, MD
Chief Infection Control . . . . Kenneth Ratzan
Director Medical/Surgical Nursing . . . . Pam Hardesty, RN
OB/GYN Womens Health. . . . . Bernard Cantor, MD
Director Radiology . . . . Manuel Viamonte, MD

Measure	Cases	This Hospital	State Average	U.S. Average	Top Hospital
Heart Attack Care					
ACE Inhibitor or ARB for LVSD[2]	99	81%	83%	82%	100%
Aspirin at Arrival[2]	184	96%	93%	92%	100%
Aspirin at Discharge[2]	313	86%	88%	90%	100%
Beta Blocker at Arrival[2]	163	91%	89%	87%	100%
Beta Blocker at Discharge[2]	339	89%	92%	90%	100%
Fibrinolytic Medication Timing[1,2]	1	0%	33%	31%	100%
PCI Within 90 Minutes of Arrival[1,2]	9	56%	52%	54%	95%
Smoking Cessation Advice[2]	97	91%	92%	88%	100%
Heart Failure Care					
ACE Inhibitor or ARB for LVSD[2]	173	80%	82%	82%	100%
Discharge Instructions[2]	305	50%	61%	61%	93%
Evaluation of LVS Function[2]	373	94%	90%	83%	99%
Smoking Cessation Advice[2]	35	91%	91%	82%	100%
Pneumonia Care					
Appropriate Initial Antibiotic[2]	128	90%	84%	83%	94%
Blood Culture Timing[2]	153	85%	88%	90%	100%
Influenza Vaccine[2]	25	40%	64%	70%	100%
Initial Antibiotic Timing[2]	193	65%	74%	80%	93%
Oxygenation Assessment[2]	219	95%	99%	99%	100%
Pneumococcal Vaccine[2]	138	53%	67%	69%	94%
Smoking Cessation Advice[2]	32	94%	90%	80%	100%
Surgical Infection Prevention					
Prophylactic Antibiotic Given[2]	547	79%	83%	77%	95%
Prophylactic Antibiotic Selection[2]	316	84%	90%	90%	100%
Prophylactic Antibiotic Stopped[2]	538	74%	70%	72%	95%
Pregnancy Care					
Inpatient Neonatal Mortality	2,158	0.19%	-	-	-
Third or Fourth Degree Laceration	1,115	1.70%	2.71%	3.63%	3.27%

Santa Rosa Medical Center

6002 Berryhill Road   Phone: 850-626-5100
Milton, FL 32570   Fax: 850-623-5083
Ownership: Proprietary   Accredited: Yes
Emergency Services: Yes   Licensed Beds: 129
Key Personnel:
CEO. . . . . Pete Gandy
Emergency Room Director. . . . . Kathy Rowe
Infection Control. . . . . Judy Wolfe
OB/GYN. . . . . Geri Coffey
Chief Radiology . . . . Jerry Womack
Director Respiratory Therapy . . . . Larry Wilkensen

NOTE: Hospital profiles are in alphabetical order by state, then city, then hospital within the city; Rankings are sorted by rate in descending order and exclude hospitals with less than 25 cases; (1) The number of cases is too small (n<25) for purposes of reliably predicting hospital performance; (2) Measure reflects the hospital's indication that its submission was based upon a sample of its relevant discharges; (3) Rate reflects fewer than the maximum possible quarters of data for the measure; (4) Inaccurate information submitted and suppressed for one or more quarters; (5) No data is available from the hospital for this measure; Please refer to the User's Guide for a full explanation of data

Measure	Cases	This Hospital	State Average	U.S. Average	Top Hospital
Heart Attack Care					
ACE Inhibitor or ARB for LVSD[1]	7	71%	83%	82%	100%
Aspirin at Arrival	52	96%	93%	92%	100%
Aspirin at Discharge[1]	24	54%	88%	90%	100%
Beta Blocker at Arrival	50	90%	89%	87%	100%
Beta Blocker at Discharge	29	76%	92%	90%	100%
Fibrinolytic Medication Timing[1]	1	0%	33%	31%	100%
PCI Within 90 Minutes of Arrival	0	-	52%	54%	95%
Smoking Cessation Advice[1]	7	100%	92%	88%	100%
Heart Failure Care					
ACE Inhibitor or ARB for LVSD	45	89%	82%	82%	100%
Discharge Instructions	122	66%	61%	61%	93%
Evaluation of LVS Function	142	91%	90%	83%	99%
Smoking Cessation Advice	48	94%	91%	82%	100%
Pneumonia Care					
Appropriate Initial Antibiotic	137	77%	84%	83%	94%
Blood Culture Timing	131	97%	88%	90%	100%
Influenza Vaccine	46	85%	64%	70%	100%
Initial Antibiotic Timing	151	78%	74%	80%	93%
Oxygenation Assessment	193	100%	99%	99%	100%
Pneumococcal Vaccine	98	82%	67%	69%	94%
Smoking Cessation Advice	67	99%	90%	80%	100%
Surgical Infection Prevention					
Prophylactic Antibiotic Given[2]	156	88%	83%	77%	95%
Prophylactic Antibiotic Selection[2]	35	89%	90%	90%	100%
Prophylactic Antibiotic Stopped[2]	153	80%	70%	72%	95%
Pregnancy Care					
Inpatient Neonatal Mortality	-	-	-	-	-
Third or Fourth Degree Laceration	-	-	2.71%	3.63%	3.27%

Memorial Hospital Miramar

1901 Sw 172nd Avenue
Miramar, FL 33029
Ownership: Voluntary non-profit - Other
Emergency Services: Yes

Phone: 954-538-4810

Accredited: Yes

Measure	Cases	This Hospital	State Average	U.S. Average	Top Hospital
Heart Attack Care					
ACE Inhibitor or ARB for LVSD[1]	3	100%	83%	82%	100%
Aspirin at Arrival	39	100%	93%	92%	100%
Aspirin at Discharge[1]	7	100%	88%	90%	100%
Beta Blocker at Arrival	39	92%	89%	87%	100%
Beta Blocker at Discharge[1]	10	100%	92%	90%	100%
Fibrinolytic Medication Timing	0	-	33%	31%	100%
PCI Within 90 Minutes of Arrival	0	-	52%	54%	95%
Smoking Cessation Advice[1]	1	100%	92%	88%	100%
Heart Failure Care					
ACE Inhibitor or ARB for LVSD[1]	24	96%	82%	82%	100%
Discharge Instructions	122	88%	61%	61%	93%
Evaluation of LVS Function	133	98%	90%	83%	99%
Smoking Cessation Advice[1]	9	89%	91%	82%	100%
Pneumonia Care					
Appropriate Initial Antibiotic	134	89%	84%	83%	94%
Blood Culture Timing	125	98%	88%	90%	100%
Influenza Vaccine	26	100%	64%	70%	100%
Initial Antibiotic Timing	150	93%	74%	80%	93%
Oxygenation Assessment	174	100%	99%	99%	100%
Pneumococcal Vaccine	92	100%	67%	69%	94%
Smoking Cessation Advice	26	100%	90%	80%	100%
Surgical Infection Prevention					
Prophylactic Antibiotic Given[2]	213	89%	83%	77%	95%
Prophylactic Antibiotic Selection[1,2]	21	95%	90%	90%	100%
Prophylactic Antibiotic Stopped[2]	210	86%	70%	72%	95%
Pregnancy Care					
Inpatient Neonatal Mortality	-	-	-	-	-
Third or Fourth Degree Laceration	-	-	2.71%	3.63%	3.27%

NCH Downtown Naples Hospital

Alternate Name: Naples Community Hospital

350 7th Street N
Naples, FL 34102
URL: www.nchmd.org
Ownership: Voluntary non-profit - Other
Emergency Services: Yes

Phone: 239-436-5000
Fax: 239-436-5048

Accredited: Yes
Licensed Beds: 446

Key Personnel:
CEO . . . . Edward A Morton
Director Catheterization Laboratory . . . . Kevin Roesch
Neurological Surgery . . . . Paul Dernbach, MD
OB/GYN Womens Health. . . . . Kevin Collins, MD

Measure	Cases	This Hospital	State Average	U.S. Average	Top Hospital
Heart Attack Care					
ACE Inhibitor or ARB for LVSD	120	91%	83%	82%	100%
Aspirin at Arrival	577	100%	93%	92%	100%
Aspirin at Discharge	700	99%	88%	90%	100%
Beta Blocker at Arrival	507	98%	89%	87%	100%
Beta Blocker at Discharge	666	98%	92%	90%	100%
Fibrinolytic Medication Timing	0	-	33%	31%	100%
PCI Within 90 Minutes of Arrival[1]	20	40%	52%	54%	95%
Smoking Cessation Advice	158	99%	92%	88%	100%
Heart Failure Care					
ACE Inhibitor or ARB for LVSD	456	80%	82%	82%	100%
Discharge Instructions	887	45%	61%	61%	93%
Evaluation of LVS Function	1,121	89%	90%	83%	99%
Smoking Cessation Advice	122	97%	91%	82%	100%
Pneumonia Care					
Appropriate Initial Antibiotic	496	88%	84%	83%	94%
Blood Culture Timing	384	85%	88%	90%	100%
Influenza Vaccine	143	28%	64%	70%	100%
Initial Antibiotic Timing	527	72%	74%	80%	93%
Oxygenation Assessment	654	100%	99%	99%	100%
Pneumococcal Vaccine	482	44%	67%	69%	94%
Smoking Cessation Advice	124	76%	90%	80%	100%
Surgical Infection Prevention					
Prophylactic Antibiotic Given	2,605	88%	83%	77%	95%
Prophylactic Antibiotic Selection	593	94%	90%	90%	100%
Prophylactic Antibiotic Stopped	2,452	80%	70%	72%	95%
Pregnancy Care					
Inpatient Neonatal Mortality	-	-	-	-	-
Third or Fourth Degree Laceration	-	-	2.71%	3.63%	3.27%

Physicians Regional Medical Center

6101 Pine Ridge Road
Naples, FL 34119
URL: www.physiciansregional.com
Ownership: Voluntary non-profit - Other
Emergency Services: Yes

Phone: 239-348-4000
Fax: 239-348-4140

Accredited: Yes
Licensed Beds: 83

Key Personnel:
CEO . . . . Robert Kay, MD
Executive Director . . . . Robert J Zehr, MD

Measure	Cases	This Hospital	State Average	U.S. Average	Top Hospital
Heart Attack Care					
ACE Inhibitor or ARB for LVSD[1]	2	100%	83%	82%	100%
Aspirin at Arrival[1]	20	95%	93%	92%	100%
Aspirin at Discharge[1]	10	100%	88%	90%	100%
Beta Blocker at Arrival[1]	22	100%	89%	87%	100%
Beta Blocker at Discharge[1]	11	100%	92%	90%	100%
Fibrinolytic Medication Timing[3]	0	-	33%	31%	100%
PCI Within 90 Minutes of Arrival	0	-	52%	54%	95%
Smoking Cessation Advice[3]	0	-	92%	88%	100%
Heart Failure Care					
ACE Inhibitor or ARB for LVSD[1]	19	100%	82%	82%	100%
Discharge Instructions[1,3]	11	27%	61%	61%	93%
Evaluation of LVS Function	60	98%	90%	83%	99%
Smoking Cessation Advice[1,3]	2	50%	91%	82%	100%
Pneumonia Care					
Appropriate Initial Antibiotic[1,3]	9	89%	84%	83%	94%
Blood Culture Timing[1,3]	7	86%	88%	90%	100%
Influenza Vaccine[5]	-	-	64%	70%	100%
Initial Antibiotic Timing	49	84%	74%	80%	93%
Oxygenation Assessment	63	100%	99%	99%	100%

NOTE: Hospital profiles are in alphabetical order by state, then city, then hospital within the city; Rankings are sorted by rate in descending order and exclude hospitals with less than 25 cases; (1) The number of cases is too small (n<25) for purposes of reliably predicting hospital performance; (2) Measure reflects the hospital's indication that its submission was based upon a sample of its relevant discharges; (3) Rate reflects fewer than the maximum possible quarters of data for the measure; (4) Inaccurate information submitted and suppressed for one or more quarters; (5) No data is available from the hospital for this measure; Please refer to the User's Guide for a full explanation of data

	Cases	This Hospital	State Average	U.S. Average	Top Hospital
Pneumococcal Vaccine[1]	35	71%	67%	69%	94%
Smoking Cessation Advice[1,3]	2	100%	90%	80%	100%
Surgical Infection Prevention					
Prophylactic Antibiotic Given[2,3]	77	74%	83%	77%	95%
Prophylactic Antibiotic Selection[5]	-	-	90%	90%	100%
Prophylactic Antibiotic Stopped[2,3]	77	95%	70%	72%	95%
Pregnancy Care					
Inpatient Neonatal Mortality[5]	0	0.00%	-	-	-
Third or Fourth Degree Laceration[5]	0	0.00%	2.71%	3.63%	3.27%

Community Hospital

Alternate Name: HCA Newport Richey Hospital
5637 Marine Parkway   Phone: 727-848-1733
New Port Richey, FL 34652   Fax: 727-845-9167
URL: www.communityhospitalnpr.com
Ownership: Proprietary   Accredited: Yes
Emergency Services: Yes   Licensed Beds: 414

Key Personnel:
CEO . . . . Ernie Meier
Emergency Room . . . . Frank Noala, MD
Emergency Room . . . . Terry Meadows, MD
Director Infection/Disease Control . . . . Michelle DeWatt
Director Respiratory Therapy . . . . Chris Stacy

Measure	Cases	This Hospital	State Average	U.S. Average	Top Hospital
Heart Attack Care					
ACE Inhibitor or ARB for LVSD	38	76%	83%	82%	100%
Aspirin at Arrival	219	94%	93%	92%	100%
Aspirin at Discharge	89	82%	88%	90%	100%
Beta Blocker at Arrival	122	89%	89%	87%	100%
Beta Blocker at Discharge	127	86%	92%	90%	100%
Fibrinolytic Medication Timing[1]	14	50%	33%	31%	100%
PCI Within 90 Minutes of Arrival	0	-	52%	54%	95%
Smoking Cessation Advice	28	100%	92%	88%	100%
Heart Failure Care					
ACE Inhibitor or ARB for LVSD	156	78%	82%	82%	100%
Discharge Instructions	346	63%	61%	61%	93%
Evaluation of LVS Function	494	84%	90%	83%	99%
Smoking Cessation Advice	72	99%	91%	82%	100%
Pneumonia Care					
Appropriate Initial Antibiotic[2]	167	90%	84%	83%	94%
Blood Culture Timing[2]	117	80%	88%	90%	100%
Influenza Vaccine	61	33%	64%	70%	100%
Initial Antibiotic Timing[2]	245	76%	74%	80%	93%
Oxygenation Assessment[2]	296	99%	99%	99%	100%
Pneumococcal Vaccine[2]	193	84%	67%	69%	94%
Smoking Cessation Advice[2]	87	100%	90%	80%	100%
Surgical Infection Prevention					
Prophylactic Antibiotic Given[2,3]	273	88%	83%	77%	95%
Prophylactic Antibiotic Selection[2]	79	87%	90%	90%	100%
Prophylactic Antibiotic Stopped[2,3]	265	66%	70%	72%	95%
Pregnancy Care					
Inpatient Neonatal Mortality	-	-	-	-	-
Third or Fourth Degree Laceration	-	-	2.71%	3.63%	3.27%

North Bay Medical Center

Alternate Name: Morton Plant North Bay Hospital
6600 Madison Street   Phone: 727-842-8468
New Port Richey, FL 34652   Fax: 727-848-8762
URL: www.mortonplant.com
Ownership: Voluntary non-profit - Private   Accredited: Yes
Emergency Services: Yes   Licensed Beds: 122
Key Personnel:
OB/GYN Womens Health . . . . Caroline Hunt
Director Respiratory Therapy . . . . David Stroizsck

Measure	Cases	This Hospital	State Average	U.S. Average	Top Hospital
Heart Attack Care					
ACE Inhibitor or ARB for LVSD[1]	9	89%	83%	82%	100%
Aspirin at Arrival	73	93%	93%	92%	100%
Aspirin at Discharge	28	86%	88%	90%	100%
Beta Blocker at Arrival	33	91%	89%	87%	100%

	Cases	This Hospital	State Average	U.S. Average	Top Hospital
Beta Blocker at Discharge	36	83%	92%	90%	100%
Fibrinolytic Medication Timing[1]	3	33%	33%	31%	100%
PCI Within 90 Minutes of Arrival	0	-	52%	54%	95%
Smoking Cessation Advice[1]	8	100%	92%	88%	100%
Heart Failure Care					
ACE Inhibitor or ARB for LVSD	71	89%	82%	82%	100%
Discharge Instructions	152	53%	61%	61%	93%
Evaluation of LVS Function	196	91%	90%	83%	99%
Smoking Cessation Advice	30	93%	91%	82%	100%
Pneumonia Care					
Appropriate Initial Antibiotic	99	81%	84%	83%	94%
Blood Culture Timing	92	92%	88%	90%	100%
Influenza Vaccine	25	40%	64%	70%	100%
Initial Antibiotic Timing	103	78%	74%	80%	93%
Oxygenation Assessment	157	100%	99%	99%	100%
Pneumococcal Vaccine	80	62%	67%	69%	94%
Smoking Cessation Advice	43	95%	90%	80%	100%
Surgical Infection Prevention					
Prophylactic Antibiotic Given[2]	111	68%	83%	77%	95%
Prophylactic Antibiotic Selection[2]	34	97%	90%	90%	100%
Prophylactic Antibiotic Stopped[2]	89	74%	70%	72%	95%
Pregnancy Care					
Inpatient Neonatal Mortality	-	-	-	-	-
Third or Fourth Degree Laceration	-	-	2.71%	3.63%	3.27%

Bert Fish Medical Center

Alternate Name: Fish Memorial Hospital
401 Palmetto Street   Phone: 386-424-5000
New Smyrna Beach, FL 32168
URL: www.bertfish.com
Ownership: Voluntary non-profit - Private   Accredited: Yes
Emergency Services: Yes   Licensed Beds: 116
Key Personnel:
Cardiology . . . . Ashraf S Elsakr, MD
General Surgery . . . . Heather M Metchick, MD
FACOG
Chief Radiology . . . . Tanya Marchand, MD

Measure	Cases	This Hospital	State Average	U.S. Average	Top Hospital
Heart Attack Care					
ACE Inhibitor or ARB for LVSD	28	82%	83%	82%	100%
Aspirin at Arrival	146	95%	93%	92%	100%
Aspirin at Discharge	65	78%	88%	90%	100%
Beta Blocker at Arrival	133	95%	89%	87%	100%
Beta Blocker at Discharge	65	95%	92%	90%	100%
Fibrinolytic Medication Timing	32	62%	33%	31%	100%
PCI Within 90 Minutes of Arrival	0	-	52%	54%	95%
Smoking Cessation Advice[1]	10	100%	92%	88%	100%
Heart Failure Care					
ACE Inhibitor or ARB for LVSD	70	76%	82%	82%	100%
Discharge Instructions	156	34%	61%	61%	93%
Evaluation of LVS Function	181	82%	90%	83%	99%
Smoking Cessation Advice[1]	15	80%	91%	82%	100%
Pneumonia Care					
Appropriate Initial Antibiotic	127	80%	84%	83%	94%
Blood Culture Timing	86	80%	88%	90%	100%
Influenza Vaccine	34	68%	64%	70%	100%
Initial Antibiotic Timing	170	86%	74%	80%	93%
Oxygenation Assessment	193	100%	99%	99%	100%
Pneumococcal Vaccine	125	78%	67%	69%	94%
Smoking Cessation Advice	43	74%	90%	80%	100%
Surgical Infection Prevention					
Prophylactic Antibiotic Given	173	77%	83%	77%	95%
Prophylactic Antibiotic Selection	48	98%	90%	90%	100%
Prophylactic Antibiotic Stopped	162	76%	70%	72%	95%
Pregnancy Care					
Inpatient Neonatal Mortality	-	-	-	-	-
Third or Fourth Degree Laceration	-	-	2.71%	3.63%	3.27%

NOTE: Hospital profiles are in alphabetical order by state, then city, then hospital within the city; Rankings are sorted by rate in descending order and exclude hospitals with less than 25 cases; (1) The number of cases is too small (n<25) for purposes of reliably predicting hospital performance; (2) Measure reflects the hospital's indication that its submission was based upon a sample of its relevant discharges; (3) Rate reflects fewer than the maximum possible quarters of data for the measure; (4) Inaccurate information submitted and suppressed for one or more quarters; (5) No data is available from the hospital for this measure; Please refer to the User's Guide for a full explanation of data

Twin Cities Hospital
2190 Highway 85 North
Niceville, FL 32578
URL: www.tchealthcare.com
Ownership: Proprietary
Emergency Services: Yes

Phone: 850-678-4131
Fax: 850-729-9473

Accredited: Yes
Licensed Beds: 65

Key Personnel:
CEO. . . . . David A Whalen
Chief Medical Staff. . . . . Mark Schroever, MD
Chief Medical Staff. . . . . William Abernathy, MD
Director Medical/Surgical Nursing . . . . Elaine Prokop, RN
Director Medical & Surgical Nursing . . . . Elaine Prokop, RN
Director Respiratory Therapy . . . . Peter Temple

Measure	Cases	This Hospital	State Average	U.S. Average	Top Hospital
Heart Attack Care					
ACE Inhibitor or ARB for LVSD	0	-	83%	82%	100%
Aspirin at Arrival[1]	7	100%	93%	92%	100%
Aspirin at Discharge[1]	1	100%	88%	90%	100%
Beta Blocker at Arrival[1]	7	86%	89%	87%	100%
Beta Blocker at Discharge[1]	1	100%	92%	90%	100%
Fibrinolytic Medication Timing	0	-	33%	31%	100%
PCI Within 90 Minutes of Arrival	0	-	52%	54%	95%
Smoking Cessation Advice[1]	1	100%	92%	88%	100%
Heart Failure Care					
ACE Inhibitor or ARB for LVSD[1]	24	92%	82%	82%	100%
Discharge Instructions	46	74%	61%	61%	93%
Evaluation of LVS Function	53	98%	90%	83%	99%
Smoking Cessation Advice[1]	8	100%	91%	82%	100%
Pneumonia Care					
Appropriate Initial Antibiotic	58	81%	84%	83%	94%
Blood Culture Timing	34	91%	88%	90%	100%
Influenza Vaccine[1]	14	93%	64%	70%	100%
Initial Antibiotic Timing	85	74%	74%	80%	93%
Oxygenation Assessment	108	100%	99%	99%	100%
Pneumococcal Vaccine	66	79%	67%	69%	94%
Smoking Cessation Advice[1]	21	100%	90%	80%	100%
Surgical Infection Prevention					
Prophylactic Antibiotic Given[3]	99	92%	83%	77%	95%
Prophylactic Antibiotic Selection	40	68%	90%	90%	100%
Prophylactic Antibiotic Stopped[3]	99	85%	70%	72%	95%
Pregnancy Care					
Inpatient Neonatal Mortality	-	-	-	-	-
Third or Fourth Degree Laceration	-	-	2.71%	3.63%	3.27%

Munroe Regional Medical Center
1500 SW 1st Avenue
Ocala, FL 34474
Ownership: Govt - Hospital District or Authority
Emergency Services: Yes

Phone: 352-351-7200
Fax: 352-351-7201
Accredited: Yes
Licensed Beds: 421

Key Personnel:
CEO. . . . . Paul Clark
Chief Medical Staff. . . . . Perin Alfred, MD
Emergency Room . . . . Vicky Nelson
Director Respiratory Therapy . . . . Karen Lappi

Measure	Cases	This Hospital	State Average	U.S. Average	Top Hospital
Heart Attack Care					
ACE Inhibitor or ARB for LVSD	170	82%	83%	82%	100%
Aspirin at Arrival	319	94%	93%	92%	100%
Aspirin at Discharge	345	95%	88%	90%	100%
Beta Blocker at Arrival	213	86%	89%	87%	100%
Beta Blocker at Discharge	397	96%	92%	90%	100%
Fibrinolytic Medication Timing	0	-	33%	31%	100%
PCI Within 90 Minutes of Arrival[1]	10	50%	52%	54%	95%
Smoking Cessation Advice	143	93%	92%	88%	100%
Heart Failure Care					
ACE Inhibitor or ARB for LVSD	229	84%	82%	82%	100%
Discharge Instructions	364	43%	61%	61%	93%
Evaluation of LVS Function	454	91%	90%	83%	99%
Smoking Cessation Advice	73	82%	91%	82%	100%
Pneumonia Care					
Appropriate Initial Antibiotic	176	86%	84%	83%	94%

Measure	Cases	This Hospital	State Average	U.S. Average	Top Hospital
Blood Culture Timing	135	89%	88%	90%	100%
Influenza Vaccine	55	84%	64%	70%	100%
Initial Antibiotic Timing	245	59%	74%	80%	93%
Oxygenation Assessment	306	100%	99%	99%	100%
Pneumococcal Vaccine	225	82%	67%	69%	94%
Smoking Cessation Advice	90	89%	90%	80%	100%
Surgical Infection Prevention					
Prophylactic Antibiotic Given	673	90%	83%	77%	95%
Prophylactic Antibiotic Selection	173	94%	90%	90%	100%
Prophylactic Antibiotic Stopped	628	81%	70%	72%	95%
Pregnancy Care					
Inpatient Neonatal Mortality	-	-	-	-	-
Third or Fourth Degree Laceration	-	-	2.71%	3.63%	3.27%

Ocala Regional Medical Center
Alternate Name: Marion Community Hospital
1431 SW 1st Avenue
PO Box 2200
Ocala, FL 34478
URL: www.ocalaregional.com
Ownership: Proprietary
Emergency Services: Yes

Phone: 352-401-1000
Fax: 352-401-1198

Accredited: Yes
Licensed Beds: 200

Key Personnel:
CEO. . . . . Steve Mahan
Chief Medical Staff. . . . . Larry Popeil
Director Cardiovascular Unit. . . . . Dawn Buss
Director Cardiac Cath Lab . . . . Gloria Nolan
Director Emergency Services. . . . . Susan Atkin
Director Medical/Surgical Nursing . . . . Faye Spencer
Director Medical/Surgical Nursing . . . . Jo McWhorter
OB/GYN Womens Health. . . . . D Raymond Arquette, MD
Director Respiratory Therapy . . . . Karin Blacquier

Measure	Cases	This Hospital	State Average	U.S. Average	Top Hospital
Heart Attack Care					
ACE Inhibitor or ARB for LVSD	106	86%	83%	82%	100%
Aspirin at Arrival	220	94%	93%	92%	100%
Aspirin at Discharge	219	95%	88%	90%	100%
Beta Blocker at Arrival	112	79%	89%	87%	100%
Beta Blocker at Discharge	260	97%	92%	90%	100%
Fibrinolytic Medication Timing	0	-	33%	31%	100%
PCI Within 90 Minutes of Arrival[1]	11	82%	52%	54%	95%
Smoking Cessation Advice	90	99%	92%	88%	100%
Heart Failure Care					
ACE Inhibitor or ARB for LVSD	204	80%	82%	82%	100%
Discharge Instructions	343	49%	61%	61%	93%
Evaluation of LVS Function	440	93%	90%	83%	99%
Smoking Cessation Advice	85	93%	91%	82%	100%
Pneumonia Care					
Appropriate Initial Antibiotic	294	90%	84%	83%	94%
Blood Culture Timing	211	82%	88%	90%	100%
Influenza Vaccine	92	84%	64%	70%	100%
Initial Antibiotic Timing	401	69%	74%	80%	93%
Oxygenation Assessment	482	100%	99%	99%	100%
Pneumococcal Vaccine	296	80%	67%	69%	94%
Smoking Cessation Advice	144	93%	90%	80%	100%
Surgical Infection Prevention					
Prophylactic Antibiotic Given	983	93%	83%	77%	95%
Prophylactic Antibiotic Selection	242	94%	90%	90%	100%
Prophylactic Antibiotic Stopped	902	92%	70%	72%	95%
Pregnancy Care					
Inpatient Neonatal Mortality	-	-	-	-	-
Third or Fourth Degree Laceration	-	-	2.71%	3.63%	3.27%

Health Central
Alternate Name: West Orange Hospital

NOTE: Hospital profiles are in alphabetical order by state, then city, then hospital within the city; Rankings are sorted by rate in descending order and exclude hospitals with less than 25 cases; (1) The number of cases is too small (n<25) for purposes of reliably predicting hospital performance; (2) Measure reflects the hospital's indication that its submission was based upon a sample of its relevant discharges; (3) Rate reflects fewer than the maximum possible quarters of data for the measure; (4) Inaccurate information submitted and suppressed for one or more quarters; (5) No data is available from the hospital for this measure; Please refer to the User's Guide for a full explanation of data

10000 W Colonial Drive
Ocoee, FL 34761
E-mail: darlenel@health-central.org
URL: www.health-central.org
Ownership: Govt - Hospital District or Authority
Emergency Services: Yes

Phone: 407-296-1000
Fax: 407-290-2118

Accredited: Yes
Licensed Beds: 171

Key Personnel:

CEO. . . . . Richard M Irwin, Jr
Emergency Room . . . . Terry Kemp
Director Medical/Surgical Nursing . . . . Joel Schmidt, RN
OB/GYN Womens Health. . . . . Jeff Feld, MD
Chief Radiology . . . . Neil Baron, MD
Director Respiratory Therapy . . . . John Thomas

Measure	Cases	This Hospital	State Average	U.S. Average	Top Hospital
Heart Attack Care					
ACE Inhibitor or ARB for LVSD[1]	11	82%	83%	82%	100%
Aspirin at Arrival	94	85%	93%	92%	100%
Aspirin at Discharge	48	88%	88%	90%	100%
Beta Blocker at Arrival	96	76%	89%	87%	100%
Beta Blocker at Discharge	53	91%	92%	90%	100%
Fibrinolytic Medication Timing	0	-	33%	31%	100%
PCI Within 90 Minutes of Arrival	0	-	52%	54%	95%
Smoking Cessation Advice[1]	11	91%	92%	88%	100%
Heart Failure Care					
ACE Inhibitor or ARB for LVSD	110	78%	82%	82%	100%
Discharge Instructions	200	39%	61%	61%	93%
Evaluation of LVS Function	268	93%	90%	83%	99%
Smoking Cessation Advice	53	85%	91%	82%	100%
Pneumonia Care					
Appropriate Initial Antibiotic	114	82%	84%	83%	94%
Blood Culture Timing	101	84%	88%	90%	100%
Influenza Vaccine[1]	22	64%	64%	70%	100%
Initial Antibiotic Timing	187	53%	74%	80%	93%
Oxygenation Assessment	202	100%	99%	99%	100%
Pneumococcal Vaccine	108	69%	67%	69%	94%
Smoking Cessation Advice	40	88%	90%	80%	100%
Surgical Infection Prevention					
Prophylactic Antibiotic Given	170	84%	83%	77%	95%
Prophylactic Antibiotic Selection	44	91%	90%	90%	100%
Prophylactic Antibiotic Stopped	167	80%	70%	72%	95%
Pregnancy Care					
Inpatient Neonatal Mortality	-	-	-	-	-
Third or Fourth Degree Laceration	-	-	2.71%	3.63%	3.27%

Raulerson Hospital

1796 Highway 441 North
Okeechobee, FL 34972
URL: www.raulersonhospital.com
Ownership: Proprietary
Emergency Services: Yes

Phone: 863-763-2151
Fax: 863-824-2991

Accredited: Yes
Licensed Beds: 101

Key Personnel:
CEO. . . . . Robert Lee

Measure	Cases	This Hospital	State Average	U.S. Average	Top Hospital
Heart Attack Care					
ACE Inhibitor or ARB for LVSD[1]	6	100%	83%	82%	100%
Aspirin at Arrival	49	88%	93%	92%	100%
Aspirin at Discharge[1]	16	94%	88%	90%	100%
Beta Blocker at Arrival	44	89%	89%	87%	100%
Beta Blocker at Discharge[1]	18	94%	92%	90%	100%
Fibrinolytic Medication Timing[1]	4	0%	33%	31%	100%
PCI Within 90 Minutes of Arrival	0	-	52%	54%	95%
Smoking Cessation Advice[1]	4	100%	92%	88%	100%
Heart Failure Care					
ACE Inhibitor or ARB for LVSD	54	89%	82%	82%	100%
Discharge Instructions	234	79%	61%	61%	93%
Evaluation of LVS Function	258	67%	90%	83%	99%
Smoking Cessation Advice	58	100%	91%	82%	100%
Pneumonia Care					
Appropriate Initial Antibiotic	149	72%	84%	83%	94%
Blood Culture Timing	102	88%	88%	90%	100%
Influenza Vaccine	49	73%	64%	70%	100%

Measure				
Initial Antibiotic Timing	189	79%	74%	80%	93%
Oxygenation Assessment	226	100%	99%	99%	100%
Pneumococcal Vaccine	143	69%	67%	69%	94%
Smoking Cessation Advice	53	100%	90%	80%	100%
Surgical Infection Prevention					
Prophylactic Antibiotic Given[3]	67	82%	83%	77%	95%
Prophylactic Antibiotic Selection	25	92%	90%	90%	100%
Prophylactic Antibiotic Stopped[3]	67	52%	70%	72%	95%
Pregnancy Care					
Inpatient Neonatal Mortality	-	-	-	-	-
Third or Fourth Degree Laceration	-	-	2.71%	3.63%	3.27%

Florida Hospital Fish Memorial

1055 Saxon Boulevard
Orange City, FL 32763
URL: www.flfishmemorial.org
Ownership: Govt - Hospital District or Authority
Emergency Services: Yes

Phone: 386-917-5000
Fax: 386-917-5425

Accredited: Yes
Licensed Beds: 139

Key Personnel:
CEO. . . . . Joe Johnson
Surgical Services Director . . . . Lynn Maltby
Director Cardiopulmonary . . . . Jan Lenhart
Cath Laboratory Supervisor . . . . Noel Rivera
Emergency Room Director. . . . . Debbie Palmer
Infection Control Coordinator . . . . Jackie Adkins
Womens Health Manager . . . . Patty Dycus
Director Surgical Services . . . . Lynn Maltby
Cardio/Pulmonary Services Director. . . . . Janet Lenhart

Measure	Cases	This Hospital	State Average	U.S. Average	Top Hospital
Heart Attack Care					
ACE Inhibitor or ARB for LVSD	31	71%	83%	82%	100%
Aspirin at Arrival	206	92%	93%	92%	100%
Aspirin at Discharge	112	87%	88%	90%	100%
Beta Blocker at Arrival	145	90%	89%	87%	100%
Beta Blocker at Discharge	109	96%	92%	90%	100%
Fibrinolytic Medication Timing	25	24%	33%	31%	100%
PCI Within 90 Minutes of Arrival[1]	1	100%	52%	54%	95%
Smoking Cessation Advice[1]	19	95%	92%	88%	100%
Heart Failure Care					
ACE Inhibitor or ARB for LVSD	123	76%	82%	82%	100%
Discharge Instructions	342	41%	61%	61%	93%
Evaluation of LVS Function	437	92%	90%	83%	99%
Smoking Cessation Advice	58	93%	91%	82%	100%
Pneumonia Care					
Appropriate Initial Antibiotic	262	88%	84%	83%	94%
Blood Culture Timing	228	89%	88%	90%	100%
Influenza Vaccine	77	53%	64%	70%	100%
Initial Antibiotic Timing	349	58%	74%	80%	93%
Oxygenation Assessment	372	100%	99%	99%	100%
Pneumococcal Vaccine	226	52%	67%	69%	94%
Smoking Cessation Advice	80	91%	90%	80%	100%
Surgical Infection Prevention					
Prophylactic Antibiotic Given	432	87%	83%	77%	95%
Prophylactic Antibiotic Selection	118	82%	90%	90%	100%
Prophylactic Antibiotic Stopped	415	76%	70%	72%	95%
Pregnancy Care					
Inpatient Neonatal Mortality	-	-	-	-	-
Third or Fourth Degree Laceration	-	-	2.71%	3.63%	3.27%

Orange Park Medical Center

Alternate Name: Humana Hospital Orange Park
2001 Kingsley Avenue
Orange Park, FL 32073
URL: www.opmedical.com
Ownership: Proprietary
Emergency Services: Yes

Phone: 904-276-8500
Fax: 904-276-8703

Accredited: Yes
Licensed Beds: 224

Key Personnel:
CEO. . . . . Robert Krieger
Emergency Room . . . . John Cole
Director Medical/Surgical Nursing . . . . Gayle Miller
OB/GYN Womens Health. . . . . Faye Barentine

NOTE: Hospital profiles are in alphabetical order by state, then city, then hospital within the city; Rankings are sorted by rate in descending order and exclude hospitals with less than 25 cases; (1) The number of cases is too small (n<25) for purposes of reliably predicting hospital performance; (2) Measure reflects the hospital's indication that its submission was based upon a sample of its relevant discharges; (3) Rate reflects fewer than the maximum possible quarters of data for the measure; (4) Inaccurate information submitted and suppressed for one or more quarters; (5) No data is available from the hospital for this measure; Please refer to the User's Guide for a full explanation of data

Measure	Cases	This Hospital	State Average	U.S. Average	Top Hospital
Heart Attack Care					
ACE Inhibitor or ARB for LVSD[1]	9	89%	83%	82%	100%
Aspirin at Arrival	84	93%	93%	92%	100%
Aspirin at Discharge	33	97%	88%	90%	100%
Beta Blocker at Arrival	65	94%	89%	87%	100%
Beta Blocker at Discharge	46	100%	92%	90%	100%
Fibrinolytic Medication Timing[1]	6	17%	33%	31%	100%
PCI Within 90 Minutes of Arrival	0	-	52%	54%	95%
Smoking Cessation Advice[1]	14	93%	92%	88%	100%
Heart Failure Care					
ACE Inhibitor or ARB for LVSD	122	86%	82%	82%	100%
Discharge Instructions	257	67%	61%	61%	93%
Evaluation of LVS Function	371	98%	90%	83%	99%
Smoking Cessation Advice	75	93%	91%	82%	100%
Pneumonia Care					
Appropriate Initial Antibiotic	303	90%	84%	83%	94%
Blood Culture Timing	447	92%	88%	90%	100%
Influenza Vaccine	118	59%	64%	70%	100%
Initial Antibiotic Timing	501	75%	74%	80%	93%
Oxygenation Assessment	669	100%	99%	99%	100%
Pneumococcal Vaccine	409	70%	67%	69%	94%
Smoking Cessation Advice	134	87%	90%	80%	100%
Surgical Infection Prevention					
Prophylactic Antibiotic Given	519	90%	83%	77%	95%
Prophylactic Antibiotic Selection	120	89%	90%	90%	100%
Prophylactic Antibiotic Stopped	498	84%	70%	72%	95%
Pregnancy Care					
Inpatient Neonatal Mortality	-	-	-	-	-
Third or Fourth Degree Laceration	-	-	2.71%	3.63%	3.27%

Florida Hospital Orlando

601 E Rollins Street
Orlando, FL 32803
URL: www.flhosp.org
Ownership: Voluntary non-profit - Church
Emergency Services: Yes

Phone: 407-303-6611
Fax: 407-200-4938

Accredited: Yes
Licensed Beds: 1,783

Key Personnel:
President . . . . Don Jernigan
Medical Staff President . . . . Robert Reynolds, MD

Measure	Cases	This Hospital	State Average	U.S. Average	Top Hospital
Heart Attack Care					
ACE Inhibitor or ARB for LVSD[2]	253	87%	83%	82%	100%
Aspirin at Arrival[2]	598	96%	93%	92%	100%
Aspirin at Discharge[2]	982	94%	88%	90%	100%
Beta Blocker at Arrival[2]	520	88%	89%	87%	100%
Beta Blocker at Discharge[2]	1,021	95%	92%	90%	100%
Fibrinolytic Medication Timing[1,2]	1	0%	33%	31%	100%
PCI Within 90 Minutes of Arrival[1,2]	15	67%	52%	54%	95%
Smoking Cessation Advice[2]	355	100%	92%	88%	100%
Heart Failure Care					
ACE Inhibitor or ARB for LVSD[2]	776	84%	82%	82%	100%
Discharge Instructions[2]	1,762	75%	61%	61%	93%
Evaluation of LVS Function[2]	2,113	94%	90%	83%	99%
Smoking Cessation Advice[2]	342	99%	91%	82%	100%
Pneumonia Care					
Appropriate Initial Antibiotic[2]	929	90%	84%	83%	94%
Blood Culture Timing[2]	951	85%	88%	90%	100%
Influenza Vaccine[4,5]	-	-	64%	70%	100%
Initial Antibiotic Timing[2]	1,482	76%	74%	80%	93%
Oxygenation Assessment[2]	1,744	100%	99%	99%	100%
Pneumococcal Vaccine[2]	894	90%	67%	69%	94%
Smoking Cessation Advice[2]	405	99%	90%	80%	100%
Surgical Infection Prevention					
Prophylactic Antibiotic Given[2]	1,434	86%	83%	77%	95%
Prophylactic Antibiotic Selection[2]	363	94%	90%	90%	100%
Prophylactic Antibiotic Stopped[2]	1,383	75%	70%	72%	95%
Pregnancy Care					
Inpatient Neonatal Mortality	-	-	-	-	-
Third or Fourth Degree Laceration	-	-	2.71%	3.63%	3.27%

Orlando Regional Healthcare

1414 Kuhl Avenue
Orlando, FL 32806
URL: www.orlandoregional.org
Ownership: Voluntary non-profit - Private
Emergency Services: Yes

Phone: 321-841-5111
Fax: 407-425-8545

Accredited: Yes
Licensed Beds: 1,572

Key Personnel:
President/CEO. . . . . John Hillenmeyer
Chief Catheterization Laboratory . . . . Trena Nunnell
Emergency Room . . . . Timothy Bullard, MD
Director Infection/Disease Control . . . . Michael Pinnell, MD
OB/GYN Womens Health. . . . . Stephen Carlan, MD
Director Respiratory Therapy . . . . Jack Fitzpatrick

Measure	Cases	This Hospital	State Average	U.S. Average	Top Hospital
Heart Attack Care					
ACE Inhibitor or ARB for LVSD	196	89%	83%	82%	100%
Aspirin at Arrival	388	93%	93%	92%	100%
Aspirin at Discharge	607	95%	88%	90%	100%
Beta Blocker at Arrival	266	86%	89%	87%	100%
Beta Blocker at Discharge	671	96%	92%	90%	100%
Fibrinolytic Medication Timing	0	-	33%	31%	100%
PCI Within 90 Minutes of Arrival[1]	23	57%	52%	54%	95%
Smoking Cessation Advice	246	96%	92%	88%	100%
Heart Failure Care					
ACE Inhibitor or ARB for LVSD	743	84%	82%	82%	100%
Discharge Instructions	1,408	37%	61%	61%	93%
Evaluation of LVS Function	1,651	99%	90%	83%	99%
Smoking Cessation Advice	334	92%	91%	82%	100%
Pneumonia Care					
Appropriate Initial Antibiotic	664	89%	84%	83%	94%
Blood Culture Timing	564	85%	88%	90%	100%
Influenza Vaccine	224	75%	64%	70%	100%
Initial Antibiotic Timing	956	65%	74%	80%	93%
Oxygenation Assessment	1,188	100%	99%	99%	100%
Pneumococcal Vaccine	581	76%	67%	69%	94%
Smoking Cessation Advice	330	89%	90%	80%	100%
Surgical Infection Prevention					
Prophylactic Antibiotic Given	3,356	93%	83%	77%	95%
Prophylactic Antibiotic Selection	847	96%	90%	90%	100%
Prophylactic Antibiotic Stopped	3,065	86%	70%	72%	95%
Pregnancy Care					
Inpatient Neonatal Mortality	-	-	-	-	-
Third or Fourth Degree Laceration	-	-	2.71%	3.63%	3.27%

Florida Hospital-Ormond Memorial

875 Sterthaus Avenue
Ormond Beach, FL 32174

Toll-Free: 888-647-0271
Phone: 386-676-6000
Fax: 386-671-5099

URL: www.fhmd.com
Ownership: Voluntary non-profit - Private
Emergency Services: Yes

Accredited: Yes
Licensed Beds: 205

Key Personnel:
CEO. . . . . Michael Gentry
Chief Medical Staff. . . . . J Timothy Tolland
Emergency Room . . . . Darlinda Copeland
Director Respiratory Therapy . . . . Tammy Collins

Measure	Cases	This Hospital	State Average	U.S. Average	Top Hospital
Heart Attack Care					
ACE Inhibitor or ARB for LVSD	96	73%	83%	82%	100%
Aspirin at Arrival	280	95%	93%	92%	100%
Aspirin at Discharge	413	94%	88%	90%	100%
Beta Blocker at Arrival	232	83%	89%	87%	100%
Beta Blocker at Discharge	419	89%	92%	90%	100%
Fibrinolytic Medication Timing[1]	4	50%	33%	31%	100%
PCI Within 90 Minutes of Arrival[1]	7	43%	52%	54%	95%
Smoking Cessation Advice	133	98%	92%	88%	100%
Heart Failure Care					
ACE Inhibitor or ARB for LVSD	211	72%	82%	82%	100%
Discharge Instructions	372	70%	61%	61%	93%
Evaluation of LVS Function	503	94%	90%	83%	99%
Smoking Cessation Advice	77	97%	91%	82%	100%

NOTE: Hospital profiles are in alphabetical order by state, then city, then hospital within the city; Rankings are sorted by rate in descending order and exclude hospitals with less than 25 cases; (1) The number of cases is too small (n<25) for purposes of reliably predicting hospital performance; (2) Measure reflects the hospital's indication that its submission was based upon a sample of its relevant discharges; (3) Rate reflects fewer than the maximum possible quarters of data for the measure; (4) Inaccurate information submitted and suppressed for one or more quarters; (5) No data is available from the hospital for this measure; Please refer to the User's Guide for a full explanation of data

Pneumonia Care					
Appropriate Initial Antibiotic	154	90%	84%	83%	94%
Blood Culture Timing	138	91%	88%	90%	100%
Influenza Vaccine[4,5]	-	-	64%	70%	100%
Initial Antibiotic Timing	218	76%	74%	80%	93%
Oxygenation Assessment	259	98%	99%	99%	100%
Pneumococcal Vaccine	171	76%	67%	69%	94%
Smoking Cessation Advice	71	87%	90%	80%	100%
Surgical Infection Prevention					
Prophylactic Antibiotic Given	866	79%	83%	77%	95%
Prophylactic Antibiotic Selection	195	93%	90%	90%	100%
Prophylactic Antibiotic Stopped	845	58%	70%	72%	95%
Pregnancy Care					
Inpatient Neonatal Mortality	-	-	-	-	-
Third or Fourth Degree Laceration	-	-	2.71%	3.63%	3.27%

Putnam Community Medical Center

Alternate Name: Putnam Community Hospital
Highway 20 West
PO Box 778
Palatka, FL 32177
URL: www.pcmcfl.com
Ownership: Proprietary
Emergency Services: Yes

Phone: 386-328-5711
Fax: 386-325-8178

Accredited: Yes
Licensed Beds: 141

Key Personnel:
CEO . . . . Bruce A Baldwin
Chief Medical Staff . . . . Michael Akhiyat, MD

Measure	Cases	This Hospital	State Average	U.S. Average	Top Hospital
Heart Attack Care					
ACE Inhibitor or ARB for LVSD[1]	9	100%	83%	82%	100%
Aspirin at Arrival	86	92%	93%	92%	100%
Aspirin at Discharge	33	94%	88%	90%	100%
Beta Blocker at Arrival	78	94%	89%	87%	100%
Beta Blocker at Discharge	43	100%	92%	90%	100%
Fibrinolytic Medication Timing[1]	7	43%	33%	31%	100%
PCI Within 90 Minutes of Arrival	0	-	52%	54%	95%
Smoking Cessation Advice[1]	11	100%	92%	88%	100%
Heart Failure Care					
ACE Inhibitor or ARB for LVSD	77	96%	82%	82%	100%
Discharge Instructions	236	81%	61%	61%	93%
Evaluation of LVS Function	275	100%	90%	83%	99%
Smoking Cessation Advice	66	100%	91%	82%	100%
Pneumonia Care					
Appropriate Initial Antibiotic	185	90%	84%	83%	94%
Blood Culture Timing	141	94%	88%	90%	100%
Influenza Vaccine	60	92%	64%	70%	100%
Initial Antibiotic Timing	275	79%	74%	80%	93%
Oxygenation Assessment	302	99%	99%	99%	100%
Pneumococcal Vaccine	182	92%	67%	69%	94%
Smoking Cessation Advice	77	100%	90%	80%	100%
Surgical Infection Prevention					
Prophylactic Antibiotic Given[3]	141	72%	83%	77%	95%
Prophylactic Antibiotic Selection	40	92%	90%	90%	100%
Prophylactic Antibiotic Stopped[3]	135	48%	70%	72%	95%
Pregnancy Care					
Inpatient Neonatal Mortality	-	-	-	-	-
Third or Fourth Degree Laceration	-	-	2.71%	3.63%	3.27%

Palm Beach Grdns Medical Center

3360 Burns Road
Palm Beach Grdns, FL 33410
URL: www.pbgmc.com
Ownership: Proprietary
Emergency Services: Yes

Phone: 561-622-1411
Fax: 561-694-7160

Accredited: Yes
Licensed Beds: 204

Key Personnel:
CEO . . . . Clint Matthews
Chief Medical Staff . . . . Michael Ravitsky, MD
Cardiac Rehabilitation . . . . Melanie Giles
Emergency Room . . . . Alberto Ortiz
Director Medical/Surgical Nursing . . . . Ruth Harris
Director Respiratory Therapy . . . . Dan Maddalino

Measure	Cases	This Hospital	State Average	U.S. Average	Top Hospital
Heart Attack Care					
ACE Inhibitor or ARB for LVSD	198	64%	83%	82%	100%
Aspirin at Arrival	364	95%	93%	92%	100%
Aspirin at Discharge	782	92%	88%	90%	100%
Beta Blocker at Arrival	333	91%	89%	87%	100%
Beta Blocker at Discharge	815	93%	92%	90%	100%
Fibrinolytic Medication Timing[1]	2	0%	33%	31%	100%
PCI Within 90 Minutes of Arrival[1]	19	74%	52%	54%	95%
Smoking Cessation Advice	219	100%	92%	88%	100%
Heart Failure Care					
ACE Inhibitor or ARB for LVSD	351	75%	82%	82%	100%
Discharge Instructions	567	85%	61%	61%	93%
Evaluation of LVS Function	672	91%	90%	83%	99%
Smoking Cessation Advice	90	99%	91%	82%	100%
Pneumonia Care					
Appropriate Initial Antibiotic	143	87%	84%	83%	94%
Blood Culture Timing	126	90%	88%	90%	100%
Influenza Vaccine	40	78%	64%	70%	100%
Initial Antibiotic Timing	166	77%	74%	80%	93%
Oxygenation Assessment	203	99%	99%	99%	100%
Pneumococcal Vaccine	132	70%	67%	69%	94%
Smoking Cessation Advice	28	96%	90%	80%	100%
Surgical Infection Prevention					
Prophylactic Antibiotic Given[2]	599	95%	83%	77%	95%
Prophylactic Antibiotic Selection[2]	129	98%	90%	90%	100%
Prophylactic Antibiotic Stopped[2]	566	42%	70%	72%	95%
Pregnancy Care					
Inpatient Neonatal Mortality	-	-	-	-	-
Third or Fourth Degree Laceration	-	-	2.71%	3.63%	3.27%

Florida Hospital Flagler

60 Memorial Medical Parkway
Palm Coast, FL 32164
Ownership: Voluntary non-profit - Private
Emergency Services: Yes

Phone: 386-586-2000
Fax: 386-586-4620
Accredited: Yes
Licensed Beds: 81

Key Personnel:
President/CEO . . . . Richard Lind
Chief Medical Staff . . . . Robert Bianco, MD
Emergency Room . . . . Maureen Sabella
VP Medical/Surgical Nursing . . . . Tammy Daniel, RN
Director Medical/Surgical Nursing . . . . Tammy Daniel, RN
Director Respiratory Therapy . . . . Dennis Valera

Measure	Cases	This Hospital	State Average	U.S. Average	Top Hospital
Heart Attack Care					
ACE Inhibitor or ARB for LVSD[1]	24	75%	83%	82%	100%
Aspirin at Arrival	177	92%	93%	92%	100%
Aspirin at Discharge	86	86%	88%	90%	100%
Beta Blocker at Arrival	165	91%	89%	87%	100%
Beta Blocker at Discharge	79	91%	92%	90%	100%
Fibrinolytic Medication Timing[1]	11	45%	33%	31%	100%
PCI Within 90 Minutes of Arrival	0	-	52%	54%	95%
Smoking Cessation Advice[1]	15	100%	92%	88%	100%
Heart Failure Care					
ACE Inhibitor or ARB for LVSD	69	83%	82%	82%	100%
Discharge Instructions	191	25%	61%	61%	93%
Evaluation of LVS Function	241	90%	90%	83%	99%
Smoking Cessation Advice	36	97%	91%	82%	100%
Pneumonia Care					
Appropriate Initial Antibiotic	92	74%	84%	83%	94%
Blood Culture Timing	85	84%	88%	90%	100%
Influenza Vaccine[1]	24	83%	64%	70%	100%
Initial Antibiotic Timing	113	86%	74%	80%	93%
Oxygenation Assessment	145	99%	99%	99%	100%
Pneumococcal Vaccine	77	69%	67%	69%	94%
Smoking Cessation Advice	37	100%	90%	80%	100%
Surgical Infection Prevention					
Prophylactic Antibiotic Given	371	75%	83%	77%	95%
Prophylactic Antibiotic Selection	96	91%	90%	90%	100%
Prophylactic Antibiotic Stopped	365	65%	70%	72%	95%
Pregnancy Care					

Inpatient Neonatal Mortality	-	-	-	-	-
Third or Fourth Degree Laceration	-	-	2.71%	3.63%	3.27%

Bay Medical Center

615 N Bonita Avenue
Panama City, FL 32401
URL: www.baymedical.org
Ownership: Govt - Hospital District or Authority
Emergency Services: Yes

Phone: 850-769-1511
Fax: 850-747-6443

Accredited: Yes
Licensed Beds: 413

Key Personnel:
President/CEO . . . . Steve Johnson
Chief Medical Staff . . . . Frederick Epstein, MD
Chief Catheterization Laboratory . . . . Frank Hedges
Manager Emergency Room Services . . . . April Smith, RN
Emergency Room . . . . Frederick Epstein, MD
Director Infection/Disease Control . . . . Nina O'Flaherty
Director Medical/Surgical Nursing . . . . Sheila Tison
OB/GYN Women's Health . . . . John Maceluch, DO
Director Surgical Services . . . . Brenda Kingdon
Chief Radiology . . . . Scott Ramey, MD
Director Respiratory Therapy . . . . Douglas Darnell, RRT

Measure	Cases	This Hospital	State Average	U.S. Average	Top Hospital
Heart Attack Care					
ACE Inhibitor or ARB for LVSD	126	74%	83%	82%	100%
Aspirin at Arrival	312	97%	93%	92%	100%
Aspirin at Discharge	359	94%	88%	90%	100%
Beta Blocker at Arrival	290	93%	89%	87%	100%
Beta Blocker at Discharge	367	94%	92%	90%	100%
Fibrinolytic Medication Timing[1]	4	0%	33%	31%	100%
PCI Within 90 Minutes of Arrival[1]	14	43%	52%	54%	95%
Smoking Cessation Advice	145	97%	92%	88%	100%
Heart Failure Care					
ACE Inhibitor or ARB for LVSD	376	81%	82%	82%	100%
Discharge Instructions	876	48%	61%	61%	93%
Evaluation of LVS Function	1,003	86%	90%	83%	99%
Smoking Cessation Advice	238	91%	91%	82%	100%
Pneumonia Care					
Appropriate Initial Antibiotic	344	81%	84%	83%	94%
Blood Culture Timing	294	78%	88%	90%	100%
Influenza Vaccine[4,5]	-	-	64%	70%	100%
Initial Antibiotic Timing	475	71%	74%	80%	93%
Oxygenation Assessment	571	100%	99%	99%	100%
Pneumococcal Vaccine	344	65%	67%	69%	94%
Smoking Cessation Advice	163	98%	90%	80%	100%
Surgical Infection Prevention					
Prophylactic Antibiotic Given	799	95%	83%	77%	95%
Prophylactic Antibiotic Selection	203	95%	90%	90%	100%
Prophylactic Antibiotic Stopped	769	80%	70%	72%	95%
Pregnancy Care					
Inpatient Neonatal Mortality	-	-	-	-	-
Third or Fourth Degree Laceration	-	-	2.71%	3.63%	3.27%

Gulf Coast Medical Center

Alternate Name: Gulf Coast Hospital
449 W 23rd St
Panama City, FL 32405
URL: www.egulfcoastmedical.com
Ownership: Proprietary
Emergency Services: Yes

Phone: 850-769-8341
Fax: 850-747-7907

Accredited: Yes
Licensed Beds: 176

Key Personnel:
CEO . . . . Todd Gallati
Chief Medical Staff . . . . Yahia Rahim, MD
Catheterization Lab . . . . Anita Jourdan
Emergency Room . . . . Ann Abrams
Infection Control . . . . Kim Turney
ICU . . . . Sirena Fritz
Medical Surgical Nursing . . . . Kay Saunders
Director OB/GYN Womens Health . . . . Patty Wehling
Director Respiratory Therapy . . . . Joe Edgecombe

Measure	Cases	This Hospital	State Average	U.S. Average	Top Hospital
Heart Attack Care					

Measure	Cases	This Hospital	State Average	U.S. Average	Top Hospital
ACE Inhibitor or ARB for LVSD[1]	3	67%	83%	82%	100%
Aspirin at Arrival[1]	16	94%	93%	92%	100%
Aspirin at Discharge[1]	5	60%	88%	90%	100%
Beta Blocker at Arrival[1]	13	100%	89%	87%	100%
Beta Blocker at Discharge[1]	8	100%	92%	90%	100%
Fibrinolytic Medication Timing	0	-	33%	31%	100%
PCI Within 90 Minutes of Arrival	0	-	52%	54%	95%
Smoking Cessation Advice[1]	1	100%	92%	88%	100%
Heart Failure Care					
ACE Inhibitor or ARB for LVSD	43	74%	82%	82%	100%
Discharge Instructions	98	40%	61%	61%	93%
Evaluation of LVS Function	132	84%	90%	83%	99%
Smoking Cessation Advice[1]	17	100%	91%	82%	100%
Pneumonia Care					
Appropriate Initial Antibiotic[2]	181	78%	84%	83%	94%
Blood Culture Timing[2]	83	73%	88%	90%	100%
Influenza Vaccine	44	55%	64%	70%	100%
Initial Antibiotic Timing[2]	269	66%	74%	80%	93%
Oxygenation Assessment[2]	304	99%	99%	99%	100%
Pneumococcal Vaccine[2]	179	45%	67%	69%	94%
Smoking Cessation Advice[2]	69	97%	90%	80%	100%
Surgical Infection Prevention					
Prophylactic Antibiotic Given[2,3]	416	70%	83%	77%	95%
Prophylactic Antibiotic Selection[2]	82	66%	90%	90%	100%
Prophylactic Antibiotic Stopped[2,3]	395	65%	70%	72%	95%
Pregnancy Care					
Inpatient Neonatal Mortality	-	-	-	-	-
Third or Fourth Degree Laceration	-	-	2.71%	3.63%	3.27%

Memorial Hospital Pembroke

Alternate Name: Pembroke Pines General Hospital
7800 Sheridan Street
Pembroke Pines, FL 33024
E-mail: info@mhs.net
URL: www.memorialpembroke.com\
Ownership: Govt - Hospital District or Authority
Emergency Services: Yes

Phone: 954-962-9650
Fax: 954-963-8471

Accredited: Yes
Licensed Beds: 149

Key Personnel:
Administrator . . . . Ken Hetladge
Chief Medical Staff . . . . Melvyn Rech, DO
Director Emergency Department Services . . . . . Jim Ball
Director Medical Surgical Services . . . . Sharon Joyns
Director Radiology . . . . India Jagan-Jones

Measure	Cases	This Hospital	State Average	U.S. Average	Top Hospital
Heart Attack Care					
ACE Inhibitor or ARB for LVSD[1]	3	100%	83%	82%	100%
Aspirin at Arrival	103	98%	93%	92%	100%
Aspirin at Discharge	32	94%	88%	90%	100%
Beta Blocker at Arrival	85	99%	89%	87%	100%
Beta Blocker at Discharge	32	100%	92%	90%	100%
Fibrinolytic Medication Timing	0	-	33%	31%	100%
PCI Within 90 Minutes of Arrival	0	-	52%	54%	95%
Smoking Cessation Advice[1]	6	100%	92%	88%	100%
Heart Failure Care					
ACE Inhibitor or ARB for LVSD	73	100%	82%	82%	100%
Discharge Instructions	237	96%	61%	61%	93%
Evaluation of LVS Function	270	100%	90%	83%	99%
Smoking Cessation Advice	46	100%	91%	82%	100%
Pneumonia Care					
Appropriate Initial Antibiotic	263	90%	84%	83%	94%
Blood Culture Timing	286	98%	88%	90%	100%
Influenza Vaccine	73	96%	64%	70%	100%
Initial Antibiotic Timing	266	92%	74%	80%	93%
Oxygenation Assessment	376	100%	99%	99%	100%
Pneumococcal Vaccine	196	97%	67%	69%	94%
Smoking Cessation Advice	68	100%	90%	80%	100%
Surgical Infection Prevention					
Prophylactic Antibiotic Given[2]	169	97%	83%	77%	95%
Prophylactic Antibiotic Selection[2]	39	97%	90%	90%	100%
Prophylactic Antibiotic Stopped[2]	155	96%	70%	72%	95%
Pregnancy Care					

NOTE: Hospital profiles are in alphabetical order by state, then city, then hospital within the city; Rankings are sorted by rate in descending order and exclude hospitals with less than 25 cases; (1) The number of cases is too small (n<25) for purposes of reliably predicting hospital performance; (2) Measure reflects the hospital's indication that its submission was based upon a sample of its relevant discharges; (3) Rate reflects fewer than the maximum possible quarters of data for the measure; (4) Inaccurate information submitted and suppressed for one or more quarters; (5) No data is available from the hospital for this measure; Please refer to the User's Guide for a full explanation of data

Inpatient Neonatal Mortality	-	-	-	-	-
Third or Fourth Degree Laceration	-	-	2.71%	3.63%	3.27%

Memorial Hospital West

703 N Flamingo Road
Pembroke Pines, FL 33028
URL: www.memorialwest.com
Ownership: Govt - Hospital District or Authority
Emergency Services: Yes

Phone: 954-436-5000
Fax: 954-433-7155

Accredited: Yes
Licensed Beds: 220

Key Personnel:
Administrator . . . . Zeff Ross
Chief Medical Staff. . . . . Beverly Greenberg, DO
Catheterization Laboratory. . . . . Dawn Annesty
Emergency Room . . . . Sue Klett
ICU . . . . Lisa Quintero
Intensive Coronary. . . . . Lisa Quintero
Medical & Surgical Nursing . . . . Fortuna Borrego
OB/GYN Womens Health. . . . . Mary Roberts
Respiratory . . . . Larry Schulman

Measure	Cases	This Hospital	State Average	U.S. Average	Top Hospital
Heart Attack Care					
ACE Inhibitor or ARB for LVSD	36	94%	83%	82%	100%
Aspirin at Arrival	264	97%	93%	92%	100%
Aspirin at Discharge	160	95%	88%	90%	100%
Beta Blocker at Arrival	167	98%	89%	87%	100%
Beta Blocker at Discharge	171	99%	92%	90%	100%
Fibrinolytic Medication Timing	0	-	33%	31%	100%
PCI Within 90 Minutes of Arrival[1]	19	89%	52%	54%	95%
Smoking Cessation Advice	56	100%	92%	88%	100%
Heart Failure Care					
ACE Inhibitor or ARB for LVSD	178	90%	82%	82%	100%
Discharge Instructions	463	84%	61%	61%	93%
Evaluation of LVS Function	523	100%	90%	83%	99%
Smoking Cessation Advice	52	100%	91%	82%	100%
Pneumonia Care					
Appropriate Initial Antibiotic	320	95%	84%	83%	94%
Blood Culture Timing	341	91%	88%	90%	100%
Influenza Vaccine	81	94%	64%	70%	100%
Initial Antibiotic Timing	436	87%	74%	80%	93%
Oxygenation Assessment	502	100%	99%	99%	100%
Pneumococcal Vaccine	264	98%	67%	69%	94%
Smoking Cessation Advice	80	100%	90%	80%	100%
Surgical Infection Prevention					
Prophylactic Antibiotic Given[2]	583	91%	83%	77%	95%
Prophylactic Antibiotic Selection[2]	41	95%	90%	90%	100%
Prophylactic Antibiotic Stopped[2]	553	83%	70%	72%	95%
Pregnancy Care					
Inpatient Neonatal Mortality	-	-	-	-	-
Third or Fourth Degree Laceration	-	-	2.71%	3.63%	3.27%

Baptist Hospital

1000 W Moreno Street
Pensacola, FL 32501
URL: www.baptisthealthcare.org
Ownership: Voluntary non-profit - Private
Emergency Services: Yes

Phone: 850-434-4011
Fax: 850-469-2307

Accredited: Yes
Licensed Beds: 546

Key Personnel:
President/CEO. . . . . Al Stubblefield
Chief Medical Staff. . . . . Craig Miller, MD
Cardiac Lab. . . . . Jim LaBahn
Catheterization Lab . . . . Donna Cain
Emergency Room . . . . Priscilla Brewer
Infection Control. . . . . Tammy Jernigan
ICU . . . . Brian Taylor
Intensive/Coronary Care . . . . Brian Taylor
Medical/Surgical Nursing . . . . Terri Wood
OB/GYN Womens Health. . . . . Linda Fricke

Measure	Cases	This Hospital	State Average	U.S. Average	Top Hospital
Heart Attack Care					
ACE Inhibitor or ARB for LVSD	54	81%	83%	82%	100%
Aspirin at Arrival	145	96%	93%	92%	100%

Measure	Cases	This Hospital	State Average	U.S. Average	Top Hospital
Aspirin at Discharge	206	96%	88%	90%	100%
Beta Blocker at Arrival	116	91%	89%	87%	100%
Beta Blocker at Discharge	204	97%	92%	90%	100%
Fibrinolytic Medication Timing	0	-	33%	31%	100%
PCI Within 90 Minutes of Arrival[1]	5	60%	52%	54%	95%
Smoking Cessation Advice	93	96%	92%	88%	100%
Heart Failure Care					
ACE Inhibitor or ARB for LVSD	136	82%	82%	82%	100%
Discharge Instructions	351	56%	61%	61%	93%
Evaluation of LVS Function	400	86%	90%	83%	99%
Smoking Cessation Advice	108	93%	91%	82%	100%
Pneumonia Care					
Appropriate Initial Antibiotic	238	89%	84%	83%	94%
Blood Culture Timing	217	82%	88%	90%	100%
Influenza Vaccine	73	71%	64%	70%	100%
Initial Antibiotic Timing	318	74%	74%	80%	93%
Oxygenation Assessment	350	100%	99%	99%	100%
Pneumococcal Vaccine	194	69%	67%	69%	94%
Smoking Cessation Advice	98	100%	90%	80%	100%
Surgical Infection Prevention					
Prophylactic Antibiotic Given	741	77%	83%	77%	95%
Prophylactic Antibiotic Selection	157	90%	90%	90%	100%
Prophylactic Antibiotic Stopped	699	63%	70%	72%	95%
Pregnancy Care					
Inpatient Neonatal Mortality	-	-	-	-	-
Third or Fourth Degree Laceration	-	-	2.71%	3.63%	3.27%

Sacred Heart Health System

5151 N 9th Avenue
Pensacola, FL 32504
URL: www.sacred-heart.org
Ownership: Voluntary non-profit - Church
Emergency Services: Yes

Phone: 850-416-7000
Fax: 850-416-6740

Accredited: Yes
Licensed Beds: 449

Key Personnel:
CEO. . . . . Patrick J Madden
Chief Medical Staff. . . . . George Dmytrenko
Emergency Room . . . . Dee Johnson
Director Infection/Disease Control . . . . Barbara Wade, MD
CCU Spvg. Nurse . . . . Ann Burns
Director Medical/Surgical Nursing . . . . John Stewart
OB/GYN Womens Health. . . . . Charles Horan
Director Radiology . . . . Ron Thompson
Director Respiratory Therapy . . . . John Stewart

Measure	Cases	This Hospital	State Average	U.S. Average	Top Hospital
Heart Attack Care					
ACE Inhibitor or ARB for LVSD[2]	74	97%	83%	82%	100%
Aspirin at Arrival[2]	226	98%	93%	92%	100%
Aspirin at Discharge[2]	312	96%	88%	90%	100%
Beta Blocker at Arrival[2]	221	98%	89%	87%	100%
Beta Blocker at Discharge[2]	310	96%	92%	90%	100%
Fibrinolytic Medication Timing[1,2]	4	50%	33%	31%	100%
PCI Within 90 Minutes of Arrival[1,2]	9	22%	52%	54%	95%
Smoking Cessation Advice[2]	128	95%	92%	88%	100%
Heart Failure Care					
ACE Inhibitor or ARB for LVSD[2]	188	95%	82%	82%	100%
Discharge Instructions[2]	342	80%	61%	61%	93%
Evaluation of LVS Function[2]	389	98%	90%	83%	99%
Smoking Cessation Advice[2]	102	98%	91%	82%	100%
Pneumonia Care					
Appropriate Initial Antibiotic[2]	219	64%	84%	83%	94%
Blood Culture Timing[2]	131	94%	88%	90%	100%
Influenza Vaccine[2]	41	66%	64%	70%	100%
Initial Antibiotic Timing[2]	228	58%	74%	80%	93%
Oxygenation Assessment[2]	299	100%	99%	99%	100%
Pneumococcal Vaccine[2]	176	62%	67%	69%	94%
Smoking Cessation Advice[2]	60	75%	90%	80%	100%
Surgical Infection Prevention					
Prophylactic Antibiotic Given[2]	349	54%	83%	77%	95%
Prophylactic Antibiotic Selection[2]	86	93%	90%	90%	100%
Prophylactic Antibiotic Stopped[2]	336	57%	70%	72%	95%
Pregnancy Care					
Inpatient Neonatal Mortality[2]	691	0.43%	-	-	-

NOTE: Hospital profiles are in alphabetical order by state, then city, then hospital within the city; Rankings are sorted by rate in descending order and exclude hospitals with less than 25 cases; (1) The number of cases is too small (n<25) for purposes of reliably predicting hospital performance; (2) Measure reflects the hospital's indication that its submission was based upon a sample of its relevant discharges; (3) Rate reflects fewer than the maximum possible quarters of data for the measure; (4) Inaccurate information submitted and suppressed for one or more quarters; (5) No data is available from the hospital for this measure; Please refer to the User's Guide for a full explanation of data

Third or Fourth Degree Laceration[2]	373	1.34%	2.71%	3.63%	3.27%

West Florida Regional Medical Center

Alternate Name: West Florida Hospital
8383 N Davis Highway
PO Box 18900
Pensacola, FL 32514
URL: www.westfloridahospital.com
Ownership: Proprietary
Emergency Services: Yes

Phone: 850-494-4000
Fax: 850-494-5216

Accredited: Yes
Licensed Beds: 531

Key Personnel:
President/CEO . . . . Dennis A Taylor
Emergency Room . . . . Margie Hobbs
Infection Control . . . . Lorraine Price
ICU . . . . Jacque Posey
Intensive/Coronary Care . . . . Jacque Posey
Respiratory/Cardiopulmonary . . . . Teresa Sieler

Measure	Cases	This Hospital	State Average	U.S. Average	Top Hospital
Heart Attack Care					
ACE Inhibitor or ARB for LVSD	46	87%	83%	82%	100%
Aspirin at Arrival	146	95%	93%	92%	100%
Aspirin at Discharge	201	99%	88%	90%	100%
Beta Blocker at Arrival	98	85%	89%	87%	100%
Beta Blocker at Discharge	210	96%	92%	90%	100%
Fibrinolytic Medication Timing	0	-	33%	31%	100%
PCI Within 90 Minutes of Arrival[1]	11	73%	52%	54%	95%
Smoking Cessation Advice	101	99%	92%	88%	100%
Heart Failure Care					
ACE Inhibitor or ARB for LVSD	127	76%	82%	82%	100%
Discharge Instructions	240	46%	61%	61%	93%
Evaluation of LVS Function	272	96%	90%	83%	99%
Smoking Cessation Advice	54	96%	91%	82%	100%
Pneumonia Care					
Appropriate Initial Antibiotic	146	84%	84%	83%	94%
Blood Culture Timing	139	97%	88%	90%	100%
Influenza Vaccine	46	78%	64%	70%	100%
Initial Antibiotic Timing	202	65%	74%	80%	93%
Oxygenation Assessment	247	100%	99%	99%	100%
Pneumococcal Vaccine	155	76%	67%	69%	94%
Smoking Cessation Advice	45	98%	90%	80%	100%
Surgical Infection Prevention					
Prophylactic Antibiotic Given[2,3]	288	64%	83%	77%	95%
Prophylactic Antibiotic Selection[2]	114	94%	90%	90%	100%
Prophylactic Antibiotic Stopped[2,3]	281	51%	70%	72%	95%
Pregnancy Care					
Inpatient Neonatal Mortality	-	-	-	-	-
Third or Fourth Degree Laceration	-	-	2.71%	3.63%	3.27%

Doctors Memorial Hospital

333 North Byron Butler Parkway
Perry, FL 32347
Ownership: Voluntary non-profit - Private
Emergency Services: No

Phone: 850-584-0800
Fax: 850-584-2524
Accredited: No
Licensed Beds: 48

Key Personnel:
CEO . . . . Rick Brown
Director Medical/Surgical Nursing . . . . Ann Gray, RN
Chief Radiology . . . . Lyn Odom
Director Respiratory Therapy . . . . Jim Mitchell

Measure	Cases	This Hospital	State Average	U.S. Average	Top Hospital
Heart Attack Care					
ACE Inhibitor or ARB for LVSD[1,2,3]	1	100%	83%	82%	100%
Aspirin at Arrival[1,2,3]	16	94%	93%	92%	100%
Aspirin at Discharge[1,2,3]	12	83%	88%	90%	100%
Beta Blocker at Arrival[1,2,3]	16	94%	89%	87%	100%
Beta Blocker at Discharge[1,2,3]	12	75%	92%	90%	100%
Fibrinolytic Medication Timing[5]	-	-	33%	31%	100%
PCI Within 90 Minutes of Arrival[5]	-	-	52%	54%	95%
Smoking Cessation Advice[5]	-	-	92%	88%	100%
Heart Failure Care					
ACE Inhibitor or ARB for LVSD[2]	28	68%	82%	82%	100%

Measure					
Discharge Instructions[1,2,3]	22	23%	61%	61%	93%
Evaluation of LVS Function[2]	74	66%	90%	83%	99%
Smoking Cessation Advice[1,2,3]	8	88%	91%	82%	100%
Pneumonia Care					
Appropriate Initial Antibiotic[1,2,3]	18	50%	84%	83%	94%
Blood Culture Timing[1,2,3]	6	100%	88%	90%	100%
Influenza Vaccine[5]	-	-	64%	70%	100%
Initial Antibiotic Timing[2]	58	79%	74%	80%	93%
Oxygenation Assessment[2]	75	97%	99%	99%	100%
Pneumococcal Vaccine[2]	37	51%	67%	69%	94%
Smoking Cessation Advice[1,2,3]	6	100%	90%	80%	100%
Surgical Infection Prevention					
Prophylactic Antibiotic Given[1,3]	7	100%	83%	77%	95%
Prophylactic Antibiotic Selection[5]	-	-	90%	90%	100%
Prophylactic Antibiotic Stopped[1,3]	7	0%	70%	72%	95%
Pregnancy Care					
Inpatient Neonatal Mortality	-	-	-	-	-
Third or Fourth Degree Laceration	-	-	2.71%	3.63%	3.27%

South Florida Baptist Hospital

301 N Alexander Street
Plant City, FL 33563
URL: www.sjbhealth.org
Ownership: Voluntary non-profit - Other
Emergency Services: Yes

Phone: 813-757-1200
Fax: 813-757-1255

Accredited: Yes
Licensed Beds: 147

Key Personnel:
President/CEO . . . . Issac Mallah
Chief Medical Staff . . . . Steve Smith, MD
Emergency Room . . . . Natalie Rivera, RN
OB/GYN Womens Health . . . . C Mahapaurya, MD
Chief Radiology . . . . Shelly Baumann, MD
Director Respiratory Therapy . . . . Fred Konzen

Measure	Cases	This Hospital	State Average	U.S. Average	Top Hospital
Heart Attack Care					
ACE Inhibitor or ARB for LVSD[1]	9	100%	83%	82%	100%
Aspirin at Arrival	33	100%	93%	92%	100%
Aspirin at Discharge[1]	14	100%	88%	90%	100%
Beta Blocker at Arrival	33	100%	89%	87%	100%
Beta Blocker at Discharge[1]	19	100%	92%	90%	100%
Fibrinolytic Medication Timing	0	-	33%	31%	100%
PCI Within 90 Minutes of Arrival	0	-	52%	54%	95%
Smoking Cessation Advice[1]	4	100%	92%	88%	100%
Heart Failure Care					
ACE Inhibitor or ARB for LVSD	63	94%	82%	82%	100%
Discharge Instructions	119	71%	61%	61%	93%
Evaluation of LVS Function	146	99%	90%	83%	99%
Smoking Cessation Advice	43	100%	91%	82%	100%
Pneumonia Care					
Appropriate Initial Antibiotic	132	86%	84%	83%	94%
Blood Culture Timing	178	94%	88%	90%	100%
Influenza Vaccine	45	62%	64%	70%	100%
Initial Antibiotic Timing	166	84%	74%	80%	93%
Oxygenation Assessment	261	100%	99%	99%	100%
Pneumococcal Vaccine	148	83%	67%	69%	94%
Smoking Cessation Advice	66	98%	90%	80%	100%
Surgical Infection Prevention					
Prophylactic Antibiotic Given[2]	114	81%	83%	77%	95%
Prophylactic Antibiotic Selection[2]	30	97%	90%	90%	100%
Prophylactic Antibiotic Stopped[2]	92	73%	70%	72%	95%
Pregnancy Care					
Inpatient Neonatal Mortality	-	-	-	-	-
Third or Fourth Degree Laceration	-	-	2.71%	3.63%	3.27%

Plantation General Hospital

Alternate Name: PGH
401 NW 42nd Avenue
Plantation, FL 33317
URL: www.plantationgeneral.com
Ownership: Proprietary
Emergency Services: Yes

Phone: 954-587-5010
Fax: 954-587-3220

Accredited: Yes
Licensed Beds: 264

Key Personnel:
CEO . . . . Anthony Degina

NOTE: Hospital profiles are in alphabetical order by state, then city, then hospital within the city; Rankings are sorted by rate in descending order and exclude hospitals with less than 25 cases; (1) The number of cases is too small (n<25) for purposes of reliably predicting hospital performance; (2) Measure reflects the hospital's indication that its submission was based upon a sample of its relevant discharges; (3) Rate reflects fewer than the maximum possible quarters of data for the measure; (4) Inaccurate information submitted and suppressed for one or more quarters; (5) No data is available from the hospital for this measure; Please refer to the User's Guide for a full explanation of data

Chief Medical Staff. . . . . Joel Jancko, MD
Women's Services . . . . Ginny Kline-Kaye
Director Cardio-Pulmonary Services . . . . Jackie Ordaz

Measure	Cases	This Hospital	State Average	U.S. Average	Top Hospital
Heart Attack Care					
ACE Inhibitor or ARB for LVSD[1]	3	100%	83%	82%	100%
Aspirin at Arrival[1]	20	90%	93%	92%	100%
Aspirin at Discharge[1]	10	80%	88%	90%	100%
Beta Blocker at Arrival[1]	21	71%	89%	87%	100%
Beta Blocker at Discharge[1]	12	75%	92%	90%	100%
Fibrinolytic Medication Timing	0	-	33%	31%	100%
PCI Within 90 Minutes of Arrival	0	-	52%	54%	95%
Smoking Cessation Advice[1]	1	0%	92%	88%	100%
Heart Failure Care					
ACE Inhibitor or ARB for LVSD	76	71%	82%	82%	100%
Discharge Instructions	131	64%	61%	61%	93%
Evaluation of LVS Function	153	86%	90%	83%	99%
Smoking Cessation Advice	37	89%	91%	82%	100%
Pneumonia Care					
Appropriate Initial Antibiotic	84	86%	84%	83%	94%
Blood Culture Timing	102	83%	88%	90%	100%
Influenza Vaccine[1]	20	10%	64%	70%	100%
Initial Antibiotic Timing	148	68%	74%	80%	93%
Oxygenation Assessment	162	99%	99%	99%	100%
Pneumococcal Vaccine	43	47%	67%	69%	94%
Smoking Cessation Advice	45	93%	90%	80%	100%
Surgical Infection Prevention					
Prophylactic Antibiotic Given[3]	146	94%	83%	77%	95%
Prophylactic Antibiotic Selection	46	96%	90%	90%	100%
Prophylactic Antibiotic Stopped[3]	146	77%	70%	72%	95%
Pregnancy Care					
Inpatient Neonatal Mortality	3,780	0.63%	-	-	-
Third or Fourth Degree Laceration	2,060	2.43%	2.71%	3.63%	3.27%

Westside Regional Medical Center

Alternate Name: Westside Regional Medical Center
8201 W Broward Boulevard
Plantation, FL 33324
URL: www.westsidehospital.com
Ownership: Proprietary
Emergency Services: Yes

Phone: 954-473-6600
Fax: 954-452-2133

Accredited: Yes
Licensed Beds: 224

Key Personnel:
CEO. . . . . Earl H Denning
Chief Medical Staff. . . . . Paul Bates, MD
Emergency Room . . . . Susan West
Director Medical/Surgical Nursing . . . . Eileen Ciotti
OB/GYN Womens Health. . . . . Jamie Mercado
Chief Radiology . . . . Wanda Fogarty, MD
Director Respiratory Therapy . . . . Steve Lamson

Measure	Cases	This Hospital	State Average	U.S. Average	Top Hospital
Heart Attack Care					
ACE Inhibitor or ARB for LVSD	68	99%	83%	82%	100%
Aspirin at Arrival	328	99%	93%	92%	100%
Aspirin at Discharge[1]	333	99%	88%	90%	100%
Beta Blocker at Arrival	307	98%	89%	87%	100%
Beta Blocker at Discharge	334	99%	92%	90%	100%
Fibrinolytic Medication Timing	0	-	33%	31%	100%
PCI Within 90 Minutes of Arrival[1]	15	60%	52%	54%	95%
Smoking Cessation Advice	64	95%	92%	88%	100%
Heart Failure Care					
ACE Inhibitor or ARB for LVSD	117	90%	82%	82%	100%
Discharge Instructions	325	71%	61%	61%	93%
Evaluation of LVS Function	394	99%	90%	83%	99%
Smoking Cessation Advice	48	98%	91%	82%	100%
Pneumonia Care					
Appropriate Initial Antibiotic	186	83%	84%	83%	94%
Blood Culture Timing	166	90%	88%	90%	100%
Influenza Vaccine	49	67%	64%	70%	100%
Initial Antibiotic Timing	249	78%	74%	80%	93%
Oxygenation Assessment	264	99%	99%	99%	100%

Measure	Cases	This Hospital	State Average	U.S. Average	Top Hospital
Pneumococcal Vaccine	146	66%	67%	69%	94%
Smoking Cessation Advice	45	100%	90%	80%	100%
Surgical Infection Prevention					
Prophylactic Antibiotic Given	540	96%	83%	77%	95%
Prophylactic Antibiotic Selection	133	94%	90%	90%	100%
Prophylactic Antibiotic Stopped	526	79%	70%	72%	95%
Pregnancy Care					
Inpatient Neonatal Mortality	-	-	-	-	-
Third or Fourth Degree Laceration	-	-	2.71%	3.63%	3.27%

Fawcett Memorial Hospital

21298 NW Olean Blvd
PO Box 494960
Port Charlotte, FL 33949
URL: www.fawcetthospital.com
Ownership: Proprietary
Emergency Services: Yes

Phone: 941-629-1181
Fax: 941-627-6142

Accredited: Yes
Licensed Beds: 238

Key Personnel:
CEO. . . . . Thomas J Rice
Chief Medical Staff. Nasir Khalidi, MD
Emergency Room . . . . Nancy Reyes
Infection Control. . . . . Vicki Pellenz
ICU . . . . Marita Annis
Medical Surgical Nursing . . . . Tammy Faircloth
CNO. . . . . Susan Griffin
Director Radiology . . . . Ellen Nicholas
Respiratory/Cardiopulmonary. . . . . Michael Mulcahy

Measure	Cases	This Hospital	State Average	U.S. Average	Top Hospital
Heart Attack Care					
ACE Inhibitor or ARB for LVSD[1]	23	78%	83%	82%	100%
Aspirin at Arrival	85	82%	93%	92%	100%
Aspirin at Discharge	50	82%	88%	90%	100%
Beta Blocker at Arrival	75	81%	89%	87%	100%
Beta Blocker at Discharge	61	90%	92%	90%	100%
Fibrinolytic Medication Timing	0	-	33%	31%	100%
PCI Within 90 Minutes of Arrival	0	-	52%	54%	95%
Smoking Cessation Advice[1]	13	92%	92%	88%	100%
Heart Failure Care					
ACE Inhibitor or ARB for LVSD	103	76%	82%	82%	100%
Discharge Instructions	246	77%	61%	61%	93%
Evaluation of LVS Function	312	84%	90%	83%	99%
Smoking Cessation Advice	38	97%	91%	82%	100%
Pneumonia Care					
Appropriate Initial Antibiotic	121	80%	84%	83%	94%
Blood Culture Timing	105	91%	88%	90%	100%
Influenza Vaccine	38	53%	64%	70%	100%
Initial Antibiotic Timing	173	80%	74%	80%	93%
Oxygenation Assessment	220	100%	99%	99%	100%
Pneumococcal Vaccine	160	72%	67%	69%	94%
Smoking Cessation Advice	44	93%	90%	80%	100%
Surgical Infection Prevention					
Prophylactic Antibiotic Given	425	91%	83%	77%	95%
Prophylactic Antibiotic Selection	87	95%	90%	90%	100%
Prophylactic Antibiotic Stopped	409	61%	70%	72%	95%
Pregnancy Care					
Inpatient Neonatal Mortality	-	-	-	-	-
Third or Fourth Degree Laceration	-	-	2.71%	3.63%	3.27%

Peace River Regional Medical Center

Alternate Name: Saint Joseph Hospital
2500 Harbor Boulevard
Port Charlotte, FL 33952
Ownership: Proprietary
Emergency Services: Yes

Phone: 941-766-4122
Fax: 941-766-4140

Accredited: Yes
Licensed Beds: 212

Key Personnel:
President/CEO. . . . . J David McCormack
Chief Medical Staff. David McAtee, DO
Catheterization Lab . . . . Dave Courson
Coordinator Emergency Room. . . . . Phil Rogers
Emergency Room . . . . Robert Leyrer, MD
Infection Control. . . . . Joyce Dulmage
ICU . . . . Carol Rothman

NOTE: Hospital profiles are in alphabetical order by state, then city, then hospital within the city; Rankings are sorted by rate in descending order and exclude hospitals with less than 25 cases; (1) The number of cases is too small (n<25) for purposes of reliably predicting hospital performance; (2) Measure reflects the hospital's indication that its submission was based upon a sample of its relevant discharges; (3) Rate reflects fewer than the maximum possible quarters of data for the measure; (4) Inaccurate information submitted and suppressed for one or more quarters; (5) No data is available from the hospital for this measure; Please refer to the User's Guide for a full explanation of data

Medical/Surgical Nursing . . . . Carolyn Quinlan
Respiratory/Cardiopulmonary. . . . . Lisa Orlick

Measure	Cases	This Hospital	State Average	U.S. Average	Top Hospital
Heart Attack Care					
ACE Inhibitor or ARB for LVSD[1]	3	100%	83%	82%	100%
Aspirin at Arrival	54	98%	93%	92%	100%
Aspirin at Discharge	28	96%	88%	90%	100%
Beta Blocker at Arrival	37	86%	89%	87%	100%
Beta Blocker at Discharge	33	100%	92%	90%	100%
Fibrinolytic Medication Timing	0	-	33%	31%	100%
PCI Within 90 Minutes of Arrival	0	-	52%	54%	95%
Smoking Cessation Advice[1]	8	100%	92%	88%	100%
Heart Failure Care					
ACE Inhibitor or ARB for LVSD	66	97%	82%	82%	100%
Discharge Instructions	175	45%	61%	61%	93%
Evaluation of LVS Function	222	99%	90%	83%	99%
Smoking Cessation Advice[1]	17	100%	91%	82%	100%
Pneumonia Care					
Appropriate Initial Antibiotic	160	79%	84%	83%	94%
Blood Culture Timing	129	91%	88%	90%	100%
Influenza Vaccine	41	90%	64%	70%	100%
Initial Antibiotic Timing	214	67%	74%	80%	93%
Oxygenation Assessment	266	99%	99%	99%	100%
Pneumococcal Vaccine	168	94%	67%	69%	94%
Smoking Cessation Advice	68	97%	90%	80%	100%
Surgical Infection Prevention					
Prophylactic Antibiotic Given[2]	401	82%	83%	77%	95%
Prophylactic Antibiotic Selection[2]	68	88%	90%	90%	100%
Prophylactic Antibiotic Stopped[2]	377	76%	70%	72%	95%
Pregnancy Care					
Inpatient Neonatal Mortality	-	-	-	-	-
Third or Fourth Degree Laceration	-	-	2.71%	3.63%	3.27%

Saint Lucie Medical Center

1800 SE Tiffany Avenue
Port Saint Lucie, FL 34952
URL: www.stluciemed.com
Ownership: Proprietary
Emergency Services: Yes

Phone: 772-335-4000
Fax: 772-398-3742

Accredited: Yes
Licensed Beds: 194

Key Personnel:
President/CEO. . . . . Gary Cantrell
Chief Medical Staff. . . . . Michael Paul, MD
Cardiac Lab . . . . Shawn Poland
Catheterization Lab . . . . Gary Guido
Emergency Room . . . . Jim Kruger
Infection Control. . . . . Suzane Perry, RN
Medical/Surgical Nursing . . . . Jesse Gabuat
OB/GYN Womens Health. . . . . Brenda Gray
Surgery Centers. . . . . Jill Logan
Respiratory/Cardiopulmonary. . . . . Shawn Poland

Measure	Cases	This Hospital	State Average	U.S. Average	Top Hospital
Heart Attack Care					
ACE Inhibitor or ARB for LVSD	26	85%	83%	82%	100%
Aspirin at Arrival	200	92%	93%	92%	100%
Aspirin at Discharge	68	82%	88%	90%	100%
Beta Blocker at Arrival	185	90%	89%	87%	100%
Beta Blocker at Discharge	79	87%	92%	90%	100%
Fibrinolytic Medication Timing	33	42%	33%	31%	100%
PCI Within 90 Minutes of Arrival	0	-	52%	54%	95%
Smoking Cessation Advice[1]	6	100%	92%	88%	100%
Heart Failure Care					
ACE Inhibitor or ARB for LVSD	185	84%	82%	82%	100%
Discharge Instructions	369	86%	61%	61%	93%
Evaluation of LVS Function	503	91%	90%	83%	99%
Smoking Cessation Advice	68	99%	91%	82%	100%
Pneumonia Care					
Appropriate Initial Antibiotic	243	86%	84%	83%	94%
Blood Culture Timing	206	89%	88%	90%	100%
Influenza Vaccine	53	55%	64%	70%	100%
Initial Antibiotic Timing	307	66%	74%	80%	93%

Measure	Cases	This Hospital	State Average	U.S. Average	Top Hospital
Oxygenation Assessment	383	100%	99%	99%	100%
Pneumococcal Vaccine	241	63%	67%	69%	94%
Smoking Cessation Advice	58	98%	90%	80%	100%
Surgical Infection Prevention					
Prophylactic Antibiotic Given[2,3]	472	90%	83%	77%	95%
Prophylactic Antibiotic Selection[2]	100	71%	90%	90%	100%
Prophylactic Antibiotic Stopped[2,3]	464	45%	70%	72%	95%
Pregnancy Care					
Inpatient Neonatal Mortality	-	-	-	-	-
Third or Fourth Degree Laceration	-	-	2.71%	3.63%	3.27%

Charlotte Regional Medical Center

Alternate Name: Medical Center Hospital
809 E Marion Avenue
Punta Gorda, FL 33950
URL: www.crmc-hma.com
Ownership: Proprietary
Emergency Services: Yes

Phone: 941-639-3131
Fax: 941-637-2454

Accredited: No
Licensed Beds: 208

Key Personnel:
President/CEO. . . . . Joshua Putter
Chief Medical Staff. . . . . John Guarino, MD
Emergency Room . . . . Darrel Billington
Respiratory/Cardiopulmonary. . . . . Donald Wilson

Measure	Cases	This Hospital	State Average	U.S. Average	Top Hospital
Heart Attack Care					
ACE Inhibitor or ARB for LVSD	85	80%	83%	82%	100%
Aspirin at Arrival	151	99%	93%	92%	100%
Aspirin at Discharge	311	95%	88%	90%	100%
Beta Blocker at Arrival	146	93%	89%	87%	100%
Beta Blocker at Discharge	332	89%	92%	90%	100%
Fibrinolytic Medication Timing[1]	1	0%	33%	31%	100%
PCI Within 90 Minutes of Arrival[1]	13	77%	52%	54%	95%
Smoking Cessation Advice	103	96%	92%	88%	100%
Heart Failure Care					
ACE Inhibitor or ARB for LVSD	253	81%	82%	82%	100%
Discharge Instructions	407	67%	61%	61%	93%
Evaluation of LVS Function	464	93%	90%	83%	99%
Smoking Cessation Advice	70	99%	91%	82%	100%
Pneumonia Care					
Appropriate Initial Antibiotic	127	85%	84%	83%	94%
Blood Culture Timing	137	95%	88%	90%	100%
Influenza Vaccine	48	58%	64%	70%	100%
Initial Antibiotic Timing	177	77%	74%	80%	93%
Oxygenation Assessment	232	99%	99%	99%	100%
Pneumococcal Vaccine	164	67%	67%	69%	94%
Smoking Cessation Advice	52	98%	90%	80%	100%
Surgical Infection Prevention					
Prophylactic Antibiotic Given[2]	464	65%	83%	77%	95%
Prophylactic Antibiotic Selection[2]	70	94%	90%	90%	100%
Prophylactic Antibiotic Stopped[2]	450	78%	70%	72%	95%
Pregnancy Care					
Inpatient Neonatal Mortality	-	-	-	-	-
Third or Fourth Degree Laceration	-	-	2.71%	3.63%	3.27%

Wuesthoff Health Systems

110 Longwood Avenue
Rockledge, FL 32955

Toll-Free: 800-742-9175
Phone: 321-636-2211
Fax: 321-690-6617

URL: www.wuesthoff.org
Ownership: Voluntary non-profit - Private
Emergency Services: Yes

Accredited: Yes
Licensed Beds: 295

Key Personnel:
Chief Medical Staff. . . . . Duff Sprawls, MD
Cardiopulmonary . . . . John Oliver
Chief Catheterization Laboratory . . . . Robert Barden, MD
Emergency Department . . . . Daniel Knell
Director Infection/Disease Control . . . . Mukul Garg, MD
CCU Spvg. Nurse . . . . Marge Miller
Director Medical/Surgical Nursing . . . . Mae Hafizi
Medical Staff Services . . . . Doreen Woods
Chief OB/GYN . . . . Snehlata Pandya, MD
Chief Radiology . . . . Robert Page, MD

NOTE: Hospital profiles are in alphabetical order by state, then city, then hospital within the city; Rankings are sorted by rate in descending order and exclude hospitals with less than 25 cases; (1) The number of cases is too small (n<25) for purposes of reliably predicting hospital performance; (2) Measure reflects the hospital's indication that its submission was based upon a sample of its relevant discharges; (3) Rate reflects fewer than the maximum possible quarters of data for the measure; (4) Inaccurate information submitted and suppressed for one or more quarters; (5) No data is available from the hospital for this measure; Please refer to the User's Guide for a full explanation of data

Director Respiratory Therapy . . . . David Knight, RRT

Measure	Cases	This Hospital	State Average	U.S. Average	Top Hospital
Heart Attack Care					
ACE Inhibitor or ARB for LVSD	68	100%	83%	82%	100%
Aspirin at Arrival	205	98%	93%	92%	100%
Aspirin at Discharge	223	99%	88%	90%	100%
Beta Blocker at Arrival	154	95%	89%	87%	100%
Beta Blocker at Discharge	255	98%	92%	90%	100%
Fibrinolytic Medication Timing[1]	1	0%	33%	31%	100%
PCI Within 90 Minutes of Arrival[1]	13	54%	52%	54%	95%
Smoking Cessation Advice	115	100%	92%	88%	100%
Heart Failure Care					
ACE Inhibitor or ARB for LVSD	180	99%	82%	82%	100%
Discharge Instructions	413	83%	61%	61%	93%
Evaluation of LVS Function	486	98%	90%	83%	99%
Smoking Cessation Advice	108	100%	91%	82%	100%
Pneumonia Care					
Appropriate Initial Antibiotic	185	84%	84%	83%	94%
Blood Culture Timing	189	92%	88%	90%	100%
Influenza Vaccine	52	94%	64%	70%	100%
Initial Antibiotic Timing	241	71%	74%	80%	93%
Oxygenation Assessment	294	100%	99%	99%	100%
Pneumococcal Vaccine	171	81%	67%	69%	94%
Smoking Cessation Advice	91	99%	90%	80%	100%
Surgical Infection Prevention					
Prophylactic Antibiotic Given[2]	664	95%	83%	77%	95%
Prophylactic Antibiotic Selection[2]	151	90%	90%	90%	100%
Prophylactic Antibiotic Stopped[2]	635	74%	70%	72%	95%
Pregnancy Care					
Inpatient Neonatal Mortality	-	-	-	-	-
Third or Fourth Degree Laceration	-	-	2.71%	3.63%	3.27%

Mease Hospital-Countryside

3231 McMullen Booth Road
Safety Harbor, FL 34695

Toll-Free: 866-632-7348
Phone: 727-725-6111
Fax: 727-725-6181

URL: www.measehospitals.com
Ownership: Voluntary non-profit - Private
Emergency Services: Yes
Accredited: Yes
Licensed Beds: 205
Key Personnel:
Administrator . . . . Jim Pfeiffer
Emergency Room . . . . Kelly Triolo, RN
Surgical Services Director . . . . Celia Larimore

Measure	Cases	This Hospital	State Average	U.S. Average	Top Hospital
Heart Attack Care					
ACE Inhibitor or ARB for LVSD[1]	19	89%	83%	82%	100%
Aspirin at Arrival	158	97%	93%	92%	100%
Aspirin at Discharge	57	88%	88%	90%	100%
Beta Blocker at Arrival	75	88%	89%	87%	100%
Beta Blocker at Discharge	88	97%	92%	90%	100%
Fibrinolytic Medication Timing	0	-	33%	31%	100%
PCI Within 90 Minutes of Arrival	0	-	52%	54%	95%
Smoking Cessation Advice[1]	9	100%	92%	88%	100%
Heart Failure Care					
ACE Inhibitor or ARB for LVSD	150	91%	82%	82%	100%
Discharge Instructions	337	68%	61%	61%	93%
Evaluation of LVS Function	434	93%	90%	83%	99%
Smoking Cessation Advice	47	98%	91%	82%	100%
Pneumonia Care					
Appropriate Initial Antibiotic	265	85%	84%	83%	94%
Blood Culture Timing	286	95%	88%	90%	100%
Influenza Vaccine	91	74%	64%	70%	100%
Initial Antibiotic Timing	281	78%	74%	80%	93%
Oxygenation Assessment	445	100%	99%	99%	100%
Pneumococcal Vaccine	296	75%	67%	69%	94%
Smoking Cessation Advice	85	98%	90%	80%	100%
Surgical Infection Prevention					
Prophylactic Antibiotic Given[2]	168	73%	83%	77%	95%
Prophylactic Antibiotic Selection[2]	61	93%	90%	90%	100%
Prophylactic Antibiotic Stopped[2]	145	78%	70%	72%	95%

Pregnancy Care					
Inpatient Neonatal Mortality	-	-	-	-	-
Third or Fourth Degree Laceration	-	-	2.71%	3.63%	3.27%

Flagler Hospital

400 Health Park Boulevard
Saint Augustine, FL 32086
URL: www.flaglerhospital.com
Ownership: Voluntary non-profit - Private
Emergency Services: Yes

Phone: 904-819-5155
Fax: 904-819-4472

Accredited: Yes
Licensed Beds: 321

Key Personnel:
President . . . . Joe Gordy
Director Medical/Surgical Nursing . . . . Cecilia Hussman
OB/GYN Womens Health. . . . . Juan Larroude

Measure	Cases	This Hospital	State Average	U.S. Average	Top Hospital
Heart Attack Care					
ACE Inhibitor or ARB for LVSD	27	74%	83%	82%	100%
Aspirin at Arrival	289	89%	93%	92%	100%
Aspirin at Discharge	257	91%	88%	90%	100%
Beta Blocker at Arrival	224	80%	89%	87%	100%
Beta Blocker at Discharge	245	86%	92%	90%	100%
Fibrinolytic Medication Timing[1]	1	0%	33%	31%	100%
PCI Within 90 Minutes of Arrival[1]	12	25%	52%	54%	95%
Smoking Cessation Advice	78	94%	92%	88%	100%
Heart Failure Care					
ACE Inhibitor or ARB for LVSD[2]	144	82%	82%	82%	100%
Discharge Instructions[2]	366	35%	61%	61%	93%
Evaluation of LVS Function[2]	458	98%	90%	83%	99%
Smoking Cessation Advice[2]	78	86%	91%	82%	100%
Pneumonia Care					
Appropriate Initial Antibiotic[2]	160	81%	84%	83%	94%
Blood Culture Timing[2]	115	86%	88%	90%	100%
Influenza Vaccine[4,5]	-	-	64%	70%	100%
Initial Antibiotic Timing[2]	216	67%	74%	80%	93%
Oxygenation Assessment[2]	265	100%	99%	99%	100%
Pneumococcal Vaccine[2]	142	65%	67%	69%	94%
Smoking Cessation Advice[2]	71	92%	90%	80%	100%
Surgical Infection Prevention					
Prophylactic Antibiotic Given[2]	259	59%	83%	77%	95%
Prophylactic Antibiotic Selection[2]	75	87%	90%	90%	100%
Prophylactic Antibiotic Stopped[2]	254	44%	70%	72%	95%
Pregnancy Care					
Inpatient Neonatal Mortality	-	-	-	-	-
Third or Fourth Degree Laceration	-	-	2.71%	3.63%	3.27%

Saint Cloud Regional Medical Center

2906 17th Street
Saint Cloud, FL 34769
Ownership: Proprietary
Emergency Services: No

Phone: 407-498-3432

Accredited: Yes

Measure	Cases	This Hospital	State Average	U.S. Average	Top Hospital
Heart Attack Care					
ACE Inhibitor or ARB for LVSD[1,3]	1	100%	83%	82%	100%
Aspirin at Arrival[1,3]	21	90%	93%	92%	100%
Aspirin at Discharge[1,3]	7	71%	88%	90%	100%
Beta Blocker at Arrival[1,3]	20	60%	89%	87%	100%
Beta Blocker at Discharge[1,3]	7	86%	92%	90%	100%
Fibrinolytic Medication Timing[3]	0	-	33%	31%	100%
PCI Within 90 Minutes of Arrival	0	-	52%	54%	95%
Smoking Cessation Advice[3]	0	-	92%	88%	100%
Heart Failure Care					
ACE Inhibitor or ARB for LVSD[3]	25	88%	82%	82%	100%
Discharge Instructions[1,3]	19	11%	61%	61%	93%
Evaluation of LVS Function[3]	80	88%	90%	83%	99%
Smoking Cessation Advice[1,3]	4	75%	91%	82%	100%
Pneumonia Care					
Appropriate Initial Antibiotic[1,3]	14	79%	84%	83%	94%
Blood Culture Timing[1,3]	12	100%	88%	90%	100%
Influenza Vaccine[5]	-	-	64%	70%	100%
Initial Antibiotic Timing[3]	84	71%	74%	80%	93%

NOTE: Hospital profiles are in alphabetical order by state, then city, then hospital within the city; Rankings are sorted by rate in descending order and exclude hospitals with less than 25 cases; (1) The number of cases is too small (n<25) for purposes of reliably predicting hospital performance; (2) Measure reflects the hospital's indication that its submission was based upon a sample of its relevant discharges; (3) Rate reflects fewer than the maximum possible quarters of data for the measure; (4) Inaccurate information submitted and suppressed for one or more quarters; (5) No data is available from the hospital for this measure; Please refer to the User's Guide for a full explanation of data

Oxygenation Assessment[3]	102	100%	99%	99%	100%
Pneumococcal Vaccine[3]	61	70%	67%	69%	94%
Smoking Cessation Advice[1,3]	8	100%	90%	80%	100%

Surgical Infection Prevention					
Prophylactic Antibiotic Given[2,3]	32	44%	83%	77%	95%
Prophylactic Antibiotic Selection[5]	-	-	90%	90%	100%
Prophylactic Antibiotic Stopped[2,3]	31	16%	70%	72%	95%

Pregnancy Care					
Inpatient Neonatal Mortality	-	-	-	-	-
Third or Fourth Degree Laceration	-	-	2.71%	3.63%	3.27%

Bayfront Medical Center

701 6th Street
Saint Petersburg, FL 33701
URL: www.bayfront.org
Ownership: Voluntary non-profit - Private
Emergency Services: Yes

Phone: 727-823-1234
Fax: 727-893-6962

Accredited: Yes
Licensed Beds: 502

Key Personnel:
CEO. . . . . Sue Brody

Measure	Cases	This Hospital	State Average	U.S. Average	Top Hospital
Heart Attack Care					
ACE Inhibitor or ARB for LVSD	26	77%	83%	82%	100%
Aspirin at Arrival	143	98%	93%	92%	100%
Aspirin at Discharge	168	91%	88%	90%	100%
Beta Blocker at Arrival	124	87%	89%	87%	100%
Beta Blocker at Discharge	168	88%	92%	90%	100%
Fibrinolytic Medication Timing[1]	2	0%	33%	31%	100%
PCI Within 90 Minutes of Arrival[1]	14	36%	52%	54%	95%
Smoking Cessation Advice	69	99%	92%	88%	100%
Heart Failure Care					
ACE Inhibitor or ARB for LVSD	134	90%	82%	82%	100%
Discharge Instructions	247	57%	61%	61%	93%
Evaluation of LVS Function	291	98%	90%	83%	99%
Smoking Cessation Advice	94	94%	91%	82%	100%
Pneumonia Care					
Appropriate Initial Antibiotic	166	95%	84%	83%	94%
Blood Culture Timing	162	86%	88%	90%	100%
Influenza Vaccine[1]	23	78%	64%	70%	100%
Initial Antibiotic Timing	218	89%	74%	80%	93%
Oxygenation Assessment	244	100%	99%	99%	100%
Pneumococcal Vaccine	115	77%	67%	69%	94%
Smoking Cessation Advice	63	94%	90%	80%	100%
Surgical Infection Prevention					
Prophylactic Antibiotic Given[2]	586	69%	83%	77%	95%
Prophylactic Antibiotic Selection[2]	64	94%	90%	90%	100%
Prophylactic Antibiotic Stopped[2]	559	66%	70%	72%	95%
Pregnancy Care					
Inpatient Neonatal Mortality	-	-	-	-	-
Third or Fourth Degree Laceration	-	-	2.71%	3.63%	3.27%

Edward White Hospital

2323 9th Avenue N
PO Box 12018
Saint Petersburg, FL 33733
URL: www.edwhitehospital.com
Ownership: Proprietary
Emergency Services: Yes

Phone: 727-323-1111
Fax: 727-328-6135

Accredited: Yes
Licensed Beds: 167

Key Personnel:
President/CEO. . . . . Roland Metivier
Emergency Room . . . . Beth Rud
Emergency Room . . . . Nagy Farag, MD
Infection Control. . . . . Michelle Haynes
ICU . . . . Claudia Leon
Medical/Surgical Nursing . . . . Roxene Riles
Director Respiratory Therapy . . . . Rick Lepak

Measure	Cases	This Hospital	State Average	U.S. Average	Top Hospital
Heart Attack Care					
ACE Inhibitor or ARB for LVSD[1]	5	100%	83%	82%	100%
Aspirin at Arrival	30	97%	93%	92%	100%
Aspirin at Discharge[1]	17	94%	88%	90%	100%

Beta Blocker at Arrival[1]	21	81%	89%	87%	100%
Beta Blocker at Discharge[1]	18	94%	92%	90%	100%
Fibrinolytic Medication Timing[1]	1	0%	33%	31%	100%
PCI Within 90 Minutes of Arrival	0	-	52%	54%	95%
Smoking Cessation Advice[1]	5	80%	92%	88%	100%

Heart Failure Care					
ACE Inhibitor or ARB for LVSD	33	82%	82%	82%	100%
Discharge Instructions	93	23%	61%	61%	93%
Evaluation of LVS Function	148	86%	90%	83%	99%
Smoking Cessation Advice[1]	21	90%	91%	82%	100%

Pneumonia Care					
Appropriate Initial Antibiotic	92	88%	84%	83%	94%
Blood Culture Timing	112	91%	88%	90%	100%
Influenza Vaccine	38	47%	64%	70%	100%
Initial Antibiotic Timing	154	92%	74%	80%	93%
Oxygenation Assessment	182	99%	99%	99%	100%
Pneumococcal Vaccine	115	53%	67%	69%	94%
Smoking Cessation Advice	45	84%	90%	80%	100%

Surgical Infection Prevention					
Prophylactic Antibiotic Given[3]	126	89%	83%	77%	95%
Prophylactic Antibiotic Selection	33	94%	90%	90%	100%
Prophylactic Antibiotic Stopped[3]	118	69%	70%	72%	95%

Pregnancy Care					
Inpatient Neonatal Mortality	-	-	-	-	-
Third or Fourth Degree Laceration	-	-	2.71%	3.63%	3.27%

Northside Hospital

6000 49th Street North
Saint Petersburg, FL 33709
URL: www.northsidehospital.com
Ownership: Proprietary
Emergency Services: Yes

Phone: 727-521-4411
Fax: 727-521-5007

Accredited: Yes
Licensed Beds: 288

Key Personnel:
President/CEO. . . . . Ward Boston III
Director Surgical Services . . . . Pat Ritter, RN

Measure	Cases	This Hospital	State Average	U.S. Average	Top Hospital
Heart Attack Care					
ACE Inhibitor or ARB for LVSD	37	95%	83%	82%	100%
Aspirin at Arrival	210	95%	93%	92%	100%
Aspirin at Discharge	257	97%	88%	90%	100%
Beta Blocker at Arrival	150	93%	89%	87%	100%
Beta Blocker at Discharge	270	96%	92%	90%	100%
Fibrinolytic Medication Timing[1]	1	100%	33%	31%	100%
PCI Within 90 Minutes of Arrival[1]	16	62%	52%	54%	95%
Smoking Cessation Advice	120	97%	92%	88%	100%
Heart Failure Care					
ACE Inhibitor or ARB for LVSD	98	83%	82%	82%	100%
Discharge Instructions	252	54%	61%	61%	93%
Evaluation of LVS Function	321	98%	90%	83%	99%
Smoking Cessation Advice	60	97%	91%	82%	100%
Pneumonia Care					
Appropriate Initial Antibiotic	275	81%	84%	83%	94%
Blood Culture Timing	222	94%	88%	90%	100%
Influenza Vaccine	73	41%	64%	70%	100%
Initial Antibiotic Timing	373	65%	74%	80%	93%
Oxygenation Assessment	411	100%	99%	99%	100%
Pneumococcal Vaccine	253	41%	67%	69%	94%
Smoking Cessation Advice	105	92%	90%	80%	100%
Surgical Infection Prevention					
Prophylactic Antibiotic Given[2,3]	228	85%	83%	77%	95%
Prophylactic Antibiotic Selection[2]	74	95%	90%	90%	100%
Prophylactic Antibiotic Stopped[2,3]	211	59%	70%	72%	95%
Pregnancy Care					
Inpatient Neonatal Mortality	-	-	-	-	-
Third or Fourth Degree Laceration	-	-	2.71%	3.63%	3.27%

NOTE: Hospital profiles are in alphabetical order by state, then city, then hospital within the city; Rankings are sorted by rate in descending order and exclude hospitals with less than 25 cases; (1) The number of cases is too small (n<25) for purposes of reliably predicting hospital performance; (2) Measure reflects the hospital's indication that its submission was based upon a sample of its relevant discharges; (3) Rate reflects fewer than the maximum possible quarters of data for the measure; (4) Inaccurate information submitted and suppressed for one or more quarters; (5) No data is available from the hospital for this measure; Please refer to the User's Guide for a full explanation of data

Palms of Pasadena Hospital

1501 Pasadena Avenue
Saint Petersburg, FL 33707
E-mail: palms@palmspasadena.com
URL: www.palmspasadena.com
Ownership: Proprietary
Emergency Services: Yes

Phone: 727-381-1000
Fax: 727-341-7009

Accredited: Yes
Licensed Beds: 307

Key Personnel:

CEO	Todd Nann
Chief Staff	Robert Wharton, MD
Director Cardiac Lab	Lynn Stilwell
Director Catheterization Lab	Lynn Stilwell
Emergency Room	Ian Aitken
Infection Control Manager	Phyllis Elliott
Medical Surgical Nursing	Rick Wilson
Director Radiology	Stephanie Poveromo
Director Respiratory Therapy	Kathy Jacobs

Measure	Cases	This Hospital	State Average	U.S. Average	Top Hospital
Heart Attack Care					
ACE Inhibitor or ARB for LVSD[1]	4	100%	83%	82%	100%
Aspirin at Arrival	44	100%	93%	92%	100%
Aspirin at Discharge[1]	20	100%	88%	90%	100%
Beta Blocker at Arrival	44	98%	89%	87%	100%
Beta Blocker at Discharge[1]	19	100%	92%	90%	100%
Fibrinolytic Medication Timing	0	-	33%	31%	100%
PCI Within 90 Minutes of Arrival	0	-	52%	54%	95%
Smoking Cessation Advice[1]	2	100%	92%	88%	100%
Heart Failure Care					
ACE Inhibitor or ARB for LVSD	42	93%	82%	82%	100%
Discharge Instructions	132	70%	61%	61%	93%
Evaluation of LVS Function	176	86%	90%	83%	99%
Smoking Cessation Advice[1]	23	78%	91%	82%	100%
Pneumonia Care					
Appropriate Initial Antibiotic	136	87%	84%	83%	94%
Blood Culture Timing	150	69%	88%	90%	100%
Influenza Vaccine[4,5]	-	-	64%	70%	100%
Initial Antibiotic Timing	199	73%	74%	80%	93%
Oxygenation Assessment	247	98%	99%	99%	100%
Pneumococcal Vaccine	188	63%	67%	69%	94%
Smoking Cessation Advice	39	77%	90%	80%	100%
Surgical Infection Prevention					
Prophylactic Antibiotic Given	336	92%	83%	77%	95%
Prophylactic Antibiotic Selection	80	91%	90%	90%	100%
Prophylactic Antibiotic Stopped	313	42%	70%	72%	95%
Pregnancy Care					
Inpatient Neonatal Mortality	-	-	-	-	-
Third or Fourth Degree Laceration	-	-	2.71%	3.63%	3.27%

Saint Anthony's Hospital

Alternate Name: Saint Joseph's/ Saint Anthony's Health System
1200 7th Avenue N
Saint Petersburg, FL 33705
URL: www.stanthonys.com
Ownership: Voluntary non-profit - Church
Emergency Services: Yes

Phone: 727-825-1100
Fax: 727-825-1302

Accredited: Yes
Licensed Beds: 405

Key Personnel:

CEO	Sue Brody
Chief Medical Staff	John Peterson, MD
Emergency Room	R Michael Smith, MD
Director Medical/Surgical Nursing	Karen Sondregger
Director Radiology	Barbara Smith

Measure	Cases	This Hospital	State Average	U.S. Average	Top Hospital
Heart Attack Care					
ACE Inhibitor or ARB for LVSD[1]	17	94%	83%	82%	100%
Aspirin at Arrival	104	93%	93%	92%	100%
Aspirin at Discharge	73	93%	88%	90%	100%
Beta Blocker at Arrival	85	93%	89%	87%	100%
Beta Blocker at Discharge	75	92%	92%	90%	100%
Fibrinolytic Medication Timing	0	-	33%	31%	100%
PCI Within 90 Minutes of Arrival	0	-	52%	54%	95%
Smoking Cessation Advice	30	100%	92%	88%	100%

Measure	Cases	This Hospital	State Average	U.S. Average	Top Hospital
Heart Failure Care					
ACE Inhibitor or ARB for LVSD	98	89%	82%	82%	100%
Discharge Instructions	217	83%	61%	61%	93%
Evaluation of LVS Function	281	87%	90%	83%	99%
Smoking Cessation Advice	69	100%	91%	82%	100%
Pneumonia Care					
Appropriate Initial Antibiotic	188	88%	84%	83%	94%
Blood Culture Timing	200	92%	88%	90%	100%
Influenza Vaccine	58	62%	64%	70%	100%
Initial Antibiotic Timing	219	75%	74%	80%	93%
Oxygenation Assessment	372	100%	99%	99%	100%
Pneumococcal Vaccine	183	64%	67%	69%	94%
Smoking Cessation Advice	112	98%	90%	80%	100%
Surgical Infection Prevention					
Prophylactic Antibiotic Given[2]	149	84%	83%	77%	95%
Prophylactic Antibiotic Selection[2]	49	84%	90%	90%	100%
Prophylactic Antibiotic Stopped[2]	136	57%	70%	72%	95%
Pregnancy Care					
Inpatient Neonatal Mortality	-	-	-	-	-
Third or Fourth Degree Laceration	-	-	2.71%	3.63%	3.27%

Saint Petersburg General Hospital

Alternate Name: Columbia Saint Petersburg Medical Center
6500 38th Avenue N
Saint Petersburg, FL 33710
URL: www.stpetemedical.com
Ownership: Proprietary
Emergency Services: Yes

Phone: 727-384-1414
Fax: 727-341-4889

Accredited: Yes
Licensed Beds: 219

Key Personnel:

CEO	Daniel J Friedrich
Chief Medical Staff	James Neiman, MD
Cardiopulmonary Vascular Services	Debby Warson
ICU	Debby Garreck
OB/GYN Womens Health	Romeo Acosta, MD
Director Radiology	Judy Gonzalez

Measure	Cases	This Hospital	State Average	U.S. Average	Top Hospital
Heart Attack Care					
ACE Inhibitor or ARB for LVSD[1]	4	75%	83%	82%	100%
Aspirin at Arrival	60	88%	93%	92%	100%
Aspirin at Discharge[1]	21	90%	88%	90%	100%
Beta Blocker at Arrival	33	97%	89%	87%	100%
Beta Blocker at Discharge[1]	24	100%	92%	90%	100%
Fibrinolytic Medication Timing	0	-	33%	31%	100%
PCI Within 90 Minutes of Arrival	0	-	52%	54%	95%
Smoking Cessation Advice[1]	5	100%	92%	88%	100%
Heart Failure Care					
ACE Inhibitor or ARB for LVSD	39	77%	82%	82%	100%
Discharge Instructions	85	42%	61%	61%	93%
Evaluation of LVS Function	134	94%	90%	83%	99%
Smoking Cessation Advice	28	86%	91%	82%	100%
Pneumonia Care					
Appropriate Initial Antibiotic	136	84%	84%	83%	94%
Blood Culture Timing	149	83%	88%	90%	100%
Influenza Vaccine	45	40%	64%	70%	100%
Initial Antibiotic Timing	228	77%	74%	80%	93%
Oxygenation Assessment	278	99%	99%	99%	100%
Pneumococcal Vaccine	162	39%	67%	69%	94%
Smoking Cessation Advice	66	89%	90%	80%	100%
Surgical Infection Prevention					
Prophylactic Antibiotic Given[3]	225	91%	83%	77%	95%
Prophylactic Antibiotic Selection	67	93%	90%	90%	100%
Prophylactic Antibiotic Stopped[3]	221	71%	70%	72%	95%
Pregnancy Care					
Inpatient Neonatal Mortality	1,587	0.06%	-	-	-
Third or Fourth Degree Laceration	1,125	1.87%	2.71%	3.63%	3.27%

Central Florida Regional Hospital

Alternate Name: Columbia Medical Center Sanford

NOTE: Hospital profiles are in alphabetical order by state, then city, then hospital within the city; Rankings are sorted by rate in descending order and exclude hospitals with less than 25 cases; (1) The number of cases is too small (n<25) for purposes of reliably predicting hospital performance; (2) Measure reflects the hospital's indication that its submission was based upon a sample of its relevant discharges; (3) Rate reflects fewer than the maximum possible quarters of data for the measure; (4) Inaccurate information submitted and suppressed for one or more quarters; (5) No data is available from the hospital for this measure; Please refer to the User's Guide for a full explanation of data

1401 W Seminole Boulevard
Sanford, FL 32771
URL: www.centralfloridaregional.com
Ownership: Proprietary
Emergency Services: Yes

Phone: 407-321-4500
Fax: 407-302-7310

Accredited: Yes
Licensed Beds: 226

Key Personnel:
CEO.................................... Rodney Smith
Emergency Room .... Linda Breum
Director Medical/Surgical Nursing .... Michelle Bourassa
OB/GYN Womens Health................. Jackie Bianco
Director Respiratory Therapy .... Jerry Lockett

Measure	Cases	This Hospital	State Average	U.S. Average	Top Hospital
Heart Attack Care					
ACE Inhibitor or ARB for LVSD	48	77%	83%	82%	100%
Aspirin at Arrival	160	96%	93%	92%	100%
Aspirin at Discharge	224	96%	88%	90%	100%
Beta Blocker at Arrival	113	89%	89%	87%	100%
Beta Blocker at Discharge	240	94%	92%	90%	100%
Fibrinolytic Medication Timing[1]	3	33%	33%	31%	100%
PCI Within 90 Minutes of Arrival[1]	6	17%	52%	54%	95%
Smoking Cessation Advice	89	97%	92%	88%	100%
Heart Failure Care					
ACE Inhibitor or ARB for LVSD	118	75%	82%	82%	100%
Discharge Instructions	283	66%	61%	61%	93%
Evaluation of LVS Function	356	91%	90%	83%	99%
Smoking Cessation Advice	97	92%	91%	82%	100%
Pneumonia Care					
Appropriate Initial Antibiotic	149	87%	84%	83%	94%
Blood Culture Timing	104	80%	88%	90%	100%
Influenza Vaccine	45	49%	64%	70%	100%
Initial Antibiotic Timing	217	56%	74%	80%	93%
Oxygenation Assessment	244	98%	99%	99%	100%
Pneumococcal Vaccine	124	47%	67%	69%	94%
Smoking Cessation Advice	68	87%	90%	80%	100%
Surgical Infection Prevention					
Prophylactic Antibiotic Given[2,3]	390	83%	83%	77%	95%
Prophylactic Antibiotic Selection[2]	100	92%	90%	90%	100%
Prophylactic Antibiotic Stopped[2,3]	364	75%	70%	72%	95%
Pregnancy Care					
Inpatient Neonatal Mortality	-	-	-	-	-
Third or Fourth Degree Laceration	-	-	2.71%	3.63%	3.27%

Doctors Hospital of Sarasota

Alternate Name: Doctor's Hospital
5731 Bee Ridge Road
Sarasota, FL 34233
URL: www.doctorsofsarasota.com
Ownership: Proprietary
Emergency Services: No

Phone: 941-342-1100
Fax: 941-377-7127

Accredited: No
Licensed Beds: 168

Key Personnel:
CEO.................................... Lindell F Om
Vice Chief Surgery........................ Richard Golub, MD

Measure	Cases	This Hospital	State Average	U.S. Average	Top Hospital
Heart Attack Care					
ACE Inhibitor or ARB for LVSD[1]	8	75%	83%	82%	100%
Aspirin at Arrival	65	89%	93%	92%	100%
Aspirin at Discharge	35	91%	88%	90%	100%
Beta Blocker at Arrival	29	79%	89%	87%	100%
Beta Blocker at Discharge	34	94%	92%	90%	100%
Fibrinolytic Medication Timing[1]	2	0%	33%	31%	100%
PCI Within 90 Minutes of Arrival	0	-	52%	54%	95%
Smoking Cessation Advice[1]	4	100%	92%	88%	100%
Heart Failure Care					
ACE Inhibitor or ARB for LVSD	65	85%	82%	82%	100%
Discharge Instructions	129	66%	61%	61%	93%
Evaluation of LVS Function	194	96%	90%	83%	99%
Smoking Cessation Advice	25	96%	91%	82%	100%
Pneumonia Care					
Appropriate Initial Antibiotic	122	87%	84%	83%	94%
Blood Culture Timing	103	87%	88%	90%	100%
Influenza Vaccine	53	70%	64%	70%	100%

Measure	Cases	This Hospital	State Average	U.S. Average	Top Hospital
Initial Antibiotic Timing	193	76%	74%	80%	93%
Oxygenation Assessment	229	100%	99%	99%	100%
Pneumococcal Vaccine	171	67%	67%	69%	94%
Smoking Cessation Advice	59	90%	90%	80%	100%
Surgical Infection Prevention					
Prophylactic Antibiotic Given[2]	226	92%	83%	77%	95%
Prophylactic Antibiotic Selection[2]	72	97%	90%	90%	100%
Prophylactic Antibiotic Stopped[2]	219	73%	70%	72%	95%
Pregnancy Care					
Inpatient Neonatal Mortality	-	-	-	-	-
Third or Fourth Degree Laceration	-	-	2.71%	3.63%	3.27%

Sarasota Memorial Health Care Systems

Alternate Name: Sarasota Memorial Hospital
1700 S Tamiami Trail
Sarasota, FL 34239

Toll-Free: 800-764-8255
Phone: 941-917-9000
Fax: 941-917-1930

E-mail: webcoordinator@smh.com
URL: www.smh.com
Ownership: Govt - Hospital District or Authority
Emergency Services: Yes

Accredited: Yes
Licensed Beds: 845

Key Personnel:
President/CEO........................ Gwen M MacKenzie, RN/MN
Chief Medical Officer .... Bernard Feinberg, MD
Catheterization Lab .... Brenda Koval
Emergency Room .... Judy Rathje
Infection Control........................ Susan Gray, RN
ICU .... Marie Barth
Intensive/Coronary Care .... Marie Barth
CNO & VP Medical/Surgical............... Lynn Whisman
OB/GYN Womens Health................. Mary Kay Capuano
Respiratory/Cardiopulmonary............. Rick Harrell

Measure	Cases	This Hospital	State Average	U.S. Average	Top Hospital
Heart Attack Care					
ACE Inhibitor or ARB for LVSD	141	87%	83%	82%	100%
Aspirin at Arrival	420	96%	93%	92%	100%
Aspirin at Discharge	528	97%	88%	90%	100%
Beta Blocker at Arrival	389	95%	89%	87%	100%
Beta Blocker at Discharge	548	94%	92%	90%	100%
Fibrinolytic Medication Timing[1]	1	0%	33%	31%	100%
PCI Within 90 Minutes of Arrival[1]	7	29%	52%	54%	95%
Smoking Cessation Advice	142	91%	92%	88%	100%
Heart Failure Care					
ACE Inhibitor or ARB for LVSD	233	84%	82%	82%	100%
Discharge Instructions	423	35%	61%	61%	93%
Evaluation of LVS Function	580	93%	90%	83%	99%
Smoking Cessation Advice	68	94%	91%	82%	100%
Pneumonia Care					
Appropriate Initial Antibiotic	221	82%	84%	83%	94%
Blood Culture Timing	222	87%	88%	90%	100%
Influenza Vaccine	57	67%	64%	70%	100%
Initial Antibiotic Timing	320	79%	74%	80%	93%
Oxygenation Assessment	421	100%	99%	99%	100%
Pneumococcal Vaccine	282	86%	67%	69%	94%
Smoking Cessation Advice	78	82%	90%	80%	100%
Surgical Infection Prevention					
Prophylactic Antibiotic Given	771	83%	83%	77%	95%
Prophylactic Antibiotic Selection	192	96%	90%	90%	100%
Prophylactic Antibiotic Stopped	754	73%	70%	72%	95%
Pregnancy Care					
Inpatient Neonatal Mortality	-	-	-	-	-
Third or Fourth Degree Laceration	-	-	2.71%	3.63%	3.27%

Sebastian River Medical Center

13695 US Highway 1
Sebastian, FL 32958
E-mail: info@srmc.hma-corp.com
URL: www.srmcenter.com
Ownership: Proprietary
Emergency Services: Yes

Phone: 772-589-3186
Fax: 772-388-3689

Accredited: Yes
Licensed Beds: 129

Key Personnel:
President/CEO........................ Kathy A Burke

NOTE: Hospital profiles are in alphabetical order by state, then city, then hospital within the city; Rankings are sorted by rate in descending order and exclude hospitals with less than 25 cases; (1) The number of cases is too small (n<25) for purposes of reliably predicting hospital performance; (2) Measure reflects the hospital's indication that its submission was based upon a sample of its relevant discharges; (3) Rate reflects fewer than the maximum possible quarters of data for the measure; (4) Inaccurate information submitted and suppressed for one or more quarters; (5) No data is available from the hospital for this measure; Please refer to the User's Guide for a full explanation of data

Chief Medical Staff. . . . . Ralph Geiger, MD
Emergency Room . . . . Debora Yarborough
Surgical Services . . . . Pattie Lefebvre
Infection Control. . . . . Denise Stidham, RN
ICU . . . . Debora Yarborough
Cardiopulmonary Director . . . . Peggy Craft

Measure	Cases	This Hospital	State Average	U.S. Average	Top Hospital
Heart Attack Care					
ACE Inhibitor or ARB for LVSD[1]	11	91%	83%	82%	100%
Aspirin at Arrival	63	98%	93%	92%	100%
Aspirin at Discharge	25	96%	88%	90%	100%
Beta Blocker at Arrival	59	95%	89%	87%	100%
Beta Blocker at Discharge[1]	24	100%	92%	90%	100%
Fibrinolytic Medication Timing[1]	2	0%	33%	31%	100%
PCI Within 90 Minutes of Arrival	0	-	52%	54%	95%
Smoking Cessation Advice[1]	3	67%	92%	88%	100%
Heart Failure Care					
ACE Inhibitor or ARB for LVSD	96	92%	82%	82%	100%
Discharge Instructions	175	62%	61%	61%	93%
Evaluation of LVS Function	153	47%	90%	83%	99%
Smoking Cessation Advice	32	91%	91%	82%	100%
Pneumonia Care					
Appropriate Initial Antibiotic	187	77%	84%	83%	94%
Blood Culture Timing	121	79%	88%	90%	100%
Influenza Vaccine	60	75%	64%	70%	100%
Initial Antibiotic Timing	188	73%	74%	80%	93%
Oxygenation Assessment	239	99%	99%	99%	100%
Pneumococcal Vaccine	198	78%	67%	69%	94%
Smoking Cessation Advice	57	86%	90%	80%	100%
Surgical Infection Prevention					
Prophylactic Antibiotic Given[2]	204	94%	83%	77%	95%
Prophylactic Antibiotic Selection[2]	46	93%	90%	90%	100%
Prophylactic Antibiotic Stopped[2]	195	93%	70%	72%	95%
Pregnancy Care					
Inpatient Neonatal Mortality	-	-	-	-	-
Third or Fourth Degree Laceration	-	-	2.71%	3.63%	3.27%

Florida Hospital Heartland Medical Center

4200 Sun 'n Lake Boulevard
PO Box 9400
Sebring, FL 33871
URL: www.fhhd.org
Ownership: Voluntary non-profit - Church
Emergency Services: Yes

Phone: 863-314-4466
Fax: 863-402-3415

Accredited: Yes
Licensed Beds: 111

Key Personnel:
President/CEO. . . . . John Harding
Emergency Room . . . . Debra Vaugh

Measure	Cases	This Hospital	State Average	U.S. Average	Top Hospital
Heart Attack Care					
ACE Inhibitor or ARB for LVSD	31	90%	83%	82%	100%
Aspirin at Arrival	119	87%	93%	92%	100%
Aspirin at Discharge	59	92%	88%	90%	100%
Beta Blocker at Arrival	90	86%	89%	87%	100%
Beta Blocker at Discharge	77	99%	92%	90%	100%
Fibrinolytic Medication Timing[1]	2	0%	33%	31%	100%
PCI Within 90 Minutes of Arrival	0	-	52%	54%	95%
Smoking Cessation Advice[1]	13	77%	92%	88%	100%
Heart Failure Care					
ACE Inhibitor or ARB for LVSD	206	71%	82%	82%	100%
Discharge Instructions	382	58%	61%	61%	93%
Evaluation of LVS Function	476	94%	90%	83%	99%
Smoking Cessation Advice	87	91%	91%	82%	100%
Pneumonia Care					
Appropriate Initial Antibiotic	193	90%	84%	83%	94%
Blood Culture Timing	137	87%	88%	90%	100%
Influenza Vaccine	57	74%	64%	70%	100%
Initial Antibiotic Timing	257	69%	74%	80%	93%
Oxygenation Assessment	287	100%	99%	99%	100%
Pneumococcal Vaccine	210	78%	67%	69%	94%
Smoking Cessation Advice	50	88%	90%	80%	100%

Surgical Infection Prevention					
Prophylactic Antibiotic Given	434	88%	83%	77%	95%
Prophylactic Antibiotic Selection	94	97%	90%	90%	100%
Prophylactic Antibiotic Stopped	418	71%	70%	72%	95%
Pregnancy Care					
Inpatient Neonatal Mortality	1,069	0.94%	-	-	-
Third or Fourth Degree Laceration	726	1.24%	2.71%	3.63%	3.27%

Highlands Regional Medical Center

3600 S Highlands Avenue
Sebring, FL 33870
URL: www.highlandsregional.com
Ownership: Proprietary
Emergency Services: Yes

Phone: 863-385-6101
Fax: 863-385-3489

Accredited: Yes
Licensed Beds: 126

Key Personnel:
CEO/Administrator. Robert G Mahaffey
Chief Medical Staff. P Chockalingam
Emergency Room . . . . Annie Haynen
Emergency Room . . . . Dorothy Reed, RN
Director Medical/Surgical Nursing . . . . Sherri Maiel, RN
Director of Pulmonary/Respiratory Care. . . . . . . Dan Chianand

Measure	Cases	This Hospital	State Average	U.S. Average	Top Hospital
Heart Attack Care					
ACE Inhibitor or ARB for LVSD[1]	5	40%	83%	82%	100%
Aspirin at Arrival	44	91%	93%	92%	100%
Aspirin at Discharge[1]	21	71%	88%	90%	100%
Beta Blocker at Arrival	39	95%	89%	87%	100%
Beta Blocker at Discharge[1]	24	75%	92%	90%	100%
Fibrinolytic Medication Timing[1]	2	0%	33%	31%	100%
PCI Within 90 Minutes of Arrival	0	-	52%	54%	95%
Smoking Cessation Advice[1]	4	100%	92%	88%	100%
Heart Failure Care					
ACE Inhibitor or ARB for LVSD	58	66%	82%	82%	100%
Discharge Instructions	160	29%	61%	61%	93%
Evaluation of LVS Function	208	83%	90%	83%	99%
Smoking Cessation Advice[1]	21	95%	91%	82%	100%
Pneumonia Care					
Appropriate Initial Antibiotic	150	71%	84%	83%	94%
Blood Culture Timing	123	93%	88%	90%	100%
Influenza Vaccine	56	46%	64%	70%	100%
Initial Antibiotic Timing	183	60%	74%	80%	93%
Oxygenation Assessment	206	100%	99%	99%	100%
Pneumococcal Vaccine	149	64%	67%	69%	94%
Smoking Cessation Advice	28	79%	90%	80%	100%
Surgical Infection Prevention					
Prophylactic Antibiotic Given[2]	135	53%	83%	77%	95%
Prophylactic Antibiotic Selection[1,2]	23	96%	90%	90%	100%
Prophylactic Antibiotic Stopped[2]	126	62%	70%	72%	95%
Pregnancy Care					
Inpatient Neonatal Mortality	-	-	-	-	-
Third or Fourth Degree Laceration	-	-	2.71%	3.63%	3.27%

Larkin Community Hospital

7031 SW 62nd Avenue
South Miami, FL 33143
E-mail: sgonzalez@larkinhospital.com
URL: www.larkinhospital.com
Ownership: Proprietary
Emergency Services: Yes

Phone: 305-284-7500
Fax: 305-284-7545

Accredited: Yes
Licensed Beds: 112

Key Personnel:
CEO. . . . . Jack J Michel, MD
Chief Medical Staff. Gustavo Leon
Emergency Room . . . . Pauline Radix
Director Infection Control . . . . Marcia Trader
Director Radiology . . . . Ellen Sconyers
Director Respiratory Therapy . . . . Lydia Nolan

Measure	Cases	This Hospital	State Average	U.S. Average	Top Hospital
Heart Attack Care					
ACE Inhibitor or ARB for LVSD[1]	3	100%	83%	82%	100%
Aspirin at Arrival	31	97%	93%	92%	100%
Aspirin at Discharge[1]	13	92%	88%	90%	100%

NOTE: Hospital profiles are in alphabetical order by state, then city, then hospital within the city; Rankings are sorted by rate in descending order and exclude hospitals with less than 25 cases; (1) The number of cases is too small (n<25) for purposes of reliably predicting hospital performance; (2) Measure reflects the hospital's indication that its submission was based upon a sample of its relevant discharges; (3) Rate reflects fewer than the maximum possible quarters of data for the measure; (4) Inaccurate information submitted and suppressed for one or more quarters; (5) No data is available from the hospital for this measure; Please refer to the User's Guide for a full explanation of data

Beta Blocker at Arrival	27	93%	89%	87%	100%
Beta Blocker at Discharge[1]	15	93%	92%	90%	100%
Fibrinolytic Medication Timing[1]	1	0%	33%	31%	100%
PCI Within 90 Minutes of Arrival	0	-	52%	54%	95%
Smoking Cessation Advice[1]	9	100%	92%	88%	100%
Heart Failure Care					
ACE Inhibitor or ARB for LVSD[1]	12	100%	82%	82%	100%
Discharge Instructions	41	98%	61%	61%	93%
Evaluation of LVS Function	73	89%	90%	83%	99%
Smoking Cessation Advice[1]	8	100%	91%	82%	100%
Pneumonia Care					
Appropriate Initial Antibiotic	65	75%	84%	83%	94%
Blood Culture Timing	83	90%	88%	90%	100%
Influenza Vaccine	29	76%	64%	70%	100%
Initial Antibiotic Timing	120	75%	74%	80%	93%
Oxygenation Assessment	135	100%	99%	99%	100%
Pneumococcal Vaccine	77	86%	67%	69%	94%
Smoking Cessation Advice	49	100%	90%	80%	100%
Surgical Infection Prevention					
Prophylactic Antibiotic Given[1]	24	100%	83%	77%	95%
Prophylactic Antibiotic Selection[1]	3	100%	90%	90%	100%
Prophylactic Antibiotic Stopped[1]	9	100%	70%	72%	95%
Pregnancy Care					
Inpatient Neonatal Mortality	-	-	-	-	-
Third or Fourth Degree Laceration	-	-	2.71%	3.63%	3.27%

Shands at Starke

Alternate Name: Bradford Hospital
922 E Call Street
Starke, FL 32091
URL: www.shands.com
Ownership: Voluntary non-profit - Private
Emergency Services: Yes

Phone: 904-368-2300
Fax: 904-368-2306

Accredited: Yes
Licensed Beds: 49

Key Personnel:
CEO . . . . Jeannie Baker
Chief Medical Staff . . . . Carl Eison
Emergency Room . . . . Dann Mann
Director Medical/Surgical Nursing . . . . Martha Epps

Measure	Cases	This Hospital	State Average	U.S. Average	Top Hospital
Heart Attack Care					
ACE Inhibitor or ARB for LVSD[3]	0	-	83%	82%	100%
Aspirin at Arrival[1,3]	3	67%	93%	92%	100%
Aspirin at Discharge[1,3]	1	100%	88%	90%	100%
Beta Blocker at Arrival[1,3]	3	0%	89%	87%	100%
Beta Blocker at Discharge[1,3]	1	100%	92%	90%	100%
Fibrinolytic Medication Timing[1,3]	1	100%	33%	31%	100%
PCI Within 90 Minutes of Arrival	0	-	52%	54%	95%
Smoking Cessation Advice[3]	0	-	92%	88%	100%
Heart Failure Care					
ACE Inhibitor or ARB for LVSD[1]	21	90%	82%	82%	100%
Discharge Instructions	43	93%	61%	61%	93%
Evaluation of LVS Function	58	93%	90%	83%	99%
Smoking Cessation Advice[1]	13	92%	91%	82%	100%
Pneumonia Care					
Appropriate Initial Antibiotic	39	82%	84%	83%	94%
Blood Culture Timing[1]	23	78%	88%	90%	100%
Influenza Vaccine[1]	6	100%	64%	70%	100%
Initial Antibiotic Timing	52	83%	74%	80%	93%
Oxygenation Assessment	64	100%	99%	99%	100%
Pneumococcal Vaccine	30	83%	67%	69%	94%
Smoking Cessation Advice[1]	8	75%	90%	80%	100%
Surgical Infection Prevention					
Prophylactic Antibiotic Given[1,3]	1	100%	83%	77%	95%
Prophylactic Antibiotic Selection[1]	1	0%	90%	90%	100%
Prophylactic Antibiotic Stopped[1,3]	1	100%	70%	72%	95%
Pregnancy Care					
Inpatient Neonatal Mortality	-	-	-	-	-
Third or Fourth Degree Laceration	-	-	2.71%	3.63%	3.27%

Martin Memorial Medical Center

Alternate Name: Martin Memorial Hospital

300 Hospital Avenue
Stuart, FL 34994
URL: www.mmhs.com
Ownership: Voluntary non-profit - Private
Emergency Services: Yes

Phone: 772-287-5200
Fax: 772-223-2801

Accredited: Yes
Licensed Beds: 236

Key Personnel:
President/CEO . . . . Richmond M Harman
Chief Medical Officer . . . . Howard M Robbins, MD
Infection Control . . . . Lynn Sullivan
Medical/Surgical Nursing . . . . Karen Ripper
OB/GYN Womens Health . . . . Kathy Rowell

Measure	Cases	This Hospital	State Average	U.S. Average	Top Hospital
Heart Attack Care					
ACE Inhibitor or ARB for LVSD	36	78%	83%	82%	100%
Aspirin at Arrival	149	95%	93%	92%	100%
Aspirin at Discharge	91	91%	88%	90%	100%
Beta Blocker at Arrival	106	90%	89%	87%	100%
Beta Blocker at Discharge	109	90%	92%	90%	100%
Fibrinolytic Medication Timing[1]	10	30%	33%	31%	100%
PCI Within 90 Minutes of Arrival[1]	5	40%	52%	54%	95%
Smoking Cessation Advice[1]	16	100%	92%	88%	100%
Heart Failure Care					
ACE Inhibitor or ARB for LVSD	101	84%	82%	82%	100%
Discharge Instructions	208	42%	61%	61%	93%
Evaluation of LVS Function	270	94%	90%	83%	99%
Smoking Cessation Advice	34	100%	91%	82%	100%
Pneumonia Care					
Appropriate Initial Antibiotic	82	87%	84%	83%	94%
Blood Culture Timing	105	85%	88%	90%	100%
Influenza Vaccine[4,5]	-	-	64%	70%	100%
Initial Antibiotic Timing	153	78%	74%	80%	93%
Oxygenation Assessment	179	100%	99%	99%	100%
Pneumococcal Vaccine	127	57%	67%	69%	94%
Smoking Cessation Advice	29	100%	90%	80%	100%
Surgical Infection Prevention					
Prophylactic Antibiotic Given	241	91%	83%	77%	95%
Prophylactic Antibiotic Selection	71	94%	90%	90%	100%
Prophylactic Antibiotic Stopped	221	72%	70%	72%	95%
Pregnancy Care					
Inpatient Neonatal Mortality	-	-	-	-	-
Third or Fourth Degree Laceration	-	-	2.71%	3.63%	3.27%

South Bay Hospital

4016 Sun City Center Boulevard
Sun City Center, FL 33573
URL: www.southbayhospital.com
Ownership: Voluntary non-profit - Other
Emergency Services: Yes

Phone: 813-634-3301
Fax: 813-634-0466

Accredited: Yes
Licensed Beds: 112

Key Personnel:
CEO . . . . Steve Rector
CNO . . . . Terrie Jefferson

Measure	Cases	This Hospital	State Average	U.S. Average	Top Hospital
Heart Attack Care					
ACE Inhibitor or ARB for LVSD[1]	13	54%	83%	82%	100%
Aspirin at Arrival	95	84%	93%	92%	100%
Aspirin at Discharge	42	79%	88%	90%	100%
Beta Blocker at Arrival	62	71%	89%	87%	100%
Beta Blocker at Discharge	53	92%	92%	90%	100%
Fibrinolytic Medication Timing	0	-	33%	31%	100%
PCI Within 90 Minutes of Arrival	0	-	52%	54%	95%
Smoking Cessation Advice[1]	3	100%	92%	88%	100%
Heart Failure Care					
ACE Inhibitor or ARB for LVSD	102	59%	82%	82%	100%
Discharge Instructions	253	49%	61%	61%	93%
Evaluation of LVS Function	338	93%	90%	83%	99%
Smoking Cessation Advice	41	95%	91%	82%	100%
Pneumonia Care					
Appropriate Initial Antibiotic	174	79%	84%	83%	94%
Blood Culture Timing	170	91%	88%	90%	100%
Influenza Vaccine	70	60%	64%	70%	100%
Initial Antibiotic Timing	238	73%	74%	80%	93%

NOTE: Hospital profiles are in alphabetical order by state, then city, then hospital within the city; Rankings are sorted by rate in descending order and exclude hospitals with less than 25 cases; (1) The number of cases is too small (n<25) for purposes of reliably predicting hospital performance; (2) Measure reflects the hospital's indication that its submission was based upon a sample of its relevant discharges; (3) Rate reflects fewer than the maximum possible quarters of data for the measure; (4) Inaccurate information submitted and suppressed for one or more quarters; (5) No data is available from the hospital for this measure; Please refer to the User's Guide for a full explanation of data

Measure	Cases	This Hospital	State Average	U.S. Average	Top Hospital
Oxygenation Assessment	286	98%	99%	99%	100%
Pneumococcal Vaccine	206	47%	67%	69%	94%
Smoking Cessation Advice	60	100%	90%	80%	100%
Surgical Infection Prevention					
Prophylactic Antibiotic Given[3]	227	87%	83%	77%	95%
Prophylactic Antibiotic Selection	66	92%	90%	90%	100%
Prophylactic Antibiotic Stopped[3]	219	61%	70%	72%	95%
Pregnancy Care					
Inpatient Neonatal Mortality	-	-	-	-	-
Third or Fourth Degree Laceration	-	-	2.71%	3.63%	3.27%

Capital Regional Medical Center

2626 Capital Medical Boulevard
Tallahassee, FL 32308
URL: www.capitalregionalmedicalcenter.com
Ownership: Proprietary
Emergency Services: Yes

Phone: 850-656-5000
Fax: 850-656-5198

Accredited: Yes
Licensed Beds: 198

Key Personnel:
CEO. . . . . Sharon Roush
Chief Medical Staff. . . . . John Thoebes, MD
Cardiac Service Line . . . . Barry Hamp
Emergency Room . . . . Susie West
Infection Control . . . . Carol Frank, RN
OB/GYN Women's Health . . . . Kathy Keane, RN
Director Respiratory Therapy . . . . Curt Varner

Measure	Cases	This Hospital	State Average	U.S. Average	Top Hospital
Heart Attack Care					
ACE Inhibitor or ARB for LVSD	39	79%	83%	82%	100%
Aspirin at Arrival	89	88%	93%	92%	100%
Aspirin at Discharge	86	88%	88%	90%	100%
Beta Blocker at Arrival	69	86%	89%	87%	100%
Beta Blocker at Discharge	95	83%	92%	90%	100%
Fibrinolytic Medication Timing	0	-	33%	31%	100%
PCI Within 90 Minutes of Arrival[1]	4	50%	52%	54%	95%
Smoking Cessation Advice	33	97%	92%	88%	100%
Heart Failure Care					
ACE Inhibitor or ARB for LVSD	158	70%	82%	82%	100%
Discharge Instructions	307	17%	61%	61%	93%
Evaluation of LVS Function	395	96%	90%	83%	99%
Smoking Cessation Advice	73	86%	91%	82%	100%
Pneumonia Care					
Appropriate Initial Antibiotic	86	80%	84%	83%	94%
Blood Culture Timing	86	84%	88%	90%	100%
Influenza Vaccine[1]	22	50%	64%	70%	100%
Initial Antibiotic Timing	139	68%	74%	80%	93%
Oxygenation Assessment	152	100%	99%	99%	100%
Pneumococcal Vaccine	77	68%	67%	69%	94%
Smoking Cessation Advice	40	90%	90%	80%	100%
Surgical Infection Prevention					
Prophylactic Antibiotic Given[3]	321	87%	83%	77%	95%
Prophylactic Antibiotic Selection	26	73%	90%	90%	100%
Prophylactic Antibiotic Stopped[3]	312	61%	70%	72%	95%
Pregnancy Care					
Inpatient Neonatal Mortality	972	0.41%	-	-	-
Third or Fourth Degree Laceration	617	3.24%	2.71%	3.63%	3.27%

Tallahassee Memorial Health Care Foundation

1300 Miccosukee Road
Tallahassee, FL 32308
URL: www.tmh.org
Ownership: Voluntary non-profit - Private
Emergency Services: Yes

Phone: 850-431-1155
Fax: 850-431-6489

Accredited: Yes
Licensed Beds: 770

Key Personnel:
President/CEO. . . . . G Mark O'Bryant
Chief Medical Officer . . . . John Mahoney, MD
Administrator Cardiology . . . . Lisa Mullee
Emergency Room . . . . Cathy Heimbecher, RN
Infection Control. . . . . Martha DeCastro, RN
Chief Medical Officer . . . . Richard I MacArthur, MD
OB/GYN Womens Health. . . . . Robin Schoeder, RN
Administrator Surgical Services . . . . Ton McLaren
Respiratory/Cardiopulmonary. . . . . Furman Cummings

Measure	Cases	This Hospital	State Average	U.S. Average	Top Hospital
Heart Attack Care					
ACE Inhibitor or ARB for LVSD	121	91%	83%	82%	100%
Aspirin at Arrival	314	96%	93%	92%	100%
Aspirin at Discharge	399	99%	88%	90%	100%
Beta Blocker at Arrival	229	96%	89%	87%	100%
Beta Blocker at Discharge	436	97%	92%	90%	100%
Fibrinolytic Medication Timing[1]	1	0%	33%	31%	100%
PCI Within 90 Minutes of Arrival[1]	17	76%	52%	54%	95%
Smoking Cessation Advice	168	98%	92%	88%	100%
Heart Failure Care					
ACE Inhibitor or ARB for LVSD	209	82%	82%	82%	100%
Discharge Instructions	355	84%	61%	61%	93%
Evaluation of LVS Function	432	97%	90%	83%	99%
Smoking Cessation Advice	88	100%	91%	82%	100%
Pneumonia Care					
Appropriate Initial Antibiotic	173	87%	84%	83%	94%
Blood Culture Timing	152	84%	88%	90%	100%
Influenza Vaccine	46	80%	64%	70%	100%
Initial Antibiotic Timing	226	62%	74%	80%	93%
Oxygenation Assessment	270	100%	99%	99%	100%
Pneumococcal Vaccine	149	92%	67%	69%	94%
Smoking Cessation Advice	66	97%	90%	80%	100%
Surgical Infection Prevention					
Prophylactic Antibiotic Given	713	92%	83%	77%	95%
Prophylactic Antibiotic Selection	180	94%	90%	90%	100%
Prophylactic Antibiotic Stopped	690	75%	70%	72%	95%
Pregnancy Care					
Inpatient Neonatal Mortality	-	-	-	-	-
Third or Fourth Degree Laceration	-	-	2.71%	3.63%	3.27%

University Hospital & Medical Center

Alternate Name: University Hospital
7201 N University Drive
Tamarac, FL 33321
URL: www.uhmchealth.com
Ownership: Proprietary
Emergency Services: Yes

Phone: 954-721-2200
Fax: 954-724-6666

Accredited: Yes
Licensed Beds: 317

Key Personnel:
CEO. . . . . James A Cruickshank
Chief Medical Staff. . . . . Nichols Katz, MD
Emergency Room . . . . Denise Eichenblat, RN
Director Medical/Surgical Nursing . . . . Marge Leeder
Chief Radiology . . . . Gaston Mendez, MD
Director Respiratory Therapy . . . . Armondo Gil

Measure	Cases	This Hospital	State Average	U.S. Average	Top Hospital
Heart Attack Care					
ACE Inhibitor or ARB for LVSD[1]	15	80%	83%	82%	100%
Aspirin at Arrival	109	87%	93%	92%	100%
Aspirin at Discharge	32	84%	88%	90%	100%
Beta Blocker at Arrival	66	86%	89%	87%	100%
Beta Blocker at Discharge	50	86%	92%	90%	100%
Fibrinolytic Medication Timing[1]	4	25%	33%	31%	100%
PCI Within 90 Minutes of Arrival	0	-	52%	54%	95%
Smoking Cessation Advice[1]	6	83%	92%	88%	100%
Heart Failure Care					
ACE Inhibitor or ARB for LVSD	97	72%	82%	82%	100%
Discharge Instructions	244	70%	61%	61%	93%
Evaluation of LVS Function	318	89%	90%	83%	99%
Smoking Cessation Advice	26	96%	91%	82%	100%
Pneumonia Care					
Appropriate Initial Antibiotic	143	89%	84%	83%	94%
Blood Culture Timing	137	86%	88%	90%	100%
Influenza Vaccine	50	70%	64%	70%	100%
Initial Antibiotic Timing	202	76%	74%	80%	93%
Oxygenation Assessment	226	97%	99%	99%	100%
Pneumococcal Vaccine	162	62%	67%	69%	94%
Smoking Cessation Advice	35	100%	90%	80%	100%
Surgical Infection Prevention					
Prophylactic Antibiotic Given[2,3]	178	90%	83%	77%	95%
Prophylactic Antibiotic Selection[2]	50	90%	90%	90%	100%

NOTE: Hospital profiles are in alphabetical order by state, then city, then hospital within the city; Rankings are sorted by rate in descending order and exclude hospitals with less than 25 cases; (1) The number of cases is too small (n<25) for purposes of reliably predicting hospital performance; (2) Measure reflects the hospital's indication that its submission was based upon a sample of its relevant discharges; (3) Rate reflects fewer than the maximum possible quarters of data for the measure; (4) Inaccurate information submitted and suppressed for one or more quarters; (5) No data is available from the hospital for this measure; Please refer to the User's Guide for a full explanation of data

Measure	Cases	This Hospital	State Average	U.S. Average	Top Hospital
Prophylactic Antibiotic Stopped[2,3]	167	71%	70%	72%	95%
Pregnancy Care					
Inpatient Neonatal Mortality	-	-	-	-	-
Third or Fourth Degree Laceration	-	-	2.71%	3.63%	3.27%

Memorial Hospital of Tampa

2901 Swann Avenue
Tampa, FL 33609
E-mail: info@memorialhospitaltampa.com
URL: www.memorialhospitaltampa.com
Ownership: Proprietary
Emergency Services: Yes

Phone: 813-873-6400
Fax: 813-874-8685

Accredited: Yes
Licensed Beds: 180

Key Personnel:
President/CEO . . . . John Mainieri
Chief Medical Staff . . . . James Hankerson
Catheterization Lab . . . . Sharon Barnett
Emergency Room . . . . Sue Neil
Infection Control . . . . Dennis Gonzales
Chief Radiology . . . . Bernard Stein, MD
Respiratory/Cardiopulmonary . . . . Ron Mitchell

Measure	Cases	This Hospital	State Average	U.S. Average	Top Hospital
Heart Attack Care					
ACE Inhibitor or ARB for LVSD[1]	3	100%	83%	82%	100%
Aspirin at Arrival[1]	22	91%	93%	92%	100%
Aspirin at Discharge[1]	8	88%	88%	90%	100%
Beta Blocker at Arrival[1]	18	94%	89%	87%	100%
Beta Blocker at Discharge[1]	8	100%	92%	90%	100%
Fibrinolytic Medication Timing	0	-	33%	31%	100%
PCI Within 90 Minutes of Arrival	0	-	52%	54%	95%
Smoking Cessation Advice[1]	3	100%	92%	88%	100%
Heart Failure Care					
ACE Inhibitor or ARB for LVSD	44	98%	82%	82%	100%
Discharge Instructions	107	94%	61%	61%	93%
Evaluation of LVS Function	144	99%	90%	83%	99%
Smoking Cessation Advice[1]	17	100%	91%	82%	100%
Pneumonia Care					
Appropriate Initial Antibiotic	139	88%	84%	83%	94%
Blood Culture Timing	144	94%	88%	90%	100%
Influenza Vaccine	32	75%	64%	70%	100%
Initial Antibiotic Timing	203	79%	74%	80%	93%
Oxygenation Assessment	208	100%	99%	99%	100%
Pneumococcal Vaccine	120	68%	67%	69%	94%
Smoking Cessation Advice	39	100%	90%	80%	100%
Surgical Infection Prevention					
Prophylactic Antibiotic Given[3]	129	81%	83%	77%	95%
Prophylactic Antibiotic Selection	36	89%	90%	90%	100%
Prophylactic Antibiotic Stopped[3]	127	64%	70%	72%	95%
Pregnancy Care					
Inpatient Neonatal Mortality	-	-	-	-	-
Third or Fourth Degree Laceration	-	-	2.71%	3.63%	3.27%

Saint Joseph's Hospital

3001 W Martin Luther King Jr Boulevard
Tampa, FL 33607
URL: www.stjosephstampa.org
Ownership: Voluntary non-profit - Church
Emergency Services: Yes

Phone: 813-870-4000
Fax: 813-870-4639

Accredited: Yes
Licensed Beds: 521

Key Personnel:
CEO . . . . Isaac Mallah
Director Same Day Surgery . . . . Paula McGuiness
Director ER . . . . Lisa Hays
Manager Infection Control . . . . Cathy Ricchezza
CCU Spvg. Nurse . . . . Karen Moyer
OB/GYN Womens Health . . . . Luciano Martinez

Measure	Cases	This Hospital	State Average	U.S. Average	Top Hospital
Heart Attack Care					
ACE Inhibitor or ARB for LVSD	178	93%	83%	82%	100%
Aspirin at Arrival	494	99%	93%	92%	100%
Aspirin at Discharge	517	96%	88%	90%	100%
Beta Blocker at Arrival	379	99%	89%	87%	100%
Beta Blocker at Discharge	529	95%	92%	90%	100%

Measure	Cases	This Hospital	State Average	U.S. Average	Top Hospital
Fibrinolytic Medication Timing	0	-	33%	31%	100%
PCI Within 90 Minutes of Arrival[1]	1	0%	52%	54%	95%
Smoking Cessation Advice	197	100%	92%	88%	100%
Heart Failure Care					
ACE Inhibitor or ARB for LVSD	422	91%	82%	82%	100%
Discharge Instructions	811	62%	61%	61%	93%
Evaluation of LVS Function	975	95%	90%	83%	99%
Smoking Cessation Advice	171	100%	91%	82%	100%
Pneumonia Care					
Appropriate Initial Antibiotic	252	87%	84%	83%	94%
Blood Culture Timing	290	70%	88%	90%	100%
Influenza Vaccine	95	76%	64%	70%	100%
Initial Antibiotic Timing	391	77%	74%	80%	93%
Oxygenation Assessment	648	100%	99%	99%	100%
Pneumococcal Vaccine	274	73%	67%	69%	94%
Smoking Cessation Advice	162	97%	90%	80%	100%
Surgical Infection Prevention					
Prophylactic Antibiotic Given[2]	225	80%	83%	77%	95%
Prophylactic Antibiotic Selection[2]	69	96%	90%	90%	100%
Prophylactic Antibiotic Stopped[2]	198	86%	70%	72%	95%
Pregnancy Care					
Inpatient Neonatal Mortality	-	-	-	-	-
Third or Fourth Degree Laceration	-	-	2.71%	3.63%	3.27%

Tampa General Healthcare

Alternate Name: Tampa General Care
2 Columbia Drive
PO Box 1289
Tampa, FL 33606
E-mail: jstone@tgh.org
URL: www.tgh.org
Ownership: Voluntary non-profit - Private
Emergency Services: Yes

Phone: 813-844-7000
Fax: 813-844-4057

Accredited: Yes

Key Personnel:
Administrator/President . . . . Ron Hytoff
Chief Catheterization Laboratory . . . . Jane Faulkner
Emergency Room . . . . James V Hillman
Director Infection/Disease Control . . . . John Sinnott, MD
Director Medical/Surgical Nursing . . . . Janet Davis, RN
OB/GYN Womens Health . . . . Michael Parsons
Chief Radiology . . . . Carlos Martinez
Director Respiratory Therapy . . . . Nancy Wood

Measure	Cases	This Hospital	State Average	U.S. Average	Top Hospital
Heart Attack Care					
ACE Inhibitor or ARB for LVSD	102	79%	83%	82%	100%
Aspirin at Arrival	252	94%	93%	92%	100%
Aspirin at Discharge	329	97%	88%	90%	100%
Beta Blocker at Arrival	198	89%	89%	87%	100%
Beta Blocker at Discharge	339	94%	92%	90%	100%
Fibrinolytic Medication Timing	0	-	33%	31%	100%
PCI Within 90 Minutes of Arrival[1]	18	50%	52%	54%	95%
Smoking Cessation Advice	137	96%	92%	88%	100%
Heart Failure Care					
ACE Inhibitor or ARB for LVSD	336	85%	82%	82%	100%
Discharge Instructions	556	71%	61%	61%	93%
Evaluation of LVS Function	605	93%	90%	83%	99%
Smoking Cessation Advice	154	99%	91%	82%	100%
Pneumonia Care					
Appropriate Initial Antibiotic	145	86%	84%	83%	94%
Blood Culture Timing	181	89%	88%	90%	100%
Influenza Vaccine	55	60%	64%	70%	100%
Initial Antibiotic Timing	255	48%	74%	80%	93%
Oxygenation Assessment	328	99%	99%	99%	100%
Pneumococcal Vaccine	110	65%	67%	69%	94%
Smoking Cessation Advice	101	96%	90%	80%	100%
Surgical Infection Prevention					
Prophylactic Antibiotic Given	1,985	81%	83%	77%	95%
Prophylactic Antibiotic Selection	517	89%	90%	90%	100%
Prophylactic Antibiotic Stopped	1,823	72%	70%	72%	95%
Pregnancy Care					
Inpatient Neonatal Mortality	5,567	0.65%	-	-	-
Third or Fourth Degree Laceration	3,699	3.43%	2.71%	3.63%	3.27%

NOTE: Hospital profiles are in alphabetical order by state, then city, then hospital within the city; Rankings are sorted by rate in descending order and exclude hospitals with less than 25 cases; (1) The number of cases is too small (n<25) for purposes of reliably predicting hospital performance; (2) Measure reflects the hospital's indication that its submission was based upon a sample of its relevant discharges; (3) Rate reflects fewer than the maximum possible quarters of data for the measure; (4) Inaccurate information submitted and suppressed for one or more quarters; (5) No data is available from the hospital for this measure; Please refer to the User's Guide for a full explanation of data

Town and Country Hospital

Alternate Name: AMI Town and Country Medical Center
6001 Webb Road
Tampa, FL 33615
Phone: 813-888-7060
Fax: 813-887-5112
E-mail: info@townandcountryhospital.com
URL: www.iasishealthcare.com
Ownership: Proprietary
Emergency Services: Yes
Accredited: Yes
Licensed Beds: 201

Key Personnel:
CEO................................... Phil Mazzuca
Chief Medical Staff....................... Edward Braun, MD
Emergency Room .... Steven Sloniger
Director Medical/Surgical Nursing .... Judy Burris
Chief Radiology .... James Quigley, MD
Director Respiratory Therapy .... Pete Hendriksen

Measure	Cases	This Hospital	State Average	U.S. Average	Top Hospital
Heart Attack Care					
ACE Inhibitor or ARB for LVSD[1]	6	83%	83%	82%	100%
Aspirin at Arrival	33	94%	93%	92%	100%
Aspirin at Discharge[1]	16	81%	88%	90%	100%
Beta Blocker at Arrival	37	86%	89%	87%	100%
Beta Blocker at Discharge[1]	23	83%	92%	90%	100%
Fibrinolytic Medication Timing[1]	1	100%	33%	31%	100%
PCI Within 90 Minutes of Arrival	0	-	52%	54%	95%
Smoking Cessation Advice[1]	4	50%	92%	88%	100%
Heart Failure Care					
ACE Inhibitor or ARB for LVSD	39	90%	82%	82%	100%
Discharge Instructions	112	32%	61%	61%	93%
Evaluation of LVS Function	154	94%	90%	83%	99%
Smoking Cessation Advice[1]	24	75%	91%	82%	100%
Pneumonia Care					
Appropriate Initial Antibiotic	112	80%	84%	83%	94%
Blood Culture Timing	88	70%	88%	90%	100%
Influenza Vaccine[4,5]	-	-	64%	70%	100%
Initial Antibiotic Timing	145	70%	74%	80%	93%
Oxygenation Assessment	160	99%	99%	99%	100%
Pneumococcal Vaccine	84	73%	67%	69%	94%
Smoking Cessation Advice	27	85%	90%	80%	100%
Surgical Infection Prevention					
Prophylactic Antibiotic Given	136	92%	83%	77%	95%
Prophylactic Antibiotic Selection	28	86%	90%	90%	100%
Prophylactic Antibiotic Stopped	128	66%	70%	72%	95%
Pregnancy Care					
Inpatient Neonatal Mortality	-	-	-	-	-
Third or Fourth Degree Laceration	-	-	2.71%	3.63%	3.27%

University Community Hospital

Alternate Name: UCH
3100 E Fletcher Avenue
Tampa, FL 33613
Phone: 813-971-6000
Fax: 813-615-7313
URL: www.uch.org
Ownership: Voluntary non-profit - Private
Emergency Services: Yes
Accredited: Yes
Licensed Beds: 551

Key Personnel:
CEO................................... Calvin Glidwell
Chief Medical Staff....................... Kurt Stonesifer, MD
Emergency Room Director.................. Mary Daegrooten
Emergency Room .... Howard Franklin, MD
Infection Control Manager .... Jackie Whittaker
ICU .... Theron Ebel, MD
Director Medical Surgical Nursing .... Mary Whillock, RN
OB/GYN Women's Health .... Margie Mueller-Boyer
Director Surgical Services .... Laura Tischler, RN
Manager Respiratory Services .... Steve Horne

Measure	Cases	This Hospital	State Average	U.S. Average	Top Hospital
Heart Attack Care					
ACE Inhibitor or ARB for LVSD	77	69%	83%	82%	100%
Aspirin at Arrival	287	95%	93%	92%	100%
Aspirin at Discharge	372	95%	88%	90%	100%
Beta Blocker at Arrival	245	92%	89%	87%	100%
Beta Blocker at Discharge	394	96%	92%	90%	100%

Measure	Cases	This Hospital	State Average	U.S. Average	Top Hospital
Fibrinolytic Medication Timing	0	-	33%	31%	100%
PCI Within 90 Minutes of Arrival[1]	20	65%	52%	54%	95%
Smoking Cessation Advice	138	98%	92%	88%	100%
Heart Failure Care					
ACE Inhibitor or ARB for LVSD	176	78%	82%	82%	100%
Discharge Instructions	351	51%	61%	61%	93%
Evaluation of LVS Function	461	94%	90%	83%	99%
Smoking Cessation Advice	68	100%	91%	82%	100%
Pneumonia Care					
Appropriate Initial Antibiotic	180	86%	84%	83%	94%
Blood Culture Timing	150	84%	88%	90%	100%
Influenza Vaccine	25	36%	64%	70%	100%
Initial Antibiotic Timing	236	61%	74%	80%	93%
Oxygenation Assessment	296	99%	99%	99%	100%
Pneumococcal Vaccine	160	42%	67%	69%	94%
Smoking Cessation Advice	56	88%	90%	80%	100%
Surgical Infection Prevention					
Prophylactic Antibiotic Given	323	69%	83%	77%	95%
Prophylactic Antibiotic Selection	90	74%	90%	90%	100%
Prophylactic Antibiotic Stopped	312	76%	70%	72%	95%
Pregnancy Care					
Inpatient Neonatal Mortality	-	-	-	-	-
Third or Fourth Degree Laceration	-	-	2.71%	3.63%	3.27%

University Community Hospital of Carrollwood

Alternate Name: Centurion Hospital of Carrollwood
7171 N Dale Mabry Highway
Tampa, FL 33614
Phone: 813-932-2222
Fax: 813-558-8011
URL: www.uchcarrollwood.com
Ownership: Voluntary non-profit - Private
Emergency Services: Yes
Accredited: Yes
Licensed Beds: 120

Key Personnel:
CEO................................... Donald Evans
Chief Medical Staff....................... Scott Bronleewe
Emergency Room .... Brenda McCartney
Chief Radiology .... Thomas Okulski, MD
Director Respiratory Therapy .... Pam Gaul

Measure	Cases	This Hospital	State Average	U.S. Average	Top Hospital
Heart Attack Care					
ACE Inhibitor or ARB for LVSD[1]	5	60%	83%	82%	100%
Aspirin at Arrival[1]	19	95%	93%	92%	100%
Aspirin at Discharge[1]	9	67%	88%	90%	100%
Beta Blocker at Arrival[1]	22	68%	89%	87%	100%
Beta Blocker at Discharge[1]	9	100%	92%	90%	100%
Fibrinolytic Medication Timing[1]	1	0%	33%	31%	100%
PCI Within 90 Minutes of Arrival	0	-	52%	54%	95%
Smoking Cessation Advice	0	-	92%	88%	100%
Heart Failure Care					
ACE Inhibitor or ARB for LVSD	42	64%	82%	82%	100%
Discharge Instructions	97	70%	61%	61%	93%
Evaluation of LVS Function	120	87%	90%	83%	99%
Smoking Cessation Advice[1]	21	100%	91%	82%	100%
Pneumonia Care					
Appropriate Initial Antibiotic	146	89%	84%	83%	94%
Blood Culture Timing	99	79%	88%	90%	100%
Influenza Vaccine[1]	12	33%	64%	70%	100%
Initial Antibiotic Timing	172	67%	74%	80%	93%
Oxygenation Assessment	193	99%	99%	99%	100%
Pneumococcal Vaccine	95	42%	67%	69%	94%
Smoking Cessation Advice	40	100%	90%	80%	100%
Surgical Infection Prevention					
Prophylactic Antibiotic Given	76	82%	83%	77%	95%
Prophylactic Antibiotic Selection	37	89%	90%	90%	100%
Prophylactic Antibiotic Stopped	72	54%	70%	72%	95%
Pregnancy Care					
Inpatient Neonatal Mortality	-	-	-	-	-
Third or Fourth Degree Laceration	-	-	2.71%	3.63%	3.27%

NOTE: Hospital profiles are in alphabetical order by state, then city, then hospital within the city; Rankings are sorted by rate in descending order and exclude hospitals with less than 25 cases; (1) The number of cases is too small (n<25) for purposes of reliably predicting hospital performance; (2) Measure reflects the hospital's indication that its submission was based upon a sample of its relevant discharges; (3) Rate reflects fewer than the maximum possible quarters of data for the measure; (4) Inaccurate information submitted and suppressed for one or more quarters; (5) No data is available from the hospital for this measure; Please refer to the User's Guide for a full explanation of data

Helen Ellis Memorial Hospital

1395 South Pinellas Avenue
Tarpon Springs, FL 34689
E-mail: heinfo@mail.uch.org
URL: www.hemh.com
Ownership: Voluntary non-profit - Other
Emergency Services: Yes

Phone: 727-942-5000
Fax: 727-942-5161

Accredited: Yes
Licensed Beds: 168

Key Personnel:
CEO . . . . Steve MacLauchlan
Chief Medical Staff . . . . John Dallman, MD
Cardiac/Catheterization Lab . . . . Cheryl Sotrop
Infection Control . . . . Paula Hartzel, RN
ICU . . . . Beth Carter
OB/GYN Womens Health . . . . Arleigh Ancheta
Director Radiology . . . . Linda Gordon
Director Cardio-Pulmonary Services . . . . Cheryl Sotrop

Measure	Cases	This Hospital	State Average	U.S. Average	Top Hospital
Heart Attack Care					
ACE Inhibitor or ARB for LVSD	31	87%	83%	82%	100%
Aspirin at Arrival	134	92%	93%	92%	100%
Aspirin at Discharge	87	68%	88%	90%	100%
Beta Blocker at Arrival	126	90%	89%	87%	100%
Beta Blocker at Discharge	96	88%	92%	90%	100%
Fibrinolytic Medication Timing	0	-	33%	31%	100%
PCI Within 90 Minutes of Arrival[1]	6	100%	52%	54%	95%
Smoking Cessation Advice	28	82%	92%	88%	100%
Heart Failure Care					
ACE Inhibitor or ARB for LVSD	122	79%	82%	82%	100%
Discharge Instructions	235	12%	61%	61%	93%
Evaluation of LVS Function	308	91%	90%	83%	99%
Smoking Cessation Advice	43	63%	91%	82%	100%
Pneumonia Care					
Appropriate Initial Antibiotic	108	84%	84%	83%	94%
Blood Culture Timing	73	89%	88%	90%	100%
Influenza Vaccine[1]	23	48%	64%	70%	100%
Initial Antibiotic Timing	139	73%	74%	80%	93%
Oxygenation Assessment	155	99%	99%	99%	100%
Pneumococcal Vaccine	97	35%	67%	69%	94%
Smoking Cessation Advice	39	64%	90%	80%	100%
Surgical Infection Prevention					
Prophylactic Antibiotic Given[2,3]	47	91%	83%	77%	95%
Prophylactic Antibiotic Selection[2]	47	81%	90%	90%	100%
Prophylactic Antibiotic Stopped[2,3]	47	55%	70%	72%	95%
Pregnancy Care					
Inpatient Neonatal Mortality	-	-	-	-	-
Third or Fourth Degree Laceration	-	-	2.71%	3.63%	3.27%

Florida Hospital Waterman

1000 Waterman Way
Tavares, FL 32778
E-mail: cindi.harrod@ahss.org
URL: www.fhwat.org
Ownership: Voluntary non-profit - Private
Emergency Services: Yes

Phone: 352-253-3333
Fax: 352-253-3927

Accredited: Yes
Licensed Beds: 204

Key Personnel:
President/CEO . . . . Kenneth R Mattison
Chief Medical Staff . . . . Rosemary Cirelli, MD
Cardiac Lab . . . . Eric Blamick
Catheterization/Special Imaging . . . . Keith Terrill
Emergency Room . . . . Heather Bentley
Director Medical/Surgical Nursing . . . . Bonnie Palmer
OB/GYN Women's Health . . . . Patty Lesmerises

Measure	Cases	This Hospital	State Average	U.S. Average	Top Hospital
Heart Attack Care					
ACE Inhibitor or ARB for LVSD	28	82%	83%	82%	100%
Aspirin at Arrival	158	89%	93%	92%	100%
Aspirin at Discharge	86	86%	88%	90%	100%
Beta Blocker at Arrival	145	83%	89%	87%	100%
Beta Blocker at Discharge	89	92%	92%	90%	100%
Fibrinolytic Medication Timing	0	-	33%	31%	100%
PCI Within 90 Minutes of Arrival	0	-	52%	54%	95%

Measure	Cases	This Hospital	State Average	U.S. Average	Top Hospital
Smoking Cessation Advice[1]	20	80%	92%	88%	100%
Heart Failure Care					
ACE Inhibitor or ARB for LVSD	234	76%	82%	82%	100%
Discharge Instructions	403	75%	61%	61%	93%
Evaluation of LVS Function	485	94%	90%	83%	99%
Smoking Cessation Advice	67	87%	91%	82%	100%
Pneumonia Care					
Appropriate Initial Antibiotic	180	77%	84%	83%	94%
Blood Culture Timing	206	88%	88%	90%	100%
Influenza Vaccine	66	79%	64%	70%	100%
Initial Antibiotic Timing	255	77%	74%	80%	93%
Oxygenation Assessment	323	100%	99%	99%	100%
Pneumococcal Vaccine	205	77%	67%	69%	94%
Smoking Cessation Advice	64	91%	90%	80%	100%
Surgical Infection Prevention					
Prophylactic Antibiotic Given	579	72%	83%	77%	95%
Prophylactic Antibiotic Selection	134	90%	90%	90%	100%
Prophylactic Antibiotic Stopped	541	64%	70%	72%	95%
Pregnancy Care					
Inpatient Neonatal Mortality	-	-	-	-	-
Third or Fourth Degree Laceration	-	-	2.71%	3.63%	3.27%

Mariners Hospital

91500 Overseas Highway
Tavernier, FL 33070
E-mail: corporatepr@baptisthealth.net
URL: www.baptisthealth.net
Ownership: Voluntary non-profit - Other
Emergency Services: Yes

Phone: 305-434-3000
Fax: 305-853-1581

Accredited: Yes
Licensed Beds: 42

Key Personnel:
President/CEO . . . . Robert H Luse
Emergency Room . . . . Tracy Murrell
Infection Control . . . . Gisele Monson
ICU . . . . Roberta Fismer, RN
Medical/Surgical Nursing . . . . Dawn Stavor, RN
Respiratory/Cardiopulmonary . . . . Susan Hayes

Measure	Cases	This Hospital	State Average	U.S. Average	Top Hospital
Heart Attack Care					
ACE Inhibitor or ARB for LVSD[1]	3	67%	83%	82%	100%
Aspirin at Arrival	32	100%	93%	92%	100%
Aspirin at Discharge[1]	7	100%	88%	90%	100%
Beta Blocker at Arrival[1]	16	94%	89%	87%	100%
Beta Blocker at Discharge[1]	6	100%	92%	90%	100%
Fibrinolytic Medication Timing	0	-	33%	31%	100%
PCI Within 90 Minutes of Arrival	0	-	52%	54%	95%
Smoking Cessation Advice[1]	3	100%	92%	88%	100%
Heart Failure Care					
ACE Inhibitor or ARB for LVSD	27	93%	82%	82%	100%
Discharge Instructions	39	100%	61%	61%	93%
Evaluation of LVS Function	46	100%	90%	83%	99%
Smoking Cessation Advice[1]	11	100%	91%	82%	100%
Pneumonia Care					
Appropriate Initial Antibiotic	60	90%	84%	83%	94%
Blood Culture Timing	47	94%	88%	90%	100%
Influenza Vaccine[1]	11	82%	64%	70%	100%
Initial Antibiotic Timing	60	93%	74%	80%	93%
Oxygenation Assessment	73	100%	99%	99%	100%
Pneumococcal Vaccine	44	93%	67%	69%	94%
Smoking Cessation Advice[1]	18	100%	90%	80%	100%
Surgical Infection Prevention					
Prophylactic Antibiotic Given[1]	13	92%	83%	77%	95%
Prophylactic Antibiotic Selection[1]	5	100%	90%	90%	100%
Prophylactic Antibiotic Stopped[1]	13	62%	70%	72%	95%
Pregnancy Care					
Inpatient Neonatal Mortality	-	-	-	-	-
Third or Fourth Degree Laceration	-	-	2.71%	3.63%	3.27%

NOTE: Hospital profiles are in alphabetical order by state, then city, then hospital within the city; Rankings are sorted by rate in descending order and exclude hospitals with less than 25 cases; (1) The number of cases is too small (n<25) for purposes of reliably predicting hospital performance; (2) Measure reflects the hospital's indication that its submission was based upon a sample of its relevant discharges; (3) Rate reflects fewer than the maximum possible quarters of data for the measure; (4) Inaccurate information submitted and suppressed for one or more quarters; (5) No data is available from the hospital for this measure; Please refer to the User's Guide for a full explanation of data

Villages Regional Hospital

1451 El Camino Real
The Villages, FL 32159
URL: www.tvrh.org
Ownership: Voluntary non-profit - Private
Emergency Services: Yes
Phone: 352-751-8000
Fax: 352-751-8975
Accredited: Yes
Licensed Beds: 60

Key Personnel:
President/CEO . . . . Louis H Bremer Jr

Measure	Cases	This Hospital	State Average	U.S. Average	Top Hospital
Heart Attack Care					
ACE Inhibitor or ARB for LVSD[1]	6	67%	83%	82%	100%
Aspirin at Arrival	64	94%	93%	92%	100%
Aspirin at Discharge[1]	18	78%	88%	90%	100%
Beta Blocker at Arrival	64	84%	89%	87%	100%
Beta Blocker at Discharge[1]	21	86%	92%	90%	100%
Fibrinolytic Medication Timing	0	-	33%	31%	100%
PCI Within 90 Minutes of Arrival	0	-	52%	54%	95%
Smoking Cessation Advice[1]	3	100%	92%	88%	100%
Heart Failure Care					
ACE Inhibitor or ARB for LVSD	93	75%	82%	82%	100%
Discharge Instructions	247	63%	61%	61%	93%
Evaluation of LVS Function	279	88%	90%	83%	99%
Smoking Cessation Advice	35	86%	91%	82%	100%
Pneumonia Care					
Appropriate Initial Antibiotic	202	88%	84%	83%	94%
Blood Culture Timing	180	84%	88%	90%	100%
Influenza Vaccine	71	79%	64%	70%	100%
Initial Antibiotic Timing	235	71%	74%	80%	93%
Oxygenation Assessment	303	99%	99%	99%	100%
Pneumococcal Vaccine	223	74%	67%	69%	94%
Smoking Cessation Advice	41	90%	90%	80%	100%
Surgical Infection Prevention					
Prophylactic Antibiotic Given	123	80%	83%	77%	95%
Prophylactic Antibiotic Selection	32	100%	90%	90%	100%
Prophylactic Antibiotic Stopped	118	69%	70%	72%	95%
Pregnancy Care					
Inpatient Neonatal Mortality	-	-	-	-	-
Third or Fourth Degree Laceration	-	-	2.71%	3.63%	3.27%

Parrish Medical Center

951 N Washington Avenue
Titusville, FL 32796
URL: www.parrishmed.com
Ownership: Govt - Hospital District or Authority
Emergency Services: Yes
Phone: 321-268-6111
Fax: 321-268-6231
Accredited: Yes
Licensed Beds: 210

Key Personnel:
CEO . . . . George Mikitarian
Chief Medical Staff . . . . Denis Perez, MD
OB/GYN Womens Health . . . . Manuel Quintana, MD
Director Radiology . . . . Debra McAlear
Director Respiratory/Cardiopulmonary . . . . Gayle Petty

Measure	Cases	This Hospital	State Average	U.S. Average	Top Hospital
Heart Attack Care					
ACE Inhibitor or ARB for LVSD	38	97%	83%	82%	100%
Aspirin at Arrival	143	94%	93%	92%	100%
Aspirin at Discharge	60	80%	88%	90%	100%
Beta Blocker at Arrival	118	96%	89%	87%	100%
Beta Blocker at Discharge	76	96%	92%	90%	100%
Fibrinolytic Medication Timing[1]	1	100%	33%	31%	100%
PCI Within 90 Minutes of Arrival	0	-	52%	54%	95%
Smoking Cessation Advice	25	100%	92%	88%	100%
Heart Failure Care					
ACE Inhibitor or ARB for LVSD	104	93%	82%	82%	100%
Discharge Instructions	182	92%	61%	61%	93%
Evaluation of LVS Function	234	94%	90%	83%	99%
Smoking Cessation Advice	39	100%	91%	82%	100%
Pneumonia Care					
Appropriate Initial Antibiotic	130	87%	84%	83%	94%
Blood Culture Timing	132	90%	88%	90%	100%
Influenza Vaccine	42	57%	64%	70%	100%
Initial Antibiotic Timing	194	74%	74%	80%	93%
Oxygenation Assessment	243	100%	99%	99%	100%
Pneumococcal Vaccine	133	74%	67%	69%	94%
Smoking Cessation Advice	49	100%	90%	80%	100%
Surgical Infection Prevention					
Prophylactic Antibiotic Given	231	90%	83%	77%	95%
Prophylactic Antibiotic Selection	59	92%	90%	90%	100%
Prophylactic Antibiotic Stopped	225	80%	70%	72%	95%
Pregnancy Care					
Inpatient Neonatal Mortality	-	-	-	-	-
Third or Fourth Degree Laceration	-	-	2.71%	3.63%	3.27%

Venice Regional Medical Center

540 The Rialto
Venice, FL 34285
URL: www.veniceregional.com
Ownership: Proprietary
Emergency Services: Yes
Phone: 941-485-7711
Fax: 941-483-7621
Accredited: Yes
Licensed Beds: 312

Key Personnel:
CEO . . . . Melody Trimble
Emergency Room . . . . Linda Caissie

Measure	Cases	This Hospital	State Average	U.S. Average	Top Hospital
Heart Attack Care					
ACE Inhibitor or ARB for LVSD[2]	74	100%	83%	82%	100%
Aspirin at Arrival[2]	311	100%	93%	92%	100%
Aspirin at Discharge[2]	260	100%	88%	90%	100%
Beta Blocker at Arrival[2]	269	99%	89%	87%	100%
Beta Blocker at Discharge[2]	320	100%	92%	90%	100%
Fibrinolytic Medication Timing[1,2]	1	0%	33%	31%	100%
PCI Within 90 Minutes of Arrival[1,2]	6	83%	52%	54%	95%
Smoking Cessation Advice[2]	81	100%	92%	88%	100%
Heart Failure Care					
ACE Inhibitor or ARB for LVSD	140	100%	82%	82%	100%
Discharge Instructions	254	93%	61%	61%	93%
Evaluation of LVS Function	323	100%	90%	83%	99%
Smoking Cessation Advice	43	100%	91%	82%	100%
Pneumonia Care					
Appropriate Initial Antibiotic	164	91%	84%	83%	94%
Blood Culture Timing	176	93%	88%	90%	100%
Influenza Vaccine	75	84%	64%	70%	100%
Initial Antibiotic Timing	263	91%	74%	80%	93%
Oxygenation Assessment	306	100%	99%	99%	100%
Pneumococcal Vaccine	241	87%	67%	69%	94%
Smoking Cessation Advice	47	100%	90%	80%	100%
Surgical Infection Prevention					
Prophylactic Antibiotic Given[2]	449	95%	83%	77%	95%
Prophylactic Antibiotic Selection[2]	93	89%	90%	90%	100%
Prophylactic Antibiotic Stopped[2]	433	87%	70%	72%	95%
Pregnancy Care					
Inpatient Neonatal Mortality	-	-	-	-	-
Third or Fourth Degree Laceration	-	-	2.71%	3.63%	3.27%

Indian River Memorial Hospital

1000 36th Street
Vero Beach, FL 32960
URL: www.irmh.com
Ownership: Govt - Hospital District or Authority
Emergency Services: No
Phone: 772-567-4311
Fax: 772-562-5628
Accredited: Yes
Licensed Beds: 335

Key Personnel:
President/CEO . . . . Jeffrey Susi
Chief Medical Staff . . . . Charles Callahand
Director Emergency Room . . . . Glenn Tremml

Measure	Cases	This Hospital	State Average	U.S. Average	Top Hospital
Heart Attack Care					
ACE Inhibitor or ARB for LVSD[1]	19	79%	83%	82%	100%
Aspirin at Arrival	134	96%	93%	92%	100%
Aspirin at Discharge	62	89%	88%	90%	100%
Beta Blocker at Arrival	144	90%	89%	87%	100%
Beta Blocker at Discharge	72	90%	92%	90%	100%
Fibrinolytic Medication Timing[1,3]	5	40%	33%	31%	100%
PCI Within 90 Minutes of Arrival	0	-	52%	54%	95%

NOTE: Hospital profiles are in alphabetical order by state, then city, then hospital within the city; Rankings are sorted by rate in descending order and exclude hospitals with less than 25 cases; (1) The number of cases is too small (n<25) for purposes of reliably predicting hospital performance; (2) Measure reflects the hospital's indication that its submission was based upon a sample of its relevant discharges; (3) Rate reflects fewer than the maximum possible quarters of data for the measure; (4) Inaccurate information submitted and suppressed for one or more quarters; (5) No data is available from the hospital for this measure; Please refer to the User's Guide for a full explanation of data

Smoking Cessation Advice[1,3]	2	100%	92%	88%	100%
Heart Failure Care					
ACE Inhibitor or ARB for LVSD	142	76%	82%	82%	100%
Discharge Instructions[3]	63	65%	61%	61%	93%
Evaluation of LVS Function	458	80%	90%	83%	99%
Smoking Cessation Advice[1,3]	15	100%	91%	82%	100%
Pneumonia Care					
Appropriate Initial Antibiotic[3]	42	79%	84%	83%	94%
Blood Culture Timing[3]	38	87%	88%	90%	100%
Influenza Vaccine[5]	-	-	64%	70%	100%
Initial Antibiotic Timing	270	72%	74%	80%	93%
Oxygenation Assessment	350	100%	99%	99%	100%
Pneumococcal Vaccine	247	37%	67%	69%	94%
Smoking Cessation Advice[1,3]	9	89%	90%	80%	100%
Surgical Infection Prevention					
Prophylactic Antibiotic Given[2,3]	59	92%	83%	77%	95%
Prophylactic Antibiotic Selection[5]	-	-	90%	90%	100%
Prophylactic Antibiotic Stopped[2,3]	58	60%	70%	72%	95%
Pregnancy Care					
Inpatient Neonatal Mortality	-	-	-	-	-
Third or Fourth Degree Laceration	-	-	2.71%	3.63%	3.27%

Florida Hospital Wauchula

Alternate Name: Walker Memorial Medical Center/Wauchula
533 W Carlton Street   Phone: 863-773-3101
PO Box 2355   Fax: 863-773-0126
Wauchula, FL 33873
Ownership: Voluntary non-profit - Private
Emergency Services: Yes   Accredited: Yes
                                        Licensed Beds: 25
Key Personnel:
CEO. . . . . John Harding

Measure	Cases	This Hospital	State Average	U.S. Average	Top Hospital
Heart Attack Care					
ACE Inhibitor or ARB for LVSD[3]	0	-	83%	82%	100%
Aspirin at Arrival[3]	0	-	93%	92%	100%
Aspirin at Discharge[3]	0	-	88%	90%	100%
Beta Blocker at Arrival[3]	0	-	89%	87%	100%
Beta Blocker at Discharge[3]	0	-	92%	90%	100%
Fibrinolytic Medication Timing[3]	0	-	33%	31%	100%
PCI Within 90 Minutes of Arrival[5]	-	-	52%	54%	95%
Smoking Cessation Advice[3]	0	-	92%	88%	100%
Heart Failure Care					
ACE Inhibitor or ARB for LVSD	0	-	82%	82%	100%
Discharge Instructions[1]	4	100%	61%	61%	93%
Evaluation of LVS Function[1]	4	75%	90%	83%	99%
Smoking Cessation Advice	0	-	91%	82%	100%
Pneumonia Care					
Appropriate Initial Antibiotic[1]	21	90%	84%	83%	94%
Blood Culture Timing[1]	21	90%	88%	90%	100%
Influenza Vaccine[1]	8	50%	64%	70%	100%
Initial Antibiotic Timing	30	83%	74%	80%	93%
Oxygenation Assessment	35	100%	99%	99%	100%
Pneumococcal Vaccine[1]	17	59%	67%	69%	94%
Smoking Cessation Advice[1]	5	100%	90%	80%	100%
Surgical Infection Prevention					
Prophylactic Antibiotic Given[5]	-	-	83%	77%	95%
Prophylactic Antibiotic Selection[5]	-	-	90%	90%	100%
Prophylactic Antibiotic Stopped[5]	-	-	70%	72%	95%
Pregnancy Care					
Inpatient Neonatal Mortality	-	-	-	-	-
Third or Fourth Degree Laceration	-	-	2.71%	3.63%	3.27%

Wellington Regional Medical Center

10101 Forest Hill Boulevard   Phone: 561-798-8500
Wellington, FL 33414   Fax: 561-753-2619
URL: www.wellingtonregional.com
Ownership: Proprietary
Emergency Services: Yes   Accredited: Yes
                                       Licensed Beds: 143
Key Personnel:
CEO. . . . . Kevin DiLallo

Measure	Cases	This Hospital	State Average	U.S. Average	Top Hospital
Heart Attack Care					
ACE Inhibitor or ARB for LVSD[1]	11	55%	83%	82%	100%
Aspirin at Arrival	51	96%	93%	92%	100%
Aspirin at Discharge[1]	24	88%	88%	90%	100%
Beta Blocker at Arrival	40	85%	89%	87%	100%
Beta Blocker at Discharge	25	84%	92%	90%	100%
Fibrinolytic Medication Timing	0	-	33%	31%	100%
PCI Within 90 Minutes of Arrival	0	-	52%	54%	95%
Smoking Cessation Advice[1]	4	75%	92%	88%	100%
Heart Failure Care					
ACE Inhibitor or ARB for LVSD	62	82%	82%	82%	100%
Discharge Instructions	208	56%	61%	61%	93%
Evaluation of LVS Function	200	81%	90%	83%	99%
Smoking Cessation Advice	33	85%	91%	82%	100%
Pneumonia Care					
Appropriate Initial Antibiotic	124	90%	84%	83%	94%
Blood Culture Timing	143	87%	88%	90%	100%
Influenza Vaccine	37	62%	64%	70%	100%
Initial Antibiotic Timing	163	83%	74%	80%	93%
Oxygenation Assessment	205	100%	99%	99%	100%
Pneumococcal Vaccine	126	56%	67%	69%	94%
Smoking Cessation Advice	46	96%	90%	80%	100%
Surgical Infection Prevention					
Prophylactic Antibiotic Given	547	79%	83%	77%	95%
Prophylactic Antibiotic Selection	137	97%	90%	90%	100%
Prophylactic Antibiotic Stopped	542	66%	70%	72%	95%
Pregnancy Care					
Inpatient Neonatal Mortality	2,652	0.04%	-	-	-
Third or Fourth Degree Laceration	1,665	3.78%	2.71%	3.63%	3.27%

Columbia Hospital

2201 45th Street   Phone: 561-842-6141
West Palm Beach, FL 33407   Fax: 561-844-8955
URL: www.columbiahospital.com
Ownership: Proprietary
Emergency Services: Yes   Accredited: Yes
                                       Licensed Beds: 250
Key Personnel:
CEO. . . . . Valerie A Jackson
Emergency Room . . . . Dennis Keown
Medical Surgical Nursing . . . . Cynthia Monroe, CNO
Director Radiology . . . . Kim Mullin
Director Respiratory/Cardiopulmonary . . . . Ethel Dosset

Measure	Cases	This Hospital	State Average	U.S. Average	Top Hospital
Heart Attack Care					
ACE Inhibitor or ARB for LVSD[1]	6	0%	83%	82%	100%
Aspirin at Arrival	65	80%	93%	92%	100%
Aspirin at Discharge	32	88%	88%	90%	100%
Beta Blocker at Arrival	47	72%	89%	87%	100%
Beta Blocker at Discharge	32	69%	92%	90%	100%
Fibrinolytic Medication Timing[1]	2	100%	33%	31%	100%
PCI Within 90 Minutes of Arrival	0	-	52%	54%	95%
Smoking Cessation Advice[1]	7	71%	92%	88%	100%
Heart Failure Care					
ACE Inhibitor or ARB for LVSD	67	63%	82%	82%	100%
Discharge Instructions	186	53%	61%	61%	93%
Evaluation of LVS Function	275	75%	90%	83%	99%
Smoking Cessation Advice	42	71%	91%	82%	100%
Pneumonia Care					
Appropriate Initial Antibiotic	62	82%	84%	83%	94%
Blood Culture Timing	80	95%	88%	90%	100%
Influenza Vaccine[1]	16	19%	64%	70%	100%
Initial Antibiotic Timing	103	83%	74%	80%	93%
Oxygenation Assessment	132	100%	99%	99%	100%
Pneumococcal Vaccine	66	47%	67%	69%	94%
Smoking Cessation Advice[1]	17	71%	90%	80%	100%
Surgical Infection Prevention					
Prophylactic Antibiotic Given	219	73%	83%	77%	95%
Prophylactic Antibiotic Selection	47	98%	90%	90%	100%
Prophylactic Antibiotic Stopped	213	54%	70%	72%	95%
Pregnancy Care					

NOTE: Hospital profiles are in alphabetical order by state, then city, then hospital within the city; Rankings are sorted by rate in descending order and exclude hospitals with less than 25 cases; (1) The number of cases is too small (n<25) for purposes of reliably predicting hospital performance; (2) Measure reflects the hospital's indication that its submission was based upon a sample of its relevant discharges; (3) Rate reflects fewer than the maximum possible quarters of data for the measure; (4) Inaccurate information submitted and suppressed for one or more quarters; (5) No data is available from the hospital for this measure; Please refer to the User's Guide for a full explanation of data

Inpatient Neonatal Mortality	-	-	-	-	-
Third or Fourth Degree Laceration	-	-	2.71%	3.63%	3.27%

Good Samaritan Medical Center

Alternate Name: Good Samaritan Medical Center

1309 N Flagler Drive
West Palm Beach, FL 33401
URL: www.goodsamaritanmc.com
Ownership: Proprietary
Emergency Services: Yes

Phone: 561-655-5511
Fax: 561-650-6127

Accredited: Yes
Licensed Beds: 341

Key Personnel:
President/CEO . . . . Trevor Fetter
Chief Medical Staff . . . . Daniel R Higgins, MD
Emergency Room . . . . David Soria, MD
Director Infection/Disease Control . . . . Arlene Merrill
OB/GYN Womens Health . . . . Moises Virelles, MD
Chief Radiology . . . . Nicholas A Rojo, MD
Director Respiratory Therapy . . . . Barbara Kelly

Measure	Cases	This Hospital	State Average	U.S. Average	Top Hospital
Heart Attack Care					
ACE Inhibitor or ARB for LVSD[1]	8	75%	83%	82%	100%
Aspirin at Arrival	51	96%	93%	92%	100%
Aspirin at Discharge[1]	23	96%	88%	90%	100%
Beta Blocker at Arrival	46	98%	89%	87%	100%
Beta Blocker at Discharge	30	100%	92%	90%	100%
Fibrinolytic Medication Timing[1]	1	0%	33%	31%	100%
PCI Within 90 Minutes of Arrival	0	-	52%	54%	95%
Smoking Cessation Advice[1]	3	100%	92%	88%	100%
Heart Failure Care					
ACE Inhibitor or ARB for LVSD	77	86%	82%	82%	100%
Discharge Instructions	206	67%	61%	61%	93%
Evaluation of LVS Function	263	95%	90%	83%	99%
Smoking Cessation Advice	27	100%	91%	82%	100%
Pneumonia Care					
Appropriate Initial Antibiotic	217	89%	84%	83%	94%
Blood Culture Timing	221	95%	88%	90%	100%
Influenza Vaccine	63	98%	64%	70%	100%
Initial Antibiotic Timing	298	84%	74%	80%	93%
Oxygenation Assessment	349	100%	99%	99%	100%
Pneumococcal Vaccine	210	94%	67%	69%	94%
Smoking Cessation Advice	61	100%	90%	80%	100%
Surgical Infection Prevention					
Prophylactic Antibiotic Given[2]	227	70%	83%	77%	95%
Prophylactic Antibiotic Selection[2]	62	97%	90%	90%	100%
Prophylactic Antibiotic Stopped[2]	219	78%	70%	72%	95%
Pregnancy Care					
Inpatient Neonatal Mortality	-	-	-	-	-
Third or Fourth Degree Laceration	-	-	2.71%	3.63%	3.27%

Saint Mary's Medical Center

901 45th Street
West Palm Beach, FL 33407
URL: www.stmarysmc.com
Ownership: Proprietary
Emergency Services: Yes

Phone: 561-644-6300
Fax: 561-882-1025

Accredited: Yes
Licensed Beds: 460

Key Personnel:
Administrator/President . . . . Steve Nathan
Chief Medical Staff . . . . David Dodson, MD
Director Catheterization Laboratory . . . . James Whittle, MD
OB/GYN Womens Health . . . . Peter A Sherman, MD
Director Radiology . . . . Nicholas Rojo, MD

Measure	Cases	This Hospital	State Average	U.S. Average	Top Hospital
Heart Attack Care					
ACE Inhibitor or ARB for LVSD[1]	3	67%	83%	82%	100%
Aspirin at Arrival	46	96%	93%	92%	100%
Aspirin at Discharge[1]	19	79%	88%	90%	100%
Beta Blocker at Arrival	45	98%	89%	87%	100%
Beta Blocker at Discharge[1]	22	86%	92%	90%	100%
Fibrinolytic Medication Timing[1]	2	0%	33%	31%	100%
PCI Within 90 Minutes of Arrival	0	-	52%	54%	95%
Smoking Cessation Advice[1]	4	100%	92%	88%	100%

Measure	Cases	This Hospital	State Average	U.S. Average	Top Hospital
Heart Failure Care					
ACE Inhibitor or ARB for LVSD	81	86%	82%	82%	100%
Discharge Instructions	168	92%	61%	61%	93%
Evaluation of LVS Function	209	95%	90%	83%	99%
Smoking Cessation Advice	46	96%	91%	82%	100%
Pneumonia Care					
Appropriate Initial Antibiotic	165	93%	84%	83%	94%
Blood Culture Timing	207	95%	88%	90%	100%
Influenza Vaccine	40	92%	64%	70%	100%
Initial Antibiotic Timing	287	78%	74%	80%	93%
Oxygenation Assessment	301	100%	99%	99%	100%
Pneumococcal Vaccine	94	90%	67%	69%	94%
Smoking Cessation Advice	95	100%	90%	80%	100%
Surgical Infection Prevention					
Prophylactic Antibiotic Given[2]	192	84%	83%	77%	95%
Prophylactic Antibiotic Selection[2]	37	89%	90%	90%	100%
Prophylactic Antibiotic Stopped[2]	185	74%	70%	72%	95%
Pregnancy Care					
Inpatient Neonatal Mortality	-	-	-	-	-
Third or Fourth Degree Laceration	-	-	2.71%	3.63%	3.27%

Cleveland Clinic Florida

Alternate Name: North Beach Community Hospital

3100 Weston Road
Weston, FL 33331

Toll-Free: 866-293-7866
Phone: 954-689-5000
Fax: 954-689-5058

URL: www.clevelandclinic.org
Ownership: Proprietary
Emergency Services: Yes

Accredited: Yes
Licensed Beds: 150

Key Personnel:
CEO . . . . Bernardo Fernandez, MD
Chief Medical Staff . . . . Eduardo Oliviera, MD
Cardiology Director . . . . Howard Bush, MD
Emergency Room . . . . Vicki Cotto, RN
Director Respiratory Therapy . . . . Laurence Smolley, MD

Measure	Cases	This Hospital	State Average	U.S. Average	Top Hospital
Heart Attack Care					
ACE Inhibitor or ARB for LVSD	41	100%	83%	82%	100%
Aspirin at Arrival	87	100%	93%	92%	100%
Aspirin at Discharge	140	100%	88%	90%	100%
Beta Blocker at Arrival	86	100%	89%	87%	100%
Beta Blocker at Discharge	142	100%	92%	90%	100%
Fibrinolytic Medication Timing	0	-	33%	31%	100%
PCI Within 90 Minutes of Arrival[1]	12	83%	52%	54%	95%
Smoking Cessation Advice	44	100%	92%	88%	100%
Heart Failure Care					
ACE Inhibitor or ARB for LVSD	97	100%	82%	82%	100%
Discharge Instructions	207	93%	61%	61%	93%
Evaluation of LVS Function	220	100%	90%	83%	99%
Smoking Cessation Advice[1]	20	100%	91%	82%	100%
Pneumonia Care					
Appropriate Initial Antibiotic	83	95%	84%	83%	94%
Blood Culture Timing	90	96%	88%	90%	100%
Influenza Vaccine	28	96%	64%	70%	100%
Initial Antibiotic Timing	84	86%	74%	80%	93%
Oxygenation Assessment	120	100%	99%	99%	100%
Pneumococcal Vaccine	71	96%	67%	69%	94%
Smoking Cessation Advice[1]	8	100%	90%	80%	100%
Surgical Infection Prevention					
Prophylactic Antibiotic Given[2]	320	97%	83%	77%	95%
Prophylactic Antibiotic Selection[2]	76	97%	90%	90%	100%
Prophylactic Antibiotic Stopped[2]	312	67%	70%	72%	95%
Pregnancy Care					
Inpatient Neonatal Mortality	-	-	-	-	-
Third or Fourth Degree Laceration	-	-	2.71%	3.63%	3.27%

Nature Coast Regional Hospital

Alternate Name: Williston Memorial Hospital

NOTE: Hospital profiles are in alphabetical order by state, then city, then hospital within the city; Rankings are sorted by rate in descending order and exclude hospitals with less than 25 cases; (1) The number of cases is too small (n<25) for purposes of reliably predicting hospital performance; (2) Measure reflects the hospital's indication that its submission was based upon a sample of its relevant discharges; (3) Rate reflects fewer than the maximum possible quarters of data for the measure; (4) Inaccurate information submitted and suppressed for one or more quarters; (5) No data is available from the hospital for this measure; Please refer to the User's Guide for a full explanation of data

125 SW 7th Street
Williston, FL 32696
E-mail: ncrh@cypress-of-fl.com
Ownership: Voluntary non-profit - Private
Emergency Services: Yes
Phone: 352-528-2801
Fax: 352-528-6149
Accredited: No
Licensed Beds: 40

Key Personnel:
CEO. . . . . Alan Bird
Chief Medical Staff. . . . . Richard Martin, MD
Emergency Room . . . . Madonna Otto, LPN
Emergency Room . . . . Karen Meyer, RN
Director Medical/Surgical Nursing . . . . Gail Pence, RN, DON
Director Medical/Surgical Nursing . . . . Beth Buckley, RN
Chief Radiology . . . . Tom Rice
Director Respiratory Therapy . . . . Nancy Campos

Measure	Cases	This Hospital	State Average	U.S. Average	Top Hospital
Heart Attack Care					
ACE Inhibitor or ARB for LVSD[3]	0	-	83%	82%	100%
Aspirin at Arrival[3]	0	-	93%	92%	100%
Aspirin at Discharge[3]	0	-	88%	90%	100%
Beta Blocker at Arrival[3]	0	-	89%	87%	100%
Beta Blocker at Discharge[3]	0	-	92%	90%	100%
Fibrinolytic Medication Timing[3]	0	-	33%	31%	100%
PCI Within 90 Minutes of Arrival	0	-	52%	54%	95%
Smoking Cessation Advice[3]	0	-	92%	88%	100%
Heart Failure Care					
ACE Inhibitor or ARB for LVSD[1]	15	87%	82%	82%	100%
Discharge Instructions[1,3]	1	0%	61%	61%	93%
Evaluation of LVS Function	41	78%	90%	83%	99%
Smoking Cessation Advice[1,3]	1	0%	91%	82%	100%
Pneumonia Care					
Appropriate Initial Antibiotic[1,3]	10	100%	84%	83%	94%
Blood Culture Timing[1,3]	4	100%	88%	90%	100%
Influenza Vaccine[5]	-	-	64%	70%	100%
Initial Antibiotic Timing	41	71%	74%	80%	93%
Oxygenation Assessment	49	100%	99%	99%	100%
Pneumococcal Vaccine[1]	21	14%	67%	69%	94%
Smoking Cessation Advice[1,3]	2	50%	90%	80%	100%
Surgical Infection Prevention					
Prophylactic Antibiotic Given[5]	-	-	83%	77%	95%
Prophylactic Antibiotic Selection[5]	-	-	90%	90%	100%
Prophylactic Antibiotic Stopped[5]	-	-	70%	72%	95%
Pregnancy Care					
Inpatient Neonatal Mortality	-	-	-	-	-
Third or Fourth Degree Laceration	-	-	2.71%	3.63%	3.27%

Winter Haven Hospital

Alternate Name: Morrow Memorial Hospital
200 Avenue F NE
Winter Haven, FL 33881
URL: www.winterhavenhospital.com
Ownership: Voluntary non-profit - Private
Emergency Services: Yes
Phone: 863-293-1121
Fax: 863-291-6028
Accredited: Yes
Licensed Beds: 579

Key Personnel:
President/CEO. . . . . Lance Anastasio
Chief Medical Staff. . . . . Peter Verril, MD
Emergency Room . . . . E Cary Pigman, MD
Director Infection/Disease Control . . . . Larry Vargo
OB/GYN Womens Health. . . . . Patricia Fearing, MD
Director Radiology . . . . Tony Patrick
Director Respiratory Therapy . . . . Kaye Larocque

Measure	Cases	This Hospital	State Average	U.S. Average	Top Hospital
Heart Attack Care					
ACE Inhibitor or ARB for LVSD	85	80%	83%	82%	100%
Aspirin at Arrival	299	97%	93%	92%	100%
Aspirin at Discharge	324	92%	88%	90%	100%
Beta Blocker at Arrival	265	89%	89%	87%	100%
Beta Blocker at Discharge	328	94%	92%	90%	100%
Fibrinolytic Medication Timing	0	-	33%	31%	100%
PCI Within 90 Minutes of Arrival[1]	12	67%	52%	54%	95%
Smoking Cessation Advice	108	99%	92%	88%	100%
Heart Failure Care					
ACE Inhibitor or ARB for LVSD	300	93%	82%	82%	100%
Discharge Instructions	436	89%	61%	61%	93%
Evaluation of LVS Function	532	96%	90%	83%	99%
Smoking Cessation Advice	72	97%	91%	82%	100%
Pneumonia Care					
Appropriate Initial Antibiotic	367	86%	84%	83%	94%
Blood Culture Timing	379	93%	88%	90%	100%
Influenza Vaccine	141	79%	64%	70%	100%
Initial Antibiotic Timing	532	77%	74%	80%	93%
Oxygenation Assessment	605	99%	99%	99%	100%
Pneumococcal Vaccine	386	78%	67%	69%	94%
Smoking Cessation Advice	114	90%	90%	80%	100%
Surgical Infection Prevention					
Prophylactic Antibiotic Given	738	92%	83%	77%	95%
Prophylactic Antibiotic Selection	198	97%	90%	90%	100%
Prophylactic Antibiotic Stopped	693	87%	70%	72%	95%
Pregnancy Care					
Inpatient Neonatal Mortality	-	-	-	-	-
Third or Fourth Degree Laceration	-	-	2.71%	3.63%	3.27%

Florida Hospital Zephyrhills

7050 Gall Boulevard
Zephyrhills, FL 33541
URL: www.fhzeph.org
Ownership: Voluntary non-profit - Church
Emergency Services: Yes
Phone: 813-788-0411
Fax: 813-783-6196
Accredited: Yes
Licensed Beds: 154

Key Personnel:
CEO. . . . . Scott Pittman
Chief Medical Staff. . . . . Paul Citrin, MD
Director Catheterization Lab. . . . . Aimee Keller
Emergency Room . . . . Barbara Neal
Infection Control. . . . . Xiomara Hewitt-Jeffrey
Director Medical/Surgical Nursing . . . . Susan McCuistion
Director OB/GYN/Women's Health. . . . . Madeline Beaumont
Director Radiology . . . . Aime Keller
Director Respiratory Therapy . . . . Cindy Bucklen

Measure	Cases	This Hospital	State Average	U.S. Average	Top Hospital
Heart Attack Care					
ACE Inhibitor or ARB for LVSD	55	69%	83%	82%	100%
Aspirin at Arrival	226	92%	93%	92%	100%
Aspirin at Discharge	185	92%	88%	90%	100%
Beta Blocker at Arrival	206	85%	89%	87%	100%
Beta Blocker at Discharge	184	89%	92%	90%	100%
Fibrinolytic Medication Timing[1]	14	14%	33%	31%	100%
PCI Within 90 Minutes of Arrival[1]	3	67%	52%	54%	95%
Smoking Cessation Advice	56	75%	92%	88%	100%
Heart Failure Care					
ACE Inhibitor or ARB for LVSD	110	82%	82%	82%	100%
Discharge Instructions	294	53%	61%	61%	93%
Evaluation of LVS Function	349	85%	90%	83%	99%
Smoking Cessation Advice	53	49%	91%	82%	100%
Pneumonia Care					
Appropriate Initial Antibiotic	176	86%	84%	83%	94%
Blood Culture Timing	101	79%	88%	90%	100%
Influenza Vaccine	59	29%	64%	70%	100%
Initial Antibiotic Timing	174	75%	74%	80%	93%
Oxygenation Assessment	233	96%	99%	99%	100%
Pneumococcal Vaccine	143	47%	67%	69%	94%
Smoking Cessation Advice	57	75%	90%	80%	100%
Surgical Infection Prevention					
Prophylactic Antibiotic Given	328	79%	83%	77%	95%
Prophylactic Antibiotic Selection	67	88%	90%	90%	100%
Prophylactic Antibiotic Stopped	308	78%	70%	72%	95%
Pregnancy Care					
Inpatient Neonatal Mortality	705	0.14%	-	-	-
Third or Fourth Degree Laceration	456	1.54%	2.71%	3.63%	3.27%

NOTE: Hospital profiles are in alphabetical order by state, then city, then hospital within the city; Rankings are sorted by rate in descending order and exclude hospitals with less than 25 cases; (1) The number of cases is too small (n<25) for purposes of reliably predicting hospital performance; (2) Measure reflects the hospital's indication that its submission was based upon a sample of its relevant discharges; (3) Rate reflects fewer than the maximum possible quarters of data for the measure; (4) Inaccurate information submitted and suppressed for one or more quarters; (5) No data is available from the hospital for this measure; Please refer to the User's Guide for a full explanation of data

Heart Attack Care

1. ACE Inhibitor or ARB for LVSD

Hospital Name	City	Rate	Cases
Atlanta Medical Center	Atlanta	100%	25
Saint Joseph Candler Hospital	Savannah	100%	55
John D Archbold Memorial Hospital	Thomasville	96%	28
Piedmont Hospital	Atlanta	94%	103
Medical College of Georgia Hospital & Clinics	Augusta	92%	59
Memorial Medical Center	Savannah	92%	91
Saint Francis Hospital	Columbus	92%	123
Grady Memorial Hospital	Atlanta	91%	103
University Hospital	Augusta	91%	113
Northeast Georgia Medical Center	Gainesville	89%	123
DeKalb Medical Center	Decatur	87%	39
Emory University Hospital	Atlanta	86%	72
Redmond Regional Medical Center	Rome	86%	140
Athens Regional Medical Center	Athens	85%	110
Southern Regional Medical Center	Riverdale	85%	26
WellStar Kennestone Hospital	Marietta	84%	159
Saint Joseph's Hospital	Atlanta	77%	324
Promina Gwinnett Health System	Lawrenceville	76%	25
Phoebe Putney Memorial Hospital	Albany	73%	128
Emory Crawford Long Hospital	Atlanta	72%	98
Medical Center of Central Georgia	Macon	58%	84
Coliseum Medical Center	Macon	55%	49

2. Aspirin at Arrival

Hospital Name	City	Rate	Cases
Colquitt Regional Medical Center	Moultrie	100%	39
John D Archbold Memorial Hospital	Thomasville	100%	122
Northside Hospital-Cherokee	Canton	100%	27
Rockdale Hospital	Conyers	100%	125
South Georgia Medical Center	Valdosta	100%	156
West Georgia Medical Center	La Grange	100%	140
Northeast Georgia Medical Center	Gainesville	99%	387
Redmond Regional Medical Center	Rome	99%	336
Atlanta Medical Center	Atlanta	98%	65
DeKalb Medical Center	Decatur	98%	171
Floyd Medical Center	Rome	98%	61
Henry Medical Center	Stockbridge	98%	164
Memorial Medical Center	Savannah	98%	233
North Fulton Regional Hospital	Roswell	98%	64
Saint Joseph's Hospital	Atlanta	98%	317
Spalding Regional Medical Center	Griffin	98%	112
Athens Regional Medical Center	Athens	97%	253
Candler Hospital	Savannah	97%	30
Emory Crawford Long Hospital	Atlanta	97%	100
Medical Center of Central Georgia	Macon	97%	121
Medical College of Georgia Hospital & Clinics	Augusta	97%	116
Oconee Regional Medical Center	Milledgeville	97%	34
Saint Joseph Candler Hospital	Savannah	97%	124
Tanner Medical Center	Villa Rica	97%	29
University Hospital	Augusta	97%	360
WellStar Douglas Hospital	Douglasville	97%	65
WellStar Kennestone Hospital	Marietta	97%	494
Newton Medical	Covington	96%	84
Northside Hospital	Atlanta	96%	49
Saint Francis Hospital	Columbus	96%	285
Tanner Medical Center	Carrollton	96%	135
Southern Regional Medical Center	Riverdale	95%	178
Dekalb Medical Center at Hillandale	Lithonia	94%	36
Emory Cartersville Medical Center	Cartersville	94%	52
Emory University Hospital	Atlanta	94%	112
Fairview Park Hospital	Dublin	94%	79
Hamilton Medical Center	Dalton	94%	97
Houston Medical Center	Warner Robins	94%	36
Northside Hospital	Cumming	94%	81
Phoebe Putney Memorial Hospital	Albany	94%	176
Piedmont Fayette Hospital	Fayetteville	94%	82
Emory Eastside Medical Center	Snellville	93%	86
Grady Memorial Hospital	Atlanta	93%	260
Saint Mary's Hospital	Athens	93%	54
Southeast Georgia Health System	Brunswick	93%	89
Tift Regional Medical Hospital	Tifton	93%	60
Doctors Hospital	Augusta	92%	39
Promina Gwinnett Health System	Lawrenceville	92%	225
South Fulton Medical Center	East Point	92%	118
Gordon Hospital	Calhoun	91%	64
Piedmont Hospital	Atlanta	91%	95
Satilla Regional Medical Center	Waycross	91%	74
Coliseum Medical Center	Macon	90%	73
Doctors Hospital	Columbus	90%	31
Meadows Regional Medical Center	Vidalia	90%	40

Hospital Name	City	Rate	Cases
BJC Medical Center	Commerce	89%	27
WellStar Cobb Hospital	Austell	89%	113
Hutcheson Medical Center	Fort Oglethorpe	88%	78
Upson Regional Medical Center	Thomaston	87%	46
East Georgia Regional Medical Center	Statesboro	86%	37
Columbus Medical Center	Columbus	85%	75
Crisp Regional Hospital	Cordele	76%	34

3. Aspirin at Discharge

Hospital Name	City	Rate	Cases
John D Archbold Memorial Hospital	Thomasville	100%	106
Rockdale Hospital	Conyers	100%	58
West Georgia Medical Center	La Grange	100%	63
Atlanta Medical Center	Atlanta	99%	67
Emory University Hospital	Atlanta	99%	244
Grady Memorial Hospital	Atlanta	99%	231
Memorial Medical Center	Savannah	99%	386
Northeast Georgia Medical Center	Gainesville	99%	560
Redmond Regional Medical Center	Rome	99%	568
Saint Joseph Candler Hospital	Savannah	99%	380
Athens Regional Medical Center	Athens	98%	345
Phoebe Putney Memorial Hospital	Albany	98%	455
Piedmont Hospital	Atlanta	98%	365
Saint Francis Hospital	Columbus	98%	361
Saint Joseph's Hospital	Atlanta	98%	1323
South Georgia Medical Center	Valdosta	98%	208
University Hospital	Augusta	98%	506
Columbus Medical Center	Columbus	97%	39
Medical College of Georgia Hospital & Clinics	Augusta	97%	159
North Fulton Regional Hospital	Roswell	96%	25
Northside Hospital	Cumming	96%	25
WellStar Kennestone Hospital	Marietta	96%	607
Emory Crawford Long Hospital	Atlanta	95%	296
Spalding Regional Medical Center	Griffin	95%	44
DeKalb Medical Center	Decatur	94%	117
Promina Gwinnett Health System	Lawrenceville	94%	81
Coliseum Medical Center	Macon	93%	123
Southeast Georgia Health System	Brunswick	92%	36
Piedmont Fayette Hospital	Fayetteville	91%	35
Gordon Hospital	Calhoun	90%	29
Medical Center of Central Georgia	Macon	90%	236
WellStar Cobb Hospital	Austell	90%	58
Tanner Medical Center	Carrollton	89%	62
Emory Eastside Medical Center	Snellville	87%	31
Fairview Park Hospital	Dublin	87%	55
Hamilton Medical Center	Dalton	86%	43
Henry Medical Center	Stockbridge	86%	71
Meadows Regional Medical Center	Vidalia	86%	37
East Georgia Regional Medical Center	Statesboro	85%	26
South Fulton Medical Center	East Point	85%	52
Tift Regional Medical Hospital	Tifton	85%	54
Newton Medical	Covington	83%	48
Saint Mary's Hospital	Athens	83%	35
Southern Regional Medical Center	Riverdale	81%	91
Hutcheson Medical Center	Fort Oglethorpe	60%	65
Satilla Regional Medical Center	Waycross	58%	31

4. Beta Blocker at Arrival

Hospital Name	City	Rate	Cases
Colquitt Regional Medical Center	Moultrie	100%	36
Rockdale Hospital	Conyers	100%	123
John D Archbold Memorial Hospital	Thomasville	99%	106
South Fulton Medical Center	East Point	99%	84
Atlanta Medical Center	Atlanta	98%	51
Memorial Medical Center	Savannah	98%	199
North Fulton Regional Hospital	Roswell	98%	58
Northside Hospital	Atlanta	98%	43
West Georgia Medical Center	La Grange	98%	110
Henry Medical Center	Stockbridge	97%	146
Medical College of Georgia Hospital & Clinics	Augusta	97%	77
Saint Francis Hospital	Columbus	97%	253
Saint Joseph's Hospital	Atlanta	97%	260
South Georgia Medical Center	Valdosta	97%	117
DeKalb Medical Center	Decatur	96%	156
Fairview Park Hospital	Dublin	96%	76
Newton Medical	Covington	96%	78
Saint Joseph Candler Hospital	Savannah	96%	91
Spalding Regional Medical Center	Griffin	96%	107
Tift Regional Medical Hospital	Tifton	96%	53
University Hospital	Augusta	96%	252
WellStar Cobb Hospital	Austell	96%	94
Emory Crawford Long Hospital	Atlanta	95%	92
Emory Eastside Medical Center	Snellville	95%	80
Emory University Hospital	Atlanta	95%	93

NOTE: Hospital profiles are in alphabetical order by state, then city, then hospital within the city; Rankings are sorted by rate in descending order and exclude hospitals with less than 25 cases; (1) The number of cases is too small (n<25) for purposes of reliably predicting hospital performance; (2) Measure reflects the hospital's indication that its submission was based upon a sample of its relevant discharges; (3) Rate reflects fewer than the maximum possible quarters of data for the measure; (4) Inaccurate information submitted and suppressed for one or more quarters; (5) No data is available from the hospital for this measure; Please refer to the User's Guide for a full explanation of data

Hospital Name	City	Rate	Cases
Hamilton Medical Center	Dalton	95%	73
Redmond Regional Medical Center	Rome	95%	242
WellStar Kennestone Hospital	Marietta	95%	382
Northeast Georgia Medical Center	Gainesville	94%	327
Promina Gwinnett Health System	Lawrenceville	94%	199
Tanner Medical Center	Carrollton	94%	111
Medical Center of Central Georgia	Macon	93%	88
Grady Memorial Hospital	Atlanta	92%	173
Saint Mary's Hospital	Athens	92%	40
Satilla Regional Medical Center	Waycross	92%	64
Dekalb Medical Center at Hillandale	Lithonia	91%	34
Piedmont Fayette Hospital	Fayetteville	91%	69
Athens Regional Medical Center	Athens	90%	164
Gordon Hospital	Calhoun	90%	63
Southern Regional Medical Center	Riverdale	90%	144
Emory Cartersville Medical Center	Cartersville	89%	38
Floyd Medical Center	Rome	89%	28
Doctors Hospital	Augusta	88%	25
Phoebe Putney Memorial Hospital	Albany	88%	162
Piedmont Hospital	Atlanta	88%	81
Coliseum Medical Center	Macon	87%	71
Oconee Regional Medical Center	Milledgeville	86%	29
Southeast Georgia Health System	Brunswick	86%	77
Tanner Medical Center	Villa Rica	86%	28
WellStar Douglas Hospital	Douglasville	85%	54
Columbus Medical Center	Columbus	84%	63
Houston Medical Center	Warner Robins	84%	32
Northside Hospital	Cumming	83%	66
Upson Regional Medical Center	Thomaston	82%	39
Meadows Regional Medical Center	Vidalia	81%	37
East Georgia Regional Medical Center	Statesboro	80%	41
BJC Medical Center	Commerce	79%	28
Hutcheson Medical Center	Fort Oglethrope	69%	68
Crisp Regional Hospital	Cordele	66%	35

5. Beta Blocker at Discharge

Hospital Name	City	Rate	Cases
Emory Eastside Medical Center	Snellville	100%	33
Medical College of Georgia Hospital & Clinics	Augusta	100%	130
Northside Hospital	Atlanta	100%	26
Rockdale Hospital	Conyers	100%	57
West Georgia Medical Center	La Grange	100%	68
Memorial Medical Center	Savannah	99%	409
Northeast Georgia Medical Center	Gainesville	99%	558
Saint Joseph Candler Hospital	Savannah	99%	401
Atlanta Medical Center	Atlanta	98%	65
Grady Memorial Hospital	Atlanta	98%	207
John D Archbold Memorial Hospital	Thomasville	98%	100
Saint Joseph's Hospital	Atlanta	98%	1275
South Fulton Medical Center	East Point	98%	52
University Hospital	Augusta	98%	447
DeKalb Medical Center	Decatur	97%	109
Piedmont Hospital	Atlanta	97%	350
Promina Gwinnett Health System	Lawrenceville	97%	91
Redmond Regional Medical Center	Rome	97%	584
Saint Francis Hospital	Columbus	97%	342
WellStar Kennestone Hospital	Marietta	97%	605
Athens Regional Medical Center	Athens	96%	332
Emory Cartersville Medical Center	Cartersville	96%	25
South Georgia Medical Center	Valdosta	96%	211
Columbus Medical Center	Columbus	95%	40
Emory University Hospital	Atlanta	95%	284
Fairview Park Hospital	Dublin	95%	59
Emory Crawford Long Hospital	Atlanta	94%	315
Medical Center of Central Georgia	Macon	94%	265
Tanner Medical Center	Carrollton	94%	63
Hamilton Medical Center	Dalton	93%	54
Phoebe Putney Memorial Hospital	Albany	93%	423
Henry Medical Center	Stockbridge	92%	73
Newton Medical	Covington	92%	49
North Fulton Regional Hospital	Roswell	92%	25
Piedmont Fayette Hospital	Fayetteville	92%	37
Southeast Georgia Health System	Brunswick	91%	43
WellStar Cobb Hospital	Austell	90%	58
Saint Mary's Hospital	Athens	89%	47
Tift Regional Medical Hospital	Tifton	89%	53
Southern Regional Medical Center	Riverdale	88%	94
Spalding Regional Medical Center	Griffin	88%	43
Gordon Hospital	Calhoun	87%	31
Coliseum Medical Center	Macon	86%	133
Satilla Regional Medical Center	Waycross	86%	28
Meadows Regional Medical Center	Vidalia	84%	37
East Georgia Regional Medical Center	Statesboro	81%	27
Hutcheson Medical Center	Fort Oglethrope	54%	59

6. Fibrinolytic Medication Timing

Hospital Name	City	Rate	Cases
Promina Gwinnett Health System	Lawrenceville	64%	47
Henry Medical Center	Stockbridge	62%	45
Southern Regional Medical Center	Riverdale	58%	36
Hamilton Medical Center	Dalton	38%	26

7. PCI Within 90 Minutes of Arrival

Hospital Name	City	Rate	Cases
WellStar Kennestone Hospital	Marietta	64%	25

8. Smoking Cessation Advice

Hospital Name	City	Rate	Cases
Athens Regional Medical Center	Athens	100%	171
DeKalb Medical Center	Decatur	100%	36
John D Archbold Memorial Hospital	Thomasville	100%	40
Northeast Georgia Medical Center	Gainesville	100%	227
Redmond Regional Medical Center	Rome	100%	284
Saint Joseph's Hospital	Atlanta	100%	466
Southern Regional Medical Center	Riverdale	100%	30
University Hospital	Augusta	100%	186
West Georgia Medical Center	La Grange	100%	36
Memorial Medical Center	Savannah	99%	169
Saint Francis Hospital	Columbus	99%	132
Saint Joseph Candler Hospital	Savannah	99%	178
Coliseum Medical Center	Macon	98%	44
Emory Crawford Long Hospital	Atlanta	98%	132
Emory University Hospital	Atlanta	98%	115
Medical Center of Central Georgia	Macon	98%	92
Medical College of Georgia Hospital & Clinics	Augusta	98%	102
Phoebe Putney Memorial Hospital	Albany	97%	207
Henry Medical Center	Stockbridge	96%	25
Piedmont Hospital	Atlanta	96%	139
WellStar Kennestone Hospital	Marietta	96%	207
South Georgia Medical Center	Valdosta	95%	85
Tanner Medical Center	Carrollton	92%	26
Hutcheson Medical Center	Fort Oglethrope	48%	25
Grady Memorial Hospital	Atlanta	44%	124

Heart Failure Care

9. ACE Inhibitor or ARB for LVSD

Hospital Name	City	Rate	Cases
Candler Hospital	Savannah	100%	126
Rockdale Hospital	Conyers	100%	84
Saint Joseph Candler Hospital	Savannah	100%	92
Atlanta Medical Center	Atlanta	99%	150
University Hospital	Augusta	98%	288
John D Archbold Memorial Hospital	Thomasville	97%	118
Tanner Medical Center	Villa Rica	94%	47
Meadows Regional Medical Center	Vidalia	93%	45
Promina Gwinnett Health System	Lawrenceville	93%	159
Saint Mary's Hospital	Athens	93%	105
Wayne Memorial Hospital	Jesup	93%	54
Emory University Hospital	Atlanta	92%	218
Memorial Medical Center	Savannah	92%	252
South Fulton Medical Center	East Point	92%	128
Newton Medical	Covington	91%	105
Smith Northview Hospital	Valdosta	91%	34
Athens Regional Medical Center	Athens	89%	94
Grady Memorial Hospital	Atlanta	89%	206
Peach Regional Medical Center	Fort Valley	89%	27
Tift Regional Medical Hospital	Tifton	89%	147
Upson Regional Medical Center	Thomaston	89%	71
Coffee Regional Medical Center	Douglas	88%	78
Henry Medical Center	Stockbridge	88%	130
North Fulton Regional Hospital	Roswell	88%	59
Northside Hospital	Atlanta	88%	86
Columbus Medical Center	Columbus	87%	106
DeKalb Medical Center	Decatur	86%	302
Dekalb Medical Center at Hillandale	Lithonia	86%	70
Medical College of Georgia Hospital & Clinics	Augusta	86%	222
Redmond Regional Medical Center	Rome	86%	314
Oconee Regional Medical Center	Milledgeville	85%	107
Spalding Regional Medical Center	Griffin	85%	146
Taylor Regional Hospital	Hawkinsville	85%	27
Doctors Hospital	Columbus	84%	91
Emory Dunwoody Medical Center	Atlanta	84%	38
Houston Medical Center	Warner Robins	84%	86
Memorial Hospital & Manor	Bainbridge	84%	31
Southern Regional Medical Center	Riverdale	83%	289
Crisp Regional Hospital	Cordele	82%	55

NOTE: Hospital profiles are in alphabetical order by state, then city, then hospital within the city; Rankings are sorted by rate in descending order and exclude hospitals with less than 25 cases; (1) The number of cases is too small (n<25) for purposes of reliably predicting hospital performance; (2) Measure reflects the hospital's indication that its submission was based upon a sample of its relevant discharges; (3) Rate reflects fewer than the maximum possible quarters of data for the measure; (4) Inaccurate information submitted and suppressed for one or more quarters; (5) No data is available from the hospital for this measure; Please refer to the User's Guide for a full explanation of data

Hospital Name	City	Rate	Cases
Emory Cartersville Medical Center	Cartersville	82%	56
Phoebe Putney Memorial Hospital	Albany	82%	182
Saint Francis Hospital	Columbus	82%	217
WellStar Cobb Hospital	Austell	82%	192
Emory Eastside Medical Center	Snellville	81%	83
Sumter Regional Hospital	Americus	81%	27
Northside Hospital-Cherokee	Canton	80%	44
South Georgia Medical Center	Valdosta	80%	126
WellStar Kennestone Hospital	Marietta	80%	332
Colquitt Regional Medical Center	Moultrie	79%	52
WellStar Douglas Hospital	Douglasville	79%	99
Emory Crawford Long Hospital	Atlanta	78%	259
Hamilton Medical Center	Dalton	78%	125
Medical Center of Central Georgia	Macon	78%	157
Piedmont Hospital	Atlanta	77%	234
West Georgia Medical Center	La Grange	77%	150
Northeast Georgia Medical Center	Gainesville	75%	217
Emory Northlake Regional Medical Center	Tucker	74%	46
Fairview Park Hospital	Dublin	74%	97
Macon Northside Hospital	Macon	74%	47
Palmyra Medical Centers	Albany	74%	58
Piedmont Fayette Hospital	Fayetteville	74%	88
Satilla Regional Medical Center	Waycross	73%	111
East Georgia Regional Medical Center	Statesboro	72%	61
Trinity Hospital of Augusta	Augusta	72%	25
Southeast Georgia Health System	Brunswick	71%	115
Coliseum Medical Center	Macon	69%	94
Walton Regional Medical Center	Monroe	69%	51
Floyd Medical Center	Rome	68%	122
Gordon Hospital	Calhoun	67%	39
Hutcheson Medical Center	Fort Oglethrope	66%	50
Doctors Hospital	Augusta	64%	73
Saint Joseph's Hospital	Atlanta	63%	420
Emanuel Medical Center	Swainsboro	62%	40
Northside Hospital	Cumming	61%	66
Tanner Medical Center	Carrollton	60%	111
Stephens County Hospital	Toccoa	48%	31
Meadows Regional Medical Center	Vidalia	68%	136
Northside Hospital	Cumming	68%	207
Oconee Regional Medical Center	Milledgeville	67%	184
Satilla Regional Medical Center	Waycross	67%	252
Northside Hospital	Atlanta	66%	185
Saint Joseph's Hospital	Atlanta	66%	634
Southeast Georgia Health Sys-Camden Campus	Saint Marys	66%	59
Taylor Regional Hospital	Hawkinsville	66%	64
Sumter Regional Hospital	Americus	65%	92
Coffee Regional Medical Center	Douglas	64%	232
Emanuel Medical Center	Swainsboro	64%	151
Northside Hospital-Cherokee	Canton	64%	96
Dorminy Medical Center	Fitzgerald	61%	33
Hart County Hospital	Hartwell	61%	66
Liberty Regional Medical Center	Hinesville	61%	36
Hutcheson Medical Center	Fort Oglethrope	60%	222
Cobb Memorial Hospital	Royston	59%	41
Habersham County Medical Center	Demorest	59%	44
Memorial Hospital & Manor	Bainbridge	59%	76
Emory Dunwoody Medical Center	Atlanta	58%	88
South Fulton Medical Center	East Point	58%	310
McDuffie Regional Medical Center	Thomson	55%	33
Saint Francis Hospital	Columbus	55%	482
Houston Medical Center	Warner Robins	53%	195
Northeast Georgia Medical Center	Gainesville	52%	474
Peach Regional Medical Center	Fort Valley	52%	67
Walton Regional Medical Center	Monroe	52%	153
Gordon Hospital	Calhoun	51%	106
Redmond Regional Medical Center	Rome	51%	574
Crisp Regional Hospital	Cordele	50%	162
Medical Center of Central Georgia	Macon	50%	241
Saint Mary's Hospital	Athens	50%	220
WellStar Kennestone Hospital	Marietta	50%	698
Coliseum Medical Center	Macon	49%	229
Union General Hospital	Blairsville	49%	61
Dekalb Medical Center at Hillandale	Lithonia	48%	136
South Georgia Medical Center	Valdosta	47%	318
Burke Medical Center	Waynesboro	46%	80
Doctors Hospital	Columbus	46%	203
Emory Crawford Long Hospital	Atlanta	46%	325
Fairview Park Hospital	Dublin	46%	224
Medical College of Georgia Hospital & Clinics	Augusta	45%	303
Piedmont Mountainside Hospital	Jasper	44%	87
Tanner Medical Center	Carrollton	43%	224
Hamilton Medical Center	Dalton	42%	327
Candler County Hospital	Metter	41%	46
Stephens County Hospital	Toccoa	41%	138
Phoebe Putney Memorial Hospital	Albany	40%	381
Emory-Adventist Hospital	Smyrna	38%	90
Tailor Telfair Regional Hospital	McRae	38%	26
Flint River Community Hospital	Montezuma	36%	44
WellStar Cobb Hospital	Austell	33%	458
Smith Northview Hospital	Valdosta	32%	79
Doctors Hospital	Augusta	30%	210
Chestatee Regional Hospital	Dahlonega	28%	29
WellStar Paulding Hospital	Dallas	28%	39
BJC Medical Center	Commerce	24%	59
Emory Cartersville Medical Center	Cartersville	21%	167
WellStar Douglas Hospital	Douglasville	21%	224
East Georgia Regional Medical Center	Statesboro	17%	180
Donalsonville Hospital	Donalsonville	12%	26
Floyd Medical Center	Rome	12%	211
Barrow Regional Medical Center	Winder	6%	65
Grady Memorial Hospital	Atlanta	1%	338

10. Discharge Instructions

Hospital Name	City	Rate	Cases
Evans Memorial Hospital	Claxton	100%	66
Wayne Memorial Hospital	Jesup	98%	103
Rockdale Hospital	Conyers	97%	306
Atlanta Medical Center	Atlanta	96%	232
Spalding Regional Medical Center	Griffin	93%	354
University Hospital	Augusta	91%	613
Dodge County Hospital	Eastman	89%	54
Hamilton Medical Center	Chatsworth	87%	63
Piedmont Fayette Hospital	Fayetteville	87%	53
Emory Eastside Medical Center	Snellville	86%	269
Emory Northlake Regional Medical Center	Tucker	85%	112
Memorial Medical Center	Savannah	85%	556
Tift Regional Medical Hospital	Tifton	84%	255
Washington County Regional Medical Center	Sandersville	84%	50
Elbert Memorial Hospital	Elberton	83%	72
Henry Medical Center	Stockbridge	83%	266
Trinity Hospital of Augusta	Augusta	83%	77
Bleckley Memorial Hospital	Cochran	82%	34
Palmyra Medical Centers	Albany	82%	106
Appling Hospital	Baxley	81%	42
West Georgia Medical Center	La Grange	81%	253
John D Archbold Memorial Hospital	Thomasville	80%	282
Piedmont Hospital	Atlanta	78%	376
Tanner Medical Center	Villa Rica	78%	100
Southeast Georgia Health System	Brunswick	77%	299
Higgins General Hospital	Bremen	75%	28
Jefferson Hospital	Louisville	75%	64
Promina Gwinnett Health System	Lawrenceville	75%	370
Newton Medical	Covington	74%	236
Colquitt Regional Medical Center	Moultrie	73%	125
Candler Hospital	Savannah	72%	366
Columbus Medical Center	Columbus	72%	314
Macon Northside Hospital	Macon	72%	109
Southern Regional Medical Center	Riverdale	72%	623
Emory University Hospital	Atlanta	71%	307
North Georgia Medical Center	Ellijay	71%	42
Perry Hospital	Perry	71%	38
Saint Joseph Candler Hospital	Savannah	71%	307
DeKalb Medical Center	Decatur	70%	500
North Fulton Regional Hospital	Roswell	70%	184
Upson Regional Medical Center	Thomaston	70%	145
Bacon County Hospital System	Alma	69%	32
Fannin Regional Hospital	Blue Ridge	69%	58
Athens Regional Medical Center	Athens	68%	260

11. Evaluation of LVS Function

Hospital Name	City	Rate	Cases
Emory University Hospital	Atlanta	100%	337
Wesley Woods Geriatric Hospital	Atlanta	100%	38
Emory Eastside Medical Center	Snellville	99%	303
Medical College of Georgia Hospital & Clinics	Augusta	99%	325
North Fulton Regional Hospital	Roswell	99%	206
Northside Hospital	Atlanta	99%	211
Promina Gwinnett Health System	Lawrenceville	99%	435
Saint Joseph's Hospital	Atlanta	99%	700
University Hospital	Augusta	99%	683
Athens Regional Medical Center	Athens	98%	281
Atlanta Medical Center	Atlanta	98%	258
Candler Hospital	Savannah	98%	425
Emory-Adventist Hospital	Smyrna	98%	99
John D Archbold Memorial Hospital	Thomasville	98%	320
Piedmont Hospital	Atlanta	98%	403
Tift Regional Medical Hospital	Tifton	98%	279
WellStar Kennestone Hospital	Marietta	98%	770

NOTE: Hospital profiles are in alphabetical order by state, then city, then hospital within the city; Rankings are sorted by rate in descending order and exclude hospitals with less than 25 cases; (1) The number of cases is too small (n<25) for purposes of reliably predicting hospital performance; (2) Measure reflects the hospital's indication that its submission was based upon a sample of its relevant discharges; (3) Rate reflects fewer than the maximum possible quarters of data for the measure; (4) Inaccurate information submitted and suppressed for one or more quarters; (5) No data is available from the hospital for this measure; Please refer to the User's Guide for a full explanation of data

Hospital Name	City	Rate	Cases
Chatuge Regional Hospital & Nursing Home	Hiawassee	97%	33
Hamilton Medical Center	Dalton	97%	390
Newton Medical	Covington	97%	268
Redmond Regional Medical Center	Rome	97%	636
Saint Joseph Candler Hospital	Savannah	97%	338
Saint Mary's Hospital	Athens	97%	242
Southeast Georgia Health System	Brunswick	97%	346
Taylor Regional Hospital	Hawkinsville	97%	76
Cobb Memorial Hospital	Royston	96%	55
Tanner Medical Center	Villa Rica	96%	106
Rockdale Hospital	Conyers	95%	346
Spalding Regional Medical Center	Griffin	95%	408
Columbus Medical Center	Columbus	94%	353
DeKalb Medical Center	Decatur	94%	580
Higgins General Hospital	Bremen	94%	36
Memorial Medical Center	Savannah	94%	606
Northside Hospital-Cherokee	Canton	94%	125
WellStar Cobb Hospital	Austell	94%	510
Dekalb Medical Center at Hillandale	Lithonia	93%	139
Emory Cartersville Medical Center	Cartersville	93%	187
Grady Memorial Hospital	Atlanta	93%	348
Medical Center of Central Georgia	Macon	93%	284
Palmyra Medical Centers	Albany	93%	123
West Georgia Medical Center	La Grange	93%	285
Colquitt Regional Medical Center	Moultrie	92%	153
Doctors Hospital	Columbus	92%	223
Emory Crawford Long Hospital	Atlanta	92%	342
Floyd Medical Center	Rome	92%	246
Habersham County Medical Center	Demorest	92%	53
Oconee Regional Medical Center	Milledgeville	92%	198
South Fulton Medical Center	East Point	92%	350
Emory Dunwoody Medical Center	Atlanta	91%	80
Northside Hospital	Cumming	91%	230
WellStar Douglas Hospital	Douglasville	91%	255
Gordon Hospital	Calhoun	90%	129
Phoebe Putney Memorial Hospital	Albany	90%	414
Tanner Medical Center	Carrollton	89%	272
WellStar Paulding Hospital	Dallas	89%	44
Emanuel Medical Center	Swainsboro	88%	164
Henry Medical Center	Stockbridge	88%	303
Piedmont Fayette Hospital	Fayetteville	88%	243
Saint Francis Hospital	Columbus	88%	560
Trinity Hospital of Augusta	Augusta	88%	96
Emory Northlake Regional Medical Center	Tucker	87%	129
Northeast Georgia Medical Center	Gainesville	87%	570
Piedmont Mountainside Hospital	Jasper	87%	102
Crisp Regional Hospital	Cordele	86%	184
Elbert Memorial Hospital	Elberton	86%	98
Fannin Regional Hospital	Blue Ridge	86%	74
Satilla Regional Medical Center	Waycross	86%	308
Wayne Memorial Hospital	Jesup	86%	124
South Georgia Medical Center	Valdosta	85%	359
Peach Regional Medical Center	Fort Valley	84%	76
Union General Hospital	Blairsville	84%	75
Walton Regional Medical Center	Monroe	84%	172
Southern Regional Medical Center	Riverdale	83%	694
Appling Hospital	Baxley	82%	44
Bacon County Hospital System	Alma	82%	39
Coliseum Medical Center	Macon	82%	253
Fairview Park Hospital	Dublin	82%	251
Macon Northside Hospital	Macon	82%	128
Sumter Regional Hospital	Americus	82%	107
Doctors Hospital	Augusta	81%	232
McDuffie Regional Medical Center	Thomson	81%	31
Meadows Regional Medical Center	Vidalia	80%	177
Upson Regional Medical Center	Thomaston	80%	171
Houston Medical Center	Warner Robins	79%	211
Perry Hospital	Perry	79%	53
Evans Memorial Hospital	Claxton	78%	59
Smith Northview Hospital	Valdosta	78%	88
Southeast Georgia Health Sys-Camden Campus	Saint Marys	77%	69
Washington County Regional Medical Center	Sandersville	75%	59
Chestatee Regional Hospital	Dahlonega	74%	43
Hutcheson Medical Center	Fort Oglethorpe	71%	250
Memorial Hospital & Manor	Bainbridge	71%	78
Memorial Hospital of Adel	Adel	71%	59
Flint River Community Hospital	Montezuma	70%	56
Coffee Regional Medical Center	Douglas	69%	254
East Georgia Regional Medical Center	Statesboro	69%	204
Hart County Hospital	Hartwell	69%	94
North Georgia Medical Center	Ellijay	67%	67
Dorminy Medical Center	Fitzgerald	66%	77
BJC Medical Center	Commerce	63%	75
Jefferson Hospital	Louisville	62%	78
Hamilton Medical Center	Chatsworth	59%	69
Liberty Regional Medical Center	Hinesville	55%	44
Stephens County Hospital	Toccoa	49%	162
Barrow Regional Medical Center	Winder	47%	51
Donalsonville Hospital	Donalsonville	45%	33
Bleckley Memorial Hospital	Cochran	32%	37
Burke Medical Center	Waynesboro	29%	86
Tailor Telfair Regional Hospital	McRae	26%	39
Dodge County Hospital	Eastman	21%	72
Candler County Hospital	Metter	15%	68
Polk Medical Center	Cedartown	14%	29

12. Smoking Cessation Advice

Hospital Name	City	Rate	Cases
Candler Hospital	Savannah	100%	59
Coliseum Medical Center	Macon	100%	58
Colquitt Regional Medical Center	Moultrie	100%	35
Dekalb Medical Center at Hillandale	Lithonia	100%	39
Doctors Hospital	Columbus	100%	45
Emory Eastside Medical Center	Snellville	100%	41
Emory University Hospital	Atlanta	100%	53
Fairview Park Hospital	Dublin	100%	54
John D Archbold Memorial Hospital	Thomasville	100%	86
Macon Northside Hospital	Macon	100%	34
Northside Hospital	Cumming	100%	44
Rockdale Hospital	Conyers	100%	42
Saint Joseph Candler Hospital	Savannah	100%	56
Southern Regional Medical Center	Riverdale	100%	166
University Hospital	Augusta	100%	108
Wayne Memorial Hospital	Jesup	100%	25
West Georgia Medical Center	La Grange	100%	55
Promina Gwinnett Health System	Lawrenceville	99%	76
Redmond Regional Medical Center	Rome	99%	139
WellStar Cobb Hospital	Austell	99%	126
Henry Medical Center	Stockbridge	98%	42
Northeast Georgia Medical Center	Gainesville	98%	84
Satilla Regional Medical Center	Waycross	98%	41
WellStar Douglas Hospital	Douglasville	98%	61
Athens Regional Medical Center	Athens	97%	62
Piedmont Hospital	Atlanta	97%	75
Saint Joseph's Hospital	Atlanta	97%	87
South Fulton Medical Center	East Point	97%	98
Spalding Regional Medical Center	Griffin	97%	111
Tift Regional Medical Hospital	Tifton	97%	62
WellStar Kennestone Hospital	Marietta	97%	174
Atlanta Medical Center	Atlanta	96%	77
Columbus Medical Center	Columbus	96%	130
DeKalb Medical Center	Decatur	96%	118
Emory Crawford Long Hospital	Atlanta	96%	73
Hamilton Medical Center	Dalton	96%	75
North Fulton Regional Hospital	Roswell	96%	27
South Georgia Medical Center	Valdosta	96%	75
Doctors Hospital	Augusta	95%	42
East Georgia Regional Medical Center	Statesboro	95%	41
Floyd Medical Center	Rome	95%	62
Meadows Regional Medical Center	Vidalia	94%	47
Northside Hospital	Atlanta	93%	30
Upson Regional Medical Center	Thomaston	91%	46
Houston Medical Center	Warner Robins	90%	72
Medical Center of Central Georgia	Macon	90%	50
Coffee Regional Medical Center	Douglas	89%	53
Crisp Regional Hospital	Cordele	89%	35
Saint Francis Hospital	Columbus	89%	123
Tanner Medical Center	Carrollton	89%	57
Emory Cartersville Medical Center	Cartersville	88%	43
Memorial Medical Center	Savannah	86%	161
Gordon Hospital	Calhoun	85%	26
Southeast Georgia Health System	Brunswick	85%	73
Oconee Regional Medical Center	Milledgeville	83%	42
Medical College of Georgia Hospital & Clinics	Augusta	81%	127
Saint Mary's Hospital	Athens	80%	66
Piedmont Mountainside Hospital	Jasper	79%	28
Newton Medical	Covington	76%	51
Phoebe Putney Memorial Hospital	Albany	76%	99
Emanuel Medical Center	Swainsboro	73%	33
Emory Northlake Regional Medical Center	Tucker	72%	32
Hutcheson Medical Center	Fort Oglethrope	57%	58
Emory-Adventist Hospital	Smyrna	41%	32
Stephens County Hospital	Toccoa	36%	28
Grady Memorial Hospital	Atlanta	25%	161

NOTE: Hospital profiles are in alphabetical order by state, then city, then hospital within the city; Rankings are sorted by rate in descending order and exclude hospitals with less than 25 cases; (1) The number of cases is too small (n<25) for purposes of reliably predicting hospital performance; (2) Measure reflects the hospital's indication that its submission was based upon a sample of its relevant discharges; (3) Rate reflects fewer than the maximum possible quarters of data for the measure; (4) Inaccurate information submitted and suppressed for one or more quarters; (5) No data is available from the hospital for this measure; Please refer to the User's Guide for a full explanation of data

Pneumonia Care

13. Appropriate Initial Antibiotic

Hospital Name	City	Rate	Cases
Chatuge Regional Hospital & Nursing Home	Hiawassee	100%	34
Upson Regional Medical Center	Thomaston	98%	91
Promina Gwinnett Health System	Lawrenceville	96%	283
Doctors Hospital	Augusta	95%	129
Northside Hospital	Atlanta	95%	181
Northside Hospital-Cherokee	Canton	94%	170
Higgins General Hospital	Bremen	93%	56
Emory Cartersville Medical Center	Cartersville	92%	199
Emory Eastside Medical Center	Snellville	92%	246
Liberty Regional Medical Center	Hinesville	92%	52
WellStar Paulding Hospital	Dallas	92%	78
John D Archbold Memorial Hospital	Thomasville	91%	132
Perry Hospital	Perry	91%	75
Spalding Regional Medical Center	Griffin	91%	224
Newton Medical	Covington	90%	153
Northside Hospital	Cumming	90%	239
University Hospital	Augusta	90%	300
Wayne Memorial Hospital	Jesup	90%	40
West Georgia Medical Center	La Grange	90%	181
Candler Hospital	Savannah	89%	217
Emory University Hospital	Atlanta	89%	55
Piedmont Hospital	Atlanta	89%	201
Saint Francis Hospital	Columbus	89%	255
Tanner Medical Center	Villa Rica	89%	104
Putnam General Hospital	Eatonton	88%	43
Rockdale Hospital	Conyers	88%	172
WellStar Douglas Hospital	Douglasville	88%	174
Chestatee Regional Hospital	Dahlonega	87%	70
Cobb Memorial Hospital	Royston	87%	52
Henry Medical Center	Stockbridge	87%	139
Houston Medical Center	Warner Robins	87%	92
Piedmont Fayette Hospital	Fayetteville	87%	31
South Georgia Medical Center	Valdosta	87%	141
Tanner Medical Center	Carrollton	87%	211
Athens Regional Medical Center	Athens	86%	107
Emory Crawford Long Hospital	Atlanta	86%	104
Fannin Regional Hospital	Blue Ridge	86%	77
Grady General Hospital	Cairo	86%	42
Habersham County Medical Center	Demorest	86%	79
Macon Northside Hospital	Macon	86%	51
Medical Center of Central Georgia	Macon	86%	80
Medical College of Georgia Hospital & Clinics	Augusta	86%	69
Northeast Georgia Medical Center	Gainesville	86%	280
Redmond Regional Medical Center	Rome	86%	276
Tift Regional Medical Hospital	Tifton	86%	138
WellStar Cobb Hospital	Austell	86%	244
Coliseum Medical Center	Macon	85%	131
Memorial Medical Center	Savannah	85%	226
Saint Joseph's Hospital	Atlanta	85%	256
Southern Regional Medical Center	Riverdale	85%	254
DeKalb Medical Center	Decatur	84%	227
Emory Dunwoody Medical Center	Atlanta	84%	44
Hamilton Medical Center	Dalton	84%	208
Monroe County Hospital	Forsyth	84%	37
Oconee Regional Medical Center	Milledgeville	84%	126
Phoebe Putney Memorial Hospital	Albany	84%	135
Satilla Regional Medical Center	Waycross	84%	166
South Fulton Medical Center	East Point	84%	182
Bacon County Hospital System	Alma	83%	35
Emanuel Medical Center	Swainsboro	83%	71
Grady Memorial Hospital	Atlanta	83%	115
Union General Hospital	Blairsville	83%	84
Walton Regional Medical Center	Monroe	83%	135
Floyd Medical Center	Rome	82%	195
North Fulton Regional Hospital	Roswell	82%	243
Saint Mary's Hospital	Athens	82%	85
Trinity Hospital of Augusta	Augusta	82%	79
Atlanta Medical Center	Atlanta	81%	47
Crisp Regional Hospital	Cordele	81%	102
Doctors Hospital	Columbus	81%	143
Palmyra Medical Centers	Albany	81%	69
WellStar Kennestone Hospital	Marietta	81%	354
Coffee Regional Medical Center	Douglas	80%	128
Dekalb Medical Center at Hillandale	Lithonia	80%	71
Gordon Hospital	Calhoun	80%	167
Hart County Hospital	Hartwell	80%	45
Meadows Regional Medical Center	Vidalia	80%	79
Saint Joseph Candler Hospital	Savannah	80%	107
Colquitt Regional Medical Center	Moultrie	79%	67
Columbus Medical Center	Columbus	79%	151

Hospital Name	City	Rate	Cases
Jefferson Hospital	Louisville	79%	47
Peach Regional Medical Center	Fort Valley	79%	39
Southeast Georgia Health System	Brunswick	79%	169
Appling Hospital	Baxley	78%	73
Smith Northview Hospital	Valdosta	78%	54
Piedmont Mountainside Hospital	Jasper	77%	149
Hamilton Medical Center	Chatsworth	76%	78
Evans Memorial Hospital	Claxton	75%	64
Burke Medical Center	Waynesboro	74%	65
Emory-Adventist Hospital	Smyrna	74%	66
Flint River Community Hospital	Montezuma	74%	34
Memorial Hospital & Manor	Bainbridge	74%	57
Washington County Regional Medical Center	Sandersville	74%	171
Emory Northlake Regional Medical Center	Tucker	73%	78
Candler County Hospital	Metter	71%	34
Elbert Memorial Hospital	Elberton	71%	73
East Georgia Regional Medical Center	Statesboro	70%	155
North Georgia Medical Center	Ellijay	70%	46
Taylor Regional Hospital	Hawkinsville	69%	52
Fairview Park Hospital	Dublin	68%	125
Southeast Georgia Health Sys-Camden Campus	Saint Marys	68%	59
Dodge County Hospital	Eastman	67%	67
Donalsonville Hospital	Donalsonville	67%	101
Sumter Regional Hospital	Americus	66%	64
Hutcheson Medical Center	Fort Oglethorpe	60%	210
Stephens County Hospital	Toccoa	60%	124
BJC Medical Center	Commerce	59%	32
Berrien County Hospital	Nashville	58%	36
McDuffie Regional Medical Center	Thomson	58%	77
Polk Medical Center	Cedartown	53%	36
Barrow Regional Medical Center	Winder	52%	82
Tailor Telfair Regional Hospital	McRae	31%	29

14. Blood Culture Timing

Hospital Name	City	Rate	Cases
Northside Hospital	Atlanta	99%	164
Fannin Regional Hospital	Blue Ridge	98%	80
Memorial Medical Center	Savannah	98%	207
Perry Hospital	Perry	98%	46
Chatuge Regional Hospital & Nursing Home	Hiawassee	97%	36
Elbert Memorial Hospital	Elberton	97%	39
Emory Dunwoody Medical Center	Atlanta	97%	37
Fairview Park Hospital	Dublin	97%	67
North Fulton Regional Hospital	Roswell	97%	240
Northside Hospital	Cumming	97%	256
Northside Hospital-Cherokee	Canton	97%	184
Palmyra Medical Centers	Albany	97%	36
Satilla Regional Medical Center	Waycross	97%	141
Stephens County Hospital	Toccoa	97%	93
Wayne Memorial Hospital	Jesup	97%	34
Emory-Adventist Hospital	Smyrna	96%	67
Saint Mary's Hospital	Athens	96%	72
Southeast Georgia Health System	Brunswick	96%	109
Crisp Regional Hospital	Cordele	95%	108
McDuffie Regional Medical Center	Thomson	95%	66
Saint Joseph Candler Hospital	Savannah	95%	105
University Hospital	Augusta	95%	400
Cobb Memorial Hospital	Royston	94%	54
Coffee Regional Medical Center	Douglas	94%	32
Doctors Hospital	Augusta	94%	94
Houston Medical Center	Warner Robins	94%	62
Saint Francis Hospital	Columbus	94%	247
Saint Joseph's Hospital	Atlanta	94%	211
South Georgia Medical Center	Valdosta	94%	53
Spalding Regional Medical Center	Griffin	94%	188
Taylor Regional Hospital	Hawkinsville	94%	32
Tift Regional Medical Hospital	Tifton	94%	66
Candler Hospital	Savannah	93%	224
Gordon Hospital	Calhoun	93%	99
Macon Northside Hospital	Macon	93%	58
Colquitt Regional Medical Center	Moultrie	92%	38
East Georgia Regional Medical Center	Statesboro	92%	74
Peach Regional Medical Center	Fort Valley	92%	36
Piedmont Mountainside Hospital	Jasper	92%	75
Rockdale Hospital	Conyers	92%	158
WellStar Paulding Hospital	Dallas	92%	59
Floyd Medical Center	Rome	91%	235
Hamilton Medical Center	Dalton	91%	163
Polk Medical Center	Cedartown	91%	32
Union General Hospital	Blairsville	91%	65
Washington County Regional Medical Center	Sandersville	91%	100
Atlanta Medical Center	Atlanta	90%	60
Emory Cartersville Medical Center	Cartersville	90%	184
Emory Eastside Medical Center	Snellville	90%	241

NOTE: Hospital profiles are in alphabetical order by state, then city, then hospital within the city; Rankings are sorted by rate in descending order and exclude hospitals with less than 25 cases; (1) The number of cases is too small (n<25) for purposes of reliably predicting hospital performance; (2) Measure reflects the hospital's indication that its submission was based upon a sample of its relevant discharges; (3) Rate reflects fewer than the maximum possible quarters of data for the measure; (4) Inaccurate information submitted and suppressed for one or more quarters; (5) No data is available from the hospital for this measure; Please refer to the User's Guide for a full explanation of data

Hospital Name	City	Rate	Cases
John D Archbold Memorial Hospital	Thomasville	90%	101
Medical Center of Central Georgia	Macon	90%	106
Piedmont Fayette Hospital	Fayetteville	90%	41
WellStar Douglas Hospital	Douglasville	90%	142
Emory University Hospital	Atlanta	89%	83
Hutcheson Medical Center	Fort Oglethrope	89%	211
WellStar Kennestone Hospital	Marietta	89%	367
Newton Medical	Covington	88%	112
Northeast Georgia Medical Center	Gainesville	88%	185
Putnam General Hospital	Eatonton	88%	33
Trinity Hospital of Augusta	Augusta	88%	77
Coliseum Medical Center	Macon	87%	109
DeKalb Medical Center	Decatur	87%	273
Liberty Regional Medical Center	Hinesville	87%	30
Redmond Regional Medical Center	Rome	87%	270
Southeast Georgia Health Sys-Camden Campus	Saint Marys	87%	31
Upson Regional Medical Center	Thomaston	87%	75
Oconee Regional Medical Center	Milledgeville	86%	146
Phoebe Putney Memorial Hospital	Albany	86%	97
Promina Gwinnett Health System	Lawrenceville	86%	289
Tanner Medical Center	Villa Rica	86%	57
West Georgia Medical Center	La Grange	86%	142
Hamilton Medical Center	Chatsworth	85%	61
Medical College of Georgia Hospital & Clinics	Augusta	85%	106
Walton Regional Medical Center	Monroe	85%	79
Meadows Regional Medical Center	Vidalia	84%	49
Piedmont Hospital	Atlanta	84%	209
Sumter Regional Hospital	Americus	84%	69
WellStar Cobb Hospital	Austell	84%	218
Athens Regional Medical Center	Athens	83%	89
Dodge County Hospital	Eastman	83%	35
Hart County Hospital	Hartwell	83%	29
Jefferson Hospital	Louisville	82%	33
Southern Regional Medical Center	Riverdale	82%	219
South Fulton Medical Center	East Point	80%	167
Emory Northlake Regional Medical Center	Tucker	78%	73
Tanner Medical Center	Carrollton	78%	113
Doctors Hospital	Columbus	77%	117
Dekalb Medical Center at Hillandale	Lithonia	75%	64
Barrow Regional Medical Center	Winder	74%	39
Habersham County Medical Center	Demorest	74%	69
Henry Medical Center	Stockbridge	74%	96
Columbus Medical Center	Columbus	73%	110
Emory Crawford Long Hospital	Atlanta	73%	113
Emanuel Medical Center	Swainsboro	69%	39
Grady Memorial Hospital	Atlanta	65%	106
Higgins General Hospital	Bremen	61%	33
Memorial Hospital & Manor	Bainbridge	61%	28
Doctors Hospital	Augusta	62%	45
Macon Northside Hospital	Macon	62%	26
Crisp Regional Hospital	Cordele	61%	31
Newton Medical	Covington	60%	53
Tanner Medical Center	Carrollton	58%	55
WellStar Kennestone Hospital	Marietta	57%	97
Trinity Hospital of Augusta	Augusta	56%	27
Walton Regional Medical Center	Monroe	56%	55
Southeast Georgia Health System	Brunswick	55%	42
Southern Regional Medical Center	Riverdale	55%	60
WellStar Douglas Hospital	Douglasville	55%	33
Houston Medical Center	Warner Robins	48%	29
Piedmont Mountainside Hospital	Jasper	48%	44
Upson Regional Medical Center	Thomaston	48%	29
Phoebe Putney Memorial Hospital	Albany	46%	35
Medical Center of Central Georgia	Macon	44%	25
Emory Crawford Long Hospital	Atlanta	38%	32
Henry Medical Center	Stockbridge	37%	30
Oconee Regional Medical Center	Milledgeville	34%	32
Meadows Regional Medical Center	Vidalia	32%	31
South Fulton Medical Center	East Point	31%	52
Medical College of Georgia Hospital & Clinics	Augusta	29%	31
Columbus Medical Center	Columbus	28%	25
Hutcheson Medical Center	Fort Oglethrope	18%	93
Hamilton Medical Center	Chatsworth	9%	32
Fairview Park Hospital	Dublin	8%	48

15. Influenza Vaccine

Hospital Name	City	Rate	Cases
Northside Hospital	Cumming	93%	58
Northside Hospital	Atlanta	92%	61
North Fulton Regional Hospital	Roswell	90%	58
Promina Gwinnett Health System	Lawrenceville	89%	62
Fannin Regional Hospital	Blue Ridge	88%	26
John D Archbold Memorial Hospital	Thomasville	88%	34
Emory Eastside Medical Center	Snellville	86%	77
Hamilton Medical Center	Dalton	84%	67
University Hospital	Augusta	83%	120
WellStar Cobb Hospital	Austell	82%	71
Northside Hospital-Cherokee	Canton	80%	41
Rockdale Hospital	Conyers	80%	59
Washington County Regional Medical Center	Sandersville	80%	35
Satilla Regional Medical Center	Waycross	79%	61
DeKalb Medical Center	Decatur	78%	85
West Georgia Medical Center	La Grange	78%	49
Floyd Medical Center	Rome	75%	72
Candler Hospital	Savannah	73%	71
Coffee Regional Medical Center	Douglas	73%	26
Coliseum Medical Center	Macon	73%	44
Piedmont Hospital	Atlanta	72%	64
Gordon Hospital	Calhoun	71%	52
Stephens County Hospital	Toccoa	71%	34
Emory-Adventist Hospital	Smyrna	69%	32
Memorial Medical Center	Savannah	69%	48
Redmond Regional Medical Center	Rome	69%	81
Saint Joseph Candler Hospital	Savannah	69%	42
South Georgia Medical Center	Valdosta	66%	29
Northeast Georgia Medical Center	Gainesville	65%	92
Saint Joseph's Hospital	Atlanta	65%	57
Doctors Hospital	Columbus	63%	35
Emory Cartersville Medical Center	Cartersville	63%	38
Athens Regional Medical Center	Athens	62%	26

16. Initial Antibiotic Timing

Hospital Name	City	Rate	Cases
Bacon County Hospital System	Alma	97%	39
Wayne Memorial Hospital	Jesup	95%	55
Habersham County Medical Center	Demorest	92%	78
Northside Hospital	Atlanta	92%	228
North Fulton Regional Hospital	Roswell	91%	302
Burke Medical Center	Waynesboro	90%	93
Cobb Memorial Hospital	Royston	90%	88
Fannin Regional Hospital	Blue Ridge	90%	124
Northeast Georgia Medical Center	Gainesville	90%	343
Northside Hospital	Cumming	90%	306
Polk Medical Center	Cedartown	90%	58
Emanuel Medical Center	Swainsboro	89%	95
Chatuge Regional Hospital & Nursing Home	Hiawassee	87%	47
Emory Cartersville Medical Center	Cartersville	87%	264
Rockdale Hospital	Conyers	87%	246
Tanner Medical Center	Villa Rica	87%	106
Upson Regional Medical Center	Thomaston	87%	138
Coffee Regional Medical Center	Douglas	86%	168
Hamilton Medical Center	Chatsworth	86%	98
Putnam General Hospital	Eatonton	86%	57
West Georgia Medical Center	La Grange	86%	259
Athens Regional Medical Center	Athens	85%	124
Berrien County Hospital	Nashville	85%	40
Gordon Hospital	Calhoun	85%	171
Grady General Hospital	Cairo	85%	40
Hart County Hospital	Hartwell	85%	65
John D Archbold Memorial Hospital	Thomasville	85%	177
McDuffie Regional Medical Center	Thomson	85%	138
Perry Hospital	Perry	85%	97
Dodge County Hospital	Eastman	84%	95
Emory Eastside Medical Center	Snellville	84%	301
Higgins General Hospital	Bremen	84%	77
Northside Hospital-Cherokee	Canton	84%	246
Southeast Georgia Health Sys-Camden Campus	Saint Marys	84%	55
Spalding Regional Medical Center	Griffin	84%	323
Donalsonville Hospital	Donalsonville	83%	99
Meadows Regional Medical Center	Vidalia	82%	118
Peach Regional Medical Center	Fort Valley	82%	39
University Hospital	Augusta	82%	524
Union General Hospital	Blairsville	81%	104
Newton Medical	Covington	80%	231
Saint Francis Hospital	Columbus	80%	342
Satilla Regional Medical Center	Waycross	80%	219
WellStar Paulding Hospital	Dallas	80%	88
Memorial Medical Center	Savannah	79%	281
Trinity Hospital of Augusta	Augusta	79%	113
Dorminy Medical Center	Fitzgerald	78%	64
Emory-Adventist Hospital	Smyrna	78%	74
Jefferson Hospital	Louisville	78%	77
Promina Gwinnett Health System	Lawrenceville	78%	377
Candler Hospital	Savannah	77%	328
Floyd Medical Center	Rome	77%	332
Piedmont Fayette Hospital	Fayetteville	77%	234
Walton Regional Medical Center	Monroe	77%	198
Washington County Regional Medical Center	Sandersville	77%	221

NOTE: Hospital profiles are in alphabetical order by state, then city, then hospital within the city; Rankings are sorted by rate in descending order and exclude hospitals with less than 25 cases; (1) The number of cases is too small (n<25) for purposes of reliably predicting hospital performance; (2) Measure reflects the hospital's indication that its submission was based upon a sample of its relevant discharges; (3) Rate reflects fewer than the maximum possible quarters of data for the measure; (4) Inaccurate information submitted and suppressed for one or more quarters; (5) No data is available from the hospital for this measure; Please refer to the User's Guide for a full explanation of data

Doctors Hospital	Columbus	76%	177
Emory Dunwoody Medical Center	Atlanta	76%	49
Saint Joseph Candler Hospital	Savannah	76%	160
Appling Hospital	Baxley	75%	113
Candler County Hospital	Metter	75%	56
Flint River Community Hospital	Montezuma	74%	53
Hutcheson Medical Center	Fort Oglethrope	74%	352
Memorial Hospital & Manor	Bainbridge	74%	70
Saint Joseph's Hospital	Atlanta	74%	318
Saint Mary's Hospital	Athens	74%	107
Stephens County Hospital	Toccoa	74%	166
Macon Northside Hospital	Macon	73%	86
Chestatee Regional Hospital	Dahlonega	72%	69
Coliseum Medical Center	Macon	72%	195
Redmond Regional Medical Center	Rome	72%	332
Tanner Medical Center	Carrollton	72%	218
WellStar Douglas Hospital	Douglasville	72%	214
Evans Memorial Hospital	Claxton	71%	96
Oconee Regional Medical Center	Milledgeville	71%	211
Sumter Regional Hospital	Americus	71%	104
Atlanta Medical Center	Atlanta	70%	96
East Georgia Regional Medical Center	Statesboro	70%	159
Elbert Memorial Hospital	Elberton	70%	81
Taylor Regional Hospital	Hawkinsville	70%	92
Columbus Medical Center	Columbus	69%	197
Barrow Regional Medical Center	Winder	68%	76
Monroe County Hospital	Forsyth	68%	40
Piedmont Hospital	Atlanta	68%	311
Southern Regional Medical Center	Riverdale	68%	314
Emory Northlake Regional Medical Center	Tucker	67%	104
Hamilton Medical Center	Dalton	67%	301
North Georgia Medical Center	Ellijay	67%	55
Piedmont Mountainside Hospital	Jasper	66%	145
Henry Medical Center	Stockbridge	65%	164
Memorial Hospital of Adel	Adel	65%	48
Smith Northview Hospital	Valdosta	65%	51
Southeast Georgia Health System	Brunswick	65%	182
Tift Regional Medical Hospital	Tifton	65%	138
Doctors Hospital	Augusta	64%	190
Medical Center of Central Georgia	Macon	64%	150
South Fulton Medical Center	East Point	64%	263
South Georgia Medical Center	Valdosta	64%	199
Dekalb Medical Center at Hillandale	Lithonia	63%	82
Emory Crawford Long Hospital	Atlanta	63%	208
WellStar Kennestone Hospital	Marietta	63%	503
DeKalb Medical Center	Decatur	61%	410
Houston Medical Center	Warner Robins	61%	133
Medical College of Georgia Hospital & Clinics	Augusta	61%	168
Phoebe Putney Memorial Hospital	Albany	60%	220
Emory University Hospital	Atlanta	59%	125
WellStar Cobb Hospital	Austell	59%	336
Fairview Park Hospital	Dublin	57%	199
Palmyra Medical Centers	Albany	57%	102
Crisp Regional Hospital	Cordele	54%	155
Liberty Regional Medical Center	Hinesville	45%	80
BJC Medical Center	Commerce	39%	57
Grady Memorial Hospital	Atlanta	32%	214

17. Oxygenation Assessment

Hospital Name	City	Rate	Cases
Appling Hospital	Baxley	100%	138
Athens Regional Medical Center	Athens	100%	170
Atlanta Medical Center	Atlanta	100%	119
BJC Medical Center	Commerce	100%	71
Bacon County Hospital System	Alma	100%	54
Barrow Regional Medical Center	Winder	100%	103
Brooks County Hospital	Quitman	100%	26
Candler County Hospital	Metter	100%	63
Candler Hospital	Savannah	100%	423
Chatuge Regional Hospital & Nursing Home	Hiawassee	100%	55
Columbus Medical Center	Columbus	100%	240
DeKalb Medical Center	Decatur	100%	504
Dekalb Medical Center at Hillandale	Lithonia	100%	95
Doctors Hospital	Augusta	100%	234
Doctors Hospital	Columbus	100%	211
Emanuel Medical Center	Swainsboro	100%	119
Emory Cartersville Medical Center	Cartersville	100%	304
Emory Crawford Long Hospital	Atlanta	100%	224
Emory Dunwoody Medical Center	Atlanta	100%	58
Emory Eastside Medical Center	Snellville	100%	394
Emory University Hospital	Atlanta	100%	149
Evans Memorial Hospital	Claxton	100%	118
Fannin Regional Hospital	Blue Ridge	100%	151
Floyd Medical Center	Rome	100%	420
Gordon Hospital	Calhoun	100%	219
Habersham County Medical Center	Demorest	100%	111
Hamilton Medical Center	Chatsworth	100%	114
Higgins General Hospital	Bremen	100%	95
Houston Medical Center	Warner Robins	100%	175
John D Archbold Memorial Hospital	Thomasville	100%	225
Liberty Regional Medical Center	Hinesville	100%	91
Macon Northside Hospital	Macon	100%	107
Meadows Regional Medical Center	Vidalia	100%	156
Medical Center of Central Georgia	Macon	100%	174
Medical College of Georgia Hospital & Clinics	Augusta	100%	190
Memorial Hospital of Adel	Adel	100%	59
Memorial Medical Center	Savannah	100%	344
Mitchell County Hospital	Camilla	100%	29
Newton Medical	Covington	100%	248
North Fulton Regional Hospital	Roswell	100%	370
Northeast Georgia Medical Center	Gainesville	100%	412
Northside Hospital	Atlanta	100%	312
Northside Hospital	Cumming	100%	397
Northside Hospital-Cherokee	Canton	100%	303
Oconee Regional Medical Center	Milledgeville	100%	236
Palmyra Medical Centers	Albany	100%	130
Peach Regional Medical Center	Fort Valley	100%	44
Phoebe Putney Memorial Hospital	Albany	100%	240
Piedmont Fayette Hospital	Fayetteville	100%	266
Piedmont Hospital	Atlanta	100%	363
Promina Gwinnett Health System	Lawrenceville	100%	450
Redmond Regional Medical Center	Rome	100%	424
Rockdale Hospital	Conyers	100%	292
Saint Francis Hospital	Columbus	100%	409
Saint Joseph Candler Hospital	Savannah	100%	215
Saint Joseph's Hospital	Atlanta	100%	397
Saint Mary's Hospital	Athens	100%	129
Satilla Regional Medical Center	Waycross	100%	270
South Fulton Medical Center	East Point	100%	309
Spalding Regional Medical Center	Griffin	100%	367
Sylvan Grove Hospital	Jackson	100%	25
Tanner Medical Center	Carrollton	100%	292
Tanner Medical Center	Villa Rica	100%	121
Taylor Regional Hospital	Hawkinsville	100%	100
Tift Regional Medical Hospital	Tifton	100%	160
Trinity Hospital of Augusta	Augusta	100%	138
Union General Hospital	Blairsville	100%	125
University Hospital	Augusta	100%	660
Upson Regional Medical Center	Thomaston	100%	171
Walton Regional Medical Center	Monroe	100%	226
Washington County Regional Medical Center	Sandersville	100%	256
Wayne Memorial Hospital	Jesup	100%	65
WellStar Cobb Hospital	Austell	100%	417
WellStar Douglas Hospital	Douglasville	100%	255
WellStar Kennestone Hospital	Marietta	100%	624
WellStar Paulding Hospital	Dallas	100%	107
West Georgia Medical Center	La Grange	100%	288
Chestatee Regional Hospital	Dahlonega	99%	102
Cobb Memorial Hospital	Royston	99%	106
Coffee Regional Medical Center	Douglas	99%	169
Dorminy Medical Center	Fitzgerald	99%	68
Elbert Memorial Hospital	Elberton	99%	111
Flint River Community Hospital	Montezuma	99%	69
Grady Memorial Hospital	Atlanta	99%	231
Hutcheson Medical Center	Fort Oglethorpe	99%	474
McDuffie Regional Medical Center	Thomson	99%	144
Memorial Hospital & Manor	Bainbridge	99%	79
North Georgia Medical Center	Ellijay	99%	69
Piedmont Mountainside Hospital	Jasper	99%	187
Polk Medical Center	Cedartown	99%	68
Putnam General Hospital	Eatonton	99%	83
South Georgia Medical Center	Valdosta	99%	240
Southern Regional Medical Center	Riverdale	99%	357
Stephens County Hospital	Toccoa	99%	190
Sumter Regional Hospital	Americus	99%	127
Coliseum Medical Center	Macon	98%	214
East Georgia Regional Medical Center	Statesboro	98%	196
Emory Northlake Regional Medical Center	Tucker	98%	118
Hamilton Medical Center	Dalton	98%	389
Henry Medical Center	Stockbridge	98%	200
Monroe County Hospital	Forsyth	98%	46
Perry Hospital	Perry	98%	129
Southeast Georgia Health System	Brunswick	98%	230
Colquitt Regional Medical Center	Moultrie	97%	109
Dodge County Hospital	Eastman	97%	111
Emory-Adventist Hospital	Smyrna	97%	101
Fairview Park Hospital	Dublin	97%	225
Hart County Hospital	Hartwell	97%	77
Southeast Georgia Health Sys-Camden Campus	Saint Marys	97%	67

NOTE: Hospital profiles are in alphabetical order by state, then city, then hospital within the city; Rankings are sorted by rate in descending order and exclude hospitals with less than 25 cases; (1) The number of cases is too small (n<25) for purposes of reliably predicting hospital performance; (2) Measure reflects the hospital's indication that its submission was based upon a sample of its relevant discharges; (3) Rate reflects fewer than the maximum possible quarters of data for the measure; (4) Inaccurate information submitted and suppressed for one or more quarters; (5) No data is available from the hospital for this measure; Please refer to the User's Guide for a full explanation of data

Tailor Telfair Regional Hospital	McRae	97%	34
Berrien County Hospital	Nashville	96%	57
Clinch Memorial Hospital	Homerville	96%	28
Grady General Hospital	Cairo	96%	55
Irwin County Hospital	Ocilla	96%	27
Smith Northview Hospital	Valdosta	96%	67
Burke Medical Center	Waynesboro	95%	110
Crisp Regional Hospital	Cordele	94%	216
Jefferson Hospital	Louisville	94%	86
Donalsonville Hospital	Donalsonville	91%	114

18. Pneumococcal Vaccine

Hospital Name	City	Rate	Cases
Chatuge Regional Hospital & Nursing Home	Hiawassee	100%	40
Tift Regional Medical Hospital	Tifton	98%	96
Emory Eastside Medical Center	Snellville	96%	243
Northside Hospital	Atlanta	94%	154
Northside Hospital	Cumming	94%	246
Tanner Medical Center	Villa Rica	94%	54
Higgins General Hospital	Bremen	92%	48
North Fulton Regional Hospital	Roswell	92%	214
Fannin Regional Hospital	Blue Ridge	91%	97
Promina Gwinnett Health System	Lawrenceville	91%	241
John D Archbold Memorial Hospital	Thomasville	90%	122
Perry Hospital	Perry	87%	75
University Hospital	Augusta	87%	399
Northside Hospital-Cherokee	Canton	85%	169
Piedmont Fayette Hospital	Fayetteville	84%	140
Spalding Regional Medical Center	Griffin	84%	201
Colquitt Regional Medical Center	Moultrie	83%	54
Crisp Regional Hospital	Cordele	83%	131
Houston Medical Center	Warner Robins	83%	89
Memorial Medical Center	Savannah	83%	136
Wayne Memorial Hospital	Jesup	82%	33
Candler Hospital	Savannah	81%	244
Habersham County Medical Center	Demorest	81%	72
Redmond Regional Medical Center	Rome	81%	285
Coliseum Medical Center	Macon	80%	123
Satilla Regional Medical Center	Waycross	80%	154
Washington County Regional Medical Center	Sandersville	80%	128
Emory University Hospital	Atlanta	78%	73
Hamilton Medical Center	Dalton	78%	217
Saint Joseph Candler Hospital	Savannah	77%	142
Evans Memorial Hospital	Claxton	76%	74
Macon Northside Hospital	Macon	76%	68
Northeast Georgia Medical Center	Gainesville	75%	244
Floyd Medical Center	Rome	74%	219
Walton Regional Medical Center	Monroe	74%	150
Doctors Hospital	Columbus	72%	103
Southern Regional Medical Center	Riverdale	72%	160
Bacon County Hospital System	Alma	71%	35
McDuffie Regional Medical Center	Thomson	71%	90
Sumter Regional Hospital	Americus	71%	72
Newton Medical	Covington	68%	143
West Georgia Medical Center	La Grange	68%	153
Cobb Memorial Hospital	Royston	67%	67
Appling Hospital	Baxley	66%	82
Elbert Memorial Hospital	Elberton	65%	63
Emanuel Medical Center	Swainsboro	65%	60
Tanner Medical Center	Carrollton	65%	172
Trinity Hospital of Augusta	Augusta	65%	82
WellStar Paulding Hospital	Dallas	65%	57
Emory Dunwoody Medical Center	Atlanta	64%	28
Gordon Hospital	Calhoun	64%	140
Union General Hospital	Blairsville	64%	81
Wesley Woods Geriatric Hospital	Atlanta	64%	39
Saint Francis Hospital	Columbus	63%	245
WellStar Cobb Hospital	Austell	63%	218
DeKalb Medical Center	Decatur	62%	237
Grady General Hospital	Cairo	62%	32
Piedmont Hospital	Atlanta	62%	181
WellStar Douglas Hospital	Douglasville	62%	117
Rockdale Hospital	Conyers	61%	154
Stephens County Hospital	Toccoa	61%	106
Athens Regional Medical Center	Athens	60%	83
Emory-Adventist Hospital	Smyrna	60%	53
Saint Mary's Hospital	Athens	60%	70
Doctors Hospital	Augusta	59%	131
Polk Medical Center	Cedartown	59%	39
Saint Joseph's Hospital	Atlanta	59%	278
Coffee Regional Medical Center	Douglas	58%	71
Memorial Hospital of Adel	Adel	58%	31
Columbus Medical Center	Columbus	56%	79
Medical Center of Central Georgia	Macon	55%	86
South Georgia Medical Center	Valdosta	55%	130
Hart County Hospital	Hartwell	54%	56
North Georgia Medical Center	Ellijay	54%	39
Upson Regional Medical Center	Thomaston	54%	90
WellStar Kennestone Hospital	Marietta	54%	333
Chestatee Regional Hospital	Dahlonega	52%	62
Dorminy Medical Center	Fitzgerald	51%	37
Henry Medical Center	Stockbridge	51%	94
Piedmont Mountainside Hospital	Jasper	51%	118
Putnam General Hospital	Eatonton	50%	56
Candler County Hospital	Metter	48%	25
South Fulton Medical Center	East Point	48%	131
Palmyra Medical Centers	Albany	47%	60
Medical College of Georgia Hospital & Clinics	Augusta	45%	87
Southeast Georgia Health System	Brunswick	45%	132
Atlanta Medical Center	Atlanta	44%	41
Emory Cartersville Medical Center	Cartersville	44%	162
Jefferson Hospital	Louisville	44%	48
Phoebe Putney Memorial Hospital	Albany	43%	127
Fairview Park Hospital	Dublin	40%	123
Oconee Regional Medical Center	Milledgeville	40%	106
Emory Crawford Long Hospital	Atlanta	39%	107
Barrow Regional Medical Center	Winder	38%	52
Southeast Georgia Health Sys-Camden Campus	Saint Marys	38%	34
Donalsonville Hospital	Donalsonville	37%	49
Emory Northlake Regional Medical Center	Tucker	37%	54
Berrien County Hospital	Nashville	36%	33
Taylor Regional Hospital	Hawkinsville	36%	56
BJC Medical Center	Commerce	34%	41
Hamilton Medical Center	Chatsworth	34%	58
Liberty Regional Medical Center	Hinesville	34%	38
Memorial Hospital & Manor	Bainbridge	34%	35
Grady Memorial Hospital	Atlanta	33%	48
Dekalb Medical Center at Hillandale	Lithonia	30%	40
Meadows Regional Medical Center	Vidalia	27%	75
Burke Medical Center	Waynesboro	22%	65
Dodge County Hospital	Eastman	20%	60
Smith Northview Hospital	Valdosta	20%	30
Flint River Community Hospital	Montezuma	14%	28
East Georgia Regional Medical Center	Statesboro	13%	84
Hutcheson Medical Center	Fort Oglethrope	13%	229
Monroe County Hospital	Forsyth	3%	38

19. Smoking Cessation Advice

Hospital Name	City	Rate	Cases
Coliseum Medical Center	Macon	100%	60
Dekalb Medical Center at Hillandale	Lithonia	100%	25
Doctors Hospital	Columbus	100%	48
Fannin Regional Hospital	Blue Ridge	100%	37
John D Archbold Memorial Hospital	Thomasville	100%	60
Macon Northside Hospital	Macon	100%	32
Northside Hospital	Atlanta	100%	52
Palmyra Medical Centers	Albany	100%	32
Promina Gwinnett Health System	Lawrenceville	100%	107
Rockdale Hospital	Conyers	100%	56
Tift Regional Medical Hospital	Tifton	100%	33
Candler Hospital	Savannah	99%	101
West Georgia Medical Center	La Grange	99%	67
Athens Regional Medical Center	Athens	98%	46
Emory Crawford Long Hospital	Atlanta	98%	54
Saint Joseph Candler Hospital	Savannah	98%	56
Colquitt Regional Medical Center	Moultrie	97%	34
Fairview Park Hospital	Dublin	97%	35
Northside Hospital	Cumming	97%	91
Appling Hospital	Baxley	96%	28
DeKalb Medical Center	Decatur	96%	113
Doctors Hospital	Augusta	96%	52
Northeast Georgia Medical Center	Gainesville	96%	96
Washington County Regional Medical Center	Sandersville	96%	51
WellStar Douglas Hospital	Douglasville	96%	80
WellStar Paulding Hospital	Dallas	96%	25
Hamilton Medical Center	Chatsworth	95%	44
Henry Medical Center	Stockbridge	95%	44
Spalding Regional Medical Center	Griffin	95%	95
WellStar Cobb Hospital	Austell	95%	111
Emory Eastside Medical Center	Snellville	94%	69
Floyd Medical Center	Rome	94%	118
Hamilton Medical Center	Dalton	94%	121
University Hospital	Augusta	94%	128
Chestatee Regional Hospital	Dahlonega	93%	29
Northside Hospital-Cherokee	Canton	93%	82
Meadows Regional Medical Center	Vidalia	92%	38
Medical Center of Central Georgia	Macon	92%	51
Piedmont Hospital	Atlanta	92%	73

NOTE: Hospital profiles are in alphabetical order by state, then city, then hospital within the city; Rankings are sorted by rate in descending order and exclude hospitals with less than 25 cases; (1) The number of cases is too small (n<25) for purposes of reliably predicting hospital performance; (2) Measure reflects the hospital's indication that its submission was based upon a sample of its relevant discharges; (3) Rate reflects fewer than the maximum possible quarters of data for the measure; (4) Inaccurate information submitted and suppressed for one or more quarters; (5) No data is available from the hospital for this measure; Please refer to the User's Guide for a full explanation of data

Hospital	City	Rate	Cases
Piedmont Mountainside Hospital	Jasper	92%	40
Redmond Regional Medical Center	Rome	92%	108
Saint Joseph's Hospital	Atlanta	92%	59
Sumter Regional Hospital	Americus	92%	25
Columbus Medical Center	Columbus	91%	89
East Georgia Regional Medical Center	Statesboro	91%	55
Emory Cartersville Medical Center	Cartersville	91%	111
WellStar Kennestone Hospital	Marietta	91%	145
Memorial Medical Center	Savannah	90%	91
Saint Francis Hospital	Columbus	90%	86
North Fulton Regional Hospital	Roswell	89%	61
Satilla Regional Medical Center	Waycross	89%	56
Southern Regional Medical Center	Riverdale	89%	100
Union General Hospital	Blairsville	89%	28
Coffee Regional Medical Center	Douglas	88%	33
South Georgia Medical Center	Valdosta	88%	50
Atlanta Medical Center	Atlanta	86%	36
Habersham County Medical Center	Demorest	86%	29
Tanner Medical Center	Villa Rica	86%	42
Emanuel Medical Center	Swainsboro	85%	40
Higgins General Hospital	Bremen	85%	26
Saint Mary's Hospital	Athens	85%	34
Barrow Regional Medical Center	Winder	83%	35
Newton Medical	Covington	83%	60
Crisp Regional Hospital	Cordele	82%	38
Gordon Hospital	Calhoun	82%	67
South Fulton Medical Center	East Point	81%	77
Walton Regional Medical Center	Monroe	81%	52
Cobb Memorial Hospital	Royston	80%	25
Upson Regional Medical Center	Thomaston	80%	46
Tanner Medical Center	Carrollton	79%	62
Houston Medical Center	Warner Robins	78%	51
Oconee Regional Medical Center	Milledgeville	77%	56
Donalsonville Hospital	Donalsonville	73%	30
Medical College of Georgia Hospital & Clinics	Augusta	67%	49
Emory Northlake Regional Medical Center	Tucker	64%	33
Phoebe Putney Memorial Hospital	Albany	60%	65
Trinity Hospital of Augusta	Augusta	60%	25
Southeast Georgia Health System	Brunswick	57%	51
Emory-Adventist Hospital	Smyrna	40%	30
Hutcheson Medical Center	Fort Oglethrope	40%	183
Stephens County Hospital	Toccoa	35%	43
Grady Memorial Hospital	Atlanta	19%	97

Hospital	City	Rate	Cases
Southern Regional Medical Center	Riverdale	82%	530
Henry Medical Center	Stockbridge	81%	149
Piedmont Mountainside Hospital	Jasper	79%	126
Cobb Memorial Hospital	Royston	78%	32
Doctors Hospital	Columbus	78%	176
East Georgia Regional Medical Center	Statesboro	78%	274
Fairview Park Hospital	Dublin	78%	92
Saint Joseph's Hospital	Atlanta	77%	262
Union General Hospital	Blairsville	77%	64
Coliseum Medical Center	Macon	76%	230
South Fulton Medical Center	East Point	76%	221
Medical College of Georgia Hospital & Clinics	Augusta	75%	257
South Georgia Medical Center	Valdosta	75%	64
Houston Medical Center	Warner Robins	74%	174
Hughston Orthopedic Hospital	Columbus	74%	1491
Sumter Regional Hospital	Americus	74%	140
Floyd Medical Center	Rome	73%	498
Medical Center of Central Georgia	Macon	71%	266
Tanner Medical Center	Carrollton	70%	401
Grady Memorial Hospital	Atlanta	69%	184
Liberty Regional Medical Center	Hinesville	68%	57
Candler Hospital	Savannah	65%	74
Walton Regional Medical Center	Monroe	65%	80
Dekalb Medical Center at Hillandale	Lithonia	64%	97
Emory Cartersville Medical Center	Cartersville	64%	143
Saint Mary's Hospital	Athens	64%	72
Southeast Georgia Health System	Brunswick	64%	463
Perry Hospital	Perry	63%	30
Upson Regional Medical Center	Thomaston	63%	35
Emory Dunwoody Medical Center	Atlanta	62%	52
Hutcheson Medical Center	Fort Oglethrope	62%	112
Satilla Regional Medical Center	Waycross	59%	63
Memorial Hospital & Manor	Bainbridge	58%	33
Athens Regional Medical Center	Athens	57%	163
Palmyra Medical Centers	Albany	55%	388
Northeast Georgia Medical Center	Gainesville	54%	79
Newton Medical	Covington	52%	48
Tift Regional Medical Hospital	Tifton	51%	136
Atlanta Medical Center	Atlanta	50%	238
Macon Northside Hospital	Macon	50%	74
Stephens County Hospital	Toccoa	48%	31
Donalsonville Hospital	Donalsonville	45%	40
BJC Medical Center	Commerce	44%	32
Barrow Regional Medical Center	Winder	44%	39
Colquitt Regional Medical Center	Moultrie	38%	45
Phoebe Putney Memorial Hospital	Albany	36%	72
Emory-Adventist Hospital	Smyrna	34%	44
Meadows Regional Medical Center	Vidalia	34%	85
Smith Northview Hospital	Valdosta	32%	59
Emory Northlake Regional Medical Center	Tucker	26%	76

Surgical Infection Prevention

20. Prophylactic Antibiotic Given

Hospital Name	City	Rate	Cases
Wayne Memorial Hospital	Jesup	97%	29
Northside Hospital	Atlanta	96%	114
Rockdale Hospital	Conyers	96%	300
Habersham County Medical Center	Demorest	94%	36
Piedmont Hospital	Atlanta	94%	436
Redmond Regional Medical Center	Rome	94%	330
Spalding Regional Medical Center	Griffin	94%	468
Taylor Regional Hospital	Hawkinsville	94%	108
Emory Eastside Medical Center	Snellville	93%	211
Northside Hospital-Cherokee	Canton	92%	38
University Hospital	Augusta	92%	1934
Hamilton Medical Center	Dalton	91%	239
Piedmont Fayette Hospital	Fayetteville	91%	87
Southeast Georgia Health Sys-Camden Campus	Saint Marys	91%	79
Promina Gwinnett Health System	Lawrenceville	90%	68
West Georgia Medical Center	La Grange	90%	86
Emory University Hospital	Atlanta	89%	575
Memorial Medical Center	Savannah	89%	215
North Fulton Regional Hospital	Roswell	89%	233
Emanuel Medical Center	Swainsboro	88%	60
DeKalb Medical Center	Decatur	87%	304
Doctors Hospital	Augusta	87%	207
Saint Francis Hospital	Columbus	87%	331
Saint Joseph Candler Hospital	Savannah	87%	113
WellStar Cobb Hospital	Austell	87%	110
WellStar Kennestone Hospital	Marietta	87%	181
Gordon Hospital	Calhoun	86%	133
Northside Hospital	Cumming	86%	63
Trinity Hospital of Augusta	Augusta	86%	125
Columbus Medical Center	Columbus	85%	260
Fannin Regional Hospital	Blue Ridge	85%	158
John D Archbold Memorial Hospital	Thomasville	85%	470
Emory Crawford Long Hospital	Atlanta	84%	551
WellStar Douglas Hospital	Douglasville	83%	29
Chestatee Regional Hospital	Dahlonega	82%	28
Oconee Regional Medical Center	Milledgeville	82%	40

21. Prophylactic Antibiotic Selection

Hospital Name	City	Rate	Cases
Gordon Hospital	Calhoun	100%	28
Hughston Orthopedic Hospital	Columbus	100%	419
Taylor Regional Hospital	Hawkinsville	100%	32
Columbus Medical Center	Columbus	98%	58
Hamilton Medical Center	Dalton	98%	40
Redmond Regional Medical Center	Rome	98%	138
Southeast Georgia Health System	Brunswick	98%	116
Trinity Hospital of Augusta	Augusta	98%	43
Emory Cartersville Medical Center	Cartersville	97%	68
Habersham County Medical Center	Demorest	97%	36
Memorial Hospital & Manor	Bainbridge	97%	29
Memorial Medical Center	Savannah	97%	75
Saint Francis Hospital	Columbus	97%	65
WellStar Douglas Hospital	Douglasville	97%	29
Chestatee Regional Hospital	Dahlonega	96%	28
Meadows Regional Medical Center	Vidalia	96%	26
Saint Joseph Candler Hospital	Savannah	96%	51
Tanner Medical Center	Carrollton	96%	83
Emory Eastside Medical Center	Snellville	95%	119
Northside Hospital	Atlanta	95%	114
South Fulton Medical Center	East Point	95%	56
Floyd Medical Center	Rome	94%	127
Spalding Regional Medical Center	Griffin	94%	126
Upson Regional Medical Center	Thomaston	94%	34
Wayne Memorial Hospital	Jesup	94%	31
Coliseum Medical Center	Macon	93%	101
Emory Northlake Regional Medical Center	Tucker	93%	28
Hutcheson Medical Center	Fort Oglethrope	93%	54
John D Archbold Memorial Hospital	Thomasville	93%	56
Northside Hospital	Cumming	93%	61
Doctors Hospital	Columbus	92%	127

NOTE: Hospital profiles are in alphabetical order by state, then city, then hospital within the city; Rankings are sorted by rate in descending order and exclude hospitals with less than 25 cases; (1) The number of cases is too small (n<25) for purposes of reliably predicting hospital performance; (2) Measure reflects the hospital's indication that its submission was based upon a sample of its relevant discharges; (3) Rate reflects fewer than the maximum possible quarters of data for the measure; (4) Inaccurate information submitted and suppressed for one or more quarters; (5) No data is available from the hospital for this measure; Please refer to the User's Guide for a full explanation of data

Hospital Name	City	Rate	Cases
Macon Northside Hospital	Macon	92%	26
Rockdale Hospital	Conyers	92%	65
Tift Regional Medical Hospital	Tifton	92%	40
University Hospital	Augusta	92%	439
WellStar Cobb Hospital	Austell	92%	113
Doctors Hospital	Augusta	91%	95
WellStar Kennestone Hospital	Marietta	91%	184
North Fulton Regional Hospital	Roswell	90%	70
Piedmont Hospital	Atlanta	90%	102
Sumter Regional Hospital	Americus	89%	35
Athens Regional Medical Center	Athens	88%	83
DeKalb Medical Center	Decatur	88%	67
Grady Memorial Hospital	Atlanta	88%	50
Henry Medical Center	Stockbridge	88%	50
Oconee Regional Medical Center	Milledgeville	88%	40
West Georgia Medical Center	La Grange	88%	74
Emory University Hospital	Atlanta	87%	84
Saint Mary's Hospital	Athens	87%	70
Stephens County Hospital	Toccoa	87%	31
Atlanta Medical Center	Atlanta	86%	65
East Georgia Regional Medical Center	Statesboro	86%	43
South Georgia Medical Center	Valdosta	86%	66
Southern Regional Medical Center	Riverdale	86%	76
Fairview Park Hospital	Dublin	85%	40
Saint Joseph's Hospital	Atlanta	84%	89
Houston Medical Center	Warner Robins	83%	48
Fannin Regional Hospital	Blue Ridge	82%	33
Dekalb Medical Center at Hillandale	Lithonia	81%	26
Medical College of Georgia Hospital & Clinics	Augusta	80%	54
Piedmont Mountainside Hospital	Jasper	80%	30
Emory Crawford Long Hospital	Atlanta	79%	89
Medical Center of Central Georgia	Macon	79%	117
Northside Hospital-Cherokee	Canton	79%	38
Palmyra Medical Centers	Albany	79%	95
Newton Medical	Covington	77%	47
Promina Gwinnett Health System	Lawrenceville	71%	68
Phoebe Putney Memorial Hospital	Albany	55%	74
Chestatee Regional Hospital	Dahlonega	69%	26
Emory-Adventist Hospital	Smyrna	69%	42
Redmond Regional Medical Center	Rome	69%	319
Athens Regional Medical Center	Athens	68%	159
Coliseum Medical Center	Macon	68%	215
South Fulton Medical Center	East Point	68%	213
Atlanta Medical Center	Atlanta	66%	232
Candler Hospital	Savannah	66%	74
Cobb Memorial Hospital	Royston	66%	32
Hughston Orthopedic Hospital	Columbus	65%	1475
WellStar Cobb Hospital	Austell	65%	110
Fannin Regional Hospital	Blue Ridge	64%	153
Saint Joseph's Hospital	Atlanta	64%	261
Emory Cartersville Medical Center	Cartersville	63%	134
Smith Northview Hospital	Valdosta	63%	57
Northside Hospital	Atlanta	62%	110
Piedmont Mountainside Hospital	Jasper	62%	120
Northside Hospital-Cherokee	Canton	61%	38
Phoebe Putney Memorial Hospital	Albany	61%	72
Columbus Medical Center	Columbus	60%	247
Medical College of Georgia Hospital & Clinics	Augusta	60%	240
Saint Joseph Candler Hospital	Savannah	60%	104
DeKalb Medical Center	Decatur	59%	290
Northside Hospital	Cumming	59%	59
Perry Hospital	Perry	59%	27
Sumter Regional Hospital	Americus	59%	130
Dekalb Medical Center at Hillandale	Lithonia	57%	93
Donalsonville Hospital	Donalsonville	57%	35
Emanuel Medical Center	Swainsboro	57%	58
WellStar Douglas Hospital	Douglasville	57%	28
Southeast Georgia Health System	Brunswick	55%	446
Palmyra Medical Centers	Albany	49%	376
Houston Medical Center	Warner Robins	48%	173
Emory Dunwoody Medical Center	Atlanta	47%	47
Medical Center of Central Georgia	Macon	47%	255
Saint Francis Hospital	Columbus	46%	324
University Hospital	Augusta	46%	1927
East Georgia Regional Medical Center	Statesboro	44%	259
Stephens County Hospital	Toccoa	42%	31
Henry Medical Center	Stockbridge	38%	149
Satilla Regional Medical Center	Waycross	32%	59
Upson Regional Medical Center	Thomaston	17%	35

22. Prophylactic Antibiotic Stopped

Hospital Name	City	Rate	Cases
Hutcheson Medical Center	Fort Oglethorpe	100%	110
Memorial Hospital & Manor	Bainbridge	100%	29
Wayne Memorial Hospital	Jesup	100%	28
Liberty Regional Medical Center	Hinesville	98%	50
Rockdale Hospital	Conyers	96%	295
Saint Mary's Hospital	Athens	96%	68
Barrow Regional Medical Center	Winder	94%	36
Northeast Georgia Medical Center	Gainesville	94%	68
Tanner Medical Center	Carrollton	93%	393
BJC Medical Center	Commerce	90%	31
Piedmont Hospital	Atlanta	88%	425
Promina Gwinnett Health System	Lawrenceville	88%	67
Union General Hospital	Blairsville	87%	61
Emory Northlake Regional Medical Center	Tucker	86%	72
Gordon Hospital	Calhoun	86%	131
Taylor Regional Hospital	Hawkinsville	86%	107
Emory University Hospital	Atlanta	85%	556
Hamilton Medical Center	Dalton	84%	228
North Fulton Regional Hospital	Roswell	84%	221
Southeast Georgia Health Sys-Camden Campus	Saint Marys	84%	74
Colquitt Regional Medical Center	Moultrie	83%	42
Floyd Medical Center	Rome	83%	494
West Georgia Medical Center	La Grange	82%	84
Emory Eastside Medical Center	Snellville	81%	201
Tift Regional Medical Hospital	Tifton	81%	125
Emory Crawford Long Hospital	Atlanta	80%	539
Macon Northside Hospital	Macon	80%	81
Oconee Regional Medical Center	Milledgeville	80%	40
Spalding Regional Medical Center	Griffin	80%	444
Meadows Regional Medical Center	Vidalia	79%	86
Fairview Park Hospital	Dublin	78%	91
WellStar Kennestone Hospital	Marietta	78%	178
Trinity Hospital of Augusta	Augusta	77%	123
Doctors Hospital	Augusta	76%	199
Piedmont Fayette Hospital	Fayetteville	76%	87
Memorial Medical Center	Savannah	75%	204
Habersham County Medical Center	Demorest	74%	35
John D Archbold Memorial Hospital	Thomasville	74%	423
Grady Memorial Hospital	Atlanta	73%	183
Newton Medical	Covington	73%	48
South Georgia Medical Center	Valdosta	73%	62
Southern Regional Medical Center	Riverdale	73%	506
Doctors Hospital	Columbus	72%	177
Walton Regional Medical Center	Monroe	70%	80

Pregnancy Care

23. Inpatient Neonatal Mortality

Hospital Name	City	Rate	Cases
Burke Medical Center	Waynesboro	0.00%	318
Dorminy Medical Center	Fitzgerald	0.00%	200
Emanuel Medical Center	Swainsboro	0.00%	204
Newton Medical	Covington	0.00%	712
Northside Hospital-Cherokee	Canton	0.00%	1101
Oconee Regional Medical Center	Milledgeville	0.00%	533
Tift Regional Medical Hospital	Tifton	0.07%	1436
Irwin County Hospital	Ocilla	0.21%	478
Northeast Georgia Medical Center	Gainesville	0.23%	3520
Satilla Regional Medical Center	Waycross	0.25%	799
Candler Hospital	Savannah	0.27%	2972
Floyd Medical Center	Rome	0.30%	2014
Donalsonville Hospital	Donalsonville	0.34%	290
Grady Memorial Hospital	Atlanta	0.36%	833
Northside Hospital	Atlanta	0.37%	18311
Henry Medical Center	Stockbridge	0.48%	414
Meadows Regional Medical Center	Vidalia	0.58%	520
Chestatee Regional Hospital	Dahlonega	0.74%	135
Appling Hospital	Baxley	0.77%	261
Medical College of Georgia Hospital & Clinics	Augusta	0.91%	110
Phoebe Putney Memorial Hospital	Albany	1.30%	3150
Memorial Medical Center	Savannah	1.59%	3203

24. Third or Fourth Degree Laceration

Hospital Name	City	Rate	Cases
Burke Medical Center	Waynesboro	0.45%	221
Dorminy Medical Center	Fitzgerald	1.00%	100
Emanuel Medical Center	Swainsboro	1.41%	142
Northside Hospital-Cherokee	Canton	1.47%	816
Memorial Medical Center	Savannah	1.67%	1732
Oconee Regional Medical Center	Milledgeville	1.86%	431
Tift Regional Medical Hospital	Tifton	2.16%	925
Northeast Georgia Medical Center	Gainesville	2.33%	2531
Grady Memorial Hospital	Atlanta	2.37%	2485
Appling Hospital	Baxley	2.41%	166
Satilla Regional Medical Center	Waycross	2.61%	574
Meadows Regional Medical Center	Vidalia	2.84%	388

NOTE: Hospital profiles are in alphabetical order by state, then city, then hospital within the city; Rankings are sorted by rate in descending order and exclude hospitals with less than 25 cases; (1) The number of cases is too small (n<25) for purposes of reliably predicting hospital performance; (2) Measure reflects the hospital's indication that its submission was based upon a sample of its relevant discharges; (3) Rate reflects fewer than the maximum possible quarters of data for the measure; (4) Inaccurate information submitted and suppressed for one or more quarters; (5) No data is available from the hospital for this measure; Please refer to the User's Guide for a full explanation of data

Phoebe Putney Memorial Hospital	Albany	2.85%	1998
Donalsonville Hospital	Donalsonville	3.19%	188
Newton Medical	Covington	3.23%	527
Candler Hospital	Savannah	3.54%	1693
Northside Hospital	Atlanta	4.59%	11482
Irwin County Hospital	Ocilla	5.45%	275
Chestatee Regional Hospital	Dahlonega	5.56%	90
Medical College of Georgia Hospital & Clinics	Augusta	6.03%	315
Henry Medical Center	Stockbridge	6.32%	570
Floyd Medical Center	Rome	7.12%	1461

NOTE: Hospital profiles are in alphabetical order by state, then city, then hospital within the city; Rankings are sorted by rate in descending order and exclude hospitals with less than 25 cases; (1) The number of cases is too small (n<25) for purposes of reliably predicting hospital performance; (2) Measure reflects the hospital's indication that its submission was based upon a sample of its relevant discharges; (3) Rate reflects fewer than the maximum possible quarters of data for the measure; (4) Inaccurate information submitted and suppressed for one or more quarters; (5) No data is available from the hospital for this measure; Please refer to the User's Guide for a full explanation of data

Memorial Hospital of Adel

706 N Parrish Avenue
Adel, GA 31620
Ownership: Proprietary
Emergency Services: Yes

Phone: 229-896-8000
Fax: 229-896-8001
Accredited: Yes
Licensed Beds: 60

Key Personnel:
CEO/President . . . . H Hawley
Chief Medical Staff . . . . Thomas Fausett
Director Infection/Disease Control . . . . Sandi Martin
Supervising Nurse CCU . . . . Bonnie Cronin, RN
Director Medical/Surgical Nursing . . . . Janet Meders, RN
Chief OB/GYN . . . . Mary Howell, MD
Director Respiratory Therapy . . . . Barbara Tippens

Measure	Cases	This Hospital	State Average	U.S. Average	Top Hospital
Heart Attack Care					
ACE Inhibitor or ARB for LVSD[1]	1	100%	78%	82%	100%
Aspirin at Arrival[1]	8	88%	91%	92%	100%
Aspirin at Discharge[1]	5	100%	87%	90%	100%
Beta Blocker at Arrival[1]	9	89%	85%	87%	100%
Beta Blocker at Discharge[1]	6	100%	87%	90%	100%
Fibrinolytic Medication Timing[3]	0	-	34%	31%	100%
PCI Within 90 Minutes of Arrival	0	-	47%	54%	95%
Smoking Cessation Advice[3]	0	-	85%	88%	100%
Heart Failure Care					
ACE Inhibitor or ARB for LVSD[1]	12	83%	81%	82%	100%
Discharge Instructions[1,3]	14	93%	59%	61%	93%
Evaluation of LVS Function	59	71%	81%	83%	99%
Smoking Cessation Advice[1,3]	5	100%	86%	82%	100%
Pneumonia Care					
Appropriate Initial Antibiotic[1,3]	6	50%	81%	83%	94%
Blood Culture Timing[1,3]	1	100%	89%	90%	100%
Influenza Vaccine[5]	-	-	60%	70%	100%
Initial Antibiotic Timing	48	65%	75%	80%	93%
Oxygenation Assessment	59	100%	99%	99%	100%
Pneumococcal Vaccine	31	58%	61%	69%	94%
Smoking Cessation Advice[1,3]	4	100%	82%	80%	100%
Surgical Infection Prevention					
Prophylactic Antibiotic Given[1,3]	8	50%	69%	77%	95%
Prophylactic Antibiotic Selection[5]	-	-	89%	90%	100%
Prophylactic Antibiotic Stopped[1,3]	8	75%	71%	72%	95%
Pregnancy Care					
Inpatient Neonatal Mortality	-	-	-	-	-
Third or Fourth Degree Laceration	-	-	3.63%	3.63%	3.27%

Palmyra Medical Centers

Alternate Name: HCA Palmyra Medical Center
2000 Palmyra Road
PO Box 1908
Albany, GA 31701
URL: www.palmyramedicalcenters.com
Ownership: Proprietary
Emergency Services: Yes

Phone: 229-434-2000
Fax: 229-434-2587

Accredited: Yes
Licensed Beds: 248

Key Personnel:
CEO . . . . Allen Golson
Infection Control . . . . Diane Daniel
Director Medical/Surgical Nursing . . . . Susan Hampson
Director Surgical Services . . . . Jackie Eschbaugh
Director Respiratory Care . . . . Brett Ford

Measure	Cases	This Hospital	State Average	U.S. Average	Top Hospital
Heart Attack Care					
ACE Inhibitor or ARB for LVSD[3]	0	-	78%	82%	100%
Aspirin at Arrival[1,3]	12	100%	91%	92%	100%
Aspirin at Discharge[1,3]	1	100%	87%	90%	100%
Beta Blocker at Arrival[1,3]	11	64%	85%	87%	100%
Beta Blocker at Discharge[1,3]	2	100%	87%	90%	100%
Fibrinolytic Medication Timing[3]	0	-	34%	31%	100%
PCI Within 90 Minutes of Arrival	0	-	47%	54%	95%
Smoking Cessation Advice[3]	0	-	85%	88%	100%
Heart Failure Care					
ACE Inhibitor or ARB for LVSD	58	74%	81%	82%	100%
Discharge Instructions	106	82%	59%	61%	93%

Measure	Cases	This Hospital	State Average	U.S. Average	Top Hospital
Evaluation of LVS Function	123	93%	81%	83%	99%
Smoking Cessation Advice[1]	24	100%	86%	82%	100%
Pneumonia Care					
Appropriate Initial Antibiotic	69	81%	81%	83%	94%
Blood Culture Timing	36	97%	89%	90%	100%
Influenza Vaccine[1]	18	67%	60%	70%	100%
Initial Antibiotic Timing	102	57%	75%	80%	93%
Oxygenation Assessment	130	100%	99%	99%	100%
Pneumococcal Vaccine	60	47%	61%	69%	94%
Smoking Cessation Advice	32	100%	82%	80%	100%
Surgical Infection Prevention					
Prophylactic Antibiotic Given	388	55%	69%	77%	95%
Prophylactic Antibiotic Selection	95	79%	89%	90%	100%
Prophylactic Antibiotic Stopped	376	49%	71%	72%	95%
Pregnancy Care					
Inpatient Neonatal Mortality	-	-	-	-	-
Third or Fourth Degree Laceration	-	-	3.63%	3.63%	3.27%

Phoebe Putney Memorial Hospital

417 3rd Avenue
Albany, GA 31701

Toll-Free: 877-312-1167
Phone: 229-312-1000
Fax: 229-312-7100

URL: www.phoebeputney.com
Ownership: Govt - Hospital District or Authority
Emergency Services: Yes

Accredited: Yes
Licensed Beds: 450

Key Personnel:
President/CEO . . . . Joel Wernick
Chief Medical Staff . . . . Hazan Rizui, MD
Emergency Room . . . . G K Derebail, MD
Director Infection/Disease Control . . . . Patsy Crosson
OB/GYN Womens Health . . . . William George
Chief Radiology . . . . MP Malbry, MD
Director Respiratory Therapy . . . . Jan Havard

Measure	Cases	This Hospital	State Average	U.S. Average	Top Hospital
Heart Attack Care					
ACE Inhibitor or ARB for LVSD	128	73%	78%	82%	100%
Aspirin at Arrival	176	94%	91%	92%	100%
Aspirin at Discharge	455	98%	87%	90%	100%
Beta Blocker at Arrival	162	88%	85%	87%	100%
Beta Blocker at Discharge	423	93%	87%	90%	100%
Fibrinolytic Medication Timing[1]	5	60%	34%	31%	100%
PCI Within 90 Minutes of Arrival[1]	22	32%	47%	54%	95%
Smoking Cessation Advice	207	97%	85%	88%	100%
Heart Failure Care					
ACE Inhibitor or ARB for LVSD	182	82%	81%	82%	100%
Discharge Instructions	381	40%	59%	61%	93%
Evaluation of LVS Function	414	90%	81%	83%	99%
Smoking Cessation Advice	99	76%	86%	82%	100%
Pneumonia Care					
Appropriate Initial Antibiotic	135	84%	81%	83%	94%
Blood Culture Timing	97	86%	89%	90%	100%
Influenza Vaccine	35	46%	60%	70%	100%
Initial Antibiotic Timing	220	60%	75%	80%	93%
Oxygenation Assessment	240	100%	99%	99%	100%
Pneumococcal Vaccine	127	43%	61%	69%	94%
Smoking Cessation Advice	65	60%	82%	80%	100%
Surgical Infection Prevention					
Prophylactic Antibiotic Given[2,3]	72	36%	69%	77%	95%
Prophylactic Antibiotic Selection[2]	74	55%	89%	90%	100%
Prophylactic Antibiotic Stopped[2,3]	72	61%	71%	72%	95%
Pregnancy Care					
Inpatient Neonatal Mortality	3,150	1.30%	-	-	-
Third or Fourth Degree Laceration	1,998	2.85%	3.63%	3.63%	3.27%

Bacon County Hospital System

302 S Wayne Street
Alma, GA 31510

Phone: 912-632-8961
Fax: 912-632-5000

URL: www.beaconcountyhealth.org
Ownership: Voluntary non-profit - Other
Emergency Services: Yes

Accredited: Yes
Licensed Beds: 50

Key Personnel:
CEO . . . . O J Booker

NOTE: Hospital profiles are in alphabetical order by state, then city, then hospital within the city; Rankings are sorted by rate in descending order and exclude hospitals with less than 25 cases; (1) The number of cases is too small (n<25) for purposes of reliably predicting hospital performance; (2) Measure reflects the hospital's indication that its submission was based upon a sample of its relevant discharges; (3) Rate reflects fewer than the maximum possible quarters of data for the measure; (4) Inaccurate information submitted and suppressed for one or more quarters; (5) No data is available from the hospital for this measure; Please refer to the User's Guide for a full explanation of data

OB/GYN Womens Health. . . . . Mary Hutchinson

Measure	Cases	This Hospital	State Average	U.S. Average	Top Hospital
Heart Attack Care					
ACE Inhibitor or ARB for LVSD[1,3]	1	100%	78%	82%	100%
Aspirin at Arrival[1,3]	2	50%	91%	92%	100%
Aspirin at Discharge[3]	0	-	87%	90%	100%
Beta Blocker at Arrival[1,3]	2	50%	85%	87%	100%
Beta Blocker at Discharge[1,3]	1	100%	87%	90%	100%
Fibrinolytic Medication Timing[3]	0	-	34%	31%	100%
PCI Within 90 Minutes of Arrival	0	-	47%	54%	95%
Smoking Cessation Advice[3]	0	-	85%	88%	100%
Heart Failure Care					
ACE Inhibitor or ARB for LVSD[1,3]	7	43%	81%	82%	100%
Discharge Instructions[3]	32	69%	59%	61%	93%
Evaluation of LVS Function[3]	39	82%	81%	83%	99%
Smoking Cessation Advice[1,3]	9	89%	86%	82%	100%
Pneumonia Care					
Appropriate Initial Antibiotic[3]	35	83%	81%	83%	94%
Blood Culture Timing[1]	18	94%	89%	90%	100%
Influenza Vaccine[1]	10	70%	60%	70%	100%
Initial Antibiotic Timing[3]	39	97%	75%	80%	93%
Oxygenation Assessment[3]	54	100%	99%	99%	100%
Pneumococcal Vaccine[3]	35	71%	61%	69%	94%
Smoking Cessation Advice[1,3]	10	100%	82%	80%	100%
Surgical Infection Prevention					
Prophylactic Antibiotic Given[5]	-	-	69%	77%	95%
Prophylactic Antibiotic Selection[5]	-	-	89%	90%	100%
Prophylactic Antibiotic Stopped[5]	-	-	71%	72%	95%
Pregnancy Care					
Inpatient Neonatal Mortality	-	-	-	-	-
Third or Fourth Degree Laceration	-	-	3.63%	3.63%	3.27%

Sumter Regional Hospital

100 Wheatley Drive   Phone: 229-924-6011
Americus, GA 31709   Fax: 229-931-1125
Ownership: Govt - Hospital District or Authority   Accredited: Yes
Emergency Services: Yes   Licensed Beds: 143
Key Personnel:
President/CEO. . . . . Jerry W Adams
Chief Medical Staff. . . . . Kirk Austin, MD
Director Medical/Surgical Nursing . . . . Susie Fussell
Chief Radiology . . . . Michael Baldwin, MD
Director Respiratory Therapy . . . . Tonja Dotson

Measure	Cases	This Hospital	State Average	U.S. Average	Top Hospital
Heart Attack Care					
ACE Inhibitor or ARB for LVSD[1]	2	50%	78%	82%	100%
Aspirin at Arrival[1]	17	88%	91%	92%	100%
Aspirin at Discharge[1]	10	80%	87%	90%	100%
Beta Blocker at Arrival[1]	16	75%	85%	87%	100%
Beta Blocker at Discharge[1]	9	78%	87%	90%	100%
Fibrinolytic Medication Timing[1]	1	0%	34%	31%	100%
PCI Within 90 Minutes of Arrival	0	-	47%	54%	95%
Smoking Cessation Advice[1]	3	100%	85%	88%	100%
Heart Failure Care					
ACE Inhibitor or ARB for LVSD	27	81%	81%	82%	100%
Discharge Instructions	92	65%	59%	61%	93%
Evaluation of LVS Function	107	82%	81%	83%	99%
Smoking Cessation Advice[1]	15	93%	86%	82%	100%
Pneumonia Care					
Appropriate Initial Antibiotic	64	66%	81%	83%	94%
Blood Culture Timing	69	84%	89%	90%	100%
Influenza Vaccine[1]	15	80%	60%	70%	100%
Initial Antibiotic Timing	104	71%	75%	80%	93%
Oxygenation Assessment	127	99%	99%	99%	100%
Pneumococcal Vaccine	72	71%	61%	69%	94%
Smoking Cessation Advice	25	92%	82%	80%	100%
Surgical Infection Prevention					
Prophylactic Antibiotic Given	140	74%	69%	77%	95%
Prophylactic Antibiotic Selection	35	89%	89%	90%	100%
Prophylactic Antibiotic Stopped	130	59%	71%	72%	95%

Measure					
Pregnancy Care					
Inpatient Neonatal Mortality	-	-	-	-	-
Third or Fourth Degree Laceration	-	-	3.63%	3.63%	3.27%

Athens Regional Medical Center

1199 Prince Avenue   Phone: 706-549-9977
Athens, GA 30606   Fax: 706-475-6774
URL: www.armc.org
Ownership: Voluntary non-profit - Other   Accredited: Yes
Emergency Services: Yes   Licensed Beds: 315
Key Personnel:
Chief Medical Staff. . . . . Dale E Green
Chief Catheterization Laboratory . . . . Hamilton Magill
CCU Spvg. Nurse . . . . Toni Lopez
Chief OB/GYN . . . . L Michael Thompson
Chief Radiology . . . . Paul Davis, Jr, DM
Director Respiratory Therapy . . . . Harry Davis

Measure	Cases	This Hospital	State Average	U.S. Average	Top Hospital
Heart Attack Care					
ACE Inhibitor or ARB for LVSD	110	85%	78%	82%	100%
Aspirin at Arrival	253	97%	91%	92%	100%
Aspirin at Discharge	345	98%	87%	90%	100%
Beta Blocker at Arrival	164	90%	85%	87%	100%
Beta Blocker at Discharge	332	96%	87%	90%	100%
Fibrinolytic Medication Timing[1]	12	58%	34%	31%	100%
PCI Within 90 Minutes of Arrival[1]	8	62%	47%	54%	95%
Smoking Cessation Advice	171	100%	85%	88%	100%
Heart Failure Care					
ACE Inhibitor or ARB for LVSD	94	89%	81%	82%	100%
Discharge Instructions	260	68%	59%	61%	93%
Evaluation of LVS Function	281	98%	81%	83%	99%
Smoking Cessation Advice	62	97%	86%	82%	100%
Pneumonia Care					
Appropriate Initial Antibiotic	107	86%	81%	83%	94%
Blood Culture Timing	89	83%	89%	90%	100%
Influenza Vaccine	26	62%	60%	70%	100%
Initial Antibiotic Timing	124	85%	75%	80%	93%
Oxygenation Assessment	170	100%	99%	99%	100%
Pneumococcal Vaccine	83	60%	61%	69%	94%
Smoking Cessation Advice	46	98%	82%	80%	100%
Surgical Infection Prevention					
Prophylactic Antibiotic Given[3]	163	57%	69%	77%	95%
Prophylactic Antibiotic Selection	83	88%	89%	90%	100%
Prophylactic Antibiotic Stopped[3]	159	68%	71%	72%	95%
Pregnancy Care					
Inpatient Neonatal Mortality	-	-	-	-	-
Third or Fourth Degree Laceration	-	-	3.63%	3.63%	3.27%

Saint Mary's Hospital

1230 Baxter Street   Toll-Free: 800-233-7864
Athens, GA 30606   Phone: 706-548-7581
    Fax: 706-354-3197
Ownership: Voluntary non-profit - Church   Accredited: Yes
Emergency Services: Yes   Licensed Beds: 196
Key Personnel:
CEO. . . . . Tom Fitz
Emergency Room . . . . Maelene Vacquez
Chief Radiology . . . . Bobby M Thomas, MD
Director Respiratory Therapy . . . . Mary Bray

Measure	Cases	This Hospital	State Average	U.S. Average	Top Hospital
Heart Attack Care					
ACE Inhibitor or ARB for LVSD[1]	18	89%	78%	82%	100%
Aspirin at Arrival	54	93%	91%	92%	100%
Aspirin at Discharge	35	83%	87%	90%	100%
Beta Blocker at Arrival	40	92%	85%	87%	100%
Beta Blocker at Discharge	47	89%	87%	90%	100%
Fibrinolytic Medication Timing[1]	13	8%	34%	31%	100%
PCI Within 90 Minutes of Arrival	0	-	47%	54%	95%
Smoking Cessation Advice[1]	19	89%	85%	88%	100%
Heart Failure Care					

NOTE: Hospital profiles are in alphabetical order by state, then city, then hospital within the city; Rankings are sorted by rate in descending order and exclude hospitals with less than 25 cases; (1) The number of cases is too small (n<25) for purposes of reliably predicting hospital performance; (2) Measure reflects the hospital's indication that its submission was based upon a sample of its relevant discharges; (3) Rate reflects fewer than the maximum possible quarters of data for the measure; (4) Inaccurate information submitted and suppressed for one or more quarters; (5) No data is available from the hospital for this measure; Please refer to the User's Guide for a full explanation of data

ACE Inhibitor or ARB for LVSD[2]	105	93%	81%	82%	100%
Discharge Instructions[2]	220	50%	59%	61%	93%
Evaluation of LVS Function[2]	242	97%	81%	83%	99%
Smoking Cessation Advice[2]	66	80%	86%	82%	100%
Pneumonia Care					
Appropriate Initial Antibiotic	85	82%	81%	83%	94%
Blood Culture Timing	72	96%	89%	90%	100%
Influenza Vaccine[1]	24	58%	60%	70%	100%
Initial Antibiotic Timing	107	74%	75%	80%	93%
Oxygenation Assessment	129	100%	99%	99%	100%
Pneumococcal Vaccine	70	60%	61%	69%	94%
Smoking Cessation Advice	34	85%	82%	80%	100%
Surgical Infection Prevention					
Prophylactic Antibiotic Given[2,3]	72	64%	69%	77%	95%
Prophylactic Antibiotic Selection[2]	70	87%	89%	90%	100%
Prophylactic Antibiotic Stopped[2,3]	68	96%	71%	72%	95%
Pregnancy Care					
Inpatient Neonatal Mortality	-	-	-	-	-
Third or Fourth Degree Laceration	-	-	3.63%	3.63%	3.27%

Atlanta Medical Center

Alternate Name: Georgia Baptist Health Care System
303 Parkway Drive NE
Atlanta, GA 30312
URL: www.atlantamedcenter.com
Ownership: Proprietary
Emergency Services: Yes

Phone: 404-265-4000
Fax: 404-265-3991

Accredited: Yes
Licensed Beds: 460

Key Personnel:
Administrator . . . . Bruce Buchanan
Chief Medical Staff . . . . Paul Krissman
Emergency Room . . . . Mark Waterman
Director Medical/Surgical Nursing . . . . Ellie Post, RN
Chief Radiology . . . . Larry Ray, MD

Measure	Cases	This Hospital	State Average	U.S. Average	Top Hospital
Heart Attack Care					
ACE Inhibitor or ARB for LVSD	25	100%	78%	82%	100%
Aspirin at Arrival	65	98%	91%	92%	100%
Aspirin at Discharge	67	99%	87%	90%	100%
Beta Blocker at Arrival	51	98%	85%	87%	100%
Beta Blocker at Discharge	65	98%	87%	90%	100%
Fibrinolytic Medication Timing	0	-	34%	31%	100%
PCI Within 90 Minutes of Arrival[1]	4	25%	47%	54%	95%
Smoking Cessation Advice[1]	24	92%	85%	88%	100%
Heart Failure Care					
ACE Inhibitor or ARB for LVSD	150	99%	81%	82%	100%
Discharge Instructions	232	96%	59%	61%	93%
Evaluation of LVS Function	258	98%	81%	83%	99%
Smoking Cessation Advice	77	96%	86%	82%	100%
Pneumonia Care					
Appropriate Initial Antibiotic	47	81%	81%	83%	94%
Blood Culture Timing	60	90%	89%	90%	100%
Influenza Vaccine[1]	20	25%	60%	70%	100%
Initial Antibiotic Timing	96	70%	75%	80%	93%
Oxygenation Assessment	119	100%	99%	99%	100%
Pneumococcal Vaccine	41	44%	61%	69%	94%
Smoking Cessation Advice	36	86%	82%	80%	100%
Surgical Infection Prevention					
Prophylactic Antibiotic Given[2]	238	50%	69%	77%	95%
Prophylactic Antibiotic Selection[2]	65	86%	89%	90%	100%
Prophylactic Antibiotic Stopped[2]	232	66%	71%	72%	95%
Pregnancy Care					
Inpatient Neonatal Mortality	-	-	-	-	-
Third or Fourth Degree Laceration	-	-	3.63%	3.63%	3.27%

Emory Crawford Long Hospital

550 Peachtree Street NE
Atlanta, GA 30308
URL: www.eusch.org
Ownership: Voluntary non-profit - Private
Emergency Services: Yes

Phone: 404-686-4411
Fax: 404-686-4619

Accredited: Yes
Licensed Beds: 583

Key Personnel:
CEO . . . . John D Henry, Sr

Chief Medical Staff . . . . Roland H Ingram, MD
Administrative Director Catheterization . . . . Linda Hardwick, RN
Emergency Room . . . . Arthur Kellerman, MD
Director Infection/Disease Control . . . . James Steinberg, MD
CCU Spvg. Nurse . . . . June Connor, RN
Director Medical/Surgical Nursing . . . . Kim Lucas, RN
OB/GYN Womens Health . . . . Camille Davis-Williams
Director Respiratory Therapy . . . . Jane Bockman

Measure	Cases	This Hospital	State Average	U.S. Average	Top Hospital
Heart Attack Care					
ACE Inhibitor or ARB for LVSD[2]	98	72%	78%	82%	100%
Aspirin at Arrival[2]	100	97%	91%	92%	100%
Aspirin at Discharge[2]	296	95%	87%	90%	100%
Beta Blocker at Arrival[2]	92	95%	85%	87%	100%
Beta Blocker at Discharge[2]	315	94%	87%	90%	100%
Fibrinolytic Medication Timing[2]	0	-	34%	31%	100%
PCI Within 90 Minutes of Arrival[1,2]	9	44%	47%	54%	95%
Smoking Cessation Advice[2]	132	98%	85%	88%	100%
Heart Failure Care					
ACE Inhibitor or ARB for LVSD[2]	259	78%	81%	82%	100%
Discharge Instructions[2]	325	46%	59%	61%	93%
Evaluation of LVS Function[2]	342	92%	81%	83%	99%
Smoking Cessation Advice[2]	73	96%	86%	82%	100%
Pneumonia Care					
Appropriate Initial Antibiotic[2]	104	86%	81%	83%	94%
Blood Culture Timing[2]	113	73%	89%	90%	100%
Influenza Vaccine[2]	32	38%	60%	70%	100%
Initial Antibiotic Timing[2]	208	63%	75%	80%	93%
Oxygenation Assessment[2]	224	100%	99%	99%	100%
Pneumococcal Vaccine[2]	107	39%	61%	69%	94%
Smoking Cessation Advice[2]	54	98%	82%	80%	100%
Surgical Infection Prevention					
Prophylactic Antibiotic Given[2]	551	84%	69%	77%	95%
Prophylactic Antibiotic Selection[2]	89	79%	89%	90%	100%
Prophylactic Antibiotic Stopped[2]	539	80%	71%	72%	95%
Pregnancy Care					
Inpatient Neonatal Mortality	-	-	-	-	-
Third or Fourth Degree Laceration	-	-	3.63%	3.63%	3.27%

Emory Dunwoody Medical Center

Alternate Name: Shallowford Community Hospital
4575 N Shallowford Road
Atlanta, GA 30338
URL: www.emorydunwoody.com
Ownership: Proprietary
Emergency Services: Yes

Phone: 770-454-2000
Fax: 770-454-4279

Accredited: Yes
Licensed Beds: 168

Key Personnel:
CEO . . . . Thomas Gilbert
Chief Medical Staff . . . . Dr. Mark Harris
Emergency Room . . . . Arthur Griffith

Measure	Cases	This Hospital	State Average	U.S. Average	Top Hospital
Heart Attack Care					
ACE Inhibitor or ARB for LVSD[1]	4	75%	78%	82%	100%
Aspirin at Arrival[1]	14	100%	91%	92%	100%
Aspirin at Discharge[1]	10	90%	87%	90%	100%
Beta Blocker at Arrival[1]	10	100%	85%	87%	100%
Beta Blocker at Discharge[1]	9	100%	87%	90%	100%
Fibrinolytic Medication Timing[1]	1	100%	34%	31%	100%
PCI Within 90 Minutes of Arrival	0	-	47%	54%	95%
Smoking Cessation Advice[1]	2	100%	85%	88%	100%
Heart Failure Care					
ACE Inhibitor or ARB for LVSD	38	84%	81%	82%	100%
Discharge Instructions	88	58%	59%	61%	93%
Evaluation of LVS Function	80	91%	81%	83%	99%
Smoking Cessation Advice[1]	21	90%	86%	82%	100%
Pneumonia Care					
Appropriate Initial Antibiotic	44	84%	81%	83%	94%
Blood Culture Timing	37	97%	89%	90%	100%
Influenza Vaccine[1]	12	58%	60%	70%	100%
Initial Antibiotic Timing	49	76%	75%	80%	93%

NOTE: Hospital profiles are in alphabetical order by state, then city, then hospital within the city; Rankings are sorted by rate in descending order and exclude hospitals with less than 25 cases; (1) The number of cases is too small (n<25) for purposes of reliably predicting hospital performance; (2) Measure reflects the hospital's indication that its submission was based upon a sample of its relevant discharges; (3) Rate reflects fewer than the maximum possible quarters of data for the measure; (4) Inaccurate information submitted and suppressed for one or more quarters; (5) No data is available from the hospital for this measure; Please refer to the User's Guide for a full explanation of data

Oxygenation Assessment	58	100%	99%	99%	100%
Pneumococcal Vaccine	28	64%	61%	69%	94%
Smoking Cessation Advice[1]	16	75%	82%	80%	100%
Surgical Infection Prevention					
Prophylactic Antibiotic Given[2,3]	52	62%	69%	77%	95%
Prophylactic Antibiotic Selection[1,2]	21	90%	89%	90%	100%
Prophylactic Antibiotic Stopped[2,3]	47	47%	71%	72%	95%
Pregnancy Care					
Inpatient Neonatal Mortality	-	-	-	-	-
Third or Fourth Degree Laceration	-	-	3.63%	3.63%	3.27%

Emory University Hospital

1364 Clifton Road, Ne
Atlanta, GA 30322
Phone: 404-686-8500
Ownership: Voluntary non-profit - Private   Accredited: Yes
Emergency Services: Yes

Measure	Cases	This Hospital	State Average	U.S. Average	Top Hospital
Heart Attack Care					
ACE Inhibitor or ARB for LVSD[2]	72	86%	78%	82%	100%
Aspirin at Arrival[2]	112	94%	91%	92%	100%
Aspirin at Discharge[2]	244	99%	87%	90%	100%
Beta Blocker at Arrival[2]	93	95%	85%	87%	100%
Beta Blocker at Discharge[2]	284	95%	87%	90%	100%
Fibrinolytic Medication Timing[1,2]	1	0%	34%	31%	100%
PCI Within 90 Minutes of Arrival[1,2]	4	25%	47%	54%	95%
Smoking Cessation Advice[2]	115	98%	85%	88%	100%
Heart Failure Care					
ACE Inhibitor or ARB for LVSD[2]	218	92%	81%	82%	100%
Discharge Instructions[2]	307	71%	59%	61%	93%
Evaluation of LVS Function[2]	337	100%	81%	83%	99%
Smoking Cessation Advice[2]	53	100%	86%	82%	100%
Pneumonia Care					
Appropriate Initial Antibiotic[2]	55	89%	81%	83%	94%
Blood Culture Timing[2]	83	89%	89%	90%	100%
Influenza Vaccine[1,2]	23	74%	60%	70%	100%
Initial Antibiotic Timing[2]	125	59%	75%	80%	93%
Oxygenation Assessment[2]	149	100%	99%	99%	100%
Pneumococcal Vaccine[2]	73	78%	61%	69%	94%
Smoking Cessation Advice[1,2]	24	100%	82%	80%	100%
Surgical Infection Prevention					
Prophylactic Antibiotic Given[2]	575	89%	69%	77%	95%
Prophylactic Antibiotic Selection[2]	84	87%	89%	90%	100%
Prophylactic Antibiotic Stopped[2]	556	85%	71%	72%	95%
Pregnancy Care					
Inpatient Neonatal Mortality	-	-	-	-	-
Third or Fourth Degree Laceration	-	-	3.63%	3.63%	3.27%

Grady Memorial Hospital

80 Jesse Hill Dr SE
Atlanta, GA 30303
URL: www.gradyhealthsystems.org
Phone: 404-616-1000
Fax: 404-616-6033
Ownership: Govt - Hospital District or Authority   Accredited: Yes
Emergency Services: Yes   Licensed Beds: 983
Key Personnel:
CEO . . . . Andrew Agwunovi
Chief of Medical Staff . . . . Curtis Lewis
Director of Cardiology/Cardiac Lab. . . . . David Harrison, MD
Emergency Room . . . . Lian Haley
Emergency Room . . . . Arthur Kellerman, MD
Chief Radiology . . . . William Small, MD
Director Respiratory Therapy . . . . Bill Hastings

Measure	Cases	This Hospital	State Average	U.S. Average	Top Hospital
Heart Attack Care					
ACE Inhibitor or ARB for LVSD[2]	103	91%	78%	82%	100%
Aspirin at Arrival[2]	260	93%	91%	92%	100%
Aspirin at Discharge[2]	231	99%	87%	90%	100%
Beta Blocker at Arrival[2]	173	92%	85%	87%	100%
Beta Blocker at Discharge[2]	207	98%	87%	90%	100%
Fibrinolytic Medication Timing[1,2]	3	33%	34%	31%	100%
PCI Within 90 Minutes of Arrival[2]	0	-	47%	54%	95%

Smoking Cessation Advice[2]	124	44%	85%	88%	100%
Heart Failure Care					
ACE Inhibitor or ARB for LVSD[2]	206	89%	81%	82%	100%
Discharge Instructions[2]	338	1%	59%	61%	93%
Evaluation of LVS Function[2]	348	93%	81%	83%	99%
Smoking Cessation Advice[2]	161	25%	86%	82%	100%
Pneumonia Care					
Appropriate Initial Antibiotic[2]	115	83%	81%	83%	94%
Blood Culture Timing[2]	106	65%	89%	90%	100%
Influenza Vaccine[1,2]	21	24%	60%	70%	100%
Initial Antibiotic Timing[2]	214	32%	75%	80%	93%
Oxygenation Assessment[2]	231	99%	99%	99%	100%
Pneumococcal Vaccine[2]	48	33%	61%	69%	94%
Smoking Cessation Advice[2]	97	19%	82%	80%	100%
Surgical Infection Prevention					
Prophylactic Antibiotic Given[2,3]	184	69%	69%	77%	95%
Prophylactic Antibiotic Selection[2]	50	88%	89%	90%	100%
Prophylactic Antibiotic Stopped[2,3]	183	73%	71%	72%	95%
Pregnancy Care					
Inpatient Neonatal Mortality[2]	833	0.36%	-	-	-
Third or Fourth Degree Laceration	2,485	2.37%	3.63%	3.63%	3.27%

Legacy Medical Center of Atlanta

501 Fairburn Road, SW
Atlanta, GA 30331
Phone: 404-505-5628
Ownership: Proprietary   Accredited: No
Emergency Services: Yes

Measure	Cases	This Hospital	State Average	U.S. Average	Top Hospital
Heart Attack Care					
ACE Inhibitor or ARB for LVSD[5]	-	-	78%	82%	100%
Aspirin at Arrival[5]	-	-	91%	92%	100%
Aspirin at Discharge[5]	-	-	87%	90%	100%
Beta Blocker at Arrival[5]	-	-	85%	87%	100%
Beta Blocker at Discharge[5]	-	-	87%	90%	100%
Fibrinolytic Medication Timing[5]	-	-	34%	31%	100%
PCI Within 90 Minutes of Arrival[5]	-	-	47%	54%	95%
Smoking Cessation Advice[5]	-	-	85%	88%	100%
Heart Failure Care					
ACE Inhibitor or ARB for LVSD[3]	0	-	81%	82%	100%
Discharge Instructions[3]	0	-	59%	61%	93%
Evaluation of LVS Function[3]	0	-	81%	83%	99%
Smoking Cessation Advice[3]	0	-	86%	82%	100%
Pneumonia Care					
Appropriate Initial Antibiotic[5]	-	-	81%	83%	94%
Blood Culture Timing[5]	-	-	89%	90%	100%
Influenza Vaccine[5]	-	-	60%	70%	100%
Initial Antibiotic Timing[5]	-	-	75%	80%	93%
Oxygenation Assessment[5]	-	-	99%	99%	100%
Pneumococcal Vaccine[5]	-	-	61%	69%	94%
Smoking Cessation Advice[5]	-	-	82%	80%	100%
Surgical Infection Prevention					
Prophylactic Antibiotic Given[5]	-	-	69%	77%	95%
Prophylactic Antibiotic Selection[5]	-	-	89%	90%	100%
Prophylactic Antibiotic Stopped[5]	-	-	71%	72%	95%
Pregnancy Care					
Inpatient Neonatal Mortality	-	-	-	-	-
Third or Fourth Degree Laceration	-	-	3.63%	3.63%	3.27%

Northside Hospital

1000 Johnson Ferry Road NE
Atlanta, GA 30342
URL: www.northside.com
Phone: 404-851-8000
Fax: 404-250-1317
Ownership: Voluntary non-profit - Private   Accredited: Yes
Emergency Services: Yes   Licensed Beds: 444
Key Personnel:
Chairman/CEO/President . . . . Sidney Kirschner
Chief Medical Staff . . . . Eimear Kennedy
Emergency Room . . . . Robert Higgins, MD
Director Infection/Disease Control . . . . Janice Fetter
Supervising Nurse CCU . . . . Lisa Thomas
Director Medical/Surgical Nursing . . . . Judy Thibadeau
OB/GYN Womens Health . . . . Jeffery Korotkin, MD

NOTE: Hospital profiles are in alphabetical order by state, then city, then hospital within the city; Rankings are sorted by rate in descending order and exclude hospitals with less than 25 cases; (1) The number of cases is too small (n<25) for purposes of reliably predicting hospital performance; (2) Measure reflects the hospital's indication that its submission was based upon a sample of its relevant discharges; (3) Rate reflects fewer than the maximum possible quarters of data for the measure; (4) Inaccurate information submitted and suppressed for one or more quarters; (5) No data is available from the hospital for this measure; Please refer to the User's Guide for a full explanation of data

Chief Radiology . . . . James Zakem, MD
Director Respiratory Therapy . . . . Len McDade

Measure	Cases	This Hospital	State Average	U.S. Average	Top Hospital
Heart Attack Care					
ACE Inhibitor or ARB for LVSD[1]	8	75%	78%	82%	100%
Aspirin at Arrival	49	96%	91%	92%	100%
Aspirin at Discharge[1]	18	89%	87%	90%	100%
Beta Blocker at Arrival	43	98%	85%	87%	100%
Beta Blocker at Discharge	26	100%	87%	90%	100%
Fibrinolytic Medication Timing[1]	1	100%	34%	31%	100%
PCI Within 90 Minutes of Arrival	0	-	47%	54%	95%
Smoking Cessation Advice[1]	3	100%	85%	88%	100%
Heart Failure Care					
ACE Inhibitor or ARB for LVSD	86	88%	81%	82%	100%
Discharge Instructions	185	66%	59%	61%	93%
Evaluation of LVS Function	211	99%	81%	83%	99%
Smoking Cessation Advice	30	93%	86%	82%	100%
Pneumonia Care					
Appropriate Initial Antibiotic	181	95%	81%	83%	94%
Blood Culture Timing	164	99%	89%	90%	100%
Influenza Vaccine	61	92%	60%	70%	100%
Initial Antibiotic Timing	228	92%	75%	80%	93%
Oxygenation Assessment	312	100%	99%	99%	100%
Pneumococcal Vaccine	154	94%	61%	69%	94%
Smoking Cessation Advice	52	100%	82%	80%	100%
Surgical Infection Prevention					
Prophylactic Antibiotic Given[2,3]	114	96%	69%	77%	95%
Prophylactic Antibiotic Selection[2]	114	95%	89%	90%	100%
Prophylactic Antibiotic Stopped[2,3]	110	62%	71%	72%	95%
Pregnancy Care					
Inpatient Neonatal Mortality	18,311	0.37%	-	-	-
Third or Fourth Degree Laceration	11,482	4.59%	3.63%	3.63%	3.27%

Piedmont Hospital

1968 Peachtree Road NW
Atlanta, GA 30309
URL: www.piedmonthospital.org
Ownership: Voluntary non-profit - Private
Emergency Services: Yes

Phone: 404-605-5000
Fax: 404-367-3551

Accredited: Yes
Licensed Beds: 500

Key Personnel:
President/CEO . . . . Richard Hubbard Jr, DO
Chief Medical Staff . . . . Dan Fergusen, MD
Emergency Room . . . . Leah Tolly
Director Infection/Disease Control . . . . Carol Mims
OB/GYN Womens Health . . . . Ramon Surez, MD
Chief Radiology . . . . Robert Halper

Measure	Cases	This Hospital	State Average	U.S. Average	Top Hospital
Heart Attack Care					
ACE Inhibitor or ARB for LVSD	103	94%	78%	82%	100%
Aspirin at Arrival	95	91%	91%	92%	100%
Aspirin at Discharge	365	98%	87%	90%	100%
Beta Blocker at Arrival	81	88%	85%	87%	100%
Beta Blocker at Discharge	350	97%	87%	90%	100%
Fibrinolytic Medication Timing	0	-	34%	31%	100%
PCI Within 90 Minutes of Arrival[1]	7	43%	47%	54%	95%
Smoking Cessation Advice	139	96%	85%	88%	100%
Heart Failure Care					
ACE Inhibitor or ARB for LVSD	234	77%	81%	82%	100%
Discharge Instructions	376	78%	59%	61%	93%
Evaluation of LVS Function	403	98%	81%	83%	99%
Smoking Cessation Advice	75	97%	86%	82%	100%
Pneumonia Care					
Appropriate Initial Antibiotic	201	89%	81%	83%	94%
Blood Culture Timing	209	84%	89%	90%	100%
Influenza Vaccine	64	72%	60%	70%	100%
Initial Antibiotic Timing	311	68%	75%	80%	93%
Oxygenation Assessment	363	100%	99%	99%	100%
Pneumococcal Vaccine	181	62%	61%	69%	94%
Smoking Cessation Advice	73	92%	82%	80%	100%
Surgical Infection Prevention					

Measure	Cases	This Hospital	State Average	U.S. Average	Top Hospital
Prophylactic Antibiotic Given	436	94%	69%	77%	95%
Prophylactic Antibiotic Selection	102	90%	89%	90%	100%
Prophylactic Antibiotic Stopped	425	88%	71%	72%	95%
Pregnancy Care					
Inpatient Neonatal Mortality	-	-	-	-	-
Third or Fourth Degree Laceration	-	-	3.63%	3.63%	3.27%

Saint Joseph's Hospital

5665 Peachtree Dunwoody Road NE
Atlanta, GA 30342
URL: www.stjosephsatlanta.org
Ownership: Voluntary non-profit - Church
Emergency Services: Yes

Phone: 404-851-7001
Fax: 404-851-7938

Accredited: Yes
Licensed Beds: 346

Key Personnel:
CEO . . . . Robin Spiegel
Chief Medical Staff . . . . Chris Shaw, MD

Measure	Cases	This Hospital	State Average	U.S. Average	Top Hospital
Heart Attack Care					
ACE Inhibitor or ARB for LVSD	324	77%	78%	82%	100%
Aspirin at Arrival	317	98%	91%	92%	100%
Aspirin at Discharge	1,323	98%	87%	90%	100%
Beta Blocker at Arrival	260	97%	85%	87%	100%
Beta Blocker at Discharge	1,275	98%	87%	90%	100%
Fibrinolytic Medication Timing[1]	1	0%	34%	31%	100%
PCI Within 90 Minutes of Arrival[1]	19	79%	47%	54%	95%
Smoking Cessation Advice	466	100%	85%	88%	100%
Heart Failure Care					
ACE Inhibitor or ARB for LVSD	420	63%	81%	82%	100%
Discharge Instructions	634	66%	59%	61%	93%
Evaluation of LVS Function	700	99%	81%	83%	99%
Smoking Cessation Advice	87	97%	86%	82%	100%
Pneumonia Care					
Appropriate Initial Antibiotic	256	85%	81%	83%	94%
Blood Culture Timing	211	94%	89%	90%	100%
Influenza Vaccine	57	65%	60%	70%	100%
Initial Antibiotic Timing	318	74%	75%	80%	93%
Oxygenation Assessment	397	100%	99%	99%	100%
Pneumococcal Vaccine	278	59%	61%	69%	94%
Smoking Cessation Advice	59	92%	82%	80%	100%
Surgical Infection Prevention					
Prophylactic Antibiotic Given[3]	262	77%	69%	77%	95%
Prophylactic Antibiotic Selection	89	84%	89%	90%	100%
Prophylactic Antibiotic Stopped[3]	261	64%	71%	72%	95%
Pregnancy Care					
Inpatient Neonatal Mortality	-	-	-	-	-
Third or Fourth Degree Laceration	-	-	3.63%	3.63%	3.27%

Wesley Woods Geriatric Hospital

1821 Clifton Road NE
Atlanta, GA 30329
E-mail: peter_basler@emoryhealthcare.org
Ownership: Voluntary non-profit - Private
Emergency Services: No

Phone: 404-712-4937
Fax: 404-728-6558

Accredited: Yes
Licensed Beds: 100

Key Personnel:
Administrator . . . . Peter A Basler
Chief Medical Officer . . . . Joseph Ouslander, MD
Infection Control . . . . Kathy Westmoreland
Respiratory/Cardiopulmonary . . . . Judith Lukjan

Measure	Cases	This Hospital	State Average	U.S. Average	Top Hospital
Heart Attack Care					
ACE Inhibitor or ARB for LVSD[3]	0	-	78%	82%	100%
Aspirin at Arrival[1,3]	2	100%	91%	92%	100%
Aspirin at Discharge[1,3]	3	100%	87%	90%	100%
Beta Blocker at Arrival[1,3]	2	0%	85%	87%	100%
Beta Blocker at Discharge[1,3]	3	100%	87%	90%	100%
Fibrinolytic Medication Timing[3]	0	-	34%	31%	100%
PCI Within 90 Minutes of Arrival[5]	-	-	47%	54%	95%
Smoking Cessation Advice[3]	0	-	85%	88%	100%
Heart Failure Care					
ACE Inhibitor or ARB for LVSD[1]	5	100%	81%	82%	100%

NOTE: Hospital profiles are in alphabetical order by state, then city, then hospital within the city; Rankings are sorted by rate in descending order and exclude hospitals with less than 25 cases; (1) The number of cases is too small (n<25) for purposes of reliably predicting hospital performance; (2) Measure reflects the hospital's indication that its submission was based upon a sample of its relevant discharges; (3) Rate reflects fewer than the maximum possible quarters of data for the measure; (4) Inaccurate information submitted and suppressed for one or more quarters; (5) No data is available from the hospital for this measure; Please refer to the User's Guide for a full explanation of data

Discharge Instructions[1]	20	60%	59%	61%	93%
Evaluation of LVS Function	38	100%	81%	83%	99%
Smoking Cessation Advice[1]	1	100%	86%	82%	100%
Pneumonia Care					
Appropriate Initial Antibiotic[1]	11	55%	81%	83%	94%
Blood Culture Timing	0	-	89%	90%	100%
Influenza Vaccine[1]	11	73%	60%	70%	100%
Initial Antibiotic Timing[1]	15	53%	75%	80%	93%
Oxygenation Assessment[1]	17	100%	99%	99%	100%
Pneumococcal Vaccine	39	64%	61%	69%	94%
Smoking Cessation Advice[1]	9	67%	82%	80%	100%
Surgical Infection Prevention					
Prophylactic Antibiotic Given[3]	0	-	69%	77%	95%
Prophylactic Antibiotic Selection	0	-	89%	90%	100%
Prophylactic Antibiotic Stopped[3]	0	-	71%	72%	95%
Pregnancy Care					
Inpatient Neonatal Mortality	-	-	-	-	-
Third or Fourth Degree Laceration	-	-	3.63%	3.63%	3.27%

Doctors Hospital

Alternate Name: Doctors Hospital of Augusta

3651 Wheeler Road
Augusta, GA 30909
URL: www.doctors-hospital.net
Ownership: Proprietary
Emergency Services: Yes

Phone: 706-651-3232
Fax: 706-651-2041

Accredited: Yes
Licensed Beds: 354

Key Personnel:
President/CEO . . . . Shayne George
President of Medical Staff . . . . Cristian Thome
Director Emergency Medicine . . . . Martha Garner
Director Medical/Surgical . . . . Brad Cheek
Director Maternal Child Services . . . . Candy Tricker
Director Surgical Services . . . . Bonnie O'Leary
Director Radiology . . . . John Doriot

Measure	Cases	This Hospital	State Average	U.S. Average	Top Hospital
Heart Attack Care					
ACE Inhibitor or ARB for LVSD[1]	6	83%	78%	82%	100%
Aspirin at Arrival	39	92%	91%	92%	100%
Aspirin at Discharge[1]	21	95%	87%	90%	100%
Beta Blocker at Arrival	25	88%	85%	87%	100%
Beta Blocker at Discharge[1]	18	94%	87%	90%	100%
Fibrinolytic Medication Timing	0	-	34%	31%	100%
PCI Within 90 Minutes of Arrival	0	-	47%	54%	95%
Smoking Cessation Advice[1]	8	100%	85%	88%	100%
Heart Failure Care					
ACE Inhibitor or ARB for LVSD	73	64%	81%	82%	100%
Discharge Instructions	210	30%	59%	61%	93%
Evaluation of LVS Function	232	81%	81%	83%	99%
Smoking Cessation Advice	42	95%	86%	82%	100%
Pneumonia Care					
Appropriate Initial Antibiotic	129	95%	81%	83%	94%
Blood Culture Timing	94	94%	89%	90%	100%
Influenza Vaccine	45	62%	60%	70%	100%
Initial Antibiotic Timing	190	64%	75%	80%	93%
Oxygenation Assessment	234	100%	99%	99%	100%
Pneumococcal Vaccine	131	59%	61%	69%	94%
Smoking Cessation Advice	52	96%	82%	80%	100%
Surgical Infection Prevention					
Prophylactic Antibiotic Given[2,3]	207	87%	69%	77%	95%
Prophylactic Antibiotic Selection[2]	95	91%	89%	90%	100%
Prophylactic Antibiotic Stopped[2,3]	199	76%	71%	72%	95%
Pregnancy Care					
Inpatient Neonatal Mortality	-	-	-	-	-
Third or Fourth Degree Laceration	-	-	3.63%	3.63%	3.27%

Medical College of Georgia Hospital & Clinics

Alternate Name: MCG Health System

1120 15th Street
Augusta, GA 30912
URL: www.mcg.edu
Ownership: Voluntary non-profit - Other
Emergency Services: Yes

Phone: 706-721-0211
Fax: 706-721-5735

Accredited: Yes
Licensed Beds: 480

Key Personnel:
President/CEO . . . . Don Snell
Interim Chief Emergency Services . . . . Richard B Schwartz, MD
Infection Control . . . . Cyndra Bystrom
Intensive Coronary . . . . Gerald Cate
Medical Surgical Nursing . . . . Angela Lambert
Chair OB/GYN Womens Health . . . . Lawrence Devoe, MD
Respiratory/Cardiopulmonary . . . . Randy Baker

Measure	Cases	This Hospital	State Average	U.S. Average	Top Hospital
Heart Attack Care					
ACE Inhibitor or ARB for LVSD	59	92%	78%	82%	100%
Aspirin at Arrival	116	97%	91%	92%	100%
Aspirin at Discharge	159	97%	87%	90%	100%
Beta Blocker at Arrival	77	97%	85%	87%	100%
Beta Blocker at Discharge	130	100%	87%	90%	100%
Fibrinolytic Medication Timing	0	-	34%	31%	100%
PCI Within 90 Minutes of Arrival[1]	2	0%	47%	54%	95%
Smoking Cessation Advice	102	98%	85%	88%	100%
Heart Failure Care					
ACE Inhibitor or ARB for LVSD[2]	222	86%	81%	82%	100%
Discharge Instructions[2]	303	45%	59%	61%	93%
Evaluation of LVS Function[2]	325	99%	81%	83%	99%
Smoking Cessation Advice[2]	127	81%	86%	82%	100%
Pneumonia Care					
Appropriate Initial Antibiotic[2]	69	86%	81%	83%	94%
Blood Culture Timing[2]	106	85%	89%	90%	100%
Influenza Vaccine[2]	31	29%	60%	70%	100%
Initial Antibiotic Timing[2]	168	61%	75%	80%	93%
Oxygenation Assessment[2]	190	100%	99%	99%	100%
Pneumococcal Vaccine[2]	87	45%	61%	69%	94%
Smoking Cessation Advice[2]	49	67%	82%	80%	100%
Surgical Infection Prevention					
Prophylactic Antibiotic Given[2,3]	257	75%	69%	77%	95%
Prophylactic Antibiotic Selection[2]	54	80%	89%	90%	100%
Prophylactic Antibiotic Stopped[2,3]	240	60%	71%	72%	95%
Pregnancy Care					
Inpatient Neonatal Mortality[2]	110	0.91%	-	-	-
Third or Fourth Degree Laceration	315	6.03%	3.63%	3.63%	3.27%

Trinity Hospital of Augusta

2260 Wrightsboro Road
Augusta, GA 30904
URL: www.trinityofaugusta.com
Ownership: Voluntary non-profit - Private
Emergency Services: Yes

Phone: 706-481-7000

Accredited: Yes
Licensed Beds: 107

Key Personnel:
President/CEO . . . . Andrew A Lasser
Emergency Room . . . . Walter Hardwood
Director Respiratory Therapy . . . . Percy Mobley

Measure	Cases	This Hospital	State Average	U.S. Average	Top Hospital
Heart Attack Care					
ACE Inhibitor or ARB for LVSD[3]	0	-	78%	82%	100%
Aspirin at Arrival[1,3]	3	100%	91%	92%	100%
Aspirin at Discharge[1,3]	3	100%	87%	90%	100%
Beta Blocker at Arrival[1,3]	3	100%	85%	87%	100%
Beta Blocker at Discharge[1,3]	3	33%	87%	90%	100%
Fibrinolytic Medication Timing[3]	0	-	34%	31%	100%
PCI Within 90 Minutes of Arrival	0	-	47%	54%	95%
Smoking Cessation Advice[3]	0	-	85%	88%	100%
Heart Failure Care					
ACE Inhibitor or ARB for LVSD	25	72%	81%	82%	100%
Discharge Instructions	77	83%	59%	61%	93%
Evaluation of LVS Function	96	88%	81%	83%	99%
Smoking Cessation Advice[1]	14	79%	86%	82%	100%
Pneumonia Care					
Appropriate Initial Antibiotic	79	82%	81%	83%	94%

NOTE: Hospital profiles are in alphabetical order by state, then city, then hospital within the city; Rankings are sorted by rate in descending order and exclude hospitals with less than 25 cases; (1) The number of cases is too small (n<25) for purposes of reliably predicting hospital performance; (2) Measure reflects the hospital's indication that its submission was based upon a sample of its relevant discharges; (3) Rate reflects fewer than the maximum possible quarters of data for the measure; (4) Inaccurate information submitted and suppressed for one or more quarters; (5) No data is available from the hospital for this measure; Please refer to the User's Guide for a full explanation of data

Blood Culture Timing	77	88%	89%	90%	100%
Influenza Vaccine	27	56%	60%	70%	100%
Initial Antibiotic Timing	113	79%	75%	80%	93%
Oxygenation Assessment	138	100%	99%	99%	100%
Pneumococcal Vaccine	82	65%	61%	69%	94%
Smoking Cessation Advice	25	60%	82%	80%	100%
Surgical Infection Prevention					
Prophylactic Antibiotic Given[2,3]	125	86%	69%	77%	95%
Prophylactic Antibiotic Selection[2]	43	98%	89%	90%	100%
Prophylactic Antibiotic Stopped[2,3]	123	77%	71%	72%	95%
Pregnancy Care					
Inpatient Neonatal Mortality	-	-	-	-	-
Third or Fourth Degree Laceration	-	-	3.63%	3.63%	3.27%

University Hospital

1350 Walton Way
Augusta, GA 30901
URL: www.universityhealth.org
Ownership: Voluntary non-profit - Other
Emergency Services: Yes

Phone: 706-722-9011
Fax: 706-774-8699

Accredited: Yes
Licensed Beds: 612

Key Personnel:
President/CEO . . . . Larry Read
Chief Medical Staff . . . . William Farr, MD
Director Emergency Room Services . . . . George Ann Phillips
Emergency Room . . . . Richard Eckert, MD
Coordinator Infection Control . . . . Vivian Ashline
OB/GYN Womens Health . . . . WG Watson, MD
Chief Radiology . . . . Jimpsey B Johnson, MD
Director Cardio-Pulmonary Services . . . . Teresa Waters

Measure	Cases	This Hospital	State Average	U.S. Average	Top Hospital
Heart Attack Care					
ACE Inhibitor or ARB for LVSD	113	91%	78%	82%	100%
Aspirin at Arrival	360	97%	91%	92%	100%
Aspirin at Discharge	506	98%	87%	90%	100%
Beta Blocker at Arrival	252	96%	85%	87%	100%
Beta Blocker at Discharge	447	98%	87%	90%	100%
Fibrinolytic Medication Timing[1]	4	0%	34%	31%	100%
PCI Within 90 Minutes of Arrival[1]	13	38%	47%	54%	95%
Smoking Cessation Advice	186	100%	85%	88%	100%
Heart Failure Care					
ACE Inhibitor or ARB for LVSD	288	98%	81%	82%	100%
Discharge Instructions	613	91%	59%	61%	93%
Evaluation of LVS Function	683	99%	81%	83%	99%
Smoking Cessation Advice	108	100%	86%	82%	100%
Pneumonia Care					
Appropriate Initial Antibiotic	300	90%	81%	83%	94%
Blood Culture Timing	400	95%	89%	90%	100%
Influenza Vaccine	120	83%	60%	70%	100%
Initial Antibiotic Timing	524	82%	75%	80%	93%
Oxygenation Assessment	660	100%	99%	99%	100%
Pneumococcal Vaccine	399	87%	61%	69%	94%
Smoking Cessation Advice	128	94%	82%	80%	100%
Surgical Infection Prevention					
Prophylactic Antibiotic Given[2]	1,934	92%	69%	77%	95%
Prophylactic Antibiotic Selection[2]	439	92%	89%	90%	100%
Prophylactic Antibiotic Stopped[2]	1,927	46%	71%	72%	95%
Pregnancy Care					
Inpatient Neonatal Mortality	-	-	-	-	-
Third or Fourth Degree Laceration	-	-	3.63%	3.63%	3.27%

WellStar Cobb Hospital

Alternate Name: Promina Cobb Hospital
3950 Austell Road
Austell, GA 30106
E-mail: generalinfo@wellstar.org
URL: www.wellstar.org
Ownership: Voluntary non-profit - Other
Emergency Services: Yes

Phone: 770-732-4000
Fax: 770-732-4015

Accredited: Yes
Licensed Beds: 322

Key Personnel:
CEO . . . . Robert Lipson
Chief Medical Staff . . . . Donald Campbell
Director Medical/Surgical Nursing . . . . Martha Hughes

OB/GYN Womens Health . . . . Mindy Fine, MD
Chief Radiology . . . . Greg Smith, MD
Director of Pulmonary Care . . . . Fred Drons

Measure	Cases	This Hospital	State Average	U.S. Average	Top Hospital
Heart Attack Care					
ACE Inhibitor or ARB for LVSD[1,2]	18	89%	78%	82%	100%
Aspirin at Arrival[2]	113	89%	91%	92%	100%
Aspirin at Discharge[2]	58	90%	87%	90%	100%
Beta Blocker at Arrival[2]	94	96%	85%	87%	100%
Beta Blocker at Discharge[2]	58	90%	87%	90%	100%
Fibrinolytic Medication Timing[1,2]	5	60%	34%	31%	100%
PCI Within 90 Minutes of Arrival[1,2]	1	100%	47%	54%	95%
Smoking Cessation Advice[1,2]	21	90%	85%	88%	100%
Heart Failure Care					
ACE Inhibitor or ARB for LVSD[2]	192	82%	81%	82%	100%
Discharge Instructions[2]	458	33%	59%	61%	93%
Evaluation of LVS Function[2]	510	94%	81%	83%	99%
Smoking Cessation Advice[2]	126	99%	86%	82%	100%
Pneumonia Care					
Appropriate Initial Antibiotic[2]	244	86%	81%	83%	94%
Blood Culture Timing[2]	218	84%	89%	90%	100%
Influenza Vaccine[2]	71	82%	60%	70%	100%
Initial Antibiotic Timing[2]	336	59%	75%	80%	93%
Oxygenation Assessment[2]	417	100%	99%	99%	100%
Pneumococcal Vaccine[2]	218	63%	61%	69%	94%
Smoking Cessation Advice[2]	111	95%	82%	80%	100%
Surgical Infection Prevention					
Prophylactic Antibiotic Given[3]	110	87%	69%	77%	95%
Prophylactic Antibiotic Selection	113	92%	89%	90%	100%
Prophylactic Antibiotic Stopped[3]	110	65%	71%	72%	95%
Pregnancy Care					
Inpatient Neonatal Mortality	-	-	-	-	-
Third or Fourth Degree Laceration	-	-	3.63%	3.63%	3.27%

Memorial Hospital & Manor

Alternate Name: Memorial Hospital
1500 E Shotwell Street
Bainbridge, GA 39817
URL: www.mh-m.org
Ownership: Govt - Hospital District or Authority
Emergency Services: Yes

Phone: 229-246-3500
Fax: 229-243-3338

Accredited: Yes
Licensed Beds: 80

Key Personnel:
CEO . . . . James G Peak
Chief Medical Staff . . . . Alan Wilson, MD
Director Infection/Disease Control . . . . Jane Chesser
Director Medical/Surgical Nursing . . . . Delores Eidson
OB/GYN Women's Health . . . . Marjorie Smith, RN
Director Respiratory Therapy . . . . Ed Newton, RRT

Measure	Cases	This Hospital	State Average	U.S. Average	Top Hospital
Heart Attack Care					
ACE Inhibitor or ARB for LVSD[1]	5	60%	78%	82%	100%
Aspirin at Arrival[1]	15	93%	91%	92%	100%
Aspirin at Discharge[1]	10	70%	87%	90%	100%
Beta Blocker at Arrival[1]	13	77%	85%	87%	100%
Beta Blocker at Discharge[1]	10	80%	87%	90%	100%
Fibrinolytic Medication Timing[1]	2	50%	34%	31%	100%
PCI Within 90 Minutes of Arrival	0	-	47%	54%	95%
Smoking Cessation Advice	0	-	85%	88%	100%
Heart Failure Care					
ACE Inhibitor or ARB for LVSD	31	84%	81%	82%	100%
Discharge Instructions	76	59%	59%	61%	93%
Evaluation of LVS Function	78	71%	81%	83%	99%
Smoking Cessation Advice[1]	14	79%	86%	82%	100%
Pneumonia Care					
Appropriate Initial Antibiotic	57	74%	81%	83%	94%
Blood Culture Timing	28	61%	89%	90%	100%
Influenza Vaccine[1]	13	46%	60%	70%	100%
Initial Antibiotic Timing	70	74%	75%	80%	93%
Oxygenation Assessment	79	99%	99%	99%	100%
Pneumococcal Vaccine	35	34%	61%	69%	94%

NOTE: Hospital profiles are in alphabetical order by state, then city, then hospital within the city; Rankings are sorted by rate in descending order and exclude hospitals with less than 25 cases; (1) The number of cases is too small (n<25) for purposes of reliably predicting hospital performance; (2) Measure reflects the hospital's indication that its submission was based upon a sample of its relevant discharges; (3) Rate reflects fewer than the maximum possible quarters of data for the measure; (4) Inaccurate information submitted and suppressed for one or more quarters; (5) No data is available from the hospital for this measure; Please refer to the User's Guide for a full explanation of data

Measure	Cases	This Hospital	State Average	U.S. Average	Top Hospital
Smoking Cessation Advice[1]	17	65%	82%	80%	100%
Surgical Infection Prevention					
Prophylactic Antibiotic Given[2,3]	33	58%	69%	77%	95%
Prophylactic Antibiotic Selection[2]	29	97%	89%	90%	100%
Prophylactic Antibiotic Stopped[2,3]	29	100%	71%	72%	95%
Pregnancy Care					
Inpatient Neonatal Mortality	-	-	-	-	-
Third or Fourth Degree Laceration	-	-	3.63%	3.63%	3.27%

Appling Hospital

PO Box 2070
Baxley, GA 31515
URL: www.appling-hospital.org
Ownership: Govt - Hospital District or Authority
Emergency Services: Yes

Phone: 912-367-9841
Fax: 912-367-7203

Accredited: Yes
Licensed Beds: 39

Key Personnel:
CEO. . . . . Dale Spell
Director Respiratory Therapy . . . . Pete Salko

Measure	Cases	This Hospital	State Average	U.S. Average	Top Hospital
Heart Attack Care					
ACE Inhibitor or ARB for LVSD[1]	1	100%	78%	82%	100%
Aspirin at Arrival[1]	9	89%	91%	92%	100%
Aspirin at Discharge[1]	1	100%	87%	90%	100%
Beta Blocker at Arrival[1]	8	100%	85%	87%	100%
Beta Blocker at Discharge[1]	2	100%	87%	90%	100%
Fibrinolytic Medication Timing	0	-	34%	31%	100%
PCI Within 90 Minutes of Arrival	0	-	47%	54%	95%
Smoking Cessation Advice[1]	1	100%	85%	88%	100%
Heart Failure Care					
ACE Inhibitor or ARB for LVSD[1]	7	86%	81%	82%	100%
Discharge Instructions	42	81%	59%	61%	93%
Evaluation of LVS Function	44	82%	81%	83%	99%
Smoking Cessation Advice[1]	10	100%	86%	82%	100%
Pneumonia Care					
Appropriate Initial Antibiotic	73	78%	81%	83%	94%
Blood Culture Timing[1]	22	86%	89%	90%	100%
Influenza Vaccine[1]	21	38%	60%	70%	100%
Initial Antibiotic Timing	113	75%	75%	80%	93%
Oxygenation Assessment	138	100%	99%	99%	100%
Pneumococcal Vaccine	82	66%	61%	69%	94%
Smoking Cessation Advice	28	96%	82%	80%	100%
Surgical Infection Prevention					
Prophylactic Antibiotic Given[1,3]	15	20%	69%	77%	95%
Prophylactic Antibiotic Selection[1]	5	40%	89%	90%	100%
Prophylactic Antibiotic Stopped[1,3]	12	100%	71%	72%	95%
Pregnancy Care					
Inpatient Neonatal Mortality	261	0.77%	-	-	-
Third or Fourth Degree Laceration	166	2.41%	3.63%	3.63%	3.27%

Union General Hospital

214 Hospital Circle
Blairsville, GA 30512
Ownership: Govt - Hospital District or Authority
Emergency Services: Yes

Phone: 706-745-2111
Fax: 706-745-7677

Accredited: Yes
Licensed Beds: 45

Key Personnel:
Administrator . . . . Rebeca Dyer
Director Medical/Surgical Nursing . . . . Tonia Albright
Chief Radiology . . . . Austin Flint, MD
Director Respiratory Therapy . . . . Tim Stepp

Measure	Cases	This Hospital	State Average	U.S. Average	Top Hospital
Heart Attack Care					
ACE Inhibitor or ARB for LVSD	0	-	78%	82%	100%
Aspirin at Arrival[1]	11	73%	91%	92%	100%
Aspirin at Discharge[1]	5	100%	87%	90%	100%
Beta Blocker at Arrival[1]	17	53%	85%	87%	100%
Beta Blocker at Discharge[1]	6	100%	87%	90%	100%
Fibrinolytic Medication Timing	0	-	34%	31%	100%
PCI Within 90 Minutes of Arrival	0	-	47%	54%	95%
Smoking Cessation Advice	0	-	85%	88%	100%
Heart Failure Care					

Measure	Cases	This Hospital	State Average	U.S. Average	Top Hospital
ACE Inhibitor or ARB for LVSD[1]	23	83%	81%	82%	100%
Discharge Instructions	61	49%	59%	61%	93%
Evaluation of LVS Function	75	84%	81%	83%	99%
Smoking Cessation Advice[1]	8	100%	86%	82%	100%
Pneumonia Care					
Appropriate Initial Antibiotic	84	83%	81%	83%	94%
Blood Culture Timing	65	91%	89%	90%	100%
Influenza Vaccine[1]	24	50%	60%	70%	100%
Initial Antibiotic Timing	104	81%	75%	80%	93%
Oxygenation Assessment	125	100%	99%	99%	100%
Pneumococcal Vaccine	81	64%	61%	69%	94%
Smoking Cessation Advice	28	89%	82%	80%	100%
Surgical Infection Prevention					
Prophylactic Antibiotic Given[2]	64	77%	69%	77%	95%
Prophylactic Antibiotic Selection[1,2]	18	94%	89%	90%	100%
Prophylactic Antibiotic Stopped[2]	61	87%	71%	72%	95%
Pregnancy Care					
Inpatient Neonatal Mortality	-	-	-	-	-
Third or Fourth Degree Laceration	-	-	3.63%	3.63%	3.27%

Early Memorial Hospital

11740 Columbia Street
Blakely, GA 39823
Ownership: Govt - Hospital District or Authority
Emergency Services: Yes

Phone: 229-723-4241
Fax: 229-723-5558

Accredited: Yes
Licensed Beds: 52

Key Personnel:
Administrator . . . . Robin Rau
President/CEO. . . . . James Storey, MD
Chief Medical Staff. . . . . Almas Yousuf
Director Medical/Surgical Nursing . . . . Stephanie Crawford
OB/GYN Womens Health. . . . . ROY Reardon, MD
Chief Radiology . . . . Norman Chadwell
Director Respiratory Therapy . . . . Pam Temples

Measure	Cases	This Hospital	State Average	U.S. Average	Top Hospital
Heart Attack Care					
ACE Inhibitor or ARB for LVSD[5]	-	-	78%	82%	100%
Aspirin at Arrival[5]	-	-	91%	92%	100%
Aspirin at Discharge[5]	-	-	87%	90%	100%
Beta Blocker at Arrival[5]	-	-	85%	87%	100%
Beta Blocker at Discharge[5]	-	-	87%	90%	100%
Fibrinolytic Medication Timing[5]	-	-	34%	31%	100%
PCI Within 90 Minutes of Arrival[5]	-	-	47%	54%	95%
Smoking Cessation Advice[5]	-	-	85%	88%	100%
Heart Failure Care					
ACE Inhibitor or ARB for LVSD[1]	2	50%	81%	82%	100%
Discharge Instructions[1]	11	91%	59%	61%	93%
Evaluation of LVS Function[1]	15	80%	81%	83%	99%
Smoking Cessation Advice[1]	1	100%	86%	82%	100%
Pneumonia Care					
Appropriate Initial Antibiotic[1,3]	12	92%	81%	83%	94%
Blood Culture Timing[1,3]	6	83%	89%	90%	100%
Influenza Vaccine[1]	3	67%	60%	70%	100%
Initial Antibiotic Timing[1,3]	13	62%	75%	80%	93%
Oxygenation Assessment[1,3]	18	100%	99%	99%	100%
Pneumococcal Vaccine[1,3]	11	27%	61%	69%	94%
Smoking Cessation Advice[1,3]	3	100%	82%	80%	100%
Surgical Infection Prevention					
Prophylactic Antibiotic Given[5]	-	-	69%	77%	95%
Prophylactic Antibiotic Selection[5]	-	-	89%	90%	100%
Prophylactic Antibiotic Stopped[5]	-	-	71%	72%	95%
Pregnancy Care					
Inpatient Neonatal Mortality	-	-	-	-	-
Third or Fourth Degree Laceration	-	-	3.63%	3.63%	3.27%

Fannin Regional Hospital

2855 Old Highway 5 N
Blue Ridge, GA 30513
Ownership: Proprietary
Emergency Services: Yes

Phone: 706-632-3711
Fax: 706-632-7216

Accredited: Yes
Licensed Beds: 50

Key Personnel:
CEO. . . . . Barry Mousa
Chief of Medical Staff. Suzanne Turner

NOTE: Hospital profiles are in alphabetical order by state, then city, then hospital within the city; Rankings are sorted by rate in descending order and exclude hospitals with less than 25 cases; (1) The number of cases is too small (n<25) for purposes of reliably predicting hospital performance; (2) Measure reflects the hospital's indication that its submission was based upon a sample of its relevant discharges; (3) Rate reflects fewer than the maximum possible quarters of data for the measure; (4) Inaccurate information submitted and suppressed for one or more quarters; (5) No data is available from the hospital for this measure; Please refer to the User's Guide for a full explanation of data

Emergency Room . . . . Annette Anderson, RN
Director Medical/Surgical Nursing . . . . Robert Pinion, RN
Manager Radiology . . . . Patricia Burley, RRT
Director Respiratory Therapy . . . . Bert Williams

Measure	Cases	This Hospital	State Average	U.S. Average	Top Hospital
Heart Attack Care					
ACE Inhibitor or ARB for LVSD	0	-	78%	82%	100%
Aspirin at Arrival[1]	9	100%	91%	92%	100%
Aspirin at Discharge[1]	3	67%	87%	90%	100%
Beta Blocker at Arrival[1]	9	100%	85%	87%	100%
Beta Blocker at Discharge[1]	3	67%	87%	90%	100%
Fibrinolytic Medication Timing	0	-	34%	31%	100%
PCI Within 90 Minutes of Arrival	0	-	47%	54%	95%
Smoking Cessation Advice	0	-	85%	88%	100%
Heart Failure Care					
ACE Inhibitor or ARB for LVSD[1]	23	91%	81%	82%	100%
Discharge Instructions	58	69%	59%	61%	93%
Evaluation of LVS Function	74	86%	81%	83%	99%
Smoking Cessation Advice[1]	12	100%	86%	82%	100%
Pneumonia Care					
Appropriate Initial Antibiotic	77	86%	81%	83%	94%
Blood Culture Timing	80	98%	89%	90%	100%
Influenza Vaccine	26	88%	60%	70%	100%
Initial Antibiotic Timing	124	90%	75%	80%	93%
Oxygenation Assessment	151	100%	99%	99%	100%
Pneumococcal Vaccine	97	91%	61%	69%	94%
Smoking Cessation Advice	37	100%	82%	80%	100%
Surgical Infection Prevention					
Prophylactic Antibiotic Given[2,3]	158	85%	69%	77%	95%
Prophylactic Antibiotic Selection[2]	33	82%	89%	90%	100%
Prophylactic Antibiotic Stopped[2,3]	153	64%	71%	72%	95%
Pregnancy Care					
Inpatient Neonatal Mortality	-	-	-	-	-
Third or Fourth Degree Laceration	-	-	3.63%	3.63%	3.27%

Higgins General Hospital
200 Allen Memorial Drive
Bremen, GA 30110
Ownership: Govt - Hospital District or Authority
Emergency Services: Yes
Key Personnel:
CEO . . . . Robbie Smith
Chief Medical Staff . . . . Sam Odgen
Chief Radiology . . . . Andrea Grace

Phone: 770-537-5851
Fax: 770-836-9870
Accredited: Yes
Licensed Beds: 57

Measure	Cases	This Hospital	State Average	U.S. Average	Top Hospital
Heart Attack Care					
ACE Inhibitor or ARB for LVSD[5]	-	-	78%	82%	100%
Aspirin at Arrival[5]	-	-	91%	92%	100%
Aspirin at Discharge[5]	-	-	87%	90%	100%
Beta Blocker at Arrival[5]	-	-	85%	87%	100%
Beta Blocker at Discharge[5]	-	-	87%	90%	100%
Fibrinolytic Medication Timing[5]	-	-	34%	31%	100%
PCI Within 90 Minutes of Arrival[5]	-	-	47%	54%	95%
Smoking Cessation Advice[5]	-	-	85%	88%	100%
Heart Failure Care					
ACE Inhibitor or ARB for LVSD[1]	16	94%	81%	82%	100%
Discharge Instructions	28	75%	59%	61%	93%
Evaluation of LVS Function	36	94%	81%	83%	99%
Smoking Cessation Advice[1]	9	67%	86%	82%	100%
Pneumonia Care					
Appropriate Initial Antibiotic	56	93%	81%	83%	94%
Blood Culture Timing	33	61%	89%	90%	100%
Influenza Vaccine[1]	21	95%	60%	70%	100%
Initial Antibiotic Timing	77	84%	75%	80%	93%
Oxygenation Assessment	95	100%	99%	99%	100%
Pneumococcal Vaccine	48	92%	61%	69%	94%
Smoking Cessation Advice	26	85%	82%	80%	100%
Surgical Infection Prevention					
Prophylactic Antibiotic Given[5]	-	-	69%	77%	95%
Prophylactic Antibiotic Selection[5]	-	-	89%	90%	100%

Prophylactic Antibiotic Stopped[5]	-	-	71%	72%	95%
Pregnancy Care					
Inpatient Neonatal Mortality	-	-	-	-	-
Third or Fourth Degree Laceration	-	-	3.63%	3.63%	3.27%

Southeast Georgia Health System
2415 Parkwood Avenue
Brunswick, GA 31520

Toll-Free: 800-537-5142
Phone: 912-466-7000
Fax: 912-466-7013

E-mail: dritchi@sghs.org
URL: www.sghs.org
Ownership: Govt - Hospital District or Authority   Accredited: Yes
Emergency Services: Yes   Licensed Beds: 278
Key Personnel:
President/CEO . . . . Gary R Colberg
Chief Medical Staff . . . . Wayne Rentz
Cardiac Lab . . . . Gerald Kilroy
Director Radiology . . . . Patrick Ebri
Respiratory Therapist . . . . Gerald Kilroy

Measure	Cases	This Hospital	State Average	U.S. Average	Top Hospital
Heart Attack Care					
ACE Inhibitor or ARB for LVSD[1,2]	11	73%	78%	82%	100%
Aspirin at Arrival[2]	89	93%	91%	92%	100%
Aspirin at Discharge[2]	36	92%	87%	90%	100%
Beta Blocker at Arrival[2]	77	86%	85%	87%	100%
Beta Blocker at Discharge[2]	43	91%	87%	90%	100%
Fibrinolytic Medication Timing[1,2]	18	28%	34%	31%	100%
PCI Within 90 Minutes of Arrival[1,2]	1	0%	47%	54%	95%
Smoking Cessation Advice[1,2]	13	77%	85%	88%	100%
Heart Failure Care					
ACE Inhibitor or ARB for LVSD	115	71%	81%	82%	100%
Discharge Instructions	299	77%	59%	61%	93%
Evaluation of LVS Function	346	97%	81%	83%	99%
Smoking Cessation Advice	73	85%	86%	82%	100%
Pneumonia Care					
Appropriate Initial Antibiotic	169	79%	81%	83%	94%
Blood Culture Timing	109	96%	89%	90%	100%
Influenza Vaccine	42	55%	60%	70%	100%
Initial Antibiotic Timing	182	65%	75%	80%	93%
Oxygenation Assessment	230	98%	99%	99%	100%
Pneumococcal Vaccine	132	45%	61%	69%	94%
Smoking Cessation Advice	51	57%	82%	80%	100%
Surgical Infection Prevention					
Prophylactic Antibiotic Given[2]	463	64%	69%	77%	95%
Prophylactic Antibiotic Selection[2]	116	98%	89%	90%	100%
Prophylactic Antibiotic Stopped[2]	446	55%	71%	72%	95%
Pregnancy Care					
Inpatient Neonatal Mortality	-	-	-	-	-
Third or Fourth Degree Laceration	-	-	3.63%	3.63%	3.27%

Grady General Hospital
1155 5th Street Southeast
Cairo, GA 39828
Ownership: Voluntary non-profit - Private
Emergency Services: Yes
Key Personnel:
CEO . . . . Glen C Davis
Chief Medical Staff . . . . Linda Walden

Phone: 229-377-1150
Fax: 229-377-7953
Accredited: Yes
Licensed Beds: 60

Measure	Cases	This Hospital	State Average	U.S. Average	Top Hospital
Heart Attack Care					
ACE Inhibitor or ARB for LVSD[1]	2	50%	78%	82%	100%
Aspirin at Arrival[1]	14	86%	91%	92%	100%
Aspirin at Discharge[1]	7	71%	87%	90%	100%
Beta Blocker at Arrival[1]	14	79%	85%	87%	100%
Beta Blocker at Discharge[1]	9	100%	87%	90%	100%
Fibrinolytic Medication Timing	0	-	34%	31%	100%
PCI Within 90 Minutes of Arrival	0	-	47%	54%	95%
Smoking Cessation Advice[1]	1	0%	85%	88%	100%
Heart Failure Care					
ACE Inhibitor or ARB for LVSD[1]	6	67%	81%	82%	100%

NOTE: Hospital profiles are in alphabetical order by state, then city, then hospital within the city; Rankings are sorted by rate in descending order and exclude hospitals with less than 25 cases; (1) The number of cases is too small (n<25) for purposes of reliably predicting hospital performance; (2) Measure reflects the hospital's indication that its submission was based upon a sample of its relevant discharges; (3) Rate reflects fewer than the maximum possible quarters of data for the measure; (4) Inaccurate information submitted and suppressed for one or more quarters; (5) No data is available from the hospital for this measure; Please refer to the User's Guide for a full explanation of data

Measure	Cases	This Hospital	State Average	U.S. Average	Top Hospital
Discharge Instructions[1]	15	47%	59%	61%	93%
Evaluation of LVS Function[1]	20	85%	81%	83%	99%
Smoking Cessation Advice[1]	3	100%	86%	82%	100%
Pneumonia Care					
Appropriate Initial Antibiotic	42	86%	81%	83%	94%
Blood Culture Timing[1]	15	67%	89%	90%	100%
Influenza Vaccine[1]	7	71%	60%	70%	100%
Initial Antibiotic Timing	40	85%	75%	80%	93%
Oxygenation Assessment	55	96%	99%	99%	100%
Pneumococcal Vaccine	32	62%	61%	69%	94%
Smoking Cessation Advice[1]	9	67%	82%	80%	100%
Surgical Infection Prevention					
Prophylactic Antibiotic Given[1,2]	15	33%	69%	77%	95%
Prophylactic Antibiotic Selection[1,2]	3	100%	89%	90%	100%
Prophylactic Antibiotic Stopped[1,2]	12	83%	71%	72%	95%
Pregnancy Care					
Inpatient Neonatal Mortality	-	-	-	-	-
Third or Fourth Degree Laceration	-	-	3.63%	3.63%	3.27%

Gordon Hospital

1035 Red Bud Road
Calhoun, GA 30701
URL: www.gordonhospital.com
Ownership: Voluntary non-profit - Church
Emergency Services: Yes

Phone: 706-602-7800
Fax: 706-629-4842

Accredited: Yes
Licensed Beds: 65

Key Personnel:
CEO . . . . Carlene Jamerson
Emergency Room . . . . Gary Moore, MD
ICU . . . . Cindy Bankhead
Medical/Surgical Nursing . . . . Stephanie Jones
Director Respiratory Therapy . . . . Judy Shanko

Measure	Cases	This Hospital	State Average	U.S. Average	Top Hospital
Heart Attack Care					
ACE Inhibitor or ARB for LVSD[1]	11	64%	78%	82%	100%
Aspirin at Arrival	64	91%	91%	92%	100%
Aspirin at Discharge	29	90%	87%	90%	100%
Beta Blocker at Arrival	63	90%	85%	87%	100%
Beta Blocker at Discharge	31	87%	87%	90%	100%
Fibrinolytic Medication Timing[1]	3	33%	34%	31%	100%
PCI Within 90 Minutes of Arrival	0	-	47%	54%	95%
Smoking Cessation Advice[1]	9	78%	85%	88%	100%
Heart Failure Care					
ACE Inhibitor or ARB for LVSD	39	67%	81%	82%	100%
Discharge Instructions	106	51%	59%	61%	93%
Evaluation of LVS Function	129	90%	81%	83%	99%
Smoking Cessation Advice	26	85%	86%	82%	100%
Pneumonia Care					
Appropriate Initial Antibiotic	167	80%	81%	83%	94%
Blood Culture Timing	99	93%	89%	90%	100%
Influenza Vaccine	52	71%	60%	70%	100%
Initial Antibiotic Timing	171	85%	75%	80%	93%
Oxygenation Assessment	219	100%	99%	99%	100%
Pneumococcal Vaccine	140	64%	61%	69%	94%
Smoking Cessation Advice	67	82%	82%	80%	100%
Surgical Infection Prevention					
Prophylactic Antibiotic Given	133	86%	69%	77%	95%
Prophylactic Antibiotic Selection	28	100%	89%	90%	100%
Prophylactic Antibiotic Stopped	131	86%	71%	72%	95%
Pregnancy Care					
Inpatient Neonatal Mortality	-	-	-	-	-
Third or Fourth Degree Laceration	-	-	3.63%	3.63%	3.27%

Mitchell County Hospital

90 E Stephens Street
Camilla, GA 31730
URL: www.archbold.org
Ownership: Voluntary non-profit - Private
Emergency Services: Yes

Phone: 229-336-5284
Fax: 229-228-8579

Accredited: Yes
Licensed Beds: 33

Key Personnel:
CEO . . . . Ron Gilliard
Chief Medical Staff . . . . Raymond J Otis Sr, MD
Emergency Room . . . . Sharon Keyton, RN

Director Medical/Surgical Nursing . . . . Beverly Backley
OB/GYN Womens Health . . . . George E Fahy, III, MD
Director Respiratory Therapy . . . . Theresa Hurst

Measure	Cases	This Hospital	State Average	U.S. Average	Top Hospital
Heart Attack Care					
ACE Inhibitor or ARB for LVSD[5]	-	-	78%	82%	100%
Aspirin at Arrival[5]	-	-	91%	92%	100%
Aspirin at Discharge[5]	-	-	87%	90%	100%
Beta Blocker at Arrival[5]	-	-	85%	87%	100%
Beta Blocker at Discharge[5]	-	-	87%	90%	100%
Fibrinolytic Medication Timing[5]	-	-	34%	31%	100%
PCI Within 90 Minutes of Arrival[5]	-	-	47%	54%	95%
Smoking Cessation Advice[5]	-	-	85%	88%	100%
Heart Failure Care					
ACE Inhibitor or ARB for LVSD[1]	2	100%	81%	82%	100%
Discharge Instructions[1]	8	50%	59%	61%	93%
Evaluation of LVS Function[1]	10	70%	81%	83%	99%
Smoking Cessation Advice[1]	4	50%	86%	82%	100%
Pneumonia Care					
Appropriate Initial Antibiotic[1]	22	91%	81%	83%	94%
Blood Culture Timing[1]	13	69%	89%	90%	100%
Influenza Vaccine[1]	5	100%	60%	70%	100%
Initial Antibiotic Timing[1]	18	67%	75%	80%	93%
Oxygenation Assessment	29	100%	99%	99%	100%
Pneumococcal Vaccine[1]	17	47%	61%	69%	94%
Smoking Cessation Advice[1]	5	60%	82%	80%	100%
Surgical Infection Prevention					
Prophylactic Antibiotic Given[5]	-	-	69%	77%	95%
Prophylactic Antibiotic Selection[5]	-	-	89%	90%	100%
Prophylactic Antibiotic Stopped[5]	-	-	71%	72%	95%
Pregnancy Care					
Inpatient Neonatal Mortality	-	-	-	-	-
Third or Fourth Degree Laceration	-	-	3.63%	3.63%	3.27%

Northside Hospital-Cherokee

201 Hospital Road
Canton, GA 30114
E-mail: Janiceb@northside.com
Ownership: Voluntary non-profit - Private
Emergency Services: Yes

Phone: 770-720-5100
Fax: 770-720-5101

Accredited: Yes
Licensed Beds: 84

Key Personnel:
President/CEO . . . . Douglas Parker
Chief Medical Staff . . . . David Edwards, MD
Emergency Room Manager . . . . Jim Chastain
Infection Control Coordinator . . . . Angela Bijens
Medical/Surgical Nursing Manager . . . . Beverly Garlanek
Women's Center Director . . . . Debbie Hulsey
Surgical Services Director . . . . Tim Hatlenig
Respiratory Services . . . . Tim Kenney

Measure	Cases	This Hospital	State Average	U.S. Average	Top Hospital
Heart Attack Care					
ACE Inhibitor or ARB for LVSD[1]	4	75%	78%	82%	100%
Aspirin at Arrival	27	100%	91%	92%	100%
Aspirin at Discharge[1]	8	100%	87%	90%	100%
Beta Blocker at Arrival[1]	24	100%	85%	87%	100%
Beta Blocker at Discharge[1]	8	100%	87%	90%	100%
Fibrinolytic Medication Timing[1]	1	0%	34%	31%	100%
PCI Within 90 Minutes of Arrival	0	-	47%	54%	95%
Smoking Cessation Advice[1]	2	100%	85%	88%	100%
Heart Failure Care					
ACE Inhibitor or ARB for LVSD[2]	44	80%	81%	82%	100%
Discharge Instructions[2]	96	64%	59%	61%	93%
Evaluation of LVS Function[2]	125	94%	81%	83%	99%
Smoking Cessation Advice[1,2]	23	87%	86%	82%	100%
Pneumonia Care					
Appropriate Initial Antibiotic	170	94%	81%	83%	94%
Blood Culture Timing	184	97%	89%	90%	100%
Influenza Vaccine	41	80%	60%	70%	100%
Initial Antibiotic Timing	246	84%	75%	80%	93%
Oxygenation Assessment	303	100%	99%	99%	100%

NOTE: Hospital profiles are in alphabetical order by state, then city, then hospital within the city; Rankings are sorted by rate in descending order and exclude hospitals with less than 25 cases; (1) The number of cases is too small (n<25) for purposes of reliably predicting hospital performance; (2) Measure reflects the hospital's indication that its submission was based upon a sample of its relevant discharges; (3) Rate reflects fewer than the maximum possible quarters of data for the measure; (4) Inaccurate information submitted and suppressed for one or more quarters; (5) No data is available from the hospital for this measure; Please refer to the User's Guide for a full explanation of data

Measure	Cases	This Hospital	State Average	U.S. Average	Top Hospital
Pneumococcal Vaccine	169	85%	61%	69%	94%
Smoking Cessation Advice	82	93%	82%	80%	100%
Surgical Infection Prevention					
Prophylactic Antibiotic Given[2,3]	38	92%	69%	77%	95%
Prophylactic Antibiotic Selection[2]	38	79%	89%	90%	100%
Prophylactic Antibiotic Stopped[2,3]	38	61%	71%	72%	95%
Pregnancy Care					
Inpatient Neonatal Mortality	1,101	0.00%	-	-	-
Third or Fourth Degree Laceration	816	1.47%	3.63%	3.63%	3.27%

Tanner Medical Center

705 Dixie Street
Carrollton, GA 30117
URL: www.tanner.org
Ownership: Govt - Hospital District or Authority
Emergency Services: Yes

Phone: 770-836-9666
Fax: 770-836-9897

Accredited: Yes
Licensed Beds: 202

Key Personnel:
President/CEO . . . . Loy M Howard
Chief Medical Staff . . . . Taylor Gordon, MD
Medical Staff Services . . . . Susan Manion-Galloway
OB/GYN Womens Health . . . . James Rash, MD
Director Surgical/Invasion Care . . . . Venita Steed
Director Cardiopulmonary . . . . Steve Odem

Measure	Cases	This Hospital	State Average	U.S. Average	Top Hospital
Heart Attack Care					
ACE Inhibitor or ARB for LVSD[1]	19	58%	78%	82%	100%
Aspirin at Arrival	135	96%	91%	92%	100%
Aspirin at Discharge	62	89%	87%	90%	100%
Beta Blocker at Arrival	111	94%	85%	87%	100%
Beta Blocker at Discharge	63	94%	87%	90%	100%
Fibrinolytic Medication Timing[1]	15	73%	34%	31%	100%
PCI Within 90 Minutes of Arrival	0	-	47%	54%	95%
Smoking Cessation Advice	26	92%	85%	88%	100%
Heart Failure Care					
ACE Inhibitor or ARB for LVSD	111	60%	81%	82%	100%
Discharge Instructions	224	43%	59%	61%	93%
Evaluation of LVS Function	272	89%	81%	83%	99%
Smoking Cessation Advice	57	89%	86%	82%	100%
Pneumonia Care					
Appropriate Initial Antibiotic	211	87%	81%	83%	94%
Blood Culture Timing	113	78%	89%	90%	100%
Influenza Vaccine	55	58%	60%	70%	100%
Initial Antibiotic Timing	218	72%	75%	80%	93%
Oxygenation Assessment	292	100%	99%	99%	100%
Pneumococcal Vaccine	172	65%	61%	69%	94%
Smoking Cessation Advice	62	79%	82%	80%	100%
Surgical Infection Prevention					
Prophylactic Antibiotic Given	401	70%	69%	77%	95%
Prophylactic Antibiotic Selection	83	96%	89%	90%	100%
Prophylactic Antibiotic Stopped	393	93%	71%	72%	95%
Pregnancy Care					
Inpatient Neonatal Mortality	-	-	-	-	-
Third or Fourth Degree Laceration	-	-	3.63%	3.63%	3.27%

Emory Cartersville Medical Center

Alternate Name: Cartersville Medical Center
960 Joe Frank Harris Parkway
Cartersville, GA 30120
URL: www.emorycartersville.com
Ownership: Proprietary
Emergency Services: Yes

Phone: 770-387-8172
Fax: 770-606-2127

Accredited: Yes
Licensed Beds: 112

Key Personnel:
CEO . . . . Keith Sandlin
Cardiac Lab . . . . Donna Roberts
Emergency Room . . . . Mary Ellen Womack
Director Medical/Surgical Nursing . . . . Natalie Stegall
OB/GYN Womens Health . . . . Toni Strawn
Respiratory/Cardiopulmonary . . . . Donna Roberts

Measure	Cases	This Hospital	State Average	U.S. Average	Top Hospital
Heart Attack Care					
ACE Inhibitor or ARB for LVSD[1]	9	78%	78%	82%	100%

Measure	Cases	This Hospital	State Average	U.S. Average	Top Hospital
Aspirin at Arrival	52	94%	91%	92%	100%
Aspirin at Discharge[1]	21	100%	87%	90%	100%
Beta Blocker at Arrival	38	89%	85%	87%	100%
Beta Blocker at Discharge	25	96%	87%	90%	100%
Fibrinolytic Medication Timing	0	-	34%	31%	100%
PCI Within 90 Minutes of Arrival	0	-	47%	54%	95%
Smoking Cessation Advice[1]	8	88%	85%	88%	100%
Heart Failure Care					
ACE Inhibitor or ARB for LVSD	56	82%	81%	82%	100%
Discharge Instructions	167	21%	59%	61%	93%
Evaluation of LVS Function	187	93%	81%	83%	99%
Smoking Cessation Advice	43	88%	86%	82%	100%
Pneumonia Care					
Appropriate Initial Antibiotic	199	92%	81%	83%	94%
Blood Culture Timing	184	90%	89%	90%	100%
Influenza Vaccine	38	63%	60%	70%	100%
Initial Antibiotic Timing	264	87%	75%	80%	93%
Oxygenation Assessment	304	100%	99%	99%	100%
Pneumococcal Vaccine	162	44%	61%	69%	94%
Smoking Cessation Advice	111	91%	82%	80%	100%
Surgical Infection Prevention					
Prophylactic Antibiotic Given[2,3]	143	64%	69%	77%	95%
Prophylactic Antibiotic Selection[2]	68	97%	89%	90%	100%
Prophylactic Antibiotic Stopped[2,3]	134	63%	71%	72%	95%
Pregnancy Care					
Inpatient Neonatal Mortality	-	-	-	-	-
Third or Fourth Degree Laceration	-	-	3.63%	3.63%	3.27%

Polk Medical Center

424 N Main Street
Cedartown, GA 30125
Ownership: Proprietary
Emergency Services: Yes

Phone: 770-748-2500
Fax: 770-749-9904
Accredited: Yes
Licensed Beds: 58

Key Personnel:
CEO . . . . Steve Hoelscher
Chief Medical Staff . . . . Neil Gordon, MD
Emergency Room . . . . Kathryn Lindsey
Infection Control . . . . Joy Lee
Medical Surgical Nursing . . . . Mimi Thompson
Director Respiratory Therapy . . . . Kathy Cox

Measure	Cases	This Hospital	State Average	U.S. Average	Top Hospital
Heart Attack Care					
ACE Inhibitor or ARB for LVSD[5]	-	-	78%	82%	100%
Aspirin at Arrival[5]	-	-	91%	92%	100%
Aspirin at Discharge[5]	-	-	87%	90%	100%
Beta Blocker at Arrival[5]	-	-	85%	87%	100%
Beta Blocker at Discharge[5]	-	-	87%	90%	100%
Fibrinolytic Medication Timing[5]	-	-	34%	31%	100%
PCI Within 90 Minutes of Arrival[5]	-	-	47%	54%	95%
Smoking Cessation Advice[5]	-	-	85%	88%	100%
Heart Failure Care					
ACE Inhibitor or ARB for LVSD	0	-	81%	82%	100%
Discharge Instructions[1]	18	22%	59%	61%	93%
Evaluation of LVS Function	29	14%	81%	83%	99%
Smoking Cessation Advice[1]	4	100%	86%	82%	100%
Pneumonia Care					
Appropriate Initial Antibiotic	36	53%	81%	83%	94%
Blood Culture Timing	32	91%	89%	90%	100%
Influenza Vaccine[1]	16	44%	60%	70%	100%
Initial Antibiotic Timing	58	90%	75%	80%	93%
Oxygenation Assessment	68	99%	99%	99%	100%
Pneumococcal Vaccine	39	59%	61%	69%	94%
Smoking Cessation Advice[1]	10	80%	82%	80%	100%
Surgical Infection Prevention					
Prophylactic Antibiotic Given[5]	-	-	69%	77%	95%
Prophylactic Antibiotic Selection[5]	-	-	89%	90%	100%
Prophylactic Antibiotic Stopped[5]	-	-	71%	72%	95%
Pregnancy Care					
Inpatient Neonatal Mortality	-	-	-	-	-
Third or Fourth Degree Laceration	-	-	3.63%	3.63%	3.27%

NOTE: Hospital profiles are in alphabetical order by state, then city, then hospital within the city; Rankings are sorted by rate in descending order and exclude hospitals with less than 25 cases; (1) The number of cases is too small (n<25) for purposes of reliably predicting hospital performance; (2) Measure reflects the hospital's indication that its submission was based upon a sample of its relevant discharges; (3) Rate reflects fewer than the maximum possible quarters of data for the measure; (4) Inaccurate information submitted and suppressed for one or more quarters; (5) No data is available from the hospital for this measure; Please refer to the User's Guide for a full explanation of data

Hamilton Medical Center

Alternate Name: Murray Medical Center
707 Old Ellijay Road
PO Box 1406
Chatsworth, GA 30705
Ownership: Voluntary non-profit - Private
Emergency Services: Yes

Phone: 706-272-6000
Fax: 706-517-2076

Accredited: Yes
Licensed Beds: 42

Key Personnel:
CEO . . . . Mickey Rabuka
Emergency Room . . . . Michelle Vandergriff
Director Radiology . . . . Brenda Holcomb
Respiratory Therapist . . . . Chip Rodgers

Measure	Cases	This Hospital	State Average	U.S. Average	Top Hospital
Heart Attack Care					
ACE Inhibitor or ARB for LVSD	0	-	78%	82%	100%
Aspirin at Arrival[1]	5	100%	91%	92%	100%
Aspirin at Discharge	0	-	87%	90%	100%
Beta Blocker at Arrival[1]	4	75%	85%	87%	100%
Beta Blocker at Discharge[1]	2	50%	87%	90%	100%
Fibrinolytic Medication Timing[1]	1	0%	34%	31%	100%
PCI Within 90 Minutes of Arrival	0	-	47%	54%	95%
Smoking Cessation Advice	0	-	85%	88%	100%
Heart Failure Care					
ACE Inhibitor or ARB for LVSD[1]	14	93%	81%	82%	100%
Discharge Instructions	63	87%	59%	61%	93%
Evaluation of LVS Function	69	59%	81%	83%	99%
Smoking Cessation Advice[1]	18	100%	86%	82%	100%
Pneumonia Care					
Appropriate Initial Antibiotic	78	76%	81%	83%	94%
Blood Culture Timing	61	85%	89%	90%	100%
Influenza Vaccine	32	9%	60%	70%	100%
Initial Antibiotic Timing	98	86%	75%	80%	93%
Oxygenation Assessment	114	100%	99%	99%	100%
Pneumococcal Vaccine	58	34%	61%	69%	94%
Smoking Cessation Advice	44	95%	82%	80%	100%
Surgical Infection Prevention					
Prophylactic Antibiotic Given[1,3]	1	100%	69%	77%	95%
Prophylactic Antibiotic Selection[1]	1	0%	89%	90%	100%
Prophylactic Antibiotic Stopped[1,3]	1	100%	71%	72%	95%
Pregnancy Care					
Inpatient Neonatal Mortality	-	-	-	-	-
Third or Fourth Degree Laceration	-	-	3.63%	3.63%	3.27%

Evans Memorial Hospital

200 N River Street
Claxton, GA 30417
Ownership: Govt - Hospital District or Authority
Emergency Services: Yes

Phone: 912-739-5000
Fax: 912-739-5106

Accredited: Yes
Licensed Beds: 49

Key Personnel:
CEO . . . . Eston Price, Jr
Chief Medical Staff . . . . Glenn J Dasher, MD
Cardiac Laboratory . . . . Michelle Sapp, RRT
Emergency Room . . . . Becky Page, RN
Emergency Room . . . . Mark Lewis, MD
Infection Control . . . . Martha Tucker
Medical Surgical Nursing . . . . Becky Page, RN
OB/GYN Womens Health . . . . Holly Hutto, RN
Director Respiratory Therapy . . . . Michelle Sapp, RRT

Measure	Cases	This Hospital	State Average	U.S. Average	Top Hospital
Heart Attack Care					
ACE Inhibitor or ARB for LVSD[1]	2	50%	78%	82%	100%
Aspirin at Arrival[1]	2	100%	91%	92%	100%
Aspirin at Discharge[1]	3	67%	87%	90%	100%
Beta Blocker at Arrival[1]	4	75%	85%	87%	100%
Beta Blocker at Discharge[1]	1	100%	87%	90%	100%
Fibrinolytic Medication Timing	0	-	34%	31%	100%
PCI Within 90 Minutes of Arrival	0	-	47%	54%	95%
Smoking Cessation Advice[1]	2	100%	85%	88%	100%
Heart Failure Care					
ACE Inhibitor or ARB for LVSD[1]	14	93%	81%	82%	100%
Discharge Instructions	66	100%	59%	61%	93%

Measure	Cases	This Hospital	State Average	U.S. Average	Top Hospital
Evaluation of LVS Function	59	78%	81%	83%	99%
Smoking Cessation Advice[1]	8	100%	86%	82%	100%
Pneumonia Care					
Appropriate Initial Antibiotic	64	75%	81%	83%	94%
Blood Culture Timing[1]	21	95%	89%	90%	100%
Influenza Vaccine[1]	20	70%	60%	70%	100%
Initial Antibiotic Timing	96	71%	75%	80%	93%
Oxygenation Assessment	118	100%	99%	99%	100%
Pneumococcal Vaccine	74	76%	61%	69%	94%
Smoking Cessation Advice[1]	21	100%	82%	80%	100%
Surgical Infection Prevention					
Prophylactic Antibiotic Given[1,3]	2	50%	69%	77%	95%
Prophylactic Antibiotic Selection[1]	2	100%	89%	90%	100%
Prophylactic Antibiotic Stopped[1,3]	2	100%	71%	72%	95%
Pregnancy Care					
Inpatient Neonatal Mortality	-	-	-	-	-
Third or Fourth Degree Laceration	-	-	3.63%	3.63%	3.27%

Bleckley Memorial Hospital

145 East Peacock Street
Cochran, GA 31014
Ownership: Govt - Hospital District or Authority
Emergency Services: Yes

Phone: 478-934-6211

Accredited: Yes

Measure	Cases	This Hospital	State Average	U.S. Average	Top Hospital
Heart Attack Care					
ACE Inhibitor or ARB for LVSD[5]	-	-	78%	82%	100%
Aspirin at Arrival[5]	-	-	91%	92%	100%
Aspirin at Discharge[5]	-	-	87%	90%	100%
Beta Blocker at Arrival[5]	-	-	85%	87%	100%
Beta Blocker at Discharge[5]	-	-	87%	90%	100%
Fibrinolytic Medication Timing[5]	-	-	34%	31%	100%
PCI Within 90 Minutes of Arrival[5]	-	-	47%	54%	95%
Smoking Cessation Advice[5]	-	-	85%	88%	100%
Heart Failure Care					
ACE Inhibitor or ARB for LVSD[1]	5	100%	81%	82%	100%
Discharge Instructions	34	82%	59%	61%	93%
Evaluation of LVS Function	37	32%	81%	83%	99%
Smoking Cessation Advice[1]	8	88%	86%	82%	100%
Pneumonia Care					
Appropriate Initial Antibiotic[1]	20	80%	81%	83%	94%
Blood Culture Timing[1]	4	100%	89%	90%	100%
Influenza Vaccine[1]	4	75%	60%	70%	100%
Initial Antibiotic Timing[1]	16	81%	75%	80%	93%
Oxygenation Assessment[1]	23	100%	99%	99%	100%
Pneumococcal Vaccine[1]	11	64%	61%	69%	94%
Smoking Cessation Advice[1]	6	100%	82%	80%	100%
Surgical Infection Prevention					
Prophylactic Antibiotic Given[5]	-	-	69%	77%	95%
Prophylactic Antibiotic Selection[5]	-	-	89%	90%	100%
Prophylactic Antibiotic Stopped[5]	-	-	71%	72%	95%
Pregnancy Care					
Inpatient Neonatal Mortality	-	-	-	-	-
Third or Fourth Degree Laceration	-	-	3.63%	3.63%	3.27%

Columbus Medical Center

710 Center Street
Columbus, GA 31901
E-mail: info@crhs.net
URL: www.columbusregional.com
Ownership: Voluntary non-profit - Other
Emergency Services: Yes

Phone: 706-571-1000
Fax: 706-571-1216

Accredited: Yes
Licensed Beds: 537

Key Personnel:
President/CEO . . . . Lance Duke
Senior VP/Chief Medical Staff . . . . Andrew Morley Jr, MD
Emergency Room . . . . Dale Miller
Director Infection/Disease Control . . . . Susan Harp
CCU Spvg. Nurse . . . . Sharon Nicks
OB/GYN Womens Health . . . . R Stauffer, MD
Chief Respiratory Therapy . . . . Alan Peiken, MD

Measure	Cases	This Hospital	State Average	U.S. Average	Top Hospital

NOTE: Hospital profiles are in alphabetical order by state, then city, then hospital within the city; Rankings are sorted by rate in descending order and exclude hospitals with less than 25 cases; (1) The number of cases is too small (n<25) for purposes of reliably predicting hospital performance; (2) Measure reflects the hospital's indication that its submission was based upon a sample of its relevant discharges; (3) Rate reflects fewer than the maximum possible quarters of data for the measure; (4) Inaccurate information submitted and suppressed for one or more quarters; (5) No data is available from the hospital for this measure; Please refer to the User's Guide for a full explanation of data

Heart Attack Care					
ACE Inhibitor or ARB for LVSD[1]	8	88%	78%	82%	100%
Aspirin at Arrival	75	85%	91%	92%	100%
Aspirin at Discharge	39	97%	87%	90%	100%
Beta Blocker at Arrival	63	84%	85%	87%	100%
Beta Blocker at Discharge	40	95%	87%	90%	100%
Fibrinolytic Medication Timing[1]	6	33%	34%	31%	100%
PCI Within 90 Minutes of Arrival	0	-	47%	54%	95%
Smoking Cessation Advice[1]	19	89%	85%	88%	100%
Heart Failure Care					
ACE Inhibitor or ARB for LVSD	106	87%	81%	82%	100%
Discharge Instructions	314	72%	59%	61%	93%
Evaluation of LVS Function	353	94%	81%	83%	99%
Smoking Cessation Advice	130	96%	86%	82%	100%
Pneumonia Care					
Appropriate Initial Antibiotic	151	79%	81%	83%	94%
Blood Culture Timing	110	73%	89%	90%	100%
Influenza Vaccine	25	28%	60%	70%	100%
Initial Antibiotic Timing	197	69%	75%	80%	93%
Oxygenation Assessment	240	100%	99%	99%	100%
Pneumococcal Vaccine	79	56%	61%	69%	94%
Smoking Cessation Advice	89	91%	82%	80%	100%
Surgical Infection Prevention					
Prophylactic Antibiotic Given[2,3]	260	85%	69%	77%	95%
Prophylactic Antibiotic Selection[2]	58	98%	89%	90%	100%
Prophylactic Antibiotic Stopped[2,3]	247	60%	71%	72%	95%
Pregnancy Care					
Inpatient Neonatal Mortality	-	-	-	-	-
Third or Fourth Degree Laceration	-	-	3.63%	3.63%	3.27%

Doctors Hospital

616 19th Street
Columbus, GA 31902
URL: www.doctorshspt.com
Ownership: Proprietary
Emergency Services: Yes

Phone: 706-494-4262
Fax: 706-327-0131

Accredited: Yes
Licensed Beds: 219

Key Personnel:
CEO . . . . Hugh Wilson
Chief Medical Staff . . . . Donna Burrell, MD
Head of Cardiology . . . . Chris Doods
Emergency Room . . . . Annie Garrard, RN
OB/GYN Womens Health. . . . . Benjamin Cheek, MD
Chief Radiology . . . . Wade Wallace, MD
Director Respiratory Therapy . . . . Natalie Simpson

Measure	Cases	This Hospital	State Average	U.S. Average	Top Hospital
Heart Attack Care					
ACE Inhibitor or ARB for LVSD[1]	5	80%	78%	82%	100%
Aspirin at Arrival	31	90%	91%	92%	100%
Aspirin at Discharge[1]	15	93%	87%	90%	100%
Beta Blocker at Arrival[1]	24	100%	85%	87%	100%
Beta Blocker at Discharge[1]	18	89%	87%	90%	100%
Fibrinolytic Medication Timing	0	-	34%	31%	100%
PCI Within 90 Minutes of Arrival	0	-	47%	54%	95%
Smoking Cessation Advice[1]	2	100%	85%	88%	100%
Heart Failure Care					
ACE Inhibitor or ARB for LVSD	91	84%	81%	82%	100%
Discharge Instructions	203	46%	59%	61%	93%
Evaluation of LVS Function	223	92%	81%	83%	99%
Smoking Cessation Advice	45	100%	86%	82%	100%
Pneumonia Care					
Appropriate Initial Antibiotic	143	81%	81%	83%	94%
Blood Culture Timing	117	77%	89%	90%	100%
Influenza Vaccine	35	63%	60%	70%	100%
Initial Antibiotic Timing	177	76%	75%	80%	93%
Oxygenation Assessment	211	100%	99%	99%	100%
Pneumococcal Vaccine	103	72%	61%	69%	94%
Smoking Cessation Advice	48	100%	82%	80%	100%
Surgical Infection Prevention					
Prophylactic Antibiotic Given[2,3]	176	78%	69%	77%	95%
Prophylactic Antibiotic Selection[2]	127	92%	89%	90%	100%
Prophylactic Antibiotic Stopped[2,3]	177	72%	71%	72%	95%

Pregnancy Care					
Inpatient Neonatal Mortality	-	-	-	-	-
Third or Fourth Degree Laceration	-	-	3.63%	3.63%	3.27%

Hughston Orthopedic Hospital

100 1st Court
Columbus, GA 31908

Toll-Free: 800-741-1517
Phone: 706-494-2100
Fax: 706-494-2446

URL: www.hughstonsports.com
Ownership: Proprietary
Emergency Services: No

Accredited: Yes
Licensed Beds: 100

Key Personnel:
President/CEO . . . . Donald Avery
Chief Medical Staff . . . . John Burkun, MD
Chief Radiology . . . . Michael Postma, MD
Director Respiratory Therapy . . . . Arthur Barker

Measure	Cases	This Hospital	State Average	U.S. Average	Top Hospital
Heart Attack Care					
ACE Inhibitor or ARB for LVSD[5]	-	-	78%	82%	100%
Aspirin at Arrival[5]	-	-	91%	92%	100%
Aspirin at Discharge[5]	-	-	87%	90%	100%
Beta Blocker at Arrival[5]	-	-	85%	87%	100%
Beta Blocker at Discharge[5]	-	-	87%	90%	100%
Fibrinolytic Medication Timing[5]	-	-	34%	31%	100%
PCI Within 90 Minutes of Arrival[5]	-	-	47%	54%	95%
Smoking Cessation Advice[5]	-	-	85%	88%	100%
Heart Failure Care					
ACE Inhibitor or ARB for LVSD[3]	0	-	81%	82%	100%
Discharge Instructions[3]	0	-	59%	61%	93%
Evaluation of LVS Function[1,3]	1	0%	81%	83%	99%
Smoking Cessation Advice[3]	0	-	86%	82%	100%
Pneumonia Care					
Appropriate Initial Antibiotic[3]	0	-	81%	83%	94%
Blood Culture Timing[3]	0	-	89%	90%	100%
Influenza Vaccine[5]	-	-	60%	70%	100%
Initial Antibiotic Timing[3]	0	-	75%	80%	93%
Oxygenation Assessment[3]	0	-	99%	99%	100%
Pneumococcal Vaccine[3]	0	-	61%	69%	94%
Smoking Cessation Advice[3]	0	-	82%	80%	100%
Surgical Infection Prevention					
Prophylactic Antibiotic Given	1,491	74%	69%	77%	95%
Prophylactic Antibiotic Selection	419	100%	89%	90%	100%
Prophylactic Antibiotic Stopped	1,475	65%	71%	72%	95%
Pregnancy Care					
Inpatient Neonatal Mortality	-	-	-	-	-
Third or Fourth Degree Laceration	-	-	3.63%	3.63%	3.27%

Saint Francis Hospital

2122 Manchester Expressway
Columbus, GA 31904
URL: wecareforlife.com
Ownership: Voluntary non-profit - Private
Emergency Services: Yes

Phone: 706-596-4000
Fax: 706-596-4481

Accredited: Yes
Licensed Beds: 376

Key Personnel:
President/CEO . . . . Michael E Garrigan
Catheterization Laboratory Director . . . . Theresa Bozd, RN
Emergency Room . . . . Cathy Homeyer
Emergency Room . . . . David Smith, MD
ICU . . . . Jeannie Smith
Cardio-Pulmonary Services Director . . . . Cindy Haines

Measure	Cases	This Hospital	State Average	U.S. Average	Top Hospital
Heart Attack Care					
ACE Inhibitor or ARB for LVSD	123	92%	78%	82%	100%
Aspirin at Arrival	285	96%	91%	92%	100%
Aspirin at Discharge	361	98%	87%	90%	100%
Beta Blocker at Arrival	253	97%	85%	87%	100%
Beta Blocker at Discharge	342	97%	87%	90%	100%
Fibrinolytic Medication Timing[1]	5	40%	34%	31%	100%
PCI Within 90 Minutes of Arrival[1]	18	56%	47%	54%	95%
Smoking Cessation Advice	132	99%	85%	88%	100%
Heart Failure Care					

NOTE: Hospital profiles are in alphabetical order by state, then city, then hospital within the city; Rankings are sorted by rate in descending order and exclude hospitals with less than 25 cases; (1) The number of cases is too small (n<25) for purposes of reliably predicting hospital performance; (2) Measure reflects the hospital's indication that its submission was based upon a sample of its relevant discharges; (3) Rate reflects fewer than the maximum possible quarters of data for the measure; (4) Inaccurate information submitted and suppressed for one or more quarters; (5) No data is available from the hospital for this measure; Please refer to the User's Guide for a full explanation of data

ACE Inhibitor or ARB for LVSD[2]	217	82%	81%	82%	100%
Discharge Instructions[2]	482	55%	59%	61%	93%
Evaluation of LVS Function[2]	560	88%	81%	83%	99%
Smoking Cessation Advice[2]	123	89%	86%	82%	100%
Pneumonia Care					
Appropriate Initial Antibiotic[2]	255	89%	81%	83%	94%
Blood Culture Timing[2]	247	94%	89%	90%	100%
Influenza Vaccine[4,5]	-	-	60%	70%	100%
Initial Antibiotic Timing[2]	342	80%	75%	80%	93%
Oxygenation Assessment[2]	409	100%	99%	99%	100%
Pneumococcal Vaccine[2]	245	63%	61%	69%	94%
Smoking Cessation Advice[2]	86	90%	82%	80%	100%
Surgical Infection Prevention					
Prophylactic Antibiotic Given[2]	331	87%	69%	77%	95%
Prophylactic Antibiotic Selection[2]	65	97%	89%	90%	100%
Prophylactic Antibiotic Stopped[2]	324	46%	71%	72%	95%
Pregnancy Care					
Inpatient Neonatal Mortality	-	-	-	-	-
Third or Fourth Degree Laceration	-	-	3.63%	3.63%	3.27%

BJC Medical Center

70 Medical Center Drive
Commerce, GA 30529
Ownership: Govt - Hospital District or Authority
Emergency Services: Yes
Phone: 706-335-1000
Fax: 706-335-7701
Accredited: Yes
Licensed Beds: 90

Key Personnel:
CEO . . . . James Yarboraugh
Chief Medical Staff . . . . Peter Mirkav
Emergency Room Coordinator . . . . Kark Brown
Emergency Room Coordinator . . . . Becky Hambrick, RN
Director Medical Surgical Nursing . . . . Jo Totherow, RN
OB/GYN Womens Health . . . . Sharrie Nash, RN
Director Radiology . . . . Ron McEver
Director Respiratory Therapy . . . . Lee Renna

Measure	Cases	This Hospital	State Average	U.S. Average	Top Hospital
Heart Attack Care					
ACE Inhibitor or ARB for LVSD[1]	8	75%	78%	82%	100%
Aspirin at Arrival	27	89%	91%	92%	100%
Aspirin at Discharge[1]	15	67%	87%	90%	100%
Beta Blocker at Arrival	28	79%	85%	87%	100%
Beta Blocker at Discharge[1]	15	80%	87%	90%	100%
Fibrinolytic Medication Timing[1]	2	0%	34%	31%	100%
PCI Within 90 Minutes of Arrival	0	-	47%	54%	95%
Smoking Cessation Advice[1]	4	100%	85%	88%	100%
Heart Failure Care					
ACE Inhibitor or ARB for LVSD[1]	18	61%	81%	82%	100%
Discharge Instructions	59	24%	59%	61%	93%
Evaluation of LVS Function	75	63%	81%	83%	99%
Smoking Cessation Advice[1]	11	82%	86%	82%	100%
Pneumonia Care					
Appropriate Initial Antibiotic	32	59%	81%	83%	94%
Blood Culture Timing[1]	15	93%	89%	90%	100%
Influenza Vaccine[1]	9	33%	60%	70%	100%
Initial Antibiotic Timing	57	39%	75%	80%	93%
Oxygenation Assessment	71	100%	99%	99%	100%
Pneumococcal Vaccine	41	34%	61%	69%	94%
Smoking Cessation Advice[1]	7	71%	82%	80%	100%
Surgical Infection Prevention					
Prophylactic Antibiotic Given[3]	32	44%	69%	77%	95%
Prophylactic Antibiotic Selection[1]	5	100%	89%	90%	100%
Prophylactic Antibiotic Stopped[3]	31	90%	71%	72%	95%
Pregnancy Care					
Inpatient Neonatal Mortality	-	-	-	-	-
Third or Fourth Degree Laceration	-	-	3.63%	3.63%	3.27%

Rockdale Hospital

1412 Milstead Avenue NE
Conyers, GA 30012
E-mail: lholbrook@rockdale.org
URL: www.rockdalehospital.org
Ownership: Govt - Hospital District or Authority
Emergency Services: Yes
Phone: 770-918-3000
Fax: 770-918-3104
Accredited: Yes
Licensed Beds: 107

Key Personnel:
CEO . . . . David Huber, MD
Chief Medical Staff . . . . Frank Patton, MD
Emergency Room . . . . Kay Neal, RN
Director Medical/Surgical Nursing . . . . Jean Fransen, RD
Director Medical/Surgical Nursing . . . . Clarence Williams
Chief Radiology . . . . Robert Price, MD
Director Respiratory Therapy . . . . Vanessa Dameron

Measure	Cases	This Hospital	State Average	U.S. Average	Top Hospital
Heart Attack Care					
ACE Inhibitor or ARB for LVSD[1]	10	100%	78%	82%	100%
Aspirin at Arrival	125	100%	91%	92%	100%
Aspirin at Discharge	58	100%	87%	90%	100%
Beta Blocker at Arrival	123	100%	85%	87%	100%
Beta Blocker at Discharge	57	100%	87%	90%	100%
Fibrinolytic Medication Timing	0	-	34%	31%	100%
PCI Within 90 Minutes of Arrival	0	-	47%	54%	95%
Smoking Cessation Advice[1]	9	100%	85%	88%	100%
Heart Failure Care					
ACE Inhibitor or ARB for LVSD	84	100%	81%	82%	100%
Discharge Instructions	306	97%	59%	61%	93%
Evaluation of LVS Function	346	95%	81%	83%	99%
Smoking Cessation Advice	42	100%	86%	82%	100%
Pneumonia Care					
Appropriate Initial Antibiotic	172	88%	81%	83%	94%
Blood Culture Timing	158	92%	89%	90%	100%
Influenza Vaccine	59	80%	60%	70%	100%
Initial Antibiotic Timing	246	87%	75%	80%	93%
Oxygenation Assessment	292	100%	99%	99%	100%
Pneumococcal Vaccine	154	61%	61%	69%	94%
Smoking Cessation Advice	56	100%	82%	80%	100%
Surgical Infection Prevention					
Prophylactic Antibiotic Given	300	96%	69%	77%	95%
Prophylactic Antibiotic Selection	65	92%	89%	90%	100%
Prophylactic Antibiotic Stopped	295	96%	71%	72%	95%
Pregnancy Care					
Inpatient Neonatal Mortality	-	-	-	-	-
Third or Fourth Degree Laceration	-	-	3.63%	3.63%	3.27%

Crisp Regional Hospital

902 7th Street N
Cordele, GA 31015
E-mail: mdhartin@hotbot.com
URL: www.crispregional.org
Ownership: Govt - Hospital District or Authority
Emergency Services: Yes
Phone: 229-276-3100
Fax: 229-276-3211
Accredited: Yes
Licensed Beds: 65

Key Personnel:
CEO . . . . Wayne Martin
Chief of Medical Staff . . . . Cristen Rischar, MD
Emergency Room . . . . Melinda Adkins
Director Respiratory Therapy . . . . Jason Hayes, 32767

Measure	Cases	This Hospital	State Average	U.S. Average	Top Hospital
Heart Attack Care					
ACE Inhibitor or ARB for LVSD[1]	3	67%	78%	82%	100%
Aspirin at Arrival	34	76%	91%	92%	100%
Aspirin at Discharge[1]	20	55%	87%	90%	100%
Beta Blocker at Arrival	35	66%	85%	87%	100%
Beta Blocker at Discharge[1]	21	86%	87%	90%	100%
Fibrinolytic Medication Timing[1]	1	100%	34%	31%	100%
PCI Within 90 Minutes of Arrival	0	-	47%	54%	95%
Smoking Cessation Advice[1]	3	67%	85%	88%	100%
Heart Failure Care					
ACE Inhibitor or ARB for LVSD	55	82%	81%	82%	100%
Discharge Instructions	162	50%	59%	61%	93%

NOTE: Hospital profiles are in alphabetical order by state, then city, then hospital within the city; Rankings are sorted by rate in descending order and exclude hospitals with less than 25 cases; (1) The number of cases is too small (n<25) for purposes of reliably predicting hospital performance; (2) Measure reflects the hospital's indication that its submission was based upon a sample of its relevant discharges; (3) Rate reflects fewer than the maximum possible quarters of data for the measure; (4) Inaccurate information submitted and suppressed for one or more quarters; (5) No data is available from the hospital for this measure; Please refer to the User's Guide for a full explanation of data

Evaluation of LVS Function	184	86%	81%	83%	99%
Smoking Cessation Advice	35	89%	86%	82%	100%
Pneumonia Care					
Appropriate Initial Antibiotic	102	81%	81%	83%	94%
Blood Culture Timing	108	95%	89%	90%	100%
Influenza Vaccine	31	61%	60%	70%	100%
Initial Antibiotic Timing	155	54%	75%	80%	93%
Oxygenation Assessment	216	94%	99%	99%	100%
Pneumococcal Vaccine	131	83%	61%	69%	94%
Smoking Cessation Advice	38	82%	82%	80%	100%
Surgical Infection Prevention					
Prophylactic Antibiotic Given[1,3]	5	60%	69%	77%	95%
Prophylactic Antibiotic Selection[1]	5	80%	89%	90%	100%
Prophylactic Antibiotic Stopped[1,3]	5	60%	71%	72%	95%
Pregnancy Care					
Inpatient Neonatal Mortality	-	-	-	-	-
Third or Fourth Degree Laceration	-	-	3.63%	3.63%	3.27%

Newton Medical

5126 Hospital Drive NE
Covington, GA 30014
URL: www.ngh.org
Ownership: Proprietary
Emergency Services: Yes

Phone: 770-786-7053
Fax: 770-787-9059

Accredited: Yes
Licensed Beds: 90

Key Personnel:
Administrator . . . . James F Weadick
Chief Medical Staff. . . . . Donald Cote, MD
Emergency Room . . . . Jill Treadwell, RN
Emergency Room . . . . Anthony T Gonter, MD
Infection Control. . . . . Judy Carman, RN
ICU . . . . Donna Persinger, RN
Intensive/Coronary Care . . . . Amy Frizzell, RN
OB/GYN Womens Health. . . . . Amanda Fitzgerald, RN
Respiratory/Cardiopulmonary. . . . . Arlin Hodges, RT

Measure	Cases	This Hospital	State Average	U.S. Average	Top Hospital
Heart Attack Care					
ACE Inhibitor or ARB for LVSD[1]	7	86%	78%	82%	100%
Aspirin at Arrival	84	96%	91%	92%	100%
Aspirin at Discharge	48	83%	87%	90%	100%
Beta Blocker at Arrival	78	96%	85%	87%	100%
Beta Blocker at Discharge	49	92%	87%	90%	100%
Fibrinolytic Medication Timing[1]	7	57%	34%	31%	100%
PCI Within 90 Minutes of Arrival	0	-	47%	54%	95%
Smoking Cessation Advice[1]	14	100%	85%	88%	100%
Heart Failure Care					
ACE Inhibitor or ARB for LVSD	105	91%	81%	82%	100%
Discharge Instructions	236	74%	59%	61%	93%
Evaluation of LVS Function	268	97%	81%	83%	99%
Smoking Cessation Advice	51	76%	86%	82%	100%
Pneumonia Care					
Appropriate Initial Antibiotic[2]	153	90%	81%	83%	94%
Blood Culture Timing[2]	112	88%	89%	90%	100%
Influenza Vaccine	53	60%	60%	70%	100%
Initial Antibiotic Timing[2]	231	80%	75%	80%	93%
Oxygenation Assessment[2]	248	100%	99%	99%	100%
Pneumococcal Vaccine[2]	143	68%	61%	69%	94%
Smoking Cessation Advice[2]	60	83%	82%	80%	100%
Surgical Infection Prevention					
Prophylactic Antibiotic Given[2,3]	48	52%	69%	77%	95%
Prophylactic Antibiotic Selection[2]	47	77%	89%	90%	100%
Prophylactic Antibiotic Stopped[2,3]	48	73%	71%	72%	95%
Pregnancy Care					
Inpatient Neonatal Mortality	712	0.00%	-	-	-
Third or Fourth Degree Laceration	527	3.23%	3.63%	3.63%	3.27%

Northside Hospital

Alternate Name: Baptist North Hospital

1200 Baptist Medical Center Drive
Cumming, GA 30041
URL: www.gbhcs.org
Ownership: Voluntary non-profit - Private
Emergency Services: Yes

Phone: 770-844-3200
Fax: 404-851-6283

Accredited: Yes
Licensed Beds: 41

Key Personnel:
CEO. . . . . Jim Litchford
Chief Medical Staff. . . . . Shannon Mize, MD
Emergency Room . . . . Cynthia Miller
Director Medical/Surgical Nursing . . . . Pat Gillian, RN
Director Respiratory Therapy . . . . Cynthia Hsia

Measure	Cases	This Hospital	State Average	U.S. Average	Top Hospital
Heart Attack Care					
ACE Inhibitor or ARB for LVSD[1]	3	67%	78%	82%	100%
Aspirin at Arrival	81	94%	91%	92%	100%
Aspirin at Discharge	25	96%	87%	90%	100%
Beta Blocker at Arrival	66	83%	85%	87%	100%
Beta Blocker at Discharge[1]	24	83%	87%	90%	100%
Fibrinolytic Medication Timing[1]	6	100%	34%	31%	100%
PCI Within 90 Minutes of Arrival	0	-	47%	54%	95%
Smoking Cessation Advice[1]	7	100%	85%	88%	100%
Heart Failure Care					
ACE Inhibitor or ARB for LVSD	66	61%	81%	82%	100%
Discharge Instructions	207	68%	59%	61%	93%
Evaluation of LVS Function	230	91%	81%	83%	99%
Smoking Cessation Advice	44	100%	86%	82%	100%
Pneumonia Care					
Appropriate Initial Antibiotic	239	90%	81%	83%	94%
Blood Culture Timing	256	97%	89%	90%	100%
Influenza Vaccine	58	93%	60%	70%	100%
Initial Antibiotic Timing	306	90%	75%	80%	93%
Oxygenation Assessment	397	100%	99%	99%	100%
Pneumococcal Vaccine	246	94%	61%	69%	94%
Smoking Cessation Advice	91	97%	82%	80%	100%
Surgical Infection Prevention					
Prophylactic Antibiotic Given[2,3]	63	86%	69%	77%	95%
Prophylactic Antibiotic Selection[2]	61	93%	89%	90%	100%
Prophylactic Antibiotic Stopped[2,3]	59	59%	71%	72%	95%
Pregnancy Care					
Inpatient Neonatal Mortality	-	-	-	-	-
Third or Fourth Degree Laceration	-	-	3.63%	3.63%	3.27%

Chestatee Regional Hospital

Alternate Name: Chestatee Hospital
227 Mountain Drive
Dahlonega, GA 30533

Ownership: Proprietary
Emergency Services: Yes

Toll-Free: 888-782-9933
Phone: 706-864-6136
Fax: 706-864-1356
Accredited: Yes
Licensed Beds: 49

Key Personnel:
CEO/President. . . . . Robert Follwell
Chief Medical Staff. . . . . Jeffrey Schermerhorn
Chief of Medical Staff. . . . . Lawrence Kulish
Emergency Room . . . . Christopher Atkins
Director Radiology . . . . Laurie Davis
Director of Pulmonary/Respiratory . . . . Steven Graham

Measure	Cases	This Hospital	State Average	U.S. Average	Top Hospital
Heart Attack Care					
ACE Inhibitor or ARB for LVSD[1]	2	50%	78%	82%	100%
Aspirin at Arrival[1]	6	100%	91%	92%	100%
Aspirin at Discharge[1]	2	50%	87%	90%	100%
Beta Blocker at Arrival[1]	7	100%	85%	87%	100%
Beta Blocker at Discharge[1]	3	100%	87%	90%	100%
Fibrinolytic Medication Timing[1]	1	0%	34%	31%	100%
PCI Within 90 Minutes of Arrival	0	-	47%	54%	95%
Smoking Cessation Advice	0	-	85%	88%	100%
Heart Failure Care					
ACE Inhibitor or ARB for LVSD[1]	11	100%	81%	82%	100%
Discharge Instructions	29	28%	59%	61%	93%
Evaluation of LVS Function	43	74%	81%	83%	99%
Smoking Cessation Advice[1]	11	73%	86%	82%	100%

NOTE: Hospital profiles are in alphabetical order by state, then city, then hospital within the city; Rankings are sorted by rate in descending order and exclude hospitals with less than 25 cases; (1) The number of cases is too small (n<25) for purposes of reliably predicting hospital performance; (2) Measure reflects the hospital's indication that its submission was based upon a sample of its relevant discharges; (3) Rate reflects fewer than the maximum possible quarters of data for the measure; (4) Inaccurate information submitted and suppressed for one or more quarters; (5) No data is available from the hospital for this measure; Please refer to the User's Guide for a full explanation of data

Pneumonia Care					
Appropriate Initial Antibiotic[2]	70	87%	81%	83%	94%
Blood Culture Timing[1,2]	22	91%	89%	90%	100%
Influenza Vaccine[1]	15	67%	60%	70%	100%
Initial Antibiotic Timing[2]	69	72%	75%	80%	93%
Oxygenation Assessment[2]	102	99%	99%	99%	100%
Pneumococcal Vaccine[2]	62	52%	61%	69%	94%
Smoking Cessation Advice[2]	29	93%	82%	80%	100%
Surgical Infection Prevention					
Prophylactic Antibiotic Given[3]	28	82%	69%	77%	95%
Prophylactic Antibiotic Selection	28	96%	89%	90%	100%
Prophylactic Antibiotic Stopped[3]	26	69%	71%	72%	95%
Pregnancy Care					
Inpatient Neonatal Mortality	135	0.74%	-	-	-
Third or Fourth Degree Laceration	90	5.56%	3.63%	3.63%	3.27%

WellStar Paulding Hospital

600 W Memorial Drive
Dallas, GA 30132
URL: www.wellstar.org
Ownership: Voluntary non-profit - Other
Emergency Services: Yes

Phone: 770-445-4411
Fax: 770-443-7057

Accredited: Yes
Licensed Beds: 219

Key Personnel:
President/CEO . . . . Rob Lipson
Chief Medical Staff . . . . Tammy J Robinson, MD
Chief Medical Staff . . . . Charles Pesson, MD
Emergency Room . . . . Melissa Drain
OB/GYN Womens Health . . . . Asber Galloway
Chief Radiology . . . . Robert Cross

Measure	Cases	This Hospital	State Average	U.S. Average	Top Hospital
Heart Attack Care					
ACE Inhibitor or ARB for LVSD[1]	4	100%	78%	82%	100%
Aspirin at Arrival[1]	13	92%	91%	92%	100%
Aspirin at Discharge[1]	7	100%	87%	90%	100%
Beta Blocker at Arrival[1]	10	90%	85%	87%	100%
Beta Blocker at Discharge[1]	7	100%	87%	90%	100%
Fibrinolytic Medication Timing	0	-	34%	31%	100%
PCI Within 90 Minutes of Arrival	0	-	47%	54%	95%
Smoking Cessation Advice[1]	1	100%	85%	88%	100%
Heart Failure Care					
ACE Inhibitor or ARB for LVSD[1]	17	82%	81%	82%	100%
Discharge Instructions	39	28%	59%	61%	93%
Evaluation of LVS Function	44	89%	81%	83%	99%
Smoking Cessation Advice[1]	10	100%	86%	82%	100%
Pneumonia Care					
Appropriate Initial Antibiotic	78	92%	81%	83%	94%
Blood Culture Timing	59	92%	89%	90%	100%
Influenza Vaccine[1]	16	75%	60%	70%	100%
Initial Antibiotic Timing	88	80%	75%	80%	93%
Oxygenation Assessment	107	100%	99%	99%	100%
Pneumococcal Vaccine	57	65%	61%	69%	94%
Smoking Cessation Advice	25	96%	82%	80%	100%
Surgical Infection Prevention					
Prophylactic Antibiotic Given[1,3]	6	67%	69%	77%	95%
Prophylactic Antibiotic Selection[1]	6	100%	89%	90%	100%
Prophylactic Antibiotic Stopped[1,3]	6	83%	71%	72%	95%
Pregnancy Care					
Inpatient Neonatal Mortality	-	-	-	-	-
Third or Fourth Degree Laceration	-	-	3.63%	3.63%	3.27%

Hamilton Medical Center

1200 Memorial Drive
Dalton, GA 30720
URL: www.hamiltonhealth.com
Ownership: Govt - Hospital District or Authority
Emergency Services: Yes

Phone: 706-272-6114
Fax: 706-272-6477

Accredited: Yes
Licensed Beds: 282

Key Personnel:
President/CEO . . . . John Bowling
Chief Medical Staff . . . . Carolton D Lancaster, MD
Emergency Room . . . . William Pullen
Emergency Room . . . . Dan Moreschi
ICU . . . . Janice Keyes, RN

OB/GYN Womens Health . . . . Brenda Guinn, RN
Respiratory/Cardiopulmonary . . . . Scott Vinsant

Measure	Cases	This Hospital	State Average	U.S. Average	Top Hospital
Heart Attack Care					
ACE Inhibitor or ARB for LVSD[1]	15	67%	78%	82%	100%
Aspirin at Arrival	97	94%	91%	92%	100%
Aspirin at Discharge	43	86%	87%	90%	100%
Beta Blocker at Arrival	73	95%	85%	87%	100%
Beta Blocker at Discharge	54	93%	87%	90%	100%
Fibrinolytic Medication Timing	26	38%	34%	31%	100%
PCI Within 90 Minutes of Arrival[1]	8	50%	47%	54%	95%
Smoking Cessation Advice[1]	17	100%	85%	88%	100%
Heart Failure Care					
ACE Inhibitor or ARB for LVSD	125	78%	81%	82%	100%
Discharge Instructions	327	42%	59%	61%	93%
Evaluation of LVS Function	390	97%	81%	83%	99%
Smoking Cessation Advice	75	96%	86%	82%	100%
Pneumonia Care					
Appropriate Initial Antibiotic	208	84%	81%	83%	94%
Blood Culture Timing	163	91%	89%	90%	100%
Influenza Vaccine	67	84%	60%	70%	100%
Initial Antibiotic Timing	301	67%	75%	80%	93%
Oxygenation Assessment	389	98%	99%	99%	100%
Pneumococcal Vaccine	217	78%	61%	69%	94%
Smoking Cessation Advice	121	94%	82%	80%	100%
Surgical Infection Prevention					
Prophylactic Antibiotic Given[2]	239	91%	69%	77%	95%
Prophylactic Antibiotic Selection[2]	40	98%	89%	90%	100%
Prophylactic Antibiotic Stopped[2]	228	84%	71%	72%	95%
Pregnancy Care					
Inpatient Neonatal Mortality	-	-	-	-	-
Third or Fourth Degree Laceration	-	-	3.63%	3.63%	3.27%

DeKalb Medical Center

2701 N Decatur Road
Decatur, GA 30033
URL: www.drhs.org
Ownership: Voluntary non-profit - Private
Emergency Services: Yes

Phone: 404-501-1000
Fax: 404-501-5147

Accredited: Yes
Licensed Beds: 523

Key Personnel:
Administrator/CEO . . . . John R Gerlach
Chief Medical Staff . . . . Rose M Taylor, MD
Chief Catheterization Laboratory . . . . Paul Kirschbaum, MD
Emergency Room . . . . James P O'Neal, MD
Director Infection/Disease Control . . . . Helen Ebaugh, RN
Director CCU . . . . Pat Horton, RN
Director Medical/Surgical Nursing . . . . Jean Kemp, RN
OB/GYN Womens Health . . . . Albert Scott, MD
Chief Radiology . . . . Gary Laskey, MD
Director Respiratory Therapy . . . . Jack Wooten

Measure	Cases	This Hospital	State Average	U.S. Average	Top Hospital
Heart Attack Care					
ACE Inhibitor or ARB for LVSD	39	87%	78%	82%	100%
Aspirin at Arrival	171	98%	91%	92%	100%
Aspirin at Discharge	117	94%	87%	90%	100%
Beta Blocker at Arrival	156	96%	85%	87%	100%
Beta Blocker at Discharge	109	97%	87%	90%	100%
Fibrinolytic Medication Timing[1]	11	36%	34%	31%	100%
PCI Within 90 Minutes of Arrival	0	-	47%	54%	95%
Smoking Cessation Advice	36	100%	85%	88%	100%
Heart Failure Care					
ACE Inhibitor or ARB for LVSD	302	86%	81%	82%	100%
Discharge Instructions	500	70%	59%	61%	93%
Evaluation of LVS Function	580	94%	81%	83%	99%
Smoking Cessation Advice	118	96%	86%	82%	100%
Pneumonia Care					
Appropriate Initial Antibiotic[2]	227	84%	81%	83%	94%
Blood Culture Timing[2]	273	87%	89%	90%	100%
Influenza Vaccine	85	78%	60%	70%	100%
Initial Antibiotic Timing[2]	410	61%	75%	80%	93%

NOTE: Hospital profiles are in alphabetical order by state, then city, then hospital within the city; Rankings are sorted by rate in descending order and exclude hospitals with less than 25 cases; (1) The number of cases is too small (n<25) for purposes of reliably predicting hospital performance; (2) Measure reflects the hospital's indication that its submission was based upon a sample of its relevant discharges; (3) Rate reflects fewer than the maximum possible quarters of data for the measure; (4) Inaccurate information submitted and suppressed for one or more quarters; (5) No data is available from the hospital for this measure; Please refer to the User's Guide for a full explanation of data

Oxygenation Assessment[2]	504	100%	99%	99%	100%
Pneumococcal Vaccine[2]	237	62%	61%	69%	94%
Smoking Cessation Advice[2]	113	96%	82%	80%	100%
Surgical Infection Prevention					
Prophylactic Antibiotic Given[2]	304	87%	69%	77%	95%
Prophylactic Antibiotic Selection[2]	67	88%	89%	90%	100%
Prophylactic Antibiotic Stopped[2]	290	59%	71%	72%	95%
Pregnancy Care					
Inpatient Neonatal Mortality	-	-	-	-	-
Third or Fourth Degree Laceration	-	-	3.63%	3.63%	3.27%

Habersham County Medical Center

Highway 441 N   Phone: 706-754-2161
Demorest, GA 30535   Fax: 706-754-7300
E-mail: tellus@hcmcmed.or
URL: www.hcmcmed.org
Ownership: Govt - Hospital District or Authority   Accredited: Yes
Emergency Services: Yes   Licensed Beds: 53
Key Personnel:
President/CEO . . . . C Richard Dwozan
Chief Medical Staff . . . . Wanda Perry
Emergency Room . . . . Marion Edwards-Drost
Emergency Room . . . . Marc Chetta, MD
Medical/Surgical Nursing . . . . Janice McKenzie
Respiratory/Cardiopulmonary . . . . MaryBelle Thomason

Measure	Cases	This Hospital	State Average	U.S. Average	Top Hospital
Heart Attack Care					
ACE Inhibitor or ARB for LVSD	0	-	78%	82%	100%
Aspirin at Arrival[1]	6	83%	91%	92%	100%
Aspirin at Discharge[1]	2	100%	87%	90%	100%
Beta Blocker at Arrival[1]	6	100%	85%	87%	100%
Beta Blocker at Discharge[1]	2	100%	87%	90%	100%
Fibrinolytic Medication Timing	0	-	34%	31%	100%
PCI Within 90 Minutes of Arrival	0	-	47%	54%	95%
Smoking Cessation Advice	0	-	85%	88%	100%
Heart Failure Care					
ACE Inhibitor or ARB for LVSD[1]	19	79%	81%	82%	100%
Discharge Instructions	44	59%	59%	61%	93%
Evaluation of LVS Function	53	92%	81%	83%	99%
Smoking Cessation Advice[1]	5	80%	86%	82%	100%
Pneumonia Care					
Appropriate Initial Antibiotic	79	86%	81%	83%	94%
Blood Culture Timing	69	74%	89%	90%	100%
Influenza Vaccine[1]	14	93%	60%	70%	100%
Initial Antibiotic Timing	78	92%	75%	80%	93%
Oxygenation Assessment	111	100%	99%	99%	100%
Pneumococcal Vaccine	72	81%	61%	69%	94%
Smoking Cessation Advice	29	86%	82%	80%	100%
Surgical Infection Prevention					
Prophylactic Antibiotic Given[2,3]	36	94%	69%	77%	95%
Prophylactic Antibiotic Selection[2]	36	97%	89%	90%	100%
Prophylactic Antibiotic Stopped[2,3]	35	74%	71%	72%	95%
Pregnancy Care					
Inpatient Neonatal Mortality	-	-	-	-	-
Third or Fourth Degree Laceration	-	-	3.63%	3.63%	3.27%

Donalsonville Hospital

102 Hospital Circle   Phone: 229-524-5217
PO Box 677   Fax: 229-524-8217
Donalsonville, GA 31745
E-mail: jmoody@surfsouth.com
Ownership: Voluntary non-profit - Private   Accredited: Yes
Emergency Services: Yes   Licensed Beds: 65
Key Personnel:
CEO . . . . Charles Orrick
Chief Medical Staff . . . . Charles Walker, MD
Emergency Room . . . . Dale Whitaker, RN
Chief Radiology . . . . Lois Curry, MD
Director Respiratory Therapy . . . . Royce M Cannington

Measure	Cases	This Hospital	State Average	U.S. Average	Top Hospital
Heart Attack Care					

Measure	Cases	This Hospital	State Average	U.S. Average	Top Hospital
ACE Inhibitor or ARB for LVSD	0	-	78%	82%	100%
Aspirin at Arrival[1]	4	50%	91%	92%	100%
Aspirin at Discharge[1]	3	67%	87%	90%	100%
Beta Blocker at Arrival[1]	4	25%	85%	87%	100%
Beta Blocker at Discharge[1]	3	33%	87%	90%	100%
Fibrinolytic Medication Timing	0	-	34%	31%	100%
PCI Within 90 Minutes of Arrival	0	-	47%	54%	95%
Smoking Cessation Advice[1]	1	0%	85%	88%	100%
Heart Failure Care					
ACE Inhibitor or ARB for LVSD[1]	2	50%	81%	82%	100%
Discharge Instructions	26	12%	59%	61%	93%
Evaluation of LVS Function	33	45%	81%	83%	99%
Smoking Cessation Advice[1]	5	80%	86%	82%	100%
Pneumonia Care					
Appropriate Initial Antibiotic	101	67%	81%	83%	94%
Blood Culture Timing[1]	3	100%	89%	90%	100%
Influenza Vaccine[1]	21	48%	60%	70%	100%
Initial Antibiotic Timing	99	83%	75%	80%	93%
Oxygenation Assessment	114	91%	99%	99%	100%
Pneumococcal Vaccine	49	37%	61%	69%	94%
Smoking Cessation Advice	30	73%	82%	80%	100%
Surgical Infection Prevention					
Prophylactic Antibiotic Given	40	45%	69%	77%	95%
Prophylactic Antibiotic Selection[1]	10	80%	89%	90%	100%
Prophylactic Antibiotic Stopped	35	57%	71%	72%	95%
Pregnancy Care					
Inpatient Neonatal Mortality	290	0.34%	-	-	-
Third or Fourth Degree Laceration	188	3.19%	3.63%	3.63%	3.27%

Coffee Regional Medical Center

Alternate Name: Coffee Regional Hospital
1101 Ocilla Road   Phone: 912-384-1900
Douglas, GA 31533   Fax: 912-389-2112
URL: www.coffeeregional.org
Ownership: Govt - Hospital District or Authority   Accredited: Yes
Emergency Services: Yes   Licensed Beds: 88
Key Personnel:
CEO . . . . George Heck
Emergency Room . . . . Jennifer Davis
Infection Control . . . . Rudean Long
ICU . . . . Betty Smith
Medical Staff Services . . . . Mindy Lott
OB/GYN . . . . Melva Brown
Surgical Services . . . . Doyle Baker
Respiratory Therapy . . . . Alicia Costew

Measure	Cases	This Hospital	State Average	U.S. Average	Top Hospital
Heart Attack Care					
ACE Inhibitor or ARB for LVSD	0	-	78%	82%	100%
Aspirin at Arrival[1]	21	81%	91%	92%	100%
Aspirin at Discharge[1]	5	60%	87%	90%	100%
Beta Blocker at Arrival[1]	22	95%	85%	87%	100%
Beta Blocker at Discharge[1]	4	100%	87%	90%	100%
Fibrinolytic Medication Timing[1]	2	100%	34%	31%	100%
PCI Within 90 Minutes of Arrival	0	-	47%	54%	95%
Smoking Cessation Advice	0	-	85%	88%	100%
Heart Failure Care					
ACE Inhibitor or ARB for LVSD	78	88%	81%	82%	100%
Discharge Instructions	232	64%	59%	61%	93%
Evaluation of LVS Function	254	69%	81%	83%	99%
Smoking Cessation Advice	53	89%	86%	82%	100%
Pneumonia Care					
Appropriate Initial Antibiotic	128	80%	81%	83%	94%
Blood Culture Timing	32	94%	89%	90%	100%
Influenza Vaccine	26	73%	60%	70%	100%
Initial Antibiotic Timing	168	86%	75%	80%	93%
Oxygenation Assessment	169	99%	99%	99%	100%
Pneumococcal Vaccine	71	58%	61%	69%	94%
Smoking Cessation Advice	33	88%	82%	80%	100%
Surgical Infection Prevention					
Prophylactic Antibiotic Given[1,3]	9	33%	69%	77%	95%
Prophylactic Antibiotic Selection[1]	9	89%	89%	90%	100%
Prophylactic Antibiotic Stopped[1,3]	9	56%	71%	72%	95%

NOTE: Hospital profiles are in alphabetical order by state, then city, then hospital within the city; Rankings are sorted by rate in descending order and exclude hospitals with less than 25 cases; (1) The number of cases is too small (n<25) for purposes of reliably predicting hospital performance; (2) Measure reflects the hospital's indication that its submission was based upon a sample of its relevant discharges; (3) Rate reflects fewer than the maximum possible quarters of data for the measure; (4) Inaccurate information submitted and suppressed for one or more quarters; (5) No data is available from the hospital for this measure; Please refer to the User's Guide for a full explanation of data

Pregnancy Care					
Inpatient Neonatal Mortality	-	-	-	-	-
Third or Fourth Degree Laceration	-	-	3.63%	3.63%	3.27%

WellStar Douglas Hospital

8954 Hospital Drive
Douglasville, GA 30134
URL: www.wellstar.org
Ownership: Voluntary non-profit - Other
Emergency Services: Yes

Phone: 770-949-1500
Fax: 770-920-6354

Accredited: Yes
Licensed Beds: 71

Key Personnel:
President/CEO . . . . Robert Lipson, MD

Measure	Cases	This Hospital	State Average	U.S. Average	Top Hospital
Heart Attack Care					
ACE Inhibitor or ARB for LVSD[1]	4	100%	78%	82%	100%
Aspirin at Arrival	65	97%	91%	92%	100%
Aspirin at Discharge[1]	19	100%	87%	90%	100%
Beta Blocker at Arrival	54	85%	85%	87%	100%
Beta Blocker at Discharge[1]	21	90%	87%	90%	100%
Fibrinolytic Medication Timing[1]	5	0%	34%	31%	100%
PCI Within 90 Minutes of Arrival	0	-	47%	54%	95%
Smoking Cessation Advice[1]	5	80%	85%	88%	100%
Heart Failure Care					
ACE Inhibitor or ARB for LVSD	99	79%	81%	82%	100%
Discharge Instructions	224	21%	59%	61%	93%
Evaluation of LVS Function	255	91%	81%	83%	99%
Smoking Cessation Advice	61	98%	86%	82%	100%
Pneumonia Care					
Appropriate Initial Antibiotic	174	88%	81%	83%	94%
Blood Culture Timing	142	90%	89%	90%	100%
Influenza Vaccine	33	55%	60%	70%	100%
Initial Antibiotic Timing	214	72%	75%	80%	93%
Oxygenation Assessment	255	100%	99%	99%	100%
Pneumococcal Vaccine	117	62%	61%	69%	94%
Smoking Cessation Advice	80	96%	82%	80%	100%
Surgical Infection Prevention					
Prophylactic Antibiotic Given[3]	29	83%	69%	77%	95%
Prophylactic Antibiotic Selection	29	97%	89%	90%	100%
Prophylactic Antibiotic Stopped[3]	28	57%	71%	72%	95%
Pregnancy Care					
Inpatient Neonatal Mortality	-	-	-	-	-
Third or Fourth Degree Laceration	-	-	3.63%	3.63%	3.27%

Fairview Park Hospital

200 Industrial Boulevard
Dublin, GA 31021
URL: www.fairviewparkhospital.com
Ownership: Proprietary
Emergency Services: Yes

Phone: 478-275-2000
Fax: 478-274-3673

Accredited: Yes
Licensed Beds: 190

Key Personnel:
CEO . . . . James Wood
Chief Medical Staff . . . . Berry Parker
Emergency Room . . . . Berry Parker
OB/GYN Womens Health . . . . Steven Palmer, MD
Chief Radiology . . . . Kenneth Bowman, MD
Director Respiratory Therapy . . . . Ken Lewis

Measure	Cases	This Hospital	State Average	U.S. Average	Top Hospital
Heart Attack Care					
ACE Inhibitor or ARB for LVSD[1]	17	82%	78%	82%	100%
Aspirin at Arrival	79	94%	91%	92%	100%
Aspirin at Discharge	55	87%	87%	90%	100%
Beta Blocker at Arrival	76	96%	85%	87%	100%
Beta Blocker at Discharge	59	95%	87%	90%	100%
Fibrinolytic Medication Timing[1]	15	60%	34%	31%	100%
PCI Within 90 Minutes of Arrival[1]	4	75%	47%	54%	95%
Smoking Cessation Advice[1]	21	100%	85%	88%	100%
Heart Failure Care					
ACE Inhibitor or ARB for LVSD	97	74%	81%	82%	100%
Discharge Instructions	224	46%	59%	61%	93%
Evaluation of LVS Function	251	82%	81%	83%	99%

Smoking Cessation Advice	54	100%	86%	82%	100%
Pneumonia Care					
Appropriate Initial Antibiotic	125	68%	81%	83%	94%
Blood Culture Timing	67	97%	89%	90%	100%
Influenza Vaccine	48	8%	60%	70%	100%
Initial Antibiotic Timing	199	57%	75%	80%	93%
Oxygenation Assessment	225	97%	99%	99%	100%
Pneumococcal Vaccine	123	40%	61%	69%	94%
Smoking Cessation Advice	35	97%	82%	80%	100%
Surgical Infection Prevention					
Prophylactic Antibiotic Given[2,3]	92	78%	69%	77%	95%
Prophylactic Antibiotic Selection[2]	40	85%	89%	90%	100%
Prophylactic Antibiotic Stopped[2,3]	91	78%	71%	72%	95%
Pregnancy Care					
Inpatient Neonatal Mortality	-	-	-	-	-
Third or Fourth Degree Laceration	-	-	3.63%	3.63%	3.27%

South Fulton Medical Center

1170 Cleveland Avenue
East Point, GA 30344
URL: www.southfultomedicalcenter.com
Ownership: Proprietary
Emergency Services: Yes

Phone: 404-466-1170
Fax: 404-466-1120

Accredited: Yes
Licensed Beds: 392

Key Personnel:
CEO . . . . Christopher Hummer
Chief Medical Staff . . . . Dr. Fernando Duralde
Chief Catheterization Laboratory . . . . Krishna Mohan
Emergency Room . . . . Gail Bundow
Director Infection/Disease Control . . . . Carol Carder
CCU Spvg. Nurse . . . . Steve Whitney
Director Medical/Surgical Nursing . . . . Carolie White, RN
OB/GYN Womens Health . . . . Gabriel F Nassar
Chief Radiology . . . . Gordon Goldstein, MD
Respiratory Therapy . . . . Carolie White, RN

Measure	Cases	This Hospital	State Average	U.S. Average	Top Hospital
Heart Attack Care					
ACE Inhibitor or ARB for LVSD[1]	18	83%	78%	82%	100%
Aspirin at Arrival	118	92%	91%	92%	100%
Aspirin at Discharge	52	85%	87%	90%	100%
Beta Blocker at Arrival	84	99%	85%	87%	100%
Beta Blocker at Discharge	52	98%	87%	90%	100%
Fibrinolytic Medication Timing[1]	12	33%	34%	31%	100%
PCI Within 90 Minutes of Arrival	0	-	47%	54%	95%
Smoking Cessation Advice[1]	19	89%	85%	88%	100%
Heart Failure Care					
ACE Inhibitor or ARB for LVSD	128	92%	81%	82%	100%
Discharge Instructions	310	58%	59%	61%	93%
Evaluation of LVS Function	350	92%	81%	83%	99%
Smoking Cessation Advice	98	97%	86%	82%	100%
Pneumonia Care					
Appropriate Initial Antibiotic	182	84%	81%	83%	94%
Blood Culture Timing	167	80%	89%	90%	100%
Influenza Vaccine	52	31%	60%	70%	100%
Initial Antibiotic Timing	263	64%	75%	80%	93%
Oxygenation Assessment	309	100%	99%	99%	100%
Pneumococcal Vaccine	131	48%	61%	69%	94%
Smoking Cessation Advice	77	81%	82%	80%	100%
Surgical Infection Prevention					
Prophylactic Antibiotic Given[2]	221	76%	69%	77%	95%
Prophylactic Antibiotic Selection[2]	56	95%	89%	90%	100%
Prophylactic Antibiotic Stopped[2]	213	68%	71%	72%	95%
Pregnancy Care					
Inpatient Neonatal Mortality	-	-	-	-	-
Third or Fourth Degree Laceration	-	-	3.63%	3.63%	3.27%

NOTE: Hospital profiles are in alphabetical order by state, then city, then hospital within the city; Rankings are sorted by rate in descending order and exclude hospitals with less than 25 cases; (1) The number of cases is too small (n<25) for purposes of reliably predicting hospital performance; (2) Measure reflects the hospital's indication that its submission was based upon a sample of its relevant discharges; (3) Rate reflects fewer than the maximum possible quarters of data for the measure; (4) Inaccurate information submitted and suppressed for one or more quarters; (5) No data is available from the hospital for this measure; Please refer to the User's Guide for a full explanation of data

Dodge County Hospital

901 Griffin Avenue
PO Box 4309
Eastman, GA 31023
URL: www.dodgecountyhospital.com
Ownership: Govt - Hospital District or Authority
Emergency Services: Yes

Phone: 478-448-4000
Fax: 478-374-9411

Accredited: Yes
Licensed Beds: 94

Key Personnel:
Interim CEO . . . . Ken Stegner
Chief of Medical Staff . . . . James Tison
Emergency Room . . . . Pauling Yown
OB/GYN Womens Health . . . . Otis Williams, MD
Chief Radiology . . . . Dr Tommy Meadows
Director of Respiratory . . . . Becky Smith

Measure	Cases	This Hospital	State Average	U.S. Average	Top Hospital
Heart Attack Care					
ACE Inhibitor or ARB for LVSD[1]	1	0%	78%	82%	100%
Aspirin at Arrival[1]	15	87%	91%	92%	100%
Aspirin at Discharge[1]	7	57%	87%	90%	100%
Beta Blocker at Arrival[1]	15	67%	85%	87%	100%
Beta Blocker at Discharge[1]	9	44%	87%	90%	100%
Fibrinolytic Medication Timing[1]	4	50%	34%	31%	100%
PCI Within 90 Minutes of Arrival	0	-	47%	54%	95%
Smoking Cessation Advice[1]	3	0%	85%	88%	100%
Heart Failure Care					
ACE Inhibitor or ARB for LVSD[1]	9	56%	81%	82%	100%
Discharge Instructions	54	89%	59%	61%	93%
Evaluation of LVS Function	72	21%	81%	83%	99%
Smoking Cessation Advice[1]	24	54%	86%	82%	100%
Pneumonia Care					
Appropriate Initial Antibiotic	67	67%	81%	83%	94%
Blood Culture Timing	35	83%	89%	90%	100%
Influenza Vaccine[4,5]	-	-	60%	70%	100%
Initial Antibiotic Timing	95	84%	75%	80%	93%
Oxygenation Assessment	111	97%	99%	99%	100%
Pneumococcal Vaccine	60	20%	61%	69%	94%
Smoking Cessation Advice[1]	21	19%	82%	80%	100%
Surgical Infection Prevention					
Prophylactic Antibiotic Given[1,3]	3	67%	69%	77%	95%
Prophylactic Antibiotic Selection[1]	3	100%	89%	90%	100%
Prophylactic Antibiotic Stopped[1,3]	3	100%	71%	72%	95%
Pregnancy Care					
Inpatient Neonatal Mortality	-	-	-	-	-
Third or Fourth Degree Laceration	-	-	3.63%	3.63%	3.27%

Putnam General Hospital

101 Lake Oconee Parkway
Eatonton, GA 31024
URL: www.putnamgeneral.com
Ownership: Govt - Hospital District or Authority
Emergency Services: Yes

Phone: 706-485-2711
Fax: 706-485-6770

Accredited: Yes
Licensed Beds: 50

Key Personnel:
CEO . . . . Darrell Oglesby
Chief Medical Staff . . . . Susan Jones, MD
Emergency Room . . . . Rakesh Kumar, MD
Chief Radiology . . . . Wilbur Baugh, MD
Director Respiratory Therapy . . . . Randy Staton

Measure	Cases	This Hospital	State Average	U.S. Average	Top Hospital
Heart Attack Care					
ACE Inhibitor or ARB for LVSD[5]	-	-	78%	82%	100%
Aspirin at Arrival[5]	-	-	91%	92%	100%
Aspirin at Discharge[5]	-	-	87%	90%	100%
Beta Blocker at Arrival[5]	-	-	85%	87%	100%
Beta Blocker at Discharge[5]	-	-	87%	90%	100%
Fibrinolytic Medication Timing[5]	-	-	34%	31%	100%
PCI Within 90 Minutes of Arrival[5]	-	-	47%	54%	95%
Smoking Cessation Advice[5]	-	-	85%	88%	100%
Heart Failure Care					
ACE Inhibitor or ARB for LVSD[5]	-	-	81%	82%	100%
Discharge Instructions[5]	-	-	59%	61%	93%
Evaluation of LVS Function[5]	-	-	81%	83%	99%

Measure	Cases	This Hospital	State Average	U.S. Average	Top Hospital
Smoking Cessation Advice[5]	-	-	86%	82%	100%
Pneumonia Care					
Appropriate Initial Antibiotic	43	88%	81%	83%	94%
Blood Culture Timing	33	88%	89%	90%	100%
Influenza Vaccine[1]	16	56%	60%	70%	100%
Initial Antibiotic Timing	57	86%	75%	80%	93%
Oxygenation Assessment	83	99%	99%	99%	100%
Pneumococcal Vaccine	56	50%	61%	69%	94%
Smoking Cessation Advice[1]	10	80%	82%	80%	100%
Surgical Infection Prevention					
Prophylactic Antibiotic Given[5]	-	-	69%	77%	95%
Prophylactic Antibiotic Selection[5]	-	-	89%	90%	100%
Prophylactic Antibiotic Stopped[5]	-	-	71%	72%	95%
Pregnancy Care					
Inpatient Neonatal Mortality	-	-	-	-	-
Third or Fourth Degree Laceration	-	-	3.63%	3.63%	3.27%

Elbert Memorial Hospital

4 Medical Drive
Elberton, GA 30635
Ownership: Govt - Hospital District or Authority
Emergency Services: Yes

Phone: 706-283-3151
Fax: 706-213-2578

Accredited: Yes
Licensed Beds: 52

Key Personnel:
CEO . . . . Mark Leneave
Medical/Surgical Nursing . . . . Donna Christian, RN
Respiratory/Cardiopulmonary . . . . Regina Holt

Measure	Cases	This Hospital	State Average	U.S. Average	Top Hospital
Heart Attack Care					
ACE Inhibitor or ARB for LVSD	0	-	78%	82%	100%
Aspirin at Arrival[1]	19	89%	91%	92%	100%
Aspirin at Discharge[1]	15	93%	87%	90%	100%
Beta Blocker at Arrival[1]	14	86%	85%	87%	100%
Beta Blocker at Discharge[1]	11	91%	87%	90%	100%
Fibrinolytic Medication Timing	0	-	34%	31%	100%
PCI Within 90 Minutes of Arrival	0	-	47%	54%	95%
Smoking Cessation Advice[1]	2	100%	85%	88%	100%
Heart Failure Care					
ACE Inhibitor or ARB for LVSD[1]	23	91%	81%	82%	100%
Discharge Instructions	72	83%	59%	61%	93%
Evaluation of LVS Function	98	86%	81%	83%	99%
Smoking Cessation Advice[1]	19	89%	86%	82%	100%
Pneumonia Care					
Appropriate Initial Antibiotic	73	71%	81%	83%	94%
Blood Culture Timing	39	97%	89%	90%	100%
Influenza Vaccine[4,5]	-	-	60%	70%	100%
Initial Antibiotic Timing	81	70%	75%	80%	93%
Oxygenation Assessment	111	99%	99%	99%	100%
Pneumococcal Vaccine	63	65%	61%	69%	94%
Smoking Cessation Advice[1]	24	96%	82%	80%	100%
Surgical Infection Prevention					
Prophylactic Antibiotic Given[1,3]	11	64%	69%	77%	95%
Prophylactic Antibiotic Selection[1]	5	100%	89%	90%	100%
Prophylactic Antibiotic Stopped[1,3]	11	82%	71%	72%	95%
Pregnancy Care					
Inpatient Neonatal Mortality	-	-	-	-	-
Third or Fourth Degree Laceration	-	-	3.63%	3.63%	3.27%

North Georgia Medical Center

1362 S Main Street
Ellijay, GA 30540
Ownership: Proprietary
Emergency Services: Yes

Phone: 706-276-4741
Fax: 706-276-3698

Accredited: Yes
Licensed Beds: 50

Key Personnel:
President/CEO . . . . Jeffrey M Dunn
Chief Medical Staff . . . . Edward Schwartz, DO
Emergency Room . . . . Michael Mudrey, DO
Infection Control . . . . Cindy Ensley, RN
ICU . . . . Laura Squires, RN
Medical Surgical Nursing . . . . Gene Carlise, RN
Director of Pulmonary/Respiratory Care . . . . Lynda Lawren

NOTE: Hospital profiles are in alphabetical order by state, then city, then hospital within the city; Rankings are sorted by rate in descending order and exclude hospitals with less than 25 cases; (1) The number of cases is too small (n<25) for purposes of reliably predicting hospital performance; (2) Measure reflects the hospital's indication that its submission was based upon a sample of its relevant discharges; (3) Rate reflects fewer than the maximum possible quarters of data for the measure; (4) Inaccurate information submitted and suppressed for one or more quarters; (5) No data is available from the hospital for this measure; Please refer to the User's Guide for a full explanation of data

Measure	Cases	This Hospital	State Average	U.S. Average	Top Hospital
Heart Attack Care					
ACE Inhibitor or ARB for LVSD[1]	1	0%	78%	82%	100%
Aspirin at Arrival[1]	5	60%	91%	92%	100%
Aspirin at Discharge[1]	4	100%	87%	90%	100%
Beta Blocker at Arrival[1]	5	20%	85%	87%	100%
Beta Blocker at Discharge[1]	3	0%	87%	90%	100%
Fibrinolytic Medication Timing	0	-	34%	31%	100%
PCI Within 90 Minutes of Arrival	0	-	47%	54%	95%
Smoking Cessation Advice	0	-	85%	88%	100%
Heart Failure Care					
ACE Inhibitor or ARB for LVSD[1]	12	50%	81%	82%	100%
Discharge Instructions	42	71%	59%	61%	93%
Evaluation of LVS Function	67	67%	81%	83%	99%
Smoking Cessation Advice[1]	7	43%	86%	82%	100%
Pneumonia Care					
Appropriate Initial Antibiotic	46	70%	81%	83%	94%
Blood Culture Timing[1]	18	83%	89%	90%	100%
Influenza Vaccine[1]	9	33%	60%	70%	100%
Initial Antibiotic Timing	55	67%	75%	80%	93%
Oxygenation Assessment	69	99%	99%	99%	100%
Pneumococcal Vaccine	39	54%	61%	69%	94%
Smoking Cessation Advice[1]	17	35%	82%	80%	100%
Surgical Infection Prevention					
Prophylactic Antibiotic Given[1,3]	10	40%	69%	77%	95%
Prophylactic Antibiotic Selection[1]	9	100%	89%	90%	100%
Prophylactic Antibiotic Stopped[1,3]	9	78%	71%	72%	95%
Pregnancy Care					
Inpatient Neonatal Mortality	-	-	-	-	-
Third or Fourth Degree Laceration	-	-	3.63%	3.63%	3.27%

Piedmont Fayette Hospital

1255 Highway 54 West
Fayetteville, GA 30214
URL: www.fayettehospital.org
Ownership: Voluntary non-profit - Private
Emergency Services: Yes

Phone: 770-719-7000
Fax: 770-719-7092

Accredited: Yes
Licensed Beds: 100

Key Personnel:
CEO/Administrator . . . . Darrel Cutts
Chief Medical Staff . . . . John Goza
Chief Cardiology . . . . George Vellanikaran
Emergency Department . . . . Mary Heath
Chief Pulmonary Therapy . . . . William Crossland

Measure	Cases	This Hospital	State Average	U.S. Average	Top Hospital
Heart Attack Care					
ACE Inhibitor or ARB for LVSD[1]	12	67%	78%	82%	100%
Aspirin at Arrival	82	94%	91%	92%	100%
Aspirin at Discharge	35	91%	87%	90%	100%
Beta Blocker at Arrival	69	91%	85%	87%	100%
Beta Blocker at Discharge	37	92%	87%	90%	100%
Fibrinolytic Medication Timing[3]	0	-	34%	31%	100%
PCI Within 90 Minutes of Arrival	0	-	47%	54%	95%
Smoking Cessation Advice[1,3]	2	100%	85%	88%	100%
Heart Failure Care					
ACE Inhibitor or ARB for LVSD	88	74%	81%	82%	100%
Discharge Instructions[3]	53	87%	59%	61%	93%
Evaluation of LVS Function	243	88%	81%	83%	99%
Smoking Cessation Advice[1,3]	10	80%	86%	82%	100%
Pneumonia Care					
Appropriate Initial Antibiotic[3]	31	87%	81%	83%	94%
Blood Culture Timing[3]	41	90%	89%	90%	100%
Influenza Vaccine[5]	-	-	60%	70%	100%
Initial Antibiotic Timing	234	77%	75%	80%	93%
Oxygenation Assessment	266	100%	99%	99%	100%
Pneumococcal Vaccine	140	84%	61%	69%	94%
Smoking Cessation Advice[1,3]	6	100%	82%	80%	100%
Surgical Infection Prevention					
Prophylactic Antibiotic Given[3]	87	91%	69%	77%	95%
Prophylactic Antibiotic Selection[5]	-	-	89%	90%	100%
Prophylactic Antibiotic Stopped[3]	87	76%	71%	72%	95%
Pregnancy Care					

Measure	Cases	This Hospital	State Average	U.S. Average	Top Hospital
Inpatient Neonatal Mortality	-	-	-	-	-
Third or Fourth Degree Laceration	-	-	3.63%	3.63%	3.27%

Dorminy Medical Center

200 Perry House Road
PO Box 1447
Fitzgerald, GA 31750
URL: www.dorminymedical.org
Ownership: Govt - Hospital District or Authority
Emergency Services: Yes

Phone: 229-424-7100
Fax: 229-424-7281

Accredited: Yes
Licensed Beds: 75

Key Personnel:
CEO . . . . Bruce Shepard
Chief Medical Staff . . . . Dr Don T Smith Jr, MD
Emergency Room . . . . Paul Webb, RN
Infection Control . . . . Dot O'Scott
ICU . . . . Dot O'Scott, RN
CNO . . . . Stacie Mims, RN
OB/GYN Womens Health . . . . William Parham, DO
Chief Radiology . . . . Luis Lopez
Director Respiratory Therapy . . . . Melanie Kimball

Measure	Cases	This Hospital	State Average	U.S. Average	Top Hospital
Heart Attack Care					
ACE Inhibitor or ARB for LVSD	0	-	78%	82%	100%
Aspirin at Arrival[1]	16	75%	91%	92%	100%
Aspirin at Discharge[1]	5	80%	87%	90%	100%
Beta Blocker at Arrival[1]	15	60%	85%	87%	100%
Beta Blocker at Discharge[1]	6	83%	87%	90%	100%
Fibrinolytic Medication Timing[1,3]	2	0%	34%	31%	100%
PCI Within 90 Minutes of Arrival	0	-	47%	54%	95%
Smoking Cessation Advice[1,3]	2	100%	85%	88%	100%
Heart Failure Care					
ACE Inhibitor or ARB for LVSD[1]	19	68%	81%	82%	100%
Discharge Instructions[3]	33	61%	59%	61%	93%
Evaluation of LVS Function	77	66%	81%	83%	99%
Smoking Cessation Advice[1,3]	5	100%	86%	82%	100%
Pneumonia Care					
Appropriate Initial Antibiotic[1,3]	19	79%	81%	83%	94%
Blood Culture Timing[1,3]	13	92%	89%	90%	100%
Influenza Vaccine[5]	-	-	60%	70%	100%
Initial Antibiotic Timing	64	78%	75%	80%	93%
Oxygenation Assessment	68	99%	99%	99%	100%
Pneumococcal Vaccine	37	51%	61%	69%	94%
Smoking Cessation Advice[1,3]	11	100%	82%	80%	100%
Surgical Infection Prevention					
Prophylactic Antibiotic Given[1,3]	2	0%	69%	77%	95%
Prophylactic Antibiotic Selection[1]	1	100%	89%	90%	100%
Prophylactic Antibiotic Stopped[1,3]	1	100%	71%	72%	95%
Pregnancy Care					
Inpatient Neonatal Mortality	200	0.00%	-	-	-
Third or Fourth Degree Laceration	100	1.00%	3.63%	3.63%	3.27%

Charlton Memorial Hospital

1203 N 3rd Street
Folkston, GA 31537
Ownership: Govt - Hospital District or Authority
Emergency Services: Yes

Phone: 912-496-2531
Fax: 912-496-3741
Accredited: No
Licensed Beds: 15

Key Personnel:
Administrator . . . . Sue Spivey
Chief Medical Staff . . . . Richard Eaton, MD
Infection Control . . . . Merita Hinnant, RN, DON
Respiratory/Cardiopulmonary . . . . Collie Lairsey

Measure	Cases	This Hospital	State Average	U.S. Average	Top Hospital
Heart Attack Care					
ACE Inhibitor or ARB for LVSD[5]	-	-	78%	82%	100%
Aspirin at Arrival[5]	-	-	91%	92%	100%
Aspirin at Discharge[5]	-	-	87%	90%	100%
Beta Blocker at Arrival[5]	-	-	85%	87%	100%
Beta Blocker at Discharge[5]	-	-	87%	90%	100%
Fibrinolytic Medication Timing[5]	-	-	34%	31%	100%
PCI Within 90 Minutes of Arrival[5]	-	-	47%	54%	95%
Smoking Cessation Advice[5]	-	-	85%	88%	100%

NOTE: Hospital profiles are in alphabetical order by state, then city, then hospital within the city; Rankings are sorted by rate in descending order and exclude hospitals with less than 25 cases; (1) The number of cases is too small (n<25) for purposes of reliably predicting hospital performance; (2) Measure reflects the hospital's indication that its submission was based upon a sample of its relevant discharges; (3) Rate reflects fewer than the maximum possible quarters of data for the measure; (4) Inaccurate information submitted and suppressed for one or more quarters; (5) No data is available from the hospital for this measure; Please refer to the User's Guide for a full explanation of data

Heart Failure Care					
ACE Inhibitor or ARB for LVSD[5]	-	-	81%	82%	100%
Discharge Instructions[5]	-	-	59%	61%	93%
Evaluation of LVS Function[5]	-	-	81%	83%	99%
Smoking Cessation Advice[5]	-	-	86%	82%	100%
Pneumonia Care					
Appropriate Initial Antibiotic[3]	0	-	81%	83%	94%
Blood Culture Timing[3]	0	-	89%	90%	100%
Influenza Vaccine	0	-	60%	70%	100%
Initial Antibiotic Timing[3]	0	-	75%	80%	93%
Oxygenation Assessment[1,3]	1	100%	99%	99%	100%
Pneumococcal Vaccine[3]	0	-	61%	69%	94%
Smoking Cessation Advice[1,3]	1	0%	82%	80%	100%
Surgical Infection Prevention					
Prophylactic Antibiotic Given[5]	-	-	69%	77%	95%
Prophylactic Antibiotic Selection[5]	-	-	89%	90%	100%
Prophylactic Antibiotic Stopped[5]	-	-	71%	72%	95%
Pregnancy Care					
Inpatient Neonatal Mortality	-	-	-	-	-
Third or Fourth Degree Laceration	-	-	3.63%	3.63%	3.27%

Monroe County Hospital

88 Martin Luther King Jr Drive
PO Box 1068
Forsyth, GA 31029
URL: www.monroehospital.org
Ownership: Govt - Hospital District or Authority
Emergency Services: Yes

Phone: 478-994-2521
Fax: 478-994-8798

Accredited: Yes
Licensed Beds: 25

Key Personnel:
President/CEO. . . . . Oliver J Booker
Chief Medical Staff. . . . . John Rogers, MD
Emergency Room . . . . Martha Morton
Emergency Room . . . . Larry Tucker
Infection Control. . . . . Christa Garner
Surgical Services. . . . . Rebecca Kilpatrick
Respiratory/Cardiopulmonary. . . . . Marcia English

Measure	Cases	This Hospital	State Average	U.S. Average	Top Hospital
Heart Attack Care					
ACE Inhibitor or ARB for LVSD[5]	-	-	78%	82%	100%
Aspirin at Arrival[5]	-	-	91%	92%	100%
Aspirin at Discharge[5]	-	-	87%	90%	100%
Beta Blocker at Arrival[5]	-	-	85%	87%	100%
Beta Blocker at Discharge[5]	-	-	87%	90%	100%
Fibrinolytic Medication Timing[5]	-	-	34%	31%	100%
PCI Within 90 Minutes of Arrival[5]	-	-	47%	54%	95%
Smoking Cessation Advice[5]	-	-	85%	88%	100%
Heart Failure Care					
ACE Inhibitor or ARB for LVSD[5]	-	-	81%	82%	100%
Discharge Instructions[5]	-	-	59%	61%	93%
Evaluation of LVS Function[5]	-	-	81%	83%	99%
Smoking Cessation Advice[5]	-	-	86%	82%	100%
Pneumonia Care					
Appropriate Initial Antibiotic	37	84%	81%	83%	94%
Blood Culture Timing[1]	15	80%	89%	90%	100%
Influenza Vaccine[1]	16	6%	60%	70%	100%
Initial Antibiotic Timing	40	68%	75%	80%	93%
Oxygenation Assessment	46	98%	99%	99%	100%
Pneumococcal Vaccine	38	3%	61%	69%	94%
Smoking Cessation Advice[1]	6	0%	82%	80%	100%
Surgical Infection Prevention					
Prophylactic Antibiotic Given[5]	-	-	69%	77%	95%
Prophylactic Antibiotic Selection[5]	-	-	89%	90%	100%
Prophylactic Antibiotic Stopped[5]	-	-	71%	72%	95%
Pregnancy Care					
Inpatient Neonatal Mortality	-	-	-	-	-
Third or Fourth Degree Laceration	-	-	3.63%	3.63%	3.27%

Hutcheson Medical Center

100 Gross Crescent Circle
Fort Oglethorpe
Fort Oglethrope, GA 30742
E-mail: dhardin@hutcheson.org
URL: www.hutcheson.org
Ownership: Govt - Hospital District or Authority
Emergency Services: Yes

Phone: 706-858-2000
Fax: 706-858-2028

Accredited: Yes
Licensed Beds: 179

Key Personnel:
CEO. . . . . Robert T Jones
Chief Medical Staff. . . . . Melissa Phillips, MD
Emergency Room . . . . Debbie Doran, RN
OB/GYN Womens Health. . . . . Sharo Klein, RN
Chief Radiology . . . . Joseph J Busch, MD
Director Respiratory Therapy . . . . Sandy McKenzie

Measure	Cases	This Hospital	State Average	U.S. Average	Top Hospital
Heart Attack Care					
ACE Inhibitor or ARB for LVSD[1]	19	47%	78%	82%	100%
Aspirin at Arrival	78	88%	91%	92%	100%
Aspirin at Discharge	65	60%	87%	90%	100%
Beta Blocker at Arrival	68	69%	85%	87%	100%
Beta Blocker at Discharge	59	54%	87%	90%	100%
Fibrinolytic Medication Timing[1]	17	12%	34%	31%	100%
PCI Within 90 Minutes of Arrival	0	-	47%	54%	95%
Smoking Cessation Advice	25	48%	85%	88%	100%
Heart Failure Care					
ACE Inhibitor or ARB for LVSD	50	66%	81%	82%	100%
Discharge Instructions	222	60%	59%	61%	93%
Evaluation of LVS Function	250	71%	81%	83%	99%
Smoking Cessation Advice	58	57%	86%	82%	100%
Pneumonia Care					
Appropriate Initial Antibiotic	210	60%	81%	83%	94%
Blood Culture Timing	211	89%	89%	90%	100%
Influenza Vaccine	93	18%	60%	70%	100%
Initial Antibiotic Timing	352	74%	75%	80%	93%
Oxygenation Assessment	474	99%	99%	99%	100%
Pneumococcal Vaccine	229	13%	61%	69%	94%
Smoking Cessation Advice	183	40%	82%	80%	100%
Surgical Infection Prevention					
Prophylactic Antibiotic Given[3]	112	62%	69%	77%	95%
Prophylactic Antibiotic Selection	54	93%	89%	90%	100%
Prophylactic Antibiotic Stopped[3]	110	100%	71%	72%	95%
Pregnancy Care					
Inpatient Neonatal Mortality	-	-	-	-	-
Third or Fourth Degree Laceration	-	-	3.63%	3.63%	3.27%

Peach Regional Medical Center

Alternate Name: Peach County Hospital
601 N Camellia Boulevard
Fort Valley, GA 31030
Ownership: Govt - Hospital District or Authority
Emergency Services: Yes

Phone: 478-825-8691
Fax: 478-825-4444
Accredited: Yes
Licensed Beds: 36

Key Personnel:
CEO. . . . . Nancy Peed
Emergency Room . . . . Francis Teed
Emergency Room . . . . Beverly Mitchell, RN
Director Medical/Surgical Nursing . . . . Mary Pope, RN
Director Respiratory Therapy . . . . Colleen Dresslar

Measure	Cases	This Hospital	State Average	U.S. Average	Top Hospital
Heart Attack Care					
ACE Inhibitor or ARB for LVSD[5]	-	-	78%	82%	100%
Aspirin at Arrival[5]	-	-	91%	92%	100%
Aspirin at Discharge[5]	-	-	87%	90%	100%
Beta Blocker at Arrival[5]	-	-	85%	87%	100%
Beta Blocker at Discharge[5]	-	-	87%	90%	100%
Fibrinolytic Medication Timing[5]	-	-	34%	31%	100%
PCI Within 90 Minutes of Arrival[5]	-	-	47%	54%	95%
Smoking Cessation Advice[5]	-	-	85%	88%	100%
Heart Failure Care					
ACE Inhibitor or ARB for LVSD	27	89%	81%	82%	100%
Discharge Instructions	67	52%	59%	61%	93%

NOTE: Hospital profiles are in alphabetical order by state, then city, then hospital within the city; Rankings are sorted by rate in descending order and exclude hospitals with less than 25 cases; (1) The number of cases is too small (n<25) for purposes of reliably predicting hospital performance; (2) Measure reflects the hospital's indication that its submission was based upon a sample of its relevant discharges; (3) Rate reflects fewer than the maximum possible quarters of data for the measure; (4) Inaccurate information submitted and suppressed for one or more quarters; (5) No data is available from the hospital for this measure; Please refer to the User's Guide for a full explanation of data

		This Hospital	State Average	U.S. Average	Top Hospital
Evaluation of LVS Function	76	84%	81%	83%	99%
Smoking Cessation Advice[1]	13	69%	86%	82%	100%
Pneumonia Care					
Appropriate Initial Antibiotic	39	79%	81%	83%	94%
Blood Culture Timing	36	92%	89%	90%	100%
Influenza Vaccine[1]	4	75%	60%	70%	100%
Initial Antibiotic Timing	39	82%	75%	80%	93%
Oxygenation Assessment	44	100%	99%	99%	100%
Pneumococcal Vaccine[1]	14	79%	61%	69%	94%
Smoking Cessation Advice[1]	15	73%	82%	80%	100%
Surgical Infection Prevention					
Prophylactic Antibiotic Given[5]	-	-	69%	77%	95%
Prophylactic Antibiotic Selection[5]	-	-	89%	90%	100%
Prophylactic Antibiotic Stopped[5]	-	-	71%	72%	95%
Pregnancy Care					
Inpatient Neonatal Mortality	-	-	-	-	-
Third or Fourth Degree Laceration	-	-	3.63%	3.63%	3.27%

Northeast Georgia Medical Center

743 Spring Street
Gainesville, GA 30501

Toll-Free: 800-282-0535
Phone: 770-535-3553
Fax: 770-718-5465

URL: www.nghs.com
Ownership: Government - Local
Emergency Services: Yes

Accredited: Yes

Key Personnel:
CEO . . . . John A Ferguson, Jr
Chief Medical Staff . . . . Jeff McIntive, MD
Cardiac Lab . . . . Martha Hemphill
Catheterization Lab . . . . Wanda Hesler
Emergency Room . . . . Sonya Hanock
Infection Control . . . . Lynn Zaricor
ICU . . . . Sheila Sullens
Intensive Coronary Care . . . . Pam Williams
OB/GYN Womens Health . . . . Pat Allen
Respiratory Therapy/Cardiopulmonary . . . . Russ Duteau

Measure	Cases	This Hospital	State Average	U.S. Average	Top Hospital
Heart Attack Care					
ACE Inhibitor or ARB for LVSD	123	89%	78%	82%	100%
Aspirin at Arrival	387	99%	91%	92%	100%
Aspirin at Discharge	560	99%	87%	90%	100%
Beta Blocker at Arrival	327	94%	85%	87%	100%
Beta Blocker at Discharge	558	99%	87%	90%	100%
Fibrinolytic Medication Timing[1]	1	0%	34%	31%	100%
PCI Within 90 Minutes of Arrival[1]	17	76%	47%	54%	95%
Smoking Cessation Advice	227	100%	85%	88%	100%
Heart Failure Care					
ACE Inhibitor or ARB for LVSD	217	75%	81%	82%	100%
Discharge Instructions	474	52%	59%	61%	93%
Evaluation of LVS Function	570	87%	81%	83%	99%
Smoking Cessation Advice	84	98%	86%	82%	100%
Pneumonia Care					
Appropriate Initial Antibiotic	280	86%	81%	83%	94%
Blood Culture Timing	185	88%	89%	90%	100%
Influenza Vaccine	92	65%	60%	70%	100%
Initial Antibiotic Timing	343	90%	75%	80%	93%
Oxygenation Assessment	412	100%	99%	99%	100%
Pneumococcal Vaccine	244	75%	61%	69%	94%
Smoking Cessation Advice	96	96%	82%	80%	100%
Surgical Infection Prevention					
Prophylactic Antibiotic Given[2,3]	79	54%	69%	77%	95%
Prophylactic Antibiotic Selection[5]	-	-	89%	90%	100%
Prophylactic Antibiotic Stopped[2,3]	68	94%	71%	72%	95%
Pregnancy Care					
Inpatient Neonatal Mortality	3,520	0.23%	-	-	-
Third or Fourth Degree Laceration	2,531	2.33%	3.63%	3.63%	3.27%

Spalding Regional Medical Center

601 South 8th Street
Griffin, GA 30224

Phone: 770-228-2721
Fax: 770-229-6953

URL: www.spaldingregional.com
Ownership: Proprietary
Emergency Services: Yes

Accredited: Yes
Licensed Beds: 160

Key Personnel:
CEO . . . . John Quinn
Chief Medical Staff . . . . Vinod C Mehta
Emergency Room . . . . James Totten
Director Respiratory Therapy . . . . George Daniel

Measure	Cases	This Hospital	State Average	U.S. Average	Top Hospital
Heart Attack Care					
ACE Inhibitor or ARB for LVSD[1]	15	87%	78%	82%	100%
Aspirin at Arrival	112	98%	91%	92%	100%
Aspirin at Discharge	44	95%	87%	90%	100%
Beta Blocker at Arrival	107	96%	85%	87%	100%
Beta Blocker at Discharge	43	88%	87%	90%	100%
Fibrinolytic Medication Timing[1]	14	57%	34%	31%	100%
PCI Within 90 Minutes of Arrival	0	-	47%	54%	95%
Smoking Cessation Advice[1]	19	100%	85%	88%	100%
Heart Failure Care					
ACE Inhibitor or ARB for LVSD	146	85%	81%	82%	100%
Discharge Instructions	354	93%	59%	61%	93%
Evaluation of LVS Function	408	95%	81%	83%	99%
Smoking Cessation Advice	111	97%	86%	82%	100%
Pneumonia Care					
Appropriate Initial Antibiotic	224	91%	81%	83%	94%
Blood Culture Timing	188	94%	89%	90%	100%
Influenza Vaccine[4,5]	-	-	60%	70%	100%
Initial Antibiotic Timing	323	84%	75%	80%	93%
Oxygenation Assessment	367	100%	99%	99%	100%
Pneumococcal Vaccine	201	84%	61%	69%	94%
Smoking Cessation Advice	95	95%	82%	80%	100%
Surgical Infection Prevention					
Prophylactic Antibiotic Given[2]	468	94%	69%	77%	95%
Prophylactic Antibiotic Selection[2]	126	94%	89%	90%	100%
Prophylactic Antibiotic Stopped[2]	444	80%	71%	72%	95%
Pregnancy Care					
Inpatient Neonatal Mortality	-	-	-	-	-
Third or Fourth Degree Laceration	-	-	3.63%	3.63%	3.27%

Hart County Hospital

138 W Gibson Street
Hartwell, GA 30643

Phone: 706-856-6100
Fax: 706-856-6294

URL: www.tycobbhealthcaresystem.org
Ownership: Govt - Hospital District or Authority
Emergency Services: Yes

Accredited: Yes
Licensed Beds: 82

Key Personnel:
CEO . . . . Jerry Wise
Chief of Medical Staff . . . . Jonathan Merril
Emergency Room . . . . Gordion Irwin
Director Medical/Surgical Nursing . . . . Carol Bowdoin
Chief Radiology . . . . Wee Whisnent
Director Respiratory Therapy . . . . Sandra Duncan

Measure	Cases	This Hospital	State Average	U.S. Average	Top Hospital
Heart Attack Care					
ACE Inhibitor or ARB for LVSD[1]	3	67%	78%	82%	100%
Aspirin at Arrival[1]	22	77%	91%	92%	100%
Aspirin at Discharge[1]	17	65%	87%	90%	100%
Beta Blocker at Arrival[1]	18	61%	85%	87%	100%
Beta Blocker at Discharge[1]	15	80%	87%	90%	100%
Fibrinolytic Medication Timing[1]	1	0%	34%	31%	100%
PCI Within 90 Minutes of Arrival	0	-	47%	54%	95%
Smoking Cessation Advice[1]	3	100%	85%	88%	100%
Heart Failure Care					
ACE Inhibitor or ARB for LVSD[1]	12	67%	81%	82%	100%
Discharge Instructions	66	61%	59%	61%	93%
Evaluation of LVS Function	94	69%	81%	83%	99%
Smoking Cessation Advice[1]	15	67%	86%	82%	100%
Pneumonia Care					

NOTE: Hospital profiles are in alphabetical order by state, then city, then hospital within the city; Rankings are sorted by rate in descending order and exclude hospitals with less than 25 cases; (1) The number of cases is too small (n<25) for purposes of reliably predicting hospital performance; (2) Measure reflects the hospital's indication that its submission was based upon a sample of its relevant discharges; (3) Rate reflects fewer than the maximum possible quarters of data for the measure; (4) Inaccurate information submitted and suppressed for one or more quarters; (5) No data is available from the hospital for this measure; Please refer to the User's Guide for a full explanation of data

Measure	Cases	This Hospital	State Average	U.S. Average	Top Hospital
Appropriate Initial Antibiotic	45	80%	81%	83%	94%
Blood Culture Timing	29	83%	89%	90%	100%
Influenza Vaccine[4,5]	-	-	60%	70%	100%
Initial Antibiotic Timing	65	85%	75%	80%	93%
Oxygenation Assessment	77	97%	99%	99%	100%
Pneumococcal Vaccine	56	54%	61%	69%	94%
Smoking Cessation Advice[1]	16	50%	82%	80%	100%
Surgical Infection Prevention					
Prophylactic Antibiotic Given[1,3]	6	50%	69%	77%	95%
Prophylactic Antibiotic Selection[1]	6	83%	89%	90%	100%
Prophylactic Antibiotic Stopped[1,3]	6	0%	71%	72%	95%
Pregnancy Care					
Inpatient Neonatal Mortality	-	-	-	-	-
Third or Fourth Degree Laceration	-	-	3.63%	3.63%	3.27%

Taylor Regional Hospital

Highway 341 N Macon Highway
Hawkinsville, GA 31036
URL: www.taylorregional.org
Ownership: Voluntary non-profit - Private
Emergency Services: Yes

Phone: 478-783-0200
Fax: 478-783-2731

Accredited: Yes
Licensed Beds: 55

Key Personnel:
President/CEO . . . . Dan Maddock
Chief Medical Staff . . . . Jack Butler
Emergency Room . . . . William Cirillo, MD
Director Surgical Services . . . . Patricia Mayo
Director Respiratory Therapy . . . . Ken Moore

Measure	Cases	This Hospital	State Average	U.S. Average	Top Hospital
Heart Attack Care					
ACE Inhibitor or ARB for LVSD[1]	2	0%	78%	82%	100%
Aspirin at Arrival[1]	21	90%	91%	92%	100%
Aspirin at Discharge[1]	7	100%	87%	90%	100%
Beta Blocker at Arrival[1]	14	86%	85%	87%	100%
Beta Blocker at Discharge[1]	6	100%	87%	90%	100%
Fibrinolytic Medication Timing[1]	4	25%	34%	31%	100%
PCI Within 90 Minutes of Arrival	0	-	47%	54%	95%
Smoking Cessation Advice	0	-	85%	88%	100%
Heart Failure Care					
ACE Inhibitor or ARB for LVSD	27	85%	81%	82%	100%
Discharge Instructions	64	66%	59%	61%	93%
Evaluation of LVS Function	76	97%	81%	83%	99%
Smoking Cessation Advice[1]	14	57%	86%	82%	100%
Pneumonia Care					
Appropriate Initial Antibiotic	52	69%	81%	83%	94%
Blood Culture Timing	32	94%	89%	90%	100%
Influenza Vaccine[1]	22	55%	60%	70%	100%
Initial Antibiotic Timing	92	70%	75%	80%	93%
Oxygenation Assessment	100	100%	99%	99%	100%
Pneumococcal Vaccine	56	36%	61%	69%	94%
Smoking Cessation Advice[1]	21	52%	82%	80%	100%
Surgical Infection Prevention					
Prophylactic Antibiotic Given[2]	108	94%	69%	77%	95%
Prophylactic Antibiotic Selection[2]	32	100%	89%	90%	100%
Prophylactic Antibiotic Stopped[2]	107	86%	71%	72%	95%
Pregnancy Care					
Inpatient Neonatal Mortality	-	-	-	-	-
Third or Fourth Degree Laceration	-	-	3.63%	3.63%	3.27%

Chatuge Regional Hospital & Nursing Home

110 S Main Street
Hiawassee, GA 30546
Ownership: Govt - Hospital District or Authority
Emergency Services: Yes

Phone: 706-896-2222
Fax: 706-896-7872
Accredited: No
Licensed Beds: 112

Key Personnel:
CEO . . . . Lewis Kelley
Chief Medical Staff . . . . Robert Stahlkuppe, MD
Emergency Room . . . . Robyen Brechbell
Emergency Room . . . . Shirl Dillard, RN
Director Medical/Surgical Nursing . . . . Joy Pippenger, RN
Director Respiratory Therapy . . . . Twila Sellers

Measure	Cases	This Hospital	State Average	U.S. Average	Top Hospital
Heart Attack Care					
ACE Inhibitor or ARB for LVSD	0	-	78%	82%	100%
Aspirin at Arrival[1]	2	100%	91%	92%	100%
Aspirin at Discharge[1]	2	100%	87%	90%	100%
Beta Blocker at Arrival[1]	2	100%	85%	87%	100%
Beta Blocker at Discharge[1]	2	100%	87%	90%	100%
Fibrinolytic Medication Timing	0	-	34%	31%	100%
PCI Within 90 Minutes of Arrival	0	-	47%	54%	95%
Smoking Cessation Advice[1]	1	0%	85%	88%	100%
Heart Failure Care					
ACE Inhibitor or ARB for LVSD[1]	7	71%	81%	82%	100%
Discharge Instructions[1]	20	60%	59%	61%	93%
Evaluation of LVS Function	33	97%	81%	83%	99%
Smoking Cessation Advice[1]	5	60%	86%	82%	100%
Pneumonia Care					
Appropriate Initial Antibiotic	34	100%	81%	83%	94%
Blood Culture Timing	36	97%	89%	90%	100%
Influenza Vaccine[1]	11	100%	60%	70%	100%
Initial Antibiotic Timing	47	87%	75%	80%	93%
Oxygenation Assessment	55	100%	99%	99%	100%
Pneumococcal Vaccine	40	100%	61%	69%	94%
Smoking Cessation Advice[1]	16	88%	82%	80%	100%
Surgical Infection Prevention					
Prophylactic Antibiotic Given[5]	-	-	69%	77%	95%
Prophylactic Antibiotic Selection[5]	-	-	89%	90%	100%
Prophylactic Antibiotic Stopped[5]	-	-	71%	72%	95%
Pregnancy Care					
Inpatient Neonatal Mortality	-	-	-	-	-
Third or Fourth Degree Laceration	-	-	3.63%	3.63%	3.27%

Liberty Regional Medical Center

Alternate Name: Liberty Memorial Hospital
462 EG Miles Parkway
Hinesville, GA 31313
E-mail: mtraylor@libertyregional.org
URL: www.libertyregional.org
Ownership: Govt - Hospital District or Authority
Emergency Services: Yes

Phone: 912-369-9400
Fax: 912-369-3653

Accredited: Yes
Licensed Beds: 25

Key Personnel:
CEO . . . . Scott Kroell
Chief Medical Staff . . . . Nizar Eskander, MD
Director Surgical Services . . . . Gabriele Nielsen, RN, CORN
Director Emergency Room . . . . Renie Weaver
Medical Director ER . . . . Jim Scow, MD
Endoscopy Lab/Director Surgical Services . . . . . Gabriele Nielsen
Director Infection Control . . . . Martha Kitchings
Director Medical Surgical Nursing . . . . Sandy Well, BSN
OB/GYN Women's Health . . . . Seth Borquaye, MD
Director Surgical Services/OR . . . . Gabriele Nielsen
Respiratory/Cardiopulmonary . . . . Tia Bacon

Measure	Cases	This Hospital	State Average	U.S. Average	Top Hospital
Heart Attack Care					
ACE Inhibitor or ARB for LVSD	0	-	78%	82%	100%
Aspirin at Arrival	0	-	91%	92%	100%
Aspirin at Discharge	0	-	87%	90%	100%
Beta Blocker at Arrival	0	-	85%	87%	100%
Beta Blocker at Discharge	0	-	87%	90%	100%
Fibrinolytic Medication Timing	0	-	34%	31%	100%
PCI Within 90 Minutes of Arrival	0	-	47%	54%	95%
Smoking Cessation Advice	0	-	85%	88%	100%
Heart Failure Care					
ACE Inhibitor or ARB for LVSD[1]	6	67%	81%	82%	100%
Discharge Instructions	36	61%	59%	61%	93%
Evaluation of LVS Function	44	55%	81%	83%	99%
Smoking Cessation Advice[1]	11	91%	86%	82%	100%
Pneumonia Care					
Appropriate Initial Antibiotic	52	92%	81%	83%	94%
Blood Culture Timing	30	87%	89%	90%	100%
Influenza Vaccine[1]	12	42%	60%	70%	100%
Initial Antibiotic Timing	80	45%	75%	80%	93%

NOTE: Hospital profiles are in alphabetical order by state, then city, then hospital within the city; Rankings are sorted by rate in descending order and exclude hospitals with less than 25 cases; (1) The number of cases is too small (n<25) for purposes of reliably predicting hospital performance; (2) Measure reflects the hospital's indication that its submission was based upon a sample of its relevant discharges; (3) Rate reflects fewer than the maximum possible quarters of data for the measure; (4) Inaccurate information submitted and suppressed for one or more quarters; (5) No data is available from the hospital for this measure; Please refer to the User's Guide for a full explanation of data

Oxygenation Assessment	91	100%	99%	99%	100%
Pneumococcal Vaccine	38	34%	61%	69%	94%
Smoking Cessation Advice[1]	17	82%	82%	80%	100%
Surgical Infection Prevention					
Prophylactic Antibiotic Given	57	68%	69%	77%	95%
Prophylactic Antibiotic Selection[1]	19	100%	89%	90%	100%
Prophylactic Antibiotic Stopped	50	98%	71%	72%	95%
Pregnancy Care					
Inpatient Neonatal Mortality	-	-	-	-	-
Third or Fourth Degree Laceration	-	-	3.63%	3.63%	3.27%

Clinch Memorial Hospital

524 Carswell Street
PO Box 516
Homerville, GA 31634
Phone: 912-487-5211
Fax: 912-487-3769
Ownership: Govt - Hospital District or Authority
Accredited: No
Emergency Services: Yes
Licensed Beds: 48

Key Personnel:

CEO. . . . . Bill Forbes
Chief Medical Staff. . . . . Samuel Cobarrubias, MD
Emergency Room . . . . Roger Huelsnitz, MD
Chief Radiology . . . . Sarah Bell
Director Respiratory Care. . . . . Kathy Oyester

Measure	Cases	This Hospital	State Average	U.S. Average	Top Hospital
Heart Attack Care					
ACE Inhibitor or ARB for LVSD[5]	-	-	78%	82%	100%
Aspirin at Arrival[5]	-	-	91%	92%	100%
Aspirin at Discharge[5]	-	-	87%	90%	100%
Beta Blocker at Arrival[5]	-	-	85%	87%	100%
Beta Blocker at Discharge[5]	-	-	87%	90%	100%
Fibrinolytic Medication Timing[5]	-	-	34%	31%	100%
PCI Within 90 Minutes of Arrival[5]	-	-	47%	54%	95%
Smoking Cessation Advice[5]	-	-	85%	88%	100%
Heart Failure Care					
ACE Inhibitor or ARB for LVSD[1]	2	50%	81%	82%	100%
Discharge Instructions[1]	16	0%	59%	61%	93%
Evaluation of LVS Function[1]	16	69%	81%	83%	99%
Smoking Cessation Advice[1]	3	67%	86%	82%	100%
Pneumonia Care					
Appropriate Initial Antibiotic[1]	20	95%	81%	83%	94%
Blood Culture Timing[1]	3	100%	89%	90%	100%
Influenza Vaccine[1]	7	43%	60%	70%	100%
Initial Antibiotic Timing[1]	16	81%	75%	80%	93%
Oxygenation Assessment	28	96%	99%	99%	100%
Pneumococcal Vaccine[1]	13	38%	61%	69%	94%
Smoking Cessation Advice[1]	2	0%	82%	80%	100%
Surgical Infection Prevention					
Prophylactic Antibiotic Given[5]	-	-	69%	77%	95%
Prophylactic Antibiotic Selection[5]	-	-	89%	90%	100%
Prophylactic Antibiotic Stopped[5]	-	-	71%	72%	95%
Pregnancy Care					
Inpatient Neonatal Mortality	-	-	-	-	-
Third or Fourth Degree Laceration	-	-	3.63%	3.63%	3.27%

Sylvan Grove Hospital

1050 McDonough Road
Jackson, GA 30233
Phone: 770-775-7861
Fax: 770-775-4478
URL: www.sylvangrovehospital.com
Ownership: Voluntary non-profit - Other
Accredited: No
Emergency Services: Yes
Licensed Beds: 25

Key Personnel:

CEO. . . . . John A Quinn
Chief Medical Staff. . . . . Shashi Madan, MD
Administrator . . . . Edward Whitehouse
Emergency Room . . . . Bernardo Maldonado, MD

Measure	Cases	This Hospital	State Average	U.S. Average	Top Hospital
Heart Attack Care					
ACE Inhibitor or ARB for LVSD[5]	-	-	78%	82%	100%
Aspirin at Arrival[5]	-	-	91%	92%	100%
Aspirin at Discharge[5]	-	-	87%	90%	100%
Beta Blocker at Arrival[5]	-	-	85%	87%	100%
Beta Blocker at Discharge[5]	-	-	87%	90%	100%
Fibrinolytic Medication Timing[5]	-	-	34%	31%	100%
PCI Within 90 Minutes of Arrival[5]	-	-	47%	54%	95%
Smoking Cessation Advice[5]	-	-	85%	88%	100%
Heart Failure Care					
ACE Inhibitor or ARB for LVSD[3]	0	-	81%	82%	100%
Discharge Instructions[1,3]	6	83%	59%	61%	93%
Evaluation of LVS Function[1,3]	10	50%	81%	83%	99%
Smoking Cessation Advice[1,3]	3	100%	86%	82%	100%
Pneumonia Care					
Appropriate Initial Antibiotic[1]	18	100%	81%	83%	94%
Blood Culture Timing[1]	12	100%	89%	90%	100%
Influenza Vaccine[1]	2	50%	60%	70%	100%
Initial Antibiotic Timing[1]	17	100%	75%	80%	93%
Oxygenation Assessment	25	100%	99%	99%	100%
Pneumococcal Vaccine[1]	11	91%	61%	69%	94%
Smoking Cessation Advice[1]	5	100%	82%	80%	100%
Surgical Infection Prevention					
Prophylactic Antibiotic Given[5]	-	-	69%	77%	95%
Prophylactic Antibiotic Selection[5]	-	-	89%	90%	100%
Prophylactic Antibiotic Stopped[5]	-	-	71%	72%	95%
Pregnancy Care					
Inpatient Neonatal Mortality	-	-	-	-	-
Third or Fourth Degree Laceration	-	-	3.63%	3.63%	3.27%

Piedmont Mountainside Hospital

Alternate Name: Pickens General Hospital
1266 E Church Street
PO Box 730
Jasper, GA 30143
Phone: 706-692-2441
Fax: 706-692-0939
E-mail: mtside@mindspring.com
URL: www.mmcjasp.com
Ownership: Voluntary non-profit - Other
Accredited: Yes
Emergency Services: Yes
Licensed Beds: 40

Key Personnel:

CEO. . . . . Earl Whiteley
Chief Medical Staff. . . . . Vincent Moliari, MD
Infection Control. . . . . Marianne Gaeland, RN
ICU . . . . Linda Hughes
Director Medical/Surgical Nursing . . . . Linda Hughes, RN
OB/GYN Womens Health. . . . . Barbara Hollinsworth, RN
Respiratory Therapy. . . . . Michael Robertson

Measure	Cases	This Hospital	State Average	U.S. Average	Top Hospital
Heart Attack Care					
ACE Inhibitor or ARB for LVSD[1]	2	100%	78%	82%	100%
Aspirin at Arrival[1]	10	100%	91%	92%	100%
Aspirin at Discharge[1]	7	86%	87%	90%	100%
Beta Blocker at Arrival[1]	12	100%	85%	87%	100%
Beta Blocker at Discharge[1]	8	100%	87%	90%	100%
Fibrinolytic Medication Timing	0	-	34%	31%	100%
PCI Within 90 Minutes of Arrival	0	-	47%	54%	95%
Smoking Cessation Advice[1]	1	100%	85%	88%	100%
Heart Failure Care					
ACE Inhibitor or ARB for LVSD[1]	14	86%	81%	82%	100%
Discharge Instructions	87	44%	59%	61%	93%
Evaluation of LVS Function	102	87%	81%	83%	99%
Smoking Cessation Advice	28	79%	86%	82%	100%
Pneumonia Care					
Appropriate Initial Antibiotic	149	77%	81%	83%	94%
Blood Culture Timing	75	92%	89%	90%	100%
Influenza Vaccine	44	48%	60%	70%	100%
Initial Antibiotic Timing	145	66%	75%	80%	93%
Oxygenation Assessment	187	99%	99%	99%	100%
Pneumococcal Vaccine	118	51%	61%	69%	94%
Smoking Cessation Advice	40	92%	82%	80%	100%
Surgical Infection Prevention					
Prophylactic Antibiotic Given	126	79%	69%	77%	95%
Prophylactic Antibiotic Selection	30	80%	89%	90%	100%
Prophylactic Antibiotic Stopped	120	62%	71%	72%	95%
Pregnancy Care					
Inpatient Neonatal Mortality	-	-	-	-	-

NOTE: Hospital profiles are in alphabetical order by state, then city, then hospital within the city; Rankings are sorted by rate in descending order and exclude hospitals with less than 25 cases; (1) The number of cases is too small (n<25) for purposes of reliably predicting hospital performance; (2) Measure reflects the hospital's indication that its submission was based upon a sample of its relevant discharges; (3) Rate reflects fewer than the maximum possible quarters of data for the measure; (4) Inaccurate information submitted and suppressed for one or more quarters; (5) No data is available from the hospital for this measure; Please refer to the User's Guide for a full explanation of data

Third or Fourth Degree Laceration	-	-	3.63%	3.63%	3.27%

Wayne Memorial Hospital

865 S 1st Street   Phone: 912-427-6811
Jesup, GA 31545   Fax: 912-530-3495
URL: www.wmhweb.com
Ownership: Govt - Hospital District or Authority   Accredited: Yes
Emergency Services: Yes   Licensed Beds: 85
Key Personnel:
Administrator/CEO . . . . Charles R Morgan, III
Chief Medical Staff . . . . Jose Delacruz, MD
Emergency Room . . . . Annette Kirksey, DON/RN
Infection Control . . . . Sue Williamson, RN
Intensive Coronary Care . . . . Deborah Wasdin, RN
Medical Surgical Nursing . . . . Lisa Mosely, RN
OB/GYN Womens Health . . . . Michelle Elder, RN
Respiratory/Cardiopulmonary . . . . Carol Hairred

Measure	Cases	This Hospital	State Average	U.S. Average	Top Hospital
Heart Attack Care					
ACE Inhibitor or ARB for LVSD[1]	2	100%	78%	82%	100%
Aspirin at Arrival[1]	22	95%	91%	92%	100%
Aspirin at Discharge[1]	9	78%	87%	90%	100%
Beta Blocker at Arrival[1]	21	86%	85%	87%	100%
Beta Blocker at Discharge[1]	9	78%	87%	90%	100%
Fibrinolytic Medication Timing	0	-	34%	31%	100%
PCI Within 90 Minutes of Arrival	0	-	47%	54%	95%
Smoking Cessation Advice[1]	1	100%	85%	88%	100%
Heart Failure Care					
ACE Inhibitor or ARB for LVSD	54	93%	81%	82%	100%
Discharge Instructions	103	98%	59%	61%	93%
Evaluation of LVS Function	124	86%	81%	83%	99%
Smoking Cessation Advice	25	100%	86%	82%	100%
Pneumonia Care					
Appropriate Initial Antibiotic	40	90%	81%	83%	94%
Blood Culture Timing	34	97%	89%	90%	100%
Influenza Vaccine[1]	7	86%	60%	70%	100%
Initial Antibiotic Timing	55	95%	75%	80%	93%
Oxygenation Assessment	65	100%	99%	99%	100%
Pneumococcal Vaccine	33	82%	61%	69%	94%
Smoking Cessation Advice[1]	18	100%	82%	80%	100%
Surgical Infection Prevention					
Prophylactic Antibiotic Given[3]	29	97%	69%	77%	95%
Prophylactic Antibiotic Selection	31	94%	89%	90%	100%
Prophylactic Antibiotic Stopped[3]	28	100%	71%	72%	95%
Pregnancy Care					
Inpatient Neonatal Mortality	-	-	-	-	-
Third or Fourth Degree Laceration	-	-	3.63%	3.63%	3.27%

West Georgia Medical Center

1514 Vernon Road   Phone: 706-882-1411
La Grange, GA 30240   Fax: 706-845-8918
E-mail: info@wghs.org
URL: www.wghs.org
Ownership: Govt - Hospital District or Authority   Accredited: Yes
Emergency Services: Yes   Licensed Beds: 276
Key Personnel:
President/CEO . . . . Gerald N Fulks
Medical/Surgical Nursing . . . . Tracy Stribling, RN
OB/GYN Womens Health . . . . Kathy Hammock
Respiratory/Cardiopulmonary . . . . Ralph Duraski

Measure	Cases	This Hospital	State Average	U.S. Average	Top Hospital
Heart Attack Care					
ACE Inhibitor or ARB for LVSD[1]	24	96%	78%	82%	100%
Aspirin at Arrival	140	100%	91%	92%	100%
Aspirin at Discharge	63	100%	87%	90%	100%
Beta Blocker at Arrival	110	98%	85%	87%	100%
Beta Blocker at Discharge	68	100%	87%	90%	100%
Fibrinolytic Medication Timing[1]	18	44%	34%	31%	100%
PCI Within 90 Minutes of Arrival[1]	1	0%	47%	54%	95%
Smoking Cessation Advice	36	100%	85%	88%	100%
Heart Failure Care					

ACE Inhibitor or ARB for LVSD	150	77%	81%	82%	100%
Discharge Instructions	253	81%	59%	61%	93%
Evaluation of LVS Function	285	93%	81%	83%	99%
Smoking Cessation Advice	55	100%	86%	82%	100%
Pneumonia Care					
Appropriate Initial Antibiotic	181	90%	81%	83%	94%
Blood Culture Timing	142	86%	89%	90%	100%
Influenza Vaccine	49	78%	60%	70%	100%
Initial Antibiotic Timing	259	86%	75%	80%	93%
Oxygenation Assessment	288	100%	99%	99%	100%
Pneumococcal Vaccine	153	68%	61%	69%	94%
Smoking Cessation Advice	67	99%	82%	80%	100%
Surgical Infection Prevention					
Prophylactic Antibiotic Given[2,3]	86	90%	69%	77%	95%
Prophylactic Antibiotic Selection[2]	74	88%	89%	90%	100%
Prophylactic Antibiotic Stopped[2,3]	84	82%	71%	72%	95%
Pregnancy Care					
Inpatient Neonatal Mortality	-	-	-	-	-
Third or Fourth Degree Laceration	-	-	3.63%	3.63%	3.27%

Promina Gwinnett Health System

Alternate Name: Gwinnett Medical Center
1000 Medical Center Boulevard   Phone: 678-442-4321
Lawrenceville, GA 30045   Fax: 770-682-2257
URL: www.gwinnetthealth.org
Ownership: Govt - Hospital District or Authority   Accredited: Yes
Emergency Services: Yes   Licensed Beds: 479
Key Personnel:
President/CEO . . . . Franklin M Rinker
Chief Medical Staff . . . . Spencer Rozin, MD
Surgical Services . . . . Mary Nash

Measure	Cases	This Hospital	State Average	U.S. Average	Top Hospital
Heart Attack Care					
ACE Inhibitor or ARB for LVSD[2]	25	76%	78%	82%	100%
Aspirin at Arrival[2]	225	92%	91%	92%	100%
Aspirin at Discharge[2]	81	94%	87%	90%	100%
Beta Blocker at Arrival[2]	199	94%	85%	87%	100%
Beta Blocker at Discharge[2]	91	97%	87%	90%	100%
Fibrinolytic Medication Timing[2]	47	64%	34%	31%	100%
PCI Within 90 Minutes of Arrival[2]	0	-	47%	54%	95%
Smoking Cessation Advice[1,2]	13	92%	85%	88%	100%
Heart Failure Care					
ACE Inhibitor or ARB for LVSD[2]	159	93%	81%	82%	100%
Discharge Instructions[2]	370	75%	59%	61%	93%
Evaluation of LVS Function[2]	435	99%	81%	83%	99%
Smoking Cessation Advice[2]	76	99%	86%	82%	100%
Pneumonia Care					
Appropriate Initial Antibiotic[2]	283	96%	81%	83%	94%
Blood Culture Timing[2]	289	86%	89%	90%	100%
Influenza Vaccine[2]	62	89%	60%	70%	100%
Initial Antibiotic Timing[2]	377	78%	75%	80%	93%
Oxygenation Assessment[2]	450	100%	99%	99%	100%
Pneumococcal Vaccine[2]	241	91%	61%	69%	94%
Smoking Cessation Advice[2]	107	100%	82%	80%	100%
Surgical Infection Prevention					
Prophylactic Antibiotic Given[2,3]	68	90%	69%	77%	95%
Prophylactic Antibiotic Selection[2]	68	71%	89%	90%	100%
Prophylactic Antibiotic Stopped[2,3]	67	88%	71%	72%	95%
Pregnancy Care					
Inpatient Neonatal Mortality	-	-	-	-	-
Third or Fourth Degree Laceration	-	-	3.63%	3.63%	3.27%

Dekalb Medical Center at Hillandale

2801 Dekalb Medical Parkway   Phone: 404-501-8040
Lithonia, GA 30058
Ownership: Govt - Hospital District or Authority   Accredited: Yes
Emergency Services: No

Measure	Cases	This Hospital	State Average	U.S. Average	Top Hospital
Heart Attack Care					
ACE Inhibitor or ARB for LVSD[1]	7	86%	78%	82%	100%

NOTE: Hospital profiles are in alphabetical order by state, then city, then hospital within the city; Rankings are sorted by rate in descending order and exclude hospitals with less than 25 cases; (1) The number of cases is too small (n<25) for purposes of reliably predicting hospital performance; (2) Measure reflects the hospital's indication that its submission was based upon a sample of its relevant discharges; (3) Rate reflects fewer than the maximum possible quarters of data for the measure; (4) Inaccurate information submitted and suppressed for one or more quarters; (5) No data is available from the hospital for this measure; Please refer to the User's Guide for a full explanation of data

Aspirin at Arrival	36	94%	91%	92%	100%
Aspirin at Discharge[1]	16	69%	87%	90%	100%
Beta Blocker at Arrival	34	91%	85%	87%	100%
Beta Blocker at Discharge[1]	17	65%	87%	90%	100%
Fibrinolytic Medication Timing[1]	6	17%	34%	31%	100%
PCI Within 90 Minutes of Arrival	0	-	47%	54%	95%
Smoking Cessation Advice[1]	2	100%	85%	88%	100%

Heart Failure Care

ACE Inhibitor or ARB for LVSD	70	86%	81%	82%	100%
Discharge Instructions	136	48%	59%	61%	93%
Evaluation of LVS Function	139	93%	81%	83%	99%
Smoking Cessation Advice	39	100%	86%	82%	100%

Pneumonia Care

Appropriate Initial Antibiotic	71	80%	81%	83%	94%
Blood Culture Timing	64	75%	89%	90%	100%
Influenza Vaccine[1]	9	11%	60%	70%	100%
Initial Antibiotic Timing	82	63%	75%	80%	93%
Oxygenation Assessment	95	100%	99%	99%	100%
Pneumococcal Vaccine	40	30%	61%	69%	94%
Smoking Cessation Advice	25	100%	82%	80%	100%

Surgical Infection Prevention

Prophylactic Antibiotic Given[2]	97	64%	69%	77%	95%
Prophylactic Antibiotic Selection[2]	26	81%	89%	90%	100%
Prophylactic Antibiotic Stopped[2]	93	57%	71%	72%	95%

Pregnancy Care

Inpatient Neonatal Mortality	-	-	-	-	-
Third or Fourth Degree Laceration	-	-	3.63%	3.63%	3.27%

Jefferson Hospital

1067 Peachtree Street
Louisville, GA 30434
Ownership: Govt - Hospital District or Authority
Emergency Services: Yes
Key Personnel:
Administrator . . . . Rita Culvern

Phone: 478-625-7000
Fax: 478-625-7446
Accredited: Yes
Licensed Beds: 37

Measure	Cases	This Hospital	State Average	U.S. Average	Top Hospital
Heart Attack Care					
ACE Inhibitor or ARB for LVSD[3]	0	-	78%	82%	100%
Aspirin at Arrival[3]	0	-	91%	92%	100%
Aspirin at Discharge[3]	0	-	87%	90%	100%
Beta Blocker at Arrival[3]	0	-	85%	87%	100%
Beta Blocker at Discharge[3]	0	-	87%	90%	100%
Fibrinolytic Medication Timing[1,3]	1	0%	34%	31%	100%
PCI Within 90 Minutes of Arrival	0	-	47%	54%	95%
Smoking Cessation Advice[3]	0	-	85%	88%	100%
Heart Failure Care					
ACE Inhibitor or ARB for LVSD[1]	16	100%	81%	82%	100%
Discharge Instructions	64	75%	59%	61%	93%
Evaluation of LVS Function	78	62%	81%	83%	99%
Smoking Cessation Advice[1]	7	43%	86%	82%	100%
Pneumonia Care					
Appropriate Initial Antibiotic	47	79%	81%	83%	94%
Blood Culture Timing	33	82%	89%	90%	100%
Influenza Vaccine[1]	12	33%	60%	70%	100%
Initial Antibiotic Timing	77	78%	75%	80%	93%
Oxygenation Assessment	86	94%	99%	99%	100%
Pneumococcal Vaccine	48	44%	61%	69%	94%
Smoking Cessation Advice[1]	17	59%	82%	80%	100%
Surgical Infection Prevention					
Prophylactic Antibiotic Given[5]	-	-	69%	77%	95%
Prophylactic Antibiotic Selection[5]	-	-	89%	90%	100%
Prophylactic Antibiotic Stopped[5]	-	-	71%	72%	95%
Pregnancy Care					
Inpatient Neonatal Mortality	-	-	-	-	-
Third or Fourth Degree Laceration	-	-	3.63%	3.63%	3.27%

Coliseum Medical Center

350 Hospital Drive
Macon, GA 31217
Ownership: Voluntary non-profit - Private
Emergency Services: Yes
Key Personnel:
President/CEO . . . . Timothy C Tobin
Emergency Room . . . . Dan Weathers, MD

Phone: 478-765-7000
Fax: 478-751-0424
Accredited: Yes
Licensed Beds: 250

Measure	Cases	This Hospital	State Average	U.S. Average	Top Hospital
Heart Attack Care					
ACE Inhibitor or ARB for LVSD	49	55%	78%	82%	100%
Aspirin at Arrival	73	90%	91%	92%	100%
Aspirin at Arrival	123	93%	87%	90%	100%
Beta Blocker at Arrival	71	87%	85%	87%	100%
Beta Blocker at Discharge	133	86%	87%	90%	100%
Fibrinolytic Medication Timing[1]	2	50%	34%	31%	100%
PCI Within 90 Minutes of Arrival[1]	3	33%	47%	54%	95%
Smoking Cessation Advice	44	98%	85%	88%	100%
Heart Failure Care					
ACE Inhibitor or ARB for LVSD	94	69%	81%	82%	100%
Discharge Instructions	229	49%	59%	61%	93%
Evaluation of LVS Function	253	82%	81%	83%	99%
Smoking Cessation Advice	58	100%	86%	82%	100%
Pneumonia Care					
Appropriate Initial Antibiotic	131	85%	81%	83%	94%
Blood Culture Timing	109	87%	89%	90%	100%
Influenza Vaccine	44	73%	60%	70%	100%
Initial Antibiotic Timing	195	72%	75%	80%	93%
Oxygenation Assessment	214	98%	99%	99%	100%
Pneumococcal Vaccine	123	80%	61%	69%	94%
Smoking Cessation Advice	60	100%	82%	80%	100%
Surgical Infection Prevention					
Prophylactic Antibiotic Given[2,3]	230	76%	69%	77%	95%
Prophylactic Antibiotic Selection[2]	101	93%	89%	90%	100%
Prophylactic Antibiotic Stopped[2,3]	215	68%	71%	72%	95%
Pregnancy Care					
Inpatient Neonatal Mortality	-	-	-	-	-
Third or Fourth Degree Laceration	-	-	3.63%	3.63%	3.27%

Macon Northside Hospital

Alternate Name: Coliseum Northside Hospital
400 Charter Boulevard
Macon, GA 31210
Ownership: Proprietary
Emergency Services: Yes
Key Personnel:
CEO . . . . Bud Costello
Chief Medical Staff . . . . Susan Oliver, MD
Emergency Room . . . . Mary Stone, RN
OB/GYN Womens Health . . . . Frank Bixler
Chief Radiology . . . . Arthur McCain, MD
Director Respiratory Therapy . . . . Susan Downing

Phone: 478-757-8200
Fax: 478-751-0424
Accredited: Yes
Licensed Beds: 103

Measure	Cases	This Hospital	State Average	U.S. Average	Top Hospital
Heart Attack Care					
ACE Inhibitor or ARB for LVSD[1]	2	100%	78%	82%	100%
Aspirin at Arrival[1]	9	89%	91%	92%	100%
Aspirin at Discharge[1]	4	100%	87%	90%	100%
Beta Blocker at Arrival[1]	4	100%	85%	87%	100%
Beta Blocker at Discharge[1]	6	83%	87%	90%	100%
Fibrinolytic Medication Timing[1]	1	0%	34%	31%	100%
PCI Within 90 Minutes of Arrival	0	-	47%	54%	95%
Smoking Cessation Advice[1]	1	100%	85%	88%	100%
Heart Failure Care					
ACE Inhibitor or ARB for LVSD	47	74%	81%	82%	100%
Discharge Instructions	109	72%	59%	61%	93%
Evaluation of LVS Function	128	82%	81%	83%	99%
Smoking Cessation Advice	34	100%	86%	82%	100%
Pneumonia Care					
Appropriate Initial Antibiotic	51	86%	81%	83%	94%
Blood Culture Timing	58	93%	89%	90%	100%
Influenza Vaccine	26	62%	60%	70%	100%

NOTE: Hospital profiles are in alphabetical order by state, then city, then hospital within the city; Rankings are sorted by rate in descending order and exclude hospitals with less than 25 cases; (1) The number of cases is too small (n<25) for purposes of reliably predicting hospital performance; (2) Measure reflects the hospital's indication that its submission was based upon a sample of its relevant discharges; (3) Rate reflects fewer than the maximum possible quarters of data for the measure; (4) Inaccurate information submitted and suppressed for one or more quarters; (5) No data is available from the hospital for this measure; Please refer to the User's Guide for a full explanation of data

Initial Antibiotic Timing	86	73%	75%	80%	93%
Oxygenation Assessment	107	100%	99%	99%	100%
Pneumococcal Vaccine	68	76%	61%	69%	94%
Smoking Cessation Advice	32	100%	82%	80%	100%
Surgical Infection Prevention					
Prophylactic Antibiotic Given[2,3]	74	50%	69%	77%	95%
Prophylactic Antibiotic Selection[2]	26	92%	89%	90%	100%
Prophylactic Antibiotic Stopped[2,3]	81	80%	71%	72%	95%
Pregnancy Care					
Inpatient Neonatal Mortality	-	-	-	-	-
Third or Fourth Degree Laceration	-	-	3.63%	3.63%	3.27%

Medical Center of Central Georgia

777 Hemlock Street
Macon, GA 31201
URL: www.mccg.org
Ownership: Govt - Hospital District or Authority
Emergency Services: Yes

Phone: 478-633-1000
Fax: 478-633-1772

Accredited: Yes
Licensed Beds: 518

Key Personnel:
Administrator/President . . . . A Donald Faulk, Jr
Chief Medical Staff. . . . . John Hudson, MD
Chief Catheterization Laboratory . . . . Steve Nola
Emergency Room . . . . Ralph C Griffin, MD
Director Infection/Disease Control . . . . Nancy Dunham
CCU Spvg. Nurse . . . . LaVonne Harn, RN
Director Medical/Surgical Nursing . . . . Lavonne Harn, RN
OB/GYN Womens Health. . . . . John Suma
Chief Radiology . . . . Lee H Hall
Director Respiratory Therapy . . . . Jim Kurish

Measure	Cases	This Hospital	State Average	U.S. Average	Top Hospital
Heart Attack Care					
ACE Inhibitor or ARB for LVSD[2]	84	58%	78%	82%	100%
Aspirin at Arrival[2]	121	97%	91%	92%	100%
Aspirin at Discharge[2]	236	90%	87%	90%	100%
Beta Blocker at Arrival[2]	88	93%	85%	87%	100%
Beta Blocker at Discharge[2]	265	94%	87%	90%	100%
Fibrinolytic Medication Timing[1,2]	1	0%	34%	31%	100%
PCI Within 90 Minutes of Arrival[1,2]	7	57%	47%	54%	95%
Smoking Cessation Advice[2]	92	98%	85%	88%	100%
Heart Failure Care					
ACE Inhibitor or ARB for LVSD[2]	157	78%	81%	82%	100%
Discharge Instructions[2]	241	50%	59%	61%	93%
Evaluation of LVS Function[2]	284	93%	81%	83%	99%
Smoking Cessation Advice[2]	50	90%	86%	82%	100%
Pneumonia Care					
Appropriate Initial Antibiotic[2]	80	86%	81%	83%	94%
Blood Culture Timing[2]	106	90%	89%	90%	100%
Influenza Vaccine[2]	25	44%	60%	70%	100%
Initial Antibiotic Timing[2]	150	64%	75%	80%	93%
Oxygenation Assessment[2]	174	100%	99%	99%	100%
Pneumococcal Vaccine[2]	86	55%	61%	69%	94%
Smoking Cessation Advice[2]	51	92%	82%	80%	100%
Surgical Infection Prevention					
Prophylactic Antibiotic Given[2,3]	266	71%	69%	77%	95%
Prophylactic Antibiotic Selection[2]	117	79%	89%	90%	100%
Prophylactic Antibiotic Stopped[2,3]	255	47%	71%	72%	95%
Pregnancy Care					
Inpatient Neonatal Mortality	-	-	-	-	-
Third or Fourth Degree Laceration	-	-	3.63%	3.63%	3.27%

WellStar Kennestone Hospital

677 Church Street
Marietta, GA 30060
URL: www.wellstar.org
Ownership: Voluntary non-profit - Other
Emergency Services: Yes

Phone: 770-793-5000

Accredited: Yes
Licensed Beds: 455

Key Personnel:
President/CEO. . . . . Paul Johnson
Chief Medical Staff. Mark Hanley
Emergency Room . . . . John Law

Measure	Cases	This Hospital	State Average	U.S. Average	Top Hospital

Heart Attack Care					
ACE Inhibitor or ARB for LVSD[2]	159	84%	78%	82%	100%
Aspirin at Arrival[2]	494	97%	91%	92%	100%
Aspirin at Discharge[2]	607	96%	87%	90%	100%
Beta Blocker at Arrival[2]	382	95%	85%	87%	100%
Beta Blocker at Discharge[2]	605	97%	87%	90%	100%
Fibrinolytic Medication Timing[2]	0	-	34%	31%	100%
PCI Within 90 Minutes of Arrival[2]	25	64%	47%	54%	95%
Smoking Cessation Advice[2]	207	96%	85%	88%	100%
Heart Failure Care					
ACE Inhibitor or ARB for LVSD[2]	332	80%	81%	82%	100%
Discharge Instructions[2]	698	50%	59%	61%	93%
Evaluation of LVS Function[2]	770	98%	81%	83%	99%
Smoking Cessation Advice[2]	174	97%	86%	82%	100%
Pneumonia Care					
Appropriate Initial Antibiotic[2]	354	81%	81%	83%	94%
Blood Culture Timing[2]	367	89%	89%	90%	100%
Influenza Vaccine[2]	97	57%	60%	70%	100%
Initial Antibiotic Timing[2]	503	63%	75%	80%	93%
Oxygenation Assessment[2]	624	100%	99%	99%	100%
Pneumococcal Vaccine[2]	333	54%	61%	69%	94%
Smoking Cessation Advice[2]	145	91%	82%	80%	100%
Surgical Infection Prevention					
Prophylactic Antibiotic Given[3]	181	87%	69%	77%	95%
Prophylactic Antibiotic Selection	184	91%	89%	90%	100%
Prophylactic Antibiotic Stopped[3]	178	78%	71%	72%	95%
Pregnancy Care					
Inpatient Neonatal Mortality	-	-	-	-	-
Third or Fourth Degree Laceration	-	-	3.63%	3.63%	3.27%

Tailor Telfair Regional Hospital

Alternate Name: Three Rivers Hospital and Medical Center
Route 1
Box 150
McRae, GA 31055
Ownership: Voluntary non-profit - Private
Emergency Services: Yes

Phone: 229-868-5621
Fax: 229-868-2574

Accredited: Yes
Licensed Beds: 25

Key Personnel:
CEO. . . . . John Hartley
Chief Medical Staff. Larth Kasir
Infection Control Manager . . . . Dolores Payne, RN
Director of Pulmonary . . . . Tracey Miller

Measure	Cases	This Hospital	State Average	U.S. Average	Top Hospital
Heart Attack Care					
ACE Inhibitor or ARB for LVSD[5]	-	-	78%	82%	100%
Aspirin at Arrival[5]	-	-	91%	92%	100%
Aspirin at Discharge[5]	-	-	87%	90%	100%
Beta Blocker at Arrival[5]	-	-	85%	87%	100%
Beta Blocker at Discharge[5]	-	-	87%	90%	100%
Fibrinolytic Medication Timing[5]	-	-	34%	31%	100%
PCI Within 90 Minutes of Arrival[5]	-	-	47%	54%	95%
Smoking Cessation Advice[5]	-	-	85%	88%	100%
Heart Failure Care					
ACE Inhibitor or ARB for LVSD[1]	1	100%	81%	82%	100%
Discharge Instructions	26	38%	59%	61%	93%
Evaluation of LVS Function	39	26%	81%	83%	99%
Smoking Cessation Advice[1]	9	67%	86%	82%	100%
Pneumonia Care					
Appropriate Initial Antibiotic	29	31%	81%	83%	94%
Blood Culture Timing[1]	6	100%	89%	90%	100%
Influenza Vaccine[1]	5	100%	60%	70%	100%
Initial Antibiotic Timing[1]	18	78%	75%	80%	93%
Oxygenation Assessment	34	97%	99%	99%	100%
Pneumococcal Vaccine[1]	20	55%	61%	69%	94%
Smoking Cessation Advice[1]	4	75%	82%	80%	100%
Surgical Infection Prevention					
Prophylactic Antibiotic Given[5]	-	-	69%	77%	95%
Prophylactic Antibiotic Selection[5]	-	-	89%	90%	100%
Prophylactic Antibiotic Stopped[5]	-	-	71%	72%	95%
Pregnancy Care					
Inpatient Neonatal Mortality	-	-	-	-	-

NOTE: Hospital profiles are in alphabetical order by state, then city, then hospital within the city; Rankings are sorted by rate in descending order and exclude hospitals with less than 25 cases; (1) The number of cases is too small (n<25) for purposes of reliably predicting hospital performance; (2) Measure reflects the hospital's indication that its submission was based upon a sample of its relevant discharges; (3) Rate reflects fewer than the maximum possible quarters of data for the measure; (4) Inaccurate information submitted and suppressed for one or more quarters; (5) No data is available from the hospital for this measure; Please refer to the User's Guide for a full explanation of data

Third or Fourth Degree Laceration	-	-	3.63%	3.63%	3.27%

Candler County Hospital

400 Cedar Street
PO Box 597
Metter, GA 30439
E-mail: cchospital@pineland.net
URL: www.candlercountyhospital.com
Ownership: Govt - Hospital District or Authority
Emergency Services: Yes

Phone: 912-685-5741
Fax: 912-685-3905

Accredited: Yes
Licensed Beds: 60

Key Personnel:
CEO. . . . . Mike Alexander
Emergency Room . . . . Dorsey Smith, MD
Infection Control. . . . . Teal Jeffers, RN
Respiratory . . . . Felicia Guilford

Measure	Cases	This Hospital	State Average	U.S. Average	Top Hospital
Heart Attack Care					
ACE Inhibitor or ARB for LVSD[3]	0	-	78%	82%	100%
Aspirin at Arrival[1,3]	1	100%	91%	92%	100%
Aspirin at Discharge[1,3]	1	100%	87%	90%	100%
Beta Blocker at Arrival[1,3]	1	100%	85%	87%	100%
Beta Blocker at Discharge[1,3]	1	100%	87%	90%	100%
Fibrinolytic Medication Timing[3]	0	-	34%	31%	100%
PCI Within 90 Minutes of Arrival	0	-	47%	54%	95%
Smoking Cessation Advice[3]	0	-	85%	88%	100%
Heart Failure Care					
ACE Inhibitor or ARB for LVSD[1]	4	100%	81%	82%	100%
Discharge Instructions	46	41%	59%	61%	93%
Evaluation of LVS Function	68	15%	81%	83%	99%
Smoking Cessation Advice[1]	13	77%	86%	82%	100%
Pneumonia Care					
Appropriate Initial Antibiotic	34	71%	81%	83%	94%
Blood Culture Timing[1]	19	100%	89%	90%	100%
Influenza Vaccine[1]	8	75%	60%	70%	100%
Initial Antibiotic Timing	56	75%	75%	80%	93%
Oxygenation Assessment	63	100%	99%	99%	100%
Pneumococcal Vaccine	25	48%	61%	69%	94%
Smoking Cessation Advice[1]	12	92%	82%	80%	100%
Surgical Infection Prevention					
Prophylactic Antibiotic Given[5]	-	-	69%	77%	95%
Prophylactic Antibiotic Selection[5]	-	-	89%	90%	100%
Prophylactic Antibiotic Stopped[5]	-	-	71%	72%	95%
Pregnancy Care					
Inpatient Neonatal Mortality	-	-	-	-	-
Third or Fourth Degree Laceration	-	-	3.63%	3.63%	3.27%

Oconee Regional Medical Center

821 N Cobb Street
Milledgeville, GA 31061
Ownership: Voluntary non-profit - Private
Emergency Services: Yes

Phone: 478-454-3500
Fax: 478-454-3555
Accredited: Yes
Licensed Beds: 160

Key Personnel:
CEO. . . . . Brian L Riddle
Chief Radiology . . . . Bill Coleman
Director Respiratory Therapy . . . . Greg Seals

Measure	Cases	This Hospital	State Average	U.S. Average	Top Hospital
Heart Attack Care					
ACE Inhibitor or ARB for LVSD[1]	7	71%	78%	82%	100%
Aspirin at Arrival	34	97%	91%	92%	100%
Aspirin at Discharge[1]	10	70%	87%	90%	100%
Beta Blocker at Arrival	29	86%	85%	87%	100%
Beta Blocker at Discharge[1]	11	64%	87%	90%	100%
Fibrinolytic Medication Timing[1]	1	0%	34%	31%	100%
PCI Within 90 Minutes of Arrival	0	-	47%	54%	95%
Smoking Cessation Advice[1]	2	100%	85%	88%	100%
Heart Failure Care					
ACE Inhibitor or ARB for LVSD	107	85%	81%	82%	100%
Discharge Instructions	184	67%	59%	61%	93%
Evaluation of LVS Function	198	92%	81%	83%	99%
Smoking Cessation Advice	42	83%	86%	82%	100%

Pneumonia Care					
Appropriate Initial Antibiotic	126	84%	81%	83%	94%
Blood Culture Timing	146	86%	89%	90%	100%
Influenza Vaccine	32	34%	60%	70%	100%
Initial Antibiotic Timing	211	71%	75%	80%	93%
Oxygenation Assessment	236	100%	99%	99%	100%
Pneumococcal Vaccine	106	40%	61%	69%	94%
Smoking Cessation Advice	56	77%	82%	80%	100%
Surgical Infection Prevention					
Prophylactic Antibiotic Given[2,3]	40	82%	69%	77%	95%
Prophylactic Antibiotic Selection[2]	40	88%	89%	90%	100%
Prophylactic Antibiotic Stopped[2,3]	40	80%	71%	72%	95%
Pregnancy Care					
Inpatient Neonatal Mortality	533	0.00%	-	-	-
Third or Fourth Degree Laceration	431	1.86%	3.63%	3.63%	3.27%

Walton Regional Medical Center

330 Alcovy Street
Monroe, GA 30655
Ownership: Proprietary
Emergency Services: Yes

Phone: 770-267-8461
Fax: 770-267-1888
Accredited: Yes
Licensed Beds: 77

Key Personnel:
CEO. . . . . Alen E George
Chief Staff . . . . Mark Shaffer
Head Emergency . . . . Ehil Meyer
Manager Radiology . . . . Brian Hatlevig
Manager Respiratory Therapy . . . . Hal Queen

Measure	Cases	This Hospital	State Average	U.S. Average	Top Hospital
Heart Attack Care					
ACE Inhibitor or ARB for LVSD[1]	2	50%	78%	82%	100%
Aspirin at Arrival[1]	17	100%	91%	92%	100%
Aspirin at Discharge[1]	6	100%	87%	90%	100%
Beta Blocker at Arrival[1]	15	73%	85%	87%	100%
Beta Blocker at Discharge[1]	8	62%	87%	90%	100%
Fibrinolytic Medication Timing	0	-	34%	31%	100%
PCI Within 90 Minutes of Arrival	0	-	47%	54%	95%
Smoking Cessation Advice[1]	1	0%	85%	88%	100%
Heart Failure Care					
ACE Inhibitor or ARB for LVSD	51	69%	81%	82%	100%
Discharge Instructions	153	52%	59%	61%	93%
Evaluation of LVS Function	172	84%	81%	83%	99%
Smoking Cessation Advice[1]	24	79%	86%	82%	100%
Pneumonia Care					
Appropriate Initial Antibiotic	135	83%	81%	83%	94%
Blood Culture Timing	79	85%	89%	90%	100%
Influenza Vaccine	55	56%	60%	70%	100%
Initial Antibiotic Timing	198	77%	75%	80%	93%
Oxygenation Assessment	226	100%	99%	99%	100%
Pneumococcal Vaccine	150	74%	61%	69%	94%
Smoking Cessation Advice	52	81%	82%	80%	100%
Surgical Infection Prevention					
Prophylactic Antibiotic Given[2]	80	65%	69%	77%	95%
Prophylactic Antibiotic Selection[1,2]	11	100%	89%	90%	100%
Prophylactic Antibiotic Stopped[2]	80	70%	71%	72%	95%
Pregnancy Care					
Inpatient Neonatal Mortality	-	-	-	-	-
Third or Fourth Degree Laceration	-	-	3.63%	3.63%	3.27%

Flint River Community Hospital

509 Sumter Street
PO Box 770
Montezuma, GA 31063
URL: www.resurgencehealthgroup.com
Ownership: Proprietary
Emergency Services: Yes

Phone: 478-472-3100
Fax: 478-472-2412

Accredited: Yes
Licensed Beds: 49

Key Personnel:
CEO. . . . . Curt Roberts
Chief Medical Staff. WM Michael McDonald, DO

Measure	Cases	This Hospital	State Average	U.S. Average	Top Hospital
Heart Attack Care					

NOTE: Hospital profiles are in alphabetical order by state, then city, then hospital within the city; Rankings are sorted by rate in descending order and exclude hospitals with less than 25 cases; (1) The number of cases is too small (n<25) for purposes of reliably predicting hospital performance; (2) Measure reflects the hospital's indication that its submission was based upon a sample of its relevant discharges; (3) Rate reflects fewer than the maximum possible quarters of data for the measure; (4) Inaccurate information submitted and suppressed for one or more quarters; (5) No data is available from the hospital for this measure; Please refer to the User's Guide for a full explanation of data

Measure	Cases	This Hospital	State Average	U.S. Average	Top Hospital
ACE Inhibitor or ARB for LVSD	0	-	78%	82%	100%
Aspirin at Arrival[1]	2	50%	91%	92%	100%
Aspirin at Discharge[1]	1	0%	87%	90%	100%
Beta Blocker at Arrival[1]	1	0%	85%	87%	100%
Beta Blocker at Discharge[1]	1	0%	87%	90%	100%
Fibrinolytic Medication Timing	0	-	34%	31%	100%
PCI Within 90 Minutes of Arrival	0	-	47%	54%	95%
Smoking Cessation Advice[1]	1	0%	85%	88%	100%
Heart Failure Care					
ACE Inhibitor or ARB for LVSD[1]	15	80%	81%	82%	100%
Discharge Instructions	44	36%	59%	61%	93%
Evaluation of LVS Function	56	70%	81%	83%	99%
Smoking Cessation Advice[1]	13	54%	86%	82%	100%
Pneumonia Care					
Appropriate Initial Antibiotic	34	74%	81%	83%	94%
Blood Culture Timing[1]	17	88%	89%	90%	100%
Influenza Vaccine[1]	14	29%	60%	70%	100%
Initial Antibiotic Timing	53	74%	75%	80%	93%
Oxygenation Assessment	69	99%	99%	99%	100%
Pneumococcal Vaccine	28	14%	61%	69%	94%
Smoking Cessation Advice[1]	11	73%	82%	80%	100%
Surgical Infection Prevention					
Prophylactic Antibiotic Given[1]	16	75%	69%	77%	95%
Prophylactic Antibiotic Selection[1]	1	100%	89%	90%	100%
Prophylactic Antibiotic Stopped[1]	15	7%	71%	72%	95%
Pregnancy Care					
Inpatient Neonatal Mortality	-	-	-	-	-
Third or Fourth Degree Laceration	-	-	3.63%	3.63%	3.27%

Jasper Mem Hosp & Retreat Nursing Home

898 College Street
Monticello, GA 31064
Ownership: Voluntary non-profit - Private
Emergency Services: Yes

Phone: 706-468-6411
Fax: 706-468-8289
Accredited: No
Licensed Beds: 75

Key Personnel:
CEO. . . . . David Owens
Chief Medical Staff. . . . . Kerry Blake, MD
Chief Radiology . . . . Janet Harrington

Measure	Cases	This Hospital	State Average	U.S. Average	Top Hospital
Heart Attack Care					
ACE Inhibitor or ARB for LVSD[5]	-	-	78%	82%	100%
Aspirin at Arrival[5]	-	-	91%	92%	100%
Aspirin at Discharge[5]	-	-	87%	90%	100%
Beta Blocker at Arrival[5]	-	-	85%	87%	100%
Beta Blocker at Discharge[5]	-	-	87%	90%	100%
Fibrinolytic Medication Timing[5]	-	-	34%	31%	100%
PCI Within 90 Minutes of Arrival[5]	-	-	47%	54%	95%
Smoking Cessation Advice[5]	-	-	85%	88%	100%
Heart Failure Care					
ACE Inhibitor or ARB for LVSD[5]	-	-	81%	82%	100%
Discharge Instructions[5]	-	-	59%	61%	93%
Evaluation of LVS Function[5]	-	-	81%	83%	99%
Smoking Cessation Advice[5]	-	-	86%	82%	100%
Pneumonia Care					
Appropriate Initial Antibiotic[5]	-	-	81%	83%	94%
Blood Culture Timing[5]	-	-	89%	90%	100%
Influenza Vaccine[5]	-	-	60%	70%	100%
Initial Antibiotic Timing[5]	-	-	75%	80%	93%
Oxygenation Assessment[5]	-	-	99%	99%	100%
Pneumococcal Vaccine[5]	-	-	61%	69%	94%
Smoking Cessation Advice[5]	-	-	82%	80%	100%
Surgical Infection Prevention					
Prophylactic Antibiotic Given[5]	-	-	69%	77%	95%
Prophylactic Antibiotic Selection[5]	-	-	89%	90%	100%
Prophylactic Antibiotic Stopped[5]	-	-	71%	72%	95%
Pregnancy Care					
Inpatient Neonatal Mortality	-	-	-	-	-
Third or Fourth Degree Laceration	-	-	3.63%	3.63%	3.27%

Colquitt Regional Medical Center

3131 S Main Street
Moultrie, GA 31768

Toll-Free: 888-262-2762
Phone: 229-985-3420
Fax: 229-890-2173

E-mail: crmc@colquittregional.com
URL: www.colquittregionad.com
Ownership: Govt - Hospital District or Authority
Emergency Services: Yes

Accredited: Yes
Licensed Beds: 99

Key Personnel:
CEO. . . . . James R Lowry, FACHE
Chief Medical Staff. . . . . Howard Nelton
Director Cardiac Laboratory . . . . Paula Howell
Catheterization Laboratory. . . . . Paula Howell
Director Emergency Services. . . . . Jason Jacobs
Director Infection Control . . . . Gail Sparkman, RN
Director Medical/Surgical Nursing . . . . Phyllis Samples, RN
OB/GYN Womens Health. . . . . Anita Edenfield, RN
Respiratory Therapy. Dena Zin

Measure	Cases	This Hospital	State Average	U.S. Average	Top Hospital
Heart Attack Care					
ACE Inhibitor or ARB for LVSD[1]	2	100%	78%	82%	100%
Aspirin at Arrival	39	100%	91%	92%	100%
Aspirin at Discharge[1]	17	100%	87%	90%	100%
Beta Blocker at Arrival	36	100%	85%	87%	100%
Beta Blocker at Discharge[1]	17	94%	87%	90%	100%
Fibrinolytic Medication Timing[1]	4	25%	34%	31%	100%
PCI Within 90 Minutes of Arrival	0	-	47%	54%	95%
Smoking Cessation Advice[1]	3	100%	85%	88%	100%
Heart Failure Care					
ACE Inhibitor or ARB for LVSD	52	79%	81%	82%	100%
Discharge Instructions	125	73%	59%	61%	93%
Evaluation of LVS Function	153	92%	81%	83%	99%
Smoking Cessation Advice	35	100%	86%	82%	100%
Pneumonia Care					
Appropriate Initial Antibiotic	67	79%	81%	83%	94%
Blood Culture Timing	38	92%	89%	90%	100%
Influenza Vaccine[1]	11	82%	60%	70%	100%
Initial Antibiotic Timing[1]	9	89%	75%	80%	93%
Oxygenation Assessment	109	97%	99%	99%	100%
Pneumococcal Vaccine	54	83%	61%	69%	94%
Smoking Cessation Advice	34	97%	82%	80%	100%
Surgical Infection Prevention					
Prophylactic Antibiotic Given[3]	45	38%	69%	77%	95%
Prophylactic Antibiotic Selection[1]	4	100%	89%	90%	100%
Prophylactic Antibiotic Stopped[3]	42	83%	71%	72%	95%
Pregnancy Care					
Inpatient Neonatal Mortality	-	-	-	-	-
Third or Fourth Degree Laceration	-	-	3.63%	3.63%	3.27%

Turning Point Hospital

3015 E Bypass SE
PO Box 1177
Moultrie, GA 31768
E-mail: tpservices@alltel.net
URL: www.turningpointcare.com
Ownership: Proprietary
Emergency Services: No

Toll-Free: 800-342-1075
Phone: 229-985-4815
Fax: 229-890-1614

Accredited: No
Licensed Beds: 59

Key Personnel:
CEO. . . . . Ben Marion

Measure	Cases	This Hospital	State Average	U.S. Average	Top Hospital
Heart Attack Care					
ACE Inhibitor or ARB for LVSD[5]	-	-	78%	82%	100%
Aspirin at Arrival[5]	-	-	91%	92%	100%
Aspirin at Discharge[5]	-	-	87%	90%	100%
Beta Blocker at Arrival[5]	-	-	85%	87%	100%
Beta Blocker at Discharge[5]	-	-	87%	90%	100%
Fibrinolytic Medication Timing[5]	-	-	34%	31%	100%
PCI Within 90 Minutes of Arrival[5]	-	-	47%	54%	95%
Smoking Cessation Advice[5]	-	-	85%	88%	100%
Heart Failure Care					
ACE Inhibitor or ARB for LVSD[5]	-	-	81%	82%	100%

NOTE: Hospital profiles are in alphabetical order by state, then city, then hospital within the city; Rankings are sorted by rate in descending order and exclude hospitals with less than 25 cases; (1) The number of cases is too small (n<25) for purposes of reliably predicting hospital performance; (2) Measure reflects the hospital's indication that its submission was based upon a sample of its relevant discharges; (3) Rate reflects fewer than the maximum possible quarters of data for the measure; (4) Inaccurate information submitted and suppressed for one or more quarters; (5) No data is available from the hospital for this measure; Please refer to the User's Guide for a full explanation of data

Measure			This Hospital	State Average	U.S. Average	Top Hospital
Discharge Instructions[5]	-	-	59%	61%	93%
Evaluation of LVS Function[5]	-	-	81%	83%	99%
Smoking Cessation Advice[5]	-	-	86%	82%	100%
Pneumonia Care						
Appropriate Initial Antibiotic[5]	-	-	81%	83%	94%
Blood Culture Timing[5]	-	-	89%	90%	100%
Influenza Vaccine[5]	-	-	60%	70%	100%
Initial Antibiotic Timing[5]	-	-	75%	80%	93%
Oxygenation Assessment[5]	-	-	99%	99%	100%
Pneumococcal Vaccine[5]	-	-	61%	69%	94%
Smoking Cessation Advice[5]	-	-	82%	80%	100%
Surgical Infection Prevention						
Prophylactic Antibiotic Given[5]	-	-	69%	77%	95%
Prophylactic Antibiotic Selection[5]	-	-	89%	90%	100%
Prophylactic Antibiotic Stopped[5]	-	-	71%	72%	95%
Pregnancy Care						
Inpatient Neonatal Mortality	-	-	-	-	-
Third or Fourth Degree Laceration	-	-	3.63%	3.63%	3.27%

Berrien County Hospital

1221 E McPherson Street
Nashville, GA 31639
E-mail: jimj@ahshospitals.com
URL: www.berrienhospital.com
Ownership: Proprietary
Emergency Services: Yes

Phone: 229-543-7100
Fax: 229-543-1724

Accredited: Yes
Licensed Beds: 71

Key Personnel:
CEO. . . . . James D Janek
Chief Medical Staff. Rick Langosch
Cardiology . . . . William W Hancock, MD
Emergency Room . . . . Kay Robertson
CCU Spvg. Nurse . . . . Phillip Simmons
Director Medical/Surgical Nursing . . . . Cheryl Chaney, RN
General Surgery . . . . Romulo P Navarro, MD
Chief Radiology . . . . Sam Wattanawanakul, MD

Measure	Cases	This Hospital	State Average	U.S. Average	Top Hospital
Heart Attack Care					
ACE Inhibitor or ARB for LVSD[1,3]	1	100%	78%	82%	100%
Aspirin at Arrival[1,3]	1	100%	91%	92%	100%
Aspirin at Discharge[1,3]	1	100%	87%	90%	100%
Beta Blocker at Arrival[1,3]	1	100%	85%	87%	100%
Beta Blocker at Discharge[1,3]	1	100%	87%	90%	100%
Fibrinolytic Medication Timing[3]	0	-	34%	31%	100%
PCI Within 90 Minutes of Arrival	0	-	47%	54%	95%
Smoking Cessation Advice[3]	0	-	85%	88%	100%
Heart Failure Care					
ACE Inhibitor or ARB for LVSD[1]	1	100%	81%	82%	100%
Discharge Instructions[1]	16	19%	59%	61%	93%
Evaluation of LVS Function[1]	23	13%	81%	83%	99%
Smoking Cessation Advice[1]	5	20%	86%	82%	100%
Pneumonia Care					
Appropriate Initial Antibiotic[2]	36	58%	81%	83%	94%
Blood Culture Timing[1,2]	9	100%	89%	90%	100%
Influenza Vaccine[1,2]	7	57%	60%	70%	100%
Initial Antibiotic Timing[2]	40	85%	75%	80%	93%
Oxygenation Assessment[2]	57	96%	99%	99%	100%
Pneumococcal Vaccine[2]	33	36%	61%	69%	94%
Smoking Cessation Advice[1,2]	14	57%	82%	80%	100%
Surgical Infection Prevention					
Prophylactic Antibiotic Given[5]	-	-	69%	77%	95%
Prophylactic Antibiotic Selection[5]	-	-	89%	90%	100%
Prophylactic Antibiotic Stopped[5]	-	-	71%	72%	95%
Pregnancy Care					
Inpatient Neonatal Mortality	-	-	-	-	-
Third or Fourth Degree Laceration	-	-	3.63%	3.63%	3.27%

Irwin County Hospital

710 N Irwin Avenue
Ocilla, GA 31774
Ownership: Govt - Hospital District or Authority
Emergency Services: Yes

Phone: 229-468-7411
Fax: 229-468-3880
Accredited: Yes
Licensed Beds: 34

Key Personnel:
CEO. . . . . Sue Spivei
Emergency Room . . . . Becky Cook
Director Medical/Surgical Nursing . . . . Barbara McDuffie
Chief Radiology . . . . Pankaj Patel
Director Respiratory Therapy . . . . Brad Van Boren

Measure	Cases	This Hospital	State Average	U.S. Average	Top Hospital
Heart Attack Care					
ACE Inhibitor or ARB for LVSD[5]	-	-	78%	82%	100%
Aspirin at Arrival[5]	-	-	91%	92%	100%
Aspirin at Discharge[5]	-	-	87%	90%	100%
Beta Blocker at Arrival[5]	-	-	85%	87%	100%
Beta Blocker at Discharge[5]	-	-	87%	90%	100%
Fibrinolytic Medication Timing[5]	-	-	34%	31%	100%
PCI Within 90 Minutes of Arrival[5]	-	-	47%	54%	95%
Smoking Cessation Advice[5]	-	-	85%	88%	100%
Heart Failure Care					
ACE Inhibitor or ARB for LVSD[1]	5	100%	81%	82%	100%
Discharge Instructions[1]	13	54%	59%	61%	93%
Evaluation of LVS Function[1]	19	63%	81%	83%	99%
Smoking Cessation Advice[1]	1	100%	86%	82%	100%
Pneumonia Care					
Appropriate Initial Antibiotic[1]	22	82%	81%	83%	94%
Blood Culture Timing[1]	5	80%	89%	90%	100%
Influenza Vaccine[1]	1	0%	60%	70%	100%
Initial Antibiotic Timing[1]	22	55%	75%	80%	93%
Oxygenation Assessment	27	96%	99%	99%	100%
Pneumococcal Vaccine[1]	13	38%	61%	69%	94%
Smoking Cessation Advice[1]	10	40%	82%	80%	100%
Surgical Infection Prevention					
Prophylactic Antibiotic Given[1,2,3]	10	90%	69%	77%	95%
Prophylactic Antibiotic Selection[1,2]	11	100%	89%	90%	100%
Prophylactic Antibiotic Stopped[1,2,3]	10	100%	71%	72%	95%
Pregnancy Care					
Inpatient Neonatal Mortality	478	0.21%	-	-	-
Third or Fourth Degree Laceration	275	5.45%	3.63%	3.63%	3.27%

Perry Hospital

1120 Morningside Drive
Perry, GA 31069
URL: www.hhc.org
Ownership: Govt - Hospital District or Authority
Emergency Services: Yes

Phone: 478-988-1627
Fax: 478-988-1613

Accredited: Yes
Licensed Beds: 45

Key Personnel:
CEO. . . . . Lora Davis
Chief Medical Staff. . . . . Horatio V Cabasares
Emergency Room . . . . Horatio V Cabasares, MD
Director Medical/Surgical Nursing . . . . Helen Parker, RN
OB/GYN Womens Health. . . . . WE Strickland, MD
Chief Radiology . . . . Gary Suhr, MD
Director Respiratory Therapy . . . . Karen Monroe

Measure	Cases	This Hospital	State Average	U.S. Average	Top Hospital
Heart Attack Care					
ACE Inhibitor or ARB for LVSD	0	-	78%	82%	100%
Aspirin at Arrival[1]	18	89%	91%	92%	100%
Aspirin at Discharge[1]	6	100%	87%	90%	100%
Beta Blocker at Arrival[1]	14	71%	85%	87%	100%
Beta Blocker at Discharge[1]	5	60%	87%	90%	100%
Fibrinolytic Medication Timing	0	-	34%	31%	100%
PCI Within 90 Minutes of Arrival	0	-	47%	54%	95%
Smoking Cessation Advice	0	-	85%	88%	100%
Heart Failure Care					
ACE Inhibitor or ARB for LVSD[1]	11	91%	81%	82%	100%
Discharge Instructions	38	71%	59%	61%	93%
Evaluation of LVS Function	53	79%	81%	83%	99%
Smoking Cessation Advice[1]	5	100%	86%	82%	100%

NOTE: Hospital profiles are in alphabetical order by state, then city, then hospital within the city; Rankings are sorted by rate in descending order and exclude hospitals with less than 25 cases; (1) The number of cases is too small (n<25) for purposes of reliably predicting hospital performance; (2) Measure reflects the hospital's indication that its submission was based upon a sample of its relevant discharges; (3) Rate reflects fewer than the maximum possible quarters of data for the measure; (4) Inaccurate information submitted and suppressed for one or more quarters; (5) No data is available from the hospital for this measure; Please refer to the User's Guide for a full explanation of data

Pneumonia Care					
Appropriate Initial Antibiotic[2]	75	91%	81%	83%	94%
Blood Culture Timing[2]	46	98%	89%	90%	100%
Influenza Vaccine[1,2]	23	70%	60%	70%	100%
Initial Antibiotic Timing[2]	97	85%	75%	80%	93%
Oxygenation Assessment[2]	129	98%	99%	99%	100%
Pneumococcal Vaccine[2]	75	87%	61%	69%	94%
Smoking Cessation Advice[1,2]	19	84%	82%	80%	100%
Surgical Infection Prevention					
Prophylactic Antibiotic Given[3]	30	63%	69%	77%	95%
Prophylactic Antibiotic Selection[1]	12	100%	89%	90%	100%
Prophylactic Antibiotic Stopped[3]	27	59%	71%	72%	95%
Pregnancy Care					
Inpatient Neonatal Mortality	-	-	-	-	-
Third or Fourth Degree Laceration	-	-	3.63%	3.63%	3.27%

Brooks County Hospital

903 N Court Street
PO Box 5000
Quitman, GA 31643
Ownership: Voluntary non-profit - Other
Emergency Services: Yes

Phone: 229-263-4171
Fax: 229-263-6318

Accredited: Yes
Licensed Beds: 35

Key Personnel:
CEO . . . . LaDon Toole
Emergency Room . . . . June Furney, RN
Infection Control . . . . Patricia Johnson
Director Medical/Surgical Nursing . . . . Nancy Williams, RN
Director Radiology . . . . Zinda McDaniel
Director Respiratory Therapy . . . . Melanie Owens

Measure	Cases	This Hospital	State Average	U.S. Average	Top Hospital
Heart Attack Care					
ACE Inhibitor or ARB for LVSD[5]	-	-	78%	82%	100%
Aspirin at Arrival[5]	-	-	91%	92%	100%
Aspirin at Discharge[5]	-	-	87%	90%	100%
Beta Blocker at Arrival[5]	-	-	85%	87%	100%
Beta Blocker at Discharge[5]	-	-	87%	90%	100%
Fibrinolytic Medication Timing[5]	-	-	34%	31%	100%
PCI Within 90 Minutes of Arrival[5]	-	-	47%	54%	95%
Smoking Cessation Advice[5]	-	-	85%	88%	100%
Heart Failure Care					
ACE Inhibitor or ARB for LVSD[1]	3	100%	81%	82%	100%
Discharge Instructions[1]	13	100%	59%	61%	93%
Evaluation of LVS Function[1]	19	84%	81%	83%	99%
Smoking Cessation Advice[1]	5	100%	86%	82%	100%
Pneumonia Care					
Appropriate Initial Antibiotic[1]	14	100%	81%	83%	94%
Blood Culture Timing[1]	9	100%	89%	90%	100%
Influenza Vaccine[1]	5	80%	60%	70%	100%
Initial Antibiotic Timing[1]	21	71%	75%	80%	93%
Oxygenation Assessment	26	100%	99%	99%	100%
Pneumococcal Vaccine[1]	13	85%	61%	69%	94%
Smoking Cessation Advice[1]	7	100%	82%	80%	100%
Surgical Infection Prevention					
Prophylactic Antibiotic Given[5]	-	-	69%	77%	95%
Prophylactic Antibiotic Selection[5]	-	-	89%	90%	100%
Prophylactic Antibiotic Stopped[5]	-	-	71%	72%	95%
Pregnancy Care					
Inpatient Neonatal Mortality	-	-	-	-	-
Third or Fourth Degree Laceration	-	-	3.63%	3.63%	3.27%

Southern Regional Medical Center

11 Upper Riverdale Road SW
Riverdale, GA 30274
URL: www.southernregional.org
Ownership: Voluntary non-profit - Private
Emergency Services: Yes

Phone: 770-991-8000
Fax: 770-991-8595

Accredited: Yes
Licensed Beds: 406

Key Personnel:
President/CEO . . . . Edward J Bonn, CHE
Chief Medical Staff . . . . Mauro Folgosa, MD
Director Heart/Vascular Services . . . . Donna Waggoner
Director Emergency Services . . . . Linda Power, RN
Director Women's Services . . . . Gael Gilbert, RN

Director Surgery Services . . . . Patricia Middleton
Director Radiology . . . . Danial Whitt

Measure	Cases	This Hospital	State Average	U.S. Average	Top Hospital
Heart Attack Care					
ACE Inhibitor or ARB for LVSD	26	85%	78%	82%	100%
Aspirin at Arrival	178	95%	91%	92%	100%
Aspirin at Discharge	91	81%	87%	90%	100%
Beta Blocker at Arrival	144	90%	85%	87%	100%
Beta Blocker at Discharge	94	88%	87%	90%	100%
Fibrinolytic Medication Timing	36	58%	34%	31%	100%
PCI Within 90 Minutes of Arrival[1]	7	14%	47%	54%	95%
Smoking Cessation Advice	30	100%	85%	88%	100%
Heart Failure Care					
ACE Inhibitor or ARB for LVSD	289	83%	81%	82%	100%
Discharge Instructions	623	72%	59%	61%	93%
Evaluation of LVS Function	694	83%	81%	83%	99%
Smoking Cessation Advice	166	100%	86%	82%	100%
Pneumonia Care					
Appropriate Initial Antibiotic	254	85%	81%	83%	94%
Blood Culture Timing	219	82%	89%	90%	100%
Influenza Vaccine	60	55%	60%	70%	100%
Initial Antibiotic Timing	314	68%	75%	80%	93%
Oxygenation Assessment	357	99%	99%	99%	100%
Pneumococcal Vaccine	160	72%	61%	69%	94%
Smoking Cessation Advice	100	89%	82%	80%	100%
Surgical Infection Prevention					
Prophylactic Antibiotic Given[2]	530	82%	69%	77%	95%
Prophylactic Antibiotic Selection[2]	76	86%	89%	90%	100%
Prophylactic Antibiotic Stopped[2]	506	73%	71%	72%	95%
Pregnancy Care					
Inpatient Neonatal Mortality	-	-	-	-	-
Third or Fourth Degree Laceration	-	-	3.63%	3.63%	3.27%

Floyd Medical Center

304 Turner McCall Boulevard
PO Box 233
Rome, GA 30162
E-mail: dnighten@floydmed.org
URL: www.floydmed.org
Ownership: Govt - Hospital District or Authority
Emergency Services: Yes

Phone: 706-509-5000
Fax: 706-509-5771

Accredited: Yes
Licensed Beds: 304

Key Personnel:
CEO . . . . Kurt Stuenkel, FACHE
Cardiac Lab . . . . Mike Cornwell
Catheterization Lab . . . . Mary Jane Hamilton
Emergency Room . . . . Kenna Baker
Intensive Coronary Care . . . . Mike Cornwell
Medical Surgical Nursing . . . . Pearl Oest, RN
OB/GYN Womens Health . . . . Phyllis Pemerton
Respiratory Therapy . . . . Robert Ropp

Measure	Cases	This Hospital	State Average	U.S. Average	Top Hospital
Heart Attack Care					
ACE Inhibitor or ARB for LVSD[1]	7	86%	78%	82%	100%
Aspirin at Arrival	61	98%	91%	92%	100%
Aspirin at Discharge[1]	18	78%	87%	90%	100%
Beta Blocker at Arrival	28	89%	85%	87%	100%
Beta Blocker at Discharge[1]	24	92%	87%	90%	100%
Fibrinolytic Medication Timing	0	-	34%	31%	100%
PCI Within 90 Minutes of Arrival	0	-	47%	54%	95%
Smoking Cessation Advice[1]	11	91%	85%	88%	100%
Heart Failure Care					
ACE Inhibitor or ARB for LVSD	122	68%	81%	82%	100%
Discharge Instructions	211	12%	59%	61%	93%
Evaluation of LVS Function	246	92%	81%	83%	99%
Smoking Cessation Advice	62	95%	86%	82%	100%
Pneumonia Care					
Appropriate Initial Antibiotic	195	82%	81%	83%	94%
Blood Culture Timing	235	91%	89%	90%	100%
Influenza Vaccine	72	75%	60%	70%	100%
Initial Antibiotic Timing	332	77%	75%	80%	93%
Oxygenation Assessment	420	100%	99%	99%	100%

NOTE: Hospital profiles are in alphabetical order by state, then city, then hospital within the city; Rankings are sorted by rate in descending order and exclude hospitals with less than 25 cases; (1) The number of cases is too small (n<25) for purposes of reliably predicting hospital performance; (2) Measure reflects the hospital's indication that its submission was based upon a sample of its relevant discharges; (3) Rate reflects fewer than the maximum possible quarters of data for the measure; (4) Inaccurate information submitted and suppressed for one or more quarters; (5) No data is available from the hospital for this measure; Please refer to the User's Guide for a full explanation of data

Measure	Cases	This Hospital	State Average	U.S. Average	Top Hospital
Pneumococcal Vaccine	219	74%	61%	69%	94%
Smoking Cessation Advice	118	94%	82%	80%	100%
Surgical Infection Prevention					
Prophylactic Antibiotic Given[2]	498	73%	69%	77%	95%
Prophylactic Antibiotic Selection[2]	127	94%	89%	90%	100%
Prophylactic Antibiotic Stopped[2]	494	83%	71%	72%	95%
Pregnancy Care					
Inpatient Neonatal Mortality[2]	2,014	0.30%	-	-	-
Third or Fourth Degree Laceration[2]	1,461	7.12%	3.63%	3.63%	3.27%

Redmond Regional Medical Center

Alternate Name: Redmond Park Hospital
501 Redmond Road
Rome, GA 30165
Ownership: Proprietary
Emergency Services: Yes

Phone: 706-291-0291
Fax: 706-291-0971
Accredited: Yes
Licensed Beds: 201

Key Personnel:
CEO . . . . James R Thomas
Chief Medical Staff . . . . Louis Lataif, MD
Emergency Room . . . . Jean Miller, RN
Chief Radiology . . . . John Goodwin
Director Respiratory Therapy . . . . Ted Porter

Measure	Cases	This Hospital	State Average	U.S. Average	Top Hospital
Heart Attack Care					
ACE Inhibitor or ARB for LVSD	140	86%	78%	82%	100%
Aspirin at Arrival	336	99%	91%	92%	100%
Aspirin at Discharge	568	99%	87%	90%	100%
Beta Blocker at Arrival	242	95%	85%	87%	100%
Beta Blocker at Discharge	584	97%	87%	90%	100%
Fibrinolytic Medication Timing	0	-	34%	31%	100%
PCI Within 90 Minutes of Arrival[1]	18	83%	47%	54%	95%
Smoking Cessation Advice	284	100%	85%	88%	100%
Heart Failure Care					
ACE Inhibitor or ARB for LVSD	314	86%	81%	82%	100%
Discharge Instructions	574	51%	59%	61%	93%
Evaluation of LVS Function	636	97%	81%	83%	99%
Smoking Cessation Advice	139	99%	86%	82%	100%
Pneumonia Care					
Appropriate Initial Antibiotic	276	86%	81%	83%	94%
Blood Culture Timing	270	87%	89%	90%	100%
Influenza Vaccine	81	69%	60%	70%	100%
Initial Antibiotic Timing	332	72%	75%	80%	93%
Oxygenation Assessment	424	100%	99%	99%	100%
Pneumococcal Vaccine	285	81%	61%	69%	94%
Smoking Cessation Advice	108	92%	82%	80%	100%
Surgical Infection Prevention					
Prophylactic Antibiotic Given[2]	330	94%	69%	77%	95%
Prophylactic Antibiotic Selection[2]	138	98%	89%	90%	100%
Prophylactic Antibiotic Stopped[2]	319	69%	71%	72%	95%
Pregnancy Care					
Inpatient Neonatal Mortality	-	-	-	-	-
Third or Fourth Degree Laceration	-	-	3.63%	3.63%	3.27%

North Fulton Regional Hospital

3000 Hospital Boulevard
Roswell, GA 30076
URL: www.northfultonregional.com
Ownership: Proprietary
Emergency Services: Yes

Phone: 770-751-2500
Fax: 770-751-2899

Accredited: Yes
Licensed Beds: 167

Key Personnel:
CEO . . . . John Holland
Chief Medical Staff . . . . John Harvey
Emergency Room . . . . John Dirves
Emergency Room . . . . Ann Abrams
Director Medical/Surgical Nursing . . . . Jean Rast
Director Surgical Nursing . . . . Cathy Gebhardt
OB/GYN Womens Health . . . . Judy Doran
Manager Radiology . . . . Randy Sprinkle

Measure	Cases	This Hospital	State Average	U.S. Average	Top Hospital
Heart Attack Care					

Measure	Cases	This Hospital	State Average	U.S. Average	Top Hospital
ACE Inhibitor or ARB for LVSD[1]	8	75%	78%	82%	100%
Aspirin at Arrival	64	98%	91%	92%	100%
Aspirin at Discharge	25	96%	87%	90%	100%
Beta Blocker at Arrival	58	98%	85%	87%	100%
Beta Blocker at Discharge	25	92%	87%	90%	100%
Fibrinolytic Medication Timing[1]	2	0%	34%	31%	100%
PCI Within 90 Minutes of Arrival	0	-	47%	54%	95%
Smoking Cessation Advice[1]	2	50%	85%	88%	100%
Heart Failure Care					
ACE Inhibitor or ARB for LVSD	59	88%	81%	82%	100%
Discharge Instructions	184	70%	59%	61%	93%
Evaluation of LVS Function	206	99%	81%	83%	99%
Smoking Cessation Advice	27	96%	86%	82%	100%
Pneumonia Care					
Appropriate Initial Antibiotic	243	82%	81%	83%	94%
Blood Culture Timing	240	97%	89%	90%	100%
Influenza Vaccine	58	90%	60%	70%	100%
Initial Antibiotic Timing	302	91%	75%	80%	93%
Oxygenation Assessment	370	100%	99%	99%	100%
Pneumococcal Vaccine	214	92%	61%	69%	94%
Smoking Cessation Advice	61	89%	82%	80%	100%
Surgical Infection Prevention					
Prophylactic Antibiotic Given[2]	233	89%	69%	77%	95%
Prophylactic Antibiotic Selection[2]	70	90%	89%	90%	100%
Prophylactic Antibiotic Stopped[2]	221	84%	71%	72%	95%
Pregnancy Care					
Inpatient Neonatal Mortality	-	-	-	-	-
Third or Fourth Degree Laceration	-	-	3.63%	3.63%	3.27%

Cobb Memorial Hospital

521 Franklin Springs St
Royston, GA 30662
URL: www.cobbmemorialhospital.com
Ownership: Voluntary non-profit - Private
Emergency Services: Yes

Phone: 706-245-5034
Fax: 706-245-1831

Accredited: Yes
Licensed Beds: 71

Key Personnel:
President/CEO . . . . H Thomas Brown
Emergency Room . . . . Debbie Barlett

Measure	Cases	This Hospital	State Average	U.S. Average	Top Hospital
Heart Attack Care					
ACE Inhibitor or ARB for LVSD[1]	3	67%	78%	82%	100%
Aspirin at Arrival[1]	12	75%	91%	92%	100%
Aspirin at Discharge[1]	6	67%	87%	90%	100%
Beta Blocker at Arrival[1]	8	88%	85%	87%	100%
Beta Blocker at Discharge[1]	5	100%	87%	90%	100%
Fibrinolytic Medication Timing[1]	3	33%	34%	31%	100%
PCI Within 90 Minutes of Arrival	0	-	47%	54%	95%
Smoking Cessation Advice	0	-	85%	88%	100%
Heart Failure Care					
ACE Inhibitor or ARB for LVSD[1]	13	92%	81%	82%	100%
Discharge Instructions	41	59%	59%	61%	93%
Evaluation of LVS Function	55	96%	81%	83%	99%
Smoking Cessation Advice[1]	16	94%	86%	82%	100%
Pneumonia Care					
Appropriate Initial Antibiotic	52	87%	81%	83%	94%
Blood Culture Timing	54	94%	89%	90%	100%
Influenza Vaccine[1]	13	54%	60%	70%	100%
Initial Antibiotic Timing	88	90%	75%	80%	93%
Oxygenation Assessment	106	99%	99%	99%	100%
Pneumococcal Vaccine	67	67%	61%	69%	94%
Smoking Cessation Advice	25	80%	82%	80%	100%
Surgical Infection Prevention					
Prophylactic Antibiotic Given[3]	32	78%	69%	77%	95%
Prophylactic Antibiotic Selection[1]	13	100%	89%	90%	100%
Prophylactic Antibiotic Stopped[3]	32	66%	71%	72%	95%
Pregnancy Care					
Inpatient Neonatal Mortality	-	-	-	-	-
Third or Fourth Degree Laceration	-	-	3.63%	3.63%	3.27%

NOTE: Hospital profiles are in alphabetical order by state, then city, then hospital within the city; Rankings are sorted by rate in descending order and exclude hospitals with less than 25 cases; (1) The number of cases is too small (n<25) for purposes of reliably predicting hospital performance; (2) Measure reflects the hospital's indication that its submission was based upon a sample of its relevant discharges; (3) Rate reflects fewer than the maximum possible quarters of data for the measure; (4) Inaccurate information submitted and suppressed for one or more quarters; (5) No data is available from the hospital for this measure; Please refer to the User's Guide for a full explanation of data

Southeast Georgia Health System-Camden Campus

2000 Dan Proctor Drive   Phone: 912-576-6401
Saint Marys, GA 31558
Ownership: Govt - Hospital District or Authority   Accredited: Yes
Emergency Services: Yes

Measure	Cases	This Hospital	State Average	U.S. Average	Top Hospital
Heart Attack Care					
ACE Inhibitor or ARB for LVSD[1]	1	100%	78%	82%	100%
Aspirin at Arrival[1]	4	75%	91%	92%	100%
Aspirin at Discharge[1]	2	50%	87%	90%	100%
Beta Blocker at Arrival[1]	4	100%	85%	87%	100%
Beta Blocker at Discharge[1]	3	100%	87%	90%	100%
Fibrinolytic Medication Timing	0	-	34%	31%	100%
PCI Within 90 Minutes of Arrival	0	-	47%	54%	95%
Smoking Cessation Advice	0	-	85%	88%	100%
Heart Failure Care					
ACE Inhibitor or ARB for LVSD[1]	22	64%	81%	82%	100%
Discharge Instructions	59	66%	59%	61%	93%
Evaluation of LVS Function	69	77%	81%	83%	99%
Smoking Cessation Advice[1]	10	90%	86%	82%	100%
Pneumonia Care					
Appropriate Initial Antibiotic	59	68%	81%	83%	94%
Blood Culture Timing	31	87%	89%	90%	100%
Influenza Vaccine[1]	17	47%	60%	70%	100%
Initial Antibiotic Timing	55	84%	75%	80%	93%
Oxygenation Assessment	67	97%	99%	99%	100%
Pneumococcal Vaccine	34	38%	61%	69%	94%
Smoking Cessation Advice[1]	15	93%	82%	80%	100%
Surgical Infection Prevention					
Prophylactic Antibiotic Given[2]	79	91%	69%	77%	95%
Prophylactic Antibiotic Selection[1,2]	16	94%	89%	90%	100%
Prophylactic Antibiotic Stopped[2]	74	84%	71%	72%	95%
Pregnancy Care					
Inpatient Neonatal Mortality	-	-	-	-	-
Third or Fourth Degree Laceration	-	-	3.63%	3.63%	3.27%

Washington County Regional Medical Center

Alternate Name: Memorial Hospital of Washington County
610 Sparta Road   Phone: 478-240-2000
Sandersville, GA 31082   Fax: 478-240-2390
Ownership: Govt - Hospital District or Authority   Accredited: Yes
Emergency Services: Yes   Licensed Beds: 116
Key Personnel:
CEO. . . . . Tom Brown
Chief Medical Staff. . . . . Jean Sumner
Chief Medical Staff. . . . . Oberto Baga
Physician Director of Cardiology . . . . Robert Wright
Director Medical/Surgical Nursing . . . . Kathy Jackson
OB/GYN Womens Health. . . . . Scott Redrick
Chief Radiology . . . . Danny McCrary
Director Respiratory Therapy . . . . Wenda Hodgef

Measure	Cases	This Hospital	State Average	U.S. Average	Top Hospital
Heart Attack Care					
ACE Inhibitor or ARB for LVSD	0	-	78%	82%	100%
Aspirin at Arrival[1]	7	57%	91%	92%	100%
Aspirin at Discharge[1]	2	100%	87%	90%	100%
Beta Blocker at Arrival[1]	5	80%	85%	87%	100%
Beta Blocker at Discharge[1]	2	100%	87%	90%	100%
Fibrinolytic Medication Timing	0	-	34%	31%	100%
PCI Within 90 Minutes of Arrival	0	-	47%	54%	95%
Smoking Cessation Advice	0	-	85%	88%	100%
Heart Failure Care					
ACE Inhibitor or ARB for LVSD[1]	16	75%	81%	82%	100%
Discharge Instructions	50	84%	59%	61%	93%
Evaluation of LVS Function	59	75%	81%	83%	99%
Smoking Cessation Advice[1]	11	100%	86%	82%	100%
Pneumonia Care					
Appropriate Initial Antibiotic	171	74%	81%	83%	94%
Blood Culture Timing	100	91%	89%	90%	100%
Influenza Vaccine	35	80%	60%	70%	100%

Measure	Cases	This Hospital	State Average	U.S. Average	Top Hospital
Initial Antibiotic Timing	221	77%	75%	80%	93%
Oxygenation Assessment	256	100%	99%	99%	100%
Pneumococcal Vaccine	128	80%	61%	69%	94%
Smoking Cessation Advice	51	96%	82%	80%	100%
Surgical Infection Prevention					
Prophylactic Antibiotic Given[1,2,3]	8	12%	69%	77%	95%
Prophylactic Antibiotic Selection[1,2]	8	12%	89%	90%	100%
Prophylactic Antibiotic Stopped[1,2,3]	8	50%	71%	72%	95%
Pregnancy Care					
Inpatient Neonatal Mortality	-	-	-	-	-
Third or Fourth Degree Laceration	-	-	3.63%	3.63%	3.27%

Candler Hospital

5353 Reynolds Street   Phone: 912-692-6000
Savannah, GA 31412
Ownership: Voluntary non-profit - Other   Accredited: Yes
Emergency Services: Yes

Measure	Cases	This Hospital	State Average	U.S. Average	Top Hospital
Heart Attack Care					
ACE Inhibitor or ARB for LVSD[1]	7	100%	78%	82%	100%
Aspirin at Arrival	30	97%	91%	92%	100%
Aspirin at Discharge[1]	18	100%	87%	90%	100%
Beta Blocker at Arrival[1]	19	100%	85%	87%	100%
Beta Blocker at Discharge[1]	21	100%	87%	90%	100%
Fibrinolytic Medication Timing	0	-	34%	31%	100%
PCI Within 90 Minutes of Arrival	0	-	47%	54%	95%
Smoking Cessation Advice[1]	4	100%	85%	88%	100%
Heart Failure Care					
ACE Inhibitor or ARB for LVSD	126	100%	81%	82%	100%
Discharge Instructions	366	72%	59%	61%	93%
Evaluation of LVS Function	425	98%	81%	83%	99%
Smoking Cessation Advice	59	100%	86%	82%	100%
Pneumonia Care					
Appropriate Initial Antibiotic	217	89%	81%	83%	94%
Blood Culture Timing	224	93%	89%	90%	100%
Influenza Vaccine	71	73%	60%	70%	100%
Initial Antibiotic Timing	328	77%	75%	80%	93%
Oxygenation Assessment	423	100%	99%	99%	100%
Pneumococcal Vaccine	244	81%	61%	69%	94%
Smoking Cessation Advice	101	99%	82%	80%	100%
Surgical Infection Prevention					
Prophylactic Antibiotic Given[2,3]	74	65%	69%	77%	95%
Prophylactic Antibiotic Selection[1,2]	22	73%	89%	90%	100%
Prophylactic Antibiotic Stopped[2,3]	74	66%	71%	72%	95%
Pregnancy Care					
Inpatient Neonatal Mortality	2,972	0.27%	-	-	-
Third or Fourth Degree Laceration	1,693	3.54%	3.63%	3.63%	3.27%

Memorial Medical Center

Alternate Name: Memorial Health University Medical Center
4700 Waters Avenue   Phone: 912-350-8000
PO Box 23089   Fax: 912-350-7073
Savannah, GA 31404
URL: www.memorialhealth.com
Ownership: Voluntary non-profit - Other   Accredited: Yes
Emergency Services: Yes   Licensed Beds: 530
Key Personnel:
President/CEO. . . . . Robert A Colvin
President Medical Staff . . . . Linda Sacks
Administrator . . . . Kathy Sydow
Administrator . . . . Julie Long
VP . . . . Andy Blalock
VP . . . . Cassandra Johnson
Senior VP/Chief Medical Officer. . . . . Ramon Mequiar, MD
Executive Director . . . . Iffath Hoskins, MD
VP . . . . Steve Stanic

Measure	Cases	This Hospital	State Average	U.S. Average	Top Hospital
Heart Attack Care					
ACE Inhibitor or ARB for LVSD	91	92%	78%	82%	100%
Aspirin at Arrival	233	98%	91%	92%	100%

Aspirin at Discharge	386	99%	87%	90%	100%
Beta Blocker at Arrival	199	98%	85%	87%	100%
Beta Blocker at Discharge	409	99%	87%	90%	100%
Fibrinolytic Medication Timing	0	-	34%	31%	100%
PCI Within 90 Minutes of Arrival[1]	18	50%	47%	54%	95%
Smoking Cessation Advice	169	99%	85%	88%	100%
Heart Failure Care					
ACE Inhibitor or ARB for LVSD	252	92%	81%	82%	100%
Discharge Instructions	556	85%	59%	61%	93%
Evaluation of LVS Function	606	94%	81%	83%	99%
Smoking Cessation Advice	161	86%	86%	82%	100%
Pneumonia Care					
Appropriate Initial Antibiotic	226	85%	81%	83%	94%
Blood Culture Timing	207	98%	89%	90%	100%
Influenza Vaccine	48	69%	60%	70%	100%
Initial Antibiotic Timing	281	79%	75%	80%	93%
Oxygenation Assessment	344	100%	99%	99%	100%
Pneumococcal Vaccine	136	83%	61%	69%	94%
Smoking Cessation Advice	91	90%	82%	80%	100%
Surgical Infection Prevention					
Prophylactic Antibiotic Given[2,3]	215	89%	69%	77%	95%
Prophylactic Antibiotic Selection[2]	75	97%	89%	90%	100%
Prophylactic Antibiotic Stopped[2,3]	204	75%	71%	72%	95%
Pregnancy Care					
Inpatient Neonatal Mortality	3,203	1.59%	-	-	-
Third or Fourth Degree Laceration	1,732	1.67%	3.63%	3.63%	3.27%

Saint Joseph Candler Hospital

11705 Mercy Boulevard
Savannah, GA 31419
URL: www.sjchs.org
Ownership: Voluntary non-profit - Other
Emergency Services: Yes

Phone: 912-925-4100
Fax: 912-819-8039

Accredited: Yes
Licensed Beds: 305

Key Personnel:
CEO . . . . Paul P Hinchey
Chief Medical Staff . . . . J Allen Meadows, MD
Emergency Room . . . . Victoria Butler
Intensive Care Unit Director . . . . Judy Peterman
OB/GYN Womens Health . . . . Cliphane McLeod, MD
Chief Radiology . . . . TA Hetherington, MD

Measure	Cases	This Hospital	State Average	U.S. Average	Top Hospital
Heart Attack Care					
ACE Inhibitor or ARB for LVSD	55	100%	78%	82%	100%
Aspirin at Arrival	124	97%	91%	92%	100%
Aspirin at Discharge	380	99%	87%	90%	100%
Beta Blocker at Arrival	91	96%	85%	87%	100%
Beta Blocker at Discharge	401	99%	87%	90%	100%
Fibrinolytic Medication Timing[1]	2	50%	34%	31%	100%
PCI Within 90 Minutes of Arrival[1]	11	45%	47%	54%	95%
Smoking Cessation Advice	178	99%	85%	88%	100%
Heart Failure Care					
ACE Inhibitor or ARB for LVSD	92	100%	81%	82%	100%
Discharge Instructions	307	71%	59%	61%	93%
Evaluation of LVS Function	338	97%	81%	83%	99%
Smoking Cessation Advice	56	100%	86%	82%	100%
Pneumonia Care					
Appropriate Initial Antibiotic	107	80%	81%	83%	94%
Blood Culture Timing	105	95%	89%	90%	100%
Influenza Vaccine	42	69%	60%	70%	100%
Initial Antibiotic Timing	160	76%	75%	80%	93%
Oxygenation Assessment	215	100%	99%	99%	100%
Pneumococcal Vaccine	142	77%	61%	69%	94%
Smoking Cessation Advice	56	98%	82%	80%	100%
Surgical Infection Prevention					
Prophylactic Antibiotic Given[2,3]	113	87%	69%	77%	95%
Prophylactic Antibiotic Selection[2]	51	96%	89%	90%	100%
Prophylactic Antibiotic Stopped[2,3]	104	60%	71%	72%	95%
Pregnancy Care					
Inpatient Neonatal Mortality	-	-	-	-	-
Third or Fourth Degree Laceration	-	-	3.63%	3.63%	3.27%

Emory-Adventist Hospital

Alternate Name: Smyrna Hospital
3949 South Cobb Drive
Smyrna, GA 30080
URL: www.ahss.org
Ownership: Voluntary non-profit - Church
Emergency Services: Yes

Phone: 770-436-3162
Fax: 770-432-4260

Accredited: Yes
Licensed Beds: 100

Key Personnel:
President/CEO . . . . Thomas L Werner
Emergency Room . . . . Eric Deal, MD
Infection Control . . . . Susan Hebert
ICU . . . . Beth Lingerfelt
Medical/Surgical Nursing . . . . Pam Warren
Respiratory/Cardiopulmonary . . . . Bert Adams

Measure	Cases	This Hospital	State Average	U.S. Average	Top Hospital
Heart Attack Care					
ACE Inhibitor or ARB for LVSD[1]	1	100%	78%	82%	100%
Aspirin at Arrival[1]	7	86%	91%	92%	100%
Aspirin at Discharge[1]	3	100%	87%	90%	100%
Beta Blocker at Arrival[1]	6	100%	85%	87%	100%
Beta Blocker at Discharge[1]	4	100%	87%	90%	100%
Fibrinolytic Medication Timing	0	-	34%	31%	100%
PCI Within 90 Minutes of Arrival	0	-	47%	54%	95%
Smoking Cessation Advice	0	-	85%	88%	100%
Heart Failure Care					
ACE Inhibitor or ARB for LVSD[1]	24	88%	81%	82%	100%
Discharge Instructions	90	38%	59%	61%	93%
Evaluation of LVS Function	99	98%	81%	83%	99%
Smoking Cessation Advice	32	41%	86%	82%	100%
Pneumonia Care					
Appropriate Initial Antibiotic	66	74%	81%	83%	94%
Blood Culture Timing	67	96%	89%	90%	100%
Influenza Vaccine	32	69%	60%	70%	100%
Initial Antibiotic Timing	74	78%	75%	80%	93%
Oxygenation Assessment	101	97%	99%	99%	100%
Pneumococcal Vaccine	53	60%	61%	69%	94%
Smoking Cessation Advice	30	40%	82%	80%	100%
Surgical Infection Prevention					
Prophylactic Antibiotic Given[3]	44	34%	69%	77%	95%
Prophylactic Antibiotic Selection[1]	11	55%	89%	90%	100%
Prophylactic Antibiotic Stopped[3]	42	69%	71%	72%	95%
Pregnancy Care					
Inpatient Neonatal Mortality	-	-	-	-	-
Third or Fourth Degree Laceration	-	-	3.63%	3.63%	3.27%

Emory Eastside Medical Center

Alternate Name: Humana Hospital-Gwinnett
1700 Medical Way
Snellville, GA 30078
Ownership: Proprietary
Emergency Services: Yes

Phone: 770-979-0200
Fax: 770-736-2395
Accredited: Yes
Licensed Beds: 131

Key Personnel:
CEO . . . . Les Beard
Emergency Room . . . . Tim Grubbs
OB/GYN Womens Health . . . . William Haberstroh
Chief Radiology . . . . Jeffrey Gould, MD

Measure	Cases	This Hospital	State Average	U.S. Average	Top Hospital
Heart Attack Care					
ACE Inhibitor or ARB for LVSD[1]	11	91%	78%	82%	100%
Aspirin at Arrival	86	93%	91%	92%	100%
Aspirin at Discharge	31	87%	87%	90%	100%
Beta Blocker at Arrival	80	95%	85%	87%	100%
Beta Blocker at Discharge	33	100%	87%	90%	100%
Fibrinolytic Medication Timing[1]	21	52%	34%	31%	100%
PCI Within 90 Minutes of Arrival	0	-	47%	54%	95%
Smoking Cessation Advice[1]	5	80%	85%	88%	100%
Heart Failure Care					
ACE Inhibitor or ARB for LVSD	83	81%	81%	82%	100%
Discharge Instructions	269	86%	59%	61%	93%
Evaluation of LVS Function	303	99%	81%	83%	99%
Smoking Cessation Advice	41	100%	86%	82%	100%

NOTE: Hospital profiles are in alphabetical order by state, then city, then hospital within the city; Rankings are sorted by rate in descending order and exclude hospitals with less than 25 cases; (1) The number of cases is too small (n<25) for purposes of reliably predicting hospital performance; (2) Measure reflects the hospital's indication that its submission was based upon a sample of its relevant discharges; (3) Rate reflects fewer than the maximum possible quarters of data for the measure; (4) Inaccurate information submitted and suppressed for one or more quarters; (5) No data is available from the hospital for this measure; Please refer to the User's Guide for a full explanation of data

Pneumonia Care					
Appropriate Initial Antibiotic	246	92%	81%	83%	94%
Blood Culture Timing	241	90%	89%	90%	100%
Influenza Vaccine	77	86%	60%	70%	100%
Initial Antibiotic Timing	301	84%	75%	80%	93%
Oxygenation Assessment	394	100%	99%	99%	100%
Pneumococcal Vaccine	243	96%	61%	69%	94%
Smoking Cessation Advice	69	94%	82%	80%	100%
Surgical Infection Prevention					
Prophylactic Antibiotic Given[2,3]	211	93%	69%	77%	95%
Prophylactic Antibiotic Selection[2]	119	95%	89%	90%	100%
Prophylactic Antibiotic Stopped[2,3]	201	81%	71%	72%	95%
Pregnancy Care					
Inpatient Neonatal Mortality	-	-	-	-	-
Third or Fourth Degree Laceration	-	-	3.63%	3.63%	3.27%

Effingham Hospital

Alternate Name: Effingham County Hospital & Extended Care Facility
459 Highway 119 S   Phone: 912-754-6451
Springfield, GA 31329   Fax: 912-754-9901
E-mail: gelowkr1@memorialhealth.com
URL: www.effinghamhospital.com
Ownership: Govt - Hospital District or Authority   Accredited: Yes
Emergency Services: Yes   Licensed Beds: 45
Key Personnel:
CEO. . . . . Terrence Finch
Chief Medical Staff. . . . . Joseph Radford, MD
Manager Cardiopulmonary. . . . . Ann Ambrose
Manager Infection Control . . . . Rebecca Rahn
Manager Surgery . . . . Patricia Parrish
Manager Radiology . . . . Ken Wimmer

Measure	Cases	This Hospital	State Average	U.S. Average	Top Hospital
Heart Attack Care					
ACE Inhibitor or ARB for LVSD[5]	-	-	78%	82%	100%
Aspirin at Arrival[5]	-	-	91%	92%	100%
Aspirin at Discharge[5]	-	-	87%	90%	100%
Beta Blocker at Arrival[5]	-	-	85%	87%	100%
Beta Blocker at Discharge[5]	-	-	87%	90%	100%
Fibrinolytic Medication Timing[5]	-	-	34%	31%	100%
PCI Within 90 Minutes of Arrival[5]	-	-	47%	54%	95%
Smoking Cessation Advice[5]	-	-	85%	88%	100%
Heart Failure Care					
ACE Inhibitor or ARB for LVSD[3]	0	-	81%	82%	100%
Discharge Instructions[1,3]	8	0%	59%	61%	93%
Evaluation of LVS Function[1,3]	8	38%	81%	83%	99%
Smoking Cessation Advice[1,3]	1	100%	86%	82%	100%
Pneumonia Care					
Appropriate Initial Antibiotic[5]	-	-	81%	83%	94%
Blood Culture Timing[5]	-	-	89%	90%	100%
Influenza Vaccine[5]	-	-	60%	70%	100%
Initial Antibiotic Timing[5]	-	-	75%	80%	93%
Oxygenation Assessment[5]	-	-	99%	99%	100%
Pneumococcal Vaccine[5]	-	-	61%	69%	94%
Smoking Cessation Advice[5]	-	-	82%	80%	100%
Surgical Infection Prevention					
Prophylactic Antibiotic Given[5]	-	-	69%	77%	95%
Prophylactic Antibiotic Selection[5]	-	-	89%	90%	100%
Prophylactic Antibiotic Stopped[5]	-	-	71%	72%	95%
Pregnancy Care					
Inpatient Neonatal Mortality	-	-	-	-	-
Third or Fourth Degree Laceration	-	-	3.63%	3.63%	3.27%

East Georgia Regional Medical Center

1499 Fair Road   Phone: 912-486-1000
Statesboro, GA 30458   Fax: 912-871-2363
URL: www.egrmc.com
Ownership: Proprietary
Emergency Services: Yes   Accredited: Yes
                                          Licensed Beds: 150
Key Personnel:
CEO/Administrator. Bob Bigley
Cardiology . . . . Anthony Chappell, MD
Cardiology . . . . Stanley Shin, MD

Measure	Cases	This Hospital	State Average	U.S. Average	Top Hospital
Heart Attack Care					
ACE Inhibitor or ARB for LVSD[1]	9	78%	78%	82%	100%
Aspirin at Arrival	37	86%	91%	92%	100%
Aspirin at Discharge	26	85%	87%	90%	100%
Beta Blocker at Arrival	41	80%	85%	87%	100%
Beta Blocker at Discharge	27	81%	87%	90%	100%
Fibrinolytic Medication Timing[1]	3	0%	34%	31%	100%
PCI Within 90 Minutes of Arrival	0	-	47%	54%	95%
Smoking Cessation Advice[1]	7	86%	85%	88%	100%
Heart Failure Care					
ACE Inhibitor or ARB for LVSD	61	72%	81%	82%	100%
Discharge Instructions	180	17%	59%	61%	93%
Evaluation of LVS Function	204	69%	81%	83%	99%
Smoking Cessation Advice	41	95%	86%	82%	100%
Pneumonia Care					
Appropriate Initial Antibiotic	155	70%	81%	83%	94%
Blood Culture Timing	74	92%	89%	90%	100%
Influenza Vaccine[4,5]	-	-	60%	70%	100%
Initial Antibiotic Timing	159	70%	75%	80%	93%
Oxygenation Assessment	196	98%	99%	99%	100%
Pneumococcal Vaccine	84	13%	61%	69%	94%
Smoking Cessation Advice	55	91%	82%	80%	100%
Surgical Infection Prevention					
Prophylactic Antibiotic Given[2]	274	78%	69%	77%	95%
Prophylactic Antibiotic Selection[2]	43	86%	89%	90%	100%
Prophylactic Antibiotic Stopped[2]	259	44%	71%	72%	95%
Pregnancy Care					
Inpatient Neonatal Mortality	-	-	-	-	-
Third or Fourth Degree Laceration	-	-	3.63%	3.63%	3.27%

Henry Medical Center

1133 Eagle's Landing Parkway   Phone: 770-389-2200
Stockbridge, GA 30281   Fax: 770-389-2093
URL: www.henrymedical.com
Ownership: Govt - Hospital District or Authority   Accredited: Yes
Emergency Services: Yes   Licensed Beds: 124
Key Personnel:
CEO. . . . . G Sam Ahern
Chief Medical Staff. . . . . Dr. Willie Cochran
Emergency Room . . . . Cheryl Minor, RN
OB/GYN Womens Health. . . . . Dodie Davis
Director Radiology . . . . Dwight Fancher
Director Respiratory/Cardiopulmonary . . . . Angela Dennis

Measure	Cases	This Hospital	State Average	U.S. Average	Top Hospital
Heart Attack Care					
ACE Inhibitor or ARB for LVSD[1]	20	70%	78%	82%	100%
Aspirin at Arrival	164	98%	91%	92%	100%
Aspirin at Discharge	71	86%	87%	90%	100%
Beta Blocker at Arrival	146	97%	85%	87%	100%
Beta Blocker at Discharge	73	92%	87%	90%	100%
Fibrinolytic Medication Timing	45	62%	34%	31%	100%
PCI Within 90 Minutes of Arrival	0	-	47%	54%	95%
Smoking Cessation Advice	25	96%	85%	88%	100%
Heart Failure Care					
ACE Inhibitor or ARB for LVSD[2]	130	88%	81%	82%	100%
Discharge Instructions[2]	266	83%	59%	61%	93%
Evaluation of LVS Function[2]	303	88%	81%	83%	99%
Smoking Cessation Advice[2]	42	98%	86%	82%	100%
Pneumonia Care					
Appropriate Initial Antibiotic[2]	139	87%	81%	83%	94%
Blood Culture Timing[2]	96	74%	89%	90%	100%
Influenza Vaccine	30	37%	60%	70%	100%
Initial Antibiotic Timing[2]	164	65%	75%	80%	93%
Oxygenation Assessment[2]	200	98%	99%	99%	100%
Pneumococcal Vaccine[2]	94	51%	61%	69%	94%
Smoking Cessation Advice[2]	44	95%	82%	80%	100%
Surgical Infection Prevention					
Prophylactic Antibiotic Given[2,3]	149	81%	69%	77%	95%
Prophylactic Antibiotic Selection[2]	50	88%	89%	90%	100%
Prophylactic Antibiotic Stopped[2,3]	149	38%	71%	72%	95%

NOTE: Hospital profiles are in alphabetical order by state, then city, then hospital within the city; Rankings are sorted by rate in descending order and exclude hospitals with less than 25 cases; (1) The number of cases is too small (n<25) for purposes of reliably predicting hospital performance; (2) Measure reflects the hospital's indication that its submission was based upon a sample of its relevant discharges; (3) Rate reflects fewer than the maximum possible quarters of data for the measure; (4) Inaccurate information submitted and suppressed for one or more quarters; (5) No data is available from the hospital for this measure; Please refer to the User's Guide for a full explanation of data

Pregnancy Care					
Inpatient Neonatal Mortality[2]	414	0.48%	-	-	-
Third or Fourth Degree Laceration[2]	570	6.32%	3.63%	3.63%	3.27%

Emanuel Medical Center

Alternate Name: Emanuel County Hospital
117 Kite Road   Phone: 478-289-1100
Swainsboro, GA 30401   Fax: 478-289-1300
Ownership: Govt - Hospital District or Authority   Accredited: Yes
Emergency Services: Yes   Licensed Beds: 120
Key Personnel:
Chief OB/GYN . . . . W Davis

Measure	Cases	This Hospital	State Average	U.S. Average	Top Hospital
Heart Attack Care					
ACE Inhibitor or ARB for LVSD[1]	1	100%	78%	82%	100%
Aspirin at Arrival[1]	3	100%	91%	92%	100%
Aspirin at Discharge[1]	1	100%	87%	90%	100%
Beta Blocker at Arrival[1]	5	60%	85%	87%	100%
Beta Blocker at Discharge[1]	2	50%	87%	90%	100%
Fibrinolytic Medication Timing	0	-	34%	31%	100%
PCI Within 90 Minutes of Arrival	0	-	47%	54%	95%
Smoking Cessation Advice	0	-	85%	88%	100%
Heart Failure Care					
ACE Inhibitor or ARB for LVSD	40	62%	81%	82%	100%
Discharge Instructions	151	64%	59%	61%	93%
Evaluation of LVS Function	164	88%	81%	83%	99%
Smoking Cessation Advice	33	73%	86%	82%	100%
Pneumonia Care					
Appropriate Initial Antibiotic	71	83%	81%	83%	94%
Blood Culture Timing	39	69%	89%	90%	100%
Influenza Vaccine[4,5]	-	-	60%	70%	100%
Initial Antibiotic Timing	95	89%	75%	80%	93%
Oxygenation Assessment	119	100%	99%	99%	100%
Pneumococcal Vaccine	60	65%	61%	69%	94%
Smoking Cessation Advice	40	85%	82%	80%	100%
Surgical Infection Prevention					
Prophylactic Antibiotic Given	60	88%	69%	77%	95%
Prophylactic Antibiotic Selection[1]	18	100%	89%	90%	100%
Prophylactic Antibiotic Stopped	58	57%	71%	72%	95%
Pregnancy Care					
Inpatient Neonatal Mortality	204	0.00%	-	-	-
Third or Fourth Degree Laceration	142	1.41%	3.63%	3.63%	3.27%

Upson Regional Medical Center

Alternate Name: Upson County Hospital
PO Box 1059   Phone: 706-647-8111
Thomaston, GA 30286   Fax: 706-646-3310
URL: www.urmc.org
Ownership: Voluntary non-profit - Private
Emergency Services: Yes   Accredited: Yes
     Licensed Beds: 115
Key Personnel:
President/CEO. . . . . Thomas D Plantz
Chief Medical Staff. . . . . Chris Colby, MD
Emergency Room . . . . Martha Bently, RN
Infection Control. . . . . Glenda Van Houten, RN
ICU . . . . Trish Morway, RN
Intensive Coronary. . . . . Trish Morway, RN
Medical Surgical Nursing . . . . Debra Dunnahoo, RN
OB/GYN/Women's Health . . . . Shari Strickland, RN
Respiratory/Cardiopulmonary. . . . . Earnestine Zellner

Measure	Cases	This Hospital	State Average	U.S. Average	Top Hospital
Heart Attack Care					
ACE Inhibitor or ARB for LVSD[1]	4	100%	78%	82%	100%
Aspirin at Arrival	46	87%	91%	92%	100%
Aspirin at Discharge[1]	20	70%	87%	90%	100%
Beta Blocker at Arrival	39	82%	85%	87%	100%
Beta Blocker at Discharge[1]	22	95%	87%	90%	100%
Fibrinolytic Medication Timing[1]	11	45%	34%	31%	100%
PCI Within 90 Minutes of Arrival	0	-	47%	54%	95%
Smoking Cessation Advice[1]	7	86%	85%	88%	100%

Heart Failure Care					
ACE Inhibitor or ARB for LVSD	71	89%	81%	82%	100%
Discharge Instructions	145	70%	59%	61%	93%
Evaluation of LVS Function	171	80%	81%	83%	99%
Smoking Cessation Advice	46	91%	86%	82%	100%
Pneumonia Care					
Appropriate Initial Antibiotic	91	98%	81%	83%	94%
Blood Culture Timing	75	87%	89%	90%	100%
Influenza Vaccine	29	48%	60%	70%	100%
Initial Antibiotic Timing	138	87%	75%	80%	93%
Oxygenation Assessment	171	100%	99%	99%	100%
Pneumococcal Vaccine	90	54%	61%	69%	94%
Smoking Cessation Advice	46	80%	82%	80%	100%
Surgical Infection Prevention					
Prophylactic Antibiotic Given[2,3]	35	63%	69%	77%	95%
Prophylactic Antibiotic Selection[2]	34	94%	89%	90%	100%
Prophylactic Antibiotic Stopped[2,3]	35	17%	71%	72%	95%
Pregnancy Care					
Inpatient Neonatal Mortality	-	-	-	-	-
Third or Fourth Degree Laceration	-	-	3.63%	3.63%	3.27%

John D Archbold Memorial Hospital

915 Gordon Avenue & Mimosa Drive   Phone: 229-723-6801
Thomasville, GA 31792   Fax: 229-228-8591
Ownership: Voluntary non-profit - Private   Accredited: Yes
Emergency Services: Yes   Licensed Beds: 224
Key Personnel:
President/CEO. . . . . James L Storey Jr, MD
Chief Medical Staff. . . . . Wesley Simmes
Emergency Room . . . . Mark Swicord
Chief Radiology . . . . Paul Carpenter, MD
Director Respiratory Therapy . . . . Bill Bitzel

Measure	Cases	This Hospital	State Average	U.S. Average	Top Hospital
Heart Attack Care					
ACE Inhibitor or ARB for LVSD	28	96%	78%	82%	100%
Aspirin at Arrival	122	100%	91%	92%	100%
Aspirin at Discharge	106	100%	87%	90%	100%
Beta Blocker at Arrival	106	99%	85%	87%	100%
Beta Blocker at Discharge	100	98%	87%	90%	100%
Fibrinolytic Medication Timing[1]	14	14%	34%	31%	100%
PCI Within 90 Minutes of Arrival[1]	4	50%	47%	54%	95%
Smoking Cessation Advice	40	100%	85%	88%	100%
Heart Failure Care					
ACE Inhibitor or ARB for LVSD[2]	118	97%	81%	82%	100%
Discharge Instructions[2]	282	80%	59%	61%	93%
Evaluation of LVS Function[2]	320	98%	81%	83%	99%
Smoking Cessation Advice[2]	86	100%	86%	82%	100%
Pneumonia Care					
Appropriate Initial Antibiotic	132	91%	81%	83%	94%
Blood Culture Timing	101	90%	89%	90%	100%
Influenza Vaccine	34	88%	60%	70%	100%
Initial Antibiotic Timing	177	85%	75%	80%	93%
Oxygenation Assessment	225	100%	99%	99%	100%
Pneumococcal Vaccine	122	90%	61%	69%	94%
Smoking Cessation Advice	60	100%	82%	80%	100%
Surgical Infection Prevention					
Prophylactic Antibiotic Given[2]	470	85%	69%	77%	95%
Prophylactic Antibiotic Selection[2]	56	93%	89%	90%	100%
Prophylactic Antibiotic Stopped[2]	423	74%	71%	72%	95%
Pregnancy Care					
Inpatient Neonatal Mortality	-	-	-	-	-
Third or Fourth Degree Laceration	-	-	3.63%	3.63%	3.27%

McDuffie Regional Medical Center

521 Hill Street SW   Phone: 706-595-1411
Thomson, GA 30824   Fax: 706-597-5377
Ownership: Govt - Hospital District or Authority   Accredited: Yes
Emergency Services: Yes   Licensed Beds: 47
Key Personnel:
CEO. . . . . Douglas C Keir
Chief Medical Staff. . . . . Joe T Wills, MD
Director of Medical Staff. . . . . April Keene

NOTE: Hospital profiles are in alphabetical order by state, then city, then hospital within the city; Rankings are sorted by rate in descending order and exclude hospitals with less than 25 cases; (1) The number of cases is too small (n<25) for purposes of reliably predicting hospital performance; (2) Measure reflects the hospital's indication that its submission was based upon a sample of its relevant discharges; (3) Rate reflects fewer than the maximum possible quarters of data for the measure; (4) Inaccurate information submitted and suppressed for one or more quarters; (5) No data is available from the hospital for this measure; Please refer to the User's Guide for a full explanation of data

Manager Emergency Room . . . . Jane Lloyd
Chief Radiology . . . . Edwin Bradshaw
Manager Pulmonary Care . . . . Donald Paster

Measure	Cases	This Hospital	State Average	U.S. Average	Top Hospital
Heart Attack Care					
ACE Inhibitor or ARB for LVSD[1,3]	1	100%	78%	82%	100%
Aspirin at Arrival[1,3]	5	80%	91%	92%	100%
Aspirin at Discharge[1,3]	3	100%	87%	90%	100%
Beta Blocker at Arrival[1,3]	5	40%	85%	87%	100%
Beta Blocker at Discharge[1,3]	4	50%	87%	90%	100%
Fibrinolytic Medication Timing[3]	0	-	34%	31%	100%
PCI Within 90 Minutes of Arrival	0	-	47%	54%	95%
Smoking Cessation Advice[3]	0	-	85%	88%	100%
Heart Failure Care					
ACE Inhibitor or ARB for LVSD[1]	12	83%	81%	82%	100%
Discharge Instructions	33	55%	59%	61%	93%
Evaluation of LVS Function	31	81%	81%	83%	99%
Smoking Cessation Advice[1]	2	100%	86%	82%	100%
Pneumonia Care					
Appropriate Initial Antibiotic[2]	77	58%	81%	83%	94%
Blood Culture Timing[2]	66	95%	89%	90%	100%
Influenza Vaccine[1]	20	70%	60%	70%	100%
Initial Antibiotic Timing[2]	138	85%	75%	80%	93%
Oxygenation Assessment[2]	144	99%	99%	99%	100%
Pneumococcal Vaccine[2]	90	71%	61%	69%	94%
Smoking Cessation Advice[1,2]	21	71%	82%	80%	100%
Surgical Infection Prevention					
Prophylactic Antibiotic Given[1,3]	12	0%	69%	77%	95%
Prophylactic Antibiotic Selection[1]	14	93%	89%	90%	100%
Prophylactic Antibiotic Stopped[1,3]	10	10%	71%	72%	95%
Pregnancy Care					
Inpatient Neonatal Mortality	-	-	-	-	-
Third or Fourth Degree Laceration	-	-	3.63%	3.63%	3.27%

Tift Regional Medical Hospital

901 E 18th Street
Tifton, GA 31794

Toll-Free: 800-648-1935
Phone: 229-382-7120
Fax: 229-353-6192

E-mail: hrdept@surfsouth.com
URL: www.tiftregional.com
Ownership: Govt - Hospital District or Authority
Emergency Services: Yes
Accredited: Yes
Licensed Beds: 191
Key Personnel:
President/CEO . . . . William T Richardson, FACHE
Chief Medical Staff . . . . Ray Moreno, MD
OB/GYN Womens Health . . . . John Dorming, MD
Director Respiratory Therapy . . . . Jerry Ethridge

Measure	Cases	This Hospital	State Average	U.S. Average	Top Hospital
Heart Attack Care					
ACE Inhibitor or ARB for LVSD[1]	19	95%	78%	82%	100%
Aspirin at Arrival	60	93%	91%	92%	100%
Aspirin at Discharge	54	85%	87%	90%	100%
Beta Blocker at Arrival	53	96%	85%	87%	100%
Beta Blocker at Discharge	53	89%	87%	90%	100%
Fibrinolytic Medication Timing	0	-	34%	31%	100%
PCI Within 90 Minutes of Arrival[1]	2	100%	47%	54%	95%
Smoking Cessation Advice[1]	20	95%	85%	88%	100%
Heart Failure Care					
ACE Inhibitor or ARB for LVSD	147	89%	81%	82%	100%
Discharge Instructions	255	84%	59%	61%	93%
Evaluation of LVS Function	279	98%	81%	83%	99%
Smoking Cessation Advice	62	97%	86%	82%	100%
Pneumonia Care					
Appropriate Initial Antibiotic	138	86%	81%	83%	94%
Blood Culture Timing	66	94%	89%	90%	100%
Influenza Vaccine[1]	21	62%	60%	70%	100%
Initial Antibiotic Timing	138	65%	75%	80%	93%
Oxygenation Assessment	160	100%	99%	99%	100%
Pneumococcal Vaccine	96	98%	61%	69%	94%

Measure	Cases	This Hospital	State Average	U.S. Average	Top Hospital
Smoking Cessation Advice	33	100%	82%	80%	100%
Surgical Infection Prevention					
Prophylactic Antibiotic Given[2,3]	136	51%	69%	77%	95%
Prophylactic Antibiotic Selection[2]	40	92%	89%	90%	100%
Prophylactic Antibiotic Stopped[2,3]	125	81%	71%	72%	95%
Pregnancy Care					
Inpatient Neonatal Mortality	1,436	0.07%	-	-	-
Third or Fourth Degree Laceration	925	2.16%	3.63%	3.63%	3.27%

Stephens County Hospital

2003 Falls Road
Toccoa, GA 30577
URL: www.stephenscountyhospital.com
Ownership: Govt - Hospital District or Authority
Emergency Services: Yes

Phone: 706-282-4200
Fax: 706-886-8045

Accredited: Yes
Licensed Beds: 96
Key Personnel:
CEO . . . . Ed Gambrell Jr
Emergency Room . . . . Vickie Ansley, RN
Chief Radiology . . . . Michelle Chitwood
Director Respiratory Therapy . . . . Jim Halsey, RRT

Measure	Cases	This Hospital	State Average	U.S. Average	Top Hospital
Heart Attack Care					
ACE Inhibitor or ARB for LVSD	0	-	78%	82%	100%
Aspirin at Arrival[1]	19	84%	91%	92%	100%
Aspirin at Discharge[1]	8	62%	87%	90%	100%
Beta Blocker at Arrival[1]	18	56%	85%	87%	100%
Beta Blocker at Discharge[1]	9	56%	87%	90%	100%
Fibrinolytic Medication Timing	0	-	34%	31%	100%
PCI Within 90 Minutes of Arrival	0	-	47%	54%	95%
Smoking Cessation Advice[1]	3	33%	85%	88%	100%
Heart Failure Care					
ACE Inhibitor or ARB for LVSD	31	48%	81%	82%	100%
Discharge Instructions	138	41%	59%	61%	93%
Evaluation of LVS Function	162	49%	81%	83%	99%
Smoking Cessation Advice	28	36%	86%	82%	100%
Pneumonia Care					
Appropriate Initial Antibiotic	124	60%	81%	83%	94%
Blood Culture Timing	93	97%	89%	90%	100%
Influenza Vaccine	34	71%	60%	70%	100%
Initial Antibiotic Timing	166	74%	75%	80%	93%
Oxygenation Assessment	190	99%	99%	99%	100%
Pneumococcal Vaccine	106	61%	61%	69%	94%
Smoking Cessation Advice	43	35%	82%	80%	100%
Surgical Infection Prevention					
Prophylactic Antibiotic Given[2,3]	31	48%	69%	77%	95%
Prophylactic Antibiotic Selection[2]	31	87%	89%	90%	100%
Prophylactic Antibiotic Stopped[2,3]	31	42%	71%	72%	95%
Pregnancy Care					
Inpatient Neonatal Mortality	-	-	-	-	-
Third or Fourth Degree Laceration	-	-	3.63%	3.63%	3.27%

Emory Northlake Regional Medical Center

Alternate Name: Northlake Regional Medical Center
1455 Montreal Road
Tucker, GA 30084
URL: www.northlakemedical.com
Ownership: Proprietary
Emergency Services: Yes

Phone: 770-270-3000
Fax: 770-270-3199

Accredited: Yes
Licensed Beds: 120
Key Personnel:
CEO . . . . Tom Gilbert
Chief Medical Staff . . . . Jeffrey Scott, MD
Emergency Room . . . . Donald Lyles, RN
Director Medical/Surgical Nursing . . . . Linda Aiken, RN
Chief Radiology . . . . Bruce Bielfelt, DO
Director Respiratory Therapy . . . . Penny Donohue

Measure	Cases	This Hospital	State Average	U.S. Average	Top Hospital
Heart Attack Care					
ACE Inhibitor or ARB for LVSD[1]	5	60%	78%	82%	100%
Aspirin at Arrival[1]	24	100%	91%	92%	100%
Aspirin at Discharge[1]	12	83%	87%	90%	100%
Beta Blocker at Arrival[1]	19	95%	85%	87%	100%

NOTE: Hospital profiles are in alphabetical order by state, then city, then hospital within the city; Rankings are sorted by rate in descending order and exclude hospitals with less than 25 cases; (1) The number of cases is too small (n<25) for purposes of reliably predicting hospital performance; (2) Measure reflects the hospital's indication that its submission was based upon a sample of its relevant discharges; (3) Rate reflects fewer than the maximum possible quarters of data for the measure; (4) Inaccurate information submitted and suppressed for one or more quarters; (5) No data is available from the hospital for this measure; Please refer to the User's Guide for a full explanation of data

Measure	Cases	This Hospital	State Average	U.S. Average	Top Hospital
Beta Blocker at Discharge[1]	12	92%	87%	90%	100%
Fibrinolytic Medication Timing[1]	1	0%	34%	31%	100%
PCI Within 90 Minutes of Arrival	0	-	47%	54%	95%
Smoking Cessation Advice[1]	2	50%	85%	88%	100%
Heart Failure Care					
ACE Inhibitor or ARB for LVSD	46	74%	81%	82%	100%
Discharge Instructions	112	85%	59%	61%	93%
Evaluation of LVS Function	129	87%	81%	83%	99%
Smoking Cessation Advice	32	72%	86%	82%	100%
Pneumonia Care					
Appropriate Initial Antibiotic	78	73%	81%	83%	94%
Blood Culture Timing	73	78%	89%	90%	100%
Influenza Vaccine[1]	20	40%	60%	70%	100%
Initial Antibiotic Timing	104	67%	75%	80%	93%
Oxygenation Assessment	118	98%	99%	99%	100%
Pneumococcal Vaccine	54	37%	61%	69%	94%
Smoking Cessation Advice	33	64%	82%	80%	100%
Surgical Infection Prevention					
Prophylactic Antibiotic Given[2,3]	76	26%	69%	77%	95%
Prophylactic Antibiotic Selection[2]	28	93%	89%	90%	100%
Prophylactic Antibiotic Stopped[2,3]	72	86%	71%	72%	95%
Pregnancy Care					
Inpatient Neonatal Mortality	-	-	-	-	-
Third or Fourth Degree Laceration	-	-	3.63%	3.63%	3.27%

Smith Northview Hospital

4280 North Valdosta Road
Valdosta, GA 31602
Ownership: Proprietary
Emergency Services: Yes

Phone: 229-671-2002

Accredited: Yes

Measure	Cases	This Hospital	State Average	U.S. Average	Top Hospital
Heart Attack Care					
ACE Inhibitor or ARB for LVSD[1]	5	60%	78%	82%	100%
Aspirin at Arrival[1]	19	100%	91%	92%	100%
Aspirin at Discharge[1]	17	100%	87%	90%	100%
Beta Blocker at Arrival[1]	23	96%	85%	87%	100%
Beta Blocker at Discharge[1]	19	89%	87%	90%	100%
Fibrinolytic Medication Timing[1]	2	0%	34%	31%	100%
PCI Within 90 Minutes of Arrival	0	-	47%	54%	95%
Smoking Cessation Advice[1]	2	50%	85%	88%	100%
Heart Failure Care					
ACE Inhibitor or ARB for LVSD[2]	34	91%	81%	82%	100%
Discharge Instructions[2]	79	32%	59%	61%	93%
Evaluation of LVS Function[2]	88	78%	81%	83%	99%
Smoking Cessation Advice[1,2]	10	20%	86%	82%	100%
Pneumonia Care					
Appropriate Initial Antibiotic	54	78%	81%	83%	94%
Blood Culture Timing[1]	17	88%	89%	90%	100%
Influenza Vaccine[1]	12	17%	60%	70%	100%
Initial Antibiotic Timing	51	65%	75%	80%	93%
Oxygenation Assessment	67	96%	99%	99%	100%
Pneumococcal Vaccine	30	20%	61%	69%	94%
Smoking Cessation Advice[1]	16	75%	82%	80%	100%
Surgical Infection Prevention					
Prophylactic Antibiotic Given[2,3]	59	32%	69%	77%	95%
Prophylactic Antibiotic Selection[1,2]	22	86%	89%	90%	100%
Prophylactic Antibiotic Stopped[2,3]	57	63%	71%	72%	95%
Pregnancy Care					
Inpatient Neonatal Mortality	-	-	-	-	-
Third or Fourth Degree Laceration	-	-	3.63%	3.63%	3.27%

South Georgia Medical Center

Pendleton Park
2501 N Patterson Street
Valdosta, GA 31603
URL: www.sgmc.org
Ownership: Govt - Hospital District or Authority
Emergency Services: Yes
Key Personnel:
CEO. . . . . James McGahee
Chief Medical Staff. . . . . Howard Jones, DO

Phone: 229-333-1000
Fax: 229-259-4423

Accredited: Yes
Licensed Beds: 288

Emergency Room . . . . Andre Shackleford
Director Medical/Surgical Nursing . . . . Chris Armstead, RN
OB/GYN Womens Health. . . . . Samuel Taylor, MD
Chief Radiology . . . . William Querin, MD
Director Respiratory Therapy . . . . Rich Griffin

Measure	Cases	This Hospital	State Average	U.S. Average	Top Hospital
Heart Attack Care					
ACE Inhibitor or ARB for LVSD[1,2]	23	78%	78%	82%	100%
Aspirin at Arrival[2]	156	100%	91%	92%	100%
Aspirin at Discharge[2]	208	98%	87%	90%	100%
Beta Blocker at Arrival[2]	117	97%	85%	87%	100%
Beta Blocker at Discharge[2]	211	96%	87%	90%	100%
Fibrinolytic Medication Timing[1,2]	11	55%	34%	31%	100%
PCI Within 90 Minutes of Arrival[1,2]	4	25%	47%	54%	95%
Smoking Cessation Advice[2]	85	95%	85%	88%	100%
Heart Failure Care					
ACE Inhibitor or ARB for LVSD	126	80%	81%	82%	100%
Discharge Instructions	318	47%	59%	61%	93%
Evaluation of LVS Function	359	85%	81%	83%	99%
Smoking Cessation Advice	75	96%	86%	82%	100%
Pneumonia Care					
Appropriate Initial Antibiotic	141	87%	81%	83%	94%
Blood Culture Timing	53	94%	89%	90%	100%
Influenza Vaccine	29	66%	60%	70%	100%
Initial Antibiotic Timing	199	64%	75%	80%	93%
Oxygenation Assessment	240	99%	99%	99%	100%
Pneumococcal Vaccine	130	55%	61%	69%	94%
Smoking Cessation Advice	50	88%	82%	80%	100%
Surgical Infection Prevention					
Prophylactic Antibiotic Given[2,3]	64	75%	69%	77%	95%
Prophylactic Antibiotic Selection[2]	66	86%	89%	90%	100%
Prophylactic Antibiotic Stopped[2,3]	62	73%	71%	72%	95%
Pregnancy Care					
Inpatient Neonatal Mortality	-	-	-	-	-
Third or Fourth Degree Laceration	-	-	3.63%	3.63%	3.27%

Meadows Regional Medical Center

Alternate Name: John M Meadows Memorial Hospital
1703 Meadows Lane
Vidalia, GA 30474
Ownership: Voluntary non-profit - Other
Emergency Services: Yes
Key Personnel:
CEO. . . . . Alan Kent
Emergency Room . . . . Marie Smith
Director Medical/Surgical Nursing . . . . Linda Aleska
Director Respiratory Therapy . . . . Payne Phillips

Phone: 912-537-8921
Fax: 912-538-5529
Accredited: Yes
Licensed Beds: 122

Measure	Cases	This Hospital	State Average	U.S. Average	Top Hospital
Heart Attack Care					
ACE Inhibitor or ARB for LVSD[1]	11	82%	78%	82%	100%
Aspirin at Arrival	40	90%	91%	92%	100%
Aspirin at Discharge	37	86%	87%	90%	100%
Beta Blocker at Arrival	37	81%	85%	87%	100%
Beta Blocker at Discharge	37	84%	87%	90%	100%
Fibrinolytic Medication Timing[1]	10	30%	34%	31%	100%
PCI Within 90 Minutes of Arrival	0	-	47%	54%	95%
Smoking Cessation Advice[1]	18	100%	85%	88%	100%
Heart Failure Care					
ACE Inhibitor or ARB for LVSD	45	93%	81%	82%	100%
Discharge Instructions	136	68%	59%	61%	93%
Evaluation of LVS Function	177	80%	81%	83%	99%
Smoking Cessation Advice	47	94%	86%	82%	100%
Pneumonia Care					
Appropriate Initial Antibiotic	79	80%	81%	83%	94%
Blood Culture Timing	49	84%	89%	90%	100%
Influenza Vaccine	31	32%	60%	70%	100%
Initial Antibiotic Timing	118	82%	75%	80%	93%
Oxygenation Assessment	156	100%	99%	99%	100%
Pneumococcal Vaccine	75	27%	61%	69%	94%
Smoking Cessation Advice	38	92%	82%	80%	100%

NOTE: Hospital profiles are in alphabetical order by state, then city, then hospital within the city; Rankings are sorted by rate in descending order and exclude hospitals with less than 25 cases; (1) The number of cases is too small (n<25) for purposes of reliably predicting hospital performance; (2) Measure reflects the hospital's indication that its submission was based upon a sample of its relevant discharges; (3) Rate reflects fewer than the maximum possible quarters of data for the measure; (4) Inaccurate information submitted and suppressed for one or more quarters; (5) No data is available from the hospital for this measure; Please refer to the User's Guide for a full explanation of data

Surgical Infection Prevention					
Prophylactic Antibiotic Given[2,3]	85	34%	69%	77%	95%
Prophylactic Antibiotic Selection[2]	26	96%	89%	90%	100%
Prophylactic Antibiotic Stopped[2,3]	86	79%	71%	72%	95%
Pregnancy Care					
Inpatient Neonatal Mortality	520	0.58%	-	-	-
Third or Fourth Degree Laceration	388	2.84%	3.63%	3.63%	3.27%

Tanner Medical Center

601 Dallas Road
Villa Rica, GA 30180
Ownership: Voluntary non-profit - Private
Emergency Services: Yes

Phone: 770-456-3000
Fax: 770-456-3390
Accredited: Yes
Licensed Beds: 52

Key Personnel:
CEO . . . . Larry Steed
Chief Medical Staff. . . . . Larry Price, MD
Emergency Room . . . . Sharon Walker
Director Medical/Surgical Nursing . . . . Sharon Walker
OB/GYN Womens Health. . . . . Larry Price, MD
Director Respiratory Therapy . . . . Deborah Lyner

Measure	Cases	This Hospital	State Average	U.S. Average	Top Hospital
Heart Attack Care					
ACE Inhibitor or ARB for LVSD[1]	4	100%	78%	82%	100%
Aspirin at Arrival	29	97%	91%	92%	100%
Aspirin at Discharge[1]	10	90%	87%	90%	100%
Beta Blocker at Arrival	28	86%	85%	87%	100%
Beta Blocker at Discharge[1]	9	89%	87%	90%	100%
Fibrinolytic Medication Timing[1]	3	67%	34%	31%	100%
PCI Within 90 Minutes of Arrival	0	-	47%	54%	95%
Smoking Cessation Advice[1]	5	100%	85%	88%	100%
Heart Failure Care					
ACE Inhibitor or ARB for LVSD	47	94%	81%	82%	100%
Discharge Instructions	100	78%	59%	61%	93%
Evaluation of LVS Function	106	96%	81%	83%	99%
Smoking Cessation Advice[1]	16	100%	86%	82%	100%
Pneumonia Care					
Appropriate Initial Antibiotic	104	89%	81%	83%	94%
Blood Culture Timing	57	86%	89%	90%	100%
Influenza Vaccine[1]	20	95%	60%	70%	100%
Initial Antibiotic Timing	106	87%	75%	80%	93%
Oxygenation Assessment	121	100%	99%	99%	100%
Pneumococcal Vaccine	54	94%	61%	69%	94%
Smoking Cessation Advice	42	86%	82%	80%	100%
Surgical Infection Prevention					
Prophylactic Antibiotic Given[1,3]	21	86%	69%	77%	95%
Prophylactic Antibiotic Selection[1]	9	100%	89%	90%	100%
Prophylactic Antibiotic Stopped[1,3]	20	90%	71%	72%	95%
Pregnancy Care					
Inpatient Neonatal Mortality	-	-	-	-	-
Third or Fourth Degree Laceration	-	-	3.63%	3.63%	3.27%

Houston Medical Center

1601 Watson Boulevard
Warner Robins, GA 31093
Ownership: Govt - Hospital District or Authority
Emergency Services: Yes

Phone: 478-922-4281
Fax: 478-542-7955
Accredited: Yes
Licensed Beds: 186

Key Personnel:
CEO. . . . . Frank J Aaron
Administrator . . . . Arthur P Christie
Emergency Room . . . . Carla Weese
OB/GYN Womens Health. . . . . Richard Heaton, MD
Chief Radiology . . . . Thomas Johnson, MD
Director Respiratory Therapy . . . . Ann Cosieod

Measure	Cases	This Hospital	State Average	U.S. Average	Top Hospital
Heart Attack Care					
ACE Inhibitor or ARB for LVSD[1]	2	100%	78%	82%	100%
Aspirin at Arrival	36	94%	91%	92%	100%
Aspirin at Discharge[1]	12	83%	87%	90%	100%
Beta Blocker at Arrival	32	84%	85%	87%	100%
Beta Blocker at Discharge[1]	9	78%	87%	90%	100%

Fibrinolytic Medication Timing[1]	8	25%	34%	31%	100%
PCI Within 90 Minutes of Arrival	0	-	47%	54%	95%
Smoking Cessation Advice[1]	2	50%	85%	88%	100%
Heart Failure Care					
ACE Inhibitor or ARB for LVSD[2]	86	84%	81%	82%	100%
Discharge Instructions[2]	195	53%	59%	61%	93%
Evaluation of LVS Function[2]	211	79%	81%	83%	99%
Smoking Cessation Advice[2]	72	90%	86%	82%	100%
Pneumonia Care					
Appropriate Initial Antibiotic[2]	92	87%	81%	83%	94%
Blood Culture Timing[2]	62	94%	89%	90%	100%
Influenza Vaccine[2]	29	48%	60%	70%	100%
Initial Antibiotic Timing[2]	133	61%	75%	80%	93%
Oxygenation Assessment[2]	175	100%	99%	99%	100%
Pneumococcal Vaccine[2]	89	83%	61%	69%	94%
Smoking Cessation Advice[2]	51	78%	82%	80%	100%
Surgical Infection Prevention					
Prophylactic Antibiotic Given[2,3]	174	74%	69%	77%	95%
Prophylactic Antibiotic Selection[2]	48	83%	89%	90%	100%
Prophylactic Antibiotic Stopped[2,3]	173	48%	71%	72%	95%
Pregnancy Care					
Inpatient Neonatal Mortality	-	-	-	-	-
Third or Fourth Degree Laceration	-	-	3.63%	3.63%	3.27%

Satilla Regional Medical Center

410 Darling Avenue
Waycross, GA 31501
Ownership: Voluntary non-profit - Other
Emergency Services: Yes

Phone: 912-283-3030
Fax: 912-287-2505
Accredited: Yes
Licensed Beds: 231

Key Personnel:
CEO. . . . . Robert Trimm
Chief Medical Staff. . . . . Wade Dye, MD
Emergency Room . . . . James Hagen Bottom, MD
Director Medical/Surgical Nursing . . . . Holli Sweat

Measure	Cases	This Hospital	State Average	U.S. Average	Top Hospital
Heart Attack Care					
ACE Inhibitor or ARB for LVSD[1]	7	71%	78%	82%	100%
Aspirin at Arrival	74	91%	91%	92%	100%
Aspirin at Discharge	31	58%	87%	90%	100%
Beta Blocker at Arrival	64	92%	85%	87%	100%
Beta Blocker at Discharge	28	86%	87%	90%	100%
Fibrinolytic Medication Timing[1]	2	50%	34%	31%	100%
PCI Within 90 Minutes of Arrival	0	-	47%	54%	95%
Smoking Cessation Advice[1]	9	89%	85%	88%	100%
Heart Failure Care					
ACE Inhibitor or ARB for LVSD	111	73%	81%	82%	100%
Discharge Instructions	252	67%	59%	61%	93%
Evaluation of LVS Function	308	86%	81%	83%	99%
Smoking Cessation Advice	41	98%	86%	82%	100%
Pneumonia Care					
Appropriate Initial Antibiotic	166	84%	81%	83%	94%
Blood Culture Timing	141	97%	89%	90%	100%
Influenza Vaccine	61	79%	60%	70%	100%
Initial Antibiotic Timing	219	80%	75%	80%	93%
Oxygenation Assessment	270	100%	99%	99%	100%
Pneumococcal Vaccine	154	80%	61%	69%	94%
Smoking Cessation Advice	56	89%	82%	80%	100%
Surgical Infection Prevention					
Prophylactic Antibiotic Given[3]	63	59%	69%	77%	95%
Prophylactic Antibiotic Selection[5]	-	-	89%	90%	100%
Prophylactic Antibiotic Stopped[3]	59	32%	71%	72%	95%
Pregnancy Care					
Inpatient Neonatal Mortality	799	0.25%	-	-	-
Third or Fourth Degree Laceration	574	2.61%	3.63%	3.63%	3.27%

NOTE: Hospital profiles are in alphabetical order by state, then city, then hospital within the city; Rankings are sorted by rate in descending order and exclude hospitals with less than 25 cases; (1) The number of cases is too small (n<25) for purposes of reliably predicting hospital performance; (2) Measure reflects the hospital's indication that its submission was based upon a sample of its relevant discharges; (3) Rate reflects fewer than the maximum possible quarters of data for the measure; (4) Inaccurate information submitted and suppressed for one or more quarters; (5) No data is available from the hospital for this measure; Please refer to the User's Guide for a full explanation of data

Burke Medical Center

351 Liberty Street
Waynesboro, GA 30830
E-mail: dhighsmith@burke.net
Ownership: Proprietary
Emergency Services: Yes

Phone: 706-554-4435
Fax: 706-554-4854

Accredited: Yes
Licensed Beds: 40

Key Personnel:
Administrator . . . . Jennifer Royale
Chief Medical Staff . . . . Shelley A Griffin, MD
Emergency Room . . . . Tammy Lane, RN
Infection Control . . . . Donna Beardon
Respiratory/Cardiopulmonary . . . . Kenny Roberts

Measure	Cases	This Hospital	State Average	U.S. Average	Top Hospital
Heart Attack Care					
ACE Inhibitor or ARB for LVSD[1]	1	0%	78%	82%	100%
Aspirin at Arrival[1]	11	73%	91%	92%	100%
Aspirin at Discharge[1]	7	71%	87%	90%	100%
Beta Blocker at Arrival[1]	11	73%	85%	87%	100%
Beta Blocker at Discharge[1]	9	100%	87%	90%	100%
Fibrinolytic Medication Timing	0	-	34%	31%	100%
PCI Within 90 Minutes of Arrival	0	-	47%	54%	95%
Smoking Cessation Advice	0	-	85%	88%	100%
Heart Failure Care					
ACE Inhibitor or ARB for LVSD[1]	9	89%	81%	82%	100%
Discharge Instructions	80	46%	59%	61%	93%
Evaluation of LVS Function	86	29%	81%	83%	99%
Smoking Cessation Advice[1]	11	45%	86%	82%	100%
Pneumonia Care					
Appropriate Initial Antibiotic	65	74%	81%	83%	94%
Blood Culture Timing[1]	23	87%	89%	90%	100%
Influenza Vaccine[1]	12	25%	60%	70%	100%
Initial Antibiotic Timing	93	90%	75%	80%	93%
Oxygenation Assessment	110	95%	99%	99%	100%
Pneumococcal Vaccine	65	22%	61%	69%	94%
Smoking Cessation Advice[1]	22	59%	82%	80%	100%
Surgical Infection Prevention					
Prophylactic Antibiotic Given[1,2,3]	3	100%	69%	77%	95%
Prophylactic Antibiotic Selection[1,2]	3	100%	89%	90%	100%
Prophylactic Antibiotic Stopped[1,2,3]	3	100%	71%	72%	95%
Pregnancy Care					
Inpatient Neonatal Mortality	318	0.00%	-	-	-
Third or Fourth Degree Laceration	221	0.45%	3.63%	3.63%	3.27%

Barrow Regional Medical Center

316 N Broad Street
Winder, GA 30680
URL: www.barrowmedical.com
Ownership: Proprietary
Emergency Services: Yes

Phone: 770-867-3400
Fax: 770-307-5215

Accredited: Yes
Licensed Beds: 56

Key Personnel:
CEO . . . . Randy Mills
Director Medical/Surgical Nursing . . . . Lynne Everett, RN
Chief Radiology . . . . Thomas Butler, MD
Director Respiratory Therapy . . . . Candy Pendergross

Measure	Cases	This Hospital	State Average	U.S. Average	Top Hospital
Heart Attack Care					
ACE Inhibitor or ARB for LVSD[1]	2	50%	78%	82%	100%
Aspirin at Arrival[1]	12	58%	91%	92%	100%
Aspirin at Discharge[1]	6	33%	87%	90%	100%
Beta Blocker at Arrival[1]	10	70%	85%	87%	100%
Beta Blocker at Discharge[1]	6	33%	87%	90%	100%
Fibrinolytic Medication Timing	0	-	34%	31%	100%
PCI Within 90 Minutes of Arrival	0	-	47%	54%	95%
Smoking Cessation Advice	0	-	85%	88%	100%
Heart Failure Care					
ACE Inhibitor or ARB for LVSD[1]	16	56%	81%	82%	100%
Discharge Instructions	65	6%	59%	61%	93%
Evaluation of LVS Function	51	47%	81%	83%	99%
Smoking Cessation Advice[1]	19	89%	86%	82%	100%
Pneumonia Care					
Appropriate Initial Antibiotic	82	52%	81%	83%	94%

Blood Culture Timing	39	74%	89%	90%	100%
Influenza Vaccine[4,5]	-	-	60%	70%	100%
Initial Antibiotic Timing	76	68%	75%	80%	93%
Oxygenation Assessment	103	100%	99%	99%	100%
Pneumococcal Vaccine	52	38%	61%	69%	94%
Smoking Cessation Advice	35	83%	82%	80%	100%
Surgical Infection Prevention					
Prophylactic Antibiotic Given[2,3]	39	44%	69%	77%	95%
Prophylactic Antibiotic Selection[1,2]	9	89%	89%	90%	100%
Prophylactic Antibiotic Stopped[2,3]	36	94%	71%	72%	95%
Pregnancy Care					
Inpatient Neonatal Mortality	-	-	-	-	-
Third or Fourth Degree Laceration	-	-	3.63%	3.63%	3.27%

NOTE: Hospital profiles are in alphabetical order by state, then city, then hospital within the city; Rankings are sorted by rate in descending order and exclude hospitals with less than 25 cases; (1) The number of cases is too small (n<25) for purposes of reliably predicting hospital performance; (2) Measure reflects the hospital's indication that its submission was based upon a sample of its relevant discharges; (3) Rate reflects fewer than the maximum possible quarters of data for the measure; (4) Inaccurate information submitted and suppressed for one or more quarters; (5) No data is available from the hospital for this measure; Please refer to the User's Guide for a full explanation of data

Heart Attack Care

1. ACE Inhibitor or ARB for LVSD

Hospital Name	City	Rate	Cases
CHRISTUS Saint Patrick Hospital	Lake Charles	100%	80
Christus Saint Frances Cabrini Hospital	Alexandria	100%	44
Heart Hospital of Lafayette	Lafayette	100%	31
Saint Tammany Parish Hospital	Covington	100%	38
Louisiana State Univ Hosp-Shreveport	Shreveport	98%	43
Lake Charles Memorial Hospital	Lake Charles	97%	29
Thibodaux Regional Medical Center	Thibodaux	97%	31
Ochsner Clinic Foundation	New Orleans	93%	81
Our Lady of the Lake Regional Medical Center	Baton Rouge	93%	88
Lafayette General Medical Center	Lafayette	92%	26
Ochsner Medical Center-Baton Rouge	Baton Rouge	90%	77
Terrebonne General Medical Center	Houma	85%	52
North Oaks Medical System	Hammond	84%	55
Rapides Regional Medical Center	Alexandria	80%	60
Christus Schumpert Health System	Shreveport	79%	33
East Jefferson General Hospital	Metairie	77%	48
West Jefferson Medical Center	Marrero	76%	80
Baton Rouge General Medical Center	Baton Rouge	74%	113
Slidell Memorial Hospital	Slidell	73%	33
Glenwood Regional Medical Center	West Monroe	72%	57
Willis Knighton Medical Center	Shreveport	68%	131
Saint Francis Medical Center	Monroe	66%	59
Lakeview Regional Medical Center	Covington	56%	25
Willis Knighton Bossier Health Center	Bossier City	48%	33

2. Aspirin at Arrival

Hospital Name	City	Rate	Cases
CHRISTUS Saint Patrick Hospital	Lake Charles	100%	177
Doctors Hospital of Opelousas	Opelousas	100%	39
Heart Hospital of Lafayette	Lafayette	100%	44
Leonard J Chabert Medical Center	Houma	100%	56
Louisiana Heart Hospital	Lacombe	100%	64
River West Medical Center	Plaquemine	100%	30
Thibodaux Regional Medical Center	Thibodaux	100%	118
Tulane University Hospital & Clinic	New Orleans	100%	50
University Medical Center	Lafayette	100%	45
Lake Charles Memorial Hospital	Lake Charles	99%	75
Ochsner Medical Center-Baton Rouge	Baton Rouge	99%	134
Our Lady of the Lake Regional Medical Center	Baton Rouge	99%	239
Saint Tammany Parish Hospital	Covington	99%	102
Beauregard Memorial Hospital	DeRidder	98%	44
Christus Saint Frances Cabrini Hospital	Alexandria	98%	128
Lincoln General Hospital	Ruston	98%	58
Louisiana State Univ Hosp-Shreveport	Shreveport	98%	117
Northshore Regional Medical Center	Slidell	98%	97
Slidell Memorial Hospital	Slidell	98%	120
Willis Knighton Medical Center	Shreveport	98%	231
Jennings American Legion Hospital	Jennings	97%	33
Opelousas General Hospital	Opelousas	97%	79
River Parishes Hospital	La Place	97%	30
Christus Schumpert Health System	Shreveport	96%	109
East Jefferson General Hospital	Metairie	96%	264
Glenwood Regional Medical Center	West Monroe	96%	137
Minden Medical Center	Minden	96%	27
North Oaks Medical System	Hammond	96%	191
West Calcasieu-Cameron Hospital	Sulphur	96%	56
West Jefferson Medical Center	Marrero	96%	279
Baton Rouge General Medical Center	Baton Rouge	95%	328
Earl K Long Medical Center	Baton Rouge	95%	77
Ochsner Clinic Foundation	New Orleans	95%	215
Saint Francis Medical Center	Monroe	95%	130
Touro Infirmary	New Orleans	95%	83
E A Conway Medical Center	Monroe	94%	84
Iberia Medical Center	New Iberia	94%	111
Our Lady of Lourdes Regional Medical Center	Lafayette	94%	124
Terrebonne General Medical Center	Houma	94%	200
Willis Knighton Bossier Health Center	Bossier City	94%	100
Lakeview Regional Medical Center	Covington	93%	69
Dauterive Hospital	New Iberia	91%	66
Lane Regional Memorial Hospital	Zachary	91%	33
Rapides Regional Medical Center	Alexandria	91%	121
Southwest Medical Center	Lafayette	90%	73
Byrd Regional Hospital	Leesville	88%	25
Lafayette General Medical Center	Lafayette	88%	125

3. Aspirin at Discharge

Hospital Name	City	Rate	Cases
CHRISTUS Saint Patrick Hospital	Lake Charles	100%	302
Christus Saint Frances Cabrini Hospital	Alexandria	100%	215
E A Conway Medical Center	Monroe	100%	44
Heart Hospital of Lafayette	Lafayette	100%	200
Louisiana Heart Hospital	Lacombe	100%	134
Lake Charles Memorial Hospital	Lake Charles	99%	108
Saint Tammany Parish Hospital	Covington	99%	115
Louisiana State Univ Hosp-Shreveport	Shreveport	98%	174
Thibodaux Regional Medical Center	Thibodaux	98%	188
Tulane University Hospital & Clinic	New Orleans	98%	55
University Medical Center	Lafayette	98%	50
Doctors Hospital of Opelousas	Opelousas	97%	29
Glenwood Regional Medical Center	West Monroe	97%	184
Lincoln General Hospital	Ruston	97%	38
Ochsner Clinic Foundation	New Orleans	97%	220
Our Lady of the Lake Regional Medical Center	Baton Rouge	97%	349
Christus Schumpert Health System	Shreveport	96%	149
Ochsner Medical Center-Baton Rouge	Baton Rouge	96%	120
Opelousas General Hospital	Opelousas	96%	70
Northshore Regional Medical Center	Slidell	95%	100
Rapides Regional Medical Center	Alexandria	95%	194
Slidell Memorial Hospital	Slidell	95%	111
Iberia Medical Center	New Iberia	94%	80
Leonard J Chabert Medical Center	Houma	94%	36
North Oaks Medical System	Hammond	94%	172
Saint Francis Medical Center	Monroe	94%	217
Terrebonne General Medical Center	Houma	94%	214
West Calcasieu-Cameron Hospital	Sulphur	94%	47
West Jefferson Medical Center	Marrero	94%	260
Willis Knighton Medical Center	Shreveport	94%	338
Lakeview Regional Medical Center	Covington	93%	75
East Jefferson General Hospital	Metairie	92%	254
Lafayette General Medical Center	Lafayette	91%	152
Touro Infirmary	New Orleans	91%	76
Earl K Long Medical Center	Baton Rouge	90%	67
Dauterive Hospital	New Iberia	89%	57
Southwest Medical Center	Lafayette	88%	85
Willis Knighton Bossier Health Center	Bossier City	88%	99
Baton Rouge General Medical Center	Baton Rouge	87%	361
Our Lady of Lourdes Regional Medical Center	Lafayette	85%	138
Beauregard Memorial Hospital	DeRidder	80%	25

4. Beta Blocker at Arrival

Hospital Name	City	Rate	Cases
CHRISTUS Saint Patrick Hospital	Lake Charles	100%	159
Heart Hospital of Lafayette	Lafayette	100%	43
Leonard J Chabert Medical Center	Houma	100%	46
Saint Tammany Parish Hospital	Covington	100%	68
Ochsner Clinic Foundation	New Orleans	99%	168
Louisiana Heart Hospital	Lacombe	98%	57
Northshore Regional Medical Center	Slidell	98%	92
Christus Saint Frances Cabrini Hospital	Alexandria	97%	115
Doctors Hospital of Opelousas	Opelousas	97%	35
Thibodaux Regional Medical Center	Thibodaux	97%	96
Tulane University Hospital & Clinic	New Orleans	97%	34
University Medical Center	Lafayette	97%	33
E A Conway Medical Center	Monroe	96%	67
East Jefferson General Hospital	Metairie	96%	240
Jennings American Legion Hospital	Jennings	96%	27
Lincoln General Hospital	Ruston	96%	55
Louisiana State Univ Hosp-Shreveport	Shreveport	96%	101
West Jefferson Medical Center	Marrero	96%	243
Christus Schumpert Health System	Shreveport	95%	94
Earl K Long Medical Center	Baton Rouge	95%	65
Lake Charles Memorial Hospital	Lake Charles	95%	56
Ochsner Medical Center-Baton Rouge	Baton Rouge	95%	110
Our Lady of the Lake Regional Medical Center	Baton Rouge	95%	216
Terrebonne General Medical Center	Houma	95%	180
Slidell Memorial Hospital	Slidell	94%	111
West Calcasieu-Cameron Hospital	Sulphur	94%	48
Baton Rouge General Medical Center	Baton Rouge	93%	287
Byrd Regional Hospital	Leesville	92%	26
Beauregard Memorial Hospital	DeRidder	91%	33
North Oaks Medical System	Hammond	91%	129
Lakeview Regional Medical Center	Covington	89%	55
Willis Knighton Medical Center	Shreveport	88%	169
Glenwood Regional Medical Center	West Monroe	87%	94
Lafayette General Medical Center	Lafayette	86%	112
Rapides Regional Medical Center	Alexandria	86%	88
River West Medical Center	Plaquemine	86%	28
Willis Knighton Bossier Health Center	Bossier City	86%	76
Opelousas General Hospital	Opelousas	85%	80
Our Lady of Lourdes Regional Medical Center	Lafayette	84%	100
Saint Francis Medical Center	Monroe	84%	128
Touro Infirmary	New Orleans	84%	79
Dauterive Hospital	New Iberia	80%	51

NOTE: Hospital profiles are in alphabetical order by state, then city, then hospital within the city; Rankings are sorted by rate in descending order and exclude hospitals with less than 25 cases; (1) The number of cases is too small (n<25) for purposes of reliably predicting hospital performance; (2) Measure reflects the hospital's indication that its submission was based upon a sample of its relevant discharges; (3) Rate reflects fewer than the maximum possible quarters of data for the measure; (4) Inaccurate information submitted and suppressed for one or more quarters; (5) No data is available from the hospital for this measure; Please refer to the User's Guide for a full explanation of data

	City	Rate	Cases
Iberia Medical Center	New Iberia	77%	75
Southwest Medical Center	Lafayette	70%	73

5. Beta Blocker at Discharge

Hospital Name	City	Rate	Cases
CHRISTUS Saint Patrick Hospital	Lake Charles	100%	288
E A Conway Medical Center	Monroe	100%	46
Heart Hospital of Lafayette	Lafayette	100%	196
Northshore Regional Medical Center	Slidell	100%	103
Saint Tammany Parish Hospital	Covington	100%	131
Tulane University Hospital & Clinic	New Orleans	100%	52
Christus Saint Frances Cabrini Hospital	Alexandria	99%	237
Louisiana Heart Hospital	Lacombe	99%	136
Louisiana State Univ Hosp-Shreveport	Shreveport	99%	174
Ochsner Clinic Foundation	New Orleans	99%	262
Thibodaux Regional Medical Center	Thibodaux	99%	177
Earl K Long Medical Center	Baton Rouge	98%	64
Leonard J Chabert Medical Center	Houma	98%	44
Doctors Hospital of Opelousas	Opelousas	97%	33
Lake Charles Memorial Hospital	Lake Charles	97%	115
North Oaks Medical System	Hammond	97%	206
Our Lady of the Lake Regional Medical Center	Baton Rouge	97%	338
West Jefferson Medical Center	Marrero	97%	265
Christus Schumpert Health System	Shreveport	96%	135
Iberia Medical Center	New Iberia	96%	85
University Medical Center	Lafayette	96%	52
West Calcasieu-Cameron Hospital	Sulphur	96%	53
Lincoln General Hospital	Ruston	95%	37
Opelousas General Hospital	Opelousas	95%	76
Terrebonne General Medical Center	Houma	95%	232
Baton Rouge General Medical Center	Baton Rouge	94%	359
Rapides Regional Medical Center	Alexandria	94%	212
Slidell Memorial Hospital	Slidell	94%	116
East Jefferson General Hospital	Metairie	93%	262
Glenwood Regional Medical Center	West Monroe	93%	201
Lafayette General Medical Center	Lafayette	93%	151
Ochsner Medical Center-Baton Rouge	Baton Rouge	93%	119
Willis Knighton Medical Center	Shreveport	92%	377
Lakeview Regional Medical Center	Covington	91%	78
Our Lady of Lourdes Regional Medical Center	Lafayette	89%	149
Beauregard Memorial Hospital	DeRidder	88%	25
Southwest Medical Center	Lafayette	86%	88
Touro Infirmary	New Orleans	85%	81
Dauterive Hospital	New Iberia	84%	56
Saint Francis Medical Center	Monroe	84%	247
Willis Knighton Bossier Health Center	Bossier City	78%	113

8. Smoking Cessation Advice

Hospital Name	City	Rate	Cases
CHRISTUS Saint Patrick Hospital	Lake Charles	100%	131
Lake Charles Memorial Hospital	Lake Charles	100%	51
Louisiana Heart Hospital	Lacombe	100%	71
North Oaks Medical System	Hammond	100%	95
Northshore Regional Medical Center	Slidell	100%	44
Opelousas General Hospital	Opelousas	100%	36
Our Lady of Lourdes Regional Medical Center	Lafayette	100%	51
Our Lady of the Lake Regional Medical Center	Baton Rouge	100%	36
Saint Francis Medical Center	Monroe	100%	79
Saint Tammany Parish Hospital	Covington	100%	41
Thibodaux Regional Medical Center	Thibodaux	100%	92
Willis Knighton Medical Center	Shreveport	100%	53
Lafayette General Medical Center	Lafayette	98%	66
Ochsner Clinic Foundation	New Orleans	98%	83
Southwest Medical Center	Lafayette	98%	42
Baton Rouge General Medical Center	Baton Rouge	97%	32
Christus Saint Frances Cabrini Hospital	Alexandria	97%	116
Rapides Regional Medical Center	Alexandria	97%	97
Christus Schumpert Health System	Shreveport	96%	57
East Jefferson General Hospital	Metairie	95%	96
Terrebonne General Medical Center	Houma	95%	110
West Jefferson Medical Center	Marrero	95%	112
Dauterive Hospital	New Iberia	93%	28
Slidell Memorial Hospital	Slidell	90%	58
Iberia Medical Center	New Iberia	89%	46
University Medical Center	Lafayette	88%	33
E A Conway Medical Center	Monroe	85%	34
Glenwood Regional Medical Center	West Monroe	84%	91
Tulane University Hospital & Clinic	New Orleans	84%	31
Earl K Long Medical Center	Baton Rouge	75%	40
Touro Infirmary	New Orleans	72%	29
Ochsner Medical Center-Baton Rouge	Baton Rouge	69%	51

Heart Failure Care

9. ACE Inhibitor or ARB for LVSD

Hospital Name	City	Rate	Cases
Acadian Medical Center	Eunice	100%	41
Saint Charles Parish Hospital	Luling	100%	51
Saint Tammany Parish Hospital	Covington	100%	153
CHRISTUS Saint Patrick Hospital	Lake Charles	99%	197
Christus Saint Frances Cabrini Hospital	Alexandria	98%	242
E A Conway Medical Center	Monroe	98%	126
Heart Hospital of Lafayette	Lafayette	98%	64
Louisiana Heart Hospital	Lacombe	96%	107
Northshore Regional Medical Center	Slidell	96%	114
Earl K Long Medical Center	Baton Rouge	95%	100
Thibodaux Regional Medical Center	Thibodaux	95%	86
Huey P Long Medical Center	Pineville	94%	48
Louisiana State Univ Hosp-Shreveport	Shreveport	94%	215
American Legion Hospital	Crowley	92%	26
Ochsner Clinic Foundation	New Orleans	92%	168
Tulane University Hospital & Clinic	New Orleans	92%	106
University Medical Center	Lafayette	92%	91
Leonard J Chabert Medical Center	Houma	91%	106
Beauregard Memorial Hospital	DeRidder	90%	41
Doctors Hospital of Opelousas	Opelousas	90%	51
Lake Charles Memorial Hospital	Lake Charles	90%	124
Ochsner Medical Center-Baton Rouge	Baton Rouge	90%	130
Winn Parish Medical Center	Winnfield	89%	28
Minden Medical Center	Minden	87%	63
Christus Schumpert Health System	Shreveport	86%	194
Iberia Medical Center	New Iberia	86%	63
Our Lady of the Lake Regional Medical Center	Baton Rouge	86%	347
River Parishes Hospital	La Place	86%	72
North Oaks Medical System	Hammond	85%	369
Teche Regional Medical Center	Morgan City	85%	46
Byrd Regional Hospital	Leesville	83%	58
Saint Francis Medical Center	Monroe	83%	169
Lafayette General Medical Center	Lafayette	82%	177
River West Medical Center	Plaquemine	82%	62
Slidell Memorial Hospital	Slidell	81%	117
Southwest Medical Center	Lafayette	81%	74
Touro Infirmary	New Orleans	81%	261
East Jefferson General Hospital	Metairie	79%	106
LSU-Bogalusa Medical Center	Bogalusa	79%	73
Saint Elizabeth Hospital	Gonzales	77%	110
Terrebonne General Medical Center	Houma	77%	158
Opelousas General Hospital	Opelousas	76%	105
Rapides Regional Medical Center	Alexandria	76%	224
Baton Rouge General Medical Center	Baton Rouge	73%	364
Our Lady of Lourdes Regional Medical Center	Lafayette	73%	141
Ville Platte Medical Center	Ville Platte	73%	77
West Calcasieu-Cameron Hospital	Sulphur	73%	48
Abbeville General Hospital	Abbeville	72%	25
West Jefferson Medical Center	Marrero	72%	335
Morehouse General Hospital	Bastrop	71%	28
Lane Regional Memorial Hospital	Zachary	70%	56
Lakeview Regional Medical Center	Covington	67%	89
Willis Knighton Medical Center	Shreveport	67%	344
Lincoln General Hospital	Ruston	66%	61
Glenwood Regional Medical Center	West Monroe	65%	133
Dauterive Hospital	New Iberia	64%	110
Savoy Medical Center	Mamou	61%	44
Natchitoches Regional Medical Center	Natchitoches	59%	51
Willis Knighton Bossier Health Center	Bossier City	46%	87

10. Discharge Instructions

Hospital Name	City	Rate	Cases
Louisiana Heart Hospital	Lacombe	100%	251
Minden Medical Center	Minden	99%	137
Doctors Hospital	Shreveport	98%	41
Jennings American Legion Hospital	Jennings	97%	30
Acadian Medical Center	Eunice	96%	95
La Salle General Hospital	Jena	96%	79
Abbeville General Hospital	Abbeville	94%	87
CHRISTUS Saint Patrick Hospital	Lake Charles	92%	358
Lake Charles Memorial Hospital	Lake Charles	92%	220
Christus Schumpert Health System	Shreveport	91%	396
Saint Elizabeth Hospital	Gonzales	91%	33
Huey P Long Medical Center	Pineville	90%	58
Teche Regional Medical Center	Morgan City	90%	139
West Calcasieu-Cameron Hospital	Sulphur	90%	68
Baton Rouge General Medical Center	Baton Rouge	89%	151
Northshore Regional Medical Center	Slidell	89%	249
Thibodaux Regional Medical Center	Thibodaux	88%	235
Winn Parish Medical Center	Winnfield	88%	50

NOTE: Hospital profiles are in alphabetical order by state, then city, then hospital within the city; Rankings are sorted by rate in descending order and exclude hospitals with less than 25 cases; (1) The number of cases is too small (n<25) for purposes of reliably predicting hospital performance; (2) Measure reflects the hospital's indication that its submission was based upon a sample of its relevant discharges; (3) Rate reflects fewer than the maximum possible quarters of data for the measure; (4) Inaccurate information submitted and suppressed for one or more quarters; (5) No data is available from the hospital for this measure; Please refer to the User's Guide for a full explanation of data

Hospital	City	Rate	Cases
Christus Saint Frances Cabrini Hospital	Alexandria	87%	468
Lallie Kemp/Regional Medical Center	Independence	87%	38
River Parishes Hospital	La Place	87%	179
Iberia Medical Center	New Iberia	85%	164
Oakdale Community Hospital	Oakdale	83%	59
Our Lady of the Lake Regional Medical Center	Baton Rouge	83%	166
Sabine Medical Center	Many	82%	67
Doctors Hospital of Opelousas	Opelousas	81%	139
Avoyelles Hospital	Marksville	80%	74
Saint Tammany Parish Hospital	Covington	78%	362
Terrebonne General Medical Center	Houma	78%	339
Tulane University Hospital & Clinic	New Orleans	78%	175
Lady of the Sea General Hospital	Cut Off	75%	48
Our Lady of Lourdes Regional Medical Center	Lafayette	74%	327
Lakeview Regional Medical Center	Covington	73%	194
Louisiana State Univ Hosp-Shreveport	Shreveport	73%	62
Opelousas General Hospital	Opelousas	72%	284
Morehouse General Hospital	Bastrop	70%	61
North Oaks Medical System	Hammond	68%	688
Jackson Parish Hospital	Jonesboro	67%	54
Lincoln General Hospital	Ruston	67%	42
Natchitoches Regional Medical Center	Natchitoches	66%	101
E A Conway Medical Center	Monroe	65%	192
Lane Regional Memorial Hospital	Zachary	65%	172
LSU-Bogalusa Medical Center	Bogalusa	63%	141
Lafayette General Medical Center	Lafayette	63%	363
Beauregard Memorial Hospital	DeRidder	60%	70
Earl K Long Medical Center	Baton Rouge	60%	149
Saint Anne General Hospital	Raceland	59%	61
Rapides Regional Medical Center	Alexandria	57%	421
Savoy Medical Center	Mamou	56%	86
Leonard J Chabert Medical Center	Houma	55%	152
Southwest Medical Center	Lafayette	55%	170
Slidell Memorial Hospital	Slidell	54%	297
East Jefferson General Hospital	Metairie	51%	234
Ochsner Medical Center-Baton Rouge	Baton Rouge	51%	210
W O Moss Regional Medical Center	Lake Charles	48%	31
Byrd Regional Hospital	Leesville	47%	145
Glenwood Regional Medical Center	West Monroe	46%	286
Ochsner Clinic Foundation	New Orleans	46%	270
Touro Infirmary	New Orleans	46%	347
Dauterive Hospital	New Iberia	45%	190
Saint Francis Medical Center	Monroe	45%	422
River West Medical Center	Plaquemine	44%	105
Ville Platte Medical Center	Ville Platte	40%	142
American Legion Hospital	Crowley	38%	76
West Jefferson Medical Center	Marrero	35%	578
Willis Knighton Medical Center	Shreveport	33%	106
Willis Knighton Bossier Health Center	Bossier City	29%	38
University Medical Center	Lafayette	23%	151
DeSoto Regional Health System	Mansfield	7%	44
Hardtner Medical Center	Olla	0%	25

Hospital	City	Rate	Cases
Lane Regional Memorial Hospital	Zachary	92%	230
Lincoln General Hospital	Ruston	92%	263
Earl K Long Medical Center	Baton Rouge	91%	156
Touro Infirmary	New Orleans	91%	462
West Jefferson Medical Center	Marrero	91%	675
Iberia Medical Center	New Iberia	90%	184
Jackson Parish Hospital	Jonesboro	90%	81
Lallie Kemp/Regional Medical Center	Independence	90%	41
Rapides Regional Medical Center	Alexandria	90%	502
River West Medical Center	Plaquemine	90%	121
Terrebonne General Medical Center	Houma	90%	385
Avoyelles Hospital	Marksville	89%	112
Natchitoches Regional Medical Center	Natchitoches	89%	123
Our Lady of Lourdes Regional Medical Center	Lafayette	89%	394
Ville Platte Medical Center	Ville Platte	89%	185
Winn Parish Medical Center	Winnfield	89%	91
East Jefferson General Hospital	Metairie	88%	284
Lakeview Regional Medical Center	Covington	88%	236
Saint Anne General Hospital	Raceland	88%	66
Southwest Medical Center	Lafayette	88%	192
Tri-Ward Rural Health Clinic	Bernice	88%	25
Willis Knighton Medical Center	Shreveport	88%	700
Oakdale Community Hospital	Oakdale	87%	85
Byrd Regional Hospital	Leesville	86%	166
Doctors Hospital of Opelousas	Opelousas	86%	172
Opelousas General Hospital	Opelousas	86%	332
Beauregard Memorial Hospital	DeRidder	85%	101
Dauterive Hospital	New Iberia	85%	209
Baton Rouge General Medical Center	Baton Rouge	84%	851
Saint Francis Medical Center	Monroe	84%	519
LSU-Bogalusa Medical Center	Bogalusa	83%	160
Willis Knighton Bossier Health Center	Bossier City	83%	184
Abbeville General Hospital	Abbeville	82%	134
Slidell Memorial Hospital	Slidell	82%	317
Acadian Medical Center	Eunice	80%	98
Springhill Medical Center	Springhill	79%	96
Lady of the Sea General Hospital	Cut Off	77%	70
Savoy Medical Center	Mamou	71%	112
Teche Regional Medical Center	Morgan City	70%	155
Citizens Medical Center	Columbia	66%	29
Homer Memorial Hospital	Homer	66%	56
DeSoto Regional Health System	Mansfield	65%	68
Doctors Hospital	Shreveport	64%	61
American Legion Hospital	Crowley	57%	102
Morehouse General Hospital	Bastrop	55%	96
Franklin Medical Center	Winnsboro	49%	61
Sabine Medical Center	Many	49%	101
Hardtner Medical Center	Olla	45%	33
Richardson Medical Center	Rayville	35%	46
Caldwell Memorial Hospital	Columbia	31%	61
West Carroll Memorial Hospital	Oak Grove	3%	99
East Carroll Parish Hospital	Lake Providence	0%	65

11. Evaluation of LVS Function

Hospital Name	City	Rate	Cases
CHRISTUS Saint Patrick Hospital	Lake Charles	100%	400
Heart Hospital of Lafayette	Lafayette	100%	135
Northshore Regional Medical Center	Slidell	100%	277
Ochsner Clinic Foundation	New Orleans	100%	288
Saint Tammany Parish Hospital	Covington	100%	401
W O Moss Regional Medical Center	Lake Charles	100%	31
Christus Saint Frances Cabrini Hospital	Alexandria	99%	533
Lake Charles Memorial Hospital	Lake Charles	99%	240
Louisiana State Univ Hosp-Shreveport	Shreveport	99%	324
Saint Charles Parish Hospital	Luling	99%	114
Christus Schumpert Health System	Shreveport	98%	484
Huey P Long Medical Center	Pineville	98%	62
La Salle General Hospital	Jena	98%	117
Louisiana Heart Hospital	Lacombe	98%	267
West Calcasieu-Cameron Hospital	Sulphur	98%	117
E A Conway Medical Center	Monroe	97%	195
Leonard J Chabert Medical Center	Houma	97%	152
Tulane University Hospital & Clinic	New Orleans	96%	176
North Oaks Medical System	Hammond	95%	816
Saint Elizabeth Hospital	Gonzales	95%	167
Thibodaux Regional Medical Center	Thibodaux	95%	279
University Medical Center	Lafayette	95%	152
Minden Medical Center	Minden	94%	180
Our Lady of the Lake Regional Medical Center	Baton Rouge	94%	873
Glenwood Regional Medical Center	West Monroe	93%	369
Lafayette General Medical Center	Lafayette	93%	404
Ochsner Medical Center-Baton Rouge	Baton Rouge	93%	211
River Parishes Hospital	La Place	93%	196
Jennings American Legion Hospital	Jennings	92%	153

12. Smoking Cessation Advice

Hospital Name	City	Rate	Cases
Huey P Long Medical Center	Pineville	100%	32
Lake Charles Memorial Hospital	Lake Charles	100%	61
Louisiana Heart Hospital	Lacombe	100%	43
Minden Medical Center	Minden	100%	32
Our Lady of Lourdes Regional Medical Center	Lafayette	100%	68
Our Lady of the Lake Regional Medical Center	Baton Rouge	100%	27
River Parishes Hospital	La Place	100%	54
Northshore Regional Medical Center	Slidell	99%	76
Saint Francis Medical Center	Monroe	99%	76
Christus Saint Frances Cabrini Hospital	Alexandria	98%	87
Thibodaux Regional Medical Center	Thibodaux	98%	42
Byrd Regional Hospital	Leesville	96%	54
LSU-Bogalusa Medical Center	Bogalusa	96%	45
Saint Tammany Parish Hospital	Covington	96%	74
CHRISTUS Saint Patrick Hospital	Lake Charles	95%	80
Leonard J Chabert Medical Center	Houma	95%	78
Doctors Hospital of Opelousas	Opelousas	94%	35
North Oaks Medical System	Hammond	94%	177
Rapides Regional Medical Center	Alexandria	94%	102
Ochsner Clinic Foundation	New Orleans	93%	57
Opelousas General Hospital	Opelousas	93%	88
Savoy Medical Center	Mamou	93%	29
Southwest Medical Center	Lafayette	93%	29
East Jefferson General Hospital	Metairie	91%	44
Christus Schumpert Health System	Shreveport	90%	87
Iberia Medical Center	New Iberia	90%	39
Abbeville General Hospital	Abbeville	88%	25
Lafayette General Medical Center	Lafayette	88%	80
Sabine Medical Center	Many	88%	25

NOTE: Hospital profiles are in alphabetical order by state, then city, then hospital within the city; Rankings are sorted by rate in descending order and exclude hospitals with less than 25 cases; (1) The number of cases is too small (n<25) for purposes of reliably predicting hospital performance; (2) Measure reflects the hospital's indication that its submission was based upon a sample of its relevant discharges; (3) Rate reflects fewer than the maximum possible quarters of data for the measure; (4) Inaccurate information submitted and suppressed for one or more quarters; (5) No data is available from the hospital for this measure; Please refer to the User's Guide for a full explanation of data

Lakeview Regional Medical Center	Covington	86%	42
Baton Rouge General Medical Center	Baton Rouge	85%	48
West Jefferson Medical Center	Marrero	85%	193
Dauterive Hospital	New Iberia	84%	61
Jackson Parish Hospital	Jonesboro	83%	29
E A Conway Medical Center	Monroe	82%	61
Lane Regional Memorial Hospital	Zachary	82%	66
Ville Platte Medical Center	Ville Platte	82%	40
American Legion Hospital	Crowley	81%	27
Avoyelles Hospital	Marksville	81%	26
Earl K Long Medical Center	Baton Rouge	80%	81
Tulane University Hospital & Clinic	New Orleans	76%	62
Terrebonne General Medical Center	Houma	75%	88
University Medical Center	Lafayette	75%	69
Glenwood Regional Medical Center	West Monroe	70%	64
Natchitoches Regional Medical Center	Natchitoches	68%	25
Slidell Memorial Hospital	Slidell	61%	59
Touro Infirmary	New Orleans	61%	80
Teche Regional Medical Center	Morgan City	59%	34
Ochsner Medical Center-Baton Rouge	Baton Rouge	46%	39

Pneumonia Care

13. Appropriate Initial Antibiotic

Hospital Name	City	Rate	Cases
Lady of the Sea General Hospital	Cut Off	93%	60
Leonard J Chabert Medical Center	Houma	93%	45
Tulane University Hospital & Clinic	New Orleans	93%	27
La Salle General Hospital	Jena	92%	38
Saint Tammany Parish Hospital	Covington	92%	173
Avoyelles Hospital	Marksville	91%	46
E A Conway Medical Center	Monroe	91%	102
Tri-Ward Rural Health Clinic	Bernice	90%	41
Christus Schumpert Health System	Shreveport	89%	158
West Calcasieu-Cameron Hospital	Sulphur	89%	46
Huey P Long Medical Center	Pineville	88%	25
North Oaks Medical System	Hammond	87%	213
River West Medical Center	Plaquemine	87%	75
Winn Parish Medical Center	Winnfield	86%	50
Baton Rouge General Medical Center	Baton Rouge	85%	39
Louisiana Heart Hospital	Lacombe	85%	26
Our Lady of the Lake Regional Medical Center	Baton Rouge	85%	46
Slidell Memorial Hospital	Slidell	85%	208
American Legion Hospital	Crowley	84%	107
Byrd Regional Hospital	Leesville	84%	134
LSU-Bogalusa Medical Center	Bogalusa	84%	124
Lane Regional Memorial Hospital	Zachary	84%	129
CHRISTUS Saint Patrick Hospital	Lake Charles	83%	196
Lafayette General Medical Center	Lafayette	83%	103
Lakeview Regional Medical Center	Covington	83%	83
Minden Medical Center	Minden	83%	63
Ochsner Clinic Foundation	New Orleans	83%	115
Saint Francis Medical Center	Monroe	83%	152
Willis Knighton Medical Center	Shreveport	83%	29
Jackson Parish Hospital	Jonesboro	82%	60
River Parishes Hospital	La Place	82%	49
Savoy Medical Center	Mamou	82%	45
Saint Anne General Hospital	Raceland	81%	27
Thibodaux Regional Medical Center	Thibodaux	81%	113
Iberia Medical Center	New Iberia	80%	88
Natchitoches Regional Medical Center	Natchitoches	80%	152
Northshore Regional Medical Center	Slidell	80%	193
Rapides Regional Medical Center	Alexandria	80%	131
Touro Infirmary	New Orleans	80%	98
Ville Platte Medical Center	Ville Platte	80%	97
West Jefferson Medical Center	Marrero	80%	169
Southwest Medical Center	Lafayette	79%	102
University Medical Center	Lafayette	78%	69
Glenwood Regional Medical Center	West Monroe	77%	98
East Jefferson General Hospital	Metairie	76%	100
Acadian Medical Center	Eunice	75%	32
Christus Saint Frances Cabrini Hospital	Alexandria	75%	174
Dauterive Hospital	New Iberia	75%	60
Lake Charles Memorial Hospital	Lake Charles	75%	158
Our Lady of Lourdes Regional Medical Center	Lafayette	74%	152
Abbeville General Hospital	Abbeville	73%	49
Doctors Hospital	Shreveport	73%	30
Earl K Long Medical Center	Baton Rouge	73%	60
Teche Regional Medical Center	Morgan City	73%	55
Opelousas General Hospital	Opelousas	71%	122
Ochsner Medical Center-Baton Rouge	Baton Rouge	70%	122
Terrebonne General Medical Center	Houma	70%	150
DeSoto Regional Health System	Mansfield	67%	48
Doctors Hospital of Opelousas	Opelousas	63%	68

Oakdale Community Hospital	Oakdale	60%	85
Morehouse General Hospital	Bastrop	53%	55
Sabine Medical Center	Many	50%	38
Beauregard Memorial Hospital	DeRidder	49%	104

14. Blood Culture Timing

Hospital Name	City	Rate	Cases
Savoy Medical Center	Mamou	100%	76
Northshore Regional Medical Center	Slidell	99%	196
Christus Schumpert Health System	Shreveport	98%	169
Winn Parish Medical Center	Winnfield	98%	48
Huey P Long Medical Center	Pineville	97%	30
North Oaks Medical System	Hammond	97%	121
River Parishes Hospital	La Place	97%	34
Leonard J Chabert Medical Center	Houma	96%	54
Rapides Regional Medical Center	Alexandria	96%	180
Lakeview Regional Medical Center	Covington	95%	65
Minden Medical Center	Minden	95%	66
Oakdale Community Hospital	Oakdale	95%	38
Saint Francis Medical Center	Monroe	95%	160
Avoyelles Hospital	Marksville	94%	68
CHRISTUS Saint Patrick Hospital	Lake Charles	94%	210
Dauterive Hospital	New Iberia	94%	50
LSU-Bogalusa Medical Center	Bogalusa	94%	72
Our Lady of Lourdes Regional Medical Center	Lafayette	94%	121
Touro Infirmary	New Orleans	94%	124
Jennings American Legion Hospital	Jennings	93%	29
La Salle General Hospital	Jena	93%	56
Beauregard Memorial Hospital	DeRidder	92%	51
E A Conway Medical Center	Monroe	92%	53
Natchitoches Regional Medical Center	Natchitoches	92%	103
River West Medical Center	Plaquemine	92%	85
Saint Tammany Parish Hospital	Covington	92%	166
Teche Regional Medical Center	Morgan City	92%	50
Abbeville General Hospital	Abbeville	91%	44
Christus Saint Frances Cabrini Hospital	Alexandria	91%	176
East Jefferson General Hospital	Metairie	91%	92
Southwest Medical Center	Lafayette	91%	45
Terrebonne General Medical Center	Houma	91%	126
Byrd Regional Hospital	Leesville	90%	83
Lake Charles Memorial Hospital	Lake Charles	90%	121
Willis Knighton Medical Center	Shreveport	90%	42
Thibodaux Regional Medical Center	Thibodaux	89%	94
Glenwood Regional Medical Center	West Monroe	88%	64
Lane Regional Memorial Hospital	Zachary	88%	166
Ochsner Medical Center-Baton Rouge	Baton Rouge	88%	113
Slidell Memorial Hospital	Slidell	88%	121
Our Lady of the Lake Regional Medical Center	Baton Rouge	87%	52
American Legion Hospital	Crowley	86%	57
Ochsner Clinic Foundation	New Orleans	86%	94
Acadian Medical Center	Eunice	85%	33
Baton Rouge General Medical Center	Baton Rouge	85%	61
Ville Platte Medical Center	Ville Platte	85%	82
West Calcasieu-Cameron Hospital	Sulphur	83%	41
West Jefferson Medical Center	Marrero	83%	123
Lady of the Sea General Hospital	Cut Off	80%	54
Opelousas General Hospital	Opelousas	80%	133
Doctors Hospital of Opelousas	Opelousas	79%	42
Earl K Long Medical Center	Baton Rouge	79%	67
Iberia Medical Center	New Iberia	79%	96
Lafayette General Medical Center	Lafayette	78%	92
University Medical Center	Lafayette	59%	46

15. Influenza Vaccine

Hospital Name	City	Rate	Cases
CHRISTUS Saint Patrick Hospital	Lake Charles	100%	51
Northshore Regional Medical Center	Slidell	100%	62
Rapides Regional Medical Center	Alexandria	96%	55
Christus Saint Frances Cabrini Hospital	Alexandria	95%	62
Minden Medical Center	Minden	93%	27
Saint Tammany Parish Hospital	Covington	92%	53
Thibodaux Regional Medical Center	Thibodaux	90%	39
Ville Platte Medical Center	Ville Platte	85%	41
Iberia Medical Center	New Iberia	84%	31
North Oaks Medical System	Hammond	84%	63
Our Lady of Lourdes Regional Medical Center	Lafayette	82%	45
Oakdale Community Hospital	Oakdale	75%	40
Saint Francis Medical Center	Monroe	70%	46
Lakeview Regional Medical Center	Covington	69%	29
Terrebonne General Medical Center	Houma	64%	45
Lafayette General Medical Center	Lafayette	63%	41
Byrd Regional Hospital	Leesville	62%	42
Glenwood Regional Medical Center	West Monroe	62%	26
Lane Regional Memorial Hospital	Zachary	60%	65

NOTE: Hospital profiles are in alphabetical order by state, then city, then hospital within the city; Rankings are sorted by rate in descending order and exclude hospitals with less than 25 cases; (1) The number of cases is too small (n<25) for purposes of reliably predicting hospital performance; (2) Measure reflects the hospital's indication that its submission was based upon a sample of its relevant discharges; (3) Rate reflects fewer than the maximum possible quarters of data for the measure; (4) Inaccurate information submitted and suppressed for one or more quarters; (5) No data is available from the hospital for this measure; Please refer to the User's Guide for a full explanation of data

Hospital Name	City	Rate	Cases
Southwest Medical Center	Lafayette	58%	31
Natchitoches Regional Medical Center	Natchitoches	51%	35
Opelousas General Hospital	Opelousas	51%	45
Slidell Memorial Hospital	Slidell	49%	67
West Jefferson Medical Center	Marrero	42%	31
East Jefferson General Hospital	Metairie	40%	30
Touro Infirmary	New Orleans	26%	38

Hospital Name	City	Rate	Cases
Leonard J Chabert Medical Center	Houma	56%	62
DeSoto Regional Health System	Mansfield	55%	42
West Jefferson Medical Center	Marrero	55%	191
Earl K Long Medical Center	Baton Rouge	54%	91
Lallie Kemp/Regional Medical Center	Independence	44%	25
Louisiana State Univ Hosp-Shreveport	Shreveport	44%	126

16. Initial Antibiotic Timing

Hospital Name	City	Rate	Cases
East Carroll Parish Hospital	Lake Providence	94%	33
Tri-Ward Rural Health Clinic	Bernice	94%	71
Avoyelles Hospital	Marksville	93%	94
Caldwell Memorial Hospital	Columbia	93%	43
Winn Parish Medical Center	Winnfield	93%	91
Jackson Parish Hospital	Jonesboro	92%	63
CHRISTUS Saint Patrick Hospital	Lake Charles	91%	256
Teche Regional Medical Center	Morgan City	91%	77
Northshore Regional Medical Center	Slidell	90%	240
Saint Tammany Parish Hospital	Covington	90%	215
Savoy Medical Center	Mamou	90%	109
Lincoln General Hospital	Ruston	89%	133
Oakdale Community Hospital	Oakdale	89%	152
Sabine Medical Center	Many	89%	63
Springhill Medical Center	Springhill	89%	64
Jennings American Legion Hospital	Jennings	88%	152
Louisiana Heart Hospital	Lacombe	88%	25
Thibodaux Regional Medical Center	Thibodaux	88%	165
Acadian Medical Center	Eunice	87%	69
Beauregard Memorial Hospital	DeRidder	87%	126
Christus Schumpert Health System	Shreveport	87%	277
Franklin Medical Center	Winnsboro	86%	90
La Salle General Hospital	Jena	86%	71
Saint Anne General Hospital	Raceland	86%	35
Abbeville General Hospital	Abbeville	85%	82
Iberia Medical Center	New Iberia	85%	142
Byrd Regional Hospital	Leesville	83%	196
Lane Regional Memorial Hospital	Zachary	83%	242
Ville Platte Medical Center	Ville Platte	83%	163
West Calcasieu-Cameron Hospital	Sulphur	83%	72
Women and Children's Hospital	Lake Charles	83%	30
Lady of the Sea General Hospital	Cut Off	82%	72
Minden Medical Center	Minden	80%	137
Natchitoches Regional Medical Center	Natchitoches	80%	230
Willis Knighton Medical Center	Shreveport	80%	381
North Oaks Medical System	Hammond	79%	334
Our Lady of the Lake Regional Medical Center	Baton Rouge	79%	312
Dauterive Hospital	New Iberia	78%	81
Saint Charles Parish Hospital	Luling	78%	63
Willis Knighton Bossier Health Center	Bossier City	78%	172
Rapides Regional Medical Center	Alexandria	77%	282
River Parishes Hospital	La Place	77%	62
Doctors Hospital	Shreveport	76%	45
Lafayette General Medical Center	Lafayette	75%	146
Saint Elizabeth Hospital	Gonzales	75%	128
Glenwood Regional Medical Center	West Monroe	74%	168
E A Conway Medical Center	Monroe	73%	108
LSU-Bogalusa Medical Center	Bogalusa	73%	122
Lake Charles Memorial Hospital	Lake Charles	73%	243
Homer Memorial Hospital	Homer	72%	57
Southwest Medical Center	Lafayette	72%	110
American Legion Hospital	Crowley	71%	163
River West Medical Center	Plaquemine	71%	116
Doctors Hospital of Opelousas	Opelousas	70%	90
Ochsner Medical Center-Baton Rouge	Baton Rouge	70%	182
Richardson Medical Center	Rayville	69%	58
Allen Parish Hospital	Kinder	68%	25
Christus Saint Frances Cabrini Hospital	Alexandria	68%	241
Citizens Medical Center	Columbia	68%	40
East Jefferson General Hospital	Metairie	68%	144
Opelousas General Hospital	Opelousas	68%	228
Huey P Long Medical Center	Pineville	67%	43
Morehouse General Hospital	Bastrop	67%	115
Baton Rouge General Medical Center	Baton Rouge	66%	512
Lakeview Regional Medical Center	Covington	66%	157
Ochsner Clinic Foundation	New Orleans	66%	131
Slidell Memorial Hospital	Slidell	66%	242
Terrebonne General Medical Center	Houma	66%	213
Saint Francis Medical Center	Monroe	65%	209
University Medical Center	Lafayette	64%	81
West Carroll Memorial Hospital	Oak Grove	63%	111
Our Lady of Lourdes Regional Medical Center	Lafayette	60%	194
Touro Infirmary	New Orleans	60%	147
Tulane University Hospital & Clinic	New Orleans	59%	27

17. Oxygenation Assessment

Hospital Name	City	Rate	Cases
Abrom Kaplan Memorial Hospital	Kaplan	100%	28
Acadian Medical Center	Eunice	100%	87
Avoyelles Hospital	Marksville	100%	121
Byrd Regional Hospital	Leesville	100%	235
CHRISTUS Saint Patrick Hospital	Lake Charles	100%	309
Christus Schumpert Health System	Shreveport	100%	342
Doctors Hospital of Opelousas	Opelousas	100%	106
Earl K Long Medical Center	Baton Rouge	100%	98
East Carroll Parish Hospital	Lake Providence	100%	35
Homer Memorial Hospital	Homer	100%	67
Huey P Long Medical Center	Pineville	100%	50
Jennings American Legion Hospital	Jennings	100%	161
Lady of the Sea General Hospital	Cut Off	100%	92
Lafayette General Medical Center	Lafayette	100%	183
Lallie Kemp/Regional Medical Center	Independence	100%	29
Lane Regional Memorial Hospital	Zachary	100%	319
Leonard J Chabert Medical Center	Houma	100%	78
Louisiana Heart Hospital	Lacombe	100%	35
Minden Medical Center	Minden	100%	177
North Oaks Medical System	Hammond	100%	407
Oakdale Community Hospital	Oakdale	100%	182
Ochsner Clinic Foundation	New Orleans	100%	173
Our Lady of the Lake Regional Medical Center	Baton Rouge	100%	378
Rapides Regional Medical Center	Alexandria	100%	316
Sabine Medical Center	Many	100%	78
Saint Charles Parish Hospital	Luling	100%	71
Saint Francis Medical Center	Monroe	100%	263
Saint Tammany Parish Hospital	Covington	100%	266
Springhill Medical Center	Springhill	100%	79
Tulane University Hospital & Clinic	New Orleans	100%	34
West Carroll Memorial Hospital	Oak Grove	100%	127
Willis Knighton Medical Center	Shreveport	100%	456
Winn Parish Medical Center	Winnfield	100%	110
Baton Rouge General Medical Center	Baton Rouge	99%	637
Beauregard Memorial Hospital	DeRidder	99%	164
Christus Saint Frances Cabrini Hospital	Alexandria	99%	318
Dauterive Hospital	New Iberia	99%	92
Glenwood Regional Medical Center	West Monroe	99%	174
Iberia Medical Center	New Iberia	99%	184
LSU-Bogalusa Medical Center	Bogalusa	99%	143
Lake Charles Memorial Hospital	Lake Charles	99%	262
Lakeview Regional Medical Center	Covington	99%	190
Natchitoches Regional Medical Center	Natchitoches	99%	282
Northshore Regional Medical Center	Slidell	99%	303
Ochsner Medical Center-Baton Rouge	Baton Rouge	99%	207
Our Lady of Lourdes Regional Medical Center	Lafayette	99%	253
River West Medical Center	Plaquemine	99%	153
Saint Elizabeth Hospital	Gonzales	99%	155
Southwest Medical Center	Lafayette	99%	123
Teche Regional Medical Center	Morgan City	99%	90
Terrebonne General Medical Center	Houma	99%	237
Thibodaux Regional Medical Center	Thibodaux	99%	198
Tri-Ward Rural Health Clinic	Bernice	99%	78
University Medical Center	Lafayette	99%	90
Ville Platte Medical Center	Ville Platte	99%	175
Willis Knighton Bossier Health Center	Bossier City	99%	201
Citizens Medical Center	Columbia	98%	54
DeSoto Regional Health System	Mansfield	98%	56
Doctors Hospital	Shreveport	98%	61
Lincoln General Hospital	Ruston	98%	145
Opelousas General Hospital	Opelousas	98%	269
Savoy Medical Center	Mamou	98%	132
Slidell Memorial Hospital	Slidell	98%	307
West Jefferson Medical Center	Marrero	98%	230
Abbeville General Hospital	Abbeville	97%	97
River Parishes Hospital	La Place	97%	74
West Calcasieu-Cameron Hospital	Sulphur	97%	88
Women and Children's Hospital	Lake Charles	97%	33
American Legion Hospital	Crowley	96%	192
East Jefferson General Hospital	Metairie	96%	178
Hardtner Medical Center	Olla	96%	26
La Salle General Hospital	Jena	96%	83
E A Conway Medical Center	Monroe	95%	119
Franklin Medical Center	Winnsboro	95%	108
Saint Anne General Hospital	Raceland	95%	38

Hospital Name	City	Rate	Cases
Touro Infirmary	New Orleans	95%	187
Allen Parish Hospital	Kinder	94%	36
Jackson Parish Hospital	Jonesboro	94%	67
Louisiana State Univ Hosp-Shreveport	Shreveport	94%	152
Richardson Medical Center	Rayville	83%	69
Morehouse General Hospital	Bastrop	78%	129
Caldwell Memorial Hospital	Columbia	71%	48

18. Pneumococcal Vaccine

Hospital Name	City	Rate	Cases
CHRISTUS Saint Patrick Hospital	Lake Charles	100%	184
Winn Parish Medical Center	Winnfield	100%	58
Northshore Regional Medical Center	Slidell	99%	181
Abbeville General Hospital	Abbeville	97%	66
Lane Regional Memorial Hospital	Zachary	95%	165
Acadian Medical Center	Eunice	93%	43
Christus Saint Frances Cabrini Hospital	Alexandria	93%	189
Christus Schumpert Health System	Shreveport	93%	223
Our Lady of Lourdes Regional Medical Center	Lafayette	92%	144
Doctors Hospital of Opelousas	Opelousas	91%	53
Rapides Regional Medical Center	Alexandria	91%	201
Iberia Medical Center	New Iberia	89%	113
Lady of the Sea General Hospital	Cut Off	89%	53
Minden Medical Center	Minden	89%	100
North Oaks Medical System	Hammond	89%	214
Ochsner Clinic Foundation	New Orleans	88%	112
Lake Charles Memorial Hospital	Lake Charles	87%	156
Saint Elizabeth Hospital	Gonzales	86%	95
Lafayette General Medical Center	Lafayette	84%	98
Sabine Medical Center	Many	84%	55
La Salle General Hospital	Jena	80%	54
Lincoln General Hospital	Ruston	80%	83
Thibodaux Regional Medical Center	Thibodaux	80%	122
Our Lady of the Lake Regional Medical Center	Baton Rouge	79%	219
Saint Tammany Parish Hospital	Covington	79%	161
Jennings American Legion Hospital	Jennings	77%	115
Oakdale Community Hospital	Oakdale	76%	107
Saint Francis Medical Center	Monroe	73%	167
American Legion Hospital	Crowley	72%	104
Byrd Regional Hospital	Leesville	72%	116
Glenwood Regional Medical Center	West Monroe	72%	123
Lakeview Regional Medical Center	Covington	72%	128
Saint Anne General Hospital	Raceland	72%	25
Tri-Ward Rural Health Clinic	Bernice	72%	54
Ville Platte Medical Center	Ville Platte	70%	101
Avoyelles Hospital	Marksville	68%	79
Baton Rouge General Medical Center	Baton Rouge	68%	320
Terrebonne General Medical Center	Houma	67%	141
West Calcasieu-Cameron Hospital	Sulphur	67%	51
Savoy Medical Center	Mamou	66%	79
Franklin Medical Center	Winnsboro	65%	74
Homer Memorial Hospital	Homer	64%	39
Beauregard Memorial Hospital	DeRidder	62%	95
Willis Knighton Bossier Health Center	Bossier City	61%	114
LSU-Bogalusa Medical Center	Bogalusa	59%	51
Opelousas General Hospital	Opelousas	59%	150
Morehouse General Hospital	Bastrop	58%	72
DeSoto Regional Health System	Mansfield	54%	35
River Parishes Hospital	La Place	54%	39
Natchitoches Regional Medical Center	Natchitoches	52%	180
Springhill Medical Center	Springhill	52%	52
West Carroll Memorial Hospital	Oak Grove	52%	89
River West Medical Center	Plaquemine	51%	61
Willis Knighton Medical Center	Shreveport	51%	280
Citizens Medical Center	Columbia	50%	32
Doctors Hospital	Shreveport	49%	41
Slidell Memorial Hospital	Slidell	48%	166
Southwest Medical Center	Lafayette	47%	68
Richardson Medical Center	Rayville	46%	35
Teche Regional Medical Center	Morgan City	44%	54
Dauterive Hospital	New Iberia	40%	53
East Jefferson General Hospital	Metairie	40%	113
Jackson Parish Hospital	Jonesboro	36%	44
Saint Charles Parish Hospital	Luling	31%	42
Touro Infirmary	New Orleans	29%	91
West Jefferson Medical Center	Marrero	29%	93
Louisiana State Univ Hosp-Shreveport	Shreveport	26%	31
Ochsner Medical Center-Baton Rouge	Baton Rouge	13%	114

19. Smoking Cessation Advice

Hospital Name	City	Rate	Cases
Beauregard Memorial Hospital	DeRidder	100%	36
Byrd Regional Hospital	Leesville	100%	69
CHRISTUS Saint Patrick Hospital	Lake Charles	100%	70

Hospital Name	City	Rate	Cases
Iberia Medical Center	New Iberia	100%	40
LSU-Bogalusa Medical Center	Bogalusa	100%	56
Lake Charles Memorial Hospital	Lake Charles	100%	57
Minden Medical Center	Minden	100%	39
Our Lady of Lourdes Regional Medical Center	Lafayette	100%	58
Saint Francis Medical Center	Monroe	100%	48
Northshore Regional Medical Center	Slidell	98%	88
Saint Tammany Parish Hospital	Covington	96%	82
Thibodaux Regional Medical Center	Thibodaux	95%	43
North Oaks Medical System	Hammond	94%	108
Christus Saint Frances Cabrini Hospital	Alexandria	93%	67
River Parishes Hospital	La Place	93%	28
Savoy Medical Center	Mamou	92%	37
Christus Schumpert Health System	Shreveport	91%	76
Lafayette General Medical Center	Lafayette	91%	56
Oakdale Community Hospital	Oakdale	90%	41
Lane Regional Memorial Hospital	Zachary	89%	90
Ville Platte Medical Center	Ville Platte	89%	56
Winn Parish Medical Center	Winnfield	89%	27
Rapides Regional Medical Center	Alexandria	88%	60
Opelousas General Hospital	Opelousas	87%	70
West Jefferson Medical Center	Marrero	82%	79
Doctors Hospital of Opelousas	Opelousas	81%	31
Lakeview Regional Medical Center	Covington	79%	47
East Jefferson General Hospital	Metairie	78%	41
River West Medical Center	Plaquemine	77%	30
Southwest Medical Center	Lafayette	77%	43
Lady of the Sea General Hospital	Cut Off	74%	27
American Legion Hospital	Crowley	73%	45
University Medical Center	Lafayette	73%	49
Baton Rouge General Medical Center	Baton Rouge	72%	29
Ochsner Clinic Foundation	New Orleans	72%	36
Ochsner Medical Center-Baton Rouge	Baton Rouge	71%	52
E A Conway Medical Center	Monroe	70%	63
Slidell Memorial Hospital	Slidell	70%	96
Earl K Long Medical Center	Baton Rouge	67%	46
Leonard J Chabert Medical Center	Houma	66%	32
Natchitoches Regional Medical Center	Natchitoches	60%	42
Terrebonne General Medical Center	Houma	52%	50
Dauterive Hospital	New Iberia	43%	30
Touro Infirmary	New Orleans	43%	35
Glenwood Regional Medical Center	West Monroe	40%	43

Surgical Infection Prevention

20. Prophylactic Antibiotic Given

Hospital Name	City	Rate	Cases
Southern Surgical Hospital	Slidell	100%	30
Woman's Hospital Foundation	Baton Rouge	96%	55
E A Conway Medical Center	Monroe	95%	250
Iberia Medical Center	New Iberia	93%	192
North Oaks Medical System	Hammond	93%	428
Women's and Children's Hospital	Lafayette	93%	262
Baton Rouge General Medical Center	Baton Rouge	92%	327
Monroe Surgical Hospital	Monroe	90%	31
Northshore Regional Medical Center	Slidell	90%	343
Huey P Long Medical Center	Pineville	89%	106
Lafayette General Medical Center	Lafayette	89%	193
Lafayette Surgical Specialty Hospital	Lafayette	89%	55
Doctors Hospital of Opelousas	Opelousas	88%	82
Heart Hospital of Lafayette	Lafayette	88%	59
Louisiana Heart Hospital	Lacombe	88%	223
Lane Regional Memorial Hospital	Zachary	87%	69
Saint Anne General Hospital	Raceland	87%	54
Women and Children's Hospital	Lake Charles	87%	326
Lake Charles Memorial Hospital	Lake Charles	86%	275
Southwest Medical Center	Lafayette	86%	144
Terrebonne General Medical Center	Houma	86%	458
Christus Schumpert Health System	Shreveport	85%	279
Lallie Kemp/Regional Medical Center	Independence	84%	67
Our Lady of Lourdes Regional Medical Center	Lafayette	84%	156
Saint Tammany Parish Hospital	Covington	84%	615
Earl K Long Medical Center	Baton Rouge	83%	167
Jennings American Legion Hospital	Jennings	83%	36
Our Lady of the Lake Regional Medical Center	Baton Rouge	83%	175
W O Moss Regional Medical Center	Lake Charles	83%	89
Beauregard Memorial Hospital	DeRidder	81%	100
Touro Infirmary	New Orleans	81%	410
Acadian Medical Center	Eunice	80%	30
West Calcasieu-Cameron Hospital	Sulphur	80%	150
Willis Knighton Medical Center	Shreveport	80%	99
Savoy Medical Center	Mamou	79%	66
East Jefferson General Hospital	Metairie	78%	215
Tulane University Hospital & Clinic	New Orleans	78%	261

NOTE: Hospital profiles are in alphabetical order by state, then city, then hospital within the city; Rankings are sorted by rate in descending order and exclude hospitals with less than 25 cases; (1) The number of cases is too small (n<25) for purposes of reliably predicting hospital performance; (2) Measure reflects the hospital's indication that its submission was based upon a sample of its relevant discharges; (3) Rate reflects fewer than the maximum possible quarters of data for the measure; (4) Inaccurate information submitted and suppressed for one or more quarters; (5) No data is available from the hospital for this measure; Please refer to the User's Guide for a full explanation of data

Hospital Name	City	Rate	Cases
Abbeville General Hospital	Abbeville	77%	83
Christus Saint Frances Cabrini Hospital	Alexandria	77%	1292
Leonard J Chabert Medical Center	Houma	77%	245
P & S Surgical Hospital	Monroe	77%	226
Teche Regional Medical Center	Morgan City	77%	43
CHRISTUS Saint Patrick Hospital	Lake Charles	76%	438
Lincoln General Hospital	Ruston	74%	31
River Parishes Hospital	La Place	74%	98
Slidell Memorial Hospital	Slidell	70%	265
Saint Francis Medical Center	Monroe	69%	213
Louisiana State Univ Hosp-Shreveport	Shreveport	68%	53
Willis Knighton Bossier Health Center	Bossier City	68%	57
LSU-Bogalusa Medical Center	Bogalusa	65%	65
Dauterive Hospital	New Iberia	64%	58
University Medical Center	Lafayette	64%	200
Ochsner Medical Center-Baton Rouge	Baton Rouge	62%	278
Glenwood Regional Medical Center	West Monroe	61%	188
Natchitoches Regional Medical Center	Natchitoches	61%	76
Green Clinic Surgical Hospital	Ruston	58%	59
West Jefferson Medical Center	Marrero	57%	328
Lakeview Regional Medical Center	Covington	55%	202
Doctors Hospital	Shreveport	54%	63
Ochsner Clinic Foundation	New Orleans	52%	623
Minden Medical Center	Minden	47%	172
Thibodaux Regional Medical Center	Thibodaux	46%	214
Morehouse General Hospital	Bastrop	45%	112
Opelousas General Hospital	Opelousas	45%	270
Physicians Surgical Specialty Hospital	Houma	44%	27
Rapides Regional Medical Center	Alexandria	44%	234
Byrd Regional Hospital	Leesville	40%	87
River West Medical Center	Plaquemine	38%	55
American Legion Hospital	Crowley	25%	144

21. Prophylactic Antibiotic Selection

Hospital Name	City	Rate	Cases
Minden Medical Center	Minden	100%	50
W O Moss Regional Medical Center	Lake Charles	100%	25
E A Conway Medical Center	Monroe	99%	80
Ochsner Clinic Foundation	New Orleans	97%	156
American Legion Hospital	Crowley	96%	45
Louisiana Heart Hospital	Lacombe	96%	82
Opelousas General Hospital	Opelousas	96%	75
Doctors Hospital of Opelousas	Opelousas	94%	36
Lafayette General Medical Center	Lafayette	92%	60
Southwest Medical Center	Lafayette	92%	66
Tulane University Hospital & Clinic	New Orleans	92%	51
Christus Schumpert Health System	Shreveport	91%	70
Glenwood Regional Medical Center	West Monroe	91%	70
Our Lady of Lourdes Regional Medical Center	Lafayette	91%	53
West Calcasieu-Cameron Hospital	Sulphur	91%	46
Women and Children's Hospital	Lake Charles	91%	104
Christus Saint Frances Cabrini Hospital	Alexandria	90%	302
Huey P Long Medical Center	Pineville	90%	41
Northshore Regional Medical Center	Slidell	90%	103
Saint Tammany Parish Hospital	Covington	89%	200
Touro Infirmary	New Orleans	89%	157
North Oaks Medical System	Hammond	88%	60
Leonard J Chabert Medical Center	Houma	87%	75
Lakeview Regional Medical Center	Covington	86%	99
Women's and Children's Hospital	Lafayette	86%	85
Iberia Medical Center	New Iberia	84%	69
Terrebonne General Medical Center	Houma	84%	57
Byrd Regional Hospital	Leesville	83%	29
Lake Charles Memorial Hospital	Lake Charles	83%	159
River Parishes Hospital	La Place	82%	34
Slidell Memorial Hospital	Slidell	82%	71
East Jefferson General Hospital	Metairie	81%	74
LSU-Bogalusa Medical Center	Bogalusa	81%	27
Ochsner Medical Center-Baton Rouge	Baton Rouge	81%	80
Saint Francis Medical Center	Monroe	80%	210
West Jefferson Medical Center	Marrero	74%	158
Abbeville General Hospital	Abbeville	73%	26
University Medical Center	Lafayette	72%	64
Earl K Long Medical Center	Baton Rouge	71%	45
Rapides Regional Medical Center	Alexandria	67%	107
Thibodaux Regional Medical Center	Thibodaux	65%	102
CHRISTUS Saint Patrick Hospital	Lake Charles	61%	122
Monroe Surgical Hospital	Monroe	41%	32
Beauregard Memorial Hospital	DeRidder	26%	35

22. Prophylactic Antibiotic Stopped

Hospital Name	City	Rate	Cases
Abbeville General Hospital	Abbeville	100%	75
Ochsner Medical Center-Baton Rouge	Baton Rouge	99%	272

Hospital Name	City	Rate	Cases
River West Medical Center	Plaquemine	96%	47
Physicians Surgical Specialty Hospital	Houma	92%	26
North Oaks Medical System	Hammond	89%	407
E A Conway Medical Center	Monroe	88%	240
Tulane University Hospital & Clinic	New Orleans	87%	260
Woman's Hospital Foundation	Baton Rouge	87%	53
Lincoln General Hospital	Ruston	86%	29
Women and Children's Hospital	Lake Charles	86%	322
Women's and Children's Hospital	Lafayette	86%	260
Earl K Long Medical Center	Baton Rouge	85%	137
Lallie Kemp/Regional Medical Center	Independence	85%	61
Acadian Medical Center	Eunice	83%	29
Leonard J Chabert Medical Center	Houma	83%	230
Lake Charles Memorial Hospital	Lake Charles	82%	253
River Parishes Hospital	La Place	81%	97
Huey P Long Medical Center	Pineville	80%	102
Heart Hospital of Lafayette	Lafayette	79%	58
Morehouse General Hospital	Bastrop	79%	110
University Medical Center	Lafayette	78%	185
Our Lady of the Lake Regional Medical Center	Baton Rouge	76%	168
Saint Francis Medical Center	Monroe	76%	209
P & S Surgical Hospital	Monroe	75%	225
Touro Infirmary	New Orleans	75%	403
Teche Regional Medical Center	Morgan City	74%	42
Green Clinic Surgical Hospital	Ruston	73%	56
Saint Anne General Hospital	Raceland	70%	53
Monroe Surgical Hospital	Monroe	68%	31
LSU-Bogalusa Medical Center	Bogalusa	67%	57
Northshore Regional Medical Center	Slidell	67%	328
Iberia Medical Center	New Iberia	65%	189
Our Lady of Lourdes Regional Medical Center	Lafayette	64%	154
Baton Rouge General Medical Center	Baton Rouge	62%	320
Terrebonne General Medical Center	Houma	62%	440
CHRISTUS Saint Patrick Hospital	Lake Charles	59%	418
Ochsner Clinic Foundation	New Orleans	59%	616
Lafayette General Medical Center	Lafayette	58%	184
Louisiana Heart Hospital	Lacombe	57%	219
Opelousas General Hospital	Opelousas	57%	236
Slidell Memorial Hospital	Slidell	57%	258
West Jefferson Medical Center	Marrero	57%	304
Willis Knighton Bossier Health Center	Bossier City	57%	49
Christus Saint Frances Cabrini Hospital	Alexandria	56%	1255
Minden Medical Center	Minden	56%	167
Thibodaux Regional Medical Center	Thibodaux	56%	190
W O Moss Regional Medical Center	Lake Charles	56%	87
Saint Tammany Parish Hospital	Covington	55%	603
Southwest Medical Center	Lafayette	55%	134
Lakeview Regional Medical Center	Covington	51%	192
Louisiana State Univ Hosp-Shreveport	Shreveport	51%	51
Glenwood Regional Medical Center	West Monroe	48%	182
Savoy Medical Center	Mamou	47%	64
Jennings American Legion Hospital	Jennings	46%	35
Willis Knighton Medical Center	Shreveport	46%	96
Christus Schumpert Health System	Shreveport	45%	267
Lafayette Surgical Specialty Hospital	Lafayette	45%	55
Doctors Hospital of Opelousas	Opelousas	44%	78
Natchitoches Regional Medical Center	Natchitoches	44%	68
Southern Surgical Hospital	Slidell	43%	30
East Jefferson General Hospital	Metairie	42%	203
Rapides Regional Medical Center	Alexandria	42%	227
Dauterive Hospital	New Iberia	40%	57
American Legion Hospital	Crowley	37%	139
Byrd Regional Hospital	Leesville	36%	66
West Calcasieu-Cameron Hospital	Sulphur	36%	150
Lane Regional Memorial Hospital	Zachary	20%	66
Beauregard Memorial Hospital	DeRidder	16%	98
Doctors Hospital	Shreveport	11%	61

Pregnancy Care

23. Inpatient Neonatal Mortality

Hospital Name	City	Rate	Cases
Saint Anne General Hospital	Raceland	0.00%	208
West Calcasieu-Cameron Hospital	Sulphur	0.00%	271
Christus Saint Frances Cabrini Hospital	Alexandria	0.09%	1135
Glenwood Regional Medical Center	West Monroe	0.09%	1113
Thibodaux Regional Medical Center	Thibodaux	0.16%	625
Northshore Regional Medical Center	Slidell	0.19%	522
Terrebonne General Medical Center	Houma	0.23%	2190
Savoy Medical Center	Mamou	0.28%	359
Leonard J Chabert Medical Center	Houma	0.43%	470
Women and Children's Hospital	Lake Charles	0.66%	1818
Women's and Children's Hospital	Lafayette	0.84%	3551
E A Conway Medical Center	Monroe	0.85%	1062

NOTE: Hospital profiles are in alphabetical order by state, then city, then hospital within the city; Rankings are sorted by rate in descending order and exclude hospitals with less than 25 cases; (1) The number of cases is too small (n<25) for purposes of reliably predicting hospital performance; (2) Measure reflects the hospital's indication that its submission was based upon a sample of its relevant discharges; (3) Rate reflects fewer than the maximum possible quarters of data for the measure; (4) Inaccurate information submitted and suppressed for one or more quarters; (5) No data is available from the hospital for this measure; Please refer to the User's Guide for a full explanation of data

Woman's Hospital Foundation	Baton Rouge	1.00%	8762
Huey P Long Medical Center	Pineville	1.11%	181
Lafayette General Medical Center	Lafayette	1.26%	1748
University Medical Center	Lafayette	1.29%	466
Louisiana State Univ Hosp-Shreveport	Shreveport	2.02%	397

24. Third or Fourth Degree Laceration

Hospital Name	City	Rate	Cases
Savoy Medical Center	Mamou	0.52%	194
West Calcasieu-Cameron Hospital	Sulphur	1.68%	179
Women and Children's Hospital	Lake Charles	2.50%	1082
Leonard J Chabert Medical Center	Houma	2.72%	294
Huey P Long Medical Center	Pineville	2.78%	108
Women's and Children's Hospital	Lafayette	2.89%	2041
Lafayette General Medical Center	Lafayette	2.94%	1054
Northshore Regional Medical Center	Slidell	2.97%	404
University Medical Center	Lafayette	3.23%	310
Terrebonne General Medical Center	Houma	3.61%	1245
Woman's Hospital Foundation	Baton Rouge	3.63%	5154
E A Conway Medical Center	Monroe	3.87%	750
Glenwood Regional Medical Center	West Monroe	3.90%	616
Louisiana State Univ Hosp-Shreveport	Shreveport	4.47%	1163
Christus Saint Frances Cabrini Hospital	Alexandria	4.55%	549
Thibodaux Regional Medical Center	Thibodaux	7.85%	293
Saint Anne General Hospital	Raceland	9.88%	81

NOTE: Hospital profiles are in alphabetical order by state, then city, then hospital within the city; Rankings are sorted by rate in descending order and exclude hospitals with less than 25 cases; (1) The number of cases is too small (n<25) for purposes of reliably predicting hospital performance; (2) Measure reflects the hospital's indication that its submission was based upon a sample of its relevant discharges; (3) Rate reflects fewer than the maximum possible quarters of data for the measure; (4) Inaccurate information submitted and suppressed for one or more quarters; (5) No data is available from the hospital for this measure; Please refer to the User's Guide for a full explanation of data

Abbeville General Hospital

118 N Hospital Drive
PO Box 580   Phone: 337-893-5466
Abbeville, LA 70511   Fax: 337-893-2801
E-mail: agh580@aol.com
URL: www.abgen.net
Ownership: Govt - Hospital District or Authority   Accredited: Yes
Emergency Services: Yes   Licensed Beds: 60
Key Personnel:
CEO. . . . . Ray Landry
Chief Medical Staff. . . . . David Craft

Measure	Cases	This Hospital	State Average	U.S. Average	Top Hospital
Heart Attack Care					
ACE Inhibitor or ARB for LVSD[1]	2	50%	84%	82%	100%
Aspirin at Arrival[1]	10	80%	91%	92%	100%
Aspirin at Discharge[1]	6	50%	87%	90%	100%
Beta Blocker at Arrival[1]	5	60%	85%	87%	100%
Beta Blocker at Discharge[1]	6	17%	88%	90%	100%
Fibrinolytic Medication Timing	0	-	32%	31%	100%
PCI Within 90 Minutes of Arrival	0	-	40%	54%	95%
Smoking Cessation Advice[1]	2	100%	88%	88%	100%
Heart Failure Care					
ACE Inhibitor or ARB for LVSD	25	72%	78%	82%	100%
Discharge Instructions	87	94%	62%	61%	93%
Evaluation of LVS Function	134	82%	81%	83%	99%
Smoking Cessation Advice	25	88%	83%	82%	100%
Pneumonia Care					
Appropriate Initial Antibiotic	49	73%	78%	83%	94%
Blood Culture Timing	44	91%	89%	90%	100%
Influenza Vaccine[1]	18	94%	58%	70%	100%
Initial Antibiotic Timing	82	85%	76%	80%	93%
Oxygenation Assessment	97	97%	98%	99%	100%
Pneumococcal Vaccine	66	97%	61%	69%	94%
Smoking Cessation Advice[1]	13	100%	78%	80%	100%
Surgical Infection Prevention					
Prophylactic Antibiotic Given[3]	83	77%	69%	77%	95%
Prophylactic Antibiotic Selection	26	73%	79%	90%	100%
Prophylactic Antibiotic Stopped[3]	75	100%	61%	72%	95%
Pregnancy Care					
Inpatient Neonatal Mortality	-	-	-	-	-
Third or Fourth Degree Laceration	-	-	3.54%	3.63%	3.27%

Christus Saint Frances Cabrini Hospital

3330 Masonic Drive   Phone: 318-448-6760
Alexandria, LA 71301   Fax: 318-448-6755
URL: www.cabrini.org
Ownership: Voluntary non-profit - Church   Accredited: Yes
Emergency Services: Yes   Licensed Beds: 232
Key Personnel:
President/CEO. . . . . Steven F Wright
Chief Radiology . . . . Carl Schofield, MD

Measure	Cases	This Hospital	State Average	U.S. Average	Top Hospital
Heart Attack Care					
ACE Inhibitor or ARB for LVSD	44	100%	84%	82%	100%
Aspirin at Arrival	128	98%	91%	92%	100%
Aspirin at Discharge	215	100%	87%	90%	100%
Beta Blocker at Arrival	115	97%	85%	87%	100%
Beta Blocker at Discharge	237	99%	88%	90%	100%
Fibrinolytic Medication Timing[1]	1	0%	32%	31%	100%
PCI Within 90 Minutes of Arrival[1]	10	60%	40%	54%	95%
Smoking Cessation Advice	116	97%	88%	88%	100%
Heart Failure Care					
ACE Inhibitor or ARB for LVSD	242	98%	78%	82%	100%
Discharge Instructions	468	87%	62%	61%	93%
Evaluation of LVS Function	533	99%	81%	83%	99%
Smoking Cessation Advice	87	98%	83%	82%	100%
Pneumonia Care					
Appropriate Initial Antibiotic	174	75%	78%	83%	94%
Blood Culture Timing	176	91%	89%	90%	100%
Influenza Vaccine	62	95%	58%	70%	100%
Initial Antibiotic Timing	241	68%	76%	80%	93%

Measure	Cases	This Hospital	State Average	U.S. Average	Top Hospital
Oxygenation Assessment	318	99%	98%	99%	100%
Pneumococcal Vaccine	189	93%	61%	69%	94%
Smoking Cessation Advice	67	93%	78%	80%	100%
Surgical Infection Prevention					
Prophylactic Antibiotic Given	1,292	77%	69%	77%	95%
Prophylactic Antibiotic Selection	302	90%	79%	90%	100%
Prophylactic Antibiotic Stopped	1,255	56%	61%	72%	95%
Pregnancy Care					
Inpatient Neonatal Mortality	1,135	0.09%	-	-	-
Third or Fourth Degree Laceration	549	4.55%	3.54%	3.63%	3.27%

Rapides Regional Medical Center

211 4th Street   Phone: 318-473-3000
Alexandria, LA 71301   Fax: 318-449-7575
URL: www.rapidesregional.com
Ownership: Proprietary   Accredited: Yes
Emergency Services: Yes   Licensed Beds: 359
Key Personnel:
Administrator/President/CEO . . . . AC Buchanan
Cardiology . . . . Ilyas Chaudhry, MD
Emergency Room . . . . Emmanuel Witherspoon, MD
Director Infection/Disease Control . . . . Grace Luneau
CCU Spvg. Nurse . . . . Marilyn Smith, RN
OB/GYN Womens Health. . . . . Benjamin R Spruill, MD
Chief Radiology . . . . Alfred A Mansour, MD
Director Respiratory Therapy . . . . Bob Jones

Measure	Cases	This Hospital	State Average	U.S. Average	Top Hospital
Heart Attack Care					
ACE Inhibitor or ARB for LVSD	60	80%	84%	82%	100%
Aspirin at Arrival	121	91%	91%	92%	100%
Aspirin at Discharge	194	95%	87%	90%	100%
Beta Blocker at Arrival	88	86%	85%	87%	100%
Beta Blocker at Discharge	212	94%	88%	90%	100%
Fibrinolytic Medication Timing	0	-	32%	31%	100%
PCI Within 90 Minutes of Arrival[1]	8	12%	40%	54%	95%
Smoking Cessation Advice	97	97%	88%	88%	100%
Heart Failure Care					
ACE Inhibitor or ARB for LVSD[2]	224	76%	78%	82%	100%
Discharge Instructions[2]	421	57%	62%	61%	93%
Evaluation of LVS Function[2]	502	90%	81%	83%	99%
Smoking Cessation Advice[2]	102	94%	83%	82%	100%
Pneumonia Care					
Appropriate Initial Antibiotic[2]	131	80%	78%	83%	94%
Blood Culture Timing[2]	180	96%	89%	90%	100%
Influenza Vaccine	55	96%	58%	70%	100%
Initial Antibiotic Timing[2]	282	77%	76%	80%	93%
Oxygenation Assessment[2]	316	100%	98%	99%	100%
Pneumococcal Vaccine[2]	201	91%	61%	69%	94%
Smoking Cessation Advice[2]	60	88%	78%	80%	100%
Surgical Infection Prevention					
Prophylactic Antibiotic Given[2,3]	234	44%	69%	77%	95%
Prophylactic Antibiotic Selection[2]	107	67%	79%	90%	100%
Prophylactic Antibiotic Stopped[2,3]	227	42%	61%	72%	95%
Pregnancy Care					
Inpatient Neonatal Mortality	-	-	-	-	-
Third or Fourth Degree Laceration	-	-	3.54%	3.63%	3.27%

Bienville Medical Center

1175 Pine Street Suite 200   Phone: 318-263-4700
Arcadia, LA 71001
Ownership: Proprietary   Accredited: No
Emergency Services: Yes

Measure	Cases	This Hospital	State Average	U.S. Average	Top Hospital
Heart Attack Care					
ACE Inhibitor or ARB for LVSD[5]	-	-	84%	82%	100%
Aspirin at Arrival[5]	-	-	91%	92%	100%
Aspirin at Discharge[5]	-	-	87%	90%	100%
Beta Blocker at Arrival[5]	-	-	85%	87%	100%
Beta Blocker at Discharge[5]	-	-	88%	90%	100%
Fibrinolytic Medication Timing[5]	-	-	32%	31%	100%

NOTE: Hospital profiles are in alphabetical order by state, then city, then hospital within the city; Rankings are sorted by rate in descending order and exclude hospitals with less than 25 cases; (1) The number of cases is too small (n<25) for purposes of reliably predicting hospital performance; (2) Measure reflects the hospital's indication that its submission was based upon a sample of its relevant discharges; (3) Rate reflects fewer than the maximum possible quarters of data for the measure; (4) Inaccurate information submitted and suppressed for one or more quarters; (5) No data is available from the hospital for this measure; Please refer to the User's Guide for a full explanation of data

Measure	Cases	This Hospital	State Average	U.S. Average	Top Hospital
PCI Within 90 Minutes of Arrival[5]	-	-	40%	54%	95%
Smoking Cessation Advice[5]	-	-	88%	88%	100%
Heart Failure Care					
ACE Inhibitor or ARB for LVSD[5]	-	-	78%	82%	100%
Discharge Instructions[5]	-	-	62%	61%	93%
Evaluation of LVS Function[5]	-	-	81%	83%	99%
Smoking Cessation Advice[5]	-	-	83%	82%	100%
Pneumonia Care					
Appropriate Initial Antibiotic[3]	0	-	78%	83%	94%
Blood Culture Timing[5]	-	-	89%	90%	100%
Influenza Vaccine[5]	-	-	58%	70%	100%
Initial Antibiotic Timing[3]	0	-	76%	80%	93%
Oxygenation Assessment[1,3]	1	100%	98%	99%	100%
Pneumococcal Vaccine[3]	0	-	61%	69%	94%
Smoking Cessation Advice[3]	0	-	78%	80%	100%
Surgical Infection Prevention					
Prophylactic Antibiotic Given[5]	-	-	69%	77%	95%
Prophylactic Antibiotic Selection[5]	-	-	79%	90%	100%
Prophylactic Antibiotic Stopped[5]	-	-	61%	72%	95%
Pregnancy Care					
Inpatient Neonatal Mortality	-	-	-	-	-
Third or Fourth Degree Laceration	-	-	3.54%	3.63%	3.27%

Morehouse General Hospital

323 W Walnut Street   Phone: 318-283-3600
PO Box 1060   Fax: 318-283-3663
Bastrop, LA 71220
URL: www.mghospital.com
Ownership: Govt - Hospital District or Authority   Accredited: No
Emergency Services: Yes   Licensed Beds: 60
Key Personnel:
Administrator . . . . William W Bing
Chief Medical Staff . . . . J M Smith, MD
Emergency Room . . . . EL Chorette, MD
Director Infection/Disease Control . . . . Melinda Jones, RN
ICU . . . . Pam Chambers, RN
Intensive/Coronary Care . . . . Pam Chambers, RN
Director Medical Surgical Nursing . . . . Katherine Tucker, RN
OB/GYN/Women's Health . . . . Lori Priestly, RN
Chief Radiology . . . . Brenton McDonald, MD
Director Respiratory Therapy . . . . James Barrett

Measure	Cases	This Hospital	State Average	U.S. Average	Top Hospital
Heart Attack Care					
ACE Inhibitor or ARB for LVSD[1]	3	67%	84%	82%	100%
Aspirin at Arrival[1]	20	75%	91%	92%	100%
Aspirin at Discharge[1]	8	62%	87%	90%	100%
Beta Blocker at Arrival[1]	17	65%	85%	87%	100%
Beta Blocker at Discharge[1]	8	75%	88%	90%	100%
Fibrinolytic Medication Timing[1]	4	75%	32%	31%	100%
PCI Within 90 Minutes of Arrival	0	-	40%	54%	95%
Smoking Cessation Advice[3]	0	-	88%	88%	100%
Heart Failure Care					
ACE Inhibitor or ARB for LVSD	28	71%	78%	82%	100%
Discharge Instructions	61	70%	62%	61%	93%
Evaluation of LVS Function	96	55%	81%	83%	99%
Smoking Cessation Advice[1]	15	80%	83%	82%	100%
Pneumonia Care					
Appropriate Initial Antibiotic	55	53%	78%	83%	94%
Blood Culture Timing[1]	20	100%	89%	90%	100%
Influenza Vaccine[1]	16	0%	58%	70%	100%
Initial Antibiotic Timing	115	67%	76%	80%	93%
Oxygenation Assessment	129	78%	98%	99%	100%
Pneumococcal Vaccine	72	58%	61%	69%	94%
Smoking Cessation Advice[1,3]	21	67%	78%	80%	100%
Surgical Infection Prevention					
Prophylactic Antibiotic Given[3]	112	45%	69%	77%	95%
Prophylactic Antibiotic Selection[1]	4	75%	79%	90%	100%
Prophylactic Antibiotic Stopped[3]	110	79%	61%	72%	95%
Pregnancy Care					
Inpatient Neonatal Mortality	-	-	-	-	-
Third or Fourth Degree Laceration	-	-	3.54%	3.63%	3.27%

Baton Rouge General Medical Center

8585 PiCardy Avenue   Phone: 225-387-7000
Baton Rouge, LA 70809   Fax: 225-381-6129
URL: www.generalhealth.org
Ownership: Voluntary non-profit - Private   Accredited: Yes
Emergency Services: Yes   Licensed Beds: 448
Key Personnel:
President/CEO . . . . William Holman
Chief Medical Officer . . . . Floyd Roberts, MD
Chief Medical Staff . . . . Benton Dupont, MD
Emergency Room . . . . Jennifer Slay
Infection Control . . . . Connie Deleo
ICU . . . . Julie Whittaker
Intensive/Coronary Care . . . . Julie Whittaker
Medical/Surgical Nursing . . . . Tammy O'Connor
OB/GYN Womens Health . . . . Cheri Barker
Respiratory/Cardiopulmonary . . . . Jim Lanoha

Measure	Cases	This Hospital	State Average	U.S. Average	Top Hospital
Heart Attack Care					
ACE Inhibitor or ARB for LVSD	113	74%	84%	82%	100%
Aspirin at Arrival	328	95%	91%	92%	100%
Aspirin at Discharge	361	87%	87%	90%	100%
Beta Blocker at Arrival	287	93%	85%	87%	100%
Beta Blocker at Discharge	359	94%	88%	90%	100%
Fibrinolytic Medication Timing[1,3]	5	40%	32%	31%	100%
PCI Within 90 Minutes of Arrival[1]	10	10%	40%	54%	95%
Smoking Cessation Advice[3]	32	97%	88%	88%	100%
Heart Failure Care					
ACE Inhibitor or ARB for LVSD	364	73%	78%	82%	100%
Discharge Instructions[3]	151	89%	62%	61%	93%
Evaluation of LVS Function	851	84%	81%	83%	99%
Smoking Cessation Advice[3]	48	85%	83%	82%	100%
Pneumonia Care					
Appropriate Initial Antibiotic[3]	39	85%	78%	83%	94%
Blood Culture Timing[3]	61	85%	89%	90%	100%
Influenza Vaccine[5]	-	-	58%	70%	100%
Initial Antibiotic Timing	512	66%	76%	80%	93%
Oxygenation Assessment	637	99%	98%	99%	100%
Pneumococcal Vaccine	320	68%	61%	69%	94%
Smoking Cessation Advice[3]	29	72%	78%	80%	100%
Surgical Infection Prevention					
Prophylactic Antibiotic Given[3]	327	92%	69%	77%	95%
Prophylactic Antibiotic Selection[5]	-	-	79%	90%	100%
Prophylactic Antibiotic Stopped[3]	320	62%	61%	72%	95%
Pregnancy Care					
Inpatient Neonatal Mortality	-	-	-	-	-
Third or Fourth Degree Laceration	-	-	3.54%	3.63%	3.27%

Earl K Long Medical Center

5825 Airline Highway   Phone: 225-356-3361
Baton Rouge, LA 70805   Fax: 225-358-1003
Ownership: Government - State   Accredited: Yes
Emergency Services: Yes   Licensed Beds: 257
Key Personnel:
Administrator . . . . Clay Dunaway
Chief Medical Director . . . . Chapman Lee, MD

Measure	Cases	This Hospital	State Average	U.S. Average	Top Hospital
Heart Attack Care					
ACE Inhibitor or ARB for LVSD[1]	20	100%	84%	82%	100%
Aspirin at Arrival	77	95%	91%	92%	100%
Aspirin at Discharge	67	90%	87%	90%	100%
Beta Blocker at Arrival	65	95%	85%	87%	100%
Beta Blocker at Discharge	64	98%	88%	90%	100%
Fibrinolytic Medication Timing[1]	7	57%	32%	31%	100%
PCI Within 90 Minutes of Arrival	0	-	40%	54%	95%
Smoking Cessation Advice	40	75%	88%	88%	100%
Heart Failure Care					
ACE Inhibitor or ARB for LVSD	100	95%	78%	82%	100%
Discharge Instructions	149	60%	62%	61%	93%
Evaluation of LVS Function	156	91%	81%	83%	99%
Smoking Cessation Advice	81	80%	83%	82%	100%

NOTE: Hospital profiles are in alphabetical order by state, then city, then hospital within the city; Rankings are sorted by rate in descending order and exclude hospitals with less than 25 cases; (1) The number of cases is too small (n<25) for purposes of reliably predicting hospital performance; (2) Measure reflects the hospital's indication that its submission was based upon a sample of its relevant discharges; (3) Rate reflects fewer than the maximum possible quarters of data for the measure; (4) Inaccurate information submitted and suppressed for one or more quarters; (5) No data is available from the hospital for this measure; Please refer to the User's Guide for a full explanation of data

Pneumonia Care					
Appropriate Initial Antibiotic	60	73%	78%	83%	94%
Blood Culture Timing	67	79%	89%	90%	100%
Influenza Vaccine[1]	11	18%	58%	70%	100%
Initial Antibiotic Timing	91	54%	76%	80%	93%
Oxygenation Assessment	98	100%	98%	99%	100%
Pneumococcal Vaccine[1]	9	11%	61%	69%	94%
Smoking Cessation Advice	46	67%	78%	80%	100%
Surgical Infection Prevention					
Prophylactic Antibiotic Given[3]	167	83%	69%	77%	95%
Prophylactic Antibiotic Selection	45	71%	79%	90%	100%
Prophylactic Antibiotic Stopped[3]	137	85%	61%	72%	95%
Pregnancy Care					
Inpatient Neonatal Mortality	-	-	-	-	-
Third or Fourth Degree Laceration	-	-	3.54%	3.63%	3.27%

Greater Baton Rouge Surgical Hospital

7855 Howell Place Blvd
Baton Rouge, LA 70807
Ownership: Voluntary non-profit - Private
Emergency Services: Yes

Phone: 225-383-7099

Accredited: No

Measure	Cases	This Hospital	State Average	U.S. Average	Top Hospital
Heart Attack Care					
ACE Inhibitor or ARB for LVSD[5]	-	-	84%	82%	100%
Aspirin at Arrival[5]	-	-	91%	92%	100%
Aspirin at Discharge[5]	-	-	87%	90%	100%
Beta Blocker at Arrival[5]	-	-	85%	87%	100%
Beta Blocker at Discharge[5]	-	-	88%	90%	100%
Fibrinolytic Medication Timing[5]	-	-	32%	31%	100%
PCI Within 90 Minutes of Arrival[5]	-	-	40%	54%	95%
Smoking Cessation Advice[5]	-	-	88%	88%	100%
Heart Failure Care					
ACE Inhibitor or ARB for LVSD[5]	-	-	78%	82%	100%
Discharge Instructions[5]	-	-	62%	61%	93%
Evaluation of LVS Function[5]	-	-	81%	83%	99%
Smoking Cessation Advice[5]	-	-	83%	82%	100%
Pneumonia Care					
Appropriate Initial Antibiotic[5]	-	-	78%	83%	94%
Blood Culture Timing[5]	-	-	89%	90%	100%
Influenza Vaccine[5]	-	-	58%	70%	100%
Initial Antibiotic Timing[5]	-	-	76%	80%	93%
Oxygenation Assessment[5]	-	-	98%	99%	100%
Pneumococcal Vaccine[5]	-	-	61%	69%	94%
Smoking Cessation Advice[5]	-	-	78%	80%	100%
Surgical Infection Prevention					
Prophylactic Antibiotic Given[1,3]	8	12%	69%	77%	95%
Prophylactic Antibiotic Selection[5]	-	-	79%	90%	100%
Prophylactic Antibiotic Stopped[1,3]	8	0%	61%	72%	95%
Pregnancy Care					
Inpatient Neonatal Mortality	-	-	-	-	-
Third or Fourth Degree Laceration	-	-	3.54%	3.63%	3.27%

Neuromedical Center Hospital

10105 Park Row Circle
Baton Rouge, LA 70810
Ownership: Proprietary
Emergency Services: No

Phone: 225-763-9900

Accredited: No

Measure	Cases	This Hospital	State Average	U.S. Average	Top Hospital
Heart Attack Care					
ACE Inhibitor or ARB for LVSD[5]	-	-	84%	82%	100%
Aspirin at Arrival[5]	-	-	91%	92%	100%
Aspirin at Discharge[5]	-	-	87%	90%	100%
Beta Blocker at Arrival[5]	-	-	85%	87%	100%
Beta Blocker at Discharge[5]	-	-	88%	90%	100%
Fibrinolytic Medication Timing[5]	-	-	32%	31%	100%
PCI Within 90 Minutes of Arrival[5]	-	-	40%	54%	95%
Smoking Cessation Advice[5]	-	-	88%	88%	100%
Heart Failure Care					
ACE Inhibitor or ARB for LVSD[5]	-	-	78%	82%	100%
Discharge Instructions[5]	-	-	62%	61%	93%

			81%	83%	99%
Evaluation of LVS Function[5]	-	-	81%	83%	99%
Smoking Cessation Advice[5]	-	-	83%	82%	100%
Pneumonia Care					
Appropriate Initial Antibiotic[5]	-	-	78%	83%	94%
Blood Culture Timing[5]	-	-	89%	90%	100%
Influenza Vaccine[5]	-	-	58%	70%	100%
Initial Antibiotic Timing[5]	-	-	76%	80%	93%
Oxygenation Assessment[5]	-	-	98%	99%	100%
Pneumococcal Vaccine[5]	-	-	61%	69%	94%
Smoking Cessation Advice[5]	-	-	78%	80%	100%
Surgical Infection Prevention					
Prophylactic Antibiotic Given[5]	-	-	69%	77%	95%
Prophylactic Antibiotic Selection[5]	-	-	79%	90%	100%
Prophylactic Antibiotic Stopped[5]	-	-	61%	72%	95%
Pregnancy Care					
Inpatient Neonatal Mortality	-	-	-	-	-
Third or Fourth Degree Laceration	-	-	3.54%	3.63%	3.27%

Ochsner Medical Center-Baton Rouge

17000 Medical Center Drive
Baton Rouge, LA 70816
Ownership: Proprietary
Emergency Services: Yes

Phone: 225-752-2470
Fax: 225-755-4883
Accredited: Yes
Licensed Beds: 201

Key Personnel:
CEO. . . . . Robert Jernigan, CHE
Chief Medical Staff. . . . . Robert Elliott, MD
Cardiac Lab . . . . Mark Green
Catheterization Lab . . . . Mark Green
Emergency Room . . . . Steven Ragusa, MD
Infection Control. . . . . Bonnie Rosenthal, RN
ICU . . . . Mary Johnson, MSN RN
Intensive Coronary Care . . . . Mary Johnson, MSN, RN
Medical Surgical Nursing . . . . Mary Johnson, MSN RN
Respiratory/Cardiopulmonary. . . . . Donna Jones, RRT

Measure	Cases	This Hospital	State Average	U.S. Average	Top Hospital
Heart Attack Care					
ACE Inhibitor or ARB for LVSD	77	90%	84%	82%	100%
Aspirin at Arrival	134	99%	91%	92%	100%
Aspirin at Discharge	120	96%	87%	90%	100%
Beta Blocker at Arrival	110	95%	85%	87%	100%
Beta Blocker at Discharge	119	93%	88%	90%	100%
Fibrinolytic Medication Timing[1]	1	0%	32%	31%	100%
PCI Within 90 Minutes of Arrival[1]	23	30%	40%	54%	95%
Smoking Cessation Advice	51	69%	88%	88%	100%
Heart Failure Care					
ACE Inhibitor or ARB for LVSD	130	90%	78%	82%	100%
Discharge Instructions	210	51%	62%	61%	93%
Evaluation of LVS Function	211	93%	81%	83%	99%
Smoking Cessation Advice	39	46%	83%	82%	100%
Pneumonia Care					
Appropriate Initial Antibiotic	122	70%	78%	83%	94%
Blood Culture Timing	113	88%	89%	90%	100%
Influenza Vaccine[4,5]	-	-	58%	70%	100%
Initial Antibiotic Timing	182	70%	76%	80%	93%
Oxygenation Assessment	207	99%	98%	99%	100%
Pneumococcal Vaccine	114	13%	61%	69%	94%
Smoking Cessation Advice	52	71%	78%	80%	100%
Surgical Infection Prevention					
Prophylactic Antibiotic Given	278	62%	69%	77%	95%
Prophylactic Antibiotic Selection	80	81%	79%	90%	100%
Prophylactic Antibiotic Stopped	272	99%	61%	72%	95%
Pregnancy Care					
Inpatient Neonatal Mortality	-	-	-	-	-
Third or Fourth Degree Laceration	-	-	3.54%	3.63%	3.27%

NOTE: Hospital profiles are in alphabetical order by state, then city, then hospital within the city; Rankings are sorted by rate in descending order and exclude hospitals with less than 25 cases; (1) The number of cases is too small (n<25) for purposes of reliably predicting hospital performance; (2) Measure reflects the hospital's indication that its submission was based upon a sample of its relevant discharges; (3) Rate reflects fewer than the maximum possible quarters of data for the measure; (4) Inaccurate information submitted and suppressed for one or more quarters; (5) No data is available from the hospital for this measure; Please refer to the User's Guide for a full explanation of data

Our Lady of the Lake Regional Medical Center

5000 Hennessy Boulevard
Baton Rouge, LA 70808
URL: www.ololrmc.com
Ownership: Voluntary non-profit - Church
Emergency Services: Yes

Phone: 225-765-6565
Fax: 225-769-3659

Accredited: Yes
Licensed Beds: 723

Key Personnel:

President/COO	Kirk G Wilson
CEO	Robert C Davidge
Chief Medical Staff	John Whitaker, MD
Chief Cardiology	Venkat R Surakanti, MD
Chief Emergency Medicine	J Thomas Miceli, MD
Director Infection/Disease Control	Darlene J Picoci
CCU Spvg. Nurse	Rose Patin
Chief Gynecology	Jane B Peek, MD
Chief Pediatric Surgery	J Robert Upp Jr, MD
Chief Radiology	Robert F Hayden, MD
Director Respiratory Therapy	James Hammerschnidt
Chief General Surgery	Peter Bostick, MD

Measure	Cases	This Hospital	State Average	U.S. Average	Top Hospital
Heart Attack Care					
ACE Inhibitor or ARB for LVSD	88	93%	84%	82%	100%
Aspirin at Arrival	239	99%	91%	92%	100%
Aspirin at Discharge	349	97%	87%	90%	100%
Beta Blocker at Arrival	216	95%	85%	87%	100%
Beta Blocker at Discharge	338	97%	88%	90%	100%
Fibrinolytic Medication Timing[1,3]	1	0%	32%	31%	100%
PCI Within 90 Minutes of Arrival[1]	15	73%	40%	54%	95%
Smoking Cessation Advice[3]	36	100%	88%	88%	100%
Heart Failure Care					
ACE Inhibitor or ARB for LVSD	347	86%	78%	82%	100%
Discharge Instructions[3]	166	83%	62%	61%	93%
Evaluation of LVS Function	873	94%	81%	83%	99%
Smoking Cessation Advice[3]	27	100%	83%	82%	100%
Pneumonia Care					
Appropriate Initial Antibiotic[3]	46	85%	78%	83%	94%
Blood Culture Timing[3]	52	87%	89%	90%	100%
Influenza Vaccine[5]	-	-	58%	70%	100%
Initial Antibiotic Timing	312	79%	76%	80%	93%
Oxygenation Assessment	378	100%	98%	99%	100%
Pneumococcal Vaccine	219	79%	61%	69%	94%
Smoking Cessation Advice[1,3]	19	100%	78%	80%	100%
Surgical Infection Prevention					
Prophylactic Antibiotic Given[3]	175	83%	69%	77%	95%
Prophylactic Antibiotic Selection[5]	-	-	79%	90%	100%
Prophylactic Antibiotic Stopped[3]	168	76%	61%	72%	95%
Pregnancy Care					
Inpatient Neonatal Mortality	-	-	-	-	-
Third or Fourth Degree Laceration	-	-	3.54%	3.63%	3.27%

Surgical Specialty Hospital

8080 Bluebonnet Blvd
Baton Rouge, LA 70810
Ownership: Proprietary
Emergency Services: No

Phone: 225-408-5500

Accredited: Yes

Measure	Cases	This Hospital	State Average	U.S. Average	Top Hospital
Heart Attack Care					
ACE Inhibitor or ARB for LVSD[5]	-	-	84%	82%	100%
Aspirin at Arrival[5]	-	-	91%	92%	100%
Aspirin at Discharge[5]	-	-	87%	90%	100%
Beta Blocker at Arrival[5]	-	-	85%	87%	100%
Beta Blocker at Discharge[5]	-	-	88%	90%	100%
Fibrinolytic Medication Timing[5]	-	-	32%	31%	100%
PCI Within 90 Minutes of Arrival[5]	-	-	40%	54%	95%
Smoking Cessation Advice[5]	-	-	88%	88%	100%
Heart Failure Care					
ACE Inhibitor or ARB for LVSD[5]	-	-	78%	82%	100%
Discharge Instructions[5]	-	-	62%	61%	93%
Evaluation of LVS Function[5]	-	-	81%	83%	99%
Smoking Cessation Advice[5]	-	-	83%	82%	100%
Pneumonia Care					

Measure	Cases	This Hospital	State Average	U.S. Average	Top Hospital
Appropriate Initial Antibiotic[5]	-	-	78%	83%	94%
Blood Culture Timing[5]	-	-	89%	90%	100%
Influenza Vaccine[5]	-	-	58%	70%	100%
Initial Antibiotic Timing[5]	-	-	76%	80%	93%
Oxygenation Assessment[5]	-	-	98%	99%	100%
Pneumococcal Vaccine[5]	-	-	61%	69%	94%
Smoking Cessation Advice[5]	-	-	78%	80%	100%
Surgical Infection Prevention					
Prophylactic Antibiotic Given[5]	-	-	69%	77%	95%
Prophylactic Antibiotic Selection[5]	-	-	79%	90%	100%
Prophylactic Antibiotic Stopped[5]	-	-	61%	72%	95%
Pregnancy Care					
Inpatient Neonatal Mortality	-	-	-	-	-
Third or Fourth Degree Laceration	-	-	3.54%	3.63%	3.27%

Vista Surgical Hospital of Baton Rouge

9032 Perkins Road
Baton Rouge, LA 70810
URL: www.vshbr.com
Ownership: Proprietary
Emergency Services: No

Phone: 225-819-4100
Fax: 225-769-7974

Accredited: No
Licensed Beds: 39

Key Personnel:

CEO/Administrator	Rene A LaBruyere

Measure	Cases	This Hospital	State Average	U.S. Average	Top Hospital
Heart Attack Care					
ACE Inhibitor or ARB for LVSD[5]	-	-	84%	82%	100%
Aspirin at Arrival[5]	-	-	91%	92%	100%
Aspirin at Discharge[5]	-	-	87%	90%	100%
Beta Blocker at Arrival[5]	-	-	85%	87%	100%
Beta Blocker at Discharge[5]	-	-	88%	90%	100%
Fibrinolytic Medication Timing[5]	-	-	32%	31%	100%
PCI Within 90 Minutes of Arrival[5]	-	-	40%	54%	95%
Smoking Cessation Advice[5]	-	-	88%	88%	100%
Heart Failure Care					
ACE Inhibitor or ARB for LVSD[5]	-	-	78%	82%	100%
Discharge Instructions[5]	-	-	62%	61%	93%
Evaluation of LVS Function[5]	-	-	81%	83%	99%
Smoking Cessation Advice[5]	-	-	83%	82%	100%
Pneumonia Care					
Appropriate Initial Antibiotic[5]	-	-	78%	83%	94%
Blood Culture Timing[5]	-	-	89%	90%	100%
Influenza Vaccine[5]	-	-	58%	70%	100%
Initial Antibiotic Timing[5]	-	-	76%	80%	93%
Oxygenation Assessment[5]	-	-	98%	99%	100%
Pneumococcal Vaccine[5]	-	-	61%	69%	94%
Smoking Cessation Advice[5]	-	-	78%	80%	100%
Surgical Infection Prevention					
Prophylactic Antibiotic Given[5]	-	-	69%	77%	95%
Prophylactic Antibiotic Selection[5]	-	-	79%	90%	100%
Prophylactic Antibiotic Stopped[5]	-	-	61%	72%	95%
Pregnancy Care					
Inpatient Neonatal Mortality	-	-	-	-	-
Third or Fourth Degree Laceration	-	-	3.54%	3.63%	3.27%

Woman's Hospital Foundation

9050 Airline Highway
PO Box 95009
Baton Rouge, LA 70815
URL: www.womans.com
Ownership: Voluntary non-profit - Other
Emergency Services: Yes

Phone: 225-927-1300
Fax: 225-924-8233

Accredited: Yes
Licensed Beds: 225

Key Personnel:

President/CEO	Teri G Fontenot
Chief Medical Staff	Charles Lawler, MD
Chief Radiology	Chester Coles, MD
Director Respiratory Therapy	Danette Legendre

Measure	Cases	This Hospital	State Average	U.S. Average	Top Hospital
Heart Attack Care					
ACE Inhibitor or ARB for LVSD[5]	-	-	84%	82%	100%
Aspirin at Arrival[5]	-	-	91%	92%	100%

NOTE: Hospital profiles are in alphabetical order by state, then city, then hospital within the city; Rankings are sorted by rate in descending order and exclude hospitals with less than 25 cases; (1) The number of cases is too small (n<25) for purposes of reliably predicting hospital performance; (2) Measure reflects the hospital's indication that its submission was based upon a sample of its relevant discharges; (3) Rate reflects fewer than the maximum possible quarters of data for the measure; (4) Inaccurate information submitted and suppressed for one or more quarters; (5) No data is available from the hospital for this measure; Please refer to the User's Guide for a full explanation of data

Measure			This Hospital	State Average	U.S. Average	Top Hospital
Aspirin at Discharge[5]	-	-	87%	90%	100%	
Beta Blocker at Arrival[5]	-	-	85%	87%	100%	
Beta Blocker at Discharge[5]	-	-	88%	90%	100%	
Fibrinolytic Medication Timing[5]	-	-	32%	31%	100%	
PCI Within 90 Minutes of Arrival[5]	-	-	40%	54%	95%	
Smoking Cessation Advice[5]	-	-	88%	88%	100%	
Heart Failure Care						
ACE Inhibitor or ARB for LVSD[5]	-	-	78%	82%	100%	
Discharge Instructions[5]	-	-	62%	61%	93%	
Evaluation of LVS Function[5]	-	-	81%	83%	99%	
Smoking Cessation Advice[5]	-	-	83%	82%	100%	
Pneumonia Care						
Appropriate Initial Antibiotic[5]	-	-	78%	83%	94%	
Blood Culture Timing[5]	-	-	89%	90%	100%	
Influenza Vaccine[5]	-	-	58%	70%	100%	
Initial Antibiotic Timing[5]	-	-	76%	80%	93%	
Oxygenation Assessment[5]	-	-	98%	99%	100%	
Pneumococcal Vaccine[5]	-	-	61%	69%	94%	
Smoking Cessation Advice[5]	-	-	78%	80%	100%	
Surgical Infection Prevention						
Prophylactic Antibiotic Given[2,3]	55	96%	69%	77%	95%	
Prophylactic Antibiotic Selection[5]	-	-	79%	90%	100%	
Prophylactic Antibiotic Stopped[2,3]	53	87%	61%	72%	95%	
Pregnancy Care						
Inpatient Neonatal Mortality	8,762	1.00%	-	-	-	
Third or Fourth Degree Laceration	5,154	3.63%	3.54%	3.63%	3.27%	

Tri-Ward Rural Health Clinic

409 1st Street
Bernice, LA 71222
Ownership: Govt - Hospital District or Authority
Emergency Services: Yes

Phone: 318-285-9066
Fax: 318-285-9039
Accredited: No
Licensed Beds: 11

Key Personnel:
Administrator/CEO/CFO. . . . . Charollette Thompson
Chief Medical Staff. . . . . R Brian Harris, MD
Emergency Room. . . . . Barbara B Jones
Infection Control. . . . . Nancy Smith, MD

Measure	Cases	This Hospital	State Average	U.S. Average	Top Hospital
Heart Attack Care					
ACE Inhibitor or ARB for LVSD[3]	0	-	84%	82%	100%
Aspirin at Arrival[1,3]	2	100%	91%	92%	100%
Aspirin at Discharge[1,3]	1	100%	87%	90%	100%
Beta Blocker at Arrival[1,3]	2	50%	85%	87%	100%
Beta Blocker at Discharge[1,3]	1	100%	88%	90%	100%
Fibrinolytic Medication Timing[3]	0	-	32%	31%	100%
PCI Within 90 Minutes of Arrival[5]	-	-	40%	54%	95%
Smoking Cessation Advice[3]	0	-	88%	88%	100%
Heart Failure Care					
ACE Inhibitor or ARB for LVSD[1]	4	75%	78%	82%	100%
Discharge Instructions[1]	14	43%	62%	61%	93%
Evaluation of LVS Function	25	88%	81%	83%	99%
Smoking Cessation Advice[1]	1	100%	83%	82%	100%
Pneumonia Care					
Appropriate Initial Antibiotic	41	90%	78%	83%	94%
Blood Culture Timing[1]	14	100%	89%	90%	100%
Influenza Vaccine[1]	14	57%	58%	70%	100%
Initial Antibiotic Timing	71	94%	76%	80%	93%
Oxygenation Assessment	78	99%	98%	99%	100%
Pneumococcal Vaccine	54	72%	61%	69%	94%
Smoking Cessation Advice[1]	16	75%	78%	80%	100%
Surgical Infection Prevention					
Prophylactic Antibiotic Given[5]	-	-	69%	77%	95%
Prophylactic Antibiotic Selection[5]	-	-	79%	90%	100%
Prophylactic Antibiotic Stopped[5]	-	-	61%	72%	95%
Pregnancy Care					
Inpatient Neonatal Mortality	-	-	-	-	-
Third or Fourth Degree Laceration	-	-	3.54%	3.63%	3.27%

LSU-Bogalusa Medical Center

433 Plaza Street
Bogalusa, LA 70427
Ownership: Government - State
Emergency Services: Yes

Phone: 985-730-6700
Fax: 985-730-6709
Accredited: Yes
Licensed Beds: 66

Key Personnel:
CEO. . . . . Kurt M Scott
Associate Administrator . . . . Regina Runfalo
Infection Control. . . . . Janice Augustine, RN

Measure	Cases	This Hospital	State Average	U.S. Average	Top Hospital
Heart Attack Care					
ACE Inhibitor or ARB for LVSD[1]	7	86%	84%	82%	100%
Aspirin at Arrival[1]	22	82%	91%	92%	100%
Aspirin at Discharge[1]	16	75%	87%	90%	100%
Beta Blocker at Arrival[1]	14	79%	85%	87%	100%
Beta Blocker at Discharge[1]	22	91%	88%	90%	100%
Fibrinolytic Medication Timing[1]	1	0%	32%	31%	100%
PCI Within 90 Minutes of Arrival	0	-	40%	54%	95%
Smoking Cessation Advice[1]	7	100%	88%	88%	100%
Heart Failure Care					
ACE Inhibitor or ARB for LVSD	73	79%	78%	82%	100%
Discharge Instructions	141	63%	62%	61%	93%
Evaluation of LVS Function	160	83%	81%	83%	99%
Smoking Cessation Advice	45	96%	83%	82%	99%
Pneumonia Care					
Appropriate Initial Antibiotic	124	84%	78%	83%	94%
Blood Culture Timing	72	94%	89%	90%	100%
Influenza Vaccine[1]	14	43%	58%	70%	100%
Initial Antibiotic Timing	122	73%	76%	80%	93%
Oxygenation Assessment	143	99%	98%	99%	100%
Pneumococcal Vaccine	51	59%	61%	69%	94%
Smoking Cessation Advice	56	100%	78%	80%	100%
Surgical Infection Prevention					
Prophylactic Antibiotic Given[3]	65	65%	69%	77%	95%
Prophylactic Antibiotic Selection	27	81%	79%	90%	100%
Prophylactic Antibiotic Stopped[3]	57	67%	61%	72%	95%
Pregnancy Care					
Inpatient Neonatal Mortality	-	-	-	-	-
Third or Fourth Degree Laceration	-	-	3.54%	3.63%	3.27%

Bossier Specialty Hospital

2105 Airline Drive
Bossier City, LA 71111
Ownership: Proprietary
Emergency Services: No

Phone: 318-549-2011

Accredited: No

Measure	Cases	This Hospital	State Average	U.S. Average	Top Hospital
Heart Attack Care					
ACE Inhibitor or ARB for LVSD[5]	-	-	84%	82%	100%
Aspirin at Arrival[5]	-	-	91%	92%	100%
Aspirin at Discharge[5]	-	-	87%	90%	100%
Beta Blocker at Arrival[5]	-	-	85%	87%	100%
Beta Blocker at Discharge[5]	-	-	88%	90%	100%
Fibrinolytic Medication Timing[5]	-	-	32%	31%	100%
PCI Within 90 Minutes of Arrival[5]	-	-	40%	54%	95%
Smoking Cessation Advice[5]	-	-	88%	88%	100%
Heart Failure Care					
ACE Inhibitor or ARB for LVSD[5]	-	-	78%	82%	100%
Discharge Instructions[5]	-	-	62%	61%	93%
Evaluation of LVS Function[5]	-	-	81%	83%	99%
Smoking Cessation Advice[5]	-	-	83%	82%	100%
Pneumonia Care					
Appropriate Initial Antibiotic[5]	-	-	78%	83%	94%
Blood Culture Timing[5]	-	-	89%	90%	100%
Influenza Vaccine[5]	-	-	58%	70%	100%
Initial Antibiotic Timing[5]	-	-	76%	80%	93%
Oxygenation Assessment[5]	-	-	98%	99%	100%
Pneumococcal Vaccine[5]	-	-	61%	69%	94%
Smoking Cessation Advice[5]	-	-	78%	80%	100%
Surgical Infection Prevention					
Prophylactic Antibiotic Given[1,3]	10	60%	69%	77%	95%

NOTE: Hospital profiles are in alphabetical order by state, then city, then hospital within the city; Rankings are sorted by rate in descending order and exclude hospitals with less than 25 cases; (1) The number of cases is too small (n<25) for purposes of reliably predicting hospital performance; (2) Measure reflects the hospital's indication that its submission was based upon a sample of its relevant discharges; (3) Rate reflects fewer than the maximum possible quarters of data for the measure; (4) Inaccurate information submitted and suppressed for one or more quarters; (5) No data is available from the hospital for this measure; Please refer to the User's Guide for a full explanation of data

Prophylactic Antibiotic Selection[5]	-	-	79%	90%	100%
Prophylactic Antibiotic Stopped[1,3]	9	67%	61%	72%	95%
Pregnancy Care					
Inpatient Neonatal Mortality	-	-	-	-	-
Third or Fourth Degree Laceration	-	-	3.54%	3.63%	3.27%

Willis Knighton Bossier Health Center

2400 Hospital Dr   Phone: 318-752-7000
Bossier City, LA 71111
Ownership: Voluntary non-profit - Private   Accredited: Yes
Emergency Services: Yes

Measure	Cases	This Hospital	State Average	U.S. Average	Top Hospital
Heart Attack Care					
ACE Inhibitor or ARB for LVSD	33	48%	84%	82%	100%
Aspirin at Arrival	100	94%	91%	92%	100%
Aspirin at Discharge	99	88%	87%	90%	100%
Beta Blocker at Arrival	76	86%	85%	87%	100%
Beta Blocker at Discharge	113	78%	88%	90%	100%
Fibrinolytic Medication Timing[3]	0	-	32%	31%	100%
PCI Within 90 Minutes of Arrival[1]	3	33%	40%	54%	95%
Smoking Cessation Advice[1,3]	8	100%	88%	88%	100%
Heart Failure Care					
ACE Inhibitor or ARB for LVSD	87	46%	78%	82%	100%
Discharge Instructions[3]	38	29%	62%	61%	93%
Evaluation of LVS Function	184	83%	81%	83%	99%
Smoking Cessation Advice[1,3]	11	100%	83%	82%	100%
Pneumonia Care					
Appropriate Initial Antibiotic[1,3]	16	81%	78%	83%	94%
Blood Culture Timing[1,3]	12	83%	89%	90%	100%
Influenza Vaccine[5]	-	-	58%	70%	100%
Initial Antibiotic Timing	172	78%	76%	80%	93%
Oxygenation Assessment	201	99%	98%	99%	100%
Pneumococcal Vaccine	114	61%	61%	69%	94%
Smoking Cessation Advice[1,3]	8	100%	78%	80%	100%
Surgical Infection Prevention					
Prophylactic Antibiotic Given[3]	57	68%	69%	77%	95%
Prophylactic Antibiotic Selection[5]	-	-	79%	90%	100%
Prophylactic Antibiotic Stopped[3]	49	57%	61%	72%	95%
Pregnancy Care					
Inpatient Neonatal Mortality	-	-	-	-	-
Third or Fourth Degree Laceration	-	-	3.54%	3.63%	3.27%

Caldwell Memorial Hospital

411 Main Street   Phone: 318-649-6111
PO Box 899   Fax: 318-649-8908
Columbia, LA 71418
Ownership: Proprietary   Accredited: No
Emergency Services: Yes   Licensed Beds: 22
Key Personnel:
CEO . . . . Jim Ritchy
Chief Medical Staff . . . . Salman Shafig, MD
Director Infection/Disease Control . . . . Mel Hart
Director Medical/Surgical Nursing . . . . Mel Hart
Chief Radiology . . . . Wildo Colon, MD

Measure	Cases	This Hospital	State Average	U.S. Average	Top Hospital
Heart Attack Care					
ACE Inhibitor or ARB for LVSD[3]	0	-	84%	82%	100%
Aspirin at Arrival[1,3]	1	0%	91%	92%	100%
Aspirin at Discharge[3]	0	-	87%	90%	100%
Beta Blocker at Arrival[1,3]	1	100%	85%	87%	100%
Beta Blocker at Discharge[3]	0	-	88%	90%	100%
Fibrinolytic Medication Timing[5]	-	-	32%	31%	100%
PCI Within 90 Minutes of Arrival[5]	-	-	40%	54%	95%
Smoking Cessation Advice[5]	-	-	88%	88%	100%
Heart Failure Care					
ACE Inhibitor or ARB for LVSD[1]	8	88%	78%	82%	100%
Discharge Instructions[1,3]	13	23%	62%	61%	93%
Evaluation of LVS Function	61	31%	81%	83%	99%
Smoking Cessation Advice[1,3]	4	25%	83%	82%	100%
Pneumonia Care					

Measure	Cases	This Hospital	State Average	U.S. Average	Top Hospital
Appropriate Initial Antibiotic[1,3]	8	25%	78%	83%	94%
Blood Culture Timing[3]	0	-	89%	90%	100%
Influenza Vaccine[5]	-	-	58%	70%	100%
Initial Antibiotic Timing	43	93%	76%	80%	93%
Oxygenation Assessment	48	71%	98%	99%	100%
Pneumococcal Vaccine[1]	24	38%	61%	69%	94%
Smoking Cessation Advice[1,3]	5	40%	78%	80%	100%
Surgical Infection Prevention					
Prophylactic Antibiotic Given[5]	-	-	69%	77%	95%
Prophylactic Antibiotic Selection[5]	-	-	79%	90%	100%
Prophylactic Antibiotic Stopped[5]	-	-	61%	72%	95%
Pregnancy Care					
Inpatient Neonatal Mortality	-	-	-	-	-
Third or Fourth Degree Laceration	-	-	3.54%	3.63%	3.27%

Citizens Medical Center

7939 US Highway 165   Phone: 318-649-6106
Columbia, LA 71418   Fax: 318-649-2080
Ownership: Govt - Hospital District or Authority   Accredited: No
Emergency Services: Yes   Licensed Beds: 40
Key Personnel:
President/CEO . . . . Thomas Bickham Jr.
Administrator . . . . Steve Barbo
Chief Medical Staff . . . . Glynda Mason
Director Infection/Disease Control . . . . Debbie Volentine

Measure	Cases	This Hospital	State Average	U.S. Average	Top Hospital
Heart Attack Care					
ACE Inhibitor or ARB for LVSD[3]	0	-	84%	82%	100%
Aspirin at Arrival[1,3]	1	100%	91%	92%	100%
Aspirin at Discharge[3]	0	-	87%	90%	100%
Beta Blocker at Arrival[1,3]	1	0%	85%	87%	100%
Beta Blocker at Discharge[3]	0	-	88%	90%	100%
Fibrinolytic Medication Timing[3]	0	-	32%	31%	100%
PCI Within 90 Minutes of Arrival	0	-	40%	54%	95%
Smoking Cessation Advice[3]	0	-	88%	88%	100%
Heart Failure Care					
ACE Inhibitor or ARB for LVSD[1]	6	50%	78%	82%	100%
Discharge Instructions[1,3]	5	20%	62%	61%	93%
Evaluation of LVS Function	29	66%	81%	83%	99%
Smoking Cessation Advice[3]	0	-	83%	82%	100%
Pneumonia Care					
Appropriate Initial Antibiotic[1,3]	3	67%	78%	83%	94%
Blood Culture Timing[1,3]	4	100%	89%	90%	100%
Influenza Vaccine[5]	-	-	58%	70%	100%
Initial Antibiotic Timing	40	68%	76%	80%	93%
Oxygenation Assessment	54	98%	98%	99%	100%
Pneumococcal Vaccine	32	50%	61%	69%	94%
Smoking Cessation Advice[1,3]	1	0%	78%	80%	100%
Surgical Infection Prevention					
Prophylactic Antibiotic Given[3]	0	-	69%	77%	95%
Prophylactic Antibiotic Selection[5]	-	-	79%	90%	100%
Prophylactic Antibiotic Stopped[3]	0	-	61%	72%	95%
Pregnancy Care					
Inpatient Neonatal Mortality	-	-	-	-	-
Third or Fourth Degree Laceration	-	-	3.54%	3.63%	3.27%

Fairway Medical Center

67252 Industry Lane   Phone: 985-809-9888
Covington, LA 70433
Ownership: Voluntary non-profit - Private   Accredited: No
Emergency Services: No
Key Personnel:
Cardiology . . . . Dorothy Banish, MD
Surgery . . . . Matthew French, MD

Measure	Cases	This Hospital	State Average	U.S. Average	Top Hospital
Heart Attack Care					
ACE Inhibitor or ARB for LVSD[5]	-	-	84%	82%	100%
Aspirin at Arrival[5]	-	-	91%	92%	100%
Aspirin at Discharge[5]	-	-	87%	90%	100%
Beta Blocker at Arrival[5]	-	-	85%	87%	100%

NOTE: Hospital profiles are in alphabetical order by state, then city, then hospital within the city; Rankings are sorted by rate in descending order and exclude hospitals with less than 25 cases; (1) The number of cases is too small (n<25) for purposes of reliably predicting hospital performance; (2) Measure reflects the hospital's indication that its submission was based upon a sample of its relevant discharges; (3) Rate reflects fewer than the maximum possible quarters of data for the measure; (4) Inaccurate information submitted and suppressed for one or more quarters; (5) No data is available from the hospital for this measure; Please refer to the User's Guide for a full explanation of data

Beta Blocker at Discharge[5]	-	-	88%	90%	100%
Fibrinolytic Medication Timing[5]	-	-	32%	31%	100%
PCI Within 90 Minutes of Arrival[5]	-	-	40%	54%	95%
Smoking Cessation Advice[5]	-	-	88%	88%	100%
Heart Failure Care					
ACE Inhibitor or ARB for LVSD[5]	-	-	78%	82%	100%
Discharge Instructions[5]	-	-	62%	61%	93%
Evaluation of LVS Function[5]	-	-	81%	83%	99%
Smoking Cessation Advice[5]	-	-	83%	82%	100%
Pneumonia Care					
Appropriate Initial Antibiotic[5]	-	-	78%	83%	94%
Blood Culture Timing[5]	-	-	89%	90%	100%
Influenza Vaccine[5]	-	-	58%	70%	100%
Initial Antibiotic Timing[5]	-	-	76%	80%	93%
Oxygenation Assessment[5]	-	-	98%	99%	100%
Pneumococcal Vaccine[5]	-	-	61%	69%	94%
Smoking Cessation Advice[5]	-	-	78%	80%	100%
Surgical Infection Prevention					
Prophylactic Antibiotic Given[1,3]	12	75%	69%	77%	95%
Prophylactic Antibiotic Selection[5]	-	-	79%	90%	100%
Prophylactic Antibiotic Stopped[1,3]	10	50%	61%	72%	95%
Pregnancy Care					
Inpatient Neonatal Mortality	-	-	-	-	-
Third or Fourth Degree Laceration	-	-	3.54%	3.63%	3.27%

Lakeview Regional Medical Center

95 East Fairway Drive
Covington, LA 70433
URL: www.lakeviewregional.com
Ownership: Proprietary
Emergency Services: Yes
Key Personnel:
CEO/Administrator . . . . Max Lauderdale

Phone: 985-867-3800
Fax: 985-867-3879

Accredited: Yes
Licensed Beds: 178

Measure	Cases	This Hospital	State Average	U.S. Average	Top Hospital
Heart Attack Care					
ACE Inhibitor or ARB for LVSD	25	56%	84%	82%	100%
Aspirin at Arrival	69	93%	91%	92%	100%
Aspirin at Discharge	75	93%	87%	90%	100%
Beta Blocker at Arrival	55	89%	85%	87%	100%
Beta Blocker at Discharge	78	91%	88%	90%	100%
Fibrinolytic Medication Timing[1]	1	0%	32%	31%	100%
PCI Within 90 Minutes of Arrival[1]	2	50%	40%	54%	95%
Smoking Cessation Advice[1]	21	95%	88%	88%	100%
Heart Failure Care					
ACE Inhibitor or ARB for LVSD	89	67%	78%	82%	100%
Discharge Instructions	194	73%	62%	61%	93%
Evaluation of LVS Function	236	88%	81%	83%	99%
Smoking Cessation Advice	42	86%	83%	82%	100%
Pneumonia Care					
Appropriate Initial Antibiotic	83	83%	78%	83%	94%
Blood Culture Timing	65	95%	89%	90%	100%
Influenza Vaccine	29	69%	58%	70%	100%
Initial Antibiotic Timing	157	66%	76%	80%	93%
Oxygenation Assessment	190	99%	98%	99%	100%
Pneumococcal Vaccine	128	72%	61%	69%	94%
Smoking Cessation Advice	47	79%	78%	80%	100%
Surgical Infection Prevention					
Prophylactic Antibiotic Given[2,3]	202	55%	69%	77%	95%
Prophylactic Antibiotic Selection[2]	99	86%	79%	90%	100%
Prophylactic Antibiotic Stopped[2,3]	192	51%	61%	72%	95%
Pregnancy Care					
Inpatient Neonatal Mortality	-	-	-	-	-
Third or Fourth Degree Laceration	-	-	3.54%	3.63%	3.27%

Saint Tammany Parish Hospital

1202 S Tyler Street
Covington, LA 70433
E-mail: marketing@stph.com
URL: www.stph.org
Ownership: Govt - Hospital District or Authority
Emergency Services: Yes
Key Personnel:
President/CEO . . . . Patti Ellish
Chief Medical Staff . . . . Robert Capitelli, MD
Emergency Room . . . . Joan Curtis, MD
Director Infection/Disease Control . . . . Karen Moise
Director Respiratory Therapy . . . . Cheryl Schoenberger

Phone: 985-898-4176
Fax: 985-898-4679

Accredited: Yes
Licensed Beds: 203

Measure	Cases	This Hospital	State Average	U.S. Average	Top Hospital
Heart Attack Care					
ACE Inhibitor or ARB for LVSD	38	100%	84%	82%	100%
Aspirin at Arrival	102	99%	91%	92%	100%
Aspirin at Discharge	115	99%	87%	90%	100%
Beta Blocker at Arrival	68	100%	85%	87%	100%
Beta Blocker at Discharge	131	100%	88%	90%	100%
Fibrinolytic Medication Timing	0	-	32%	31%	100%
PCI Within 90 Minutes of Arrival[1]	5	60%	40%	54%	95%
Smoking Cessation Advice	41	100%	88%	88%	100%
Heart Failure Care					
ACE Inhibitor or ARB for LVSD	153	100%	78%	82%	100%
Discharge Instructions	362	78%	62%	61%	93%
Evaluation of LVS Function	401	100%	81%	83%	99%
Smoking Cessation Advice	74	96%	83%	82%	100%
Pneumonia Care					
Appropriate Initial Antibiotic	173	92%	78%	83%	94%
Blood Culture Timing	166	92%	89%	90%	100%
Influenza Vaccine	53	92%	58%	70%	100%
Initial Antibiotic Timing	215	90%	76%	80%	93%
Oxygenation Assessment	266	100%	98%	99%	100%
Pneumococcal Vaccine	161	79%	61%	69%	94%
Smoking Cessation Advice	82	96%	78%	80%	100%
Surgical Infection Prevention					
Prophylactic Antibiotic Given[3]	615	84%	69%	77%	95%
Prophylactic Antibiotic Selection	200	89%	79%	90%	100%
Prophylactic Antibiotic Stopped[3]	603	55%	61%	72%	95%
Pregnancy Care					
Inpatient Neonatal Mortality	-	-	-	-	-
Third or Fourth Degree Laceration	-	-	3.54%	3.63%	3.27%

American Legion Hospital

1305 Crowley Rayne Highway
Crowley, LA 70526
Ownership: Voluntary non-profit - Private
Emergency Services: Yes

Phone: 337-783-3222

Accredited: No

Measure	Cases	This Hospital	State Average	U.S. Average	Top Hospital
Heart Attack Care					
ACE Inhibitor or ARB for LVSD[1,3]	1	100%	84%	82%	100%
Aspirin at Arrival[1,3]	5	100%	91%	92%	100%
Aspirin at Discharge[1,3]	4	100%	87%	90%	100%
Beta Blocker at Arrival[1,3]	5	80%	85%	87%	100%
Beta Blocker at Discharge[1,3]	4	100%	88%	90%	100%
Fibrinolytic Medication Timing[3]	0	-	32%	31%	100%
PCI Within 90 Minutes of Arrival	0	-	40%	54%	95%
Smoking Cessation Advice[1,3]	1	100%	88%	88%	100%
Heart Failure Care					
ACE Inhibitor or ARB for LVSD	26	92%	78%	82%	100%
Discharge Instructions	76	38%	62%	61%	93%
Evaluation of LVS Function	102	57%	81%	83%	99%
Smoking Cessation Advice	27	81%	83%	82%	100%
Pneumonia Care					
Appropriate Initial Antibiotic	107	84%	78%	83%	94%
Blood Culture Timing	57	86%	89%	90%	100%
Influenza Vaccine[1]	24	38%	58%	70%	100%
Initial Antibiotic Timing	163	71%	76%	80%	93%
Oxygenation Assessment	192	96%	98%	99%	100%

NOTE: Hospital profiles are in alphabetical order by state, then city, then hospital within the city; Rankings are sorted by rate in descending order and exclude hospitals with less than 25 cases; (1) The number of cases is too small (n<25) for purposes of reliably predicting hospital performance; (2) Measure reflects the hospital's indication that its submission was based upon a sample of its relevant discharges; (3) Rate reflects fewer than the maximum possible quarters of data for the measure; (4) Inaccurate information submitted and suppressed for one or more quarters; (5) No data is available from the hospital for this measure; Please refer to the User's Guide for a full explanation of data

		This Hospital	State Average	U.S. Average	Top Hospital
Pneumococcal Vaccine	104	72%	61%	69%	94%
Smoking Cessation Advice	45	73%	78%	80%	100%
Surgical Infection Prevention					
Prophylactic Antibiotic Given[3]	144	25%	69%	77%	95%
Prophylactic Antibiotic Selection	45	96%	79%	90%	100%
Prophylactic Antibiotic Stopped[3]	139	37%	61%	72%	95%
Pregnancy Care					
Inpatient Neonatal Mortality	-	-	-	-	-
Third or Fourth Degree Laceration	-	-	3.54%	3.63%	3.27%

Lady of the Sea General Hospital

200 W 134 Place
Cut Off, LA 70345
URL: www.losgh.org
Ownership: Govt - Hospital District or Authority
Emergency Services: Yes

Phone: 985-632-6401
Fax: 985-632-8310

Accredited: No
Licensed Beds: 49

Key Personnel:
Administrator/CEO . . . . Raymond L Ford
Emergency Room . . . . William Crenshaw, LVN
Director Infection/Disease Control . . . . Helene Durham, RN
Director Medical/Surgical Nursing . . . . Cindy Mayeur, RN
Chief Radiology . . . . Jose Rivero, MD

Measure	Cases	This Hospital	State Average	U.S. Average	Top Hospital
Heart Attack Care					
ACE Inhibitor or ARB for LVSD[3]	0	-	84%	82%	100%
Aspirin at Arrival[1,3]	12	83%	91%	92%	100%
Aspirin at Discharge[1,3]	4	75%	87%	90%	100%
Beta Blocker at Arrival[1,3]	10	100%	85%	87%	100%
Beta Blocker at Discharge[1,3]	4	100%	88%	90%	100%
Fibrinolytic Medication Timing[3]	0	-	32%	31%	100%
PCI Within 90 Minutes of Arrival	0	-	40%	54%	95%
Smoking Cessation Advice[1,3]	1	0%	88%	88%	100%
Heart Failure Care					
ACE Inhibitor or ARB for LVSD[1]	18	89%	78%	82%	100%
Discharge Instructions	48	75%	62%	61%	93%
Evaluation of LVS Function	70	77%	81%	83%	99%
Smoking Cessation Advice[1]	11	73%	83%	82%	100%
Pneumonia Care					
Appropriate Initial Antibiotic	60	93%	78%	83%	94%
Blood Culture Timing	54	80%	89%	90%	100%
Influenza Vaccine[1]	14	100%	58%	70%	100%
Initial Antibiotic Timing	72	82%	76%	80%	93%
Oxygenation Assessment	92	100%	98%	99%	100%
Pneumococcal Vaccine	53	89%	61%	69%	94%
Smoking Cessation Advice	27	74%	78%	80%	100%
Surgical Infection Prevention					
Prophylactic Antibiotic Given[5]	-	-	69%	77%	95%
Prophylactic Antibiotic Selection[5]	-	-	79%	90%	100%
Prophylactic Antibiotic Stopped[5]	-	-	61%	72%	95%
Pregnancy Care					
Inpatient Neonatal Mortality	-	-	-	-	-
Third or Fourth Degree Laceration	-	-	3.54%	3.63%	3.27%

Beauregard Memorial Hospital

600 S Pine Street
PO Box 730
DeRidder, LA 70634
URL: www.beauregard.org
Ownership: Govt - Hospital District or Authority
Emergency Services: Yes

Phone: 337-462-7100
Fax: 337-462-7479

Accredited: Yes
Licensed Beds: 60

Key Personnel:
Chief Medical Staff. . . . . David Brown, MD
Catheterization Lab . . . . Lee Pinkley, RN
Emergency Room . . . . Sharon Manitzas, RN
Infection Control. . . . . Jo Blankenship
ICU . . . . Lee Pinkley, RN
Medical/Surgical Nursing . . . . Lynn Mulero
Respiratory/Cardiopulmonary. . . . . Alan Slaydon

Measure	Cases	This Hospital	State Average	U.S. Average	Top Hospital
Heart Attack Care					
ACE Inhibitor or ARB for LVSD[1]	5	100%	84%	82%	100%

Measure	Cases	This Hospital	State Average	U.S. Average	Top Hospital
Aspirin at Arrival	44	98%	91%	92%	100%
Aspirin at Discharge	25	80%	87%	90%	100%
Beta Blocker at Arrival	33	91%	85%	87%	100%
Beta Blocker at Discharge	25	88%	88%	90%	100%
Fibrinolytic Medication Timing[1]	11	27%	32%	31%	100%
PCI Within 90 Minutes of Arrival	0	-	40%	54%	95%
Smoking Cessation Advice[1]	7	86%	88%	88%	100%
Heart Failure Care					
ACE Inhibitor or ARB for LVSD	41	90%	78%	82%	100%
Discharge Instructions	70	60%	62%	61%	93%
Evaluation of LVS Function	101	85%	81%	83%	99%
Smoking Cessation Advice[1]	17	88%	83%	82%	100%
Pneumonia Care					
Appropriate Initial Antibiotic	104	49%	78%	83%	94%
Blood Culture Timing	51	92%	89%	90%	100%
Influenza Vaccine[4,5]	-	-	58%	70%	100%
Initial Antibiotic Timing	126	87%	76%	80%	93%
Oxygenation Assessment	164	99%	98%	99%	100%
Pneumococcal Vaccine	95	62%	61%	69%	94%
Smoking Cessation Advice	36	100%	78%	80%	100%
Surgical Infection Prevention					
Prophylactic Antibiotic Given[3]	100	81%	69%	77%	95%
Prophylactic Antibiotic Selection	35	26%	79%	90%	100%
Prophylactic Antibiotic Stopped[3]	98	16%	61%	72%	95%
Pregnancy Care					
Inpatient Neonatal Mortality	-	-	-	-	-
Third or Fourth Degree Laceration	-	-	3.54%	3.63%	3.27%

Acadian Medical Center

3501 Highway 190
Eunice, LA 70535
Ownership: Proprietary
Emergency Services: Yes

Phone: 337-457-5244

Accredited: Yes

Measure	Cases	This Hospital	State Average	U.S. Average	Top Hospital
Heart Attack Care					
ACE Inhibitor or ARB for LVSD[1]	1	100%	84%	82%	100%
Aspirin at Arrival[1]	1	100%	91%	92%	100%
Aspirin at Discharge[1]	2	100%	87%	90%	100%
Beta Blocker at Arrival[1]	1	100%	85%	87%	100%
Beta Blocker at Discharge[1]	2	100%	88%	90%	100%
Fibrinolytic Medication Timing[1]	4	75%	32%	31%	100%
PCI Within 90 Minutes of Arrival	0	-	40%	54%	95%
Smoking Cessation Advice	0	-	88%	88%	100%
Heart Failure Care					
ACE Inhibitor or ARB for LVSD	41	100%	78%	82%	100%
Discharge Instructions	95	96%	62%	61%	93%
Evaluation of LVS Function	98	80%	81%	83%	99%
Smoking Cessation Advice[1]	24	100%	83%	82%	100%
Pneumonia Care					
Appropriate Initial Antibiotic	32	75%	78%	83%	94%
Blood Culture Timing	33	85%	89%	90%	100%
Influenza Vaccine[1]	14	93%	58%	70%	100%
Initial Antibiotic Timing	69	87%	76%	80%	93%
Oxygenation Assessment	87	100%	98%	99%	100%
Pneumococcal Vaccine	43	93%	61%	69%	94%
Smoking Cessation Advice[1]	22	100%	78%	80%	100%
Surgical Infection Prevention					
Prophylactic Antibiotic Given[3]	30	80%	69%	77%	95%
Prophylactic Antibiotic Selection[1]	13	77%	79%	90%	100%
Prophylactic Antibiotic Stopped[3]	29	83%	61%	72%	95%
Pregnancy Care					
Inpatient Neonatal Mortality	-	-	-	-	-
Third or Fourth Degree Laceration	-	-	3.54%	3.63%	3.27%

NOTE: Hospital profiles are in alphabetical order by state, then city, then hospital within the city; Rankings are sorted by rate in descending order and exclude hospitals with less than 25 cases; (1) The number of cases is too small (n<25) for purposes of reliably predicting hospital performance; (2) Measure reflects the hospital's indication that its submission was based upon a sample of its relevant discharges; (3) Rate reflects fewer than the maximum possible quarters of data for the measure; (4) Inaccurate information submitted and suppressed for one or more quarters; (5) No data is available from the hospital for this measure; Please refer to the User's Guide for a full explanation of data

Saint Elizabeth Hospital

1125 W Highway 30
Gonzales, LA 70737
URL: www.steh.com
Ownership: Voluntary non-profit - Church
Emergency Services: Yes

Phone: 225-647-5090
Fax: 225-647-7408

Accredited: Yes
Licensed Beds: 95

Key Personnel:

CEO . . . . Dolores Lejeune
Chief Medical Staff . . . . John Fraiche, MD
Emergency Room . . . . Leslie Norman
Infection Control . . . . Susan Waguespack
Respiratory/Cardiopulmonary . . . . Victor Vidaurre

Measure	Cases	This Hospital	State Average	U.S. Average	Top Hospital
Heart Attack Care					
ACE Inhibitor or ARB for LVSD[1]	6	67%	84%	82%	100%
Aspirin at Arrival[1]	23	91%	91%	92%	100%
Aspirin at Discharge[1]	12	83%	87%	90%	100%
Beta Blocker at Arrival[1]	21	90%	85%	87%	100%
Beta Blocker at Discharge[1]	11	91%	88%	90%	100%
Fibrinolytic Medication Timing[1,3]	1	100%	32%	31%	100%
PCI Within 90 Minutes of Arrival	0	-	40%	54%	95%
Smoking Cessation Advice[3]	0	-	88%	88%	100%
Heart Failure Care					
ACE Inhibitor or ARB for LVSD	110	77%	78%	82%	100%
Discharge Instructions[3]	33	91%	62%	61%	93%
Evaluation of LVS Function	167	95%	81%	83%	99%
Smoking Cessation Advice[1,3]	6	100%	83%	82%	100%
Pneumonia Care					
Appropriate Initial Antibiotic[1,3]	21	90%	78%	83%	94%
Blood Culture Timing[1,3]	23	96%	89%	90%	100%
Influenza Vaccine[5]	-	-	58%	70%	100%
Initial Antibiotic Timing	128	75%	76%	80%	93%
Oxygenation Assessment	155	99%	98%	99%	100%
Pneumococcal Vaccine	95	86%	61%	69%	94%
Smoking Cessation Advice[1,3]	11	91%	78%	80%	100%
Surgical Infection Prevention					
Prophylactic Antibiotic Given[1,3]	11	91%	69%	77%	95%
Prophylactic Antibiotic Selection[5]	-	-	79%	90%	100%
Prophylactic Antibiotic Stopped[1,3]	11	0%	61%	72%	95%
Pregnancy Care					
Inpatient Neonatal Mortality	-	-	-	-	-
Third or Fourth Degree Laceration	-	-	3.54%	3.63%	3.27%

Meadowcrest Hospital

Alternate Name: Ochsner Medical Center
2500 Belle Chasse Highway
Gretna, LA 70056
E-mail: belinda.smith@tenethealth.com
URL: www.meadowcresthosp.com
Ownership: Voluntary non-profit - Private
Emergency Services: Yes

Phone: 504-392-3131
Fax: 504-391-5498

Accredited: No
Licensed Beds: 221

Key Personnel:

CEO . . . . Phillip E Sowa
Chief Medical Staff . . . . Michael Puente, MD
Cardiac Lab . . . . Wayne Taylor
Emergency Room Director . . . . Glenn Landry, RN
ICU . . . . Glenn Landry, RN
Intensive/Coronary Care . . . . Glenn Landry, RN
Medical Surgical Nursing . . . . Brenda Bankston, RN
OB/GYN/Women's Health . . . . Joan Rooney, RN

Measure	Cases	This Hospital	State Average	U.S. Average	Top Hospital
Heart Attack Care					
ACE Inhibitor or ARB for LVSD[5]	-	-	84%	82%	100%
Aspirin at Arrival[5]	-	-	91%	92%	100%
Aspirin at Discharge[5]	-	-	87%	90%	100%
Beta Blocker at Arrival[5]	-	-	85%	87%	100%
Beta Blocker at Discharge[5]	-	-	88%	90%	100%
Fibrinolytic Medication Timing[5]	-	-	32%	31%	100%
PCI Within 90 Minutes of Arrival[5]	-	-	40%	54%	95%
Smoking Cessation Advice[5]	-	-	88%	88%	100%
Heart Failure Care					

Measure		This Hospital	State Average	U.S. Average	Top Hospital
ACE Inhibitor or ARB for LVSD[5]	-	-	78%	82%	100%
Discharge Instructions[5]	-	-	62%	61%	93%
Evaluation of LVS Function[5]	-	-	81%	83%	99%
Smoking Cessation Advice[5]	-	-	83%	82%	100%
Pneumonia Care					
Appropriate Initial Antibiotic[5]	-	-	78%	83%	94%
Blood Culture Timing[5]	-	-	89%	90%	100%
Influenza Vaccine[5]	-	-	58%	70%	100%
Initial Antibiotic Timing[5]	-	-	76%	80%	93%
Oxygenation Assessment[5]	-	-	98%	99%	100%
Pneumococcal Vaccine[5]	-	-	61%	69%	94%
Smoking Cessation Advice[5]	-	-	78%	80%	100%
Surgical Infection Prevention					
Prophylactic Antibiotic Given[5]	-	-	69%	77%	95%
Prophylactic Antibiotic Selection[5]	-	-	79%	90%	100%
Prophylactic Antibiotic Stopped[5]	-	-	61%	72%	95%
Pregnancy Care					
Inpatient Neonatal Mortality	-	-	-	-	-
Third or Fourth Degree Laceration	-	-	3.54%	3.63%	3.27%

North Oaks Medical System

Alternate Name: Seventh Ward General Hospital
15790 Medical Center Drive
Hammond, LA 70403
E-mail: nohs@northoaks.org
URL: www.northoaks.org
Ownership: Govt - Hospital District or Authority
Emergency Services: Yes

Phone: 985-345-2700
Fax: 985-230-6482

Accredited: Yes
Licensed Beds: 354

Key Personnel:

CEO . . . . James E Cathey Jr
Chief Medical Officer . . . . James Nelson, MD

Measure	Cases	This Hospital	State Average	U.S. Average	Top Hospital
Heart Attack Care					
ACE Inhibitor or ARB for LVSD	55	84%	84%	82%	100%
Aspirin at Arrival	191	96%	91%	92%	100%
Aspirin at Discharge	172	94%	87%	90%	100%
Beta Blocker at Arrival	129	91%	85%	87%	100%
Beta Blocker at Discharge	206	97%	88%	90%	100%
Fibrinolytic Medication Timing[1]	1	0%	32%	31%	100%
PCI Within 90 Minutes of Arrival[1]	9	44%	40%	54%	95%
Smoking Cessation Advice	95	100%	88%	88%	100%
Heart Failure Care					
ACE Inhibitor or ARB for LVSD	369	85%	78%	82%	100%
Discharge Instructions	688	68%	62%	61%	93%
Evaluation of LVS Function	816	95%	81%	83%	99%
Smoking Cessation Advice	177	94%	83%	82%	100%
Pneumonia Care					
Appropriate Initial Antibiotic[2]	213	87%	78%	83%	94%
Blood Culture Timing[2]	121	97%	89%	90%	100%
Influenza Vaccine	63	84%	58%	70%	100%
Initial Antibiotic Timing[2]	334	79%	76%	80%	93%
Oxygenation Assessment[2]	407	100%	98%	99%	100%
Pneumococcal Vaccine[2]	214	89%	61%	69%	94%
Smoking Cessation Advice[2]	108	94%	78%	80%	100%
Surgical Infection Prevention					
Prophylactic Antibiotic Given[2]	428	93%	69%	77%	95%
Prophylactic Antibiotic Selection[2]	60	88%	79%	90%	100%
Prophylactic Antibiotic Stopped[2]	407	89%	61%	72%	95%
Pregnancy Care					
Inpatient Neonatal Mortality	-	-	-	-	-
Third or Fourth Degree Laceration	-	-	3.54%	3.63%	3.27%

Homer Memorial Hospital

620 E College Street
Homer, LA 71040
Ownership: Government - Local
Emergency Services: Yes

Phone: 318-927-2024
Fax: 318-927-3158
Accredited: No
Licensed Beds: 60

Key Personnel:

CEO . . . . Doug Efferson
Chief of Medical Staff . . . . DK Haynes
Emergency Room . . . . Debra Woodard
Respiratory Care . . . . Melissa Gibson

NOTE: Hospital profiles are in alphabetical order by state, then city, then hospital within the city; Rankings are sorted by rate in descending order and exclude hospitals with less than 25 cases; (1) The number of cases is too small (n<25) for purposes of reliably predicting hospital performance; (2) Measure reflects the hospital's indication that its submission was based upon a sample of its relevant discharges; (3) Rate reflects fewer than the maximum possible quarters of data for the measure; (4) Inaccurate information submitted and suppressed for one or more quarters; (5) No data is available from the hospital for this measure; Please refer to the User's Guide for a full explanation of data

Measure	Cases	This Hospital	State Average	U.S. Average	Top Hospital
Heart Attack Care					
ACE Inhibitor or ARB for LVSD[1]	3	67%	84%	82%	100%
Aspirin at Arrival[1]	16	94%	91%	92%	100%
Aspirin at Discharge[1]	7	86%	87%	90%	100%
Beta Blocker at Arrival[1]	10	90%	85%	87%	100%
Beta Blocker at Discharge[1]	5	100%	88%	90%	100%
Fibrinolytic Medication Timing[1,3]	5	40%	32%	31%	100%
PCI Within 90 Minutes of Arrival	0	-	40%	54%	95%
Smoking Cessation Advice[1,3]	3	33%	88%	88%	100%
Heart Failure Care					
ACE Inhibitor or ARB for LVSD[1,2]	4	100%	78%	82%	100%
Discharge Instructions[1,2,3]	17	12%	62%	61%	93%
Evaluation of LVS Function[2]	56	66%	81%	83%	99%
Smoking Cessation Advice[1,2,3]	6	50%	83%	82%	100%
Pneumonia Care					
Appropriate Initial Antibiotic[1,2,3]	11	18%	78%	83%	94%
Blood Culture Timing[1,2,3]	7	86%	89%	90%	100%
Influenza Vaccine[5]	-	-	58%	70%	100%
Initial Antibiotic Timing[2]	57	72%	76%	80%	93%
Oxygenation Assessment[2]	67	100%	98%	99%	100%
Pneumococcal Vaccine[2]	39	64%	61%	69%	94%
Smoking Cessation Advice[1,2,3]	3	100%	78%	80%	100%
Surgical Infection Prevention					
Prophylactic Antibiotic Given[1,3]	1	0%	69%	77%	95%
Prophylactic Antibiotic Selection[5]	-	-	79%	90%	100%
Prophylactic Antibiotic Stopped[1,3]	1	100%	61%	72%	95%
Pregnancy Care					
Inpatient Neonatal Mortality	-	-	-	-	-
Third or Fourth Degree Laceration	-	-	3.54%	3.63%	3.27%

Leonard J Chabert Medical Center

Alternate Name: South Louisiana Medical Center
1978 Industrial Boulevard
Houma, LA 70363
E-mail: trahanda@cmc.lhca.state.la.us
URL: www.lsuhsc.edu/hcsd
Ownership: Govt - Hospital District or Authority   Accredited: Yes
Emergency Services: Yes   Licensed Beds: 147
Key Personnel:
Administrator . . . . Daniel Trahan
CEO. . . . . Donald R Smithburg

Measure	Cases	This Hospital	State Average	U.S. Average	Top Hospital
Heart Attack Care					
ACE Inhibitor or ARB for LVSD[1]	12	83%	84%	82%	100%
Aspirin at Arrival	56	100%	91%	92%	100%
Aspirin at Discharge	36	94%	87%	90%	100%
Beta Blocker at Arrival	46	100%	85%	87%	100%
Beta Blocker at Discharge	44	98%	88%	90%	100%
Fibrinolytic Medication Timing[1]	1	0%	32%	31%	100%
PCI Within 90 Minutes of Arrival	0	-	40%	54%	95%
Smoking Cessation Advice[1]	24	92%	88%	88%	100%
Heart Failure Care					
ACE Inhibitor or ARB for LVSD	106	91%	78%	82%	100%
Discharge Instructions	152	55%	62%	61%	93%
Evaluation of LVS Function	152	97%	81%	83%	99%
Smoking Cessation Advice	78	95%	83%	82%	100%
Pneumonia Care					
Appropriate Initial Antibiotic	45	93%	78%	83%	94%
Blood Culture Timing	54	96%	89%	90%	100%
Influenza Vaccine[1]	15	53%	58%	70%	100%
Initial Antibiotic Timing	62	56%	76%	80%	93%
Oxygenation Assessment	78	100%	98%	99%	100%
Pneumococcal Vaccine[1]	11	64%	61%	69%	94%
Smoking Cessation Advice	32	66%	78%	80%	100%
Surgical Infection Prevention					
Prophylactic Antibiotic Given[3]	245	77%	69%	77%	95%
Prophylactic Antibiotic Selection	75	87%	79%	90%	100%
Prophylactic Antibiotic Stopped[3]	230	83%	61%	72%	95%
Pregnancy Care					
Inpatient Neonatal Mortality	470	0.43%	-	-	-

Third or Fourth Degree Laceration	294	2.72%	3.54%	3.63%	3.27%

Physicians Surgical Specialty Hospital

218 Corporate Drive   Phone: 504-853-1390
Houma, LA 70360
Ownership: Proprietary   Accredited: No
Emergency Services: No

Measure	Cases	This Hospital	State Average	U.S. Average	Top Hospital
Heart Attack Care					
ACE Inhibitor or ARB for LVSD[5]	-	-	84%	82%	100%
Aspirin at Arrival[5]	-	-	91%	92%	100%
Aspirin at Discharge[5]	-	-	87%	90%	100%
Beta Blocker at Arrival[5]	-	-	85%	87%	100%
Beta Blocker at Discharge[5]	-	-	88%	90%	100%
Fibrinolytic Medication Timing[5]	-	-	32%	31%	100%
PCI Within 90 Minutes of Arrival[5]	-	-	40%	54%	95%
Smoking Cessation Advice[5]	-	-	88%	88%	100%
Heart Failure Care					
ACE Inhibitor or ARB for LVSD[5]	-	-	78%	82%	100%
Discharge Instructions[5]	-	-	62%	61%	93%
Evaluation of LVS Function[5]	-	-	81%	83%	99%
Smoking Cessation Advice[5]	-	-	83%	82%	100%
Pneumonia Care					
Appropriate Initial Antibiotic[5]	-	-	78%	83%	94%
Blood Culture Timing[5]	-	-	89%	90%	100%
Influenza Vaccine[5]	-	-	58%	70%	100%
Initial Antibiotic Timing[3]	0	-	76%	80%	93%
Oxygenation Assessment[1,3]	1	100%	98%	99%	100%
Pneumococcal Vaccine[1,3]	1	0%	61%	69%	94%
Smoking Cessation Advice[5]	-	-	78%	80%	100%
Surgical Infection Prevention					
Prophylactic Antibiotic Given[3]	27	44%	69%	77%	95%
Prophylactic Antibiotic Selection[5]	-	-	79%	90%	100%
Prophylactic Antibiotic Stopped[3]	26	92%	61%	72%	95%
Pregnancy Care					
Inpatient Neonatal Mortality	-	-	-	-	-
Third or Fourth Degree Laceration	-	-	3.54%	3.63%	3.27%

Terrebonne General Medical Center

8166 Main Street   Toll-Free: 888-543-TGMC
Houma, LA 70360   Phone: 985-873-4141
                            Fax: 985-873-4215

E-mail: com relations@cajunnet.com
URL: www.tgmc.com
Ownership: Govt - Hospital District or Authority   Accredited: Yes
Emergency Services: Yes   Licensed Beds: 321
Key Personnel:
President/CEO. . . . . Phyllis Peoples
Chief Medical Staff. . . . . Robert Davis, MD
Director Catheterization Laboratory . . . . Gary Chaisson
Chief Catheterization Laboratory . . . . William Ladd, MD
Director Infection/Disease Control . . . . Gustavia Growe
CCU Spvg. Nurse . . . . Teresita Melancon
Chief OB/GYN . . . . Christine Albrecht, MD
Chief Radiology . . . . Joe Fontenot, MD
Director Respiratory Therapy . . . . Mike Folse

Measure	Cases	This Hospital	State Average	U.S. Average	Top Hospital
Heart Attack Care					
ACE Inhibitor or ARB for LVSD	52	85%	84%	82%	100%
Aspirin at Arrival	200	94%	91%	92%	100%
Aspirin at Discharge	214	94%	87%	90%	100%
Beta Blocker at Arrival	180	95%	85%	87%	100%
Beta Blocker at Discharge	232	95%	88%	90%	100%
Fibrinolytic Medication Timing	0	-	32%	31%	100%
PCI Within 90 Minutes of Arrival[1]	20	55%	40%	54%	95%
Smoking Cessation Advice	110	95%	88%	88%	100%
Heart Failure Care					
ACE Inhibitor or ARB for LVSD	158	77%	78%	82%	100%
Discharge Instructions	339	78%	62%	61%	93%
Evaluation of LVS Function	385	90%	81%	83%	99%

NOTE: Hospital profiles are in alphabetical order by state, then city, then hospital within the city; Rankings are sorted by rate in descending order and exclude hospitals with less than 25 cases; (1) The number of cases is too small (n<25) for purposes of reliably predicting hospital performance; (2) Measure reflects the hospital's indication that its submission was based upon a sample of its relevant discharges; (3) Rate reflects fewer than the maximum possible quarters of data for the measure; (4) Inaccurate information submitted and suppressed for one or more quarters; (5) No data is available from the hospital for this measure; Please refer to the User's Guide for a full explanation of data

Smoking Cessation Advice	88	75%	83%	82%	100%
Pneumonia Care					
Appropriate Initial Antibiotic	150	70%	78%	83%	94%
Blood Culture Timing	126	91%	89%	90%	100%
Influenza Vaccine	45	64%	58%	70%	100%
Initial Antibiotic Timing	213	66%	76%	80%	93%
Oxygenation Assessment	237	99%	98%	99%	100%
Pneumococcal Vaccine	141	67%	61%	69%	94%
Smoking Cessation Advice	50	52%	78%	80%	100%
Surgical Infection Prevention					
Prophylactic Antibiotic Given[2,3]	458	86%	69%	77%	95%
Prophylactic Antibiotic Selection[2]	57	84%	79%	90%	100%
Prophylactic Antibiotic Stopped[2,3]	440	62%	61%	72%	95%
Pregnancy Care					
Inpatient Neonatal Mortality	2,190	0.23%	-	-	-
Third or Fourth Degree Laceration	1,245	3.61%	3.54%	3.63%	3.27%

Lallie Kemp/Regional Medical Center

52579 Highway 51 S
Independence, LA 70443

Toll-Free: 800-259-9521
Phone: 985-878-9421
Fax: 985-878-1306

URL: www.lsuhospitals.org
Ownership: Government - State
Emergency Services: Yes

Accredited: No
Licensed Beds: 90

Key Personnel:
President/CEO . . . . LeVern S. Meades
Chief Medical Staff . . . . Kathleen Willis, MD
Emergency Room . . . . Michael Kotler
Director Medical/Surgical Nursing . . . . Connie Liuzza, RN
OB/GYN Womens Health . . . . Maria Alleman, MD
Director Respiratory Therapy . . . . Pat Conley

Measure	Cases	This Hospital	State Average	U.S. Average	Top Hospital
Heart Attack Care					
ACE Inhibitor or ARB for LVSD[1,3]	1	100%	84%	82%	100%
Aspirin at Arrival[1,3]	2	100%	91%	92%	100%
Aspirin at Discharge[1,3]	1	0%	87%	90%	100%
Beta Blocker at Arrival[1,3]	1	100%	85%	87%	100%
Beta Blocker at Discharge[1,3]	1	100%	88%	90%	100%
Fibrinolytic Medication Timing[3]	0	-	32%	31%	100%
PCI Within 90 Minutes of Arrival[5]	-	-	40%	54%	95%
Smoking Cessation Advice[1,3]	1	100%	88%	88%	100%
Heart Failure Care					
ACE Inhibitor or ARB for LVSD[1]	22	82%	78%	82%	100%
Discharge Instructions	38	87%	62%	61%	93%
Evaluation of LVS Function	41	90%	81%	83%	99%
Smoking Cessation Advice[1]	19	95%	83%	82%	100%
Pneumonia Care					
Appropriate Initial Antibiotic[1]	24	67%	78%	83%	94%
Blood Culture Timing[1]	15	93%	89%	90%	100%
Influenza Vaccine[1]	5	0%	58%	70%	100%
Initial Antibiotic Timing	25	44%	76%	80%	93%
Oxygenation Assessment	29	100%	98%	99%	100%
Pneumococcal Vaccine[1]	10	40%	61%	69%	94%
Smoking Cessation Advice[1]	13	100%	78%	80%	100%
Surgical Infection Prevention					
Prophylactic Antibiotic Given[3]	67	84%	69%	77%	95%
Prophylactic Antibiotic Selection[1]	21	95%	79%	90%	100%
Prophylactic Antibiotic Stopped[3]	61	85%	61%	72%	95%
Pregnancy Care					
Inpatient Neonatal Mortality	-	-	-	-	-
Third or Fourth Degree Laceration	-	-	3.54%	3.63%	3.27%

Villa Feliciana Medical Complex

Highway 10
PO Box 438
Jackson, LA 70748
Ownership: Government - State
Emergency Services: No

Phone: 225-634-4000
Fax: 225-634-4191

Accredited: No
Licensed Beds: 225

Key Personnel:
Administrator . . . . James E Bradham
Infection Control . . . . Jessica Holden
Respiratory/Cardiopulmonary . . . . Kusandra Taylor

Measure	Cases	This Hospital	State Average	U.S. Average	Top Hospital
Heart Attack Care					
ACE Inhibitor or ARB for LVSD[5]	-	-	84%	82%	100%
Aspirin at Arrival[5]	-	-	91%	92%	100%
Aspirin at Discharge[5]	-	-	87%	90%	100%
Beta Blocker at Arrival[5]	-	-	85%	87%	100%
Beta Blocker at Discharge[5]	-	-	88%	90%	100%
Fibrinolytic Medication Timing[5]	-	-	32%	31%	100%
PCI Within 90 Minutes of Arrival[5]	-	-	40%	54%	95%
Smoking Cessation Advice[5]	-	-	88%	88%	100%
Heart Failure Care					
ACE Inhibitor or ARB for LVSD[5]	-	-	78%	82%	100%
Discharge Instructions[5]	-	-	62%	61%	93%
Evaluation of LVS Function[5]	-	-	81%	83%	99%
Smoking Cessation Advice[5]	-	-	83%	82%	100%
Pneumonia Care					
Appropriate Initial Antibiotic[5]	-	-	78%	83%	94%
Blood Culture Timing[5]	-	-	89%	90%	100%
Influenza Vaccine[5]	-	-	58%	70%	100%
Initial Antibiotic Timing[1,3]	1	100%	76%	80%	93%
Oxygenation Assessment[1,3]	8	100%	98%	99%	100%
Pneumococcal Vaccine[3]	0	-	61%	69%	94%
Smoking Cessation Advice[5]	-	-	78%	80%	100%
Surgical Infection Prevention					
Prophylactic Antibiotic Given[5]	-	-	69%	77%	95%
Prophylactic Antibiotic Selection[5]	-	-	79%	90%	100%
Prophylactic Antibiotic Stopped[5]	-	-	61%	72%	95%
Pregnancy Care					
Inpatient Neonatal Mortality	-	-	-	-	-
Third or Fourth Degree Laceration	-	-	3.54%	3.63%	3.27%

La Salle General Hospital

187 Ninth Street
Jena, LA 71342
E-mail: information@lasallegeneralhospital.com
URL: www.lasallegeneralhospital.com
Ownership: Govt - Hospital District or Authority
Emergency Services: Yes

Phone: 318-992-9200
Fax: 318-992-9245

Accredited: No
Licensed Beds: 60

Key Personnel:
CEO . . . . Mary Mossett
Chief Medical Staff . . . . Sinit Srookul
Emergency Room . . . . G Rohr
Chief of Respiratory Therapy . . . . Ben Hernanded

Measure	Cases	This Hospital	State Average	U.S. Average	Top Hospital
Heart Attack Care					
ACE Inhibitor or ARB for LVSD[1,3]	1	100%	84%	82%	100%
Aspirin at Arrival[1,3]	7	100%	91%	92%	100%
Aspirin at Discharge[1,3]	4	100%	87%	90%	100%
Beta Blocker at Arrival[1,3]	5	60%	85%	87%	100%
Beta Blocker at Discharge[1,3]	5	80%	88%	90%	100%
Fibrinolytic Medication Timing[3]	0	-	32%	31%	100%
PCI Within 90 Minutes of Arrival	0	-	40%	54%	95%
Smoking Cessation Advice[3]	0	-	88%	88%	100%
Heart Failure Care					
ACE Inhibitor or ARB for LVSD[1,2]	24	83%	78%	82%	100%
Discharge Instructions[2]	79	96%	62%	61%	93%
Evaluation of LVS Function[2]	117	98%	81%	83%	99%
Smoking Cessation Advice[1,2]	18	83%	83%	82%	100%
Pneumonia Care					
Appropriate Initial Antibiotic[2]	38	92%	78%	83%	94%
Blood Culture Timing[2]	56	93%	89%	90%	100%
Influenza Vaccine[1,2]	12	75%	58%	70%	100%
Initial Antibiotic Timing[2]	71	86%	76%	80%	93%
Oxygenation Assessment[2]	83	96%	98%	99%	100%
Pneumococcal Vaccine[2]	54	80%	61%	69%	94%
Smoking Cessation Advice[1,2]	15	87%	78%	80%	100%
Surgical Infection Prevention					
Prophylactic Antibiotic Given[5]	-	-	69%	77%	95%
Prophylactic Antibiotic Selection[5]	-	-	79%	90%	100%
Prophylactic Antibiotic Stopped[5]	-	-	61%	72%	95%
Pregnancy Care					

NOTE: Hospital profiles are in alphabetical order by state, then city, then hospital within the city; Rankings are sorted by rate in descending order and exclude hospitals with less than 25 cases; (1) The number of cases is too small (n<25) for purposes of reliably predicting hospital performance; (2) Measure reflects the hospital's indication that its submission was based upon a sample of its relevant discharges; (3) Rate reflects fewer than the maximum possible quarters of data for the measure; (4) Inaccurate information submitted and suppressed for one or more quarters; (5) No data is available from the hospital for this measure; Please refer to the User's Guide for a full explanation of data

Inpatient Neonatal Mortality	-	-	-	-	-
Third or Fourth Degree Laceration	-	-	3.54%	3.63%	3.27%

Jennings American Legion Hospital

1634 Elton Road
Jennings, LA 70546
E-mail: webmail@jalh.com
URL: www.jalh.com
Ownership: Voluntary non-profit - Private
Emergency Services: Yes

Phone: 337-616-7000
Fax: 337-616-7044

Accredited: Yes
Licensed Beds: 178

Key Personnel:
CEO . . . . Terry W Osborne
Chief Medical Staff . . . . Arshavir Michael, MD
Emergency Room . . . . Faye Kershaw
Infection Control . . . . Connie Sittig
ICU . . . . Tricia Semar
Chief Respiratory Therapy . . . . Tom Kopp

Measure	Cases	This Hospital	State Average	U.S. Average	Top Hospital
Heart Attack Care					
ACE Inhibitor or ARB for LVSD[1]	2	100%	84%	82%	100%
Aspirin at Arrival	33	97%	91%	92%	100%
Aspirin at Discharge[1]	14	93%	87%	90%	100%
Beta Blocker at Arrival	27	96%	85%	87%	100%
Beta Blocker at Discharge[1]	19	100%	88%	90%	100%
Fibrinolytic Medication Timing[3]	0	-	32%	31%	100%
PCI Within 90 Minutes of Arrival	0	-	40%	54%	95%
Smoking Cessation Advice[1,3]	2	100%	88%	88%	100%
Heart Failure Care					
ACE Inhibitor or ARB for LVSD[1]	24	100%	78%	82%	100%
Discharge Instructions[3]	30	97%	62%	61%	93%
Evaluation of LVS Function	153	92%	81%	83%	99%
Smoking Cessation Advice[1,3]	7	86%	83%	82%	100%
Pneumonia Care					
Appropriate Initial Antibiotic[1,3]	18	89%	78%	83%	94%
Blood Culture Timing[3]	29	93%	89%	90%	100%
Influenza Vaccine[5]	-	-	58%	70%	100%
Initial Antibiotic Timing	152	88%	76%	80%	93%
Oxygenation Assessment	161	100%	98%	99%	100%
Pneumococcal Vaccine	115	77%	61%	69%	94%
Smoking Cessation Advice[1,3]	5	80%	78%	80%	100%
Surgical Infection Prevention					
Prophylactic Antibiotic Given[3]	36	83%	69%	77%	95%
Prophylactic Antibiotic Selection[5]	-	-	79%	90%	100%
Prophylactic Antibiotic Stopped[3]	35	46%	61%	72%	95%
Pregnancy Care					
Inpatient Neonatal Mortality	-	-	-	-	-
Third or Fourth Degree Laceration	-	-	3.54%	3.63%	3.27%

Jackson Parish Hospital

165 Beech Springs Road
Jonesboro, LA 71251
E-mail: nashw@stfran.com
URL: www.jacksonparishhospital.com
Ownership: Govt - Hospital District or Authority
Emergency Services: Yes

Phone: 318-259-4435
Fax: 318-395-4259

Accredited: No
Licensed Beds: 49

Key Personnel:
CEO . . . . LJ Pecot
Chief Medical Staff . . . . Rebecca Crouch, MD
Emergency Room . . . . Ann Standley
Infection Control . . . . Mary Lynn McBride

Measure	Cases	This Hospital	State Average	U.S. Average	Top Hospital
Heart Attack Care					
ACE Inhibitor or ARB for LVSD[5]	-	-	84%	82%	100%
Aspirin at Arrival[5]	-	-	91%	92%	100%
Aspirin at Discharge[5]	-	-	87%	90%	100%
Beta Blocker at Arrival[5]	-	-	85%	87%	100%
Beta Blocker at Discharge[5]	-	-	88%	90%	100%
Fibrinolytic Medication Timing[5]	-	-	32%	31%	100%
PCI Within 90 Minutes of Arrival[5]	-	-	40%	54%	95%
Smoking Cessation Advice[5]	-	-	88%	88%	100%
Heart Failure Care					

Measure	Cases	This Hospital	State Average	U.S. Average	Top Hospital
ACE Inhibitor or ARB for LVSD[1]	15	80%	78%	82%	100%
Discharge Instructions	54	67%	62%	61%	93%
Evaluation of LVS Function	81	90%	81%	83%	99%
Smoking Cessation Advice	29	83%	83%	82%	100%
Pneumonia Care					
Appropriate Initial Antibiotic	60	82%	78%	83%	94%
Blood Culture Timing[1]	19	95%	89%	90%	100%
Influenza Vaccine[1]	10	30%	58%	70%	100%
Initial Antibiotic Timing	63	92%	76%	80%	93%
Oxygenation Assessment	67	94%	98%	99%	100%
Pneumococcal Vaccine	44	36%	61%	69%	94%
Smoking Cessation Advice[1]	14	86%	78%	80%	100%
Surgical Infection Prevention					
Prophylactic Antibiotic Given[5]	-	-	69%	77%	95%
Prophylactic Antibiotic Selection[5]	-	-	79%	90%	100%
Prophylactic Antibiotic Stopped[5]	-	-	61%	72%	95%
Pregnancy Care					
Inpatient Neonatal Mortality	-	-	-	-	-
Third or Fourth Degree Laceration	-	-	3.54%	3.63%	3.27%

Abrom Kaplan Memorial Hospital

1310 W 7th Street
Kaplan, LA 70548
Ownership: Govt - Hospital District or Authority
Emergency Services: Yes

Phone: 337-643-8300
Fax: 337-643-5309

Accredited: No
Licensed Beds: 50

Key Personnel:
Administrator . . . . Lyman Trahan
Chief of Medical Staff . . . . Randell Faulk
Emergency Room . . . . Kitty Lormand, RN
Director Infection/Disease Control . . . . Terry Williams
Director Medical/Surgical Nursing . . . . Terry Williams
Director of Pulmonary/Respiratory Care . . . . Sharon Reel

Measure	Cases	This Hospital	State Average	U.S. Average	Top Hospital
Heart Attack Care					
ACE Inhibitor or ARB for LVSD[3]	0	-	84%	82%	100%
Aspirin at Arrival[1,3]	1	0%	91%	92%	100%
Aspirin at Discharge[1,3]	1	0%	87%	90%	100%
Beta Blocker at Arrival[1,3]	1	0%	85%	87%	100%
Beta Blocker at Discharge[1,3]	1	0%	88%	90%	100%
Fibrinolytic Medication Timing[3]	0	-	32%	31%	100%
PCI Within 90 Minutes of Arrival	0	-	40%	54%	95%
Smoking Cessation Advice[3]	0	-	88%	88%	100%
Heart Failure Care					
ACE Inhibitor or ARB for LVSD[1]	2	50%	78%	82%	100%
Discharge Instructions[1]	11	27%	62%	61%	93%
Evaluation of LVS Function[1]	19	53%	81%	83%	99%
Smoking Cessation Advice[1]	1	100%	83%	82%	100%
Pneumonia Care					
Appropriate Initial Antibiotic[1]	12	83%	78%	83%	94%
Blood Culture Timing[1]	14	86%	89%	90%	100%
Influenza Vaccine[1]	3	67%	58%	70%	100%
Initial Antibiotic Timing[1]	23	74%	76%	80%	93%
Oxygenation Assessment	28	100%	98%	99%	100%
Pneumococcal Vaccine[1]	19	53%	61%	69%	94%
Smoking Cessation Advice[1]	5	40%	78%	80%	100%
Surgical Infection Prevention					
Prophylactic Antibiotic Given[1,3]	9	11%	69%	77%	95%
Prophylactic Antibiotic Selection[1]	2	100%	79%	90%	100%
Prophylactic Antibiotic Stopped[1,3]	8	62%	61%	72%	95%
Pregnancy Care					
Inpatient Neonatal Mortality	-	-	-	-	-
Third or Fourth Degree Laceration	-	-	3.54%	3.63%	3.27%

Kenner Regional Medical Center

Alternate Name: Ochsner Medical Center-Kenner
180 W Esplanade Avenue
Kenner, LA 70065
URL: www.kennerregional.com
Ownership: Voluntary non-profit - Private
Emergency Services: Yes

Phone: 504-468-8600
Fax: 504-464-8139

Accredited: No
Licensed Beds: 203

Key Personnel:
Administrator/CEO . . . . Paolo Zambito, RN

NOTE: Hospital profiles are in alphabetical order by state, then city, then hospital within the city; Rankings are sorted by rate in descending order and exclude hospitals with less than 25 cases; (1) The number of cases is too small (n<25) for purposes of reliably predicting hospital performance; (2) Measure reflects the hospital's indication that its submission was based upon a sample of its relevant discharges; (3) Rate reflects fewer than the maximum possible quarters of data for the measure; (4) Inaccurate information submitted and suppressed for one or more quarters; (5) No data is available from the hospital for this measure; Please refer to the User's Guide for a full explanation of data

Chief Medical Staff . . . . Melissa Ponthieux
Emergency Room . . . . Marylann Smith
Emergency Room . . . . Elizabeth Allen, RN
Director Respiratory Therapy . . . . Carry Dufresne

Measure	Cases	This Hospital	State Average	U.S. Average	Top Hospital
Heart Attack Care					
ACE Inhibitor or ARB for LVSD[5]	-	-	84%	82%	100%
Aspirin at Arrival[5]	-	-	91%	92%	100%
Aspirin at Discharge[5]	-	-	87%	90%	100%
Beta Blocker at Arrival[5]	-	-	85%	87%	100%
Beta Blocker at Discharge[5]	-	-	88%	90%	100%
Fibrinolytic Medication Timing[5]	-	-	32%	31%	100%
PCI Within 90 Minutes of Arrival[5]	-	-	40%	54%	95%
Smoking Cessation Advice[5]	-	-	88%	88%	100%
Heart Failure Care					
ACE Inhibitor or ARB for LVSD[5]	-	-	78%	82%	100%
Discharge Instructions[5]	-	-	62%	61%	93%
Evaluation of LVS Function[5]	-	-	81%	83%	99%
Smoking Cessation Advice[5]	-	-	83%	82%	100%
Pneumonia Care					
Appropriate Initial Antibiotic[5]	-	-	78%	83%	94%
Blood Culture Timing[5]	-	-	89%	90%	100%
Influenza Vaccine[5]	-	-	58%	70%	100%
Initial Antibiotic Timing[5]	-	-	76%	80%	93%
Oxygenation Assessment[5]	-	-	98%	99%	100%
Pneumococcal Vaccine[5]	-	-	61%	69%	94%
Smoking Cessation Advice[5]	-	-	78%	80%	100%
Surgical Infection Prevention					
Prophylactic Antibiotic Given[5]	-	-	69%	77%	95%
Prophylactic Antibiotic Selection[5]	-	-	79%	90%	100%
Prophylactic Antibiotic Stopped[5]	-	-	61%	72%	95%
Pregnancy Care					
Inpatient Neonatal Mortality	-	-	-	-	-
Third or Fourth Degree Laceration	-	-	3.54%	3.63%	3.27%

Allen Parish Hospital

108 N 6th Street
PO Box 1670
Kinder, LA 70648
E-mail: allenph@yahoo.com
Ownership: Govt - Hospital District or Authority
Emergency Services: No

Toll-Free: 800-737-2537
Phone: 337-738-2527
Fax: 337-738-2901

Accredited: No
Licensed Beds: 49

Key Personnel:
Administrator/CEO . . . . Scott Barrilleaux
Chief Medical Staff . . . . Peggy Allemand, MD
Emergency Room . . . . Levie Johnson
Director Infection/Disease Control . . . . Paige Fontenot
Manager Radiology . . . . Terry Robin
Director Respiratory Therapy . . . . Robert Christopher

Measure	Cases	This Hospital	State Average	U.S. Average	Top Hospital
Heart Attack Care					
ACE Inhibitor or ARB for LVSD[3]	0	-	84%	82%	100%
Aspirin at Arrival[1,3]	1	100%	91%	92%	100%
Aspirin at Discharge[1,3]	1	100%	87%	90%	100%
Beta Blocker at Arrival[1,3]	1	100%	85%	87%	100%
Beta Blocker at Discharge[1,3]	1	100%	88%	90%	100%
Fibrinolytic Medication Timing[5]	-	-	32%	31%	100%
PCI Within 90 Minutes of Arrival[5]	-	-	40%	54%	95%
Smoking Cessation Advice[5]	-	-	88%	88%	100%
Heart Failure Care					
ACE Inhibitor or ARB for LVSD[1]	3	100%	78%	82%	100%
Discharge Instructions[1,3]	2	0%	62%	61%	93%
Evaluation of LVS Function[1]	22	50%	81%	83%	99%
Smoking Cessation Advice[3]	0	-	83%	82%	100%
Pneumonia Care					
Appropriate Initial Antibiotic[1,3]	1	100%	78%	83%	94%
Blood Culture Timing[1,3]	3	100%	89%	90%	100%
Influenza Vaccine[5]	-	-	58%	70%	100%
Initial Antibiotic Timing	25	68%	76%	80%	93%
Oxygenation Assessment	36	94%	98%	99%	100%

Measure	Cases	This Hospital	State Average	U.S. Average	Top Hospital
Pneumococcal Vaccine[1]	23	0%	61%	69%	94%
Smoking Cessation Advice[3]	0	-	78%	80%	100%
Surgical Infection Prevention					
Prophylactic Antibiotic Given[5]	-	-	69%	77%	95%
Prophylactic Antibiotic Selection[5]	-	-	79%	90%	100%
Prophylactic Antibiotic Stopped[5]	-	-	61%	72%	95%
Pregnancy Care					
Inpatient Neonatal Mortality	-	-	-	-	-
Third or Fourth Degree Laceration	-	-	3.54%	3.63%	3.27%

Louisiana Heart Hospital

64030 Highway 434
Lacombe, LA 70445
URL: www.louisianahearthospital.com
Ownership: Proprietary
Emergency Services: Yes

Phone: 985-690-7500
Fax: 985-690-7530

Accredited: Yes
Licensed Beds: 58

Key Personnel:
Administrator/CEO . . . . Bill Fox

Measure	Cases	This Hospital	State Average	U.S. Average	Top Hospital
Heart Attack Care					
ACE Inhibitor or ARB for LVSD[1]	20	100%	84%	82%	100%
Aspirin at Arrival	64	100%	91%	92%	100%
Aspirin at Discharge	134	100%	87%	90%	100%
Beta Blocker at Arrival	57	98%	85%	87%	100%
Beta Blocker at Discharge	136	99%	88%	90%	100%
Fibrinolytic Medication Timing	0	-	32%	31%	100%
PCI Within 90 Minutes of Arrival[1]	5	80%	40%	54%	95%
Smoking Cessation Advice	71	100%	88%	88%	100%
Heart Failure Care					
ACE Inhibitor or ARB for LVSD	107	96%	78%	82%	100%
Discharge Instructions	251	100%	62%	61%	93%
Evaluation of LVS Function	267	98%	81%	83%	99%
Smoking Cessation Advice	43	100%	83%	82%	100%
Pneumonia Care					
Appropriate Initial Antibiotic	26	85%	78%	83%	94%
Blood Culture Timing[1]	20	85%	89%	90%	100%
Influenza Vaccine[4,5]	-	-	58%	70%	100%
Initial Antibiotic Timing	25	88%	76%	80%	93%
Oxygenation Assessment	35	100%	98%	99%	100%
Pneumococcal Vaccine[1]	19	89%	61%	69%	94%
Smoking Cessation Advice[1]	12	92%	78%	80%	100%
Surgical Infection Prevention					
Prophylactic Antibiotic Given[2,3]	223	88%	69%	77%	95%
Prophylactic Antibiotic Selection[2]	82	96%	79%	90%	100%
Prophylactic Antibiotic Stopped[2,3]	219	57%	61%	72%	95%
Pregnancy Care					
Inpatient Neonatal Mortality	-	-	-	-	-
Third or Fourth Degree Laceration	-	-	3.54%	3.63%	3.27%

Heart Hospital of Lafayette

1105 Kaliste Saloom
Lafayette, LA 70508
E-mail: info@hearthospitaloflafayette.com
URL: www.hearthospitaloflafayette.com
Ownership: Proprietary
Emergency Services: Yes

Phone: 337-521-1000
Fax: 337-521-1006

Accredited: Yes
Licensed Beds: 24

Key Personnel:
Chief of Medical Staff . . . . Edgar Feinberg, MD
Cardiology . . . . Elizabeth Reinhardt
Infection Control . . . . Vicky Manuel
Surgical Services . . . . John Horn
Respiratory . . . . Mike Hebert

Measure	Cases	This Hospital	State Average	U.S. Average	Top Hospital
Heart Attack Care					
ACE Inhibitor or ARB for LVSD	31	100%	84%	82%	100%
Aspirin at Arrival	44	100%	91%	92%	100%
Aspirin at Discharge	200	100%	87%	90%	100%
Beta Blocker at Arrival	43	100%	85%	87%	100%
Beta Blocker at Discharge	196	100%	88%	90%	100%
Fibrinolytic Medication Timing[3]	0	-	32%	31%	100%

NOTE: Hospital profiles are in alphabetical order by state, then city, then hospital within the city; Rankings are sorted by rate in descending order and exclude hospitals with less than 25 cases; (1) The number of cases is too small (n<25) for purposes of reliably predicting hospital performance; (2) Measure reflects the hospital's indication that its submission was based upon a sample of its relevant discharges; (3) Rate reflects fewer than the maximum possible quarters of data for the measure; (4) Inaccurate information submitted and suppressed for one or more quarters; (5) No data is available from the hospital for this measure; Please refer to the User's Guide for a full explanation of data

		This Hospital	State Average	U.S. Average	Top Hospital
PCI Within 90 Minutes of Arrival[1]	7	14%	40%	54%	95%
Smoking Cessation Advice[1,3]	21	100%	88%	88%	100%
Heart Failure Care					
ACE Inhibitor or ARB for LVSD	64	98%	78%	82%	100%
Discharge Instructions[1,3]	22	100%	62%	61%	93%
Evaluation of LVS Function	135	100%	81%	83%	99%
Smoking Cessation Advice[1,3]	9	100%	83%	82%	100%
Pneumonia Care					
Appropriate Initial Antibiotic[2,3]	0	-	78%	83%	94%
Blood Culture Timing[2,3]	0	-	89%	90%	100%
Influenza Vaccine[5]	-	-	58%	70%	100%
Initial Antibiotic Timing[1,2,3]	3	67%	76%	80%	93%
Oxygenation Assessment[1,2,3]	3	100%	98%	99%	100%
Pneumococcal Vaccine[1,2,3]	2	50%	61%	69%	94%
Smoking Cessation Advice[2,3]	0	-	78%	80%	100%
Surgical Infection Prevention					
Prophylactic Antibiotic Given[3]	59	88%	69%	77%	95%
Prophylactic Antibiotic Selection[5]	-	-	79%	90%	100%
Prophylactic Antibiotic Stopped[3]	58	79%	61%	72%	95%
Pregnancy Care					
Inpatient Neonatal Mortality	-	-	-	-	-
Third or Fourth Degree Laceration	-	-	3.54%	3.63%	3.27%

Lafayette General Medical Center

1214 Coolidge Boulevard
Lafayette, LA 70503
URL: www.lafayettegeneral.org
Ownership: Voluntary non-profit - Other
Emergency Services: Yes

Phone: 337-289-7991
Fax: 337-289-8466

Accredited: Yes
Licensed Beds: 297

Key Personnel:
President/CEO . . . . James Thaw
Director of Cardiology/Cardiac Lab. . . . . Charlie Olinger
Emergency Room . . . . Karen Wible
Director Medical/Surgical Nursing . . . . Sylvia Oats
OB/GYN Womens Health. . . . . Sylvia Oats
Surgical Services . . . . Dani Marine
Director Radiology . . . . Paul Thibodeaux
Respiratory Care . . . . Jina Cook

Measure	Cases	This Hospital	State Average	U.S. Average	Top Hospital
Heart Attack Care					
ACE Inhibitor or ARB for LVSD	26	92%	84%	82%	100%
Aspirin at Arrival	125	88%	91%	92%	100%
Aspirin at Discharge	152	91%	87%	90%	100%
Beta Blocker at Arrival	112	86%	85%	87%	100%
Beta Blocker at Discharge	151	93%	88%	90%	100%
Fibrinolytic Medication Timing[1]	2	0%	32%	31%	100%
PCI Within 90 Minutes of Arrival[1]	9	44%	40%	54%	95%
Smoking Cessation Advice	66	98%	88%	88%	100%
Heart Failure Care					
ACE Inhibitor or ARB for LVSD[2]	177	82%	78%	82%	100%
Discharge Instructions[2]	363	63%	62%	61%	93%
Evaluation of LVS Function[2]	404	93%	81%	83%	99%
Smoking Cessation Advice[2]	80	88%	83%	82%	100%
Pneumonia Care					
Appropriate Initial Antibiotic[2]	103	83%	78%	83%	94%
Blood Culture Timing[2]	92	78%	89%	90%	100%
Influenza Vaccine[2]	41	63%	58%	70%	100%
Initial Antibiotic Timing[2]	146	75%	76%	80%	93%
Oxygenation Assessment[2]	183	100%	98%	99%	100%
Pneumococcal Vaccine[2]	98	84%	61%	69%	94%
Smoking Cessation Advice[2]	56	91%	78%	80%	100%
Surgical Infection Prevention					
Prophylactic Antibiotic Given[2,3]	193	89%	69%	77%	95%
Prophylactic Antibiotic Selection[2]	60	92%	79%	90%	100%
Prophylactic Antibiotic Stopped[2,3]	184	58%	61%	72%	95%
Pregnancy Care					
Inpatient Neonatal Mortality	1,748	1.26%	-	-	-
Third or Fourth Degree Laceration	1,054	2.94%	3.54%	3.63%	3.27%

Lafayette General Surgical Hospital

1000 W Pinhook Rd Suite 100
Lafayette, LA 70503
Ownership: Voluntary non-profit - Private
Emergency Services: No

Phone: 337-289-8095

Accredited: No

Measure	Cases	This Hospital	State Average	U.S. Average	Top Hospital
Heart Attack Care					
ACE Inhibitor or ARB for LVSD[5]	-	-	84%	82%	100%
Aspirin at Arrival[5]	-	-	91%	92%	100%
Aspirin at Discharge[5]	-	-	87%	90%	100%
Beta Blocker at Arrival[5]	-	-	85%	87%	100%
Beta Blocker at Discharge[5]	-	-	88%	90%	100%
Fibrinolytic Medication Timing[5]	-	-	32%	31%	100%
PCI Within 90 Minutes of Arrival[5]	-	-	40%	54%	95%
Smoking Cessation Advice[5]	-	-	88%	88%	100%
Heart Failure Care					
ACE Inhibitor or ARB for LVSD[5]	-	-	78%	82%	100%
Discharge Instructions[5]	-	-	62%	61%	93%
Evaluation of LVS Function[5]	-	-	81%	83%	99%
Smoking Cessation Advice[5]	-	-	83%	82%	100%
Pneumonia Care					
Appropriate Initial Antibiotic[5]	-	-	78%	83%	94%
Blood Culture Timing[5]	-	-	89%	90%	100%
Influenza Vaccine[5]	-	-	58%	70%	100%
Initial Antibiotic Timing[5]	-	-	76%	80%	93%
Oxygenation Assessment[5]	-	-	98%	99%	100%
Pneumococcal Vaccine[5]	-	-	61%	69%	94%
Smoking Cessation Advice[5]	-	-	78%	80%	100%
Surgical Infection Prevention					
Prophylactic Antibiotic Given[5]	-	-	69%	77%	95%
Prophylactic Antibiotic Selection[5]	-	-	79%	90%	100%
Prophylactic Antibiotic Stopped[5]	-	-	61%	72%	95%
Pregnancy Care					
Inpatient Neonatal Mortality	-	-	-	-	-
Third or Fourth Degree Laceration	-	-	3.54%	3.63%	3.27%

Lafayette Surgical Specialty Hospital

1101 Kaliste Saloom Rd
Lafayette, LA 70505
Ownership: Proprietary
Emergency Services: No

Phone: 337-769-4100

Accredited: Yes

Measure	Cases	This Hospital	State Average	U.S. Average	Top Hospital
Heart Attack Care					
ACE Inhibitor or ARB for LVSD[5]	-	-	84%	82%	100%
Aspirin at Arrival[5]	-	-	91%	92%	100%
Aspirin at Discharge[5]	-	-	87%	90%	100%
Beta Blocker at Arrival[5]	-	-	85%	87%	100%
Beta Blocker at Discharge[5]	-	-	88%	90%	100%
Fibrinolytic Medication Timing[5]	-	-	32%	31%	100%
PCI Within 90 Minutes of Arrival[5]	-	-	40%	54%	95%
Smoking Cessation Advice[5]	-	-	88%	88%	100%
Heart Failure Care					
ACE Inhibitor or ARB for LVSD[5]	-	-	78%	82%	100%
Discharge Instructions[5]	-	-	62%	61%	93%
Evaluation of LVS Function[5]	-	-	81%	83%	99%
Smoking Cessation Advice[5]	-	-	83%	82%	100%
Pneumonia Care					
Appropriate Initial Antibiotic[5]	-	-	78%	83%	94%
Blood Culture Timing[5]	-	-	89%	90%	100%
Influenza Vaccine[5]	-	-	58%	70%	100%
Initial Antibiotic Timing[5]	-	-	76%	80%	93%
Oxygenation Assessment[5]	-	-	98%	99%	100%
Pneumococcal Vaccine[5]	-	-	61%	69%	94%
Smoking Cessation Advice[5]	-	-	78%	80%	100%
Surgical Infection Prevention					
Prophylactic Antibiotic Given	55	89%	69%	77%	95%
Prophylactic Antibiotic Selection[1]	12	83%	79%	90%	100%
Prophylactic Antibiotic Stopped	55	45%	61%	72%	95%
Pregnancy Care					
Inpatient Neonatal Mortality	-	-	-	-	-

NOTE: Hospital profiles are in alphabetical order by state, then city, then hospital within the city; Rankings are sorted by rate in descending order and exclude hospitals with less than 25 cases; (1) The number of cases is too small (n<25) for purposes of reliably predicting hospital performance; (2) Measure reflects the hospital's indication that its submission was based upon a sample of its relevant discharges; (3) Rate reflects fewer than the maximum possible quarters of data for the measure; (4) Inaccurate information submitted and suppressed for one or more quarters; (5) No data is available from the hospital for this measure; Please refer to the User's Guide for a full explanation of data

Third or Fourth Degree Laceration	-	-	3.54%	3.63%	3.27%

Our Lady of Lourdes Regional Medical Center

611 Saint Landry Street   Phone: 337-289-2000
Lafayette, LA 70506   Fax: 337-289-2796
E-mail: info@lourdes.net
URL: www.lourdes.net
Ownership: Voluntary non-profit - Church   Accredited: Yes
Emergency Services: Yes   Licensed Beds: 293
Key Personnel:
President/CEO . . . . Bud Barrow
Cardiology . . . . Sharon Richard
Director Emergency Department . . . . David McManus, MD
Emergency Room . . . . Carol Aubrey
Infection Control. . . . . Lena Hackney
Director Radiology . . . . Victor H Gunderson, MD
Director Respiratory Therapy . . . . Mary Nelson
Surgery Department Chairman . . . . Christopher Fontenot, MD
Vice Chief Surgery. . . . . Philip Gachassin, MD

Measure	Cases	This Hospital	State Average	U.S. Average	Top Hospital
Heart Attack Care					
ACE Inhibitor or ARB for LVSD[1]	20	90%	84%	82%	100%
Aspirin at Arrival	124	94%	91%	92%	100%
Aspirin at Discharge	138	85%	87%	90%	100%
Beta Blocker at Arrival	100	84%	85%	87%	100%
Beta Blocker at Discharge	149	89%	88%	90%	100%
Fibrinolytic Medication Timing[1]	2	50%	32%	31%	100%
PCI Within 90 Minutes of Arrival[1]	5	0%	40%	54%	95%
Smoking Cessation Advice	51	100%	88%	88%	100%
Heart Failure Care					
ACE Inhibitor or ARB for LVSD	141	73%	78%	82%	100%
Discharge Instructions	327	74%	62%	61%	93%
Evaluation of LVS Function	394	89%	81%	83%	99%
Smoking Cessation Advice	68	100%	83%	82%	100%
Pneumonia Care					
Appropriate Initial Antibiotic	152	74%	78%	83%	94%
Blood Culture Timing	121	94%	89%	90%	100%
Influenza Vaccine	45	82%	58%	70%	100%
Initial Antibiotic Timing	194	60%	76%	80%	93%
Oxygenation Assessment	253	99%	98%	99%	100%
Pneumococcal Vaccine	144	92%	61%	69%	94%
Smoking Cessation Advice	58	100%	78%	80%	100%
Surgical Infection Prevention					
Prophylactic Antibiotic Given[2,3]	156	84%	69%	77%	95%
Prophylactic Antibiotic Selection[2]	53	91%	79%	90%	100%
Prophylactic Antibiotic Stopped[2,3]	154	64%	61%	72%	95%
Pregnancy Care					
Inpatient Neonatal Mortality	-	-	-	-	-
Third or Fourth Degree Laceration	-	-	3.54%	3.63%	3.27%

Park Place Surgical Hospital

901 Wilson Street   Phone: 337-237-8119
Lafayette, LA 70503
Ownership: Proprietary   Accredited: No
Emergency Services: No

Measure	Cases	This Hospital	State Average	U.S. Average	Top Hospital
Heart Attack Care					
ACE Inhibitor or ARB for LVSD[5]	-	-	84%	82%	100%
Aspirin at Arrival[5]	-	-	91%	92%	100%
Aspirin at Discharge[5]	-	-	87%	90%	100%
Beta Blocker at Arrival[5]	-	-	85%	87%	100%
Beta Blocker at Discharge[5]	-	-	88%	90%	100%
Fibrinolytic Medication Timing[5]	-	-	32%	31%	100%
PCI Within 90 Minutes of Arrival[5]	-	-	40%	54%	95%
Smoking Cessation Advice[5]	-	-	88%	88%	100%
Heart Failure Care					
ACE Inhibitor or ARB for LVSD[5]	-	-	78%	82%	100%
Discharge Instructions[5]	-	-	62%	61%	93%
Evaluation of LVS Function[5]	-	-	81%	83%	99%
Smoking Cessation Advice[5]	-	-	83%	82%	100%

Measure	Cases	This Hospital	State Average	U.S. Average	Top Hospital
Pneumonia Care					
Appropriate Initial Antibiotic[5]	-	-	78%	83%	94%
Blood Culture Timing[5]	-	-	89%	90%	100%
Influenza Vaccine[5]	-	-	58%	70%	100%
Initial Antibiotic Timing[5]	-	-	76%	80%	93%
Oxygenation Assessment[5]	-	-	98%	99%	100%
Pneumococcal Vaccine[5]	-	-	61%	69%	94%
Smoking Cessation Advice[5]	-	-	78%	80%	100%
Surgical Infection Prevention					
Prophylactic Antibiotic Given[1,3]	12	42%	69%	77%	95%
Prophylactic Antibiotic Selection[5]	-	-	79%	90%	100%
Prophylactic Antibiotic Stopped[1,3]	7	57%	61%	72%	95%
Pregnancy Care					
Inpatient Neonatal Mortality	-	-	-	-	-
Third or Fourth Degree Laceration	-	-	3.54%	3.63%	3.27%

Southpark Community Hospital

314 Youngsville Highway   Phone: 337-769-2080
Lafayette, LA 70508
Ownership: Proprietary   Accredited: No
Emergency Services: No

Measure	Cases	This Hospital	State Average	U.S. Average	Top Hospital
Heart Attack Care					
ACE Inhibitor or ARB for LVSD[5]	-	-	84%	82%	100%
Aspirin at Arrival[5]	-	-	91%	92%	100%
Aspirin at Discharge[5]	-	-	87%	90%	100%
Beta Blocker at Arrival[5]	-	-	85%	87%	100%
Beta Blocker at Discharge[5]	-	-	88%	90%	100%
Fibrinolytic Medication Timing[5]	-	-	32%	31%	100%
PCI Within 90 Minutes of Arrival[5]	-	-	40%	54%	95%
Smoking Cessation Advice[5]	-	-	88%	88%	100%
Heart Failure Care					
ACE Inhibitor or ARB for LVSD[1,3]	2	0%	78%	82%	100%
Discharge Instructions[1,3]	9	0%	62%	61%	93%
Evaluation of LVS Function[1,3]	16	19%	81%	83%	99%
Smoking Cessation Advice[3]	0	-	83%	82%	100%
Pneumonia Care					
Appropriate Initial Antibiotic[1,3]	1	0%	78%	83%	94%
Blood Culture Timing[1,3]	2	100%	89%	90%	100%
Influenza Vaccine[5]	-	-	58%	70%	100%
Initial Antibiotic Timing[3]	0	-	76%	80%	93%
Oxygenation Assessment[1,3]	4	100%	98%	99%	100%
Pneumococcal Vaccine[1,3]	3	0%	61%	69%	94%
Smoking Cessation Advice[3]	0	-	78%	80%	100%
Surgical Infection Prevention					
Prophylactic Antibiotic Given[3]	0	-	69%	77%	95%
Prophylactic Antibiotic Selection	0	-	79%	90%	100%
Prophylactic Antibiotic Stopped[3]	0	-	61%	72%	95%
Pregnancy Care					
Inpatient Neonatal Mortality	-	-	-	-	-
Third or Fourth Degree Laceration	-	-	3.54%	3.63%	3.27%

Southwest Medical Center

2810 Ambassador Caffery Parkway   Phone: 337-981-2949
Lafayette, LA 70506   Fax: 337-989-6781
URL: www.southwestmc.com
Ownership: Proprietary   Accredited: Yes
Emergency Services: Yes   Licensed Beds: 135
Key Personnel:
CEO/Administrator . . . . Kyle J Viator

Measure	Cases	This Hospital	State Average	U.S. Average	Top Hospital
Heart Attack Care					
ACE Inhibitor or ARB for LVSD[1]	17	88%	84%	82%	100%
Aspirin at Arrival	73	90%	91%	92%	100%
Aspirin at Discharge	85	88%	87%	90%	100%
Beta Blocker at Arrival	73	70%	85%	87%	100%
Beta Blocker at Discharge	88	86%	88%	90%	100%
Fibrinolytic Medication Timing	0	-	32%	31%	100%
PCI Within 90 Minutes of Arrival[1]	5	40%	40%	54%	95%
Smoking Cessation Advice	42	98%	88%	88%	100%

NOTE: Hospital profiles are in alphabetical order by state, then city, then hospital within the city; Rankings are sorted by rate in descending order and exclude hospitals with less than 25 cases; (1) The number of cases is too small (n<25) for purposes of reliably predicting hospital performance; (2) Measure reflects the hospital's indication that its submission was based upon a sample of its relevant discharges; (3) Rate reflects fewer than the maximum possible quarters of data for the measure; (4) Inaccurate information submitted and suppressed for one or more quarters; (5) No data is available from the hospital for this measure; Please refer to the User's Guide for a full explanation of data

Heart Failure Care					
ACE Inhibitor or ARB for LVSD	74	81%	78%	82%	100%
Discharge Instructions	170	55%	62%	61%	93%
Evaluation of LVS Function	192	88%	81%	83%	99%
Smoking Cessation Advice	29	93%	83%	82%	100%
Pneumonia Care					
Appropriate Initial Antibiotic	102	79%	78%	83%	94%
Blood Culture Timing	45	91%	89%	90%	100%
Influenza Vaccine	31	58%	58%	70%	100%
Initial Antibiotic Timing	110	72%	76%	80%	93%
Oxygenation Assessment	123	99%	98%	99%	100%
Pneumococcal Vaccine	68	47%	61%	69%	94%
Smoking Cessation Advice	43	77%	78%	80%	100%
Surgical Infection Prevention					
Prophylactic Antibiotic Given[2,3]	144	86%	69%	77%	95%
Prophylactic Antibiotic Selection[2]	66	92%	79%	90%	100%
Prophylactic Antibiotic Stopped[2,3]	134	55%	61%	72%	95%
Pregnancy Care					
Inpatient Neonatal Mortality	-	-	-	-	-
Third or Fourth Degree Laceration	-	-	3.54%	3.63%	3.27%

University Medical Center

2390 W Congress Street
PO Box 69300
Lafayette, LA 70603
E-mail: ldorse1@lsuhsc.edu
URL: www.umcip.lsumc.edu
Ownership: Government - State
Emergency Services: Yes

Phone: 337-261-6000
Fax: 337-261-6660

Accredited: Yes
Licensed Beds: 208

Key Personnel:
President/CEO.........................Larry Dorsey
Chief Medical Staff....................James Falterman, MD
Cardiac Lab..........................Carolyn Pons
Catheterization Lab....................Elzie Cormier
Emergency Room......................Mary Menard
Infection Control......................Becky McNeese, RN
ICU...............................Laurence Vincent, RN
Medical/Surgical Nursing...............Mary Broussard, RN
OB/GYN Womens Health................Barbara Power, RN
Respiratory/Cardiopulmonary............Peggy Pennison

Measure	Cases	This Hospital	State Average	U.S. Average	Top Hospital
Heart Attack Care					
ACE Inhibitor or ARB for LVSD[1]	11	91%	84%	82%	100%
Aspirin at Arrival	45	100%	91%	92%	100%
Aspirin at Discharge	50	98%	87%	90%	100%
Beta Blocker at Arrival	33	97%	85%	87%	100%
Beta Blocker at Discharge	52	96%	88%	90%	100%
Fibrinolytic Medication Timing[1]	8	12%	32%	31%	100%
PCI Within 90 Minutes of Arrival[1]	1	0%	40%	54%	95%
Smoking Cessation Advice	33	88%	88%	88%	100%
Heart Failure Care					
ACE Inhibitor or ARB for LVSD	91	92%	78%	82%	100%
Discharge Instructions	151	23%	62%	61%	93%
Evaluation of LVS Function	152	95%	81%	83%	99%
Smoking Cessation Advice	69	75%	83%	82%	100%
Pneumonia Care					
Appropriate Initial Antibiotic	69	78%	78%	83%	94%
Blood Culture Timing	46	59%	89%	90%	100%
Influenza Vaccine[1]	10	10%	58%	70%	100%
Initial Antibiotic Timing	81	64%	76%	80%	93%
Oxygenation Assessment	90	99%	98%	99%	100%
Pneumococcal Vaccine[1]	7	14%	61%	69%	94%
Smoking Cessation Advice	49	73%	78%	80%	100%
Surgical Infection Prevention					
Prophylactic Antibiotic Given[3]	200	64%	69%	77%	95%
Prophylactic Antibiotic Selection	64	72%	79%	90%	100%
Prophylactic Antibiotic Stopped[3]	185	78%	61%	72%	95%
Pregnancy Care					
Inpatient Neonatal Mortality	466	1.29%	-	-	-
Third or Fourth Degree Laceration	310	3.23%	3.54%	3.63%	3.27%

Women's and Children's Hospital

Alternate Name: Womens Hospital of Acadiana
4600 Ambassador Caffery Parkway
Lafayette, LA 70508
URL: www.womens-childrens.com
Ownership: Proprietary
Emergency Services: Yes

Phone: 337-521-9100
Fax: 337-521-9102

Accredited: Yes
Licensed Beds: 157

Key Personnel:
CEO................................Kathy J Bobbs
Chief Medical Staff....................Susan Silverman

Measure	Cases	This Hospital	State Average	U.S. Average	Top Hospital
Heart Attack Care					
ACE Inhibitor or ARB for LVSD[5]	-	-	84%	82%	100%
Aspirin at Arrival[5]	-	-	91%	92%	100%
Aspirin at Discharge[5]	-	-	87%	90%	100%
Beta Blocker at Arrival[5]	-	-	85%	87%	100%
Beta Blocker at Discharge[5]	-	-	88%	90%	100%
Fibrinolytic Medication Timing[5]	-	-	32%	31%	100%
PCI Within 90 Minutes of Arrival[5]	-	-	40%	54%	95%
Smoking Cessation Advice[5]	-	-	88%	88%	100%
Heart Failure Care					
ACE Inhibitor or ARB for LVSD[5]	-	-	78%	82%	100%
Discharge Instructions[5]	-	-	62%	61%	93%
Evaluation of LVS Function[5]	-	-	81%	83%	99%
Smoking Cessation Advice[5]	-	-	83%	82%	100%
Pneumonia Care					
Appropriate Initial Antibiotic[1,3]	2	50%	78%	83%	94%
Blood Culture Timing[1,3]	1	100%	89%	90%	100%
Influenza Vaccine[5]	-	-	58%	70%	100%
Initial Antibiotic Timing[1,3]	1	0%	76%	80%	93%
Oxygenation Assessment[1,3]	2	100%	98%	99%	100%
Pneumococcal Vaccine[3]	0	-	61%	69%	94%
Smoking Cessation Advice[1,3]	2	50%	78%	80%	100%
Surgical Infection Prevention					
Prophylactic Antibiotic Given[3]	262	93%	69%	77%	95%
Prophylactic Antibiotic Selection[3]	85	86%	79%	90%	100%
Prophylactic Antibiotic Stopped[3]	260	86%	61%	72%	95%
Pregnancy Care					
Inpatient Neonatal Mortality	3,551	0.84%	-	-	-
Third or Fourth Degree Laceration	2,041	2.89%	3.54%	3.63%	3.27%

CHRISTUS Saint Patrick Hospital

524 S Ryan Street
Lake Charles, LA 70601
URL: www.stpatrickhospital.org
Ownership: Voluntary non-profit - Church
Emergency Services: Yes

Phone: 337-436-2511
Fax: 337-491-7157

Accredited: Yes
Licensed Beds: 290

Key Personnel:
President..............................Bernard Leger
CEO................................Ellen Jones
Chief Medical Staff....................Walter Divers, MD
Emergency Room......................Howard Rigg, MD
Infection Control Officer.................Carol Spence
Director Medical/Surgical Nursing..........Dorothy Corrigan
OB/GYN Womens Health.................Johnny Biddle, MD
Chief Radiology.......................John R Romero, III, DP
Manager Respiratory Therapy.............Debbie Glasepeal

Measure	Cases	This Hospital	State Average	U.S. Average	Top Hospital
Heart Attack Care					
ACE Inhibitor or ARB for LVSD	80	100%	84%	82%	100%
Aspirin at Arrival	177	100%	91%	92%	100%
Aspirin at Discharge	302	100%	87%	90%	100%
Beta Blocker at Arrival	159	100%	85%	87%	100%
Beta Blocker at Discharge	288	100%	88%	90%	100%
Fibrinolytic Medication Timing[1]	1	100%	32%	31%	100%
PCI Within 90 Minutes of Arrival[1]	13	85%	40%	54%	95%
Smoking Cessation Advice	131	100%	88%	88%	100%
Heart Failure Care					
ACE Inhibitor or ARB for LVSD	197	99%	78%	82%	100%
Discharge Instructions	358	92%	62%	61%	93%
Evaluation of LVS Function	400	100%	81%	83%	99%

NOTE: Hospital profiles are in alphabetical order by state, then city, then hospital within the city; Rankings are sorted by rate in descending order and exclude hospitals with less than 25 cases; (1) The number of cases is too small (n<25) for purposes of reliably predicting hospital performance; (2) Measure reflects the hospital's indication that its submission was based upon a sample of its relevant discharges; (3) Rate reflects fewer than the maximum possible quarters of data for the measure; (4) Inaccurate information submitted and suppressed for one or more quarters; (5) No data is available from the hospital for this measure; Please refer to the User's Guide for a full explanation of data

	80	95%	83%	82%	100%
Smoking Cessation Advice	80	95%	83%	82%	100%
Pneumonia Care					
Appropriate Initial Antibiotic	196	83%	78%	83%	94%
Blood Culture Timing	210	94%	89%	90%	100%
Influenza Vaccine	51	100%	58%	70%	100%
Initial Antibiotic Timing	256	91%	76%	80%	93%
Oxygenation Assessment	309	100%	98%	99%	100%
Pneumococcal Vaccine	184	100%	61%	69%	94%
Smoking Cessation Advice	70	100%	78%	80%	100%
Surgical Infection Prevention					
Prophylactic Antibiotic Given	438	76%	69%	77%	95%
Prophylactic Antibiotic Selection	122	61%	79%	90%	100%
Prophylactic Antibiotic Stopped	418	59%	61%	72%	95%
Pregnancy Care					
Inpatient Neonatal Mortality	-	-	-	-	-
Third or Fourth Degree Laceration	-	-	3.54%	3.63%	3.27%

Lake Charles Memorial Hospital

1701 Oak Park Boulevard
Lake Charles, LA 70601
URL: www.lcmh.com
Ownership: Voluntary non-profit - Other
Emergency Services: Yes

Phone: 337-494-3000
Fax: 337-494-3299

Accredited: Yes
Licensed Beds: 324

Key Personnel:
President . . . . Elton L Williams
Chief Medical Staff . . . . Alan LeBato, MD
Director Catheterization Laboratory . . . . Julia Yates, RN
CCU Spvg. Nurse . . . . Gerald Bryant, RN
Chief OB/GYN . . . . David Darbonne
Director Radiology . . . . Gene Lampson

Measure	Cases	This Hospital	State Average	U.S. Average	Top Hospital
Heart Attack Care					
ACE Inhibitor or ARB for LVSD	29	97%	84%	82%	100%
Aspirin at Arrival	75	99%	91%	92%	100%
Aspirin at Discharge	108	99%	87%	90%	100%
Beta Blocker at Arrival	56	95%	85%	87%	100%
Beta Blocker at Discharge	115	97%	88%	90%	100%
Fibrinolytic Medication Timing	0	-	32%	31%	100%
PCI Within 90 Minutes of Arrival[1]	4	50%	40%	54%	95%
Smoking Cessation Advice	51	100%	88%	88%	100%
Heart Failure Care					
ACE Inhibitor or ARB for LVSD	124	90%	78%	82%	100%
Discharge Instructions	220	92%	62%	61%	93%
Evaluation of LVS Function	240	99%	81%	83%	99%
Smoking Cessation Advice	61	100%	83%	82%	100%
Pneumonia Care					
Appropriate Initial Antibiotic	158	75%	78%	83%	94%
Blood Culture Timing	121	90%	89%	90%	100%
Influenza Vaccine[4,5]	-	-	58%	70%	100%
Initial Antibiotic Timing	243	73%	76%	80%	93%
Oxygenation Assessment	262	99%	98%	99%	100%
Pneumococcal Vaccine	156	87%	61%	69%	94%
Smoking Cessation Advice	57	100%	78%	80%	100%
Surgical Infection Prevention					
Prophylactic Antibiotic Given[3]	275	86%	69%	77%	95%
Prophylactic Antibiotic Selection	159	83%	79%	90%	100%
Prophylactic Antibiotic Stopped[3]	253	82%	61%	72%	95%
Pregnancy Care					
Inpatient Neonatal Mortality	-	-	-	-	-
Third or Fourth Degree Laceration	-	-	3.54%	3.63%	3.27%

W O Moss Regional Medical Center

Alternate Name: Walter Olin Moss Regional Hospital
1000 Walters Street
Lake Charles, LA 70607
Ownership: Government - State
Emergency Services: Yes

Phone: 337-475-8100
Fax: 337-475-8104
Accredited: No
Licensed Beds: 108

Key Personnel:
Administrator . . . . Patrick Robinson, MD
Chief Medical Staff . . . . Patrick Robinson, MD
Emergency Room . . . . Eulogio Tan, MD
Director Infection/Disease Control . . . . Rhonda Sullivan, RN

CCU Spvg. Nurse . . . . Chad Higginbotham, RN
Director Medical/Surgical Nursing . . . . Ginger Holmes, RN
OB/GYN Womens Health . . . . Ben Darby, MD
Director of Pulmonary/Respiratory Care . . . . Lana Gammage

Measure	Cases	This Hospital	State Average	U.S. Average	Top Hospital
Heart Attack Care					
ACE Inhibitor or ARB for LVSD[3]	0	-	84%	82%	100%
Aspirin at Arrival[1,3]	1	100%	91%	92%	100%
Aspirin at Discharge[3]	0	-	87%	90%	100%
Beta Blocker at Arrival[1,3]	1	100%	85%	87%	100%
Beta Blocker at Discharge[3]	0	-	88%	90%	100%
Fibrinolytic Medication Timing[3]	0	-	32%	31%	100%
PCI Within 90 Minutes of Arrival	0	-	40%	54%	95%
Smoking Cessation Advice[3]	0	-	88%	88%	100%
Heart Failure Care					
ACE Inhibitor or ARB for LVSD[1]	18	89%	78%	82%	100%
Discharge Instructions	31	48%	62%	61%	93%
Evaluation of LVS Function	31	100%	81%	83%	99%
Smoking Cessation Advice[1]	11	64%	83%	82%	100%
Pneumonia Care					
Appropriate Initial Antibiotic[1]	15	100%	78%	83%	94%
Blood Culture Timing[1]	8	50%	89%	90%	100%
Influenza Vaccine[1]	2	0%	58%	70%	100%
Initial Antibiotic Timing[1]	14	93%	76%	80%	93%
Oxygenation Assessment[1]	16	100%	98%	99%	100%
Pneumococcal Vaccine[1]	1	0%	61%	69%	94%
Smoking Cessation Advice[1]	4	25%	78%	80%	100%
Surgical Infection Prevention					
Prophylactic Antibiotic Given	89	83%	69%	77%	95%
Prophylactic Antibiotic Selection	25	100%	79%	90%	100%
Prophylactic Antibiotic Stopped	87	56%	61%	72%	95%
Pregnancy Care					
Inpatient Neonatal Mortality	-	-	-	-	-
Third or Fourth Degree Laceration	-	-	3.54%	3.63%	3.27%

Women and Children's Hospital

Alternate Name: Lake Area Medical Center
4200 Nelson Road
Lake Charles, LA 70605
E-mail: info@women-childrens.com
URL: www.women-childrens.com
Ownership: Proprietary
Emergency Services: Yes

Phone: 337-474-6370
Fax: 337-475-4143

Accredited: Yes
Licensed Beds: 80

Key Personnel:
CEO . . . . Bill Willis
Chief Medical Staff . . . . Jim Jancuska
Infection Control . . . . Sissy Horn, RN
ICU . . . . Donna Mead, RN
Director OB/GYN . . . . Stanley Kordisch, MD
Director of Pulmonary/Respiratory Care . . . . Tammy Six

Measure	Cases	This Hospital	State Average	U.S. Average	Top Hospital
Heart Attack Care					
ACE Inhibitor or ARB for LVSD[3]	0	-	84%	82%	100%
Aspirin at Arrival[1,3]	1	100%	91%	92%	100%
Aspirin at Discharge[1,3]	1	100%	87%	90%	100%
Beta Blocker at Arrival[1,3]	2	100%	85%	87%	100%
Beta Blocker at Discharge[1,3]	1	100%	88%	90%	100%
Fibrinolytic Medication Timing[3]	0	-	32%	31%	100%
PCI Within 90 Minutes of Arrival[5]	-	-	40%	54%	95%
Smoking Cessation Advice[3]	0	-	88%	88%	100%
Heart Failure Care					
ACE Inhibitor or ARB for LVSD[1]	6	83%	78%	82%	100%
Discharge Instructions[1]	14	100%	62%	61%	93%
Evaluation of LVS Function[1]	14	100%	81%	83%	99%
Smoking Cessation Advice[1]	4	100%	83%	82%	100%
Pneumonia Care					
Appropriate Initial Antibiotic[1]	22	100%	78%	83%	94%
Blood Culture Timing[1]	12	100%	89%	90%	100%
Influenza Vaccine[1]	6	0%	58%	70%	100%
Initial Antibiotic Timing	30	83%	76%	80%	93%

NOTE: Hospital profiles are in alphabetical order by state, then city, then hospital within the city; Rankings are sorted by rate in descending order and exclude hospitals with less than 25 cases; (1) The number of cases is too small (n<25) for purposes of reliably predicting hospital performance; (2) Measure reflects the hospital's indication that its submission was based upon a sample of its relevant discharges; (3) Rate reflects fewer than the maximum possible quarters of data for the measure; (4) Inaccurate information submitted and suppressed for one or more quarters; (5) No data is available from the hospital for this measure; Please refer to the User's Guide for a full explanation of data

Oxygenation Assessment	33	97%	98%	99%	100%
Pneumococcal Vaccine[1]	12	83%	61%	69%	94%
Smoking Cessation Advice[1]	12	92%	78%	80%	100%
Surgical Infection Prevention					
Prophylactic Antibiotic Given	326	87%	69%	77%	95%
Prophylactic Antibiotic Selection	104	91%	79%	90%	100%
Prophylactic Antibiotic Stopped	322	86%	61%	72%	95%
Pregnancy Care					
Inpatient Neonatal Mortality	1,818	0.66%	-	-	-
Third or Fourth Degree Laceration	1,082	2.50%	3.54%	3.63%	3.27%

East Carroll Parish Hospital

226 N Hood Street
Lake Providence, LA 71254
Ownership: Govt - Hospital District or Authority
Emergency Services: Yes
Key Personnel:
Administrator/CEO . . . . LaDonna Englerth
Chief Medical Staff . . . . Don Bailey
Director Infection/Disease Control . . . . Francis Jordan

Phone: 318-559-4023
Fax: 318-559-3761
Accredited: No
Licensed Beds: 29

Measure	Cases	This Hospital	State Average	U.S. Average	Top Hospital
Heart Attack Care					
ACE Inhibitor or ARB for LVSD[3]	0	-	84%	82%	100%
Aspirin at Arrival[3]	0	-	91%	92%	100%
Aspirin at Discharge[3]	0	-	87%	90%	100%
Beta Blocker at Arrival[3]	0	-	85%	87%	100%
Beta Blocker at Discharge[3]	0	-	88%	90%	100%
Fibrinolytic Medication Timing[5]	-	-	32%	31%	100%
PCI Within 90 Minutes of Arrival[5]	-	-	40%	54%	95%
Smoking Cessation Advice[5]	-	-	88%	88%	100%
Heart Failure Care					
ACE Inhibitor or ARB for LVSD	0	-	78%	82%	100%
Discharge Instructions[1,3]	10	0%	62%	61%	93%
Evaluation of LVS Function	65	0%	81%	83%	99%
Smoking Cessation Advice[1,3]	4	25%	83%	82%	100%
Pneumonia Care					
Appropriate Initial Antibiotic[1,3]	3	100%	78%	83%	94%
Blood Culture Timing[3]	0	-	89%	90%	100%
Influenza Vaccine[4,5]	-	-	58%	70%	100%
Initial Antibiotic Timing	33	94%	76%	80%	93%
Oxygenation Assessment	35	100%	98%	99%	100%
Pneumococcal Vaccine[1]	14	0%	61%	69%	94%
Smoking Cessation Advice[3]	0	-	78%	80%	100%
Surgical Infection Prevention					
Prophylactic Antibiotic Given[5]	-	-	69%	77%	95%
Prophylactic Antibiotic Selection[5]	-	-	79%	90%	100%
Prophylactic Antibiotic Stopped[5]	-	-	61%	72%	95%
Pregnancy Care					
Inpatient Neonatal Mortality	-	-	-	-	-
Third or Fourth Degree Laceration	-	-	3.54%	3.63%	3.27%

River Parishes Hospital

Alternate Name: River Parishes Medical Center
500 Rue De Sante
La Place, LA 70068
URL: www.riverparisheshospital.com
Ownership: Proprietary
Emergency Services: Yes
Key Personnel:
Administrator/CEO . . . . Scott Boudreaux

Phone: 985-652-7000
Fax: 985-652-5161

Accredited: Yes
Licensed Beds: 102

Measure	Cases	This Hospital	State Average	U.S. Average	Top Hospital
Heart Attack Care					
ACE Inhibitor or ARB for LVSD[1]	6	83%	84%	82%	100%
Aspirin at Arrival	30	97%	91%	92%	100%
Aspirin at Discharge[1]	23	87%	87%	90%	100%
Beta Blocker at Arrival[1]	24	83%	85%	87%	100%
Beta Blocker at Discharge[1]	22	82%	88%	90%	100%
Fibrinolytic Medication Timing[1]	3	33%	32%	31%	100%
PCI Within 90 Minutes of Arrival	0	-	40%	54%	95%
Smoking Cessation Advice[1]	7	100%	88%	88%	100%

Measure	Cases	This Hospital	State Average	U.S. Average	Top Hospital
Heart Failure Care					
ACE Inhibitor or ARB for LVSD	72	86%	78%	82%	100%
Discharge Instructions	179	87%	62%	61%	93%
Evaluation of LVS Function	196	93%	81%	83%	99%
Smoking Cessation Advice	54	100%	83%	82%	100%
Pneumonia Care					
Appropriate Initial Antibiotic	49	82%	78%	83%	94%
Blood Culture Timing	34	97%	89%	90%	100%
Influenza Vaccine[1]	11	45%	58%	70%	100%
Initial Antibiotic Timing	62	77%	76%	80%	93%
Oxygenation Assessment	74	97%	98%	99%	100%
Pneumococcal Vaccine	39	54%	61%	69%	94%
Smoking Cessation Advice	28	93%	78%	80%	100%
Surgical Infection Prevention					
Prophylactic Antibiotic Given[2,3]	98	74%	69%	77%	95%
Prophylactic Antibiotic Selection[2]	34	82%	79%	90%	100%
Prophylactic Antibiotic Stopped[2,3]	97	81%	61%	72%	95%
Pregnancy Care					
Inpatient Neonatal Mortality	-	-	-	-	-
Third or Fourth Degree Laceration	-	-	3.54%	3.63%	3.27%

Byrd Regional Hospital

1020 Fertitta Boulevard
Leesville, LA 71446
E-mail: lmaricle@hq.chs.net
URL: www.byrdregional.com
Ownership: Proprietary
Emergency Services: Yes
Key Personnel:
CEO . . . . Roger LeDoux
Chief Medical Staff . . . . Reymond Meadan, MD
Catheterization Lab . . . . Sherri Bennett
Emergency Room . . . . Angelika Dixon, RN
Infection Control . . . . Sherry Bennett, RN
ICU . . . . Angelika Dixon, RN
OB/GYN Women's Health . . . . Cindy Andries, RN
Director Radiology . . . . Gord Hessie
Respiratory/Cardiopulmonary . . . . Charissa Cart, RRT

Phone: 337-239-9041
Fax: 337-239-5360

Accredited: Yes
Licensed Beds: 60

Measure	Cases	This Hospital	State Average	U.S. Average	Top Hospital
Heart Attack Care					
ACE Inhibitor or ARB for LVSD[1]	5	100%	84%	82%	100%
Aspirin at Arrival	25	88%	91%	92%	100%
Aspirin at Discharge[1]	11	82%	87%	90%	100%
Beta Blocker at Arrival	26	92%	85%	87%	100%
Beta Blocker at Discharge[1]	14	86%	88%	90%	100%
Fibrinolytic Medication Timing[1]	8	38%	32%	31%	100%
PCI Within 90 Minutes of Arrival	0	-	40%	54%	95%
Smoking Cessation Advice[1]	5	100%	88%	88%	100%
Heart Failure Care					
ACE Inhibitor or ARB for LVSD	58	83%	78%	82%	100%
Discharge Instructions	145	47%	62%	61%	93%
Evaluation of LVS Function	166	86%	81%	83%	99%
Smoking Cessation Advice	54	96%	83%	82%	100%
Pneumonia Care					
Appropriate Initial Antibiotic	134	84%	78%	83%	94%
Blood Culture Timing	83	90%	89%	90%	100%
Influenza Vaccine	42	62%	58%	70%	100%
Initial Antibiotic Timing	196	83%	76%	80%	93%
Oxygenation Assessment	235	100%	98%	99%	100%
Pneumococcal Vaccine	116	72%	61%	69%	94%
Smoking Cessation Advice	69	100%	78%	80%	100%
Surgical Infection Prevention					
Prophylactic Antibiotic Given[2,3]	87	40%	69%	77%	95%
Prophylactic Antibiotic Selection[2]	29	83%	79%	90%	100%
Prophylactic Antibiotic Stopped[2,3]	66	36%	61%	72%	95%
Pregnancy Care					
Inpatient Neonatal Mortality	-	-	-	-	-
Third or Fourth Degree Laceration	-	-	3.54%	3.63%	3.27%

NOTE: Hospital profiles are in alphabetical order by state, then city, then hospital within the city; Rankings are sorted by rate in descending order and exclude hospitals with less than 25 cases; (1) The number of cases is too small (n<25) for purposes of reliably predicting hospital performance; (2) Measure reflects the hospital's indication that its submission was based upon a sample of its relevant discharges; (3) Rate reflects fewer than the maximum possible quarters of data for the measure; (4) Inaccurate information submitted and suppressed for one or more quarters; (5) No data is available from the hospital for this measure; Please refer to the User's Guide for a full explanation of data

Saint Charles Parish Hospital

1057 Paul Maillard Road
Luling, LA 70070
URL: www.stch.net
Ownership: Govt - Hospital District or Authority   Accredited: Yes
Emergency Services: Yes

Phone: 985-785-6242
Fax: 985-785-3642

Key Personnel:

CEO. . . . . Fred Martinez, Jr
Chief Medical Staff. . . . . Martin Belanger
Emergency Room . . . . Mitzi Tregre
Infection Control. Donna Bologna
Respiratory/Cardiopulmonary. . . . . Doug McIntrye

Measure	Cases	This Hospital	State Average	U.S. Average	Top Hospital
Heart Attack Care					
ACE Inhibitor or ARB for LVSD[1]	5	100%	84%	82%	100%
Aspirin at Arrival[1]	21	86%	91%	92%	100%
Aspirin at Discharge[1]	14	100%	87%	90%	100%
Beta Blocker at Arrival[1]	20	80%	85%	87%	100%
Beta Blocker at Discharge[1]	16	81%	88%	90%	100%
Fibrinolytic Medication Timing[3]	0	-	32%	31%	100%
PCI Within 90 Minutes of Arrival	0	-	40%	54%	95%
Smoking Cessation Advice[3]	0	-	88%	88%	100%
Heart Failure Care					
ACE Inhibitor or ARB for LVSD	51	100%	78%	82%	100%
Discharge Instructions[1,3]	15	80%	62%	61%	93%
Evaluation of LVS Function	114	99%	81%	83%	99%
Smoking Cessation Advice[1,3]	2	100%	83%	82%	100%
Pneumonia Care					
Appropriate Initial Antibiotic[1,3]	9	56%	78%	83%	94%
Blood Culture Timing[1,3]	8	75%	89%	90%	100%
Influenza Vaccine[5]	-	-	58%	70%	100%
Initial Antibiotic Timing	63	78%	76%	80%	93%
Oxygenation Assessment	71	100%	98%	99%	100%
Pneumococcal Vaccine	42	31%	61%	69%	94%
Smoking Cessation Advice[1,3]	3	100%	78%	80%	100%
Surgical Infection Prevention					
Prophylactic Antibiotic Given[1,3]	3	100%	69%	77%	95%
Prophylactic Antibiotic Selection[5]	-	-	79%	90%	100%
Prophylactic Antibiotic Stopped[1,3]	2	50%	61%	72%	95%
Pregnancy Care					
Inpatient Neonatal Mortality	-	-	-	-	-
Third or Fourth Degree Laceration	-	-	3.54%	3.63%	3.27%

Savoy Medical Center

801 Poinciana Avenue
Mamou, LA 70554
URL: www.savoymedical.com
Ownership: Proprietary
Emergency Services: Yes

Phone: 337-468-5261
Fax: 337-468-3342

Accredited: Yes
Licensed Beds: 205

Key Personnel:

Administrator/CEO. . . . . Gerald A Fosnoff
Emergency Room Director. . . . . Vickie Sagg
ICU Director. . . . . Vickie Sagg

Measure	Cases	This Hospital	State Average	U.S. Average	Top Hospital
Heart Attack Care					
ACE Inhibitor or ARB for LVSD[1]	2	100%	84%	82%	100%
Aspirin at Arrival[1]	9	89%	91%	92%	100%
Aspirin at Discharge[1]	5	80%	87%	90%	100%
Beta Blocker at Arrival[1]	8	88%	85%	87%	100%
Beta Blocker at Discharge[1]	4	75%	88%	90%	100%
Fibrinolytic Medication Timing[1]	1	100%	32%	31%	100%
PCI Within 90 Minutes of Arrival	0	-	40%	54%	95%
Smoking Cessation Advice[1]	2	100%	88%	88%	100%
Heart Failure Care					
ACE Inhibitor or ARB for LVSD	44	61%	78%	82%	100%
Discharge Instructions	86	56%	62%	61%	93%
Evaluation of LVS Function	112	71%	81%	83%	99%
Smoking Cessation Advice	29	93%	83%	82%	100%
Pneumonia Care					
Appropriate Initial Antibiotic	45	82%	78%	83%	94%
Blood Culture Timing	76	100%	89%	90%	100%

Measure	Cases	This Hospital	State Average	U.S. Average	Top Hospital
Influenza Vaccine[1]	21	52%	58%	70%	100%
Initial Antibiotic Timing	109	90%	76%	80%	93%
Oxygenation Assessment	132	98%	98%	99%	100%
Pneumococcal Vaccine	79	66%	61%	69%	94%
Smoking Cessation Advice	37	92%	78%	80%	100%
Surgical Infection Prevention					
Prophylactic Antibiotic Given[2,3]	66	79%	69%	77%	95%
Prophylactic Antibiotic Selection[1,2]	21	86%	79%	90%	100%
Prophylactic Antibiotic Stopped[2,3]	64	47%	61%	72%	95%
Pregnancy Care					
Inpatient Neonatal Mortality	359	0.28%	-	-	-
Third or Fourth Degree Laceration	194	0.52%	3.54%	3.63%	3.27%

DeSoto Regional Health System

Alternate Name: De Soto General Hospital
207 Jefferson Street
Mansfield, LA 71052
E-mail: lhishaw@bellsouth.net
URL: www.desotoregional.com
Ownership: Proprietary
Emergency Services: Yes

Phone: 318-872-4610
Fax: 318-872-1502

Accredited: No
Licensed Beds: 57

Key Personnel:

Administrator/CEO. . . . . Scott Stafford
Chief of Medical Staff. Leigh Dillard, MD
Emergency Room . . . . Nell Norwood
Respiratory Care . . . . Lynn Martin

Measure	Cases	This Hospital	State Average	U.S. Average	Top Hospital
Heart Attack Care					
ACE Inhibitor or ARB for LVSD[1,3]	2	100%	84%	82%	100%
Aspirin at Arrival[1,3]	8	50%	91%	92%	100%
Aspirin at Discharge[1,3]	5	0%	87%	90%	100%
Beta Blocker at Arrival[1,3]	6	67%	85%	87%	100%
Beta Blocker at Discharge[1,3]	4	50%	88%	90%	100%
Fibrinolytic Medication Timing[1,3]	1	0%	32%	31%	100%
PCI Within 90 Minutes of Arrival	0	-	40%	54%	95%
Smoking Cessation Advice[1,3]	1	0%	88%	88%	100%
Heart Failure Care					
ACE Inhibitor or ARB for LVSD[1,3]	22	86%	78%	82%	100%
Discharge Instructions[3]	44	7%	62%	61%	93%
Evaluation of LVS Function[3]	68	65%	81%	83%	99%
Smoking Cessation Advice[1,3]	14	14%	83%	82%	100%
Pneumonia Care					
Appropriate Initial Antibiotic[3]	48	67%	78%	83%	94%
Blood Culture Timing[1,3]	16	81%	89%	90%	100%
Influenza Vaccine[5]	-	-	58%	70%	100%
Initial Antibiotic Timing[3]	42	55%	76%	80%	93%
Oxygenation Assessment[3]	56	98%	98%	99%	100%
Pneumococcal Vaccine[3]	35	54%	61%	69%	94%
Smoking Cessation Advice[1,3]	9	22%	78%	80%	100%
Surgical Infection Prevention					
Prophylactic Antibiotic Given[3]	0	-	69%	77%	95%
Prophylactic Antibiotic Selection	0	-	79%	90%	100%
Prophylactic Antibiotic Stopped[3]	0	-	61%	72%	95%
Pregnancy Care					
Inpatient Neonatal Mortality	-	-	-	-	-
Third or Fourth Degree Laceration	-	-	3.54%	3.63%	3.27%

Sabine Medical Center

240 Highland Drive
Many, LA 71449
Ownership: Proprietary
Emergency Services: Yes

Phone: 318-256-5691
Fax: 318-256-7540
Accredited: Yes
Licensed Beds: 44

Key Personnel:

Administrator/CEO. . . . . Patrick Gandy
Chief Medical Staff. Jack Corley, MD

Measure	Cases	This Hospital	State Average	U.S. Average	Top Hospital
Heart Attack Care					
ACE Inhibitor or ARB for LVSD[1]	2	100%	84%	82%	100%
Aspirin at Arrival[1]	24	71%	91%	92%	100%
Aspirin at Discharge[1]	16	75%	87%	90%	100%

NOTE: Hospital profiles are in alphabetical order by state, then city, then hospital within the city; Rankings are sorted by rate in descending order and exclude hospitals with less than 25 cases; (1) The number of cases is too small (n<25) for purposes of reliably predicting hospital performance; (2) Measure reflects the hospital's indication that its submission was based upon a sample of its relevant discharges; (3) Rate reflects fewer than the maximum possible quarters of data for the measure; (4) Inaccurate information submitted and suppressed for one or more quarters; (5) No data is available from the hospital for this measure; Please refer to the User's Guide for a full explanation of data

Measure	Cases	This Hospital	State Average	U.S. Average	Top Hospital
Beta Blocker at Arrival[1]	14	57%	85%	87%	100%
Beta Blocker at Discharge[1]	14	93%	88%	90%	100%
Fibrinolytic Medication Timing	0	-	32%	31%	100%
PCI Within 90 Minutes of Arrival	0	-	40%	54%	95%
Smoking Cessation Advice[1]	3	67%	88%	88%	100%
Heart Failure Care					
ACE Inhibitor or ARB for LVSD[1]	14	79%	78%	82%	100%
Discharge Instructions	67	82%	62%	61%	93%
Evaluation of LVS Function	101	49%	81%	83%	99%
Smoking Cessation Advice	25	88%	83%	82%	100%
Pneumonia Care					
Appropriate Initial Antibiotic	38	50%	78%	83%	94%
Blood Culture Timing[1]	22	91%	89%	90%	100%
Influenza Vaccine[1]	11	91%	58%	70%	100%
Initial Antibiotic Timing	63	89%	76%	80%	93%
Oxygenation Assessment	78	100%	98%	99%	100%
Pneumococcal Vaccine	55	84%	61%	69%	94%
Smoking Cessation Advice[1]	11	91%	78%	80%	100%
Surgical Infection Prevention					
Prophylactic Antibiotic Given[1,3]	6	50%	69%	77%	95%
Prophylactic Antibiotic Selection[1]	1	0%	79%	90%	100%
Prophylactic Antibiotic Stopped[1,3]	5	100%	61%	72%	95%
Pregnancy Care					
Inpatient Neonatal Mortality	-	-	-	-	-
Third or Fourth Degree Laceration	-	-	3.54%	3.63%	3.27%

Avoyelles Hospital

4231 Highway 1192
PO Box 249
Marksville, LA 71351
URL: www.avoyelleshospital.com
Ownership: Proprietary
Emergency Services: Yes

Phone: 318-253-8611
Fax: 318-240-6077

Accredited: Yes
Licensed Beds: 55

Key Personnel:
CEO . . . . David M Mitchel
Chief Medical Staff . . . . Allen McClure, MD
Emergency Room . . . . Cheryl Moreau, RN
Infection Control . . . . Jeanie Tessin
ICU . . . . Donna Foret
Medical/Surgical Nursing . . . . Elizabeth Mire
Respiratory/Cardiopulmonary . . . . Billy Tingle

Measure	Cases	This Hospital	State Average	U.S. Average	Top Hospital
Heart Attack Care					
ACE Inhibitor or ARB for LVSD[3]	0	-	84%	82%	100%
Aspirin at Arrival[1,3]	2	50%	91%	92%	100%
Aspirin at Discharge[1,3]	2	100%	87%	90%	100%
Beta Blocker at Arrival[3]	0	-	85%	87%	100%
Beta Blocker at Discharge[1,3]	2	0%	88%	90%	100%
Fibrinolytic Medication Timing[3]	0	-	32%	31%	100%
PCI Within 90 Minutes of Arrival	0	-	40%	54%	95%
Smoking Cessation Advice[3]	0	-	88%	88%	100%
Heart Failure Care					
ACE Inhibitor or ARB for LVSD[1]	24	88%	78%	82%	100%
Discharge Instructions	74	80%	62%	61%	93%
Evaluation of LVS Function	112	89%	81%	83%	99%
Smoking Cessation Advice	26	81%	83%	82%	100%
Pneumonia Care					
Appropriate Initial Antibiotic	46	91%	78%	83%	94%
Blood Culture Timing	68	94%	89%	90%	100%
Influenza Vaccine[1]	21	57%	58%	70%	100%
Initial Antibiotic Timing	94	93%	76%	80%	93%
Oxygenation Assessment	121	100%	98%	99%	100%
Pneumococcal Vaccine	79	68%	61%	69%	94%
Smoking Cessation Advice[1]	19	74%	78%	80%	100%
Surgical Infection Prevention					
Prophylactic Antibiotic Given[1,2,3]	2	100%	69%	77%	95%
Prophylactic Antibiotic Selection[5]	-	-	79%	90%	100%
Prophylactic Antibiotic Stopped[1,2,3]	2	0%	61%	72%	95%
Pregnancy Care					
Inpatient Neonatal Mortality	-	-	-	-	-
Third or Fourth Degree Laceration	-	-	3.54%	3.63%	3.27%

West Jefferson Medical Center

1101 Medical Center Boulevard
Marrero, LA 70072
URL: www.wjmc.org
Ownership: Govt - Hospital District or Authority
Emergency Services: Yes

Phone: 504-347-5511
Fax: 504-349-6299

Accredited: Yes
Licensed Beds: 462

Key Personnel:
President/CEO . . . . A Gary Muller, FACHE
Chief Medical Officer . . . . Alferd Abaunza
Emergency Room . . . . Robert Chugden, MD
ER Coordinator . . . . Connie Revelsn, RN
Infection Control . . . . Teri Bergeron
ICU . . . . Juanita Farris, RN
Intensive Coronary . . . . Juanita Farris, RN
Med/Surg Nursing . . . . Pat Judd, RN
Chairman Dept of Obstetrics/Gynecology . . . . . Juan Labadie, MD
Chief Radiology . . . . Jimmie Mains, MD
Respiratory/Cardiopulmonary . . . . Rebecca Vidrine

Measure	Cases	This Hospital	State Average	U.S. Average	Top Hospital
Heart Attack Care					
ACE Inhibitor or ARB for LVSD	80	76%	84%	82%	100%
Aspirin at Arrival	279	96%	91%	92%	100%
Aspirin at Discharge	260	94%	87%	90%	100%
Beta Blocker at Arrival	243	96%	85%	87%	100%
Beta Blocker at Discharge	265	97%	88%	90%	100%
Fibrinolytic Medication Timing[1]	1	0%	32%	31%	100%
PCI Within 90 Minutes of Arrival[1]	6	17%	40%	54%	95%
Smoking Cessation Advice	112	95%	88%	88%	100%
Heart Failure Care					
ACE Inhibitor or ARB for LVSD	335	72%	78%	82%	100%
Discharge Instructions	578	35%	62%	61%	93%
Evaluation of LVS Function	675	91%	81%	83%	99%
Smoking Cessation Advice	193	85%	83%	82%	100%
Pneumonia Care					
Appropriate Initial Antibiotic	169	80%	78%	83%	94%
Blood Culture Timing	123	83%	89%	90%	100%
Influenza Vaccine	31	42%	58%	70%	100%
Initial Antibiotic Timing	191	55%	76%	80%	93%
Oxygenation Assessment	230	98%	98%	99%	100%
Pneumococcal Vaccine	93	29%	61%	69%	94%
Smoking Cessation Advice	79	82%	78%	80%	100%
Surgical Infection Prevention					
Prophylactic Antibiotic Given[2,3]	328	57%	69%	77%	95%
Prophylactic Antibiotic Selection[2]	158	74%	79%	90%	100%
Prophylactic Antibiotic Stopped[2,3]	304	57%	61%	72%	95%
Pregnancy Care					
Inpatient Neonatal Mortality	-	-	-	-	-
Third or Fourth Degree Laceration	-	-	3.54%	3.63%	3.27%

East Jefferson General Hospital

4200 Houma Boulevard
Metairie, LA 70006
URL: www.EastJeffHospital.org
Ownership: Govt - Hospital District or Authority
Emergency Services: Yes

Phone: 504-454-5655
Fax: 504-889-7114

Accredited: Yes
Licensed Beds: 448

Key Personnel:
Administrator/CEO . . . . Mark Peters
Chief Radiology . . . . Floyd Scales, MD
Director Respiratory Therapy . . . . Audie Hymel
VP Surgical Services . . . . Judy Bauer

Measure	Cases	This Hospital	State Average	U.S. Average	Top Hospital
Heart Attack Care					
ACE Inhibitor or ARB for LVSD[2]	48	77%	84%	82%	100%
Aspirin at Arrival[2]	264	96%	91%	92%	100%
Aspirin at Discharge[2]	254	92%	87%	90%	100%
Beta Blocker at Arrival[2]	240	96%	85%	87%	100%
Beta Blocker at Discharge[2]	262	93%	88%	90%	100%
Fibrinolytic Medication Timing[2]	0	-	32%	31%	100%
PCI Within 90 Minutes of Arrival[1,2]	18	28%	40%	54%	95%
Smoking Cessation Advice[2]	96	95%	88%	88%	100%
Heart Failure Care					

NOTE: Hospital profiles are in alphabetical order by state, then city, then hospital within the city; Rankings are sorted by rate in descending order and exclude hospitals with less than 25 cases; (1) The number of cases is too small (n<25) for purposes of reliably predicting hospital performance; (2) Measure reflects the hospital's indication that its submission was based upon a sample of its relevant discharges; (3) Rate reflects fewer than the maximum possible quarters of data for the measure; (4) Inaccurate information submitted and suppressed for one or more quarters; (5) No data is available from the hospital for this measure; Please refer to the User's Guide for a full explanation of data

Measure	Cases	This Hospital	State Average	U.S. Average	Top Hospital
ACE Inhibitor or ARB for LVSD[2]	106	79%	78%	82%	100%
Discharge Instructions[2]	234	51%	62%	61%	93%
Evaluation of LVS Function[2]	284	88%	81%	83%	99%
Smoking Cessation Advice[2]	44	91%	83%	82%	100%
Pneumonia Care					
Appropriate Initial Antibiotic[2]	100	76%	78%	83%	94%
Blood Culture Timing[2]	92	91%	89%	90%	100%
Influenza Vaccine	30	40%	58%	70%	100%
Initial Antibiotic Timing[2]	144	68%	76%	80%	93%
Oxygenation Assessment[2]	178	96%	98%	99%	100%
Pneumococcal Vaccine[2]	113	40%	61%	69%	94%
Smoking Cessation Advice[2]	41	78%	78%	80%	100%
Surgical Infection Prevention					
Prophylactic Antibiotic Given[2,3]	215	78%	69%	77%	95%
Prophylactic Antibiotic Selection[2]	74	81%	79%	90%	100%
Prophylactic Antibiotic Stopped[2,3]	203	42%	61%	72%	95%
Pregnancy Care					
Inpatient Neonatal Mortality	-	-	-	-	-
Third or Fourth Degree Laceration	-	-	3.54%	3.63%	3.27%

Community Specialty Hosp of N Louisiana

108 Meadowbrook   Phone: 318-377-5555
Minden, LA 71055
Ownership: Government - Federal   Accredited: No
Emergency Services: Yes

Measure	Cases	This Hospital	State Average	U.S. Average	Top Hospital
Heart Attack Care					
ACE Inhibitor or ARB for LVSD[5]	-	-	84%	82%	100%
Aspirin at Arrival[5]	-	-	91%	92%	100%
Aspirin at Discharge[5]	-	-	87%	90%	100%
Beta Blocker at Arrival[5]	-	-	85%	87%	100%
Beta Blocker at Discharge[5]	-	-	88%	90%	100%
Fibrinolytic Medication Timing[5]	-	-	32%	31%	100%
PCI Within 90 Minutes of Arrival[5]	-	-	40%	54%	95%
Smoking Cessation Advice[5]	-	-	88%	88%	100%
Heart Failure Care					
ACE Inhibitor or ARB for LVSD[5]	-	-	78%	82%	100%
Discharge Instructions[5]	-	-	62%	61%	93%
Evaluation of LVS Function[5]	-	-	81%	83%	99%
Smoking Cessation Advice[5]	-	-	83%	82%	100%
Pneumonia Care					
Appropriate Initial Antibiotic[5]	-	-	78%	83%	94%
Blood Culture Timing[5]	-	-	89%	90%	100%
Influenza Vaccine[5]	-	-	58%	70%	100%
Initial Antibiotic Timing[5]	-	-	76%	80%	93%
Oxygenation Assessment[5]	-	-	98%	99%	100%
Pneumococcal Vaccine[5]	-	-	61%	69%	94%
Smoking Cessation Advice[5]	-	-	78%	80%	100%
Surgical Infection Prevention					
Prophylactic Antibiotic Given[5]	-	-	69%	77%	95%
Prophylactic Antibiotic Selection[5]	-	-	79%	90%	100%
Prophylactic Antibiotic Stopped[5]	-	-	61%	72%	95%
Pregnancy Care					
Inpatient Neonatal Mortality	-	-	-	-	-
Third or Fourth Degree Laceration	-	-	3.54%	3.63%	3.27%

Minden Medical Center

1 Medical Plaza   Phone: 318-377-2321
Minden, LA 71055   Fax: 318-371-5606
URL: www.mindenmedicalcenter.com
Ownership: Proprietary   Accredited: Yes
Emergency Services: Yes   Licensed Beds: 159
Key Personnel:
CEO . . . . George E French, III
Chief Medical Staff . . . . James O Hudson
Director Respiratory Therapy . . . . Cynthia Williams

Measure	Cases	This Hospital	State Average	U.S. Average	Top Hospital
Heart Attack Care					
ACE Inhibitor or ARB for LVSD[1]	6	100%	84%	82%	100%
Aspirin at Arrival	27	96%	91%	92%	100%

Measure	Cases	This Hospital	State Average	U.S. Average	Top Hospital
Aspirin at Discharge[1]	21	100%	87%	90%	100%
Beta Blocker at Arrival[1]	20	95%	85%	87%	100%
Beta Blocker at Discharge[1]	19	100%	88%	90%	100%
Fibrinolytic Medication Timing[1]	1	0%	32%	31%	100%
PCI Within 90 Minutes of Arrival[1]	1	100%	40%	54%	95%
Smoking Cessation Advice[1]	3	100%	88%	88%	100%
Heart Failure Care					
ACE Inhibitor or ARB for LVSD	63	87%	78%	82%	100%
Discharge Instructions	137	99%	62%	61%	93%
Evaluation of LVS Function	180	94%	81%	83%	99%
Smoking Cessation Advice	32	100%	83%	82%	100%
Pneumonia Care					
Appropriate Initial Antibiotic	63	83%	78%	83%	94%
Blood Culture Timing	66	95%	89%	90%	100%
Influenza Vaccine	27	93%	58%	70%	100%
Initial Antibiotic Timing	137	80%	76%	80%	93%
Oxygenation Assessment	177	100%	98%	99%	100%
Pneumococcal Vaccine	100	89%	61%	69%	94%
Smoking Cessation Advice	39	100%	78%	80%	100%
Surgical Infection Prevention					
Prophylactic Antibiotic Given[3]	172	47%	69%	77%	95%
Prophylactic Antibiotic Selection	50	100%	79%	90%	100%
Prophylactic Antibiotic Stopped[3]	167	56%	61%	72%	95%
Pregnancy Care					
Inpatient Neonatal Mortality	-	-	-	-	-
Third or Fourth Degree Laceration	-	-	3.54%	3.63%	3.27%

E A Conway Medical Center

4864 Jackson Street   Phone: 318-330-7000
PO Box 1881   Fax: 318-330-7446
Monroe, LA 71202
URL: www.conway.lsuhsc.edu
Ownership: Government - State   Accredited: Yes
Emergency Services: Yes   Licensed Beds: 153
Key Personnel:
Administrator . . . . H Aryon McGuire

Measure	Cases	This Hospital	State Average	U.S. Average	Top Hospital
Heart Attack Care					
ACE Inhibitor or ARB for LVSD[1]	10	100%	84%	82%	100%
Aspirin at Arrival	84	94%	91%	92%	100%
Aspirin at Discharge	44	100%	87%	90%	100%
Beta Blocker at Arrival	67	96%	85%	87%	100%
Beta Blocker at Discharge	46	100%	88%	90%	100%
Fibrinolytic Medication Timing[1]	10	50%	32%	31%	100%
PCI Within 90 Minutes of Arrival	0	-	40%	54%	95%
Smoking Cessation Advice	34	85%	88%	88%	100%
Heart Failure Care					
ACE Inhibitor or ARB for LVSD	126	98%	78%	82%	100%
Discharge Instructions	192	65%	62%	61%	93%
Evaluation of LVS Function	195	97%	81%	83%	99%
Smoking Cessation Advice	61	82%	83%	82%	100%
Pneumonia Care					
Appropriate Initial Antibiotic	102	91%	78%	83%	94%
Blood Culture Timing	53	92%	89%	90%	100%
Influenza Vaccine[1]	17	29%	58%	70%	100%
Initial Antibiotic Timing	108	73%	76%	80%	93%
Oxygenation Assessment	119	95%	98%	99%	100%
Pneumococcal Vaccine[1]	12	83%	61%	69%	94%
Smoking Cessation Advice	63	70%	78%	80%	100%
Surgical Infection Prevention					
Prophylactic Antibiotic Given	250	95%	69%	77%	95%
Prophylactic Antibiotic Selection	80	99%	79%	90%	100%
Prophylactic Antibiotic Stopped	240	88%	61%	72%	95%
Pregnancy Care					
Inpatient Neonatal Mortality	1,062	0.85%	-	-	-
Third or Fourth Degree Laceration	750	3.87%	3.54%	3.63%	3.27%

NOTE: Hospital profiles are in alphabetical order by state, then city, then hospital within the city; Rankings are sorted by rate in descending order and exclude hospitals with less than 25 cases; (1) The number of cases is too small (n<25) for purposes of reliably predicting hospital performance; (2) Measure reflects the hospital's indication that its submission was based upon a sample of its relevant discharges; (3) Rate reflects fewer than the maximum possible quarters of data for the measure; (4) Inaccurate information submitted and suppressed for one or more quarters; (5) No data is available from the hospital for this measure; Please refer to the User's Guide for a full explanation of data

| Third or Fourth Degree Laceration | - | - | 3.54% | 3.63% | 3.27% |

Monroe Surgical Hospital

2408 Broadmoor Blvd
Monroe, LA 71201
Ownership: Proprietary
Emergency Services: No

Phone: 318-410-0002

Accredited: Yes

Measure	Cases	This Hospital	State Average	U.S. Average	Top Hospital
Heart Attack Care					
ACE Inhibitor or ARB for LVSD[5]	-	-	84%	82%	100%
Aspirin at Arrival[5]	-	-	91%	92%	100%
Aspirin at Discharge[5]	-	-	87%	90%	100%
Beta Blocker at Arrival[5]	-	-	85%	87%	100%
Beta Blocker at Discharge[5]	-	-	88%	90%	100%
Fibrinolytic Medication Timing[5]	-	-	32%	31%	100%
PCI Within 90 Minutes of Arrival[5]	-	-	40%	54%	95%
Smoking Cessation Advice[5]	-	-	88%	88%	100%
Heart Failure Care					
ACE Inhibitor or ARB for LVSD[3]	0	-	78%	82%	100%
Discharge Instructions[1,3]	1	100%	62%	61%	93%
Evaluation of LVS Function[1,3]	1	0%	81%	83%	99%
Smoking Cessation Advice[3]	0	-	83%	82%	100%
Pneumonia Care					
Appropriate Initial Antibiotic[2,3]	0	-	78%	83%	94%
Blood Culture Timing[2,3]	0	-	89%	90%	100%
Influenza Vaccine[1,2]	4	25%	58%	70%	100%
Initial Antibiotic Timing[2,3]	0	-	76%	80%	93%
Oxygenation Assessment[1,2,3]	6	100%	98%	99%	100%
Pneumococcal Vaccine[1,2,3]	3	33%	61%	69%	94%
Smoking Cessation Advice[2,3]	0	-	78%	80%	100%
Surgical Infection Prevention					
Prophylactic Antibiotic Given[3]	31	90%	69%	77%	95%
Prophylactic Antibiotic Selection	32	41%	79%	90%	100%
Prophylactic Antibiotic Stopped[3]	31	68%	61%	72%	95%
Pregnancy Care					
Inpatient Neonatal Mortality	-	-	-	-	-
Third or Fourth Degree Laceration	-	-	3.54%	3.63%	3.27%

P & S Surgical Hospital

312 Grammont Saint Suite 101
Monroe, LA 71201
Ownership: Proprietary
Emergency Services: No

Phone: 318-388-4040

Accredited: No

Measure	Cases	This Hospital	State Average	U.S. Average	Top Hospital
Heart Attack Care					
ACE Inhibitor or ARB for LVSD[5]	-	-	84%	82%	100%
Aspirin at Arrival[5]	-	-	91%	92%	100%
Aspirin at Discharge[5]	-	-	87%	90%	100%
Beta Blocker at Arrival[5]	-	-	85%	87%	100%
Beta Blocker at Discharge[5]	-	-	88%	90%	100%
Fibrinolytic Medication Timing[5]	-	-	32%	31%	100%
PCI Within 90 Minutes of Arrival[5]	-	-	40%	54%	95%
Smoking Cessation Advice[5]	-	-	88%	88%	100%
Heart Failure Care					
ACE Inhibitor or ARB for LVSD[5]	-	-	78%	82%	100%
Discharge Instructions[5]	-	-	62%	61%	93%
Evaluation of LVS Function[5]	-	-	81%	83%	99%
Smoking Cessation Advice[5]	-	-	83%	82%	100%
Pneumonia Care					
Appropriate Initial Antibiotic[5]	-	-	78%	83%	94%
Blood Culture Timing[5]	-	-	89%	90%	100%
Influenza Vaccine[5]	-	-	58%	70%	100%
Initial Antibiotic Timing[5]	-	-	76%	80%	93%
Oxygenation Assessment[5]	-	-	98%	99%	100%
Pneumococcal Vaccine[5]	-	-	61%	69%	94%
Smoking Cessation Advice[5]	-	-	78%	80%	100%
Surgical Infection Prevention					
Prophylactic Antibiotic Given[2]	226	77%	69%	77%	95%
Prophylactic Antibiotic Selection[5]	-	-	79%	90%	100%
Prophylactic Antibiotic Stopped[2]	225	75%	61%	72%	95%
Pregnancy Care					
Inpatient Neonatal Mortality	-	-	-	-	-

Saint Francis Medical Center

309 Jackson Street
Monroe, LA 71210
URL: www.stfran.com
Ownership: Voluntary non-profit - Church
Emergency Services: Yes

Phone: 318-327-4000
Fax: 318-327-4142

Accredited: Yes
Licensed Beds: 339

Key Personnel:
CEO . . . . Scott Westor
Emergency Room . . . . Teresa Daniel
Director Medical/Surgical Nursing . . . . Sabrina Webb, RN
Respiratory Care . . . . Marie Easterling

Measure	Cases	This Hospital	State Average	U.S. Average	Top Hospital
Heart Attack Care					
ACE Inhibitor or ARB for LVSD	59	66%	84%	82%	100%
Aspirin at Arrival	130	95%	91%	92%	100%
Aspirin at Discharge	217	94%	87%	90%	100%
Beta Blocker at Arrival	128	84%	85%	87%	100%
Beta Blocker at Discharge	247	84%	88%	90%	100%
Fibrinolytic Medication Timing[1]	1	100%	32%	31%	100%
PCI Within 90 Minutes of Arrival[1]	6	17%	40%	54%	95%
Smoking Cessation Advice	79	100%	88%	88%	100%
Heart Failure Care					
ACE Inhibitor or ARB for LVSD	169	83%	78%	82%	100%
Discharge Instructions	422	45%	62%	61%	93%
Evaluation of LVS Function	519	84%	81%	83%	99%
Smoking Cessation Advice	76	99%	83%	82%	100%
Pneumonia Care					
Appropriate Initial Antibiotic	152	83%	78%	83%	94%
Blood Culture Timing	160	95%	89%	90%	100%
Influenza Vaccine	46	70%	58%	70%	100%
Initial Antibiotic Timing	209	65%	76%	80%	93%
Oxygenation Assessment	263	100%	98%	99%	100%
Pneumococcal Vaccine	167	73%	61%	69%	94%
Smoking Cessation Advice	48	100%	78%	80%	100%
Surgical Infection Prevention					
Prophylactic Antibiotic Given[3]	213	69%	69%	77%	95%
Prophylactic Antibiotic Selection	210	80%	79%	90%	100%
Prophylactic Antibiotic Stopped[3]	209	76%	61%	72%	95%
Pregnancy Care					
Inpatient Neonatal Mortality	-	-	-	-	-
Third or Fourth Degree Laceration	-	-	3.54%	3.63%	3.27%

Teche Regional Medical Center

Alternate Name: Lakewood Medical Center
1125 Marturite Street
Morgan City, LA 70380
URL: www.techeregional.com
Ownership: Proprietary
Emergency Services: Yes

Phone: 985-384-2200
Fax: 985-380-4546

Accredited: Yes
Licensed Beds: 149

Key Personnel:
CEO . . . . Scott Smith
Chief of Medical Staff . . . . Natalie Dishman
Emergency Room Director . . . . Cerri Gianluca, MD
Infection/Disease Control . . . . Brenda Topham
Surgical Services . . . . Tammy Clement
Chief of Radiology . . . . Dave Berger
Respiratory . . . . Raymond Pisani

Measure	Cases	This Hospital	State Average	U.S. Average	Top Hospital
Heart Attack Care					
ACE Inhibitor or ARB for LVSD[1]	8	100%	84%	82%	100%
Aspirin at Arrival[1]	22	100%	91%	92%	100%
Aspirin at Discharge[1]	11	100%	87%	90%	100%
Beta Blocker at Arrival[1]	24	100%	85%	87%	100%
Beta Blocker at Discharge[1]	15	87%	88%	90%	100%
Fibrinolytic Medication Timing	0	-	32%	31%	100%
PCI Within 90 Minutes of Arrival	0	-	40%	54%	95%
Smoking Cessation Advice[1]	2	100%	88%	88%	100%
Heart Failure Care					
ACE Inhibitor or ARB for LVSD	46	85%	78%	82%	100%

NOTE: Hospital profiles are in alphabetical order by state, then city, then hospital within the city; Rankings are sorted by rate in descending order and exclude hospitals with less than 25 cases; (1) The number of cases is too small (n<25) for purposes of reliably predicting hospital performance; (2) Measure reflects the hospital's indication that its submission was based upon a sample of its relevant discharges; (3) Rate reflects fewer than the maximum possible quarters of data for the measure; (4) Inaccurate information submitted and suppressed for one or more quarters; (5) No data is available from the hospital for this measure; Please refer to the User's Guide for a full explanation of data

Measure	Cases	This Hospital	State Average	U.S. Average	Top Hospital
Discharge Instructions	139	90%	62%	61%	93%
Evaluation of LVS Function	155	70%	81%	83%	99%
Smoking Cessation Advice	34	59%	83%	82%	100%
Pneumonia Care					
Appropriate Initial Antibiotic	55	73%	78%	83%	94%
Blood Culture Timing	50	92%	89%	90%	100%
Influenza Vaccine[1]	19	63%	58%	70%	100%
Initial Antibiotic Timing	77	91%	76%	80%	93%
Oxygenation Assessment	90	99%	98%	99%	100%
Pneumococcal Vaccine	54	44%	61%	69%	94%
Smoking Cessation Advice[1]	21	52%	78%	80%	100%
Surgical Infection Prevention					
Prophylactic Antibiotic Given[3]	43	77%	69%	77%	95%
Prophylactic Antibiotic Selection[1]	15	67%	79%	90%	100%
Prophylactic Antibiotic Stopped[3]	42	74%	61%	72%	95%
Pregnancy Care					
Inpatient Neonatal Mortality	-	-	-	-	-
Third or Fourth Degree Laceration	-	-	3.54%	3.63%	3.27%

Assumption Community Hospital

Alternate Name: Assumption General Hospital
135 Highway 402
Napoleonville, LA 70390
Ownership: Voluntary non-profit - Church
Emergency Services: Yes

Phone: 985-369-3600
Fax: 985-369-4271
Accredited: No
Licensed Beds: 15

Key Personnel:
Administrator/CEO...................... Wayne M Arboneaux
Chief Medical Director .... Tony Sun, MD
Director Respiratory Therapy .... Warren Arboneaux

Measure	Cases	This Hospital	State Average	U.S. Average	Top Hospital
Heart Attack Care					
ACE Inhibitor or ARB for LVSD[5]	-	-	84%	82%	100%
Aspirin at Arrival[5]	-	-	91%	92%	100%
Aspirin at Discharge[5]	-	-	87%	90%	100%
Beta Blocker at Arrival[5]	-	-	85%	87%	100%
Beta Blocker at Discharge[5]	-	-	88%	90%	100%
Fibrinolytic Medication Timing[5]	-	-	32%	31%	100%
PCI Within 90 Minutes of Arrival[5]	-	-	40%	54%	95%
Smoking Cessation Advice[5]	-	-	88%	88%	100%
Heart Failure Care					
ACE Inhibitor or ARB for LVSD[5]	-	-	78%	82%	100%
Discharge Instructions[5]	-	-	62%	61%	93%
Evaluation of LVS Function[5]	-	-	81%	83%	99%
Smoking Cessation Advice[5]	-	-	83%	82%	100%
Pneumonia Care					
Appropriate Initial Antibiotic[5]	-	-	78%	83%	94%
Blood Culture Timing[5]	-	-	89%	90%	100%
Influenza Vaccine[5]	-	-	58%	70%	100%
Initial Antibiotic Timing[5]	-	-	76%	80%	93%
Oxygenation Assessment[5]	-	-	98%	99%	100%
Pneumococcal Vaccine[5]	-	-	61%	69%	94%
Smoking Cessation Advice[5]	-	-	78%	80%	100%
Surgical Infection Prevention					
Prophylactic Antibiotic Given[5]	-	-	69%	77%	95%
Prophylactic Antibiotic Selection[5]	-	-	79%	90%	100%
Prophylactic Antibiotic Stopped[5]	-	-	61%	72%	95%
Pregnancy Care					
Inpatient Neonatal Mortality	-	-	-	-	-
Third or Fourth Degree Laceration	-	-	3.54%	3.63%	3.27%

Natchitoches Regional Medical Center

501 Keyser Avenue
Natchitoches, LA 71457
URL: www.natchitocheshospital.org
Ownership: Govt - Hospital District or Authority
Emergency Services: Yes

Phone: 318-214-4200
Fax: 318-214-4354
Accredited: Yes
Licensed Beds: 99

Key Personnel:
Administrator/CEO...................... Mark Marley
Chief of Medical Staff.................... Otis Barnum
Respiratory/Cardiopulmonary.............. Danita Olivier

Measure	Cases	This Hospital	State Average	U.S. Average	Top Hospital
Heart Attack Care					
ACE Inhibitor or ARB for LVSD[1]	3	33%	84%	82%	100%
Aspirin at Arrival[1]	21	95%	91%	92%	100%
Aspirin at Discharge[1]	3	33%	87%	90%	100%
Beta Blocker at Arrival[1]	20	85%	85%	87%	100%
Beta Blocker at Discharge[1]	4	100%	88%	90%	100%
Fibrinolytic Medication Timing[1]	7	43%	32%	31%	100%
PCI Within 90 Minutes of Arrival	0	-	40%	54%	95%
Smoking Cessation Advice[1]	1	100%	88%	88%	100%
Heart Failure Care					
ACE Inhibitor or ARB for LVSD	51	59%	78%	82%	100%
Discharge Instructions	101	66%	62%	61%	93%
Evaluation of LVS Function	123	89%	81%	83%	99%
Smoking Cessation Advice	25	68%	83%	82%	100%
Pneumonia Care					
Appropriate Initial Antibiotic	152	80%	78%	83%	94%
Blood Culture Timing	103	92%	89%	90%	100%
Influenza Vaccine	35	51%	58%	70%	100%
Initial Antibiotic Timing	230	80%	76%	80%	93%
Oxygenation Assessment	282	99%	98%	99%	100%
Pneumococcal Vaccine	180	52%	61%	69%	94%
Smoking Cessation Advice	42	60%	78%	80%	100%
Surgical Infection Prevention					
Prophylactic Antibiotic Given	76	61%	69%	77%	95%
Prophylactic Antibiotic Selection[1]	16	56%	79%	90%	100%
Prophylactic Antibiotic Stopped	68	44%	61%	72%	95%
Pregnancy Care					
Inpatient Neonatal Mortality	-	-	-	-	-
Third or Fourth Degree Laceration	-	-	3.54%	3.63%	3.27%

Dauterive Hospital

600 North Lewis Avenue
New Iberia, LA 70563
URL: www.dauterivehospital.com
Ownership: Proprietary
Emergency Services: Yes

Phone: 337-365-7311
Fax: 337-374-4104
Accredited: Yes
Licensed Beds: 107

Key Personnel:
Interim CEO............................ Cheryl A Wilson
Chief Medical Staff...................... Kurt O'Brien
Catheterization Lab Supervisor .... Cynthia Dubois
Emergency Room Medical Director .... Kevin J Chamas, MD
Director Infection/Disease Control .... Tara Dubois, RN
OB/GYN Womens Health.................. Gilbert Pellerin, Jr, MD
Chief Radiology .... Barry Verret
Director Respiratory Therapy .... Katie Hebert

Measure	Cases	This Hospital	State Average	U.S. Average	Top Hospital
Heart Attack Care					
ACE Inhibitor or ARB for LVSD[1]	15	87%	84%	82%	100%
Aspirin at Arrival	66	91%	91%	92%	100%
Aspirin at Discharge	57	89%	87%	90%	100%
Beta Blocker at Arrival	51	80%	85%	87%	100%
Beta Blocker at Discharge	56	84%	88%	90%	100%
Fibrinolytic Medication Timing	0	-	32%	31%	100%
PCI Within 90 Minutes of Arrival[1]	2	50%	40%	54%	95%
Smoking Cessation Advice	28	93%	88%	88%	100%
Heart Failure Care					
ACE Inhibitor or ARB for LVSD	110	64%	78%	82%	100%
Discharge Instructions	190	45%	62%	61%	93%
Evaluation of LVS Function	209	85%	81%	83%	99%
Smoking Cessation Advice	61	84%	83%	82%	100%
Pneumonia Care					
Appropriate Initial Antibiotic	60	75%	78%	83%	94%
Blood Culture Timing	50	94%	89%	90%	100%
Influenza Vaccine[1]	20	50%	58%	70%	100%
Initial Antibiotic Timing	81	78%	76%	80%	93%
Oxygenation Assessment	92	99%	98%	99%	100%
Pneumococcal Vaccine	53	40%	61%	69%	94%
Smoking Cessation Advice	30	43%	78%	80%	100%
Surgical Infection Prevention					
Prophylactic Antibiotic Given[2,3]	58	64%	69%	77%	95%

NOTE: Hospital profiles are in alphabetical order by state, then city, then hospital within the city; Rankings are sorted by rate in descending order and exclude hospitals with less than 25 cases; (1) The number of cases is too small (n<25) for purposes of reliably predicting hospital performance; (2) Measure reflects the hospital's indication that its submission was based upon a sample of its relevant discharges; (3) Rate reflects fewer than the maximum possible quarters of data for the measure; (4) Inaccurate information submitted and suppressed for one or more quarters; (5) No data is available from the hospital for this measure; Please refer to the User's Guide for a full explanation of data

Prophylactic Antibiotic Selection[1,2]	23	87%	79%	90%	100%
Prophylactic Antibiotic Stopped[2,3]	57	40%	61%	72%	95%
Pregnancy Care					
Inpatient Neonatal Mortality	-	-	-	-	-
Third or Fourth Degree Laceration	-	-	3.54%	3.63%	3.27%

Iberia Medical Center

Alternate Name: Iberia General Hospital & Medical Center
2315 E Main Street   Phone: 337-364-0441
New Iberia, LA 70560   Fax: 337-374-7641
URL: www.iberiamedicalcenter.com
Ownership: Govt - Hospital District or Authority   Accredited: Yes
Emergency Services: Yes   Licensed Beds: 101
Key Personnel:
Chief Medical Staff . . . . Kenneth Ritter

Measure	Cases	This Hospital	State Average	U.S. Average	Top Hospital
Heart Attack Care					
ACE Inhibitor or ARB for LVSD[1]	24	92%	84%	82%	100%
Aspirin at Arrival	111	94%	91%	92%	100%
Aspirin at Discharge	80	94%	87%	90%	100%
Beta Blocker at Arrival	75	77%	85%	87%	100%
Beta Blocker at Discharge	85	96%	88%	90%	100%
Fibrinolytic Medication Timing	0	-	32%	31%	100%
PCI Within 90 Minutes of Arrival	0	-	40%	54%	95%
Smoking Cessation Advice	46	89%	88%	88%	100%
Heart Failure Care					
ACE Inhibitor or ARB for LVSD	63	86%	78%	82%	100%
Discharge Instructions	164	85%	62%	61%	93%
Evaluation of LVS Function	184	90%	81%	83%	99%
Smoking Cessation Advice	39	90%	83%	82%	100%
Pneumonia Care					
Appropriate Initial Antibiotic	88	80%	78%	83%	94%
Blood Culture Timing	96	79%	89%	90%	100%
Influenza Vaccine	31	84%	58%	70%	100%
Initial Antibiotic Timing	142	85%	76%	80%	93%
Oxygenation Assessment	184	99%	98%	99%	100%
Pneumococcal Vaccine	113	89%	61%	69%	94%
Smoking Cessation Advice	40	100%	78%	80%	100%
Surgical Infection Prevention					
Prophylactic Antibiotic Given[3]	192	93%	69%	77%	95%
Prophylactic Antibiotic Selection	69	84%	79%	90%	100%
Prophylactic Antibiotic Stopped[3]	189	65%	61%	72%	95%
Pregnancy Care					
Inpatient Neonatal Mortality	-	-	-	-	-
Third or Fourth Degree Laceration	-	-	3.54%	3.63%	3.27%

Lindy Boggs Medical Center

301 North Jefferson Davis Pkwy   Phone: 504-483-5103
New Orleans, LA 70119
Ownership: Proprietary   Accredited: Yes
Emergency Services: Yes

Measure	Cases	This Hospital	State Average	U.S. Average	Top Hospital
Heart Attack Care					
ACE Inhibitor or ARB for LVSD[5]	-	-	84%	82%	100%
Aspirin at Arrival[5]	-	-	91%	92%	100%
Aspirin at Discharge[5]	-	-	87%	90%	100%
Beta Blocker at Arrival[5]	-	-	85%	87%	100%
Beta Blocker at Discharge[5]	-	-	88%	90%	100%
Fibrinolytic Medication Timing[5]	-	-	32%	31%	100%
PCI Within 90 Minutes of Arrival[5]	-	-	40%	54%	95%
Smoking Cessation Advice[5]	-	-	88%	88%	100%
Heart Failure Care					
ACE Inhibitor or ARB for LVSD[5]	-	-	78%	82%	100%
Discharge Instructions[5]	-	-	62%	61%	93%
Evaluation of LVS Function[5]	-	-	81%	83%	99%
Smoking Cessation Advice[5]	-	-	83%	82%	100%
Pneumonia Care					
Appropriate Initial Antibiotic[5]	-	-	78%	83%	94%
Blood Culture Timing[5]	-	-	89%	90%	100%
Influenza Vaccine[5]	-	-	58%	70%	100%

Initial Antibiotic Timing[5]	-	-	76%	80%	93%
Oxygenation Assessment[5]	-	-	98%	99%	100%
Pneumococcal Vaccine[5]	-	-	61%	69%	94%
Smoking Cessation Advice[5]	-	-	78%	80%	100%
Surgical Infection Prevention					
Prophylactic Antibiotic Given[5]	-	-	69%	77%	95%
Prophylactic Antibiotic Selection[5]	-	-	79%	90%	100%
Prophylactic Antibiotic Stopped[5]	-	-	61%	72%	95%
Pregnancy Care					
Inpatient Neonatal Mortality	-	-	-	-	-
Third or Fourth Degree Laceration	-	-	3.54%	3.63%	3.27%

Medical Center of Louisiana at New Orleans

2021 Perdido St 4th Floor   Phone: 504-903-0289
New Orleans, LA 70112
Ownership: Government - State   Accredited: Yes
Emergency Services: Yes

Measure	Cases	This Hospital	State Average	U.S. Average	Top Hospital
Heart Attack Care					
ACE Inhibitor or ARB for LVSD[5]	-	-	84%	82%	100%
Aspirin at Arrival[5]	-	-	91%	92%	100%
Aspirin at Discharge[5]	-	-	87%	90%	100%
Beta Blocker at Arrival[5]	-	-	85%	87%	100%
Beta Blocker at Discharge[5]	-	-	88%	90%	100%
Fibrinolytic Medication Timing[5]	-	-	32%	31%	100%
PCI Within 90 Minutes of Arrival[5]	-	-	40%	54%	95%
Smoking Cessation Advice[5]	-	-	88%	88%	100%
Heart Failure Care					
ACE Inhibitor or ARB for LVSD[5]	-	-	78%	82%	100%
Discharge Instructions[5]	-	-	62%	61%	93%
Evaluation of LVS Function[5]	-	-	81%	83%	99%
Smoking Cessation Advice[5]	-	-	83%	82%	100%
Pneumonia Care					
Appropriate Initial Antibiotic[5]	-	-	78%	83%	94%
Blood Culture Timing[5]	-	-	89%	90%	100%
Influenza Vaccine[5]	-	-	58%	70%	100%
Initial Antibiotic Timing[5]	-	-	76%	80%	93%
Oxygenation Assessment[5]	-	-	98%	99%	100%
Pneumococcal Vaccine[5]	-	-	61%	69%	94%
Smoking Cessation Advice[5]	-	-	78%	80%	100%
Surgical Infection Prevention					
Prophylactic Antibiotic Given[1,3]	7	43%	69%	77%	95%
Prophylactic Antibiotic Selection[1]	5	40%	79%	90%	100%
Prophylactic Antibiotic Stopped[1,3]	7	57%	61%	72%	95%
Pregnancy Care					
Inpatient Neonatal Mortality	-	-	-	-	-
Third or Fourth Degree Laceration	-	-	3.54%	3.63%	3.27%

Methodist Hospital

5620 Read Boulevard   Phone: 504-244-5474
New Orleans, LA 70127
Ownership: Voluntary non-profit - Private   Accredited: Yes
Emergency Services: Yes

Measure	Cases	This Hospital	State Average	U.S. Average	Top Hospital
Heart Attack Care					
ACE Inhibitor or ARB for LVSD[5]	-	-	84%	82%	100%
Aspirin at Arrival[5]	-	-	91%	92%	100%
Aspirin at Discharge[5]	-	-	87%	90%	100%
Beta Blocker at Arrival[5]	-	-	85%	87%	100%
Beta Blocker at Discharge[5]	-	-	88%	90%	100%
Fibrinolytic Medication Timing[5]	-	-	32%	31%	100%
PCI Within 90 Minutes of Arrival[5]	-	-	40%	54%	95%
Smoking Cessation Advice[5]	-	-	88%	88%	100%
Heart Failure Care					
ACE Inhibitor or ARB for LVSD[5]	-	-	78%	82%	100%
Discharge Instructions[5]	-	-	62%	61%	93%
Evaluation of LVS Function[5]	-	-	81%	83%	99%
Smoking Cessation Advice[5]	-	-	83%	82%	100%
Pneumonia Care					
Appropriate Initial Antibiotic[5]	-	-	78%	83%	94%

NOTE: Hospital profiles are in alphabetical order by state, then city, then hospital within the city; Rankings are sorted by rate in descending order and exclude hospitals with less than 25 cases; (1) The number of cases is too small (n<25) for purposes of reliably predicting hospital performance; (2) Measure reflects the hospital's indication that its submission was based upon a sample of its relevant discharges; (3) Rate reflects fewer than the maximum possible quarters of data for the measure; (4) Inaccurate information submitted and suppressed for one or more quarters; (5) No data is available from the hospital for this measure; Please refer to the User's Guide for a full explanation of data

Blood Culture Timing[5]	-	-	89%	90%	100%
Influenza Vaccine[5]	-	-	58%	70%	100%
Initial Antibiotic Timing[5]	-	-	76%	80%	93%
Oxygenation Assessment[5]	-	-	98%	99%	100%
Pneumococcal Vaccine[5]	-	-	61%	69%	94%
Smoking Cessation Advice[5]	-	-	78%	80%	100%
Surgical Infection Prevention					
Prophylactic Antibiotic Given[5]	-	-	69%	77%	95%
Prophylactic Antibiotic Selection[5]	-	-	79%	90%	100%
Prophylactic Antibiotic Stopped[5]	-	-	61%	72%	95%
Pregnancy Care					
Inpatient Neonatal Mortality	-	-	-	-	-
Third or Fourth Degree Laceration	-	-	3.54%	3.63%	3.27%

Ochsner Baptist Medical Center

2700 Napoleon Avenue   Phone: 504-899-9311
New Orleans, LA 70115
Ownership: Voluntary non-profit - Private
Emergency Services: Yes   Accredited: Yes

Measure	Cases	This Hospital	State Average	U.S. Average	Top Hospital
Heart Attack Care					
ACE Inhibitor or ARB for LVSD[5]	-	-	84%	82%	100%
Aspirin at Arrival[5]	-	-	91%	92%	100%
Aspirin at Discharge[5]	-	-	87%	90%	100%
Beta Blocker at Arrival[5]	-	-	85%	87%	100%
Beta Blocker at Discharge[5]	-	-	88%	90%	100%
Fibrinolytic Medication Timing[5]	-	-	32%	31%	100%
PCI Within 90 Minutes of Arrival[5]	-	-	40%	54%	95%
Smoking Cessation Advice[5]	-	-	88%	88%	100%
Heart Failure Care					
ACE Inhibitor or ARB for LVSD[5]	-	-	78%	82%	100%
Discharge Instructions[5]	-	-	62%	61%	93%
Evaluation of LVS Function[5]	-	-	81%	83%	99%
Smoking Cessation Advice[5]	-	-	83%	82%	100%
Pneumonia Care					
Appropriate Initial Antibiotic[5]	-	-	78%	83%	94%
Blood Culture Timing[5]	-	-	89%	90%	100%
Influenza Vaccine[5]	-	-	58%	70%	100%
Initial Antibiotic Timing[5]	-	-	76%	80%	93%
Oxygenation Assessment[5]	-	-	98%	99%	100%
Pneumococcal Vaccine[5]	-	-	61%	69%	94%
Smoking Cessation Advice[5]	-	-	78%	80%	100%
Surgical Infection Prevention					
Prophylactic Antibiotic Given[5]	-	-	69%	77%	95%
Prophylactic Antibiotic Selection[5]	-	-	79%	90%	100%
Prophylactic Antibiotic Stopped[5]	-	-	61%	72%	95%
Pregnancy Care					
Inpatient Neonatal Mortality	-	-	-	-	-
Third or Fourth Degree Laceration	-	-	3.54%	3.63%	3.27%

Ochsner Clinic Foundation

1514 Jefferson Highway   Toll-Free: 800-928-6247
New Orleans, LA 70121   Phone: 504-842-3000
                                  Fax: 504-842-5856
URL: www.ochsner.org
Ownership: Voluntary non-profit - Private   Accredited: Yes
Emergency Services: Yes   Licensed Beds: 460
Key Personnel:
President/COO.........................Warner Thomas
CEO..................................Patrick J Quinlan, MD
Chief Medical Staff..................Richard Guthrie, MD
Cardiac Lab..........................Mark French
Catheterization Lab..................Mark French
Emergency Room.......................Nancy Davis, RN
Infection Control....................Eric McMillen
ICU..................................Ed Spears, RN
Intensive/Coronary Care..............Mark French
Medical/Surgical Nursing.............Nancy Davis, RN
Respiratory/Cardiopulmonary..........Mark French

Measure	Cases	This Hospital	State Average	U.S. Average	Top Hospital

Measure	Cases	This Hospital	State Average	U.S. Average	Top Hospital
Heart Attack Care					
ACE Inhibitor or ARB for LVSD	81	93%	84%	82%	100%
Aspirin at Arrival	215	95%	91%	92%	100%
Aspirin at Discharge	220	97%	87%	90%	100%
Beta Blocker at Arrival	168	99%	85%	87%	100%
Beta Blocker at Discharge	262	99%	88%	90%	100%
Fibrinolytic Medication Timing	0	-	32%	31%	100%
PCI Within 90 Minutes of Arrival[1]	10	100%	40%	54%	95%
Smoking Cessation Advice	83	98%	88%	88%	100%
Heart Failure Care					
ACE Inhibitor or ARB for LVSD	168	92%	78%	82%	100%
Discharge Instructions	270	46%	62%	61%	93%
Evaluation of LVS Function	288	100%	81%	83%	99%
Smoking Cessation Advice	57	93%	83%	82%	100%
Pneumonia Care					
Appropriate Initial Antibiotic	115	83%	78%	83%	94%
Blood Culture Timing	94	86%	89%	90%	100%
Influenza Vaccine[4,5]	-	-	58%	70%	100%
Initial Antibiotic Timing	131	66%	76%	80%	93%
Oxygenation Assessment	173	100%	98%	99%	100%
Pneumococcal Vaccine	112	88%	61%	69%	94%
Smoking Cessation Advice	36	72%	78%	80%	100%
Surgical Infection Prevention					
Prophylactic Antibiotic Given[3]	623	52%	69%	77%	95%
Prophylactic Antibiotic Selection	156	97%	79%	90%	100%
Prophylactic Antibiotic Stopped[3]	616	59%	61%	72%	95%
Pregnancy Care					
Inpatient Neonatal Mortality	-	-	-	-	-
Third or Fourth Degree Laceration	-	-	3.54%	3.63%	3.27%

Touro Infirmary

1401 Foucher Street   Phone: 504-897-7011
New Orleans, LA 70115   Fax: 504-897-8106
E-mail: rhodesd@touro.com
URL: www.touro.com
Ownership: Voluntary non-profit - Private   Accredited: Yes
Emergency Services: Yes   Licensed Beds: 465
Key Personnel:
President/CEO........................Leslie Hirsch
Chief Medical Staff.................Sal Caputto, MD
Catheterization Lab.................Raja Dhurandhar, MD
Emergency Room......................Vicky Hebert, MD
Infection Control...................Carol Scioneaux
ICU.................................Charles C Smith, III, DP
Intensive/Coronary Care.............Judy Mysing
Medical/Surgical Nursing............Brenda Bankston
Director Medical/Surgical Nursing...Brenda Bankston
OB/GYN Womens Health................Jack Jacob, MD
Respiratory/Cardiopulmonary.........Bobbie McWilliams

Measure	Cases	This Hospital	State Average	U.S. Average	Top Hospital
Heart Attack Care					
ACE Inhibitor or ARB for LVSD[1]	24	67%	84%	82%	100%
Aspirin at Arrival	83	95%	91%	92%	100%
Aspirin at Discharge	76	91%	87%	90%	100%
Beta Blocker at Arrival	79	84%	85%	87%	100%
Beta Blocker at Discharge	81	85%	88%	90%	100%
Fibrinolytic Medication Timing[1,3]	7	14%	32%	31%	100%
PCI Within 90 Minutes of Arrival[1]	3	33%	40%	54%	95%
Smoking Cessation Advice[3]	29	72%	88%	88%	100%
Heart Failure Care					
ACE Inhibitor or ARB for LVSD	261	81%	78%	82%	100%
Discharge Instructions[3]	347	46%	62%	61%	93%
Evaluation of LVS Function	462	91%	81%	83%	99%
Smoking Cessation Advice[3]	80	61%	83%	82%	100%
Pneumonia Care					
Appropriate Initial Antibiotic[3]	98	80%	78%	83%	94%
Blood Culture Timing	124	94%	89%	90%	100%
Influenza Vaccine	38	26%	58%	70%	100%
Initial Antibiotic Timing	147	60%	76%	80%	93%
Oxygenation Assessment	187	95%	98%	99%	100%
Pneumococcal Vaccine	91	29%	61%	69%	94%
Smoking Cessation Advice[3]	35	43%	78%	80%	100%

NOTE: Hospital profiles are in alphabetical order by state, then city, then hospital within the city; Rankings are sorted by rate in descending order and exclude hospitals with less than 25 cases; (1) The number of cases is too small (n<25) for purposes of reliably predicting hospital performance; (2) Measure reflects the hospital's indication that its submission was based upon a sample of its relevant discharges; (3) Rate reflects fewer than the maximum possible quarters of data for the measure; (4) Inaccurate information submitted and suppressed for one or more quarters; (5) No data is available from the hospital for this measure; Please refer to the User's Guide for a full explanation of data

Surgical Infection Prevention					
Prophylactic Antibiotic Given[3]	410	81%	69%	77%	95%
Prophylactic Antibiotic Selection	157	89%	79%	90%	100%
Prophylactic Antibiotic Stopped[3]	403	75%	61%	72%	95%
Pregnancy Care					
Inpatient Neonatal Mortality	-	-	-	-	-
Third or Fourth Degree Laceration	-	-	3.54%	3.63%	3.27%

Tulane University Hospital & Clinic

1415 Tulane Avenue
New Orleans, LA 70112
URL: www.tuhc.com
Ownership: Proprietary
Emergency Services: Yes

Phone: 504-988-5800
Fax: 504-988-6077

Accredited: Yes
Licensed Beds: 341

Key Personnel:
President/CEO. . . . . Jim Montgomery
Emergency Room . . . . Tom Serviss

Measure	Cases	This Hospital	State Average	U.S. Average	Top Hospital
Heart Attack Care					
ACE Inhibitor or ARB for LVSD[1]	17	94%	84%	82%	100%
Aspirin at Arrival	50	100%	91%	92%	100%
Aspirin at Discharge	55	98%	87%	90%	100%
Beta Blocker at Arrival	34	97%	85%	87%	100%
Beta Blocker at Discharge	52	100%	88%	90%	100%
Fibrinolytic Medication Timing	0	-	32%	31%	100%
PCI Within 90 Minutes of Arrival[1]	10	10%	40%	54%	95%
Smoking Cessation Advice	31	84%	88%	88%	100%
Heart Failure Care					
ACE Inhibitor or ARB for LVSD	106	92%	78%	82%	100%
Discharge Instructions	175	78%	62%	61%	93%
Evaluation of LVS Function	176	96%	81%	83%	99%
Smoking Cessation Advice	62	76%	83%	82%	100%
Pneumonia Care					
Appropriate Initial Antibiotic	27	93%	78%	83%	94%
Blood Culture Timing[1]	24	79%	89%	90%	100%
Influenza Vaccine[1]	5	40%	58%	70%	100%
Initial Antibiotic Timing	27	59%	76%	80%	93%
Oxygenation Assessment	34	100%	98%	99%	100%
Pneumococcal Vaccine[1]	6	50%	61%	69%	94%
Smoking Cessation Advice[1]	17	53%	78%	80%	100%
Surgical Infection Prevention					
Prophylactic Antibiotic Given[2]	261	78%	69%	77%	95%
Prophylactic Antibiotic Selection[2]	51	92%	79%	90%	100%
Prophylactic Antibiotic Stopped[2]	260	87%	61%	72%	95%
Pregnancy Care					
Inpatient Neonatal Mortality	-	-	-	-	-
Third or Fourth Degree Laceration	-	-	3.54%	3.63%	3.27%

West Carroll Memorial Hospital

706 Ross Street
Oak Grove, LA 71263
Ownership: Voluntary non-profit - Other
Emergency Services: Yes

Phone: 318-428-3237
Fax: 318-428-6180
Accredited: No
Licensed Beds: 21

Key Personnel:
Administrator/CEO . . . . Randall Morris

Measure	Cases	This Hospital	State Average	U.S. Average	Top Hospital
Heart Attack Care					
ACE Inhibitor or ARB for LVSD[5]	-	-	84%	82%	100%
Aspirin at Arrival[5]	-	-	91%	92%	100%
Aspirin at Discharge[5]	-	-	87%	90%	100%
Beta Blocker at Arrival[5]	-	-	85%	87%	100%
Beta Blocker at Discharge[5]	-	-	88%	90%	100%
Fibrinolytic Medication Timing[5]	-	-	32%	31%	100%
PCI Within 90 Minutes of Arrival[5]	-	-	40%	54%	95%
Smoking Cessation Advice[5]	-	-	88%	88%	100%
Heart Failure Care					
ACE Inhibitor or ARB for LVSD[1]	2	0%	78%	82%	100%
Discharge Instructions[1,3]	21	38%	62%	61%	93%
Evaluation of LVS Function	99	3%	81%	83%	99%
Smoking Cessation Advice[1,3]	3	0%	83%	82%	100%

Pneumonia Care					
Appropriate Initial Antibiotic[1,3]	7	86%	78%	83%	94%
Blood Culture Timing[1,3]	2	100%	89%	90%	100%
Influenza Vaccine[5]	-	-	58%	70%	100%
Initial Antibiotic Timing	111	63%	76%	80%	93%
Oxygenation Assessment	127	100%	98%	99%	100%
Pneumococcal Vaccine	89	52%	61%	69%	94%
Smoking Cessation Advice[1,3]	2	0%	78%	80%	100%
Surgical Infection Prevention					
Prophylactic Antibiotic Given[5]	-	-	69%	77%	95%
Prophylactic Antibiotic Selection[5]	-	-	79%	90%	100%
Prophylactic Antibiotic Stopped[5]	-	-	61%	72%	95%
Pregnancy Care					
Inpatient Neonatal Mortality	-	-	-	-	-
Third or Fourth Degree Laceration	-	-	3.54%	3.63%	3.27%

Oakdale Community Hospital

Alternate Name: Humana Hospital-Oakdale
130 N Hospital Drive
Oakdale, LA 71463
URL: www.oakdalecommunityhospital.com
Ownership: Voluntary non-profit - Other
Emergency Services: Yes

Phone: 318-335-3700
Fax: 318-215-3024

Accredited: Yes
Licensed Beds: 60

Key Personnel:
Administrator/CEO . . . . HJ Gaspard
Emergency Room . . . . Cindy Saxon
Director Infection/Disease Control . . . . Paula Carter, RN
Director Medical/Surgical Nursing . . . . Rita Drake, RN
Chief Radiology . . . . Mustafa Kajan, MD
Director Respiratory Therapy . . . . James Bordelon

Measure	Cases	This Hospital	State Average	U.S. Average	Top Hospital
Heart Attack Care					
ACE Inhibitor or ARB for LVSD[3]	0	-	84%	82%	100%
Aspirin at Arrival[1,3]	3	100%	91%	92%	100%
Aspirin at Discharge[3]	0	-	87%	90%	100%
Beta Blocker at Arrival[1,3]	3	100%	85%	87%	100%
Beta Blocker at Discharge[3]	0	-	88%	90%	100%
Fibrinolytic Medication Timing[3]	0	-	32%	31%	100%
PCI Within 90 Minutes of Arrival	0	-	40%	54%	95%
Smoking Cessation Advice[3]	0	-	88%	88%	100%
Heart Failure Care					
ACE Inhibitor or ARB for LVSD[1]	22	68%	78%	82%	100%
Discharge Instructions	59	83%	62%	61%	93%
Evaluation of LVS Function	85	87%	81%	83%	99%
Smoking Cessation Advice[1]	11	100%	83%	82%	100%
Pneumonia Care					
Appropriate Initial Antibiotic	85	60%	78%	83%	94%
Blood Culture Timing	38	95%	89%	90%	100%
Influenza Vaccine	40	75%	58%	70%	100%
Initial Antibiotic Timing	152	89%	76%	80%	93%
Oxygenation Assessment	182	100%	98%	99%	100%
Pneumococcal Vaccine	107	76%	61%	69%	94%
Smoking Cessation Advice	41	90%	78%	80%	100%
Surgical Infection Prevention					
Prophylactic Antibiotic Given[1,3]	5	80%	69%	77%	95%
Prophylactic Antibiotic Selection[1]	2	100%	79%	90%	100%
Prophylactic Antibiotic Stopped[1,3]	5	0%	61%	72%	95%
Pregnancy Care					
Inpatient Neonatal Mortality	-	-	-	-	-
Third or Fourth Degree Laceration	-	-	3.54%	3.63%	3.27%

Hardtner Medical Center

1102 N Pine Road
Olla, LA 71465
E-mail: admin@hardtnermedical.com
URL: www.hardtnermedical.com
Ownership: Govt - Hospital District or Authority
Emergency Services: Yes

Phone: 318-495-3131
Fax: 318-495-3229

Accredited: No
Licensed Beds: 35

Key Personnel:
President/CEO. . . . . Paul G Matthews
Chief of Medical Staff. . . . . Kenneth P Mauterer, MD
Emergency Room Director. . . . . Brian Krier, MD

NOTE: Hospital profiles are in alphabetical order by state, then city, then hospital within the city; Rankings are sorted by rate in descending order and exclude hospitals with less than 25 cases; (1) The number of cases is too small (n<25) for purposes of reliably predicting hospital performance; (2) Measure reflects the hospital's indication that its submission was based upon a sample of its relevant discharges; (3) Rate reflects fewer than the maximum possible quarters of data for the measure; (4) Inaccurate information submitted and suppressed for one or more quarters; (5) No data is available from the hospital for this measure; Please refer to the User's Guide for a full explanation of data

Infection Control. . . . . Genae Butler, RN
Respiratory/Cardiopulmonary. . . . . Joyce King

Measure	Cases	This Hospital	State Average	U.S. Average	Top Hospital
Heart Attack Care					
ACE Inhibitor or ARB for LVSD[5]	-	-	84%	82%	100%
Aspirin at Arrival[5]	-	-	91%	92%	100%
Aspirin at Discharge[5]	-	-	87%	90%	100%
Beta Blocker at Arrival[5]	-	-	85%	87%	100%
Beta Blocker at Discharge[5]	-	-	88%	90%	100%
Fibrinolytic Medication Timing[5]	-	-	32%	31%	100%
PCI Within 90 Minutes of Arrival[5]	-	-	40%	54%	95%
Smoking Cessation Advice[5]	-	-	88%	88%	100%
Heart Failure Care					
ACE Inhibitor or ARB for LVSD[1]	7	14%	78%	82%	100%
Discharge Instructions	25	0%	62%	61%	93%
Evaluation of LVS Function	33	45%	81%	83%	99%
Smoking Cessation Advice[1]	11	100%	83%	82%	100%
Pneumonia Care					
Appropriate Initial Antibiotic[1]	20	85%	78%	83%	94%
Blood Culture Timing[1]	4	75%	89%	90%	100%
Influenza Vaccine[1]	7	57%	58%	70%	100%
Initial Antibiotic Timing[1]	20	65%	76%	80%	93%
Oxygenation Assessment	26	96%	98%	99%	100%
Pneumococcal Vaccine[1]	21	48%	61%	69%	94%
Smoking Cessation Advice[1]	5	100%	78%	80%	100%
Surgical Infection Prevention					
Prophylactic Antibiotic Given[5]	-	-	69%	77%	95%
Prophylactic Antibiotic Selection[5]	-	-	79%	90%	100%
Prophylactic Antibiotic Stopped[5]	-	-	61%	72%	95%
Pregnancy Care					
Inpatient Neonatal Mortality	-	-	-	-	-
Third or Fourth Degree Laceration	-	-	3.54%	3.63%	3.27%

Doctors Hospital of Opelousas

3983 I 49 South Service Road   Phone: 337-948-2100
Opelousas, LA 70570   Fax: 337-948-2173
E-mail: sbranton@prhc.net
URL: www.doctorshospital.com
Ownership: Proprietary   Accredited: Yes
Emergency Services: Yes   Licensed Beds: 165
Key Personnel:
CEO. . . . . Mark Caton
Chief Medical Staff. . . . . Dr Gary Porbusky
Emergency Room . . . . Dr John Barton, MD
Director Infection/Disease Control . . . . Yvonne Noel, RN
ICU . . . . Glenn LeBlanc
Supervising Nurse CCU. . . . . Glenn LeBlanc, RN
Medical Surgical Nursing . . . . Mary Ellen Devillier
CEO. . . . . Don Stelly
Director Respiratory Therapy . . . . Mark Aucoin

Measure	Cases	This Hospital	State Average	U.S. Average	Top Hospital
Heart Attack Care					
ACE Inhibitor or ARB for LVSD[1]	6	100%	84%	82%	100%
Aspirin at Arrival	39	100%	91%	92%	100%
Aspirin at Discharge	29	97%	87%	90%	100%
Beta Blocker at Arrival	35	97%	85%	87%	100%
Beta Blocker at Discharge	33	97%	88%	90%	100%
Fibrinolytic Medication Timing	0	-	32%	31%	100%
PCI Within 90 Minutes of Arrival	0	-	40%	54%	95%
Smoking Cessation Advice[1]	17	94%	88%	88%	100%
Heart Failure Care					
ACE Inhibitor or ARB for LVSD	51	90%	78%	82%	100%
Discharge Instructions	139	81%	62%	61%	93%
Evaluation of LVS Function	172	86%	81%	83%	99%
Smoking Cessation Advice	35	94%	83%	82%	100%
Pneumonia Care					
Appropriate Initial Antibiotic	68	63%	78%	83%	94%
Blood Culture Timing	42	79%	89%	90%	100%
Influenza Vaccine[4,5]	-	-	58%	70%	100%
Initial Antibiotic Timing	90	70%	76%	80%	93%

Measure	Cases	This Hospital	State Average	U.S. Average	Top Hospital
Oxygenation Assessment	106	100%	98%	99%	100%
Pneumococcal Vaccine	53	91%	61%	69%	94%
Smoking Cessation Advice	31	81%	78%	80%	100%
Surgical Infection Prevention					
Prophylactic Antibiotic Given[3]	82	88%	69%	77%	95%
Prophylactic Antibiotic Selection	36	94%	79%	90%	100%
Prophylactic Antibiotic Stopped[3]	78	44%	61%	72%	95%
Pregnancy Care					
Inpatient Neonatal Mortality	-	-	-	-	-
Third or Fourth Degree Laceration	-	-	3.54%	3.63%	3.27%

Opelousas General Hospital

539 E Prudhomme Street   Phone: 337-948-3011
Opelousas, LA 70570   Fax: 337-948-5126
URL: www.opelousasgeneral.com
Ownership: Govt - Hospital District or Authority   Accredited: Yes
Emergency Services: Yes   Licensed Beds: 180
Key Personnel:
President/CEO. . . . . William F Barrow, II
Chief Medical Staff. . . . . Gary Blanchard, MD
Catheterization Lab . . . . Desiree Robinson
Emergency Room . . . . Mark Olivier, MD
Director Infection/Disease Control . . . . Laurie Going
ICU . . . . Jackie Harbour, RN
OB/GYN Womens Health. . . . . Ann Ruffino, RN

Measure	Cases	This Hospital	State Average	U.S. Average	Top Hospital
Heart Attack Care					
ACE Inhibitor or ARB for LVSD[1]	11	64%	84%	82%	100%
Aspirin at Arrival	79	97%	91%	92%	100%
Aspirin at Discharge	70	96%	87%	90%	100%
Beta Blocker at Arrival	80	85%	85%	87%	100%
Beta Blocker at Discharge	76	95%	88%	90%	100%
Fibrinolytic Medication Timing	0	-	32%	31%	100%
PCI Within 90 Minutes of Arrival[1]	6	33%	40%	54%	95%
Smoking Cessation Advice	36	100%	88%	88%	100%
Heart Failure Care					
ACE Inhibitor or ARB for LVSD	105	76%	78%	82%	100%
Discharge Instructions	284	72%	62%	61%	93%
Evaluation of LVS Function	332	86%	81%	83%	99%
Smoking Cessation Advice	88	93%	83%	82%	100%
Pneumonia Care					
Appropriate Initial Antibiotic	122	71%	78%	83%	94%
Blood Culture Timing	133	80%	89%	90%	100%
Influenza Vaccine	45	51%	58%	70%	100%
Initial Antibiotic Timing	228	68%	76%	80%	93%
Oxygenation Assessment	269	98%	98%	99%	100%
Pneumococcal Vaccine	150	59%	61%	69%	94%
Smoking Cessation Advice	70	87%	78%	80%	100%
Surgical Infection Prevention					
Prophylactic Antibiotic Given[3]	270	45%	69%	77%	95%
Prophylactic Antibiotic Selection	75	96%	79%	90%	100%
Prophylactic Antibiotic Stopped[3]	236	57%	61%	72%	95%
Pregnancy Care					
Inpatient Neonatal Mortality	-	-	-	-	-
Third or Fourth Degree Laceration	-	-	3.54%	3.63%	3.27%

Huey P Long Medical Center

352 Hospital Boulevard   Phone: 318-448-0811
Pineville, LA 71361   Fax: 318-473-6360
E-mail: j.morga2@lsumc.edu
URL: www.lsuhsc.edu/hcsd
Ownership: Government - State   Accredited: Yes
Emergency Services: Yes   Licensed Beds: 137
Key Personnel:
Administrator/CEO. . . . . James E Morgan
Chief Medical Staff. . . . . David Barnard, MD

Measure	Cases	This Hospital	State Average	U.S. Average	Top Hospital
Heart Attack Care					
ACE Inhibitor or ARB for LVSD[1]	3	67%	84%	82%	100%
Aspirin at Arrival[1]	14	100%	91%	92%	100%
Aspirin at Discharge[1]	10	90%	87%	90%	100%

NOTE: Hospital profiles are in alphabetical order by state, then city, then hospital within the city; Rankings are sorted by rate in descending order and exclude hospitals with less than 25 cases; (1) The number of cases is too small (n<25) for purposes of reliably predicting hospital performance; (2) Measure reflects the hospital's indication that its submission was based upon a sample of its relevant discharges; (3) Rate reflects fewer than the maximum possible quarters of data for the measure; (4) Inaccurate information submitted and suppressed for one or more quarters; (5) No data is available from the hospital for this measure; Please refer to the User's Guide for a full explanation of data

Measure	Cases	This Hospital	State Average	U.S. Average	Top Hospital
Beta Blocker at Arrival[1]	13	92%	85%	87%	100%
Beta Blocker at Discharge[1]	9	89%	88%	90%	100%
Fibrinolytic Medication Timing[1]	1	100%	32%	31%	100%
PCI Within 90 Minutes of Arrival	0	-	40%	54%	95%
Smoking Cessation Advice[1]	7	100%	88%	88%	100%
Heart Failure Care					
ACE Inhibitor or ARB for LVSD	48	94%	78%	82%	100%
Discharge Instructions	58	90%	62%	61%	93%
Evaluation of LVS Function	62	98%	81%	83%	99%
Smoking Cessation Advice	32	100%	83%	82%	100%
Pneumonia Care					
Appropriate Initial Antibiotic	25	88%	78%	83%	94%
Blood Culture Timing	30	97%	89%	90%	100%
Influenza Vaccine[1]	5	0%	58%	70%	100%
Initial Antibiotic Timing	43	67%	76%	80%	93%
Oxygenation Assessment	50	100%	98%	99%	100%
Pneumococcal Vaccine[1]	6	67%	61%	69%	94%
Smoking Cessation Advice[1]	20	95%	78%	80%	100%
Surgical Infection Prevention					
Prophylactic Antibiotic Given[3]	106	89%	69%	77%	95%
Prophylactic Antibiotic Selection	41	90%	79%	90%	100%
Prophylactic Antibiotic Stopped[3]	102	80%	61%	72%	95%
Pregnancy Care					
Inpatient Neonatal Mortality	181	1.11%	-	-	-
Third or Fourth Degree Laceration	108	2.78%	3.54%	3.63%	3.27%

River West Medical Center

59355 River West Drive
PO Box 737
Plaquemine, LA 70764
URL: www.riverwest.mc.com
Ownership: Proprietary
Emergency Services: Yes

Phone: 225-687-9222
Fax: 225-687-1454

Accredited: Yes
Licensed Beds: 80

Key Personnel:
CEO . . . . Scott Smith
Manager Catheterization Lab . . . . Barry Dison, RN
Emergency Room . . . . Sandra Delas, RN
Infection Control . . . . Debbie Courtade, RN
Manager Med Surg Nursing . . . . Wanda Ventress
Surgery Director . . . . Misty Bradford, RN
Director Radiology . . . . Kari Prince
Respiratory/Cardiopulmonary . . . . Ray Warner

Measure	Cases	This Hospital	State Average	U.S. Average	Top Hospital
Heart Attack Care					
ACE Inhibitor or ARB for LVSD[1]	8	88%	84%	82%	100%
Aspirin at Arrival	30	100%	91%	92%	100%
Aspirin at Discharge[1]	22	95%	87%	90%	100%
Beta Blocker at Arrival	28	86%	85%	87%	100%
Beta Blocker at Discharge[1]	23	91%	88%	90%	100%
Fibrinolytic Medication Timing[1]	1	0%	32%	31%	100%
PCI Within 90 Minutes of Arrival	0	-	40%	54%	95%
Smoking Cessation Advice[1]	7	100%	88%	88%	100%
Heart Failure Care					
ACE Inhibitor or ARB for LVSD	62	82%	78%	82%	100%
Discharge Instructions	105	44%	62%	61%	93%
Evaluation of LVS Function	121	90%	81%	83%	99%
Smoking Cessation Advice[1]	23	78%	83%	82%	100%
Pneumonia Care					
Appropriate Initial Antibiotic	75	87%	78%	83%	94%
Blood Culture Timing	85	92%	89%	90%	100%
Influenza Vaccine[1]	17	53%	58%	70%	100%
Initial Antibiotic Timing	116	71%	76%	80%	93%
Oxygenation Assessment	153	99%	98%	99%	100%
Pneumococcal Vaccine	61	51%	61%	69%	94%
Smoking Cessation Advice	30	77%	78%	80%	100%
Surgical Infection Prevention					
Prophylactic Antibiotic Given[2,3]	55	38%	69%	77%	95%
Prophylactic Antibiotic Selection[1,2]	20	70%	79%	90%	100%
Prophylactic Antibiotic Stopped[2,3]	47	96%	61%	72%	95%
Pregnancy Care					
Inpatient Neonatal Mortality	-	-	-	-	-
Third or Fourth Degree Laceration	-	-	3.54%	3.63%	3.27%

Saint Anne General Hospital

4608 Highway 1
Raceland, LA 70394
E-mail: administration@stannegeneral.com
URL: www.stannegeneral.com
Ownership: Voluntary non-profit - Other
Emergency Services: Yes

Phone: 985-537-6841
Fax: 985-537-8272

Accredited: No
Licensed Beds: 45

Key Personnel:
Administrator/CEO . . . . Milton Bourgeois, Jr
Emergency Room Manager . . . . Adele Dantin
OB/GYN . . . . Lucia Champagne

Measure	Cases	This Hospital	State Average	U.S. Average	Top Hospital
Heart Attack Care					
ACE Inhibitor or ARB for LVSD[1,3]	3	100%	84%	82%	100%
Aspirin at Arrival[1,3]	5	100%	91%	92%	100%
Aspirin at Discharge[1,3]	5	100%	87%	90%	100%
Beta Blocker at Arrival[1,3]	5	80%	85%	87%	100%
Beta Blocker at Discharge[1,3]	5	40%	88%	90%	100%
Fibrinolytic Medication Timing[1,3]	1	0%	32%	31%	100%
PCI Within 90 Minutes of Arrival[5]	-	-	40%	54%	95%
Smoking Cessation Advice[3]	0	-	88%	88%	100%
Heart Failure Care					
ACE Inhibitor or ARB for LVSD[1]	19	63%	78%	82%	100%
Discharge Instructions	61	59%	62%	61%	93%
Evaluation of LVS Function	66	88%	81%	83%	99%
Smoking Cessation Advice[1]	9	89%	83%	82%	100%
Pneumonia Care					
Appropriate Initial Antibiotic	27	81%	78%	83%	94%
Blood Culture Timing[1]	14	93%	89%	90%	100%
Influenza Vaccine[1]	10	90%	58%	70%	100%
Initial Antibiotic Timing	35	86%	76%	80%	93%
Oxygenation Assessment	38	95%	98%	99%	100%
Pneumococcal Vaccine	25	72%	61%	69%	94%
Smoking Cessation Advice[1]	9	67%	78%	80%	100%
Surgical Infection Prevention					
Prophylactic Antibiotic Given[3]	54	87%	69%	77%	95%
Prophylactic Antibiotic Selection[1]	16	0%	79%	90%	100%
Prophylactic Antibiotic Stopped[3]	53	70%	61%	72%	95%
Pregnancy Care					
Inpatient Neonatal Mortality	208	0.00%	-	-	-
Third or Fourth Degree Laceration	81	9.88%	3.54%	3.63%	3.27%

Richardson Medical Center

Alternate Name: Richland Parish Hospital Service District
254 Highway 3048 Christian Dr
Rayville, LA 71269
E-mail: info@richardsonmed.org
URL: www.richardsonmedicalcenter.org
Ownership: Govt - Hospital District or Authority
Emergency Services: Yes

Phone: 318-728-4181
Fax: 318-728-8248

Accredited: No
Licensed Beds: 49

Key Personnel:
Administrator . . . . Bill Klamfoth
Chief Medical Staff . . . . Dan LaFleur, MD
Director Infection/Disease Control . . . . Betty Hill, RN
Chief Radiology . . . . Craig P Folse, MD
Director Respiratory Therapy . . . . Kathryn Thompson

Measure	Cases	This Hospital	State Average	U.S. Average	Top Hospital
Heart Attack Care					
ACE Inhibitor or ARB for LVSD[2,3]	0	-	84%	82%	100%
Aspirin at Arrival[1,2,3]	7	100%	91%	92%	100%
Aspirin at Discharge[1,2,3]	3	67%	87%	90%	100%
Beta Blocker at Arrival[1,2,3]	7	71%	85%	87%	100%
Beta Blocker at Discharge[1,2,3]	3	100%	88%	90%	100%
Fibrinolytic Medication Timing[2,3]	0	-	32%	31%	100%
PCI Within 90 Minutes of Arrival[2]	0	-	40%	54%	95%
Smoking Cessation Advice[2,3]	0	-	88%	88%	100%
Heart Failure Care					
ACE Inhibitor or ARB for LVSD[1,2]	4	50%	78%	82%	100%
Discharge Instructions[1,2,3]	6	0%	62%	61%	93%
Evaluation of LVS Function[2]	46	35%	81%	83%	99%
Smoking Cessation Advice[1,2,3]	1	0%	83%	82%	100%

NOTE: Hospital profiles are in alphabetical order by state, then city, then hospital within the city; Rankings are sorted by rate in descending order and exclude hospitals with less than 25 cases; (1) The number of cases is too small (n<25) for purposes of reliably predicting hospital performance; (2) Measure reflects the hospital's indication that its submission was based upon a sample of its relevant discharges; (3) Rate reflects fewer than the maximum possible quarters of data for the measure; (4) Inaccurate information submitted and suppressed for one or more quarters; (5) No data is available from the hospital for this measure; Please refer to the User's Guide for a full explanation of data

Pneumonia Care					
Appropriate Initial Antibiotic[1,2,3]	4	25%	78%	83%	94%
Blood Culture Timing[1,2,3]	4	100%	89%	90%	100%
Influenza Vaccine[5]	-	-	58%	70%	100%
Initial Antibiotic Timing[2]	58	69%	76%	80%	93%
Oxygenation Assessment[2]	69	83%	98%	99%	100%
Pneumococcal Vaccine[2]	35	46%	61%	69%	94%
Smoking Cessation Advice[2,3]	0	-	78%	80%	100%
Surgical Infection Prevention					
Prophylactic Antibiotic Given[1,3]	3	33%	69%	77%	95%
Prophylactic Antibiotic Selection[5]	-	-	79%	90%	100%
Prophylactic Antibiotic Stopped[1,3]	2	100%	61%	72%	95%
Pregnancy Care					
Inpatient Neonatal Mortality	-	-	-	-	-
Third or Fourth Degree Laceration	-	-	3.54%	3.63%	3.27%

Green Clinic Surgical Hospital

1118 Farmerville Street   Phone: 318-232-7700
Ruston, LA 71270
Ownership: Voluntary non-profit - Private   Accredited: No
Emergency Services: No

Measure	Cases	This Hospital	State Average	U.S. Average	Top Hospital
Heart Attack Care					
ACE Inhibitor or ARB for LVSD[3]	0	-	84%	82%	100%
Aspirin at Arrival[1,3]	1	100%	91%	92%	100%
Aspirin at Discharge[3]	0	-	87%	90%	100%
Beta Blocker at Arrival[1,3]	1	100%	85%	87%	100%
Beta Blocker at Discharge[3]	0	-	88%	90%	100%
Fibrinolytic Medication Timing[5]	-	-	32%	31%	100%
PCI Within 90 Minutes of Arrival[5]	-	-	40%	54%	95%
Smoking Cessation Advice[5]	-	-	88%	88%	100%
Heart Failure Care					
ACE Inhibitor or ARB for LVSD[1,3]	3	0%	78%	82%	100%
Discharge Instructions[1,3]	2	0%	62%	61%	93%
Evaluation of LVS Function[1,3]	5	80%	81%	83%	99%
Smoking Cessation Advice[3]	0	-	83%	82%	100%
Pneumonia Care					
Appropriate Initial Antibiotic[3]	0	-	78%	83%	94%
Blood Culture Timing[3]	0	-	89%	90%	100%
Influenza Vaccine[5]	-	-	58%	70%	100%
Initial Antibiotic Timing[1,3]	1	100%	76%	80%	93%
Oxygenation Assessment[1,3]	2	100%	98%	99%	100%
Pneumococcal Vaccine[1,3]	2	0%	61%	69%	94%
Smoking Cessation Advice[3]	0	-	78%	80%	100%
Surgical Infection Prevention					
Prophylactic Antibiotic Given[3]	59	58%	69%	77%	95%
Prophylactic Antibiotic Selection[5]	-	-	79%	90%	100%
Prophylactic Antibiotic Stopped[3]	56	73%	61%	72%	95%
Pregnancy Care					
Inpatient Neonatal Mortality	-	-	-	-	-
Third or Fourth Degree Laceration	-	-	3.54%	3.63%	3.27%

Lincoln General Hospital

401 East Vaughn Avenue   Phone: 318-254-2100
Ruston, LA 71270   Fax: 318-254-2728
URL: www.lincolnhealth.com
Ownership: Voluntary non-profit - Other   Accredited: Yes
Emergency Services: Yes   Licensed Beds: 160
Key Personnel:
Administrator/CEO . . . . Thomas J Stone
Chief Medical Staff . . . . William Tanner, MD
Director Cardiology . . . . Alan Brazzell
Catheterization Lab . . . . Sue Campbell
Emergency Room . . . . Eva Morris
Director Infection Control . . . . Carrie McCullin, RNC
ICU . . . . Belinda Gray
Intensive/Coronary Care . . . . Belinda Gray
Director Surgical Services . . . . Gayle Smith, RN
Director OB/GYN Womens Health . . . . Pam R Collingsworth
Outpatient Surgery Manager . . . . Ann Hough
Director Respiratory/Cardiopulmonary . . . . . . Barbara Elmore

Measure	Cases	This Hospital	State Average	U.S. Average	Top Hospital
Heart Attack Care					
ACE Inhibitor or ARB for LVSD[1]	5	100%	84%	82%	100%
Aspirin at Arrival	58	98%	91%	92%	100%
Aspirin at Discharge	38	97%	87%	90%	100%
Beta Blocker at Arrival	55	96%	85%	87%	100%
Beta Blocker at Discharge	37	95%	88%	90%	100%
Fibrinolytic Medication Timing[1,3]	1	100%	32%	31%	100%
PCI Within 90 Minutes of Arrival	0	-	40%	54%	95%
Smoking Cessation Advice[1,3]	1	100%	88%	88%	100%
Heart Failure Care					
ACE Inhibitor or ARB for LVSD	61	66%	78%	82%	100%
Discharge Instructions[3]	42	67%	62%	61%	93%
Evaluation of LVS Function	263	92%	81%	83%	99%
Smoking Cessation Advice[1,3]	11	100%	83%	82%	100%
Pneumonia Care					
Appropriate Initial Antibiotic[1,3]	18	89%	78%	83%	94%
Blood Culture Timing[1,3]	18	72%	89%	90%	100%
Influenza Vaccine[5]	-	-	58%	70%	100%
Initial Antibiotic Timing	133	89%	76%	80%	93%
Oxygenation Assessment	145	98%	98%	99%	100%
Pneumococcal Vaccine	83	80%	61%	69%	94%
Smoking Cessation Advice[1,3]	6	100%	78%	80%	100%
Surgical Infection Prevention					
Prophylactic Antibiotic Given[3]	31	74%	69%	77%	95%
Prophylactic Antibiotic Selection[5]	-	-	79%	90%	100%
Prophylactic Antibiotic Stopped[3]	29	86%	61%	72%	95%
Pregnancy Care					
Inpatient Neonatal Mortality	-	-	-	-	-
Third or Fourth Degree Laceration	-	-	3.54%	3.63%	3.27%

Christus Schumpert Health System

Alternate Name: Schumpert Medical Center
One Saint Mary Place   Phone: 318-681-4500
Shreveport, LA 71101   Fax: 318-681-4424
E-mail: sally.croom@christushealth.org
URL: www.christusschumpert.org
Ownership: Voluntary non-profit - Church   Accredited: Yes
Emergency Services: Yes   Licensed Beds: 809
Key Personnel:
Administrator/CEO . . . . Charles J Paine
Chief Medical Staff . . . . Sanders Hearne, MD
Director of Catheterization . . . . Arnie Young
Emergency Room . . . . EL Edwards, MD
Director Infection/Disease Control . . . . Kathy Brooks
OB/GYN Womens Health . . . . EB Robinson, MD
Director Respiratory Therapy . . . . George Speckman

Measure	Cases	This Hospital	State Average	U.S. Average	Top Hospital
Heart Attack Care					
ACE Inhibitor or ARB for LVSD	33	79%	84%	82%	100%
Aspirin at Arrival	109	96%	91%	92%	100%
Aspirin at Discharge	149	96%	87%	90%	100%
Beta Blocker at Arrival	94	95%	85%	87%	100%
Beta Blocker at Discharge	135	96%	88%	90%	100%
Fibrinolytic Medication Timing[1]	3	0%	32%	31%	100%
PCI Within 90 Minutes of Arrival[1]	6	33%	40%	54%	95%
Smoking Cessation Advice	57	96%	88%	88%	100%
Heart Failure Care					
ACE Inhibitor or ARB for LVSD	194	86%	78%	82%	100%
Discharge Instructions	396	91%	62%	61%	93%
Evaluation of LVS Function	484	98%	81%	83%	99%
Smoking Cessation Advice	87	90%	83%	82%	100%
Pneumonia Care					
Appropriate Initial Antibiotic	158	89%	78%	83%	94%
Blood Culture Timing	169	98%	89%	90%	100%
Influenza Vaccine[4,5]	-	-	58%	70%	100%
Initial Antibiotic Timing	277	87%	76%	80%	93%
Oxygenation Assessment	342	100%	98%	99%	100%
Pneumococcal Vaccine	223	93%	61%	69%	94%
Smoking Cessation Advice	76	91%	78%	80%	100%
Surgical Infection Prevention					

NOTE: Hospital profiles are in alphabetical order by state, then city, then hospital within the city; Rankings are sorted by rate in descending order and exclude hospitals with less than 25 cases; (1) The number of cases is too small (n<25) for purposes of reliably predicting hospital performance; (2) Measure reflects the hospital's indication that its submission was based upon a sample of its relevant discharges; (3) Rate reflects fewer than the maximum possible quarters of data for the measure; (4) Inaccurate information submitted and suppressed for one or more quarters; (5) No data is available from the hospital for this measure; Please refer to the User's Guide for a full explanation of data

Prophylactic Antibiotic Given	279	85%	69%	77%	95%
Prophylactic Antibiotic Selection	70	91%	79%	90%	100%
Prophylactic Antibiotic Stopped	267	45%	61%	72%	95%
Pregnancy Care					
Inpatient Neonatal Mortality	-	-	-	-	-
Third or Fourth Degree Laceration	-	-	3.54%	3.63%	3.27%

Doctors Hospital

1130 Louisiana Avenue   Phone: 318-227-1211
Shreveport, LA 71101   Fax: 318-678-4112
URL: www.doctorshospitalshreveport.com
Ownership: Proprietary   Accredited: Yes
Emergency Services: Yes   Licensed Beds: 118
Key Personnel:
CEO. . . . . Charles Boyd
Chief Medical Director . . . . Gary B Mazzanti, MD
OB/GYN. . . . . Paula E Rembent, MD
Respiratory Care . . . . Dennis Yates

Measure	Cases	This Hospital	State Average	U.S. Average	Top Hospital
Heart Attack Care					
ACE Inhibitor or ARB for LVSD[1]	2	50%	84%	82%	100%
Aspirin at Arrival[1]	6	100%	91%	92%	100%
Aspirin at Discharge[1]	6	100%	87%	90%	100%
Beta Blocker at Arrival[1]	6	83%	85%	87%	100%
Beta Blocker at Discharge[1]	6	83%	88%	90%	100%
Fibrinolytic Medication Timing	0	-	32%	31%	100%
PCI Within 90 Minutes of Arrival	0	-	40%	54%	95%
Smoking Cessation Advice	0	-	88%	88%	100%
Heart Failure Care					
ACE Inhibitor or ARB for LVSD[1]	20	75%	78%	82%	100%
Discharge Instructions	41	98%	62%	61%	93%
Evaluation of LVS Function	61	64%	81%	83%	99%
Smoking Cessation Advice[1]	15	100%	83%	82%	100%
Pneumonia Care					
Appropriate Initial Antibiotic	30	73%	78%	83%	94%
Blood Culture Timing[1]	15	80%	89%	90%	100%
Influenza Vaccine[1]	8	12%	58%	70%	100%
Initial Antibiotic Timing	45	76%	76%	80%	93%
Oxygenation Assessment	61	98%	98%	99%	100%
Pneumococcal Vaccine	41	49%	61%	69%	94%
Smoking Cessation Advice[1]	7	100%	78%	80%	100%
Surgical Infection Prevention					
Prophylactic Antibiotic Given[3]	63	54%	69%	77%	95%
Prophylactic Antibiotic Selection[1]	13	46%	79%	90%	100%
Prophylactic Antibiotic Stopped[3]	61	11%	61%	72%	95%
Pregnancy Care					
Inpatient Neonatal Mortality	-	-	-	-	-
Third or Fourth Degree Laceration	-	-	3.54%	3.63%	3.27%

Louisiana State Univ Hosp-Shreveport

1501 Kings Highway   Phone: 318-675-5000
Shreveport, LA 71130   Fax: 318-675-5666
URL: www.lsumc.edu
Ownership: Government - State   Accredited: Yes
Emergency Services: Yes   Licensed Beds: 650
Key Personnel:
President/CEO. . . . . Benjamin Rush, MD
Chief Medical Staff. . . . . Ronald George
Chief Catheterization Laboratory . . . . Don Fadley
Emergency Room . . . . Steven Conrad
Director Infection/Disease Control . . . . Robert Penn
Director Medical/Surgical Nursing . . . . Jodi Alphin
OB/GYN Womens Health. . . . . Steve N London, MD
Chief Radiology . . . . James Lecky, MD

Measure	Cases	This Hospital	State Average	U.S. Average	Top Hospital
Heart Attack Care					
ACE Inhibitor or ARB for LVSD	43	98%	84%	82%	100%
Aspirin at Arrival	117	98%	91%	92%	100%
Aspirin at Discharge	174	98%	87%	90%	100%
Beta Blocker at Arrival	101	96%	85%	87%	100%
Beta Blocker at Discharge	174	99%	88%	90%	100%

Fibrinolytic Medication Timing[3]	0	-	32%	31%	100%
PCI Within 90 Minutes of Arrival[1]	5	0%	40%	54%	95%
Smoking Cessation Advice[1,3]	22	86%	88%	88%	100%
Heart Failure Care					
ACE Inhibitor or ARB for LVSD[2]	215	94%	78%	82%	100%
Discharge Instructions[2,3]	62	73%	62%	61%	93%
Evaluation of LVS Function[2]	324	99%	81%	83%	99%
Smoking Cessation Advice[1,2,3]	19	89%	83%	82%	100%
Pneumonia Care					
Appropriate Initial Antibiotic[1,2,3]	14	71%	78%	83%	94%
Blood Culture Timing[1,2,3]	17	88%	89%	90%	100%
Influenza Vaccine[5]	-	-	58%	70%	100%
Initial Antibiotic Timing[2]	126	44%	76%	80%	93%
Oxygenation Assessment[2]	152	94%	98%	99%	100%
Pneumococcal Vaccine[2]	31	26%	61%	69%	94%
Smoking Cessation Advice[1,2,3]	12	75%	78%	80%	100%
Surgical Infection Prevention					
Prophylactic Antibiotic Given[2,3]	53	68%	69%	77%	95%
Prophylactic Antibiotic Selection[5]	-	-	79%	90%	100%
Prophylactic Antibiotic Stopped[2,3]	51	51%	61%	72%	95%
Pregnancy Care					
Inpatient Neonatal Mortality[2]	397	2.02%	-	-	-
Third or Fourth Degree Laceration	1,163	4.47%	3.54%	3.63%	3.27%

Willis Knighton Medical Center

2600 Greenwood Road   Phone: 318-212-4000
Shreveport, LA 71103
Ownership: Voluntary non-profit - Private   Accredited: Yes
Emergency Services: Yes

Measure	Cases	This Hospital	State Average	U.S. Average	Top Hospital
Heart Attack Care					
ACE Inhibitor or ARB for LVSD	131	68%	84%	82%	100%
Aspirin at Arrival	231	98%	91%	92%	100%
Aspirin at Discharge	338	94%	87%	90%	100%
Beta Blocker at Arrival	169	88%	85%	87%	100%
Beta Blocker at Discharge	377	92%	88%	90%	100%
Fibrinolytic Medication Timing[1,3]	1	0%	32%	31%	100%
PCI Within 90 Minutes of Arrival[1]	11	18%	40%	54%	95%
Smoking Cessation Advice[3]	53	100%	88%	88%	100%
Heart Failure Care					
ACE Inhibitor or ARB for LVSD	344	67%	78%	82%	100%
Discharge Instructions[3]	106	33%	62%	61%	93%
Evaluation of LVS Function	700	88%	81%	83%	99%
Smoking Cessation Advice[1,3]	22	100%	83%	82%	100%
Pneumonia Care					
Appropriate Initial Antibiotic[3]	29	83%	78%	83%	94%
Blood Culture Timing[3]	42	90%	89%	90%	100%
Influenza Vaccine[5]	-	-	58%	70%	100%
Initial Antibiotic Timing	381	80%	76%	80%	93%
Oxygenation Assessment	456	100%	98%	99%	100%
Pneumococcal Vaccine	280	51%	61%	69%	94%
Smoking Cessation Advice[1,3]	17	94%	78%	80%	100%
Surgical Infection Prevention					
Prophylactic Antibiotic Given[3]	99	80%	69%	77%	95%
Prophylactic Antibiotic Selection[5]	-	-	79%	90%	100%
Prophylactic Antibiotic Stopped[3]	96	46%	61%	72%	95%
Pregnancy Care					
Inpatient Neonatal Mortality	-	-	-	-	-
Third or Fourth Degree Laceration	-	-	3.54%	3.63%	3.27%

Doctors' Hospital of Slidell

989 Robert Blvd   Phone: 504-690-8200
Slidell, LA 70458
Ownership: Voluntary non-profit - Private   Accredited: No
Emergency Services: No

Measure	Cases	This Hospital	State Average	U.S. Average	Top Hospital
Heart Attack Care					
ACE Inhibitor or ARB for LVSD[5]	-	-	84%	82%	100%
Aspirin at Arrival[5]	-	-	91%	92%	100%
Aspirin at Discharge[5]	-	-	87%	90%	100%

NOTE: Hospital profiles are in alphabetical order by state, then city, then hospital within the city; Rankings are sorted by rate in descending order and exclude hospitals with less than 25 cases; (1) The number of cases is too small (n<25) for purposes of reliably predicting hospital performance; (2) Measure reflects the hospital's indication that its submission was based upon a sample of its relevant discharges; (3) Rate reflects fewer than the maximum possible quarters of data for the measure; (4) Inaccurate information submitted and suppressed for one or more quarters; (5) No data is available from the hospital for this measure; Please refer to the User's Guide for a full explanation of data

Beta Blocker at Arrival[5]	-	-	85%	87%	100%
Beta Blocker at Discharge[5]	-	-	88%	90%	100%
Fibrinolytic Medication Timing[5]	-	-	32%	31%	100%
PCI Within 90 Minutes of Arrival[5]	-	-	40%	54%	95%
Smoking Cessation Advice[5]	-	-	88%	88%	100%
Heart Failure Care					
ACE Inhibitor or ARB for LVSD[5]	-	-	78%	82%	100%
Discharge Instructions[5]	-	-	62%	61%	93%
Evaluation of LVS Function[5]	-	-	81%	83%	99%
Smoking Cessation Advice[5]	-	-	83%	82%	100%
Pneumonia Care					
Appropriate Initial Antibiotic[1,3]	1	100%	78%	83%	94%
Blood Culture Timing[3]	0	-	89%	90%	100%
Influenza Vaccine[5]	-	-	58%	70%	100%
Initial Antibiotic Timing[1,3]	1	100%	76%	80%	93%
Oxygenation Assessment[1,3]	2	100%	98%	99%	100%
Pneumococcal Vaccine[3]	0	-	61%	69%	94%
Smoking Cessation Advice[1,3]	1	0%	78%	80%	100%
Surgical Infection Prevention					
Prophylactic Antibiotic Given[1,2,3]	17	76%	69%	77%	95%
Prophylactic Antibiotic Selection[5]	-	-	79%	90%	100%
Prophylactic Antibiotic Stopped[1,2,3]	17	71%	61%	72%	95%
Pregnancy Care					
Inpatient Neonatal Mortality	-	-	-	-	-
Third or Fourth Degree Laceration	-	-	3.54%	3.63%	3.27%

Northshore Regional Medical Center

100 Medical Center Drive
Slidell, LA 70461
E-mail: rita.koder@tenethealth.com
URL: www.northshoremedctr.com
Ownership: Proprietary
Emergency Services: Yes

Phone: 985-649-7070
Fax: 985-646-5552

Accredited: Yes
Licensed Beds: 58

Key Personnel:
CEO . . . . George Terry

Measure	Cases	This Hospital	State Average	U.S. Average	Top Hospital
Heart Attack Care					
ACE Inhibitor or ARB for LVSD[1]	22	95%	84%	82%	100%
Aspirin at Arrival	97	98%	91%	92%	100%
Aspirin at Discharge	100	95%	87%	90%	100%
Beta Blocker at Arrival	92	98%	85%	87%	100%
Beta Blocker at Discharge	103	100%	88%	90%	100%
Fibrinolytic Medication Timing[1]	4	25%	32%	31%	100%
PCI Within 90 Minutes of Arrival[1]	2	100%	40%	54%	95%
Smoking Cessation Advice	44	100%	88%	88%	100%
Heart Failure Care					
ACE Inhibitor or ARB for LVSD	114	96%	78%	82%	100%
Discharge Instructions	249	89%	62%	61%	93%
Evaluation of LVS Function	277	100%	81%	83%	99%
Smoking Cessation Advice	76	99%	83%	82%	100%
Pneumonia Care					
Appropriate Initial Antibiotic	193	80%	78%	83%	94%
Blood Culture Timing	196	99%	89%	90%	100%
Influenza Vaccine	62	100%	58%	70%	100%
Initial Antibiotic Timing	240	90%	76%	80%	93%
Oxygenation Assessment	303	99%	98%	99%	100%
Pneumococcal Vaccine	181	99%	61%	69%	94%
Smoking Cessation Advice	88	98%	78%	80%	100%
Surgical Infection Prevention					
Prophylactic Antibiotic Given[2]	343	90%	69%	77%	95%
Prophylactic Antibiotic Selection[2]	103	90%	79%	90%	100%
Prophylactic Antibiotic Stopped[2]	328	67%	61%	72%	95%
Pregnancy Care					
Inpatient Neonatal Mortality	522	0.19%	-	-	-
Third or Fourth Degree Laceration	404	2.97%	3.54%	3.63%	3.27%

Slidell Memorial Hospital

1001 Gause Boulevard
Slidell, LA 70458
URL: www.sliddelmemorial.org
Ownership: Govt - Hospital District or Authority
Emergency Services: Yes

Phone: 985-643-2200
Fax: 985-649-8778

Accredited: Yes
Licensed Beds: 182

Key Personnel:
Administrator/CEO . . . . Robert L Hawley, Jr
Chief of Medical Staff . . . . Diana Clavin, MD
Director Emergency Room . . . . Kumar Amaraneni, MD
Chief Radiology . . . . Kishore Kamath
Director of Pulmonary/Respiratory Care . . . . . . Brook Coelemt, MD

Measure	Cases	This Hospital	State Average	U.S. Average	Top Hospital
Heart Attack Care					
ACE Inhibitor or ARB for LVSD	33	73%	84%	82%	100%
Aspirin at Arrival	120	98%	91%	92%	100%
Aspirin at Discharge	111	95%	87%	90%	100%
Beta Blocker at Arrival	111	94%	85%	87%	100%
Beta Blocker at Discharge	116	94%	88%	90%	100%
Fibrinolytic Medication Timing	0	-	32%	31%	100%
PCI Within 90 Minutes of Arrival[1]	1	0%	40%	54%	95%
Smoking Cessation Advice	58	90%	88%	88%	100%
Heart Failure Care					
ACE Inhibitor or ARB for LVSD	117	81%	78%	82%	100%
Discharge Instructions	297	54%	62%	61%	93%
Evaluation of LVS Function	317	82%	81%	83%	99%
Smoking Cessation Advice	59	61%	83%	82%	100%
Pneumonia Care					
Appropriate Initial Antibiotic	208	85%	78%	83%	94%
Blood Culture Timing	121	88%	89%	90%	100%
Influenza Vaccine	67	49%	58%	70%	100%
Initial Antibiotic Timing	242	66%	76%	80%	93%
Oxygenation Assessment	307	98%	98%	99%	100%
Pneumococcal Vaccine	166	48%	61%	69%	94%
Smoking Cessation Advice	96	70%	78%	80%	100%
Surgical Infection Prevention					
Prophylactic Antibiotic Given	265	70%	69%	77%	95%
Prophylactic Antibiotic Selection	71	82%	79%	90%	100%
Prophylactic Antibiotic Stopped	258	57%	61%	72%	95%
Pregnancy Care					
Inpatient Neonatal Mortality	-	-	-	-	-
Third or Fourth Degree Laceration	-	-	3.54%	3.63%	3.27%

Southern Surgical Hospital

1700 W Lindberg Drive
Slidell, LA 70458
Ownership: Proprietary
Emergency Services: Yes

Phone: 985-641-0600

Accredited: Yes

Key Personnel:
Cardiology . . . . Sergio Barrios, MD
Pulmonary . . . . Lasandra Barton, MD
Infection Control . . . . Michael Hill, MD

Measure	Cases	This Hospital	State Average	U.S. Average	Top Hospital
Heart Attack Care					
ACE Inhibitor or ARB for LVSD[5]	-	-	84%	82%	100%
Aspirin at Arrival[5]	-	-	91%	92%	100%
Aspirin at Discharge[5]	-	-	87%	90%	100%
Beta Blocker at Arrival[5]	-	-	85%	87%	100%
Beta Blocker at Discharge[5]	-	-	88%	90%	100%
Fibrinolytic Medication Timing[5]	-	-	32%	31%	100%
PCI Within 90 Minutes of Arrival[5]	-	-	40%	54%	95%
Smoking Cessation Advice[5]	-	-	88%	88%	100%
Heart Failure Care					
ACE Inhibitor or ARB for LVSD[5]	-	-	78%	82%	100%
Discharge Instructions[5]	-	-	62%	61%	93%
Evaluation of LVS Function[5]	-	-	81%	83%	99%
Smoking Cessation Advice[5]	-	-	83%	82%	100%
Pneumonia Care					
Appropriate Initial Antibiotic[5]	-	-	78%	83%	94%
Blood Culture Timing[5]	-	-	89%	90%	100%
Influenza Vaccine[5]	-	-	58%	70%	100%

NOTE: Hospital profiles are in alphabetical order by state, then city, then hospital within the city; Rankings are sorted by rate in descending order and exclude hospitals with less than 25 cases; (1) The number of cases is too small (n<25) for purposes of reliably predicting hospital performance; (2) Measure reflects the hospital's indication that its submission was based upon a sample of its relevant discharges; (3) Rate reflects fewer than the maximum possible quarters of data for the measure; (4) Inaccurate information submitted and suppressed for one or more quarters; (5) No data is available from the hospital for this measure; Please refer to the User's Guide for a full explanation of data

Initial Antibiotic Timing[5]	-	-	76%	80%	93%
Oxygenation Assessment[5]	-	-	98%	99%	100%
Pneumococcal Vaccine[5]	-	-	61%	69%	94%
Smoking Cessation Advice[5]	-	-	78%	80%	100%
Surgical Infection Prevention					
Prophylactic Antibiotic Given[3]	30	100%	69%	77%	95%
Prophylactic Antibiotic Selection[5]		-	79%	90%	100%
Prophylactic Antibiotic Stopped[3]	30	43%	61%	72%	95%
Pregnancy Care					
Inpatient Neonatal Mortality	-	-	-	-	-
Third or Fourth Degree Laceration	-	-	3.54%	3.63%	3.27%

Springhill Medical Center

2001 Doctors Drive
Springhill, LA 71075
E-mail: derek.melancon@emailsmc.com
URL: www.smccare.com
Ownership: Proprietary
Emergency Services: Yes

Phone: 318-539-1000
Fax: 318-539-4085

Accredited: Yes
Licensed Beds: 60

Key Personnel:
CEO . . . . Todd Blanchard
Director Cardiology . . . . Albert N Krause, MD
Pulmonology . . . . Robert Holladay, MD
Chief Radiology . . . . Robert Edwards, MD
Director of Pulmonary/Respiratory Care . . . . Veronica Scott

Measure	Cases	This Hospital	State Average	U.S. Average	Top Hospital
Heart Attack Care					
ACE Inhibitor or ARB for LVSD[1]	1	0%	84%	82%	100%
Aspirin at Arrival[1]	9	89%	91%	92%	100%
Aspirin at Discharge[1]	5	80%	87%	90%	100%
Beta Blocker at Arrival[1]	8	50%	85%	87%	100%
Beta Blocker at Discharge[1]	5	60%	88%	90%	100%
Fibrinolytic Medication Timing[3]	0	-	32%	31%	100%
PCI Within 90 Minutes of Arrival	0	-	40%	54%	95%
Smoking Cessation Advice[3]	0	-	88%	88%	100%
Heart Failure Care					
ACE Inhibitor or ARB for LVSD[1]	16	75%	78%	82%	100%
Discharge Instructions[1,3]	17	47%	62%	61%	93%
Evaluation of LVS Function	96	79%	81%	83%	99%
Smoking Cessation Advice[1,3]	5	80%	83%	82%	100%
Pneumonia Care					
Appropriate Initial Antibiotic[1,3]	7	86%	78%	83%	94%
Blood Culture Timing[1,3]	7	86%	89%	90%	100%
Influenza Vaccine[5]	-	-	58%	70%	100%
Initial Antibiotic Timing	64	89%	76%	80%	93%
Oxygenation Assessment	79	100%	98%	99%	100%
Pneumococcal Vaccine	52	52%	61%	69%	94%
Smoking Cessation Advice[1,3]	3	100%	78%	80%	100%
Surgical Infection Prevention					
Prophylactic Antibiotic Given[1,3]	2	100%	69%	77%	95%
Prophylactic Antibiotic Selection[5]	-	-	79%	90%	100%
Prophylactic Antibiotic Stopped[1,3]	2	50%	61%	72%	95%
Pregnancy Care					
Inpatient Neonatal Mortality	-	-	-	-	-
Third or Fourth Degree Laceration	-	-	3.54%	3.63%	3.27%

West Calcasieu-Cameron Hospital

701 Cypress Street
Sulphur, LA 70663
E-mail: info@wcch.com
URL: www.wcch.com
Ownership: Govt - Hospital District or Authority
Emergency Services: Yes

Phone: 337-527-7034
Fax: 337-527-4163

Accredited: Yes
Licensed Beds: 120

Key Personnel:
Administrator/CEO . . . . Bill Hankins
Chief Medical Staff . . . . Josen Gonzales
Emergency Room . . . . Tim Quattrone, MD
Director Infection/Disease Control . . . . Jolie Khoury
Director Medical/Surgical Nursing . . . . Theresa Woods
OB/GYN Womens Health . . . . Ben Darby, MD
Chief Radiology . . . . JW Peloquin
Director Respiratory Therapy . . . . Gary Taylor

Measure	Cases	This Hospital	State Average	U.S. Average	Top Hospital
Heart Attack Care					
ACE Inhibitor or ARB for LVSD[1]	18	89%	84%	82%	100%
Aspirin at Arrival	56	96%	91%	92%	100%
Aspirin at Discharge	47	94%	87%	90%	100%
Beta Blocker at Arrival	48	94%	85%	87%	100%
Beta Blocker at Discharge	53	96%	88%	90%	100%
Fibrinolytic Medication Timing[1,3]	3	0%	32%	31%	100%
PCI Within 90 Minutes of Arrival[1]	1	0%	40%	54%	95%
Smoking Cessation Advice[1,3]	23	91%	88%	88%	100%
Heart Failure Care					
ACE Inhibitor or ARB for LVSD	48	73%	78%	82%	100%
Discharge Instructions[3]	68	90%	62%	61%	93%
Evaluation of LVS Function	117	98%	81%	83%	99%
Smoking Cessation Advice[1,3]	17	100%	83%	82%	100%
Pneumonia Care					
Appropriate Initial Antibiotic[3]	46	89%	78%	83%	94%
Blood Culture Timing	41	83%	89%	90%	100%
Influenza Vaccine[1]	14	79%	58%	70%	100%
Initial Antibiotic Timing	72	83%	76%	80%	93%
Oxygenation Assessment	88	97%	98%	99%	100%
Pneumococcal Vaccine	51	67%	61%	69%	94%
Smoking Cessation Advice[1,3]	20	90%	78%	80%	100%
Surgical Infection Prevention					
Prophylactic Antibiotic Given[3]	150	80%	69%	77%	95%
Prophylactic Antibiotic Selection	46	91%	79%	90%	100%
Prophylactic Antibiotic Stopped[3]	150	36%	61%	72%	95%
Pregnancy Care					
Inpatient Neonatal Mortality	271	0.00%	-	-	-
Third or Fourth Degree Laceration	179	1.68%	3.54%	3.63%	3.27%

Thibodaux Regional Medical Center

602 N Acadia Road
Thibodaux, LA 70301

Toll-Free: 800-822-8442
Phone: 985-447-5500
Fax: 985-449-2533

E-mail: info@thibodaux.com
URL: www.thibodaux.com
Ownership: Government - Federal
Emergency Services: Yes

Accredited: Yes
Licensed Beds: 185

Key Personnel:
CEO . . . . Greg Stock
Chief Medical Staff . . . . Leo Hebert
Emergency Room . . . . Missy Keiffe
Director Infection/Disease Control . . . . Rita Cade
CCU Spvg. Nurse . . . . Missy Keiffe
OB/GYN Womens Health . . . . John Milek
Chief Radiology . . . . Greg Dobard, MD
Director Respiratory Therapy . . . . Ann Parker

Measure	Cases	This Hospital	State Average	U.S. Average	Top Hospital
Heart Attack Care					
ACE Inhibitor or ARB for LVSD	31	97%	84%	82%	100%
Aspirin at Arrival	118	100%	91%	92%	100%
Aspirin at Discharge	188	98%	87%	90%	100%
Beta Blocker at Arrival	96	97%	85%	87%	100%
Beta Blocker at Discharge	177	99%	88%	90%	100%
Fibrinolytic Medication Timing[1]	1	0%	32%	31%	100%
PCI Within 90 Minutes of Arrival[1]	4	75%	40%	54%	95%
Smoking Cessation Advice	92	100%	88%	88%	100%
Heart Failure Care					
ACE Inhibitor or ARB for LVSD	86	95%	78%	82%	100%
Discharge Instructions	235	88%	62%	61%	93%
Evaluation of LVS Function	279	95%	81%	83%	99%
Smoking Cessation Advice	42	98%	83%	82%	100%
Pneumonia Care					
Appropriate Initial Antibiotic	113	81%	78%	83%	94%
Blood Culture Timing	94	89%	89%	90%	100%
Influenza Vaccine	39	90%	58%	70%	100%
Initial Antibiotic Timing	165	88%	76%	80%	93%
Oxygenation Assessment	198	99%	98%	99%	100%
Pneumococcal Vaccine	122	80%	61%	69%	94%
Smoking Cessation Advice	43	95%	78%	80%	100%

NOTE: Hospital profiles are in alphabetical order by state, then city, then hospital within the city; Rankings are sorted by rate in descending order and exclude hospitals with less than 25 cases; (1) The number of cases is too small (n<25) for purposes of reliably predicting hospital performance; (2) Measure reflects the hospital's indication that its submission was based upon a sample of its relevant discharges; (3) Rate reflects fewer than the maximum possible quarters of data for the measure; (4) Inaccurate information submitted and suppressed for one or more quarters; (5) No data is available from the hospital for this measure; Please refer to the User's Guide for a full explanation of data

Surgical Infection Prevention					
Prophylactic Antibiotic Given[3]	214	46%	69%	77%	95%
Prophylactic Antibiotic Selection	102	65%	79%	90%	100%
Prophylactic Antibiotic Stopped[3]	190	56%	61%	72%	95%
Pregnancy Care					
Inpatient Neonatal Mortality	625	0.16%	-	-	-
Third or Fourth Degree Laceration	293	7.85%	3.54%	3.63%	3.27%

Ville Platte Medical Center

800 E Main Street
Ville Platte, LA 70586
E-mail: dana.mcdaniel@lpnt.net
URL: www.vpmc.com
Ownership: Proprietary
Emergency Services: Yes

Phone: 337-363-5684
Fax: 337-363-9488

Accredited: Yes
Licensed Beds: 102

Key Personnel:
CEO. . . . . Steven Downs
Chief Staff . . . . Charles Monier, MD
Cardiac Lab Supervisor . . . . Jeanett LeDay, RN
Director Emergency Room. . . . . Lisa Johnson, RN
ICU Supervisor. . . . . Karleen Vidrine
Obstetrics Supervisor. . . . . Karen Fontenot, RN
Director Radiology . . . . Steven Pitre

Measure	Cases	This Hospital	State Average	U.S. Average	Top Hospital
Heart Attack Care					
ACE Inhibitor or ARB for LVSD[1]	1	100%	84%	82%	100%
Aspirin at Arrival[1]	18	94%	91%	92%	100%
Aspirin at Discharge[1]	11	64%	87%	90%	100%
Beta Blocker at Arrival[1]	12	92%	85%	87%	100%
Beta Blocker at Discharge[1]	9	89%	88%	90%	100%
Fibrinolytic Medication Timing[1]	5	0%	32%	31%	100%
PCI Within 90 Minutes of Arrival	0	-	40%	54%	95%
Smoking Cessation Advice[1]	2	50%	88%	88%	100%
Heart Failure Care					
ACE Inhibitor or ARB for LVSD	77	73%	78%	82%	100%
Discharge Instructions	142	40%	62%	61%	93%
Evaluation of LVS Function	185	89%	81%	83%	99%
Smoking Cessation Advice	40	82%	83%	82%	100%
Pneumonia Care					
Appropriate Initial Antibiotic	97	80%	78%	83%	94%
Blood Culture Timing	82	85%	89%	90%	100%
Influenza Vaccine	41	85%	58%	70%	100%
Initial Antibiotic Timing	163	83%	76%	80%	93%
Oxygenation Assessment	175	99%	98%	99%	100%
Pneumococcal Vaccine	101	70%	61%	69%	94%
Smoking Cessation Advice	56	89%	78%	80%	100%
Surgical Infection Prevention					
Prophylactic Antibiotic Given[1,2,3]	11	27%	69%	77%	95%
Prophylactic Antibiotic Selection[1,2]	5	60%	79%	90%	100%
Prophylactic Antibiotic Stopped[1,2,3]	11	82%	61%	72%	95%
Pregnancy Care					
Inpatient Neonatal Mortality	-	-	-	-	-
Third or Fourth Degree Laceration	-	-	3.54%	3.63%	3.27%

Glenwood Regional Medical Center

Alternate Name: GRMC Glenwood Hospital
503 McMillian Road
West Monroe, LA 71291
URL: www.grmc.com
Ownership: Voluntary non-profit - Private
Emergency Services: Yes

Phone: 318-329-4200
Fax: 318-329-4710

Accredited: Yes
Licensed Beds: 244

Key Personnel:
Interim President/CEO . . . . Brian Spraberry
Chief Medical Staff. John Maxwell, MD
Director Cardiology Services . . . . Richard Ford
Director Emergency Room. . . . . Kim Koengay
Director Infection Control . . . . Teresa Reagan
Director Intensive Coronary . . . . Becky McCann
Director Medical Surgical Nursing . . . . Paula Phillips
Director Surgical Services . . . . Tanya French
Director Radiology . . . . Chuck Miles
Director Respiratory Therapy . . . . Ray Guess

Measure	Cases	This Hospital	State Average	U.S. Average	Top Hospital
Heart Attack Care					
ACE Inhibitor or ARB for LVSD	57	72%	84%	82%	100%
Aspirin at Arrival	137	96%	91%	92%	100%
Aspirin at Discharge	184	97%	87%	90%	100%
Beta Blocker at Arrival	94	87%	85%	87%	100%
Beta Blocker at Discharge	201	93%	88%	90%	100%
Fibrinolytic Medication Timing	0	-	32%	31%	100%
PCI Within 90 Minutes of Arrival	0	-	40%	54%	95%
Smoking Cessation Advice	91	84%	88%	88%	100%
Heart Failure Care					
ACE Inhibitor or ARB for LVSD	133	65%	78%	82%	100%
Discharge Instructions	286	46%	62%	61%	93%
Evaluation of LVS Function	369	93%	81%	83%	99%
Smoking Cessation Advice	64	70%	83%	82%	100%
Pneumonia Care					
Appropriate Initial Antibiotic	98	77%	78%	83%	94%
Blood Culture Timing	64	88%	89%	90%	100%
Influenza Vaccine	26	62%	58%	70%	100%
Initial Antibiotic Timing	168	74%	76%	80%	93%
Oxygenation Assessment	174	99%	98%	99%	100%
Pneumococcal Vaccine	123	72%	61%	69%	94%
Smoking Cessation Advice	43	40%	78%	80%	100%
Surgical Infection Prevention					
Prophylactic Antibiotic Given[3]	188	61%	69%	77%	95%
Prophylactic Antibiotic Selection	70	91%	79%	90%	100%
Prophylactic Antibiotic Stopped[3]	182	48%	61%	72%	95%
Pregnancy Care					
Inpatient Neonatal Mortality	1,113	0.09%	-	-	-
Third or Fourth Degree Laceration	616	3.90%	3.54%	3.63%	3.27%

Ouachita Community Hospital

1275 Glennwood Drive
West Monroe, LA 71291
Ownership: Voluntary non-profit - Private
Emergency Services: No

Phone: 318-332-1339

Accredited: Yes

Measure	Cases	This Hospital	State Average	U.S. Average	Top Hospital
Heart Attack Care					
ACE Inhibitor or ARB for LVSD[5]	-	-	84%	82%	100%
Aspirin at Arrival[5]	-	-	91%	92%	100%
Aspirin at Discharge[5]	-	-	87%	90%	100%
Beta Blocker at Arrival[5]	-	-	85%	87%	100%
Beta Blocker at Discharge[5]	-	-	88%	90%	100%
Fibrinolytic Medication Timing[5]	-	-	32%	31%	100%
PCI Within 90 Minutes of Arrival[5]	-	-	40%	54%	95%
Smoking Cessation Advice[5]	-	-	88%	88%	100%
Heart Failure Care					
ACE Inhibitor or ARB for LVSD[5]	-	-	78%	82%	100%
Discharge Instructions[5]	-	-	62%	61%	93%
Evaluation of LVS Function[5]	-	-	81%	83%	99%
Smoking Cessation Advice[5]	-	-	83%	82%	100%
Pneumonia Care					
Appropriate Initial Antibiotic[5]	-	-	78%	83%	94%
Blood Culture Timing[5]	-	-	89%	90%	100%
Influenza Vaccine[5]	-	-	58%	70%	100%
Initial Antibiotic Timing[5]	-	-	76%	80%	93%
Oxygenation Assessment[5]	-	-	98%	99%	100%
Pneumococcal Vaccine[5]	-	-	61%	69%	94%
Smoking Cessation Advice[5]	-	-	78%	80%	100%
Surgical Infection Prevention					
Prophylactic Antibiotic Given[1,3]	14	14%	69%	77%	95%
Prophylactic Antibiotic Selection[5]	-	-	79%	90%	100%
Prophylactic Antibiotic Stopped[1,3]	14	43%	61%	72%	95%
Pregnancy Care					
Inpatient Neonatal Mortality	-	-	-	-	-
Third or Fourth Degree Laceration	-	-	3.54%	3.63%	3.27%

Winn Parish Medical Center

Alternate Name: Humana Hospital-Winn Parish

301 W Boundary Street
Winnfield, LA 71483
Ownership: Proprietary
Emergency Services: Yes
Key Personnel:
Administrator/CEO . . . . Bobby Jordan

Phone: 318-648-3000
Fax: 318-628-2035
Accredited: Yes
Licensed Beds: 60

Measure	Cases	This Hospital	State Average	U.S. Average	Top Hospital
Heart Attack Care					
ACE Inhibitor or ARB for LVSD[1]	1	0%	84%	82%	100%
Aspirin at Arrival[1]	2	50%	91%	92%	100%
Aspirin at Discharge	0	-	87%	90%	100%
Beta Blocker at Arrival[1]	1	0%	85%	87%	100%
Beta Blocker at Discharge	0	-	88%	90%	100%
Fibrinolytic Medication Timing	0	-	32%	31%	100%
PCI Within 90 Minutes of Arrival	0	-	40%	54%	95%
Smoking Cessation Advice	0	-	88%	88%	100%
Heart Failure Care					
ACE Inhibitor or ARB for LVSD	28	89%	78%	82%	100%
Discharge Instructions	50	88%	62%	61%	93%
Evaluation of LVS Function	91	89%	81%	83%	99%
Smoking Cessation Advice[1]	16	94%	83%	82%	100%
Pneumonia Care					
Appropriate Initial Antibiotic	50	86%	78%	83%	94%
Blood Culture Timing	48	98%	89%	90%	100%
Influenza Vaccine[1]	17	100%	58%	70%	100%
Initial Antibiotic Timing	91	93%	76%	80%	93%
Oxygenation Assessment	110	100%	98%	99%	100%
Pneumococcal Vaccine	58	100%	61%	69%	94%
Smoking Cessation Advice	27	89%	78%	80%	100%
Surgical Infection Prevention					
Prophylactic Antibiotic Given[1,2,3]	2	50%	69%	77%	95%
Prophylactic Antibiotic Selection[1,2]	1	100%	79%	90%	100%
Prophylactic Antibiotic Stopped[1,2,3]	1	0%	61%	72%	95%
Pregnancy Care					
Inpatient Neonatal Mortality	-	-	-	-	-
Third or Fourth Degree Laceration	-	-	3.54%	3.63%	3.27%

Franklin Medical Center

Alternate Name: Franklin Parish Hospital
2106 Loop Road
PO Box 1300
Winnsboro, LA 71295
Ownership: Govt - Hospital District or Authority
Emergency Services: Yes
Key Personnel:
President/CEO . . . . Leon J Belila
Chief Medical Staff . . . . Dr Jimmy Coughran
Cardiac Lab . . . . Dr Roger Smith
Emergency Room . . . . Brenda Yates
Infection Control . . . . Debi Elrod
CCU Spvg. Nurse . . . . Jo Young, RN
Director Respiratory Therapy . . . . Sherry Harrell

Phone: 318-435-9411
Fax: 318-435-3842
Accredited: No
Licensed Beds: 59

Measure	Cases	This Hospital	State Average	U.S. Average	Top Hospital
Heart Attack Care					
ACE Inhibitor or ARB for LVSD	0	-	84%	82%	100%
Aspirin at Arrival[1]	17	65%	91%	92%	100%
Aspirin at Discharge[1]	9	67%	87%	90%	100%
Beta Blocker at Arrival[1]	16	69%	85%	87%	100%
Beta Blocker at Discharge[1]	14	79%	88%	90%	100%
Fibrinolytic Medication Timing[3]	0	-	32%	31%	100%
PCI Within 90 Minutes of Arrival	0	-	40%	54%	95%
Smoking Cessation Advice[1,3]	1	0%	88%	88%	100%
Heart Failure Care					
ACE Inhibitor or ARB for LVSD[1]	8	88%	78%	82%	100%
Discharge Instructions[1,3]	14	36%	62%	61%	93%
Evaluation of LVS Function	61	49%	81%	83%	99%
Smoking Cessation Advice[1,3]	3	0%	83%	82%	100%
Pneumonia Care					
Appropriate Initial Antibiotic[1,3]	1	100%	78%	83%	94%
Blood Culture Timing[1,3]	5	60%	89%	90%	100%
Influenza Vaccine[5]	-	-	58%	70%	100%

Initial Antibiotic Timing	90	86%	76%	80%	93%
Oxygenation Assessment	108	95%	98%	99%	100%
Pneumococcal Vaccine	74	65%	61%	69%	94%
Smoking Cessation Advice[1,3]	2	100%	78%	80%	100%
Surgical Infection Prevention					
Prophylactic Antibiotic Given[1,3]	7	14%	69%	77%	95%
Prophylactic Antibiotic Selection[5]	-	-	79%	90%	100%
Prophylactic Antibiotic Stopped[1,3]	7	71%	61%	72%	95%
Pregnancy Care					
Inpatient Neonatal Mortality	-	-	-	-	-
Third or Fourth Degree Laceration	-	-	3.54%	3.63%	3.27%

Lane Regional Memorial Hospital

6300 Main Street
Zachary, LA 70791
URL: www.lanehospital.org
Ownership: Govt - Hospital District or Authority
Emergency Services: Yes
Key Personnel:
CEO . . . . Randall Olson
Chief Medical Staff . . . . Clayton Brown, MD
ICU . . . . Billy Conerly, RN

Phone: 225-658-4000
Fax: 225-658-4287
Accredited: Yes
Licensed Beds: 137

Measure	Cases	This Hospital	State Average	U.S. Average	Top Hospital
Heart Attack Care					
ACE Inhibitor or ARB for LVSD[1]	1	100%	84%	82%	100%
Aspirin at Arrival	33	91%	91%	92%	100%
Aspirin at Discharge[1]	15	87%	87%	90%	100%
Beta Blocker at Arrival[1]	21	86%	85%	87%	100%
Beta Blocker at Discharge[1]	19	79%	88%	90%	100%
Fibrinolytic Medication Timing[1]	2	50%	32%	31%	100%
PCI Within 90 Minutes of Arrival	0	-	40%	54%	95%
Smoking Cessation Advice[1]	7	86%	88%	88%	100%
Heart Failure Care					
ACE Inhibitor or ARB for LVSD	56	70%	78%	82%	100%
Discharge Instructions	172	65%	62%	61%	93%
Evaluation of LVS Function	230	92%	81%	83%	99%
Smoking Cessation Advice	66	82%	83%	82%	100%
Pneumonia Care					
Appropriate Initial Antibiotic	129	84%	78%	83%	94%
Blood Culture Timing	166	88%	89%	90%	100%
Influenza Vaccine	65	60%	58%	70%	100%
Initial Antibiotic Timing	242	83%	76%	80%	93%
Oxygenation Assessment	319	100%	98%	99%	100%
Pneumococcal Vaccine	165	95%	61%	69%	94%
Smoking Cessation Advice	90	89%	78%	80%	100%
Surgical Infection Prevention					
Prophylactic Antibiotic Given[3]	69	87%	69%	77%	95%
Prophylactic Antibiotic Selection[1]	19	84%	79%	90%	100%
Prophylactic Antibiotic Stopped[3]	66	20%	61%	72%	95%
Pregnancy Care					
Inpatient Neonatal Mortality	-	-	-	-	-
Third or Fourth Degree Laceration	-	-	3.54%	3.63%	3.27%

NOTE: Hospital profiles are in alphabetical order by state, then city, then hospital within the city; Rankings are sorted by rate in descending order and exclude hospitals with less than 25 cases; (1) The number of cases is too small (n<25) for purposes of reliably predicting hospital performance; (2) Measure reflects the hospital's indication that its submission was based upon a sample of its relevant discharges; (3) Rate reflects fewer than the maximum possible quarters of data for the measure; (4) Inaccurate information submitted and suppressed for one or more quarters; (5) No data is available from the hospital for this measure; Please refer to the User's Guide for a full explanation of data

Heart Attack Care

1. ACE Inhibitor or ARB for LVSD

Hospital Name	City	Rate	Cases
Jeff Anderson Regional Medical Center	Meridian	100%	36
Rush Foundation Hospital	Meridian	97%	32
Forrest County General Hospital	Hattiesburg	96%	71
Wesley Medical Center	Hattiesburg	96%	27
Singing River Hospital	Pascagoula	93%	67
Baptist Memorial Hospital Desoto	Southaven	92%	52
North Mississippi Medical Center	Tupelo	92%	208
Saint Dominic Jackson Memorial Hospital	Jackson	90%	69
Memorial Hospital at Gulfport	Gulfport	87%	99
University of Mississippi Medical Center	Jackson	85%	40
Mississippi Baptist Health Systems	Jackson	84%	101
River Region Health System	Vicksburg	83%	35
Magnolia Regional Health Center	Corinth	80%	30
Northwest Mississippi Regional Medical Center	Clarksdale	70%	27
Southwest Mississippi Regional Medical Center	McComb	70%	27
Central Mississippi Medical Center	Jackson	64%	33

2. Aspirin at Arrival

Hospital Name	City	Rate	Cases
Jeff Anderson Regional Medical Center	Meridian	99%	109
North Mississippi Medical Center	Tupelo	99%	360
Saint Dominic Jackson Memorial Hospital	Jackson	99%	153
Delta Regional Medical Center	Greenville	98%	105
Forrest County General Hospital	Hattiesburg	98%	315
Mississippi Baptist Health Systems	Jackson	98%	200
Natchez Regional Medical Center	Natchez	98%	52
University of Mississippi Medical Center	Jackson	98%	121
Baptist Memorial Hospital Desoto	Southaven	97%	269
Rush Foundation Hospital	Meridian	97%	79
Singing River Hospital	Pascagoula	97%	263
Wesley Medical Center	Hattiesburg	97%	94
Baptist Memorial Hospital-North Mississippi	Oxford	96%	119
River Region Health System	Vicksburg	96%	130
Memorial Hospital at Gulfport	Gulfport	94%	177
Baptist Memorial Hospital-Golden Triangle	Columbus	93%	91
Central Mississippi Medical Center	Jackson	93%	124
Magnolia Regional Health Center	Corinth	93%	112
Bolivar Medical Center	Cleveland	90%	51
South Central Regional Medical Center	Laurel	90%	112
Greenwood LeFlore Hospital	Greenwood	88%	52
Northwest Mississippi Regional Medical Center	Clarksdale	85%	68
Grenada Lake Medical Center	Grenada	81%	31
Southwest Mississippi Regional Medical Center	McComb	81%	79
Natchez Community Hospital	Natchez	79%	29
Madison County Medical Center	Canton	71%	34

3. Aspirin at Discharge

Hospital Name	City	Rate	Cases
North Mississippi Medical Center	Tupelo	100%	781
Rush Foundation Hospital	Meridian	100%	116
Baptist Memorial Hospital-Golden Triangle	Columbus	99%	93
Jeff Anderson Regional Medical Center	Meridian	99%	153
Memorial Hospital at Gulfport	Gulfport	99%	298
Wesley Medical Center	Hattiesburg	99%	132
University of Mississippi Medical Center	Jackson	98%	135
Forrest County General Hospital	Hattiesburg	97%	497
Saint Dominic Jackson Memorial Hospital	Jackson	97%	272
Mississippi Baptist Health Systems	Jackson	96%	382
Singing River Hospital	Pascagoula	96%	258
Baptist Memorial Hospital Desoto	Southaven	95%	279
River Region Health System	Vicksburg	95%	141
Southwest Mississippi Regional Medical Center	McComb	94%	94
Baptist Memorial Hospital-North Mississippi	Oxford	93%	148
Magnolia Regional Health Center	Corinth	93%	108
Central Mississippi Medical Center	Jackson	88%	115
Northwest Mississippi Regional Medical Center	Clarksdale	88%	49
Delta Regional Medical Center	Greenville	87%	124
South Central Regional Medical Center	Laurel	85%	53
Natchez Regional Medical Center	Natchez	78%	45
Greenwood LeFlore Hospital	Greenwood	73%	26

4. Beta Blocker at Arrival

Hospital Name	City	Rate	Cases
Jeff Anderson Regional Medical Center	Meridian	99%	102
Rush Foundation Hospital	Meridian	99%	68
Natchez Regional Medical Center	Natchez	98%	47
North Mississippi Medical Center	Tupelo	97%	310
Wesley Medical Center	Hattiesburg	97%	74

Hospital Name	City	Rate	Cases
Forrest County General Hospital	Hattiesburg	96%	183
Singing River Hospital	Pascagoula	95%	217
University of Mississippi Medical Center	Jackson	95%	97
Baptist Memorial Hospital-North Mississippi	Oxford	92%	101
Saint Dominic Jackson Memorial Hospital	Jackson	91%	134
Baptist Memorial Hospital-Golden Triangle	Columbus	89%	75
Mississippi Baptist Health Systems	Jackson	89%	172
River Region Health System	Vicksburg	87%	83
Delta Regional Medical Center	Greenville	86%	71
Greenwood LeFlore Hospital	Greenwood	86%	49
Baptist Memorial Hospital Desoto	Southaven	84%	202
Magnolia Regional Health Center	Corinth	82%	94
Memorial Hospital at Gulfport	Gulfport	81%	134
South Central Regional Medical Center	Laurel	80%	105
Central Mississippi Medical Center	Jackson	79%	108
Grenada Lake Medical Center	Grenada	79%	28
Bolivar Medical Center	Cleveland	70%	47
Madison County Medical Center	Canton	69%	32
Southwest Mississippi Regional Medical Center	McComb	69%	54
Northwest Mississippi Regional Medical Center	Clarksdale	66%	70

5. Beta Blocker at Discharge

Hospital Name	City	Rate	Cases
Wesley Medical Center	Hattiesburg	100%	122
Jeff Anderson Regional Medical Center	Meridian	99%	172
North Mississippi Medical Center	Tupelo	99%	722
Rush Foundation Hospital	Meridian	98%	107
University of Mississippi Medical Center	Jackson	98%	150
Forrest County General Hospital	Hattiesburg	97%	514
Saint Dominic Jackson Memorial Hospital	Jackson	96%	270
Mississippi Baptist Health Systems	Jackson	94%	400
Baptist Memorial Hospital-North Mississippi	Oxford	93%	147
Singing River Hospital	Pascagoula	93%	243
Memorial Hospital at Gulfport	Gulfport	92%	329
Northwest Mississippi Regional Medical Center	Clarksdale	92%	51
River Region Health System	Vicksburg	92%	142
Southwest Mississippi Regional Medical Center	McComb	92%	104
Baptist Memorial Hospital Desoto	Southaven	90%	290
Baptist Memorial Hospital-Golden Triangle	Columbus	87%	86
Magnolia Regional Health Center	Corinth	86%	112
Central Mississippi Medical Center	Jackson	85%	123
Natchez Regional Medical Center	Natchez	84%	50
Delta Regional Medical Center	Greenville	82%	113
Greenwood LeFlore Hospital	Greenwood	82%	28
South Central Regional Medical Center	Laurel	82%	55

8. Smoking Cessation Advice

Hospital Name	City	Rate	Cases
Baptist Memorial Hospital-North Mississippi	Oxford	100%	67
Forrest County General Hospital	Hattiesburg	100%	225
Saint Dominic Jackson Memorial Hospital	Jackson	100%	84
Singing River Hospital	Pascagoula	100%	109
Wesley Medical Center	Hattiesburg	100%	47
Baptist Memorial Hospital Desoto	Southaven	99%	130
North Mississippi Medical Center	Tupelo	99%	347
Central Mississippi Medical Center	Jackson	98%	53
Mississippi Baptist Health Systems	Jackson	98%	154
University of Mississippi Medical Center	Jackson	98%	107
Baptist Memorial Hospital-Golden Triangle	Columbus	97%	35
Jeff Anderson Regional Medical Center	Meridian	97%	65
River Region Health System	Vicksburg	97%	66
Southwest Mississippi Regional Medical Center	McComb	97%	36
Memorial Hospital at Gulfport	Gulfport	96%	159
Rush Foundation Hospital	Meridian	93%	55
Delta Regional Medical Center	Greenville	92%	48
Magnolia Regional Health Center	Corinth	74%	39

Heart Failure Care

9. ACE Inhibitor or ARB for LVSD

Hospital Name	City	Rate	Cases
Jeff Anderson Regional Medical Center	Meridian	99%	102
Wesley Medical Center	Hattiesburg	99%	121
Baptist Memorial Hospital-Union County	New Albany	97%	30
King's Daughters Medical Center	Brookhaven	96%	55
Mississippi Baptist Health Systems	Jackson	96%	329
Delta Regional Medical Center	Greenville	95%	44
Rush Foundation Hospital	Meridian	93%	89
Riley Memorial Hospital	Meridian	92%	53
Clay County Medical Center	West Point	91%	57
Forrest County General Hospital	Hattiesburg	91%	224
River Region Health System	Vicksburg	91%	162
Singing River Hospital	Pascagoula	91%	259

NOTE: Hospital profiles are in alphabetical order by state, then city, then hospital within the city; Rankings are sorted by rate in descending order and exclude hospitals with less than 25 cases; (1) The number of cases is too small (n<25) for purposes of reliably predicting hospital performance; (2) Measure reflects the hospital's indication that its submission was based upon a sample of its relevant discharges; (3) Rate reflects fewer than the maximum possible quarters of data for the measure; (4) Inaccurate information submitted and suppressed for one or more quarters; (5) No data is available from the hospital for this measure; Please refer to the User's Guide for a full explanation of data

Baptist Memorial Hospital Desoto	Southaven	90%	156
Magee General Hospital	Magee	90%	29
North Mississippi Medical Center	Tupelo	90%	430
Garden Park Medical Center	Gulfport	88%	32
Natchez Community Hospital	Natchez	87%	76
North Mississippi Medical Center-Eupora	Eupora	87%	30
Baptist Memorial Hospital-Golden Triangle	Columbus	86%	63
Saint Dominic Jackson Memorial Hospital	Jackson	86%	145
University of Mississippi Medical Center	Jackson	86%	242
Rankin Medical Center	Brandon	84%	70
Natchez Regional Medical Center	Natchez	82%	51
Wayne General Hospital	Waynesboro	81%	53
Marion General Hospital	Columbia	79%	42
Grenada Lake Medical Center	Grenada	77%	73
Memorial Hospital at Gulfport	Gulfport	77%	275
Northwest Mississippi Regional Medical Center	Clarksdale	77%	183
Baptist Memorial Hospital-North Mississippi	Oxford	76%	127
Biloxi Regional Medical Center	Biloxi	76%	147
Bolivar Medical Center	Cleveland	76%	157
Central Mississippi Medical Center	Jackson	71%	128
Southwest Mississippi Regional Medical Center	McComb	70%	113
South Central Regional Medical Center	Laurel	69%	75
Greenwood LeFlore Hospital	Greenwood	68%	99
Magnolia Regional Health Center	Corinth	68%	148
Madison County Medical Center	Canton	63%	27
South Sunflower County Hospital	Indianola	62%	34

10. Discharge Instructions

Hospital Name	City	Rate	Cases
Baptist Memorial Hospital-Union County	New Albany	100%	84
North Mississippi Medical Center	Tupelo	97%	645
Winston Medical Center	Louisville	97%	29
Riley Memorial Hospital	Meridian	95%	125
Singing River Hospital	Pascagoula	95%	494
Delta Regional Medical Center	Greenville	90%	144
Rush Foundation Hospital	Meridian	86%	186
Wesley Medical Center	Hattiesburg	86%	220
Mississippi Baptist Health Systems	Jackson	83%	675
Baptist Memorial Hospital Desoto	Southaven	82%	460
Baptist Memorial Hospital-North Mississippi	Oxford	82%	233
Saint Dominic Jackson Memorial Hospital	Jackson	81%	284
Calhoun Health Services	Calhoun City	80%	44
Marion General Hospital	Columbia	79%	71
Baptist Memorial Hospital-Golden Triangle	Columbus	75%	142
Bolivar Medical Center	Cleveland	75%	288
Garden Park Medical Center	Gulfport	75%	115
Clay County Medical Center	West Point	73%	26
Forrest County General Hospital	Hattiesburg	72%	505
King's Daughters Medical Center	Brookhaven	70%	135
Neshoba County General Hospital	Philadelphia	64%	59
Southwest Mississippi Regional Medical Center	McComb	64%	255
River Region Health System	Vicksburg	63%	395
Rankin Medical Center	Brandon	62%	145
Scott Regioanl Hospital	Morton	62%	26
Gilmore Memorial Hospital	Amory	61%	67
Northwest Mississippi Regional Medical Center	Clarksdale	61%	318
Gulf Coast Medical Center/Gulf Oaks Hospital	Biloxi	58%	40
Magee General Hospital	Magee	56%	63
Hancock Medical Center	Bay Saint Louis	55%	51
Jeff Anderson Regional Medical Center	Meridian	54%	311
Magnolia Regional Health Center	Corinth	52%	225
Central Mississippi Medical Center	Jackson	51%	206
University of Mississippi Medical Center	Jackson	46%	304
South Central Regional Medical Center	Laurel	45%	149
Biloxi Regional Medical Center	Biloxi	42%	259
Memorial Hospital at Gulfport	Gulfport	42%	616
Field Memorial Community Hospital	Centreville	37%	60
Natchez Community Hospital	Natchez	37%	177
Oktibbeha County Hospital	Starkville	33%	54
Grenada Lake Medical Center	Grenada	30%	135
River Oaks Hospital	Jackson	30%	104
Walthall County General Hospital	Tylertown	30%	40
Natchez Regional Medical Center	Natchez	21%	159
Greenwood LeFlore Hospital	Greenwood	20%	244
Montfort Jones Memorial Hospital	Kosciusko	8%	65
Madison County Medical Center	Canton	2%	84

11. Evaluation of LVS Function

Hospital Name	City	Rate	Cases
Baptist Memorial Hospital-Booneville	Booneville	100%	59
Wesley Medical Center	Hattiesburg	100%	261
Jeff Anderson Regional Medical Center	Meridian	99%	368
Baptist Memorial Hospital-Union County	New Albany	98%	105
Magee General Hospital	Magee	98%	83

Baptist Memorial Hospital-North Mississippi	Oxford	97%	273
Delta Regional Medical Center	Greenville	97%	154
Mississippi Baptist Health Systems	Jackson	97%	760
River Region Health System	Vicksburg	97%	466
Rush Foundation Hospital	Meridian	97%	208
University of Mississippi Medical Center	Jackson	97%	310
Baptist Memorial Hospital Desoto	Southaven	96%	538
Forrest County General Hospital	Hattiesburg	95%	572
Magnolia Regional Health Center	Corinth	95%	272
North Mississippi Medical Center	Tupelo	95%	725
Singing River Hospital	Pascagoula	95%	532
King's Daughters Medical Center	Brookhaven	94%	155
Grenada Lake Medical Center	Grenada	93%	169
Rankin Medical Center	Brandon	93%	194
Riley Memorial Hospital	Meridian	93%	150
Winston Medical Center	Louisville	93%	41
Baptist Memorial Hospital-Golden Triangle	Columbus	92%	164
Biloxi Regional Medical Center	Biloxi	92%	288
Natchez Community Hospital	Natchez	92%	200
Central Mississippi Medical Center	Jackson	91%	249
Northwest Mississippi Regional Medical Center	Clarksdale	91%	343
Garden Park Medical Center	Gulfport	90%	121
Gulf Coast Medical Center/Gulf Oaks Hospital	Biloxi	90%	50
Memorial Hospital at Gulfport	Gulfport	90%	703
Saint Dominic Jackson Memorial Hospital	Jackson	89%	312
Wayne General Hospital	Waynesboro	89%	73
Franklin County Memorial Hospital	Meadville	88%	41
Hancock Medical Center	Bay Saint Louis	88%	59
North Mississippi Medical Center-Eupora	Eupora	88%	81
Bolivar Medical Center	Cleveland	87%	371
Marion General Hospital	Columbia	87%	87
Neshoba County General Hospital	Philadelphia	87%	68
George County Hospital	Lucedale	86%	87
South Sunflower County Hospital	Indianola	86%	79
Trace Regional Hospital	Houston	84%	50
Gilmore Memorial Hospital	Amory	81%	101
North Mississippi Medical Center-Iuka	Iuka	81%	120
North Sunflower County Hospital	Ruleville	81%	27
South Central Regional Medical Center	Laurel	81%	177
Calhoun Health Services	Calhoun City	80%	51
North Oak Regional Medical Center	Senatobia	79%	80
River Oaks Hospital	Jackson	79%	122
Greenwood LeFlore Hospital	Greenwood	78%	279
Natchez Regional Medical Center	Natchez	76%	187
Clay County Medical Center	West Point	74%	129
Simpson General Hospital	Mendenhall	74%	27
Oktibbeha County Hospital	Starkville	73%	60
Southwest Mississippi Regional Medical Center	McComb	72%	297
Beacham Memorial Hospital	Magnolia	71%	76
Tippah County Hospital	Ripley	71%	42
Newton Regional Hospital	Newton	67%	54
Madison County Medical Center	Canton	63%	95
Tri-Lakes Medical Center	Batesville	63%	110
Montfort Jones Memorial Hospital	Kosciusko	62%	74
Alliance Healthcare System	Holly Springs	57%	47
Field Memorial Community Hospital	Centreville	52%	73
Yalobusha General Hospital	Water Valley	48%	33
Scott Regioanl Hospital	Morton	47%	38
Walthall County General Hospital	Tylertown	43%	63
Laird Hospital	Union	34%	41

12. Smoking Cessation Advice

Hospital Name	City	Rate	Cases
Forrest County General Hospital	Hattiesburg	100%	108
Garden Park Medical Center	Gulfport	100%	35
North Mississippi Medical Center	Tupelo	100%	210
River Region Health System	Vicksburg	100%	98
Singing River Hospital	Pascagoula	100%	129
Southwest Mississippi Regional Medical Center	McComb	100%	53
Biloxi Regional Medical Center	Biloxi	99%	90
Bolivar Medical Center	Cleveland	99%	95
Northwest Mississippi Regional Medical Center	Clarksdale	99%	84
Saint Dominic Jackson Memorial Hospital	Jackson	98%	42
Wesley Medical Center	Hattiesburg	98%	64
Baptist Memorial Hospital Desoto	Southaven	97%	130
Baptist Memorial Hospital-North Mississippi	Oxford	97%	64
Central Mississippi Medical Center	Jackson	97%	67
Mississippi Baptist Health Systems	Jackson	97%	134
South Central Regional Medical Center	Laurel	97%	34
Jeff Anderson Regional Medical Center	Meridian	96%	52
Baptist Memorial Hospital-Golden Triangle	Columbus	94%	31
Riley Memorial Hospital	Meridian	94%	34
Field Memorial Community Hospital	Centreville	93%	27
Memorial Hospital at Gulfport	Gulfport	93%	180

NOTE: Hospital profiles are in alphabetical order by state, then city, then hospital within the city; Rankings are sorted by rate in descending order and exclude hospitals with less than 25 cases; (1) The number of cases is too small (n<25) for purposes of reliably predicting hospital performance; (2) Measure reflects the hospital's indication that its submission was based upon a sample of its relevant discharges; (3) Rate reflects fewer than the maximum possible quarters of data for the measure; (4) Inaccurate information submitted and suppressed for one or more quarters; (5) No data is available from the hospital for this measure; Please refer to the User's Guide for a full explanation of data

Rankin Medical Center	Brandon	92%	50
Greenwood LeFlore Hospital	Greenwood	90%	59
Rush Foundation Hospital	Meridian	90%	50
Magnolia Regional Health Center	Corinth	89%	55
Delta Regional Medical Center	Greenville	88%	26
University of Mississippi Medical Center	Jackson	88%	114
Natchez Community Hospital	Natchez	80%	41
Grenada Lake Medical Center	Grenada	79%	43
Natchez Regional Medical Center	Natchez	50%	26

Pneumonia Care

13. Appropriate Initial Antibiotic

Hospital Name	City	Rate	Cases
Marion General Hospital	Columbia	97%	72
Magee General Hospital	Magee	95%	112
King's Daughters Medical Center	Brookhaven	93%	68
Rankin Medical Center	Brandon	93%	99
Delta Regional Medical Center	Greenville	90%	98
Scott Regioanl Hospital	Morton	90%	99
Neshoba County General Hospital	Philadelphia	89%	36
Forrest County General Hospital	Hattiesburg	88%	236
Bolivar Medical Center	Cleveland	87%	89
Gilmore Memorial Hospital	Amory	87%	90
Memorial Hospital at Gulfport	Gulfport	87%	171
South Central Regional Medical Center	Laurel	87%	156
Wesley Medical Center	Hattiesburg	87%	131
Saint Dominic Jackson Memorial Hospital	Jackson	86%	90
Baptist Memorial Hospital Desoto	Southaven	84%	234
Greenwood LeFlore Hospital	Greenwood	84%	73
North Mississippi Medical Center	Tupelo	84%	206
Singing River Hospital	Pascagoula	84%	245
Gulf Coast Medical Center/Gulf Oaks Hospital	Biloxi	83%	48
University of Mississippi Medical Center	Jackson	83%	59
Winston Medical Center	Louisville	83%	29
Baptist Memorial Hospital-North Mississippi	Oxford	82%	131
Rush Foundation Hospital	Meridian	82%	76
Baptist Memorial Hospital-Golden Triangle	Columbus	81%	142
Mississippi Baptist Health Systems	Jackson	81%	77
Grenada Lake Medical Center	Grenada	78%	76
Lackey Memorial Hospital	Forest	78%	54
River Region Health System	Vicksburg	78%	181
Garden Park Medical Center	Gulfport	77%	64
Magnolia Regional Health Center	Corinth	77%	182
Hancock Medical Center	Bay Saint Louis	76%	63
Walthall County General Hospital	Tylertown	75%	44
Baptist Memorial Hospital-Union County	New Albany	74%	80
Central Mississippi Medical Center	Jackson	73%	111
Montfort Jones Memorial Hospital	Kosciusko	73%	63
River Oaks Hospital	Jackson	73%	115
Southwest Mississippi Regional Medical Center	McComb	71%	139
Jeff Anderson Regional Medical Center	Meridian	70%	172
Oktibbeha County Hospital	Starkville	70%	86
Natchez Regional Medical Center	Natchez	66%	68
Natchez Community Hospital	Natchez	58%	130
Riley Memorial Hospital	Meridian	56%	70
Biloxi Regional Medical Center	Biloxi	54%	111
Northwest Mississippi Regional Medical Center	Clarksdale	45%	55

14. Blood Culture Timing

Hospital Name	City	Rate	Cases
Marion General Hospital	Columbia	100%	44
Magee General Hospital	Magee	97%	88
Memorial Hospital at Gulfport	Gulfport	97%	150
Mississippi Baptist Health Systems	Jackson	96%	51
Rush Foundation Hospital	Meridian	96%	46
Wesley Medical Center	Hattiesburg	96%	113
Gilmore Memorial Hospital	Amory	95%	66
River Oaks Hospital	Jackson	95%	56
River Region Health System	Vicksburg	95%	147
Baptist Memorial Hospital-North Mississippi	Oxford	94%	109
Riley Memorial Hospital	Meridian	94%	62
Natchez Community Hospital	Natchez	92%	95
Rankin Medical Center	Brandon	92%	60
Baptist Memorial Hospital-Union County	New Albany	91%	47
Forrest County General Hospital	Hattiesburg	91%	246
King's Daughters Medical Center	Brookhaven	91%	55
Biloxi Regional Medical Center	Biloxi	90%	88
Jeff Anderson Regional Medical Center	Meridian	90%	88
Neshoba County General Hospital	Philadelphia	90%	30
Oktibbeha County Hospital	Starkville	90%	67
Southwest Mississippi Regional Medical Center	McComb	90%	92
Baptist Memorial Hospital-Golden Triangle	Columbus	89%	120
Grenada Lake Medical Center	Grenada	89%	63

Magnolia Regional Health Center	Corinth	89%	114
Greenwood LeFlore Hospital	Greenwood	88%	52
North Mississippi Medical Center	Tupelo	88%	158
Delta Regional Medical Center	Greenville	87%	127
Saint Dominic Jackson Memorial Hospital	Jackson	87%	84
Baptist Memorial Hospital Desoto	Southaven	86%	173
Bolivar Medical Center	Cleveland	86%	64
Garden Park Medical Center	Gulfport	86%	28
Singing River Hospital	Pascagoula	86%	183
South Central Regional Medical Center	Laurel	86%	92
Central Mississippi Medical Center	Jackson	85%	86
Hancock Medical Center	Bay Saint Louis	84%	38
Natchez Regional Medical Center	Natchez	84%	55
University of Mississippi Medical Center	Jackson	84%	69

15. Influenza Vaccine

Hospital Name	City	Rate	Cases
Wesley Medical Center	Hattiesburg	97%	32
Magee General Hospital	Magee	94%	35
River Region Health System	Vicksburg	93%	58
Baptist Memorial Hospital Desoto	Southaven	90%	51
Delta Regional Medical Center	Greenville	90%	50
Central Mississippi Medical Center	Jackson	88%	32
Baptist Memorial Hospital-North Mississippi	Oxford	83%	52
Hancock Medical Center	Bay Saint Louis	81%	31
King's Daughters Medical Center	Brookhaven	81%	27
Singing River Hospital	Pascagoula	81%	68
Forrest County General Hospital	Hattiesburg	66%	67
Magnolia Regional Health Center	Corinth	59%	46
North Mississippi Medical Center	Tupelo	59%	88
Memorial Hospital at Gulfport	Gulfport	56%	48
Biloxi Regional Medical Center	Biloxi	55%	29
South Central Regional Medical Center	Laurel	47%	34
Scott Regioanl Hospital	Morton	45%	31
River Oaks Hospital	Jackson	35%	26
Southwest Mississippi Regional Medical Center	McComb	11%	35

16. Initial Antibiotic Timing

Hospital Name	City	Rate	Cases
Neshoba County General Hospital	Philadelphia	98%	40
Magee General Hospital	Magee	97%	173
Baptist Memorial Hospital-Booneville	Booneville	96%	85
Gulf Coast Medical Center/Gulf Oaks Hospital	Biloxi	96%	49
Yalobusha General Hospital	Water Valley	96%	25
North Mississippi Medical Center-Eupora	Eupora	94%	128
Clay County Medical Center	West Point	92%	78
Trace Regional Hospital	Houston	92%	74
Wayne General Hospital	Waynesboro	92%	62
Franklin County Memorial Hospital	Meadville	91%	33
Singing River Hospital	Pascagoula	91%	293
Marion General Hospital	Columbia	90%	91
Rankin Medical Center	Brandon	90%	109
South Central Regional Medical Center	Laurel	90%	191
River Region Health System	Vicksburg	89%	221
Walthall County General Hospital	Tylertown	89%	46
Hancock Medical Center	Bay Saint Louis	88%	59
Gilmore Memorial Hospital	Amory	87%	98
Baptist Memorial Hospital-North Mississippi	Oxford	86%	161
Baptist Memorial Hospital-Union County	New Albany	86%	83
George County Hospital	Lucedale	86%	63
Rush Foundation Hospital	Meridian	86%	63
Wesley Medical Center	Hattiesburg	86%	138
Beacham Memorial Hospital	Magnolia	85%	80
Greenwood LeFlore Hospital	Greenwood	85%	108
Winston Medical Center	Louisville	85%	33
Tippah County Hospital	Ripley	84%	64
Lackey Memorial Hospital	Forest	83%	60
Scott Regioanl Hospital	Morton	83%	132
King's Daughters Medical Center	Brookhaven	82%	94
Grenada Lake Medical Center	Grenada	81%	107
Tri-Lakes Medical Center	Batesville	81%	64
North Oak Regional Medical Center	Senatobia	80%	41
Oktibbeha County Hospital	Starkville	79%	103
Saint Dominic Jackson Memorial Hospital	Jackson	79%	110
Magnolia Regional Health Center	Corinth	78%	208
North Mississippi Medical Center-Iuka	Iuka	78%	51
North Sunflower County Hospital	Ruleville	78%	49
Southwest Mississippi Regional Medical Center	McComb	78%	181
Natchez Regional Medical Center	Natchez	76%	111
North Mississippi Medical Center	Tupelo	76%	251
Bolivar Medical Center	Cleveland	75%	110
Delta Regional Medical Center	Greenville	75%	142
Forrest County General Hospital	Hattiesburg	73%	329
Madison County Medical Center	Canton	73%	30

NOTE: Hospital profiles are in alphabetical order by state, then city, then hospital within the city; Rankings are sorted by rate in descending order and exclude hospitals with less than 25 cases; (1) The number of cases is too small (n<25) for purposes of reliably predicting hospital performance; (2) Measure reflects the hospital's indication that its submission was based upon a sample of its relevant discharges; (3) Rate reflects fewer than the maximum possible quarters of data for the measure; (4) Inaccurate information submitted and suppressed for one or more quarters; (5) No data is available from the hospital for this measure; Please refer to the User's Guide for a full explanation of data

Natchez Community Hospital	Natchez	72%	168
River Oaks Hospital	Jackson	72%	118
South Sunflower County Hospital	Indianola	71%	63
Mississippi Baptist Health Systems	Jackson	70%	123
Montfort Jones Memorial Hospital	Kosciusko	70%	64
Riley Memorial Hospital	Meridian	70%	89
Baptist Memorial Hospital-Golden Triangle	Columbus	69%	158
Biloxi Regional Medical Center	Biloxi	69%	138
Alliance Healthcare System	Holly Springs	68%	34
Jeff Anderson Regional Medical Center	Meridian	67%	287
Garden Park Medical Center	Gulfport	65%	81
Central Mississippi Medical Center	Jackson	62%	157
Baptist Memorial Hospital Desoto	Southaven	59%	237
University of Mississippi Medical Center	Jackson	59%	106
Northwest Mississippi Regional Medical Center	Clarksdale	58%	55
Covington County Hospital	Collins	56%	34
Memorial Hospital at Gulfport	Gulfport	45%	271

17. Oxygenation Assessment

Hospital Name	City	Rate	Cases
Baptist Memorial Hospital Desoto	Southaven	100%	279
Baptist Memorial Hospital-Booneville	Booneville	100%	97
Baptist Memorial Hospital-North Mississippi	Oxford	100%	216
Baptist Memorial Hospital-Union County	New Albany	100%	90
Bolivar Medical Center	Cleveland	100%	133
Calhoun Health Services	Calhoun City	100%	26
Field Memorial Community Hospital	Centreville	100%	32
Franklin County Memorial Hospital	Meadville	100%	41
Garden Park Medical Center	Gulfport	100%	84
Gilmore Memorial Hospital	Amory	100%	120
Greenwood LeFlore Hospital	Greenwood	100%	128
Grenada Lake Medical Center	Grenada	100%	121
Gulf Coast Medical Center/Gulf Oaks Hospital	Biloxi	100%	58
King's Daughters Medical Center	Brookhaven	100%	125
Marion General Hospital	Columbia	100%	99
Montfort Jones Memorial Hospital	Kosciusko	100%	87
Neshoba County General Hospital	Philadelphia	100%	47
North Mississippi Medical Center	Tupelo	100%	370
North Sunflower County Hospital	Ruleville	100%	59
Northwest Mississippi Regional Medical Center	Clarksdale	100%	70
Rankin Medical Center	Brandon	100%	134
River Oaks Hospital	Jackson	100%	160
Saint Dominic Jackson Memorial Hospital	Jackson	100%	145
Scott Regioanl Hospital	Morton	100%	136
Singing River Hospital	Pascagoula	100%	352
Trace Regional Hospital	Houston	100%	86
Wayne General Hospital	Waynesboro	100%	79
Wesley Medical Center	Hattiesburg	100%	190
Winston Medical Center	Louisville	100%	44
Baptist Memorial Hospital-Golden Triangle	Columbus	99%	194
Biloxi Regional Medical Center	Biloxi	99%	169
Magee General Hospital	Magee	99%	191
Magnolia Regional Health Center	Corinth	99%	242
Mississippi Baptist Health Systems	Jackson	99%	150
River Region Health System	Vicksburg	99%	275
Southwest Mississippi Regional Medical Center	McComb	99%	225
University of Mississippi Medical Center	Jackson	99%	137
Alliance Healthcare System	Holly Springs	98%	43
Central Mississippi Medical Center	Jackson	98%	187
Covington County Hospital	Collins	98%	43
Delta Regional Medical Center	Greenville	98%	167
Hancock Medical Center	Bay Saint Louis	98%	66
Jeff Anderson Regional Medical Center	Meridian	98%	352
Memorial Hospital at Gulfport	Gulfport	98%	336
Natchez Community Hospital	Natchez	98%	190
Natchez Regional Medical Center	Natchez	98%	129
North Mississippi Medical Center-Eupora	Eupora	98%	181
Riley Memorial Hospital	Meridian	98%	118
Tippah County Hospital	Ripley	98%	91
Tri-Lakes Medical Center	Batesville	98%	80
Clay County Medical Center	West Point	97%	91
Forrest County General Hospital	Hattiesburg	97%	432
North Mississippi Medical Center-Iuka	Iuka	97%	65
Rush Foundation Hospital	Meridian	97%	91
George County Hospital	Lucedale	96%	85
North Oak Regional Medical Center	Senatobia	96%	47
South Central Regional Medical Center	Laurel	96%	210
Lackey Memorial Hospital	Forest	91%	68
Oktibbeha County Hospital	Starkville	91%	121
Beacham Memorial Hospital	Magnolia	89%	104
Madison County Medical Center	Canton	88%	33
South Sunflower County Hospital	Indianola	83%	87
Yalobusha General Hospital	Water Valley	83%	29
Laird Hospital	Union	82%	51

Walthall County General Hospital	Tylertown	79%	63

18. Pneumococcal Vaccine

Hospital Name	City	Rate	Cases
Wesley Medical Center	Hattiesburg	98%	104
Rankin Medical Center	Brandon	97%	63
River Region Health System	Vicksburg	96%	135
Baptist Memorial Hospital-Booneville	Booneville	94%	66
Magee General Hospital	Magee	94%	121
Scott Regioanl Hospital	Morton	92%	49
North Mississippi Medical Center	Tupelo	91%	251
Grenada Lake Medical Center	Grenada	90%	49
Marion General Hospital	Columbia	90%	51
Montfort Jones Memorial Hospital	Kosciusko	90%	49
Baptist Memorial Hospital-Union County	New Albany	88%	51
Neshoba County General Hospital	Philadelphia	88%	26
Baptist Memorial Hospital-North Mississippi	Oxford	87%	134
Baptist Memorial Hospital Desoto	Southaven	86%	140
Riley Memorial Hospital	Meridian	84%	58
Delta Regional Medical Center	Greenville	83%	94
Hancock Medical Center	Bay Saint Louis	82%	28
Singing River Hospital	Pascagoula	80%	183
Central Mississippi Medical Center	Jackson	79%	89
Wayne General Hospital	Waynesboro	79%	39
Forrest County General Hospital	Hattiesburg	77%	207
Gilmore Memorial Hospital	Amory	75%	67
Rush Foundation Hospital	Meridian	75%	44
Baptist Memorial Hospital-Golden Triangle	Columbus	74%	93
Oktibbeha County Hospital	Starkville	74%	66
Garden Park Medical Center	Gulfport	73%	33
King's Daughters Medical Center	Brookhaven	73%	70
Biloxi Regional Medical Center	Biloxi	72%	85
Magnolia Regional Health Center	Corinth	71%	118
North Sunflower County Hospital	Ruleville	71%	38
Saint Dominic Jackson Memorial Hospital	Jackson	71%	79
North Mississippi Medical Center-Eupora	Eupora	70%	106
Mississippi Baptist Health Systems	Jackson	68%	90
Clay County Medical Center	West Point	67%	60
South Sunflower County Hospital	Indianola	67%	52
Trace Regional Hospital	Houston	67%	54
Memorial Hospital at Gulfport	Gulfport	64%	174
Gulf Coast Medical Center/Gulf Oaks Hospital	Biloxi	62%	29
North Mississippi Medical Center-Iuka	Iuka	61%	28
Lackey Memorial Hospital	Forest	59%	29
Tippah County Hospital	Ripley	59%	58
Southwest Mississippi Regional Medical Center	McComb	58%	128
Jeff Anderson Regional Medical Center	Meridian	57%	221
Bolivar Medical Center	Cleveland	53%	64
Natchez Regional Medical Center	Natchez	51%	85
River Oaks Hospital	Jackson	49%	68
Natchez Community Hospital	Natchez	48%	96
Greenwood LeFlore Hospital	Greenwood	45%	65
South Central Regional Medical Center	Laurel	44%	116
Beacham Memorial Hospital	Magnolia	25%	64
Northwest Mississippi Regional Medical Center	Clarksdale	18%	28
George County Hospital	Lucedale	17%	53
Tri-Lakes Medical Center	Batesville	15%	34
University of Mississippi Medical Center	Jackson	5%	37
Walthall County General Hospital	Tylertown	3%	32

19. Smoking Cessation Advice

Hospital Name	City	Rate	Cases
Forrest County General Hospital	Hattiesburg	100%	117
Hancock Medical Center	Bay Saint Louis	100%	29
Singing River Hospital	Pascagoula	100%	93
Wesley Medical Center	Hattiesburg	100%	52
Baptist Memorial Hospital Desoto	Southaven	99%	108
North Mississippi Medical Center	Tupelo	98%	112
South Central Regional Medical Center	Laurel	98%	49
Baptist Memorial Hospital-North Mississippi	Oxford	97%	60
Bolivar Medical Center	Cleveland	97%	35
Baptist Memorial Hospital-Golden Triangle	Columbus	96%	51
King's Daughters Medical Center	Brookhaven	96%	26
River Region Health System	Vicksburg	95%	86
Magee General Hospital	Magee	94%	35
Rankin Medical Center	Brandon	94%	51
Southwest Mississippi Regional Medical Center	McComb	94%	48
Jeff Anderson Regional Medical Center	Meridian	93%	60
Scott Regioanl Hospital	Morton	93%	46
Riley Memorial Hospital	Meridian	92%	25
Delta Regional Medical Center	Greenville	91%	35
Greenwood LeFlore Hospital	Greenwood	91%	35
Central Mississippi Medical Center	Jackson	90%	50
Marion General Hospital	Columbia	90%	29

NOTE: Hospital profiles are in alphabetical order by state, then city, then hospital within the city; Rankings are sorted by rate in descending order and exclude hospitals with less than 25 cases; (1) The number of cases is too small (n<25) for purposes of reliably predicting hospital performance; (2) Measure reflects the hospital's indication that its submission was based upon a sample of its relevant discharges; (3) Rate reflects fewer than the maximum possible quarters of data for the measure; (4) Inaccurate information submitted and suppressed for one or more quarters; (5) No data is available from the hospital for this measure; Please refer to the User's Guide for a full explanation of data

Rush Foundation Hospital	Meridian	89%	28
Biloxi Regional Medical Center	Biloxi	86%	76
Memorial Hospital at Gulfport	Gulfport	82%	109
Natchez Community Hospital	Natchez	81%	47
Gilmore Memorial Hospital	Amory	79%	33
University of Mississippi Medical Center	Jackson	79%	53
Magnolia Regional Health Center	Corinth	76%	58
Mississippi Baptist Health Systems	Jackson	68%	28
River Oaks Hospital	Jackson	63%	43
Grenada Lake Medical Center	Grenada	57%	28
Natchez Regional Medical Center	Natchez	42%	33

Surgical Infection Prevention

20. Prophylactic Antibiotic Given

Hospital Name	City	Rate	Cases
Gulf Coast Medical Center/Gulf Oaks Hospital	Biloxi	95%	99
Baptist Memorial Hospital-Union County	New Albany	94%	126
Delta Regional Medical Center	Greenville	93%	129
North Mississippi Medical Center	Tupelo	92%	951
Wesley Medical Center	Hattiesburg	92%	1007
Baptist Memorial Hospital Desoto	Southaven	90%	455
Central Mississippi Medical Center	Jackson	90%	432
Baptist Memorial Hospital-Golden Triangle	Columbus	89%	516
Garden Park Medical Center	Gulfport	89%	140
Grenada Lake Medical Center	Grenada	89%	141
Southwest Mississippi Regional Medical Center	McComb	89%	475
Baptist Memorial Hospital-North Mississippi	Oxford	88%	442
University of Mississippi Medical Center	Jackson	88%	326
Natchez Regional Medical Center	Natchez	87%	164
Natchez Community Hospital	Natchez	86%	94
Rankin Medical Center	Brandon	86%	69
Singing River Hospital	Pascagoula	86%	175
Woman's Hospital at River Oaks	Jackson	86%	339
King's Daughters Medical Center	Brookhaven	85%	86
Biloxi Regional Medical Center	Biloxi	84%	206
Bolivar Medical Center	Cleveland	84%	100
Magnolia Regional Health Center	Corinth	83%	288
Forrest County General Hospital	Hattiesburg	82%	320
Gilmore Memorial Hospital	Amory	80%	176
River Region Health System	Vicksburg	80%	406
Northwest Mississippi Regional Medical Center	Clarksdale	78%	129
South Central Regional Medical Center	Laurel	78%	490
Mississippi Baptist Health Systems	Jackson	77%	305
Jeff Anderson Regional Medical Center	Meridian	73%	377
Rush Foundation Hospital	Meridian	73%	174
Saint Dominic Jackson Memorial Hospital	Jackson	72%	268
Memorial Hospital at Gulfport	Gulfport	70%	449
Clay County Medical Center	West Point	68%	37
Riley Memorial Hospital	Meridian	67%	114
River Oaks Hospital	Jackson	60%	823
Oktibbeha County Hospital	Starkville	56%	305
Greenwood LeFlore Hospital	Greenwood	53%	193
Madison County Medical Center	Canton	18%	39

21. Prophylactic Antibiotic Selection

Hospital Name	City	Rate	Cases
Baptist Memorial Hospital Desoto	Southaven	98%	58
Central Mississippi Medical Center	Jackson	97%	63
Grenada Lake Medical Center	Grenada	96%	28
Garden Park Medical Center	Gulfport	95%	81
Northwest Mississippi Regional Medical Center	Clarksdale	95%	40
Southwest Mississippi Regional Medical Center	McComb	95%	98
Baptist Memorial Hospital-Union County	New Albany	94%	34
Bolivar Medical Center	Cleveland	94%	32
Delta Regional Medical Center	Greenville	94%	64
Greenwood LeFlore Hospital	Greenwood	94%	62
Magnolia Regional Health Center	Corinth	94%	80
University of Mississippi Medical Center	Jackson	94%	206
King's Daughters Medical Center	Brookhaven	93%	27
Jeff Anderson Regional Medical Center	Meridian	92%	142
Memorial Hospital at Gulfport	Gulfport	92%	145
Natchez Regional Medical Center	Natchez	92%	49
South Central Regional Medical Center	Laurel	92%	117
Gulf Coast Medical Center/Gulf Oaks Hospital	Biloxi	91%	35
River Region Health System	Vicksburg	91%	99
Wesley Medical Center	Hattiesburg	91%	250
Mississippi Baptist Health Systems	Jackson	90%	73
Saint Dominic Jackson Memorial Hospital	Jackson	90%	69
Singing River Hospital	Pascagoula	89%	175
Gilmore Memorial Hospital	Amory	88%	43
Baptist Memorial Hospital-Golden Triangle	Columbus	85%	156
Baptist Memorial Hospital-North Mississippi	Oxford	85%	61
North Mississippi Medical Center	Tupelo	84%	255

River Oaks Hospital	Jackson	80%	69
Biloxi Regional Medical Center	Biloxi	78%	36
Rush Foundation Hospital	Meridian	78%	60
Forrest County General Hospital	Hattiesburg	76%	130
Oktibbeha County Hospital	Starkville	68%	88

22. Prophylactic Antibiotic Stopped

Hospital Name	City	Rate	Cases
Grenada Lake Medical Center	Grenada	93%	129
Delta Regional Medical Center	Greenville	84%	116
Woman's Hospital at River Oaks	Jackson	84%	337
Wesley Medical Center	Hattiesburg	83%	995
Gilmore Memorial Hospital	Amory	81%	175
Gulf Coast Medical Center/Gulf Oaks Hospital	Biloxi	81%	99
King's Daughters Medical Center	Brookhaven	80%	84
Oktibbeha County Hospital	Starkville	80%	296
Southwest Mississippi Regional Medical Center	McComb	80%	467
Clay County Medical Center	West Point	79%	33
Mississippi Baptist Health Systems	Jackson	79%	295
Baptist Memorial Hospital-Golden Triangle	Columbus	78%	495
Natchez Regional Medical Center	Natchez	78%	160
Memorial Hospital at Gulfport	Gulfport	76%	443
River Oaks Hospital	Jackson	76%	814
Singing River Hospital	Pascagoula	76%	172
University of Mississippi Medical Center	Jackson	76%	320
Baptist Memorial Hospital Desoto	Southaven	75%	428
Rankin Medical Center	Brandon	75%	65
Riley Memorial Hospital	Meridian	75%	107
Baptist Memorial Hospital-North Mississippi	Oxford	72%	401
Natchez Community Hospital	Natchez	72%	87
North Mississippi Medical Center	Tupelo	72%	903
Jeff Anderson Regional Medical Center	Meridian	70%	361
Baptist Memorial Hospital-Union County	New Albany	68%	116
Biloxi Regional Medical Center	Biloxi	67%	188
Central Mississippi Medical Center	Jackson	66%	419
Saint Dominic Jackson Memorial Hospital	Jackson	66%	254
River Region Health System	Vicksburg	64%	386
Rush Foundation Hospital	Meridian	64%	165
Northwest Mississippi Regional Medical Center	Clarksdale	57%	126
Madison County Medical Center	Canton	56%	36
Forrest County General Hospital	Hattiesburg	55%	313
Bolivar Medical Center	Cleveland	48%	96
Greenwood LeFlore Hospital	Greenwood	45%	185
Garden Park Medical Center	Gulfport	39%	135
South Central Regional Medical Center	Laurel	26%	485
Magnolia Regional Health Center	Corinth	16%	284

Pregnancy Care

23. Inpatient Neonatal Mortality

Hospital Name	City	Rate	Cases
Natchez Regional Medical Center	Natchez	0.00%	247
Delta Regional Medical Center	Greenville	0.13%	746
Clay County Medical Center	West Point	0.19%	517
South Sunflower County Hospital	Indianola	0.24%	413
Baptist Memorial Hospital-Union County	New Albany	0.29%	1049
Woman's Hospital at River Oaks	Jackson	0.33%	1530
Grenada Lake Medical Center	Grenada	0.44%	226
North Mississippi Medical Center	Tupelo	1.04%	483
University of Mississippi Medical Center	Jackson	2.32%	3925

24. Third or Fourth Degree Laceration

Hospital Name	City	Rate	Cases
Natchez Regional Medical Center	Natchez	0.71%	425
Clay County Medical Center	West Point	0.90%	332
Baptist Memorial Hospital-Union County	New Albany	1.46%	751
University of Mississippi Medical Center	Jackson	1.70%	2349
Delta Regional Medical Center	Greenville	1.89%	529
South Sunflower County Hospital	Indianola	2.68%	261
Grenada Lake Medical Center	Grenada	2.88%	416
Woman's Hospital at River Oaks	Jackson	4.03%	769
North Mississippi Medical Center	Tupelo	6.35%	315

NOTE: Hospital profiles are in alphabetical order by state, then city, then hospital within the city; Rankings are sorted by rate in descending order and exclude hospitals with less than 25 cases; (1) The number of cases is too small (n<25) for purposes of reliably predicting hospital performance; (2) Measure reflects the hospital's indication that its submission was based upon a sample of its relevant discharges; (3) Rate reflects fewer than the maximum possible quarters of data for the measure; (4) Inaccurate information submitted and suppressed for one or more quarters; (5) No data is available from the hospital for this measure; Please refer to the User's Guide for a full explanation of data

Gilmore Memorial Hospital

1105 Earl Frye Boulevard
PO Box 459
Amory, MS 38821
URL: www.gilmorehealth.com
Ownership: Proprietary
Emergency Services: Yes

Phone: 662-256-7111
Fax: 662-256-3133

Accredited: Yes
Licensed Beds: 95

Key Personnel:
President/CEO . . . . Danny Spreitler
Chief Medical Staff . . . . Woodrow Brand, III, MD
Cardiac Lab . . . . Bert Mize
Emergency Room . . . . Shelby Howell, MD
Emergency Room . . . . Tammy Lyle
Medical Surgical Nursing . . . . Tammy Lyle
OB/GYN Womens Health . . . . Hollie Glenn
Respiratory/Cardiopulmonary . . . . Bert Mize

Measure	Cases	This Hospital	State Average	U.S. Average	Top Hospital
Heart Attack Care					
ACE Inhibitor or ARB for LVSD[1]	1	100%	80%	82%	100%
Aspirin at Arrival[1]	13	92%	86%	92%	100%
Aspirin at Discharge[1]	4	100%	84%	90%	100%
Beta Blocker at Arrival[1]	11	91%	74%	87%	100%
Beta Blocker at Discharge[1]	6	100%	81%	90%	100%
Fibrinolytic Medication Timing[1]	1	100%	32%	31%	100%
PCI Within 90 Minutes of Arrival	0	-	46%	54%	95%
Smoking Cessation Advice[1]	2	100%	88%	88%	100%
Heart Failure Care					
ACE Inhibitor or ARB for LVSD[1]	16	75%	76%	82%	100%
Discharge Instructions	67	61%	55%	61%	93%
Evaluation of LVS Function	101	81%	78%	83%	99%
Smoking Cessation Advice[1]	14	93%	80%	82%	100%
Pneumonia Care					
Appropriate Initial Antibiotic	90	87%	78%	83%	94%
Blood Culture Timing	66	95%	89%	90%	100%
Influenza Vaccine[1]	17	59%	64%	70%	100%
Initial Antibiotic Timing	98	87%	79%	80%	93%
Oxygenation Assessment	120	100%	97%	99%	100%
Pneumococcal Vaccine	67	75%	62%	69%	94%
Smoking Cessation Advice	33	79%	77%	80%	100%
Surgical Infection Prevention					
Prophylactic Antibiotic Given[2]	176	80%	76%	77%	95%
Prophylactic Antibiotic Selection[2]	43	88%	83%	90%	100%
Prophylactic Antibiotic Stopped[2]	175	81%	70%	72%	95%
Pregnancy Care					
Inpatient Neonatal Mortality	-	-	-	-	-
Third or Fourth Degree Laceration	-	-	2.26%	3.63%	3.27%

Tri-Lakes Medical Center

305 Medical Center Drive
Batesville, MS 38606
URL: www.trilakesmedical.com
Ownership: Voluntary non-profit - Private
Emergency Services: Yes

Phone: 662-563-5611
Fax: 662-563-0155

Accredited: No
Licensed Beds: 110

Key Personnel:
CEO . . . . Barry Morrison

Measure	Cases	This Hospital	State Average	U.S. Average	Top Hospital
Heart Attack Care					
ACE Inhibitor or ARB for LVSD	0	-	80%	82%	100%
Aspirin at Arrival[1]	6	100%	86%	92%	100%
Aspirin at Discharge[1]	1	100%	84%	90%	100%
Beta Blocker at Arrival[1]	3	33%	74%	87%	100%
Beta Blocker at Discharge[1]	1	100%	81%	90%	100%
Fibrinolytic Medication Timing[3]	0	-	32%	31%	100%
PCI Within 90 Minutes of Arrival	0	-	46%	54%	95%
Smoking Cessation Advice[3]	0	-	88%	88%	100%
Heart Failure Care					
ACE Inhibitor or ARB for LVSD[1]	14	57%	76%	82%	100%
Discharge Instructions[1,3]	23	48%	55%	61%	93%
Evaluation of LVS Function	110	63%	78%	83%	99%
Smoking Cessation Advice[1,3]	5	60%	80%	82%	100%
Pneumonia Care					

Appropriate Initial Antibiotic[1,3]	11	91%	78%	83%	94%
Blood Culture Timing[1,3]	7	71%	89%	90%	100%
Influenza Vaccine[5]	-	-	64%	70%	100%
Initial Antibiotic Timing	64	81%	79%	80%	93%
Oxygenation Assessment	80	98%	97%	99%	100%
Pneumococcal Vaccine	34	15%	62%	69%	94%
Smoking Cessation Advice[1,3]	5	20%	77%	80%	100%
Surgical Infection Prevention					
Prophylactic Antibiotic Given[1,3]	3	33%	76%	77%	95%
Prophylactic Antibiotic Selection[5]	-	-	83%	90%	100%
Prophylactic Antibiotic Stopped[1,3]	3	100%	70%	72%	95%
Pregnancy Care					
Inpatient Neonatal Mortality	-	-	-	-	-
Third or Fourth Degree Laceration	-	-	2.26%	3.63%	3.27%

Hancock Medical Center

PO Box 2790
Bay Saint Louis, MS 39521
Ownership: Government - Local
Emergency Services: Yes

Phone: 228-467-8600
Fax: 228-467-8799
Accredited: No
Licensed Beds: 104

Key Personnel:
Administrator/CEO . . . . Hal W Leftwich
Chief Medical Staff . . . . Tad Carter
Emergency Room . . . . Jeffrey L Giddens
Emergency Room . . . . Jeffrey Giddins, MD
Director Infection/Disease Control . . . . Cecilia Burke, RN
Chief Radiology . . . . Laura Justice, MD
Director of Pulmonary/Respiratory Care . . . . . . Sayeed Aziz

Measure	Cases	This Hospital	State Average	U.S. Average	Top Hospital
Heart Attack Care					
ACE Inhibitor or ARB for LVSD[5]	-	-	80%	82%	100%
Aspirin at Arrival[5]	-	-	86%	92%	100%
Aspirin at Discharge[5]	-	-	84%	90%	100%
Beta Blocker at Arrival[5]	-	-	74%	87%	100%
Beta Blocker at Discharge[5]	-	-	81%	90%	100%
Fibrinolytic Medication Timing[5]	-	-	32%	31%	100%
PCI Within 90 Minutes of Arrival[5]	-	-	46%	54%	95%
Smoking Cessation Advice[5]	-	-	88%	88%	100%
Heart Failure Care					
ACE Inhibitor or ARB for LVSD[5]	-	-	76%	82%	100%
Discharge Instructions[5]	-	-	55%	61%	93%
Evaluation of LVS Function[5]	-	-	78%	83%	99%
Smoking Cessation Advice[5]	-	-	80%	82%	100%
Pneumonia Care					
Appropriate Initial Antibiotic[5]	-	-	78%	83%	94%
Blood Culture Timing[5]	-	-	89%	90%	100%
Influenza Vaccine[5]	-	-	64%	70%	100%
Initial Antibiotic Timing[5]	-	-	79%	80%	93%
Oxygenation Assessment[5]	-	-	97%	99%	100%
Pneumococcal Vaccine[5]	-	-	62%	69%	94%
Smoking Cessation Advice[5]	-	-	77%	80%	100%
Surgical Infection Prevention					
Prophylactic Antibiotic Given[5]	-	-	76%	77%	95%
Prophylactic Antibiotic Selection[5]	-	-	83%	90%	100%
Prophylactic Antibiotic Stopped[5]	-	-	70%	72%	95%
Pregnancy Care					
Inpatient Neonatal Mortality	-	-	-	-	-
Third or Fourth Degree Laceration	-	-	2.26%	3.63%	3.27%

Hancock Medical Center

149 Drinkwater Blvd
Bay Saint Louis, MS 39521
Ownership: Proprietary
Emergency Services: Yes

Phone: 228-467-8744

Accredited: No

Measure	Cases	This Hospital	State Average	U.S. Average	Top Hospital
Heart Attack Care					
ACE Inhibitor or ARB for LVSD[5]	-	-	80%	82%	100%
Aspirin at Arrival[5]	-	-	86%	92%	100%
Aspirin at Discharge[5]	-	-	84%	90%	100%
Beta Blocker at Arrival[5]	-	-	74%	87%	100%

NOTE: Hospital profiles are in alphabetical order by state, then city, then hospital within the city; Rankings are sorted by rate in descending order and exclude hospitals with less than 25 cases; (1) The number of cases is too small (n<25) for purposes of reliably predicting hospital performance; (2) Measure reflects the hospital's indication that its submission was based upon a sample of its relevant discharges; (3) Rate reflects fewer than the maximum possible quarters of data for the measure; (4) Inaccurate information submitted and suppressed for one or more quarters; (5) No data is available from the hospital for this measure; Please refer to the User's Guide for a full explanation of data

Beta Blocker at Discharge[5]	-	-	81%	90%	100%
Fibrinolytic Medication Timing[5]	-	-	32%	31%	100%
PCI Within 90 Minutes of Arrival[5]	-	-	46%	54%	95%
Smoking Cessation Advice[5]	-	-	88%	88%	100%
Heart Failure Care					
ACE Inhibitor or ARB for LVSD[1,3]	23	65%	76%	82%	100%
Discharge Instructions[3]	51	55%	55%	61%	93%
Evaluation of LVS Function[3]	59	88%	78%	83%	99%
Smoking Cessation Advice[1,3]	20	100%	80%	82%	100%
Pneumonia Care					
Appropriate Initial Antibiotic[3]	63	76%	78%	83%	94%
Blood Culture Timing	38	84%	89%	90%	100%
Influenza Vaccine	31	81%	64%	70%	100%
Initial Antibiotic Timing[3]	59	88%	79%	80%	93%
Oxygenation Assessment[3]	66	98%	97%	99%	100%
Pneumococcal Vaccine[3]	28	82%	62%	69%	94%
Smoking Cessation Advice[3]	29	100%	77%	80%	100%
Surgical Infection Prevention					
Prophylactic Antibiotic Given[1,3]	4	100%	76%	77%	95%
Prophylactic Antibiotic Selection[1]	4	25%	83%	90%	100%
Prophylactic Antibiotic Stopped[1,3]	4	50%	70%	72%	95%
Pregnancy Care					
Inpatient Neonatal Mortality	-	-	-	-	-
Third or Fourth Degree Laceration	-	-	2.26%	3.63%	3.27%

Jasper General Hospital
15 A S 6th Street
Bay Springs, MS 39422
Ownership: Govt - Hospital District or Authority
Emergency Services: No
Key Personnel:
CEO . . . . Kenneth Posey

Phone: 601-764-2101
Fax: 601-764-4789
Accredited: No
Licensed Beds: 22

Measure	Cases	This Hospital	State Average	U.S. Average	Top Hospital
Heart Attack Care					
ACE Inhibitor or ARB for LVSD[5]	-	-	80%	82%	100%
Aspirin at Arrival[5]	-	-	86%	92%	100%
Aspirin at Discharge[5]	-	-	84%	90%	100%
Beta Blocker at Arrival[5]	-	-	74%	87%	100%
Beta Blocker at Discharge[5]	-	-	81%	90%	100%
Fibrinolytic Medication Timing[5]	-	-	32%	31%	100%
PCI Within 90 Minutes of Arrival[5]	-	-	46%	54%	95%
Smoking Cessation Advice[5]	-	-	88%	88%	100%
Heart Failure Care					
ACE Inhibitor or ARB for LVSD[5]	-	-	76%	82%	100%
Discharge Instructions[5]	-	-	55%	61%	93%
Evaluation of LVS Function[5]	-	-	78%	83%	99%
Smoking Cessation Advice[5]	-	-	80%	82%	100%
Pneumonia Care					
Appropriate Initial Antibiotic[1,3]	1	0%	78%	83%	94%
Blood Culture Timing[3]	0	-	89%	90%	100%
Influenza Vaccine[5]	-	-	64%	70%	100%
Initial Antibiotic Timing[1,3]	2	100%	79%	80%	93%
Oxygenation Assessment[1,3]	4	100%	97%	99%	100%
Pneumococcal Vaccine[1,3]	3	33%	62%	69%	94%
Smoking Cessation Advice[3]	0	-	77%	80%	100%
Surgical Infection Prevention					
Prophylactic Antibiotic Given[5]	-	-	76%	77%	95%
Prophylactic Antibiotic Selection[5]	-	-	83%	90%	100%
Prophylactic Antibiotic Stopped[5]	-	-	70%	72%	95%
Pregnancy Care					
Inpatient Neonatal Mortality	-	-	-	-	-
Third or Fourth Degree Laceration	-	-	2.26%	3.63%	3.27%

Biloxi Regional Medical Center
150 Reynoir Street
PO Box 128
Biloxi, MS 39533
URL: www.hmabrmc.com
Ownership: Proprietary
Emergency Services: Yes
Key Personnel:
Administrator . . . . Robert L Hammond
Chief Medical Staff . . . . Edward Shumski, MD
Emergency Room . . . . IraFaye Tremmel
Emergency Room . . . . Jim Mitchell, DO
Infection Control . . . . Pam McVey
ICU . . . . Jenny Kostmayer
Medical & Surgical Nursing . . . . Donna Griggs
OB/GYN Womens Health. . . . . Beth Mellish
Respiratory Therapy. . . . . Wanda Beville

Phone: 228-432-1571
Fax: 228-436-1205

Accredited: Yes
Licensed Beds: 153

Measure	Cases	This Hospital	State Average	U.S. Average	Top Hospital
Heart Attack Care					
ACE Inhibitor or ARB for LVSD[1]	5	80%	80%	82%	100%
Aspirin at Arrival[1]	13	85%	86%	92%	100%
Aspirin at Discharge[1]	4	100%	84%	90%	100%
Beta Blocker at Arrival[1]	5	20%	74%	87%	100%
Beta Blocker at Discharge[1]	8	100%	81%	90%	100%
Fibrinolytic Medication Timing	0	-	32%	31%	100%
PCI Within 90 Minutes of Arrival	0	-	46%	54%	95%
Smoking Cessation Advice[1]	3	100%	88%	88%	100%
Heart Failure Care					
ACE Inhibitor or ARB for LVSD	147	76%	76%	82%	100%
Discharge Instructions	259	42%	55%	61%	93%
Evaluation of LVS Function	288	92%	78%	83%	99%
Smoking Cessation Advice	90	99%	80%	82%	100%
Pneumonia Care					
Appropriate Initial Antibiotic	111	54%	78%	83%	94%
Blood Culture Timing	88	90%	89%	90%	100%
Influenza Vaccine	29	55%	64%	70%	100%
Initial Antibiotic Timing	138	69%	79%	80%	93%
Oxygenation Assessment	169	99%	97%	99%	100%
Pneumococcal Vaccine	85	72%	62%	69%	94%
Smoking Cessation Advice	76	86%	77%	80%	100%
Surgical Infection Prevention					
Prophylactic Antibiotic Given[2]	206	84%	76%	77%	95%
Prophylactic Antibiotic Selection[2]	36	78%	83%	90%	100%
Prophylactic Antibiotic Stopped[2]	188	67%	70%	72%	95%
Pregnancy Care					
Inpatient Neonatal Mortality	-	-	-	-	-
Third or Fourth Degree Laceration	-	-	2.26%	3.63%	3.27%

Gulf Coast Medical Center/Gulf Oaks Hospital
PO Box 4518
Biloxi, MS 39531
URL: www.gulfcoastmedicalcenter.com
Ownership: Government - State
Emergency Services: Yes
Key Personnel:
Administrator/CEO. . . . . Rick Carter
Chief Medical Staff. . . . . Paul Matherne
Emergency Room . . . . Christa Bell, RN
Director Infection/Disease Control . . . . Carolyn Fisher
ICU . . . . Christa Bell
Intensive Coronary Care . . . . Christa Bell
OB/GYN Womens Health. . . . . Shahira Hanna, MD
Director Respiratory Therapy . . . . Terry Bradley

Phone: 228-388-0211
Fax: 228-388-0358

Accredited: Yes
Licensed Beds: 189

Measure	Cases	This Hospital	State Average	U.S. Average	Top Hospital
Heart Attack Care					
ACE Inhibitor or ARB for LVSD[1]	1	0%	80%	82%	100%
Aspirin at Arrival[1]	10	90%	86%	92%	100%
Aspirin at Discharge[1]	3	100%	84%	90%	100%
Beta Blocker at Arrival[1]	13	62%	74%	87%	100%
Beta Blocker at Discharge[1]	5	100%	81%	90%	100%
Fibrinolytic Medication Timing	0	-	32%	31%	100%

NOTE: Hospital profiles are in alphabetical order by state, then city, then hospital within the city; Rankings are sorted by rate in descending order and exclude hospitals with less than 25 cases; (1) The number of cases is too small (n<25) for purposes of reliably predicting hospital performance; (2) Measure reflects the hospital's indication that its submission was based upon a sample of its relevant discharges; (3) Rate reflects fewer than the maximum possible quarters of data for the measure; (4) Inaccurate information submitted and suppressed for one or more quarters; (5) No data is available from the hospital for this measure; Please refer to the User's Guide for a full explanation of data

Measure	Cases	This Hospital	State Average	U.S. Average	Top Hospital
PCI Within 90 Minutes of Arrival	0	-	46%	54%	95%
Smoking Cessation Advice[1]	1	100%	88%	88%	100%
Heart Failure Care					
ACE Inhibitor or ARB for LVSD[1]	11	64%	76%	82%	100%
Discharge Instructions	40	58%	55%	61%	93%
Evaluation of LVS Function	50	90%	78%	83%	99%
Smoking Cessation Advice[1]	6	83%	80%	82%	100%
Pneumonia Care					
Appropriate Initial Antibiotic	48	83%	78%	83%	94%
Blood Culture Timing[1]	21	86%	89%	90%	100%
Influenza Vaccine[1]	13	46%	64%	70%	100%
Initial Antibiotic Timing	49	96%	79%	80%	93%
Oxygenation Assessment	58	100%	97%	99%	100%
Pneumococcal Vaccine	29	62%	62%	69%	94%
Smoking Cessation Advice[1]	11	73%	77%	80%	100%
Surgical Infection Prevention					
Prophylactic Antibiotic Given[2]	99	95%	76%	77%	95%
Prophylactic Antibiotic Selection[2]	35	91%	83%	90%	100%
Prophylactic Antibiotic Stopped[2]	99	81%	70%	72%	95%
Pregnancy Care					
Inpatient Neonatal Mortality	-	-	-	-	-
Third or Fourth Degree Laceration	-	-	2.26%	3.63%	3.27%

Baptist Memorial Hospital-Booneville

100 Hospital Street   Phone: 662-720-5000
Booneville, MS 38829   Fax: 662-720-5005
URL: www.baptistonline.org/facilities/booneville
Ownership: Voluntary non-profit - Church   Accredited: Yes
Emergency Services: Yes   Licensed Beds: 114
Key Personnel:
Administration/CEO . . . . Larkin Kennedy
President . . . . Dr Nathan Baldwin
Infection Control . . . . Doris Box, RN
CCU . . . . Jean Pannell, RN
Medical/Surgical Nursing . . . . Brandi Taylor
Respiratory/Cardiopulmonary . . . . Barry Yeaber

Measure	Cases	This Hospital	State Average	U.S. Average	Top Hospital
Heart Attack Care					
ACE Inhibitor or ARB for LVSD[1]	2	100%	80%	82%	100%
Aspirin at Arrival[1]	6	83%	86%	92%	100%
Aspirin at Discharge[1]	4	100%	84%	90%	100%
Beta Blocker at Arrival[1]	3	67%	74%	87%	100%
Beta Blocker at Discharge[1]	3	100%	81%	90%	100%
Fibrinolytic Medication Timing[3]	0	-	32%	31%	100%
PCI Within 90 Minutes of Arrival	0	-	46%	54%	95%
Smoking Cessation Advice[3]	0	-	88%	88%	100%
Heart Failure Care					
ACE Inhibitor or ARB for LVSD[1]	14	100%	76%	82%	100%
Discharge Instructions[1,3]	2	100%	55%	61%	93%
Evaluation of LVS Function	59	100%	78%	83%	99%
Smoking Cessation Advice[1,3]	2	100%	80%	82%	100%
Pneumonia Care					
Appropriate Initial Antibiotic[1,3]	12	100%	78%	83%	94%
Blood Culture Timing[1,3]	17	94%	89%	90%	100%
Influenza Vaccine[5]	-	-	64%	70%	100%
Initial Antibiotic Timing	85	96%	79%	80%	93%
Oxygenation Assessment	97	100%	97%	99%	100%
Pneumococcal Vaccine	66	94%	62%	69%	94%
Smoking Cessation Advice[1,3]	4	100%	77%	80%	100%
Surgical Infection Prevention					
Prophylactic Antibiotic Given[3]	0	-	76%	77%	95%
Prophylactic Antibiotic Selection[5]	-	-	83%	90%	100%
Prophylactic Antibiotic Stopped[3]	0	-	70%	72%	95%
Pregnancy Care					
Inpatient Neonatal Mortality	-	-	-	-	-
Third or Fourth Degree Laceration	-	-	2.26%	3.63%	3.27%

Rankin Medical Center

350 Crossgates Boulevard   Phone: 601-825-2811
Brandon, MS 39042   Fax: 601-824-8530
URL: www.rankinmedcenter.com
Ownership: Proprietary   Accredited: Yes
Emergency Services: Yes   Licensed Beds: 134
Key Personnel:
Chief Medical Staff . . . . Dr James Jefferson
Director Surgical Services . . . . Diane Smith
Emergency Room . . . . Patricia Irby
Director Infection/Disease Control . . . . Marie Bagwell
ICU . . . . Glenda Shorter
Director Medical/Surgical Nursing . . . . Melissa Knight
CNO . . . . Corie Ramsey
Director Respiratory Therapy . . . . Vickie Byrd

Measure	Cases	This Hospital	State Average	U.S. Average	Top Hospital
Heart Attack Care					
ACE Inhibitor or ARB for LVSD[1]	1	100%	80%	82%	100%
Aspirin at Arrival[1]	17	94%	86%	92%	100%
Aspirin at Discharge[1]	7	71%	84%	90%	100%
Beta Blocker at Arrival[1]	16	94%	74%	87%	100%
Beta Blocker at Discharge[1]	7	86%	81%	90%	100%
Fibrinolytic Medication Timing	0	-	32%	31%	100%
PCI Within 90 Minutes of Arrival	0	-	46%	54%	95%
Smoking Cessation Advice[1]	2	50%	88%	88%	100%
Heart Failure Care					
ACE Inhibitor or ARB for LVSD	70	84%	76%	82%	100%
Discharge Instructions	145	62%	55%	61%	93%
Evaluation of LVS Function	194	93%	78%	83%	99%
Smoking Cessation Advice	50	92%	80%	82%	100%
Pneumonia Care					
Appropriate Initial Antibiotic	99	93%	78%	83%	94%
Blood Culture Timing	60	92%	89%	90%	100%
Influenza Vaccine[4,5]	-	-	64%	70%	100%
Initial Antibiotic Timing	109	90%	79%	80%	93%
Oxygenation Assessment	134	100%	97%	99%	100%
Pneumococcal Vaccine	63	97%	62%	69%	94%
Smoking Cessation Advice	51	94%	77%	80%	100%
Surgical Infection Prevention					
Prophylactic Antibiotic Given[2]	69	86%	76%	77%	95%
Prophylactic Antibiotic Selection[1,2]	19	74%	83%	90%	100%
Prophylactic Antibiotic Stopped[2]	65	75%	70%	72%	95%
Pregnancy Care					
Inpatient Neonatal Mortality	-	-	-	-	-
Third or Fourth Degree Laceration	-	-	2.26%	3.63%	3.27%

King's Daughters Medical Center

Highway 51 N   Phone: 601-833-6011
Brookhaven, MS 39601   Fax: 601-835-9380
E-mail: ccraig@kdmc.org
Ownership: Voluntary non-profit - Other   Accredited: Yes
Emergency Services: Yes   Licensed Beds: 122
Key Personnel:
CEO . . . . Phillip Gradey
Emergency Room . . . . Jane Jones
Director Infection/Disease Control . . . . Cathy Bridge, RN
Director Medical/Surgical Nursing . . . . Tammy Livingston, RN
Director of Pulmonary/Respiratory . . . . Holar Larkin

Measure	Cases	This Hospital	State Average	U.S. Average	Top Hospital
Heart Attack Care					
ACE Inhibitor or ARB for LVSD[1]	2	100%	80%	82%	100%
Aspirin at Arrival[1]	13	100%	86%	92%	100%
Aspirin at Discharge[1]	5	80%	84%	90%	100%
Beta Blocker at Arrival[1]	10	80%	74%	87%	100%
Beta Blocker at Discharge[1]	8	88%	81%	90%	100%
Fibrinolytic Medication Timing	0	-	32%	31%	100%
PCI Within 90 Minutes of Arrival	0	-	46%	54%	95%
Smoking Cessation Advice	0	-	88%	88%	100%
Heart Failure Care					
ACE Inhibitor or ARB for LVSD	55	96%	76%	82%	100%
Discharge Instructions	135	70%	55%	61%	93%

NOTE: Hospital profiles are in alphabetical order by state, then city, then hospital within the city; Rankings are sorted by rate in descending order and exclude hospitals with less than 25 cases; (1) The number of cases is too small (n<25) for purposes of reliably predicting hospital performance; (2) Measure reflects the hospital's indication that its submission was based upon a sample of its relevant discharges; (3) Rate reflects fewer than the maximum possible quarters of data for the measure; (4) Inaccurate information submitted and suppressed for one or more quarters; (5) No data is available from the hospital for this measure; Please refer to the User's Guide for a full explanation of data

Evaluation of LVS Function	155	94%	78%	83%	99%
Smoking Cessation Advice[1]	24	100%	80%	82%	100%

Pneumonia Care

Appropriate Initial Antibiotic	68	93%	78%	83%	94%
Blood Culture Timing	55	91%	89%	90%	100%
Influenza Vaccine	27	81%	64%	70%	100%
Initial Antibiotic Timing	94	82%	79%	80%	93%
Oxygenation Assessment	125	100%	97%	99%	100%
Pneumococcal Vaccine	70	73%	62%	69%	94%
Smoking Cessation Advice	26	96%	77%	80%	100%

Surgical Infection Prevention

Prophylactic Antibiotic Given[3]	86	85%	76%	77%	95%
Prophylactic Antibiotic Selection	27	93%	83%	90%	100%
Prophylactic Antibiotic Stopped[3]	84	80%	70%	72%	95%

Pregnancy Care

Inpatient Neonatal Mortality	-	-	-	-	-
Third or Fourth Degree Laceration	-	-	2.26%	3.63%	3.27%

Calhoun Health Services

140 Burke/Calhoun City Road   Phone: 662-628-6611
Calhoun City, MS 38916   Fax: 662-628-6300
URL: www.nmhs.net
Ownership: Government - Local   Accredited: No
Emergency Services: Yes   Licensed Beds: 30
Key Personnel:
CEO . . . . James Franklin
Chief Medical Staff . . . . Guy Sarmer, MD
Respiratory Care . . . . Daney Whitt

Measure	Cases	This Hospital	State Average	U.S. Average	Top Hospital
Heart Attack Care					
ACE Inhibitor or ARB for LVSD	0	-	80%	82%	100%
Aspirin at Arrival[1]	6	83%	86%	92%	100%
Aspirin at Discharge[1]	6	67%	84%	90%	100%
Beta Blocker at Arrival[1]	4	100%	74%	87%	100%
Beta Blocker at Discharge[1]	6	83%	81%	90%	100%
Fibrinolytic Medication Timing	0	-	32%	31%	100%
PCI Within 90 Minutes of Arrival	0	-	46%	54%	95%
Smoking Cessation Advice	0	-	88%	88%	100%
Heart Failure Care					
ACE Inhibitor or ARB for LVSD[1]	11	82%	76%	82%	100%
Discharge Instructions	44	80%	55%	61%	93%
Evaluation of LVS Function	51	80%	78%	83%	99%
Smoking Cessation Advice[1]	17	88%	80%	82%	100%
Pneumonia Care					
Appropriate Initial Antibiotic[1]	16	88%	78%	83%	94%
Blood Culture Timing[1]	13	92%	89%	90%	100%
Influenza Vaccine[1]	3	100%	64%	70%	100%
Initial Antibiotic Timing[1]	19	95%	79%	80%	93%
Oxygenation Assessment	26	100%	97%	99%	100%
Pneumococcal Vaccine[1]	13	92%	62%	69%	94%
Smoking Cessation Advice[1]	12	100%	77%	80%	100%
Surgical Infection Prevention					
Prophylactic Antibiotic Given[5]	-	-	76%	77%	95%
Prophylactic Antibiotic Selection[5]	-	-	83%	90%	100%
Prophylactic Antibiotic Stopped[5]	-	-	70%	72%	95%
Pregnancy Care					
Inpatient Neonatal Mortality	-	-	-	-	-
Third or Fourth Degree Laceration	-	-	2.26%	3.63%	3.27%

Madison County Medical Center

Alternate Name: Madison General Hospital
1421 E Peace St   Phone: 601-859-1331
Canton, MS 39046   Fax: 601-855-5100
Ownership: Proprietary   Accredited: No
Emergency Services: Yes   Licensed Beds: 127
Key Personnel:
President/CEO . . . . Joseph D Weaver
Chief Medical Staff . . . . Sanjib Shrestha, MD
Cardiology . . . . Anurag Mehta, MD
Emergency Room . . . . Parvesh Goel, MD
Medical/Surgical Nursing . . . . Carol Clark, RN
OB/GYN Womens Health . . . . Wesley Prater, MD

Surgical Services . . . . Garth Murray, MD
Chief Radiology . . . . Richard Kuebler, MD
Director Respiratory Therapy . . . . Mary Sumler

Measure	Cases	This Hospital	State Average	U.S. Average	Top Hospital
Heart Attack Care					
ACE Inhibitor or ARB for LVSD[1]	2	100%	80%	82%	100%
Aspirin at Arrival	34	71%	86%	92%	100%
Aspirin at Discharge[1]	17	71%	84%	90%	100%
Beta Blocker at Arrival	32	69%	74%	87%	100%
Beta Blocker at Discharge[1]	17	71%	81%	90%	100%
Fibrinolytic Medication Timing	0	-	32%	31%	100%
PCI Within 90 Minutes of Arrival	0	-	46%	54%	95%
Smoking Cessation Advice[1]	3	67%	88%	88%	100%
Heart Failure Care					
ACE Inhibitor or ARB for LVSD	27	63%	76%	82%	100%
Discharge Instructions	84	2%	55%	61%	93%
Evaluation of LVS Function	95	63%	78%	83%	99%
Smoking Cessation Advice[1]	20	70%	80%	82%	100%
Pneumonia Care					
Appropriate Initial Antibiotic[1]	18	83%	78%	83%	94%
Blood Culture Timing[1]	9	78%	89%	90%	100%
Influenza Vaccine[1]	6	33%	64%	70%	100%
Initial Antibiotic Timing	30	73%	79%	80%	93%
Oxygenation Assessment	33	88%	97%	99%	100%
Pneumococcal Vaccine[1]	13	23%	62%	69%	94%
Smoking Cessation Advice[1]	6	50%	77%	80%	100%
Surgical Infection Prevention					
Prophylactic Antibiotic Given[2]	39	18%	76%	77%	95%
Prophylactic Antibiotic Selection[1,2]	10	50%	83%	90%	100%
Prophylactic Antibiotic Stopped[2]	36	56%	70%	72%	95%
Pregnancy Care					
Inpatient Neonatal Mortality	-	-	-	-	-
Third or Fourth Degree Laceration	-	-	2.26%	3.63%	3.27%

Field Memorial Community Hospital

270 W Main Street   Phone: 601-645-5221
Centreville, MS 39631   Fax: 601-645-5842
Ownership: Government - Local   Accredited: Yes
Emergency Services: Yes   Licensed Beds: 25
Key Personnel:
President/CEO . . . . Brock Slabach
Chief Medical Staff . . . . Robert Lewis
Emergency Room . . . . Dr Rich Field
Infection Control . . . . LaVerne McDaniel, RN
Respiratory/Cardiopulmonary . . . . Paula Huff

Measure	Cases	This Hospital	State Average	U.S. Average	Top Hospital
Heart Attack Care					
ACE Inhibitor or ARB for LVSD[1]	3	67%	80%	82%	100%
Aspirin at Arrival[1]	17	82%	86%	92%	100%
Aspirin at Discharge[1]	10	70%	84%	90%	100%
Beta Blocker at Arrival[1]	10	100%	74%	87%	100%
Beta Blocker at Discharge[1]	10	90%	81%	90%	100%
Fibrinolytic Medication Timing[1]	1	0%	32%	31%	100%
PCI Within 90 Minutes of Arrival[5]	-	-	46%	54%	95%
Smoking Cessation Advice[1]	5	100%	88%	88%	100%
Heart Failure Care					
ACE Inhibitor or ARB for LVSD[1]	24	67%	76%	82%	100%
Discharge Instructions	60	37%	55%	61%	93%
Evaluation of LVS Function	73	52%	78%	83%	99%
Smoking Cessation Advice	27	93%	80%	82%	100%
Pneumonia Care					
Appropriate Initial Antibiotic[1]	17	100%	78%	83%	94%
Blood Culture Timing[1]	5	100%	89%	90%	100%
Influenza Vaccine[1]	8	88%	64%	70%	100%
Initial Antibiotic Timing[1]	22	91%	79%	80%	93%
Oxygenation Assessment	32	100%	97%	99%	100%
Pneumococcal Vaccine[1]	22	27%	62%	69%	94%
Smoking Cessation Advice[1]	9	89%	77%	80%	100%
Surgical Infection Prevention					
Prophylactic Antibiotic Given[5]	-	-	76%	77%	95%

NOTE: Hospital profiles are in alphabetical order by state, then city, then hospital within the city; Rankings are sorted by rate in descending order and exclude hospitals with less than 25 cases; (1) The number of cases is too small (n<25) for purposes of reliably predicting hospital performance; (2) Measure reflects the hospital's indication that its submission was based upon a sample of its relevant discharges; (3) Rate reflects fewer than the maximum possible quarters of data for the measure; (4) Inaccurate information submitted and suppressed for one or more quarters; (5) No data is available from the hospital for this measure; Please refer to the User's Guide for a full explanation of data

Prophylactic Antibiotic Selection[5]	-	-	83%	90%	100%
Prophylactic Antibiotic Stopped[5]	-	-	70%	72%	95%

Pregnancy Care					
Inpatient Neonatal Mortality	-	-	-	-	-
Third or Fourth Degree Laceration	-	-	2.26%	3.63%	3.27%

Northwest Mississippi Regional Medical Center

1970 Hospital Drive
PO Box 1218
Clarksdale, MS 38614
URL: www.nwmsregionalmedcenter.com
Ownership: Proprietary   Accredited: Yes
Emergency Services: Yes   Licensed Beds: 195
Key Personnel:
President/CEO. . . . . W Douglas Arnold
Chief Medical Staff. Vernon Thomas Hughes, DO
Cardiac Lab . . . . Steve Gressmire
Catheterization Lab . . . . Steve Gressmire
Emergency Room . . . . Rob Stiles
Infection Control. . . . . Mae Bramlett
ICU . . . . Loreather Stacker
Medical Surgical Nursing . . . . Lorean Willingham
OB/GYN/Women's Health . . . . Dana Barton
Respiratory/Cardiopulmonary. . . . . Chuck Bell

Measure	Cases	This Hospital	State Average	U.S. Average	Top Hospital
Heart Attack Care					
ACE Inhibitor or ARB for LVSD	27	70%	80%	82%	100%
Aspirin at Arrival	68	85%	86%	92%	100%
Aspirin at Discharge	49	88%	84%	90%	100%
Beta Blocker at Arrival	70	66%	74%	87%	100%
Beta Blocker at Discharge	51	92%	81%	90%	100%
Fibrinolytic Medication Timing[1]	7	14%	32%	31%	100%
PCI Within 90 Minutes of Arrival	0	-	46%	54%	95%
Smoking Cessation Advice[1]	18	100%	88%	88%	100%
Heart Failure Care					
ACE Inhibitor or ARB for LVSD	183	77%	76%	82%	100%
Discharge Instructions	318	61%	55%	61%	93%
Evaluation of LVS Function	343	91%	78%	83%	99%
Smoking Cessation Advice	84	99%	80%	82%	100%
Pneumonia Care					
Appropriate Initial Antibiotic	55	45%	78%	83%	94%
Blood Culture Timing[1]	21	95%	89%	90%	100%
Influenza Vaccine[1]	4	0%	64%	70%	100%
Initial Antibiotic Timing	55	58%	79%	80%	93%
Oxygenation Assessment	70	100%	97%	99%	100%
Pneumococcal Vaccine	28	18%	62%	69%	94%
Smoking Cessation Advice[1]	23	100%	77%	80%	100%
Surgical Infection Prevention					
Prophylactic Antibiotic Given[2]	129	78%	76%	77%	95%
Prophylactic Antibiotic Selection[2]	40	95%	83%	90%	100%
Prophylactic Antibiotic Stopped[2]	126	57%	70%	72%	95%
Pregnancy Care					
Inpatient Neonatal Mortality	-	-	-	-	-
Third or Fourth Degree Laceration	-	-	2.26%	3.63%	3.27%

Bolivar Medical Center

PO Box 1380
Cleveland, MS 38732
Ownership: Proprietary   Phone: 662-846-0061
Emergency Services: Yes   Fax: 662-846-2380
    Accredited: Yes
    Licensed Beds: 150
Key Personnel:
CEO. . . . . Lowell Benton
Emergency Room . . . . Donna Parrot
ICU . . . . Lisa Ellis

Measure	Cases	This Hospital	State Average	U.S. Average	Top Hospital
Heart Attack Care					
ACE Inhibitor or ARB for LVSD[1]	12	67%	80%	82%	100%
Aspirin at Arrival	51	90%	86%	92%	100%
Aspirin at Discharge[1]	22	64%	84%	90%	100%
Beta Blocker at Arrival	47	70%	74%	87%	100%
Beta Blocker at Discharge[1]	24	67%	81%	90%	100%

Fibrinolytic Medication Timing[1]	5	60%	32%	31%	100%
PCI Within 90 Minutes of Arrival	0	-	46%	54%	95%
Smoking Cessation Advice[1]	5	100%	88%	88%	100%
Heart Failure Care					
ACE Inhibitor or ARB for LVSD	157	76%	76%	82%	100%
Discharge Instructions	288	75%	55%	61%	93%
Evaluation of LVS Function	371	87%	78%	83%	99%
Smoking Cessation Advice	95	99%	80%	82%	100%
Pneumonia Care					
Appropriate Initial Antibiotic	89	87%	78%	83%	94%
Blood Culture Timing	64	86%	89%	90%	100%
Influenza Vaccine[1]	16	56%	64%	70%	100%
Initial Antibiotic Timing	110	75%	79%	80%	93%
Oxygenation Assessment	133	100%	97%	99%	100%
Pneumococcal Vaccine	64	53%	62%	69%	94%
Smoking Cessation Advice	35	97%	77%	80%	100%
Surgical Infection Prevention					
Prophylactic Antibiotic Given[3]	100	84%	76%	77%	95%
Prophylactic Antibiotic Selection	32	94%	83%	90%	100%
Prophylactic Antibiotic Stopped[3]	96	48%	70%	72%	95%
Pregnancy Care					
Inpatient Neonatal Mortality	-	-	-	-	-
Third or Fourth Degree Laceration	-	-	2.26%	3.63%	3.27%

Covington County Hospital

701 Holly Avenue
Collins, MS 39428
Ownership: Government - Local   Phone: 601-765-6711
Emergency Services: Yes   Fax: 601-698-0180
    Accredited: No
    Licensed Beds: 82
Key Personnel:
CEO/President. . . . . Clay Johnson
Chief Medical Staff. Ward Johnson
Emergency Room . . . . Lynn Scott
Emergency Room . . . . Betty Mason, RN
Director Infection/Disease Control . . . . Audie Lawson
Director Medical/Surgical Nursing . . . . Carolyn Walker, RN
Chief Radiology . . . . Jane Bullock

Measure	Cases	This Hospital	State Average	U.S. Average	Top Hospital
Heart Attack Care					
ACE Inhibitor or ARB for LVSD[3]	0	-	80%	82%	100%
Aspirin at Arrival[1,3]	1	0%	86%	92%	100%
Aspirin at Discharge[3]	0	-	84%	90%	100%
Beta Blocker at Arrival[1,3]	1	0%	74%	87%	100%
Beta Blocker at Discharge[3]	0	-	81%	90%	100%
Fibrinolytic Medication Timing[3]	0	-	32%	31%	100%
PCI Within 90 Minutes of Arrival	0	-	46%	54%	95%
Smoking Cessation Advice[3]	0	-	88%	88%	100%
Heart Failure Care					
ACE Inhibitor or ARB for LVSD[1,3]	16	69%	76%	82%	100%
Discharge Instructions[1,3]	12	25%	55%	61%	93%
Evaluation of LVS Function[1,3]	18	89%	78%	83%	99%
Smoking Cessation Advice[1,3]	3	100%	80%	82%	100%
Pneumonia Care					
Appropriate Initial Antibiotic[1,3]	3	67%	78%	83%	94%
Blood Culture Timing[1]	9	89%	89%	90%	100%
Influenza Vaccine[1]	6	0%	64%	70%	100%
Initial Antibiotic Timing[3]	34	56%	79%	80%	93%
Oxygenation Assessment[3]	43	98%	97%	99%	100%
Pneumococcal Vaccine[1,3]	21	5%	62%	69%	94%
Smoking Cessation Advice[1,3]	7	14%	77%	80%	100%
Surgical Infection Prevention					
Prophylactic Antibiotic Given[5]	-	-	76%	77%	95%
Prophylactic Antibiotic Selection[5]	-	-	83%	90%	100%
Prophylactic Antibiotic Stopped[5]	-	-	70%	72%	95%
Pregnancy Care					
Inpatient Neonatal Mortality	-	-	-	-	-
Third or Fourth Degree Laceration	-	-	2.26%	3.63%	3.27%

NOTE: Hospital profiles are in alphabetical order by state, then city, then hospital within the city; Rankings are sorted by rate in descending order and exclude hospitals with less than 25 cases; (1) The number of cases is too small (n<25) for purposes of reliably predicting hospital performance; (2) Measure reflects the hospital's indication that its submission was based upon a sample of its relevant discharges; (3) Rate reflects fewer than the maximum possible quarters of data for the measure; (4) Inaccurate information submitted and suppressed for one or more quarters; (5) No data is available from the hospital for this measure; Please refer to the User's Guide for a full explanation of data

Marion General Hospital

1560 Sumrall Rd P O Box 630
Columbia, MS 39429
Ownership: Government - Local
Emergency Services: Yes

Phone: 601-736-6303

Accredited: No

Measure	Cases	This Hospital	State Average	U.S. Average	Top Hospital
Heart Attack Care					
ACE Inhibitor or ARB for LVSD	0	-	80%	82%	100%
Aspirin at Arrival[1]	16	81%	86%	92%	100%
Aspirin at Discharge[1]	10	80%	84%	90%	100%
Beta Blocker at Arrival[1]	11	82%	74%	87%	100%
Beta Blocker at Discharge[1]	10	90%	81%	90%	100%
Fibrinolytic Medication Timing[1]	3	0%	32%	31%	100%
PCI Within 90 Minutes of Arrival	0	-	46%	54%	95%
Smoking Cessation Advice[1]	3	67%	88%	88%	100%
Heart Failure Care					
ACE Inhibitor or ARB for LVSD	42	79%	76%	82%	100%
Discharge Instructions	71	79%	55%	61%	93%
Evaluation of LVS Function	87	87%	78%	83%	99%
Smoking Cessation Advice[1]	20	85%	80%	82%	100%
Pneumonia Care					
Appropriate Initial Antibiotic	72	97%	78%	83%	94%
Blood Culture Timing	44	100%	89%	90%	100%
Influenza Vaccine[1]	13	46%	64%	70%	100%
Initial Antibiotic Timing	91	90%	79%	80%	93%
Oxygenation Assessment	99	100%	97%	99%	100%
Pneumococcal Vaccine	51	90%	62%	69%	94%
Smoking Cessation Advice	29	90%	77%	80%	100%
Surgical Infection Prevention					
Prophylactic Antibiotic Given[3]	0	-	76%	77%	95%
Prophylactic Antibiotic Selection	0	-	83%	90%	100%
Prophylactic Antibiotic Stopped[3]	0	-	70%	72%	95%
Pregnancy Care					
Inpatient Neonatal Mortality	-	-	-	-	-
Third or Fourth Degree Laceration	-	-	2.26%	3.63%	3.27%

Baptist Memorial Hospital-Golden Triangle

Alternate Name: Golden Triangle Regional Medical Center
2520 5th Street North
Columbus, MS 39705
URL: www.bmhcc.org
Ownership: Voluntary non-profit - Church
Emergency Services: Yes

Phone: 662-244-1000
Fax: 662-244-1564

Accredited: Yes
Licensed Beds: 479

Key Personnel:
President/CEO . . . . Stephen C Reynolds
Chief Medical Staff . . . . James Woodard, MD
Director Radiology . . . . Barry McAllister
Director Respiratory Therapy . . . . Linda Barrett

Measure	Cases	This Hospital	State Average	U.S. Average	Top Hospital
Heart Attack Care					
ACE Inhibitor or ARB for LVSD[1]	21	76%	80%	82%	100%
Aspirin at Arrival	91	93%	86%	92%	100%
Aspirin at Discharge	93	99%	84%	90%	100%
Beta Blocker at Arrival	75	89%	74%	87%	100%
Beta Blocker at Discharge	86	87%	81%	90%	100%
Fibrinolytic Medication Timing[1]	9	44%	32%	31%	100%
PCI Within 90 Minutes of Arrival[1]	6	50%	46%	54%	95%
Smoking Cessation Advice	35	97%	88%	88%	100%
Heart Failure Care					
ACE Inhibitor or ARB for LVSD	63	86%	76%	82%	100%
Discharge Instructions	142	75%	55%	61%	93%
Evaluation of LVS Function	164	92%	78%	83%	99%
Smoking Cessation Advice	31	94%	80%	82%	100%
Pneumonia Care					
Appropriate Initial Antibiotic	142	81%	78%	83%	94%
Blood Culture Timing	120	89%	89%	90%	100%
Influenza Vaccine[1]	22	91%	64%	70%	100%
Initial Antibiotic Timing	158	69%	79%	80%	93%
Oxygenation Assessment	194	99%	97%	99%	100%
Pneumococcal Vaccine	93	74%	62%	69%	94%

Smoking Cessation Advice	51	96%	77%	80%	100%
Surgical Infection Prevention					
Prophylactic Antibiotic Given	516	89%	76%	77%	95%
Prophylactic Antibiotic Selection	156	85%	83%	90%	100%
Prophylactic Antibiotic Stopped	495	78%	70%	72%	95%
Pregnancy Care					
Inpatient Neonatal Mortality	-	-	-	-	-
Third or Fourth Degree Laceration	-	-	2.26%	3.63%	3.27%

Magnolia Regional Health Center

Alternate Name: Magnolia Hospital
611 Alcorn Drive
Corinth, MS 38834
URL: www.mrhc.org
Ownership: Government - Local
Emergency Services: Yes

Phone: 662-293-1300
Fax: 662-293-4285

Accredited: Yes
Licensed Beds: 178

Key Personnel:
CEO . . . . Diane Boatman
Cardiac Lab . . . . Tommy Bain
Emergency Room . . . . Wendell Jourdan
Infection Control . . . . Elwanda Whiteker
Intensive/Coronary Care . . . . Rick Crane
Respiratory/Cardiopulmonary . . . . Mike Cooper

Measure	Cases	This Hospital	State Average	U.S. Average	Top Hospital
Heart Attack Care					
ACE Inhibitor or ARB for LVSD	30	80%	80%	82%	100%
Aspirin at Arrival	112	93%	86%	92%	100%
Aspirin at Discharge	108	93%	84%	90%	100%
Beta Blocker at Arrival	94	82%	74%	87%	100%
Beta Blocker at Discharge	112	86%	81%	90%	100%
Fibrinolytic Medication Timing[1]	23	57%	32%	31%	100%
PCI Within 90 Minutes of Arrival[1]	1	100%	46%	54%	95%
Smoking Cessation Advice	39	74%	88%	88%	100%
Heart Failure Care					
ACE Inhibitor or ARB for LVSD	148	68%	76%	82%	100%
Discharge Instructions	225	52%	55%	61%	93%
Evaluation of LVS Function	272	95%	78%	83%	99%
Smoking Cessation Advice	55	89%	80%	82%	100%
Pneumonia Care					
Appropriate Initial Antibiotic	182	77%	78%	83%	94%
Blood Culture Timing	114	89%	89%	90%	100%
Influenza Vaccine	46	59%	64%	70%	100%
Initial Antibiotic Timing	208	78%	79%	80%	93%
Oxygenation Assessment	242	99%	97%	99%	100%
Pneumococcal Vaccine	118	71%	62%	69%	94%
Smoking Cessation Advice	58	76%	77%	80%	100%
Surgical Infection Prevention					
Prophylactic Antibiotic Given	288	83%	76%	77%	95%
Prophylactic Antibiotic Selection	80	94%	83%	90%	100%
Prophylactic Antibiotic Stopped	284	16%	70%	72%	95%
Pregnancy Care					
Inpatient Neonatal Mortality	-	-	-	-	-
Third or Fourth Degree Laceration	-	-	2.26%	3.63%	3.27%

North Mississippi Medical Center-Eupora

500 Veterans Memorial Blvd
Eupora, MS 39744
URL: www.nmhs.net/eupora
Ownership: Voluntary non-profit - Other
Emergency Services: Yes

Phone: 662-258-6221

Accredited: Yes
Licensed Beds: 43

Key Personnel:
Administrator . . . . Harold H Whitaker IV, MD
Chief Medical Staff . . . . Charles Ozborn, MD
Emergency Room . . . . Evelyn Easley, RN
Director Infection/Disease Control . . . . Sherrie Johnson, RN
Director Medical/Surgical Nursing . . . . Sherrie Johnson
Chief Radiology . . . . Danny Burney
Director Respiratory Therapy . . . . David Fields

Measure	Cases	This Hospital	State Average	U.S. Average	Top Hospital
Heart Attack Care					
ACE Inhibitor or ARB for LVSD[1,3]	1	100%	80%	82%	100%

NOTE: Hospital profiles are in alphabetical order by state, then city, then hospital within the city; Rankings are sorted by rate in descending order and exclude hospitals with less than 25 cases; (1) The number of cases is too small (n<25) for purposes of reliably predicting hospital performance; (2) Measure reflects the hospital's indication that its submission was based upon a sample of its relevant discharges; (3) Rate reflects fewer than the maximum possible quarters of data for the measure; (4) Inaccurate information submitted and suppressed for one or more quarters; (5) No data is available from the hospital for this measure; Please refer to the User's Guide for a full explanation of data

Measure	Cases	This Hospital	State Average	U.S. Average	Top Hospital
Aspirin at Arrival[1,3]	2	100%	86%	92%	100%
Aspirin at Discharge[3]	0	-	84%	90%	100%
Beta Blocker at Arrival[1,3]	2	100%	74%	87%	100%
Beta Blocker at Discharge[1,3]	1	100%	81%	90%	100%
Fibrinolytic Medication Timing[3]	0	-	32%	31%	100%
PCI Within 90 Minutes of Arrival	0	-	46%	54%	95%
Smoking Cessation Advice[3]	0	-	88%	88%	100%
Heart Failure Care					
ACE Inhibitor or ARB for LVSD	30	87%	76%	82%	100%
Discharge Instructions[1,3]	20	60%	55%	61%	93%
Evaluation of LVS Function	81	88%	78%	83%	99%
Smoking Cessation Advice[1,3]	6	83%	80%	82%	100%
Pneumonia Care					
Appropriate Initial Antibiotic[1,3]	19	63%	78%	83%	94%
Blood Culture Timing[1,3]	12	100%	89%	90%	100%
Influenza Vaccine[5]	-	-	64%	70%	100%
Initial Antibiotic Timing	128	94%	79%	80%	93%
Oxygenation Assessment	181	98%	97%	99%	100%
Pneumococcal Vaccine	106	70%	62%	69%	94%
Smoking Cessation Advice[1,3]	7	43%	77%	80%	100%
Surgical Infection Prevention					
Prophylactic Antibiotic Given[3]	0	-	76%	77%	95%
Prophylactic Antibiotic Selection[5]	-	-	83%	90%	100%
Prophylactic Antibiotic Stopped[3]	0	-	70%	72%	95%
Pregnancy Care					
Inpatient Neonatal Mortality	-	-	-	-	-
Third or Fourth Degree Laceration	-	-	2.26%	3.63%	3.27%

Jefferson County Hospital

809 S Main
Fayette, MS 39069
Ownership: Government - Local
Emergency Services: Yes

Phone: 601-786-3401
Fax: 601-786-3400
Accredited: No
Licensed Beds: 30

Key Personnel:
CEO/President . . . . Jerry Kinbee
Emergency Room . . . . Ado Wilson

Measure	Cases	This Hospital	State Average	U.S. Average	Top Hospital
Heart Attack Care					
ACE Inhibitor or ARB for LVSD[5]	-	-	80%	82%	100%
Aspirin at Arrival[5]	-	-	86%	92%	100%
Aspirin at Discharge[5]	-	-	84%	90%	100%
Beta Blocker at Arrival[5]	-	-	74%	87%	100%
Beta Blocker at Discharge[5]	-	-	81%	90%	100%
Fibrinolytic Medication Timing[5]	-	-	32%	31%	100%
PCI Within 90 Minutes of Arrival[5]	-	-	46%	54%	95%
Smoking Cessation Advice[5]	-	-	88%	88%	100%
Heart Failure Care					
ACE Inhibitor or ARB for LVSD[2]	0	-	76%	82%	100%
Discharge Instructions[1,2,3]	2	100%	55%	61%	93%
Evaluation of LVS Function[1,2]	19	0%	78%	83%	99%
Smoking Cessation Advice[1,2,3]	1	100%	80%	82%	100%
Pneumonia Care					
Appropriate Initial Antibiotic[1,2,3]	2	0%	78%	83%	94%
Blood Culture Timing[2,3]	0	-	89%	90%	100%
Influenza Vaccine[5]	-	-	64%	70%	100%
Initial Antibiotic Timing[1,2]	3	67%	79%	80%	93%
Oxygenation Assessment[1,2]	16	81%	97%	99%	100%
Pneumococcal Vaccine[1,2]	6	0%	62%	69%	94%
Smoking Cessation Advice[2,3]	0	-	77%	80%	100%
Surgical Infection Prevention					
Prophylactic Antibiotic Given[5]	-	-	76%	77%	95%
Prophylactic Antibiotic Selection[5]	-	-	83%	90%	100%
Prophylactic Antibiotic Stopped[5]	-	-	70%	72%	95%
Pregnancy Care					
Inpatient Neonatal Mortality	-	-	-	-	-
Third or Fourth Degree Laceration	-	-	2.26%	3.63%	3.27%

Lackey Memorial Hospital

330 N Broad Street
Forest, MS 39074
URL: www.selackey.com
Ownership: Voluntary non-profit - Private
Emergency Services: Yes

Phone: 601-469-4151
Fax: 601-469-3681

Accredited: No
Licensed Beds: 74

Key Personnel:
Administrator . . . . Donna Riser
Chief Medical Staff . . . . John P Lee

Measure	Cases	This Hospital	State Average	U.S. Average	Top Hospital
Heart Attack Care					
ACE Inhibitor or ARB for LVSD[3]	0	-	80%	82%	100%
Aspirin at Arrival[3]	0	-	86%	92%	100%
Aspirin at Discharge[3]	0	-	84%	90%	100%
Beta Blocker at Arrival[3]	0	-	74%	87%	100%
Beta Blocker at Discharge[3]	0	-	81%	90%	100%
Fibrinolytic Medication Timing[3]	0	-	32%	31%	100%
PCI Within 90 Minutes of Arrival[5]	-	-	46%	54%	95%
Smoking Cessation Advice[3]	0	-	88%	88%	100%
Heart Failure Care					
ACE Inhibitor or ARB for LVSD[1,3]	4	100%	76%	82%	100%
Discharge Instructions[1,3]	12	0%	55%	61%	93%
Evaluation of LVS Function[1,3]	18	67%	78%	83%	99%
Smoking Cessation Advice[3]	0	-	80%	82%	100%
Pneumonia Care					
Appropriate Initial Antibiotic	54	78%	78%	83%	94%
Blood Culture Timing[1]	8	88%	89%	90%	100%
Influenza Vaccine[1]	14	71%	64%	70%	100%
Initial Antibiotic Timing	60	83%	79%	80%	93%
Oxygenation Assessment	68	91%	97%	99%	100%
Pneumococcal Vaccine	29	59%	62%	69%	94%
Smoking Cessation Advice[1]	23	13%	77%	80%	100%
Surgical Infection Prevention					
Prophylactic Antibiotic Given[5]	-	-	76%	77%	95%
Prophylactic Antibiotic Selection[5]	-	-	83%	90%	100%
Prophylactic Antibiotic Stopped[5]	-	-	70%	72%	95%
Pregnancy Care					
Inpatient Neonatal Mortality	-	-	-	-	-
Third or Fourth Degree Laceration	-	-	2.26%	3.63%	3.27%

Delta Regional Medical Center

PO Box 5247
Greenville, MS 38704
URL: deltaregional.com
Ownership: Government - Local
Emergency Services: Yes

Phone: 662-378-3783
Fax: 662-725-2189

Accredited: Yes
Licensed Beds: 398

Key Personnel:
CEO . . . . L Ray Humphreys, FACHE
Director, Cardiac Catheterization Lab. . . . . Michelle Britton
Director, Infection Control. . . . . Sharon Henderson
Director, Surgery . . . . Sue Peets, RN
Director Respiratory Care. . . . . Elrgah Johnson

Measure	Cases	This Hospital	State Average	U.S. Average	Top Hospital
Heart Attack Care					
ACE Inhibitor or ARB for LVSD[1]	16	100%	80%	82%	100%
Aspirin at Arrival	105	98%	86%	92%	100%
Aspirin at Discharge	124	87%	84%	90%	100%
Beta Blocker at Arrival	71	86%	74%	87%	100%
Beta Blocker at Discharge	113	82%	81%	90%	100%
Fibrinolytic Medication Timing[1]	8	25%	32%	31%	100%
PCI Within 90 Minutes of Arrival	0	-	46%	54%	95%
Smoking Cessation Advice	48	92%	88%	88%	100%
Heart Failure Care					
ACE Inhibitor or ARB for LVSD[2,3]	44	95%	76%	82%	100%
Discharge Instructions[2,3]	144	90%	55%	61%	93%
Evaluation of LVS Function[2,3]	154	97%	78%	83%	99%
Smoking Cessation Advice[2,3]	26	88%	80%	82%	100%
Pneumonia Care					
Appropriate Initial Antibiotic	98	90%	78%	83%	94%
Blood Culture Timing	127	87%	89%	90%	100%
Influenza Vaccine	50	90%	64%	70%	100%

NOTE: Hospital profiles are in alphabetical order by state, then city, then hospital within the city; Rankings are sorted by rate in descending order and exclude hospitals with less than 25 cases; (1) The number of cases is too small (n<25) for purposes of reliably predicting hospital performance; (2) Measure reflects the hospital's indication that its submission was based upon a sample of its relevant discharges; (3) Rate reflects fewer than the maximum possible quarters of data for the measure; (4) Inaccurate information submitted and suppressed for one or more quarters; (5) No data is available from the hospital for this measure; Please refer to the User's Guide for a full explanation of data

Initial Antibiotic Timing	142	75%	79%	80%	93%
Oxygenation Assessment	167	98%	97%	99%	100%
Pneumococcal Vaccine	94	83%	62%	69%	94%
Smoking Cessation Advice	35	91%	77%	80%	100%

Surgical Infection Prevention

Prophylactic Antibiotic Given[2,3]	129	93%	76%	77%	95%
Prophylactic Antibiotic Selection[2]	64	94%	83%	90%	100%
Prophylactic Antibiotic Stopped[2,3]	116	84%	70%	72%	95%

Pregnancy Care

Inpatient Neonatal Mortality	746	0.13%	-	-	-
Third or Fourth Degree Laceration	529	1.89%	2.26%	3.63%	3.27%

Greenwood LeFlore Hospital

1401 River Road
Greenwood, MS 38935
E-mail: humanresources@glh.org
URL: www.glh.org
Ownership: Government - Local
Emergency Services: Yes

Phone: 662-459-7000
Fax: 662-459-7117

Accredited: Yes
Licensed Beds: 260

Key Personnel:
Executive Director . . . . Jerry W Adams

Measure	Cases	This Hospital	State Average	U.S. Average	Top Hospital
Heart Attack Care					
ACE Inhibitor or ARB for LVSD[1]	9	67%	80%	82%	100%
Aspirin at Arrival	52	88%	86%	92%	100%
Aspirin at Discharge	26	73%	84%	90%	100%
Beta Blocker at Arrival	49	86%	74%	87%	100%
Beta Blocker at Discharge	28	82%	81%	90%	100%
Fibrinolytic Medication Timing[1]	8	12%	32%	31%	100%
PCI Within 90 Minutes of Arrival	0	-	46%	54%	95%
Smoking Cessation Advice[1]	6	100%	88%	88%	100%
Heart Failure Care					
ACE Inhibitor or ARB for LVSD	99	68%	76%	82%	100%
Discharge Instructions	244	20%	55%	61%	93%
Evaluation of LVS Function	279	78%	78%	83%	99%
Smoking Cessation Advice	59	90%	80%	82%	100%
Pneumonia Care					
Appropriate Initial Antibiotic	73	84%	78%	83%	94%
Blood Culture Timing	52	88%	89%	90%	100%
Influenza Vaccine[1]	18	44%	64%	70%	100%
Initial Antibiotic Timing	108	85%	79%	80%	93%
Oxygenation Assessment	128	100%	97%	99%	100%
Pneumococcal Vaccine	65	45%	62%	69%	94%
Smoking Cessation Advice	35	91%	77%	80%	100%
Surgical Infection Prevention					
Prophylactic Antibiotic Given	193	53%	76%	77%	95%
Prophylactic Antibiotic Selection	62	94%	83%	90%	100%
Prophylactic Antibiotic Stopped	185	45%	70%	72%	95%
Pregnancy Care					
Inpatient Neonatal Mortality	-	-	-	-	-
Third or Fourth Degree Laceration	-	-	2.26%	3.63%	3.27%

Grenada Lake Medical Center

960 Avent Drive
Grenada, MS 38901
Ownership: Government - Local
Emergency Services: Yes

Phone: 662-227-7000
Fax: 662-227-7453
Accredited: Yes
Licensed Beds: 156

Key Personnel:
President/CEO. . . . . Charles Denton
Director of Cardiology/Cardiac Lab. . . . . John Seibel, MD
Director Radiology . . . . Murray Dozier

Measure	Cases	This Hospital	State Average	U.S. Average	Top Hospital
Heart Attack Care					
ACE Inhibitor or ARB for LVSD[1]	6	67%	80%	82%	100%
Aspirin at Arrival	31	81%	86%	92%	100%
Aspirin at Discharge[1]	12	75%	84%	90%	100%
Beta Blocker at Arrival	28	79%	74%	87%	100%
Beta Blocker at Discharge[1]	16	62%	81%	90%	100%
Fibrinolytic Medication Timing[1]	4	25%	32%	31%	100%
PCI Within 90 Minutes of Arrival	0	-	46%	54%	95%

Smoking Cessation Advice[1]	6	83%	88%	88%	100%

Heart Failure Care

ACE Inhibitor or ARB for LVSD	73	77%	76%	82%	100%
Discharge Instructions	135	30%	55%	61%	93%
Evaluation of LVS Function	169	93%	78%	83%	99%
Smoking Cessation Advice	43	79%	80%	82%	100%

Pneumonia Care

Appropriate Initial Antibiotic	76	78%	78%	83%	94%
Blood Culture Timing	63	89%	89%	90%	100%
Influenza Vaccine[1]	13	100%	64%	70%	100%
Initial Antibiotic Timing	107	81%	79%	80%	93%
Oxygenation Assessment	121	100%	97%	99%	100%
Pneumococcal Vaccine	49	90%	62%	69%	94%
Smoking Cessation Advice	28	57%	77%	80%	100%

Surgical Infection Prevention

Prophylactic Antibiotic Given[2]	141	89%	76%	77%	95%
Prophylactic Antibiotic Selection[2]	28	96%	83%	90%	100%
Prophylactic Antibiotic Stopped[2]	129	93%	70%	72%	95%

Pregnancy Care

Inpatient Neonatal Mortality	226	0.44%	-	-	-
Third or Fourth Degree Laceration	416	2.88%	2.26%	3.63%	3.27%

Garden Park Medical Center

15200 Community Road
Gulfport, MS 39501
Ownership: Proprietary
Emergency Services: Yes

Phone: 601-864-4210

Accredited: Yes

Measure	Cases	This Hospital	State Average	U.S. Average	Top Hospital
Heart Attack Care					
ACE Inhibitor or ARB for LVSD[1]	2	100%	80%	82%	100%
Aspirin at Arrival[1]	24	88%	86%	92%	100%
Aspirin at Discharge[1]	4	100%	84%	90%	100%
Beta Blocker at Arrival[1]	14	64%	74%	87%	100%
Beta Blocker at Discharge[1]	3	67%	81%	90%	100%
Fibrinolytic Medication Timing	0	-	32%	31%	100%
PCI Within 90 Minutes of Arrival	0	-	46%	54%	95%
Smoking Cessation Advice[1]	2	100%	88%	88%	100%
Heart Failure Care					
ACE Inhibitor or ARB for LVSD	32	88%	76%	82%	100%
Discharge Instructions	115	75%	55%	61%	93%
Evaluation of LVS Function	121	90%	78%	83%	99%
Smoking Cessation Advice	35	100%	80%	82%	100%
Pneumonia Care					
Appropriate Initial Antibiotic	64	77%	78%	83%	94%
Blood Culture Timing	28	86%	89%	90%	100%
Influenza Vaccine[1]	15	73%	64%	70%	100%
Initial Antibiotic Timing	81	65%	79%	80%	93%
Oxygenation Assessment	84	100%	97%	99%	100%
Pneumococcal Vaccine	33	73%	62%	69%	94%
Smoking Cessation Advice[1]	20	100%	77%	80%	100%
Surgical Infection Prevention					
Prophylactic Antibiotic Given[2,3]	140	89%	76%	77%	95%
Prophylactic Antibiotic Selection[2]	81	95%	83%	90%	100%
Prophylactic Antibiotic Stopped[2,3]	135	39%	70%	72%	95%
Pregnancy Care					
Inpatient Neonatal Mortality	-	-	-	-	-
Third or Fourth Degree Laceration	-	-	2.26%	3.63%	3.27%

Memorial Hospital at Gulfport

4500 13th Street
PO Box 1810
Gulfport, MS 39501
URL: www.gulfportmemorial.com
Ownership: Government - Local
Emergency Services: Yes

Phone: 228-867-4000
Fax: 228-865-3378

Accredited: Yes
Licensed Beds: 445

Key Personnel:
President/CEO. . . . . Gary Marchand
Emergency Room . . . . George Ward, MD
Director Medical/Surgical Nursing . . . . Jennifer Dumal
OB/GYN Womens Health. . . . . Richard Colson, MD
Chief Radiology . . . . Frank Schmidt, MD
Chief of Pulmonary. . . . . Tania Wescovich

NOTE: Hospital profiles are in alphabetical order by state, then city, then hospital within the city; Rankings are sorted by rate in descending order and exclude hospitals with less than 25 cases; (1) The number of cases is too small (n<25) for purposes of reliably predicting hospital performance; (2) Measure reflects the hospital's indication that its submission was based upon a sample of its relevant discharges; (3) Rate reflects fewer than the maximum possible quarters of data for the measure; (4) Inaccurate information submitted and suppressed for one or more quarters; (5) No data is available from the hospital for this measure; Please refer to the User's Guide for a full explanation of data

Measure	Cases	This Hospital	State Average	U.S. Average	Top Hospital
Heart Attack Care					
ACE Inhibitor or ARB for LVSD	99	87%	80%	82%	100%
Aspirin at Arrival	177	94%	86%	92%	100%
Aspirin at Discharge	298	99%	84%	90%	100%
Beta Blocker at Arrival	134	81%	74%	87%	100%
Beta Blocker at Discharge	329	92%	81%	90%	100%
Fibrinolytic Medication Timing[1]	4	50%	32%	31%	100%
PCI Within 90 Minutes of Arrival[1]	10	40%	46%	54%	95%
Smoking Cessation Advice	159	96%	88%	88%	100%
Heart Failure Care					
ACE Inhibitor or ARB for LVSD	275	77%	76%	82%	100%
Discharge Instructions	616	42%	55%	61%	93%
Evaluation of LVS Function	703	90%	78%	83%	99%
Smoking Cessation Advice	180	93%	80%	82%	100%
Pneumonia Care					
Appropriate Initial Antibiotic	171	87%	78%	83%	94%
Blood Culture Timing	150	97%	89%	90%	100%
Influenza Vaccine	48	56%	64%	70%	100%
Initial Antibiotic Timing	271	45%	79%	80%	93%
Oxygenation Assessment	336	98%	97%	99%	100%
Pneumococcal Vaccine	174	64%	62%	69%	94%
Smoking Cessation Advice	109	82%	77%	80%	100%
Surgical Infection Prevention					
Prophylactic Antibiotic Given[3]	449	70%	76%	77%	95%
Prophylactic Antibiotic Selection	145	92%	83%	90%	100%
Prophylactic Antibiotic Stopped[3]	443	76%	70%	72%	95%
Pregnancy Care					
Inpatient Neonatal Mortality	-	-	-	-	-
Third or Fourth Degree Laceration	-	-	2.26%	3.63%	3.27%

Forrest County General Hospital

Alternate Name: Forrest General Hospital
6051 US Highway 49 S
Hattiesburg, MS 39401
URL: www.forrestgeneral.com
Ownership: Government - Local
Emergency Services: Yes
Phone: 601-288-7000
Fax: 601-288-4441

Accredited: Yes
Licensed Beds: 537

Key Personnel:
President . . . . William C Oliver
Director Cardiac Catheterization Lab . . . . Sandra K Jones
Director Surgical Services . . . . K A Russum
Director Emergency Services . . . . Jan Walker, RN
Infection Prevention Officer . . . . Cathy Blythe
ICU . . . . Leanne Davis
Medical/Surgical Nursing . . . . Carol Gould
OB/GYN Womens Health. . . . . Carol Gould
Director of Surgical Services . . . . Kathryn Russum
Director Respiratory Care. . . . . Kathy Ehlers

Measure	Cases	This Hospital	State Average	U.S. Average	Top Hospital
Heart Attack Care					
ACE Inhibitor or ARB for LVSD	71	96%	80%	82%	100%
Aspirin at Arrival	315	98%	86%	92%	100%
Aspirin at Discharge	497	97%	84%	90%	100%
Beta Blocker at Arrival	183	96%	74%	87%	100%
Beta Blocker at Discharge	514	97%	81%	90%	100%
Fibrinolytic Medication Timing[1]	2	0%	32%	31%	100%
PCI Within 90 Minutes of Arrival[1]	9	67%	46%	54%	95%
Smoking Cessation Advice	225	100%	88%	88%	100%
Heart Failure Care					
ACE Inhibitor or ARB for LVSD	224	91%	76%	82%	100%
Discharge Instructions	505	72%	55%	61%	93%
Evaluation of LVS Function	572	95%	78%	83%	99%
Smoking Cessation Advice	108	100%	80%	82%	100%
Pneumonia Care					
Appropriate Initial Antibiotic	236	88%	78%	83%	94%
Blood Culture Timing	246	91%	89%	90%	100%
Influenza Vaccine	67	66%	64%	70%	100%
Initial Antibiotic Timing	329	73%	79%	80%	93%
Oxygenation Assessment	432	97%	97%	99%	100%
Pneumococcal Vaccine	207	77%	62%	69%	94%

Measure	Cases	This Hospital	State Average	U.S. Average	Top Hospital
Smoking Cessation Advice	117	100%	77%	80%	100%
Surgical Infection Prevention					
Prophylactic Antibiotic Given[3]	320	82%	76%	77%	95%
Prophylactic Antibiotic Selection	130	76%	83%	90%	100%
Prophylactic Antibiotic Stopped[3]	313	55%	70%	72%	95%
Pregnancy Care					
Inpatient Neonatal Mortality	-	-	-	-	-
Third or Fourth Degree Laceration	-	-	2.26%	3.63%	3.27%

Wesley Medical Center

5001 Hardy Street
Hattiesburg, MS 39402
URL: www.wesley.com
Ownership: Proprietary
Emergency Services: Yes
Phone: 601-268-8000
Fax: 601-268-5008

Accredited: Yes
Licensed Beds: 211

Key Personnel:
CEO. . . . . Ronald T Seal
Director Medical/Surgical Nursing . . . . Phyllis Tingle
OB/GYN Womens Health. . . . . Joseph Washburne
Chief Radiology . . . . Craig Howard
Director Respiratory Therapy . . . . Stan Grantham

Measure	Cases	This Hospital	State Average	U.S. Average	Top Hospital
Heart Attack Care					
ACE Inhibitor or ARB for LVSD	27	96%	80%	82%	100%
Aspirin at Arrival	94	97%	86%	92%	100%
Aspirin at Discharge	132	99%	84%	90%	100%
Beta Blocker at Arrival	74	97%	74%	87%	100%
Beta Blocker at Discharge	122	100%	81%	90%	100%
Fibrinolytic Medication Timing[1]	3	0%	32%	31%	100%
PCI Within 90 Minutes of Arrival[1]	2	100%	46%	54%	95%
Smoking Cessation Advice	47	100%	88%	88%	100%
Heart Failure Care					
ACE Inhibitor or ARB for LVSD	121	99%	76%	82%	100%
Discharge Instructions	220	86%	55%	61%	93%
Evaluation of LVS Function	261	100%	78%	83%	99%
Smoking Cessation Advice	64	98%	80%	82%	100%
Pneumonia Care					
Appropriate Initial Antibiotic	131	87%	78%	83%	94%
Blood Culture Timing	113	96%	89%	90%	100%
Influenza Vaccine	32	97%	64%	70%	100%
Initial Antibiotic Timing	138	86%	79%	80%	93%
Oxygenation Assessment	190	100%	97%	99%	100%
Pneumococcal Vaccine	104	98%	62%	69%	94%
Smoking Cessation Advice	52	100%	77%	80%	100%
Surgical Infection Prevention					
Prophylactic Antibiotic Given	1,007	92%	76%	77%	95%
Prophylactic Antibiotic Selection	250	91%	83%	90%	100%
Prophylactic Antibiotic Stopped	995	83%	70%	72%	95%
Pregnancy Care					
Inpatient Neonatal Mortality	-	-	-	-	-
Third or Fourth Degree Laceration	-	-	2.26%	3.63%	3.27%

Alliance Healthcare System

Alternate Name: Memorial Hospital Holly Springs
1430 Highway 4 E
Holly Springs, MS 38635
Ownership: Voluntary non-profit - Private
Emergency Services: No
Phone: 662-252-1212
Fax: 662-252-5537
Accredited: No
Licensed Beds: 40

Key Personnel:
Administrator/CEO. . . . . Perry E Williams, SR

Measure	Cases	This Hospital	State Average	U.S. Average	Top Hospital
Heart Attack Care					
ACE Inhibitor or ARB for LVSD[3]	0	-	80%	82%	100%
Aspirin at Arrival[1,3]	2	100%	86%	92%	100%
Aspirin at Discharge[1,3]	2	50%	84%	90%	100%
Beta Blocker at Arrival[1,3]	2	100%	74%	87%	100%
Beta Blocker at Discharge[1,3]	2	100%	81%	90%	100%
Fibrinolytic Medication Timing[3]	0	-	32%	31%	100%
PCI Within 90 Minutes of Arrival	0	-	46%	54%	95%
Smoking Cessation Advice[3]	0	-	88%	88%	100%

NOTE: Hospital profiles are in alphabetical order by state, then city, then hospital within the city; Rankings are sorted by rate in descending order and exclude hospitals with less than 25 cases; (1) The number of cases is too small (n<25) for purposes of reliably predicting hospital performance; (2) Measure reflects the hospital's indication that its submission was based upon a sample of its relevant discharges; (3) Rate reflects fewer than the maximum possible quarters of data for the measure; (4) Inaccurate information submitted and suppressed for one or more quarters; (5) No data is available from the hospital for this measure; Please refer to the User's Guide for a full explanation of data

(continued)

Measure	Cases	This Hospital	State Average	U.S. Average	Top Hospital
Heart Failure Care					
ACE Inhibitor or ARB for LVSD[1]	6	83%	76%	82%	100%
Discharge Instructions[1,3]	9	0%	55%	61%	93%
Evaluation of LVS Function	47	57%	78%	83%	99%
Smoking Cessation Advice[1,3]	1	0%	80%	82%	100%
Pneumonia Care					
Appropriate Initial Antibiotic[1,3]	2	100%	78%	83%	94%
Blood Culture Timing[1,3]	2	50%	89%	90%	100%
Influenza Vaccine[5]	-	-	64%	70%	100%
Initial Antibiotic Timing	34	68%	79%	80%	93%
Oxygenation Assessment	43	98%	97%	99%	100%
Pneumococcal Vaccine[1]	22	50%	62%	69%	94%
Smoking Cessation Advice[1,3]	1	0%	77%	80%	100%
Surgical Infection Prevention					
Prophylactic Antibiotic Given[1,3]	1	0%	76%	77%	95%
Prophylactic Antibiotic Selection[5]	-	-	83%	90%	100%
Prophylactic Antibiotic Stopped[1,3]	1	100%	70%	72%	95%
Pregnancy Care					
Inpatient Neonatal Mortality	-	-	-	-	-
Third or Fourth Degree Laceration	-	-	2.26%	3.63%	3.27%

Trace Regional Hospital

Alternate Name: Houston Community Hospital
Highway 8 E   Phone: 662-456-3700
Houston, MS 38851   Fax: 662-456-5417
Ownership: Proprietary   Accredited: Yes
Emergency Services: Yes   Licensed Beds: 84
Key Personnel:
President/CEO.........................Gary Staten
Emergency Room ....Curtis Cunningham

Measure	Cases	This Hospital	State Average	U.S. Average	Top Hospital
Heart Attack Care					
ACE Inhibitor or ARB for LVSD[1]	1	100%	80%	82%	100%
Aspirin at Arrival[1]	13	92%	86%	92%	100%
Aspirin at Discharge[1]	10	100%	84%	90%	100%
Beta Blocker at Arrival[1]	8	88%	74%	87%	100%
Beta Blocker at Discharge[1]	9	89%	81%	90%	100%
Fibrinolytic Medication Timing[3]	0	-	32%	31%	100%
PCI Within 90 Minutes of Arrival	0	-	46%	54%	95%
Smoking Cessation Advice[3]	0	-	88%	88%	100%
Heart Failure Care					
ACE Inhibitor or ARB for LVSD[1]	7	86%	76%	82%	100%
Discharge Instructions[1,3]	8	38%	55%	61%	93%
Evaluation of LVS Function	50	84%	78%	83%	99%
Smoking Cessation Advice[3]	0	-	80%	82%	100%
Pneumonia Care					
Appropriate Initial Antibiotic[1,3]	2	100%	78%	83%	94%
Blood Culture Timing[1,3]	3	67%	89%	90%	100%
Influenza Vaccine[5]	-	-	64%	70%	100%
Initial Antibiotic Timing	74	92%	79%	80%	93%
Oxygenation Assessment	86	100%	97%	99%	100%
Pneumococcal Vaccine	54	67%	62%	69%	94%
Smoking Cessation Advice[1,3]	2	50%	77%	80%	100%
Surgical Infection Prevention					
Prophylactic Antibiotic Given[5]	-	-	76%	77%	95%
Prophylactic Antibiotic Selection[5]	-	-	83%	90%	100%
Prophylactic Antibiotic Stopped[5]	-	-	70%	72%	95%
Pregnancy Care					
Inpatient Neonatal Mortality	-	-	-	-	-
Third or Fourth Degree Laceration	-	-	2.26%	3.63%	3.27%

South Sunflower County Hospital

121 E Baker Street   Phone: 662-887-5235
Indianola, MS 38751   Fax: 662-887-4111
Ownership: Government - Local   Accredited: Yes
Emergency Services: Yes   Licensed Beds: 69
Key Personnel:
Administrator ....H J Blessitt

Measure	Cases	This Hospital	State Average	U.S. Average	Top Hospital
Heart Attack Care					

Measure	Cases	This Hospital	State Average	U.S. Average	Top Hospital
ACE Inhibitor or ARB for LVSD[1]	4	50%	80%	82%	100%
Aspirin at Arrival[1]	21	57%	86%	92%	100%
Aspirin at Discharge[1]	17	53%	84%	90%	100%
Beta Blocker at Arrival[1]	17	53%	74%	87%	100%
Beta Blocker at Discharge[1]	17	71%	81%	90%	100%
Fibrinolytic Medication Timing[3]	0	-	32%	31%	100%
PCI Within 90 Minutes of Arrival	0	-	46%	54%	95%
Smoking Cessation Advice[1,3]	1	100%	88%	88%	100%
Heart Failure Care					
ACE Inhibitor or ARB for LVSD	34	62%	76%	82%	100%
Discharge Instructions[1,3]	19	0%	55%	61%	93%
Evaluation of LVS Function	79	86%	78%	83%	99%
Smoking Cessation Advice[1,3]	6	50%	80%	82%	100%
Pneumonia Care					
Appropriate Initial Antibiotic[1,3]	7	86%	78%	83%	94%
Blood Culture Timing[3]	0	-	89%	90%	100%
Influenza Vaccine[5]	-	-	64%	70%	100%
Initial Antibiotic Timing	63	71%	79%	80%	93%
Oxygenation Assessment	87	83%	97%	99%	100%
Pneumococcal Vaccine	52	67%	62%	69%	94%
Smoking Cessation Advice[1,3]	2	0%	77%	80%	100%
Surgical Infection Prevention					
Prophylactic Antibiotic Given[1,3]	8	100%	76%	77%	95%
Prophylactic Antibiotic Selection[5]	-	-	83%	90%	100%
Prophylactic Antibiotic Stopped[1,3]	8	88%	70%	72%	95%
Pregnancy Care					
Inpatient Neonatal Mortality	413	0.24%	-	-	-
Third or Fourth Degree Laceration	261	2.68%	2.26%	3.63%	3.27%

North Mississippi Medical Center-Iuka

1777 Curtis Drive   Toll-Free: 800-843-3375
Iuka, MS 38852   Phone: 662-423-6051
                                     Fax: 662-423-4515
URL: www.nmhs.net/iuka
Ownership: Voluntary non-profit - Private
Emergency Services: Yes   Accredited: Yes
                                     Licensed Beds: 48
Key Personnel:
President/CEO.........................John Heer
Administrator ....James R Carter Jr
Chief Medical Officer ....Ken Davis, MD

Measure	Cases	This Hospital	State Average	U.S. Average	Top Hospital
Heart Attack Care					
ACE Inhibitor or ARB for LVSD[1]	1	100%	80%	82%	100%
Aspirin at Arrival[1]	8	50%	86%	92%	100%
Aspirin at Discharge[1]	6	67%	84%	90%	100%
Beta Blocker at Arrival[1]	8	62%	74%	87%	100%
Beta Blocker at Discharge[1]	7	57%	81%	90%	100%
Fibrinolytic Medication Timing[3]	0	-	32%	31%	100%
PCI Within 90 Minutes of Arrival	0	-	46%	54%	95%
Smoking Cessation Advice[3]	0	-	88%	88%	100%
Heart Failure Care					
ACE Inhibitor or ARB for LVSD[1]	8	88%	76%	82%	100%
Discharge Instructions[1,3]	23	74%	55%	61%	93%
Evaluation of LVS Function	120	81%	78%	83%	99%
Smoking Cessation Advice[1,3]	5	100%	80%	82%	100%
Pneumonia Care					
Appropriate Initial Antibiotic[1,3]	6	83%	78%	83%	94%
Blood Culture Timing[1,3]	2	100%	89%	90%	100%
Influenza Vaccine[5]	-	-	64%	70%	100%
Initial Antibiotic Timing	51	78%	79%	80%	93%
Oxygenation Assessment	65	97%	97%	99%	100%
Pneumococcal Vaccine	28	61%	62%	69%	94%
Smoking Cessation Advice[1,3]	3	100%	77%	80%	100%
Surgical Infection Prevention					
Prophylactic Antibiotic Given[5]	-	-	76%	77%	95%
Prophylactic Antibiotic Selection[5]	-	-	83%	90%	100%
Prophylactic Antibiotic Stopped[6]	-	-	70%	72%	95%
Pregnancy Care					
Inpatient Neonatal Mortality	-	-	-	-	-
Third or Fourth Degree Laceration	-	-	2.26%	3.63%	3.27%

NOTE: Hospital profiles are in alphabetical order by state, then city, then hospital within the city; Rankings are sorted by rate in descending order and exclude hospitals with less than 25 cases; (1) The number of cases is too small (n<25) for purposes of reliably predicting hospital performance; (2) Measure reflects the hospital's indication that its submission was based upon a sample of its relevant discharges; (3) Rate reflects fewer than the maximum possible quarters of data for the measure; (4) Inaccurate information submitted and suppressed for one or more quarters; (5) No data is available from the hospital for this measure; Please refer to the User's Guide for a full explanation of data

Central Mississippi Medical Center

1850 Chadwick Drive
Jackson, MS 39204
URL: www.centralmississippimedicalcenter.com
Ownership: Proprietary
Emergency Services: Yes

Phone: 601-376-2561
Fax: 601-376-2975

Accredited: Yes
Licensed Beds: 473

Key Personnel:

President/CEO	Cam Welton
Chief Medical Staff	Barbara J Proctor, MD
Director Infection/Disease Control	Jo P Wilson, MD
Director Medical/Surgical Nursing	Joan Causey, RN
OB/GYN Womens Health	Chris Ball, MD
Chief Radiology	Waymond L Rone, MD
Director Respiratory Therapy	Steve Buckley

Measure	Cases	This Hospital	State Average	U.S. Average	Top Hospital
Heart Attack Care					
ACE Inhibitor or ARB for LVSD	33	64%	80%	82%	100%
Aspirin at Arrival	124	93%	86%	92%	100%
Aspirin at Discharge	115	88%	84%	90%	100%
Beta Blocker at Arrival	108	79%	74%	87%	100%
Beta Blocker at Discharge	123	85%	81%	90%	100%
Fibrinolytic Medication Timing[1]	8	88%	32%	31%	100%
PCI Within 90 Minutes of Arrival[1]	5	0%	46%	54%	95%
Smoking Cessation Advice	53	98%	88%	88%	100%
Heart Failure Care					
ACE Inhibitor or ARB for LVSD	128	71%	76%	82%	100%
Discharge Instructions	206	51%	55%	61%	93%
Evaluation of LVS Function	249	91%	78%	83%	99%
Smoking Cessation Advice	67	97%	80%	82%	100%
Pneumonia Care					
Appropriate Initial Antibiotic	111	73%	78%	83%	94%
Blood Culture Timing	86	85%	89%	90%	100%
Influenza Vaccine	32	88%	64%	70%	100%
Initial Antibiotic Timing	157	62%	79%	80%	93%
Oxygenation Assessment	187	98%	97%	99%	100%
Pneumococcal Vaccine	89	79%	62%	69%	94%
Smoking Cessation Advice	50	90%	77%	80%	100%
Surgical Infection Prevention					
Prophylactic Antibiotic Given[2]	432	90%	76%	77%	95%
Prophylactic Antibiotic Selection[2]	63	97%	83%	90%	100%
Prophylactic Antibiotic Stopped[2]	419	66%	70%	72%	95%
Pregnancy Care					
Inpatient Neonatal Mortality	-	-	-	-	-
Third or Fourth Degree Laceration	-	-	2.26%	3.63%	3.27%

Mississippi Baptist Health Systems

1225 N State Street
Jackson, MS 39202

URL: www.mbmc.org
Ownership: Voluntary non-profit - Private
Emergency Services: Yes

Toll-Free: 800-948-6262
Phone: 601-968-1000
Fax: 601-968-1383

Accredited: Yes
Licensed Beds: 564

Key Personnel:

CEO	Kurt Mepzmer
Chief Medical Staff	R Deaver Collins, MD
Chief Catheterization Laboratory	Dave Dear, MD
Emergency Room	Jeffery Glover, MD
CCU Spvg. Nurse	Julie Porter, RN
Director Medical/Surgical Nursing	Debbie Logan
OB/GYN Womens Health	Thomas Wiley, MD
Chief Radiology	Edward Phillips, MD
Director Respiratory Therapy	Robert Wall

Measure	Cases	This Hospital	State Average	U.S. Average	Top Hospital
Heart Attack Care					
ACE Inhibitor or ARB for LVSD	101	84%	80%	82%	100%
Aspirin at Arrival	200	98%	86%	92%	100%
Aspirin at Discharge	382	96%	84%	90%	100%
Beta Blocker at Arrival	172	89%	74%	87%	100%
Beta Blocker at Discharge	400	94%	81%	90%	100%
Fibrinolytic Medication Timing	0	-	32%	31%	100%
PCI Within 90 Minutes of Arrival[1]	14	14%	46%	54%	95%

Measure	Cases	This Hospital	State Average	U.S. Average	Top Hospital
Smoking Cessation Advice	154	98%	88%	88%	100%
Heart Failure Care					
ACE Inhibitor or ARB for LVSD	329	96%	76%	82%	100%
Discharge Instructions	675	83%	55%	61%	93%
Evaluation of LVS Function	760	97%	78%	83%	99%
Smoking Cessation Advice	134	97%	80%	82%	100%
Pneumonia Care					
Appropriate Initial Antibiotic[2]	77	81%	78%	83%	94%
Blood Culture Timing[2]	51	96%	89%	90%	100%
Influenza Vaccine[1,2]	23	74%	64%	70%	100%
Initial Antibiotic Timing[2]	123	70%	79%	80%	93%
Oxygenation Assessment[2]	150	99%	97%	99%	100%
Pneumococcal Vaccine[2]	90	68%	62%	69%	94%
Smoking Cessation Advice[2]	28	68%	77%	80%	100%
Surgical Infection Prevention					
Prophylactic Antibiotic Given[2]	305	77%	76%	77%	95%
Prophylactic Antibiotic Selection[2]	73	90%	83%	90%	100%
Prophylactic Antibiotic Stopped[2]	295	79%	70%	72%	95%
Pregnancy Care					
Inpatient Neonatal Mortality	-	-	-	-	-
Third or Fourth Degree Laceration	-	-	2.26%	3.63%	3.27%

Mississippi Methodist Rehab Center

1350 E Woodrow Wilson Dr
Jackson, MS 39216
Ownership: Voluntary non-profit - Private
Emergency Services: No

Phone: 601-981-2611

Accredited: Yes

Measure	Cases	This Hospital	State Average	U.S. Average	Top Hospital
Heart Attack Care					
ACE Inhibitor or ARB for LVSD[5]	-	-	80%	82%	100%
Aspirin at Arrival[5]	-	-	86%	92%	100%
Aspirin at Discharge[5]	-	-	84%	90%	100%
Beta Blocker at Arrival[5]	-	-	74%	87%	100%
Beta Blocker at Discharge[5]	-	-	81%	90%	100%
Fibrinolytic Medication Timing[5]	-	-	32%	31%	100%
PCI Within 90 Minutes of Arrival[5]	-	-	46%	54%	95%
Smoking Cessation Advice[5]	-	-	88%	88%	100%
Heart Failure Care					
ACE Inhibitor or ARB for LVSD[5]	-	-	76%	82%	100%
Discharge Instructions[5]	-	-	55%	61%	93%
Evaluation of LVS Function[5]	-	-	78%	83%	99%
Smoking Cessation Advice[5]	-	-	80%	82%	100%
Pneumonia Care					
Appropriate Initial Antibiotic[5]	-	-	78%	83%	94%
Blood Culture Timing[5]	-	-	89%	90%	100%
Influenza Vaccine[5]	-	-	64%	70%	100%
Initial Antibiotic Timing[3]	0	-	79%	80%	93%
Oxygenation Assessment[1,3]	1	100%	97%	99%	100%
Pneumococcal Vaccine[3]	0	-	62%	69%	94%
Smoking Cessation Advice[5]	-	-	77%	80%	100%
Surgical Infection Prevention					
Prophylactic Antibiotic Given[5]	-	-	76%	77%	95%
Prophylactic Antibiotic Selection[5]	-	-	83%	90%	100%
Prophylactic Antibiotic Stopped[5]	-	-	70%	72%	95%
Pregnancy Care					
Inpatient Neonatal Mortality	-	-	-	-	-
Third or Fourth Degree Laceration	-	-	2.26%	3.63%	3.27%

Regency Hospital of Jackson

969 Lakeland Drive, 6th Floor
Jackson, MS 39216
Ownership: Proprietary
Emergency Services: No

Phone: 601-364-6200

Accredited: No

Measure	Cases	This Hospital	State Average	U.S. Average	Top Hospital
Heart Attack Care					
ACE Inhibitor or ARB for LVSD[5]	-	-	80%	82%	100%
Aspirin at Arrival[5]	-	-	86%	92%	100%
Aspirin at Discharge[5]	-	-	84%	90%	100%
Beta Blocker at Arrival[5]	-	-	74%	87%	100%
Beta Blocker at Discharge[5]	-	-	81%	90%	100%

Measure			This Hospital	State Average	U.S. Average	Top Hospital
Fibrinolytic Medication Timing[5]	-	-	32%	31%	100%	
PCI Within 90 Minutes of Arrival[5]	-	-	46%	54%	95%	
Smoking Cessation Advice[5]	-	-	88%	88%	100%	
Heart Failure Care						
ACE Inhibitor or ARB for LVSD[5]	-	-	76%	82%	100%	
Discharge Instructions[5]	-	-	55%	61%	93%	
Evaluation of LVS Function[5]	-	-	78%	83%	99%	
Smoking Cessation Advice[5]	-	-	80%	82%	100%	
Pneumonia Care						
Appropriate Initial Antibiotic[3]	0	-	78%	83%	94%	
Blood Culture Timing[3]	0	-	89%	90%	100%	
Influenza Vaccine[5]	-	-	64%	70%	100%	
Initial Antibiotic Timing[3]	0	-	79%	80%	93%	
Oxygenation Assessment[3]	0	-	97%	99%	100%	
Pneumococcal Vaccine[3]	0	-	62%	69%	94%	
Smoking Cessation Advice[3]	0	-	77%	80%	100%	
Surgical Infection Prevention						
Prophylactic Antibiotic Given[5]	-	-	76%	77%	95%	
Prophylactic Antibiotic Selection[5]	-	-	83%	90%	100%	
Prophylactic Antibiotic Stopped[5]	-	-	70%	72%	95%	
Pregnancy Care						
Inpatient Neonatal Mortality	-	-	-	-	-	
Third or Fourth Degree Laceration	-	-	2.26%	3.63%	3.27%	

River Oaks Hospital

1030 River Oaks Drive
Jackson, MS 39232
URL: www.riveroakshospital.org
Ownership: Proprietary
Emergency Services: Yes

Phone: 601-932-1030
Fax: 601-936-2275

Accredited: Yes
Licensed Beds: 110

Key Personnel:
President/CEO . . . . Davis Richards
Chief Medical Staff . . . . Peter Neglen, MD
Catheterization Lab . . . . Greg Ross
Director Emergency Room . . . . Tony Rucker
Infection Control . . . . Peggy Shute
ICU . . . . Chad Colbert
Medical/Surgical Nursing . . . . Shery Cook
Women's Health Coordinator . . . . Becky Humphreys
Director Radiology . . . . Beverly Greenhill
Respiratory/Cardiopulmonary . . . . Larry Johnson

Measure	Cases	This Hospital	State Average	U.S. Average	Top Hospital
Heart Attack Care					
ACE Inhibitor or ARB for LVSD[1]	1	100%	80%	82%	100%
Aspirin at Arrival[1]	19	89%	86%	92%	100%
Aspirin at Discharge[1]	9	78%	84%	90%	100%
Beta Blocker at Arrival[1]	15	93%	74%	87%	100%
Beta Blocker at Discharge[1]	7	71%	81%	90%	100%
Fibrinolytic Medication Timing[1]	4	0%	32%	31%	100%
PCI Within 90 Minutes of Arrival	0	-	46%	54%	95%
Smoking Cessation Advice[1]	3	33%	88%	88%	100%
Heart Failure Care					
ACE Inhibitor or ARB for LVSD[1]	20	55%	76%	82%	100%
Discharge Instructions	104	30%	55%	61%	93%
Evaluation of LVS Function	122	79%	78%	83%	99%
Smoking Cessation Advice[1]	20	70%	80%	82%	100%
Pneumonia Care					
Appropriate Initial Antibiotic	115	73%	78%	83%	94%
Blood Culture Timing	56	95%	89%	90%	100%
Influenza Vaccine	26	35%	64%	70%	100%
Initial Antibiotic Timing	118	72%	79%	80%	93%
Oxygenation Assessment	160	100%	97%	99%	100%
Pneumococcal Vaccine	68	49%	62%	69%	94%
Smoking Cessation Advice	43	63%	77%	80%	100%
Surgical Infection Prevention					
Prophylactic Antibiotic Given[2]	823	60%	76%	77%	95%
Prophylactic Antibiotic Selection[2]	69	80%	83%	90%	100%
Prophylactic Antibiotic Stopped[2]	814	76%	70%	72%	95%
Pregnancy Care					
Inpatient Neonatal Mortality	-	-	-	-	-
Third or Fourth Degree Laceration	-	-	2.26%	3.63%	3.27%

Saint Dominic Jackson Memorial Hospital

969 Lakeland Drive
Jackson, MS 39216
URL: www.stdom.com
Ownership: Voluntary non-profit - Other
Emergency Services: Yes

Phone: 601-200-2000
Fax: 601-200-0890

Accredited: Yes
Licensed Beds: 571

Key Personnel:
President . . . . Claude W Harbarger

Measure	Cases	This Hospital	State Average	U.S. Average	Top Hospital
Heart Attack Care					
ACE Inhibitor or ARB for LVSD	69	90%	80%	82%	100%
Aspirin at Arrival	153	99%	86%	92%	100%
Aspirin at Discharge	272	97%	84%	90%	100%
Beta Blocker at Arrival	134	91%	74%	87%	100%
Beta Blocker at Discharge	270	96%	81%	90%	100%
Fibrinolytic Medication Timing[1]	2	0%	32%	31%	100%
PCI Within 90 Minutes of Arrival[1]	5	40%	46%	54%	95%
Smoking Cessation Advice	84	100%	88%	88%	100%
Heart Failure Care					
ACE Inhibitor or ARB for LVSD	145	86%	76%	82%	100%
Discharge Instructions	284	81%	55%	61%	93%
Evaluation of LVS Function	312	89%	78%	83%	99%
Smoking Cessation Advice	42	98%	80%	82%	100%
Pneumonia Care					
Appropriate Initial Antibiotic[2]	90	86%	78%	83%	94%
Blood Culture Timing[2]	84	87%	89%	90%	100%
Influenza Vaccine[4,5]	-	-	64%	70%	100%
Initial Antibiotic Timing[2]	110	79%	79%	80%	93%
Oxygenation Assessment[2]	145	100%	97%	99%	100%
Pneumococcal Vaccine[2]	79	71%	62%	69%	94%
Smoking Cessation Advice[1,2]	24	96%	77%	80%	100%
Surgical Infection Prevention					
Prophylactic Antibiotic Given[2]	268	72%	76%	77%	95%
Prophylactic Antibiotic Selection[2]	69	90%	83%	90%	100%
Prophylactic Antibiotic Stopped[2]	254	66%	70%	72%	95%
Pregnancy Care					
Inpatient Neonatal Mortality	-	-	-	-	-
Third or Fourth Degree Laceration	-	-	2.26%	3.63%	3.27%

University of Mississippi Medical Center

2500 N State Street
Jackson, MS 39216
URL: www.umc.edu
Ownership: Government - State
Emergency Services: Yes

Phone: 601-984-1000
Fax: 601-984-1973

Accredited: Yes
Licensed Beds: 665

Key Personnel:
CEO . . . . Daniel Jones
Chief Medical Staff . . . . Joe Files, MD
Director Respiratory Therapy . . . . Gail Carlson

Measure	Cases	This Hospital	State Average	U.S. Average	Top Hospital
Heart Attack Care					
ACE Inhibitor or ARB for LVSD	40	85%	80%	82%	100%
Aspirin at Arrival	121	98%	86%	92%	100%
Aspirin at Discharge	135	98%	84%	90%	100%
Beta Blocker at Arrival	97	95%	74%	87%	100%
Beta Blocker at Discharge	150	98%	81%	90%	100%
Fibrinolytic Medication Timing	0	-	32%	31%	100%
PCI Within 90 Minutes of Arrival[1]	8	50%	46%	54%	95%
Smoking Cessation Advice	107	98%	88%	88%	100%
Heart Failure Care					
ACE Inhibitor or ARB for LVSD	242	86%	76%	82%	100%
Discharge Instructions	304	46%	55%	61%	93%
Evaluation of LVS Function	310	97%	78%	83%	99%
Smoking Cessation Advice	114	88%	80%	82%	100%
Pneumonia Care					
Appropriate Initial Antibiotic	59	83%	78%	83%	94%
Blood Culture Timing	69	84%	89%	90%	100%
Influenza Vaccine[1]	18	6%	64%	70%	100%
Initial Antibiotic Timing	106	59%	79%	80%	93%
Oxygenation Assessment	137	99%	97%	99%	100%

NOTE: Hospital profiles are in alphabetical order by state, then city, then hospital within the city; Rankings are sorted by rate in descending order and exclude hospitals with less than 25 cases; (1) The number of cases is too small (n<25) for purposes of reliably predicting hospital performance; (2) Measure reflects the hospital's indication that its submission was based upon a sample of its relevant discharges; (3) Rate reflects fewer than the maximum possible quarters of data for the measure; (4) Inaccurate information submitted and suppressed for one or more quarters; (5) No data is available from the hospital for this measure; Please refer to the User's Guide for a full explanation of data

Pneumococcal Vaccine	37	5%	62%	69%	94%
Smoking Cessation Advice	53	79%	77%	80%	100%
Surgical Infection Prevention					
Prophylactic Antibiotic Given[2,3]	326	88%	76%	77%	95%
Prophylactic Antibiotic Selection[2]	206	94%	83%	90%	100%
Prophylactic Antibiotic Stopped[2,3]	320	76%	70%	72%	95%
Pregnancy Care					
Inpatient Neonatal Mortality	3,925	2.32%	-	-	-
Third or Fourth Degree Laceration	2,349	1.70%	2.26%	3.63%	3.27%

Woman's Hospital at River Oaks

Alternate Name: Woman's Hospital
1026 N Flowood Drive
Jackson, MS 39232
URL: www.womanshospitalone.com
Ownership: Proprietary
Emergency Services: No

Phone: 601-932-1000
Fax: 601-936-3086

Accredited: Yes
Licensed Beds: 111

Key Personnel:
President/CEO . . . . Jack Cleary
Chief Medical Staff . . . . Ed Barham, MD
Infection Control Director . . . . Peggy Shute
Surgery Director . . . . Carmen Polk
Director Radiology . . . . Beverly Greenhill

Measure	Cases	This Hospital	State Average	U.S. Average	Top Hospital
Heart Attack Care					
ACE Inhibitor or ARB for LVSD[5]	-	-	80%	82%	100%
Aspirin at Arrival[5]	-	-	86%	92%	100%
Aspirin at Discharge[5]	-	-	84%	90%	100%
Beta Blocker at Arrival[5]	-	-	74%	87%	100%
Beta Blocker at Discharge[5]	-	-	81%	90%	100%
Fibrinolytic Medication Timing[5]	-	-	32%	31%	100%
PCI Within 90 Minutes of Arrival[5]	-	-	46%	54%	95%
Smoking Cessation Advice[5]	-	-	88%	88%	100%
Heart Failure Care					
ACE Inhibitor or ARB for LVSD[5]	-	-	76%	82%	100%
Discharge Instructions[5]	-	-	55%	61%	93%
Evaluation of LVS Function[5]	-	-	78%	83%	99%
Smoking Cessation Advice[5]	-	-	80%	82%	100%
Pneumonia Care					
Appropriate Initial Antibiotic[5]	-	-	78%	83%	94%
Blood Culture Timing[5]	-	-	89%	90%	100%
Influenza Vaccine[5]	-	-	64%	70%	100%
Initial Antibiotic Timing[5]	-	-	79%	80%	93%
Oxygenation Assessment[5]	-	-	97%	99%	100%
Pneumococcal Vaccine[5]	-	-	62%	69%	94%
Smoking Cessation Advice[5]	-	-	77%	80%	100%
Surgical Infection Prevention					
Prophylactic Antibiotic Given[2]	339	86%	76%	77%	95%
Prophylactic Antibiotic Selection[1,2]	18	78%	83%	90%	100%
Prophylactic Antibiotic Stopped[2]	337	84%	70%	72%	95%
Pregnancy Care					
Inpatient Neonatal Mortality	1,530	0.33%	-	-	-
Third or Fourth Degree Laceration	769	4.03%	2.26%	3.63%	3.27%

Kilmichael Hospital

301 Lamar Avenue
Kilmichael, MS 39747
Ownership: Govt - Hospital District or Authority
Emergency Services: No

Phone: 662-262-4311
Fax: 662-262-5586
Accredited: No
Licensed Beds: 19

Key Personnel:
President/CEO . . . . Calvin Johnson
Chief Medical Staff . . . . Katrina Poe, MD
Emergency Room . . . . LC Henson, MD

Measure	Cases	This Hospital	State Average	U.S. Average	Top Hospital
Heart Attack Care					
ACE Inhibitor or ARB for LVSD[5]	-	-	80%	82%	100%
Aspirin at Arrival[5]	-	-	86%	92%	100%
Aspirin at Discharge[5]	-	-	84%	90%	100%
Beta Blocker at Arrival[5]	-	-	74%	87%	100%
Beta Blocker at Discharge[5]	-	-	81%	90%	100%

Fibrinolytic Medication Timing[5]	-	-	32%	31%	100%
PCI Within 90 Minutes of Arrival[5]	-	-	46%	54%	95%
Smoking Cessation Advice[5]	-	-	88%	88%	100%
Heart Failure Care					
ACE Inhibitor or ARB for LVSD[3]	0	-	76%	82%	100%
Discharge Instructions[1,3]	6	50%	55%	61%	93%
Evaluation of LVS Function[1,3]	20	0%	78%	83%	99%
Smoking Cessation Advice[1,3]	1	0%	80%	82%	100%
Pneumonia Care					
Appropriate Initial Antibiotic[3]	0	-	78%	83%	94%
Blood Culture Timing[3]	0	-	89%	90%	100%
Influenza Vaccine[5]	-	-	64%	70%	100%
Initial Antibiotic Timing[1]	11	100%	79%	80%	93%
Oxygenation Assessment[1]	20	100%	97%	99%	100%
Pneumococcal Vaccine[1]	16	6%	62%	69%	94%
Smoking Cessation Advice[3]	0	-	77%	80%	100%
Surgical Infection Prevention					
Prophylactic Antibiotic Given[5]	-	-	76%	77%	95%
Prophylactic Antibiotic Selection[5]	-	-	83%	90%	100%
Prophylactic Antibiotic Stopped[5]	-	-	70%	72%	95%
Pregnancy Care					
Inpatient Neonatal Mortality	-	-	-	-	-
Third or Fourth Degree Laceration	-	-	2.26%	3.63%	3.27%

Montfort Jones Memorial Hospital

PO Box 887
Kosciusko, MS 39090
Ownership: Government - Local
Emergency Services: Yes

Phone: 662-289-4322
Fax: 662-289-6080
Accredited: No
Licensed Beds: 72

Key Personnel:
Administrator . . . . Thomas Bland
Chief Medical Staff . . . . D Stanley Hartness, MD
Emergency Room . . . . Cynthia Lassiter, RN
Chief Radiology . . . . Ronnie Christian, MD
Director Respiratory Therapy . . . . Ronnie Summers

Measure	Cases	This Hospital	State Average	U.S. Average	Top Hospital
Heart Attack Care					
ACE Inhibitor or ARB for LVSD[1,2]	2	100%	80%	82%	100%
Aspirin at Arrival[1,2]	16	100%	86%	92%	100%
Aspirin at Discharge[1,2]	2	100%	84%	90%	100%
Beta Blocker at Arrival[1,2]	18	72%	74%	87%	100%
Beta Blocker at Discharge[1,2]	3	100%	81%	90%	100%
Fibrinolytic Medication Timing[2]	0	-	32%	31%	100%
PCI Within 90 Minutes of Arrival[2]	0	-	46%	54%	95%
Smoking Cessation Advice[1,2]	1	0%	88%	88%	100%
Heart Failure Care					
ACE Inhibitor or ARB for LVSD[1,2]	23	70%	76%	82%	100%
Discharge Instructions[2]	65	8%	55%	61%	93%
Evaluation of LVS Function[2]	74	62%	78%	83%	99%
Smoking Cessation Advice[1,2]	9	33%	80%	82%	100%
Pneumonia Care					
Appropriate Initial Antibiotic[2]	63	73%	78%	83%	94%
Blood Culture Timing[1,2]	19	84%	89%	90%	100%
Influenza Vaccine[1]	21	86%	64%	70%	100%
Initial Antibiotic Timing[2]	64	70%	79%	80%	93%
Oxygenation Assessment[2]	87	100%	97%	99%	100%
Pneumococcal Vaccine[2]	49	90%	62%	69%	94%
Smoking Cessation Advice[1,2]	18	39%	77%	80%	100%
Surgical Infection Prevention					
Prophylactic Antibiotic Given[1,2]	4	50%	76%	77%	95%
Prophylactic Antibiotic Selection[1,2]	1	0%	83%	90%	100%
Prophylactic Antibiotic Stopped[1,2]	3	33%	70%	72%	95%
Pregnancy Care					
Inpatient Neonatal Mortality	-	-	-	-	-
Third or Fourth Degree Laceration	-	-	2.26%	3.63%	3.27%

South Central Regional Medical Center

Alternate Name: Jones County Community Hospital

NOTE: Hospital profiles are in alphabetical order by state, then city, then hospital within the city; Rankings are sorted by rate in descending order and exclude hospitals with less than 25 cases; (1) The number of cases is too small (n<25) for purposes of reliably predicting hospital performance; (2) Measure reflects the hospital's indication that its submission was based upon a sample of its relevant discharges; (3) Rate reflects fewer than the maximum possible quarters of data for the measure; (4) Inaccurate information submitted and suppressed for one or more quarters; (5) No data is available from the hospital for this measure; Please refer to the User's Guide for a full explanation of data

1220 Jefferson Street
PO Box 607
Laurel, MS 39441
URL: www.scrmc.com
Ownership: Government - Local
Emergency Services: Yes

Phone: 601-426-4000
Fax: 601-426-4729

Accredited: Yes
Licensed Beds: 285

Key Personnel:
Executive Director . . . . Doug Higginbotham
Chief Medical Staff. . . . . Stephen Johnson, MD
Cardiac Lab . . . . Edwin Todd
Catheterization Lab . . . . Paula Prestwood, RN
Emergency Room . . . . Mack Knight, RN
Emergency Room . . . . Michael LaRochelle, DO
ICU . . . . Pam Ninu, RN
Medical/Surgical Nursing . . . . Connie Landrum
OB/GYN Womens Health. . . . . Vicke Walters, RN
Respiratory/Cardiopulmonary. . . . . Edwin Todd

Measure	Cases	This Hospital	State Average	U.S. Average	Top Hospital
Heart Attack Care					
ACE Inhibitor or ARB for LVSD[1]	16	75%	80%	82%	100%
Aspirin at Arrival	112	90%	86%	92%	100%
Aspirin at Discharge	53	85%	84%	90%	100%
Beta Blocker at Arrival	105	80%	74%	87%	100%
Beta Blocker at Discharge	55	82%	81%	90%	100%
Fibrinolytic Medication Timing[1]	10	70%	32%	31%	100%
PCI Within 90 Minutes of Arrival	0	-	46%	54%	95%
Smoking Cessation Advice[1]	12	92%	88%	88%	100%
Heart Failure Care					
ACE Inhibitor or ARB for LVSD	75	69%	76%	82%	100%
Discharge Instructions	149	45%	55%	61%	93%
Evaluation of LVS Function	177	81%	78%	83%	99%
Smoking Cessation Advice	34	97%	80%	82%	100%
Pneumonia Care					
Appropriate Initial Antibiotic	156	87%	78%	83%	94%
Blood Culture Timing	92	86%	89%	90%	100%
Influenza Vaccine	34	47%	64%	70%	100%
Initial Antibiotic Timing	191	90%	79%	80%	93%
Oxygenation Assessment	210	96%	97%	99%	100%
Pneumococcal Vaccine	116	44%	62%	69%	94%
Smoking Cessation Advice	49	98%	77%	80%	100%
Surgical Infection Prevention					
Prophylactic Antibiotic Given	490	78%	76%	77%	95%
Prophylactic Antibiotic Selection	117	92%	83%	90%	100%
Prophylactic Antibiotic Stopped	485	26%	70%	72%	95%
Pregnancy Care					
Inpatient Neonatal Mortality	-	-	-	-	-
Third or Fourth Degree Laceration	-	-	2.26%	3.63%	3.27%

Winston Medical Center

562 East Main Street
PO Box 967
Louisville, MS 39339
E-mail: info@winstonmedical.org
URL: www.winstonmedical.org
Ownership: Voluntary non-profit - Private
Emergency Services: Yes

Phone: 662-773-6211
Fax: 662-773-6223

Accredited: No
Licensed Beds: 185

Key Personnel:
Administrator . . . . W Dale Saulters

Measure	Cases	This Hospital	State Average	U.S. Average	Top Hospital
Heart Attack Care					
ACE Inhibitor or ARB for LVSD[3]	0	-	80%	82%	100%
Aspirin at Arrival[1,3]	1	100%	86%	92%	100%
Aspirin at Discharge[1,3]	1	0%	84%	90%	100%
Beta Blocker at Arrival[1,3]	1	100%	74%	87%	100%
Beta Blocker at Discharge[1,3]	1	100%	81%	90%	100%
Fibrinolytic Medication Timing[3]	0	-	32%	31%	100%
PCI Within 90 Minutes of Arrival[5]	-	-	46%	54%	95%
Smoking Cessation Advice[3]	0	-	88%	88%	100%
Heart Failure Care					
ACE Inhibitor or ARB for LVSD[1]	8	75%	76%	82%	100%
Discharge Instructions	29	97%	55%	61%	93%

Measure	Cases	This Hospital	State Average	U.S. Average	Top Hospital
Evaluation of LVS Function	41	93%	78%	83%	99%
Smoking Cessation Advice[1]	9	78%	80%	82%	100%
Pneumonia Care					
Appropriate Initial Antibiotic	29	83%	78%	83%	94%
Blood Culture Timing[1]	14	93%	89%	90%	100%
Influenza Vaccine[1]	10	90%	64%	70%	100%
Initial Antibiotic Timing	33	85%	79%	80%	93%
Oxygenation Assessment	44	100%	97%	99%	100%
Pneumococcal Vaccine[1]	23	87%	62%	69%	94%
Smoking Cessation Advice[1]	8	88%	77%	80%	100%
Surgical Infection Prevention					
Prophylactic Antibiotic Given[5]	-	-	76%	77%	95%
Prophylactic Antibiotic Selection[5]	-	-	83%	90%	100%
Prophylactic Antibiotic Stopped[5]	-	-	70%	72%	95%
Pregnancy Care					
Inpatient Neonatal Mortality	-	-	-	-	-
Third or Fourth Degree Laceration	-	-	2.26%	3.63%	3.27%

George County Hospital

859 Winter Street
Lucedale, MS 39452
E-mail: hospital@ametro.nrt
Ownership: Government - Local
Emergency Services: Yes

Phone: 601-947-3161
Fax: 601-947-9206

Accredited: No
Licensed Beds: 53

Key Personnel:
CEO/President. . . . . Dabby Braynon
Chief Medical Staff. . . . . Kevin O'Hes
Emergency Room . . . . John Van Derwood, MD
Director Infection/Disease Control . . . . Retha Gunter, RN
CCU Spvg. Nurse . . . . Mark Scott
Director Medical/Surgical Nursing . . . . Mark Scott, RN
OB/GYN Womens Health. . . . . Denise Teasley, MD
Chief Radiology . . . . Sandy Sellers
Director Respiratory Therapy . . . . Lendon Elmore

Measure	Cases	This Hospital	State Average	U.S. Average	Top Hospital
Heart Attack Care					
ACE Inhibitor or ARB for LVSD[1]	1	100%	80%	82%	100%
Aspirin at Arrival[1]	15	93%	86%	92%	100%
Aspirin at Discharge[1]	6	100%	84%	90%	100%
Beta Blocker at Arrival[1]	12	67%	74%	87%	100%
Beta Blocker at Discharge[1]	6	83%	81%	90%	100%
Fibrinolytic Medication Timing[3]	0	-	32%	31%	100%
PCI Within 90 Minutes of Arrival	0	-	46%	54%	95%
Smoking Cessation Advice[3]	0	-	88%	88%	100%
Heart Failure Care					
ACE Inhibitor or ARB for LVSD[1]	21	81%	76%	82%	100%
Discharge Instructions[1,3]	9	44%	55%	61%	93%
Evaluation of LVS Function	87	86%	78%	83%	99%
Smoking Cessation Advice[1,3]	1	0%	80%	82%	100%
Pneumonia Care					
Appropriate Initial Antibiotic[1,3]	7	71%	78%	83%	94%
Blood Culture Timing[1,3]	9	100%	89%	90%	100%
Influenza Vaccine[5]	-	-	64%	70%	100%
Initial Antibiotic Timing	63	86%	79%	80%	93%
Oxygenation Assessment	85	96%	97%	99%	100%
Pneumococcal Vaccine	53	17%	62%	69%	94%
Smoking Cessation Advice[1,3]	2	50%	77%	80%	100%
Surgical Infection Prevention					
Prophylactic Antibiotic Given[1,2,3]	4	75%	76%	77%	95%
Prophylactic Antibiotic Selection[5]	-	-	83%	90%	100%
Prophylactic Antibiotic Stopped[1,2,3]	3	67%	70%	72%	95%
Pregnancy Care					
Inpatient Neonatal Mortality	-	-	-	-	-
Third or Fourth Degree Laceration	-	-	2.26%	3.63%	3.27%

Magee General Hospital

300 3rd Avenue SE
Magee, MS 39111
Ownership: Voluntary non-profit - Private
Emergency Services: Yes

Phone: 601-849-5070
Fax: 601-849-7397
Accredited: No
Licensed Beds: 64

Key Personnel:
CEO. . . . . Althea Crumpton

NOTE: Hospital profiles are in alphabetical order by state, then city, then hospital within the city; Rankings are sorted by rate in descending order and exclude hospitals with less than 25 cases; (1) The number of cases is too small (n<25) for purposes of reliably predicting hospital performance; (2) Measure reflects the hospital's indication that its submission was based upon a sample of its relevant discharges; (3) Rate reflects fewer than the maximum possible quarters of data for the measure; (4) Inaccurate information submitted and suppressed for one or more quarters; (5) No data is available from the hospital for this measure; Please refer to the User's Guide for a full explanation of data

Chief Medical Staff. . . . . Dr. RS. Runnels
Emergency Room . . . . Dr. RS Runnels

Measure	Cases	This Hospital	State Average	U.S. Average	Top Hospital
Heart Attack Care					
ACE Inhibitor or ARB for LVSD[1]	1	100%	80%	82%	100%
Aspirin at Arrival[1]	8	75%	86%	92%	100%
Aspirin at Discharge[1]	3	100%	84%	90%	100%
Beta Blocker at Arrival[1]	8	75%	74%	87%	100%
Beta Blocker at Discharge[1]	4	100%	81%	90%	100%
Fibrinolytic Medication Timing	0	-	32%	31%	100%
PCI Within 90 Minutes of Arrival	0	-	46%	54%	95%
Smoking Cessation Advice	0	-	88%	88%	100%
Heart Failure Care					
ACE Inhibitor or ARB for LVSD	29	90%	76%	82%	100%
Discharge Instructions	63	56%	55%	61%	93%
Evaluation of LVS Function	83	98%	78%	83%	99%
Smoking Cessation Advice[1]	20	95%	80%	82%	100%
Pneumonia Care					
Appropriate Initial Antibiotic	112	95%	78%	83%	94%
Blood Culture Timing	88	97%	89%	90%	100%
Influenza Vaccine	35	94%	64%	70%	100%
Initial Antibiotic Timing	173	97%	79%	80%	93%
Oxygenation Assessment	191	99%	97%	99%	100%
Pneumococcal Vaccine	121	94%	62%	69%	94%
Smoking Cessation Advice	35	94%	77%	80%	100%
Surgical Infection Prevention					
Prophylactic Antibiotic Given[5]	-	-	76%	77%	95%
Prophylactic Antibiotic Selection[5]	-	-	83%	90%	100%
Prophylactic Antibiotic Stopped[5]	-	-	70%	72%	95%
Pregnancy Care					
Inpatient Neonatal Mortality	-	-	-	-	-
Third or Fourth Degree Laceration	-	-	2.26%	3.63%	3.27%

Beacham Memorial Hospital

205 N Cherry Street
Magnolia, MS 39652
URL: www.beachammemorial.com
Ownership: Voluntary non-profit - Private
Emergency Services: No

Phone: 601-783-2353
Fax: 601-783-9003

Accredited: No
Licensed Beds: 37

Key Personnel:
Administrator/CEO. . . . . Guy Geller
Respiratory Therapist. . . . . Denise Weatherspoon

Measure	Cases	This Hospital	State Average	U.S. Average	Top Hospital
Heart Attack Care					
ACE Inhibitor or ARB for LVSD	0	-	80%	82%	100%
Aspirin at Arrival[1]	5	80%	86%	92%	100%
Aspirin at Discharge[1]	4	75%	84%	90%	100%
Beta Blocker at Arrival[1]	5	40%	74%	87%	100%
Beta Blocker at Discharge[1]	4	50%	81%	90%	100%
Fibrinolytic Medication Timing[3]	0	-	32%	31%	100%
PCI Within 90 Minutes of Arrival	0	-	46%	54%	95%
Smoking Cessation Advice[3]	0	-	88%	88%	100%
Heart Failure Care					
ACE Inhibitor or ARB for LVSD[1]	15	67%	76%	82%	100%
Discharge Instructions[1,3]	10	50%	55%	61%	93%
Evaluation of LVS Function	76	71%	78%	83%	99%
Smoking Cessation Advice[1,3]	2	0%	80%	82%	100%
Pneumonia Care					
Appropriate Initial Antibiotic[1,3]	3	67%	78%	83%	94%
Blood Culture Timing[3]	0	-	89%	90%	100%
Influenza Vaccine[5]	-	-	64%	70%	100%
Initial Antibiotic Timing	80	85%	79%	80%	93%
Oxygenation Assessment	104	89%	97%	99%	100%
Pneumococcal Vaccine	64	25%	62%	69%	94%
Smoking Cessation Advice[3]	0	-	77%	80%	100%
Surgical Infection Prevention					
Prophylactic Antibiotic Given[5]	-	-	76%	77%	95%
Prophylactic Antibiotic Selection[5]	-	-	83%	90%	100%
Prophylactic Antibiotic Stopped[5]	-	-	70%	72%	95%
Pregnancy Care					

Inpatient Neonatal Mortality	-	-	-	-	-
Third or Fourth Degree Laceration	-	-	2.26%	3.63%	3.27%

Southwest Mississippi Regional Medical Center

215 Marion Avenue
McComb, MS 39648
E-mail: pubrel@smrmc.com
URL: www.smrmc.com
Ownership: Government - Local
Emergency Services: Yes

Phone: 601-249-5500
Fax: 601-249-1748

Accredited: Yes
Licensed Beds: 160

Key Personnel:
Administrator . . . . Norman M Price
Chief Medical Staff. Brian Remley, MD
Cardiovascular Institute . . . . Phillip Pandolf
Emergency Room . . . . Scott Smith, MD
Director Infection/Disease Control . . . . Charles Dykes, RN
Medical/Surgical Nursing . . . . Lavoyce Boggs
OB/GYN Womens Health. . . . . Sonya Travis
Chief Radiology . . . . Charles Regan
Director Respiratory Therapy . . . . James Greer

Measure	Cases	This Hospital	State Average	U.S. Average	Top Hospital
Heart Attack Care					
ACE Inhibitor or ARB for LVSD	27	70%	80%	82%	100%
Aspirin at Arrival	79	81%	86%	92%	100%
Aspirin at Discharge	94	94%	84%	90%	100%
Beta Blocker at Arrival	54	69%	74%	87%	100%
Beta Blocker at Discharge	104	92%	81%	90%	100%
Fibrinolytic Medication Timing[1]	1	0%	32%	31%	100%
PCI Within 90 Minutes of Arrival[1]	4	25%	46%	54%	95%
Smoking Cessation Advice	36	97%	88%	88%	100%
Heart Failure Care					
ACE Inhibitor or ARB for LVSD	113	70%	76%	82%	100%
Discharge Instructions	255	64%	55%	61%	93%
Evaluation of LVS Function	297	72%	78%	83%	99%
Smoking Cessation Advice	53	100%	80%	82%	100%
Pneumonia Care					
Appropriate Initial Antibiotic	139	71%	78%	83%	94%
Blood Culture Timing	92	90%	89%	90%	100%
Influenza Vaccine	35	11%	64%	70%	100%
Initial Antibiotic Timing	181	78%	79%	80%	93%
Oxygenation Assessment	225	99%	97%	99%	100%
Pneumococcal Vaccine	128	58%	62%	69%	94%
Smoking Cessation Advice	48	94%	77%	80%	100%
Surgical Infection Prevention					
Prophylactic Antibiotic Given	475	89%	76%	77%	95%
Prophylactic Antibiotic Selection	98	95%	83%	90%	100%
Prophylactic Antibiotic Stopped	467	80%	70%	72%	95%
Pregnancy Care					
Inpatient Neonatal Mortality	-	-	-	-	-
Third or Fourth Degree Laceration	-	-	2.26%	3.63%	3.27%

Franklin County Memorial Hospital

40 Union Church Road
PO Box 636
Meadville, MS 39653
URL: www.fcmh.net
Ownership: Government - Local
Emergency Services: Yes

Phone: 601-384-5801
Fax: 601-384-4100

Accredited: No
Licensed Beds: 53

Key Personnel:
Administrator . . . . G Lance Moak
Chief Medical Staff. Melanie Herrel, MD
Utilization Review/Infection Control . . . . Doylene Cupit
Respiratory Therapy Director . . . . Syd Jordan

Measure	Cases	This Hospital	State Average	U.S. Average	Top Hospital
Heart Attack Care					
ACE Inhibitor or ARB for LVSD	0	-	80%	82%	100%
Aspirin at Arrival[1]	2	100%	86%	92%	100%
Aspirin at Discharge[1]	1	100%	84%	90%	100%
Beta Blocker at Arrival[1]	2	100%	74%	87%	100%
Beta Blocker at Discharge[1]	1	100%	81%	90%	100%
Fibrinolytic Medication Timing[3]	0	-	32%	31%	100%

NOTE: Hospital profiles are in alphabetical order by state, then city, then hospital within the city; Rankings are sorted by rate in descending order and exclude hospitals with less than 25 cases; (1) The number of cases is too small (n<25) for purposes of reliably predicting hospital performance; (2) Measure reflects the hospital's indication that its submission was based upon a sample of its relevant discharges; (3) Rate reflects fewer than the maximum possible quarters of data for the measure; (4) Inaccurate information submitted and suppressed for one or more quarters; (5) No data is available from the hospital for this measure; Please refer to the User's Guide for a full explanation of data

Measure		This Hospital	State Average	U.S. Average	Top Hospital
PCI Within 90 Minutes of Arrival	0	-	46%	54%	95%
Smoking Cessation Advice[3]	0	-	88%	88%	100%
Heart Failure Care					
ACE Inhibitor or ARB for LVSD[1]	14	57%	76%	82%	100%
Discharge Instructions[1,3]	9	44%	55%	61%	93%
Evaluation of LVS Function	41	88%	78%	83%	99%
Smoking Cessation Advice[1,3]	1	100%	80%	82%	100%
Pneumonia Care					
Appropriate Initial Antibiotic[1,3]	7	29%	78%	83%	94%
Blood Culture Timing[3]	0	-	89%	90%	100%
Influenza Vaccine[5]	-	-	64%	70%	100%
Initial Antibiotic Timing	33	91%	79%	80%	93%
Oxygenation Assessment	41	100%	97%	99%	100%
Pneumococcal Vaccine[1]	22	91%	62%	69%	94%
Smoking Cessation Advice[1,3]	1	100%	77%	80%	100%
Surgical Infection Prevention					
Prophylactic Antibiotic Given[5]	-	-	76%	77%	95%
Prophylactic Antibiotic Selection[5]	-	-	83%	90%	100%
Prophylactic Antibiotic Stopped[5]	-	-	70%	72%	95%
Pregnancy Care					
Inpatient Neonatal Mortality	-	-	-	-	-
Third or Fourth Degree Laceration	-	-	2.26%	3.63%	3.27%

Simpson General Hospital

1842 Simpson Highway 149
Mendenhall, MS 39114
Ownership: Government - Local
Emergency Services: Yes

Phone: 601-847-2221
Fax: 601-847-5872
Accredited: No
Licensed Beds: 49

Key Personnel:
CEO. . . . . Michael Nester
Chief Medical Staff. . . . . W G Munn
Director Infection/Disease Control . . . . Joyce Pearson, RN
Director Respiratory Therapy . . . . Michelle Barrett

Measure	Cases	This Hospital	State Average	U.S. Average	Top Hospital
Heart Attack Care					
ACE Inhibitor or ARB for LVSD[5]	-	-	80%	82%	100%
Aspirin at Arrival[5]	-	-	86%	92%	100%
Aspirin at Discharge[5]	-	-	84%	90%	100%
Beta Blocker at Arrival[5]	-	-	74%	87%	100%
Beta Blocker at Discharge[5]	-	-	81%	90%	100%
Fibrinolytic Medication Timing[5]	-	-	32%	31%	100%
PCI Within 90 Minutes of Arrival[5]	-	-	46%	54%	95%
Smoking Cessation Advice[5]	-	-	88%	88%	100%
Heart Failure Care					
ACE Inhibitor or ARB for LVSD[1]	6	67%	76%	82%	100%
Discharge Instructions[1]	15	47%	55%	61%	93%
Evaluation of LVS Function	27	74%	78%	83%	99%
Smoking Cessation Advice[1]	11	82%	80%	82%	100%
Pneumonia Care					
Appropriate Initial Antibiotic[1]	15	20%	78%	83%	94%
Blood Culture Timing[1]	4	75%	89%	90%	100%
Influenza Vaccine[1]	8	0%	64%	70%	100%
Initial Antibiotic Timing[1]	11	64%	79%	80%	93%
Oxygenation Assessment[1]	19	79%	97%	99%	100%
Pneumococcal Vaccine[1]	15	13%	62%	69%	94%
Smoking Cessation Advice[1]	5	60%	77%	80%	100%
Surgical Infection Prevention					
Prophylactic Antibiotic Given[5]	-	-	76%	77%	95%
Prophylactic Antibiotic Selection[5]	-	-	83%	90%	100%
Prophylactic Antibiotic Stopped[5]	-	-	70%	72%	95%
Pregnancy Care					
Inpatient Neonatal Mortality	-	-	-	-	-
Third or Fourth Degree Laceration	-	-	2.26%	3.63%	3.27%

Alliance Health Center

5000 Highway 39 N
Meridian, MS 39301

Toll-Free: 877-853-3094
Phone: 601-483-6211
Fax: 601-696-4898

E-mail: bpatterson@psysolutions.com
URL: www.AllianceHealthCenter.com
Ownership: Proprietary
Emergency Services: Yes

Accredited: Yes
Licensed Beds: 134

Key Personnel:
CEO. . . . . Bill Patterson
Chief Medical Staff. . . . . Terry Jordan, MD
Infection Control. Brenda Thompson

Measure	Cases	This Hospital	State Average	U.S. Average	Top Hospital
Heart Attack Care					
ACE Inhibitor or ARB for LVSD[5]	-	-	80%	82%	100%
Aspirin at Arrival[5]	-	-	86%	92%	100%
Aspirin at Discharge[5]	-	-	84%	90%	100%
Beta Blocker at Arrival[5]	-	-	74%	87%	100%
Beta Blocker at Discharge[5]	-	-	81%	90%	100%
Fibrinolytic Medication Timing[5]	-	-	32%	31%	100%
PCI Within 90 Minutes of Arrival[5]	-	-	46%	54%	95%
Smoking Cessation Advice[5]	-	-	88%	88%	100%
Heart Failure Care					
ACE Inhibitor or ARB for LVSD[5]	-	-	76%	82%	100%
Discharge Instructions[5]	-	-	55%	61%	93%
Evaluation of LVS Function[5]	-	-	78%	83%	99%
Smoking Cessation Advice[5]	-	-	80%	82%	100%
Pneumonia Care					
Appropriate Initial Antibiotic[5]	-	-	78%	83%	94%
Blood Culture Timing[5]	-	-	89%	90%	100%
Influenza Vaccine[5]	-	-	64%	70%	100%
Initial Antibiotic Timing[5]	-	-	79%	80%	93%
Oxygenation Assessment[5]	-	-	97%	99%	100%
Pneumococcal Vaccine[5]	-	-	62%	69%	94%
Smoking Cessation Advice[5]	-	-	77%	80%	100%
Surgical Infection Prevention					
Prophylactic Antibiotic Given[5]	-	-	76%	77%	95%
Prophylactic Antibiotic Selection[5]	-	-	83%	90%	100%
Prophylactic Antibiotic Stopped[5]	-	-	70%	72%	95%
Pregnancy Care					
Inpatient Neonatal Mortality	-	-	-	-	-
Third or Fourth Degree Laceration	-	-	2.26%	3.63%	3.27%

Jeff Anderson Regional Medical Center

2124 14th Street
Meridian, MS 39301
Ownership: Voluntary non-profit - Private
Emergency Services: Yes

Phone: 601-553-6000
Fax: 601-553-6834
Accredited: Yes
Licensed Beds: 260

Key Personnel:
CEO. . . . . Mark D McPhail
Emergency Room . . . . Ramona Jackson, RN
Director Medical/Surgical Nursing . . . . Betty Clark, RN
Director Respiratory Therapy . . . . Brenda Roberson

Measure	Cases	This Hospital	State Average	U.S. Average	Top Hospital
Heart Attack Care					
ACE Inhibitor or ARB for LVSD	36	100%	80%	82%	100%
Aspirin at Arrival	109	99%	86%	92%	100%
Aspirin at Discharge	153	99%	84%	90%	100%
Beta Blocker at Arrival	102	99%	74%	87%	100%
Beta Blocker at Discharge	172	99%	81%	90%	100%
Fibrinolytic Medication Timing	0	-	32%	31%	100%
PCI Within 90 Minutes of Arrival[1]	2	0%	46%	54%	95%
Smoking Cessation Advice	65	97%	88%	88%	100%
Heart Failure Care					
ACE Inhibitor or ARB for LVSD	102	99%	76%	82%	100%
Discharge Instructions	311	54%	55%	61%	93%
Evaluation of LVS Function	368	99%	78%	83%	99%
Smoking Cessation Advice	52	96%	80%	82%	100%
Pneumonia Care					
Appropriate Initial Antibiotic	172	70%	78%	83%	94%
Blood Culture Timing	88	90%	89%	90%	100%

NOTE: Hospital profiles are in alphabetical order by state, then city, then hospital within the city; Rankings are sorted by rate in descending order and exclude hospitals with less than 25 cases; (1) The number of cases is too small (n<25) for purposes of reliably predicting hospital performance; (2) Measure reflects the hospital's indication that its submission was based upon a sample of its relevant discharges; (3) Rate reflects fewer than the maximum possible quarters of data for the measure; (4) Inaccurate information submitted and suppressed for one or more quarters; (5) No data is available from the hospital for this measure; Please refer to the User's Guide for a full explanation of data

Influenza Vaccine[4,5]	-	-	64%	70%	100%
Initial Antibiotic Timing	287	67%	79%	80%	93%
Oxygenation Assessment	352	98%	97%	99%	100%
Pneumococcal Vaccine	221	57%	62%	69%	94%
Smoking Cessation Advice	60	93%	77%	80%	100%
Surgical Infection Prevention					
Prophylactic Antibiotic Given[3]	377	73%	76%	77%	95%
Prophylactic Antibiotic Selection	142	92%	83%	90%	100%
Prophylactic Antibiotic Stopped[3]	361	70%	70%	72%	95%
Pregnancy Care					
Inpatient Neonatal Mortality	-	-	-	-	-
Third or Fourth Degree Laceration	-	-	2.26%	3.63%	3.27%

Riley Memorial Hospital

1102 Constitution Avenue
Meridian, MS 39301

Toll-Free: 800-248-1199
Phone: 601-693-2511
Fax: 601-484-3130

URL: www.rileyhosp.com
Ownership: Proprietary
Emergency Services: Yes

Accredited: Yes
Licensed Beds: 140

Key Personnel:
CEO. . . . . Steve Nicholas
Director Emergency Room. . . . . Burt Turcotte

Measure	Cases	This Hospital	State Average	U.S. Average	Top Hospital
Heart Attack Care					
ACE Inhibitor or ARB for LVSD[1]	7	100%	80%	82%	100%
Aspirin at Arrival[1]	20	95%	86%	92%	100%
Aspirin at Discharge[1]	15	100%	84%	90%	100%
Beta Blocker at Arrival[1]	21	90%	74%	87%	100%
Beta Blocker at Discharge[1]	15	93%	81%	90%	100%
Fibrinolytic Medication Timing	0	-	32%	31%	100%
PCI Within 90 Minutes of Arrival	0	-	46%	54%	95%
Smoking Cessation Advice[1]	4	100%	88%	88%	100%
Heart Failure Care					
ACE Inhibitor or ARB for LVSD	53	92%	76%	82%	100%
Discharge Instructions	125	95%	55%	61%	93%
Evaluation of LVS Function	150	93%	78%	83%	99%
Smoking Cessation Advice	34	94%	80%	82%	100%
Pneumonia Care					
Appropriate Initial Antibiotic	70	56%	78%	83%	94%
Blood Culture Timing	62	94%	89%	90%	100%
Influenza Vaccine[1]	15	80%	64%	70%	100%
Initial Antibiotic Timing	89	70%	79%	80%	93%
Oxygenation Assessment	118	98%	97%	99%	100%
Pneumococcal Vaccine	58	84%	62%	69%	94%
Smoking Cessation Advice	25	92%	77%	80%	100%
Surgical Infection Prevention					
Prophylactic Antibiotic Given[2]	114	67%	76%	77%	95%
Prophylactic Antibiotic Selection[1,2]	23	78%	83%	90%	100%
Prophylactic Antibiotic Stopped[2]	107	75%	70%	72%	95%
Pregnancy Care					
Inpatient Neonatal Mortality	-	-	-	-	-
Third or Fourth Degree Laceration	-	-	2.26%	3.63%	3.27%

Rush Foundation Hospital

1314 19th Avenue
Meridian, MS 39301
URL: www.rushhealthsystems.org
Ownership: Voluntary non-profit - Private
Emergency Services: Yes

Phone: 601-483-0011
Fax: 601-485-8079

Accredited: Yes
Licensed Beds: 215

Key Personnel:
CEO. . . . . Wallce Strickland
Chief Medical Staff. . . . . Scott Bell
Chief Catheterization Laboratory . . . . Allen Duplantis, MD
Emergency Room . . . . Walt Willis, MD
Director Infection/Disease Control . . . . Cherry Flanigan
CCU Spvg. Nurse . . . . Charlotte Keeton
OB/GYN Womens Health. . . . . Fred Grant, MD
Director Respiratory Therapy . . . . James Rush

Measure	Cases	This Hospital	State Average	U.S. Average	Top Hospital
Heart Attack Care					

ACE Inhibitor or ARB for LVSD	32	97%	80%	82%	100%
Aspirin at Arrival	79	97%	86%	92%	100%
Aspirin at Discharge	116	100%	84%	90%	100%
Beta Blocker at Arrival	68	99%	74%	87%	100%
Beta Blocker at Discharge	107	98%	81%	90%	100%
Fibrinolytic Medication Timing	0	-	32%	31%	100%
PCI Within 90 Minutes of Arrival[1]	5	80%	46%	54%	95%
Smoking Cessation Advice	55	93%	88%	88%	100%
Heart Failure Care					
ACE Inhibitor or ARB for LVSD	89	93%	76%	82%	100%
Discharge Instructions	186	86%	55%	61%	93%
Evaluation of LVS Function	208	97%	78%	83%	99%
Smoking Cessation Advice	50	90%	80%	82%	100%
Pneumonia Care					
Appropriate Initial Antibiotic	76	82%	78%	83%	94%
Blood Culture Timing	46	96%	89%	90%	100%
Influenza Vaccine[1]	16	94%	64%	70%	100%
Initial Antibiotic Timing	63	86%	79%	80%	93%
Oxygenation Assessment	91	97%	97%	99%	100%
Pneumococcal Vaccine	44	75%	62%	69%	94%
Smoking Cessation Advice	28	89%	77%	80%	100%
Surgical Infection Prevention					
Prophylactic Antibiotic Given[2,3]	174	73%	76%	77%	95%
Prophylactic Antibiotic Selection[2]	60	78%	83%	90%	100%
Prophylactic Antibiotic Stopped[2,3]	165	64%	70%	72%	95%
Pregnancy Care					
Inpatient Neonatal Mortality	-	-	-	-	-
Third or Fourth Degree Laceration	-	-	2.26%	3.63%	3.27%

Scott Regioanl Hospital

317 Highway 13 South
PO Box 259
Morton, MS 39117
Ownership: Voluntary non-profit - Private
Emergency Services: No

Phone: 601-732-6301
Fax: 601-732-8970

Accredited: No
Licensed Beds: 40

Key Personnel:
CEO. . . . . Paul Black
Chief Medical Staff. . . . . Michael Edwards

Measure	Cases	This Hospital	State Average	U.S. Average	Top Hospital
Heart Attack Care					
ACE Inhibitor or ARB for LVSD	0	-	80%	82%	100%
Aspirin at Arrival[1]	2	50%	86%	92%	100%
Aspirin at Discharge[1]	1	0%	84%	90%	100%
Beta Blocker at Arrival[1]	2	0%	74%	87%	100%
Beta Blocker at Discharge[1]	1	0%	81%	90%	100%
Fibrinolytic Medication Timing	0	-	32%	31%	100%
PCI Within 90 Minutes of Arrival	0	-	46%	54%	95%
Smoking Cessation Advice	0	-	88%	88%	100%
Heart Failure Care					
ACE Inhibitor or ARB for LVSD[1]	1	0%	76%	82%	100%
Discharge Instructions	26	62%	55%	61%	93%
Evaluation of LVS Function	38	47%	78%	83%	99%
Smoking Cessation Advice[1]	9	78%	80%	82%	100%
Pneumonia Care					
Appropriate Initial Antibiotic	99	90%	78%	83%	94%
Blood Culture Timing[1]	2	100%	89%	90%	100%
Influenza Vaccine	31	45%	64%	70%	100%
Initial Antibiotic Timing	132	83%	79%	80%	93%
Oxygenation Assessment	136	100%	97%	99%	100%
Pneumococcal Vaccine	49	92%	62%	69%	94%
Smoking Cessation Advice	46	93%	77%	80%	100%
Surgical Infection Prevention					
Prophylactic Antibiotic Given[5]	-	-	76%	77%	95%
Prophylactic Antibiotic Selection[5]	-	-	83%	90%	100%
Prophylactic Antibiotic Stopped[5]	-	-	70%	72%	95%
Pregnancy Care					
Inpatient Neonatal Mortality	-	-	-	-	-
Third or Fourth Degree Laceration	-	-	2.26%	3.63%	3.27%

NOTE: Hospital profiles are in alphabetical order by state, then city, then hospital within the city; Rankings are sorted by rate in descending order and exclude hospitals with less than 25 cases; (1) The number of cases is too small (n<25) for purposes of reliably predicting hospital performance; (2) Measure reflects the hospital's indication that its submission was based upon a sample of its relevant discharges; (3) Rate reflects fewer than the maximum possible quarters of data for the measure; (4) Inaccurate information submitted and suppressed for one or more quarters; (5) No data is available from the hospital for this measure; Please refer to the User's Guide for a full explanation of data

Natchez Community Hospital

129 Jefferson Davis Boulevard
Natchez, MS 39120
Ownership: Proprietary
Emergency Services: Yes

Phone: 601-445-6200
Fax: 601-445-6233
Accredited: Yes
Licensed Beds: 101

Key Personnel:
CEO . . . . J Allen Tyra
Chief Medical Staff . . . . Jennifer Russ
Emergency Room . . . . Tracy Laird
Director of Respiratory . . . . Jimmy Dickey

Measure	Cases	This Hospital	State Average	U.S. Average	Top Hospital
Heart Attack Care					
ACE Inhibitor or ARB for LVSD[1]	1	0%	80%	82%	100%
Aspirin at Arrival	29	79%	86%	92%	100%
Aspirin at Discharge[1]	16	62%	84%	90%	100%
Beta Blocker at Arrival[1]	22	59%	74%	87%	100%
Beta Blocker at Discharge[1]	17	76%	81%	90%	100%
Fibrinolytic Medication Timing[1]	1	0%	32%	31%	100%
PCI Within 90 Minutes of Arrival	0	-	46%	54%	95%
Smoking Cessation Advice[1]	7	57%	88%	88%	100%
Heart Failure Care					
ACE Inhibitor or ARB for LVSD	76	87%	76%	82%	100%
Discharge Instructions	177	37%	55%	61%	93%
Evaluation of LVS Function	200	92%	78%	83%	99%
Smoking Cessation Advice	41	80%	80%	82%	100%
Pneumonia Care					
Appropriate Initial Antibiotic	130	58%	78%	83%	94%
Blood Culture Timing	95	92%	89%	90%	100%
Influenza Vaccine[1]	24	46%	64%	70%	100%
Initial Antibiotic Timing	168	72%	79%	80%	93%
Oxygenation Assessment	190	98%	97%	99%	100%
Pneumococcal Vaccine	96	48%	62%	69%	94%
Smoking Cessation Advice	47	81%	77%	80%	100%
Surgical Infection Prevention					
Prophylactic Antibiotic Given[2]	94	86%	76%	77%	95%
Prophylactic Antibiotic Selection[1,2]	24	75%	83%	90%	100%
Prophylactic Antibiotic Stopped[2]	87	72%	70%	72%	95%
Pregnancy Care					
Inpatient Neonatal Mortality	-	-	-	-	-
Third or Fourth Degree Laceration	-	-	2.26%	3.63%	3.27%

Natchez Regional Medical Center

Alternate Name: Jefferson Davis Memorial Hospital
Seargent S Prentiss Drive
Natchez, MS 39121
Ownership: Government - Local
Emergency Services: Yes

Phone: 601-443-2723
Fax: 601-443-2891
Accredited: Yes
Licensed Beds: 205

Key Personnel:
Administrator . . . . Jack Houghton
Cardiac Lab . . . . Lisa Moise
Emergency Room . . . . Rosie Williams
Infection Control . . . . Lana Morgan
ICU . . . . Catherine Ratcliffe
Director Respiratory Therapy . . . . Joseph Hudson

Measure	Cases	This Hospital	State Average	U.S. Average	Top Hospital
Heart Attack Care					
ACE Inhibitor or ARB for LVSD[1]	9	33%	80%	82%	100%
Aspirin at Arrival	52	98%	86%	92%	100%
Aspirin at Discharge	45	78%	84%	90%	100%
Beta Blocker at Arrival	47	98%	74%	87%	100%
Beta Blocker at Discharge	50	84%	81%	90%	100%
Fibrinolytic Medication Timing[1]	5	0%	32%	31%	100%
PCI Within 90 Minutes of Arrival[1]	2	50%	46%	54%	95%
Smoking Cessation Advice[1]	21	71%	88%	88%	100%
Heart Failure Care					
ACE Inhibitor or ARB for LVSD	51	82%	76%	82%	100%
Discharge Instructions	159	21%	55%	61%	93%
Evaluation of LVS Function	187	76%	78%	83%	99%
Smoking Cessation Advice	26	50%	80%	82%	100%
Pneumonia Care					
Appropriate Initial Antibiotic	68	66%	78%	83%	94%

Measure	Cases	This Hospital	State Average	U.S. Average	Top Hospital
Blood Culture Timing	55	84%	89%	90%	100%
Influenza Vaccine[1]	15	60%	64%	70%	100%
Initial Antibiotic Timing	111	76%	79%	80%	93%
Oxygenation Assessment	129	98%	97%	99%	100%
Pneumococcal Vaccine	85	51%	62%	69%	94%
Smoking Cessation Advice	33	42%	77%	80%	100%
Surgical Infection Prevention					
Prophylactic Antibiotic Given[2]	164	87%	76%	77%	95%
Prophylactic Antibiotic Selection[2]	49	92%	83%	90%	100%
Prophylactic Antibiotic Stopped[2]	160	78%	70%	72%	95%
Pregnancy Care					
Inpatient Neonatal Mortality[2]	247	0.00%	-	-	-
Third or Fourth Degree Laceration	425	0.71%	2.26%	3.63%	3.27%

Baptist Memorial Hospital-Union County

200 Highway 30 W
New Albany, MS 38652
Ownership: Voluntary non-profit - Church
Emergency Services: Yes

Phone: 662-538-7631
Fax: 662-538-2572
Accredited: Yes
Licensed Beds: 153

Key Personnel:
CEO . . . . Mitch Johnson
Chief Medical Staff . . . . David Williams, MD
Emergency Room . . . . Debra Taylor
Infection Control . . . . Doris Box
CCU Supervisor . . . . Barbara Freeman
Medical Surgical Nursing . . . . Yvonne Thompson
Respiratory Therapy . . . . Terry Kirk

Measure	Cases	This Hospital	State Average	U.S. Average	Top Hospital
Heart Attack Care					
ACE Inhibitor or ARB for LVSD[1]	4	75%	80%	82%	100%
Aspirin at Arrival[1]	13	100%	86%	92%	100%
Aspirin at Discharge[1]	10	90%	84%	90%	100%
Beta Blocker at Arrival[1]	10	90%	74%	87%	100%
Beta Blocker at Discharge[1]	6	83%	81%	90%	100%
Fibrinolytic Medication Timing	0	-	32%	31%	100%
PCI Within 90 Minutes of Arrival	0	-	46%	54%	95%
Smoking Cessation Advice[1]	3	100%	88%	88%	100%
Heart Failure Care					
ACE Inhibitor or ARB for LVSD	30	97%	76%	82%	100%
Discharge Instructions	84	100%	55%	61%	93%
Evaluation of LVS Function	105	98%	78%	83%	99%
Smoking Cessation Advice[1]	15	93%	80%	82%	100%
Pneumonia Care					
Appropriate Initial Antibiotic	80	74%	78%	83%	94%
Blood Culture Timing	47	91%	89%	90%	100%
Influenza Vaccine[1]	17	94%	64%	70%	100%
Initial Antibiotic Timing	83	86%	79%	80%	93%
Oxygenation Assessment	90	100%	97%	99%	100%
Pneumococcal Vaccine	51	88%	62%	69%	94%
Smoking Cessation Advice[1]	22	95%	77%	80%	100%
Surgical Infection Prevention					
Prophylactic Antibiotic Given[2,3]	126	94%	76%	77%	95%
Prophylactic Antibiotic Selection[2]	34	94%	83%	90%	100%
Prophylactic Antibiotic Stopped[2,3]	116	68%	70%	72%	95%
Pregnancy Care					
Inpatient Neonatal Mortality	1,049	0.29%	-	-	-
Third or Fourth Degree Laceration	751	1.46%	2.26%	3.63%	3.27%

Newton Regional Hospital

Alternate Name: Rush Hospital-Newton
208 S Main Street
Newton, MS 39345
E-mail: newtonrh@newtonregionalhospital.com
URL: www.newtonregionalhospital.com
Ownership: Voluntary non-profit - Private
Emergency Services: No

Phone: 601-683-2031
Fax: 601-683-6963

Accredited: No
Licensed Beds: 49

Key Personnel:
Administrator . . . . Tim Thomas
Chief Medical Staff . . . . Stephen A Tramill, DO
Infection Control . . . . Michael Miller

Measure	Cases	This Hospital	State Average	U.S. Average	Top Hospital

NOTE: Hospital profiles are in alphabetical order by state, then city, then hospital within the city; Rankings are sorted by rate in descending order and exclude hospitals with less than 25 cases; (1) The number of cases is too small (n<25) for purposes of reliably predicting hospital performance; (2) Measure reflects the hospital's indication that its submission was based upon a sample of its relevant discharges; (3) Rate reflects fewer than the maximum possible quarters of data for the measure; (4) Inaccurate information submitted and suppressed for one or more quarters; (5) No data is available from the hospital for this measure; Please refer to the User's Guide for a full explanation of data

Heart Attack Care					
ACE Inhibitor or ARB for LVSD[3]	0	-	80%	82%	100%
Aspirin at Arrival[1,3]	4	100%	86%	92%	100%
Aspirin at Discharge[1,3]	1	100%	84%	90%	100%
Beta Blocker at Arrival[1,3]	2	50%	74%	87%	100%
Beta Blocker at Discharge[1,3]	1	100%	81%	90%	100%
Fibrinolytic Medication Timing[3]	0	-	32%	31%	100%
PCI Within 90 Minutes of Arrival	0	-	46%	54%	95%
Smoking Cessation Advice[3]	0	-	88%	88%	100%
Heart Failure Care					
ACE Inhibitor or ARB for LVSD[1]	14	57%	76%	82%	100%
Discharge Instructions[1,3]	12	92%	55%	61%	93%
Evaluation of LVS Function	54	67%	78%	83%	99%
Smoking Cessation Advice[1,3]	2	100%	80%	82%	100%
Pneumonia Care					
Appropriate Initial Antibiotic[1,3]	1	100%	78%	83%	94%
Blood Culture Timing[3]	0	-	89%	90%	100%
Influenza Vaccine[5]	-	-	64%	70%	100%
Initial Antibiotic Timing[1]	20	80%	79%	80%	93%
Oxygenation Assessment[1]	24	100%	97%	99%	100%
Pneumococcal Vaccine[1]	15	60%	62%	69%	94%
Smoking Cessation Advice[1,3]	1	100%	77%	80%	100%
Surgical Infection Prevention					
Prophylactic Antibiotic Given[5]	-	-	76%	77%	95%
Prophylactic Antibiotic Selection[5]	-	-	83%	90%	100%
Prophylactic Antibiotic Stopped[5]	-	-	70%	72%	95%
Pregnancy Care					
Inpatient Neonatal Mortality	-	-	-	-	-
Third or Fourth Degree Laceration	-	-	2.26%	3.63%	3.27%

Baptist Memorial Hospital-North Mississippi

2301 S Lamar
Oxford, MS 38655
URL: www.baptistonline.org/facilities/oxford
Ownership: Voluntary non-profit - Private
Emergency Services: Yes

Phone: 662-232-8100
Fax: 662-232-8391

Accredited: Yes
Licensed Beds: 204

Measure	Cases	This Hospital	State Average	U.S. Average	Top Hospital
Heart Attack Care					
ACE Inhibitor or ARB for LVSD[1]	20	85%	80%	82%	100%
Aspirin at Arrival	119	96%	86%	92%	100%
Aspirin at Discharge	148	93%	84%	90%	100%
Beta Blocker at Arrival	101	92%	74%	87%	100%
Beta Blocker at Discharge	147	93%	81%	90%	100%
Fibrinolytic Medication Timing[1]	17	71%	32%	31%	100%
PCI Within 90 Minutes of Arrival	0	-	46%	54%	95%
Smoking Cessation Advice	67	100%	88%	88%	100%
Heart Failure Care					
ACE Inhibitor or ARB for LVSD	127	76%	76%	82%	100%
Discharge Instructions	233	82%	55%	61%	93%
Evaluation of LVS Function	273	97%	78%	83%	99%
Smoking Cessation Advice	64	97%	80%	82%	100%
Pneumonia Care					
Appropriate Initial Antibiotic	131	82%	78%	83%	94%
Blood Culture Timing	109	94%	89%	90%	100%
Influenza Vaccine	52	83%	64%	70%	100%
Initial Antibiotic Timing	161	86%	79%	80%	93%
Oxygenation Assessment	216	100%	97%	99%	100%
Pneumococcal Vaccine	134	87%	62%	69%	94%
Smoking Cessation Advice	60	97%	77%	80%	100%
Surgical Infection Prevention					
Prophylactic Antibiotic Given[2]	442	88%	76%	77%	95%
Prophylactic Antibiotic Selection[2]	61	85%	83%	90%	100%
Prophylactic Antibiotic Stopped[2]	401	72%	70%	72%	95%
Pregnancy Care					
Inpatient Neonatal Mortality	-	-	-	-	-
Third or Fourth Degree Laceration	-	-	2.26%	3.63%	3.27%

Singing River Hospital

2809 Denny Avenue
Pascagoula, MS 39581
URL: www.srhshealth.com
Ownership: Government - Local
Emergency Services: Yes

Phone: 228-809-5000
Fax: 228-809-5064

Accredited: Yes
Licensed Beds: 415

Key Personnel:
President/CEO . . . . Chris Anderson
Chief Medical Staff . . . . Steve Demetropoulos
Cardiac Laboratory . . . . Glenda Smith
Catheterization Laboratory . . . . Jan Brantley
Emergency Room . . . . Charles Howard
OB/GYN Womens Health . . . . Cynthia Bowlin
Respiratory . . . . Pam Nelson

Measure	Cases	This Hospital	State Average	U.S. Average	Top Hospital
Heart Attack Care					
ACE Inhibitor or ARB for LVSD	67	93%	80%	82%	100%
Aspirin at Arrival	263	97%	86%	92%	100%
Aspirin at Discharge	258	96%	84%	90%	100%
Beta Blocker at Arrival	217	95%	74%	87%	100%
Beta Blocker at Discharge	243	93%	81%	90%	100%
Fibrinolytic Medication Timing	0	-	32%	31%	100%
PCI Within 90 Minutes of Arrival[1]	10	50%	46%	54%	95%
Smoking Cessation Advice	109	100%	88%	88%	100%
Heart Failure Care					
ACE Inhibitor or ARB for LVSD	259	91%	76%	82%	100%
Discharge Instructions	494	95%	55%	61%	93%
Evaluation of LVS Function	532	95%	78%	83%	99%
Smoking Cessation Advice	129	100%	80%	82%	100%
Pneumonia Care					
Appropriate Initial Antibiotic	245	84%	78%	83%	94%
Blood Culture Timing	183	86%	89%	90%	100%
Influenza Vaccine	68	81%	64%	70%	100%
Initial Antibiotic Timing	293	91%	79%	80%	93%
Oxygenation Assessment	352	100%	97%	99%	100%
Pneumococcal Vaccine	183	80%	62%	69%	94%
Smoking Cessation Advice	93	100%	77%	80%	100%
Surgical Infection Prevention					
Prophylactic Antibiotic Given[3]	175	86%	76%	77%	95%
Prophylactic Antibiotic Selection[3]	175	89%	83%	90%	100%
Prophylactic Antibiotic Stopped[3]	172	76%	70%	72%	95%
Pregnancy Care					
Inpatient Neonatal Mortality	-	-	-	-	-
Third or Fourth Degree Laceration	-	-	2.26%	3.63%	3.27%

Choctaw Health Center

Route 7
PO Box 6010
Philadelphia, MS 39350
E-mail: info@choctaw.org
URL: www.choctaw.org
Ownership: Government - Federal
Emergency Services: Yes

Phone: 601-389-6261
Fax: 601-656-5091

Accredited: Yes
Licensed Beds: 35

Key Personnel:
President/CEO . . . . James Wallace
Chief Medical Staff . . . . Joann Coaten
Infection Control . . . . Jackie Holley
Medical/Surgical Nursing . . . . Cynthia Clemons
OB/GYN Womens Health . . . . Jamie Hilyer

Measure	Cases	This Hospital	State Average	U.S. Average	Top Hospital
Heart Attack Care					
ACE Inhibitor or ARB for LVSD[5]	-	-	80%	82%	100%
Aspirin at Arrival[5]	-	-	86%	92%	100%
Aspirin at Discharge[5]	-	-	84%	90%	100%
Beta Blocker at Arrival[5]	-	-	74%	87%	100%
Beta Blocker at Discharge[5]	-	-	81%	90%	100%
Fibrinolytic Medication Timing[5]	-	-	32%	31%	100%
PCI Within 90 Minutes of Arrival[5]	-	-	46%	54%	95%
Smoking Cessation Advice[5]	-	-	88%	88%	100%
Heart Failure Care					
ACE Inhibitor or ARB for LVSD[1,3]	1	0%	76%	82%	100%

NOTE: Hospital profiles are in alphabetical order by state, then city, then hospital within the city; Rankings are sorted by rate in descending order and exclude hospitals with less than 25 cases; (1) The number of cases is too small (n<25) for purposes of reliably predicting hospital performance; (2) Measure reflects the hospital's indication that its submission was based upon a sample of its relevant discharges; (3) Rate reflects fewer than the maximum possible quarters of data for the measure; (4) Inaccurate information submitted and suppressed for one or more quarters; (5) No data is available from the hospital for this measure; Please refer to the User's Guide for a full explanation of data

Discharge Instructions[5]	-	-	55%	61%	93%
Evaluation of LVS Function[1,3]	5	80%	78%	83%	99%
Smoking Cessation Advice[5]	-	-	80%	82%	100%
Pneumonia Care					
Appropriate Initial Antibiotic[3]	0	-	78%	83%	94%
Blood Culture Timing[3]	0	-	89%	90%	100%
Influenza Vaccine[5]	-	-	64%	70%	100%
Initial Antibiotic Timing[1,3]	4	0%	79%	80%	93%
Oxygenation Assessment[1,3]	5	100%	97%	99%	100%
Pneumococcal Vaccine[1,3]	2	100%	62%	69%	94%
Smoking Cessation Advice[3]	0	-	77%	80%	100%
Surgical Infection Prevention					
Prophylactic Antibiotic Given[5]	-	-	76%	77%	95%
Prophylactic Antibiotic Selection[5]	-	-	83%	90%	100%
Prophylactic Antibiotic Stopped[5]	-	-	70%	72%	95%
Pregnancy Care					
Inpatient Neonatal Mortality	-	-	-	-	-
Third or Fourth Degree Laceration	-	-	2.26%	3.63%	3.27%

Neshoba County General Hospital

Highway 19 S   Phone: 601-663-1200
Philadelphia, MS 39350   Fax: 601-663-1497
Ownership: Government - Local   Accredited: No
Emergency Services: Yes   Licensed Beds: 82
Key Personnel:
Administrator . . . . Lawrence Graeber
Chief Medical Staff. . . . . AP Soriano, MD
Emergency Room . . . . Todd Willis, MD
Director Infection/Disease Control . . . . Beth Burns
Chief Radiology . . . . Jim Barlow, MD
Director Respiratory Therapy . . . . Margaret Posey

Measure	Cases	This Hospital	State Average	U.S. Average	Top Hospital
Heart Attack Care					
ACE Inhibitor or ARB for LVSD[3]	0	-	80%	82%	100%
Aspirin at Arrival[1,3]	3	67%	86%	92%	100%
Aspirin at Discharge[1,3]	3	67%	84%	90%	100%
Beta Blocker at Arrival[1,3]	2	0%	74%	87%	100%
Beta Blocker at Discharge[1,3]	2	0%	81%	90%	100%
Fibrinolytic Medication Timing[3]	0	-	32%	31%	100%
PCI Within 90 Minutes of Arrival	0	-	46%	54%	95%
Smoking Cessation Advice[3]	0	-	88%	88%	100%
Heart Failure Care					
ACE Inhibitor or ARB for LVSD[1]	21	71%	76%	82%	100%
Discharge Instructions	59	64%	55%	61%	93%
Evaluation of LVS Function	68	87%	78%	83%	99%
Smoking Cessation Advice[1]	15	87%	80%	82%	100%
Pneumonia Care					
Appropriate Initial Antibiotic	36	89%	78%	83%	94%
Blood Culture Timing	30	90%	89%	90%	100%
Influenza Vaccine[1]	18	72%	64%	70%	100%
Initial Antibiotic Timing	40	98%	79%	80%	93%
Oxygenation Assessment	47	100%	97%	99%	100%
Pneumococcal Vaccine	26	88%	62%	69%	94%
Smoking Cessation Advice[1]	11	100%	77%	80%	100%
Surgical Infection Prevention					
Prophylactic Antibiotic Given[1,3]	1	100%	76%	77%	95%
Prophylactic Antibiotic Selection	0	-	83%	90%	100%
Prophylactic Antibiotic Stopped[1,3]	1	100%	70%	72%	95%
Pregnancy Care					
Inpatient Neonatal Mortality	-	-	-	-	-
Third or Fourth Degree Laceration	-	-	2.26%	3.63%	3.27%

Highland Community Hospital

801 Goodyear Boulevard   Phone: 601-798-4711
Picayune, GF 39466   Fax: 601-749-3187
URL: www.highlandch.com
Ownership: Proprietary   Accredited: No
Emergency Services: Yes   Licensed Beds: 95
Key Personnel:
Administrator . . . . Steve Grimm
Chief of Medical Staff. . . . . Robert Lopez
Director Emergency Department . . . . Debbie Farmer

Director Cardiology . . . . Pam O'Flynn
Director Surgical Services . . . . Debbie Green
Director Radiology . . . . Pam O'Flynn

Measure	Cases	This Hospital	State Average	U.S. Average	Top Hospital
Heart Attack Care					
ACE Inhibitor or ARB for LVSD	0	-	80%	82%	100%
Aspirin at Arrival[1]	22	100%	86%	92%	100%
Aspirin at Discharge[1]	10	100%	84%	90%	100%
Beta Blocker at Arrival	26	96%	74%	87%	100%
Beta Blocker at Discharge[1]	14	100%	81%	90%	100%
Fibrinolytic Medication Timing[3]	0	-	32%	31%	100%
PCI Within 90 Minutes of Arrival	0	-	46%	54%	95%
Smoking Cessation Advice[3]	0	-	88%	88%	100%
Heart Failure Care					
ACE Inhibitor or ARB for LVSD[1]	14	100%	76%	82%	100%
Discharge Instructions[1,3]	13	77%	55%	61%	93%
Evaluation of LVS Function	100	44%	78%	83%	99%
Smoking Cessation Advice[1,3]	1	100%	80%	82%	100%
Pneumonia Care					
Appropriate Initial Antibiotic[1,3]	23	87%	78%	83%	94%
Blood Culture Timing[1,3]	14	86%	89%	90%	100%
Influenza Vaccine[5]	-	-	64%	70%	100%
Initial Antibiotic Timing	169	73%	79%	80%	93%
Oxygenation Assessment	209	100%	97%	99%	100%
Pneumococcal Vaccine	102	30%	62%	69%	94%
Smoking Cessation Advice[1,3]	8	88%	77%	80%	100%
Surgical Infection Prevention					
Prophylactic Antibiotic Given[1,3]	2	100%	76%	77%	95%
Prophylactic Antibiotic Selection[5]	-	-	83%	90%	100%
Prophylactic Antibiotic Stopped[1,3]	2	100%	70%	72%	95%
Pregnancy Care					
Inpatient Neonatal Mortality	-	-	-	-	-
Third or Fourth Degree Laceration	-	-	2.26%	3.63%	3.27%

Pearl River County Hospital and Nursing Home

Alternate Name: Pearl River Medical Complex
305 W Moody Street   Phone: 601-795-4543
PO Box 392   Fax: 601-795-4238
Poplarville, MS 39470
E-mail: lfc829@aol.com
Ownership: Government - Local   Accredited: No
Emergency Services: No   Licensed Beds: 30
Key Personnel:
CEO. . . . . Dorthy Bilbo
Chief Medical Staff. . . . . John Aaron
Director Infection/Disease Control . . . . Christie Ladner
ICU Supervising Nurse. Begerly Amacker
Chief Radiology . . . . Jim Carlisle
Director Respiratory Therapy . . . . Lywanda Whotten

Measure	Cases	This Hospital	State Average	U.S. Average	Top Hospital
Heart Attack Care					
ACE Inhibitor or ARB for LVSD[5]	-	-	80%	82%	100%
Aspirin at Arrival[5]	-	-	86%	92%	100%
Aspirin at Discharge[5]	-	-	84%	90%	100%
Beta Blocker at Arrival[5]	-	-	74%	87%	100%
Beta Blocker at Discharge[5]	-	-	81%	90%	100%
Fibrinolytic Medication Timing[5]	-	-	32%	31%	100%
PCI Within 90 Minutes of Arrival[5]	-	-	46%	54%	95%
Smoking Cessation Advice[5]	-	-	88%	88%	100%
Heart Failure Care					
ACE Inhibitor or ARB for LVSD[3]	0	-	76%	82%	100%
Discharge Instructions[5]	-	-	55%	61%	93%
Evaluation of LVS Function[1,3]	4	75%	78%	83%	99%
Smoking Cessation Advice[5]	-	-	80%	82%	100%
Pneumonia Care					
Appropriate Initial Antibiotic[3]	0	-	78%	83%	94%
Blood Culture Timing[1,3]	1	100%	89%	90%	100%
Influenza Vaccine[5]	-	-	64%	70%	100%
Initial Antibiotic Timing[1]	10	80%	79%	80%	93%
Oxygenation Assessment[1]	13	100%	97%	99%	100%

NOTE: Hospital profiles are in alphabetical order by state, then city, then hospital within the city; Rankings are sorted by rate in descending order and exclude hospitals with less than 25 cases; (1) The number of cases is too small (n<25) for purposes of reliably predicting hospital performance; (2) Measure reflects the hospital's indication that its submission was based upon a sample of its relevant discharges; (3) Rate reflects fewer than the maximum possible quarters of data for the measure; (4) Inaccurate information submitted and suppressed for one or more quarters; (5) No data is available from the hospital for this measure; Please refer to the User's Guide for a full explanation of data

Pneumococcal Vaccine[1]	5	80%	62%	69%	94%
Smoking Cessation Advice[3]	0	-	77%	80%	100%
Surgical Infection Prevention					
Prophylactic Antibiotic Given[5]	-	-	76%	77%	95%
Prophylactic Antibiotic Selection[5]	-	-	83%	90%	100%
Prophylactic Antibiotic Stopped[5]	-	-	70%	72%	95%
Pregnancy Care					
Inpatient Neonatal Mortality	-	-	-	-	-
Third or Fourth Degree Laceration	-	-	2.26%	3.63%	3.27%

Claiborne County Hospital

123 McComb Avenue
Port Gibson, MS 39150
E-mail: chospi7707@aol.com
Ownership: Government - Local
Emergency Services: Yes

Phone: 601-437-5141
Fax: 601-437-5145

Accredited: No
Licensed Beds: 32

Key Personnel:
Administrator/CEO . . . . Wanda Fleming
Chief Medical Staff . . . . Roy Barnes
Emergency Room . . . . Genette Edwards, RN
Director Infection/Disease Control . . . . Sandra Sampson
Director Respiratory Therapy . . . . Sadrick Mckenzie

Measure	Cases	This Hospital	State Average	U.S. Average	Top Hospital
Heart Attack Care					
ACE Inhibitor or ARB for LVSD[5]	-	-	80%	82%	100%
Aspirin at Arrival[5]	-	-	86%	92%	100%
Aspirin at Discharge[5]	-	-	84%	90%	100%
Beta Blocker at Arrival[5]	-	-	74%	87%	100%
Beta Blocker at Discharge[5]	-	-	81%	90%	100%
Fibrinolytic Medication Timing[5]	-	-	32%	31%	100%
PCI Within 90 Minutes of Arrival[5]	-	-	46%	54%	95%
Smoking Cessation Advice[5]	-	-	88%	88%	100%
Heart Failure Care					
ACE Inhibitor or ARB for LVSD[5]	-	-	76%	82%	100%
Discharge Instructions[5]	-	-	55%	61%	93%
Evaluation of LVS Function[5]	-	-	78%	83%	99%
Smoking Cessation Advice[5]	-	-	80%	82%	100%
Pneumonia Care					
Appropriate Initial Antibiotic[5]	-	-	78%	83%	94%
Blood Culture Timing[5]	-	-	89%	90%	100%
Influenza Vaccine[5]	-	-	64%	70%	100%
Initial Antibiotic Timing[5]	-	-	79%	80%	93%
Oxygenation Assessment[5]	-	-	97%	99%	100%
Pneumococcal Vaccine[5]	-	-	62%	69%	94%
Smoking Cessation Advice[5]	-	-	77%	80%	100%
Surgical Infection Prevention					
Prophylactic Antibiotic Given[5]	-	-	76%	77%	95%
Prophylactic Antibiotic Selection[5]	-	-	83%	90%	100%
Prophylactic Antibiotic Stopped[5]	-	-	70%	72%	95%
Pregnancy Care					
Inpatient Neonatal Mortality	-	-	-	-	-
Third or Fourth Degree Laceration	-	-	2.26%	3.63%	3.27%

Jefferson Davis Community Hospital

1102 Rose Street
Prentiss, MS 39474
URL: www.jdchnet.org
Ownership: Voluntary non-profit - Private
Emergency Services: Yes

Phone: 601-792-4276
Fax: 601-792-2947

Accredited: No
Licensed Beds: 41

Key Personnel:
CEO . . . . Mary Cardis
Chief Medical Staff . . . . Calor Berg
Emergency Room . . . . Lisa Berry, RN

Measure	Cases	This Hospital	State Average	U.S. Average	Top Hospital
Heart Attack Care					
ACE Inhibitor or ARB for LVSD[5]	-	-	80%	82%	100%
Aspirin at Arrival[5]	-	-	86%	92%	100%
Aspirin at Discharge[5]	-	-	84%	90%	100%
Beta Blocker at Arrival[5]	-	-	74%	87%	100%
Beta Blocker at Discharge[5]	-	-	81%	90%	100%

Measure	Cases	This Hospital	State Average	U.S. Average	Top Hospital
Fibrinolytic Medication Timing[5]	-	-	32%	31%	100%
PCI Within 90 Minutes of Arrival[5]	-	-	46%	54%	95%
Smoking Cessation Advice[5]	-	-	88%	88%	100%
Heart Failure Care					
ACE Inhibitor or ARB for LVSD[1,3]	7	100%	76%	82%	100%
Discharge Instructions[1,3]	17	35%	55%	61%	93%
Evaluation of LVS Function[1,3]	16	56%	78%	83%	99%
Smoking Cessation Advice[1,3]	8	75%	80%	82%	100%
Pneumonia Care					
Appropriate Initial Antibiotic[1,3]	14	93%	78%	83%	94%
Blood Culture Timing[1]	8	75%	89%	90%	100%
Influenza Vaccine[1]	5	80%	64%	70%	100%
Initial Antibiotic Timing[1,3]	20	80%	79%	80%	93%
Oxygenation Assessment[1,3]	22	100%	97%	99%	100%
Pneumococcal Vaccine[1,3]	14	79%	62%	69%	94%
Smoking Cessation Advice[1,3]	7	57%	77%	80%	100%
Surgical Infection Prevention					
Prophylactic Antibiotic Given[5]	-	-	76%	77%	95%
Prophylactic Antibiotic Selection[5]	-	-	83%	90%	100%
Prophylactic Antibiotic Stopped[5]	-	-	70%	72%	95%
Pregnancy Care					
Inpatient Neonatal Mortality	-	-	-	-	-
Third or Fourth Degree Laceration	-	-	2.26%	3.63%	3.27%

H C Watkins Memorial Hospital

605 S Archusa Avenue
Quitman, MS 39355
Ownership: Voluntary non-profit - Private
Emergency Services: Yes

Phone: 601-776-6925
Fax: 601-776-7158
Accredited: No
Licensed Beds: 32

Key Personnel:
Administrator/CEO . . . . Fred Truesdale
Chief Medical Staff . . . . IV Zamora, MD
Emergency Room . . . . OW Byrd, MD
Director Infection/Disease Control . . . . Sherry Zahn, RN
Director Medical/Surgical Nursing . . . . Sheri Zahn, RN

Measure	Cases	This Hospital	State Average	U.S. Average	Top Hospital
Heart Attack Care					
ACE Inhibitor or ARB for LVSD[5]	-	-	80%	82%	100%
Aspirin at Arrival[5]	-	-	86%	92%	100%
Aspirin at Discharge[5]	-	-	84%	90%	100%
Beta Blocker at Arrival[5]	-	-	74%	87%	100%
Beta Blocker at Discharge[5]	-	-	81%	90%	100%
Fibrinolytic Medication Timing[5]	-	-	32%	31%	100%
PCI Within 90 Minutes of Arrival[5]	-	-	46%	54%	95%
Smoking Cessation Advice[5]	-	-	88%	88%	100%
Heart Failure Care					
ACE Inhibitor or ARB for LVSD[1,3]	1	100%	76%	82%	100%
Discharge Instructions[1,3]	4	0%	55%	61%	93%
Evaluation of LVS Function[1,3]	10	30%	78%	83%	99%
Smoking Cessation Advice[1,3]	2	100%	80%	82%	100%
Pneumonia Care					
Appropriate Initial Antibiotic[1,3]	11	27%	78%	83%	94%
Blood Culture Timing[1,3]	2	100%	89%	90%	100%
Influenza Vaccine[5]	-	-	64%	70%	100%
Initial Antibiotic Timing[1,3]	8	38%	79%	80%	93%
Oxygenation Assessment[1,3]	17	94%	97%	99%	100%
Pneumococcal Vaccine[1,3]	12	25%	62%	69%	94%
Smoking Cessation Advice[1,3]	2	0%	77%	80%	100%
Surgical Infection Prevention					
Prophylactic Antibiotic Given[5]	-	-	76%	77%	95%
Prophylactic Antibiotic Selection[5]	-	-	83%	90%	100%
Prophylactic Antibiotic Stopped[5]	-	-	70%	72%	95%
Pregnancy Care					
Inpatient Neonatal Mortality	-	-	-	-	-
Third or Fourth Degree Laceration	-	-	2.26%	3.63%	3.27%

NOTE: Hospital profiles are in alphabetical order by state, then city, then hospital within the city; Rankings are sorted by rate in descending order and exclude hospitals with less than 25 cases; (1) The number of cases is too small (n<25) for purposes of reliably predicting hospital performance; (2) Measure reflects the hospital's indication that its submission was based upon a sample of its relevant discharges; (3) Rate reflects fewer than the maximum possible quarters of data for the measure; (4) Inaccurate information submitted and suppressed for one or more quarters; (5) No data is available from the hospital for this measure; Please refer to the User's Guide for a full explanation of data

Tippah County Hospital

1005 City Avenue N
Ripley, MS 38663
Ownership: Government - Local
Emergency Services: Yes

Phone: 662-837-9221
Fax: 662-837-2110
Accredited: Yes
Licensed Beds: 110

Key Personnel:
Chief Medical Staff. . . . . Charles M Elliot, MD
Emergency Room . . . . Paula Jones, RN
Emergency Room . . . . Pam Bates, RN,DON
Infection Control . . . . Joey Gray, RN
Respiratory/Cardiopulmonary. . . . . Pam Manley, CRRT

Measure	Cases	This Hospital	State Average	U.S. Average	Top Hospital
Heart Attack Care					
ACE Inhibitor or ARB for LVSD[3]	0	-	80%	82%	100%
Aspirin at Arrival[1,3]	2	100%	86%	92%	100%
Aspirin at Discharge[1,3]	2	100%	84%	90%	100%
Beta Blocker at Arrival[1,3]	1	0%	74%	87%	100%
Beta Blocker at Discharge[1,3]	2	0%	81%	90%	100%
Fibrinolytic Medication Timing[5]	-	-	32%	31%	100%
PCI Within 90 Minutes of Arrival[5]	-	-	46%	54%	95%
Smoking Cessation Advice[5]	-	-	88%	88%	100%
Heart Failure Care					
ACE Inhibitor or ARB for LVSD[1]	15	73%	76%	82%	100%
Discharge Instructions[1,3]	9	44%	55%	61%	93%
Evaluation of LVS Function	42	71%	78%	83%	99%
Smoking Cessation Advice[1,3]	3	33%	80%	82%	100%
Pneumonia Care					
Appropriate Initial Antibiotic[1,3]	1	100%	78%	83%	94%
Blood Culture Timing[1,3]	7	86%	89%	90%	100%
Influenza Vaccine[4,5]	-	-	64%	70%	100%
Initial Antibiotic Timing	64	84%	79%	80%	93%
Oxygenation Assessment	91	98%	97%	99%	100%
Pneumococcal Vaccine	58	59%	62%	69%	94%
Smoking Cessation Advice[3]	0	-	77%	80%	100%
Surgical Infection Prevention					
Prophylactic Antibiotic Given[3]	0	-	76%	77%	95%
Prophylactic Antibiotic Selection[5]	-	-	83%	90%	100%
Prophylactic Antibiotic Stopped[3]	0	-	70%	72%	95%
Pregnancy Care					
Inpatient Neonatal Mortality	-	-	-	-	-
Third or Fourth Degree Laceration	-	-	2.26%	3.63%	3.27%

Sharkey Issaquena Community Hospital

47 South 4 St
Rolling Fork, MS 39159
Ownership: Government - Local
Emergency Services: Yes

Phone: 662-873-4395

Accredited: No

Measure	Cases	This Hospital	State Average	U.S. Average	Top Hospital
Heart Attack Care					
ACE Inhibitor or ARB for LVSD[5]	-	-	80%	82%	100%
Aspirin at Arrival[5]	-	-	86%	92%	100%
Aspirin at Discharge[5]	-	-	84%	90%	100%
Beta Blocker at Arrival[5]	-	-	74%	87%	100%
Beta Blocker at Discharge[5]	-	-	81%	90%	100%
Fibrinolytic Medication Timing[5]	-	-	32%	31%	100%
PCI Within 90 Minutes of Arrival[5]	-	-	46%	54%	95%
Smoking Cessation Advice[5]	-	-	88%	88%	100%
Heart Failure Care					
ACE Inhibitor or ARB for LVSD[1,3]	1	0%	76%	82%	100%
Discharge Instructions[1,3]	2	0%	55%	61%	93%
Evaluation of LVS Function[1,3]	14	7%	78%	83%	99%
Smoking Cessation Advice[3]	0	-	80%	82%	100%
Pneumonia Care					
Appropriate Initial Antibiotic[3]	0	-	78%	83%	94%
Blood Culture Timing[3]	0	-	89%	90%	100%
Influenza Vaccine[5]	-	-	64%	70%	100%
Initial Antibiotic Timing[1]	6	83%	79%	80%	93%
Oxygenation Assessment[1]	6	100%	97%	99%	100%
Pneumococcal Vaccine[1]	5	0%	62%	69%	94%
Smoking Cessation Advice[3]	0	-	77%	80%	100%

Measure		This Hospital	State Average	U.S. Average	Top Hospital
Surgical Infection Prevention					
Prophylactic Antibiotic Given[5]	-	-	76%	77%	95%
Prophylactic Antibiotic Selection[5]	-	-	83%	90%	100%
Prophylactic Antibiotic Stopped[5]	-	-	70%	72%	95%
Pregnancy Care					
Inpatient Neonatal Mortality	-	-	-	-	-
Third or Fourth Degree Laceration	-	-	2.26%	3.63%	3.27%

North Sunflower County Hospital

840 N Oak Avenue
PO Box 369
Ruleville, MS 38771
Ownership: Government - Local
Emergency Services: Yes

Phone: 662-756-2711
Fax: 662-756-4114

Accredited: No
Licensed Beds: 44

Key Personnel:
Administrator . . . . Douglass D Dailey
Chief Medical Staff. . . . . Adelo Aquino, MD
Director Infection/Disease Control . . . . Marianne Eastland
Chief Radiology . . . . Vincent Luciano
Director Respiratory Therapy . . . . Keleigh Nichols

Measure	Cases	This Hospital	State Average	U.S. Average	Top Hospital
Heart Attack Care					
ACE Inhibitor or ARB for LVSD[5]	-	-	80%	82%	100%
Aspirin at Arrival[5]	-	-	86%	92%	100%
Aspirin at Discharge[5]	-	-	84%	90%	100%
Beta Blocker at Arrival[5]	-	-	74%	87%	100%
Beta Blocker at Discharge[5]	-	-	81%	90%	100%
Fibrinolytic Medication Timing[5]	-	-	32%	31%	100%
PCI Within 90 Minutes of Arrival[5]	-	-	46%	54%	95%
Smoking Cessation Advice[5]	-	-	88%	88%	100%
Heart Failure Care					
ACE Inhibitor or ARB for LVSD[1]	9	89%	76%	82%	100%
Discharge Instructions[1]	13	23%	55%	61%	93%
Evaluation of LVS Function	27	81%	78%	83%	99%
Smoking Cessation Advice[1]	2	100%	80%	82%	100%
Pneumonia Care					
Appropriate Initial Antibiotic[1]	20	80%	78%	83%	94%
Blood Culture Timing[1]	18	83%	89%	90%	100%
Influenza Vaccine[1]	10	60%	64%	70%	100%
Initial Antibiotic Timing	49	78%	79%	80%	93%
Oxygenation Assessment	59	100%	97%	99%	100%
Pneumococcal Vaccine	38	71%	62%	69%	94%
Smoking Cessation Advice[1]	6	100%	77%	80%	100%
Surgical Infection Prevention					
Prophylactic Antibiotic Given[5]	-	-	76%	77%	95%
Prophylactic Antibiotic Selection[5]	-	-	83%	90%	100%
Prophylactic Antibiotic Stopped[5]	-	-	70%	72%	95%
Pregnancy Care					
Inpatient Neonatal Mortality	-	-	-	-	-
Third or Fourth Degree Laceration	-	-	2.26%	3.63%	3.27%

North Oak Regional Medical Center

Alternate Name: Senatobia Community Hospital
401 Getwell Drive
Senatobia, MS 38668
Ownership: Proprietary
Emergency Services: Yes

Phone: 662-562-3100
Fax: 662-560-6295
Accredited: Yes
Licensed Beds: 76

Measure	Cases	This Hospital	State Average	U.S. Average	Top Hospital
Heart Attack Care					
ACE Inhibitor or ARB for LVSD[3]	0	-	80%	82%	100%
Aspirin at Arrival[1,3]	2	50%	86%	92%	100%
Aspirin at Discharge[1,3]	1	100%	84%	90%	100%
Beta Blocker at Arrival[1,3]	4	25%	74%	87%	100%
Beta Blocker at Discharge[1,3]	3	33%	81%	90%	100%
Fibrinolytic Medication Timing[3]	0	-	32%	31%	100%
PCI Within 90 Minutes of Arrival	0	-	46%	54%	95%
Smoking Cessation Advice[3]	0	-	88%	88%	100%
Heart Failure Care					
ACE Inhibitor or ARB for LVSD[1]	5	40%	76%	82%	100%
Discharge Instructions[1,3]	18	83%	55%	61%	93%

NOTE: Hospital profiles are in alphabetical order by state, then city, then hospital within the city; Rankings are sorted by rate in descending order and exclude hospitals with less than 25 cases; (1) The number of cases is too small (n<25) for purposes of reliably predicting hospital performance; (2) Measure reflects the hospital's indication that its submission was based upon a sample of its relevant discharges; (3) Rate reflects fewer than the maximum possible quarters of data for the measure; (4) Inaccurate information submitted and suppressed for one or more quarters; (5) No data is available from the hospital for this measure; Please refer to the User's Guide for a full explanation of data

Evaluation of LVS Function	80	79%	78%	83%	99%
Smoking Cessation Advice[1,3]	1	100%	80%	82%	100%
Pneumonia Care					
Appropriate Initial Antibiotic[1,3]	1	100%	78%	83%	94%
Blood Culture Timing[1,3]	1	100%	89%	90%	100%
Influenza Vaccine[4,5]	-	-	64%	70%	100%
Initial Antibiotic Timing	41	80%	79%	80%	93%
Oxygenation Assessment	47	96%	97%	99%	100%
Pneumococcal Vaccine[1]	24	83%	62%	69%	94%
Smoking Cessation Advice[3]	0	-	77%	80%	100%
Surgical Infection Prevention					
Prophylactic Antibiotic Given[1,3]	6	67%	76%	77%	95%
Prophylactic Antibiotic Selection[5]	-	-	83%	90%	100%
Prophylactic Antibiotic Stopped[1,3]	6	67%	70%	72%	95%
Pregnancy Care					
Inpatient Neonatal Mortality	-	-	-	-	-
Third or Fourth Degree Laceration	-	-	2.26%	3.63%	3.27%

Baptist Memorial Hospital Desoto

7601 Southcrest Parkway
Southaven, MS 38671
URL: www.baptistonline.org
Ownership: Voluntary non-profit - Private
Emergency Services: Yes

Phone: 662-772-4000
Fax: 662-349-4570

Accredited: Yes
Licensed Beds: 199

Key Personnel:
CEO . . . . Randy King
Emergency Room . . . . Stanley Thomson

Measure	Cases	This Hospital	State Average	U.S. Average	Top Hospital
Heart Attack Care					
ACE Inhibitor or ARB for LVSD	52	92%	80%	82%	100%
Aspirin at Arrival	269	97%	86%	92%	100%
Aspirin at Discharge	279	95%	84%	90%	100%
Beta Blocker at Arrival	202	84%	74%	87%	100%
Beta Blocker at Discharge	290	90%	81%	90%	100%
Fibrinolytic Medication Timing[1]	4	50%	32%	31%	100%
PCI Within 90 Minutes of Arrival[1]	14	36%	46%	54%	95%
Smoking Cessation Advice	130	99%	88%	88%	100%
Heart Failure Care					
ACE Inhibitor or ARB for LVSD	156	90%	76%	82%	100%
Discharge Instructions	460	82%	55%	61%	93%
Evaluation of LVS Function	538	96%	78%	83%	99%
Smoking Cessation Advice	130	97%	80%	82%	100%
Pneumonia Care					
Appropriate Initial Antibiotic	234	84%	78%	83%	94%
Blood Culture Timing	173	86%	89%	90%	100%
Influenza Vaccine	51	90%	64%	70%	100%
Initial Antibiotic Timing	237	59%	79%	80%	93%
Oxygenation Assessment	279	100%	97%	99%	100%
Pneumococcal Vaccine	140	86%	62%	69%	94%
Smoking Cessation Advice	108	99%	77%	80%	100%
Surgical Infection Prevention					
Prophylactic Antibiotic Given[2]	455	90%	76%	77%	95%
Prophylactic Antibiotic Selection[2]	58	98%	83%	90%	100%
Prophylactic Antibiotic Stopped[2]	428	75%	70%	72%	95%
Pregnancy Care					
Inpatient Neonatal Mortality	-	-	-	-	-
Third or Fourth Degree Laceration	-	-	2.26%	3.63%	3.27%

Oktibbeha County Hospital

400 Hospital Road
Starkville, MS 39759
URL: www.och.org
Ownership: Government - Local
Emergency Services: Yes

Phone: 662-323-4320
Fax: 662-338-3345

Accredited: Yes
Licensed Beds: 96

Key Personnel:
CEO . . . . Arthur C Kelly
Chief Medical Staff . . . . Linda Blake
Director Cardiac Lab . . . . Elizabeth Varco, RN
Supervisor Emergency Room . . . . Eddie Coats, RN
Director Infection Control . . . . Carolyn Arnold, RN
CCU Spvg. Nurse . . . . Cheryl Guyton, RN
Director Radiology . . . . Glynn Stone

Director Respiratory/Cardiopulmonary . . . . Wes Andrews

Measure	Cases	This Hospital	State Average	U.S. Average	Top Hospital
Heart Attack Care					
ACE Inhibitor or ARB for LVSD[1,3]	1	100%	80%	82%	100%
Aspirin at Arrival[1,3]	3	100%	86%	92%	100%
Aspirin at Discharge[1,3]	3	100%	84%	90%	100%
Beta Blocker at Arrival[1,3]	3	67%	74%	87%	100%
Beta Blocker at Discharge[1,3]	2	100%	81%	90%	100%
Fibrinolytic Medication Timing[3]	0	-	32%	31%	100%
PCI Within 90 Minutes of Arrival[5]	-	-	46%	54%	95%
Smoking Cessation Advice[3]	0	-	88%	88%	100%
Heart Failure Care					
ACE Inhibitor or ARB for LVSD[1]	20	80%	76%	82%	100%
Discharge Instructions	54	33%	55%	61%	93%
Evaluation of LVS Function	60	73%	78%	83%	99%
Smoking Cessation Advice[1]	7	29%	80%	82%	100%
Pneumonia Care					
Appropriate Initial Antibiotic	86	70%	78%	83%	94%
Blood Culture Timing	67	90%	89%	90%	100%
Influenza Vaccine[1]	17	76%	64%	70%	100%
Initial Antibiotic Timing	103	79%	79%	80%	93%
Oxygenation Assessment	121	91%	97%	99%	100%
Pneumococcal Vaccine	66	74%	62%	69%	94%
Smoking Cessation Advice[1]	18	78%	77%	80%	100%
Surgical Infection Prevention					
Prophylactic Antibiotic Given	305	56%	76%	77%	95%
Prophylactic Antibiotic Selection	88	68%	83%	90%	100%
Prophylactic Antibiotic Stopped	296	80%	70%	72%	95%
Pregnancy Care					
Inpatient Neonatal Mortality	-	-	-	-	-
Third or Fourth Degree Laceration	-	-	2.26%	3.63%	3.27%

North Mississippi Medical Center

830 S Gloster Street
Tupelo, MS 38801

Toll-Free: 800-843-3375
Phone: 662-377-3000
Fax: 662-377-3552

URL: www.nmhs.net/nmmc
Ownership: Voluntary non-profit - Private
Emergency Services: Yes

Accredited: Yes
Licensed Beds: 650

Key Personnel:
President . . . . Chuck Stokes
Chief Medical Officer . . . . Ken Davis, MD
OB/GYN Womens Health. . . . . Charles Robertson, MD
Director Respiratory Therapy . . . . Ron Pittman

Measure	Cases	This Hospital	State Average	U.S. Average	Top Hospital
Heart Attack Care					
ACE Inhibitor or ARB for LVSD	208	92%	80%	82%	100%
Aspirin at Arrival	360	99%	86%	92%	100%
Aspirin at Discharge	781	100%	84%	90%	100%
Beta Blocker at Arrival	310	97%	74%	87%	100%
Beta Blocker at Discharge	722	99%	81%	90%	100%
Fibrinolytic Medication Timing[1]	6	33%	32%	31%	100%
PCI Within 90 Minutes of Arrival[1]	22	45%	46%	54%	95%
Smoking Cessation Advice	347	99%	88%	88%	100%
Heart Failure Care					
ACE Inhibitor or ARB for LVSD	430	90%	76%	82%	100%
Discharge Instructions	645	97%	55%	61%	93%
Evaluation of LVS Function	725	95%	78%	83%	99%
Smoking Cessation Advice	210	100%	80%	82%	100%
Pneumonia Care					
Appropriate Initial Antibiotic	206	84%	78%	83%	94%
Blood Culture Timing	158	88%	89%	90%	100%
Influenza Vaccine	88	59%	64%	70%	100%
Initial Antibiotic Timing	251	76%	79%	80%	93%
Oxygenation Assessment	370	100%	97%	99%	100%
Pneumococcal Vaccine	251	91%	62%	69%	94%
Smoking Cessation Advice	112	98%	77%	80%	100%
Surgical Infection Prevention					
Prophylactic Antibiotic Given[2]	951	92%	76%	77%	95%
Prophylactic Antibiotic Selection[2]	255	84%	83%	90%	100%

Prophylactic Antibiotic Stopped[2]	903	72%	70%	72%	95%
Pregnancy Care					
Inpatient Neonatal Mortality[2]	483	1.04%	-	-	-
Third or Fourth Degree Laceration[2]	315	6.35%	2.26%	3.63%	3.27%

Walthall County General Hospital

100 Hospital Drive
Tylertown, MS 39667
Ownership: Government - Local
Emergency Services: No

Phone: 601-876-2122

Accredited: No

Measure	Cases	This Hospital	State Average	U.S. Average	Top Hospital
Heart Attack Care					
ACE Inhibitor or ARB for LVSD[3]	0	-	80%	82%	100%
Aspirin at Arrival[1,3]	2	50%	86%	92%	100%
Aspirin at Discharge[1,3]	2	100%	84%	90%	100%
Beta Blocker at Arrival[1,3]	2	100%	74%	87%	100%
Beta Blocker at Discharge[1,3]	3	67%	81%	90%	100%
Fibrinolytic Medication Timing[3]	0	-	32%	31%	100%
PCI Within 90 Minutes of Arrival	0	-	46%	54%	95%
Smoking Cessation Advice[3]	0	-	88%	88%	100%
Heart Failure Care					
ACE Inhibitor or ARB for LVSD[1]	3	67%	76%	82%	100%
Discharge Instructions	40	30%	55%	61%	93%
Evaluation of LVS Function	63	43%	78%	83%	99%
Smoking Cessation Advice[1]	7	29%	80%	82%	100%
Pneumonia Care					
Appropriate Initial Antibiotic	44	75%	78%	83%	94%
Blood Culture Timing[1]	6	100%	89%	90%	100%
Influenza Vaccine[1]	12	17%	64%	70%	100%
Initial Antibiotic Timing	46	89%	79%	80%	93%
Oxygenation Assessment	63	79%	97%	99%	100%
Pneumococcal Vaccine	32	3%	62%	69%	94%
Smoking Cessation Advice[1]	13	23%	77%	80%	100%
Surgical Infection Prevention					
Prophylactic Antibiotic Given[5]	-	-	76%	77%	95%
Prophylactic Antibiotic Selection[5]	-	-	83%	90%	100%
Prophylactic Antibiotic Stopped[5]	-	-	70%	72%	95%
Pregnancy Care					
Inpatient Neonatal Mortality	-	-	-	-	-
Third or Fourth Degree Laceration	-	-	2.26%	3.63%	3.27%

Laird Hospital

25117 Highway 15
Union, MS 39365
Ownership: Voluntary non-profit - Other
Emergency Services: Yes

Phone: 601-774-8214
Fax: 601-774-1573
Accredited: Yes
Licensed Beds: 50

Key Personnel:
CEO . . . . Tomy Bartlett
Emergency Room . . . . OJ Briseno, MD
Director Medical/Surgical Nursing . . . . Noel Palmer, RN
Director Respiratory Therapy . . . . Christy Battle

Measure	Cases	This Hospital	State Average	U.S. Average	Top Hospital
Heart Attack Care					
ACE Inhibitor or ARB for LVSD[1]	1	0%	80%	82%	100%
Aspirin at Arrival[1]	5	80%	86%	92%	100%
Aspirin at Discharge[1]	4	75%	84%	90%	100%
Beta Blocker at Arrival[1]	5	60%	74%	87%	100%
Beta Blocker at Discharge[1]	4	100%	81%	90%	100%
Fibrinolytic Medication Timing	0	-	32%	31%	100%
PCI Within 90 Minutes of Arrival	0	-	46%	54%	95%
Smoking Cessation Advice	0	-	88%	88%	100%
Heart Failure Care					
ACE Inhibitor or ARB for LVSD[1]	4	75%	76%	82%	100%
Discharge Instructions[1]	21	33%	55%	61%	93%
Evaluation of LVS Function	41	34%	78%	83%	99%
Smoking Cessation Advice[1]	6	0%	80%	82%	100%
Pneumonia Care					
Appropriate Initial Antibiotic[1]	20	95%	78%	83%	94%
Blood Culture Timing[1]	3	67%	89%	90%	100%

Measure	Cases	This Hospital	State Average	U.S. Average	Top Hospital
Influenza Vaccine[1]	7	71%	64%	70%	100%
Initial Antibiotic Timing[1]	12	100%	79%	80%	93%
Oxygenation Assessment	51	82%	97%	99%	100%
Pneumococcal Vaccine[1]	23	65%	62%	69%	94%
Smoking Cessation Advice[1]	11	36%	77%	80%	100%
Surgical Infection Prevention					
Prophylactic Antibiotic Given[5]	-	-	76%	77%	95%
Prophylactic Antibiotic Selection[5]	-	-	83%	90%	100%
Prophylactic Antibiotic Stopped[5]	-	-	70%	72%	95%
Pregnancy Care					
Inpatient Neonatal Mortality	-	-	-	-	-
Third or Fourth Degree Laceration	-	-	2.26%	3.63%	3.27%

River Region Health System

2100 Hwy 61 N
Vicksburg, MS 39183
Ownership: Proprietary
Emergency Services: Yes

Phone: 601-883-5136

Accredited: Yes

Measure	Cases	This Hospital	State Average	U.S. Average	Top Hospital
Heart Attack Care					
ACE Inhibitor or ARB for LVSD	35	83%	80%	82%	100%
Aspirin at Arrival	130	96%	86%	92%	100%
Aspirin at Discharge	141	95%	84%	90%	100%
Beta Blocker at Arrival	83	87%	74%	87%	100%
Beta Blocker at Discharge	142	92%	81%	90%	100%
Fibrinolytic Medication Timing[1]	19	58%	32%	31%	100%
PCI Within 90 Minutes of Arrival[1]	7	29%	46%	54%	95%
Smoking Cessation Advice	66	97%	88%	88%	100%
Heart Failure Care					
ACE Inhibitor or ARB for LVSD	162	91%	76%	82%	100%
Discharge Instructions	395	63%	55%	61%	93%
Evaluation of LVS Function	466	97%	78%	83%	99%
Smoking Cessation Advice	98	100%	80%	82%	100%
Pneumonia Care					
Appropriate Initial Antibiotic	181	78%	78%	83%	94%
Blood Culture Timing	147	95%	89%	90%	100%
Influenza Vaccine	58	93%	64%	70%	100%
Initial Antibiotic Timing	221	89%	79%	80%	93%
Oxygenation Assessment	275	99%	97%	99%	100%
Pneumococcal Vaccine	135	96%	62%	69%	94%
Smoking Cessation Advice	86	95%	77%	80%	100%
Surgical Infection Prevention					
Prophylactic Antibiotic Given	406	80%	76%	77%	95%
Prophylactic Antibiotic Selection	99	91%	83%	90%	100%
Prophylactic Antibiotic Stopped	386	64%	70%	72%	95%
Pregnancy Care					
Inpatient Neonatal Mortality	-	-	-	-	-
Third or Fourth Degree Laceration	-	-	2.26%	3.63%	3.27%

Yalobusha General Hospital

PO Box 728
Water Valley, MS 38965
Ownership: Government - Local
Emergency Services: No

Phone: 662-473-1411
Fax: 662-473-4922
Accredited: No
Licensed Beds: 91

Key Personnel:
CEO . . . . Perry Varner
Chief of Medical Staff . . . . Joe Walker
Director of Respiratory . . . . Susan Hammond

Measure	Cases	This Hospital	State Average	U.S. Average	Top Hospital
Heart Attack Care					
ACE Inhibitor or ARB for LVSD[1,3]	1	0%	80%	82%	100%
Aspirin at Arrival[1,3]	1	0%	86%	92%	100%
Aspirin at Discharge[1,3]	1	0%	84%	90%	100%
Beta Blocker at Arrival[1,3]	1	0%	74%	87%	100%
Beta Blocker at Discharge[1,3]	1	0%	81%	90%	100%
Fibrinolytic Medication Timing[5]	-	-	32%	31%	100%
PCI Within 90 Minutes of Arrival[5]	-	-	46%	54%	95%
Smoking Cessation Advice[5]	-	-	88%	88%	100%
Heart Failure Care					
ACE Inhibitor or ARB for LVSD[1]	4	50%	76%	82%	100%

NOTE: Hospital profiles are in alphabetical order by state, then city, then hospital within the city; Rankings are sorted by rate in descending order and exclude hospitals with less than 25 cases; (1) The number of cases is too small (n<25) for purposes of reliably predicting hospital performance; (2) Measure reflects the hospital's indication that its submission was based upon a sample of its relevant discharges; (3) Rate reflects fewer than the maximum possible quarters of data for the measure; (4) Inaccurate information submitted and suppressed for one or more quarters; (5) No data is available from the hospital for this measure; Please refer to the User's Guide for a full explanation of data

	Cases	This Hospital	State Average	U.S. Average	Top Hospital
Discharge Instructions[1,3]	7	14%	55%	61%	93%
Evaluation of LVS Function	33	48%	78%	83%	99%
Smoking Cessation Advice[3]	0	-	80%	82%	100%
Pneumonia Care					
Appropriate Initial Antibiotic[1,3]	3	100%	78%	83%	94%
Blood Culture Timing[3]	0	-	89%	90%	100%
Influenza Vaccine[5]	-	-	64%	70%	100%
Initial Antibiotic Timing	25	96%	79%	80%	93%
Oxygenation Assessment	29	83%	97%	99%	100%
Pneumococcal Vaccine[1]	22	27%	62%	69%	94%
Smoking Cessation Advice[1,3]	3	100%	77%	80%	100%
Surgical Infection Prevention					
Prophylactic Antibiotic Given[5]	-	-	76%	77%	95%
Prophylactic Antibiotic Selection[5]	-	-	83%	90%	100%
Prophylactic Antibiotic Stopped[5]	-	-	70%	72%	95%
Pregnancy Care					
Inpatient Neonatal Mortality	-	-	-	-	-
Third or Fourth Degree Laceration	-	-	2.26%	3.63%	3.27%

Wayne General Hospital

950 Matthew Drive   Phone: 601-735-5151
Waynesboro, MS 39367   Fax: 601-735-7150
Ownership: Government - Local   Accredited: Yes
Emergency Services: Yes   Licensed Beds: 80
Key Personnel:
Administrator . . . . Donald Hemeter
Chief of Medical Staff . . . . Tod Stokley
Emergency Room . . . . Jennifer Myeras
Emergency Room . . . . Bobbie Cooksey
Director Infection/Disease Control . . . . Paulette Cooley

Measure	Cases	This Hospital	State Average	U.S. Average	Top Hospital
Heart Attack Care					
ACE Inhibitor or ARB for LVSD[1]	1	100%	80%	82%	100%
Aspirin at Arrival[1]	9	67%	86%	92%	100%
Aspirin at Discharge[1]	5	60%	84%	90%	100%
Beta Blocker at Arrival[1]	9	56%	74%	87%	100%
Beta Blocker at Discharge[1]	5	40%	81%	90%	100%
Fibrinolytic Medication Timing[3]	0	-	32%	31%	100%
PCI Within 90 Minutes of Arrival	0	-	46%	54%	95%
Smoking Cessation Advice[3]	0	-	88%	88%	100%
Heart Failure Care					
ACE Inhibitor or ARB for LVSD	53	81%	76%	82%	100%
Discharge Instructions[1,3]	19	63%	55%	61%	93%
Evaluation of LVS Function	73	89%	78%	83%	99%
Smoking Cessation Advice[1,3]	1	0%	80%	82%	100%
Pneumonia Care					
Appropriate Initial Antibiotic[1,3]	7	86%	78%	83%	94%
Blood Culture Timing[1,3]	6	83%	89%	90%	100%
Influenza Vaccine[5]	-	-	64%	70%	100%
Initial Antibiotic Timing	62	92%	79%	80%	93%
Oxygenation Assessment	79	100%	97%	99%	100%
Pneumococcal Vaccine	39	79%	62%	69%	94%
Smoking Cessation Advice[1,3]	3	100%	77%	80%	100%
Surgical Infection Prevention					
Prophylactic Antibiotic Given[1,3]	4	0%	76%	77%	95%
Prophylactic Antibiotic Selection[5]	-	-	83%	90%	100%
Prophylactic Antibiotic Stopped[1,3]	3	33%	70%	72%	95%
Pregnancy Care					
Inpatient Neonatal Mortality	-	-	-	-	-
Third or Fourth Degree Laceration	-	-	2.26%	3.63%	3.27%

Clay County Medical Center

835 Medical Center Drive   Phone: 662-495-2300
West Point, MS 39773   Fax: 662-495-2361
URL: www.nmhs.net
Ownership: Government - Local   Accredited: Yes
Emergency Services: Yes   Licensed Beds: 60
Key Personnel:
Administrator . . . . David M Reid
Chief Medical Staff . . . . Charlotte Magnussen
Director Infection/Disease Control . . . . Paula Bryan
Director Medical/Surgical Nursing . . . . Jane Windle

Director Respiratory Therapy . . . . Georgia Williams

Measure	Cases	This Hospital	State Average	U.S. Average	Top Hospital
Heart Attack Care					
ACE Inhibitor or ARB for LVSD[1]	1	100%	80%	82%	100%
Aspirin at Arrival[1]	3	100%	86%	92%	100%
Aspirin at Discharge[1]	4	100%	84%	90%	100%
Beta Blocker at Arrival[1]	4	100%	74%	87%	100%
Beta Blocker at Discharge[1]	3	100%	81%	90%	100%
Fibrinolytic Medication Timing[3]	0	-	32%	31%	100%
PCI Within 90 Minutes of Arrival	0	-	46%	54%	95%
Smoking Cessation Advice[3]	0	-	88%	88%	100%
Heart Failure Care					
ACE Inhibitor or ARB for LVSD	57	91%	76%	82%	100%
Discharge Instructions[3]	26	73%	55%	61%	93%
Evaluation of LVS Function	129	74%	78%	83%	99%
Smoking Cessation Advice[1,3]	5	100%	80%	82%	100%
Pneumonia Care					
Appropriate Initial Antibiotic[1,3]	12	92%	78%	83%	94%
Blood Culture Timing[1,3]	12	83%	89%	90%	100%
Influenza Vaccine[5]	-	-	64%	70%	100%
Initial Antibiotic Timing	78	92%	79%	80%	93%
Oxygenation Assessment	91	97%	97%	99%	100%
Pneumococcal Vaccine	60	67%	62%	69%	94%
Smoking Cessation Advice[1,3]	2	100%	77%	80%	100%
Surgical Infection Prevention					
Prophylactic Antibiotic Given[2,3]	37	68%	76%	77%	95%
Prophylactic Antibiotic Selection[5]	-	-	83%	90%	100%
Prophylactic Antibiotic Stopped[2,3]	33	79%	70%	72%	95%
Pregnancy Care					
Inpatient Neonatal Mortality	517	0.19%	-	-	-
Third or Fourth Degree Laceration	332	0.90%	2.26%	3.63%	3.27%

Whitfield Medical Surgical Hospital

3350 Highway 468   Phone: 601-351-8023
Box 157-A   Fax: 601-351-8364
Whitfield, MS 39193
E-mail: mikula@msh.state.ms.us
Ownership: Government - State
Emergency Services: No   Accredited: Yes
     Licensed Beds: 43
Key Personnel:
Administrator . . . . Diana Mikula
Chief Medical Staff . . . . Dan Coughlin, MD
Infection Control . . . . Judy Pearce
Medical Surgical Nursing . . . . Janice Moore, RN

Measure	Cases	This Hospital	State Average	U.S. Average	Top Hospital
Heart Attack Care					
ACE Inhibitor or ARB for LVSD[3]	0	-	80%	82%	100%
Aspirin at Arrival[1,3]	1	100%	86%	92%	100%
Aspirin at Discharge[1,3]	1	100%	84%	90%	100%
Beta Blocker at Arrival[1,3]	1	100%	74%	87%	100%
Beta Blocker at Discharge[3]	0	-	81%	90%	100%
Fibrinolytic Medication Timing[5]	-	-	32%	31%	100%
PCI Within 90 Minutes of Arrival[5]	-	-	46%	54%	95%
Smoking Cessation Advice[5]	-	-	88%	88%	100%
Heart Failure Care					
ACE Inhibitor or ARB for LVSD[1,3]	2	100%	76%	82%	100%
Discharge Instructions[5]	-	-	55%	61%	93%
Evaluation of LVS Function[1,3]	2	100%	78%	83%	99%
Smoking Cessation Advice[5]	-	-	80%	82%	100%
Pneumonia Care					
Appropriate Initial Antibiotic[3]	0	-	78%	83%	94%
Blood Culture Timing[3]	0	-	89%	90%	100%
Influenza Vaccine[5]	-	-	64%	70%	100%
Initial Antibiotic Timing[1]	18	100%	79%	80%	93%
Oxygenation Assessment[1]	19	100%	97%	99%	100%
Pneumococcal Vaccine[1]	7	86%	62%	69%	94%
Smoking Cessation Advice[3]	0	-	77%	80%	100%
Surgical Infection Prevention					
Prophylactic Antibiotic Given[5]	-	-	76%	77%	95%
Prophylactic Antibiotic Selection[5]	-	-	83%	90%	100%

NOTE: Hospital profiles are in alphabetical order by state, then city, then hospital within the city; Rankings are sorted by rate in descending order and exclude hospitals with less than 25 cases; (1) The number of cases is too small (n<25) for purposes of reliably predicting hospital performance; (2) Measure reflects the hospital's indication that its submission was based upon a sample of its relevant discharges; (3) Rate reflects fewer than the maximum possible quarters of data for the measure; (4) Inaccurate information submitted and suppressed for one or more quarters; (5) No data is available from the hospital for this measure; Please refer to the User's Guide for a full explanation of data

Prophylactic Antibiotic Stopped[5]	-	-	70%	72%	95%
Pregnancy Care					
Inpatient Neonatal Mortality	-	-	-	-	-
Third or Fourth Degree Laceration	-	-	2.26%	3.63%	3.27%

NOTE: Hospital profiles are in alphabetical order by state, then city, then hospital within the city; Rankings are sorted by rate in descending order and exclude hospitals with less than 25 cases; (1) The number of cases is too small (n<25) for purposes of reliably predicting hospital performance; (2) Measure reflects the hospital's indication that its submission was based upon a sample of its relevant discharges; (3) Rate reflects fewer than the maximum possible quarters of data for the measure; (4) Inaccurate information submitted and suppressed for one or more quarters; (5) No data is available from the hospital for this measure; Please refer to the User's Guide for a full explanation of data

Heart Attack Care

1. ACE Inhibitor or ARB for LVSD

Hospital Name	City	Rate	Cases
Hospital Damas	Ponce	100%	42
Manati Medical Center Doctor Otero Lopez	Manati	100%	32
Hospital De La Concepcion	San German	98%	43
Hospital San Cristobal	Coto Laurel	94%	31
Cardiovascular Center of Puerto Rico	Rio Piedras	90%	77
UPR Carolina	Carolina	88%	142
San Luke's Memorial Hospital	Ponce	87%	30
Hospital San Pablo	Bayamon	78%	89
Auxilio Mutuo Hospital	San Juan	73%	33
Hospital Doctor Cayetano Coll Y Toste	Arecibo	68%	37
Hospital Metropolitano Doctor Tito Mattei	Yauco	67%	43
Ramon E Betances Hospital	Mayaguez	66%	50
Hospital Comunitario Buen Samaritano	Aguadilla	50%	42

2. Aspirin at Arrival

Hospital Name	City	Rate	Cases
Hospital Wilma N Vazquez	Vega Baja	100%	33
Manati Medical Center Doctor Otero Lopez	Manati	99%	195
Hospital Universitario Doctor Ramon Ruiz Arnau	Bayamon	98%	41
Cardiovascular Center of Puerto Rico	Rio Piedras	97%	69
Hospital Metropolitano	San German	97%	31
Hima Humacao	Humacao	96%	55
Hospital Doctor Susoni	Arecibo	96%	53
Hospital Menonita De Cayey	Cayey	96%	49
Ryder Memorial Hospital	Humacao	96%	27
Hospital Damas	Ponce	95%	132
Ramon E Betances Hospital	Mayaguez	95%	78
Hospital San Francisco	San Juan	94%	36
San Luke's Memorial Hospital	Ponce	94%	187
Ashford Presbyterian Community Hospital	San Juan	93%	45
Hospital De La Concepcion	San German	93%	111
UPR Carolina	Carolina	93%	238
Hospital Doctor Cayetano Coll Y Toste	Arecibo	92%	77
Hospital Metropolitano Doctor Tito Mattei	Yauco	91%	270
Auxilio Mutuo Hospital	San Juan	85%	132
Hospital San Cristobal	Coto Laurel	85%	67
Hospital Comunitario Buen Samaritano	Aguadilla	79%	136
Hospital San Juan Bautista Medical Center	Caguas	79%	150
Hospital Episcopal Cristo Redentor	Guayama	77%	53
Hospital San Pablo	Bayamon	75%	238
Bella Vista Hospital	Mayaguez	74%	54
Hospital Doctor Pila	Ponce	71%	167

3. Aspirin at Discharge

Hospital Name	City	Rate	Cases
Hima Humacao	Humacao	100%	48
Hospital Metropolitano	San German	100%	33
Manati Medical Center Doctor Otero Lopez	Manati	100%	91
Cardiovascular Center of Puerto Rico	Rio Piedras	99%	259
Hospital Damas	Ponce	96%	124
Hospital Pavia Santurce	Fernandez Juncos	93%	205
Hospital De La Concepcion	San German	90%	102
Hospital Doctor Cayetano Coll Y Toste	Arecibo	90%	80
San Luke's Memorial Hospital	Ponce	88%	105
UPR Carolina	Carolina	86%	175
Auxilio Mutuo Hospital	San Juan	85%	138
Hospital Doctor Susoni	Arecibo	80%	46
Hospital Menonita De Cayey	Cayey	80%	30
Ramon E Betances Hospital	Mayaguez	80%	110
Bella Vista Hospital	Mayaguez	72%	39
Hospital Metropolitano Doctor Tito Mattei	Yauco	70%	283
Hospital Comunitario Buen Samaritano	Aguadilla	42%	118

4. Beta Blocker at Arrival

Hospital Name	City	Rate	Cases
Hospital San Cristobal	Coto Laurel	99%	69
Cardiovascular Center of Puerto Rico	Rio Piedras	97%	70
Hospital Metropolitano	San German	97%	31
Hima Humacao	Humacao	96%	51
Manati Medical Center Doctor Otero Lopez	Manati	95%	162
Hospital Interamericano de Medicina	Caguas	94%	71
Hospital Damas	Ponce	92%	125
Hospital De La Concepcion	San German	91%	104
Hospital Universitario Doctor Ramon Ruiz Arnau	Bayamon	90%	41
Ashford Presbyterian Community Hospital	San Juan	89%	46
Ryder Memorial Hospital	Humacao	89%	27
UPR Carolina	Carolina	88%	190
Hospital San Francisco	San Juan	85%	34

Hospital Doctor Susoni	Arecibo	81%	42
Hospital Menonita De Cayey	Cayey	80%	51
Ramon E Betances Hospital	Mayaguez	80%	79
Hospital Metropolitano Doctor Tito Mattei	Yauco	78%	238
Hospital Comunitario Buen Samaritano	Aguadilla	75%	134
Auxilio Mutuo Hospital	San Juan	73%	105
Hospital Doctor Cayetano Coll Y Toste	Arecibo	68%	74
San Juan Municipal Hospital	Rio Piedras	68%	25
Hospital Episcopal Cristo Redentor	Guayama	66%	58
San Luke's Memorial Hospital	Ponce	62%	190
Bella Vista Hospital	Mayaguez	53%	51

5. Beta Blocker at Discharge

Hospital Name	City	Rate	Cases
Hima Humacao	Humacao	100%	48
Hospital Damas	Ponce	97%	139
Cardiovascular Center of Puerto Rico	Rio Piedras	96%	226
Hospital De La Concepcion	San German	95%	110
Hospital San Cristobal	Coto Laurel	95%	73
Manati Medical Center Doctor Otero Lopez	Manati	95%	77
Hospital Metropolitano	San German	91%	35
UPR Carolina	Carolina	90%	173
San Luke's Memorial Hospital	Ponce	85%	110
Hospital Menonita De Cayey	Cayey	83%	41
Auxilio Mutuo Hospital	San Juan	81%	150
San Juan Municipal Hospital	Rio Piedras	81%	26
Hospital Doctor Cayetano Coll Y Toste	Arecibo	79%	80
Ramon E Betances Hospital	Mayaguez	78%	113
Hospital Metropolitano Doctor Tito Mattei	Yauco	72%	261
Bella Vista Hospital	Mayaguez	60%	47
Hospital Doctor Susoni	Arecibo	59%	39
Hospital Comunitario Buen Samaritano	Aguadilla	52%	118

6. Fibrinolytic Medication Timing

Hospital Name	City	Rate	Cases
Hospital Doctor Pila	Ponce	24%	33

8. Smoking Cessation Advice

Hospital Name	City	Rate	Cases
Hospital Doctor Cayetano Coll Y Toste	Arecibo	100%	27
Manati Medical Center Doctor Otero Lopez	Manati	100%	35
Hospital Pavia Santurce	Fernandez Juncos	98%	60
Hospital San Pablo	Bayamon	98%	59
Ramon E Betances Hospital	Mayaguez	96%	25
Hospital Metropolitano Doctor Tito Mattei	Yauco	93%	108
UPR Carolina	Carolina	90%	40
Cardiovascular Center of Puerto Rico	Rio Piedras	89%	55
Hospital San Juan Bautista Medical Center	Caguas	61%	31

Heart Failure Care

9. ACE Inhibitor or ARB for LVSD

Hospital Name	City	Rate	Cases
Ashford Presbyterian Community Hospital	San Juan	100%	33
Hima Humacao	Humacao	100%	31
Manati Medical Center Doctor Otero Lopez	Manati	100%	150
Metropolitan Hospital	San Juan	100%	42
Hospital De La Concepcion	San German	99%	70
Cardiovascular Center of Puerto Rico	Rio Piedras	97%	239
Hospital Damas	Ponce	95%	73
Hospital Interamericano de Medicina	Caguas	94%	81
Hospital Menonita De Cayey	Cayey	93%	60
UPR Carolina	Carolina	93%	101
Hospital San Cristobal	Coto Laurel	92%	25
San Luke's Memorial Hospital	Ponce	92%	65
Hima-San Pablo Fajardo	Fajardo	89%	65
Hospital Pavia Santurce	Fernandez Juncos	89%	84
Hospital Doctor Cayetano Coll Y Toste	Arecibo	82%	101
Hospital Episcopal Cristo Redentor	Guayama	82%	28
Bella Vista Hospital	Mayaguez	75%	36
Hospital San Pablo	Bayamon	75%	185
Hospital Metropolitano Doctor Tito Mattei	Yauco	73%	55
Hospital Perea	Mayaguez	68%	25
Ramon E Betances Hospital	Mayaguez	66%	65
Auxilio Mutuo Hospital	San Juan	64%	86
Hospital Comunitario Buen Samaritano	Aguadilla	44%	89

10. Discharge Instructions

Hospital Name	City	Rate	Cases
Ashford Presbyterian Community Hospital	San Juan	100%	69
Clinica Espanola	Mayaguez	100%	25
Doctors Center Hospital	Manati	100%	35

NOTE: Hospital profiles are in alphabetical order by state, then city, then hospital within the city; Rankings are sorted by rate in descending order and exclude hospitals with less than 25 cases; (1) The number of cases is too small (n<25) for purposes of reliably predicting hospital performance; (2) Measure reflects the hospital's indication that its submission was based upon a sample of its relevant discharges; (3) Rate reflects fewer than the maximum possible quarters of data for the measure; (4) Inaccurate information submitted and suppressed for one or more quarters; (5) No data is available from the hospital for this measure; Please refer to the User's Guide for a full explanation of data

Hospital Damas	Ponce	100%	210
Hospital De La Concepcion	San German	100%	178
Hospital Metropolitano	San German	100%	52
Hospital Pavia Santurce	Fernandez Juncos	100%	215
Hospital Santa Rosa	Guayama	100%	29
Hospital Universitario Doctor Ramon Ruiz Arnau	Bayamon	100%	58
Hospital Wilma N Vazquez	Vega Baja	100%	46
Lafayette Hospital	Arroyo	100%	41
Manati Medical Center Doctor Otero Lopez	Manati	100%	493
Mennonite General Hospital	Aibonito	100%	63
Hospital Interamericano de Medicina	Caguas	99%	112
Metropolitan Hospital	San Juan	98%	232
Hima-San Pablo Fajardo	Fajardo	95%	107
San Juan Municipal Hospital	Rio Piedras	95%	43
Cardiovascular Center of Puerto Rico	Rio Piedras	94%	373
Hima Humacao	Humacao	93%	122
Hospital San Juan Bautista Medical Center	Caguas	84%	134
Bella Vista Hospital	Mayaguez	82%	140
Hospital Doctor Cayetano Coll Y Toste	Arecibo	82%	160
Ramon E Betances Hospital	Mayaguez	77%	146
San Luke's Memorial Hospital	Ponce	71%	171
Hospital Episcopal Cristo Redentor	Guayama	69%	88
Hospital San Cristobal	Coto Laurel	69%	42
Hospital Perea	Mayaguez	64%	42
Hospital Comunitario Buen Samaritano	Aguadilla	63%	259
Hospital Del Maestro	San Juan	57%	106
Hospital Doctor Dominguez	Humacao	49%	41
Hospital Menonita De Cayey	Cayey	41%	224
Auxilio Mutuo Hospital	San Juan	35%	302
Hospital San Carlos Borromeo	Moca	32%	25
Hospital Doctor Susoni	Arecibo	28%	65
UPR Carolina	Carolina	27%	318
Hospital Metropolitano Doctor Tito Mattei	Yauco	18%	228
Hospital San Francisco	San Juan	0%	79

11. Evaluation of LVS Function

Hospital Name	City	Rate	Cases
Hospital Metropolitano	San German	100%	52
Hospital Santa Rosa	Guayama	100%	29
Hospital Universitario Doctor Ramon Ruiz Arnau	Bayamon	100%	59
Hospital Wilma N Vazquez	Vega Baja	100%	46
Lafayette Hospital	Arroyo	100%	41
Manati Medical Center Doctor Otero Lopez	Manati	100%	493
UPR Carolina	Carolina	100%	319
Hospital Metropolitano Doctor Tito Mattei	Yauco	99%	226
Hospital De La Concepcion	San German	96%	175
Ashford Presbyterian Community Hospital	San Juan	93%	68
Hima Humacao	Humacao	93%	122
Doctors Center Hospital	Manati	89%	35
Hospital Damas	Ponce	89%	211
Hospital Interamericano de Medicina	Caguas	89%	112
Cardiovascular Center of Puerto Rico	Rio Piedras	87%	373
Hospital Doctor Cayetano Coll Y Toste	Arecibo	86%	152
Hima-San Pablo Fajardo	Fajardo	85%	110
Hospital Doctor Pila	Ponce	85%	103
Ramon E Betances Hospital	Mayaguez	84%	146
Auxilio Mutuo Hospital	San Juan	82%	304
Ryder Memorial Hospital	Humacao	81%	48
Clinica Espanola	Mayaguez	80%	25
Hospital Doctor Susoni	Arecibo	76%	46
San Luke's Memorial Hospital	Ponce	74%	170
Hospital Episcopal Cristo Redentor	Guayama	72%	88
Bella Vista Hospital	Mayaguez	65%	142
Hospital Menonita De Cayey	Cayey	65%	222
Hospital Comunitario Buen Samaritano	Aguadilla	62%	260
Hospital Doctor Dominguez	Humacao	62%	26
Hospital San Carlos Borromeo	Moca	60%	25
Hospital San Francisco	San Juan	59%	80
San Juan Municipal Hospital	Rio Piedras	59%	41
Hospital Del Maestro	San Juan	58%	106
Mennonite General Hospital	Aibonito	57%	63
Hospital San Juan Bautista Medical Center	Caguas	54%	134

12. Smoking Cessation Advice

Hospital Name	City	Rate	Cases
Hospital Damas	Ponce	100%	26
Hospital Doctor Cayetano Coll Y Toste	Arecibo	100%	31
Hospital Pavia Santurce	Fernandez Juncos	100%	32
Manati Medical Center Doctor Otero Lopez	Manati	100%	59
Metropolitan Hospital	San Juan	98%	58
Hospital Menonita De Cayey	Cayey	97%	30
Hospital San Pablo	Bayamon	97%	37
Hospital Metropolitano Doctor Tito Mattei	Yauco	90%	69
Hospital Comunitario Buen Samaritano	Aguadilla	87%	39

UPR Carolina	Carolina	82%	38
Hospital San Juan Bautista Medical Center	Caguas	78%	27

Pneumonia Care

13. Appropriate Initial Antibiotic

Hospital Name	City	Rate	Cases
Hospital Metropolitano	San German	94%	33
Hima Humacao	Humacao	88%	141
Hospital Menonita De Cayey	Cayey	85%	55
Hospital Doctor Dominguez	Humacao	83%	59
Hospital San Francisco	San Juan	81%	75
Mennonite General Hospital	Aibonito	80%	30
Ashford Presbyterian Community Hospital	San Juan	79%	85
Bella Vista Hospital	Mayaguez	79%	121
San Luke's Memorial Hospital	Ponce	79%	121
Hospital Comunitario Buen Samaritano	Aguadilla	77%	113
Hospital Pavia Hato Rey	Hato Rey	73%	52
Hospital Damas	Ponce	71%	70
Hospital Perea	Mayaguez	70%	40
Hospital San Pablo	Bayamon	69%	202
Hospital Doctor Susoni	Arecibo	67%	64
Hospital San Gerardo	Rio Piedras	66%	32
Hospital Metropolitano Doctor Tito Mattei	Yauco	64%	119
Hospital Doctor Cayetano Coll Y Toste	Arecibo	62%	73
Ramon E Betances Hospital	Mayaguez	62%	48
Auxilio Mutuo Hospital	San Juan	61%	137
Hospital Doctor Pila	Ponce	60%	111
Hospital Pavia Santurce	Fernandez Juncos	60%	204
Hospital Universitario Doctor Ramon Ruiz Arnau	Bayamon	57%	127
Lafayette Hospital	Arroyo	57%	28
UPR Carolina	Carolina	57%	292
Hospital Del Maestro	San Juan	55%	76
Hospital Episcopal Cristo Redentor	Guayama	55%	42
Hospital San Juan Bautista Medical Center	Caguas	51%	80
Hima-San Pablo Fajardo	Fajardo	48%	75

14. Blood Culture Timing

Hospital Name	City	Rate	Cases
Ryder Memorial Hospital	Humacao	97%	29
Hospital Del Maestro	San Juan	93%	72
Hospital Metropolitano Doctor Tito Mattei	Yauco	92%	65
Hima Humacao	Humacao	89%	80
Metropolitan Hospital	San Juan	88%	119
Hospital Damas	Ponce	87%	60
Hospital Comunitario Buen Samaritano	Aguadilla	84%	85
Ramon E Betances Hospital	Mayaguez	79%	29
Hima-San Pablo Fajardo	Fajardo	78%	36
Hospital Doctor Cayetano Coll Y Toste	Arecibo	78%	64
Mennonite General Hospital	Aibonito	75%	28
San Luke's Memorial Hospital	Ponce	75%	64
Auxilio Mutuo Hospital	San Juan	71%	213
Hospital Doctor Susoni	Arecibo	71%	38
UPR Carolina	Carolina	69%	84
Ashford Presbyterian Community Hospital	San Juan	66%	71
Bella Vista Hospital	Mayaguez	66%	112
Hospital Universitario Doctor Ramon Ruiz Arnau	Bayamon	64%	154
Hospital Doctor Pila	Ponce	61%	59
Hospital Menonita De Cayey	Cayey	52%	25
Hospital San Francisco	San Juan	45%	42

15. Influenza Vaccine

Hospital Name	City	Rate	Cases
Manati Medical Center Doctor Otero Lopez	Manati	56%	57
Auxilio Mutuo Hospital	San Juan	47%	45
Hima Humacao	Humacao	34%	35
UPR Carolina	Carolina	11%	46
Bella Vista Hospital	Mayaguez	9%	35
Hospital Metropolitano Doctor Tito Mattei	Yauco	8%	26

16. Initial Antibiotic Timing

Hospital Name	City	Rate	Cases
Manati Medical Center Doctor Otero Lopez	Manati	92%	393
San Juan Municipal Hospital	Rio Piedras	78%	37
Hospital Wilma N Vazquez	Vega Baja	67%	27
Hospital Damas	Ponce	64%	83
Hima Humacao	Humacao	63%	151
Hospital Del Maestro	San Juan	62%	76
Hospital San Pablo	Bayamon	55%	285
Hima-San Pablo Fajardo	Fajardo	54%	78
Lafayette Hospital	Arroyo	52%	29
Hospital Universitario Doctor Ramon Ruiz Arnau	Bayamon	51%	150

NOTE: Hospital profiles are in alphabetical order by state, then city, then hospital within the city; Rankings are sorted by rate in descending order and exclude hospitals with less than 25 cases; (1) The number of cases is too small (n<25) for purposes of reliably predicting hospital performance; (2) Measure reflects the hospital's indication that its submission was based upon a sample of its relevant discharges; (3) Rate reflects fewer than the maximum possible quarters of data for the measure; (4) Inaccurate information submitted and suppressed for one or more quarters; (5) No data is available from the hospital for this measure; Please refer to the User's Guide for a full explanation of data

San Luke's Memorial Hospital	Ponce	51%	123
Hospital Pavia Hato Rey	Hato Rey	46%	54
Auxilio Mutuo Hospital	San Juan	45%	248
Bella Vista Hospital	Mayaguez	43%	148
Hospital Doctor Cayetano Coll Y Toste	Arecibo	42%	81
Hospital Doctor Susoni	Arecibo	41%	66
Mennonite General Hospital	Aibonito	41%	27
Hospital Episcopal Cristo Redentor	Guayama	40%	47
UPR Carolina	Carolina	39%	372
Hospital Menonita De Cayey	Cayey	34%	68
Hospital Comunitario Buen Samaritano	Aguadilla	30%	115
Hospital San Francisco	San Juan	29%	68
Ryder Memorial Hospital	Humacao	27%	26
Doctors Center Hospital	Manati	21%	28
Hospital Perea	Mayaguez	20%	40
Hospital Metropolitano Doctor Tito Mattei	Yauco	12%	145
Hospital Doctor Dominguez	Humacao	10%	58

17. Oxygenation Assessment

Hospital Name	City	Rate	Cases
Ashford Presbyterian Community Hospital	San Juan	100%	100
Bella Vista Hospital	Mayaguez	100%	165
Doctors Center Hospital	Manati	100%	28
Hospital Metropolitano	San German	100%	35
Hospital San Cristobal	Coto Laurel	100%	50
Hospital Universitario Doctor Ramon Ruiz Arnau	Bayamon	100%	155
Manati Medical Center Doctor Otero Lopez	Manati	100%	394
Ryder Memorial Hospital	Humacao	100%	29
San Luke's Memorial Hospital	Ponce	100%	124
Hima Humacao	Humacao	99%	155
Hospital Del Maestro	San Juan	99%	83
Hospital San Juan Bautista Medical Center	Caguas	99%	99
Hospital San Pablo	Bayamon	98%	291
Hospital Comunitario Buen Samaritano	Aguadilla	97%	118
Lafayette Hospital	Arroyo	97%	29
Mennonite General Hospital	Aibonito	97%	33
Ramon E Betances Hospital	Mayaguez	97%	74
San Juan Municipal Hospital	Rio Piedras	97%	58
UPR Carolina	Carolina	97%	409
Hospital Menonita De Cayey	Cayey	96%	73
Hospital Interamericano de Medicina	Caguas	95%	180
Hospital Pavia Santurce	Fernandez Juncos	94%	218
Hima-San Pablo Fajardo	Fajardo	93%	83
Hospital Doctor Pila	Ponce	93%	150
Hospital De La Concepcion	San German	92%	124
Hospital Doctor Dominguez	Humacao	92%	79
Hospital San Francisco	San Juan	92%	91
Hospital Damas	Ponce	90%	94
Hospital Episcopal Cristo Redentor	Guayama	90%	49
Hospital Pavia Hato Rey	Hato Rey	90%	59
Hospital Doctor Cayetano Coll Y Toste	Arecibo	87%	83
Hospital Metropolitano Doctor Tito Mattei	Yauco	87%	154
Hospital San Gerardo	Rio Piedras	82%	33
Auxilio Mutuo Hospital	San Juan	81%	268
Hospital Doctor Susoni	Arecibo	77%	69
Hospital Wilma N Vazquez	Vega Baja	76%	29

18. Pneumococcal Vaccine

Hospital Name	City	Rate	Cases
San Luke's Memorial Hospital	Ponce	88%	67
Hospital Doctor Cayetano Coll Y Toste	Arecibo	71%	52
Hospital Universitario Doctor Ramon Ruiz Arnau	Bayamon	56%	50
Auxilio Mutuo Hospital	San Juan	49%	144
Hospital Doctor Pila	Ponce	47%	79
Hospital Perea	Mayaguez	45%	31
Ramon E Betances Hospital	Mayaguez	41%	34
Manati Medical Center Doctor Otero Lopez	Manati	40%	232
Hospital Menonita De Cayey	Cayey	39%	36
Hospital Episcopal Cristo Redentor	Guayama	36%	25
Hima Humacao	Humacao	34%	91
Hospital Metropolitano Doctor Tito Mattei	Yauco	25%	84
Hospital Del Maestro	San Juan	24%	45
Ryder Memorial Hospital	Humacao	24%	25
Hospital Damas	Ponce	20%	56
Hospital San Pablo	Bayamon	17%	202
Hospital Doctor Dominguez	Humacao	14%	49
Hospital San Francisco	San Juan	14%	58
Hima-San Pablo Fajardo	Fajardo	10%	48
Hospital De La Concepcion	San German	10%	73
Hospital Doctor Susoni	Arecibo	10%	42
UPR Carolina	Carolina	9%	206
Hospital Comunitario Buen Samaritano	Aguadilla	6%	64
Bella Vista Hospital	Mayaguez	5%	96

19. Smoking Cessation Advice

Hospital Name	City	Rate	Cases
Hospital Doctor Cayetano Coll Y Toste	Arecibo	100%	26
Hospital Interamericano de Medicina	Caguas	100%	34
Hospital Universitario Doctor Ramon Ruiz Arnau	Bayamon	100%	28
Manati Medical Center Doctor Otero Lopez	Manati	100%	135
San Juan Municipal Hospital	Rio Piedras	100%	32
Hospital San Pablo	Bayamon	98%	53
Metropolitan Hospital	San Juan	98%	47
Hospital Metropolitano Doctor Tito Mattei	Yauco	93%	29
Hospital Pavia Santurce	Fernandez Juncos	89%	27
UPR Carolina	Carolina	80%	80

Surgical Infection Prevention

20. Prophylactic Antibiotic Given

Hospital Name	City	Rate	Cases
Hospital San Pablo	Bayamon	84%	603
Auxilio Mutuo Hospital	San Juan	77%	171
UPR Carolina	Carolina	77%	112
Cardiovascular Center of Puerto Rico	Rio Piedras	76%	748
Hospital Comunitario Buen Samaritano	Aguadilla	74%	27
Hospital Matilde Brenes	Bayamon	73%	30
University District Hospital	Rio Piedras	73%	237
Ashford Presbyterian Community Hospital	San Juan	72%	368
San Luke's Memorial Hospital	Ponce	68%	137
Hospital Damas	Ponce	64%	195
Doctor I Gonzalez Martinez Oncologic Hospital	San Juan	62%	332
Hospital Menonita De Cayey	Cayey	60%	55
Hospital Doctor Pila	Ponce	57%	88
Bella Vista Hospital	Mayaguez	56%	313
Hospital Doctor Cayetano Coll Y Toste	Arecibo	47%	78
Doctors Center Hospital	Manati	45%	29
Hospital Doctor Susoni	Arecibo	44%	50
Hospital Metropolitano Doctor Tito Mattei	Yauco	36%	55
Hima-San Pablo Fajardo	Fajardo	26%	43
Hospital Episcopal Cristo Redentor	Guayama	14%	63

21. Prophylactic Antibiotic Selection

Hospital Name	City	Rate	Cases
Hospital De La Concepcion	San German	100%	27
UPR Carolina	Carolina	100%	27
Auxilio Mutuo Hospital	San Juan	99%	89
Hospital Interamericano de Medicina	Caguas	98%	118
Ashford Presbyterian Community Hospital	San Juan	97%	108
Cardiovascular Center of Puerto Rico	Rio Piedras	97%	307
Doctor I Gonzalez Martinez Oncologic Hospital	San Juan	97%	88
Hospital Menonita De Cayey	Cayey	97%	31
San Luke's Memorial Hospital	Ponce	97%	34
Bella Vista Hospital	Mayaguez	96%	51
Hospital San Pablo	Bayamon	91%	70
Hospital Pavia Santurce	Fernandez Juncos	89%	151
Hospital Damas	Ponce	88%	75
Hospital Doctor Pila	Ponce	85%	27
University District Hospital	Rio Piedras	84%	67

22. Prophylactic Antibiotic Stopped

Hospital Name	City	Rate	Cases
Auxilio Mutuo Hospital	San Juan	100%	158
Hima-San Pablo Fajardo	Fajardo	100%	36
Hospital Comunitario Buen Samaritano	Aguadilla	100%	26
Hospital Doctor Susoni	Arecibo	100%	33
Hospital Interamericano de Medicina	Caguas	100%	172
Hospital Metropolitano Doctor Tito Mattei	Yauco	100%	31
Hospital San Cristobal	Coto Laurel	100%	55
San Juan Municipal Hospital	Rio Piedras	100%	28
Cardiovascular Center of Puerto Rico	Rio Piedras	99%	742
Hospital Doctor Pila	Ponce	95%	88
Hospital Menonita De Cayey	Cayey	89%	54
Hospital Matilde Brenes	Bayamon	88%	32
Hospital De La Concepcion	San German	79%	70
UPR Carolina	Carolina	73%	101
University District Hospital	Rio Piedras	69%	231
San Luke's Memorial Hospital	Ponce	65%	137
Hospital Damas	Ponce	52%	193
Hospital Episcopal Cristo Redentor	Guayama	52%	63
Hospital Doctor Cayetano Coll Y Toste	Arecibo	45%	78
Doctor I Gonzalez Martinez Oncologic Hospital	San Juan	24%	328
Doctors Center Hospital	Manati	24%	29
Bella Vista Hospital	Mayaguez	6%	303

NOTE: Hospital profiles are in alphabetical order by state, then city, then hospital within the city; Rankings are sorted by rate in descending order and exclude hospitals with less than 25 cases; (1) The number of cases is too small (n<25) for purposes of reliably predicting hospital performance; (2) Measure reflects the hospital's indication that its submission was based upon a sample of its relevant discharges; (3) Rate reflects fewer than the maximum possible quarters of data for the measure; (4) Inaccurate information submitted and suppressed for one or more quarters; (5) No data is available from the hospital for this measure; Please refer to the User's Guide for a full explanation of data

24. Third or Fourth Degree Laceration

Hospital Name	City	Rate	Cases
Ashford Presbyterian Community Hospital	San Juan	7.04%	1222

Hospital Comunitario Buen Samaritano

Carr. 2 Km 1.4 Ave. Severiano Cuevas #18   Phone: 787-658-0000
Aguadilla, PR 00603
Ownership: Voluntary non-profit - Private   Accredited: Yes
Emergency Services: Yes

Measure	Cases	This Hospital	State Average	U.S. Average	Top Hospital
Heart Attack Care					
ACE Inhibitor or ARB for LVSD	42	50%	81%	82%	100%
Aspirin at Arrival	136	79%	90%	92%	100%
Aspirin at Discharge	118	42%	82%	90%	100%
Beta Blocker at Arrival	134	75%	81%	87%	100%
Beta Blocker at Discharge	118	52%	80%	90%	100%
Fibrinolytic Medication Timing[1]	2	0%	27%	31%	100%
PCI Within 90 Minutes of Arrival	0	-	0%	54%	95%
Smoking Cessation Advice[1]	18	72%	88%	88%	100%
Heart Failure Care					
ACE Inhibitor or ARB for LVSD	89	44%	84%	82%	100%
Discharge Instructions	259	63%	72%	61%	93%
Evaluation of LVS Function	260	62%	78%	83%	99%
Smoking Cessation Advice	39	87%	92%	82%	100%
Pneumonia Care					
Appropriate Initial Antibiotic	113	77%	68%	83%	94%
Blood Culture Timing	85	84%	71%	90%	100%
Influenza Vaccine[1]	16	0%	38%	70%	100%
Initial Antibiotic Timing	115	30%	46%	80%	93%
Oxygenation Assessment	118	97%	93%	99%	100%
Pneumococcal Vaccine	64	6%	34%	69%	94%
Smoking Cessation Advice[1]	20	85%	89%	80%	100%
Surgical Infection Prevention					
Prophylactic Antibiotic Given[3]	27	74%	55%	77%	95%
Prophylactic Antibiotic Selection[1]	2	100%	90%	90%	100%
Prophylactic Antibiotic Stopped[3]	26	100%	78%	72%	95%
Pregnancy Care					
Inpatient Neonatal Mortality	-	-	-	-	-
Third or Fourth Degree Laceration	-	-	-	3.63%	3.27%

Mennonite General Hospital

PO Box 1379   Phone: 787-735-8001
Aibonito, PR 00705   Fax: 787-735-7111
Ownership: Voluntary non-profit - Other   Accredited: No
Emergency Services: Yes   Licensed Beds: 150
Key Personnel:
CEO . . . . Domingo Torrez Zaya
Chief Medical Staff . . . . Roberto Alvaves
Emergency Room . . . . Jorge Calderon
Director Infection/Disease Control . . . . Ana Amelia Camacho
Director Medical/Surgical Nursing . . . . Josefa Santiago
OB/GYN Womens Health . . . . Josa A Colon
Chief Radiology . . . . Silverio Perez
Director Respiratory Therapy . . . . Minerva Marrero

Measure	Cases	This Hospital	State Average	U.S. Average	Top Hospital
Heart Attack Care					
ACE Inhibitor or ARB for LVSD[1,2,3]	1	100%	81%	82%	100%
Aspirin at Arrival[1,2,3]	20	95%	90%	92%	100%
Aspirin at Discharge[1,2,3]	5	60%	82%	90%	100%
Beta Blocker at Arrival[1,2,3]	20	70%	81%	87%	100%
Beta Blocker at Discharge[1,2,3]	5	40%	80%	90%	100%
Fibrinolytic Medication Timing[2,3]	0	-	27%	31%	100%
PCI Within 90 Minutes of Arrival[2]	0	-	0%	54%	95%
Smoking Cessation Advice[1,2,3]	1	100%	88%	88%	100%
Heart Failure Care					
ACE Inhibitor or ARB for LVSD[1,2,3]	11	73%	84%	82%	100%
Discharge Instructions[2,3]	63	100%	72%	61%	93%
Evaluation of LVS Function[2,3]	63	57%	78%	83%	99%
Smoking Cessation Advice[1,2,3]	7	100%	92%	82%	100%
Pneumonia Care					
Appropriate Initial Antibiotic[2,3]	30	80%	68%	83%	94%
Blood Culture Timing[2]	28	75%	71%	90%	100%
Influenza Vaccine[1,2]	1	0%	38%	70%	100%
Initial Antibiotic Timing[2,3]	27	41%	46%	80%	93%

Measure	Cases	This Hospital	State Average	U.S. Average	Top Hospital
Oxygenation Assessment[2,3]	33	97%	93%	99%	100%
Pneumococcal Vaccine[1,2,3]	20	35%	34%	69%	94%
Smoking Cessation Advice[1,2,3]	9	100%	89%	80%	100%
Surgical Infection Prevention					
Prophylactic Antibiotic Given[5]	-	-	55%	77%	95%
Prophylactic Antibiotic Selection[5]	-	-	90%	90%	100%
Prophylactic Antibiotic Stopped[5]	-	-	78%	72%	95%
Pregnancy Care					
Inpatient Neonatal Mortality	-	-	-	-	-
Third or Fourth Degree Laceration	-	-	-	3.63%	3.27%

Hospital Doctor Cayetano Coll Y Toste

Carretera 129 Km.1 Avenida San Luis   Phone: 787-650-7272
Arecibo, PR 00613
Ownership: Proprietary   Accredited: Yes
Emergency Services: Yes

Measure	Cases	This Hospital	State Average	U.S. Average	Top Hospital
Heart Attack Care					
ACE Inhibitor or ARB for LVSD[2,3]	37	68%	81%	82%	100%
Aspirin at Arrival[2,3]	77	92%	90%	92%	100%
Aspirin at Discharge[2,3]	80	90%	82%	90%	100%
Beta Blocker at Arrival[2,3]	74	68%	81%	87%	100%
Beta Blocker at Discharge[2,3]	80	79%	80%	90%	100%
Fibrinolytic Medication Timing[1,2,3]	24	33%	27%	31%	100%
PCI Within 90 Minutes of Arrival[2]	0	-	0%	54%	95%
Smoking Cessation Advice[2,3]	27	100%	88%	88%	100%
Heart Failure Care					
ACE Inhibitor or ARB for LVSD[2,3]	101	82%	84%	82%	100%
Discharge Instructions[2,3]	160	82%	72%	61%	93%
Evaluation of LVS Function[2,3]	152	86%	78%	83%	99%
Smoking Cessation Advice[2,3]	31	100%	92%	82%	100%
Pneumonia Care					
Appropriate Initial Antibiotic[2,3]	73	62%	68%	83%	94%
Blood Culture Timing[2]	64	78%	71%	90%	100%
Influenza Vaccine[1]	22	73%	38%	70%	100%
Initial Antibiotic Timing[2,3]	81	42%	46%	80%	93%
Oxygenation Assessment[2,3]	83	87%	93%	99%	100%
Pneumococcal Vaccine[2,3]	52	71%	34%	69%	94%
Smoking Cessation Advice[2,3]	26	100%	89%	80%	100%
Surgical Infection Prevention					
Prophylactic Antibiotic Given[3]	78	47%	55%	77%	95%
Prophylactic Antibiotic Selection[5]	-	-	90%	90%	100%
Prophylactic Antibiotic Stopped[3]	78	45%	78%	72%	95%
Pregnancy Care					
Inpatient Neonatal Mortality	-	-	-	-	-
Third or Fourth Degree Laceration	-	-	-	3.63%	3.27%

Hospital Doctor Susoni

55 Palma Street   Phone: 787-878-1010
Arecibo, PR 00614   Fax: 787-650-1040
Ownership: Voluntary non-profit - Private   Accredited: No
Emergency Services: Yes   Licensed Beds: 185
Key Personnel:
President/CEO . . . . Homer Perez
Chief Medical Staff . . . . Manuel Somohano, MD
Director Medical/Surgical Nursing . . . . Sonia Acevedo
OB/GYN Womens Health . . . . Jose Rodriguez
Chief Radiology . . . . Jorge Perez
Director Respiratory Therapy . . . . Sol Ortega

Measure	Cases	This Hospital	State Average	U.S. Average	Top Hospital
Heart Attack Care					
ACE Inhibitor or ARB for LVSD[1,2,3]	18	56%	81%	82%	100%
Aspirin at Arrival[2,3]	53	96%	90%	92%	100%
Aspirin at Discharge[2,3]	46	80%	82%	90%	100%
Beta Blocker at Arrival[2,3]	42	81%	81%	87%	100%
Beta Blocker at Discharge[2,3]	39	59%	80%	90%	100%
Fibrinolytic Medication Timing[1,2,3]	14	36%	27%	31%	100%
PCI Within 90 Minutes of Arrival[2]	0	-	0%	54%	95%
Smoking Cessation Advice[1,2,3]	4	100%	88%	88%	100%
Heart Failure Care					

NOTE: Hospital profiles are in alphabetical order by state, then city, then hospital within the city; Rankings are sorted by rate in descending order and exclude hospitals with less than 25 cases; (1) The number of cases is too small (n<25) for purposes of reliably predicting hospital performance; (2) Measure reflects the hospital's indication that its submission was based upon a sample of its relevant discharges; (3) Rate reflects fewer than the maximum possible quarters of data for the measure; (4) Inaccurate information submitted and suppressed for one or more quarters; (5) No data is available from the hospital for this measure; Please refer to the User's Guide for a full explanation of data

ACE Inhibitor or ARB for LVSD[1,2,3]	23	91%	84%	82%	100%
Discharge Instructions[2,3]	65	28%	72%	61%	93%
Evaluation of LVS Function[2,3]	46	76%	78%	83%	99%
Smoking Cessation Advice[1,2,3]	6	100%	92%	82%	100%
Pneumonia Care					
Appropriate Initial Antibiotic[2,3]	64	67%	68%	83%	94%
Blood Culture Timing[2]	38	71%	71%	90%	100%
Influenza Vaccine[1]	19	5%	38%	70%	100%
Initial Antibiotic Timing[2,3]	66	41%	46%	80%	93%
Oxygenation Assessment[2,3]	69	77%	93%	99%	100%
Pneumococcal Vaccine[2,3]	42	10%	34%	69%	94%
Smoking Cessation Advice[1,2,3]	6	100%	89%	80%	100%
Surgical Infection Prevention					
Prophylactic Antibiotic Given[2,3]	50	44%	55%	77%	95%
Prophylactic Antibiotic Selection[1,2]	6	100%	90%	90%	100%
Prophylactic Antibiotic Stopped[2,3]	33	100%	78%	72%	95%
Pregnancy Care					
Inpatient Neonatal Mortality	-	-	-	-	-
Third or Fourth Degree Laceration	-	-	-	3.63%	3.27%

Lafayette Hospital

Central Lafayette
PO Box 207
Arroyo, PR 00714
Ownership: Proprietary
Emergency Services: Yes

Phone: 787-839-3232
Fax: 787-839-4330

Accredited: No
Licensed Beds: 66

Key Personnel:
President/CEO . . . . Francisco A Vazquez
Chief Medical Staff . . . . Jorge Rodles, Dr
Emergency Room . . . . Jofe Rivira

Measure	Cases	This Hospital	State Average	U.S. Average	Top Hospital
Heart Attack Care					
ACE Inhibitor or ARB for LVSD[1]	6	100%	81%	82%	100%
Aspirin at Arrival[1]	23	91%	90%	92%	100%
Aspirin at Discharge[1]	12	75%	82%	90%	100%
Beta Blocker at Arrival[1]	15	80%	81%	87%	100%
Beta Blocker at Discharge[1]	9	78%	80%	90%	100%
Fibrinolytic Medication Timing	0	-	27%	31%	100%
PCI Within 90 Minutes of Arrival	0	-	0%	54%	95%
Smoking Cessation Advice[1]	2	100%	88%	88%	100%
Heart Failure Care					
ACE Inhibitor or ARB for LVSD[1]	17	100%	84%	82%	100%
Discharge Instructions	41	100%	72%	61%	93%
Evaluation of LVS Function	41	100%	78%	83%	99%
Smoking Cessation Advice[1]	2	100%	92%	82%	100%
Pneumonia Care					
Appropriate Initial Antibiotic[2]	28	57%	68%	83%	94%
Blood Culture Timing[1,2]	16	81%	71%	90%	100%
Influenza Vaccine[1]	4	100%	38%	70%	100%
Initial Antibiotic Timing[2]	29	52%	46%	80%	93%
Oxygenation Assessment[2]	29	97%	93%	99%	100%
Pneumococcal Vaccine[1,2]	24	83%	34%	69%	94%
Smoking Cessation Advice[1,2]	7	100%	89%	80%	100%
Surgical Infection Prevention					
Prophylactic Antibiotic Given[5]	-	-	55%	77%	95%
Prophylactic Antibiotic Selection[5]	-	-	90%	90%	100%
Prophylactic Antibiotic Stopped[5]	-	-	78%	72%	95%
Pregnancy Care					
Inpatient Neonatal Mortality	-	-	-	-	-
Third or Fourth Degree Laceration	-	-	-	3.63%	3.27%

Hospital Hermanos Melendez

Route 2 Km 11.8
Bayamon, PR 00960
Ownership: Proprietary
Emergency Services: Yes

Phone: 787-798-8181
Fax: 787-269-0085

Accredited: Yes
Licensed Beds: 211

Key Personnel:
Administrator . . . . Tomas Martinez
Chief Medical Staff . . . . Antonio Reyes-Beltran
OB/GYN Womens Health . . . . Manuel Nater, MD

Measure	Cases	This Hospital	State Average	U.S. Average	Top Hospital
Heart Attack Care					
ACE Inhibitor or ARB for LVSD[5]	-	-	81%	82%	100%
Aspirin at Arrival[5]	-	-	90%	92%	100%
Aspirin at Discharge[5]	-	-	82%	90%	100%
Beta Blocker at Arrival[5]	-	-	81%	87%	100%
Beta Blocker at Discharge[5]	-	-	80%	90%	100%
Fibrinolytic Medication Timing[5]	-	-	27%	31%	100%
PCI Within 90 Minutes of Arrival[5]	-	-	0%	54%	95%
Smoking Cessation Advice[5]	-	-	88%	88%	100%
Heart Failure Care					
ACE Inhibitor or ARB for LVSD[5]	-	-	84%	82%	100%
Discharge Instructions[5]	-	-	72%	61%	93%
Evaluation of LVS Function[5]	-	-	78%	83%	99%
Smoking Cessation Advice[5]	-	-	92%	82%	100%
Pneumonia Care					
Appropriate Initial Antibiotic[5]	-	-	68%	83%	94%
Blood Culture Timing[5]	-	-	71%	90%	100%
Influenza Vaccine[5]	-	-	38%	70%	100%
Initial Antibiotic Timing[5]	-	-	46%	80%	93%
Oxygenation Assessment[5]	-	-	93%	99%	100%
Pneumococcal Vaccine[5]	-	-	34%	69%	94%
Smoking Cessation Advice[5]	-	-	89%	80%	100%
Surgical Infection Prevention					
Prophylactic Antibiotic Given[5]	-	-	55%	77%	95%
Prophylactic Antibiotic Selection[5]	-	-	90%	90%	100%
Prophylactic Antibiotic Stopped[5]	-	-	78%	72%	95%
Pregnancy Care					
Inpatient Neonatal Mortality	-	-	-	-	-
Third or Fourth Degree Laceration	-	-	-	3.63%	3.27%

Hospital Matilde Brenes

9 J Street Extension Hermanas Davila
Bayamon, PR 00960
Ownership: Government - Federal
Emergency Services: Yes

Phone: 787-622-5420
Fax: 787-622-5432

Accredited: No
Licensed Beds: 106

Key Personnel:
Administrator . . . . Patricia Vilaro

Measure	Cases	This Hospital	State Average	U.S. Average	Top Hospital
Heart Attack Care					
ACE Inhibitor or ARB for LVSD[1,2,3]	3	67%	81%	82%	100%
Aspirin at Arrival[1,2,3]	10	100%	90%	92%	100%
Aspirin at Discharge[1,2,3]	14	71%	82%	90%	100%
Beta Blocker at Arrival[1,2,3]	8	88%	81%	87%	100%
Beta Blocker at Discharge[1,2,3]	12	75%	80%	90%	100%
Fibrinolytic Medication Timing[2,3]	0	-	27%	31%	100%
PCI Within 90 Minutes of Arrival[2]	0	-	0%	54%	95%
Smoking Cessation Advice[5]	-	-	88%	88%	100%
Heart Failure Care					
ACE Inhibitor or ARB for LVSD[1,2,3]	11	55%	84%	82%	100%
Discharge Instructions[5]	-	-	72%	61%	93%
Evaluation of LVS Function[1,2,3]	20	95%	78%	83%	99%
Smoking Cessation Advice[1,2,3]	2	50%	92%	82%	100%
Pneumonia Care					
Appropriate Initial Antibiotic[5]	-	-	68%	83%	94%
Blood Culture Timing[5]	-	-	71%	90%	100%
Influenza Vaccine[5]	-	-	38%	70%	100%
Initial Antibiotic Timing[1,2,3]	12	33%	46%	80%	93%
Oxygenation Assessment[1,2,3]	18	100%	93%	99%	100%
Pneumococcal Vaccine[1,2,3]	15	7%	34%	69%	94%
Smoking Cessation Advice[1,2,3]	6	50%	89%	80%	100%
Surgical Infection Prevention					
Prophylactic Antibiotic Given[2,3]	30	73%	55%	77%	95%
Prophylactic Antibiotic Selection[5]	-	-	90%	90%	100%
Prophylactic Antibiotic Stopped[2,3]	32	88%	78%	72%	95%
Pregnancy Care					
Inpatient Neonatal Mortality	-	-	-	-	-
Third or Fourth Degree Laceration	-	-	-	3.63%	3.27%

NOTE: Hospital profiles are in alphabetical order by state, then city, then hospital within the city; Rankings are sorted by rate in descending order and exclude hospitals with less than 25 cases; (1) The number of cases is too small (n<25) for purposes of reliably predicting hospital performance; (2) Measure reflects the hospital's indication that its submission was based upon a sample of its relevant discharges; (3) Rate reflects fewer than the maximum possible quarters of data for the measure; (4) Inaccurate information submitted and suppressed for one or more quarters; (5) No data is available from the hospital for this measure; Please refer to the User's Guide for a full explanation of data

Hospital San Pablo

PO Box 236
Bayamon, PR 00960
Ownership: Proprietary
Emergency Services: Yes
Key Personnel:
Administrator . . . . Jorge Madta

Phone: 787-740-4747
Fax: 787-798-5495
Accredited: Yes
Licensed Beds: 420

Measure	Cases	This Hospital	State Average	U.S. Average	Top Hospital
Heart Attack Care					
ACE Inhibitor or ARB for LVSD[2,3]	89	78%	81%	82%	100%
Aspirin at Arrival[2,3]	238	75%	90%	92%	100%
Aspirin at Discharge[5]	-	-	82%	90%	100%
Beta Blocker at Arrival[5]	-	-	81%	87%	100%
Beta Blocker at Discharge[5]	-	-	80%	90%	100%
Fibrinolytic Medication Timing[1,2,3]	2	50%	27%	31%	100%
PCI Within 90 Minutes of Arrival[1,2]	3	0%	0%	54%	95%
Smoking Cessation Advice[2,3]	59	98%	88%	88%	100%
Heart Failure Care					
ACE Inhibitor or ARB for LVSD[2,3]	185	75%	84%	82%	100%
Discharge Instructions[5]	-	-	72%	61%	93%
Evaluation of LVS Function[5]	-	-	78%	83%	99%
Smoking Cessation Advice[2,3]	37	97%	92%	82%	100%
Pneumonia Care					
Appropriate Initial Antibiotic[2,3]	202	69%	68%	83%	94%
Blood Culture Timing[5]	-	-	71%	90%	100%
Influenza Vaccine[5]	-	-	38%	70%	100%
Initial Antibiotic Timing[2,3]	285	55%	46%	80%	93%
Oxygenation Assessment[2,3]	291	98%	93%	99%	100%
Pneumococcal Vaccine[2,3]	202	17%	34%	69%	94%
Smoking Cessation Advice[2,3]	53	98%	89%	80%	100%
Surgical Infection Prevention					
Prophylactic Antibiotic Given[2,3]	603	84%	55%	77%	95%
Prophylactic Antibiotic Selection[2]	70	91%	90%	90%	100%
Prophylactic Antibiotic Stopped[5]	-	-	78%	72%	95%
Pregnancy Care					
Inpatient Neonatal Mortality	-	-	-	-	-
Third or Fourth Degree Laceration	-	-	-	3.63%	3.27%

Hospital Universitario Doctor Ramon Ruiz Arnau

Avenue Laurel, Urb Santa Juanita
Bayamon, PR 00956
Ownership: Government - State
Emergency Services: No
Key Personnel:
President/CEO. . . . . Nilda E Diaz Fontan
Chief Medical Staff. . . . . Robert Hunter
Emergency Room . . . . Eva Y Calderon, MD
Director Infection/Disease Control . . . . Ana M Rodriguez
CCU Spvg. Nurse . . . . Maria Torres Davilla
OB/GYN Womens Health. . . . . Blas Santamaria, MD
Chief Radiology . . . . Lorraine Vazquez
Director Respiratory Therapy . . . . Alvin Ramirez

Phone: 787-787-5151
Fax: 787-787-7979
Accredited: Yes
Licensed Beds: 415

Measure	Cases	This Hospital	State Average	U.S. Average	Top Hospital
Heart Attack Care					
ACE Inhibitor or ARB for LVSD[1,3]	12	75%	81%	82%	100%
Aspirin at Arrival[3]	41	98%	90%	92%	100%
Aspirin at Discharge[1,3]	22	50%	82%	90%	100%
Beta Blocker at Arrival[3]	41	90%	81%	87%	100%
Beta Blocker at Discharge[1,3]	21	52%	80%	90%	100%
Fibrinolytic Medication Timing[1,3]	7	29%	27%	31%	100%
PCI Within 90 Minutes of Arrival[5]	-	-	0%	54%	95%
Smoking Cessation Advice[1,3]	9	100%	88%	88%	100%
Heart Failure Care					
ACE Inhibitor or ARB for LVSD[1,3]	21	100%	84%	82%	100%
Discharge Instructions[3]	58	100%	72%	61%	93%
Evaluation of LVS Function[3]	59	100%	78%	83%	99%
Smoking Cessation Advice[1,3]	11	100%	92%	82%	100%
Pneumonia Care					
Appropriate Initial Antibiotic[3]	127	57%	68%	83%	94%
Blood Culture Timing	154	64%	71%	90%	100%
Influenza Vaccine[1]	21	29%	38%	70%	100%

Initial Antibiotic Timing[3]	150	51%	46%	80%	93%
Oxygenation Assessment[3]	155	100%	93%	99%	100%
Pneumococcal Vaccine[3]	50	56%	34%	69%	94%
Smoking Cessation Advice[3]	28	100%	89%	80%	100%
Surgical Infection Prevention					
Prophylactic Antibiotic Given[1,3]	2	0%	55%	77%	95%
Prophylactic Antibiotic Selection[1]	2	100%	90%	90%	100%
Prophylactic Antibiotic Stopped[1,3]	2	100%	78%	72%	95%
Pregnancy Care					
Inpatient Neonatal Mortality	-	-	-	-	-
Third or Fourth Degree Laceration	-	-	-	3.63%	3.27%

Hospital Interamericano de Medicina

Ave Luis Munoz Marin
Caguas, PR 00725
Ownership: Government - State
Emergency Services: Yes

Phone: 787-653-3434

Accredited: Yes

Measure	Cases	This Hospital	State Average	U.S. Average	Top Hospital
Heart Attack Care					
ACE Inhibitor or ARB for LVSD[5]	-	-	81%	82%	100%
Aspirin at Arrival[5]	-	-	90%	92%	100%
Aspirin at Discharge[5]	-	-	82%	90%	100%
Beta Blocker at Arrival[3]	71	94%	81%	87%	100%
Beta Blocker at Discharge[5]	-	-	80%	90%	100%
Fibrinolytic Medication Timing[3]	0	-	27%	31%	100%
PCI Within 90 Minutes of Arrival[5]	-	-	0%	54%	95%
Smoking Cessation Advice[1,3]	12	100%	88%	88%	100%
Heart Failure Care					
ACE Inhibitor or ARB for LVSD[3]	81	94%	84%	82%	100%
Discharge Instructions[3]	112	99%	72%	61%	93%
Evaluation of LVS Function[3]	112	89%	78%	83%	99%
Smoking Cessation Advice[1,3]	23	100%	92%	82%	100%
Pneumonia Care					
Appropriate Initial Antibiotic[5]	-	-	68%	83%	94%
Blood Culture Timing[5]	-	-	71%	90%	100%
Influenza Vaccine[5]	-	-	38%	70%	100%
Initial Antibiotic Timing[5]	-	-	46%	80%	93%
Oxygenation Assessment[2,3]	180	95%	93%	99%	100%
Pneumococcal Vaccine[5]	-	-	34%	69%	94%
Smoking Cessation Advice[2,3]	34	100%	89%	80%	100%
Surgical Infection Prevention					
Prophylactic Antibiotic Given[5]	-	-	55%	77%	95%
Prophylactic Antibiotic Selection	118	98%	90%	90%	100%
Prophylactic Antibiotic Stopped[3]	172	100%	78%	72%	95%
Pregnancy Care					
Inpatient Neonatal Mortality	-	-	-	-	-
Third or Fourth Degree Laceration	-	-	-	3.63%	3.27%

Hospital San Juan Bautista Medical Center

Carr 172 Urb Turabo Gardens
Caguas, PR 00725
Ownership: Govt - Hospital District or Authority
Emergency Services: Yes

Phone: 787-744-3141

Accredited: Yes

Measure	Cases	This Hospital	State Average	U.S. Average	Top Hospital
Heart Attack Care					
ACE Inhibitor or ARB for LVSD[1,3]	21	71%	81%	82%	100%
Aspirin at Arrival[3]	150	79%	90%	92%	100%
Aspirin at Discharge[5]	-	-	82%	90%	100%
Beta Blocker at Arrival[5]	-	-	81%	87%	100%
Beta Blocker at Discharge[5]	-	-	80%	90%	100%
Fibrinolytic Medication Timing[5]	-	-	27%	31%	100%
PCI Within 90 Minutes of Arrival	0	-	0%	54%	95%
Smoking Cessation Advice[3]	31	61%	88%	88%	100%
Heart Failure Care					
ACE Inhibitor or ARB for LVSD[1,3]	15	60%	84%	82%	100%
Discharge Instructions[3]	134	84%	72%	61%	93%
Evaluation of LVS Function[3]	134	54%	78%	83%	99%
Smoking Cessation Advice[3]	27	78%	92%	82%	100%
Pneumonia Care					
Appropriate Initial Antibiotic[3]	80	51%	68%	83%	94%

NOTE: Hospital profiles are in alphabetical order by state, then city, then hospital within the city; Rankings are sorted by rate in descending order and exclude hospitals with less than 25 cases; (1) The number of cases is too small (n<25) for purposes of reliably predicting hospital performance; (2) Measure reflects the hospital's indication that its submission was based upon a sample of its relevant discharges; (3) Rate reflects fewer than the maximum possible quarters of data for the measure; (4) Inaccurate information submitted and suppressed for one or more quarters; (5) No data is available from the hospital for this measure; Please refer to the User's Guide for a full explanation of data

Measure				
Blood Culture Timing[1]	24	33%	71%	90%	100%
Influenza Vaccine[1]	13	15%	38%	70%	100%
Initial Antibiotic Timing[5]	-	-	46%	80%	93%
Oxygenation Assessment[3]	99	99%	93%	99%	100%
Pneumococcal Vaccine[5]	-	-	34%	69%	94%
Smoking Cessation Advice[1,3]	20	40%	89%	80%	100%
Surgical Infection Prevention					
Prophylactic Antibiotic Given[5]	-	-	55%	77%	95%
Prophylactic Antibiotic Selection[5]	-	-	90%	90%	100%
Prophylactic Antibiotic Stopped[5]	-	-	78%	72%	95%
Pregnancy Care					
Inpatient Neonatal Mortality	-	-	-	-	-
Third or Fourth Degree Laceration	-	-	-	3.63%	3.27%

UPR Carolina

Ave 65th Infanteria Box 3747
Carolina, PR 00985
Ownership: Proprietary
Emergency Services: No

Phone: 787-757-1800

Accredited: Yes

Measure	Cases	This Hospital	State Average	U.S. Average	Top Hospital
Heart Attack Care					
ACE Inhibitor or ARB for LVSD[2]	142	88%	81%	82%	100%
Aspirin at Arrival[2]	238	93%	90%	92%	100%
Aspirin at Discharge[2]	175	86%	82%	90%	100%
Beta Blocker at Arrival[2]	190	88%	81%	87%	100%
Beta Blocker at Discharge[2]	173	90%	80%	90%	100%
Fibrinolytic Medication Timing[1,2]	21	38%	27%	31%	100%
PCI Within 90 Minutes of Arrival[2]	0	-	0%	54%	95%
Smoking Cessation Advice[2]	40	90%	88%	88%	100%
Heart Failure Care					
ACE Inhibitor or ARB for LVSD	101	93%	84%	82%	100%
Discharge Instructions	318	27%	72%	61%	93%
Evaluation of LVS Function	319	100%	78%	83%	99%
Smoking Cessation Advice	38	82%	92%	82%	100%
Pneumonia Care					
Appropriate Initial Antibiotic	292	57%	68%	83%	94%
Blood Culture Timing	84	69%	71%	90%	100%
Influenza Vaccine	46	11%	38%	70%	100%
Initial Antibiotic Timing	372	39%	46%	80%	93%
Oxygenation Assessment	409	97%	93%	99%	100%
Pneumococcal Vaccine	206	9%	34%	69%	94%
Smoking Cessation Advice	80	80%	89%	80%	100%
Surgical Infection Prevention					
Prophylactic Antibiotic Given	112	77%	55%	77%	95%
Prophylactic Antibiotic Selection	27	100%	90%	90%	100%
Prophylactic Antibiotic Stopped	101	73%	78%	72%	95%
Pregnancy Care					
Inpatient Neonatal Mortality	-	-	-	-	-
Third or Fourth Degree Laceration	-	-	-	3.63%	3.27%

Castaner General Hospital

Saint 135 Km 64 2
Castaner, PR 00631
Ownership: Government - Local
Emergency Services: Yes

Phone: 787-829-5010

Accredited: No

Measure	Cases	This Hospital	State Average	U.S. Average	Top Hospital
Heart Attack Care					
ACE Inhibitor or ARB for LVSD[5]	-	-	81%	82%	100%
Aspirin at Arrival[5]	-	-	90%	92%	100%
Aspirin at Discharge[5]	-	-	82%	90%	100%
Beta Blocker at Arrival[5]	-	-	81%	87%	100%
Beta Blocker at Discharge[5]	-	-	80%	90%	100%
Fibrinolytic Medication Timing[5]	-	-	27%	31%	100%
PCI Within 90 Minutes of Arrival[5]	-	-	0%	54%	95%
Smoking Cessation Advice[5]	-	-	88%	88%	100%
Heart Failure Care					
ACE Inhibitor or ARB for LVSD[3]	0	-	84%	82%	100%
Discharge Instructions[1,3]	2	0%	72%	61%	93%
Evaluation of LVS Function[1,3]	2	0%	78%	83%	99%
Smoking Cessation Advice[3]	0	-	92%	82%	100%

Measure				
Pneumonia Care					
Appropriate Initial Antibiotic[5]	-	-	68%	83%	94%
Blood Culture Timing[5]	-	-	71%	90%	100%
Influenza Vaccine[5]	-	-	38%	70%	100%
Initial Antibiotic Timing[5]	-	-	46%	80%	93%
Oxygenation Assessment[5]	-	-	93%	99%	100%
Pneumococcal Vaccine[5]	-	-	34%	69%	94%
Smoking Cessation Advice[5]	-	-	89%	80%	100%
Surgical Infection Prevention					
Prophylactic Antibiotic Given[5]	-	-	55%	77%	95%
Prophylactic Antibiotic Selection[5]	-	-	90%	90%	100%
Prophylactic Antibiotic Stopped[5]	-	-	78%	72%	95%
Pregnancy Care					
Inpatient Neonatal Mortality	-	-	-	-	-
Third or Fourth Degree Laceration	-	-	-	3.63%	3.27%

Hospital Menonita De Cayey

4 H Mendoza Street
Cayey, PR 00736
Ownership: Voluntary non-profit - Private
Emergency Services: No
Key Personnel:
Administrator . . . . Pedro Melendez
Chief Medical Staff . . . . Sandra Vazquez
Emergency Room . . . . Ruben Mendez, MD
Director Infection/Disease Control . . . . Carmen E Flores, RN
Director Medical/Surgical Nursing . . . . Maria Colon, RN
OB/GYN Womens Health . . . . Floreni Perez
Chief Radiology . . . . Silverio Perez, MD
Director Respiratory Therapy . . . . Mayra Febus

Phone: 787-263-1001
Fax: 787-535-1034
Accredited: No
Licensed Beds: 118

Measure	Cases	This Hospital	State Average	U.S. Average	Top Hospital
Heart Attack Care					
ACE Inhibitor or ARB for LVSD[1,2]	2	100%	81%	82%	100%
Aspirin at Arrival[2]	49	96%	90%	92%	100%
Aspirin at Discharge[2]	30	80%	82%	90%	100%
Beta Blocker at Arrival[2]	51	80%	81%	87%	100%
Beta Blocker at Discharge[2]	41	83%	80%	90%	100%
Fibrinolytic Medication Timing[1,2]	5	0%	27%	31%	100%
PCI Within 90 Minutes of Arrival[2]	0	-	0%	54%	95%
Smoking Cessation Advice[1,2]	8	100%	88%	88%	100%
Heart Failure Care					
ACE Inhibitor or ARB for LVSD[2]	60	93%	84%	82%	100%
Discharge Instructions[2]	224	41%	72%	61%	93%
Evaluation of LVS Function[2]	222	65%	78%	83%	99%
Smoking Cessation Advice[2]	30	97%	92%	82%	100%
Pneumonia Care					
Appropriate Initial Antibiotic[2]	55	85%	68%	83%	94%
Blood Culture Timing[2]	25	52%	71%	90%	100%
Influenza Vaccine[1,2]	13	54%	38%	70%	100%
Initial Antibiotic Timing[2]	68	34%	46%	80%	93%
Oxygenation Assessment[2]	73	96%	93%	99%	100%
Pneumococcal Vaccine[2]	36	39%	34%	69%	94%
Smoking Cessation Advice[1,2]	17	94%	89%	80%	100%
Surgical Infection Prevention					
Prophylactic Antibiotic Given[2,3]	55	60%	55%	77%	95%
Prophylactic Antibiotic Selection[2]	31	97%	90%	90%	100%
Prophylactic Antibiotic Stopped[2,3]	54	89%	78%	72%	95%
Pregnancy Care					
Inpatient Neonatal Mortality	-	-	-	-	-
Third or Fourth Degree Laceration	-	-	-	3.63%	3.27%

Hospital San Cristobal

Carr 506 Km 1 0
Coto Laurel, PR 00780
Ownership: Voluntary non-profit - Private
Emergency Services: Yes

Phone: 787-848-2100

Accredited: No

Measure	Cases	This Hospital	State Average	U.S. Average	Top Hospital
Heart Attack Care					
ACE Inhibitor or ARB for LVSD	31	94%	81%	82%	100%
Aspirin at Arrival	67	85%	90%	92%	100%

NOTE: Hospital profiles are in alphabetical order by state, then city, then hospital within the city; Rankings are sorted by rate in descending order and exclude hospitals with less than 25 cases; (1) The number of cases is too small (n<25) for purposes of reliably predicting hospital performance; (2) Measure reflects the hospital's indication that its submission was based upon a sample of its relevant discharges; (3) Rate reflects fewer than the maximum possible quarters of data for the measure; (4) Inaccurate information submitted and suppressed for one or more quarters; (5) No data is available from the hospital for this measure; Please refer to the User's Guide for a full explanation of data

Measure	Cases	This Hospital	State Average	U.S. Average	Top Hospital
Aspirin at Discharge[5]	-	-	82%	90%	100%
Beta Blocker at Arrival	69	99%	81%	87%	100%
Beta Blocker at Discharge	73	95%	80%	90%	100%
Fibrinolytic Medication Timing[1]	2	50%	27%	31%	100%
PCI Within 90 Minutes of Arrival	0	-	0%	54%	95%
Smoking Cessation Advice[1]	18	100%	88%	88%	100%
Heart Failure Care					
ACE Inhibitor or ARB for LVSD	25	92%	84%	82%	100%
Discharge Instructions	42	69%	72%	61%	93%
Evaluation of LVS Function[5]	-	-	78%	83%	99%
Smoking Cessation Advice[1]	14	93%	92%	82%	100%
Pneumonia Care					
Appropriate Initial Antibiotic[5]	-	-	68%	83%	94%
Blood Culture Timing[5]	-	-	71%	90%	100%
Influenza Vaccine	0	-	38%	70%	100%
Initial Antibiotic Timing[5]	-	-	46%	80%	93%
Oxygenation Assessment	50	100%	93%	99%	100%
Pneumococcal Vaccine[5]	-	-	34%	69%	94%
Smoking Cessation Advice[1]	14	93%	89%	80%	100%
Surgical Infection Prevention					
Prophylactic Antibiotic Given[5]	-	-	55%	77%	95%
Prophylactic Antibiotic Selection	0	-	90%	90%	100%
Prophylactic Antibiotic Stopped	55	100%	78%	72%	95%
Pregnancy Care					
Inpatient Neonatal Mortality	-	-	-	-	-
Third or Fourth Degree Laceration	-	-	-	3.63%	3.27%

Hima-San Pablo Fajardo

General Valero Ave#404
Fajardo, PR 00738
Ownership: Proprietary
Emergency Services: Yes

Phone: 787-655-0505

Accredited: Yes

Measure	Cases	This Hospital	State Average	U.S. Average	Top Hospital
Heart Attack Care					
ACE Inhibitor or ARB for LVSD[1,3]	7	86%	81%	82%	100%
Aspirin at Arrival[1,3]	21	86%	90%	92%	100%
Aspirin at Discharge[1,3]	12	92%	82%	90%	100%
Beta Blocker at Arrival[1,3]	17	82%	81%	87%	100%
Beta Blocker at Discharge[1,3]	11	100%	80%	90%	100%
Fibrinolytic Medication Timing[1,3]	1	0%	27%	31%	100%
PCI Within 90 Minutes of Arrival	0	-	0%	54%	95%
Smoking Cessation Advice[1,3]	1	100%	88%	88%	100%
Heart Failure Care					
ACE Inhibitor or ARB for LVSD	65	89%	84%	82%	100%
Discharge Instructions	107	95%	72%	61%	93%
Evaluation of LVS Function	110	85%	78%	83%	99%
Smoking Cessation Advice[1]	3	100%	92%	82%	100%
Pneumonia Care					
Appropriate Initial Antibiotic	75	48%	68%	83%	94%
Blood Culture Timing	36	78%	71%	90%	100%
Influenza Vaccine[1]	1	0%	38%	70%	100%
Initial Antibiotic Timing	78	54%	46%	80%	93%
Oxygenation Assessment	83	93%	93%	99%	100%
Pneumococcal Vaccine	48	10%	34%	69%	94%
Smoking Cessation Advice[1]	6	100%	89%	80%	100%
Surgical Infection Prevention					
Prophylactic Antibiotic Given	43	26%	55%	77%	95%
Prophylactic Antibiotic Selection	0	-	90%	90%	100%
Prophylactic Antibiotic Stopped	36	100%	78%	72%	95%
Pregnancy Care					
Inpatient Neonatal Mortality	-	-	-	-	-
Third or Fourth Degree Laceration	-	-	-	3.63%	3.27%

Hospital Pavia Santurce

Calle Profesor Augusto Rodriguez #1462
Fernandez Juncos, PR 00910
Ownership: Voluntary non-profit - Private
Emergency Services: Yes

Phone: 787-727-6060

Accredited: Yes

Measure	Cases	This Hospital	State Average	U.S. Average	Top Hospital
Heart Attack Care					

Measure	Cases	This Hospital	State Average	U.S. Average	Top Hospital
ACE Inhibitor or ARB for LVSD[5]	-	-	81%	82%	100%
Aspirin at Arrival[5]	-	-	90%	92%	100%
Aspirin at Discharge	205	93%	82%	90%	100%
Beta Blocker at Arrival[5]	-	-	81%	87%	100%
Beta Blocker at Discharge[5]	-	-	80%	90%	100%
Fibrinolytic Medication Timing	0	-	27%	31%	100%
PCI Within 90 Minutes of Arrival	0	-	0%	54%	95%
Smoking Cessation Advice	60	98%	88%	88%	100%
Heart Failure Care					
ACE Inhibitor or ARB for LVSD	84	89%	84%	82%	100%
Discharge Instructions	215	100%	72%	61%	93%
Evaluation of LVS Function[5]	-	-	78%	83%	99%
Smoking Cessation Advice	32	100%	92%	82%	100%
Pneumonia Care					
Appropriate Initial Antibiotic	204	60%	68%	83%	94%
Blood Culture Timing[5]	-	-	71%	90%	100%
Influenza Vaccine[4,5]	-	-	38%	70%	100%
Initial Antibiotic Timing[5]	-	-	46%	80%	93%
Oxygenation Assessment	218	94%	93%	99%	100%
Pneumococcal Vaccine[5]	-	-	34%	69%	94%
Smoking Cessation Advice	27	89%	89%	80%	100%
Surgical Infection Prevention					
Prophylactic Antibiotic Given[5]	-	-	55%	77%	95%
Prophylactic Antibiotic Selection	151	89%	90%	90%	100%
Prophylactic Antibiotic Stopped[5]	-	-	78%	72%	95%
Pregnancy Care					
Inpatient Neonatal Mortality	-	-	-	-	-
Third or Fourth Degree Laceration	-	-	-	3.63%	3.27%

Hospital Episcopal Cristo Redentor

Alternate Name: Hospital De Area Doctor Buitrago
Urb La Hacienda
Guayama, PR 00784
Ownership: Proprietary
Emergency Services: Yes

Phone: 787-864-4300
Fax: 787-864-4466
Accredited: Yes
Licensed Beds: 161

Key Personnel:
Administrator . . . . Jose J Core
Chief Medical Staff. . . . . Jorge Del Pozo
Emergency Room . . . . Jose Anglero Ramos
Director Infection/Disease Control . . . . Carlos Leon Valiente
CCU Spvg. Nurse . . . . Jozita Carrasquillo
OB/GYN Womens Health. . . . . Edward Hernandez
Chief Radiology . . . . Jose Pratt
Director Respiratory Therapy . . . . Rafael J Perez Brache

Measure	Cases	This Hospital	State Average	U.S. Average	Top Hospital
Heart Attack Care					
ACE Inhibitor or ARB for LVSD[1]	8	88%	81%	82%	100%
Aspirin at Arrival	53	77%	90%	92%	100%
Aspirin at Discharge[1]	18	72%	82%	90%	100%
Beta Blocker at Arrival	58	66%	81%	87%	100%
Beta Blocker at Discharge[1]	20	80%	80%	90%	100%
Fibrinolytic Medication Timing	0	-	27%	31%	100%
PCI Within 90 Minutes of Arrival	0	-	0%	54%	95%
Smoking Cessation Advice[1]	1	100%	88%	88%	100%
Heart Failure Care					
ACE Inhibitor or ARB for LVSD[2]	28	82%	84%	82%	100%
Discharge Instructions[2]	88	69%	72%	61%	93%
Evaluation of LVS Function[2]	88	72%	78%	83%	99%
Smoking Cessation Advice[1,2]	16	94%	92%	82%	100%
Pneumonia Care					
Appropriate Initial Antibiotic	42	55%	68%	83%	94%
Blood Culture Timing[1]	11	82%	71%	90%	100%
Influenza Vaccine[1]	7	14%	38%	70%	100%
Initial Antibiotic Timing	47	40%	46%	80%	93%
Oxygenation Assessment	49	90%	93%	99%	100%
Pneumococcal Vaccine	25	36%	34%	69%	94%
Smoking Cessation Advice[1]	4	75%	89%	80%	100%
Surgical Infection Prevention					
Prophylactic Antibiotic Given	63	14%	55%	77%	95%
Prophylactic Antibiotic Selection[1]	21	95%	90%	90%	100%
Prophylactic Antibiotic Stopped	63	52%	78%	72%	95%
Pregnancy Care					

NOTE: Hospital profiles are in alphabetical order by state, then city, then hospital within the city; Rankings are sorted by rate in descending order and exclude hospitals with less than 25 cases; (1) The number of cases is too small (n<25) for purposes of reliably predicting hospital performance; (2) Measure reflects the hospital's indication that its submission was based upon a sample of its relevant discharges; (3) Rate reflects fewer than the maximum possible quarters of data for the measure; (4) Inaccurate information submitted and suppressed for one or more quarters; (5) No data is available from the hospital for this measure; Please refer to the User's Guide for a full explanation of data

Measure				
Inpatient Neonatal Mortality	-	-	-	-	-
Third or Fourth Degree Laceration	-	-	-	3.63%	3.27%

Hospital Santa Rosa

Alternate Name: Santa Rosa Clinic
PO Box 10008
Guayama, PR 00785
Ownership: Voluntary non-profit - Other
Emergency Services: Yes

Phone: 787-864-0101
Fax: 787-866-0489
Accredited: No
Licensed Beds: 99

Key Personnel:
CEO . . . . Herson Lomorales

Measure	Cases	This Hospital	State Average	U.S. Average	Top Hospital
Heart Attack Care					
ACE Inhibitor or ARB for LVSD[1,2]	1	100%	81%	82%	100%
Aspirin at Arrival[1,2]	9	89%	90%	92%	100%
Aspirin at Discharge[1,2]	3	100%	82%	90%	100%
Beta Blocker at Arrival[1,2]	10	100%	81%	87%	100%
Beta Blocker at Discharge[1,2]	9	100%	80%	90%	100%
Fibrinolytic Medication Timing[5]	-	-	27%	31%	100%
PCI Within 90 Minutes of Arrival[5]	-	-	0%	54%	95%
Smoking Cessation Advice[1,2]	5	100%	88%	88%	100%
Heart Failure Care					
ACE Inhibitor or ARB for LVSD[1,2]	11	100%	84%	82%	100%
Discharge Instructions[2]	29	100%	72%	61%	93%
Evaluation of LVS Function[2]	29	100%	78%	83%	99%
Smoking Cessation Advice[1,2]	5	100%	92%	82%	100%
Pneumonia Care					
Appropriate Initial Antibiotic[1,2]	13	77%	68%	83%	94%
Blood Culture Timing[2]	0	-	71%	90%	100%
Influenza Vaccine[4,5]	-	-	38%	70%	100%
Initial Antibiotic Timing[5]	-	-	46%	80%	93%
Oxygenation Assessment[1,2]	18	100%	93%	99%	100%
Pneumococcal Vaccine[1,2]	13	46%	34%	69%	94%
Smoking Cessation Advice[1,2]	3	100%	89%	80%	100%
Surgical Infection Prevention					
Prophylactic Antibiotic Given[1,2,3]	4	50%	55%	77%	95%
Prophylactic Antibiotic Selection[1,2]	1	100%	90%	90%	100%
Prophylactic Antibiotic Stopped[1,2,3]	4	50%	78%	72%	95%
Pregnancy Care					
Inpatient Neonatal Mortality	-	-	-	-	-
Third or Fourth Degree Laceration	-	-	-	3.63%	3.27%

Auxilio Mutuo Hospital

Ponce De Leon Avenue
PO Box 191227
San Juan, PR 00918
E-mail: jgalarce@auxilio.com
URL: www.auxiliopr.com
Ownership: Voluntary non-profit - Private
Emergency Services: Yes

Phone: 787-758-2000
Fax: 787-771-7951

Accredited: Yes
Licensed Beds: 510

Key Personnel:
President/CEO . . . . Enrique Fierres
Chief Medical Staff . . . . Angel Rodriguez
Chief Catheterization Laboratory . . . . Efrain Feliciano, MD
Emergency Room . . . . Wilfredo Rendon, MD
Director Infection/Disease Control . . . . Quirico Canario-Brea, MD
CCU Spvg. Nurse . . . . Digna Cartagena
OB/GYN Womens Health . . . . Adrian Colon Laracuente
Chief Radiology . . . . Fernando Salduondo, MD
Director Respiratory Therapy . . . . Angel L Rivera, MD

Measure	Cases	This Hospital	State Average	U.S. Average	Top Hospital
Heart Attack Care					
ACE Inhibitor or ARB for LVSD[3]	33	73%	81%	82%	100%
Aspirin at Arrival[3]	132	85%	90%	92%	100%
Aspirin at Discharge[3]	138	85%	82%	90%	100%
Beta Blocker at Arrival[3]	105	73%	81%	87%	100%
Beta Blocker at Discharge[3]	150	81%	80%	90%	100%
Fibrinolytic Medication Timing[3]	0	-	27%	31%	100%
PCI Within 90 Minutes of Arrival[1]	2	0%	0%	54%	95%
Smoking Cessation Advice[1,3]	16	81%	88%	88%	100%
Heart Failure Care					

Measure	Cases	This Hospital	State Average	U.S. Average	Top Hospital
ACE Inhibitor or ARB for LVSD[3]	86	64%	84%	82%	100%
Discharge Instructions[3]	302	35%	72%	61%	93%
Evaluation of LVS Function[3]	304	82%	78%	83%	99%
Smoking Cessation Advice[1,3]	11	91%	92%	82%	100%
Pneumonia Care					
Appropriate Initial Antibiotic[3]	137	61%	68%	83%	94%
Blood Culture Timing	213	71%	71%	90%	100%
Influenza Vaccine	45	47%	38%	70%	100%
Initial Antibiotic Timing[3]	248	45%	46%	80%	93%
Oxygenation Assessment[3]	268	81%	93%	99%	100%
Pneumococcal Vaccine[3]	144	49%	34%	69%	94%
Smoking Cessation Advice[1,3]	12	42%	89%	80%	100%
Surgical Infection Prevention					
Prophylactic Antibiotic Given[2,3]	171	77%	55%	77%	95%
Prophylactic Antibiotic Selection[2]	89	99%	90%	90%	100%
Prophylactic Antibiotic Stopped[2,3]	158	100%	78%	72%	95%
Pregnancy Care					
Inpatient Neonatal Mortality	-	-	-	-	-
Third or Fourth Degree Laceration	-	-	-	3.63%	3.27%

Hospital Pavia Hato Rey

Ave Ponce De Leon 435
Hato Rey, PR 00919
Ownership: Voluntary non-profit - Private
Emergency Services: Yes

Phone: 787-754-0909

Accredited: Yes

Measure	Cases	This Hospital	State Average	U.S. Average	Top Hospital
Heart Attack Care					
ACE Inhibitor or ARB for LVSD[5]	-	-	81%	82%	100%
Aspirin at Arrival[5]	-	-	90%	92%	100%
Aspirin at Discharge[5]	-	-	82%	90%	100%
Beta Blocker at Arrival[1,3]	11	91%	81%	87%	100%
Beta Blocker at Discharge[5]	-	-	80%	90%	100%
Fibrinolytic Medication Timing[3]	0	-	27%	31%	100%
PCI Within 90 Minutes of Arrival	0	-	0%	54%	95%
Smoking Cessation Advice[1,3]	1	100%	88%	88%	100%
Heart Failure Care					
ACE Inhibitor or ARB for LVSD[5]	-	-	84%	82%	100%
Discharge Instructions[5]	-	-	72%	61%	93%
Evaluation of LVS Function[5]	-	-	78%	83%	99%
Smoking Cessation Advice[1,3]	12	92%	92%	82%	100%
Pneumonia Care					
Appropriate Initial Antibiotic[3]	52	73%	68%	83%	94%
Blood Culture Timing[1,3]	14	71%	71%	90%	100%
Influenza Vaccine[5]	-	-	38%	70%	100%
Initial Antibiotic Timing[3]	54	46%	46%	80%	93%
Oxygenation Assessment[3]	59	90%	93%	99%	100%
Pneumococcal Vaccine[5]	-	-	34%	69%	94%
Smoking Cessation Advice[1,3]	17	88%	89%	80%	100%
Surgical Infection Prevention					
Prophylactic Antibiotic Given[5]	-	-	55%	77%	95%
Prophylactic Antibiotic Selection[5]	-	-	90%	90%	100%
Prophylactic Antibiotic Stopped[5]	-	-	78%	72%	95%
Pregnancy Care					
Inpatient Neonatal Mortality	-	-	-	-	-
Third or Fourth Degree Laceration	-	-	-	3.63%	3.27%

Hima Humacao

Ave Font Martelo #3
Humacao, PR 00792
Ownership: Proprietary
Emergency Services: Yes

Phone: 787-656-2424

Accredited: Yes

Measure	Cases	This Hospital	State Average	U.S. Average	Top Hospital
Heart Attack Care					
ACE Inhibitor or ARB for LVSD[1,3]	13	100%	81%	82%	100%
Aspirin at Arrival[3]	55	96%	90%	92%	100%
Aspirin at Discharge[3]	48	100%	82%	90%	100%
Beta Blocker at Arrival[3]	51	96%	81%	87%	100%
Beta Blocker at Discharge[3]	48	100%	80%	90%	100%
Fibrinolytic Medication Timing[1,3]	1	0%	27%	31%	100%
PCI Within 90 Minutes of Arrival[5]	-	-	0%	54%	95%

NOTE: Hospital profiles are in alphabetical order by state, then city, then hospital within the city; Rankings are sorted by rate in descending order and exclude hospitals with less than 25 cases; (1) The number of cases is too small (n<25) for purposes of reliably predicting hospital performance; (2) Measure reflects the hospital's indication that its submission was based upon a sample of its relevant discharges; (3) Rate reflects fewer than the maximum possible quarters of data for the measure; (4) Inaccurate information submitted and suppressed for one or more quarters; (5) No data is available from the hospital for this measure; Please refer to the User's Guide for a full explanation of data

Measure		This Hospital	State Average	U.S. Average	Top Hospital
Smoking Cessation Advice[1,3]	10	100%	88%	88%	100%
Heart Failure Care					
ACE Inhibitor or ARB for LVSD[3]	31	100%	84%	82%	100%
Discharge Instructions[3]	122	93%	72%	61%	93%
Evaluation of LVS Function[3]	122	93%	78%	83%	99%
Smoking Cessation Advice[1,3]	12	100%	92%	82%	100%
Pneumonia Care					
Appropriate Initial Antibiotic[3]	141	88%	68%	83%	94%
Blood Culture Timing[3]	80	89%	71%	90%	100%
Influenza Vaccine	35	34%	38%	70%	100%
Initial Antibiotic Timing[3]	151	63%	46%	80%	93%
Oxygenation Assessment[3]	155	99%	93%	99%	100%
Pneumococcal Vaccine[3]	91	34%	34%	69%	94%
Smoking Cessation Advice[1,3]	23	100%	89%	80%	100%
Surgical Infection Prevention					
Prophylactic Antibiotic Given[5]	-	-	55%	77%	95%
Prophylactic Antibiotic Selection[5]	-	-	90%	90%	100%
Prophylactic Antibiotic Stopped[5]	-	-	78%	72%	95%
Pregnancy Care					
Inpatient Neonatal Mortality	-	-	-	-	-
Third or Fourth Degree Laceration	-	-	-	3.63%	3.27%

Hospital Doctor Dominguez

300 Font Martelo Avenue
Humacao, PR 00792
Ownership: Voluntary non-profit - Private
Emergency Services: Yes

Phone: 787-852-0505
Fax: 787-850-4230
Accredited: No
Licensed Beds: 60

Key Personnel:
Administrator . . . . Neffer E Carrillo
Chief Medical Staff. . . . . Carmelo Herrero, MD
Emergency Room . . . . Ana P Perez, MD
Director Infection/Disease Control . . . . Agripino Lugo, MD
OB/GYN Womens Health. . . . . Rafael Viceas, MD
Chief Radiology . . . . Jose A Nassar, MD
Director Respiratory Therapy . . . . Ahmed Bajandad, MD

Measure	Cases	This Hospital	State Average	U.S. Average	Top Hospital
Heart Attack Care					
ACE Inhibitor or ARB for LVSD[1,3]	8	100%	81%	82%	100%
Aspirin at Arrival[1,3]	16	81%	90%	92%	100%
Aspirin at Discharge[1,3]	21	100%	82%	90%	100%
Beta Blocker at Arrival[1,3]	16	75%	81%	87%	100%
Beta Blocker at Discharge[1,3]	20	95%	80%	90%	100%
Fibrinolytic Medication Timing[1,3]	12	33%	27%	31%	100%
PCI Within 90 Minutes of Arrival	0	-	0%	54%	95%
Smoking Cessation Advice[1,3]	5	80%	88%	88%	100%
Heart Failure Care					
ACE Inhibitor or ARB for LVSD[1,3]	9	100%	84%	82%	100%
Discharge Instructions[3]	41	49%	72%	61%	93%
Evaluation of LVS Function[3]	26	62%	78%	83%	99%
Smoking Cessation Advice[1,3]	5	100%	92%	82%	100%
Pneumonia Care					
Appropriate Initial Antibiotic[3]	59	83%	68%	83%	94%
Blood Culture Timing[1]	8	75%	71%	90%	100%
Influenza Vaccine[1]	20	5%	38%	70%	100%
Initial Antibiotic Timing[3]	58	10%	46%	80%	93%
Oxygenation Assessment[3]	79	92%	93%	99%	100%
Pneumococcal Vaccine[3]	49	14%	34%	69%	94%
Smoking Cessation Advice[1,3]	12	100%	89%	80%	100%
Surgical Infection Prevention					
Prophylactic Antibiotic Given[5]	-	-	55%	77%	95%
Prophylactic Antibiotic Selection[5]	-	-	90%	90%	100%
Prophylactic Antibiotic Stopped[5]	-	-	78%	72%	95%
Pregnancy Care					
Inpatient Neonatal Mortality	-	-	-	-	-
Third or Fourth Degree Laceration	-	-	-	3.63%	3.27%

Ryder Memorial Hospital

355 Font Martelo Street
Box 859
Humacao, PR 00919
Ownership: Voluntary non-profit - Private
Emergency Services: Yes

Phone: 787-852-0768
Fax: 787-656-0737

Accredited: No
Licensed Beds: 144

Key Personnel:
CEO . . . . Nemuel Artiles
Chief Medical Staff . . . . Juan Gonsalez, MD
Director of Cardiology/Cardiac Lab . . . . Wistremondo Dones, MD
Emergency Room . . . . Juan Hernandez
Director of Pulmonary/Respiratory Care . . . . . . Elizabeth Rodrigueb

Measure	Cases	This Hospital	State Average	U.S. Average	Top Hospital
Heart Attack Care					
ACE Inhibitor or ARB for LVSD[1,3]	4	100%	81%	82%	100%
Aspirin at Arrival[3]	27	96%	90%	92%	100%
Aspirin at Discharge[1,3]	22	86%	82%	90%	100%
Beta Blocker at Arrival[3]	27	89%	81%	87%	100%
Beta Blocker at Discharge[1,3]	23	87%	80%	90%	100%
Fibrinolytic Medication Timing[1,3]	1	100%	27%	31%	100%
PCI Within 90 Minutes of Arrival	0	-	0%	54%	95%
Smoking Cessation Advice[5]	-	-	88%	88%	100%
Heart Failure Care					
ACE Inhibitor or ARB for LVSD[1,3]	7	86%	84%	82%	100%
Discharge Instructions[5]	-	-	72%	61%	93%
Evaluation of LVS Function[3]	48	81%	78%	83%	99%
Smoking Cessation Advice[5]	-	-	92%	82%	100%
Pneumonia Care					
Appropriate Initial Antibiotic[5]	-	-	68%	83%	94%
Blood Culture Timing[3]	29	97%	71%	90%	100%
Influenza Vaccine[5]	-	-	38%	70%	100%
Initial Antibiotic Timing[3]	26	27%	46%	80%	93%
Oxygenation Assessment[3]	29	100%	93%	99%	100%
Pneumococcal Vaccine[3]	25	24%	34%	69%	94%
Smoking Cessation Advice[5]	-	-	89%	80%	100%
Surgical Infection Prevention					
Prophylactic Antibiotic Given[5]	-	-	55%	77%	95%
Prophylactic Antibiotic Selection[1]	10	100%	90%	90%	100%
Prophylactic Antibiotic Stopped[1,3]	15	100%	78%	72%	95%
Pregnancy Care					
Inpatient Neonatal Mortality	-	-	-	-	-
Third or Fourth Degree Laceration	-	-	-	3.63%	3.27%

Doctors Center Hospital

State Road No 2, Km 47 7
Manati, PR 00674
Ownership: Proprietary
Emergency Services: Yes

Phone: 787-854-3322

Accredited: No

Measure	Cases	This Hospital	State Average	U.S. Average	Top Hospital
Heart Attack Care					
ACE Inhibitor or ARB for LVSD[1,2,3]	3	100%	81%	82%	100%
Aspirin at Arrival[1,2,3]	12	100%	90%	92%	100%
Aspirin at Discharge[1,2,3]	5	100%	82%	90%	100%
Beta Blocker at Arrival[1,2,3]	11	73%	81%	87%	100%
Beta Blocker at Discharge[1,2,3]	5	80%	80%	90%	100%
Fibrinolytic Medication Timing[2,3]	0	-	27%	31%	100%
PCI Within 90 Minutes of Arrival[2]	0	-	0%	54%	95%
Smoking Cessation Advice[1,2,3]	1	0%	88%	88%	100%
Heart Failure Care					
ACE Inhibitor or ARB for LVSD[1,2,3]	13	100%	84%	82%	100%
Discharge Instructions[2,3]	35	100%	72%	61%	93%
Evaluation of LVS Function[2,3]	35	89%	78%	83%	99%
Smoking Cessation Advice[1,2,3]	1	100%	92%	82%	100%
Pneumonia Care					
Appropriate Initial Antibiotic[1,2,3]	19	79%	68%	83%	94%
Blood Culture Timing[1,2,3]	16	38%	71%	90%	100%
Influenza Vaccine[5]	-	-	38%	70%	100%
Initial Antibiotic Timing[2,3]	28	21%	46%	80%	93%
Oxygenation Assessment[2,3]	28	100%	93%	99%	100%
Pneumococcal Vaccine[5]	-	-	34%	69%	94%

NOTE: Hospital profiles are in alphabetical order by state, then city, then hospital within the city; Rankings are sorted by rate in descending order and exclude hospitals with less than 25 cases; (1) The number of cases is too small (n<25) for purposes of reliably predicting hospital performance; (2) Measure reflects the hospital's indication that its submission was based upon a sample of its relevant discharges; (3) Rate reflects fewer than the maximum possible quarters of data for the measure; (4) Inaccurate information submitted and suppressed for one or more quarters; (5) No data is available from the hospital for this measure; Please refer to the User's Guide for a full explanation of data

Smoking Cessation Advice[1,2,3]	3	100%	89%	80%	100%
Surgical Infection Prevention					
Prophylactic Antibiotic Given[2,3]	29	45%	55%	77%	95%
Prophylactic Antibiotic Selection[1,2]	17	35%	90%	90%	100%
Prophylactic Antibiotic Stopped[2,3]	29	24%	78%	72%	95%
Pregnancy Care					
Inpatient Neonatal Mortality	-	-	-	-	-
Third or Fourth Degree Laceration	-	-	-	3.63%	3.27%

Manati Medical Center Doctor Otero Lopez

Calle Hernandez Carrion Urb Atenas   Phone: 787-621-3700
Manati, PR 00674
Ownership: Proprietary   Accredited: Yes
Emergency Services: Yes

Measure	Cases	This Hospital	State Average	U.S. Average	Top Hospital
Heart Attack Care					
ACE Inhibitor or ARB for LVSD	32	100%	81%	82%	100%
Aspirin at Arrival	195	99%	90%	92%	100%
Aspirin at Discharge	91	100%	82%	90%	100%
Beta Blocker at Arrival	162	95%	81%	87%	100%
Beta Blocker at Discharge	77	95%	80%	90%	100%
Fibrinolytic Medication Timing[5]	-	-	27%	31%	100%
PCI Within 90 Minutes of Arrival[5]	-	-	0%	54%	95%
Smoking Cessation Advice	35	100%	88%	88%	100%
Heart Failure Care					
ACE Inhibitor or ARB for LVSD	150	100%	84%	82%	100%
Discharge Instructions	493	100%	72%	61%	93%
Evaluation of LVS Function	493	100%	78%	83%	99%
Smoking Cessation Advice	59	100%	92%	82%	100%
Pneumonia Care					
Appropriate Initial Antibiotic[5]	-	-	68%	83%	94%
Blood Culture Timing[5]	-	-	71%	90%	100%
Influenza Vaccine	57	56%	38%	70%	100%
Initial Antibiotic Timing	393	92%	46%	80%	93%
Oxygenation Assessment	394	100%	93%	99%	100%
Pneumococcal Vaccine	232	40%	34%	69%	94%
Smoking Cessation Advice	135	100%	89%	80%	100%
Surgical Infection Prevention					
Prophylactic Antibiotic Given[5]	-	-	55%	77%	95%
Prophylactic Antibiotic Selection[1]	22	91%	90%	90%	100%
Prophylactic Antibiotic Stopped[1]	22	95%	78%	72%	95%
Pregnancy Care					
Inpatient Neonatal Mortality	-	-	-	-	-
Third or Fourth Degree Laceration	-	-	-	3.63%	3.27%

Professional Hospital

Road #2 Km 49 5 #3 Interseccion 685   Phone: 787-884-0505
Manati, PR 00674
Ownership: Voluntary non-profit - Private   Accredited: No
Emergency Services: Yes

Measure	Cases	This Hospital	State Average	U.S. Average	Top Hospital
Heart Attack Care					
ACE Inhibitor or ARB for LVSD[5]	-	-	81%	82%	100%
Aspirin at Arrival[5]	-	-	90%	92%	100%
Aspirin at Discharge[5]	-	-	82%	90%	100%
Beta Blocker at Arrival[5]	-	-	81%	87%	100%
Beta Blocker at Discharge[5]	-	-	80%	90%	100%
Fibrinolytic Medication Timing[5]	-	-	27%	31%	100%
PCI Within 90 Minutes of Arrival[5]	-	-	0%	54%	95%
Smoking Cessation Advice[5]	-	-	88%	88%	100%
Heart Failure Care					
ACE Inhibitor or ARB for LVSD[5]	-	-	84%	82%	100%
Discharge Instructions[5]	-	-	72%	61%	93%
Evaluation of LVS Function[5]	-	-	78%	83%	99%
Smoking Cessation Advice[5]	-	-	92%	82%	100%
Pneumonia Care					
Appropriate Initial Antibiotic[5]	-	-	68%	83%	94%
Blood Culture Timing[5]	-	-	71%	90%	100%
Influenza Vaccine[5]	-	-	38%	70%	100%
Initial Antibiotic Timing[5]	-	-	46%	80%	93%

Oxygenation Assessment[5]	-	-	93%	99%	100%
Pneumococcal Vaccine[5]	-	-	34%	69%	94%
Smoking Cessation Advice[5]	-	-	89%	80%	100%
Surgical Infection Prevention					
Prophylactic Antibiotic Given[1,3]	13	38%	55%	77%	95%
Prophylactic Antibiotic Selection[5]	-	-	90%	90%	100%
Prophylactic Antibiotic Stopped[1,3]	13	8%	78%	72%	95%
Pregnancy Care					
Inpatient Neonatal Mortality	-	-	-	-	-
Third or Fourth Degree Laceration	-	-	-	3.63%	3.27%

Bella Vista Hospital

PO Box 1750   Phone: 787-834-2350
Mayaguez, PR 00681   Fax: 787-831-6315
Ownership: Voluntary non-profit - Church   Accredited: Yes
Emergency Services: Yes   Licensed Beds: 199
Key Personnel:
Administrator/CEO . . . . Jesus Nieves
Cardiology . . . . Carlos Rosario, MD
Chief Catheterization Laboratory . . . . Edgar Vazquez, MD
Emergency Room Director. . . . . Sony Moretta, MD
Director Infection/Disease Control . . . . Haydee Cuadrado
Chief OB/GYN . . . . Adalgiza Suriel, MD
Director Respiratory Therapy . . . . Iris M Cruz

Measure	Cases	This Hospital	State Average	U.S. Average	Top Hospital
Heart Attack Care					
ACE Inhibitor or ARB for LVSD[1,3]	15	80%	81%	82%	100%
Aspirin at Arrival[3]	54	74%	90%	92%	100%
Aspirin at Discharge[3]	39	72%	82%	90%	100%
Beta Blocker at Arrival[3]	51	53%	81%	87%	100%
Beta Blocker at Discharge[3]	47	60%	80%	90%	100%
Fibrinolytic Medication Timing[1,3]	5	60%	27%	31%	100%
PCI Within 90 Minutes of Arrival	0	-	0%	54%	95%
Smoking Cessation Advice[1,3]	4	50%	88%	88%	100%
Heart Failure Care					
ACE Inhibitor or ARB for LVSD[3]	36	75%	84%	82%	100%
Discharge Instructions[3]	140	82%	72%	61%	93%
Evaluation of LVS Function[3]	142	65%	78%	83%	99%
Smoking Cessation Advice[1,3]	3	67%	92%	82%	100%
Pneumonia Care					
Appropriate Initial Antibiotic[3]	121	79%	68%	83%	94%
Blood Culture Timing	112	66%	71%	90%	100%
Influenza Vaccine	35	9%	38%	70%	100%
Initial Antibiotic Timing[3]	148	43%	46%	80%	93%
Oxygenation Assessment[3]	165	100%	93%	99%	100%
Pneumococcal Vaccine[3]	96	5%	34%	69%	94%
Smoking Cessation Advice[1,3]	9	89%	89%	80%	100%
Surgical Infection Prevention					
Prophylactic Antibiotic Given[3]	313	56%	55%	77%	95%
Prophylactic Antibiotic Selection	51	96%	90%	90%	100%
Prophylactic Antibiotic Stopped[3]	303	6%	78%	72%	95%
Pregnancy Care					
Inpatient Neonatal Mortality	-	-	-	-	-
Third or Fourth Degree Laceration	-	-	-	3.63%	3.27%

Clinica Espanola

PO Box 4190   Phone: 787-832-0404
Mayaguez, PR 00681   Fax: 787-832-2094
Ownership: Proprietary   Accredited: No
Emergency Services: Yes   Licensed Beds: 89
Key Personnel:
Administrator/President . . . . Emigdio Inigo-Agostini, MD
Chief Medical Staff. . . . . Emiglio Inigo-Fas
Emergency Room . . . . Jesus Anthony, MD
Director of Pulmonary/Respiratory Care . . . . George Cole

Measure	Cases	This Hospital	State Average	U.S. Average	Top Hospital
Heart Attack Care					
ACE Inhibitor or ARB for LVSD[2,3]	0	-	81%	82%	100%
Aspirin at Arrival[2,3]	0	-	90%	92%	100%
Aspirin at Discharge[1,2,3]	1	100%	82%	90%	100%

NOTE: Hospital profiles are in alphabetical order by state, then city, then hospital within the city; Rankings are sorted by rate in descending order and exclude hospitals with less than 25 cases; (1) The number of cases is too small (n<25) for purposes of reliably predicting hospital performance; (2) Measure reflects the hospital's indication that its submission was based upon a sample of its relevant discharges; (3) Rate reflects fewer than the maximum possible quarters of data for the measure; (4) Inaccurate information submitted and suppressed for one or more quarters; (5) No data is available from the hospital for this measure; Please refer to the User's Guide for a full explanation of data

Beta Blocker at Arrival[2,3]	0	-	81%	87%	100%
Beta Blocker at Discharge[1,2,3]	1	100%	80%	90%	100%
Fibrinolytic Medication Timing[2,3]	0	-	27%	31%	100%
PCI Within 90 Minutes of Arrival[5]	-	-	0%	54%	95%
Smoking Cessation Advice[1,2,3]	1	100%	88%	88%	100%
Heart Failure Care					
ACE Inhibitor or ARB for LVSD[1,2]	20	100%	84%	82%	100%
Discharge Instructions[2]	25	100%	72%	61%	93%
Evaluation of LVS Function[2]	25	80%	78%	83%	99%
Smoking Cessation Advice[1,2]	7	100%	92%	82%	100%
Pneumonia Care					
Appropriate Initial Antibiotic[1,2]	12	67%	68%	83%	94%
Blood Culture Timing[1,2]	8	50%	71%	90%	100%
Influenza Vaccine[1]	3	100%	38%	70%	100%
Initial Antibiotic Timing[1,2]	11	91%	46%	80%	93%
Oxygenation Assessment[1,2]	14	79%	93%	99%	100%
Pneumococcal Vaccine[1,2]	11	100%	34%	69%	94%
Smoking Cessation Advice[1,2]	2	100%	89%	80%	100%
Surgical Infection Prevention					
Prophylactic Antibiotic Given[5]	-	-	55%	77%	95%
Prophylactic Antibiotic Selection[5]	-	-	90%	90%	100%
Prophylactic Antibiotic Stopped[5]	-	-	78%	72%	95%
Pregnancy Care					
Inpatient Neonatal Mortality	-	-	-	-	-
Third or Fourth Degree Laceration	-	-	-	3.63%	3.27%

Hospital Perea

15 Drive Basora Street
Mayaguez, PR 00681
URL: www.hospitalperea.com
Ownership: Voluntary non-profit - Private
Emergency Services: Yes

Phone: 787-834-0101
Fax: 787-265-2455

Accredited: No
Licensed Beds: 103

Key Personnel:
CEO . . . . Rafael Alvarado, MHSA
Chief Medical Staff . . . . Humberto Olivencia
Catheterization Lab . . . . Aida Muniz
Emergency Room . . . . Zoe Pizarro
Infection Control . . . . Carmen Tomassini, RN
ICU . . . . Janet Crespo, RN
OB/GYN/Women's Health . . . . Aida Vega, RN
Respiratory Supervisor . . . . Gerardo Roman

Measure	Cases	This Hospital	State Average	U.S. Average	Top Hospital
Heart Attack Care					
ACE Inhibitor or ARB for LVSD[1,2]	8	25%	81%	82%	100%
Aspirin at Arrival[5]	-	-	90%	92%	100%
Aspirin at Discharge[1,2]	23	61%	82%	90%	100%
Beta Blocker at Arrival[1,2]	18	72%	81%	87%	100%
Beta Blocker at Discharge[1,2]	22	55%	80%	90%	100%
Fibrinolytic Medication Timing[1,2]	2	0%	27%	31%	100%
PCI Within 90 Minutes of Arrival[2]	0	-	0%	54%	95%
Smoking Cessation Advice[1,2]	1	0%	88%	88%	100%
Heart Failure Care					
ACE Inhibitor or ARB for LVSD[2]	25	68%	84%	82%	100%
Discharge Instructions[2]	42	64%	72%	61%	93%
Evaluation of LVS Function[5]	-	-	78%	83%	99%
Smoking Cessation Advice[1,2]	9	33%	92%	82%	100%
Pneumonia Care					
Appropriate Initial Antibiotic[2]	40	70%	68%	83%	94%
Blood Culture Timing[5]	-	-	71%	90%	100%
Influenza Vaccine[5]	-	-	38%	70%	100%
Initial Antibiotic Timing[2]	40	20%	46%	80%	93%
Oxygenation Assessment[5]	-	-	93%	99%	100%
Pneumococcal Vaccine[2]	31	45%	34%	69%	94%
Smoking Cessation Advice[1,2]	5	60%	89%	80%	100%
Surgical Infection Prevention					
Prophylactic Antibiotic Given[2,3]	0	-	55%	77%	95%
Prophylactic Antibiotic Selection[2]	0	-	90%	90%	100%
Prophylactic Antibiotic Stopped[2,3]	0	-	78%	72%	95%
Pregnancy Care					
Inpatient Neonatal Mortality	-	-	-	-	-
Third or Fourth Degree Laceration	-	-	-	3.63%	3.27%

Ramon E Betances Hospital

Alternate Name: Advanced Cardiology Center
Centro Medico, 410 Carr. 2
Mayaguez, PR 00680
Ownership: Proprietary
Emergency Services: Yes

Phone: 787-834-8687
Fax: 787-834-3010
Accredited: Yes
Licensed Beds: 391

Key Personnel:
CEO . . . . Maria del Pilar Rodri
Chief Medical Staff . . . . Franklyn Plaguez, MD
Chief Catheterization Laboratory . . . . Marcos Velazquez, MD
Emergency Room . . . . Virgilio Cora, MD
Director Infection/Disease Control . . . . Emilia Arrocho, RN
CCU Spvg. Nurse . . . . Ramonita Mendez, RN
Director Medical/Surgical Nursing . . . . Alcides Ramos, RN
OB/GYN Womens Health . . . . Vilma Gonzalez, MD
Chief Radiology . . . . Angel R Colon
Director Respiratory Therapy . . . . Antonio Padua, MD

Measure	Cases	This Hospital	State Average	U.S. Average	Top Hospital
Heart Attack Care					
ACE Inhibitor or ARB for LVSD	50	66%	81%	82%	100%
Aspirin at Arrival	78	95%	90%	92%	100%
Aspirin at Discharge	110	80%	82%	90%	100%
Beta Blocker at Arrival	79	80%	81%	87%	100%
Beta Blocker at Discharge	113	78%	80%	90%	100%
Fibrinolytic Medication Timing	0	-	27%	31%	100%
PCI Within 90 Minutes of Arrival[1]	1	0%	0%	54%	95%
Smoking Cessation Advice	25	96%	88%	88%	100%
Heart Failure Care					
ACE Inhibitor or ARB for LVSD	65	66%	84%	82%	100%
Discharge Instructions	146	77%	72%	61%	93%
Evaluation of LVS Function	146	84%	78%	83%	99%
Smoking Cessation Advice[1]	21	100%	92%	82%	100%
Pneumonia Care					
Appropriate Initial Antibiotic	48	62%	68%	83%	94%
Blood Culture Timing	29	79%	71%	90%	100%
Influenza Vaccine[1]	11	36%	38%	70%	100%
Initial Antibiotic Timing[5]	-	-	46%	80%	93%
Oxygenation Assessment	74	97%	93%	99%	100%
Pneumococcal Vaccine	34	41%	34%	69%	94%
Smoking Cessation Advice[1]	10	100%	89%	80%	100%
Surgical Infection Prevention					
Prophylactic Antibiotic Given[5]	-	-	55%	77%	95%
Prophylactic Antibiotic Selection[5]	-	-	90%	90%	100%
Prophylactic Antibiotic Stopped[5]	-	-	78%	72%	95%
Pregnancy Care					
Inpatient Neonatal Mortality	-	-	-	-	-
Third or Fourth Degree Laceration	-	-	-	3.63%	3.27%

Hospital San Carlos Borromeo

Calle Concepcion Vera Ayala #550 S
Moca, PR 00676
Ownership: Voluntary non-profit - Private
Emergency Services: Yes

Phone: 787-877-8000

Accredited: No

Measure	Cases	This Hospital	State Average	U.S. Average	Top Hospital
Heart Attack Care					
ACE Inhibitor or ARB for LVSD[1,3]	5	60%	81%	82%	100%
Aspirin at Arrival[1,3]	16	81%	90%	92%	100%
Aspirin at Discharge[1,3]	18	61%	82%	90%	100%
Beta Blocker at Arrival[1,3]	19	68%	81%	87%	100%
Beta Blocker at Discharge[1,3]	20	75%	80%	90%	100%
Fibrinolytic Medication Timing[1,3]	3	0%	27%	31%	100%
PCI Within 90 Minutes of Arrival	0	-	0%	54%	95%
Smoking Cessation Advice[1,3]	2	100%	88%	88%	100%
Heart Failure Care					
ACE Inhibitor or ARB for LVSD[1,3]	8	50%	84%	82%	100%
Discharge Instructions[3]	25	32%	72%	61%	93%
Evaluation of LVS Function[3]	25	60%	78%	83%	99%
Smoking Cessation Advice[1,3]	1	100%	92%	82%	100%
Pneumonia Care					
Appropriate Initial Antibiotic[1,3]	10	70%	68%	83%	94%
Blood Culture Timing[1]	12	83%	71%	90%	100%

NOTE: Hospital profiles are in alphabetical order by state, then city, then hospital within the city; Rankings are sorted by rate in descending order and exclude hospitals with less than 25 cases; (1) The number of cases is too small (n<25) for purposes of reliably predicting hospital performance; (2) Measure reflects the hospital's indication that its submission was based upon a sample of its relevant discharges; (3) Rate reflects fewer than the maximum possible quarters of data for the measure; (4) Inaccurate information submitted and suppressed for one or more quarters; (5) No data is available from the hospital for this measure; Please refer to the User's Guide for a full explanation of data

Measure					
Influenza Vaccine[1]	1	0%	38%	70%	100%
Initial Antibiotic Timing[1,3]	14	29%	46%	80%	93%
Oxygenation Assessment[1,3]	14	64%	93%	99%	100%
Pneumococcal Vaccine[1,3]	10	20%	34%	69%	94%
Smoking Cessation Advice[1,3]	1	100%	89%	80%	100%
Surgical Infection Prevention					
Prophylactic Antibiotic Given[5]	-	-	55%	77%	95%
Prophylactic Antibiotic Selection[5]	-	-	90%	90%	100%
Prophylactic Antibiotic Stopped[5]	-	-	78%	72%	95%
Pregnancy Care					
Inpatient Neonatal Mortality	-	-	-	-	-
Third or Fourth Degree Laceration	-	-	-	3.63%	3.27%

Hospital Damas

2213 Ponce By Pass
Ponce, PR 00731
E-mail: recursoshumanos@hospitaldamas.com
Ownership: Voluntary non-profit - Private
Emergency Services: Yes

Phone: 787-840-8686
Fax: 787-813-0592

Accredited: Yes
Licensed Beds: 306

Key Personnel:
Director Cardiology Department . . . . Jose Gomez Riviera, MD
Chief Catheterization Laboratory . . . . Jorge Jovane, MD
Emergency Room . . . . Dr. Colon Gran
OB/GYN/Women's Health . . . . Jose Cintron-Villaro, MD
Chief Radiology . . . . German Chavez, MD
Director Respiratory Therapy . . . . Hector Rosado, MD

Measure	Cases	This Hospital	State Average	U.S. Average	Top Hospital
Heart Attack Care					
ACE Inhibitor or ARB for LVSD	42	100%	81%	82%	100%
Aspirin at Arrival	132	95%	90%	92%	100%
Aspirin at Discharge	124	96%	82%	90%	100%
Beta Blocker at Arrival	125	92%	81%	87%	100%
Beta Blocker at Discharge	139	97%	80%	90%	100%
Fibrinolytic Medication Timing[1]	19	47%	27%	31%	100%
PCI Within 90 Minutes of Arrival	0	-	0%	54%	95%
Smoking Cessation Advice[1]	15	93%	88%	88%	100%
Heart Failure Care					
ACE Inhibitor or ARB for LVSD	73	95%	84%	82%	100%
Discharge Instructions	210	100%	72%	61%	93%
Evaluation of LVS Function	211	89%	78%	83%	99%
Smoking Cessation Advice	26	100%	92%	82%	100%
Pneumonia Care					
Appropriate Initial Antibiotic	70	71%	68%	83%	94%
Blood Culture Timing	60	87%	71%	90%	100%
Influenza Vaccine[4,5]	-	-	38%	70%	100%
Initial Antibiotic Timing	83	64%	46%	80%	93%
Oxygenation Assessment	94	90%	93%	99%	100%
Pneumococcal Vaccine	56	20%	34%	69%	94%
Smoking Cessation Advice[1]	12	100%	89%	80%	100%
Surgical Infection Prevention					
Prophylactic Antibiotic Given[3]	195	64%	55%	77%	95%
Prophylactic Antibiotic Selection	75	88%	90%	90%	100%
Prophylactic Antibiotic Stopped[3]	193	52%	78%	72%	95%
Pregnancy Care					
Inpatient Neonatal Mortality	-	-	-	-	-
Third or Fourth Degree Laceration	-	-	-	3.63%	3.27%

Hospital Doctor Pila

Alternate Name: Pilas Hospital, Dr.
Avenue Las Americas
Ponce, PR 00733
Ownership: Voluntary non-profit - Private
Emergency Services: Yes

Phone: 787-848-5600
Fax: 787-841-3454
Accredited: Yes
Licensed Beds: 183

Key Personnel:
CEO/Executive Director . . . . Alfonso Vazquez
Chief Medical Staff. . . . . Luis Rodriguez Herna
Emergency Room . . . . Jesus Marin de Gracia
Director Infection/Disease Control . . . . Ana Cintron
Director Medical/Surgical Nursing . . . . Melba Febus
OB/GYN Womens Health. . . . . Miguel Pereira
Director Respiratory Therapy . . . . Diana Acosta

Measure	Cases	This Hospital	State Average	U.S. Average	Top Hospital
Heart Attack Care					
ACE Inhibitor or ARB for LVSD[5]	-	-	81%	82%	100%
Aspirin at Arrival[2]	167	71%	90%	92%	100%
Aspirin at Discharge[5]	-	-	82%	90%	100%
Beta Blocker at Arrival[5]	-	-	81%	87%	100%
Beta Blocker at Discharge[5]	-	-	80%	90%	100%
Fibrinolytic Medication Timing[2]	33	24%	27%	31%	100%
PCI Within 90 Minutes of Arrival[5]	-	-	0%	54%	95%
Smoking Cessation Advice[5]	-	-	88%	88%	100%
Heart Failure Care					
ACE Inhibitor or ARB for LVSD[5]	-	-	84%	82%	100%
Discharge Instructions[5]	-	-	72%	61%	93%
Evaluation of LVS Function[2]	103	85%	78%	83%	99%
Smoking Cessation Advice[5]	-	-	92%	82%	100%
Pneumonia Care					
Appropriate Initial Antibiotic[2]	111	60%	68%	83%	94%
Blood Culture Timing[2]	59	61%	71%	90%	100%
Influenza Vaccine[5]	-	-	38%	70%	100%
Initial Antibiotic Timing[5]	-	-	46%	80%	93%
Oxygenation Assessment[2]	150	93%	93%	99%	100%
Pneumococcal Vaccine[2]	79	47%	34%	69%	94%
Smoking Cessation Advice[5]	-	-	89%	80%	100%
Surgical Infection Prevention					
Prophylactic Antibiotic Given[3]	88	57%	55%	77%	95%
Prophylactic Antibiotic Selection	27	85%	90%	90%	100%
Prophylactic Antibiotic Stopped[3]	88	95%	78%	72%	95%
Pregnancy Care					
Inpatient Neonatal Mortality	-	-	-	-	-
Third or Fourth Degree Laceration	-	-	-	3.63%	3.27%

Hospital Oncologico Andres Grillasca

Ave Tito Castro Carr 14 Antiguo Centro Medico   Phone: 787-848-0800
Ponce, PR 00733
Ownership: Voluntary non-profit - Private   Accredited: Yes
Emergency Services: Yes

Measure	Cases	This Hospital	State Average	U.S. Average	Top Hospital
Heart Attack Care					
ACE Inhibitor or ARB for LVSD[5]	-	-	81%	82%	100%
Aspirin at Arrival[5]	-	-	90%	92%	100%
Aspirin at Discharge[5]	-	-	82%	90%	100%
Beta Blocker at Arrival[5]	-	-	81%	87%	100%
Beta Blocker at Discharge[5]	-	-	80%	90%	100%
Fibrinolytic Medication Timing[5]	-	-	27%	31%	100%
PCI Within 90 Minutes of Arrival[5]	-	-	0%	54%	95%
Smoking Cessation Advice[5]	-	-	88%	88%	100%
Heart Failure Care					
ACE Inhibitor or ARB for LVSD[5]	-	-	84%	82%	100%
Discharge Instructions[5]	-	-	72%	61%	93%
Evaluation of LVS Function[5]	-	-	78%	83%	99%
Smoking Cessation Advice[5]	-	-	92%	82%	100%
Pneumonia Care					
Appropriate Initial Antibiotic[3]	0	-	68%	83%	94%
Blood Culture Timing[1,3]	2	100%	71%	90%	100%
Influenza Vaccine[1]	1	100%	38%	70%	100%
Initial Antibiotic Timing[1,3]	2	100%	46%	80%	93%
Oxygenation Assessment[1,3]	2	100%	93%	99%	100%
Pneumococcal Vaccine[1,3]	1	0%	34%	69%	94%
Smoking Cessation Advice[1,3]	1	100%	89%	80%	100%
Surgical Infection Prevention					
Prophylactic Antibiotic Given[1,3]	14	29%	55%	77%	95%
Prophylactic Antibiotic Selection[1]	3	33%	90%	90%	100%
Prophylactic Antibiotic Stopped[1,3]	16	100%	78%	72%	95%
Pregnancy Care					
Inpatient Neonatal Mortality	-	-	-	-	-
Third or Fourth Degree Laceration	-	-	-	3.63%	3.27%

NOTE: Hospital profiles are in alphabetical order by state, then city, then hospital within the city; Rankings are sorted by rate in descending order and exclude hospitals with less than 25 cases; (1) The number of cases is too small (n<25) for purposes of reliably predicting hospital performance; (2) Measure reflects the hospital's indication that its submission was based upon a sample of its relevant discharges; (3) Rate reflects fewer than the maximum possible quarters of data for the measure; (4) Inaccurate information submitted and suppressed for one or more quarters; (5) No data is available from the hospital for this measure; Please refer to the User's Guide for a full explanation of data

San Luke's Memorial Hospital

Tito Castro Ave #917   Phone: 787-844-2080
Ponce, PR 00731
Ownership: Voluntary non-profit - Church   Accredited: Yes
Emergency Services: Yes

Measure	Cases	This Hospital	State Average	U.S. Average	Top Hospital
Heart Attack Care					
ACE Inhibitor or ARB for LVSD	30	87%	81%	82%	100%
Aspirin at Arrival	187	94%	90%	92%	100%
Aspirin at Discharge	105	88%	82%	90%	100%
Beta Blocker at Arrival	190	62%	81%	87%	100%
Beta Blocker at Discharge	110	85%	80%	90%	100%
Fibrinolytic Medication Timing[1]	10	10%	27%	31%	100%
PCI Within 90 Minutes of Arrival	0	-	0%	54%	95%
Smoking Cessation Advice[1]	16	100%	88%	88%	100%
Heart Failure Care					
ACE Inhibitor or ARB for LVSD	65	92%	84%	82%	100%
Discharge Instructions	171	71%	72%	61%	93%
Evaluation of LVS Function	170	74%	78%	83%	99%
Smoking Cessation Advice[1]	22	100%	92%	82%	100%
Pneumonia Care					
Appropriate Initial Antibiotic	121	79%	68%	83%	94%
Blood Culture Timing	64	75%	71%	90%	100%
Influenza Vaccine[4,5]	-	-	38%	70%	100%
Initial Antibiotic Timing	123	51%	46%	80%	93%
Oxygenation Assessment	124	100%	93%	99%	100%
Pneumococcal Vaccine	67	88%	34%	69%	94%
Smoking Cessation Advice[1]	19	100%	89%	80%	100%
Surgical Infection Prevention					
Prophylactic Antibiotic Given	137	68%	55%	77%	95%
Prophylactic Antibiotic Selection	34	97%	90%	90%	100%
Prophylactic Antibiotic Stopped	137	65%	78%	72%	95%
Pregnancy Care					
Inpatient Neonatal Mortality	-	-	-	-	-
Third or Fourth Degree Laceration	-	-	-	3.63%	3.27%

Cardiovascular Center of Puerto Rico

Avenida Americo Miranda   Phone: 787-754-8500
Entrada Principal, Centro Medico   Fax: 787-999-0860
Rio Piedras, PR 00936
URL: www.cardiovascular.gobierno.pr
Ownership: Government - State   Accredited: Yes
Emergency Services: Yes   Licensed Beds: 122
Key Personnel:
Executive Director . . . . Carlos G Melendez

Measure	Cases	This Hospital	State Average	U.S. Average	Top Hospital
Heart Attack Care					
ACE Inhibitor or ARB for LVSD	77	90%	81%	82%	100%
Aspirin at Arrival	69	97%	90%	92%	100%
Aspirin at Discharge	259	99%	82%	90%	100%
Beta Blocker at Arrival	70	97%	81%	87%	100%
Beta Blocker at Discharge	226	96%	80%	90%	100%
Fibrinolytic Medication Timing	0	-	27%	31%	100%
PCI Within 90 Minutes of Arrival	0	-	0%	54%	95%
Smoking Cessation Advice	55	89%	88%	88%	100%
Heart Failure Care					
ACE Inhibitor or ARB for LVSD	239	97%	84%	82%	100%
Discharge Instructions	373	94%	72%	61%	93%
Evaluation of LVS Function	373	87%	78%	83%	99%
Smoking Cessation Advice[1]	18	83%	92%	82%	100%
Pneumonia Care					
Appropriate Initial Antibiotic[5]	-	-	68%	83%	94%
Blood Culture Timing[5]	-	-	71%	90%	100%
Influenza Vaccine[5]	-	-	38%	70%	100%
Initial Antibiotic Timing[5]	-	-	46%	80%	93%
Oxygenation Assessment[5]	-	-	93%	99%	100%
Pneumococcal Vaccine[5]	-	-	34%	69%	94%
Smoking Cessation Advice[5]	-	-	89%	80%	100%
Surgical Infection Prevention					
Prophylactic Antibiotic Given	748	76%	55%	77%	95%

Measure	Cases	This Hospital	State Average	U.S. Average	Top Hospital
Prophylactic Antibiotic Selection	307	97%	90%	90%	100%
Prophylactic Antibiotic Stopped	742	99%	78%	72%	95%
Pregnancy Care					
Inpatient Neonatal Mortality	-	-	-	-	-
Third or Fourth Degree Laceration	-	-	-	3.63%	3.27%

Hospital San Gerardo

Road No 844 Km 0 5 Po Cupey Bajo   Phone: 787-761-8383
Rio Piedras, PR 00928
Ownership: Proprietary   Accredited: No
Emergency Services: Yes

Measure	Cases	This Hospital	State Average	U.S. Average	Top Hospital
Heart Attack Care					
ACE Inhibitor or ARB for LVSD[3]	0	-	81%	82%	100%
Aspirin at Arrival[1,3]	7	71%	90%	92%	100%
Aspirin at Discharge[1,3]	4	50%	82%	90%	100%
Beta Blocker at Arrival[1,3]	7	29%	81%	87%	100%
Beta Blocker at Discharge[1,3]	4	25%	80%	90%	100%
Fibrinolytic Medication Timing[3]	0	-	27%	31%	100%
PCI Within 90 Minutes of Arrival	0	-	0%	54%	95%
Smoking Cessation Advice[1,3]	2	100%	88%	88%	100%
Heart Failure Care					
ACE Inhibitor or ARB for LVSD[1,2,3]	1	0%	84%	82%	100%
Discharge Instructions[1,2,3]	10	70%	72%	61%	93%
Evaluation of LVS Function[1,2,3]	11	9%	78%	83%	99%
Smoking Cessation Advice[2,3]	0	-	92%	82%	100%
Pneumonia Care					
Appropriate Initial Antibiotic[2,3]	32	66%	68%	83%	94%
Blood Culture Timing[2,3]	0	-	71%	90%	100%
Influenza Vaccine[5]	-	-	38%	70%	100%
Initial Antibiotic Timing[1,2,3]	19	47%	46%	80%	93%
Oxygenation Assessment[2,3]	33	82%	93%	99%	100%
Pneumococcal Vaccine[1,2,3]	21	0%	34%	69%	94%
Smoking Cessation Advice[1,2,3]	1	100%	89%	80%	100%
Surgical Infection Prevention					
Prophylactic Antibiotic Given[5]	-	-	55%	77%	95%
Prophylactic Antibiotic Selection[5]	-	-	90%	90%	100%
Prophylactic Antibiotic Stopped[5]	-	-	78%	72%	95%
Pregnancy Care					
Inpatient Neonatal Mortality	-	-	-	-	-
Third or Fourth Degree Laceration	-	-	-	3.63%	3.27%

San Juan Municipal Hospital

Barrio Monacillos, Centro Medico   Phone: 787-756-8535
Rio Piedras, PR 00936
Ownership: Voluntary non-profit - Other   Accredited: Yes
Emergency Services: No

Measure	Cases	This Hospital	State Average	U.S. Average	Top Hospital
Heart Attack Care					
ACE Inhibitor or ARB for LVSD[1]	8	75%	81%	82%	100%
Aspirin at Arrival[1]	22	91%	90%	92%	100%
Aspirin at Discharge[1]	22	68%	82%	90%	100%
Beta Blocker at Arrival	25	68%	81%	87%	100%
Beta Blocker at Discharge	26	81%	80%	90%	100%
Fibrinolytic Medication Timing[5]	-	-	27%	31%	100%
PCI Within 90 Minutes of Arrival[5]	-	-	0%	54%	95%
Smoking Cessation Advice[1]	13	100%	88%	88%	100%
Heart Failure Care					
ACE Inhibitor or ARB for LVSD[1]	14	93%	84%	82%	100%
Discharge Instructions	43	95%	72%	61%	93%
Evaluation of LVS Function	41	59%	78%	83%	99%
Smoking Cessation Advice[1]	17	100%	92%	82%	100%
Pneumonia Care					
Appropriate Initial Antibiotic[5]	-	-	68%	83%	94%
Blood Culture Timing[5]	-	-	71%	90%	100%
Influenza Vaccine[5]	-	-	38%	70%	100%
Initial Antibiotic Timing	37	78%	46%	80%	93%
Oxygenation Assessment	58	97%	93%	99%	100%
Pneumococcal Vaccine[1]	20	5%	34%	69%	94%
Smoking Cessation Advice	32	100%	89%	80%	100%

NOTE: Hospital profiles are in alphabetical order by state, then city, then hospital within the city; Rankings are sorted by rate in descending order and exclude hospitals with less than 25 cases; (1) The number of cases is too small (n<25) for purposes of reliably predicting hospital performance; (2) Measure reflects the hospital's indication that its submission was based upon a sample of its relevant discharges; (3) Rate reflects fewer than the maximum possible quarters of data for the measure; (4) Inaccurate information submitted and suppressed for one or more quarters; (5) No data is available from the hospital for this measure; Please refer to the User's Guide for a full explanation of data

Surgical Infection Prevention					
Prophylactic Antibiotic Given[5]	-	-	55%	77%	95%
Prophylactic Antibiotic Selection[5]	-	-	90%	90%	100%
Prophylactic Antibiotic Stopped[3]	28	100%	78%	72%	95%
Pregnancy Care					
Inpatient Neonatal Mortality	-	-	-	-	-
Third or Fourth Degree Laceration	-	-	-	3.63%	3.27%

University District Hospital

Barrio Monacillos Centromedico   Phone: 787-754-0101
Rio Piedras, PR 00927
Ownership: Government - State   Accredited: Yes
Emergency Services: Yes

Measure	Cases	This Hospital	State Average	U.S. Average	Top Hospital
Heart Attack Care					
ACE Inhibitor or ARB for LVSD[1,3]	1	0%	81%	82%	100%
Aspirin at Arrival[1,3]	1	100%	90%	92%	100%
Aspirin at Discharge[1,3]	1	100%	82%	90%	100%
Beta Blocker at Arrival[1,3]	1	100%	81%	87%	100%
Beta Blocker at Discharge[1,3]	1	100%	80%	90%	100%
Fibrinolytic Medication Timing[3]	0	-	27%	31%	100%
PCI Within 90 Minutes of Arrival	0	-	0%	54%	95%
Smoking Cessation Advice[1,3]	1	0%	88%	88%	100%
Heart Failure Care					
ACE Inhibitor or ARB for LVSD[1,3]	3	67%	84%	82%	100%
Discharge Instructions[1,3]	6	0%	72%	61%	93%
Evaluation of LVS Function[1,3]	6	83%	78%	83%	99%
Smoking Cessation Advice[1,3]	4	75%	92%	82%	100%
Pneumonia Care					
Appropriate Initial Antibiotic[1]	7	29%	68%	83%	94%
Blood Culture Timing[1]	1	0%	71%	90%	100%
Influenza Vaccine	0	-	38%	70%	100%
Initial Antibiotic Timing[1]	9	33%	46%	80%	93%
Oxygenation Assessment[1]	9	89%	93%	99%	100%
Pneumococcal Vaccine[1]	1	0%	34%	69%	94%
Smoking Cessation Advice[1]	3	33%	89%	80%	100%
Surgical Infection Prevention					
Prophylactic Antibiotic Given	237	73%	55%	77%	95%
Prophylactic Antibiotic Selection	67	84%	90%	90%	100%
Prophylactic Antibiotic Stopped	231	69%	78%	72%	95%
Pregnancy Care					
Inpatient Neonatal Mortality	-	-	-	-	-
Third or Fourth Degree Laceration	-	-	-	3.63%	3.27%

Hospital De La Concepcion

Avenida Universidad Interamericana #41   Phone: 787-892-1860
San German, PR 00683   Fax: 787-892-6465
Ownership: Proprietary   Accredited: Yes
Emergency Services: Yes   Licensed Beds: 167
Key Personnel:
President/CEO......................... Jaime F Maestre Grau
Chief Medical Staff...................... Francisco Jaume
Emergency Room .... Jose V Carrillo Monllor
ICU Director........................... Anibal Lugo
Intensive/Cornary Care Supervisor .... Maria L Lebron
OB/GYN/Womens Health................. Lourdes Ramirez
Chief Radiology .... Manuel R Prats Vega
Respiratory Therapy Director .... Ruth Enid Morales

Measure	Cases	This Hospital	State Average	U.S. Average	Top Hospital
Heart Attack Care					
ACE Inhibitor or ARB for LVSD[2,3]	43	98%	81%	82%	100%
Aspirin at Arrival[2,3]	111	93%	90%	92%	100%
Aspirin at Discharge[2,3]	102	90%	82%	90%	100%
Beta Blocker at Arrival[2,3]	104	91%	81%	87%	100%
Beta Blocker at Discharge[2,3]	110	95%	80%	90%	100%
Fibrinolytic Medication Timing[5]	-	-	27%	31%	100%
PCI Within 90 Minutes of Arrival[2]	0	-	0%	54%	95%
Smoking Cessation Advice[1,2,3]	16	100%	88%	88%	100%
Heart Failure Care					
ACE Inhibitor or ARB for LVSD[2,3]	70	99%	84%	82%	100%

Discharge Instructions[2,3]	178	100%	72%	61%	93%
Evaluation of LVS Function[2,3]	175	96%	78%	83%	99%
Smoking Cessation Advice[5]	-	-	92%	82%	100%
Pneumonia Care					
Appropriate Initial Antibiotic[1,2,3]	5	40%	68%	83%	94%
Blood Culture Timing[5]	-	-	71%	90%	100%
Influenza Vaccine[4,5]	-	-	38%	70%	100%
Initial Antibiotic Timing[1,2,3]	5	20%	46%	80%	93%
Oxygenation Assessment[2,3]	124	92%	93%	99%	100%
Pneumococcal Vaccine[2,3]	73	10%	34%	69%	94%
Smoking Cessation Advice[1,2,3]	10	70%	89%	80%	100%
Surgical Infection Prevention					
Prophylactic Antibiotic Given[5]	-	-	55%	77%	95%
Prophylactic Antibiotic Selection[2]	27	100%	90%	90%	100%
Prophylactic Antibiotic Stopped[2,3]	70	79%	78%	72%	95%
Pregnancy Care					
Inpatient Neonatal Mortality	-	-	-	-	-
Third or Fourth Degree Laceration	-	-	-	3.63%	3.27%

Hospital Metropolitano

Alternate Name: San German Area Hospital
PO Box 63   Phone: 787-892-5300
San German, PR 00683   Fax: 787-892-1362
Ownership: Voluntary non-profit - Private Accredited: No
Emergency Services: Yes   Licensed Beds: 42
Key Personnel:
CEO................................ Jorge Martines
Chief Medical Staff................. Edgar H Moreno, MD
Emergency Room .... Rosalia Ayala, RN
Emergency Room .... Raymond Tossas, MD
Infection Control.................. Elga E Gonzalez, RN
ICU .... Maria Ramirez, RN
Respiratory/Cardiopulmonary.............. Julio Irizarry

Measure	Cases	This Hospital	State Average	U.S. Average	Top Hospital
Heart Attack Care					
ACE Inhibitor or ARB for LVSD[1,2]	17	94%	81%	82%	100%
Aspirin at Arrival[2]	31	97%	90%	92%	100%
Aspirin at Discharge[2]	33	100%	82%	90%	100%
Beta Blocker at Arrival[2]	31	97%	81%	87%	100%
Beta Blocker at Discharge[2]	35	91%	80%	90%	100%
Fibrinolytic Medication Timing[2]	0	-	27%	31%	100%
PCI Within 90 Minutes of Arrival[2]	0	-	0%	54%	95%
Smoking Cessation Advice[1,2]	13	100%	88%	88%	100%
Heart Failure Care					
ACE Inhibitor or ARB for LVSD[1,2]	19	100%	84%	82%	100%
Discharge Instructions[2]	52	100%	72%	61%	93%
Evaluation of LVS Function[2]	52	100%	78%	83%	99%
Smoking Cessation Advice[1,2]	16	100%	92%	82%	100%
Pneumonia Care					
Appropriate Initial Antibiotic[2]	33	94%	68%	83%	94%
Blood Culture Timing[5]	-	-	71%	90%	100%
Influenza Vaccine[1,2]	7	100%	38%	70%	100%
Initial Antibiotic Timing[5]	-	-	46%	80%	93%
Oxygenation Assessment[2]	35	100%	93%	99%	100%
Pneumococcal Vaccine[1,2]	19	100%	34%	69%	94%
Smoking Cessation Advice[1,2]	6	100%	89%	80%	100%
Surgical Infection Prevention					
Prophylactic Antibiotic Given[1,2,3]	8	88%	55%	77%	95%
Prophylactic Antibiotic Selection[5]	-	-	90%	90%	100%
Prophylactic Antibiotic Stopped[1,2,3]	8	100%	78%	72%	95%
Pregnancy Care					
Inpatient Neonatal Mortality	-	-	-	-	-
Third or Fourth Degree Laceration	-	-	-	3.63%	3.27%

Admin de Servicios Medicos Puerto Rico

Monacillo Ward Building # 1 Centro Medico   Phone: 787-777-3400
San Juan, PR 00922
Ownership: Government - Local   Accredited: Yes
Emergency Services: Yes

Measure	Cases	This Hospital	State Average	U.S. Average	Top Hospital

NOTE: Hospital profiles are in alphabetical order by state, then city, then hospital within the city; Rankings are sorted by rate in descending order and exclude hospitals with less than 25 cases; (1) The number of cases is too small (n<25) for purposes of reliably predicting hospital performance; (2) Measure reflects the hospital's indication that its submission was based upon a sample of its relevant discharges; (3) Rate reflects fewer than the maximum possible quarters of data for the measure; (4) Inaccurate information submitted and suppressed for one or more quarters; (5) No data is available from the hospital for this measure; Please refer to the User's Guide for a full explanation of data

Heart Attack Care					
ACE Inhibitor or ARB for LVSD[5]	-	-	81%	82%	100%
Aspirin at Arrival[5]	-	-	90%	92%	100%
Aspirin at Discharge[5]	-	-	82%	90%	100%
Beta Blocker at Arrival[5]	-	-	81%	87%	100%
Beta Blocker at Discharge[5]	-	-	80%	90%	100%
Fibrinolytic Medication Timing[5]	-	-	27%	31%	100%
PCI Within 90 Minutes of Arrival[5]	-	-	0%	54%	95%
Smoking Cessation Advice[5]	-	-	88%	88%	100%
Heart Failure Care					
ACE Inhibitor or ARB for LVSD[5]	-	-	84%	82%	100%
Discharge Instructions[5]	-	-	72%	61%	93%
Evaluation of LVS Function[5]	-	-	78%	83%	99%
Smoking Cessation Advice[5]	-	-	92%	82%	100%
Pneumonia Care					
Appropriate Initial Antibiotic[5]	-	-	68%	83%	94%
Blood Culture Timing[5]	-	-	71%	90%	100%
Influenza Vaccine[5]	-	-	38%	70%	100%
Initial Antibiotic Timing[5]	-	-	46%	80%	93%
Oxygenation Assessment[5]	-	-	93%	99%	100%
Pneumococcal Vaccine[5]	-	-	34%	69%	94%
Smoking Cessation Advice[5]	-	-	89%	80%	100%
Surgical Infection Prevention					
Prophylactic Antibiotic Given[5]	-	-	55%	77%	95%
Prophylactic Antibiotic Selection[5]	-	-	90%	90%	100%
Prophylactic Antibiotic Stopped[5]	-	-	78%	72%	95%
Pregnancy Care					
Inpatient Neonatal Mortality	-	-	-	-	-
Third or Fourth Degree Laceration	-	-	-	3.63%	3.27%

Ashford Presbyterian Community Hospital

Alternate Name: Presbyterian Community Hospital
1451 Ashford Avenue
San Juan, PR 00902
URL: www.presbypr.com
Ownership: Voluntary non-profit - Other
Emergency Services: Yes

Phone: 787-721-2160
Fax: 787-723-3797

Accredited: Yes
Licensed Beds: 207

Key Personnel:
CEO. . . . . Pedro J Gonzales, MHSH
Cardiology . . . . Josue Mercado, MD
Manager Emergency Room . . . . Eva Betancourt
Emergency Room . . . . Carlos Alvarez, MD
Director Infection/Disease Control . . . . Hilda Aleman, BSN
CCU Director . . . . Josue Mercado, MD
Director OB/GYN Womens Health . . . . Edgardo Aprinte, MD
Surgical Services . . . . Nancy Casares
Respiratory Therapy. . . . . Kiomary Negron

Measure	Cases	This Hospital	State Average	U.S. Average	Top Hospital
Heart Attack Care					
ACE Inhibitor or ARB for LVSD[1,3]	10	100%	81%	82%	100%
Aspirin at Arrival[3]	45	93%	90%	92%	100%
Aspirin at Discharge[1,3]	24	71%	82%	90%	100%
Beta Blocker at Arrival[3]	46	89%	81%	87%	100%
Beta Blocker at Discharge[1,3]	23	91%	80%	90%	100%
Fibrinolytic Medication Timing[3]	0	-	27%	31%	100%
PCI Within 90 Minutes of Arrival[5]	-	-	0%	54%	95%
Smoking Cessation Advice[1,3]	4	100%	88%	88%	100%
Heart Failure Care					
ACE Inhibitor or ARB for LVSD[3]	33	100%	84%	82%	100%
Discharge Instructions[3]	69	100%	72%	61%	93%
Evaluation of LVS Function[3]	68	93%	78%	83%	99%
Smoking Cessation Advice[5]	-	-	92%	82%	100%
Pneumonia Care					
Appropriate Initial Antibiotic[3]	85	79%	68%	83%	94%
Blood Culture Timing	71	66%	71%	90%	100%
Influenza Vaccine[5]	-	-	38%	70%	100%
Initial Antibiotic Timing[5]	-	-	46%	80%	93%
Oxygenation Assessment[3]	100	100%	93%	99%	100%
Pneumococcal Vaccine[5]	-	-	34%	69%	94%
Smoking Cessation Advice[1,3]	7	71%	89%	80%	100%
Surgical Infection Prevention					
Prophylactic Antibiotic Given[3]	368	72%	55%	77%	95%
Prophylactic Antibiotic Selection	108	97%	90%	90%	100%
Prophylactic Antibiotic Stopped[5]	-	-	78%	72%	95%
Pregnancy Care					
Inpatient Neonatal Mortality[5]	0	0.00%	-	-	-
Third or Fourth Degree Laceration	1,222	7.04%	-	3.63%	3.27%

Doctor I Gonzalez Martinez Oncologic Hospital

Alternate Name: Martinez Oncologic Hospital, I. G.
PO Box 191811
San Juan, PR 00919
Ownership: Voluntary non-profit - Private
Emergency Services: No

Phone: 787-765-2382
Fax: 787-751-7940

Accredited: Yes
Licensed Beds: 143

Key Personnel:
CEO. . . . . Milagros Bargas
Chief Medical Staff. . . . . Carlos Chevere
Director Infection/Disease Control . . . . Francisca Marin, RN
CCU Spvg. Nurse . . . . Elizabeth De Jesus, RN
Director Medical/Surgical Nursing . . . . Elizabeth DeJesus, MSN
OB/GYN Womens Health. . . . . Gilberto Marrero
Chief Radiology . . . . Jose Riviera, MD
Director Respiratory Therapy . . . . Lourdes Medina, MD

Measure	Cases	This Hospital	State Average	U.S. Average	Top Hospital
Heart Attack Care					
ACE Inhibitor or ARB for LVSD[5]	-	-	81%	82%	100%
Aspirin at Arrival[5]	-	-	90%	92%	100%
Aspirin at Discharge[5]	-	-	82%	90%	100%
Beta Blocker at Arrival[5]	-	-	81%	87%	100%
Beta Blocker at Discharge[5]	-	-	80%	90%	100%
Fibrinolytic Medication Timing[5]	-	-	27%	31%	100%
PCI Within 90 Minutes of Arrival[5]	-	-	0%	54%	95%
Smoking Cessation Advice[5]	-	-	88%	88%	100%
Heart Failure Care					
ACE Inhibitor or ARB for LVSD[5]	-	-	84%	82%	100%
Discharge Instructions[5]	-	-	72%	61%	93%
Evaluation of LVS Function[5]	-	-	78%	83%	99%
Smoking Cessation Advice[5]	-	-	92%	82%	100%
Pneumonia Care					
Appropriate Initial Antibiotic[1,3]	1	100%	68%	83%	94%
Blood Culture Timing[5]	-	-	71%	90%	100%
Influenza Vaccine[5]	-	-	38%	70%	100%
Initial Antibiotic Timing[5]	-	-	46%	80%	93%
Oxygenation Assessment[1,3]	3	100%	93%	99%	100%
Pneumococcal Vaccine[5]	-	-	34%	69%	94%
Smoking Cessation Advice[5]	-	-	89%	80%	100%
Surgical Infection Prevention					
Prophylactic Antibiotic Given[2]	332	62%	55%	77%	95%
Prophylactic Antibiotic Selection[2]	88	97%	90%	90%	100%
Prophylactic Antibiotic Stopped[2]	328	24%	78%	72%	95%
Pregnancy Care					
Inpatient Neonatal Mortality	-	-	-	-	-
Third or Fourth Degree Laceration	-	-	-	3.63%	3.27%

Hospital Del Maestro

Domenech Avenue
San Juan, PR 00918
E-mail: info@maestrofacmed.com
URL: www.maestrofacmed.com
Ownership: Voluntary non-profit - Other
Emergency Services: Yes

Phone: 787-758-8383
Fax: 787-758-0105

Accredited: Yes
Licensed Beds: 255

Key Personnel:
CEO. . . . . Milton Maldonado
Chief Medical Staff. . . . . Jose Montalvo
Chief Catheterization Laboratory . . . . Jose Cardona, MD
Emergency Room . . . . Luis Sarzalejo, MD
Director Infection/Disease Control . . . . Carlos Leon Valiente, MD
OB/GYN Womens Health. . . . . Enrique Cruzado, MD
Chief Radiology . . . . Jose Taveras, MD
Director Respiratory Therapy . . . . Rene Colon

Measure	Cases	This Hospital	State Average	U.S. Average	Top Hospital
Heart Attack Care					
ACE Inhibitor or ARB for LVSD[1,3]	3	67%	81%	82%	100%

NOTE: Hospital profiles are in alphabetical order by state, then city, then hospital within the city; Rankings are sorted by rate in descending order and exclude hospitals with less than 25 cases; (1) The number of cases is too small (n<25) for purposes of reliably predicting hospital performance; (2) Measure reflects the hospital's indication that its submission was based upon a sample of its relevant discharges; (3) Rate reflects fewer than the maximum possible quarters of data for the measure; (4) Inaccurate information submitted and suppressed for one or more quarters; (5) No data is available from the hospital for this measure; Please refer to the User's Guide for a full explanation of data

Measure	Cases	This Hospital	State Average	U.S. Average	Top Hospital
Aspirin at Arrival[1,3]	13	77%	90%	92%	100%
Aspirin at Discharge[1,3]	15	67%	82%	90%	100%
Beta Blocker at Arrival[1,3]	15	60%	81%	87%	100%
Beta Blocker at Discharge[1,3]	16	56%	80%	90%	100%
Fibrinolytic Medication Timing[3]	0	-	27%	31%	100%
PCI Within 90 Minutes of Arrival	0	-	0%	54%	95%
Smoking Cessation Advice[1,3]	7	100%	88%	88%	100%
Heart Failure Care					
ACE Inhibitor or ARB for LVSD[1,2,3]	15	100%	84%	82%	100%
Discharge Instructions[2,3]	106	57%	72%	61%	93%
Evaluation of LVS Function[2,3]	106	58%	78%	83%	99%
Smoking Cessation Advice[1,2,3]	15	93%	92%	82%	100%
Pneumonia Care					
Appropriate Initial Antibiotic[3]	76	55%	68%	83%	94%
Blood Culture Timing[3]	72	93%	71%	90%	100%
Influenza Vaccine[5]	-	-	38%	70%	100%
Initial Antibiotic Timing[3]	76	62%	46%	80%	93%
Oxygenation Assessment[3]	83	99%	93%	99%	100%
Pneumococcal Vaccine[3]	45	24%	34%	69%	94%
Smoking Cessation Advice[1,3]	12	92%	89%	80%	100%
Surgical Infection Prevention					
Prophylactic Antibiotic Given[5]	-	-	55%	77%	95%
Prophylactic Antibiotic Selection[5]	-	-	90%	90%	100%
Prophylactic Antibiotic Stopped[5]	-	-	78%	72%	95%
Pregnancy Care					
Inpatient Neonatal Mortality	-	-	-	-	-
Third or Fourth Degree Laceration	-	-	-	3.63%	3.27%

Hospital San Francisco

371 De Diego Ave
San Juan, PR 00929
Ownership: Proprietary
Emergency Services: Yes

Phone: 787-767-2528

Accredited: Yes

Measure	Cases	This Hospital	State Average	U.S. Average	Top Hospital
Heart Attack Care					
ACE Inhibitor or ARB for LVSD[1]	5	100%	81%	82%	100%
Aspirin at Arrival	36	94%	90%	92%	100%
Aspirin at Discharge[1]	17	94%	82%	90%	100%
Beta Blocker at Arrival	34	85%	81%	87%	100%
Beta Blocker at Discharge[1]	18	100%	80%	90%	100%
Fibrinolytic Medication Timing[1]	4	0%	27%	31%	100%
PCI Within 90 Minutes of Arrival	0	-	0%	54%	95%
Smoking Cessation Advice[1]	4	100%	88%	88%	100%
Heart Failure Care					
ACE Inhibitor or ARB for LVSD[1]	20	85%	84%	82%	100%
Discharge Instructions	79	0%	72%	61%	93%
Evaluation of LVS Function	80	59%	78%	83%	99%
Smoking Cessation Advice[1]	9	100%	92%	82%	100%
Pneumonia Care					
Appropriate Initial Antibiotic[2]	75	81%	68%	83%	94%
Blood Culture Timing[2]	42	45%	71%	90%	100%
Influenza Vaccine[1,2]	8	25%	38%	70%	100%
Initial Antibiotic Timing[2]	68	29%	46%	80%	93%
Oxygenation Assessment[2]	91	92%	93%	99%	100%
Pneumococcal Vaccine[2]	58	14%	34%	69%	94%
Smoking Cessation Advice[1,2]	5	100%	89%	80%	100%
Surgical Infection Prevention					
Prophylactic Antibiotic Given[1,2,3]	20	30%	55%	77%	95%
Prophylactic Antibiotic Selection[1,2]	20	80%	90%	90%	100%
Prophylactic Antibiotic Stopped[1,2,3]	20	100%	78%	72%	95%
Pregnancy Care					
Inpatient Neonatal Mortality	-	-	-	-	-
Third or Fourth Degree Laceration	-	-	-	3.63%	3.27%

Metropolitan Hospital

Carretera #1785 Urb Las Lomas
San Juan, PR 00922
Ownership: Proprietary
Emergency Services: Yes

Phone: 787-793-5013

Accredited: Yes

Measure	Cases	This Hospital	State Average	U.S. Average	Top Hospital

---

Measure	Cases	This Hospital	State Average	U.S. Average	Top Hospital
Heart Attack Care					
ACE Inhibitor or ARB for LVSD[5]	-	-	81%	82%	100%
Aspirin at Arrival[1,2]	22	100%	90%	92%	100%
Aspirin at Discharge[5]	-	-	82%	90%	100%
Beta Blocker at Arrival[1,2]	22	100%	81%	87%	100%
Beta Blocker at Discharge[5]	-	-	80%	90%	100%
Fibrinolytic Medication Timing[5]	-	-	27%	31%	100%
PCI Within 90 Minutes of Arrival[2]	0	-	0%	54%	95%
Smoking Cessation Advice[1,2]	10	100%	88%	88%	100%
Heart Failure Care					
ACE Inhibitor or ARB for LVSD[2]	42	100%	84%	82%	100%
Discharge Instructions[2]	232	98%	72%	61%	93%
Evaluation of LVS Function[5]	-	-	78%	83%	99%
Smoking Cessation Advice[2]	58	98%	92%	82%	100%
Pneumonia Care					
Appropriate Initial Antibiotic[5]	-	-	68%	83%	94%
Blood Culture Timing[2]	119	88%	71%	90%	100%
Influenza Vaccine[4,5]	-	-	38%	70%	100%
Initial Antibiotic Timing[5]	-	-	46%	80%	93%
Oxygenation Assessment[5]	-	-	93%	99%	100%
Pneumococcal Vaccine[5]	-	-	34%	69%	94%
Smoking Cessation Advice[2]	47	98%	89%	80%	100%
Surgical Infection Prevention					
Prophylactic Antibiotic Given[5]	-	-	55%	77%	95%
Prophylactic Antibiotic Selection[5]	-	-	90%	90%	100%
Prophylactic Antibiotic Stopped[1,2]	6	100%	78%	72%	95%
Pregnancy Care					
Inpatient Neonatal Mortality	-	-	-	-	-
Third or Fourth Degree Laceration	-	-	-	3.63%	3.27%

Hospital Wilma N Vazquez

Carr. 2 Km 39.5 Road Number 2
Vega Baja, PR 00694
Ownership: Voluntary non-profit - Private
Emergency Services: Yes

Phone: 787-858-1580

Accredited: No

Measure	Cases	This Hospital	State Average	U.S. Average	Top Hospital
Heart Attack Care					
ACE Inhibitor or ARB for LVSD[1,2]	4	100%	81%	82%	100%
Aspirin at Arrival[2]	33	100%	90%	92%	100%
Aspirin at Discharge[1,2]	23	100%	82%	90%	100%
Beta Blocker at Arrival[1,2]	23	96%	81%	87%	100%
Beta Blocker at Discharge[1,2]	18	100%	80%	90%	100%
Fibrinolytic Medication Timing[5]	-	-	27%	31%	100%
PCI Within 90 Minutes of Arrival[2]	0	-	0%	54%	95%
Smoking Cessation Advice[1,2]	1	100%	88%	88%	100%
Heart Failure Care					
ACE Inhibitor or ARB for LVSD[1,2]	4	100%	84%	82%	100%
Discharge Instructions[2]	46	100%	72%	61%	93%
Evaluation of LVS Function[2]	46	100%	78%	83%	99%
Smoking Cessation Advice[1,2]	1	100%	92%	82%	100%
Pneumonia Care					
Appropriate Initial Antibiotic[1,2]	18	44%	68%	83%	94%
Blood Culture Timing[5]	-	-	71%	90%	100%
Influenza Vaccine[1,2]	4	100%	38%	70%	100%
Initial Antibiotic Timing[2]	27	67%	46%	80%	93%
Oxygenation Assessment[2]	29	76%	93%	99%	100%
Pneumococcal Vaccine[1,2]	18	89%	34%	69%	94%
Smoking Cessation Advice[1,2]	2	100%	89%	80%	100%
Surgical Infection Prevention					
Prophylactic Antibiotic Given[5]	-	-	55%	77%	95%
Prophylactic Antibiotic Selection[5]	-	-	90%	90%	100%
Prophylactic Antibiotic Stopped[5]	-	-	78%	72%	95%
Pregnancy Care					
Inpatient Neonatal Mortality	-	-	-	-	-
Third or Fourth Degree Laceration	-	-	-	3.63%	3.27%

NOTE: Hospital profiles are in alphabetical order by state, then city, then hospital within the city; Rankings are sorted by rate in descending order and exclude hospitals with less than 25 cases; (1) The number of cases is too small (n<25) for purposes of reliably predicting hospital performance; (2) Measure reflects the hospital's indication that its submission was based upon a sample of its relevant discharges; (3) Rate reflects fewer than the maximum possible quarters of data for the measure; (4) Inaccurate information submitted and suppressed for one or more quarters; (5) No data is available from the hospital for this measure; Please refer to the User's Guide for a full explanation of data

Hospital Metropolitano Doctor Tito Mattei

PO Box 68
Yauco, PR 00698
URL: www.hmyauco.com
Ownership: Proprietary
Emergency Services: Yes

Phone: 787-856-2105
Fax: 787-856-4250

Accredited: Yes
Licensed Beds: 186

Key Personnel:

President/CEO . . . . Pedro F Barez, FACHE
Chief Medical Staff . . . . Manuel Ramirez Soto, MD
Cardiology Director . . . . Anibal Lugo, MD
Emergency Room . . . . Daniel Ortiz
Infection Control . . . . Luis Lugo, MD
OB/GYN Womens Health . . . . Norman Torres, MD
Surgical Services . . . . Anibal Torres, MD
Chief Radiology . . . . Tomas Irizarry, MD
Director Respiratory Therapy . . . . Hernan Orengo

Measure	Cases	This Hospital	State Average	U.S. Average	Top Hospital
Heart Attack Care					
ACE Inhibitor or ARB for LVSD	43	67%	81%	82%	100%
Aspirin at Arrival	270	91%	90%	92%	100%
Aspirin at Discharge	283	70%	82%	90%	100%
Beta Blocker at Arrival	238	78%	81%	87%	100%
Beta Blocker at Discharge	261	72%	80%	90%	100%
Fibrinolytic Medication Timing[1]	6	33%	27%	31%	100%
PCI Within 90 Minutes of Arrival	0	-	0%	54%	95%
Smoking Cessation Advice	108	93%	88%	88%	100%
Heart Failure Care					
ACE Inhibitor or ARB for LVSD	55	73%	84%	82%	100%
Discharge Instructions	228	18%	72%	61%	93%
Evaluation of LVS Function	226	99%	78%	83%	99%
Smoking Cessation Advice	69	90%	92%	82%	100%
Pneumonia Care					
Appropriate Initial Antibiotic	119	64%	68%	83%	94%
Blood Culture Timing	65	92%	71%	90%	100%
Influenza Vaccine	26	8%	38%	70%	100%
Initial Antibiotic Timing	145	12%	46%	80%	93%
Oxygenation Assessment	154	87%	93%	99%	100%
Pneumococcal Vaccine	84	25%	34%	69%	94%
Smoking Cessation Advice	29	93%	89%	80%	100%
Surgical Infection Prevention					
Prophylactic Antibiotic Given[3]	55	36%	55%	77%	95%
Prophylactic Antibiotic Selection	0	-	90%	90%	100%
Prophylactic Antibiotic Stopped[3]	31	100%	78%	72%	95%
Pregnancy Care					
Inpatient Neonatal Mortality	-	-	-	-	-
Third or Fourth Degree Laceration	-	-	-	3.63%	3.27%

NOTE: Hospital profiles are in alphabetical order by state, then city, then hospital within the city; Rankings are sorted by rate in descending order and exclude hospitals with less than 25 cases; (1) The number of cases is too small (n<25) for purposes of reliably predicting hospital performance; (2) Measure reflects the hospital's indication that its submission was based upon a sample of its relevant discharges; (3) Rate reflects fewer than the maximum possible quarters of data for the measure; (4) Inaccurate information submitted and suppressed for one or more quarters; (5) No data is available from the hospital for this measure; Please refer to the User's Guide for a full explanation of data

Heart Attack Care

1. ACE Inhibitor or ARB for LVSD

Hospital Name	City	Rate	Cases
Aiken Regional Medical Centers	Aiken	100%	36
Anderson Area Medical Center	Anderson	100%	54
Self Regional Healthcare Center	Greenwood	100%	53
Saint Francis Hospital	Greenville	97%	37
Providence Hosp/Providence Heart Inst	Columbia	92%	59
Palmetto Health Richland Hospital	Columbia	91%	85
Grand Strand Regional Medical Center	Myrtle Beach	89%	106
Piedmont Medical Center	Rock Hill	89%	92
Greenville Memorial Medical Campus	Greenville	88%	220
McLeod Regional Medical Center-Pee Dee	Florence	87%	188
Roper Hospital	Charleston	86%	51
Spartanburg Regional Health Care System	Spartanburg	86%	160
Medical University of S Carolina Med Ctr.	Charleston	85%	60
Trident Medical Center	Charleston	82%	76
Carolinas Hospital System-Florence	Florence	73%	49
Lexington Medical Center	West Columbia	68%	28

2. Aspirin at Arrival

Hospital Name	City	Rate	Cases
Anderson Area Medical Center	Anderson	100%	322
Conway Medical Center	Conway	100%	85
Grand Strand Regional Medical Center	Myrtle Beach	100%	322
Hilton Head Regional Medical Center	Hilton Head Isl	100%	80
Saint Francis Hospital	Greenville	100%	139
Aiken Regional Medical Centers	Aiken	99%	126
Medical University of S Carolina Med Ctr.	Charleston	99%	122
Piedmont Medical Center	Rock Hill	99%	298
Self Regional Healthcare Center	Greenwood	99%	175
Loris Community Hospital	Loris	98%	56
Mary Black Memorial Hospital	Spartanburg	98%	42
McLeod Regional Medical Center-Pee Dee	Florence	98%	323
Palmetto Health Baptist Columbia	Columbia	98%	60
Greenville Memorial Medical Campus	Greenville	97%	492
Roper Hospital	Charleston	97%	147
Spartanburg Regional Health Care System	Spartanburg	97%	406
Providence Hosp/Providence Heart Inst	Columbia	96%	171
Regional Med Ctr of Orangeburg & Calhoun	Orangeburg	96%	114
Trident Medical Center	Charleston	96%	205
Carolinas Hospital System-Florence	Florence	95%	144
Georgetown Memorial Hospital	Georgetown	95%	81
Lexington Medical Center	West Columbia	95%	183
Palmetto Health Richland Hospital	Columbia	94%	185
Beaufort Memorial Hospital	Beaufort	93%	72
Marion County Medical Center	Marion	93%	54
Oconee Memorial Hospital	Seneca	93%	44
Palmetto Baptist Medical Center Easley	Easley	93%	68
Waccamaw Community Hospital	Murrells Inlet	93%	59
Laurens County Hospital	Clinton	90%	31
Springs Memorial Hospital	Lancaster	90%	123
Carolina Pines Regional Medical Center	Hartsville	86%	37
Upstate Carolina Medical Center	Gaffney	84%	32
Tuomey Regional Medical Center	Sumter	81%	53
Kershaw County Medical Center	Camden	78%	41

3. Aspirin at Discharge

Hospital Name	City	Rate	Cases
Aiken Regional Medical Centers	Aiken	100%	134
Anderson Area Medical Center	Anderson	100%	326
Medical University of S Carolina Med Ctr.	Charleston	100%	266
Hilton Head Regional Medical Center	Hilton Head Isl	99%	93
Saint Francis Hospital	Greenville	99%	171
Spartanburg Regional Health Care System	Spartanburg	99%	557
Grand Strand Regional Medical Center	Myrtle Beach	98%	416
Greenville Memorial Medical Campus	Greenville	98%	658
McLeod Regional Medical Center-Pee Dee	Florence	98%	503
Palmetto Health Richland Hospital	Columbia	98%	363
Piedmont Medical Center	Rock Hill	98%	347
Providence Hosp/Providence Heart Inst	Columbia	98%	302
Self Regional Healthcare Center	Greenwood	98%	180
Palmetto Health Baptist Columbia	Columbia	97%	33
Roper Hospital	Charleston	97%	297
Lexington Medical Center	West Columbia	95%	91
Trident Medical Center	Charleston	95%	326
Carolinas Hospital System-Florence	Florence	94%	192
Loris Community Hospital	Loris	94%	34
Marion County Medical Center	Marion	94%	35
Beaufort Memorial Hospital	Beaufort	92%	38
Palmetto Baptist Medical Center Easley	Easley	92%	40
Regional Med Ctr of Orangeburg & Calhoun	Orangeburg	91%	57

Georgetown Memorial Hospital	Georgetown	90%	60
Conway Medical Center	Conway	87%	39
Waccamaw Community Hospital	Murrells Inlet	84%	31
Springs Memorial Hospital	Lancaster	81%	75
Tuomey Regional Medical Center	Sumter	77%	30

4. Beta Blocker at Arrival

Hospital Name	City	Rate	Cases
Anderson Area Medical Center	Anderson	100%	272
Palmetto Health Baptist Columbia	Columbia	100%	43
Saint Francis Hospital	Greenville	100%	102
Beaufort Memorial Hospital	Beaufort	99%	68
Medical University of S Carolina Med Ctr.	Charleston	99%	114
Grand Strand Regional Medical Center	Myrtle Beach	98%	273
Loris Community Hospital	Loris	98%	52
Spartanburg Regional Health Care System	Spartanburg	98%	315
Roper Hospital	Charleston	97%	129
Conway Medical Center	Conway	96%	75
Hilton Head Regional Medical Center	Hilton Head Isl	96%	54
Marion County Medical Center	Marion	96%	48
Aiken Regional Medical Centers	Aiken	95%	85
McLeod Regional Medical Center-Pee Dee	Florence	95%	253
Greenville Memorial Medical Campus	Greenville	94%	383
Providence Hosp/Providence Heart Inst	Columbia	94%	162
Self Regional Healthcare Center	Greenwood	94%	132
Carolinas Hospital System-Florence	Florence	93%	109
Mary Black Memorial Hospital	Spartanburg	93%	45
Palmetto Baptist Medical Center Easley	Easley	93%	46
Piedmont Medical Center	Rock Hill	93%	280
Regional Med Ctr of Orangeburg & Calhoun	Orangeburg	93%	82
Georgetown Memorial Hospital	Georgetown	92%	74
Palmetto Health Richland Hospital	Columbia	92%	131
Waccamaw Community Hospital	Murrells Inlet	91%	54
Oconee Memorial Hospital	Seneca	89%	28
Lexington Medical Center	West Columbia	87%	131
Springs Memorial Hospital	Lancaster	86%	105
Trident Medical Center	Charleston	85%	186
Tuomey Regional Medical Center	Sumter	85%	33
Kershaw County Medical Center	Camden	82%	38
Carolina Pines Regional Medical Center	Hartsville	81%	32
Laurens County Hospital	Clinton	77%	30
Upstate Carolina Medical Center	Gaffney	62%	29

5. Beta Blocker at Discharge

Hospital Name	City	Rate	Cases
Aiken Regional Medical Centers	Aiken	100%	125
Anderson Area Medical Center	Anderson	100%	309
Palmetto Health Baptist Columbia	Columbia	100%	34
Waccamaw Community Hospital	Murrells Inlet	100%	32
Grand Strand Regional Medical Center	Myrtle Beach	99%	413
McLeod Regional Medical Center-Pee Dee	Florence	99%	609
Medical University of S Carolina Med Ctr.	Charleston	99%	276
Saint Francis Hospital	Greenville	99%	193
Spartanburg Regional Health Care System	Spartanburg	99%	603
Carolinas Hospital System-Florence	Florence	98%	205
Hilton Head Regional Medical Center	Hilton Head Isl	98%	92
Self Regional Healthcare Center	Greenwood	98%	186
Greenville Memorial Medical Campus	Greenville	97%	744
Lexington Medical Center	West Columbia	97%	92
Piedmont Medical Center	Rock Hill	97%	338
Palmetto Health Richland Hospital	Columbia	96%	344
Regional Med Ctr of Orangeburg & Calhoun	Orangeburg	96%	67
Beaufort Memorial Hospital	Beaufort	95%	37
Conway Medical Center	Conway	95%	37
Palmetto Baptist Medical Center Easley	Easley	95%	44
Providence Hosp/Providence Heart Inst	Columbia	95%	292
Roper Hospital	Charleston	95%	270
Loris Community Hospital	Loris	94%	35
Marion County Medical Center	Marion	92%	38
Trident Medical Center	Charleston	92%	317
Tuomey Regional Medical Center	Sumter	91%	45
Georgetown Memorial Hospital	Georgetown	90%	60
Springs Memorial Hospital	Lancaster	84%	77

6. Fibrinolytic Medication Timing

Hospital Name	City	Rate	Cases
Oconee Memorial Hospital	Seneca	45%	29

7. PCI Within 90 Minutes of Arrival

Hospital Name	City	Rate	Cases
Grand Strand Regional Medical Center	Myrtle Beach	83%	29
Greenville Memorial Medical Campus	Greenville	68%	34
Spartanburg Regional Health Care System	Spartanburg	68%	25

NOTE: Hospital profiles are in alphabetical order by state, then city, then hospital within the city; Rankings are sorted by rate in descending order and exclude hospitals with less than 25 cases; (1) The number of cases is too small (n<25) for purposes of reliably predicting hospital performance; (2) Measure reflects the hospital's indication that its submission was based upon a sample of its relevant discharges; (3) Rate reflects fewer than the maximum possible quarters of data for the measure; (4) Inaccurate information submitted and suppressed for one or more quarters; (5) No data is available from the hospital for this measure; Please refer to the User's Guide for a full explanation of data

8. Smoking Cessation Advice

Hospital Name	City	Rate	Cases
Anderson Area Medical Center	Anderson	100%	138
Georgetown Memorial Hospital	Georgetown	100%	30
Greenville Memorial Medical Campus	Greenville	100%	404
McLeod Regional Medical Center-Pee Dee	Florence	100%	270
Palmetto Health Richland Hospital	Columbia	100%	191
Providence Hosp/Providence Heart Inst	Columbia	100%	124
Saint Francis Hospital	Greenville	100%	65
Spartanburg Regional Health Care System	Spartanburg	100%	307
Grand Strand Regional Medical Center	Myrtle Beach	99%	167
Piedmont Medical Center	Rock Hill	99%	151
Self Regional Healthcare Center	Greenwood	99%	74
Medical University of S Carolina Med Ctr	Charleston	98%	112
Carolinas Hospital System-Florence	Florence	97%	73
Springs Memorial Hospital	Lancaster	97%	31
Trident Medical Center	Charleston	96%	135
Aiken Regional Medical Centers	Aiken	95%	60
Hilton Head Regional Medical Center	Hilton Head Isl	93%	29
Roper Hospital	Charleston	86%	104

Heart Failure Care

9. ACE Inhibitor or ARB for LVSD

Hospital Name	City	Rate	Cases
Aiken Regional Medical Centers	Aiken	99%	138
Saint Francis Hospital	Greenville	99%	160
Palmetto Baptist Medical Center Easley	Easley	98%	48
Spartanburg Regional Health Care System	Spartanburg	98%	286
Chesterfield General Hospital	Cheraw	97%	39
Marlboro Park Hospital	Bennettsville	97%	31
Waccamaw Community Hospital	Murrells Inlet	96%	54
Greenville Memorial Medical Campus	Greenville	94%	395
Palmetto Health Baptist Columbia	Columbia	93%	87
Roper Hospital	Charleston	93%	297
Wilson Medical Center	Darlington	93%	27
Self Regional Healthcare Center	Greenwood	92%	193
Conway Medical Center	Conway	91%	86
Laurens County Hospital	Clinton	90%	31
Mary Black Memorial Hospital	Spartanburg	90%	63
Providence Hosp/Providence Heart Inst	Columbia	90%	181
Anderson Area Medical Center	Anderson	89%	212
Bon Secours Saint Francis Hospital	Charleston	89%	45
Grand Strand Regional Medical Center	Myrtle Beach	89%	181
Marion County Medical Center	Marion	89%	100
Loris Community Hospital	Loris	88%	59
McLeod Regional Medical Center-Pee Dee	Florence	88%	355
Carolinas Hospital System-Florence	Florence	87%	210
Medical University of S Carolina Med Ctr	Charleston	87%	290
Palmetto Health Richland Hospital	Columbia	87%	279
Tuomey Regional Medical Center	Sumter	87%	206
Allen Bennett Memorial Hospital	Greer	86%	36
Beaufort Memorial Hospital	Beaufort	86%	118
East Cooper Regional Medical Center	Mount Pleasant	85%	26
Piedmont Medical Center	Rock Hill	84%	160
Clarendon Memorial Hospital	Manning	83%	35
Georgetown Memorial Hospital	Georgetown	83%	102
Regional Med Ctr of Orangeburg & Calhoun	Orangeburg	82%	119
Hilton Head Regional Medical Center	Hilton Head Isl	79%	78
Carolina Pines Regional Medical Center	Hartsville	78%	109
Colleton Medical Center	Walterboro	78%	83
McLeod Medical Center Dillon	Dillon	78%	46
Kershaw County Medical Center	Camden	77%	90
Trident Medical Center	Charleston	77%	248
Wallace Thomson Hospital	Union	77%	30
Lexington Medical Center	West Columbia	76%	105
Newberry County Memorial Hospital	Newberry	74%	42
Oconee Memorial Hospital	Seneca	72%	71
Springs Memorial Hospital	Lancaster	72%	103
Upstate Carolina Medical Center	Gaffney	69%	36
Carolinas Hospital System-Lake City	Lake City	67%	27
Chester Regional Medical Center	Chester	64%	39

10. Discharge Instructions

Hospital Name	City	Rate	Cases
Grand Strand Regional Medical Center	Myrtle Beach	99%	479
Providence Hosp/Providence Heart Inst	Columbia	96%	277
Carolinas Hospital System-Lake City	Lake City	91%	55
Conway Medical Center	Conway	90%	49
Spartanburg Regional Health Care System	Spartanburg	90%	631
Loris Community Hospital	Loris	89%	165
East Cooper Regional Medical Center	Mount Pleasant	88%	75
Cannon Memorial Hospital	Pickens	87%	31

Hospital Name	City	Rate	Cases
Medical University of S Carolina Med Ctr	Charleston	86%	449
Palmetto Health Baptist Columbia	Columbia	86%	198
Palmetto Baptist Medical Center Easley	Easley	85%	117
Clarendon Memorial Hospital	Manning	84%	103
Newberry County Memorial Hospital	Newberry	83%	119
McLeod Regional Medical Center-Pee Dee	Florence	82%	679
Bon Secours Saint Francis Hospital	Charleston	81%	137
Springs Memorial Hospital	Lancaster	81%	189
Allen Bennett Memorial Hospital	Greer	78%	76
Georgetown Memorial Hospital	Georgetown	77%	209
Saint Francis Hospital	Greenville	76%	325
Anderson Area Medical Center	Anderson	75%	448
McLeod Medical Center Dillon	Dillon	75%	36
Piedmont Medical Center	Rock Hill	75%	293
Roper Hospital	Charleston	75%	602
Palmetto Health Richland Hospital	Columbia	74%	472
Beaufort Memorial Hospital	Beaufort	73%	243
Hillcrest Hospital	Simpsonville	71%	41
Greenville Memorial Medical Campus	Greenville	70%	694
Waccamaw Community Hospital	Murrells Inlet	69%	153
Bamberg County Memorial Hospital	Bamberg	67%	46
Edgefield County Hospital	Edgefield	67%	45
Chesterfield General Hospital	Cheraw	66%	87
Marion County Medical Center	Marion	66%	221
Self Regional Healthcare Center	Greenwood	66%	333
Carolinas Hospital System-Florence	Florence	64%	394
Coastal Carolina Medical Center	Hardeeville	62%	39
Laurens County Hospital	Clinton	62%	66
Carolina Pines Regional Medical Center	Hartsville	60%	226
Lexington Medical Center	West Columbia	59%	217
Hilton Head Regional Medical Center	Hilton Head Isl	58%	155
Marlboro Park Hospital	Bennettsville	58%	73
Mary Black Memorial Hospital	Spartanburg	57%	141
Oconee Memorial Hospital	Seneca	57%	162
Kershaw County Medical Center	Camden	56%	200
Chester Regional Medical Center	Chester	54%	123
Upstate Carolina Medical Center	Gaffney	54%	110
Regional Med Ctr of Orangeburg & Calhoun	Orangeburg	53%	373
Tuomey Regional Medical Center	Sumter	51%	472
Aiken Regional Medical Centers	Aiken	47%	226
Wallace Thomson Hospital	Union	46%	145
Colleton Medical Center	Walterboro	42%	265
Trident Medical Center	Charleston	38%	591
Fairfield Memorial Hospital	Winnsboro	18%	34
Williamsburg Regional Hospital	Kingstree	17%	29
Hampton Regional Medical Center	Varnville	0%	25

11. Evaluation of LVS Function

Hospital Name	City	Rate	Cases
Saint Francis Hospital	Greenville	100%	372
Spartanburg Regional Health Care System	Spartanburg	100%	737
Aiken Regional Medical Centers	Aiken	99%	276
Grand Strand Regional Medical Center	Myrtle Beach	99%	534
Lexington Medical Center	West Columbia	99%	268
Medical University of S Carolina Med Ctr	Charleston	99%	475
Palmetto Health Richland Hospital	Columbia	99%	530
Piedmont Medical Center	Rock Hill	99%	355
Providence Hosp/Providence Heart Inst	Columbia	99%	326
Carolina Pines Regional Medical Center	Hartsville	98%	252
Greenville Memorial Medical Campus	Greenville	98%	800
Mary Black Memorial Hospital	Spartanburg	98%	174
Palmetto Health Baptist Columbia	Columbia	98%	232
Roper Hospital	Charleston	98%	705
Wilson Medical Center	Darlington	98%	49
Carolinas Hospital System-Florence	Florence	97%	477
Georgetown Memorial Hospital	Georgetown	97%	237
Self Regional Healthcare Center	Greenwood	97%	380
Anderson Area Medical Center	Anderson	96%	567
Kershaw County Medical Center	Camden	96%	252
Bon Secours Saint Francis Hospital	Charleston	95%	167
Palmetto Baptist Medical Center Easley	Easley	95%	147
Springs Memorial Hospital	Lancaster	95%	256
Allen Bennett Memorial Hospital	Greer	94%	104
Colleton Medical Center	Walterboro	94%	287
Hillcrest Hospital	Simpsonville	94%	54
Hilton Head Regional Medical Center	Hilton Head Isl	94%	199
Marion County Medical Center	Marion	94%	248
Loris Community Hospital	Loris	93%	175
McLeod Regional Medical Center-Pee Dee	Florence	93%	747
Carolinas Hospital System-Lake City	Lake City	92%	64
Conway Medical Center	Conway	92%	260
Waccamaw Community Hospital	Murrells Inlet	92%	178
Chesterfield General Hospital	Cheraw	91%	101
Chester Regional Medical Center	Chester	89%	146

NOTE: Hospital profiles are in alphabetical order by state, then city, then hospital within the city; Rankings are sorted by rate in descending order and exclude hospitals with less than 25 cases; (1) The number of cases is too small (n<25) for purposes of reliably predicting hospital performance; (2) Measure reflects the hospital's indication that its submission was based upon a sample of its relevant discharges; (3) Rate reflects fewer than the maximum possible quarters of data for the measure; (4) Inaccurate information submitted and suppressed for one or more quarters; (5) No data is available from the hospital for this measure; Please refer to the User's Guide for a full explanation of data

Regional Med Ctr of Orangeburg & Calhoun	Orangeburg	89%	412
Trident Medical Center	Charleston	87%	671
Tuomey Regional Medical Center	Sumter	85%	571
Upstate Carolina Medical Center	Gaffney	84%	141
Beaufort Memorial Hospital	Beaufort	83%	264
Clarendon Memorial Hospital	Manning	83%	112
East Cooper Regional Medical Center	Mount Pleasant	82%	94
Oconee Memorial Hospital	Seneca	82%	203
Marlboro Park Hospital	Bennettsville	81%	79
Barnwell County Hospital	Barnwell	78%	46
Cannon Memorial Hospital	Pickens	78%	37
Laurens County Hospital	Clinton	78%	112
Bamberg County Memorial Hospital	Bamberg	77%	53
Newberry County Memorial Hospital	Newberry	77%	144
McLeod Medical Center Dillon	Dillon	76%	178
Edgefield County Hospital	Edgefield	68%	59
Wallace Thomson Hospital	Union	67%	163
Williamsburg Regional Hospital	Kingstree	65%	31
Coastal Carolina Medical Center	Hardeeville	63%	41
Fairfield Memorial Hospital	Winnsboro	63%	41
Hampton Regional Medical Center	Varnville	48%	25

12. Smoking Cessation Advice

Hospital Name	City	Rate	Cases
Anderson Area Medical Center	Anderson	100%	124
Grand Strand Regional Medical Center	Myrtle Beach	100%	97
Oconee Memorial Hospital	Seneca	100%	28
Palmetto Baptist Medical Center Easley	Easley	100%	34
Piedmont Medical Center	Rock Hill	100%	85
Providence Hosp/Providence Heart Inst	Columbia	100%	67
Saint Francis Hospital	Greenville	100%	97
Self Regional Healthcare Center	Greenwood	100%	85
Springs Memorial Hospital	Lancaster	100%	57
Carolinas Hospital System-Florence	Florence	99%	98
McLeod Regional Medical Center-Pee Dee	Florence	99%	174
Palmetto Health Richland Hospital	Columbia	99%	176
Regional Med Ctr of Orangeburg & Calhoun	Orangeburg	99%	98
Spartanburg Regional Health Care System	Spartanburg	99%	184
Aiken Regional Medical Centers	Aiken	98%	42
Georgetown Memorial Hospital	Georgetown	96%	50
Greenville Memorial Medical Campus	Greenville	96%	195
Colleton Medical Center	Walterboro	95%	56
Mary Black Memorial Hospital	Spartanburg	95%	43
Palmetto Health Baptist Columbia	Columbia	95%	63
Medical University of S Carolina Med Ctr	Charleston	94%	131
Waccamaw Community Hospital	Murrells Inlet	94%	35
Lexington Medical Center	West Columbia	93%	58
Marion County Medical Center	Marion	93%	69
Newberry County Memorial Hospital	Newberry	93%	27
Trident Medical Center	Charleston	93%	121
Tuomey Regional Medical Center	Sumter	92%	135
Beaufort Memorial Hospital	Beaufort	91%	46
Kershaw County Medical Center	Camden	89%	62
Loris Community Hospital	Loris	89%	45
Bon Secours Saint Francis Hospital	Charleston	85%	26
Marlboro Park Hospital	Bennettsville	85%	26
Carolina Pines Regional Medical Center	Hartsville	84%	62
Roper Hospital	Charleston	84%	128
Carolinas Hospital System-Lake City	Lake City	72%	25
Chester Regional Medical Center	Chester	70%	44
Upstate Carolina Medical Center	Gaffney	68%	37
Wallace Thomson Hospital	Union	52%	29

Pneumonia Care

13. Appropriate Initial Antibiotic

Hospital Name	City	Rate	Cases
Carolinas Hospital System-Lake City	Lake City	97%	64
Hilton Head Regional Medical Center	Hilton Head Isl	96%	98
Hillcrest Hospital	Simpsonville	94%	85
Allen Bennett Memorial Hospital	Greer	93%	123
Greenville Memorial Medical Campus	Greenville	93%	294
Anderson Area Medical Center	Anderson	92%	443
Bon Secours Saint Francis Hospital	Charleston	92%	138
Saint Francis Hospital	Greenville	92%	225
Spartanburg Regional Health Care System	Spartanburg	92%	325
Palmetto Baptist Medical Center Easley	Easley	91%	127
Georgetown Memorial Hospital	Georgetown	90%	84
Hampton Regional Medical Center	Varnville	90%	29
Trident Medical Center	Charleston	90%	277
East Cooper Regional Medical Center	Mount Pleasant	89%	103
Kershaw County Medical Center	Camden	89%	161
Oconee Memorial Hospital	Seneca	89%	248
Aiken Regional Medical Centers	Aiken	88%	104

Grand Strand Regional Medical Center	Myrtle Beach	88%	182
Medical University of S Carolina Med Ctr	Charleston	88%	107
Palmetto Health Richland Hospital	Columbia	88%	130
Carolina Pines Regional Medical Center	Hartsville	87%	196
Mary Black Memorial Hospital	Spartanburg	87%	107
Cannon Memorial Hospital	Pickens	86%	81
McLeod Regional Medical Center-Pee Dee	Florence	86%	235
Roper Hospital	Charleston	85%	155
Beaufort Memorial Hospital	Beaufort	84%	92
Self Regional Healthcare Center	Greenwood	84%	187
Coastal Carolina Medical Center	Hardeeville	83%	30
Piedmont Medical Center	Rock Hill	83%	336
Providence Hosp/Providence Heart Inst	Columbia	83%	150
Waccamaw Community Hospital	Murrells Inlet	83%	103
Laurens County Hospital	Clinton	82%	122
Lexington Medical Center	West Columbia	82%	122
Chesterfield General Hospital	Cheraw	81%	98
Clarendon Memorial Hospital	Manning	81%	132
Palmetto Health Baptist Columbia	Columbia	81%	172
Tuomey Regional Medical Center	Sumter	79%	162
Regional Med Ctr of Orangeburg & Calhoun	Orangeburg	78%	184
Carolinas Hospital System-Florence	Florence	77%	190
Loris Community Hospital	Loris	77%	82
Marlboro Park Hospital	Bennettsville	77%	70
Fairfield Memorial Hospital	Winnsboro	76%	38
Edgefield County Hospital	Edgefield	75%	40
Newberry County Memorial Hospital	Newberry	75%	64
Marion County Medical Center	Marion	74%	57
Springs Memorial Hospital	Lancaster	71%	148
Colleton Medical Center	Walterboro	67%	83
Upstate Carolina Medical Center	Gaffney	66%	109
Bamberg County Memorial Hospital	Bamberg	64%	45
Chester Regional Medical Center	Chester	64%	94
Wallace Thomson Hospital	Union	61%	82
Williamsburg Regional Hospital	Kingstree	56%	32

14. Blood Culture Timing

Hospital Name	City	Rate	Cases
Hillcrest Hospital	Simpsonville	100%	48
Allen Bennett Memorial Hospital	Greer	99%	74
Medical University of S Carolina Med Ctr	Charleston	99%	145
Anderson Area Medical Center	Anderson	98%	567
Carolinas Hospital System-Florence	Florence	97%	172
Colleton Medical Center	Walterboro	97%	59
Roper Hospital	Charleston	97%	139
McLeod Regional Medical Center-Pee Dee	Florence	96%	244
Saint Francis Hospital	Greenville	96%	232
Self Regional Healthcare Center	Greenwood	96%	212
Upstate Carolina Medical Center	Gaffney	96%	113
Carolina Pines Regional Medical Center	Hartsville	95%	175
Greenville Memorial Medical Campus	Greenville	95%	268
Loris Community Hospital	Loris	95%	59
Spartanburg Regional Health Care System	Spartanburg	95%	346
Georgetown Memorial Hospital	Georgetown	94%	118
Palmetto Baptist Medical Center Easley	Easley	94%	125
Palmetto Health Baptist Columbia	Columbia	94%	175
Regional Med Ctr of Orangeburg & Calhoun	Orangeburg	94%	204
Palmetto Health Richland Hospital	Columbia	93%	121
Aiken Regional Medical Centers	Aiken	92%	116
Bon Secours Saint Francis Hospital	Charleston	92%	131
Cannon Memorial Hospital	Pickens	92%	91
Lexington Medical Center	West Columbia	92%	98
Conway Medical Center	Conway	91%	33
Oconee Memorial Hospital	Seneca	91%	127
Carolinas Hospital System-Lake City	Lake City	90%	42
Clarendon Memorial Hospital	Manning	90%	87
Hilton Head Regional Medical Center	Hilton Head Isl	90%	92
Marlboro Park Hospital	Bennettsville	90%	50
Waccamaw Community Hospital	Murrells Inlet	90%	94
Chester Regional Medical Center	Chester	89%	37
East Cooper Regional Medical Center	Mount Pleasant	87%	97
Chesterfield General Hospital	Cheraw	86%	86
Mary Black Memorial Hospital	Spartanburg	86%	122
Kershaw County Medical Center	Camden	85%	114
Laurens County Hospital	Clinton	85%	86
Tuomey Regional Medical Center	Sumter	85%	117
Wallace Thomson Hospital	Union	85%	47
Bamberg County Memorial Hospital	Bamberg	84%	32
Grand Strand Regional Medical Center	Myrtle Beach	84%	197
Marion County Medical Center	Marion	84%	58
Newberry County Memorial Hospital	Newberry	84%	50
Springs Memorial Hospital	Lancaster	84%	89
Trident Medical Center	Charleston	83%	208
Piedmont Medical Center	Rock Hill	79%	291

NOTE: Hospital profiles are in alphabetical order by state, then city, then hospital within the city; Rankings are sorted by rate in descending order and exclude hospitals with less than 25 cases; (1) The number of cases is too small (n<25) for purposes of reliably predicting hospital performance; (2) Measure reflects the hospital's indication that its submission was based upon a sample of its relevant discharges; (3) Rate reflects fewer than the maximum possible quarters of data for the measure; (4) Inaccurate information submitted and suppressed for one or more quarters; (5) No data is available from the hospital for this measure; Please refer to the User's Guide for a full explanation of data

Beaufort Memorial Hospital	Beaufort	77%	48

15. Influenza Vaccine

Hospital Name	City	Rate	Cases
Palmetto Baptist Medical Center Easley	Easley	100%	25
Springs Memorial Hospital	Lancaster	100%	40
Saint Francis Hospital	Greenville	97%	73
Lexington Medical Center	West Columbia	92%	26
Providence Hosp/Providence Heart Inst	Columbia	92%	51
Bon Secours Saint Francis Hospital	Charleston	90%	48
McLeod Regional Medical Center-Pee Dee	Florence	90%	63
Piedmont Medical Center	Rock Hill	90%	102
Spartanburg Regional Health Care System	Spartanburg	89%	82
Allen Bennett Memorial Hospital	Greer	88%	34
Roper Hospital	Charleston	87%	75
Aiken Regional Medical Centers	Aiken	85%	34
Medical University of S Carolina Med Ctr	Charleston	84%	32
Greenville Memorial Medical Campus	Greenville	83%	98
Palmetto Health Richland Hospital	Columbia	83%	30
Waccamaw Community Hospital	Murrells Inlet	83%	36
Mary Black Memorial Hospital	Spartanburg	81%	42
Loris Community Hospital	Loris	79%	28
Self Regional Healthcare Center	Greenwood	79%	62
Anderson Area Medical Center	Anderson	77%	156
East Cooper Regional Medical Center	Mount Pleasant	76%	34
Tuomey Regional Medical Center	Sumter	76%	34
Hilton Head Regional Medical Center	Hilton Head Isl	74%	27
Carolinas Hospital System-Florence	Florence	73%	45
Laurens County Hospital	Clinton	73%	30
Palmetto Health Baptist Columbia	Columbia	73%	52
Oconee Memorial Hospital	Seneca	72%	90
Grand Strand Regional Medical Center	Myrtle Beach	64%	74
Kershaw County Medical Center	Camden	62%	48
Chesterfield General Hospital	Cheraw	61%	31
Regional Med Ctr of Orangeburg & Calhoun	Orangeburg	58%	48
Carolina Pines Regional Medical Center	Hartsville	57%	49
Trident Medical Center	Charleston	51%	91
Georgetown Memorial Hospital	Georgetown	37%	30

16. Initial Antibiotic Timing

Hospital Name	City	Rate	Cases
Edgefield County Hospital	Edgefield	100%	47
Aiken Regional Medical Centers	Aiken	94%	164
Chesterfield General Hospital	Cheraw	94%	132
Hilton Head Regional Medical Center	Hilton Head Isl	94%	108
Fairfield Memorial Hospital	Winnsboro	93%	43
Waccamaw Community Hospital	Murrells Inlet	93%	166
Allen Bennett Memorial Hospital	Greer	92%	148
Newberry County Memorial Hospital	Newberry	92%	88
Carolina Pines Regional Medical Center	Hartsville	90%	292
Oconee Memorial Hospital	Seneca	90%	349
Colleton Medical Center	Walterboro	88%	127
Conway Medical Center	Conway	88%	248
Carolinas Hospital System-Lake City	Lake City	87%	70
Georgetown Memorial Hospital	Georgetown	87%	162
Regional Med Ctr of Orangeburg & Calhoun	Orangeburg	87%	303
Springs Memorial Hospital	Lancaster	87%	187
Bon Secours Saint Francis Hospital	Charleston	86%	181
East Cooper Regional Medical Center	Mount Pleasant	85%	139
Grand Strand Regional Medical Center	Myrtle Beach	85%	277
Hillcrest Hospital	Simpsonville	85%	109
McLeod Medical Center Dillon	Dillon	85%	93
Mary Black Memorial Hospital	Spartanburg	84%	152
Roper Hospital	Charleston	84%	248
Clarendon Memorial Hospital	Manning	83%	156
Saint Francis Hospital	Greenville	83%	318
Bamberg County Memorial Hospital	Bamberg	82%	57
Barnwell County Hospital	Barnwell	82%	93
Laurens County Hospital	Clinton	82%	131
Spartanburg Regional Health Care System	Spartanburg	82%	499
Upstate Carolina Medical Center	Gaffney	82%	164
Cannon Memorial Hospital	Pickens	81%	100
Loris Community Hospital	Loris	81%	93
Palmetto Health Baptist Columbia	Columbia	81%	222
Carolinas Hospital System-Florence	Florence	79%	277
McLeod Regional Medical Center-Pee Dee	Florence	79%	319
Self Regional Healthcare Center	Greenwood	79%	274
Williamsburg Regional Hospital	Kingstree	79%	38
Anderson Area Medical Center	Anderson	78%	715
Marlboro Park Hospital	Bennettsville	77%	75
Palmetto Baptist Medical Center Easley	Easley	77%	201
Piedmont Medical Center	Rock Hill	77%	511
Wallace Thomson Hospital	Union	77%	111
Lexington Medical Center	West Columbia	76%	138

Hospital Name	City	Rate	Cases
Medical University of S Carolina Med Ctr	Charleston	76%	210
Kershaw County Medical Center	Camden	73%	230
Marion County Medical Center	Marion	73%	85
Wilson Medical Center	Darlington	72%	29
Palmetto Health Richland Hospital	Columbia	70%	195
Beaufort Memorial Hospital	Beaufort	67%	87
Greenville Memorial Medical Campus	Greenville	67%	456
Tuomey Regional Medical Center	Sumter	66%	241
Chester Regional Medical Center	Chester	65%	101
Providence Hosp/Providence Heart Inst	Columbia	64%	164
Trident Medical Center	Charleston	54%	402

17. Oxygenation Assessment

Hospital Name	City	Rate	Cases
Aiken Regional Medical Centers	Aiken	100%	197
Allen Bennett Memorial Hospital	Greer	100%	187
Bon Secours Saint Francis Hospital	Charleston	100%	219
Cannon Memorial Hospital	Pickens	100%	140
Carolina Pines Regional Medical Center	Hartsville	100%	336
Carolinas Hospital System-Lake City	Lake City	100%	73
Conway Medical Center	Conway	100%	294
East Cooper Regional Medical Center	Mount Pleasant	100%	169
Edgefield County Hospital	Edgefield	100%	60
Fairfield Memorial Hospital	Winnsboro	100%	49
Georgetown Memorial Hospital	Georgetown	100%	188
Grand Strand Regional Medical Center	Myrtle Beach	100%	349
Greenville Memorial Medical Campus	Greenville	100%	552
Hampton Regional Medical Center	Varnville	100%	32
Hilton Head Regional Medical Center	Hilton Head Isl	100%	167
Kershaw County Medical Center	Camden	100%	293
Laurens County Hospital	Clinton	100%	181
Lexington Medical Center	West Columbia	100%	184
Loris Community Hospital	Loris	100%	140
Marion County Medical Center	Marion	100%	112
Mary Black Memorial Hospital	Spartanburg	100%	205
McLeod Medical Center Dillon	Dillon	100%	133
Medical University of S Carolina Med Ctr	Charleston	100%	249
Newberry County Memorial Hospital	Newberry	100%	92
Oconee Memorial Hospital	Seneca	100%	488
Palmetto Baptist Medical Center Easley	Easley	100%	233
Palmetto Health Baptist Columbia	Columbia	100%	274
Palmetto Health Richland Hospital	Columbia	100%	249
Piedmont Medical Center	Rock Hill	100%	584
Providence Hosp/Providence Heart Inst	Columbia	100%	221
Regional Med Ctr of Orangeburg & Calhoun	Orangeburg	100%	360
Roper Hospital	Charleston	100%	309
Saint Francis Hospital	Greenville	100%	415
Spartanburg Regional Health Care System	Spartanburg	100%	604
Trident Medical Center	Charleston	100%	527
Tuomey Regional Medical Center	Sumter	100%	292
Waccamaw Community Hospital	Murrells Inlet	100%	198
Wilson Medical Center	Darlington	100%	33
Anderson Area Medical Center	Anderson	99%	868
Bamberg County Memorial Hospital	Bamberg	99%	83
Chesterfield General Hospital	Cheraw	99%	154
Clarendon Memorial Hospital	Manning	99%	193
Colleton Medical Center	Walterboro	99%	150
Hillcrest Hospital	Simpsonville	99%	129
Marlboro Park Hospital	Bennettsville	99%	91
McLeod Regional Medical Center-Pee Dee	Florence	99%	421
Self Regional Healthcare Center	Greenwood	99%	345
Springs Memorial Hospital	Lancaster	99%	200
Upstate Carolina Medical Center	Gaffney	99%	218
Wallace Thomson Hospital	Union	99%	140
Barnwell County Hospital	Barnwell	98%	118
Beaufort Memorial Hospital	Beaufort	98%	106
Carolinas Hospital System-Florence	Florence	98%	336
Chester Regional Medical Center	Chester	98%	109
Coastal Carolina Medical Center	Hardeeville	97%	38
Williamsburg Regional Hospital	Kingstree	93%	44

18. Pneumococcal Vaccine

Hospital Name	City	Rate	Cases
Palmetto Baptist Medical Center Easley	Easley	99%	144
Aiken Regional Medical Centers	Aiken	97%	120
Lexington Medical Center	West Columbia	95%	94
Spartanburg Regional Health Care System	Spartanburg	95%	356
East Cooper Regional Medical Center	Mount Pleasant	94%	111
Waccamaw Community Hospital	Murrells Inlet	93%	128
Mary Black Memorial Hospital	Spartanburg	92%	130
Anderson Area Medical Center	Anderson	91%	558
Edgefield County Hospital	Edgefield	91%	46
Hillcrest Hospital	Simpsonville	89%	81
Cannon Memorial Hospital	Pickens	88%	86

NOTE: Hospital profiles are in alphabetical order by state, then city, then hospital within the city; Rankings are sorted by rate in descending order and exclude hospitals with less than 25 cases; (1) The number of cases is too small (n<25) for purposes of reliably predicting hospital performance; (2) Measure reflects the hospital's indication that its submission was based upon a sample of its relevant discharges; (3) Rate reflects fewer than the maximum possible quarters of data for the measure; (4) Inaccurate information submitted and suppressed for one or more quarters; (5) No data is available from the hospital for this measure; Please refer to the User's Guide for a full explanation of data

Piedmont Medical Center	Rock Hill	88%	315
Springs Memorial Hospital	Lancaster	88%	108
Allen Bennett Memorial Hospital	Greer	87%	119
Carolinas Hospital System-Lake City	Lake City	86%	35
Saint Francis Hospital	Greenville	86%	292
Georgetown Memorial Hospital	Georgetown	85%	109
McLeod Regional Medical Center-Pee Dee	Florence	85%	227
Palmetto Health Baptist Columbia	Columbia	85%	144
Bon Secours Saint Francis Hospital	Charleston	84%	138
Palmetto Health Richland Hospital	Columbia	84%	112
Providence Hosp/Providence Heart Inst	Columbia	84%	142
Upstate Carolina Medical Center	Gaffney	83%	124
Greenville Memorial Medical Campus	Greenville	82%	301
Carolinas Hospital System-Florence	Florence	81%	187
Grand Strand Regional Medical Center	Myrtle Beach	81%	242
Hilton Head Regional Medical Center	Hilton Head Isl	78%	125
Self Regional Healthcare Center	Greenwood	78%	210
Roper Hospital	Charleston	77%	226
Tuomey Regional Medical Center	Sumter	77%	145
Chesterfield General Hospital	Cheraw	74%	93
Loris Community Hospital	Loris	74%	92
Marion County Medical Center	Marion	74%	50
Oconee Memorial Hospital	Seneca	73%	291
Clarendon Memorial Hospital	Manning	71%	95
Conway Medical Center	Conway	71%	145
Laurens County Hospital	Clinton	71%	105
Medical University of S Carolina Med Ctr	Charleston	71%	87
Newberry County Memorial Hospital	Newberry	71%	58
Wallace Thomson Hospital	Union	70%	79
Carolina Pines Regional Medical Center	Hartsville	69%	169
Colleton Medical Center	Walterboro	69%	78
Regional Med Ctr of Orangeburg & Calhoun	Orangeburg	68%	174
Bamberg County Memorial Hospital	Bamberg	65%	49
Kershaw County Medical Center	Camden	64%	183
Hampton Regional Medical Center	Varnville	58%	26
Trident Medical Center	Charleston	54%	297
Chester Regional Medical Center	Chester	53%	60
Beaufort Memorial Hospital	Beaufort	47%	57
Marlboro Park Hospital	Bennettsville	47%	49
Fairfield Memorial Hospital	Winnsboro	44%	32
McLeod Medical Center Dillon	Dillon	34%	56
Barnwell County Hospital	Barnwell	29%	63
Williamsburg Regional Hospital	Kingstree	15%	27

19. Smoking Cessation Advice

Hospital Name	City	Rate	Cases
Aiken Regional Medical Centers	Aiken	100%	39
Anderson Area Medical Center	Anderson	100%	219
Carolinas Hospital System-Florence	Florence	100%	87
Hillcrest Hospital	Simpsonville	100%	32
Oconee Memorial Hospital	Seneca	100%	137
Palmetto Health Richland Hospital	Columbia	100%	88
Providence Hosp/Providence Heart Inst	Columbia	100%	59
Saint Francis Hospital	Greenville	100%	94
Spartanburg Regional Health Care System	Spartanburg	100%	173
Springs Memorial Hospital	Lancaster	100%	63
Waccamaw Community Hospital	Murrells Inlet	100%	44
McLeod Regional Medical Center-Pee Dee	Florence	99%	129
Piedmont Medical Center	Rock Hill	99%	151
Self Regional Healthcare Center	Greenwood	99%	86
Grand Strand Regional Medical Center	Myrtle Beach	98%	116
Marion County Medical Center	Marion	98%	44
Regional Med Ctr of Orangeburg & Calhoun	Orangeburg	98%	88
Clarendon Memorial Hospital	Manning	97%	36
Mary Black Memorial Hospital	Spartanburg	97%	65
Allen Bennett Memorial Hospital	Greer	96%	55
Loris Community Hospital	Loris	96%	48
Georgetown Memorial Hospital	Georgetown	95%	43
Greenville Memorial Medical Campus	Greenville	94%	174
Palmetto Baptist Medical Center Easley	Easley	92%	59
Trident Medical Center	Charleston	92%	140
Tuomey Regional Medical Center	Sumter	92%	75
Beaufort Memorial Hospital	Beaufort	91%	34
Carolina Pines Regional Medical Center	Hartsville	90%	101
Cannon Memorial Hospital	Pickens	88%	34
Palmetto Health Baptist Columbia	Columbia	88%	83
Marlboro Park Hospital	Bennettsville	86%	28
Lexington Medical Center	West Columbia	83%	47
Bon Secours Saint Francis Hospital	Charleston	82%	51
Medical University of S Carolina Med Ctr	Charleston	81%	81
Upstate Carolina Medical Center	Gaffney	80%	66
Chester Regional Medical Center	Chester	78%	37
Chesterfield General Hospital	Cheraw	76%	46
Colleton Medical Center	Walterboro	75%	28

Kershaw County Medical Center	Camden	73%	66
Roper Hospital	Charleston	65%	83
Laurens County Hospital	Clinton	50%	38
Wallace Thomson Hospital	Union	42%	36

Surgical Infection Prevention

20. Prophylactic Antibiotic Given

Hospital Name	City	Rate	Cases
Bon Secours Saint Francis Hospital	Charleston	97%	497
McLeod Regional Medical Center-Pee Dee	Florence	96%	255
Saint Francis Hospital	Greenville	96%	323
Medical University of S Carolina Med Ctr.	Charleston	95%	693
Palmetto Baptist Medical Center Easley	Easley	95%	259
Palmetto Health Richland Hospital	Columbia	95%	1725
Self Regional Healthcare Center.	Greenwood	95%	812
Spartanburg Regional Health Care System	Spartanburg	95%	1545
Waccamaw Community Hospital	Murrells Inlet	95%	295
Loris Community Hospital	Loris	94%	195
Roper Hospital	Charleston	94%	365
Conway Medical Center.	Conway	93%	41
Grand Strand Regional Medical Center.	Myrtle Beach	93%	363
Greenville Memorial Medical Campus.	Greenville	93%	253
Piedmont Medical Center.	Rock Hill	93%	796
Palmetto Health Baptist Columbia	Columbia	92%	1182
Upstate Carolina Medical Center.	Gaffney	92%	110
Aiken Regional Medical Centers	Aiken	91%	574
Anderson Area Medical Center.	Anderson	90%	582
Carolina Pines Regional Medical Center.	Hartsville	90%	150
Georgetown Memorial Hospital	Georgetown	90%	328
Kershaw County Medical Center	Camden	90%	209
Carolinas Hospital System-Florence	Florence	89%	674
Providence Hosp/Providence Heart Inst	Columbia	89%	268
Beaufort Memorial Hospital	Beaufort	88%	542
Lexington Medical Center	West Columbia	88%	205
Oconee Memorial Hospital	Seneca	88%	186
Hillcrest Hospital	Simpsonville	87%	69
Mary Black Memorial Hospital	Spartanburg	87%	635
Marion County Medical Center	Marion	86%	153
Regional Med Ctr of Orangeburg & Calhoun	Orangeburg	86%	194
Hilton Head Regional Medical Center.	Hilton Head Isl	84%	238
Colleton Medical Center	Walterboro	83%	167
Allen Bennett Memorial Hospital.	Greer	82%	94
East Cooper Regional Medical Center.	Mount Pleasant	82%	222
Newberry County Memorial Hospital.	Newberry	80%	83
Tuomey Regional Medical Center	Sumter	78%	426
Trident Medical Center.	Charleston	75%	517
Laurens County Hospital	Clinton	73%	172
Chester Regional Medical Center.	Chester	68%	28
Springs Memorial Hospital.	Lancaster	68%	121
Clarendon Memorial Hospital	Manning	49%	86
Wallace Thomson Hospital.	Union	31%	29

21. Prophylactic Antibiotic Selection

Hospital Name	City	Rate	Cases
Kershaw County Medical Center	Camden	100%	50
Oconee Memorial Hospital	Seneca	100%	33
Bon Secours Saint Francis Hospital	Charleston	99%	99
Saint Francis Hospital.	Greenville	99%	85
Tuomey Regional Medical Center	Sumter	99%	117
Aiken Regional Medical Centers	Aiken	98%	128
Colleton Medical Center	Walterboro	98%	41
Beaufort Memorial Hospital	Beaufort	97%	155
Grand Strand Regional Medical Center.	Myrtle Beach	97%	224
Hilton Head Regional Medical Center.	Hilton Head Isl	97%	37
Self Regional Healthcare Center.	Greenwood	97%	63
Mary Black Memorial Hospital	Spartanburg	96%	171
Roper Hospital	Charleston	96%	85
Carolinas Hospital System-Florence	Florence	95%	167
McLeod Regional Medical Center-Pee Dee	Florence	95%	66
Palmetto Health Baptist Columbia	Columbia	95%	302
Allen Bennett Memorial Hospital	Greer	94%	32
Georgetown Memorial Hospital	Georgetown	94%	77
Greenville Memorial Medical Campus.	Greenville	94%	88
Palmetto Health Richland Hospital	Columbia	93%	478
Piedmont Medical Center.	Rock Hill	93%	81
Upstate Carolina Medical Center.	Gaffney	93%	27
Regional Med Ctr of Orangeburg & Calhoun	Orangeburg	92%	59
Carolina Pines Regional Medical Center	Hartsville	91%	34
Palmetto Baptist Medical Center Easley	Easley	90%	70
Clarendon Memorial Hospital	Manning	89%	28
Loris Community Hospital	Loris	89%	38
Laurens County Hospital	Clinton	88%	40
Spartanburg Regional Health Care System	Spartanburg	88%	310

Anderson Area Medical Center	Anderson	86%	64
Trident Medical Center	Charleston	86%	351
East Cooper Regional Medical Center	Mount Pleasant	83%	48
Lexington Medical Center	West Columbia	83%	48
Waccamaw Community Hospital	Murrells Inlet	76%	67
Medical University of S Carolina Med Ctr	Charleston	74%	169
Springs Memorial Hospital	Lancaster	66%	38

22. Prophylactic Antibiotic Stopped

Hospital Name	City	Rate	Cases
Wallace Thomson Hospital	Union	96%	27
East Cooper Regional Medical Center	Mount Pleasant	93%	224
Saint Francis Hospital	Greenville	93%	310
Palmetto Health Baptist Columbia	Columbia	91%	1154
Allen Bennett Memorial Hospital	Greer	90%	89
Bon Secours Saint Francis Hospital	Charleston	90%	487
Greenville Memorial Medical Campus	Greenville	90%	239
Roper Hospital	Charleston	90%	353
Self Regional Healthcare Center	Greenwood	89%	790
Clarendon Memorial Hospital	Manning	88%	84
Regional Med Ctr of Orangeburg & Calhoun	Orangeburg	87%	182
Hilton Head Regional Medical Center	Hilton Head Isl	86%	232
Palmetto Baptist Medical Center Easley	Easley	86%	246
Piedmont Medical Center	Rock Hill	86%	785
Anderson Area Medical Center	Anderson	85%	531
Medical University of S Carolina Med Ctr	Charleston	85%	665
Loris Community Hospital	Loris	84%	191
Palmetto Health Richland Hospital	Columbia	84%	1671
Upstate Carolina Medical Center	Gaffney	84%	102
Aiken Regional Medical Centers	Aiken	81%	538
Spartanburg Regional Health Care System	Spartanburg	81%	1478
Tuomey Regional Medical Center	Sumter	81%	417
McLeod Regional Medical Center-Pee Dee	Florence	80%	245
Beaufort Memorial Hospital	Beaufort	79%	535
Carolinas Hospital System-Florence	Florence	79%	658
Waccamaw Community Hospital	Murrells Inlet	79%	290
Hillcrest Hospital	Simpsonville	78%	69
Mary Black Memorial Hospital	Spartanburg	78%	616
Oconee Memorial Hospital	Seneca	77%	175
Conway Medical Center	Conway	76%	38
Laurens County Hospital	Clinton	71%	168
Carolina Pines Regional Medical Center	Hartsville	70%	145
Colleton Medical Center	Walterboro	69%	154
Providence Hosp/Providence Heart Inst	Columbia	69%	261
Trident Medical Center	Charleston	68%	496
Grand Strand Regional Medical Center	Myrtle Beach	67%	354
Newberry County Memorial Hospital	Newberry	65%	83
Lexington Medical Center	West Columbia	59%	201
Kershaw County Medical Center	Camden	54%	205
Springs Memorial Hospital	Lancaster	52%	112
Marion County Medical Center	Marion	37%	145
Georgetown Memorial Hospital	Georgetown	34%	319
Chester Regional Medical Center	Chester	18%	28

Pregnancy Care

23. Inpatient Neonatal Mortality

Hospital Name	City	Rate	Cases
Bamberg County Memorial Hospital	Bamberg	0.00%	60
Roper Hospital	Charleston	0.00%	666
Trident Medical Center	Charleston	0.03%	3533
Bon Secours Saint Francis Hospital	Charleston	0.12%	1707
Palmetto Health Baptist Columbia	Columbia	0.20%	3946
Medical University of S Carolina Med Ctr	Charleston	2.52%	634

24. Third or Fourth Degree Laceration

Hospital Name	City	Rate	Cases
Bamberg County Memorial Hospital	Bamberg	1.59%	63
Trident Medical Center	Charleston	1.91%	2511
Roper Hospital	Charleston	3.15%	444
Bon Secours Saint Francis Hospital	Charleston	3.28%	1159
Medical University of S Carolina Med Ctr	Charleston	3.29%	1643
Palmetto Health Baptist Columbia	Columbia	3.47%	2364

NOTE: Hospital profiles are in alphabetical order by state, then city, then hospital within the city; Rankings are sorted by rate in descending order and exclude hospitals with less than 25 cases; (1) The number of cases is too small (n<25) for purposes of reliably predicting hospital performance; (2) Measure reflects the hospital's indication that its submission was based upon a sample of its relevant discharges; (3) Rate reflects fewer than the maximum possible quarters of data for the measure; (4) Inaccurate information submitted and suppressed for one or more quarters; (5) No data is available from the hospital for this measure; Please refer to the User's Guide for a full explanation of data

Abbeville County Memorial Hospital

901 W Greenwood Street
Highway 72 W
Abbeville, SC 29620
Ownership: Voluntary non-profit - Other
Emergency Services: Yes

Phone: 864-459-5011
Fax: 864-366-3317

Accredited: Yes
Licensed Beds: 52

Key Personnel:
President/CEO . . . . Alvin Hoover
Cardiac Lab . . . . Brenda Holtzclaw
Emergency Room . . . . Benjamin Lewis
Emergency Room . . . . Debbie Erwin
Infection Control . . . . Debbie Erwin
ICU . . . . Angie Miller
Medical/Surgical Nursing . . . . Angie Miller
Respiratory/Cardiopulmonary . . . . Mark Rolin

Measure	Cases	This Hospital	State Average	U.S. Average	Top Hospital
Heart Attack Care					
ACE Inhibitor or ARB for LVSD[1,3]	1	100%	84%	82%	100%
Aspirin at Arrival[1,3]	9	89%	92%	92%	100%
Aspirin at Discharge[1,3]	1	100%	87%	90%	100%
Beta Blocker at Arrival[1,3]	7	100%	87%	87%	100%
Beta Blocker at Discharge[1,3]	1	100%	92%	90%	100%
Fibrinolytic Medication Timing[3]	0	-	34%	31%	100%
PCI Within 90 Minutes of Arrival	0	-	58%	54%	95%
Smoking Cessation Advice[3]	0	-	89%	88%	100%
Heart Failure Care					
ACE Inhibitor or ARB for LVSD[1,3]	4	75%	85%	82%	100%
Discharge Instructions[1,3]	16	81%	66%	61%	93%
Evaluation of LVS Function[1,3]	17	94%	89%	83%	99%
Smoking Cessation Advice[1,3]	5	60%	85%	82%	100%
Pneumonia Care					
Appropriate Initial Antibiotic[1,3]	10	90%	83%	83%	94%
Blood Culture Timing[1,3]	7	86%	91%	90%	100%
Influenza Vaccine[5]	-	-	77%	70%	100%
Initial Antibiotic Timing[1,3]	14	93%	81%	80%	93%
Oxygenation Assessment[1,3]	17	100%	99%	99%	100%
Pneumococcal Vaccine[1,3]	8	75%	75%	69%	94%
Smoking Cessation Advice[1,3]	4	25%	83%	80%	100%
Surgical Infection Prevention					
Prophylactic Antibiotic Given[5]	-	-	78%	77%	95%
Prophylactic Antibiotic Selection[5]	-	-	92%	90%	100%
Prophylactic Antibiotic Stopped[5]	-	-	78%	72%	95%
Pregnancy Care					
Inpatient Neonatal Mortality	-	-	-	-	-
Third or Fourth Degree Laceration	-	-	-	3.63%	3.27%

Aiken Regional Medical Centers

Alternate Name: HCA Aiken Regional Medical Center
302 University Parkway
PO Box 1117
Aiken, SC 29802
URL: www.aikenregional.com
Ownership: Proprietary
Emergency Services: Yes

Toll-Free: 800-245-3679
Phone: 803-641-5000
Fax: 803-641-5179

Accredited: Yes
Licensed Beds: 230

Key Personnel:
CEO . . . . K D Justin
Chief Medical Staff . . . . Donald McCartney
Emergency Room . . . . John Arnold
Director Medical/Surgical Nursing . . . . Maggie Longshore
OB/GYN Womens Health . . . . Jonathan Collins
Chief Radiology . . . . Jack Cannon
Director Respiratory Therapy . . . . Susan Hosenbach

Measure	Cases	This Hospital	State Average	U.S. Average	Top Hospital
Heart Attack Care					
ACE Inhibitor or ARB for LVSD	36	100%	84%	82%	100%
Aspirin at Arrival	126	99%	92%	92%	100%
Aspirin at Discharge	134	100%	87%	90%	100%
Beta Blocker at Arrival	85	95%	87%	87%	100%
Beta Blocker at Discharge	125	100%	92%	90%	100%
Fibrinolytic Medication Timing	0	-	34%	31%	100%
PCI Within 90 Minutes of Arrival[1]	9	56%	58%	54%	95%

Measure	Cases	This Hospital	State Average	U.S. Average	Top Hospital
Smoking Cessation Advice	60	95%	89%	88%	100%
Heart Failure Care					
ACE Inhibitor or ARB for LVSD	138	99%	85%	82%	100%
Discharge Instructions	226	47%	66%	61%	93%
Evaluation of LVS Function	276	99%	89%	83%	99%
Smoking Cessation Advice	42	98%	85%	82%	100%
Pneumonia Care					
Appropriate Initial Antibiotic	104	88%	83%	83%	94%
Blood Culture Timing	116	92%	91%	90%	100%
Influenza Vaccine	34	85%	77%	70%	100%
Initial Antibiotic Timing	164	94%	81%	80%	93%
Oxygenation Assessment	197	100%	99%	99%	100%
Pneumococcal Vaccine	120	97%	75%	69%	94%
Smoking Cessation Advice	39	100%	83%	80%	100%
Surgical Infection Prevention					
Prophylactic Antibiotic Given	574	91%	78%	77%	95%
Prophylactic Antibiotic Selection	128	98%	92%	90%	100%
Prophylactic Antibiotic Stopped	538	81%	78%	72%	95%
Pregnancy Care					
Inpatient Neonatal Mortality	-	-	-	-	-
Third or Fourth Degree Laceration	-	-	-	3.63%	3.27%

Anderson Area Medical Center

Alternate Name: Anmed Health
800 N Fant Street
Anderson, SC 29621
URL: www.anmed.com
Ownership: Voluntary non-profit - Private
Emergency Services: Yes

Phone: 864-512-1000
Fax: 864-512-1952

Accredited: Yes
Licensed Beds: 461

Key Personnel:
Administrator/President . . . . John A Miller Jr
Chief Medical Staff . . . . Harold Morse, MD
Chief Catheterization Laboratory . . . . John Ware, MD
Emergency Room . . . . M Tillirson, MD
Director Infection/Disease Control . . . . Thomas Crocker, MD
CCU Spvg. Nurse . . . . Elaine Reimels
OB/GYN Womens Health . . . . James Herbert, MD
Chief Radiology . . . . Carl Geier, MD
Director Respiratory Therapy . . . . Miles Cheatham

Measure	Cases	This Hospital	State Average	U.S. Average	Top Hospital
Heart Attack Care					
ACE Inhibitor or ARB for LVSD	54	100%	84%	82%	100%[5]
Aspirin at Arrival	322	100%	92%	92%	100%
Aspirin at Discharge	326	100%	87%	90%	100%
Beta Blocker at Arrival	272	100%	87%	87%	100%
Beta Blocker at Discharge	309	100%	92%	90%	100%
Fibrinolytic Medication Timing	0	-	34%	31%	100%
PCI Within 90 Minutes of Arrival[1]	23	96%	58%	54%	95%
Smoking Cessation Advice	138	100%	89%	88%	100%
Heart Failure Care					
ACE Inhibitor or ARB for LVSD	212	89%	85%	82%	100%
Discharge Instructions	448	75%	66%	61%	93%
Evaluation of LVS Function	567	96%	89%	83%	99%
Smoking Cessation Advice	124	100%	85%	82%	100%
Pneumonia Care					
Appropriate Initial Antibiotic	443	92%	83%	83%	94%
Blood Culture Timing	567	98%	91%	90%	100%
Influenza Vaccine	156	77%	77%	70%	100%
Initial Antibiotic Timing	715	78%	81%	80%	93%
Oxygenation Assessment	868	99%	99%	99%	100%
Pneumococcal Vaccine	558	91%	75%	69%	94%
Smoking Cessation Advice	219	100%	83%	80%	100%
Surgical Infection Prevention					
Prophylactic Antibiotic Given[2,3]	582	90%	78%	77%	95%
Prophylactic Antibiotic Selection[2]	64	86%	92%	90%	100%
Prophylactic Antibiotic Stopped[2,3]	531	85%	78%	72%	95%
Pregnancy Care					
Inpatient Neonatal Mortality	-	-	-	-	-
Third or Fourth Degree Laceration	-	-	-	3.63%	3.27%

NOTE: Hospital profiles are in alphabetical order by state, then city, then hospital within the city; Rankings are sorted by rate in descending order and exclude hospitals with less than 25 cases; (1) The number of cases is too small (n<25) for purposes of reliably predicting hospital performance; (2) Measure reflects the hospital's indication that its submission was based upon a sample of its relevant discharges; (3) Rate reflects fewer than the maximum possible quarters of data for the measure; (4) Inaccurate information submitted and suppressed for one or more quarters; (5) No data is available from the hospital for this measure; Please refer to the User's Guide for a full explanation of data

Bamberg County Memorial Hospital

N & McGee Streets
Bamberg, SC 29003
Ownership: Government - Local
Emergency Services: Yes

Phone: 803-245-4321
Fax: 803-245-6272
Accredited: Yes
Licensed Beds: 59

Key Personnel:
Administrator . . . . Warren E Hammett
Director Infection/Disease Control . . . . Jennifer Reynolds
Director Respiratory Therapy . . . . Peggy Lemon

Measure	Cases	This Hospital	State Average	U.S. Average	Top Hospital
Heart Attack Care					
ACE Inhibitor or ARB for LVSD[3]	0	-	84%	82%	100%
Aspirin at Arrival[1,3]	3	100%	92%	92%	100%
Aspirin at Discharge[3]	0	-	87%	90%	100%
Beta Blocker at Arrival[1,3]	3	100%	87%	87%	100%
Beta Blocker at Discharge[1,3]	2	100%	92%	90%	100%
Fibrinolytic Medication Timing[3]	0	-	34%	31%	100%
PCI Within 90 Minutes of Arrival	0	-	58%	54%	95%
Smoking Cessation Advice[3]	0	-	89%	88%	100%
Heart Failure Care					
ACE Inhibitor or ARB for LVSD[1]	12	75%	85%	82%	100%
Discharge Instructions	46	67%	66%	61%	93%
Evaluation of LVS Function	53	77%	89%	83%	99%
Smoking Cessation Advice[1]	7	14%	85%	82%	100%
Pneumonia Care					
Appropriate Initial Antibiotic	45	64%	83%	83%	94%
Blood Culture Timing	32	84%	91%	90%	100%
Influenza Vaccine[1]	14	79%	77%	70%	100%
Initial Antibiotic Timing	57	82%	81%	80%	93%
Oxygenation Assessment	83	99%	99%	99%	100%
Pneumococcal Vaccine	49	65%	75%	69%	94%
Smoking Cessation Advice[1]	20	70%	83%	80%	100%
Surgical Infection Prevention					
Prophylactic Antibiotic Given[5]	-	-	78%	77%	95%
Prophylactic Antibiotic Selection[5]	-	-	92%	90%	100%
Prophylactic Antibiotic Stopped[5]	-	-	78%	72%	95%
Pregnancy Care					
Inpatient Neonatal Mortality	60	0.00%	-	-	-
Third or Fourth Degree Laceration	63	1.59%	-	3.63%	3.27%

Barnwell County Hospital

811 Reynolds Road
Barnwell, SC 29812
Ownership: Government - Local
Emergency Services: Yes

Phone: 803-259-1000
Fax: 803-541-4387
Accredited: Yes
Licensed Beds: 53

Key Personnel:
CEO. . . . . Robert Walters
Chief Medical Staff. . . . . S Richard, MD
Emergency Room . . . . Afsar Waraich, MD
Director Infection/Disease Control . . . . Allene Townes, RN
Director Medical/Surgical Nursing . . . . Tony Kirkland
Chief Radiology . . . . Jenny Mayo, RT
Director Respiratory Therapy . . . . Rovella Thillith

Measure	Cases	This Hospital	State Average	U.S. Average	Top Hospital
Heart Attack Care					
ACE Inhibitor or ARB for LVSD	0	-	84%	82%	100%
Aspirin at Arrival[1]	13	92%	92%	92%	100%
Aspirin at Discharge[1]	8	88%	87%	90%	100%
Beta Blocker at Arrival[1]	7	100%	87%	87%	100%
Beta Blocker at Discharge[1]	9	89%	92%	90%	100%
Fibrinolytic Medication Timing[3]	0	-	34%	31%	100%
PCI Within 90 Minutes of Arrival	0	-	58%	54%	95%
Smoking Cessation Advice[1,3]	1	100%	89%	88%	100%
Heart Failure Care					
ACE Inhibitor or ARB for LVSD[1]	12	92%	85%	82%	100%
Discharge Instructions[1,3]	5	40%	66%	61%	93%
Evaluation of LVS Function	46	78%	89%	83%	99%
Smoking Cessation Advice[1,3]	2	50%	85%	82%	100%
Pneumonia Care					
Appropriate Initial Antibiotic[1,3]	6	67%	83%	83%	94%
Blood Culture Timing[1,3]	12	83%	91%	90%	100%

Measure	Cases	This Hospital	State Average	U.S. Average	Top Hospital
Influenza Vaccine[4,5]	-	-	77%	70%	100%
Initial Antibiotic Timing	93	82%	81%	80%	93%
Oxygenation Assessment	118	98%	99%	99%	100%
Pneumococcal Vaccine	63	29%	75%	69%	94%
Smoking Cessation Advice[1,3]	2	0%	83%	80%	100%
Surgical Infection Prevention					
Prophylactic Antibiotic Given[1,3]	1	0%	78%	77%	95%
Prophylactic Antibiotic Selection[5]	-	-	92%	90%	100%
Prophylactic Antibiotic Stopped[1,3]	1	100%	78%	72%	95%
Pregnancy Care					
Inpatient Neonatal Mortality	-	-	-	-	-
Third or Fourth Degree Laceration	-	-	-	3.63%	3.27%

Beaufort Memorial Hospital

955 Ribaut Road
Beaufort, SC 29902

Toll-Free: 877-532-6472
Phone: 843-522-5200
Fax: 843-522-5671

URL: www.bmhsc.org
Ownership: Government - Local
Emergency Services: Yes

Accredited: Yes
Licensed Beds: 170

Key Personnel:
CEO. . . . . David E Brown
Chief Medical Staff. . . . . Brad Collins, MD
Chief of Medical Staff. . . . . Curt Gambla
Head Emergency Room. . . . . Kevin Kramer
Emergency Room . . . . Connie Gowdowns, RN

Measure	Cases	This Hospital	State Average	U.S. Average	Top Hospital
Heart Attack Care					
ACE Inhibitor or ARB for LVSD[1]	14	100%	84%	82%	100%
Aspirin at Arrival	72	93%	92%	92%	100%
Aspirin at Discharge	38	92%	87%	90%	100%
Beta Blocker at Arrival	68	99%	87%	87%	100%
Beta Blocker at Discharge	37	95%	92%	90%	100%
Fibrinolytic Medication Timing	0	-	34%	31%	100%
PCI Within 90 Minutes of Arrival	0	-	58%	54%	95%
Smoking Cessation Advice[1]	10	100%	89%	88%	100%
Heart Failure Care					
ACE Inhibitor or ARB for LVSD	118	86%	85%	82%	100%
Discharge Instructions	243	73%	66%	61%	93%
Evaluation of LVS Function	264	83%	89%	83%	99%
Smoking Cessation Advice	46	91%	85%	82%	100%
Pneumonia Care					
Appropriate Initial Antibiotic	92	84%	83%	83%	94%
Blood Culture Timing	48	77%	91%	90%	100%
Influenza Vaccine[1]	14	50%	77%	70%	100%
Initial Antibiotic Timing	87	67%	81%	80%	93%
Oxygenation Assessment	106	98%	99%	99%	100%
Pneumococcal Vaccine	57	47%	75%	69%	94%
Smoking Cessation Advice	34	91%	83%	80%	100%
Surgical Infection Prevention					
Prophylactic Antibiotic Given	542	88%	78%	77%	95%
Prophylactic Antibiotic Selection	155	97%	92%	90%	100%
Prophylactic Antibiotic Stopped	535	79%	78%	72%	95%
Pregnancy Care					
Inpatient Neonatal Mortality	-	-	-	-	-
Third or Fourth Degree Laceration	-	-	-	3.63%	3.27%

Marlboro Park Hospital

PO Box 738
Bennettsville, SC 29512
Ownership: Proprietary
Emergency Services: Yes

Phone: 843-479-2881
Fax: 843-479-5860
Accredited: Yes
Licensed Beds: 109

Key Personnel:
President/CEO. . . . . Mark W Caton
Chief Medical Staff. . . . . Dell A Dembosky, MD
Infection Control. . . . . Doug Stanton
ICU . . . . Jane Hodkin
Medical/Surgical Nursing . . . . Valarie Quick
OB/GYN Womens Health. . . . . Kathleen Carter

Measure	Cases	This Hospital	State Average	U.S. Average	Top Hospital
Heart Attack Care					

NOTE: Hospital profiles are in alphabetical order by state, then city, then hospital within the city; Rankings are sorted by rate in descending order and exclude hospitals with less than 25 cases; (1) The number of cases is too small (n<25) for purposes of reliably predicting hospital performance; (2) Measure reflects the hospital's indication that its submission was based upon a sample of its relevant discharges; (3) Rate reflects fewer than the maximum possible quarters of data for the measure; (4) Inaccurate information submitted and suppressed for one or more quarters; (5) No data is available from the hospital for this measure; Please refer to the User's Guide for a full explanation of data

ACE Inhibitor or ARB for LVSD[1]	2	100%	84%	82%	100%
Aspirin at Arrival[1]	7	100%	92%	92%	100%
Aspirin at Discharge[1]	1	100%	87%	90%	100%
Beta Blocker at Arrival[1]	7	86%	87%	87%	100%
Beta Blocker at Discharge[1]	3	100%	92%	90%	100%
Fibrinolytic Medication Timing[1]	2	0%	34%	31%	100%
PCI Within 90 Minutes of Arrival	0	-	58%	54%	95%
Smoking Cessation Advice[1]	1	100%	89%	88%	100%
Heart Failure Care					
ACE Inhibitor or ARB for LVSD	31	97%	85%	82%	100%
Discharge Instructions	73	58%	66%	61%	93%
Evaluation of LVS Function	79	81%	89%	83%	99%
Smoking Cessation Advice	26	85%	85%	82%	100%
Pneumonia Care					
Appropriate Initial Antibiotic	70	77%	83%	83%	94%
Blood Culture Timing	50	90%	91%	90%	100%
Influenza Vaccine[1]	17	65%	77%	70%	100%
Initial Antibiotic Timing	75	77%	81%	80%	93%
Oxygenation Assessment	91	99%	99%	99%	100%
Pneumococcal Vaccine	49	47%	75%	69%	94%
Smoking Cessation Advice	28	86%	83%	80%	100%
Surgical Infection Prevention					
Prophylactic Antibiotic Given[1,2,3]	17	47%	78%	77%	95%
Prophylactic Antibiotic Selection[1,2]	5	80%	92%	90%	100%
Prophylactic Antibiotic Stopped[1,3]	11	91%	78%	72%	95%
Pregnancy Care					
Inpatient Neonatal Mortality	-	-	-	-	-
Third or Fourth Degree Laceration	-	-	-	3.63%	3.27%

Kershaw County Medical Center

Alternate Name: Kershaw County Memorial Hospital
Haile & Roberts Streets
PO Box 7003
Camden, SC 29020
Ownership: Government - Local
Emergency Services: Yes

Phone: 803-432-4311
Fax: 803-713-6369

Accredited: Yes
Licensed Beds: 209

Key Personnel:
President/CEO . . . . Donnie J Weeks
Chief Medical Staff . . . . J Carl Kearse, MD
Emergency Room . . . . Tommy Norris, MD
CCU Spvg. Nurse . . . . Susan Outen, RN
OB/GYN Womens Health . . . . John Moore, MD
Chief Radiology . . . . Don Copley, MD
Director Respiratory Therapy . . . . Barbara Skipper, RN

Measure	Cases	This Hospital	State Average	U.S. Average	Top Hospital
Heart Attack Care					
ACE Inhibitor or ARB for LVSD[1]	5	60%	84%	82%	100%
Aspirin at Arrival	41	78%	92%	92%	100%
Aspirin at Discharge[1]	17	71%	87%	90%	100%
Beta Blocker at Arrival	38	82%	87%	87%	100%
Beta Blocker at Discharge[1]	19	79%	92%	90%	100%
Fibrinolytic Medication Timing[1]	5	40%	34%	31%	100%
PCI Within 90 Minutes of Arrival	0	-	58%	54%	95%
Smoking Cessation Advice[1]	4	50%	89%	88%	100%
Heart Failure Care					
ACE Inhibitor or ARB for LVSD	90	77%	85%	82%	100%
Discharge Instructions	200	56%	66%	61%	93%
Evaluation of LVS Function	252	96%	89%	83%	99%
Smoking Cessation Advice	62	89%	85%	82%	100%
Pneumonia Care					
Appropriate Initial Antibiotic	161	89%	83%	83%	94%
Blood Culture Timing	114	85%	91%	90%	100%
Influenza Vaccine	48	62%	77%	70%	100%
Initial Antibiotic Timing	230	73%	81%	80%	93%
Oxygenation Assessment	293	100%	99%	99%	100%
Pneumococcal Vaccine	183	64%	75%	69%	94%
Smoking Cessation Advice	66	73%	83%	80%	100%
Surgical Infection Prevention					
Prophylactic Antibiotic Given	209	90%	78%	77%	95%
Prophylactic Antibiotic Selection	50	100%	92%	90%	100%
Prophylactic Antibiotic Stopped	205	54%	78%	72%	95%
Pregnancy Care					

| Inpatient Neonatal Mortality | - | - | - | - | - |
| Third or Fourth Degree Laceration | - | - | - | 3.63% | 3.27% |

Bon Secours Saint Francis Hospital

2095 Henry Tecklenburg Drive
Charleston, SC 29414

Toll-Free: 800-720-8333
Phone: 843-402-1000
Fax: 843-720-5761

URL: www.stfrancishealth.org
Ownership: Voluntary non-profit - Church
Emergency Services: Yes

Accredited: Yes
Licensed Beds: 141

Key Personnel:
President/CEO . . . . Michael C Tarwater
Chief Medical Staff . . . . William B Ellison Jr, MD
Director Cardiac Surgery . . . . James J Morris, MD
Emergency Room . . . . Wanda Brockmeyer
Director Infection/Disease Control . . . . Timothy West, MD
Director Medical/Surgical Nursing . . . . Allison Walters
OB/GYN Womens Health . . . . Wyman Frumptons, MD
Surgical Services . . . . Allison Walters, RN

Measure	Cases	This Hospital	State Average	U.S. Average	Top Hospital
Heart Attack Care					
ACE Inhibitor or ARB for LVSD[1]	1	0%	84%	82%	100%
Aspirin at Arrival[1]	22	91%	92%	92%	100%
Aspirin at Discharge[1]	6	100%	87%	90%	100%
Beta Blocker at Arrival[1]	21	76%	87%	87%	100%
Beta Blocker at Discharge[1]	5	100%	92%	90%	100%
Fibrinolytic Medication Timing	0	-	34%	31%	100%
PCI Within 90 Minutes of Arrival	0	-	58%	54%	95%
Smoking Cessation Advice[1]	1	100%	89%	88%	100%
Heart Failure Care					
ACE Inhibitor or ARB for LVSD	45	89%	85%	82%	100%
Discharge Instructions	137	81%	66%	61%	93%
Evaluation of LVS Function	167	95%	89%	83%	99%
Smoking Cessation Advice	26	85%	85%	82%	100%
Pneumonia Care					
Appropriate Initial Antibiotic	138	92%	83%	83%	94%
Blood Culture Timing	131	92%	91%	90%	100%
Influenza Vaccine	48	90%	77%	70%	100%
Initial Antibiotic Timing	181	86%	81%	80%	93%
Oxygenation Assessment	219	100%	99%	99%	100%
Pneumococcal Vaccine	138	84%	75%	69%	94%
Smoking Cessation Advice	51	82%	83%	80%	100%
Surgical Infection Prevention					
Prophylactic Antibiotic Given	497	97%	78%	77%	95%
Prophylactic Antibiotic Selection	99	99%	92%	90%	100%
Prophylactic Antibiotic Stopped	487	90%	78%	72%	95%
Pregnancy Care					
Inpatient Neonatal Mortality	1,707	0.12%	-	-	-
Third or Fourth Degree Laceration	1,159	3.28%	-	3.63%	3.27%

Charleston Memorial Hospital

326 Calhoun Street
Charleston, SC 29401
URL: www.musc.edu/medcenter/cmh
Ownership: Government - State
Emergency Services: Yes

Phone: 843-792-2300
Fax: 843-577-2926

Accredited: Yes
Licensed Beds: 113

Key Personnel:
President/CEO . . . . Thomas F Moore
Chief Medical Staff . . . . John Heffner, MD
Emergency Room . . . . Ellen Ruja, RN
Emergency Room . . . . James Tolley, MD
Infection Control . . . . Betty W Harley
Chief Radiology . . . . Judy A Ware
Respiratory Therapy . . . . Marian Colwell

Measure	Cases	This Hospital	State Average	U.S. Average	Top Hospital
Heart Attack Care					
ACE Inhibitor or ARB for LVSD[5]	-	-	84%	82%	100%
Aspirin at Arrival[5]	-	-	92%	92%	100%
Aspirin at Discharge[5]	-	-	87%	90%	100%
Beta Blocker at Arrival[5]	-	-	87%	87%	100%
Beta Blocker at Discharge[5]	-	-	92%	90%	100%

NOTE: Hospital profiles are in alphabetical order by state, then city, then hospital within the city; Rankings are sorted by rate in descending order and exclude hospitals with less than 25 cases; (1) The number of cases is too small (n<25) for purposes of reliably predicting hospital performance; (2) Measure reflects the hospital's indication that its submission was based upon a sample of its relevant discharges; (3) Rate reflects fewer than the maximum possible quarters of data for the measure; (4) Inaccurate information submitted and suppressed for one or more quarters; (5) No data is available from the hospital for this measure; Please refer to the User's Guide for a full explanation of data

Fibrinolytic Medication Timing[5]	-	-	34%	31%	100%
PCI Within 90 Minutes of Arrival[5]	-	-	58%	54%	95%
Smoking Cessation Advice[5]	-	-	89%	88%	100%
Heart Failure Care					
ACE Inhibitor or ARB for LVSD[5]	-	-	85%	82%	100%
Discharge Instructions[5]	-	-	66%	61%	93%
Evaluation of LVS Function[5]	-	-	89%	83%	99%
Smoking Cessation Advice[5]	-	-	85%	82%	100%
Pneumonia Care					
Appropriate Initial Antibiotic[5]	-	-	83%	83%	94%
Blood Culture Timing[5]	-	-	91%	90%	100%
Influenza Vaccine[5]	-	-	77%	70%	100%
Initial Antibiotic Timing[5]	-	-	81%	80%	93%
Oxygenation Assessment[5]	-	-	99%	99%	100%
Pneumococcal Vaccine[5]	-	-	75%	69%	94%
Smoking Cessation Advice[5]	-	-	83%	80%	100%
Surgical Infection Prevention					
Prophylactic Antibiotic Given[5]	-	-	78%	77%	95%
Prophylactic Antibiotic Selection[5]	-	-	92%	90%	100%
Prophylactic Antibiotic Stopped[5]	-	-	78%	72%	95%
Pregnancy Care					
Inpatient Neonatal Mortality	-	-	-	-	-
Third or Fourth Degree Laceration	-	-	-	3.63%	3.27%

Medical University of S Carolina Med Ctr

Alternate Name: Medical University Hospital
171 Ashley Avenue
Charleston, SC 29425

Toll-Free: 800-424-MUSC
Phone: 843-792-4120
Fax: 843-792-6682

URL: www.musc.edu
Ownership: Government - State
Emergency Services: Yes

Accredited: Yes
Licensed Beds: 596

Key Personnel:
President . . . . Raymond Greenberg
CEO. . . . . W Stuart Smith
Chief Medical Staff. . . . . Patrick Cawley
Cardiology . . . . Fred Crawford
Emergency Room . . . . Ralph P Shealy, MD
Director Infection/Disease Control . . . . Linda Formby
OB/GYN Womens Health. . . . . Peter Van Dorsten, MD
Chief Radiology . . . . Jeremy Young, MD
Director Respiratory Therapy . . . . June Darby

Measure	Cases	This Hospital	State Average	U.S. Average	Top Hospital
Heart Attack Care					
ACE Inhibitor or ARB for LVSD[2]	60	85%	84%	82%	100%
Aspirin at Arrival[2]	122	99%	92%	92%	100%
Aspirin at Discharge[2]	266	100%	87%	90%	100%
Beta Blocker at Arrival[2]	114	99%	87%	87%	100%
Beta Blocker at Discharge[2]	276	99%	92%	90%	100%
Fibrinolytic Medication Timing[2]	0	-	34%	31%	100%
PCI Within 90 Minutes of Arrival[1,2]	11	55%	58%	54%	95%
Smoking Cessation Advice[2]	112	98%	89%	88%	100%
Heart Failure Care					
ACE Inhibitor or ARB for LVSD[2]	290	87%	85%	82%	100%
Discharge Instructions[2]	449	86%	66%	61%	93%
Evaluation of LVS Function[2]	475	99%	89%	83%	99%
Smoking Cessation Advice[2]	131	94%	85%	82%	100%
Pneumonia Care					
Appropriate Initial Antibiotic	107	88%	83%	83%	94%
Blood Culture Timing	145	99%	91%	90%	100%
Influenza Vaccine	32	84%	77%	70%	100%
Initial Antibiotic Timing	210	76%	81%	80%	93%
Oxygenation Assessment	249	100%	99%	99%	100%
Pneumococcal Vaccine	87	71%	75%	69%	94%
Smoking Cessation Advice	81	81%	83%	80%	100%
Surgical Infection Prevention					
Prophylactic Antibiotic Given[2]	693	95%	78%	77%	95%
Prophylactic Antibiotic Selection[2]	169	74%	92%	90%	100%
Prophylactic Antibiotic Stopped[2]	665	85%	78%	72%	95%
Pregnancy Care					
Inpatient Neonatal Mortality[2]	634	2.52%	-	-	-
Third or Fourth Degree Laceration	1,643	3.29%	-	3.63%	3.27%

Roper Hospital

316 Calhoun Street
Charleston, SC 29401
URL: www.carolinashealthcare.org
Ownership: Voluntary non-profit - Private
Emergency Services: Yes

Phone: 843-724-2000
Fax: 843-724-1987

Accredited: Yes
Licensed Beds: 453

Key Personnel:
CEO. . . . . Matthew J Severance

Measure	Cases	This Hospital	State Average	U.S. Average	Top Hospital
Heart Attack Care					
ACE Inhibitor or ARB for LVSD	51	86%	84%	82%	100%
Aspirin at Arrival	147	97%	92%	92%	100%
Aspirin at Discharge	297	97%	87%	90%	100%
Beta Blocker at Arrival	129	97%	87%	87%	100%
Beta Blocker at Discharge	270	95%	92%	90%	100%
Fibrinolytic Medication Timing	0	-	34%	31%	100%
PCI Within 90 Minutes of Arrival[1]	15	60%	58%	54%	95%
Smoking Cessation Advice	104	86%	89%	88%	100%
Heart Failure Care					
ACE Inhibitor or ARB for LVSD	297	93%	85%	82%	100%
Discharge Instructions	602	75%	66%	61%	93%
Evaluation of LVS Function	705	98%	89%	83%	99%
Smoking Cessation Advice	128	84%	85%	82%	100%
Pneumonia Care					
Appropriate Initial Antibiotic	155	85%	83%	83%	94%
Blood Culture Timing	139	97%	91%	90%	100%
Influenza Vaccine	75	87%	77%	70%	100%
Initial Antibiotic Timing	248	84%	81%	80%	93%
Oxygenation Assessment	309	100%	99%	99%	100%
Pneumococcal Vaccine	226	77%	75%	69%	94%
Smoking Cessation Advice	83	65%	83%	80%	100%
Surgical Infection Prevention					
Prophylactic Antibiotic Given[2]	365	94%	78%	77%	95%
Prophylactic Antibiotic Selection[2]	85	96%	92%	90%	100%
Prophylactic Antibiotic Stopped[2]	353	90%	78%	72%	95%
Pregnancy Care					
Inpatient Neonatal Mortality	666	0.00%	-	-	-
Third or Fourth Degree Laceration	444	3.15%	-	3.63%	3.27%

Trident Medical Center

9330 Medical Plaza Drive
Charleston, SC 29406
URL: www.tridenthealthsystem.com
Ownership: Proprietary
Emergency Services: Yes

Phone: 843-797-8860
Fax: 843-797-4958

Accredited: Yes
Licensed Beds: 296

Key Personnel:
President/CEO. . . . . Michael P Joyce
Chief Medical Staff. . . . . William Cook, MD
Chief Catheterization Laboratory . . . . M Coker, MD
Emergency Room . . . . Baird Oldfield, MD
Director Infection/Disease Control . . . . Ann Hutson
Director Medical/Surgical Nursing . . . . Rosina Feagin
OB/GYN Womens Health. . . . . Christopher Accetta, MD
Chief Radiology . . . . Al Wilson, MD
Director Respiratory Therapy . . . . Lynn Fortenberry

Measure	Cases	This Hospital	State Average	U.S. Average	Top Hospital
Heart Attack Care					
ACE Inhibitor or ARB for LVSD	76	82%	84%	82%	100%
Aspirin at Arrival	205	96%	92%	92%	100%
Aspirin at Discharge	326	95%	87%	90%	100%
Beta Blocker at Arrival	186	85%	87%	87%	100%
Beta Blocker at Discharge	317	92%	92%	90%	100%
Fibrinolytic Medication Timing	0	-	34%	31%	100%
PCI Within 90 Minutes of Arrival[1]	17	59%	58%	54%	95%
Smoking Cessation Advice	135	96%	89%	88%	100%
Heart Failure Care					
ACE Inhibitor or ARB for LVSD	248	77%	85%	82%	100%
Discharge Instructions	591	38%	66%	61%	93%
Evaluation of LVS Function	671	87%	89%	83%	99%
Smoking Cessation Advice	121	93%	85%	82%	100%
Pneumonia Care					

NOTE: Hospital profiles are in alphabetical order by state, then city, then hospital within the city; Rankings are sorted by rate in descending order and exclude hospitals with less than 25 cases; (1) The number of cases is too small (n<25) for purposes of reliably predicting hospital performance; (2) Measure reflects the hospital's indication that its submission was based upon a sample of its relevant discharges; (3) Rate reflects fewer than the maximum possible quarters of data for the measure; (4) Inaccurate information submitted and suppressed for one or more quarters; (5) No data is available from the hospital for this measure; Please refer to the User's Guide for a full explanation of data

Appropriate Initial Antibiotic	277	90%	83%	83%	94%
Blood Culture Timing	208	83%	91%	90%	100%
Influenza Vaccine	91	51%	77%	70%	100%
Initial Antibiotic Timing	402	54%	81%	80%	93%
Oxygenation Assessment	527	100%	99%	99%	100%
Pneumococcal Vaccine	297	54%	75%	69%	94%
Smoking Cessation Advice	140	92%	83%	80%	100%
Surgical Infection Prevention					
Prophylactic Antibiotic Given[2,3]	517	75%	78%	77%	95%
Prophylactic Antibiotic Selection[2]	351	86%	92%	90%	100%
Prophylactic Antibiotic Stopped[2,3]	496	68%	78%	72%	95%
Pregnancy Care					
Inpatient Neonatal Mortality	3,533	0.03%	-	-	-
Third or Fourth Degree Laceration	2,511	1.91%	-	3.63%	3.27%

Chesterfield General Hospital

711 Chesterfield Highway   Phone: 843-537-7881
Cheraw, SC 29520   Fax: 843-320-3491
URL: www.chesterfieldgeneral.com
Ownership: Proprietary
Emergency Services: Yes   Accredited: Yes
    Licensed Beds: 59
Key Personnel:
CEO. . . . . Vance Reynolds

Measure	Cases	This Hospital	State Average	U.S. Average	Top Hospital
Heart Attack Care					
ACE Inhibitor or ARB for LVSD[3]	0	-	84%	82%	100%
Aspirin at Arrival[1,3]	6	100%	92%	92%	100%
Aspirin at Discharge[1,3]	5	100%	87%	90%	100%
Beta Blocker at Arrival[1,3]	5	100%	87%	87%	100%
Beta Blocker at Discharge[1,3]	5	100%	92%	90%	100%
Fibrinolytic Medication Timing[3]	0	-	34%	31%	100%
PCI Within 90 Minutes of Arrival	0	-	58%	54%	95%
Smoking Cessation Advice[3]	0	-	89%	88%	100%
Heart Failure Care					
ACE Inhibitor or ARB for LVSD	39	97%	85%	82%	100%
Discharge Instructions	87	66%	66%	61%	93%
Evaluation of LVS Function	101	91%	89%	83%	99%
Smoking Cessation Advice[1]	14	64%	85%	82%	100%
Pneumonia Care					
Appropriate Initial Antibiotic	98	81%	83%	83%	94%
Blood Culture Timing	86	86%	91%	90%	100%
Influenza Vaccine	31	61%	77%	70%	100%
Initial Antibiotic Timing	132	94%	81%	80%	93%
Oxygenation Assessment	154	99%	99%	99%	100%
Pneumococcal Vaccine	93	74%	75%	69%	94%
Smoking Cessation Advice	46	76%	83%	80%	100%
Surgical Infection Prevention					
Prophylactic Antibiotic Given[1,2,3]	22	45%	78%	77%	95%
Prophylactic Antibiotic Selection[1,2]	6	100%	92%	90%	100%
Prophylactic Antibiotic Stopped[1,2,3]	15	100%	78%	72%	95%
Pregnancy Care					
Inpatient Neonatal Mortality	-	-	-	-	-
Third or Fourth Degree Laceration	-	-	-	3.63%	3.27%

Chester Regional Medical Center

One Medical Park Drive   Phone: 803-581-3151
Chester, SC 29706   Fax: 803-581-2565
E-mail: whbundy@infoave.net
URL: www.chapital.org
Ownership: Proprietary
Emergency Services: Yes   Accredited: Yes
    Licensed Beds: 82
Key Personnel:
President . . . . HL Perry Pepper
Chief Medical Staff. . . . . Jennifer Edwards
Emergency Room . . . . Isom Lowman
Director Infection Control . . . . Amy Shehane
Director Medical/Surgical Nursing . . . . Brenda Worthy
Manager OB/GYN Womens Health . . . . Joane Young
Director Radiology . . . . Glenda Allen

Measure	Cases	This Hospital	State Average	U.S. Average	Top Hospital

Measure	Cases	This Hospital	State Average	U.S. Average	Top Hospital
Heart Attack Care					
ACE Inhibitor or ARB for LVSD[1]	5	20%	84%	82%	100%
Aspirin at Arrival[1]	17	71%	92%	92%	100%
Aspirin at Discharge[1]	6	67%	87%	90%	100%
Beta Blocker at Arrival[1]	17	76%	87%	87%	100%
Beta Blocker at Discharge[1]	7	86%	92%	90%	100%
Fibrinolytic Medication Timing[1]	1	0%	34%	31%	100%
PCI Within 90 Minutes of Arrival	0	-	58%	54%	95%
Smoking Cessation Advice	0	-	89%	88%	100%
Heart Failure Care					
ACE Inhibitor or ARB for LVSD	39	64%	85%	82%	100%
Discharge Instructions	123	54%	66%	61%	93%
Evaluation of LVS Function	146	89%	89%	83%	99%
Smoking Cessation Advice	44	70%	85%	82%	100%
Pneumonia Care					
Appropriate Initial Antibiotic	94	64%	83%	83%	94%
Blood Culture Timing	37	89%	91%	90%	100%
Influenza Vaccine[1]	17	29%	77%	70%	100%
Initial Antibiotic Timing	101	65%	81%	80%	93%
Oxygenation Assessment	109	98%	99%	99%	100%
Pneumococcal Vaccine	60	53%	75%	69%	94%
Smoking Cessation Advice	37	78%	83%	80%	100%
Surgical Infection Prevention					
Prophylactic Antibiotic Given[2]	28	68%	78%	77%	95%
Prophylactic Antibiotic Selection[1,2]	9	89%	92%	90%	100%
Prophylactic Antibiotic Stopped[2]	28	18%	78%	72%	95%
Pregnancy Care					
Inpatient Neonatal Mortality	-	-	-	-	-
Third or Fourth Degree Laceration	-	-	-	3.63%	3.27%

Laurens County Hospital

US Highway 76 W   Phone: 864-833-9100
Clinton, SC 29325   Fax: 863-833-9471
E-mail: lroper@lchcs.org
URL: www.lchcs.org
Ownership: Govt - Hospital District or Authority   Accredited: Yes
Emergency Services: Yes   Licensed Beds: 76

Measure	Cases	This Hospital	State Average	U.S. Average	Top Hospital
Heart Attack Care					
ACE Inhibitor or ARB for LVSD[1]	3	67%	84%	82%	100%
Aspirin at Arrival	31	90%	92%	92%	100%
Aspirin at Discharge[1]	12	75%	87%	90%	100%
Beta Blocker at Arrival	30	77%	87%	87%	100%
Beta Blocker at Discharge[1]	13	69%	92%	90%	100%
Fibrinolytic Medication Timing[1]	3	0%	34%	31%	100%
PCI Within 90 Minutes of Arrival	0	-	58%	54%	95%
Smoking Cessation Advice[1]	3	67%	89%	88%	100%
Heart Failure Care					
ACE Inhibitor or ARB for LVSD	31	90%	85%	82%	100%
Discharge Instructions	66	62%	66%	61%	93%
Evaluation of LVS Function	112	78%	89%	83%	99%
Smoking Cessation Advice[1]	24	67%	85%	82%	100%
Pneumonia Care					
Appropriate Initial Antibiotic	122	82%	83%	83%	94%
Blood Culture Timing	86	85%	91%	90%	100%
Influenza Vaccine	30	73%	77%	70%	100%
Initial Antibiotic Timing	131	82%	81%	80%	93%
Oxygenation Assessment	181	100%	99%	99%	100%
Pneumococcal Vaccine	105	71%	75%	69%	94%
Smoking Cessation Advice	38	50%	83%	80%	100%
Surgical Infection Prevention					
Prophylactic Antibiotic Given	172	73%	78%	77%	95%
Prophylactic Antibiotic Selection	40	88%	92%	90%	100%
Prophylactic Antibiotic Stopped	168	71%	78%	72%	95%
Pregnancy Care					
Inpatient Neonatal Mortality	-	-	-	-	-
Third or Fourth Degree Laceration	-	-	-	3.63%	3.27%

NOTE: Hospital profiles are in alphabetical order by state, then city, then hospital within the city; Rankings are sorted by rate in descending order and exclude hospitals with less than 25 cases; (1) The number of cases is too small (n<25) for purposes of reliably predicting hospital performance; (2) Measure reflects the hospital's indication that its submission was based upon a sample of its relevant discharges; (3) Rate reflects fewer than the maximum possible quarters of data for the measure; (4) Inaccurate information submitted and suppressed for one or more quarters; (5) No data is available from the hospital for this measure; Please refer to the User's Guide for a full explanation of data

Palmetto Health Baptist Columbia

Taylor at Marion Street   Phone: 803-771-5010
Columbia, SC 29220   Fax: 803-434-3127
URL: www.palmettohealth.org
Ownership: Government - Federal   Accredited: Yes
Emergency Services: Yes   Licensed Beds: 489

Key Personnel:
President/CEO . . . . Charles D Beaman, Jr
Chief Catheterization Laboratory . . . . S Stanley Juk, Jr, DM
Emergency Room . . . . Donald Moore, MD
Director Infection/Disease Control . . . . Gwen Floyd
CCU Spvg. Nurse . . . . Shelby Reece, RN
Director Medical/Surgical Nursing . . . . Shelby Reece, RN
OB/GYN Womens Health . . . . M Bert Hutchinson, MD
Chief Radiology . . . . Mark A Lovern, MD
Director Respiratory Therapy . . . . Bob Cook

Measure	Cases	This Hospital	State Average	U.S. Average	Top Hospital
Heart Attack Care					
ACE Inhibitor or ARB for LVSD[1]	5	100%	84%	82%	100%
Aspirin at Arrival	60	98%	92%	92%	100%
Aspirin at Discharge	33	97%	87%	90%	100%
Beta Blocker at Arrival	43	100%	87%	87%	100%
Beta Blocker at Discharge	34	100%	92%	90%	100%
Fibrinolytic Medication Timing	0	-	34%	31%	100%
PCI Within 90 Minutes of Arrival	0	-	58%	54%	95%
Smoking Cessation Advice[1]	5	80%	89%	88%	100%
Heart Failure Care					
ACE Inhibitor or ARB for LVSD	87	93%	85%	82%	100%
Discharge Instructions	198	86%	66%	61%	93%
Evaluation of LVS Function	232	98%	89%	83%	99%
Smoking Cessation Advice	63	95%	85%	82%	100%
Pneumonia Care					
Appropriate Initial Antibiotic	172	81%	83%	83%	94%
Blood Culture Timing	175	94%	91%	90%	100%
Influenza Vaccine	52	73%	77%	70%	100%
Initial Antibiotic Timing	222	81%	81%	80%	93%
Oxygenation Assessment	274	100%	99%	99%	100%
Pneumococcal Vaccine	144	85%	75%	69%	94%
Smoking Cessation Advice	83	88%	83%	80%	100%
Surgical Infection Prevention					
Prophylactic Antibiotic Given	1,182	92%	78%	77%	95%
Prophylactic Antibiotic Selection	302	95%	92%	90%	100%
Prophylactic Antibiotic Stopped	1,154	91%	78%	72%	95%
Pregnancy Care					
Inpatient Neonatal Mortality	3,946	0.20%	-	-	-
Third or Fourth Degree Laceration	2,364	3.47%	-	3.63%	3.27%

Palmetto Health Richland Hospital

5 Richland Medical Park   Phone: 803-434-7000
Columbia, SC 29203   Fax: 803-434-2885
Ownership: Government - Federal   Accredited: Yes
Emergency Services: No   Licensed Beds: 649

Key Personnel:
Administrator/President . . . . Kester S Freeman, Jr
Director Infection/Disease Control . . . . Charles S Bryan, MD
Director Medical/Surgical Nursing . . . . Lindy Beaver
Director Respiratory Therapy . . . . Sandra Cassell

Measure	Cases	This Hospital	State Average	U.S. Average	Top Hospital
Heart Attack Care					
ACE Inhibitor or ARB for LVSD	85	91%	84%	82%	100%
Aspirin at Arrival	185	94%	92%	92%	100%
Aspirin at Discharge	363	98%	87%	90%	100%
Beta Blocker at Arrival	131	92%	87%	87%	100%
Beta Blocker at Discharge	344	96%	92%	90%	100%
Fibrinolytic Medication Timing[1]	2	0%	34%	31%	100%
PCI Within 90 Minutes of Arrival[1]	8	25%	58%	54%	95%
Smoking Cessation Advice	191	100%	89%	88%	100%
Heart Failure Care					
ACE Inhibitor or ARB for LVSD	279	87%	85%	82%	100%
Discharge Instructions	472	74%	66%	61%	93%
Evaluation of LVS Function	530	99%	89%	83%	99%

Measure	Cases	This Hospital	State Average	U.S. Average	Top Hospital
Smoking Cessation Advice	176	99%	85%	82%	100%
Pneumonia Care					
Appropriate Initial Antibiotic	130	88%	83%	83%	94%
Blood Culture Timing	121	93%	91%	90%	100%
Influenza Vaccine	30	83%	77%	70%	100%
Initial Antibiotic Timing	195	70%	81%	80%	93%
Oxygenation Assessment	249	100%	99%	99%	100%
Pneumococcal Vaccine	112	84%	75%	69%	94%
Smoking Cessation Advice	88	100%	83%	80%	100%
Surgical Infection Prevention					
Prophylactic Antibiotic Given	1,725	95%	78%	77%	95%
Prophylactic Antibiotic Selection	478	93%	92%	90%	100%
Prophylactic Antibiotic Stopped	1,671	84%	78%	72%	95%
Pregnancy Care					
Inpatient Neonatal Mortality	-	-	-	-	-
Third or Fourth Degree Laceration	-	-	-	3.63%	3.27%

Providence Hosp/Providence Heart Inst

2435 Forest Drive   Toll-Free: 800-262-5682
Columbia, SC 29204   Phone: 803-256-5300
    Fax: 803-256-5935

E-mail: info@provhosp.com
URL: www.providencehospitals.com
Ownership: Voluntary non-profit - Church   Accredited: Yes
Emergency Services: Yes   Licensed Beds: 239

Key Personnel:
President/CEO . . . . Sr Judith Ann Karam, CSA
Emergency Room . . . . Pat Griffith
Emergency Room . . . . Diane Kerenick
Chief Radiology . . . . Maxine Bass
Director Respiratory Therapy . . . . Tom Charles

Measure	Cases	This Hospital	State Average	U.S. Average	Top Hospital
Heart Attack Care					
ACE Inhibitor or ARB for LVSD[2]	59	92%	84%	82%	100%
Aspirin at Arrival[2]	171	96%	92%	92%	100%
Aspirin at Discharge[2]	302	98%	87%	90%	100%
Beta Blocker at Arrival[2]	162	94%	87%	87%	100%
Beta Blocker at Discharge[2]	292	95%	92%	90%	100%
Fibrinolytic Medication Timing[2]	0	-	34%	31%	100%
PCI Within 90 Minutes of Arrival[1,2]	12	25%	58%	54%	95%
Smoking Cessation Advice[2]	124	100%	89%	88%	100%
Heart Failure Care					
ACE Inhibitor or ARB for LVSD[2]	181	90%	85%	82%	100%
Discharge Instructions[2]	277	96%	66%	61%	93%
Evaluation of LVS Function[2]	326	99%	89%	83%	99%
Smoking Cessation Advice[2]	67	100%	85%	82%	100%
Pneumonia Care					
Appropriate Initial Antibiotic[2]	150	83%	83%	83%	94%
Blood Culture Timing[1,2,3]	20	100%	91%	90%	100%
Influenza Vaccine	51	92%	77%	70%	100%
Initial Antibiotic Timing[2]	164	64%	81%	80%	93%
Oxygenation Assessment[2]	221	100%	99%	99%	100%
Pneumococcal Vaccine[2]	142	84%	75%	69%	94%
Smoking Cessation Advice[2]	59	100%	83%	80%	100%
Surgical Infection Prevention					
Prophylactic Antibiotic Given[2]	268	89%	78%	77%	95%
Prophylactic Antibiotic Selection[5]	-	-	92%	90%	100%
Prophylactic Antibiotic Stopped[2]	261	69%	78%	72%	95%
Pregnancy Care					
Inpatient Neonatal Mortality	-	-	-	-	-
Third or Fourth Degree Laceration	-	-	-	3.63%	3.27%

Conway Medical Center

300 Singleton Ridge Road   Phone: 843-347-7111
Conway, SC 29526   Fax: 843-347-8056
Ownership: Voluntary non-profit - Private   Accredited: Yes
Emergency Services: Yes   Licensed Beds: 160

Key Personnel:
CEO . . . . Phillip Clayton
Emergency Room . . . . Barbara Bryant, RN

NOTE: Hospital profiles are in alphabetical order by state, then city, then hospital within the city; Rankings are sorted by rate in descending order and exclude hospitals with less than 25 cases; (1) The number of cases is too small (n<25) for purposes of reliably predicting hospital performance; (2) Measure reflects the hospital's indication that its submission was based upon a sample of its relevant discharges; (3) Rate reflects fewer than the maximum possible quarters of data for the measure; (4) Inaccurate information submitted and suppressed for one or more quarters; (5) No data is available from the hospital for this measure; Please refer to the User's Guide for a full explanation of data

Measure	Cases	This Hospital	State Average	U.S. Average	Top Hospital
Heart Attack Care					
ACE Inhibitor or ARB for LVSD[1]	8	100%	84%	82%	100%
Aspirin at Arrival	85	100%	92%	92%	100%
Aspirin at Discharge	39	87%	87%	90%	100%
Beta Blocker at Arrival	75	96%	87%	87%	100%
Beta Blocker at Discharge	37	95%	92%	90%	100%
Fibrinolytic Medication Timing[1,3]	10	80%	34%	31%	100%
PCI Within 90 Minutes of Arrival	0	-	58%	54%	95%
Smoking Cessation Advice[1,3]	5	100%	89%	88%	100%
Heart Failure Care					
ACE Inhibitor or ARB for LVSD	86	91%	85%	82%	100%
Discharge Instructions[3]	49	90%	66%	61%	93%
Evaluation of LVS Function	260	92%	89%	83%	99%
Smoking Cessation Advice[1,3]	12	100%	85%	82%	100%
Pneumonia Care					
Appropriate Initial Antibiotic[1,3]	17	82%	83%	83%	94%
Blood Culture Timing[3]	33	91%	91%	90%	100%
Influenza Vaccine[5]	-	-	77%	70%	100%
Initial Antibiotic Timing	248	88%	81%	80%	93%
Oxygenation Assessment	294	100%	99%	99%	100%
Pneumococcal Vaccine	145	71%	75%	69%	94%
Smoking Cessation Advice[1,3]	15	100%	83%	80%	100%
Surgical Infection Prevention					
Prophylactic Antibiotic Given[2,3]	41	93%	78%	77%	95%
Prophylactic Antibiotic Selection[5]	-	-	92%	90%	100%
Prophylactic Antibiotic Stopped[2,3]	38	76%	78%	72%	95%
Pregnancy Care					
Inpatient Neonatal Mortality	-	-	-	-	-
Third or Fourth Degree Laceration	-	-	-	3.63%	3.27%

Wilson Medical Center

Alternate Name: Mcleod Medical Center-Darlington
701 Cashua Ferry Road
Darlington, SC 29532
URL: www.mcleodhealth.org
Ownership: Voluntary non-profit - Private
Emergency Services: No

Phone: 843-777-1100
Fax: 843-777-1146

Accredited: Yes
Licensed Beds: 50

Key Personnel:
Administrator . . . . Tom Hartley
Chief Medical Staff. . . . . Tom Dickinson, MD
Emergency Room . . . . Richard Rogers
Director Infection/Disease Control . . . . Nancy Vivian
Director Medical/Surgical Nursing . . . . Pat Jarvis
Director Respiratory Therapy . . . . Faye Streett

Measure	Cases	This Hospital	State Average	U.S. Average	Top Hospital
Heart Attack Care					
ACE Inhibitor or ARB for LVSD[1,3]	1	100%	84%	82%	100%
Aspirin at Arrival[1,3]	1	100%	92%	92%	100%
Aspirin at Discharge[3]	0	-	87%	90%	100%
Beta Blocker at Arrival[3]	0	-	87%	87%	100%
Beta Blocker at Discharge[1,3]	1	100%	92%	90%	100%
Fibrinolytic Medication Timing[3]	0	-	34%	31%	100%
PCI Within 90 Minutes of Arrival	0	-	58%	54%	95%
Smoking Cessation Advice[3]	0	-	89%	88%	100%
Heart Failure Care					
ACE Inhibitor or ARB for LVSD	27	93%	85%	82%	100%
Discharge Instructions[1,3]	6	17%	66%	61%	93%
Evaluation of LVS Function	49	98%	89%	83%	99%
Smoking Cessation Advice[1,3]	1	100%	85%	82%	100%
Pneumonia Care					
Appropriate Initial Antibiotic[1,3]	1	100%	83%	83%	94%
Blood Culture Timing[3]	0	-	91%	90%	100%
Influenza Vaccine[4,5]	-	-	77%	70%	100%
Initial Antibiotic Timing	29	72%	81%	80%	93%
Oxygenation Assessment	33	100%	99%	99%	100%
Pneumococcal Vaccine[1]	21	90%	75%	69%	94%
Smoking Cessation Advice[1,3]	1	100%	83%	80%	100%
Surgical Infection Prevention					
Prophylactic Antibiotic Given[5]	-	-	78%	77%	95%
Prophylactic Antibiotic Selection[5]	-	-	92%	90%	100%

Prophylactic Antibiotic Stopped[5]	-	-	78%	72%	95%
Pregnancy Care					
Inpatient Neonatal Mortality	-	-	-	-	-
Third or Fourth Degree Laceration	-	-	-	3.63%	3.27%

McLeod Medical Center Dillon

Alternate Name: Saint Eugene Community Hospital
301 E Jackson Street
Dillon, SC 29536
URL: www.mcleodhealth.org
Ownership: Voluntary non-profit - Private
Emergency Services: Yes

Phone: 843-774-4111
Fax: 843-774-1563

Accredited: Yes
Licensed Beds: 92

Key Personnel:
Administrator/President . . . . Donald Sundoval
Chief Medical Staff. . . . . Yvonne Ramirez-Welden, MD
Emergency Room . . . . Lance Davis, MD
Director Infection/Disease Control . . . . Mary Kay Bagnal
Director Medical/Surgical Nursing . . . . Michele Britt, RN
OB/GYN Womens Health. . . . . Juan Cornejo, MD
Chief Radiology . . . . Mathew J Cerny, MD

Measure	Cases	This Hospital	State Average	U.S. Average	Top Hospital
Heart Attack Care					
ACE Inhibitor or ARB for LVSD[1]	5	80%	84%	82%	100%
Aspirin at Arrival[1]	21	90%	92%	92%	100%
Aspirin at Discharge[1]	15	80%	87%	90%	100%
Beta Blocker at Arrival[1]	14	93%	87%	87%	100%
Beta Blocker at Discharge[1]	18	94%	92%	90%	100%
Fibrinolytic Medication Timing[1,3]	1	0%	34%	31%	100%
PCI Within 90 Minutes of Arrival	0	-	58%	54%	95%
Smoking Cessation Advice[1,3]	1	100%	89%	88%	100%
Heart Failure Care					
ACE Inhibitor or ARB for LVSD	46	78%	85%	82%	100%
Discharge Instructions[3]	36	75%	66%	61%	93%
Evaluation of LVS Function	178	76%	89%	83%	99%
Smoking Cessation Advice[1,3]	4	100%	85%	82%	100%
Pneumonia Care					
Appropriate Initial Antibiotic[1,3]	12	67%	83%	83%	94%
Blood Culture Timing[1,3]	11	82%	91%	90%	100%
Influenza Vaccine[5]	-	-	77%	70%	100%
Initial Antibiotic Timing	93	85%	81%	80%	93%
Oxygenation Assessment	133	100%	99%	99%	100%
Pneumococcal Vaccine	56	34%	75%	69%	94%
Smoking Cessation Advice[1,3]	5	100%	83%	80%	100%
Surgical Infection Prevention					
Prophylactic Antibiotic Given[1,2,3]	14	100%	78%	77%	95%
Prophylactic Antibiotic Selection[5]	-	-	92%	90%	100%
Prophylactic Antibiotic Stopped[1,2,3]	13	62%	78%	72%	95%
Pregnancy Care					
Inpatient Neonatal Mortality	-	-	-	-	-
Third or Fourth Degree Laceration	-	-	-	3.63%	3.27%

Palmetto Baptist Medical Center Easley

Alternate Name: Baptist Medical Center-Easley
200 Fleetwood Drive
PO Box 2129
Easley, SC 29640
URL: www.palmettohealth.org
Ownership: Voluntary non-profit - Private
Emergency Services: Yes

Phone: 864-855-7200
Fax: 864-442-7890

Accredited: Yes
Licensed Beds: 96

Key Personnel:
CEO. . . . . Charles Beaman
Chief Medical Staff. . . . . Hubert Bowick, MD
Emergency Room . . . . Brad Howard, MD
Director Infection/Disease Control . . . . Julie Chastain
CCU Spvg. Nurse . . . . Sandy Myers
Director Medical/Surgical Nursing . . . . Mary Ann Hunter, MD
Director Pulmonary Therapy . . . . John Clordy

Measure	Cases	This Hospital	State Average	U.S. Average	Top Hospital
Heart Attack Care					
ACE Inhibitor or ARB for LVSD[1]	12	100%	84%	82%	100%

NOTE: Hospital profiles are in alphabetical order by state, then city, then hospital within the city; Rankings are sorted by rate in descending order and exclude hospitals with less than 25 cases; (1) The number of cases is too small (n<25) for purposes of reliably predicting hospital performance; (2) Measure reflects the hospital's indication that its submission was based upon a sample of its relevant discharges; (3) Rate reflects fewer than the maximum possible quarters of data for the measure; (4) Inaccurate information submitted and suppressed for one or more quarters; (5) No data is available from the hospital for this measure; Please refer to the User's Guide for a full explanation of data

Aspirin at Arrival	68	93%	92%	92%	100%
Aspirin at Discharge	40	92%	87%	90%	100%
Beta Blocker at Arrival	46	93%	87%	87%	100%
Beta Blocker at Discharge	44	95%	92%	90%	100%
Fibrinolytic Medication Timing[1]	5	40%	34%	31%	100%
PCI Within 90 Minutes of Arrival	0	-	58%	54%	95%
Smoking Cessation Advice[1]	16	88%	89%	88%	100%
Heart Failure Care					
ACE Inhibitor or ARB for LVSD	48	98%	85%	82%	100%
Discharge Instructions	117	85%	66%	61%	93%
Evaluation of LVS Function	147	95%	89%	83%	99%
Smoking Cessation Advice	34	100%	85%	82%	100%
Pneumonia Care					
Appropriate Initial Antibiotic	127	91%	83%	83%	94%
Blood Culture Timing	125	94%	91%	90%	100%
Influenza Vaccine	25	100%	77%	70%	100%
Initial Antibiotic Timing	201	77%	81%	80%	93%
Oxygenation Assessment	233	100%	99%	99%	100%
Pneumococcal Vaccine	144	99%	75%	69%	94%
Smoking Cessation Advice	59	92%	83%	80%	100%
Surgical Infection Prevention					
Prophylactic Antibiotic Given	259	95%	78%	77%	95%
Prophylactic Antibiotic Selection	70	90%	92%	90%	100%
Prophylactic Antibiotic Stopped	246	86%	78%	72%	95%
Pregnancy Care					
Inpatient Neonatal Mortality	-	-	-	-	-
Third or Fourth Degree Laceration	-	-	-	3.63%	3.27%

Edgefield County Hospital

300 Bridge medical Plaza
Edgefield, SC 29824
Ownership: Government - Local
Emergency Services: Yes

Phone: 803-637-3174
Fax: 803-637-3174
Accredited: Yes
Licensed Beds: 40

Key Personnel:
CEO/President . . . . Sam Gregory
Chief Medical Staff . . . . Joseph Sell
Chief of Medical Staff . . . . George Rainsord
Emergency Room . . . . Paul Espinoza
Director of Pulmonary/Respiratory Care . . . . Barry Powers

Measure	Cases	This Hospital	State Average	U.S. Average	Top Hospital
Heart Attack Care					
ACE Inhibitor or ARB for LVSD[1]	1	100%	84%	82%	100%
Aspirin at Arrival[1]	2	100%	92%	92%	100%
Aspirin at Discharge[1]	3	67%	87%	90%	100%
Beta Blocker at Arrival[1]	3	67%	87%	87%	100%
Beta Blocker at Discharge[1]	3	67%	92%	90%	100%
Fibrinolytic Medication Timing	0	-	34%	31%	100%
PCI Within 90 Minutes of Arrival	0	-	58%	54%	95%
Smoking Cessation Advice[1]	1	100%	89%	88%	100%
Heart Failure Care					
ACE Inhibitor or ARB for LVSD[1]	13	85%	85%	82%	100%
Discharge Instructions	45	67%	66%	61%	93%
Evaluation of LVS Function	59	68%	89%	83%	99%
Smoking Cessation Advice[1]	15	73%	85%	82%	100%
Pneumonia Care					
Appropriate Initial Antibiotic	40	75%	83%	83%	94%
Blood Culture Timing[1]	24	100%	91%	90%	100%
Influenza Vaccine[1]	18	89%	77%	70%	100%
Initial Antibiotic Timing	47	100%	81%	80%	93%
Oxygenation Assessment	60	100%	99%	99%	100%
Pneumococcal Vaccine	46	91%	75%	69%	94%
Smoking Cessation Advice[1]	9	44%	83%	80%	100%
Surgical infection Prevention					
Prophylactic Antibiotic Given[5]	-	-	78%	77%	95%
Prophylactic Antibiotic Selection[5]	-	-	92%	90%	100%
Prophylactic Antibiotic Stopped[5]	-	-	78%	72%	95%
Pregnancy Care					
Inpatient Neonatal Mortality	-	-	-	-	-
Third or Fourth Degree Laceration	-	-	-	3.63%	3.27%

Carolinas Hospital System-Florence

Alternate Name: Florence General Hospital
805 Pamplico Highway
Florence, SC 29505
E-mail: info@carolinashospital.com
URL: www.carolinashospital.com
Ownership: Proprietary
Emergency Services: Yes

Phone: 843-674-5000
Fax: 843-674-2647

Accredited: Yes
Licensed Beds: 372

Key Personnel:
CEO . . . . James O'Loughlin
Chief Medical Staff . . . . Richard Davis, MD
Cardiology . . . . Rilla Hemmingsen, RN
Emergency Room . . . . William Cauthen, MD
Director Infection/Disease Control . . . . Sue Ann Avin, RN
CCU Spvg. Nurse . . . . Leslie Phelps, RN
OB/GYN Womens Health . . . . Thomas W Phillips, MD
Surgical Services . . . . David Ferguson
Chief Radiology . . . . Robert Whitesides, MD
Director Respiratory Therapy . . . . Sandy Byrdic

Measure	Cases	This Hospital	State Average	U.S. Average	Top Hospital
Heart Attack Care					
ACE Inhibitor or ARB for LVSD	49	73%	84%	82%	100%
Aspirin at Arrival	144	95%	92%	92%	100%
Aspirin at Discharge	192	94%	87%	90%	100%
Beta Blocker at Arrival	109	93%	87%	87%	100%
Beta Blocker at Discharge	205	98%	92%	90%	100%
Fibrinolytic Medication Timing	0	-	34%	31%	100%
PCI Within 90 Minutes of Arrival[1]	3	67%	58%	54%	95%
Smoking Cessation Advice	73	97%	89%	88%	100%
Heart Failure Care					
ACE Inhibitor or ARB for LVSD	210	87%	85%	82%	100%
Discharge Instructions	394	64%	66%	61%	93%
Evaluation of LVS Function	477	97%	89%	83%	99%
Smoking Cessation Advice	98	99%	85%	82%	100%
Pneumonia Care					
Appropriate Initial Antibiotic	190	77%	83%	83%	94%
Blood Culture Timing	172	97%	91%	90%	100%
Influenza Vaccine	45	73%	77%	70%	100%
Initial Antibiotic Timing	277	79%	81%	80%	93%
Oxygenation Assessment	336	98%	99%	99%	100%
Pneumococcal Vaccine	187	81%	75%	69%	94%
Smoking Cessation Advice	87	100%	83%	80%	100%
Surgical Infection Prevention					
Prophylactic Antibiotic Given	674	89%	78%	77%	95%
Prophylactic Antibiotic Selection	167	95%	92%	90%	100%
Prophylactic Antibiotic Stopped	658	79%	78%	72%	95%
Pregnancy Care					
Inpatient Neonatal Mortality	-	-	-	-	-
Third or Fourth Degree Laceration	-	-	-	3.63%	3.27%

McLeod Regional Medical Center-Pee Dee

555 E Cheves Street
Florence, SC 29506
URL: www.mcleodhealth.org
Ownership: Voluntary non-profit - Private
Emergency Services: Yes

Phone: 843-777-2000
Fax: 843-777-2810

Accredited: Yes
Licensed Beds: 371

Key Personnel:
President/CEO . . . . J Bruce Barragan
Chief Medical Staff . . . . Richard Ervin, MD
Chief Catheterization Laboratory . . . . Joe Kmonicek, MD
Emergency Room . . . . Hart Smith, RN
Director Infection/Disease Control . . . . Vicky Zelenka, RN
CCU Spvg. Nurse . . . . Daphne Bazen, RN
Director Medical/Surgical Nursing . . . . Beki Cooley, RN
OB/GYN Womens Health . . . . Edward O'Dell, MD
Chief Radiology . . . . Raymond L Thomas
Director Respiratory Therapy . . . . Thomas Charles

Measure	Cases	This Hospital	State Average	U.S. Average	Top Hospital
Heart Attack Care					
ACE Inhibitor or ARB for LVSD	188	87%	84%	82%	100%
Aspirin at Arrival	323	98%	92%	92%	100%
Aspirin at Discharge	503	98%	87%	90%	100%

NOTE: Hospital profiles are in alphabetical order by state, then city, then hospital within the city; Rankings are sorted by rate in descending order and exclude hospitals with less than 25 cases; (1) The number of cases is too small (n<25) for purposes of reliably predicting hospital performance; (2) Measure reflects the hospital's indication that its submission was based upon a sample of its relevant discharges; (3) Rate reflects fewer than the maximum possible quarters of data for the measure; (4) Inaccurate information submitted and suppressed for one or more quarters; (5) No data is available from the hospital for this measure; Please refer to the User's Guide for a full explanation of data

Measure	Cases	This Hospital	State Average	U.S. Average	Top Hospital
Beta Blocker at Arrival	253	95%	87%	87%	100%
Beta Blocker at Discharge	609	99%	92%	90%	100%
Fibrinolytic Medication Timing[1]	3	67%	34%	31%	100%
PCI Within 90 Minutes of Arrival[1]	14	79%	58%	54%	95%
Smoking Cessation Advice	270	100%	89%	88%	100%
Heart Failure Care					
ACE Inhibitor or ARB for LVSD	355	88%	85%	82%	100%
Discharge Instructions	679	82%	66%	61%	93%
Evaluation of LVS Function	747	93%	89%	83%	99%
Smoking Cessation Advice	174	99%	85%	82%	100%
Pneumonia Care					
Appropriate Initial Antibiotic	235	86%	83%	83%	94%
Blood Culture Timing	244	96%	91%	90%	100%
Influenza Vaccine	63	90%	77%	70%	100%
Initial Antibiotic Timing	319	79%	81%	80%	93%
Oxygenation Assessment	421	99%	99%	99%	100%
Pneumococcal Vaccine	227	85%	75%	69%	94%
Smoking Cessation Advice	129	99%	83%	80%	100%
Surgical Infection Prevention					
Prophylactic Antibiotic Given[2]	255	96%	78%	77%	95%
Prophylactic Antibiotic Selection[2]	66	95%	92%	90%	100%
Prophylactic Antibiotic Stopped[2]	245	80%	78%	72%	95%
Pregnancy Care					
Inpatient Neonatal Mortality	-	-	-	-	-
Third or Fourth Degree Laceration	-	-	-	3.63%	3.27%

Upstate Carolina Medical Center

Alternate Name: Upstate Carolina Memorial Center

1530 N Limestone Street
Gaffney, SC 29340
Ownership: Proprietary
Emergency Services: Yes

Phone: 864-487-4271
Fax: 864-489-0585
Accredited: Yes
Licensed Beds: 125

Key Personnel:
CEO . . . . Jo Howell
Chief Medical Staff . . . . Donald McIntosh, MD
Emergency Room . . . . Dan Karns, MD
Director Infection/Disease Control . . . . Sherri Almond
ICU Director . . . . Gerry Wicklund
Director Medical/Surgical Nursing . . . . Tessa Downs
Director Respiratory Therapy . . . . Shannon Wylie

Measure	Cases	This Hospital	State Average	U.S. Average	Top Hospital
Heart Attack Care					
ACE Inhibitor or ARB for LVSD[1]	1	100%	84%	82%	100%
Aspirin at Arrival	32	84%	92%	92%	100%
Aspirin at Discharge[1]	12	92%	87%	90%	100%
Beta Blocker at Arrival	29	62%	87%	87%	100%
Beta Blocker at Discharge[1]	12	92%	92%	90%	100%
Fibrinolytic Medication Timing	0	-	34%	31%	100%
PCI Within 90 Minutes of Arrival	0	-	58%	54%	95%
Smoking Cessation Advice[1]	4	25%	89%	88%	100%
Heart Failure Care					
ACE Inhibitor or ARB for LVSD	36	69%	85%	82%	100%
Discharge Instructions	110	54%	66%	61%	93%
Evaluation of LVS Function	141	84%	89%	83%	99%
Smoking Cessation Advice	37	68%	85%	82%	100%
Pneumonia Care					
Appropriate Initial Antibiotic	109	66%	83%	83%	94%
Blood Culture Timing	113	96%	91%	90%	100%
Influenza Vaccine[4,5]	-	-	77%	70%	100%
Initial Antibiotic Timing	164	82%	81%	80%	93%
Oxygenation Assessment	218	99%	99%	99%	100%
Pneumococcal Vaccine	124	83%	75%	69%	94%
Smoking Cessation Advice	66	80%	83%	80%	100%
Surgical Infection Prevention					
Prophylactic Antibiotic Given[2]	110	92%	78%	77%	95%
Prophylactic Antibiotic Selection[2]	27	93%	92%	90%	100%
Prophylactic Antibiotic Stopped[2]	102	84%	78%	72%	95%
Pregnancy Care					
Inpatient Neonatal Mortality	-	-	-	-	-
Third or Fourth Degree Laceration	-	-	-	3.63%	3.27%

Georgetown Memorial Hospital

606 Black River Road
Georgetown, SC 29442
E-mail: georgettem@gmhsc.com
Ownership: Voluntary non-profit - Private
Emergency Services: Yes

Phone: 843-527-7000
Fax: 843-520-7887

Accredited: Yes
Licensed Beds: 142

Key Personnel:
Administrator . . . . Paul D Gatens, Sr
Chief Medical Staff . . . . Faron J Kemp, MD
Chief Catheterization Laboratory . . . . Craig Lieberman, MD
Emergency Room . . . . William D Richmond, MD
Director Infection/Disease Control . . . . Erma Miller, RN
Director Medical/Surgical Nursing . . . . Crystal Reid, RN
OB/GYN Womens Health . . . . Cynthia G Bindner, MD
Chief Radiology . . . . Robert O Jones, MD
Director Respiratory Therapy . . . . Julie Pope

Measure	Cases	This Hospital	State Average	U.S. Average	Top Hospital
Heart Attack Care					
ACE Inhibitor or ARB for LVSD[1]	14	86%	84%	82%	100%
Aspirin at Arrival	81	95%	92%	92%	100%
Aspirin at Discharge	60	90%	87%	90%	100%
Beta Blocker at Arrival	74	92%	87%	87%	100%
Beta Blocker at Discharge	60	90%	92%	90%	100%
Fibrinolytic Medication Timing	0	-	34%	31%	100%
PCI Within 90 Minutes of Arrival	0	-	58%	54%	95%
Smoking Cessation Advice	30	100%	89%	88%	100%
Heart Failure Care					
ACE Inhibitor or ARB for LVSD	102	83%	85%	82%	100%
Discharge Instructions	209	77%	66%	61%	93%
Evaluation of LVS Function	237	97%	89%	83%	99%
Smoking Cessation Advice	50	96%	85%	82%	100%
Pneumonia Care					
Appropriate Initial Antibiotic	84	90%	83%	83%	94%
Blood Culture Timing	118	94%	91%	90%	100%
Influenza Vaccine	30	37%	77%	70%	100%
Initial Antibiotic Timing	162	87%	81%	80%	93%
Oxygenation Assessment	188	100%	99%	99%	100%
Pneumococcal Vaccine	109	85%	75%	69%	94%
Smoking Cessation Advice	43	95%	83%	80%	100%
Surgical Infection Prevention					
Prophylactic Antibiotic Given	328	90%	78%	77%	95%
Prophylactic Antibiotic Selection	77	94%	92%	90%	100%
Prophylactic Antibiotic Stopped	319	34%	78%	72%	95%
Pregnancy Care					
Inpatient Neonatal Mortality	-	-	-	-	-
Third or Fourth Degree Laceration	-	-	-	3.63%	3.27%

Greenville Memorial Medical Campus

Alternate Name: Greenville Memorial Hospital

701 Grove Road
Greenville, SC 29605

Toll-Free: 877-447-4636
Phone: 864-455-7000
Fax: 864-455-6218

URL: www.ghs.org
Ownership: Government - State
Emergency Services: Yes

Accredited: Yes
Licensed Beds: 710

Key Personnel:
President/CEO . . . . Frank Pinckney

Measure	Cases	This Hospital	State Average	U.S. Average	Top Hospital
Heart Attack Care					
ACE Inhibitor or ARB for LVSD	220	88%	84%	82%	100%
Aspirin at Arrival	492	97%	92%	92%	100%
Aspirin at Discharge	658	98%	87%	90%	100%
Beta Blocker at Arrival	383	94%	87%	87%	100%
Beta Blocker at Discharge	744	97%	92%	90%	100%
Fibrinolytic Medication Timing[1]	1	100%	34%	31%	100%
PCI Within 90 Minutes of Arrival	34	68%	58%	54%	95%
Smoking Cessation Advice	404	100%	89%	88%	100%
Heart Failure Care					
ACE Inhibitor or ARB for LVSD	395	94%	85%	82%	100%
Discharge Instructions	694	70%	66%	61%	93%
Evaluation of LVS Function	800	98%	89%	83%	99%

NOTE: Hospital profiles are in alphabetical order by state, then city, then hospital within the city; Rankings are sorted by rate in descending order and exclude hospitals with less than 25 cases; (1) The number of cases is too small (n<25) for purposes of reliably predicting hospital performance; (2) Measure reflects the hospital's indication that its submission was based upon a sample of its relevant discharges; (3) Rate reflects fewer than the maximum possible quarters of data for the measure; (4) Inaccurate information submitted and suppressed for one or more quarters; (5) No data is available from the hospital for this measure; Please refer to the User's Guide for a full explanation of data

Smoking Cessation Advice	195	96%	85%	82%	100%
Pneumonia Care					
Appropriate Initial Antibiotic	294	93%	83%	83%	94%
Blood Culture Timing	268	95%	91%	90%	100%
Influenza Vaccine	98	83%	77%	70%	100%
Initial Antibiotic Timing	456	67%	81%	80%	93%
Oxygenation Assessment	552	100%	99%	99%	100%
Pneumococcal Vaccine	301	82%	75%	69%	94%
Smoking Cessation Advice	174	94%	83%	80%	100%
Surgical Infection Prevention					
Prophylactic Antibiotic Given[2,3]	253	93%	78%	77%	95%
Prophylactic Antibiotic Selection[2]	88	94%	92%	90%	100%
Prophylactic Antibiotic Stopped[2,3]	239	90%	78%	72%	95%
Pregnancy Care					
Inpatient Neonatal Mortality	-	-	-	-	-
Third or Fourth Degree Laceration	-	-	-	3.63%	3.27%

Saint Francis Hospital

Alternate Name: Saint Francis Health System
One Saint Francis Drive   Phone: 864-255-1000
Greenville, SC 29601   Fax: 864-255-1034
URL: www.stfrancishealth.org
Ownership: Voluntary non-profit - Church   Accredited: Yes
Emergency Services: Yes   Licensed Beds: 257
Key Personnel:
CEO . . . . Valinda Rutledge
Chief Medical Staff . . . . MaryJo Cagle
Emergency Room . . . . Scott Pietras
Emergency Room . . . . Antoinette Ruff, RN
OB/GYN Womens Health . . . . Mary Cagle, MD
Chief Radiology . . . . Jeff Schramek, MD
Respiratory Care . . . . Susie Morlin

Measure	Cases	This Hospital	State Average	U.S. Average	Top Hospital
Heart Attack Care					
ACE Inhibitor or ARB for LVSD	37	97%	84%	82%	100%
Aspirin at Arrival	139	100%	92%	92%	100%
Aspirin at Discharge	171	99%	87%	90%	100%
Beta Blocker at Arrival	102	100%	87%	87%	100%
Beta Blocker at Discharge	193	99%	92%	90%	100%
Fibrinolytic Medication Timing[1]	2	100%	34%	31%	100%
PCI Within 90 Minutes of Arrival[1]	5	100%	58%	54%	95%
Smoking Cessation Advice	65	100%	89%	88%	100%
Heart Failure Care					
ACE Inhibitor or ARB for LVSD	160	99%	85%	82%	100%
Discharge Instructions	325	76%	66%	61%	93%
Evaluation of LVS Function	372	100%	89%	83%	99%
Smoking Cessation Advice	97	100%	85%	82%	100%
Pneumonia Care					
Appropriate Initial Antibiotic	225	92%	83%	83%	94%
Blood Culture Timing	232	96%	91%	90%	100%
Influenza Vaccine	73	97%	77%	70%	100%
Initial Antibiotic Timing	318	83%	81%	80%	93%
Oxygenation Assessment	415	100%	99%	99%	100%
Pneumococcal Vaccine	292	86%	75%	69%	94%
Smoking Cessation Advice	94	100%	83%	80%	100%
Surgical Infection Prevention					
Prophylactic Antibiotic Given[2]	323	96%	78%	77%	95%
Prophylactic Antibiotic Selection[2]	85	99%	92%	90%	100%
Prophylactic Antibiotic Stopped[2]	310	93%	78%	72%	95%
Pregnancy Care					
Inpatient Neonatal Mortality	-	-	-	-	-
Third or Fourth Degree Laceration	-	-	-	3.63%	3.27%

Self Regional Healthcare Center

Alternate Name: Self Memorial Hospital
1325 Spring Street   Phone: 864-725-4111
Greenwood, SC 29646   Fax: 864-725-4711
URL: www.selfregional.org
Ownership: Voluntary non-profit - Other   Accredited: Yes
Emergency Services: Yes   Licensed Beds: 421
Key Personnel:
President/CEO . . . . M John Heydel

Chief Medical Staff . . . . Julius Leary, MD
Chief Catheterization Laboratory . . . . Ennis James, MD
Emergency Room Medical Director . . . . J W Logan, MD
Infection Control . . . . Dorrell Antley
ICU . . . . Jackie Thornton
Intensive Coronary . . . . Jackie Thornton
Nurse Manager OB/GYN Womens Health . . . . . Monica Blochowiak, RN
Clinical Director Respiratory . . . . Ron Deeder

Measure	Cases	This Hospital	State Average	U.S. Average	Top Hospital
Heart Attack Care					
ACE Inhibitor or ARB for LVSD	53	100%	84%	82%	100%
Aspirin at Arrival	175	99%	92%	92%	100%
Aspirin at Discharge	180	98%	87%	90%	100%
Beta Blocker at Arrival	132	94%	87%	87%	100%
Beta Blocker at Discharge	186	98%	92%	90%	100%
Fibrinolytic Medication Timing[1]	5	40%	34%	31%	100%
PCI Within 90 Minutes of Arrival[1]	13	8%	58%	54%	95%
Smoking Cessation Advice	74	99%	89%	88%	100%
Heart Failure Care					
ACE Inhibitor or ARB for LVSD	193	92%	85%	82%	100%
Discharge Instructions	333	66%	66%	61%	93%
Evaluation of LVS Function	380	97%	89%	83%	99%
Smoking Cessation Advice	85	100%	85%	82%	100%
Pneumonia Care					
Appropriate Initial Antibiotic	187	84%	83%	83%	94%
Blood Culture Timing	212	96%	91%	90%	100%
Influenza Vaccine	62	79%	77%	70%	100%
Initial Antibiotic Timing	274	79%	81%	80%	93%
Oxygenation Assessment	345	99%	99%	99%	100%
Pneumococcal Vaccine	210	78%	75%	69%	94%
Smoking Cessation Advice	86	99%	83%	80%	100%
Surgical Infection Prevention					
Prophylactic Antibiotic Given[2]	812	95%	78%	77%	95%
Prophylactic Antibiotic Selection[2]	63	97%	92%	90%	100%
Prophylactic Antibiotic Stopped[2]	790	89%	78%	72%	95%
Pregnancy Care					
Inpatient Neonatal Mortality	-	-	-	-	-
Third or Fourth Degree Laceration	-	-	-	3.63%	3.27%

Allen Bennett Memorial Hospital

313 Memorial Drive   Phone: 864-848-8200
Greer, SC 29652   Fax: 864-455-6218
E-mail: mmassey@ghs.org
URL: www.ghs.org
Ownership: Government - State   Accredited: Yes
Emergency Services: Yes   Licensed Beds: 58
Key Personnel:
Administrator . . . . Michael W Massey
Chief Medical Staff . . . . John Sanders
Emergency Room . . . . Kevin Gregg, MD
Director Infection/Disease Control . . . . Belvin Holman, RN
Head Nurse CCU . . . . Eleanor Bell
Director Medical/Surgical Nursing . . . . Lee Gilreath
OB/GYN Womens Health . . . . George Helmrich, MD
Chief Respiratory Therapy . . . . Clara Puras

Measure	Cases	This Hospital	State Average	U.S. Average	Top Hospital
Heart Attack Care					
ACE Inhibitor or ARB for LVSD[3]	0	-	84%	82%	100%
Aspirin at Arrival[1,3]	1	100%	92%	92%	100%
Aspirin at Discharge[3]	0	-	87%	90%	100%
Beta Blocker at Arrival[1,3]	1	100%	87%	87%	100%
Beta Blocker at Discharge[3]	0	-	92%	90%	100%
Fibrinolytic Medication Timing[3]	0	-	34%	31%	100%
PCI Within 90 Minutes of Arrival[5]	-	-	58%	54%	95%
Smoking Cessation Advice[3]	0	-	89%	88%	100%
Heart Failure Care					
ACE Inhibitor or ARB for LVSD	36	86%	85%	82%	100%
Discharge Instructions	76	78%	66%	61%	93%
Evaluation of LVS Function	104	94%	89%	83%	99%
Smoking Cessation Advice[1]	18	94%	85%	82%	100%
Pneumonia Care					

NOTE: Hospital profiles are in alphabetical order by state, then city, then hospital within the city; Rankings are sorted by rate in descending order and exclude hospitals with less than 25 cases; (1) The number of cases is too small (n<25) for purposes of reliably predicting hospital performance; (2) Measure reflects the hospital's indication that its submission was based upon a sample of its relevant discharges; (3) Rate reflects fewer than the maximum possible quarters of data for the measure; (4) Inaccurate information submitted and suppressed for one or more quarters; (5) No data is available from the hospital for this measure; Please refer to the User's Guide for a full explanation of data

Appropriate Initial Antibiotic	123	93%	83%	83%	94%
Blood Culture Timing	74	99%	91%	90%	100%
Influenza Vaccine	34	88%	77%	70%	100%
Initial Antibiotic Timing	148	92%	81%	80%	93%
Oxygenation Assessment	187	100%	99%	99%	100%
Pneumococcal Vaccine	119	87%	75%	69%	94%
Smoking Cessation Advice	55	96%	83%	80%	100%
Surgical Infection Prevention					
Prophylactic Antibiotic Given[2,3]	94	82%	78%	77%	95%
Prophylactic Antibiotic Selection[2]	32	94%	92%	90%	100%
Prophylactic Antibiotic Stopped[2,3]	89	90%	78%	72%	95%
Pregnancy Care					
Inpatient Neonatal Mortality	-	-	-	-	-
Third or Fourth Degree Laceration	-	-	-	3.63%	3.27%

Coastal Carolina Medical Center

1000 Medical Center Drive
Hardeeville, SC 29927   Phone: 843-784-8000
Ownership: Proprietary   Accredited: No
Emergency Services: Yes

Measure	Cases	This Hospital	State Average	U.S. Average	Top Hospital
Heart Attack Care					
ACE Inhibitor or ARB for LVSD	0	-	84%	82%	100%
Aspirin at Arrival[1]	4	50%	92%	92%	100%
Aspirin at Discharge[1]	1	100%	87%	90%	100%
Beta Blocker at Arrival[1]	3	100%	87%	87%	100%
Beta Blocker at Discharge[1]	1	100%	92%	90%	100%
Fibrinolytic Medication Timing	0	-	34%	31%	100%
PCI Within 90 Minutes of Arrival	0	-	58%	54%	95%
Smoking Cessation Advice[1]	1	0%	89%	88%	100%
Heart Failure Care					
ACE Inhibitor or ARB for LVSD[1]	6	100%	85%	82%	100%
Discharge Instructions	39	62%	66%	61%	93%
Evaluation of LVS Function	41	63%	89%	83%	99%
Smoking Cessation Advice[1]	6	83%	85%	82%	100%
Pneumonia Care					
Appropriate Initial Antibiotic	30	83%	83%	83%	94%
Blood Culture Timing[1]	24	96%	91%	90%	100%
Influenza Vaccine[1]	7	86%	77%	70%	100%
Initial Antibiotic Timing[1]	18	67%	81%	80%	93%
Oxygenation Assessment	38	97%	99%	99%	100%
Pneumococcal Vaccine[1]	21	71%	75%	69%	94%
Smoking Cessation Advice[1]	3	33%	83%	80%	100%
Surgical Infection Prevention					
Prophylactic Antibiotic Given[1,3]	13	54%	78%	77%	95%
Prophylactic Antibiotic Selection[1]	5	100%	92%	90%	100%
Prophylactic Antibiotic Stopped[1,3]	12	58%	78%	72%	95%
Pregnancy Care					
Inpatient Neonatal Mortality	-	-	-	-	-
Third or Fourth Degree Laceration	-	-	-	3.63%	3.27%

Carolina Pines Regional Medical Center

Alternate Name: Byerly Hospital
1304 W Bobo Newsom Highway   Phone: 843-339-2100
Hartsville, SC 29550   Fax: 843-339-4116
Ownership: Proprietary   Accredited: Yes
Emergency Services: Yes   Licensed Beds: 116
Key Personnel:
Administrator . . . . David Setchel
Chief Medical Staff . . . . KC Evans, MD
Emergency Room . . . . James Balvich, MD
Director Infection/Disease Control . . . . Shari Carter, RN
Director Medical/Surgical Nursing . . . . Carol Mozingo
Chief Radiology . . . . Greg Connor, MD
Director Respiratory Therapy . . . . Jamie Guin

Measure	Cases	This Hospital	State Average	U.S. Average	Top Hospital
Heart Attack Care					
ACE Inhibitor or ARB for LVSD[1]	2	50%	84%	82%	100%
Aspirin at Arrival	37	86%	92%	92%	100%
Aspirin at Discharge[1]	16	81%	87%	90%	100%

Beta Blocker at Arrival	32	81%	87%	87%	100%
Beta Blocker at Discharge[1]	18	78%	92%	90%	100%
Fibrinolytic Medication Timing[1]	4	75%	34%	31%	100%
PCI Within 90 Minutes of Arrival	0	-	58%	54%	95%
Smoking Cessation Advice[1]	4	100%	89%	88%	100%
Heart Failure Care					
ACE Inhibitor or ARB for LVSD	109	78%	85%	82%	100%
Discharge Instructions	226	60%	66%	61%	93%
Evaluation of LVS Function	252	98%	89%	83%	99%
Smoking Cessation Advice	62	84%	85%	82%	100%
Pneumonia Care					
Appropriate Initial Antibiotic	196	87%	83%	83%	94%
Blood Culture Timing	175	95%	91%	90%	100%
Influenza Vaccine	49	57%	77%	70%	100%
Initial Antibiotic Timing	292	90%	81%	80%	93%
Oxygenation Assessment	336	100%	99%	99%	100%
Pneumococcal Vaccine	169	69%	75%	69%	94%
Smoking Cessation Advice	101	90%	83%	80%	100%
Surgical Infection Prevention					
Prophylactic Antibiotic Given[2]	150	90%	78%	77%	95%
Prophylactic Antibiotic Selection[2]	34	91%	92%	90%	100%
Prophylactic Antibiotic Stopped[2]	145	70%	78%	72%	95%
Pregnancy Care					
Inpatient Neonatal Mortality	-	-	-	-	-
Third or Fourth Degree Laceration	-	-	-	3.63%	3.27%

Hilton Head Regional Medical Center

25 Hospital Center Blvd
Hilton Head Isl, SC 29926   Phone: 843-681-6122
URL: www.hiltonheadmedCentercom   Fax: 843-689-3670
Ownership: Proprietary   Accredited: Yes
Emergency Services: Yes   Licensed Beds: 93
Key Personnel:
President . . . . Elizabeth Lamkin
CEO . . . . Erik W Olson
Chairman Department of Surgery . . . . Thomas Rzeczycki, MD

Measure	Cases	This Hospital	State Average	U.S. Average	Top Hospital
Heart Attack Care					
ACE Inhibitor or ARB for LVSD[1]	14	79%	84%	82%	100%
Aspirin at Arrival	80	100%	92%	92%	100%
Aspirin at Discharge	93	99%	87%	90%	100%
Beta Blocker at Arrival	54	96%	87%	87%	100%
Beta Blocker at Discharge	92	98%	92%	90%	100%
Fibrinolytic Medication Timing	0	-	34%	31%	100%
PCI Within 90 Minutes of Arrival[1]	5	20%	58%	54%	95%
Smoking Cessation Advice	29	93%	89%	88%	100%
Heart Failure Care					
ACE Inhibitor or ARB for LVSD	78	79%	85%	82%	100%
Discharge Instructions	155	58%	66%	61%	93%
Evaluation of LVS Function	199	94%	89%	83%	99%
Smoking Cessation Advice[1]	21	86%	85%	82%	100%
Pneumonia Care					
Appropriate Initial Antibiotic	98	96%	83%	83%	94%
Blood Culture Timing	92	90%	91%	90%	100%
Influenza Vaccine	27	74%	77%	70%	100%
Initial Antibiotic Timing	108	94%	81%	80%	93%
Oxygenation Assessment	167	100%	99%	99%	100%
Pneumococcal Vaccine	125	78%	75%	69%	94%
Smoking Cessation Advice[1]	23	96%	83%	80%	100%
Surgical Infection Prevention					
Prophylactic Antibiotic Given[2]	238	84%	78%	77%	95%
Prophylactic Antibiotic Selection[2]	37	97%	92%	90%	100%
Prophylactic Antibiotic Stopped[2]	232	86%	78%	72%	95%
Pregnancy Care					
Inpatient Neonatal Mortality	-	-	-	-	-
Third or Fourth Degree Laceration	-	-	-	3.63%	3.27%

Williamsburg Regional Hospital
Alternate Name: Williamsburg County Memorial Hospital

NOTE: Hospital profiles are in alphabetical order by state, then city, then hospital within the city; Rankings are sorted by rate in descending order and exclude hospitals with less than 25 cases; (1) The number of cases is too small (n<25) for purposes of reliably predicting hospital performance; (2) Measure reflects the hospital's indication that its submission is based upon a sample of its relevant discharges; (3) Rate reflects fewer than the maximum possible quarters of data for the measure; (4) Inaccurate information submitted and suppressed for one or more quarters; (5) No data is available from the hospital for this measure; Please refer to the User's Guide for a full explanation of data

500 Nelson Boulevard
Kingstree, SC 29556
URL: www.w-rh.org
Ownership: Govt - Hospital District or Authority
Emergency Services: Yes

Phone: 843-355-8888
Fax: 843-355-0128

Accredited: Yes
Licensed Beds: 78

Key Personnel:

CEO. . . . . John C Hales, FACHE
Chief Medical Staff. . . . . Dr Frank Trefry
Emergency Room . . . . Mindi Huckabee, RN
Emergency Room . . . . Frank A Tretny, MD
Infection Control. . . . . Jeanie Brown, RN
ICU . . . . Pam Ziegenhorn, RN
Medical Surgical Nursing . . . . Pam Ziegenhorn, RN
OB/GYN/Women's Health . . . . Alice Carter, RN
Director of Surgical Services . . . . Jeannie Brown

Measure	Cases	This Hospital	State Average	U.S. Average	Top Hospital
Heart Attack Care					
ACE Inhibitor or ARB for LVSD[1,3]	1	100%	84%	82%	100%
Aspirin at Arrival[1,3]	5	80%	92%	92%	100%
Aspirin at Discharge[1,3]	3	100%	87%	90%	100%
Beta Blocker at Arrival[1,3]	5	20%	87%	87%	100%
Beta Blocker at Discharge[1,3]	3	33%	92%	90%	100%
Fibrinolytic Medication Timing[1,3]	1	0%	34%	31%	100%
PCI Within 90 Minutes of Arrival	0	-	58%	54%	95%
Smoking Cessation Advice[3]	0	-	89%	88%	100%
Heart Failure Care					
ACE Inhibitor or ARB for LVSD[1,3]	14	86%	85%	82%	100%
Discharge Instructions[3]	29	17%	66%	61%	93%
Evaluation of LVS Function[3]	31	65%	89%	83%	99%
Smoking Cessation Advice[1,3]	4	50%	85%	82%	100%
Pneumonia Care					
Appropriate Initial Antibiotic[3]	32	56%	83%	83%	94%
Blood Culture Timing[1,3]	15	93%	91%	90%	100%
Influenza Vaccine[5]	-	-	77%	70%	100%
Initial Antibiotic Timing[3]	38	79%	81%	80%	93%
Oxygenation Assessment[3]	44	93%	99%	99%	100%
Pneumococcal Vaccine[3]	27	15%	75%	69%	94%
Smoking Cessation Advice[1,3]	5	40%	83%	80%	100%
Surgical Infection Prevention					
Prophylactic Antibiotic Given[1,3]	1	0%	78%	77%	95%
Prophylactic Antibiotic Selection[5]	-	-	92%	90%	100%
Prophylactic Antibiotic Stopped[3]	0	-	78%	72%	95%
Pregnancy Care					
Inpatient Neonatal Mortality	-	-	-	-	-
Third or Fourth Degree Laceration	-	-	-	3.63%	3.27%

Carolinas Hospital System-Lake City

Alternate Name: Lake City Community Hospital
258 N Ron McNair Boulevard
Lake City, SC 29560
Ownership: Govt - Hospital District or Authority
Emergency Services: Yes

Phone: 843-394-2036
Fax: 843-674-2198

Accredited: Yes
Licensed Beds: 48

Key Personnel:

CEO. . . . . Clarence Bowman
Chief Medical Staff. . . . . Iris Hanna
Emergency Room . . . . Randall Davis
Director Infection/Disease Control . . . . Cindy Moon
Director Medical/Surgical Nursing . . . . Russ Garland
Director Respiratory Therapy . . . . Russ Garland

Measure	Cases	This Hospital	State Average	U.S. Average	Top Hospital
Heart Attack Care					
ACE Inhibitor or ARB for LVSD[1]	1	100%	84%	82%	100%
Aspirin at Arrival[1]	4	100%	92%	92%	100%
Aspirin at Discharge	0	-	87%	90%	100%
Beta Blocker at Arrival[1]	5	20%	87%	87%	100%
Beta Blocker at Discharge[1]	2	50%	92%	90%	100%
Fibrinolytic Medication Timing	0	-	34%	31%	100%
PCI Within 90 Minutes of Arrival	0	-	58%	54%	95%
Smoking Cessation Advice	0	-	89%	88%	100%
Heart Failure Care					
ACE Inhibitor or ARB for LVSD	27	67%	85%	82%	100%

Measure		This Hospital	State Average	U.S. Average	Top Hospital
Discharge Instructions	55	91%	66%	61%	93%
Evaluation of LVS Function	64	92%	89%	83%	99%
Smoking Cessation Advice	25	72%	85%	82%	100%
Pneumonia Care					
Appropriate Initial Antibiotic	64	97%	83%	83%	94%
Blood Culture Timing	42	90%	91%	90%	100%
Influenza Vaccine[1]	8	100%	77%	70%	100%
Initial Antibiotic Timing	70	87%	81%	80%	93%
Oxygenation Assessment	73	100%	99%	99%	100%
Pneumococcal Vaccine	35	86%	75%	69%	94%
Smoking Cessation Advice[1]	13	85%	83%	80%	100%
Surgical Infection Prevention					
Prophylactic Antibiotic Given[1,3]	2	50%	78%	77%	95%
Prophylactic Antibiotic Selection	0	-	92%	90%	100%
Prophylactic Antibiotic Stopped[1,3]	2	100%	78%	72%	95%
Pregnancy Care					
Inpatient Neonatal Mortality	-	-	-	-	-
Third or Fourth Degree Laceration	-	-	-	3.63%	3.27%

Springs Memorial Hospital

Alternate Name: Elliott White Springs Memorial Hospital
800 W Meeting Street
Lancaster, SC 29720
Ownership: Proprietary
Emergency Services: Yes

Phone: 803-286-1481
Fax: 803-286-1367
Accredited: Yes
Licensed Beds: 194

Key Personnel:

CEO. . . . . Daniel E McKay
Chief Medical Staff. . . . . RS Glickenberger, MD
Emergency Room . . . . A Midkiff, MD
Director Infection/Disease Control . . . . Sharon Jowers
CCU Spvg. Nurse . . . . Teresa Neal
Director Medical/Surgical Nursing . . . . Teresa Neal
OB/GYN Womens Health. . . . . RE Townsend, MD
Chief Radiology . . . . JS Webster, MD
Director Respiratory Therapy . . . . Judy Robinson

Measure	Cases	This Hospital	State Average	U.S. Average	Top Hospital
Heart Attack Care					
ACE Inhibitor or ARB for LVSD[1]	21	76%	84%	82%	100%
Aspirin at Arrival	123	90%	92%	92%	100%
Aspirin at Discharge	75	81%	87%	90%	100%
Beta Blocker at Arrival	105	86%	87%	87%	100%
Beta Blocker at Discharge	77	84%	92%	90%	100%
Fibrinolytic Medication Timing[1]	10	50%	34%	31%	100%
PCI Within 90 Minutes of Arrival	0	-	58%	54%	95%
Smoking Cessation Advice	31	97%	89%	88%	100%
Heart Failure Care					
ACE Inhibitor or ARB for LVSD	103	72%	85%	82%	100%
Discharge Instructions	189	81%	66%	61%	93%
Evaluation of LVS Function	256	95%	89%	83%	99%
Smoking Cessation Advice	57	100%	85%	82%	100%
Pneumonia Care					
Appropriate Initial Antibiotic	148	71%	83%	83%	94%
Blood Culture Timing	89	84%	91%	90%	100%
Influenza Vaccine	40	100%	77%	70%	100%
Initial Antibiotic Timing	187	87%	81%	80%	93%
Oxygenation Assessment	200	99%	99%	99%	100%
Pneumococcal Vaccine	108	88%	75%	69%	94%
Smoking Cessation Advice	63	100%	83%	80%	100%
Surgical Infection Prevention					
Prophylactic Antibiotic Given[2,3]	121	68%	78%	77%	95%
Prophylactic Antibiotic Selection[2]	38	66%	92%	90%	100%
Prophylactic Antibiotic Stopped[2,3]	112	52%	78%	72%	95%
Pregnancy Care					
Inpatient Neonatal Mortality	-	-	-	-	-
Third or Fourth Degree Laceration	-	-	-	3.63%	3.27%

NOTE: Hospital profiles are in alphabetical order by state, then city, then hospital within the city; Rankings are sorted by rate in descending order and exclude hospitals with less than 25 cases; (1) The number of cases is too small (n<25) for purposes of reliably predicting hospital performance; (2) Measure reflects the hospital's indication that its submission was based upon a sample of its relevant discharges; (3) Rate reflects fewer than the maximum possible quarters of data for the measure; (4) Inaccurate information submitted and suppressed for one or more quarters; (5) No data is available from the hospital for this measure; Please refer to the User's Guide for a full explanation of data

Loris Community Hospital

3655 Mitchell Street
Box 690001
Loris, SC 29569
URL: www.lorishealth.org
Ownership: Govt - Hospital District or Authority
Emergency Services: Yes

Phone: 843-716-7000
Fax: 843-716-7195

Accredited: Yes
Licensed Beds: 105

Key Personnel:

Administrator/CEO . . . . J Timothy Browne
Chief Medical Staff . . . . Gavin Leask
Emergency Room . . . . Steve Harvey, MD
Director Infection/Disease Control . . . . Linda Mills, RN
CCU Spvg. Nurse . . . . Frances Fowler, RN
Surgical Services . . . . Garnett Irby
Director Respiratory Therapy . . . . Von Baker

Measure	Cases	This Hospital	State Average	U.S. Average	Top Hospital
Heart Attack Care					
ACE Inhibitor or ARB for LVSD[1]	6	83%	84%	82%	100%
Aspirin at Arrival	56	98%	92%	92%	100%
Aspirin at Discharge	34	94%	87%	90%	100%
Beta Blocker at Arrival	52	98%	87%	87%	100%
Beta Blocker at Discharge	35	94%	92%	90%	100%
Fibrinolytic Medication Timing	0	-	34%	31%	100%
PCI Within 90 Minutes of Arrival	0	-	58%	54%	95%
Smoking Cessation Advice[1]	8	88%	89%	88%	100%
Heart Failure Care					
ACE Inhibitor or ARB for LVSD	59	88%	85%	82%	100%
Discharge Instructions	165	89%	66%	61%	93%
Evaluation of LVS Function	175	93%	89%	83%	99%
Smoking Cessation Advice	45	89%	85%	82%	100%
Pneumonia Care					
Appropriate Initial Antibiotic	82	77%	83%	83%	94%
Blood Culture Timing	59	95%	91%	90%	100%
Influenza Vaccine	28	79%	77%	70%	100%
Initial Antibiotic Timing	93	81%	81%	80%	93%
Oxygenation Assessment	140	100%	99%	99%	100%
Pneumococcal Vaccine	92	74%	75%	69%	94%
Smoking Cessation Advice	48	96%	83%	80%	100%
Surgical Infection Prevention					
Prophylactic Antibiotic Given	195	94%	78%	77%	95%
Prophylactic Antibiotic Selection	38	89%	92%	90%	100%
Prophylactic Antibiotic Stopped	191	84%	78%	72%	95%
Pregnancy Care					
Inpatient Neonatal Mortality	-	-	-	-	-
Third or Fourth Degree Laceration	-	-	-	3.63%	3.27%

Clarendon Memorial Hospital

10 Hospital Street
Manning, SC 29102
E-mail: cmhosp@ftc-I.net
URL: www.clarendonmemorial.com
Ownership: Govt - Hospital District or Authority
Emergency Services: Yes

Phone: 803-435-8463
Fax: 803-435-3256

Accredited: Yes
Licensed Beds: 56

Key Personnel:

CEO . . . . Edward R Frye, Jr
Chief Medical Staff . . . . Beryl Bchus-Keith, MD
Director ER . . . . Marsha Nelson, RN
Emergency Room . . . . Ken Johnson, MD
Director Infection/Disease Control . . . . Vicki Myers
CCU Spvg. Nurse . . . . Mary Beth Anderson
Director Medical/Surgical Nursing . . . . Tony Perritt
OB/GYN Womens Health . . . . Robert Ridgeway
Chief Radiology . . . . Michael Faulstich, MD
Director Respiratory Therapy . . . . Bruce Baker

Measure	Cases	This Hospital	State Average	U.S. Average	Top Hospital
Heart Attack Care					
ACE Inhibitor or ARB for LVSD[1]	1	0%	84%	82%	100%
Aspirin at Arrival[1]	10	70%	92%	92%	100%
Aspirin at Discharge[1]	5	40%	87%	90%	100%
Beta Blocker at Arrival[1]	6	50%	87%	87%	100%
Beta Blocker at Discharge[1]	5	60%	92%	90%	100%

Measure	Cases	This Hospital	State Average	U.S. Average	Top Hospital
Fibrinolytic Medication Timing	0	-	34%	31%	100%
PCI Within 90 Minutes of Arrival	0	-	58%	54%	95%
Smoking Cessation Advice	0	-	89%	88%	100%
Heart Failure Care					
ACE Inhibitor or ARB for LVSD	35	83%	85%	82%	100%
Discharge Instructions	103	84%	66%	61%	93%
Evaluation of LVS Function	112	83%	89%	83%	99%
Smoking Cessation Advice[1]	24	92%	85%	82%	100%
Pneumonia Care					
Appropriate Initial Antibiotic	132	81%	83%	83%	94%
Blood Culture Timing	87	90%	91%	90%	100%
Influenza Vaccine[4,5]	-	-	77%	70%	100%
Initial Antibiotic Timing	156	83%	81%	80%	93%
Oxygenation Assessment	193	99%	99%	99%	100%
Pneumococcal Vaccine	95	71%	75%	69%	94%
Smoking Cessation Advice	36	97%	83%	80%	100%
Surgical Infection Prevention					
Prophylactic Antibiotic Given[3]	86	49%	78%	77%	95%
Prophylactic Antibiotic Selection	28	89%	92%	90%	100%
Prophylactic Antibiotic Stopped[3]	84	88%	78%	72%	95%
Pregnancy Care					
Inpatient Neonatal Mortality	-	-	-	-	-
Third or Fourth Degree Laceration	-	-	-	3.63%	3.27%

Marion County Medical Center

Highway 76 Between Marion & Mullins
Marion, SC 29574
Ownership: Voluntary non-profit - Other
Emergency Services: Yes

Phone: 843-431-2000
Fax: 843-431-2414
Accredited: Yes
Licensed Beds: 124

Key Personnel:

CEO . . . . Harold E Tucker
Chief Medical Staff . . . . JB Berry, Jr, DM
Emergency Room . . . . Daniel Phillips, MD
Director Infection/Disease Control . . . . Sharon Elvington, MD
CCU Spvg. Nurse . . . . Dawn Williams, RN
OB/GYN Womens Health . . . . Donald Wu, MD
Chief Radiology . . . . Arturo E Macasinag, MD
Director Respiratory Therapy . . . . Mike Siders

Measure	Cases	This Hospital	State Average	U.S. Average	Top Hospital
Heart Attack Care					
ACE Inhibitor or ARB for LVSD[1]	10	90%	84%	82%	100%
Aspirin at Arrival	54	93%	92%	92%	100%
Aspirin at Discharge	35	94%	87%	90%	100%
Beta Blocker at Arrival	48	96%	87%	87%	100%
Beta Blocker at Discharge	38	92%	92%	90%	100%
Fibrinolytic Medication Timing[1]	1	0%	34%	31%	100%
PCI Within 90 Minutes of Arrival	0	-	58%	54%	95%
Smoking Cessation Advice[1]	3	100%	89%	88%	100%
Heart Failure Care					
ACE Inhibitor or ARB for LVSD	100	89%	85%	82%	100%
Discharge Instructions	221	66%	66%	61%	93%
Evaluation of LVS Function	248	94%	89%	83%	99%
Smoking Cessation Advice	69	93%	85%	82%	100%
Pneumonia Care					
Appropriate Initial Antibiotic	57	74%	83%	83%	94%
Blood Culture Timing	58	84%	91%	90%	100%
Influenza Vaccine[1]	19	74%	77%	70%	100%
Initial Antibiotic Timing	85	73%	81%	80%	93%
Oxygenation Assessment	112	100%	99%	99%	100%
Pneumococcal Vaccine	50	74%	75%	69%	94%
Smoking Cessation Advice	44	98%	83%	80%	100%
Surgical Infection Prevention					
Prophylactic Antibiotic Given[2]	153	86%	78%	77%	95%
Prophylactic Antibiotic Selection[1,2]	24	100%	92%	90%	100%
Prophylactic Antibiotic Stopped[2]	145	37%	78%	72%	95%
Pregnancy Care					
Inpatient Neonatal Mortality	-	-	-	-	-
Third or Fourth Degree Laceration	-	-	-	3.63%	3.27%

East Cooper Regional Medical Center

Alternate Name: AMI East Cooper Community Hospital

NOTE: Hospital profiles are in alphabetical order by state, then city, then hospital within the city; Rankings are sorted by rate in descending order and exclude hospitals with less than 25 cases; (1) The number of cases is too small (n<25) for purposes of reliably predicting hospital performance; (2) Measure reflects the hospital's indication that its submission was based upon a sample of its relevant discharges; (3) Rate reflects fewer than the maximum possible quarters of data for the measure; (4) Inaccurate information submitted and suppressed for one or more quarters; (5) No data is available from the hospital for this measure; Please refer to the User's Guide for a full explanation of data

1200 Johnnie Dodds Boulevard
Mount Pleasant, SC 29464
Ownership: Proprietary
Emergency Services: Yes

Phone: 843-881-0100
Fax: 843-881-4396
Accredited: Yes
Licensed Beds: 100

Key Personnel:

CEO . . . . Jack Dusenbery
Chief Medical Staff . . . . William Wilson
Emergency Room . . . . Zack Phillips

Measure	Cases	This Hospital	State Average	U.S. Average	Top Hospital
Heart Attack Care					
ACE Inhibitor or ARB for LVSD[1]	1	100%	84%	82%	100%
Aspirin at Arrival[1]	4	100%	92%	92%	100%
Aspirin at Discharge[1]	3	67%	87%	90%	100%
Beta Blocker at Arrival[1]	6	100%	87%	87%	100%
Beta Blocker at Discharge[1]	5	100%	92%	90%	100%
Fibrinolytic Medication Timing	0	-	34%	31%	100%
PCI Within 90 Minutes of Arrival	0	-	58%	54%	95%
Smoking Cessation Advice	0	-	89%	88%	100%
Heart Failure Care					
ACE Inhibitor or ARB for LVSD	26	85%	85%	82%	100%
Discharge Instructions	75	88%	66%	61%	93%
Evaluation of LVS Function	94	82%	89%	83%	99%
Smoking Cessation Advice[1]	7	100%	85%	82%	100%
Pneumonia Care					
Appropriate Initial Antibiotic	103	89%	83%	83%	94%
Blood Culture Timing	97	87%	91%	90%	100%
Influenza Vaccine	34	76%	77%	70%	100%
Initial Antibiotic Timing	139	85%	81%	80%	93%
Oxygenation Assessment	169	100%	99%	99%	100%
Pneumococcal Vaccine	111	94%	75%	69%	94%
Smoking Cessation Advice[1]	16	100%	83%	80%	100%
Surgical Infection Prevention					
Prophylactic Antibiotic Given[2]	222	82%	78%	77%	95%
Prophylactic Antibiotic Selection[2]	48	83%	92%	90%	100%
Prophylactic Antibiotic Stopped[2]	224	93%	78%	72%	95%
Pregnancy Care					
Inpatient Neonatal Mortality	-	-	-	-	-
Third or Fourth Degree Laceration	-	-	-	3.63%	3.27%

Waccamaw Community Hospital

4070 Highway 17 By-Pass
PO Box 3350
Murrells Inlet, SC 29576
URL: www.gmhsc.com
Ownership: Voluntary non-profit - Private
Emergency Services: Yes

Accredited: Yes
Licensed Beds: 83

Key Personnel:

CEO. . . . . Bruce P Bailey
Administrator . . . . Gayle L Resetar
Chief Medical Staff. William Richmend
Director Cardiology . . . . Robert Pugh
Director Emergency Room. . . . . William D Richmend
Director Respiratory . . . . Shrrel Brown

Measure	Cases	This Hospital	State Average	U.S. Average	Top Hospital
Heart Attack Care					
ACE Inhibitor or ARB for LVSD[1]	6	83%	84%	82%	100%
Aspirin at Arrival	59	93%	92%	92%	100%
Aspirin at Discharge	31	84%	87%	90%	100%
Beta Blocker at Arrival	54	91%	87%	87%	100%
Beta Blocker at Discharge	32	100%	92%	90%	100%
Fibrinolytic Medication Timing	0	-	34%	31%	100%
PCI Within 90 Minutes of Arrival	0	-	58%	54%	95%
Smoking Cessation Advice[1]	10	100%	89%	88%	100%
Heart Failure Care					
ACE Inhibitor or ARB for LVSD	54	96%	85%	82%	100%
Discharge Instructions	153	69%	66%	61%	93%
Evaluation of LVS Function	178	92%	89%	83%	99%
Smoking Cessation Advice	35	94%	85%	82%	100%
Pneumonia Care					
Appropriate Initial Antibiotic	103	83%	83%	83%	94%
Blood Culture Timing	94	90%	91%	90%	100%

Measure	Cases	This Hospital	State Average	U.S. Average	Top Hospital
Influenza Vaccine	36	83%	77%	70%	100%
Initial Antibiotic Timing	166	93%	81%	80%	93%
Oxygenation Assessment	198	100%	99%	99%	100%
Pneumococcal Vaccine	128	93%	75%	69%	94%
Smoking Cessation Advice	44	100%	83%	80%	100%
Surgical Infection Prevention					
Prophylactic Antibiotic Given	295	95%	78%	77%	95%
Prophylactic Antibiotic Selection	67	76%	92%	90%	100%
Prophylactic Antibiotic Stopped	290	79%	78%	72%	95%
Pregnancy Care					
Inpatient Neonatal Mortality	-	-	-	-	-
Third or Fourth Degree Laceration	-	-	-	3.63%	3.27%

Grand Strand Regional Medical Center

Alternate Name: Grand Strand Regional Medical Center
809 82nd Parkway
Myrtle Beach, SC 29572
URL: www.grandstrandmed.com
Ownership: Proprietary
Emergency Services: Yes

Phone: 843-692-1000
Fax: 843-692-1109

Accredited: Yes
Licensed Beds: 219

Key Personnel:

President/CEO . . . . Doug White
Chief Medical Staff . . . . RIchard Wunder, MD
Chief Catheterization Laboratory . . . . Don Gibson
Emergency Room . . . . Jim Hunter, MD
Director Infection/Disease Control . . . . Winona McLamb
Director Medical/Surgical Nursing . . . . Joyce Gardner
Chief Radiology . . . . Robert Speir, MD
Director Respiratory Therapy . . . . Don Gibson

Measure	Cases	This Hospital	State Average	U.S. Average	Top Hospital
Heart Attack Care					
ACE Inhibitor or ARB for LVSD	106	89%	84%	82%	100%
Aspirin at Arrival	322	100%	92%	92%	100%
Aspirin at Discharge	416	98%	87%	90%	100%
Beta Blocker at Arrival	273	98%	87%	87%	100%
Beta Blocker at Discharge	413	99%	92%	90%	100%
Fibrinolytic Medication Timing[1]	3	67%	34%	31%	100%
PCI Within 90 Minutes of Arrival	29	83%	58%	54%	95%
Smoking Cessation Advice	167	99%	89%	88%	100%
Heart Failure Care					
ACE Inhibitor or ARB for LVSD	181	89%	85%	82%	100%
Discharge Instructions	479	99%	66%	61%	93%
Evaluation of LVS Function	534	99%	89%	83%	99%
Smoking Cessation Advice	97	100%	85%	82%	100%
Pneumonia Care					
Appropriate Initial Antibiotic	182	88%	83%	83%	94%
Blood Culture Timing	197	84%	91%	90%	100%
Influenza Vaccine	74	64%	77%	70%	100%
Initial Antibiotic Timing	277	85%	81%	80%	93%
Oxygenation Assessment	349	100%	99%	99%	100%
Pneumococcal Vaccine	242	81%	75%	69%	94%
Smoking Cessation Advice	116	98%	83%	80%	100%
Surgical Infection Prevention					
Prophylactic Antibiotic Given[2,3]	363	93%	78%	77%	95%
Prophylactic Antibiotic Selection[2]	224	97%	92%	90%	100%
Prophylactic Antibiotic Stopped[2,3]	354	67%	78%	72%	95%
Pregnancy Care					
Inpatient Neonatal Mortality	-	-	-	-	-
Third or Fourth Degree Laceration	-	-	-	3.63%	3.27%

Newberry County Memorial Hospital

2669 Kinard Street
Newberry, SC 29108
URL: www.newberryhospital.org
Ownership: Government - Local
Emergency Services: Yes

Phone: 803-276-7570
Fax: 803-276-6885

Accredited: Yes
Licensed Beds: 102

Key Personnel:

Administrator/CEO . . . . Lynn W Beasley
Emergency Room . . . . Ronald W Price, MD
Infection Control . . . . Lindy Beaver, RN
ICU Supervising Nurse. . . . . Kay Traylor
Intensive Coronary . . . . Kay Traylor

NOTE: Hospital profiles are in alphabetical order by state, then city, then hospital within the city; Rankings are sorted by rate in descending order and exclude hospitals with less than 25 cases; (1) The number of cases is too small (n<25) for purposes of reliably predicting hospital performance; (2) Measure reflects the hospital's indication that its submission was based upon a sample of its relevant discharges; (3) Rate reflects fewer than the maximum possible quarters of data for the measure; (4) Inaccurate information submitted and suppressed for one or more quarters; (5) No data is available from the hospital for this measure; Please refer to the User's Guide for a full explanation of data

Director Medical/Surgical Nursing . . . . Kay Traylor, RN
Chief Radiology . . . . Lawrence Lough, MD
Director Respiratory Therapy . . . . Brenda Gallman

Measure	Cases	This Hospital	State Average	U.S. Average	Top Hospital
Heart Attack Care					
ACE Inhibitor or ARB for LVSD[1]	3	100%	84%	82%	100%
Aspirin at Arrival[1]	13	92%	92%	92%	100%
Aspirin at Discharge[1]	7	57%	87%	90%	100%
Beta Blocker at Arrival[1]	9	100%	87%	87%	100%
Beta Blocker at Discharge[1]	9	100%	92%	90%	100%
Fibrinolytic Medication Timing	0	-	34%	31%	100%
PCI Within 90 Minutes of Arrival	0	-	58%	54%	95%
Smoking Cessation Advice	0	-	89%	88%	100%
Heart Failure Care					
ACE Inhibitor or ARB for LVSD	42	74%	85%	82%	100%
Discharge Instructions	119	83%	66%	61%	93%
Evaluation of LVS Function	144	77%	89%	83%	99%
Smoking Cessation Advice	27	93%	85%	82%	100%
Pneumonia Care					
Appropriate Initial Antibiotic	64	75%	83%	83%	94%
Blood Culture Timing	50	84%	91%	90%	100%
Influenza Vaccine[1]	18	83%	77%	70%	100%
Initial Antibiotic Timing	88	92%	81%	80%	93%
Oxygenation Assessment	92	100%	99%	99%	100%
Pneumococcal Vaccine	58	71%	75%	69%	94%
Smoking Cessation Advice[1]	22	91%	83%	80%	100%
Surgical Infection Prevention					
Prophylactic Antibiotic Given[2]	83	80%	78%	77%	95%
Prophylactic Antibiotic Selection[1,2]	19	84%	92%	90%	100%
Prophylactic Antibiotic Stopped[2]	83	65%	78%	72%	95%
Pregnancy Care					
Inpatient Neonatal Mortality	-	-	-	-	-
Third or Fourth Degree Laceration	-	-	-	3.63%	3.27%

Regional Med Ctr of Orangeburg & Calhoun

3000 Saint Matthews Road
Orangeburg, SC 29118   Phone: 803-533-2200
Ownership: Government - Local   Fax: 803-395-2304
Emergency Services: Yes   Accredited: Yes
Key Personnel: Licensed Beds: 286
CEO . . . . Thomas C Dandridge
Chief Medical Staff . . . . John Hutto
Emergency Room . . . . Robert Swetnam, MD
Infection Control . . . . Sonya Ehrnhardt
Administrative Radiology Director . . . . Sandra Connor
Director Respiratory Therapy . . . . Kathy Williams

Measure	Cases	This Hospital	State Average	U.S. Average	Top Hospital
Heart Attack Care					
ACE Inhibitor or ARB for LVSD[1]	16	81%	84%	82%	100%
Aspirin at Arrival	114	96%	92%	92%	100%
Aspirin at Discharge	57	91%	87%	90%	100%
Beta Blocker at Arrival	82	93%	87%	87%	100%
Beta Blocker at Discharge	67	96%	92%	90%	100%
Fibrinolytic Medication Timing[1]	11	55%	34%	31%	100%
PCI Within 90 Minutes of Arrival	0	-	58%	54%	95%
Smoking Cessation Advice[1]	16	94%	89%	88%	100%
Heart Failure Care					
ACE Inhibitor or ARB for LVSD	119	82%	85%	82%	100%
Discharge Instructions	373	53%	66%	61%	93%
Evaluation of LVS Function	412	89%	89%	83%	99%
Smoking Cessation Advice	98	99%	85%	82%	100%
Pneumonia Care					
Appropriate Initial Antibiotic	184	78%	83%	83%	94%
Blood Culture Timing	204	94%	91%	90%	100%
Influenza Vaccine	48	58%	77%	70%	100%
Initial Antibiotic Timing	303	87%	81%	80%	93%
Oxygenation Assessment	360	100%	99%	99%	100%
Pneumococcal Vaccine	174	68%	75%	69%	94%
Smoking Cessation Advice	88	98%	83%	80%	100%
Surgical Infection Prevention					

Prophylactic Antibiotic Given[3]	194	86%	78%	77%	95%
Prophylactic Antibiotic Selection	59	92%	92%	90%	100%
Prophylactic Antibiotic Stopped[3]	182	87%	78%	72%	95%
Pregnancy Care					
Inpatient Neonatal Mortality	-	-	-	-	-
Third or Fourth Degree Laceration	-	-	-	3.63%	3.27%

Cannon Memorial Hospital

123 W G Acker Drive
PO Box 188   Phone: 864-878-4791
Pickens, SC 29671   Fax: 864-878-8354
URL: www.cannonhospital.org
Ownership: Voluntary non-profit - Private   Accredited: Yes
Emergency Services: Yes   Licensed Beds: 55
Key Personnel:
President/CEO . . . . Norman G Rentz
Chief Medical Staff . . . . Martha Seaborn
Emergency Room . . . . Michael L Dillard, MD
Director Infection/Disease Control . . . . Donna Anderson, RN
CCU Spvg. Nurse . . . . Jean Watson, RN
Medical/Surgical Nursing . . . . Norah Kertis, RN
Respiratory Cardiopulmonary . . . . Gary Grahn, RT

Measure	Cases	This Hospital	State Average	U.S. Average	Top Hospital
Heart Attack Care					
ACE Inhibitor or ARB for LVSD[1]	1	100%	84%	82%	100%
Aspirin at Arrival[1]	13	77%	92%	92%	100%
Aspirin at Discharge[1]	5	80%	87%	90%	100%
Beta Blocker at Arrival[1]	12	83%	87%	87%	100%
Beta Blocker at Discharge[1]	6	100%	92%	90%	100%
Fibrinolytic Medication Timing[1]	5	20%	34%	31%	100%
PCI Within 90 Minutes of Arrival	0	-	58%	54%	95%
Smoking Cessation Advice[1]	1	100%	89%	88%	100%
Heart Failure Care					
ACE Inhibitor or ARB for LVSD[1]	11	100%	85%	82%	100%
Discharge Instructions	31	87%	66%	61%	93%
Evaluation of LVS Function	37	78%	89%	83%	99%
Smoking Cessation Advice[1]	5	100%	85%	82%	100%
Pneumonia Care					
Appropriate Initial Antibiotic	81	86%	83%	83%	94%
Blood Culture Timing	91	92%	91%	90%	100%
Influenza Vaccine[1]	24	100%	77%	70%	100%
Initial Antibiotic Timing	100	81%	81%	80%	93%
Oxygenation Assessment	140	100%	99%	99%	100%
Pneumococcal Vaccine	86	88%	75%	69%	94%
Smoking Cessation Advice	34	88%	83%	80%	100%
Surgical Infection Prevention					
Prophylactic Antibiotic Given[1,3]	24	79%	78%	77%	95%
Prophylactic Antibiotic Selection[1]	10	100%	92%	90%	100%
Prophylactic Antibiotic Stopped[1,3]	24	92%	78%	72%	95%
Pregnancy Care					
Inpatient Neonatal Mortality	-	-	-	-	-
Third or Fourth Degree Laceration	-	-	-	3.63%	3.27%

Piedmont Medical Center

222 S Herlong Avenue
Rock Hill, SC 29732   Toll-Free: 800-578-4555
                                         Phone: 803-329-1234
                                         Fax: 803-329-0979
URL: www.piedmontmedicalcenter.com
Ownership: Proprietary   Accredited: Yes
Emergency Services: Yes   Licensed Beds: 268
Key Personnel:
CEO . . . . Charles Miller
Chief Medical Staff . . . . Dave Jenkins, MD
Emergency Room . . . . Wilma Jenkins
Director Medical/Surgical Nursing . . . . Pat Dye
OB/GYN Womens Health . . . . Ted Garcia, MD
Chief Radiology . . . . Howard Snider, MD
Director Respiratory Therapy . . . . John Reeds

Measure	Cases	This Hospital	State Average	U.S. Average	Top Hospital
Heart Attack Care					
ACE Inhibitor or ARB for LVSD	92	89%	84%	82%	100%

NOTE: Hospital profiles are in alphabetical order by state, then city, then hospital within the city; Rankings are sorted by rate in descending order and exclude hospitals with less than 25 cases; (1) The number of cases is too small (n<25) for purposes of reliably predicting hospital performance; (2) Measure reflects the hospital's indication that its submission was based upon a sample of its relevant discharges; (3) Rate reflects fewer than the maximum possible quarters of data for the measure; (4) Inaccurate information submitted and suppressed for one or more quarters; (5) No data is available from the hospital for this measure; Please refer to the User's Guide for a full explanation of data

Measure	Cases	This Hospital	State Average	U.S. Average	Top Hospital
Aspirin at Arrival	298	99%	92%	92%	100%
Aspirin at Discharge	347	98%	87%	90%	100%
Beta Blocker at Arrival	280	93%	87%	87%	100%
Beta Blocker at Discharge	338	97%	92%	90%	100%
Fibrinolytic Medication Timing[1]	1	0%	34%	31%	100%
PCI Within 90 Minutes of Arrival[1]	19	63%	58%	54%	95%
Smoking Cessation Advice	151	99%	89%	88%	100%
Heart Failure Care					
ACE Inhibitor or ARB for LVSD	160	84%	85%	82%	100%
Discharge Instructions	293	75%	66%	61%	93%
Evaluation of LVS Function	355	99%	89%	83%	99%
Smoking Cessation Advice	85	100%	85%	82%	100%
Pneumonia Care					
Appropriate Initial Antibiotic	336	83%	83%	83%	94%
Blood Culture Timing	291	79%	91%	90%	100%
Influenza Vaccine	102	90%	77%	70%	100%
Initial Antibiotic Timing	511	77%	81%	80%	93%
Oxygenation Assessment	584	100%	99%	99%	100%
Pneumococcal Vaccine	315	88%	75%	69%	94%
Smoking Cessation Advice	151	99%	83%	80%	100%
Surgical Infection Prevention					
Prophylactic Antibiotic Given[2]	796	93%	78%	77%	95%
Prophylactic Antibiotic Selection[2]	81	93%	92%	90%	100%
Prophylactic Antibiotic Stopped[2]	785	86%	78%	72%	95%
Pregnancy Care					
Inpatient Neonatal Mortality	-	-	-	-	-
Third or Fourth Degree Laceration	-	-	-	3.63%	3.27%

Oconee Memorial Hospital

298 Memorial Drive
Seneca, SC 29672
URL: www.oconeememorial.org
Ownership: Voluntary non-profit - Private
Emergency Services: Yes

Phone: 864-882-3351
Fax: 864-885-7391

Accredited: Yes
Licensed Beds: 160

Key Personnel:
President/CEO . . . . WH Hudson
Chief Medical Staff . . . . Tauqueer Alan
Emergency Room . . . . Patrick Johannes

Measure	Cases	This Hospital	State Average	U.S. Average	Top Hospital
Heart Attack Care					
ACE Inhibitor or ARB for LVSD[1]	10	90%	84%	82%	100%
Aspirin at Arrival	44	93%	92%	92%	100%
Aspirin at Discharge[1]	21	95%	87%	90%	100%
Beta Blocker at Arrival	28	89%	87%	87%	100%
Beta Blocker at Discharge[1]	23	83%	92%	90%	100%
Fibrinolytic Medication Timing	29	45%	34%	31%	100%
PCI Within 90 Minutes of Arrival	0	-	58%	54%	95%
Smoking Cessation Advice[1]	11	100%	89%	88%	100%
Heart Failure Care					
ACE Inhibitor or ARB for LVSD	71	72%	85%	82%	100%
Discharge Instructions	162	57%	66%	61%	93%
Evaluation of LVS Function	203	82%	89%	83%	99%
Smoking Cessation Advice	28	100%	85%	82%	100%
Pneumonia Care					
Appropriate Initial Antibiotic	248	89%	83%	83%	94%
Blood Culture Timing	127	91%	91%	90%	100%
Influenza Vaccine	90	72%	77%	70%	100%
Initial Antibiotic Timing	349	90%	81%	80%	93%
Oxygenation Assessment	488	100%	99%	99%	100%
Pneumococcal Vaccine	291	73%	75%	69%	94%
Smoking Cessation Advice	137	100%	83%	80%	100%
Surgical Infection Prevention					
Prophylactic Antibiotic Given[3]	186	88%	78%	77%	95%
Prophylactic Antibiotic Selection	33	100%	92%	90%	100%
Prophylactic Antibiotic Stopped[3]	175	77%	78%	72%	95%
Pregnancy Care					
Inpatient Neonatal Mortality	-	-	-	-	-
Third or Fourth Degree Laceration	-	-	-	3.63%	3.27%

Hillcrest Hospital

729 S E Main Street
Simpsonville, SC 29681
Ownership: Government - State
Emergency Services: Yes

Phone: 864-967-6100
Fax: 864-967-6147
Accredited: Yes
Licensed Beds: 56

Key Personnel:
Administrator . . . . Mark Slyter
Chief Medical Staff . . . . David C Silkiner, MD
Coordinator Infection Control . . . . Judy Major

Measure	Cases	This Hospital	State Average	U.S. Average	Top Hospital
Heart Attack Care					
ACE Inhibitor or ARB for LVSD[1]	4	75%	84%	82%	100%
Aspirin at Arrival[1]	17	88%	92%	92%	100%
Aspirin at Discharge[1]	5	100%	87%	90%	100%
Beta Blocker at Arrival[1]	9	78%	87%	87%	100%
Beta Blocker at Discharge[1]	11	91%	92%	90%	100%
Fibrinolytic Medication Timing	0	-	34%	31%	100%
PCI Within 90 Minutes of Arrival	0	-	58%	54%	95%
Smoking Cessation Advice[1]	1	100%	89%	88%	100%
Heart Failure Care					
ACE Inhibitor or ARB for LVSD[1]	19	84%	85%	82%	100%
Discharge Instructions	41	71%	66%	61%	93%
Evaluation of LVS Function	54	94%	89%	83%	99%
Smoking Cessation Advice[1]	9	100%	85%	82%	100%
Pneumonia Care					
Appropriate Initial Antibiotic	85	94%	83%	83%	94%
Blood Culture Timing	48	100%	91%	90%	100%
Influenza Vaccine[1]	18	83%	77%	70%	100%
Initial Antibiotic Timing	109	85%	81%	80%	93%
Oxygenation Assessment	129	99%	99%	99%	100%
Pneumococcal Vaccine	81	89%	75%	69%	94%
Smoking Cessation Advice	32	100%	83%	80%	100%
Surgical Infection Prevention					
Prophylactic Antibiotic Given[2,3]	69	87%	78%	77%	95%
Prophylactic Antibiotic Selection[1,2]	20	100%	92%	90%	100%
Prophylactic Antibiotic Stopped[2,3]	69	78%	78%	72%	95%
Pregnancy Care					
Inpatient Neonatal Mortality	-	-	-	-	-
Third or Fourth Degree Laceration	-	-	-	3.63%	3.27%

Mary Black Memorial Hospital

1700 Skylyn Drive
PO Box 3217
Spartanburg, SC 29307
E-mail: webmaster@maryblack.org
URL: www.maryblackhealthsystem.com
Ownership: Voluntary non-profit - Other
Emergency Services: Yes

Phone: 864-573-3000
Fax: 864-573-3454

Accredited: Yes
Licensed Beds: 226

Key Personnel:
CEO . . . . Glenn A Robinson
Chief Medical Staff . . . . Vickie Shehan
Head of Emergency Room . . . . Cathy Trammell
Director Medical/Surgical Nursing . . . . Teri Keel, RN
OB/GYN Womens Health . . . . David Mainman
Chief Radiology . . . . Penelope Galbraith, MD
Director Respiratory Therapy . . . . Berry Jennings

Measure	Cases	This Hospital	State Average	U.S. Average	Top Hospital
Heart Attack Care					
ACE Inhibitor or ARB for LVSD[1]	5	100%	84%	82%	100%
Aspirin at Arrival	42	98%	92%	92%	100%
Aspirin at Discharge[1]	20	85%	87%	90%	100%
Beta Blocker at Arrival	45	93%	87%	87%	100%
Beta Blocker at Discharge[1]	19	89%	92%	90%	100%
Fibrinolytic Medication Timing[1]	1	0%	34%	31%	100%
PCI Within 90 Minutes of Arrival	0	-	58%	54%	95%
Smoking Cessation Advice[1]	2	100%	89%	88%	100%
Heart Failure Care					
ACE Inhibitor or ARB for LVSD	63	90%	85%	82%	100%
Discharge Instructions	141	57%	66%	61%	93%
Evaluation of LVS Function	174	98%	89%	83%	99%
Smoking Cessation Advice	43	95%	85%	82%	100%

NOTE: Hospital profiles are in alphabetical order by state, then city, then hospital within the city; Rankings are sorted by rate in descending order and exclude hospitals with less than 25 cases; (1) The number of cases is too small (n<25) for purposes of reliably predicting hospital performance; (2) Measure reflects the hospital's indication that its submission was based upon a sample of its relevant discharges; (3) Rate reflects fewer than the maximum possible quarters of data for the measure; (4) Inaccurate information submitted and suppressed for one or more quarters; (5) No data is available from the hospital for this measure; Please refer to the User's Guide for a full explanation of data

Pneumonia Care					
Appropriate Initial Antibiotic	107	87%	83%	83%	94%
Blood Culture Timing	122	86%	91%	90%	100%
Influenza Vaccine	42	81%	77%	70%	100%
Initial Antibiotic Timing	152	84%	81%	80%	93%
Oxygenation Assessment	205	100%	99%	99%	100%
Pneumococcal Vaccine	130	92%	75%	69%	94%
Smoking Cessation Advice	65	97%	83%	80%	100%
Surgical Infection Prevention					
Prophylactic Antibiotic Given	635	87%	78%	77%	95%
Prophylactic Antibiotic Selection	171	96%	92%	90%	100%
Prophylactic Antibiotic Stopped	616	78%	78%	72%	95%
Pregnancy Care					
Inpatient Neonatal Mortality	-	-	-	-	-
Third or Fourth Degree Laceration	-	-	-	3.63%	3.27%

Spartanburg Regional Health Care System

101 East Wood Street   Phone: 864-560-6000
Spartanburg, SC 29303   Fax: 864-560-6001
URL: www.srhs.com
Ownership: Govt - Hospital District or Authority   Accredited: Yes
Emergency Services: Yes   Licensed Beds: 588
Key Personnel:
President/CEO. . . . . Ingo Angermeier
Chief Medical Staff. Robert Riehle, MD
Executive Director Cardiology . . . . David Parks
Chief Catheterization Laboratory . . . . David Parks
Director Emergency Services. . . . . Gwen Burley
Director Infection Control . . . . Lynn Cromer
OB/GYN Womens Health. . . . . Dean Davis, MD

Measure	Cases	This Hospital	State Average	U.S. Average	Top Hospital
Heart Attack Care					
ACE Inhibitor or ARB for LVSD	160	86%	84%	82%	100%
Aspirin at Arrival	406	97%	92%	92%	100%
Aspirin at Discharge	557	99%	87%	90%	100%
Beta Blocker at Arrival	315	98%	87%	87%	100%
Beta Blocker at Discharge	603	99%	92%	90%	100%
Fibrinolytic Medication Timing[1]	3	67%	34%	31%	100%
PCI Within 90 Minutes of Arrival	25	68%	58%	54%	95%
Smoking Cessation Advice	307	100%	89%	88%	100%
Heart Failure Care					
ACE Inhibitor or ARB for LVSD	286	98%	85%	82%	100%
Discharge Instructions	631	90%	66%	61%	93%
Evaluation of LVS Function	737	100%	89%	83%	99%
Smoking Cessation Advice	184	99%	85%	82%	100%
Pneumonia Care					
Appropriate Initial Antibiotic	325	92%	83%	83%	94%
Blood Culture Timing	346	95%	91%	90%	100%
Influenza Vaccine	82	89%	77%	70%	100%
Initial Antibiotic Timing	499	82%	81%	80%	93%
Oxygenation Assessment	604	100%	99%	99%	100%
Pneumococcal Vaccine	356	95%	75%	69%	94%
Smoking Cessation Advice	173	100%	83%	80%	100%
Surgical Infection Prevention					
Prophylactic Antibiotic Given[2]	1,545	95%	78%	77%	95%
Prophylactic Antibiotic Selection[2]	310	88%	92%	90%	100%
Prophylactic Antibiotic Stopped[2]	1,478	81%	78%	72%	95%
Pregnancy Care					
Inpatient Neonatal Mortality	-	-	-	-	-
Third or Fourth Degree Laceration	-	-	-	3.63%	3.27%

Tuomey Regional Medical Center

129 N Washington   Phone: 803-774-9000
Sumter, SC 29150   Fax: 803-774-9494
URL: www.tuomey.com
Ownership: Voluntary non-profit - Private   Accredited: Yes
Emergency Services: Yes   Licensed Beds: 266
Key Personnel:
CEO. . . . . Jay Cox
Chief Medical Staff. Mark Crabbe
Emergency Room . . . . Mitchell Logan-Owens
Emergency Room . . . . Paul Schumacher

Director Radiology . . . . Bill Smith
Director of Pulmonary/Respiratory Care. . . . . . . Sonya McDaniel

Measure	Cases	This Hospital	State Average	U.S. Average	Top Hospital
Heart Attack Care					
ACE Inhibitor or ARB for LVSD[1]	17	100%	84%	82%	100%
Aspirin at Arrival	53	81%	92%	92%	100%
Aspirin at Discharge	30	77%	87%	90%	100%
Beta Blocker at Arrival	33	85%	87%	87%	100%
Beta Blocker at Discharge	45	91%	92%	90%	100%
Fibrinolytic Medication Timing	0	-	34%	31%	100%
PCI Within 90 Minutes of Arrival	0	-	58%	54%	95%
Smoking Cessation Advice[1]	10	90%	89%	88%	100%
Heart Failure Care					
ACE Inhibitor or ARB for LVSD	206	87%	85%	82%	100%
Discharge Instructions	472	51%	66%	61%	93%
Evaluation of LVS Function	571	85%	89%	83%	99%
Smoking Cessation Advice	135	92%	85%	82%	100%
Pneumonia Care					
Appropriate Initial Antibiotic	162	79%	83%	83%	94%
Blood Culture Timing	117	85%	91%	90%	100%
Influenza Vaccine	34	76%	77%	70%	100%
Initial Antibiotic Timing	241	66%	81%	80%	93%
Oxygenation Assessment	292	100%	99%	99%	100%
Pneumococcal Vaccine	145	77%	75%	69%	94%
Smoking Cessation Advice	75	92%	83%	80%	100%
Surgical Infection Prevention					
Prophylactic Antibiotic Given	426	78%	78%	77%	95%
Prophylactic Antibiotic Selection	117	99%	92%	90%	100%
Prophylactic Antibiotic Stopped	417	81%	78%	72%	95%
Pregnancy Care					
Inpatient Neonatal Mortality	-	-	-	-	-
Third or Fourth Degree Laceration	-	-	-	3.63%	3.27%

Wallace Thomson Hospital

322 W S Street   Phone: 864-427-0351
PO Box 789   Fax: 864-429-2653
Union, SC 29379
URL: www.wallacethomson.com
Ownership: Govt - Hospital District or Authority   Accredited: Yes
Emergency Services: Yes   Licensed Beds: 143
Key Personnel:
CEO. . . . . Karen Fiducia
Chief Medical Staff. Kenneth Hill
Director of Cardiology/Cardiac Lab. . . . . Ad Bolds
Emergency Room . . . . Ann Brannan

Measure	Cases	This Hospital	State Average	U.S. Average	Top Hospital
Heart Attack Care					
ACE Inhibitor or ARB for LVSD	0	-	84%	82%	100%
Aspirin at Arrival[1]	21	71%	92%	92%	100%
Aspirin at Discharge[1]	9	67%	87%	90%	100%
Beta Blocker at Arrival[1]	15	80%	87%	87%	100%
Beta Blocker at Discharge[1]	9	78%	92%	90%	100%
Fibrinolytic Medication Timing	0	-	34%	31%	100%
PCI Within 90 Minutes of Arrival	0	-	58%	54%	95%
Smoking Cessation Advice[1]	2	0%	89%	88%	100%
Heart Failure Care					
ACE Inhibitor or ARB for LVSD	30	77%	85%	82%	100%
Discharge Instructions	145	46%	66%	61%	93%
Evaluation of LVS Function	163	67%	89%	83%	99%
Smoking Cessation Advice	29	52%	85%	82%	100%
Pneumonia Care					
Appropriate Initial Antibiotic	82	61%	83%	83%	94%
Blood Culture Timing	47	85%	91%	90%	100%
Influenza Vaccine[1]	22	68%	77%	70%	100%
Initial Antibiotic Timing	111	77%	81%	80%	93%
Oxygenation Assessment	140	99%	99%	99%	100%
Pneumococcal Vaccine	79	70%	75%	69%	94%
Smoking Cessation Advice	36	42%	83%	80%	100%
Surgical Infection Prevention					
Prophylactic Antibiotic Given[3]	29	31%	78%	77%	95%

NOTE: Hospital profiles are in alphabetical order by state, then city, then hospital within the city; Rankings are sorted by rate in descending order and exclude hospitals with less than 25 cases; (1) The number of cases is too small (n<25) for purposes of reliably predicting hospital performance; (2) Measure reflects the hospital's indication that its submission was based upon a sample of its relevant discharges; (3) Rate reflects fewer than the maximum possible quarters of data for the measure; (4) Inaccurate information submitted and suppressed for one or more quarters; (5) No data is available from the hospital for this measure; Please refer to the User's Guide for a full explanation of data

Prophylactic Antibiotic Selection[1]	13	85%	92%	90%	100%
Prophylactic Antibiotic Stopped[3]	27	96%	78%	72%	95%
Pregnancy Care					
Inpatient Neonatal Mortality	-	-	-	-	-
Third or Fourth Degree Laceration	-	-	-	3.63%	3.27%

Hampton Regional Medical Center

Alternate Name: Hampton General Hospital
595 Carolina Avenue West
Varnville, SC 29944

Toll-Free: 800-575-1435
Phone: 803-943-2771
Fax: 803-943-1241

Ownership: Govt - Hospital District or Authority
Emergency Services: Yes

Accredited: No
Licensed Beds: 68

Key Personnel:
President/CEO . . . . Dave H Hamill
Chief Medical Staff . . . . Glenn W Welcker, MD
Infection Control . . . . Lauren Ginn
Surgery Director . . . . Donna Blocker
Cardiopulmonary Director . . . . Diane Langdale

Measure	Cases	This Hospital	State Average	U.S. Average	Top Hospital
Heart Attack Care					
ACE Inhibitor or ARB for LVSD[1,3]	1	100%	84%	82%	100%
Aspirin at Arrival[1,3]	4	75%	92%	92%	100%
Aspirin at Discharge[1,3]	3	67%	87%	90%	100%
Beta Blocker at Arrival[1,3]	3	67%	87%	87%	100%
Beta Blocker at Discharge[1,3]	3	100%	92%	90%	100%
Fibrinolytic Medication Timing[1,3]	1	0%	34%	31%	100%
PCI Within 90 Minutes of Arrival	0	-	58%	54%	95%
Smoking Cessation Advice[3]	0	-	89%	88%	100%
Heart Failure Care					
ACE Inhibitor or ARB for LVSD[1]	6	50%	85%	82%	100%
Discharge Instructions	25	0%	66%	61%	93%
Evaluation of LVS Function	25	48%	89%	83%	99%
Smoking Cessation Advice[1]	3	0%	85%	82%	100%
Pneumonia Care					
Appropriate Initial Antibiotic	29	90%	83%	83%	94%
Blood Culture Timing[1]	7	100%	91%	90%	100%
Influenza Vaccine[1]	7	86%	77%	70%	100%
Initial Antibiotic Timing[1]	12	92%	81%	80%	93%
Oxygenation Assessment	32	100%	99%	99%	100%
Pneumococcal Vaccine	26	58%	75%	69%	94%
Smoking Cessation Advice[1]	7	43%	83%	80%	100%
Surgical Infection Prevention					
Prophylactic Antibiotic Given[1,3]	1	0%	78%	77%	95%
Prophylactic Antibiotic Selection[1]	2	100%	92%	90%	100%
Prophylactic Antibiotic Stopped[1,3]	1	100%	78%	72%	95%
Pregnancy Care					
Inpatient Neonatal Mortality	-	-	-	-	-
Third or Fourth Degree Laceration	-	-	-	3.63%	3.27%

Colleton Medical Center

501 Robertson Boulevard
Walterboro, SC 29488
Ownership: Proprietary
Emergency Services: Yes

Phone: 843-549-6371
Fax: 843-549-7562
Accredited: Yes
Licensed Beds: 131

Key Personnel:
Administrator . . . . Rebecca Brewer
Chief Medical Staff . . . . Frank Biggers
Emergency Room . . . . D Meacher, MD
Director Infection/Disease Control . . . . Gail Sartain
Chief Radiology . . . . Bob Abbott
Director Respiratory Therapy . . . . Diane Langdale

Measure	Cases	This Hospital	State Average	U.S. Average	Top Hospital
Heart Attack Care					
ACE Inhibitor or ARB for LVSD[1]	4	75%	84%	82%	100%
Aspirin at Arrival[1]	12	67%	92%	92%	100%
Aspirin at Discharge[1]	8	88%	87%	90%	100%
Beta Blocker at Arrival[1]	7	71%	87%	87%	100%
Beta Blocker at Discharge[1]	6	100%	92%	90%	100%
Fibrinolytic Medication Timing[1]	1	0%	34%	31%	100%

PCI Within 90 Minutes of Arrival	0	-	58%	54%	95%
Smoking Cessation Advice[1]	1	100%	89%	88%	100%
Heart Failure Care					
ACE Inhibitor or ARB for LVSD	83	78%	85%	82%	100%
Discharge Instructions	265	42%	66%	61%	93%
Evaluation of LVS Function	287	94%	89%	83%	99%
Smoking Cessation Advice	56	95%	85%	82%	100%
Pneumonia Care					
Appropriate Initial Antibiotic	83	67%	83%	83%	94%
Blood Culture Timing	59	97%	91%	90%	100%
Influenza Vaccine[1]	24	79%	77%	70%	100%
Initial Antibiotic Timing	127	88%	81%	80%	93%
Oxygenation Assessment	150	99%	99%	99%	100%
Pneumococcal Vaccine	78	69%	75%	69%	94%
Smoking Cessation Advice	28	75%	83%	80%	100%
Surgical Infection Prevention					
Prophylactic Antibiotic Given	167	83%	78%	77%	95%
Prophylactic Antibiotic Selection	41	98%	92%	90%	100%
Prophylactic Antibiotic Stopped	154	69%	78%	72%	95%
Pregnancy Care					
Inpatient Neonatal Mortality	-	-	-	-	-
Third or Fourth Degree Laceration	-	-	-	3.63%	3.27%

Lexington Medical Center

2720 Sunset Boulevard
West Columbia, SC 29169
E-mail: magregory@lexhealth.org
URL: www.lexmed.com
Ownership: Government - Local
Emergency Services: Yes

Phone: 803-791-2000
Fax: 803-791-2660

Accredited: Yes
Licensed Beds: 346

Key Personnel:
CEO . . . . Michael J Biediger
Chief Medical Staff . . . . Steven A Madden, MD
OB/GYN Womens Health . . . . Miriam A Wilcox, MD
Chief Radiology . . . . Charles Hood
Director Respiratory Therapy . . . . Robin Stephens

Measure	Cases	This Hospital	State Average	U.S. Average	Top Hospital
Heart Attack Care					
ACE Inhibitor or ARB for LVSD	28	68%	84%	82%	100%
Aspirin at Arrival	183	95%	92%	92%	100%
Aspirin at Discharge	91	95%	87%	90%	100%
Beta Blocker at Arrival	131	87%	87%	87%	100%
Beta Blocker at Discharge	92	97%	92%	90%	100%
Fibrinolytic Medication Timing	0	-	34%	31%	100%
PCI Within 90 Minutes of Arrival	0	-	58%	54%	95%
Smoking Cessation Advice[1]	24	79%	89%	88%	100%
Heart Failure Care					
ACE Inhibitor or ARB for LVSD	105	76%	85%	82%	100%
Discharge Instructions	217	59%	66%	61%	93%
Evaluation of LVS Function	268	99%	89%	83%	99%
Smoking Cessation Advice	58	93%	85%	82%	100%
Pneumonia Care					
Appropriate Initial Antibiotic	122	82%	83%	83%	94%
Blood Culture Timing	98	92%	91%	90%	100%
Influenza Vaccine	26	92%	77%	70%	100%
Initial Antibiotic Timing	138	76%	81%	80%	93%
Oxygenation Assessment	184	100%	99%	99%	100%
Pneumococcal Vaccine	94	95%	75%	69%	94%
Smoking Cessation Advice	47	83%	83%	80%	100%
Surgical Infection Prevention					
Prophylactic Antibiotic Given	205	88%	78%	77%	95%
Prophylactic Antibiotic Selection	48	83%	92%	90%	100%
Prophylactic Antibiotic Stopped	201	59%	78%	72%	95%
Pregnancy Care					
Inpatient Neonatal Mortality	-	-	-	-	-
Third or Fourth Degree Laceration	-	-	-	3.63%	3.27%

NOTE: Hospital profiles are in alphabetical order by state, then city, then hospital within the city; Rankings are sorted by rate in descending order and exclude hospitals with less than 25 cases; (1) The number of cases is too small (n<25) for purposes of reliably predicting hospital performance; (2) Measure reflects the hospital's indication that its submission was based upon a sample of its relevant discharges; (3) Rate reflects fewer than the maximum possible quarters of data for the measure; (4) Inaccurate information submitted and suppressed for one or more quarters; (5) No data is available from the hospital for this measure; Please refer to the User's Guide for a full explanation of data

Fairfield Memorial Hospital

102 US Highway 321 By-Pass N
PO Box 620
Winnsboro, SC 29180
URL: www.fairfieldmemorial.com
Ownership: Government - Local
Emergency Services: No

Phone: 803-635-5548
Fax: 803-635-5612

Accredited: Yes
Licensed Beds: 25

Key Personnel:

President/CEO . . . . J L Dozier Jr, FACHE
Chief of Medical Staff . . . . Steven Barnett, MD
Cardiac Lab . . . . Mike Williams
Emergency Room . . . . Larry Cantey, MD
Infection Control . . . . Janet Bussie, RN
Medical/Surgical Nursing . . . . Janet Bussie, RN
Surgical Services . . . . Shirley Hall, RN
Respiratory/Cardiopulmonary . . . . Mike Williams

Measure	Cases	This Hospital	State Average	U.S. Average	Top Hospital
Heart Attack Care					
ACE Inhibitor or ARB for LVSD[3]	0	-	84%	82%	100%
Aspirin at Arrival[1,3]	2	100%	92%	92%	100%
Aspirin at Discharge[1,3]	1	0%	87%	90%	100%
Beta Blocker at Arrival[1,3]	1	100%	87%	87%	100%
Beta Blocker at Discharge[1,3]	1	100%	92%	90%	100%
Fibrinolytic Medication Timing[3]	0	-	34%	31%	100%
PCI Within 90 Minutes of Arrival[5]	-	-	58%	54%	95%
Smoking Cessation Advice[3]	0	-	89%	88%	100%
Heart Failure Care					
ACE Inhibitor or ARB for LVSD[1]	6	83%	85%	82%	100%
Discharge Instructions	34	18%	66%	61%	93%
Evaluation of LVS Function	41	63%	89%	83%	99%
Smoking Cessation Advice[1]	2	50%	85%	82%	100%
Pneumonia Care					
Appropriate Initial Antibiotic	38	76%	83%	83%	94%
Blood Culture Timing[1]	20	85%	91%	90%	100%
Influenza Vaccine[1]	7	43%	77%	70%	100%
Initial Antibiotic Timing	43	93%	81%	80%	93%
Oxygenation Assessment	49	100%	99%	99%	100%
Pneumococcal Vaccine	32	44%	75%	69%	94%
Smoking Cessation Advice[1]	12	42%	83%	80%	100%
Surgical Infection Prevention					
Prophylactic Antibiotic Given[5]	-	-	78%	77%	95%
Prophylactic Antibiotic Selection[5]	-	-	92%	90%	100%
Prophylactic Antibiotic Stopped[5]	-	-	78%	72%	95%
Pregnancy Care					
Inpatient Neonatal Mortality	-	-	-	-	-
Third or Fourth Degree Laceration	-	-	-	3.63%	3.27%

NOTE: Hospital profiles are in alphabetical order by state, then city, then hospital within the city; Rankings are sorted by rate in descending order and exclude hospitals with less than 25 cases; (1) The number of cases is too small (n<25) for purposes of reliably predicting hospital performance; (2) Measure reflects the hospital's indication that its submission was based upon a sample of its relevant discharges; (3) Rate reflects fewer than the maximum possible quarters of data for the measure; (4) Inaccurate information submitted and suppressed for one or more quarters; (5) No data is available from the hospital for this measure; Please refer to the User's Guide for a full explanation of data

Heart Attack Care

1. ACE inhibitor or ARB for LVSD

Hospital Name	City	Rate	Cases
Abilene Regional Medical Center	Abilene	100%	33
Baylor Medical Center at Garland	Garland	100%	36
Baylor Regional Medical Center at Plano	Plano	100%	35
Christus Saint John Hospital	Houston	100%	31
Detar Hospital Navarro	Victoria	100%	35
Doctors Hospital	Dallas	100%	28
Kingwood Medical Center	Kingwood	100%	27
Richardson Medical Center	Richardson	100%	35
Saint Joseph Medical Center	Houston	100%	38
Valley Baptist Medical Center	Harlingen	100%	65
Charlton Methodist Hospital	Dallas	98%	44
Seton Medical Center	Austin	98%	56
Baylor Medical Center at Irving	Irving	97%	36
Plaza Medical Center	Fort Worth	97%	58
Christus Santa Rosa Hospital-City Centre	San Antonio	96%	28
Good Shepherd Medical Center	Longview	96%	48
Harris Methodist HEB Hospital	Bedford	96%	25
North Hills Hospital	N Richland Hills	96%	25
Paris Regional Medical Center-South Campus	Paris	96%	54
Scott & White	Temple	96%	91
Brownsville Medical Center	Brownsville	95%	57
Clear Lake Regional Medical Center	Webster	95%	97
Medical Center of Arlington	Arlington	95%	44
Midland Memorial Hospital	Midland	95%	44
Baylor University Medical Center	Dallas	94%	171
East Houston Regional Medical Center	Houston	94%	32
Memorial Hermann Baptist Beaumont	Beaumont	94%	33
Memorial Hermann Healthcare System	Houston	94%	174
Memorial Hermann-Texas Medical Center	Houston	94%	85
Harris County Hospital District	Houston	93%	68
North Austin Medical Center	Austin	93%	42
Houston Northwest Medical Center	Houston	92%	91
Memorial Hermann Memorial City	Houston	92%	64
Methodist Medical Center	Dallas	92%	65
Texoma Medical Center	Denison	92%	39
Christus Saint Michael Health System	Texarkana	91%	125
Medical Center of Plano	Plano	91%	34
Methodist Hospital	Houston	91%	152
Presbyterian Hospital of Denton	Denton	91%	33
Saint Luke's Episcopal Hospital	Houston	91%	120
United Regional Healthcare System	Wichita Falls	91%	64
Wadley Regional Medical Center	Texarkana	91%	47
West Houston Medical Center	Houston	90%	39
Heart Hospital of Austin	Austin	89%	105
Presbyterian Hospital of Plano	Plano	89%	28
Woodland Heights Medical Center	Lufkin	89%	38
Texsan Heart Hospital	San Antonio	88%	48
Conroe Regional Medical Center	Conroe	87%	75
Corpus Christi Medical Center-Bay Area	Corpus Christi	87%	31
San Jacinto Methodist Hospital	Baytown	87%	47
Mother Frances Hospital-Tyler	Tyler	86%	111
Presbyterian Hospital of Dallas	Dallas	86%	49
Saint Joseph Regional Health Center	Bryan	86%	71
Baylor All Saints Med Ctr at Forth Worth	Fort Worth	85%	52
Parkland Health & Hospital System	Dallas	85%	65
Valley Regional Medical Center	Brownsville	85%	46
Northwest Texas Healthcare System	Amarillo	84%	57
Shannon Medical Center	San Angelo	84%	63
South Austin Hospital	Austin	84%	100
Christus Saint Elizabeth Hospital	Beaumont	83%	88
Columbia Spring Branch Medical Center	Houston	83%	35
Arlington Memorial Hospital	Arlington	82%	65
East Texas Medical Center-Tyler	Tyler	82%	66
Saint David's Rehabiltation Center	Austin	82%	34
Doctors Hospital Parkway+Tidwell	Houston	81%	27
Hillcrest Baptist Medical Center	Waco	81%	32
Medical Center Hospital	Odessa	81%	124
Tomball Regional Hospital	Tomball	81%	36
University of Texas Medical Branch Hospitals	Galveston	80%	98
Harris Methodist Continued Care Hospital	Fort Worth	79%	108
Wilson N Jones Medical Center	Sherman	79%	52
Christus Spohn Memorial Hospital	Corpus Christi	78%	116
Hendrick Medical Center	Abilene	78%	51
Medical Center of Southeast Texas	Port Arthur	78%	27
John Peter Smith Hospital	Fort Worth	77%	39
Medical Center of Mesquite	Mesquite	77%	26
Providence Health Center	Waco	76%	49
Covenant Medical Center	Lubbock	75%	132
Methodist Hospital	San Antonio	75%	116
UT Southwestern Saint Paul Hospital	Dallas	75%	36
Bayshore Medical Center	Pasadena	74%	35
University Hospital	San Antonio	74%	46
Memorial Health System of East Texas-Lufkin	Lufkin	72%	39
Del Sol Medical Center	El Paso	71%	34
University Medical Center	Lubbock	71%	49
Doctors Hospital at Renaissance	Edinburg	69%	51
Providence Memorial Hospital	El Paso	68%	34
Laredo Medical Center	Laredo	67%	27
Baptist Medical Center	San Antonio	66%	50
Lubbock Heart Hospital	Lubbock	66%	29
Rio Grande Regional Hospital	McAllen	59%	46
McAllen Medical Center	McAllen	54%	71

2. Aspirin at Arrival

Hospital Name	City	Rate	Cases
Abilene Regional Medical Center	Abilene	100%	66
Baylor Medical Center at Garland	Garland	100%	200
Baylor Medical Center at Irving	Irving	100%	211
Baylor Regional Medical Center at Grapevine	Grapevine	100%	172
Baylor Regional Medical Center at Plano	Plano	100%	87
Brackenridge Hospital	Austin	100%	89
Christus Santa Rosa Hospital-City Centre	San Antonio	100%	161
Citizens Medical Center	Victoria	100%	133
Conroe Regional Medical Center	Conroe	100%	225
Good Shepherd Medical Center	Longview	100%	244
Harlingen Medical Center	Harlingen	100%	65
Heart Hospital of Austin	Austin	100%	111
Lake Pointe Medical Center	Rowlett	100%	52
Medical Center of Arlington	Arlington	100%	240
Memorial Herman Baptist Orange Hospital	Orange	100%	39
Memorial Herman Katy Hospital	Katy	100%	75
Memorial Hermann-Texas Medical Center	Houston	100%	260
Nix Healthcare System	San Antonio	100%	39
Northeast Medical Center	Bonham	100%	27
Plaza Medical Center	Fort Worth	100%	133
Presbyterian Hospital of Plano	Plano	100%	133
Providence Memorial Hospital	El Paso	100%	136
Scott & White	Temple	100%	339
Texsan Heart Hospital	San Antonio	100%	75
Thomason General Hospital	El Paso	100%	86
Valley Baptist Medical Center	Harlingen	100%	285
Arlington Memorial Hospital	Arlington	99%	217
Baptist-Saint Anthony's Health System	Amarillo	99%	169
Christus Saint John Hospital	Houston	99%	119
Christus Saint Michael Health System	Texarkana	99%	321
Corpus Christi Medical Center-Bay Area	Corpus Christi	99%	174
Denton Regional Medical Center	Denton	99%	128
Doctors Hospital	Dallas	99%	141
Harris County Hospital District	Houston	99%	204
Kingwood Medical Center	Kingwood	99%	136
Medical Center of Plano	Plano	99%	139
Medical City Dallas	Dallas	99%	112
Methodist Medical Center	Dallas	99%	173
North Central Medical Center	McKinney	99%	142
Richardson Medical Center	Richardson	99%	104
Round Rock Medical Center	Round Rock	99%	125
Saint Luke's Episcopal Hospital	Houston	99%	433
San Angelo Community Medical Center	San Angelo	99%	76
San Jacinto Methodist Hospital	Baytown	99%	217
Seton Medical Center	Austin	99%	189
Sierra Medical Center	El Paso	99%	127
University Hospital	San Antonio	99%	122
Baylor University Medical Center	Dallas	98%	313
Brazosport Memorial Hospital	Lake Jackson	98%	48
Centennial Medical Center	Frisco	98%	62
Central Texas Medical Center	San Marcos	98%	47
Charlton Methodist Hospital	Dallas	98%	234
Clear Lake Regional Medical Center	Webster	98%	372
College Station Medical Center	College Station	98%	51
Cypress Fairbanks Medical Center and Hospital	Houston	98%	101
Del Sol Medical Center	El Paso	98%	207
Detar Hospital Navarro	Victoria	98%	82
East Texas Medical Center-Athens	Athens	98%	86
Harris Methodist Erath County	Stephenville	98%	42
Harris Methodist HEB Hospital	Bedford	98%	191
Harris Methodist Southwest	Fort Worth	98%	87
Las Palmas Medical Center	El Paso	98%	59
Longview Regional Medical Center	Longview	98%	80
Memorial Hermann Healthcare System	Houston	98%	752
Memorial Hermann Memorial City	Houston	98%	196
Mesquite Community Hospital	Mesquite	98%	53
Methodist Willowbrook Hospital	Houston	98%	97
Midland Memorial Hospital	Midland	98%	187
Mother Frances Hospital-Tyler	Tyler	98%	323

NOTE: Hospital profiles are in alphabetical order by state, then city, then hospital within the city; Rankings are sorted by rate in descending order and exclude hospitals with less than 25 cases; (1) The number of cases is too small (n<25) for purposes of reliably predicting hospital performance; (2) Measure reflects the hospital's indication that its submission was based upon a sample of its relevant discharges; (3) Rate reflects fewer than the maximum possible quarters of data for the measure; (4) Inaccurate information submitted and suppressed for one or more quarters; (5) No data is available from the hospital for this measure; Please refer to the User's Guide for a full explanation of data

Hospital Name	City	Rate	Cases
North Hills Hospital	N Richland Hills	98%	162
Saint David's Rehabiltation Center	Austin	98%	146
Saint Joseph Medical Center	Houston	98%	122
Saint Joseph Regional Health Center	Bryan	98%	184
Shannon Medical Center	San Angelo	98%	125
UT Southwestern Saint Paul Hospital	Dallas	98%	117
Wadley Regional Medical Center	Texarkana	98%	164
Alice Regional Hospital	Alice	97%	76
Brownsville Medical Center	Brownsville	97%	205
Cleveland Regional Medical Center	Cleveland	97%	29
Hillcrest Baptist Medical Center	Waco	97%	169
Huguley Memorial Medical Center	Burleson	97%	186
McKenna Memorial Hospital	New Braunfels	97%	39
Medical Center of Lewisville	Lewisville	97%	60
Methodist Sugar Land Hospital	Sugar Land	97%	30
Oakbend Medical Center	Richmond	97%	36
Paris Regional Medical Center-South Campus	Paris	97%	119
Parkland Health & Hospital System	Dallas	97%	253
Presbyterian Hospital of Dallas	Dallas	97%	214
Presbyterian Hospital of Denton	Denton	97%	130
South Austin Hospital	Austin	97%	252
South Texas Regional Medical Center	Jourdanton	97%	31
Starr County Memorial Hospital	Rio Grande City	97%	35
Texoma Medical Center	Denison	97%	116
Trinity Medical Center	Carrollton	97%	35
United Regional Healthcare System	Wichita Falls	97%	199
University of Texas Medical Branch Hospitals	Galveston	97%	214
Christus Saint Catherine Hospital	Katy	96%	47
Christus Spohn Memorial Hospital	Corpus Christi	96%	402
Doctors Hospital of Laredo	Laredo	96%	48
Harris Methodist Continued Care Hospital	Fort Worth	96%	476
Houston Northwest Medical Center	Houston	96%	306
Lubbock Heart Hospital	Lubbock	96%	78
Mainland Medical Center	Texas City	96%	110
North Austin Medical Center	Austin	96%	159
Northwest Texas Healthcare System	Amarillo	96%	205
Palestine Regional Medical Center	Palestine	96%	51
Woodland Heights Medical Center	Lufkin	96%	92
Baptist Medical Center	San Antonio	95%	239
Baylor All Saints Med Ctr at Forth Worth	Fort Worth	95%	175
Christus Saint Elizabeth Hospital	Beaumont	95%	352
Covenant Medical Center	Lubbock	95%	225
East Texas Medical Center-Tyler	Tyler	95%	106
Marshall Regional Medical Center	Marshall	95%	39
Medical Center Hospital	Odessa	95%	276
RHD Memorial Medical Center	Dallas	95%	104
Wilson N Jones Medical Center	Sherman	95%	172
East Houston Regional Medical Center	Houston	94%	156
Hendrick Medical Center	Abilene	94%	214
Medical Center at Terrell	Terrell	94%	54
Memorial Hermann Baptist Beaumont	Beaumont	94%	130
Methodist Hospital	San Antonio	94%	558
Nacogdoches Memorial Hospital	Nacogdoches	94%	54
Saint Luke's Community Med Ctr-The Woodlands	The Woodlands	94%	89
Twelve Oaks Hospital	Houston	94%	31
University Medical Center	Lubbock	94%	233
University of Texas Health Center at Tyler	Tyler	94%	47
West Houston Medical Center	Houston	94%	156
Doctors Hospital at Renaissance	Edinburg	93%	119
Harris Methodist Northwest	Azle	93%	30
Memorial Hermann Fort Bend Hospital	Missouri City	93%	29
Methodist Hospital	Houston	93%	280
Metroplex Hospital	Killeen	93%	42
Providence Health Center	Waco	93%	251
Rio Grande Regional Hospital	McAllen	93%	166
Southwest General Hospital	San Antonio	93%	45
Tomball Regional Hospital	Tomball	93%	168
Gulf Coast Medical Center	Wharton	92%	25
Knapp Medical Center	Weslaco	92%	73
Medical Center of Southeast Texas	Port Arthur	92%	101
Memorial Health System of East Texas-Lufkin	Lufkin	92%	88
Renaissance Hospital-East Texas	Groves	92%	25
Columbia Spring Branch Medical Center	Houston	91%	113
Fort Duncan Medical Center	Eagle Pass	91%	34
John Peter Smith Hospital	Fort Worth	91%	199
Mission Hospital	Mission	91%	116
Valley Regional Medical Center	Brownsville	91%	145
Walls Regional Hospital	Cleburne	91%	32
Bayshore Medical Center	Pasadena	90%	212
Laredo Medical Center	Laredo	90%	146
Matagorda County Hospital District	Bay City	90%	31
McAllen Medical Center	McAllen	90%	241
Medical Center at Lancaster	Lancaster	90%	41
Campbell Health System	Weatherford	89%	27
Park Plaza Hospital	Houston	89%	38

Hospital Name	City	Rate	Cases
Medical Center of Mesquite	Mesquite	88%	164
Northeast Medical Center Hospital	Humble	88%	154
Edinburg Regional Medical Center	Edinburg	87%	46
Val Verde Regional Medical Center	Del Rio	87%	30
Nacogdoches Medical Center Hospital	Nacogdoches	86%	81
Presbyterian Hospital of Greenville	Greenville	86%	69
Hopkins County Memorial Hospital	Sulphur Springs	84%	31
Guadalupe Valley Hospital	Seguin	83%	29
Navarro Regional Hospital	Corsicana	83%	35
Alliance Hospital	Odessa	82%	33
Connally Memorial Medical Center	Floresville	82%	34
Doctors Hospital Parkway+Tidwell	Houston	80%	103

3. Aspirin at Discharge

Hospital Name	City	Rate	Cases
Baylor Heart and Vascular Center	Dallas	100%	140
Baylor Regional Medical Center at Plano	Plano	100%	122
Brackenridge Hospital	Austin	100%	90
Centennial Medical Center	Frisco	100%	71
Citizens Medical Center	Victoria	100%	157
Cypress Fairbanks Medical Center and Hospital	Houston	100%	78
Detar Hospital Navarro	Victoria	100%	159
Good Shepherd Medical Center	Longview	100%	292
Harlingen Medical Center	Harlingen	100%	72
Harris Methodist HEB Hospital	Bedford	100%	185
Medical Center of Arlington	Arlington	100%	220
Methodist Medical Center	Dallas	100%	216
Nix Healthcare System	San Antonio	100%	43
North Hills Hospital	N Richland Hills	100%	137
San Angelo Community Medical Center	San Angelo	100%	84
Scott & White	Temple	100%	571
Starr County Memorial Hospital	Rio Grande City	100%	25
Valley Baptist Medical Center	Harlingen	100%	256
Abilene Regional Medical Center	Abilene	99%	152
Charlton Methodist Hospital	Dallas	99%	194
Conroe Regional Medical Center	Conroe	99%	270
Harris Methodist Continued Care Hospital	Fort Worth	99%	620
Heart Hospital of Austin	Austin	99%	454
Kingwood Medical Center	Kingwood	99%	83
Memorial Hermann Baptist Beaumont	Beaumont	99%	169
Northwest Texas Healthcare System	Amarillo	99%	298
Plaza Medical Center	Fort Worth	99%	335
Presbyterian Hospital of Dallas	Dallas	99%	290
Seton Medical Center	Austin	99%	326
Arlington Memorial Hospital	Arlington	98%	210
Baylor Medical Center at Garland	Garland	98%	189
Baylor Regional Medical Center at Grapevine	Grapevine	98%	162
Christus Saint Elizabeth Hospital	Beaumont	98%	432
Christus Saint John Hospital	Houston	98%	101
Christus Santa Rosa Hospital-City Centre	San Antonio	98%	160
College Station Medical Center	College Station	98%	61
Doctors Hospital	Dallas	98%	130
Longview Regional Medical Center	Longview	98%	82
Paris Regional Medical Center-South Campus	Paris	98%	163
Parkland Health & Hospital System	Dallas	98%	207
Richardson Medical Center	Richardson	98%	93
Saint David's Rehabiltation Center	Austin	98%	166
Saint Joseph Regional Health Center	Bryan	98%	247
Texoma Medical Center	Denison	98%	130
Texsan Heart Hospital	San Antonio	98%	321
Thomason General Hospital	El Paso	98%	54
University Hospital	San Antonio	98%	151
University of Texas Medical Branch Hospitals	Galveston	98%	271
Baylor Medical Center at Irving	Irving	97%	198
Baylor University Medical Center	Dallas	97%	545
Brownsville Medical Center	Brownsville	97%	177
Christus Saint Michael Health System	Texarkana	97%	363
Clear Lake Regional Medical Center	Webster	97%	409
East Texas Medical Center-Tyler	Tyler	97%	275
Harris County Hospital District	Houston	97%	228
Huguley Memorial Medical Center	Burleson	97%	167
Lubbock Heart Hospital	Lubbock	97%	180
Medical Center at Terrell	Terrell	97%	32
Memorial Hermann Healthcare System	Houston	97%	793
North Austin Medical Center	Austin	97%	172
North Central Medical Center	McKinney	97%	147
Providence Memorial Hospital	El Paso	97%	132
Saint Joseph Medical Center	Houston	97%	119
Saint Luke's Episcopal Hospital	Houston	97%	648
South Austin Hospital	Austin	97%	232
UT Southwestern Saint Paul Hospital	Dallas	97%	118
West Houston Medical Center	Houston	97%	148
Baylor All Saints Med Ctr at Forth Worth	Fort Worth	96%	185
Christus Spohn Memorial Hospital	Corpus Christi	96%	529

Hospital Name	City	Rate	Cases
Denton Regional Medical Center	Denton	96%	202
Hendrick Medical Center	Abilene	96%	318
Houston Northwest Medical Center	Houston	96%	333
Medical Center of Plano	Plano	96%	132
Medical City Dallas	Dallas	96%	136
Memorial Hermann Memorial City	Houston	96%	281
Methodist Hospital	Houston	96%	628
Park Plaza Hospital	Houston	96%	27
Shannon Medical Center	San Angelo	96%	121
Sierra Medical Center	El Paso	96%	121
Tomball Regional Hospital	Tomball	96%	161
University Medical Center	Lubbock	96%	263
Baptist-Saint Anthony's Health System	Amarillo	95%	257
Corpus Christi Medical Center-Bay Area	Corpus Christi	95%	242
East Texas Medical Center-Athens	Athens	95%	39
Harris Methodist Southwest	Fort Worth	95%	61
Memorial Herman Katy Hospital	Katy	95%	43
Memorial Hermann-Texas Medical Center	Houston	95%	472
Mother Frances Hospital-Tyler	Tyler	95%	501
Medical Center Hospital	Odessa	94%	380
Medical Center of Southeast Texas	Port Arthur	94%	107
Methodist Hospital	San Antonio	94%	614
Presbyterian Hospital of Denton	Denton	94%	158
Woodland Heights Medical Center	Lufkin	94%	122
Covenant Medical Center	Lubbock	93%	531
Hillcrest Baptist Medical Center	Waco	93%	199
John Peter Smith Hospital	Fort Worth	93%	149
Las Palmas Medical Center	El Paso	93%	71
Mainland Medical Center	Texas City	93%	60
Round Rock Medical Center	Round Rock	93%	126
United Regional Healthcare System	Wichita Falls	93%	301
Wadley Regional Medical Center	Texarkana	93%	171
Alliance Hospital	Odessa	92%	106
Central Texas Medical Center	San Marcos	92%	25
East Houston Regional Medical Center	Houston	92%	106
McKenna Memorial Hospital	New Braunfels	92%	26
Presbyterian Hospital of Plano	Plano	92%	178
Renaissance Hospital-East Texas	Groves	92%	25
University of Texas Health Center at Tyler	Tyler	92%	51
Baptist Medical Center	San Antonio	91%	262
McAllen Medical Center	McAllen	91%	233
Wilson N Jones Medical Center	Sherman	91%	160
Doctors Hospital of Laredo	Laredo	90%	29
Metroplex Hospital	Killeen	90%	31
Midland Memorial Hospital	Midland	90%	202
Del Sol Medical Center	El Paso	89%	189
Knapp Medical Center	Weslaco	89%	27
Palestine Regional Medical Center	Palestine	89%	27
Providence Health Center	Waco	89%	312
San Jacinto Methodist Hospital	Baytown	89%	152
Alice Regional Hospital	Alice	88%	33
Bayshore Medical Center	Pasadena	88%	194
Doctors Hospital at Renaissance	Edinburg	88%	203
Laredo Medical Center	Laredo	87%	136
Methodist Willowbrook Hospital	Houston	87%	68
Rio Grande Regional Hospital	McAllen	87%	175
Valley Regional Medical Center	Brownsville	87%	133
Nacogdoches Medical Center Hospital	Nacogdoches	86%	77
Saint Luke's Community Med Ctr-The Woodlands	The Woodlands	86%	83
Memorial Health System of East Texas-Lufkin	Lufkin	85%	131
Northeast Medical Center Hospital	Humble	85%	61
Columbia Spring Branch Medical Center	Houston	84%	114
Twelve Oaks Hospital	Houston	84%	32
Nacogdoches Memorial Hospital	Nacogdoches	83%	72
Physicians Specialty Hospital of El Paso	El Paso	82%	28
Mission Hospital	Mission	79%	99
RHD Memorial Medical Center	Dallas	79%	87
Medical Center of Mesquite	Mesquite	76%	172
Presbyterian Hospital of Greenville	Greenville	72%	32
Doctors Hospital Parkway+Tidwell	Houston	66%	100
Edinburg Regional Medical Center	Edinburg	55%	31

4. Beta Blocker at Arrival

Hospital Name	City	Rate	Cases
Abilene Regional Medical Center	Abilene	100%	58
Baylor Medical Center at Garland	Garland	100%	183
Baylor Regional Medical Center at Plano	Plano	100%	77
Citizens Medical Center	Victoria	100%	112
College Station Medical Center	College Station	100%	33
Harlingen Medical Center	Harlingen	100%	64
Harris Methodist Southwest	Fort Worth	100%	78
Memorial Herman Katy Hospital	Katy	100%	68
Memorial Hermann-Texas Medical Center	Houston	100%	238
North Hills Hospital	N Richland Hills	100%	131
Plaza Medical Center	Fort Worth	100%	119
Richardson Medical Center	Richardson	100%	84
Baylor Medical Center at Irving	Irving	99%	192
Baylor Regional Medical Center at Grapevine	Grapevine	99%	161
Brackenridge Hospital	Austin	99%	76
Brownsville Medical Center	Brownsville	99%	174
Doctors Hospital	Dallas	99%	119
Good Shepherd Medical Center	Longview	99%	208
Hillcrest Baptist Medical Center	Waco	99%	150
Medical Center of Arlington	Arlington	99%	167
Medical Center of Plano	Plano	99%	109
Methodist Medical Center	Dallas	99%	146
Scott & White	Temple	99%	311
Valley Baptist Medical Center	Harlingen	99%	245
Baptist-Saint Anthony's Health System	Amarillo	98%	156
Christus Saint John Hospital	Houston	98%	121
Christus Santa Rosa Hospital-City Centre	San Antonio	98%	143
Denton Regional Medical Center	Denton	98%	114
Lake Pointe Medical Center	Rowlett	98%	50
McKenna Memorial Hospital	New Braunfels	98%	40
Mother Frances Hospital-Tyler	Tyler	98%	210
Palestine Regional Medical Center	Palestine	98%	47
Presbyterian Hospital of Plano	Plano	98%	108
Saint Luke's Episcopal Hospital	Houston	98%	389
San Angelo Community Medical Center	San Angelo	98%	64
Seton Medical Center	Austin	98%	162
University of Texas Medical Branch Hospitals	Galveston	98%	182
Alice Regional Hospital	Alice	97%	60
Baylor University Medical Center	Dallas	97%	227
Centennial Medical Center	Frisco	97%	59
Charlton Methodist Hospital	Dallas	97%	163
Detar Hospital Navarro	Victoria	97%	62
Longview Regional Medical Center	Longview	97%	72
Memorial Herman Baptist Orange Hospital	Orange	97%	38
Memorial Hermann Healthcare System	Houston	97%	629
Memorial Hermann Memorial City	Houston	97%	127
Nix Healthcare System	San Antonio	97%	37
Oakbend Medical Center	Richmond	97%	35
Round Rock Medical Center	Round Rock	97%	105
Texsan Heart Hospital	San Antonio	97%	64
Arlington Memorial Hospital	Arlington	96%	185
Harris County Hospital District	Houston	96%	155
Heart Hospital of Austin	Austin	96%	96
Kings Daughters Hospital	Temple	96%	25
Northwest Texas Healthcare System	Amarillo	96%	180
Paris Regional Medical Center-South Campus	Paris	96%	105
Saint David's Rehabiltation Center	Austin	96%	104
San Jacinto Methodist Hospital	Baytown	96%	198
Thomason General Hospital	El Paso	96%	81
Woodland Heights Medical Center	Lufkin	96%	82
Baptist Medical Center	San Antonio	95%	154
Baylor All Saints Med Ctr at Forth Worth	Fort Worth	95%	150
Central Texas Medical Center	San Marcos	95%	43
Christus Saint Catherine Hospital	Katy	95%	42
Christus Saint Michael Health System	Texarkana	95%	257
Clear Lake Regional Medical Center	Webster	95%	315
Conroe Regional Medical Center	Conroe	95%	149
Harris Methodist HEB Hospital	Bedford	95%	133
Huguley Memorial Medical Center	Burleson	95%	146
Las Palmas Medical Center	El Paso	95%	41
Medical City Dallas	Dallas	95%	102
Metroplex Hospital	Killeen	95%	39
North Central Medical Center	McKinney	95%	116
Presbyterian Hospital of Dallas	Dallas	95%	179
Texoma Medical Center	Denison	95%	102
United Regional Healthcare System	Wichita Falls	95%	185
Christus Spohn Memorial Hospital	Corpus Christi	94%	369
Methodist Hospital	Houston	94%	212
Presbyterian Hospital of Denton	Denton	94%	104
Saint Joseph Medical Center	Houston	94%	83
Saint Joseph Regional Health Center	Bryan	94%	140
University of Texas Health Center at Tyler	Tyler	94%	32
Wadley Regional Medical Center	Texarkana	94%	148
Cypress Fairbanks Medical Center and Hospital	Houston	93%	85
Doctors Hospital of Laredo	Laredo	93%	43
East Texas Medical Center-Athens	Athens	93%	85
Harris Methodist Continued Care Hospital	Fort Worth	93%	393
Houston Northwest Medical Center	Houston	93%	247
Kingwood Medical Center	Kingwood	93%	111
Methodist Willowbrook Hospital	Houston	93%	87
Mission Hospital	Mission	93%	96
Parkland Health & Hospital System	Dallas	93%	226
Providence Memorial Hospital	El Paso	93%	106
UT Southwestern Saint Paul Hospital	Dallas	93%	107
Corpus Christi Medical Center-Bay Area	Corpus Christi	92%	160

NOTE: Hospital profiles are in alphabetical order by state, then city, then hospital within the city; Rankings are sorted by rate in descending order and exclude hospitals with less than 25 cases; (1) The number of cases is too small (n<25) for purposes of reliably predicting hospital performance; (2) Measure reflects the hospital's indication that its submission was based upon a sample of its relevant discharges; (3) Rate reflects fewer than the maximum possible quarters of data for the measure; (4) Inaccurate information submitted and suppressed for one or more quarters; (5) No data is available from the hospital for this measure; Please refer to the User's Guide for a full explanation of data

Hospital Name	City	Rate	Cases
East Texas Medical Center-Tyler	Tyler	92%	93
Medical Center of Lewisville	Lewisville	92%	52
RHD Memorial Medical Center	Dallas	92%	108
Shannon Medical Center	San Angelo	92%	105
University Medical Center	Lubbock	92%	161
Val Verde Regional Medical Center	Del Rio	92%	26
West Houston Medical Center	Houston	92%	99
Del Sol Medical Center	El Paso	91%	139
Harris Methodist Erath County	Stephenville	91%	34
North Austin Medical Center	Austin	91%	81
Starr County Memorial Hospital	Rio Grande City	91%	34
Memorial Hermann Baptist Beaumont	Beaumont	90%	101
Mesquite Community Hospital	Mesquite	90%	52
South Austin Hospital	Austin	90%	172
Christus Saint Elizabeth Hospital	Beaumont	89%	301
Columbia Spring Branch Medical Center	Houston	89%	97
Medical Center at Lancaster	Lancaster	89%	28
Memorial Health System of East Texas-Lufkin	Lufkin	89%	89
Methodist Hospital	San Antonio	89%	412
Sierra Medical Center	El Paso	89%	87
Trinity Medical Center	Carrollton	89%	35
East Houston Regional Medical Center	Houston	88%	130
Mainland Medical Center	Texas City	88%	113
Medical Center Hospital	Odessa	88%	222
Northeast Medical Center	Bonham	88%	25
Providence Health Center	Waco	88%	199
Medical Center of Mesquite	Mesquite	87%	169
Midland Memorial Hospital	Midland	87%	135
University Hospital	San Antonio	87%	91
Bayshore Medical Center	Pasadena	86%	162
Brazosport Memorial Hospital	Lake Jackson	86%	51
John Peter Smith Hospital	Fort Worth	86%	185
McAllen Medical Center	McAllen	86%	147
Wilson N Jones Medical Center	Sherman	86%	153
Hendrick Medical Center	Abilene	85%	172
Marshall Regional Medical Center	Marshall	85%	39
Medical Center at Terrell	Terrell	85%	48
Campbell Health System	Weatherford	84%	31
Navarro Regional Hospital	Corsicana	84%	25
Renaissance Hospital-East Texas	Groves	84%	25
Covenant Medical Center	Lubbock	83%	189
Medical Center of Southeast Texas	Port Arthur	83%	92
Rio Grande Regional Hospital	McAllen	82%	104
Southwest General Hospital	San Antonio	82%	34
Hopkins County Memorial Hospital	Sulphur Springs	81%	27
Knapp Medical Center	Weslaco	81%	43
Park Plaza Hospital	Houston	81%	27
Nacogdoches Medical Center Hospital	Nacogdoches	80%	69
Northeast Medical Center Hospital	Humble	80%	111
Tomball Regional Hospital	Tomball	79%	149
Valley Regional Medical Center	Brownsville	79%	121
Saint Luke's Community Med Ctr-The Woodlands	The Woodlands	78%	89
Edinburg Regional Medical Center	Edinburg	77%	35
Lubbock Heart Hospital	Lubbock	76%	66
Doctors Hospital at Renaissance	Edinburg	75%	113
Nacogdoches Memorial Hospital	Nacogdoches	74%	54
Laredo Medical Center	Laredo	72%	57
Twelve Oaks Hospital	Houston	72%	32
South Texas Regional Medical Center	Jourdanton	71%	28
Presbyterian Hospital of Greenville	Greenville	70%	66
Alliance Hospital	Odessa	62%	32
Fort Duncan Medical Center	Eagle Pass	61%	28
Connally Memorial Medical Center	Floresville	56%	34
Doctors Hospital Parkway+Tidwell	Houston	56%	80

5. Beta Blocker at Discharge

Hospital Name	City	Rate	Cases
Charlton Methodist Hospital	Dallas	100%	228
Citizens Medical Center	Victoria	100%	147
College Station Medical Center	College Station	100%	61
Doctors Hospital	Dallas	100%	122
Harlingen Medical Center	Harlingen	100%	67
Harris Methodist Southwest	Fort Worth	100%	59
Medical Center of Arlington	Arlington	100%	208
Nix Healthcare System	San Antonio	100%	42
North Hills Hospital	N Richland Hills	100%	138
San Angelo Community Medical Center	San Angelo	100%	82
Scott & White	Temple	100%	567
Abilene Regional Medical Center	Abilene	99%	138
Baylor Heart and Vascular Center	Dallas	99%	136
Baylor Medical Center at Garland	Garland	99%	190
Baylor Medical Center at Irving	Irving	99%	183
Brackenridge Hospital	Austin	99%	86
Centennial Medical Center	Frisco	99%	72

Hospital Name	City	Rate	Cases
Denton Regional Medical Center	Denton	99%	198
Detar Hospital Navarro	Victoria	99%	173
Kingwood Medical Center	Kingwood	99%	83
Medical City Dallas	Dallas	99%	128
Methodist Medical Center	Dallas	99%	216
Paris Regional Medical Center-South Campus	Paris	99%	155
Parkland Health & Hospital System	Dallas	99%	227
Plaza Medical Center	Fort Worth	99%	352
Shannon Medical Center	San Angelo	99%	146
Valley Baptist Medical Center	Harlingen	99%	251
Baptist-Saint Anthony's Health System	Amarillo	98%	262
Baylor All Saints Med Ctr at Forth Worth	Fort Worth	98%	182
Baylor Regional Medical Center at Plano	Plano	98%	122
Baylor University Medical Center	Dallas	98%	509
Brownsville Medical Center	Brownsville	98%	178
Christus Saint John Hospital	Houston	98%	100
Christus Santa Rosa Hospital-City Centre	San Antonio	98%	164
Good Shepherd Medical Center	Longview	98%	257
Harris Methodist Continued Care Hospital	Fort Worth	98%	640
Huguley Memorial Medical Center	Burleson	98%	179
Memorial Herman Katy Hospital	Katy	98%	46
Methodist Hospital	Houston	98%	643
Richardson Medical Center	Richardson	98%	85
Seton Medical Center	Austin	98%	293
South Austin Hospital	Austin	98%	204
University Hospital	San Antonio	98%	141
University of Texas Medical Branch Hospitals	Galveston	98%	283
Arlington Memorial Hospital	Arlington	97%	200
Christus Saint Michael Health System	Texarkana	97%	356
Clear Lake Regional Medical Center	Webster	97%	390
Harris Methodist HEB Hospital	Bedford	97%	186
Hillcrest Baptist Medical Center	Waco	97%	192
Houston Northwest Medical Center	Houston	97%	321
Medical Center at Terrell	Terrell	97%	31
Memorial Hermann Healthcare System	Houston	97%	781
Memorial Hermann Memorial City	Houston	97%	284
Metroplex Hospital	Killeen	97%	33
Northwest Texas Healthcare System	Amarillo	97%	294
Presbyterian Hospital of Dallas	Dallas	97%	287
Saint David's Rehabiltation Center	Austin	97%	172
Saint Joseph Medical Center	Houston	97%	100
Saint Luke's Episcopal Hospital	Houston	97%	670
Thomason General Hospital	El Paso	97%	63
West Houston Medical Center	Houston	97%	143
Alice Regional Hospital	Alice	96%	27
Baylor Regional Medical Center at Grapevine	Grapevine	96%	150
Christus Saint Catherine Hospital	Katy	96%	27
Christus Spohn Memorial Hospital	Corpus Christi	96%	552
Conroe Regional Medical Center	Conroe	96%	243
Cypress Fairbanks Medical Center and Hospital	Houston	96%	70
Heart Hospital of Austin	Austin	96%	426
John Peter Smith Hospital	Fort Worth	96%	166
Longview Regional Medical Center	Longview	96%	83
McKenna Memorial Hospital	New Braunfels	96%	26
Memorial Hermann Baptist Beaumont	Beaumont	96%	169
Mother Frances Hospital-Tyler	Tyler	96%	290
North Austin Medical Center	Austin	96%	164
North Central Medical Center	McKinney	96%	150
Park Plaza Hospital	Houston	96%	28
Presbyterian Hospital of Denton	Denton	96%	161
Presbyterian Hospital of Plano	Plano	96%	170
Texoma Medical Center	Denison	96%	138
UT Southwestern Saint Paul Hospital	Dallas	96%	115
Woodland Heights Medical Center	Lufkin	96%	114
Harris County Hospital District	Houston	95%	229
Las Palmas Medical Center	El Paso	95%	58
Medical Center of Plano	Plano	95%	154
Memorial Hermann-Texas Medical Center	Houston	95%	454
Methodist Hospital	San Antonio	95%	657
Saint Joseph Regional Health Center	Bryan	95%	235
Texsan Heart Hospital	San Antonio	95%	306
United Regional Healthcare System	Wichita Falls	95%	291
Baptist Medical Center	San Antonio	94%	273
Christus Saint Elizabeth Hospital	Beaumont	94%	430
Del Sol Medical Center	El Paso	94%	159
Medical Center of Southeast Texas	Port Arthur	94%	106
San Jacinto Methodist Hospital	Baytown	94%	166
University Medical Center	Lubbock	94%	261
Wadley Regional Medical Center	Texarkana	94%	172
East Texas Medical Center-Tyler	Tyler	93%	276
Round Rock Medical Center	Round Rock	93%	117
University of Texas Health Center at Tyler	Tyler	93%	58
Corpus Christi Medical Center-Bay Area	Corpus Christi	92%	248
Covenant Medical Center	Lubbock	92%	541
East Houston Regional Medical Center	Houston	92%	106

NOTE: Hospital profiles are in alphabetical order by state, then city, then hospital within the city; Rankings are sorted by rate in descending order and exclude hospitals with less than 25 cases; (1) The number of cases is too small (n<25) for purposes of reliably predicting hospital performance; (2) Measure reflects the hospital's indication that its submission was based upon a sample of its relevant discharges; (3) Rate reflects fewer than the maximum possible quarters of data for the measure; (4) Inaccurate information submitted and suppressed for one or more quarters; (5) No data is available from the hospital for this measure; Please refer to the User's Guide for a full explanation of data

Methodist Willowbrook Hospital	Houston	92%	75
Tomball Regional Hospital	Tomball	92%	155
Mainland Medical Center	Texas City	91%	69
Medical Center Hospital	Odessa	91%	354
Palestine Regional Medical Center	Palestine	91%	33
Providence Health Center	Waco	91%	305
Columbia Spring Branch Medical Center	Houston	90%	121
Knapp Medical Center	Weslaco	90%	31
Nacogdoches Medical Center Hospital	Nacogdoches	89%	73
Renaissance Hospital-East Texas	Groves	89%	27
Central Texas Medical Center	San Marcos	88%	26
East Texas Medical Center-Athens	Athens	88%	41
Hendrick Medical Center	Abilene	88%	326
Marshall Regional Medical Center	Marshall	88%	25
Memorial Health System of East Texas-Lufkin	Lufkin	88%	128
Providence Memorial Hospital	El Paso	88%	122
Starr County Memorial Hospital	Rio Grande City	88%	25
Bayshore Medical Center	Pasadena	87%	188
Midland Memorial Hospital	Midland	87%	215
Northeast Medical Center Hospital	Humble	87%	53
Rio Grande Regional Hospital	McAllen	87%	174
Wilson N Jones Medical Center	Sherman	87%	165
Doctors Hospital of Laredo	Laredo	86%	28
Mission Hospital	Mission	86%	85
Valley Regional Medical Center	Brownsville	86%	134
Medical Center of Mesquite	Mesquite	84%	174
Saint Luke's Community Med Ctr-The Woodlands	The Woodlands	84%	77
Alliance Hospital	Odessa	83%	105
McAllen Medical Center	McAllen	83%	262
RHD Memorial Medical Center	Dallas	83%	95
Sierra Medical Center	El Paso	83%	119
Doctors Hospital at Renaissance	Edinburg	81%	212
Presbyterian Hospital of Greenville	Greenville	81%	32
Nacogdoches Memorial Hospital	Nacogdoches	80%	75
Lubbock Heart Hospital	Lubbock	79%	158
Laredo Medical Center	Laredo	72%	123
Twelve Oaks Hospital	Houston	71%	34
Doctors Hospital Parkway+Tidwell	Houston	65%	97
Edinburg Regional Medical Center	Edinburg	65%	31
Physicians Specialty Hospital of El Paso	El Paso	61%	28

6. Fibrinolytic Medication Timing

Hospital Name	City	Rate	Cases
Memorial Hermann Healthcare System	Houston	23%	39

7. PCI Within 90 Minutes of Arrival

Hospital Name	City	Rate	Cases
Memorial Hermann-Texas Medical Center	Houston	96%	26
Houston Northwest Medical Center	Houston	92%	25
Harris Methodist Continued Care Hospital	Fort Worth	70%	33
Memorial Hermann Healthcare System	Houston	44%	25
Methodist Hospital	San Antonio	24%	25

8. Smoking Cessation Advice

Hospital Name	City	Rate	Cases
Abilene Regional Medical Center	Abilene	100%	57
Baylor All Saints Med Ctr at Forth Worth	Fort Worth	100%	58
Baylor Heart and Vascular Center	Dallas	100%	53
Baylor Medical Center at Irving	Irving	100%	75
Baylor University Medical Center	Dallas	100%	236
Brackenridge Hospital	Austin	100%	51
Charlton Methodist Hospital	Dallas	100%	81
Christus Saint Michael Health System	Texarkana	100%	150
Christus Spohn Memorial Hospital	Corpus Christi	100%	175
Citizens Medical Center	Victoria	100%	44
Covenant Medical Center	Lubbock	100%	214
Cypress Fairbanks Medical Center and Hospital	Houston	100%	26
Detar Hospital Navarro	Victoria	100%	62
Harris Methodist HEB Hospital	Bedford	100%	70
Huguley Memorial Medical Center	Burleson	100%	78
Kingwood Medical Center	Kingwood	100%	47
Las Palmas Medical Center	El Paso	100%	28
Longview Regional Medical Center	Longview	100%	34
Medical Center of Southeast Texas	Port Arthur	100%	32
Methodist Medical Center	Dallas	100%	93
Mother Frances Hospital-Tyler	Tyler	100%	216
North Central Medical Center	McKinney	100%	60
North Hills Hospital	N Richland Hills	100%	53
Plaza Medical Center	Fort Worth	100%	145
RHD Memorial Medical Center	Dallas	100%	34
Saint David's Rehabiltation Center	Austin	100%	81
San Angelo Community Medical Center	San Angelo	100%	28
San Jacinto Methodist Hospital	Baytown	100%	52

Scott & White	Temple	100%	208
South Austin Hospital	Austin	100%	89
Texoma Medical Center	Denison	100%	52
Thomason General Hospital	El Paso	100%	25
UT Southwestern Saint Paul Hospital	Dallas	100%	32
Valley Baptist Medical Center	Harlingen	100%	57
Valley Regional Medical Center	Brownsville	100%	36
Woodland Heights Medical Center	Lufkin	100%	47
Bayshore Medical Center	Pasadena	99%	87
Christus Saint Elizabeth Hospital	Beaumont	99%	188
Conroe Regional Medical Center	Conroe	99%	138
Houston Northwest Medical Center	Houston	99%	145
Medical Center of Arlington	Arlington	99%	96
Memorial Hermann Healthcare System	Houston	99%	244
Memorial Hermann Memorial City	Houston	99%	97
West Houston Medical Center	Houston	99%	67
Baptist Medical Center	San Antonio	98%	84
Baylor Medical Center at Garland	Garland	98%	66
Christus Saint John Hospital	Houston	98%	50
Christus Santa Rosa Hospital-City Centre	San Antonio	98%	49
Clear Lake Regional Medical Center	Webster	98%	168
Columbia Spring Branch Medical Center	Houston	98%	54
Doctors Hospital	Dallas	98%	45
Medical Center of Plano	Plano	98%	45
Memorial Hermann-Texas Medical Center	Houston	98%	290
Presbyterian Hospital of Dallas	Dallas	98%	103
Presbyterian Hospital of Plano	Plano	98%	57
Round Rock Medical Center	Round Rock	98%	52
Saint Luke's Episcopal Hospital	Houston	98%	175
Baptist-Saint Anthony's Health System	Amarillo	97%	93
Brownsville Medical Center	Brownsville	97%	31
Good Shepherd Medical Center	Longview	97%	111
Methodist Hospital	San Antonio	97%	239
Midland Memorial Hospital	Midland	97%	74
Nacogdoches Medical Center Hospital	Nacogdoches	97%	29
Northwest Texas Healthcare System	Amarillo	97%	157
Paris Regional Medical Center-South Campus	Paris	97%	65
Providence Memorial Hospital	El Paso	97%	32
Saint Joseph Medical Center	Houston	97%	39
Texsan Heart Hospital	San Antonio	97%	95
University of Texas Medical Branch Hospitals	Galveston	97%	119
Wadley Regional Medical Center	Texarkana	97%	64
Del Sol Medical Center	El Paso	96%	67
Denton Regional Medical Center	Denton	96%	77
Medical City Dallas	Dallas	96%	52
Methodist Willowbrook Hospital	Houston	96%	25
Mission Hospital	Mission	96%	25
North Austin Medical Center	Austin	96%	81
Providence Health Center	Waco	96%	113
Seton Medical Center	Austin	96%	93
Harris Methodist Continued Care Hospital	Fort Worth	94%	288
Hillcrest Baptist Medical Center	Waco	94%	87
Parkland Health & Hospital System	Dallas	94%	98
Presbyterian Hospital of Denton	Denton	94%	68
Rio Grande Regional Hospital	McAllen	94%	33
Arlington Memorial Hospital	Arlington	93%	81
East Houston Regional Medical Center	Houston	93%	55
Heart Hospital of Austin	Austin	93%	174
Hendrick Medical Center	Abilene	93%	134
Sierra Medical Center	El Paso	93%	30
Baylor Regional Medical Center at Grapevine	Grapevine	92%	60
Methodist Hospital	Houston	92%	200
United Regional Healthcare System	Wichita Falls	92%	119
Centennial Medical Center	Frisco	90%	31
Saint Joseph Regional Health Center	Bryan	89%	82
University Medical Center	Lubbock	89%	117
Corpus Christi Medical Center-Bay Area	Corpus Christi	87%	82
Medical Center Hospital	Odessa	87%	143
University of Texas Health Center at Tyler	Tyler	86%	28
Harris County Hospital District	Houston	84%	100
McAllen Medical Center	McAllen	84%	69
Doctors Hospital at Renaissance	Edinburg	80%	35
East Texas Medical Center-Tyler	Tyler	79%	110
John Peter Smith Hospital	Fort Worth	70%	103
Laredo Medical Center	Laredo	67%	51
Medical Center of Mesquite	Mesquite	62%	72
University Hospital	San Antonio	42%	65

Heart Failure Care

9. ACE Inhibitor or ARB for LVSD

Hospital Name	City	Rate	Cases
Baylor Heart and Vascular Center	Dallas	100%	234
Baylor Medical Center-Ellis County	Waxahachie	100%	25

NOTE: Hospital profiles are in alphabetical order by state, then city, then hospital within the city; Rankings are sorted by rate in descending order and exclude hospitals with less than 25 cases; (1) The number of cases is too small (n<25) for purposes of reliably predicting hospital performance; (2) Measure reflects the hospital's indication that its submission was based upon a sample of its relevant discharges; (3) Rate reflects fewer than the maximum possible quarters of data for the measure; (4) Inaccurate information submitted and suppressed for one or more quarters; (5) No data is available from the hospital for this measure; Please refer to the User's Guide for a full explanation of data

Hospital	City	Rate	Cases
Christus Saint John Hospital	Houston	100%	87
Citizens Medical Center	Victoria	100%	88
Harlingen Medical Center	Harlingen	100%	38
Harris Methodist Southwest	Fort Worth	100%	57
Lake Pointe Medical Center	Rowlett	100%	43
North Hills Hospital	N Richland Hills	100%	83
Valley Baptist Medical Center	Harlingen	100%	228
Walls Regional Hospital	Cleburne	100%	61
Brackenridge Hospital	Austin	99%	108
Detar Hospital Navarro	Victoria	99%	72
Brownsville Medical Center	Brownsville	98%	100
Christus Saint Catherine Hospital	Katy	98%	49
Christus Spohn Hospital Beeville	Beeville	98%	49
Harris Methodist Continued Care Hospital	Fort Worth	98%	338
Harris Methodist HEB Hospital	Bedford	98%	93
Memorial Herman Katy Hospital	Katy	98%	63
Memorial Hermann-Texas Medical Center	Houston	98%	316
Pampa Regional Medical Center	Pampa	98%	42
Richardson Medical Center	Richardson	98%	59
Seton Medical Center	Austin	98%	244
Abilene Regional Medical Center	Abilene	97%	68
Good Shepherd Medical Center	Longview	97%	124
Methodist Medical Center	Dallas	97%	284
Baylor Medical Center at Irving	Irving	96%	136
Baylor Regional Medical Center at Grapevine	Grapevine	96%	46
Charlton Methodist Hospital	Dallas	96%	250
College Station Medical Center	College Station	96%	52
Hopkins County Memorial Hospital	Sulphur Springs	96%	46
Memorial Herman Baptist Orange Hospital	Orange	96%	54
Memorial Hermann Fort Bend Hospital	Missouri City	96%	50
Memorial Hermann Healthcare System	Houston	96%	745
Palestine Regional Medical Center	Palestine	96%	51
Scott & White	Temple	96%	267
West Houston Medical Center	Houston	96%	159
Baylor Regional Medical Center at Plano	Plano	95%	177
Christus Santa Rosa Hospital-City Centre	San Antonio	95%	129
Huguley Memorial Medical Center	Burleson	95%	75
Mother Frances Hospital-Tyler	Tyler	95%	238
Saint Joseph Medical Center	Houston	95%	171
University of Texas Health Center at Tyler	Tyler	95%	82
Uvalde Memorial Hospital	Uvalde	95%	44
Woodland Heights Medical Center	Lufkin	95%	119
Alice Regional Hospital	Alice	94%	64
Brownwood Regional Medical Center	Brownwood	94%	50
Doctors Hospital	Dallas	94%	144
Gulf Coast Medical Center	Wharton	94%	31
Texoma Medical Center	Denison	94%	88
Baylor Medical Center at Garland	Garland	93%	122
Baylor University Medical Center	Dallas	93%	446
Ennis Regional Medical Center	Ennis	93%	30
Henderson Memorial Hospital	Henderson	93%	28
Marshall Regional Medical Center	Marshall	93%	57
Conroe Regional Medical Center	Conroe	91%	190
Medical Center of Arlington	Arlington	91%	87
Memorial Hermann Memorial City	Houston	91%	206
Navarro Regional Hospital	Corsicana	91%	56
Presbyterian Hospital of Kaufman	Kaufman	91%	33
Christus Saint Michael Health System	Texarkana	90%	324
Kingwood Medical Center	Kingwood	90%	96
Mainland Medical Center	Texas City	90%	143
Plaza Medical Center	Fort Worth	90%	172
Shannon Medical Center	San Angelo	90%	92
Thomason General Hospital	El Paso	90%	87
Christus Saint Elizabeth Hospital	Beaumont	89%	348
Huntsville Memorial Hospital	Huntsville	89%	37
Medical City Dallas	Dallas	89%	243
Parkland Health & Hospital System	Dallas	89%	521
Presbyterian Hospital of Plano	Plano	89%	46
Tomball Regional Hospital	Tomball	89%	127
John Peter Smith Hospital	Fort Worth	88%	318
Las Colinas Medical Center	Irving	88%	33
Saint David's Rehabiltation Center	Austin	88%	175
East Houston Regional Medical Center	Houston	87%	149
Memorial Hermann Baptist Beaumont	Beaumont	87%	155
University Hospital	San Antonio	87%	191
Val Verde Regional Medical Center	Del Rio	87%	38
Harris County Hospital District	Houston	86%	406
Longview Regional Medical Center	Longview	86%	59
Midland Memorial Hospital	Midland	86%	135
Providence Memorial Hospital	El Paso	86%	151
Round Rock Medical Center	Round Rock	86%	50
Trinity Medical Center	Carrollton	86%	50
Wadley Regional Medical Center	Texarkana	86%	177
Wilson N Jones Medical Center	Sherman	86%	147
Denton Regional Medical Center	Denton	85%	79
Heart Hospital of Austin	Austin	85%	232
Hendrick Medical Center	Abilene	85%	188
Medical Center Hospital	Odessa	85%	188
Paris Regional Medical Center-South Campus	Paris	85%	121
South Austin Hospital	Austin	85%	199
South Texas Regional Medical Center	Jourdanton	85%	27
Clear Lake Regional Medical Center	Webster	84%	219
Cypress Fairbanks Medical Center and Hospital	Houston	84%	81
Doctors Hospital of Laredo	Laredo	84%	62
East Texas Medical Center-Clarksville	Clarksville	84%	38
Medical Center of Southeast Texas	Port Arthur	84%	97
Mesquite Community Hospital	Mesquite	84%	92
Methodist Hospital	Houston	84%	425
Methodist Willowbrook Hospital	Houston	84%	55
Presbyterian Hospital of Dallas	Dallas	84%	300
UT Southwestern Saint Paul Hospital	Dallas	84%	210
University Medical Center	Lubbock	84%	125
Medical Center of Lewisville	Lewisville	83%	69
Northwest Texas Healthcare System	Amarillo	83%	144
Texsan Heart Hospital	San Antonio	83%	119
United Regional Healthcare System	Wichita Falls	83%	116
Baylor All Saints Med Ctr at Forth Worth	Fort Worth	82%	197
Palo Pinto General Hospital	Mineral Wells	82%	28
Arlington Memorial Hospital	Arlington	81%	197
Columbia Spring Branch Medical Center	Houston	81%	119
McKenna Memorial Hospital	New Braunfels	81%	36
Nacogdoches Memorial Hospital	Nacogdoches	81%	114
Park Plaza Hospital	Houston	81%	115
Scenic Mountain Medical Center	Big Spring	81%	26
Valley Regional Medical Center	Brownsville	81%	70
Christus Spohn Memorial Hospital	Corpus Christi	80%	466
Medical Center of Plano	Plano	80%	131
Saint Joseph Regional Health Center	Bryan	80%	336
Titus Regional Medical Center	Mount Pleasant	80%	40
Corpus Christi Medical Center-Bay Area	Corpus Christi	79%	153
East Texas Medical Center-Athens	Athens	79%	68
Matagorda County Hospital District	Bay City	79%	28
Houston Northwest Medical Center	Houston	78%	263
Providence Health Center	Waco	78%	166
Central Texas Medical Center	San Marcos	77%	52
Las Palmas Medical Center	El Paso	77%	65
North Austin Medical Center	Austin	77%	107
University of Texas Medical Branch Hospitals	Galveston	77%	243
Alliance Hospital	Odessa	76%	70
Guadalupe Valley Hospital	Seguin	76%	50
Memorial Health System of East Texas-Lufkin	Lufkin	76%	107
Methodist Hospital	San Antonio	76%	546
Baptist-Saint Anthony's Health System	Amarillo	75%	72
Metroplex Hospital	Killeen	75%	83
Mission Hospital	Mission	75%	60
Presbyterian Hospital of Denton	Denton	75%	73
Saint Luke's Community Med Ctr-The Woodlands	The Woodlands	75%	48
San Jacinto Methodist Hospital	Baytown	75%	115
Twelve Oaks Hospital	Houston	75%	85
Fort Duncan Medical Center	Eagle Pass	74%	78
Georgetown Healthcare System	Georgetown	74%	27
Northeast Medical Center Hospital	Humble	74%	149
Del Sol Medical Center	El Paso	73%	150
Sierra Medical Center	El Paso	73%	206
Southwest General Hospital	San Antonio	73%	52
Medical Center at Terrell	Terrell	72%	36
East Texas Medical Center-Tyler	Tyler	71%	188
Oakbend Medical Center	Richmond	71%	70
RHD Memorial Medical Center	Dallas	71%	55
Doctors Hospital at Renaissance	Edinburg	70%	193
North Central Medical Center	McKinney	70%	81
Physicians Specialty Hospital of El Paso	El Paso	70%	40
Baptist Medical Center	San Antonio	68%	113
Knapp Medical Center	Weslaco	68%	104
Bayshore Medical Center	Pasadena	67%	149
Centennial Medical Center	Frisco	67%	27
Doctors Hospital Parkway+Tidwell	Houston	67%	123
Hillcrest Baptist Medical Center	Waco	67%	102
Medical Center of Mesquite	Mesquite	67%	132
Nacogdoches Medical Center Hospital	Nacogdoches	67%	45
Rio Grande Regional Hospital	McAllen	67%	131
Saint Luke's Episcopal Hospital	Houston	67%	754
Covenant Medical Center	Lubbock	66%	314
Atlanta Memorial Hospital	Atlanta	65%	43
Cleveland Regional Medical Center	Cleveland	65%	46
Medical Center at Lancaster	Lancaster	65%	57
Memorial Medical Center Livingston	Livingston	65%	46
Christus Spohn Hospital Kleberg	Kingsville	64%	50
McAllen Medical Center	McAllen	64%	135
Presbyterian Hospital of Greenville	Greenville	64%	143

NOTE: Hospital profiles are in alphabetical order by state, then city, then hospital within the city; Rankings are sorted by rate in descending order and exclude hospitals with less than 25 cases; (1) The number of cases is too small (n<25) for purposes of reliably predicting hospital performance; (2) Measure reflects the hospital's indication that its submission was based upon a sample of its relevant discharges; (3) Rate reflects fewer than the maximum possible quarters of data for the measure; (4) Inaccurate information submitted and suppressed for one or more quarters; (5) No data is available from the hospital for this measure; Please refer to the User's Guide for a full explanation of data

Hospital Name	City	Rate	Cases
Brazosport Memorial Hospital	Lake Jackson	58%	57
Laredo Medical Center	Laredo	58%	113
Lubbock Heart Hospital	Lubbock	57%	89
Campbell Health System	Weatherford	54%	26
Edinburg Regional Medical Center	Edinburg	44%	43

10. Discharge Instructions

Hospital Name	City	Rate	Cases
Abilene Regional Medical Center	Abilene	100%	136
Baylor Heart and Vascular Center	Dallas	100%	266
Bellville General Hospital	Bellville	100%	29
Bowie Memorial Hospital	Bowie	100%	42
Citizens Medical Center	Victoria	100%	247
Cuero Community Hospital	Cuero	100%	50
Detar Hospital Navarro	Victoria	100%	197
Palo Pinto General Hospital	Mineral Wells	100%	90
Tomball Regional Hospital	Tomball	100%	84
Valley Baptist Medical Center	Harlingen	100%	635
Harris Methodist Southwest	Fort Worth	99%	161
Longview Regional Medical Center	Longview	99%	148
Walls Regional Hospital	Cleburne	99%	135
Alice Regional Hospital	Alice	98%	40
East Texas Medical Center-Athens	Athens	98%	232
Nix Healthcare System	San Antonio	98%	64
Rolling Plains Memorial Hospital	Sweetwater	98%	42
Goodall-Witcher Healthcare Foundation	Clifton	97%	39
Lake Granbury Medical Center	Granbury	97%	32
Memorial Herman Baptist Orange Hospital	Orange	97%	108
Methodist Medical Center	Dallas	97%	508
Christus Santa Rosa Hospital-City Centre	San Antonio	96%	554
Harlingen Medical Center	Harlingen	96%	146
Memorial Hermann Fort Bend Hospital	Missouri City	96%	114
Baylor Regional Medical Center at Plano	Plano	95%	65
Presbyterian Hospital of Kaufman	Kaufman	95%	125
Brownsville Medical Center	Brownsville	94%	263
Good Shepherd Medical Center	Longview	94%	261
Harris Methodist Erath County	Stephenville	94%	62
Mother Frances Hospital-Tyler	Tyler	94%	511
Denton Regional Medical Center	Denton	93%	220
Lake Pointe Medical Center	Rowlett	93%	97
Harris Methodist Northwest	Azle	92%	73
Valley Regional Medical Center	Brownsville	92%	227
Frio Hospital	Pearsall	91%	34
Oakbend Medical Center	Richmond	91%	144
Presbyterian Hospital of Winnsboro	Winnsboro	91%	32
Wilbarger General Hospital	Vernon	91%	43
Christus Saint Elizabeth Hospital	Beaumont	90%	812
Doctors Hospital	Dallas	90%	292
Baylor University Medical Center	Dallas	88%	805
Campbell Health System	Weatherford	88%	25
Marshall Regional Medical Center	Marshall	88%	102
Memorial Hermann Baptist Beaumont	Beaumont	88%	81
Presbyterian Hospital of Plano	Plano	88%	146
Shelby Regional Medical Center	Center	88%	34
Memorial Herman Katy Hospital	Katy	87%	106
Baylor Medical Center at Irving	Irving	86%	288
Hopkins County Memorial Hospital	Sulphur Springs	86%	110
Kings Daughters Hospital	Temple	86%	35
Memorial Hermann-Texas Medical Center	Houston	86%	518
Christus Saint Catherine Hospital	Katy	85%	130
Christus Spohn Hospital Kleberg	Kingsville	85%	152
Falls Community Hospital	Marlin	85%	85
Graham Regional Medical Center	Graham	85%	59
Hill Country Memorial Hospital	Fredericksburg	85%	59
Palestine Regional Medical Center	Palestine	85%	115
Wise Regional Health System	Decatur	85%	52
Del Sol Medical Center	El Paso	84%	378
Presbyterian Hospital of Dallas	Dallas	84%	505
Texoma Medical Center	Denison	84%	172
Baylor Medical Center at Garland	Garland	83%	345
Baylor Medical Center-Ellis County	Waxahachie	83%	66
Northwest Texas Healthcare System	Amarillo	83%	264
Plaza Medical Center	Fort Worth	83%	341
Thomason General Hospital	El Paso	83%	183
Brackenridge Hospital	Austin	82%	236
Christus Spohn Hospital Beeville	Beeville	82%	38
Seton Medical Center	Austin	82%	491
Wilson N Jones Medical Center	Sherman	82%	65
Uvalde Memorial Hospital	Uvalde	81%	79
Christus Saint Michael Health System	Texarkana	80%	515
Trinity Medical Center	Brenham	80%	35
Baylor All Saints Med Ctr at Forth Worth	Fort Worth	79%	387
Baptist Medical Center	San Antonio	78%	344
Baylor Regional Medical Center at Grapevine	Grapevine	77%	128

Hospital Name	City	Rate	Cases
Charlton Methodist Hospital	Dallas	77%	449
Val Verde Regional Medical Center	Del Rio	77%	105
Christus Jasper Memorial Hospital	Jasper	76%	55
Park Plaza Hospital	Houston	76%	295
Saint Joseph Medical Center	Houston	76%	322
San Angelo Community Medical Center	San Angelo	76%	105
Woodland Heights Medical Center	Lufkin	76%	207
Harris Methodist HEB Hospital	Bedford	75%	220
Methodist Hospital	Houston	75%	765
South Texas Regional Medical Center	Jourdanton	75%	141
Brazosport Memorial Hospital	Lake Jackson	74%	117
Christus Spohn Memorial Hospital	Corpus Christi	74%	1028
Kingwood Medical Center	Kingwood	74%	251
Medical Center of Arlington	Arlington	74%	234
San Jacinto Methodist Hospital	Baytown	74%	264
Christus Saint John Hospital	Houston	73%	177
Harris Methodist Continued Care Hospital	Fort Worth	72%	686
Wadley Regional Medical Center	Texarkana	72%	317
Guadalupe Valley Hospital	Seguin	71%	121
Las Palmas Medical Center	El Paso	71%	183
Memorial Medical Center	Port Lavaca	70%	43
Methodist Sugar Land Hospital	Sugar Land	70%	69
College Station Medical Center	College Station	69%	93
Memorial Health System of East Texas-Lufkin	Lufkin	69%	35
Methodist Willowbrook Hospital	Houston	69%	32
Providence Memorial Hospital	El Paso	69%	377
Fort Duncan Medical Center	Eagle Pass	68%	217
Northeast Medical Center	Bonham	68%	31
Arlington Memorial Hospital	Arlington	67%	386
Henderson Memorial Hospital	Henderson	67%	96
McKenna Memorial Hospital	New Braunfels	67%	123
Medical Center of Southeast Texas	Port Arthur	67%	236
Parkview Regional Hospital	Mexia	67%	136
Richardson Medical Center	Richardson	67%	105
Rio Grande Regional Hospital	McAllen	67%	369
Saint Luke's Episcopal Hospital	Houston	67%	1297
Medical Center Hospital	Odessa	66%	341
Sid Peterson Memorial Hospital	Kerrville	66%	107
North Central Medical Center	McKinney	65%	188
North Austin Medical Center	Austin	64%	237
Odessa Regional Hospital	Odessa	64%	25
Scott & White	Temple	64%	442
Shannon Medical Center	San Angelo	64%	33
Comanche County Medical Center	Comanche	63%	52
East Texas Medical Center-Clarksville	Clarksville	63%	27
East Texas Medical Center-Crockett	Crockett	63%	76
Huntsville Memorial Hospital	Huntsville	63%	65
Brownwood Regional Medical Center	Brownwood	62%	121
Conroe Regional Medical Center	Conroe	62%	498
Medical Center of Mesquite	Mesquite	62%	346
Seton Northwest Hospital	Austin	62%	39
Texsan Heart Hospital	San Antonio	62%	156
Central Texas Medical Center	San Marcos	61%	28
East Houston Regional Medical Center	Houston	61%	332
Huguley Memorial Medical Center	Burleson	61%	280
Medical Center at Terrell	Terrell	61%	88
Metroplex Hospital	Killeen	61%	213
Navarro Regional Hospital	Corsicana	61%	114
Parkland Health & Hospital System	Dallas	61%	790
Providence Health Center	Waco	61%	378
Saint David's Rehabiltation Center	Austin	61%	421
Heart Hospital of Austin	Austin	60%	320
Memorial Hermann Memorial City	Houston	60%	378
East Texas Medical Center-Carthage	Carthage	59%	32
McAllen Medical Center	McAllen	59%	271
Mesquite Community Hospital	Mesquite	59%	202
Cypress Fairbanks Medical Center and Hospital	Houston	58%	197
East Texas Medical Center-Quitman	Quitman	58%	55
Knapp Medical Center	Weslaco	58%	295
Laird Memorial Hospital	Kilgore	58%	55
Las Colinas Medical Center	Irving	58%	76
Harris County Hospital District	Houston	57%	678
Hendrick Medical Center	Abilene	57%	336
Midland Memorial Hospital	Midland	57%	303
Rollins Brook Community Hospital	Lampasas	57%	30
South Austin Hospital	Austin	57%	351
Trinity Medical Center	Carrollton	57%	111
Hill Regional Hospital	Hillsboro	56%	86
Houston Northwest Medical Center	Houston	56%	487
RHD Memorial Medical Center	Dallas	56%	114
West Houston Medical Center	Houston	56%	311
Ennis Regional Medical Center	Ennis	55%	73
Memorial Hermann Healthcare System	Houston	55%	1575
North Hills Hospital	N Richland Hills	55%	197
Smithville Regional Hospital	Smithville	55%	51

NOTE: Hospital profiles are in alphabetical order by state, then city, then hospital within the city; Rankings are sorted by rate in descending order and exclude hospitals with less than 25 cases; (1) The number of cases is too small (n<25) for purposes of reliably predicting hospital performance; (2) Measure reflects the hospital's indication that its submission was based upon a sample of its relevant discharges; (3) Rate reflects fewer than the maximum possible quarters of data for the measure; (4) Inaccurate information submitted and suppressed for one or more quarters; (5) No data is available from the hospital for this measure; Please refer to the User's Guide for a full explanation of data

Hospital	City	Rate	Cases
Coleman County Medical Center	Coleman	54%	26
East Texas Medical Center-Pittsburg	Pittsburg	54%	54
Mainland Medical Center	Texas City	54%	301
Methodist Hospital	San Antonio	54%	1224
Round Rock Medical Center	Round Rock	54%	114
Columbia Spring Branch Medical Center	Houston	53%	227
Hillcrest Baptist Medical Center	Waco	53%	210
Medical Center of Lewisville	Lewisville	53%	203
Saint Joseph Regional Health Center	Bryan	53%	514
Baptist-Saint Anthony's Health System	Amarillo	52%	229
Medical Center of Plano	Plano	52%	260
Zale-Lipshy University Hospital	Dallas	52%	29
Laredo Medical Center	Laredo	51%	265
El Campo Memorial Hospital	El Campo	50%	46
University Medical Center	Lubbock	49%	239
Medical City Dallas	Dallas	47%	412
Nacogdoches Medical Center Hospital	Nacogdoches	47%	112
Hamilton General Hospital	Hamilton	46%	74
Paris Regional Medical Center-South Campus	Paris	46%	217
Georgetown Healthcare System	Georgetown	45%	60
Presbyterian Hospital of Denton	Denton	45%	209
Seton Highland Lakes	Burnet	45%	40
University of Texas Medical Branch Hospitals	Galveston	45%	311
Clear Lake Regional Medical Center	Webster	44%	386
Corpus Christi Medical Center-Bay Area	Corpus Christi	44%	388
UT Southwestern Saint Paul Hospital	Dallas	44%	368
Edinburg Regional Medical Center	Edinburg	43%	130
Angleton-Danbury Medical Center	Angleton	42%	31
Atlanta Memorial Hospital	Atlanta	42%	97
Doctors Hospital at Renaissance	Edinburg	42%	359
Pampa Regional Medical Center	Pampa	42%	73
Presbyterian Hospital of Allen	Allen	42%	50
United Regional Healthcare System	Wichita Falls	42%	262
Alliance Hospital	Odessa	41%	46
Mission Hospital	Mission	40%	230
Childress Regional Medical Center	Childress	38%	26
Doctors Hospital of Laredo	Laredo	37%	200
Lubbock Heart Hospital	Lubbock	37%	71
Matagorda County Hospital District	Bay City	37%	76
Northeast Medical Center Hospital	Humble	37%	416
Gulf Coast Medical Center	Wharton	36%	75
Sierra Medical Center	El Paso	35%	425
Nacogdoches Memorial Hospital	Nacogdoches	34%	50
Covenant Medical Center	Lubbock	33%	665
Seton Edgar B Davis Memorial Hospital	Luling	32%	25
Yoakum Community Hospital	Yoakum	31%	42
Bayshore Medical Center	Pasadena	30%	432
Centennial Medical Center	Frisco	30%	60
Scenic Mountain Medical Center	Big Spring	29%	115
East Texas Medical Center-Tyler	Tyler	25%	293
Southwest General Hospital	San Antonio	25%	243
Titus Regional Medical Center	Mount Pleasant	22%	27
University of Texas Health Center at Tyler	Tyler	19%	161
Pecos County Memorial Hosptial	Fort Stockton	18%	33
Doctors Hospital Parkway+Tidwell	Houston	17%	64
John Peter Smith Hospital	Fort Worth	14%	485
Big Bend Regional Medical Center	Alpine	12%	26
North Texas Medical Center	Gainesville	12%	73
Cleveland Regional Medical Center	Cleveland	6%	112
University Hospital	San Antonio	5%	296
Presbyterian Hospital of Greenville	Greenville	1%	267
Brownfield Regional Medical Center	Brownfield	0%	36
Memorial Hospital	Gonzales	0%	38

11. Evaluation of LVS Function

Hospital Name	City	Rate	Cases
Abilene Regional Medical Center	Abilene	100%	166
Baylor Heart and Vascular Center	Dallas	100%	268
Christus Saint Catherine Hospital	Katy	100%	155
Christus Saint John Hospital	Houston	100%	210
Citizens Medical Center	Victoria	100%	296
Clear Lake Regional Medical Center	Webster	100%	526
Graham Regional Medical Center	Graham	100%	68
Kings Daughters Hospital	Temple	100%	39
Lake Pointe Medical Center	Rowlett	100%	147
Longview Regional Medical Center	Longview	100%	168
Memorial Herman Katy Hospital	Katy	100%	150
Parkland Health & Hospital System	Dallas	100%	820
Seton Northwest Hospital	Austin	100%	45
Texsan Heart Hospital	San Antonio	100%	172
Valley Baptist Medical Center	Harlingen	100%	713
Walls Regional Hospital	Cleburne	100%	176
Baylor Medical Center at Irving	Irving	99%	324
Baylor Regional Medical Center at Plano	Plano	99%	266

Hospital	City	Rate	Cases
Baylor University Medical Center	Dallas	99%	944
Brackenridge Hospital	Austin	99%	249
Christus Santa Rosa Hospital-City Centre	San Antonio	99%	602
College Station Medical Center	College Station	99%	103
John Peter Smith Hospital	Fort Worth	99%	505
Memorial Hermann Healthcare System	Houston	99%	1905
Memorial Hermann Memorial City	Houston	99%	461
Memorial Hermann-Texas Medical Center	Houston	99%	562
North Hills Hospital	N Richland Hills	99%	266
Plaza Medical Center	Fort Worth	99%	379
University of Texas Medical Branch Hospitals	Galveston	99%	337
Alice Regional Hospital	Alice	98%	240
Bowie Memorial Hospital	Bowie	98%	52
Detar Hospital Navarro	Victoria	98%	296
Doctors Hospital	Dallas	98%	365
Memorial Herman Baptist Orange Hospital	Orange	98%	141
Memorial Hermann Fort Bend Hospital	Missouri City	98%	131
Methodist Hospital	Houston	98%	842
Methodist Medical Center	Dallas	98%	529
Mother Frances Hospital-Tyler	Tyler	98%	641
Presbyterian Hospital of Plano	Plano	98%	172
Saint David's Rehabiltation Center	Austin	98%	492
South Austin Hospital	Austin	98%	405
West Houston Medical Center	Houston	98%	383
Brazosport Memorial Hospital	Lake Jackson	97%	142
Charlton Methodist Hospital	Dallas	97%	552
Christus Saint Michael Health System	Texarkana	97%	660
Cypress Fairbanks Medical Center and Hospital	Houston	97%	262
Harlingen Medical Center	Harlingen	97%	168
Harris County Hospital District	Houston	97%	697
Huguley Memorial Medical Center	Burleson	97%	345
Kingwood Medical Center	Kingwood	97%	305
Marshall Regional Medical Center	Marshall	97%	124
San Angelo Community Medical Center	San Angelo	97%	149
Seton Medical Center	Austin	97%	584
Thomason General Hospital	El Paso	97%	185
Tomball Regional Hospital	Tomball	97%	413
UT Southwestern Saint Paul Hospital	Dallas	97%	397
Woodland Heights Medical Center	Lufkin	97%	276
Brownsville Medical Center	Brownsville	96%	253
Christus Spohn Memorial Hospital	Corpus Christi	96%	1190
Conroe Regional Medical Center	Conroe	96%	482
Falls Community Hospital	Marlin	96%	105
Heart Hospital of Austin	Austin	96%	361
Hendrick Medical Center	Abilene	96%	411
Mainland Medical Center	Texas City	96%	359
Medical Center of Arlington	Arlington	96%	282
Medical Center of Lewisville	Lewisville	96%	223
Memorial Hermann Baptist Beaumont	Beaumont	96%	373
Nix Healthcare System	San Antonio	96%	83
North Austin Medical Center	Austin	96%	277
Presbyterian Hospital of Dallas	Dallas	96%	650
Rolling Plains Memorial Hospital	Sweetwater	96%	57
Saint Joseph Medical Center	Houston	96%	379
University Hospital	San Antonio	96%	309
Uvalde Memorial Hospital	Uvalde	96%	99
Baylor All Saints Med Ctr at Forth Worth	Fort Worth	95%	459
Baylor Medical Center at Garland	Garland	95%	426
Baylor Medical Center-Ellis County	Waxahachie	95%	88
Christus Jasper Memorial Hospital	Jasper	95%	79
Christus Spohn Hospital Beeville	Beeville	95%	222
Columbia Spring Branch Medical Center	Houston	95%	300
East Texas Medical Center-Carthage	Carthage	95%	40
Paris Regional Medical Center-South Campus	Paris	95%	292
Richardson Medical Center	Richardson	95%	147
Scott & White	Temple	95%	566
Southwest General Hospital	San Antonio	95%	293
Wise Regional Health System	Decatur	95%	58
Baylor Regional Medical Center at Grapevine	Grapevine	94%	150
Cozby-Germany Hospital	Grand Saline	94%	34
Cuero Community Hospital	Cuero	94%	77
East Texas Medical Center-Jacksonville	Jacksonville	94%	64
Medical Center of Plano	Plano	94%	356
Medical City Dallas	Dallas	94%	479
Methodist Sugar Land Hospital	Sugar Land	94%	87
Presbyterian Hospital of Allen	Allen	94%	62
Round Rock Medical Center	Round Rock	94%	145
Wilbarger General Hospital	Vernon	94%	51
Christus Saint Elizabeth Hospital	Beaumont	93%	928
Frio Hospital	Pearsall	93%	29
Harris Methodist Erath County	Stephenville	93%	71
Harris Methodist Northwest	Azle	93%	91
North Central Medical Center	McKinney	93%	256
Presbyterian Hospital of Greenville	Greenville	93%	338
Presbyterian Hospital of Winnsboro	Winnsboro	93%	45

NOTE: Hospital profiles are in alphabetical order by state, then city, then hospital within the city; Rankings are sorted by rate in descending order and exclude hospitals with less than 25 cases; (1) The number of cases is too small (n<25) for purposes of reliably predicting hospital performance; (2) Measure reflects the hospital's indication that its submission was based upon a sample of its relevant discharges; (3) Rate reflects fewer than the maximum possible quarters of data for the measure; (4) Inaccurate information submitted and suppressed for one or more quarters; (5) No data is available from the hospital for this measure; Please refer to the User's Guide for a full explanation of data

Texoma Medical Center	Denison	93%	207
Trinity Medical Center	Carrollton	93%	143
Central Texas Medical Center	San Marcos	92%	132
Dallas Southwest Medical Center	Dallas	92%	36
Denton Regional Medical Center	Denton	92%	272
Gulf Coast Medical Center	Wharton	92%	88
Harris Methodist Continued Care Hospital	Fort Worth	92%	849
Harris Methodist HEB Hospital	Bedford	92%	274
Las Colinas Medical Center	Irving	92%	78
Medical Center of Southeast Texas	Port Arthur	92%	283
Navarro Regional Hospital	Corsicana	92%	162
Park Plaza Hospital	Houston	92%	339
Parkview Regional Hospital	Mexia	92%	158
Columbus Community Hospital	Columbus	91%	34
East Texas Medical Center-Athens	Athens	91%	280
Glen Rose Medical Center	Glen Rose	91%	34
Good Shepherd Medical Center	Longview	91%	318
Laredo Medical Center	Laredo	91%	292
Saint Luke's Episcopal Hospital	Houston	91%	1426
Valley Regional Medical Center	Brownsville	91%	246
Doctors Hospital at Renaissance	Edinburg	90%	425
El Campo Memorial Hospital	El Campo	90%	59
Harris Methodist Southwest	Fort Worth	90%	231
Houston Northwest Medical Center	Houston	90%	568
Knapp Medical Center	Weslaco	90%	337
Medical Center Hospital	Odessa	90%	362
Mesquite Community Hospital	Mesquite	90%	248
Methodist Willowbrook Hospital	Houston	90%	193
Metroplex Hospital	Killeen	90%	249
Saint Joseph Regional Health Center	Bryan	90%	589
San Jacinto Methodist Hospital	Baytown	90%	314
Sierra Medical Center	El Paso	90%	490
United Regional Healthcare System	Wichita Falls	90%	323
Wadley Regional Medical Center	Texarkana	90%	423
Zale-Lipshy University Hospital	Dallas	90%	29
Palestine Regional Medical Center	Palestine	89%	153
Providence Memorial Hospital	El Paso	89%	406
Baptist Medical Center	San Antonio	88%	431
Baptist-Saint Anthony's Health System	Amarillo	88%	274
Centennial Medical Center	Frisco	88%	81
Corpus Christi Medical Center-Bay Area	Corpus Christi	88%	455
East Houston Regional Medical Center	Houston	88%	369
East Texas Medical Center-Clarksville	Clarksville	88%	138
East Texas Medical Center-Tyler	Tyler	88%	383
Llano Memorial Hospital	Llano	88%	40
Northwest Texas Healthcare System	Amarillo	88%	326
Providence Health Center	Waco	88%	483
Shannon Medical Center	San Angelo	88%	220
University Medical Center	Lubbock	88%	285
University of Texas Health Center at Tyler	Tyler	88%	186
Bayshore Medical Center	Pasadena	87%	592
Hillcrest Baptist Medical Center	Waco	87%	283
Lubbock Heart Hospital	Lubbock	87%	275
Methodist Hospital	San Antonio	87%	1525
Presbyterian Hospital of Kaufman	Kaufman	87%	149
South Texas Regional Medical Center	Jourdanton	87%	165
Hill Country Memorial Hospital	Fredericksburg	86%	83
Las Palmas Medical Center	El Paso	86%	205
Northeast Medical Center Hospital	Humble	86%	503
Saint Luke's Community Med Ctr-The Woodlands	The Woodlands	86%	107
Covenant Medical Center	Lubbock	85%	802
Wilson N Jones Medical Center	Sherman	85%	403
Arlington Memorial Hospital	Arlington	84%	473
Childress Regional Medical Center	Childress	84%	31
East Texas Medical Center-Crockett	Crockett	84%	107
Medical Arts Hospital	Lamesa	84%	51
Physicians Specialty Hospital of El Paso	El Paso	84%	81
Stephens Memorial Hospital	Breckenridge	84%	68
Angleton-Danbury Medical Center	Angleton	83%	47
Bellville General Hospital	Bellville	83%	36
Cleveland Regional Medical Center	Cleveland	83%	141
Memorial Hospital	Dumas	83%	41
Presbyterian Hospital of Denton	Denton	83%	275
Matagorda County Hospital District	Bay City	82%	100
McAllen Medical Center	McAllen	82%	307
Nacogdoches Medical Center Hospital	Nacogdoches	82%	134
Yoakum Community Hospital	Yoakum	82%	60
Del Sol Medical Center	El Paso	81%	429
Edinburg Regional Medical Center	Edinburg	81%	154
Oakbend Medical Center	Richmond	81%	180
Twelve Oaks Hospital	Houston	81%	179
Brownwood Regional Medical Center	Brownwood	80%	162
Doctors Hospital Parkway+Tidwell	Houston	80%	287
Lake Granbury Medical Center	Granbury	80%	40
Midland Memorial Hospital	Midland	80%	333
Nacogdoches Memorial Hospital	Nacogdoches	80%	281
RHD Memorial Medical Center	Dallas	80%	137
Scenic Mountain Medical Center	Big Spring	80%	148
Sid Peterson Memorial Hospital	Kerrville	80%	117
Atlanta Memorial Hospital	Atlanta	79%	112
Christus Spohn Hospital Kleberg	Kingsville	79%	179
Hill Regional Hospital	Hillsboro	79%	122
Memorial Health System of East Texas-Lufkin	Lufkin	78%	274
Shelby Regional Medical Center	Center	78%	46
Goodall-Witcher Healthcare Foundation	Clifton	77%	65
Hopkins County Memorial Hospital	Sulphur Springs	77%	143
Memorial Medical Center Livingston	Livingston	77%	107
Odessa Regional Hospital	Odessa	77%	26
Titus Regional Medical Center	Mount Pleasant	77%	130
Rio Grande Regional Hospital	McAllen	76%	417
Seton Edgar B Davis Memorial Hospital	Luling	76%	42
Henderson Memorial Hospital	Henderson	75%	125
Comanche County Medical Center	Comanche	74%	86
East Texas Medical Center-Quitman	Quitman	74%	80
North Bay Hospital	Aransas Pass	74%	27
Doctors Hospital of Laredo	Laredo	73%	226
Ennis Regional Medical Center	Ennis	73%	99
Laird Memorial Hospital	Kilgore	73%	74
McKenna Memorial Hospital	New Braunfels	73%	165
Medical Center at Lancaster	Lancaster	73%	176
Mission Hospital	Mission	73%	275
Pampa Regional Medical Center	Pampa	73%	107
Huntsville Memorial Hospital	Huntsville	72%	85
Georgetown Healthcare System	Georgetown	71%	87
Alliance Hospital	Odessa	70%	223
East Texas Medical Center-Gilmer	Gilmer	70%	88
Tyler County Hospital	Woodville	70%	54
Val Verde Regional Medical Center	Del Rio	70%	125
Memorial Hospital	Gonzales	69%	51
Smithville Regional Hospital	Smithville	69%	80
Coleman County Medical Center	Coleman	67%	36
Guadalupe Valley Hospital	Seguin	67%	193
Medical Center of Mesquite	Mesquite	67%	394
Northeast Medical Center	Bonham	67%	63
Trinity Medical Center	Brenham	67%	54
Campbell Health System	Weatherford	65%	130
Saint Marks Medical Center	La Grange	65%	77
East Texas Medical Center-Mount Vernon	Mount Vernon	62%	26
Lavaca Medical Center	Hallettsville	61%	44
Hamilton General Hospital	Hamilton	60%	107
Palo Pinto General Hospital	Mineral Wells	60%	105
Starr County Memorial Hospital	Rio Grande City	59%	69
Renaissance Hospital-East Texas	Groves	58%	71
Seton Highland Lakes	Burnet	56%	48
Medical Center at Terrell	Terrell	53%	118
East Texas Medical Center-Trinity	Trinity	52%	48
Eastland Memorial Hospital	Eastland	52%	71
North Texas Medical Center	Gainesville	51%	103
East Texas Medical Center-Pittsburg	Pittsburg	49%	79
Southwestern General Hospital	El Paso	48%	31
Big Bend Regional Medical Center	Alpine	47%	30
Memorial Medical Center	Port Lavaca	45%	51
Renaissance Hospital Houston	Houston	44%	48
East Texas Medical Center-Fairfield	Fairfield	43%	67
Brownfield Regional Medical Center	Brownfield	42%	40
Coryell Memorial Hospital	Gatesville	41%	34
Covenant Hospital Plainview	Plainview	40%	60
Fort Duncan Medical Center	Eagle Pass	39%	220
Hereford Regional Medical Center	Hereford	35%	31
Lamb Healthcare Center	Littlefield	35%	37
Rollins Brook Community Hospital	Lampasas	25%	55
Coon Memorial Hospital	Dalhart	24%	29
Good Shephard Medical Center-Linden	Linden	21%	28
D M Cogdell Memorial Hospital	Snyder	18%	40
Pecos County Memorial Hosptial	Fort Stockton	16%	38
Colorado Fayette Medical Center	Weimar	15%	46
Otto Kaiser Memorial Hospital	Kenedy	13%	31
Covenant Hospital Levelland	Levelland	4%	25
Dimmit County Memorial Hospital	Carrizo Springs	0%	40

12. Smoking Cessation Advice

Hospital Name	City	Rate	Cases
Abilene Regional Medical Center	Abilene	100%	49
Baylor Heart and Vascular Center	Dallas	100%	50
Baylor Medical Center at Garland	Garland	100%	82
Baylor University Medical Center	Dallas	100%	249
Brownwood Regional Medical Center	Brownwood	100%	35
Christus Saint John Hospital	Houston	100%	36
Christus Saint Michael Health System	Texarkana	100%	96

NOTE: Hospital profiles are in alphabetical order by state, then city, then hospital within the city; Rankings are sorted by rate in descending order and exclude hospitals with less than 25 cases; (1) The number of cases is too small (n<25) for purposes of reliably predicting hospital performance; (2) Measure reflects the hospital's indication that its submission was based upon a sample of its relevant discharges; (3) Rate reflects fewer than the maximum possible quarters of data for the measure; (4) Inaccurate information submitted and suppressed for one or more quarters; (5) No data is available from the hospital for this measure; Please refer to the User's Guide for a full explanation of data

Christus Santa Rosa Hospital-City Centre	San Antonio	100%	90
Christus Spohn Hospital Kleberg	Kingsville	100%	43
Denton Regional Medical Center	Denton	100%	52
Detar Hospital Navarro	Victoria	100%	47
East Texas Medical Center-Athens	Athens	100%	53
Falls Community Hospital	Marlin	100%	25
Good Shepherd Medical Center	Longview	100%	60
Kingwood Medical Center	Kingwood	100%	63
Las Palmas Medical Center	El Paso	100%	30
Longview Regional Medical Center	Longview	100%	32
Medical Center of Southeast Texas	Port Arthur	100%	52
Memorial Herman Baptist Orange Hospital	Orange	100%	32
Memorial Hermann Memorial City	Houston	100%	57
Memorial Hermann-Texas Medical Center	Houston	100%	180
Mesquite Community Hospital	Mesquite	100%	78
Methodist Medical Center	Dallas	100%	131
North Central Medical Center	McKinney	100%	46
Park Plaza Hospital	Houston	100%	75
Southwest General Hospital	San Antonio	100%	72
Thomason General Hospital	El Paso	100%	92
UT Southwestern Saint Paul Hospital	Dallas	100%	67
Valley Baptist Medical Center	Harlingen	100%	54
Valley Regional Medical Center	Brownsville	100%	39
Walls Regional Hospital	Cleburne	100%	30
Woodland Heights Medical Center	Lufkin	100%	38
Christus Spohn Memorial Hospital	Corpus Christi	99%	192
Houston Northwest Medical Center	Houston	99%	119
Huguley Memorial Medical Center	Burleson	99%	91
Mother Frances Hospital-Tyler	Tyler	99%	110
Northeast Medical Center Hospital	Humble	99%	88
Saint David's Rehabiltation Center	Austin	99%	110
South Austin Hospital	Austin	99%	92
Baptist-Saint Anthony's Health System	Amarillo	98%	50
Baylor Medical Center at Irving	Irving	98%	57
Charlton Methodist Hospital	Dallas	98%	149
Covenant Medical Center	Lubbock	98%	127
Harris Methodist HEB Hospital	Bedford	98%	50
Mission Hospital	Mission	98%	52
North Hills Hospital	N Richland Hills	98%	50
Presbyterian Hospital of Dallas	Dallas	98%	123
Saint Joseph Medical Center	Houston	98%	84
Scott & White	Temple	98%	104
West Houston Medical Center	Houston	98%	93
Citizens Medical Center	Victoria	97%	33
Conroe Regional Medical Center	Conroe	97%	154
Cypress Fairbanks Medical Center and Hospital	Houston	97%	36
Mainland Medical Center	Texas City	97%	66
Memorial Hermann Healthcare System	Houston	97%	395
Presbyterian Hospital of Plano	Plano	97%	36
RHD Memorial Medical Center	Dallas	97%	39
San Jacinto Methodist Hospital	Baytown	97%	62
Bayshore Medical Center	Pasadena	96%	138
Brackenridge Hospital	Austin	96%	109
Christus Saint Elizabeth Hospital	Beaumont	96%	236
East Houston Regional Medical Center	Houston	96%	109
Medical Center of Arlington	Arlington	96%	48
Medical Center of Plano	Plano	96%	57
Memorial Hermann Baptist Beaumont	Beaumont	96%	28
Parkland Health & Hospital System	Dallas	96%	366
San Angelo Community Medical Center	San Angelo	96%	26
Del Sol Medical Center	El Paso	95%	76
Medical City Dallas	Dallas	95%	86
Presbyterian Hospital of Kaufman	Kaufman	95%	37
Saint Joseph Regional Health Center	Bryan	95%	128
Baptist Medical Center	San Antonio	94%	71
Columbia Spring Branch Medical Center	Houston	94%	67
Northwest Texas Healthcare System	Amarillo	94%	94
Plaza Medical Center	Fort Worth	94%	83
Doctors Hospital	Dallas	93%	75
North Austin Medical Center	Austin	93%	72
Providence Memorial Hospital	El Paso	93%	28
South Texas Regional Medical Center	Jourdanton	93%	27
Methodist Hospital	San Antonio	92%	232
Texoma Medical Center	Denison	92%	40
Baylor All Saints Med Ctr at Forth Worth	Fort Worth	91%	91
Rio Grande Regional Hospital	McAllen	91%	54
Harris Methodist Southwest	Fort Worth	90%	42
Hendrick Medical Center	Abilene	90%	78
Providence Health Center	Waco	90%	77
Clear Lake Regional Medical Center	Webster	89%	74
Presbyterian Hospital of Greenville	Greenville	89%	62
Seton Medical Center	Austin	89%	97
University of Texas Health Center at Tyler	Tyler	89%	47
Methodist Hospital	Houston	88%	121
University of Texas Medical Branch Hospitals	Galveston	88%	100

Arlington Memorial Hospital	Arlington	87%	95
Wadley Regional Medical Center	Texarkana	87%	71
East Texas Medical Center-Crockett	Crockett	86%	28
Medical Center of Lewisville	Lewisville	86%	42
Harris Methodist Continued Care Hospital	Fort Worth	85%	143
Saint Luke's Episcopal Hospital	Houston	85%	201
Scenic Mountain Medical Center	Big Spring	85%	26
Hopkins County Memorial Hospital	Sulphur Springs	83%	29
Paris Regional Medical Center-South Campus	Paris	82%	55
Sierra Medical Center	El Paso	82%	60
Presbyterian Hospital of Denton	Denton	81%	52
Doctors Hospital at Renaissance	Edinburg	80%	56
Heart Hospital of Austin	Austin	80%	65
Medical Center Hospital	Odessa	80%	94
Medical Center of Mesquite	Mesquite	80%	102
Cleveland Regional Medical Center	Cleveland	79%	38
Fort Duncan Medical Center	Eagle Pass	79%	39
Harris County Hospital District	Houston	79%	247
Doctors Hospital of Laredo	Laredo	77%	30
Metroplex Hospital	Killeen	77%	48
United Regional Healthcare System	Wichita Falls	77%	62
Laredo Medical Center	Laredo	76%	33
Hillcrest Baptist Medical Center	Waco	75%	68
Midland Memorial Hospital	Midland	75%	59
John Peter Smith Hospital	Fort Worth	70%	214
University Medical Center	Lubbock	68%	74
Knapp Medical Center	Weslaco	66%	32
Corpus Christi Medical Center-Bay Area	Corpus Christi	64%	67
East Texas Medical Center-Tyler	Tyler	60%	77
Brazosport Memorial Hospital	Lake Jackson	54%	28
Atlanta Memorial Hospital	Atlanta	36%	25
University Hospital	San Antonio	35%	106

Pneumonia Care

13. Appropriate Initial Antibiotic

Hospital Name	City	Rate	Cases
Graham Regional Medical Center	Graham	98%	51
Mitchell County Hospital	Colorado City	97%	30
Llano Memorial Hospital	Llano	95%	66
Saint David's Rehabiltation Center	Austin	95%	183
Seton Northwest Hospital	Austin	95%	128
Baylor Medical Center at Irving	Irving	94%	173
Childress Regional Medical Center	Childress	94%	32
College Station Medical Center	College Station	94%	54
East Texas Medical Center-Carthage	Carthage	94%	54
Medical Center of Arlington	Arlington	94%	207
Saint Joseph Medical Center	Houston	93%	179
Texoma Medical Center	Denison	93%	169
Cypress Fairbanks Medical Center and Hospital	Houston	92%	202
Good Shepherd Medical Center	Longview	92%	90
Kings Daughters Hospital	Temple	92%	49
Memorial Hermann-Texas Medical Center	Houston	92%	73
North Austin Medical Center	Austin	92%	119
Valley Regional Medical Center	Brownsville	92%	135
West Houston Medical Center	Houston	92%	147
Abilene Regional Medical Center	Abilene	91%	65
Baylor Medical Center-Ellis County	Waxahachie	91%	106
Baylor Regional Medical Center at Grapevine	Grapevine	91%	136
Doctors Hospital	Dallas	91%	193
North Central Medical Center	McKinney	91%	189
North Hills Hospital	N Richland Hills	91%	180
Seton Medical Center	Austin	91%	81
Thomason General Hospital	El Paso	91%	125
Christus Saint Catherine Hospital	Katy	90%	151
Comanche County Medical Center	Comanche	90%	41
Frio Hospital	Pearsall	90%	31
Kingwood Medical Center	Kingwood	90%	181
Matagorda County Hospital District	Bay City	90%	42
Medical Center of Plano	Plano	90%	136
Seton Highland Lakes	Burnet	90%	59
Walls Regional Hospital	Cleburne	90%	156
Wise Regional Health System	Decatur	90%	49
Baylor Medical Center at Garland	Garland	89%	179
Baylor University Medical Center	Dallas	89%	396
Christus Spohn Hospital Kleberg	Kingsville	89%	167
Citizens Medical Center	Victoria	89%	94
Cozby-Germany Hospital	Grand Saline	89%	35
Houston Northwest Medical Center	Houston	89%	237
Lake Pointe Medical Center	Rowlett	89%	100
Longview Regional Medical Center	Longview	89%	131
Medical City Dallas	Dallas	89%	124
Paris Regional Medical Center-South Campus	Paris	89%	182
Park Plaza Hospital	Houston	89%	95

NOTE: Hospital profiles are in alphabetical order by state, then city, then hospital within the city; Rankings are sorted by rate in descending order and exclude hospitals with less than 25 cases; (1) The number of cases is too small (n<25) for purposes of reliably predicting hospital performance; (2) Measure reflects the hospital's indication that its submission was based upon a sample of its relevant discharges; (3) Rate reflects fewer than the maximum possible quarters of data for the measure; (4) Inaccurate information submitted and suppressed for one or more quarters; (5) No data is available from the hospital for this measure; Please refer to the User's Guide for a full explanation of data

Hospital	City	Rate	Cases
Presbyterian Hospital of Dallas	Dallas	89%	249
Wadley Regional Medical Center	Texarkana	89%	123
Baptist Medical Center	San Antonio	88%	166
Baylor All Saints Med Ctr at Forth Worth	Fort Worth	88%	214
Christus Saint Michael Health System	Texarkana	88%	253
Detar Hospital Navarro	Victoria	88%	93
Gulf Coast Medical Center	Wharton	88%	50
Harlingen Medical Center	Harlingen	88%	101
Hill Regional Hospital	Hillsboro	88%	69
Memorial Hermann Fort Bend Hospital	Missouri City	88%	81
Methodist Willowbrook Hospital	Houston	88%	120
Palestine Regional Medical Center	Palestine	88%	80
Pampa Regional Medical Center	Pampa	88%	74
Permian General Hospital	Andrews	88%	25
Seton Edgar B Davis Memorial Hospital	Luling	88%	34
South Texas Regional Medical Center	Jourdanton	88%	119
Arlington Memorial Hospital	Arlington	87%	244
Conroe Regional Medical Center	Conroe	87%	260
Denton Regional Medical Center	Denton	87%	118
Guadalupe Valley Hospital	Seguin	87%	47
Harris County Hospital District	Houston	87%	247
Harris Methodist Continued Care Hospital	Fort Worth	87%	417
Lake Granbury Medical Center	Granbury	87%	68
Providence Health Center	Waco	87%	217
Round Rock Medical Center	Round Rock	87%	172
South Austin Hospital	Austin	87%	183
Christus Santa Rosa Hospital-City Centre	San Antonio	86%	192
Clear Lake Regional Medical Center	Webster	86%	178
East Texas Medical Center-Athens	Athens	86%	130
East Texas Medical Center-Quitman	Quitman	86%	43
Harris Methodist Northwest	Azle	86%	139
Mesquite Community Hospital	Mesquite	86%	153
Methodist Hospital	Houston	86%	209
Mother Frances Hospital Jacksonville	Jacksonville	86%	35
Presbyterian Hospital of Allen	Allen	86%	70
Smithville Regional Hospital	Smithville	86%	83
Harris Methodist HEB Hospital	Bedford	85%	194
Las Colinas Medical Center	Irving	85%	52
Memorial Herman Katy Hospital	Katy	85%	102
Saint Joseph Regional Health Center	Bryan	85%	172
Saint Luke's Episcopal Hospital	Houston	85%	255
Scott & White	Temple	85%	183
Sierra Medical Center	El Paso	85%	209
University of Texas Health Center at Tyler	Tyler	85%	110
Valley Baptist Medical Center	Harlingen	85%	332
Brackenridge Hospital	Austin	84%	108
Christus Saint John Hospital	Houston	84%	160
Mainland Medical Center	Texas City	84%	140
Mother Frances Hospital-Tyler	Tyler	84%	268
Navarro Regional Hospital	Corsicana	84%	81
San Angelo Community Medical Center	San Angelo	84%	123
Trinity Medical Center	Carrollton	84%	167
Christus Saint Elizabeth Hospital	Beaumont	83%	406
Christus Spohn Memorial Hospital	Corpus Christi	83%	537
Edinburg Regional Medical Center	Edinburg	83%	78
Huntsville Memorial Hospital	Huntsville	83%	99
McAllen Medical Center	McAllen	83%	87
Memorial Hermann Baptist Beaumont	Beaumont	83%	29
Memorial Hermann Memorial City	Houston	83%	162
Methodist Hospital	San Antonio	83%	575
Richardson Medical Center	Richardson	83%	109
University Hospital	San Antonio	83%	88
University of Texas Medical Branch Hospitals	Galveston	83%	100
Cleveland Regional Medical Center	Cleveland	82%	96
Ennis Regional Medical Center	Ennis	82%	67
Medical Center of Lewisville	Lewisville	82%	118
Memorial Hospital	Gonzales	82%	33
Methodist Medical Center	Dallas	82%	173
Northeast Medical Center Hospital	Humble	82%	197
Parkland Health & Hospital System	Dallas	82%	182
East Texas Medical Center-Pittsburg	Pittsburg	81%	27
Georgetown Healthcare System	Georgetown	81%	81
Harris Methodist Southwest	Fort Worth	81%	165
Henderson Memorial Hospital	Henderson	81%	80
Northeast Medical Center	Bonham	81%	32
San Jacinto Methodist Hospital	Baytown	81%	140
United Regional Healthcare System	Wichita Falls	81%	166
Bowie Memorial Hospital	Bowie	80%	74
Charlton Methodist Hospital	Dallas	80%	169
Doctors Hospital at Renaissance	Edinburg	80%	85
Hill Country Memorial Hospital	Fredericksburg	80%	110
Huguley Memorial Medical Center	Burleson	80%	226
Medical Center Hospital	Odessa	80%	181
Metroplex Hospital	Killeen	80%	61
Presbyterian Hospital of Kaufman	Kaufman	80%	76
Sid Peterson Memorial Hospital	Kerrville	80%	142
Wilson N Jones Medical Center	Sherman	80%	25
Centennial Medical Center	Frisco	79%	66
East Houston Regional Medical Center	Houston	79%	170
Hendrick Medical Center	Abilene	79%	218
Medical Center at Terrell	Terrell	79%	80
Nix Healthcare System	San Antonio	79%	68
Presbyterian Hospital of Plano	Plano	79%	115
RHD Memorial Medical Center	Dallas	79%	97
Rio Grande Regional Hospital	McAllen	79%	146
Baptist-Saint Anthony's Health System	Amarillo	78%	97
Big Bend Regional Medical Center	Alpine	78%	95
Covenant Medical Center	Lubbock	78%	329
Memorial Herman Baptist Orange Hospital	Orange	78%	96
Southwest General Hospital	San Antonio	78%	114
John Peter Smith Hospital	Fort Worth	77%	276
Knapp Medical Center	Weslaco	77%	189
Lavaca Medical Center	Hallettsville	77%	39
UT Southwestern Saint Paul Hospital	Dallas	77%	99
Hamilton General Hospital	Hamilton	76%	86
Hillcrest Baptist Medical Center	Waco	76%	99
McKenna Memorial Hospital	New Braunfels	76%	135
Northwest Texas Healthcare System	Amarillo	76%	245
Presbyterian Hospital of Denton	Denton	76%	130
University Medical Center	Lubbock	76%	88
Brownsville Medical Center	Brownsville	75%	107
Cuero Community Hospital	Cuero	75%	83
Doctors Hospital of Laredo	Laredo	75%	64
Falls Community Hospital	Marlin	75%	97
Goodall-Witcher Healthcare Foundation	Clifton	75%	55
Laredo Medical Center	Laredo	75%	111
Mission Hospital	Mission	75%	177
Plaza Medical Center	Fort Worth	75%	133
Presbyterian Hospital of Greenville	Greenville	75%	178
Trinity Medical Center	Brenham	75%	32
Christus Jasper Memorial Hospital	Jasper	74%	46
Columbia Spring Branch Medical Center	Houston	74%	127
Fort Duncan Medical Center	Eagle Pass	74%	110
Oakbend Medical Center	Richmond	74%	156
Providence Memorial Hospital	El Paso	74%	291
Bayshore Medical Center	Pasadena	73%	262
East Texas Medical Center-Tyler	Tyler	73%	52
Tomball Regional Hospital	Tomball	73%	41
Wilbarger General Hospital	Vernon	73%	37
Anson General Hospital	Anson	72%	25
Brownwood Regional Medical Center	Brownwood	72%	130
Corpus Christi Medical Center-Bay Area	Corpus Christi	72%	204
Las Palmas Medical Center	El Paso	72%	81
Marshall Regional Medical Center	Marshall	72%	129
Memorial Hermann Healthcare System	Houston	72%	957
Odessa Regional Hospital	Odessa	72%	47
Palo Pinto General Hospital	Mineral Wells	72%	101
Parkview Regional Hospital	Mexia	72%	107
Shannon Medical Center	San Angelo	72%	29
Shelby Regional Medical Center	Center	72%	82
Brazosport Memorial Hospital	Lake Jackson	71%	121
Coleman County Medical Center	Coleman	71%	52
Rolling Plains Memorial Hospital	Sweetwater	71%	77
Uvalde Memorial Hospital	Uvalde	71%	51
Woodland Heights Medical Center	Lufkin	71%	122
Hopkins County Memorial Hospital	Sulphur Springs	69%	139
Nacogdoches Medical Center Hospital	Nacogdoches	69%	93
Rollins Brook Community Hospital	Lampasas	69%	35
Angleton-Danbury Medical Center	Angleton	68%	73
East Texas Medical Center-Crockett	Crockett	67%	48
Titus Regional Medical Center	Mount Pleasant	67%	27
El Campo Memorial Hospital	El Campo	66%	44
Atlanta Memorial Hospital	Atlanta	65%	63
Midland Memorial Hospital	Midland	65%	200
Del Sol Medical Center	El Paso	64%	333
Medical Center of Southeast Texas	Port Arthur	63%	135
North Texas Medical Center	Gainesville	63%	46
Pecos County Memorial Hosptial	Fort Stockton	61%	54
Methodist Sugar Land Hospital	Sugar Land	60%	73
Harris Methodist Erath County	Stephenville	58%	83
Laird Memorial Hospital	Kilgore	58%	62
Scenic Mountain Medical Center	Big Spring	58%	64
Heart Hospital of Austin	Austin	56%	25
Highland Community Hospital	Lubbock	56%	34
Memorial Medical Center	Port Lavaca	52%	64
Val Verde Regional Medical Center	Del Rio	51%	55
Medical Center of Mesquite	Mesquite	50%	161
Bellville General Hospital	Bellville	48%	29
Lamb Healthcare Center	Littlefield	42%	38
Dolly Vinsant Memorial Hospital	San Benito	41%	29

NOTE: Hospital profiles are in alphabetical order by state, then city, then hospital within the city; Rankings are sorted by rate in descending order and exclude hospitals with less than 25 cases; (1) The number of cases is too small (n<25) for purposes of reliably predicting hospital performance; (2) Measure reflects the hospital's indication that its submission was based upon a sample of its relevant discharges; (3) Rate reflects fewer than the maximum possible quarters of data for the measure; (4) Inaccurate information submitted and suppressed for one or more quarters; (5) No data is available from the hospital for this measure; Please refer to the User's Guide for a full explanation of data

14. Blood Culture Timing

Hospital Name	City	Rate	Cases
Coleman County Medical Center	Coleman	100%	43
El Campo Memorial Hospital	El Campo	100%	31
Memorial Health System of East Texas-Lufkin	Lufkin	100%	35
Memorial Hermann Fort Bend Hospital	Missouri City	100%	73
Nix Healthcare System	San Antonio	100%	25
North Texas Medical Center	Gainesville	100%	31
W J Mangold Memorial Hospital	Lockney	100%	28
Christus Saint John Hospital	Houston	99%	135
Detar Hospital Navarro	Victoria	99%	88
South Texas Regional Medical Center	Jourdanton	99%	109
Walls Regional Hospital	Cleburne	99%	124
Falls Community Hospital	Marlin	98%	62
Mainland Medical Center	Texas City	98%	128
Presbyterian Hospital of Allen	Allen	98%	51
Presbyterian Hospital of Plano	Plano	98%	93
Saint Joseph Medical Center	Houston	98%	167
Cuero Community Hospital	Cuero	97%	39
Lake Pointe Medical Center	Rowlett	97%	166
Memorial Hermann Baptist Beaumont	Beaumont	97%	34
Nacogdoches Medical Center Hospital	Nacogdoches	97%	89
Presbyterian Hospital of Winnsboro	Winnsboro	97%	30
Texoma Medical Center	Denison	97%	133
Baylor Medical Center at Garland	Garland	96%	172
Centennial Medical Center	Frisco	96%	56
Citizens Medical Center	Victoria	96%	79
Clear Lake Regional Medical Center	Webster	96%	213
East Texas Medical Center-Crockett	Crockett	96%	25
Medical Center of Plano	Plano	96%	148
Memorial Herman Katy Hospital	Katy	96%	112
Presbyterian Hospital of Denton	Denton	96%	119
San Angelo Community Medical Center	San Angelo	96%	129
Shannon Medical Center	San Angelo	96%	28
Christus Saint Michael Health System	Texarkana	95%	227
Christus Santa Rosa Hospital-City Centre	San Antonio	95%	167
College Station Medical Center	College Station	95%	43
Doctors Hospital	Dallas	95%	171
East Texas Medical Center-Athens	Athens	95%	79
Edinburg Regional Medical Center	Edinburg	95%	43
Graham Regional Medical Center	Graham	95%	43
Harris Methodist Continued Care Hospital	Fort Worth	95%	648
Harris Methodist Erath County	Stephenville	95%	91
Memorial Hermann Memorial City	Houston	95%	157
Methodist Medical Center	Dallas	95%	209
Oakbend Medical Center	Richmond	95%	138
Pampa Regional Medical Center	Pampa	95%	40
Park Plaza Hospital	Houston	95%	153
Parkview Regional Hospital	Mexia	95%	74
Presbyterian Hospital of Dallas	Dallas	95%	260
Presbyterian Hospital of Kaufman	Kaufman	95%	64
Richardson Medical Center	Richardson	95%	103
Round Rock Medical Center	Round Rock	95%	136
Saint David's Rehabiltation Center	Austin	95%	206
Trinity Medical Center	Carrollton	95%	130
University of Texas Health Center at Tyler	Tyler	95%	78
Angleton-Danbury Medical Center	Angleton	94%	34
Christus Spohn Hospital Kleberg	Kingsville	94%	63
Covenant Medical Center	Lubbock	94%	477
East Houston Regional Medical Center	Houston	94%	139
Goodall-Witcher Healthcare Foundation	Clifton	94%	49
Medical City Dallas	Dallas	94%	131
Memorial Hermann-Texas Medical Center	Houston	94%	114
Methodist Hospital	Houston	94%	277
North Austin Medical Center	Austin	94%	140
Paris Regional Medical Center-South Campus	Paris	94%	153
RHD Memorial Medical Center	Dallas	94%	126
Rio Grande Regional Hospital	McAllen	94%	125
South Austin Hospital	Austin	94%	179
Wise Regional Health System	Decatur	94%	53
Baptist Medical Center	San Antonio	93%	260
Baylor Medical Center-Ellis County	Waxahachie	93%	96
Columbia Spring Branch Medical Center	Houston	93%	149
Guadalupe Valley Hospital	Seguin	93%	56
Harris Methodist Northwest	Azle	93%	114
Houston Northwest Medical Center	Houston	93%	180
Marshall Regional Medical Center	Marshall	93%	60
North Hills Hospital	N Richland Hills	93%	216
Pecos County Memorial Hosptial	Fort Stockton	93%	27
Scott & White	Temple	93%	229
Seton Highland Lakes	Burnet	93%	30
Valley Regional Medical Center	Brownsville	93%	113
Baylor All Saints Med Ctr at Forth Worth	Fort Worth	92%	198
Brownwood Regional Medical Center	Brownwood	92%	135
Christus Saint Catherine Hospital	Katy	92%	78
Doctors Hospital at Renaissance	Edinburg	92%	65
Gulf Coast Medical Center	Wharton	92%	38
Harlingen Medical Center	Harlingen	92%	99
Harris Methodist HEB Hospital	Bedford	92%	212
Hillcrest Baptist Medical Center	Waco	92%	87
Huntsville Memorial Hospital	Huntsville	92%	53
Longview Regional Medical Center	Longview	92%	126
Matagorda County Hospital District	Bay City	92%	36
Seton Edgar B Davis Memorial Hospital	Luling	92%	38
Seton Medical Center	Austin	92%	66
Arlington Memorial Hospital	Arlington	91%	264
Baylor University Medical Center	Dallas	91%	373
Del Sol Medical Center	El Paso	91%	239
Knapp Medical Center	Weslaco	91%	151
Methodist Sugar Land Hospital	Sugar Land	91%	81
Plaza Medical Center	Fort Worth	91%	137
Uvalde Memorial Hospital	Uvalde	91%	44
Big Bend Regional Medical Center	Alpine	90%	52
Charlton Methodist Hospital	Dallas	90%	156
Denton Regional Medical Center	Denton	90%	136
Georgetown Healthcare System	Georgetown	90%	62
Harris Methodist Southwest	Fort Worth	90%	187
Las Colinas Medical Center	Irving	90%	40
McKenna Memorial Hospital	New Braunfels	90%	90
Medical Center of Mesquite	Mesquite	90%	103
Memorial Hermann Healthcare System	Houston	90%	875
Methodist Willowbrook Hospital	Houston	90%	118
Metroplex Hospital	Killeen	90%	51
San Jacinto Methodist Hospital	Baytown	90%	88
Shelby Regional Medical Center	Center	90%	48
Woodland Heights Medical Center	Lufkin	90%	73
Conroe Regional Medical Center	Conroe	89%	210
Corpus Christi Medical Center-Bay Area	Corpus Christi	89%	185
Hill Regional Hospital	Hillsboro	89%	37
McAllen Medical Center	McAllen	89%	79
Mission Hospital	Mission	89%	115
Mother Frances Hospital Jacksonville	Jacksonville	89%	37
Sid Peterson Memorial Hospital	Kerrville	89%	105
UT Southwestern Saint Paul Hospital	Dallas	89%	113
Valley Baptist Medical Center	Harlingen	89%	251
Alice Regional Hospital	Alice	88%	33
Baylor Medical Center at Irving	Irving	88%	194
Cypress Fairbanks Medical Center and Hospital	Houston	88%	219
Medical Center of Arlington	Arlington	88%	237
Midland Memorial Hospital	Midland	88%	102
Mother Frances Hospital-Tyler	Tyler	88%	242
North Central Medical Center	McKinney	88%	176
Palestine Regional Medical Center	Palestine	88%	86
Saint Luke's Episcopal Hospital	Houston	88%	265
Val Verde Regional Medical Center	Del Rio	88%	40
Christus Saint Elizabeth Hospital	Beaumont	87%	392
Hendrick Medical Center	Abilene	87%	175
Las Palmas Medical Center	El Paso	87%	87
Medical Center at Terrell	Terrell	87%	71
Mesquite Community Hospital	Mesquite	87%	126
Baptist-Saint Anthony's Health System	Amarillo	86%	70
Good Shepherd Medical Center	Longview	86%	91
Henderson Memorial Hospital	Henderson	86%	56
Northeast Medical Center Hospital	Humble	86%	172
Providence Health Center	Waco	86%	182
Scenic Mountain Medical Center	Big Spring	86%	35
Bayshore Medical Center	Pasadena	85%	231
Brackenridge Hospital	Austin	85%	86
Christus Spohn Memorial Hospital	Corpus Christi	85%	513
Hill Country Memorial Hospital	Fredericksburg	85%	82
Hopkins County Memorial Hospital	Sulphur Springs	85%	66
John Peter Smith Hospital	Fort Worth	85%	255
Llano Memorial Hospital	Llano	85%	81
Medical Center Hospital	Odessa	85%	114
Palo Pinto General Hospital	Mineral Wells	85%	27
Rolling Plains Memorial Hospital	Sweetwater	85%	40
Saint Joseph Regional Health Center	Bryan	85%	169
Sierra Medical Center	El Paso	85%	195
University of Texas Medical Branch Hospitals	Galveston	85%	61
Baylor Regional Medical Center at Grapevine	Grapevine	84%	118
Brazosport Memorial Hospital	Lake Jackson	84%	94
Kingwood Medical Center	Kingwood	84%	158
Memorial Herman Baptist Orange Hospital	Orange	84%	62
Northeast Medical Center	Bonham	84%	56
Smithville Regional Hospital	Smithville	84%	62
Southwest General Hospital	San Antonio	84%	117
Thomason General Hospital	El Paso	84%	101
East Texas Medical Center-Carthage	Carthage	83%	35
Huguley Memorial Medical Center	Burleson	83%	193

NOTE: Hospital profiles are in alphabetical order by state, then city, then hospital within the city; Rankings are sorted by rate in descending order and exclude hospitals with less than 25 cases; (1) The number of cases is too small (n<25) for purposes of reliably predicting hospital performance; (2) Measure reflects the hospital's indication that its submission was based upon a sample of its relevant discharges; (3) Rate reflects fewer than the maximum possible quarters of data for the measure; (4) Inaccurate information submitted and suppressed for one or more quarters; (5) No data is available from the hospital for this measure; Please refer to the User's Guide for a full explanation of data

Methodist Hospital	San Antonio	83%	615
University Medical Center	Lubbock	83%	69
Cozby-Germany Hospital	Grand Saline	82%	40
Harris County Hospital District	Houston	82%	237
Providence Memorial Hospital	El Paso	82%	202
Seton Northwest Hospital	Austin	82%	96
Trinity Medical Center	Brenham	82%	33
United Regional Healthcare System	Wichita Falls	82%	138
Abilene Regional Medical Center	Abilene	81%	31
Brownsville Medical Center	Brownsville	81%	89
East Texas Medical Center-Quitman	Quitman	81%	37
East Texas Medical Center-Tyler	Tyler	81%	37
Lake Granbury Medical Center	Granbury	81%	64
Frio Hospital	Pearsall	80%	25
Kings Daughters Hospital	Temple	80%	35
Laird Memorial Hospital	Kilgore	80%	44
Medical Center of Lewisville	Lewisville	80%	98
Navarro Regional Hospital	Corsicana	80%	81
Christus Jasper Memorial Hospital	Jasper	79%	38
Cleveland Regional Medical Center	Cleveland	79%	72
Ennis Regional Medical Center	Ennis	79%	52
Northwest Texas Healthcare System	Amarillo	79%	137
Parkland Health & Hospital System	Dallas	79%	239
Wadley Regional Medical Center	Texarkana	79%	121
West Houston Medical Center	Houston	79%	175
University Hospital	San Antonio	78%	67
Presbyterian Hospital of Greenville	Greenville	77%	151
Wilson N Jones Medical Center	Sherman	76%	37
Medical Center of Southeast Texas	Port Arthur	75%	52
Laredo Medical Center	Laredo	74%	84
Tomball Regional Hospital	Tomball	74%	34
Odessa Regional Hospital	Odessa	73%	30
Fort Duncan Medical Center	Eagle Pass	67%	67
Doctors Hospital of Laredo	Laredo	64%	67

15. Influenza Vaccine

Hospital Name	City	Rate	Cases
Christus Saint John Hospital	Houston	100%	35
Coleman County Medical Center	Coleman	100%	29
Llano Memorial Hospital	Llano	100%	37
Northeast Medical Center	Bonham	100%	29
Texoma Medical Center	Denison	100%	43
South Texas Regional Medical Center	Jourdanton	98%	49
Goodall-Witcher Healthcare Foundation	Clifton	97%	33
Longview Regional Medical Center	Longview	97%	34
Memorial Hermann-Texas Medical Center	Houston	97%	30
Presbyterian Hospital of Kaufman	Kaufman	97%	33
Marshall Regional Medical Center	Marshall	96%	25
Trinity Medical Center	Carrollton	96%	46
Presbyterian Hospital of Dallas	Dallas	95%	83
Baylor Medical Center-Ellis County	Waxahachie	93%	29
Methodist Medical Center	Dallas	93%	56
Christus Saint Elizabeth Hospital	Beaumont	92%	114
Parkland Health & Hospital System	Dallas	92%	50
Woodland Heights Medical Center	Lufkin	92%	37
Rio Grande Regional Hospital	McAllen	91%	43
Clear Lake Regional Medical Center	Webster	90%	72
Kingwood Medical Center	Kingwood	90%	61
Baylor University Medical Center	Dallas	89%	142
Christus Saint Michael Health System	Texarkana	89%	66
Harris Methodist HEB Hospital	Bedford	89%	71
Hendrick Medical Center	Abilene	89%	70
Walls Regional Hospital	Cleburne	89%	44
Charlton Methodist Hospital	Dallas	88%	50
Palestine Regional Medical Center	Palestine	88%	25
RHD Memorial Medical Center	Dallas	88%	43
Brownwood Regional Medical Center	Brownwood	87%	70
Cypress Fairbanks Medical Center and Hospital	Houston	87%	76
Baylor All Saints Med Ctr at Forth Worth	Fort Worth	86%	69
Saint Joseph Medical Center	Houston	86%	44
Bayshore Medical Center	Pasadena	85%	72
Good Shepherd Medical Center	Longview	85%	27
Harris Methodist Continued Care Hospital	Fort Worth	85%	180
Harris Methodist Northwest	Azle	84%	44
Harris Methodist Southwest	Fort Worth	84%	63
Sierra Medical Center	El Paso	84%	76
Detar Hospital Navarro	Victoria	83%	36
Harris Methodist Erath County	Stephenville	83%	42
Thomason General Hospital	El Paso	83%	29
University of Texas Health Center at Tyler	Tyler	83%	35
Hill Country Memorial Hospital	Fredericksburg	82%	38
Nacogdoches Medical Center Hospital	Nacogdoches	82%	33
Arlington Memorial Hospital	Arlington	81%	62
Baylor Regional Medical Center at Grapevine	Grapevine	81%	37

Mainland Medical Center	Texas City	81%	42
Memorial Hermann Memorial City	Houston	81%	53
Columbia Spring Branch Medical Center	Houston	79%	42
South Austin Hospital	Austin	79%	57
Round Rock Medical Center	Round Rock	78%	36
Baptist Medical Center	San Antonio	77%	100
Big Bend Regional Medical Center	Alpine	77%	31
Saint David's Rehabiltation Center	Austin	77%	62
Doctors Hospital	Dallas	76%	54
North Austin Medical Center	Austin	76%	37
Wadley Regional Medical Center	Texarkana	76%	49
Baylor Medical Center at Irving	Irving	75%	64
West Houston Medical Center	Houston	75%	48
Brazosport Memorial Hospital	Lake Jackson	74%	34
East Texas Medical Center-Athens	Athens	73%	33
Huguley Memorial Medical Center	Burleson	73%	73
Paris Regional Medical Center-South Campus	Paris	72%	82
Conroe Regional Medical Center	Conroe	71%	62
Covenant Medical Center	Lubbock	70%	186
Hopkins County Memorial Hospital	Sulphur Springs	70%	37
Methodist Hospital	Houston	70%	64
Mother Frances Hospital-Tyler	Tyler	70%	109
Midland Memorial Hospital	Midland	68%	47
Medical Center of Arlington	Arlington	67%	69
Shelby Regional Medical Center	Center	64%	25
Medical Center of Lewisville	Lewisville	63%	51
North Hills Hospital	N Richland Hills	63%	59
Harlingen Medical Center	Harlingen	62%	42
Pampa Regional Medical Center	Pampa	62%	29
Houston Northwest Medical Center	Houston	61%	72
McAllen Medical Center	McAllen	60%	25
Presbyterian Hospital of Denton	Denton	60%	57
Presbyterian Hospital of Greenville	Greenville	60%	68
San Angelo Community Medical Center	San Angelo	60%	57
Navarro Regional Hospital	Corsicana	59%	32
United Regional Healthcare System	Wichita Falls	59%	44
Corpus Christi Medical Center-Bay Area	Corpus Christi	58%	79
McKenna Memorial Hospital	New Braunfels	58%	40
Northwest Texas Healthcare System	Amarillo	58%	52
Plaza Medical Center	Fort Worth	57%	51
Hamilton General Hospital	Hamilton	56%	36
Medical Center of Mesquite	Mesquite	56%	45
Presbyterian Hospital of Plano	Plano	56%	27
Denton Regional Medical Center	Denton	55%	58
Methodist Hospital	San Antonio	55%	231
Mesquite Community Hospital	Mesquite	54%	39
North Central Medical Center	McKinney	54%	46
Baylor Medical Center at Garland	Garland	52%	50
East Houston Regional Medical Center	Houston	52%	40
Laredo Medical Center	Laredo	52%	27
UT Southwestern Saint Paul Hospital	Dallas	51%	35
Ennis Regional Medical Center	Ennis	48%	25
Medical City Dallas	Dallas	48%	44
Northeast Medical Center Hospital	Humble	48%	54
Richardson Medical Center	Richardson	44%	27
Saint Joseph Regional Health Center	Bryan	44%	66
Medical Center Hospital	Odessa	43%	58
San Jacinto Methodist Hospital	Baytown	43%	28
Valley Baptist Medical Center	Harlingen	42%	86
Baptist-Saint Anthony's Health System	Amarillo	41%	27
Del Sol Medical Center	El Paso	39%	88
Smithville Regional Hospital	Smithville	39%	28
Citizens Medical Center	Victoria	38%	50
Medical Center of Southeast Texas	Port Arthur	31%	26
Brownsville Medical Center	Brownsville	30%	47
Mission Hospital	Mission	29%	58
Providence Health Center	Waco	26%	69
Valley Regional Medical Center	Brownsville	23%	43
Guadalupe Valley Hospital	Seguin	8%	25
John Peter Smith Hospital	Fort Worth	2%	58
Medical Center of Plano	Plano	0%	58

16. Initial Antibiotic Timing

Hospital Name	City	Rate	Cases
Anson General Hospital	Anson	100%	29
Presbyterian Hospital of Kaufman	Kaufman	98%	89
Shelby Regional Medical Center	Center	98%	84
Harris Methodist Northwest	Azle	97%	161
Hill Regional Hospital	Hillsboro	97%	86
Memorial Hermann Fort Bend Hospital	Missouri City	97%	94
Mother Frances Hospital Jacksonville	Jacksonville	97%	35
W J Mangold Memorial Hospital	Lockney	97%	31
Cuero Community Hospital	Cuero	96%	103
Bowie Memorial Hospital	Bowie	95%	111

NOTE: Hospital profiles are in alphabetical order by state, then city, then hospital within the city; Rankings are sorted by rate in descending order and exclude hospitals with less than 25 cases; (1) The number of cases is too small (n<25) for purposes of reliably predicting hospital performance; (2) Measure reflects the hospital's indication that its submission was based upon a sample of its relevant discharges; (3) Rate reflects fewer than the maximum possible quarters of data for the measure; (4) Inaccurate information submitted and suppressed for one or more quarters; (5) No data is available from the hospital for this measure; Please refer to the User's Guide for a full explanation of data

Hospital	City	Rate	Cases
Christus Spohn Hospital Beeville	Beeville	95%	96
Nix Healthcare System	San Antonio	95%	58
Walls Regional Hospital	Cleburne	95%	164
Centennial Medical Center	Frisco	94%	68
Cozby-Germany Hospital	Grand Saline	94%	64
Frio Hospital	Pearsall	94%	36
Brownfield Regional Medical Center	Brownfield	93%	41
Campbell Health System	Weatherford	93%	158
Glen Rose Medical Center	Glen Rose	93%	94
Graham Regional Medical Center	Graham	93%	86
Lake Pointe Medical Center	Rowlett	93%	207
North Central Medical Center	McKinney	93%	263
Baylor Regional Medical Center at Plano	Plano	92%	75
Christus Saint John Hospital	Houston	92%	165
Coleman County Medical Center	Coleman	92%	36
Laird Memorial Hospital	Kilgore	92%	86
Memorial Herman Katy Hospital	Katy	92%	145
Mitchell County Hospital	Colorado City	92%	50
Baylor All Saints Med Ctr at Forth Worth	Fort Worth	91%	257
Baylor Medical Center-Ellis County	Waxahachie	91%	139
Big Bend Regional Medical Center	Alpine	91%	113
East Texas Medical Center-Quitman	Quitman	91%	57
Lavaca Medical Center	Hallettsville	91%	69
Medical Center of Arlington	Arlington	91%	298
Presbyterian Hospital of Allen	Allen	91%	65
Presbyterian Hospital of Winnsboro	Winnsboro	91%	35
Richardson Medical Center	Richardson	91%	159
Stephens Memorial Hospital	Breckenridge	91%	43
Baylor Medical Center at Irving	Irving	90%	265
College Station Medical Center	College Station	90%	60
Covenant Hospital Levelland	Levelland	90%	30
East Texas Medical Center-Crockett	Crockett	90%	70
East Texas Medical Center-Jacksonville	Jacksonville	90%	90
Christus Saint Catherine Hospital	Katy	89%	143
Columbus Community Hospital	Columbus	89%	37
Harris Methodist Continued Care Hospital	Fort Worth	89%	776
Harris Methodist Erath County	Stephenville	89%	122
Harris Methodist HEB Hospital	Bedford	89%	257
Nocona General Hospital	Nocona	89%	44
Presbyterian Hospital of Dallas	Dallas	89%	351
Sid Peterson Memorial Hospital	Kerrville	89%	224
East Texas Medical Center-Carthage	Carthage	88%	50
Falls Community Hospital	Marlin	88%	144
Hamilton General Hospital	Hamilton	88%	93
Mainland Medical Center	Texas City	88%	192
Pampa Regional Medical Center	Pampa	88%	103
Parkview Regional Hospital	Mexia	88%	151
Rollins Brook Community Hospital	Lampasas	88%	50
Smithville Regional Hospital	Smithville	88%	129
Arlington Memorial Hospital	Arlington	87%	346
Bellville General Hospital	Bellville	87%	47
Columbia Spring Branch Medical Center	Houston	87%	253
East Texas Medical Center-Clarksville	Clarksville	87%	116
Harris Methodist Southwest	Fort Worth	87%	237
Saint Joseph Medical Center	Houston	87%	239
Scenic Mountain Medical Center	Big Spring	87%	68
Woodland Heights Medical Center	Lufkin	87%	141
Baylor Regional Medical Center at Grapevine	Grapevine	86%	159
Goodall-Witcher Healthcare Foundation	Clifton	86%	83
Llano Memorial Hospital	Llano	86%	133
Longview Regional Medical Center	Longview	86%	175
Marshall Regional Medical Center	Marshall	86%	111
Matagorda County Hospital District	Bay City	86%	58
Memorial Hospital	Dumas	86%	50
Tyler County Hospital	Woodville	86%	63
Baylor Medical Center at Garland	Garland	85%	202
Gulf Coast Medical Center	Wharton	85%	71
Henderson Memorial Hospital	Henderson	85%	108
Kings Daughters Hospital	Temple	85%	59
Lake Granbury Medical Center	Granbury	85%	79
Methodist Willowbrook Hospital	Houston	85%	140
Pecos County Memorial Hosptial	Fort Stockton	85%	59
Christus Spohn Hospital Kleberg	Kingsville	84%	204
Citizens Medical Center	Victoria	84%	150
Harlingen Medical Center	Harlingen	84%	153
Methodist Hospital	Houston	84%	403
Methodist Sugar Land Hospital	Sugar Land	84%	111
North Texas Medical Center	Gainesville	84%	57
Oakbend Medical Center	Richmond	84%	221
Trinity Medical Center	Carrollton	84%	185
Alice Regional Hospital	Alice	83%	213
Brazosport Memorial Hospital	Lake Jackson	83%	160
Coryell Memorial Hospital	Gatesville	83%	78
Detar Hospital Navarro	Victoria	83%	118
East Texas Medical Center-Athens	Athens	83%	187
Las Colinas Medical Center	Irving	83%	63
Medical Center of Plano	Plano	83%	211
Reeves County Hospital	Pecos	83%	36
Renaissance Hospital Houston	Houston	83%	29
Texoma Medical Center	Denison	83%	212
Trinity Medical Center	Brenham	83%	48
Wilson N Jones Medical Center	Sherman	83%	248
Yoakum Community Hospital	Yoakum	83%	30
Charlton Methodist Hospital	Dallas	82%	291
Childress Regional Medical Center	Childress	82%	55
Christus Saint Michael Health System	Texarkana	82%	358
Cypress Fairbanks Medical Center and Hospital	Houston	82%	265
Eastland Memorial Hospital	Eastland	82%	114
Lamb Healthcare Center	Littlefield	82%	44
Memorial Hermann Baptist Beaumont	Beaumont	82%	250
North Hills Hospital	N Richland Hills	82%	240
Palestine Regional Medical Center	Palestine	82%	130
Presbyterian Hospital of Plano	Plano	82%	120
Saint David's Rehabiltation Center	Austin	82%	276
Christus Saint Elizabeth Hospital	Beaumont	81%	564
Denton Regional Medical Center	Denton	81%	200
Memorial Hermann Memorial City	Houston	81%	234
Mesquite Community Hospital	Mesquite	81%	175
Seton Edgar B Davis Memorial Hospital	Luling	81%	47
Southwest General Hospital	San Antonio	81%	152
Baptist Medical Center	San Antonio	80%	376
Brownwood Regional Medical Center	Brownwood	80%	225
Christus Santa Rosa Hospital-City Centre	San Antonio	80%	257
Hereford Regional Medical Center	Hereford	80%	44
Medical Center at Terrell	Terrell	80%	112
Methodist Medical Center	Dallas	80%	266
Presbyterian Hospital of Denton	Denton	80%	181
Scott & White	Temple	80%	317
Wise Regional Health System	Decatur	80%	61
Baylor University Medical Center	Dallas	79%	573
Clear Lake Regional Medical Center	Webster	79%	267
Colorado Fayette Medical Center	Weimar	79%	48
El Campo Memorial Hospital	El Campo	79%	70
Good Shepherd Medical Center	Longview	79%	141
Highland Community Hospital	Lubbock	79%	34
Hill Country Memorial Hospital	Fredericksburg	79%	160
Kell West Regional Hospital	Wichita Falls	79%	34
Medical City Dallas	Dallas	79%	189
Nacogdoches Medical Center Hospital	Nacogdoches	79%	130
RHD Memorial Medical Center	Dallas	79%	163
Seton Highland Lakes	Burnet	79%	57
South Texas Regional Medical Center	Jourdanton	79%	162
Uvalde Memorial Hospital	Uvalde	79%	73
Central Texas Medical Center	San Marcos	78%	123
Comanche County Medical Center	Comanche	78%	49
East Texas Medical Center-Pittsburg	Pittsburg	78%	32
Guadalupe Valley Hospital	Seguin	78%	91
Memorial Hermann Healthcare System	Houston	78%	1245
Saint Joseph Regional Health System	Bryan	78%	228
San Angelo Community Medical Center	San Angelo	78%	190
Wadley Regional Medical Center	Texarkana	78%	207
Conroe Regional Medical Center	Conroe	77%	337
Doctors Hospital	Dallas	77%	225
Ennis Regional Medical Center	Ennis	77%	96
Huguley Memorial Medical Center	Burleson	77%	308
North Bay Hospital	Aransas Pass	77%	30
Northeast Medical Center	Bonham	77%	53
Providence Health Center	Waco	77%	261
Round Rock Medical Center	Round Rock	77%	206
Seton Northwest Hospital	Austin	77%	152
East Houston Regional Medical Center	Houston	76%	223
Georgetown Healthcare System	Georgetown	76%	99
Hillcrest Baptist Medical Center	Waco	76%	136
Kingwood Medical Center	Kingwood	76%	249
Las Palmas Medical Center	El Paso	76%	136
McKenna Memorial Hospital	New Braunfels	76%	164
Memorial Hermann-Texas Medical Center	Houston	76%	135
Paris Regional Medical Center-South Campus	Paris	76%	272
United Regional Healthcare System	Wichita Falls	76%	222
Valley Baptist Medical Center	Harlingen	76%	369
Cleveland Regional Medical Center	Cleveland	75%	128
Huntsville Memorial Hospital	Huntsville	75%	91
Navarro Regional Hospital	Corsicana	75%	136
Covenant Medical Center	Lubbock	74%	616
Medical Center Hospital	Odessa	74%	188
Mother Frances Hospital-Tyler	Tyler	74%	328
Park Plaza Hospital	Houston	74%	210
Saint Marks Medical Center	La Grange	74%	105
San Jacinto Methodist Hospital	Baytown	74%	184
Shannon Medical Center	San Angelo	74%	255

NOTE: Hospital profiles are in alphabetical order by state, then city, then hospital within the city; Rankings are sorted by rate in descending order and exclude hospitals with less than 25 cases; (1) The number of cases is too small (n<25) for purposes of reliably predicting hospital performance; (2) Measure reflects the hospital's indication that its submission was based upon a sample of its relevant discharges; (3) Rate reflects fewer than the maximum possible quarters of data for the measure; (4) Inaccurate information submitted and suppressed for one or more quarters; (5) No data is available from the hospital for this measure; Please refer to the User's Guide for a full explanation of data

Hendrick Medical Center	Abilene	73%	259
Hopkins County Memorial Hospital	Sulphur Springs	73%	164
Memorial Medical Center	Port Lavaca	73%	48
Odessa Regional Hospital	Odessa	73%	44
Rolling Plains Memorial Hospital	Sweetwater	73%	102
University Medical Center	Lubbock	73%	129
Abilene Regional Medical Center	Abilene	72%	67
Christus Spohn Memorial Hospital	Corpus Christi	72%	801
D M Cogdell Memorial Hospital	Snyder	72%	39
Laredo Medical Center	Laredo	72%	140
Medical Arts Hospital	Lamesa	72%	58
Seton Medical Center	Austin	72%	135
Valley Regional Medical Center	Brownsville	72%	183
Brackenridge Hospital	Austin	71%	144
Covenant Hospital Plainview	Plainview	71%	49
Dolly Vinsant Memorial Hospital	San Benito	71%	34
East Texas Medical Center-Fairfield	Fairfield	71%	34
Memorial Medical Center Livingston	Livingston	71%	86
North Austin Medical Center	Austin	71%	177
Rio Grande Regional Hospital	McAllen	71%	238
Tomball Regional Hospital	Tomball	71%	249
Corpus Christi Medical Center-Bay Area	Corpus Christi	70%	297
Palo Pinto General Hospital	Mineral Wells	70%	103
Providence Memorial Hospital	El Paso	70%	361
Saint Luke's Episcopal Hospital	Houston	70%	358
South Austin Hospital	Austin	70%	230
Bayshore Medical Center	Pasadena	69%	369
Northwest Texas Healthcare System	Amarillo	69%	229
Plaza Medical Center	Fort Worth	69%	191
Presbyterian Hospital of Greenville	Greenville	69%	221
UT Southwestern Saint Paul Hospital	Dallas	69%	151
Alliance Hospital	Odessa	68%	56
Atlanta Memorial Hospital	Atlanta	68%	90
Christus Jasper Memorial Hospital	Jasper	68%	69
Memorial Herman Baptist Orange Hospital	Orange	68%	107
Wilbarger General Hospital	Vernon	68%	38
Del Sol Medical Center	El Paso	67%	451
Methodist Hospital	San Antonio	67%	955
Sierra Medical Center	El Paso	67%	303
Dimmit County Memorial Hospital	Carrizo Springs	66%	29
Fort Duncan Medical Center	Eagle Pass	66%	116
Renaissance Hospital-East Texas	Groves	66%	44
Doctors Hospital of Laredo	Laredo	65%	121
Houston Northwest Medical Center	Houston	64%	353
Medical Center of Lewisville	Lewisville	64%	192
Nacogdoches Memorial Hospital	Nacogdoches	64%	160
Saint Luke's Community Med Ctr-The Woodlands	The Woodlands	64%	105
Heart Hospital of Austin	Austin	63%	30
Knapp Medical Center	Weslaco	63%	278
Thomason General Hospital	El Paso	63%	145
West Houston Medical Center	Houston	63%	236
Medical Center of Mesquite	Mesquite	62%	192
Memorial Health System of East Texas-Lufkin	Lufkin	62%	251
Twelve Oaks Hospital	Houston	62%	53
Metroplex Hospital	Killeen	61%	84
University of Texas Health Center at Tyler	Tyler	61%	199
Angleton-Danbury Medical Center	Angleton	60%	78
Doctors Hospital Parkway+Tidwell	Houston	60%	126
Midland Memorial Hospital	Midland	60%	205
Brownsville Medical Center	Brownsville	59%	169
Southwestern General Hospital	El Paso	59%	32
Starr County Memorial Hospital	Rio Grande City	59%	46
East Texas Medical Center-Gilmer	Gilmer	58%	65
Baptist-Saint Anthony's Health System	Amarillo	57%	159
East Texas Medical Center-Tyler	Tyler	57%	81
Memorial Hospital	Gonzales	57%	53
Edinburg Regional Medical Center	Edinburg	56%	90
Mission Hospital	Mission	56%	224
Northeast Medical Center Hospital	Humble	56%	278
Connally Memorial Medical Center	Floresville	55%	42
Val Verde Regional Medical Center	Del Rio	55%	65
McAllen Medical Center	McAllen	54%	133
Medical Center of Southeast Texas	Port Arthur	54%	134
Coon Memorial Hospital	Dalhart	53%	30
Titus Regional Medical Center	Mount Pleasant	53%	221
Medical Center at Lancaster	Lancaster	49%	49
Harris County Hospital District	Houston	48%	332
University Hospital	San Antonio	47%	109
Doctors Hospital at Renaissance	Edinburg	46%	112
East Texas Medical Center-Trinity	Trinity	46%	41
University of Texas Medical Branch Hospitals	Galveston	41%	143
John Peter Smith Hospital	Fort Worth	40%	339
Parkland Health & Hospital System	Dallas	39%	315
Physicians Specialty Hospital of El Paso	El Paso	36%	80

17. Oxygenation Assessment

Hospital Name	City	Rate	Cases
Abilene Regional Medical Center	Abilene	100%	87
Alliance Hospital	Odessa	100%	71
Arlington Memorial Hospital	Arlington	100%	396
Baptist Medical Center	San Antonio	100%	441
Baptist-Saint Anthony's Health System	Amarillo	100%	175
Baylor All Saints Med Ctr at Forth Worth	Fort Worth	100%	300
Baylor Medical Center at Garland	Garland	100%	281
Baylor Medical Center at Irving	Irving	100%	299
Baylor Medical Center-Ellis County	Waxahachie	100%	167
Baylor Regional Medical Center at Grapevine	Grapevine	100%	201
Baylor Regional Medical Center at Plano	Plano	100%	106
Baylor University Medical Center	Dallas	100%	691
Big Bend Regional Medical Center	Alpine	100%	121
Bowie Memorial Hospital	Bowie	100%	134
Brownfield Regional Medical Center	Brownfield	100%	45
Brownwood Regional Medical Center	Brownwood	100%	272
Campbell Health System	Weatherford	100%	214
Centennial Medical Center	Frisco	100%	96
Charlton Methodist Hospital	Dallas	100%	312
Childress Regional Medical Center	Childress	100%	67
Christus Jasper Memorial Hospital	Jasper	100%	78
Christus Saint Catherine Hospital	Katy	100%	159
Christus Saint John Hospital	Houston	100%	191
Christus Saint Michael Health System	Texarkana	100%	413
Christus Santa Rosa Hospital-City Centre	San Antonio	100%	281
Christus Spohn Memorial Hospital	Corpus Christi	100%	939
Citizens Medical Center	Victoria	100%	175
Coleman County Medical Center	Coleman	100%	96
College Station Medical Center	College Station	100%	75
Colorado Fayette Medical Center	Weimar	100%	57
Comanche County Medical Center	Comanche	100%	60
Connally Memorial Medical Center	Floresville	100%	52
Coon Memorial Hospital	Dalhart	100%	36
Coryell Memorial Hospital	Gatesville	100%	98
Covenant Hospital Plainview	Plainview	100%	63
Covenant Medical Center	Lubbock	100%	726
Cozby-Germany Hospital	Grand Saline	100%	74
Cuero Community Hospital	Cuero	100%	119
Cypress Fairbanks Medical Center and Hospital	Houston	100%	379
Denton Regional Medical Center	Denton	100%	239
Detar Hospital Navarro	Victoria	100%	152
Doctors Hospital	Dallas	100%	284
Doctors Hospital at Renaissance	Edinburg	100%	153
Doctors Hospital of Laredo	Laredo	100%	127
Dolly Vinsant Memorial Hospital	San Benito	100%	40
East Texas Medical Center-Carthage	Carthage	100%	69
East Texas Medical Center-Gilmer	Gilmer	100%	93
East Texas Medical Center-Jacksonville	Jacksonville	100%	106
East Texas Medical Center-Pittsburg	Pittsburg	100%	40
East Texas Medical Center-Quitman	Quitman	100%	75
East Texas Medical Center-Trinity	Trinity	100%	51
East Texas Medical Center-Tyler	Tyler	100%	101
El Campo Memorial Hospital	El Campo	100%	77
Falls Community Hospital	Marlin	100%	165
Frio Hospital	Pearsall	100%	44
Glen Rose Medical Center	Glen Rose	100%	114
Graham Regional Medical Center	Graham	100%	101
Guadalupe Valley Hospital	Seguin	100%	103
Harlingen Medical Center	Harlingen	100%	165
Harris Methodist Continued Care Hospital	Fort Worth	100%	903
Harris Methodist HEB Hospital	Bedford	100%	327
Harris Methodist Northwest	Azle	100%	210
Harris Methodist Southwest	Fort Worth	100%	292
Henderson Memorial Hospital	Henderson	100%	128
Hendrick Medical Center	Abilene	100%	317
Hereford Regional Medical Center	Hereford	100%	53
Highland Community Hospital	Lubbock	100%	40
Hill Country Memorial Hospital	Fredericksburg	100%	195
Hill Regional Hospital	Hillsboro	100%	101
Hillcrest Baptist Medical Center	Waco	100%	188
Hopkins County Memorial Hospital	Sulphur Springs	100%	209
Houston Northwest Medical Center	Houston	100%	417
John Peter Smith Hospital	Fort Worth	100%	389
Kell West Regional Hospital	Wichita Falls	100%	39
Kings Daughters Hospital	Temple	100%	62
Laird Memorial Hospital	Kilgore	100%	95
Lake Granbury Medical Center	Granbury	100%	108
Lake Pointe Medical Center	Rowlett	100%	290
Laredo Medical Center	Laredo	100%	154
Las Colinas Medical Center	Irving	100%	65
Lavaca Medical Center	Hallettsville	100%	82
Llano Memorial Hospital	Llano	100%	152

NOTE: Hospital profiles are in alphabetical order by state, then city, then hospital within the city; Rankings are sorted by rate in descending order and exclude hospitals with less than 25 cases; (1) The number of cases is too small (n<25) for purposes of reliably predicting hospital performance; (2) Measure reflects the hospital's indication that its submission was based upon a sample of its relevant discharges; (3) Rate reflects fewer than the maximum possible quarters of data for the measure; (4) Inaccurate information submitted and suppressed for one or more quarters; (5) No data is available from the hospital for this measure; Please refer to the User's Guide for a full explanation of data

Hospital	City	Rate	Cases
McKenna Memorial Hospital	New Braunfels	100%	196
Medical Arts Hospital	Lamesa	100%	69
Medical Center Hospital	Odessa	100%	240
Medical Center at Lancaster	Lancaster	100%	75
Medical Center at Terrell	Terrell	100%	137
Medical Center of Arlington	Arlington	100%	371
Medical Center of Mesquite	Mesquite	100%	251
Medical Center of Plano	Plano	100%	259
Medical City Dallas	Dallas	100%	235
Memorial Herman Baptist Orange Hospital	Orange	100%	121
Memorial Hermann Katy Hospital	Katy	100%	180
Memorial Hermann Baptist Beaumont	Beaumont	100%	282
Memorial Hermann Fort Bend Hospital	Missouri City	100%	116
Memorial Hermann Healthcare System	Houston	100%	1468
Memorial Hermann Memorial City	Houston	100%	286
Memorial Hermann-Texas Medical Center	Houston	100%	173
Memorial Hospital	Gonzales	100%	56
Mesquite Community Hospital	Mesquite	100%	204
Methodist Hospital	Houston	100%	448
Methodist Medical Center	Dallas	100%	312
Methodist Sugar Land Hospital	Sugar Land	100%	140
Metroplex Hospital	Killeen	100%	101
Midland Memorial Hospital	Midland	100%	257
Mitchell County Hospital	Colorado City	100%	62
Mother Frances Hospital Jacksonville	Jacksonville	100%	43
Mother Frances Hospital-Tyler	Tyler	100%	448
Nacogdoches Medical Center Hospital	Nacogdoches	100%	162
Nix Healthcare System	San Antonio	100%	93
North Austin Medical Center	Austin	100%	219
North Central Medical Center	McKinney	100%	330
North Hills Hospital	N Richland Hills	100%	299
Northeast Medical Center	Bonham	100%	77
Northwest Texas Healthcare System	Amarillo	100%	281
Odessa Regional Hospital	Odessa	100%	52
Otto Kaiser Memorial Hospital	Kenedy	100%	25
Palestine Regional Medical Center	Palestine	100%	165
Palo Pinto General Hospital	Mineral Wells	100%	117
Park Plaza Hospital	Houston	100%	255
Parkview Regional Hospital	Mexia	100%	175
Pecos County Memorial Hosptial	Fort Stockton	100%	76
Physicians Specialty Hospital of El Paso	El Paso	100%	109
Presbyterian Hospital of Allen	Allen	100%	87
Presbyterian Hospital of Dallas	Dallas	100%	412
Presbyterian Hospital of Denton	Denton	100%	253
Presbyterian Hospital of Kaufman	Kaufman	100%	116
Presbyterian Hospital of Plano	Plano	100%	150
Presbyterian Hospital of Winnsboro	Winnsboro	100%	51
Providence Health Center	Waco	100%	322
Providence Memorial Hospital	El Paso	100%	436
RHD Memorial Medical Center	Dallas	100%	212
Reeves County Hospital	Pecos	100%	40
Renaissance Hospital-East Texas	Groves	100%	63
Richardson Medical Center	Richardson	100%	192
Rolling Plains Memorial Hospital	Sweetwater	100%	111
Rollins Brook Community Hospital	Lampasas	100%	70
Round Rock Medical Center	Round Rock	100%	222
Saint David's Rehabiltation Center	Austin	100%	321
Saint Luke's Episcopal Hospital	Houston	100%	470
San Angelo Community Medical Center	San Angelo	100%	224
San Jacinto Methodist Hospital	Baytown	100%	221
Scenic Mountain Medical Center	Big Spring	100%	80
Scott & White	Temple	100%	416
Seton Edgar B Davis Memorial Hospital	Luling	100%	54
Seton Highland Lakes	Burnet	100%	73
Seton Medical Center	Austin	100%	145
Seton Southwest Healthcare Center	Austin	100%	26
Seymour Hospital	Seymour	100%	32
Shannon Medical Center	San Angelo	100%	308
Sid Peterson Memorial Hospital	Kerrville	100%	269
Smithville Regional Hospital	Smithville	100%	148
South Austin Hospital	Austin	100%	303
South Texas Regional Medical Center	Jourdanton	100%	182
Southwestern General Hospital	El Paso	100%	39
Stephens Memorial Hospital	Breckenridge	100%	57
Texoma Medical Center	Denison	100%	236
Thomason General Hospital	El Paso	100%	156
Tomball Regional Hospital	Tomball	100%	310
Trinity Medical Center	Brenham	100%	65
Twelve Oaks Hospital	Houston	100%	70
Tyler County Hospital	Woodville	100%	70
United Regional Healthcare System	Wichita Falls	100%	272
University Hospital	San Antonio	100%	137
University Medical Center	Lubbock	100%	158
University of Texas Health Center at Tyler	Tyler	100%	225
Uvalde Memorial Hospital	Uvalde	100%	87
Valley Baptist Medical Center	Harlingen	100%	440
W J Mangold Memorial Hospital	Lockney	100%	57
Wadley Regional Medical Center	Texarkana	100%	227
Walls Regional Hospital	Cleburne	100%	216
Wilbarger General Hospital	Vernon	100%	47
Wise Regional Health System	Decatur	100%	74
Woodland Heights Medical Center	Lufkin	100%	169
Yoakum Community Hospital	Yoakum	100%	34
Alice Regional Hospital	Alice	99%	235
Brackenridge Hospital	Austin	99%	152
Central Texas Medical Center	San Marcos	99%	158
Christus Saint Elizabeth Hospital	Beaumont	99%	636
Christus Spohn Hospital Beeville	Beeville	99%	115
Clear Lake Regional Medical Center	Webster	99%	338
Conroe Regional Medical Center	Conroe	99%	383
Corpus Christi Medical Center-Bay Area	Corpus Christi	99%	377
Del Sol Medical Center	El Paso	99%	535
East Texas Medical Center-Athens	Athens	99%	208
East Texas Medical Center-Clarksville	Clarksville	99%	145
Edinburg Regional Medical Center	Edinburg	99%	120
Ennis Regional Medical Center	Ennis	99%	107
Georgetown Healthcare System	Georgetown	99%	140
Good Shepherd Medical Center	Longview	99%	167
Goodall-Witcher Healthcare Foundation	Clifton	99%	118
Harris Methodist Erath County	Stephenville	99%	160
Longview Regional Medical Center	Longview	99%	197
Mainland Medical Center	Texas City	99%	227
Marshall Regional Medical Center	Marshall	99%	133
Methodist Hospital	San Antonio	99%	1147
Methodist Willowbrook Hospital	Houston	99%	189
Navarro Regional Hospital	Corsicana	99%	164
North Texas Medical Center	Gainesville	99%	70
Northeast Medical Center Hospital	Humble	99%	324
Pampa Regional Medical Center	Pampa	99%	119
Paris Regional Medical Center-South Campus	Paris	99%	348
Parkland Health & Hospital System	Dallas	99%	368
Plaza Medical Center	Fort Worth	99%	241
Presbyterian Hospital of Greenville	Greenville	99%	292
Saint Joseph Medical Center	Houston	99%	258
Saint Luke's Community Med Ctr-The Woodlands	The Woodlands	99%	145
Seton Northwest Hospital	Austin	99%	168
Shelby Regional Medical Center	Center	99%	105
Sierra Medical Center	El Paso	99%	380
Southwest General Hospital	San Antonio	99%	182
Trinity Medical Center	Carrollton	99%	228
UT Southwestern Saint Paul Hospital	Dallas	99%	231
West Houston Medical Center	Houston	99%	288
Wilson N Jones Medical Center	Sherman	99%	288
Angleton-Danbury Medical Center	Angleton	98%	99
Brazosport Memorial Hospital	Lake Jackson	98%	192
Cleveland Regional Medical Center	Cleveland	98%	144
Columbia Spring Branch Medical Center	Houston	98%	266
Columbus Community Hospital	Columbus	98%	43
East Houston Regional Medical Center	Houston	98%	245
East Texas Medical Center-Crockett	Crockett	98%	87
East Texas Medical Center-Fairfield	Fairfield	98%	47
Harris County Hospital District	Houston	98%	371
Huguley Memorial Medical Center	Burleson	98%	371
Kingwood Medical Center	Kingwood	98%	300
Lamb Healthcare Center	Littlefield	98%	64
Las Palmas Medical Center	El Paso	98%	178
Matagorda County Hospital District	Bay City	98%	83
Medical Center of Southeast Texas	Port Arthur	98%	165
Memorial Hospital	Dumas	98%	54
Memorial Medical Center	Port Lavaca	98%	65
Mission Hospital	Mission	98%	243
Nacogdoches Memorial Hospital	Nacogdoches	98%	185
Saint Marks Medical Center	La Grange	98%	118
Starr County Memorial Hospital	Rio Grande City	98%	61
University of Texas Medical Branch Hospitals	Galveston	98%	177
Val Verde Regional Medical Center	Del Rio	98%	81
Valley Regional Medical Center	Brownsville	98%	206
Bayshore Medical Center	Pasadena	97%	445
Brownsville Medical Center	Brownsville	97%	198
Christus Spohn Hospital Kleberg	Kingsville	97%	226
Heart Hospital of Austin	Austin	97%	35
Huntsville Memorial Hospital	Huntsville	97%	103
McAllen Medical Center	McAllen	97%	156
Medical Center of Lewisville	Lewisville	97%	218
Memorial Health System of East Texas-Lufkin	Lufkin	97%	272
Oakbend Medical Center	Richmond	97%	257
Renaissance Hospital Houston	Houston	97%	35
Saint Joseph Regional Health Center	Bryan	97%	315
Fort Duncan Medical Center	Eagle Pass	96%	126
Hamilton General Hospital	Hamilton	96%	128

NOTE: Hospital profiles are in alphabetical order by state, then city, then hospital within the city; Rankings are sorted by rate in descending order and exclude hospitals with less than 25 cases; (1) The number of cases is too small (n<25) for purposes of reliably predicting hospital performance; (2) Measure reflects the hospital's indication that its submission was based upon a sample of its relevant discharges; (3) Rate reflects fewer than the maximum possible quarters of data for the measure; (4) Inaccurate information submitted and suppressed for one or more quarters; (5) No data is available from the hospital for this measure; Please refer to the User's Guide for a full explanation of data

Hospital Name	City	Rate	Cases
Knapp Medical Center	Weslaco	96%	309
Nocona General Hospital	Nocona	96%	45
Rio Grande Regional Hospital	McAllen	96%	259
Anson General Hospital	Anson	95%	38
Covenant Hospital Levelland	Levelland	95%	43
Doctors Hospital Parkway+Tidwell	Houston	95%	132
Gulf Coast Medical Center	Wharton	95%	80
Memorial Medical Center Livingston	Livingston	95%	87
Dimmit County Memorial Hospital	Carrizo Springs	94%	36
North Bay Hospital	Aransas Pass	94%	36
Permian General Hospital	Andrews	94%	34
Atlanta Memorial Hospital	Atlanta	93%	107
Bellville General Hospital	Bellville	91%	56
D M Cogdell Memorial Hospital	Snyder	83%	54
Eastland Memorial Hospital	Eastland	83%	121
Titus Regional Medical Center	Mount Pleasant	77%	253

18. Pneumococcal Vaccine

Hospital Name	City	Rate	Cases
Cuero Community Hospital	Cuero	100%	81
Nix Healthcare System	San Antonio	100%	68
Stephens Memorial Hospital	Breckenridge	100%	43
Wilbarger General Hospital	Vernon	100%	28
Lake Pointe Medical Center	Rowlett	99%	170
Texoma Medical Center	Denison	99%	153
Graham Regional Medical Center	Graham	98%	80
Memorial Herman Katy Hospital	Katy	98%	103
Presbyterian Hospital of Winnsboro	Winnsboro	98%	41
Detar Hospital Navarro	Victoria	97%	107
Longview Regional Medical Center	Longview	97%	116
Methodist Medical Center	Dallas	97%	143
Christus Santa Rosa Hospital-City Centre	San Antonio	96%	143
Palestine Regional Medical Center	Palestine	96%	98
South Texas Regional Medical Center	Jourdanton	96%	100
Christus Saint John Hospital	Houston	95%	119
Falls Community Hospital	Marlin	95%	81
Glen Rose Medical Center	Glen Rose	95%	65
Llano Memorial Hospital	Llano	95%	107
Walls Regional Hospital	Cleburne	95%	124
Baylor Medical Center at Irving	Irving	94%	176
East Texas Medical Center-Quitman	Quitman	94%	51
Memorial Hermann Fort Bend Hospital	Missouri City	94%	64
Charlton Methodist Hospital	Dallas	93%	146
Christus Saint Catherine Hospital	Katy	93%	86
Presbyterian Hospital of Dallas	Dallas	93%	273
Rolling Plains Memorial Hospital	Sweetwater	93%	74
Woodland Heights Medical Center	Lufkin	93%	109
Alice Regional Hospital	Alice	92%	137
Baylor All Saints Med Ctr at Forth Worth	Fort Worth	92%	172
Baylor Medical Center at Garland	Garland	92%	152
Bowie Memorial Hospital	Bowie	92%	97
Harris Methodist HEB Hospital	Bedford	92%	200
Uvalde Memorial Hospital	Uvalde	92%	52
Big Bend Regional Medical Center	Alpine	91%	79
College Station Medical Center	College Station	91%	44
Connally Memorial Medical Center	Floresville	91%	43
Coryell Memorial Hospital	Gatesville	91%	76
Kings Daughters Hospital	Temple	91%	44
Lavaca Medical Center	Hallettsville	91%	58
Methodist Willowbrook Hospital	Houston	91%	100
Providence Memorial Hospital	El Paso	91%	274
Arlington Memorial Hospital	Arlington	90%	230
Baylor Medical Center-Ellis County	Waxahachie	90%	83
Clear Lake Regional Medical Center	Webster	90%	197
Coleman County Medical Center	Coleman	90%	73
Columbus Community Hospital	Columbus	90%	30
Comanche County Medical Center	Comanche	90%	40
Huguley Memorial Medical Center	Burleson	90%	181
Pecos County Memorial Hospital	Fort Stockton	90%	41
Presbyterian Hospital of Kaufman	Kaufman	90%	77
Cypress Fairbanks Medical Center and Hospital	Houston	89%	189
Gulf Coast Medical Center	Wharton	89%	47
Kingwood Medical Center	Kingwood	89%	163
Northeast Medical Center	Bonham	89%	54
San Jacinto Methodist Hospital	Baytown	89%	110
Nocona General Hospital	Nocona	88%	33
Trinity Medical Center	Carrollton	88%	92
Christus Saint Elizabeth Hospital	Beaumont	87%	339
Christus Saint Michael Health System	Texarkana	87%	252
Harris Methodist Erath County	Stephenville	87%	92
Harris Methodist Southwest	Fort Worth	87%	172
Hendrick Medical Center	Abilene	87%	179
Hill Country Memorial Hospital	Fredericksburg	87%	149
Medical Arts Hospital	Lamesa	87%	39
Memorial Hermann-Texas Medical Center	Houston	87%	60
Methodist Sugar Land Hospital	Sugar Land	87%	90
Saint Joseph Medical Center	Houston	87%	122
Baylor Regional Medical Center at Grapevine	Grapevine	86%	105
Baylor Regional Medical Center at Plano	Plano	86%	58
Baylor University Medical Center	Dallas	86%	367
Christus Spohn Hospital Kleberg	Kingsville	86%	121
Harris Methodist Continued Care Hospital	Fort Worth	86%	525
Marshall Regional Medical Center	Marshall	86%	83
Presbyterian Hospital of Plano	Plano	86%	66
Shannon Medical Center	San Angelo	86%	222
Sierra Medical Center	El Paso	86%	268
Goodall-Witcher Healthcare Foundation	Clifton	85%	92
North Hills Hospital	N Richland Hills	85%	177
Presbyterian Hospital of Allen	Allen	85%	46
RHD Memorial Medical Center	Dallas	85%	126
Methodist Hospital	Houston	84%	234
Seton Northwest Hospital	Austin	84%	82
Seymour Hospital	Seymour	84%	25
Sid Peterson Memorial Hospital	Kerrville	84%	180
University of Texas Health Center at Tyler	Tyler	84%	122
Bayshore Medical Center	Pasadena	83%	241
Brazosport Memorial Hospital	Lake Jackson	83%	111
Brownwood Regional Medical Center	Brownwood	83%	162
Central Texas Medical Center	San Marcos	83%	92
Childress Regional Medical Center	Childress	83%	41
Columbia Spring Branch Medical Center	Houston	83%	157
Lake Granbury Medical Center	Granbury	83%	69
Medical Center of Plano	Plano	83%	167
Memorial Hermann Healthcare System	Houston	83%	820
San Angelo Community Medical Center	San Angelo	83%	156
W J Mangold Memorial Hospital	Lockney	83%	36
West Houston Medical Center	Houston	83%	173
Christus Spohn Hospital Beeville	Beeville	82%	66
Harlingen Medical Center	Harlingen	82%	108
Hill Regional Hospital	Hillsboro	82%	67
Las Colinas Medical Center	Irving	82%	44
Scott & White	Temple	82%	293
Seton Highland Lakes	Burnet	82%	50
Citizens Medical Center	Victoria	81%	111
Navarro Regional Hospital	Corsicana	81%	101
East Texas Medical Center-Carthage	Carthage	80%	40
El Campo Memorial Hospital	El Campo	80%	50
Parkland Health & Hospital System	Dallas	80%	70
East Texas Medical Center-Jacksonville	Jacksonville	79%	61
Memorial Herman Baptist Orange Hospital	Orange	79%	57
Wadley Regional Medical Center	Texarkana	79%	146
Christus Spohn Memorial Hospital	Corpus Christi	78%	533
Covenant Medical Center	Lubbock	78%	473
Harris Methodist Northwest	Azle	78%	131
Mainland Medical Center	Texas City	78%	129
Round Rock Medical Center	Round Rock	78%	121
Conroe Regional Medical Center	Conroe	77%	216
Medical Center at Terrell	Terrell	77%	83
Mesquite Community Hospital	Mesquite	77%	77
North Austin Medical Center	Austin	77%	129
Abilene Regional Medical Center	Abilene	76%	54
Metroplex Hospital	Killeen	76%	51
Saint David's Rehabiltation Center	Austin	76%	188
Thomason General Hospital	El Paso	76%	62
Atlanta Memorial Hospital	Atlanta	75%	63
Huntsville Memorial Hospital	Huntsville	75%	65
Memorial Hermann Memorial City	Houston	75%	171
Rio Grande Regional Hospital	McAllen	75%	168
Doctors Hospital	Dallas	74%	172
Baptist-Saint Anthony's Health System	Amarillo	73%	109
Parkview Regional Hospital	Mexia	73%	94
Richardson Medical Center	Richardson	73%	114
Seton Medical Center	Austin	73%	91
Hamilton General Hospital	Hamilton	72%	98
Henderson Memorial Hospital	Henderson	72%	76
Laird Memorial Hospital	Kilgore	72%	57
McAllen Medical Center	McAllen	72%	85
Memorial Hermann Baptist Beaumont	Beaumont	72%	149
Nacogdoches Medical Center Hospital	Nacogdoches	72%	111
Shelby Regional Medical Center	Center	72%	61
Tomball Regional Hospital	Tomball	72%	156
United Regional Healthcare System	Wichita Falls	72%	156
Baptist Medical Center	San Antonio	71%	289
Centennial Medical Center	Frisco	71%	48
Memorial Health System of East Texas-Lufkin	Lufkin	71%	172
Mitchell County Hospital	Colorado City	71%	35
Park Plaza Hospital	Houston	71%	142
Rollins Brook Community Hospital	Lampasas	71%	59
Anson General Hospital	Anson	70%	27

NOTE: Hospital profiles are in alphabetical order by state, then city, then hospital within the city; Rankings are sorted by rate in descending order and exclude hospitals with less than 25 cases; (1) The number of cases is too small (n<25) for purposes of reliably predicting hospital performance; (2) Measure reflects the hospital's indication that its submission was based upon a sample of its relevant discharges; (3) Rate reflects fewer than the maximum possible quarters of data for the measure; (4) Inaccurate information submitted and suppressed for one or more quarters; (5) No data is available from the hospital for this measure; Please refer to the User's Guide for a full explanation of data

Hospital Name	City	Rate	Cases
Georgetown Healthcare System	Georgetown	70%	96
Houston Northwest Medical Center	Houston	70%	199
Corpus Christi Medical Center-Bay Area	Corpus Christi	69%	262
East Houston Regional Medical Center	Houston	69%	113
Eastland Memorial Hospital	Eastland	69%	83
Palo Pinto General Hospital	Mineral Wells	69%	70
Paris Regional Medical Center-South Campus	Paris	69%	207
Seton Edgar B Davis Memorial Hospital	Luling	69%	35
Trinity Medical Center	Brenham	69%	32
Saint Luke's Episcopal Hospital	Houston	68%	252
Midland Memorial Hospital	Midland	67%	156
Southwest General Hospital	San Antonio	67%	90
Hopkins County Memorial Hospital	Sulphur Springs	66%	139
Wilson N Jones Medical Center	Sherman	66%	184
East Texas Medical Center-Athens	Athens	65%	125
Northwest Texas Healthcare System	Amarillo	64%	123
Presbyterian Hospital of Denton	Denton	64%	152
South Austin Hospital	Austin	64%	159
Valley Baptist Medical Center	Harlingen	64%	287
Saint Luke's Community Med Ctr-The Woodlands	The Woodlands	63%	71
Christus Jasper Memorial Hospital	Jasper	62%	53
Denton Regional Medical Center	Denton	62%	141
East Texas Medical Center-Clarksville	Clarksville	62%	91
East Texas Medical Center-Gilmer	Gilmer	62%	47
Matagorda County Hospital District	Bay City	62%	45
Memorial Hospital	Dumas	62%	26
Plaza Medical Center	Fort Worth	62%	133
Fort Duncan Medical Center	Eagle Pass	61%	79
Mother Frances Hospital-Tyler	Tyler	60%	289
UT Southwestern Saint Paul Hospital	Dallas	60%	92
Good Shepherd Medical Center	Longview	59%	102
Knapp Medical Center	Weslaco	59%	213
North Central Medical Center	McKinney	59%	199
North Texas Medical Center	Gainesville	59%	39
Northeast Medical Center Hospital	Humble	59%	153
Oakbend Medical Center	Richmond	59%	150
Pampa Regional Medical Center	Pampa	59%	73
Cleveland Regional Medical Center	Cleveland	58%	66
Colorado Fayette Medical Center	Weimar	58%	40
East Texas Medical Center-Crockett	Crockett	58%	65
Medical Center of Lewisville	Lewisville	58%	122
Memorial Medical Center	Port Lavaca	58%	36
Presbyterian Hospital of Greenville	Greenville	58%	162
Saint Joseph Regional Health Center	Bryan	58%	183
Covenant Hospital Plainview	Plainview	57%	42
Medical City Dallas	Dallas	57%	138
Medical Center of Arlington	Arlington	56%	195
Scenic Mountain Medical Center	Big Spring	56%	39
Valley Regional Medical Center	Brownsville	56%	131
Edinburg Regional Medical Center	Edinburg	55%	73
McKenna Memorial Hospital	New Braunfels	54%	125
Las Palmas Medical Center	El Paso	53%	112
Tyler County Hospital	Woodville	53%	45
Nacogdoches Memorial Hospital	Nacogdoches	52%	117
Doctors Hospital of Laredo	Laredo	51%	78
Laredo Medical Center	Laredo	49%	88
Methodist Hospital	San Antonio	48%	646
Ennis Regional Medical Center	Ennis	46%	68
Brackenridge Hospital	Austin	44%	39
Cozby-Germany Hospital	Grand Saline	44%	50
Hillcrest Baptist Medical Center	Waco	44%	96
Medical Center of Mesquite	Mesquite	44%	136
Bellville General Hospital	Bellville	43%	35
East Texas Medical Center-Fairfield	Fairfield	43%	30
Memorial Medical Center Livingston	Livingston	43%	49
Val Verde Regional Medical Center	Del Rio	43%	51
Medical Center Hospital	Odessa	42%	139
Medical Center of Southeast Texas	Port Arthur	41%	97
Smithville Regional Hospital	Smithville	41%	93
University Medical Center	Lubbock	40%	65
Guadalupe Valley Hospital	Seguin	36%	72
Harris County Hospital District	Houston	36%	96
University of Texas Medical Branch Hospitals	Galveston	36%	80
Saint Marks Medical Center	La Grange	35%	94
East Texas Medical Center-Tyler	Tyler	34%	68
Alliance Hospital	Odessa	33%	48
Del Sol Medical Center	El Paso	33%	315
East Texas Medical Center-Trinity	Trinity	32%	31
University Hospital	San Antonio	31%	29
Brownsville Medical Center	Brownsville	30%	128
Providence Health Center	Waco	28%	213
Reeves County Hospital	Pecos	27%	26
Mission Hospital	Mission	26%	153
Angleton-Danbury Medical Center	Angleton	25%	53
Lamb Healthcare Center	Littlefield	25%	44
Memorial Hospital	Gonzales	20%	41
Titus Regional Medical Center	Mount Pleasant	20%	136
Campbell Health System	Weatherford	19%	128
Doctors Hospital at Renaissance	Edinburg	18%	102
Hereford Regional Medical Center	Hereford	18%	34
Renaissance Hospital-East Texas	Groves	17%	35
John Peter Smith Hospital	Fort Worth	16%	61
Brownfield Regional Medical Center	Brownfield	13%	31
Twelve Oaks Hospital	Houston	12%	26
Medical Center at Lancaster	Lancaster	11%	28
Doctors Hospital Parkway+Tidwell	Houston	10%	58
Starr County Memorial Hospital	Rio Grande City	10%	42
Physicians Specialty Hospital of El Paso	El Paso	0%	66

19. Smoking Cessation Advice

Hospital Name	City	Rate	Cases
Abilene Regional Medical Center	Abilene	100%	36
Arlington Memorial Hospital	Arlington	100%	109
Baylor Medical Center at Garland	Garland	100%	62
Bowie Memorial Hospital	Bowie	100%	30
Christus Saint Catherine Hospital	Katy	100%	28
Christus Saint John Hospital	Houston	100%	34
Christus Saint Michael Health System	Texarkana	100%	125
Christus Santa Rosa Hospital-City Centre	San Antonio	100%	54
Christus Spohn Hospital Kleberg	Kingsville	100%	39
Detar Hospital Navarro	Victoria	100%	44
Harris Methodist Erath County	Stephenville	100%	40
Kingwood Medical Center	Kingwood	100%	90
Lake Pointe Medical Center	Rowlett	100%	64
Las Palmas Medical Center	El Paso	100%	33
Longview Regional Medical Center	Longview	100%	41
Medical Center of Arlington	Arlington	100%	76
Medical Center of Southeast Texas	Port Arthur	100%	35
Memorial Herman Baptist Orange Hospital	Orange	100%	38
Memorial Herman Katy Hospital	Katy	100%	39
Memorial Hermann Fort Bend Hospital	Missouri City	100%	25
Methodist Medical Center	Dallas	100%	98
Mother Frances Hospital-Tyler	Tyler	100%	101
Park Plaza Hospital	Houston	100%	40
Presbyterian Hospital of Plano	Plano	100%	37
San Angelo Community Medical Center	San Angelo	100%	32
Shelby Regional Medical Center	Center	100%	27
South Austin Hospital	Austin	100%	86
Texoma Medical Center	Denison	100%	52
Thomason General Hospital	El Paso	100%	64
Trinity Medical Center	Carrollton	100%	68
UT Southwestern Saint Paul Hospital	Dallas	100%	32
Valley Baptist Medical Center	Harlingen	100%	45
Walls Regional Hospital	Cleburne	100%	55
Woodland Heights Medical Center	Lufkin	100%	44
Baylor Medical Center at Irving	Irving	99%	70
Baylor University Medical Center	Dallas	99%	170
Charlton Methodist Hospital	Dallas	99%	73
Harris Methodist HEB Hospital	Bedford	99%	88
Harris Methodist Northwest	Azle	99%	70
Baptist-Saint Anthony's Health System	Amarillo	98%	41
Christus Spohn Memorial Hospital	Corpus Christi	98%	208
Mesquite Community Hospital	Mesquite	98%	80
Cleveland Regional Medical Center	Cleveland	97%	58
Conroe Regional Medical Center	Conroe	97%	130
Covenant Medical Center	Lubbock	97%	158
Huguley Memorial Medical Center	Burleson	97%	116
Memorial Hermann-Texas Medical Center	Houston	97%	58
Mission Hospital	Mission	97%	36
Navarro Regional Hospital	Corsicana	97%	34
North Central Medical Center	McKinney	97%	59
Presbyterian Hospital of Allen	Allen	97%	30
Presbyterian Hospital of Kaufman	Kaufman	97%	36
Richardson Medical Center	Richardson	97%	34
Round Rock Medical Center	Round Rock	97%	61
Saint David's Rehabiltation Center	Austin	97%	87
San Jacinto Methodist Hospital	Baytown	97%	59
Valley Regional Medical Center	Brownsville	97%	34
Baylor Regional Medical Center at Grapevine	Grapevine	96%	51
Bayshore Medical Center	Pasadena	96%	130
Denton Regional Medical Center	Denton	96%	55
Falls Community Hospital	Marlin	96%	53
Northeast Medical Center Hospital	Humble	96%	68
Parkview Regional Hospital	Mexia	96%	45
Providence Health Center	Waco	96%	71
Southwest General Hospital	San Antonio	96%	48
Cypress Fairbanks Medical Center and Hospital	Houston	95%	66
Harris Methodist Southwest	Fort Worth	95%	42
Memorial Hermann Healthcare System	Houston	95%	320

NOTE: Hospital profiles are in alphabetical order by state, then city, then hospital within the city; Rankings are sorted by rate in descending order and exclude hospitals with less than 25 cases; (1) The number of cases is too small (n<25) for purposes of reliably predicting hospital performance; (2) Measure reflects the hospital's indication that its submission was based upon a sample of its relevant discharges; (3) Rate reflects fewer than the maximum possible quarters of data for the measure; (4) Inaccurate information submitted and suppressed for one or more quarters; (5) No data is available from the hospital for this measure; Please refer to the User's Guide for a full explanation of data

Hospital Name	City	Rate	Cases
Presbyterian Hospital of Dallas	Dallas	95%	66
West Houston Medical Center	Houston	95%	65
Clear Lake Regional Medical Center	Webster	94%	100
Medical Center of Plano	Plano	94%	49
North Austin Medical Center	Austin	94%	48
North Hills Hospital	N Richland Hills	94%	81
Sid Peterson Memorial Hospital	Kerrville	94%	49
Del Sol Medical Center	El Paso	93%	123
East Texas Medical Center-Athens	Athens	93%	57
Houston Northwest Medical Center	Houston	93%	94
Memorial Hermann Memorial City	Houston	93%	45
RHD Memorial Medical Center	Dallas	93%	43
Scott & White	Temple	93%	91
Baylor All Saints Med Ctr at Forth Worth	Fort Worth	92%	65
Edinburg Regional Medical Center	Edinburg	92%	25
Medical Center of Mesquite	Mesquite	92%	59
Marshall Regional Medical Center	Marshall	91%	35
Baptist Medical Center	San Antonio	90%	83
East Houston Regional Medical Center	Houston	90%	93
Good Shepherd Medical Center	Longview	90%	51
Lake Granbury Medical Center	Granbury	90%	29
Mainland Medical Center	Texas City	90%	62
Methodist Hospital	Houston	90%	73
Palestine Regional Medical Center	Palestine	90%	29
Saint Joseph Medical Center	Houston	90%	67
South Texas Regional Medical Center	Jourdanton	90%	41
University of Texas Health Center at Tyler	Tyler	90%	68
Christus Saint Elizabeth Hospital	Beaumont	89%	179
Northwest Texas Healthcare System	Amarillo	89%	103
Columbia Spring Branch Medical Center	Houston	88%	57
Oakbend Medical Center	Richmond	88%	40
Brownwood Regional Medical Center	Brownwood	87%	68
Hendrick Medical Center	Abilene	86%	86
Saint Luke's Episcopal Hospital	Houston	86%	69
Citizens Medical Center	Victoria	85%	33
Hopkins County Memorial Hospital	Sulphur Springs	85%	54
Llano Memorial Hospital	Llano	85%	27
Medical Center of Lewisville	Lewisville	85%	52
Presbyterian Hospital of Greenville	Greenville	85%	88
Saint Joseph Regional Health Center	Bryan	85%	80
Wadley Regional Medical Center	Texarkana	85%	67
Doctors Hospital	Dallas	84%	68
Harris Methodist Continued Care Hospital	Fort Worth	84%	193
Medical Center at Terrell	Terrell	84%	31
Parkland Health & Hospital System	Dallas	84%	180
United Regional Healthcare System	Wichita Falls	84%	88
Methodist Hospital	San Antonio	83%	235
Metroplex Hospital	Killeen	82%	34
Plaza Medical Center	Fort Worth	82%	44
Rio Grande Regional Hospital	McAllen	82%	28
Baylor Medical Center-Ellis County	Waxahachie	81%	36
McKenna Memorial Hospital	New Braunfels	81%	37
Hill Regional Hospital	Hillsboro	80%	25
Paris Regional Medical Center-South Campus	Paris	80%	98
Hillcrest Baptist Medical Center	Waco	79%	68
Presbyterian Hospital of Denton	Denton	79%	56
Scenic Mountain Medical Center	Big Spring	79%	29
Seton Northwest Hospital	Austin	79%	43
Medical City Dallas	Dallas	78%	46
Nacogdoches Medical Center Hospital	Nacogdoches	78%	32
University of Texas Medical Branch Hospitals	Galveston	77%	47
Sierra Medical Center	El Paso	76%	63
Brazosport Memorial Hospital	Lake Jackson	73%	44
Hill Country Memorial Hospital	Fredericksburg	73%	26
Midland Memorial Hospital	Midland	71%	58
Seton Medical Center	Austin	71%	28
Smithville Regional Hospital	Smithville	71%	28
Brackenridge Hospital	Austin	70%	56
Knapp Medical Center	Weslaco	70%	30
Pampa Regional Medical Center	Pampa	70%	27
Corpus Christi Medical Center-Bay Area	Corpus Christi	68%	71
Harris County Hospital District	Houston	67%	144
Palo Pinto General Hospital	Mineral Wells	67%	42
Providence Memorial Hospital	El Paso	62%	39
University Medical Center	Lubbock	62%	32
Atlanta Memorial Hospital	Atlanta	54%	26
East Texas Medical Center-Tyler	Tyler	47%	38
John Peter Smith Hospital	Fort Worth	47%	175
Medical Center Hospital	Odessa	39%	76
University Hospital	San Antonio	29%	42

Surgical Infection Prevention

20. Prophylactic Antibiotic Given

Hospital Name	City	Rate	Cases
Austin Surgical Hospital	Austin	99%	67
Baylor Heart and Vascular Center	Dallas	99%	176
Baylor Regional Medical Center at Plano	Plano	98%	124
Charlton Methodist Hospital	Dallas	98%	139
Baylor All Saints Med Ctr at Forth Worth	Fort Worth	97%	1383
Baylor Medical Center-Ellis County	Waxahachie	97%	306
College Station Medical Center	College Station	97%	270
Texas Orthopedic Hospital	Houston	97%	690
Baylor Medical Center at Irving	Irving	96%	760
Baylor Regional Medical Center at Grapevine	Grapevine	96%	805
Methodist Medical Center	Dallas	96%	194
Baylor Medical Center at Garland	Garland	95%	721
Presbyterian Hospital of Denton	Denton	95%	451
Baylor University Medical Center	Dallas	94%	3530
Brownsville Surgical Hospital	Brownsville	94%	62
Detar Hospital Navarro	Victoria	94%	450
Harris Methodist Erath County	Stephenville	94%	99
Huntsville Memorial Hospital	Huntsville	94%	166
Matagorda County Hospital District	Bay City	94%	63
Centennial Medical Center	Frisco	92%	142
Christus Saint Michael Health System	Texarkana	92%	1260
Las Palmas Medical Center	El Paso	92%	211
Womans Hospital of Texas	Houston	92%	943
Conroe Regional Medical Center	Conroe	91%	291
Paris Regional Medical Center-South Campus	Paris	91%	508
Physicians Centre	Bryan	91%	57
Central Texas Medical Center	San Marcos	90%	59
Presbyterian Hospital of Dallas	Dallas	90%	263
Walls Regional Hospital	Cleburne	90%	108
Citizens Medical Center	Victoria	89%	447
Harris Methodist Continued Care Hospital	Fort Worth	89%	248
Lake Granbury Medical Center	Granbury	89%	103
Parkland Health & Hospital System	Dallas	89%	142
Physicians Surgical Hospital at Quail Creek	Amarillo	89%	35
Shannon Medical Center	San Angelo	89%	218
Texoma Medical Center	Denison	89%	374
Texsan Heart Hospital	San Antonio	89%	361
Cornerstone Regional Hospital	Edinburg	88%	51
El Paso Specialty Hospital	El Paso	88%	341
Gulf Coast Medical Center	Wharton	88%	145
Hendrick Medical Center	Abilene	88%	276
Houston Northwest Medical Center	Houston	88%	881
Navarro Regional Hospital	Corsicana	88%	120
Plaza Medical Center	Fort Worth	88%	304
Presbyterian Plano Ctr for Diag & Surgery	Plano	88%	42
Saint Joseph Regional Health Center	Bryan	88%	1051
Sid Peterson Memorial Hospital	Kerrville	88%	363
Wise Regional Health System	Decatur	88%	41
Woodland Heights Medical Center	Lufkin	88%	424
Abilene Regional Medical Center	Abilene	87%	633
Baptist Medical Center	San Antonio	87%	498
Childress Regional Medical Center	Childress	87%	46
Denton Regional Medical Center	Denton	87%	223
Medical City Dallas	Dallas	87%	376
Palo Pinto General Hospital	Mineral Wells	87%	93
Tomball Regional Hospital	Tomball	87%	55
Christus Spohn Hospital Kleberg	Kingsville	86%	64
Huguley Memorial Medical Center	Burleson	86%	407
Memorial Health System of East Texas-Lufkin	Lufkin	86%	97
Providence Memorial Hospital	El Paso	86%	327
Saint Joseph Medical Center	Houston	86%	792
Valley Regional Medical Center	Brownsville	86%	137
Baptist-Saint Anthony's Health System	Amarillo	85%	310
Christus Jasper Memorial Hospital	Jasper	85%	46
Cypress Fairbanks Medical Center and Hospital	Houston	85%	119
Harlingen Medical Center	Harlingen	85%	258
Harris Methodist Southwest	Fort Worth	85%	110
Hill Country Memorial Hospital	Fredericksburg	85%	459
Methodist Willowbrook Hospital	Houston	85%	196
Midland Memorial Hospital	Midland	85%	320
Saint David's Rehabiltation Center	Austin	85%	278
San Angelo Community Medical Center	San Angelo	85%	432
Arlington Memorial Hospital	Arlington	84%	180
Memorial Hermann Baptist Beaumont	Beaumont	84%	104
Memorial Hermann Fort Bend Hospital	Missouri City	84%	50
Baylor Medical Center at Frisco	Frisco	83%	58
Christus Santa Rosa Hospital-City Centre	San Antonio	83%	1183
Medical Center of Arlington	Arlington	83%	186
Medical Center of Plano	Plano	83%	194
Scott & White	Temple	83%	1772

Hospital Name	City	Rate	Cases
Heart Hospital of Austin	Austin	82%	106
Kings Daughters Hospital	Temple	82%	93
Memorial Herman Katy Hospital	Katy	82%	249
Nacogdoches Memorial Hospital	Nacogdoches	81%	75
Northwest Texas Healthcare System	Amarillo	81%	979
Alliance Hospital	Odessa	80%	71
Longview Regional Medical Center	Longview	80%	379
Mother Frances Hospital Jacksonville	Jacksonville	80%	40
East Texas Medical Center-Athens	Athens	79%	124
McKenna Memorial Hospital	New Braunfels	79%	121
Mesquite Community Hospital	Mesquite	79%	297
Pampa Regional Medical Center	Pampa	79%	107
Valley Baptist Medical Center	Harlingen	79%	197
Christus Saint John Hospital	Houston	78%	348
Methodist Hospital	Houston	78%	429
Presbyterian Hospital of Kaufman	Kaufman	78%	55
Round Rock Medical Center	Round Rock	78%	172
University Medical Center	Lubbock	78%	176
Christus Spohn Memorial Hospital	Corpus Christi	77%	1444
John Peter Smith Hospital	Fort Worth	77%	487
Memorial Hermann Healthcare System	Houston	77%	2534
Memorial Medical Center Livingston	Livingston	77%	30
Sierra Medical Center	El Paso	77%	320
The Hospital at Westlake Medical Center	Austin	77%	30
Thomason General Hospital	El Paso	77%	173
Trinity Medical Center	Brenham	77%	78
Clear Lake Regional Medical Center	Webster	76%	238
Doctors Hospital at Renaissance	Edinburg	76%	372
West Houston Medical Center	Houston	76%	188
Doctors Hospital	Dallas	75%	244
Las Colinas Medical Center	Irving	75%	92
Brackenridge Hospital	Austin	74%	135
Harris Methodist HEB Hospital	Bedford	74%	180
North Austin Medical Center	Austin	74%	233
Presbyterian Hospital of Plano	Plano	74%	180
South Austin Hospital	Austin	74%	262
Val Verde Regional Medical Center	Del Rio	74%	100
Knapp Medical Center	Weslaco	73%	174
Lake Pointe Medical Center	Rowlett	73%	164
Northeast Medical Center Hospital	Humble	73%	230
San Jacinto Methodist Hospital	Baytown	73%	182
Harris County Hospital District	Houston	72%	296
Mainland Medical Center	Texas City	72%	132
Memorial Hermann-Texas Medical Center	Houston	72%	641
Presbyterian Hospital of Greenville	Greenville	72%	264
Zale-Lipshy University Hospital	Dallas	72%	83
Covenant Medical Center	Lubbock	71%	272
Harris Methodist Southlake Ctr for Diag	Southlake	71%	31
Seton Medical Center	Austin	71%	232
University Hospital	San Antonio	71%	204
University of Texas Health Center at Tyler	Tyler	71%	87
East Houston Regional Medical Center	Houston	70%	105
Georgetown Healthcare System	Georgetown	70%	115
Henderson Memorial Hospital	Henderson	70%	40
Nacogdoches Medical Center Hospital	Nacogdoches	70%	346
Seton Southwest Healthcare Center	Austin	70%	37
USMD Hospital at Arlington	Arlington	70%	46
UT Southwestern Saint Paul Hospital	Dallas	70%	235
Corpus Christi Medical Center-Bay Area	Corpus Christi	69%	291
Odessa Regional Hospital	Odessa	69%	140
RHD Memorial Medical Center	Dallas	69%	105
Trinity Medical Center	Carrollton	69%	183
Brazosport Memorial Hospital	Lake Jackson	68%	91
Brownsville Medical Center	Brownsville	68%	150
Christus Saint Catherine Hospital	Katy	68%	155
Park Plaza Hospital	Houston	68%	158
Providence Health Center	Waco	68%	196
Spine Hospital of South Texas	San Antonio	68%	81
Medical Center Hospital	Odessa	67%	483
Oakbend Medical Center	Richmond	67%	166
Columbia Spring Branch Medical Center	Houston	66%	158
Rio Grande Regional Hospital	McAllen	66%	125
Seton Northwest Hospital	Austin	66%	113
Hillcrest Baptist Medical Center	Waco	65%	222
Mother Frances Hospital-Tyler	Tyler	65%	255
North Texas Medical Center	Gainesville	65%	81
Christus Saint Elizabeth Hospital	Beaumont	64%	1358
Del Sol Medical Center	El Paso	64%	129
Good Shepherd Medical Center	Longview	64%	70
Richardson Medical Center	Richardson	64%	182
Medical Center of Southeast Texas	Port Arthur	63%	259
North Central Medical Center	McKinney	63%	143
Methodist Hospital	San Antonio	62%	460
Guadalupe Valley Hospital	Seguin	61%	200
Methodist Sugar Land Hospital	Sugar Land	61%	148
Wadley Regional Medical Center	Texarkana	61%	311
Permian General Hospital	Andrews	60%	67
Lubbock Heart Hospital	Lubbock	59%	32
Laredo Medical Center	Laredo	58%	384
McAllen Medical Center	McAllen	58%	251
Nix Healthcare System	San Antonio	55%	164
Marshall Regional Medical Center	Marshall	54%	161
Angleton-Danbury Medical Center	Angleton	53%	170
Medical Center of Lewisville	Lewisville	53%	135
Memorial Hermann Memorial City	Houston	53%	792
Saint Luke's Community Med Ctr-The Woodlands	The Woodlands	53%	38
Saint Luke's Episcopal Hospital	Houston	53%	310
Uvalde Memorial Hospital	Uvalde	53%	59
Campbell Health System	Weatherford	52%	90
Harris Methodist Northwest	Azle	52%	52
North Hills Hospital	N Richland Hills	52%	197
Metroplex Hospital	Killeen	51%	215
Kingwood Medical Center	Kingwood	49%	70
University of Texas Medical Branch Hospitals	Galveston	49%	348
Connally Memorial Medical Center	Floresville	48%	25
Presbyterian Hospital of Allen	Allen	48%	93
Hopkins County Memorial Hospital	Sulphur Springs	47%	153
Titus Regional Medical Center	Mount Pleasant	47%	51
Medical Center of Mesquite	Mesquite	46%	206
South Texas Regional Medical Center	Jourdanton	46%	59
Tops Surgical Specialty Hospital	Houston	46%	26
Wilson N Jones Medical Center	Sherman	46%	56
Brownwood Regional Medical Center	Brownwood	44%	272
Doctors Hospital of Laredo	Laredo	43%	184
Ennis Regional Medical Center	Ennis	43%	72
Highland Community Hospital	Lubbock	43%	81
Palestine Regional Medical Center	Palestine	42%	270
Fort Duncan Medical Center	Eagle Pass	40%	53
Mission Hospital	Mission	40%	172
Bayshore Medical Center	Pasadena	39%	202
Twelve Oaks Hospital	Houston	38%	37
East Texas Medical Center-Tyler	Tyler	36%	159
Edinburg Regional Medical Center	Edinburg	36%	55
Memorial Herman Baptist Orange Hospital	Orange	35%	65
United Regional Healthcare System	Wichita Falls	32%	276
Cleveland Regional Medical Center	Cleveland	30%	54
Southwest General Hospital	San Antonio	23%	190
Scenic Mountain Medical Center	Big Spring	18%	40
Physicians Specialty Hospital of El Paso	El Paso	11%	37

21. Prophylactic Antibiotic Selection

Hospital Name	City	Rate	Cases
Baylor Heart and Vascular Center	Dallas	100%	48
Brownsville Medical Center	Brownsville	100%	39
Charlton Methodist Hospital	Dallas	100%	39
El Paso Specialty Hospital	El Paso	100%	109
Ennis Regional Medical Center	Ennis	100%	26
Heart Hospital of Austin	Austin	100%	36
Highland Community Hospital	Lubbock	100%	29
Texas Orthopedic Hospital	Houston	100%	223
Texsan Heart Hospital	San Antonio	100%	143
Valley Regional Medical Center	Brownsville	100%	57
Baylor Medical Center at Garland	Garland	99%	162
Las Palmas Medical Center	El Paso	99%	94
Presbyterian Hospital of Dallas	Dallas	99%	94
Denton Regional Medical Center	Denton	98%	109
Parkland Health & Hospital System	Dallas	98%	144
Presbyterian Hospital of Denton	Denton	98%	120
Sierra Medical Center	El Paso	98%	81
Thomason General Hospital	El Paso	98%	42
Baylor All Saints Med Ctr at Forth Worth	Fort Worth	97%	329
Baylor Medical Center at Irving	Irving	97%	176
Knapp Medical Center	Weslaco	97%	73
Seton Northwest Hospital	Austin	97%	30
Texoma Medical Center	Denison	97%	124
The Hospital at Westlake Medical Center	Austin	97%	30
Baptist Medical Center	San Antonio	96%	117
Baylor Medical Center-Ellis County	Waxahachie	96%	76
Corpus Christi Medical Center-Bay Area	Corpus Christi	96%	156
Detar Hospital Navarro	Victoria	96%	113
Hill Country Memorial Hospital	Fredericksburg	96%	108
Pampa Regional Medical Center	Pampa	96%	25
Providence Memorial Hospital	El Paso	96%	78
Round Rock Medical Center	Round Rock	96%	79
Saint Joseph Regional Health Center	Bryan	96%	257
Seton Medical Center	Austin	96%	81
Harris Methodist Continued Care Hospital	Fort Worth	95%	82
Palo Pinto General Hospital	Mineral Wells	95%	41
Presbyterian Hospital of Plano	Plano	95%	55

NOTE: Hospital profiles are in alphabetical order by state, then city, then hospital within the city; Rankings are sorted by rate in descending order and exclude hospitals with less than 25 cases; (1) The number of cases is too small (n<25) for purposes of reliably predicting hospital performance; (2) Measure reflects the hospital's indication that its submission was based upon a sample of its relevant discharges; (3) Rate reflects fewer than the maximum possible quarters of data for the measure; (4) Inaccurate information submitted and suppressed for one or more quarters; (5) No data is available from the hospital for this measure; Please refer to the User's Guide for a full explanation of data

Hospital Name	City	Rate	Cases
Sid Peterson Memorial Hospital	Kerrville	95%	131
Christus Saint Catherine Hospital	Katy	94%	31
Christus Santa Rosa Hospital-City Centre	San Antonio	94%	335
Citizens Medical Center	Victoria	94%	172
Cypress Fairbanks Medical Center and Hospital	Houston	94%	33
Georgetown Healthcare System	Georgetown	94%	51
Hendrick Medical Center	Abilene	94%	69
Methodist Medical Center	Dallas	94%	65
Rio Grande Regional Hospital	McAllen	94%	49
Saint Joseph Medical Center	Houston	94%	179
Wadley Regional Medical Center	Texarkana	94%	124
Walls Regional Hospital	Cleburne	94%	36
Christus Spohn Memorial Hospital	Corpus Christi	93%	533
Harlingen Medical Center	Harlingen	93%	86
Memorial Hermann Healthcare System	Houston	93%	815
Navarro Regional Hospital	Corsicana	93%	28
North Austin Medical Center	Austin	93%	111
Permian General Hospital	Andrews	93%	28
Saint David's Rehabiltation Center	Austin	93%	135
South Austin Hospital	Austin	93%	122
UT Southwestern Saint Paul Hospital	Dallas	93%	73
University Hospital	San Antonio	93%	43
Baylor Regional Medical Center at Grapevine	Grapevine	92%	184
Brackenridge Hospital	Austin	92%	40
College Station Medical Center	College Station	92%	75
Doctors Hospital of Laredo	Laredo	92%	36
Hillcrest Baptist Medical Center	Waco	92%	78
Methodist Hospital	San Antonio	92%	219
Providence Health Center	Waco	92%	72
United Regional Healthcare System	Wichita Falls	92%	87
Womans Hospital of Texas	Houston	92%	298
Zale-Lipshy University Hospital	Dallas	92%	38
Brazosport Memorial Hospital	Lake Jackson	91%	33
Gulf Coast Medical Center	Wharton	91%	35
Harris Methodist HEB Hospital	Bedford	91%	58
Huntsville Memorial Hospital	Huntsville	91%	33
Las Colinas Medical Center	Irving	91%	43
Medical Center of Arlington	Arlington	91%	87
Memorial Hermann-Texas Medical Center	Houston	91%	186
Palestine Regional Medical Center	Palestine	91%	90
Christus Saint Michael Health System	Texarkana	90%	296
Medical City Dallas	Dallas	90%	173
Park Plaza Hospital	Houston	90%	42
Valley Baptist Medical Center	Harlingen	90%	59
Cleveland Regional Medical Center	Cleveland	89%	27
Good Shepherd Medical Center	Longview	89%	74
McKenna Memorial Hospital	New Braunfels	89%	118
Medical Center of Plano	Plano	89%	93
Metroplex Hospital	Killeen	89%	84
Oakbend Medical Center	Richmond	89%	63
Arlington Memorial Hospital	Arlington	88%	58
Baylor Medical Center at Frisco	Frisco	88%	25
Baylor University Medical Center	Dallas	88%	877
Centennial Medical Center	Frisco	88%	34
Conroe Regional Medical Center	Conroe	88%	168
Lake Pointe Medical Center	Rowlett	88%	41
McAllen Medical Center	McAllen	88%	57
Memorial Herman Katy Hospital	Katy	88%	92
Mission Hospital	Mission	88%	56
Paris Regional Medical Center-South Campus	Paris	88%	157
Scott & White	Temple	88%	436
Southwest General Hospital	San Antonio	88%	51
Baptist-Saint Anthony's Health System	Amarillo	87%	82
Midland Memorial Hospital	Midland	87%	97
Odessa Regional Hospital	Odessa	87%	54
Richardson Medical Center	Richardson	87%	53
Saint Luke's Episcopal Hospital	Houston	87%	102
Angleton-Danbury Medical Center	Angleton	86%	37
John Peter Smith Hospital	Fort Worth	86%	100
Medical Center Hospital	Odessa	86%	140
Nix Healthcare System	San Antonio	86%	43
Plaza Medical Center	Fort Worth	86%	152
San Jacinto Methodist Hospital	Baytown	86%	37
Henderson Memorial Hospital	Henderson	85%	39
Lake Granbury Medical Center	Granbury	85%	34
Mother Frances Hospital-Tyler	Tyler	85%	82
Woodland Heights Medical Center	Lufkin	85%	110
Del Sol Medical Center	El Paso	84%	49
Laredo Medical Center	Laredo	84%	102
Longview Regional Medical Center	Longview	83%	101
Medical Center of Mesquite	Mesquite	83%	48
Memorial Hermann Memorial City	Houston	83%	83
University Medical Center	Lubbock	83%	63
Abilene Regional Medical Center	Abilene	82%	174
Columbia Spring Branch Medical Center	Houston	82%	66
Medical Center of Lewisville	Lewisville	81%	63
Mesquite Community Hospital	Mesquite	81%	69
Northwest Texas Healthcare System	Amarillo	81%	211
Harris Methodist Southwest	Fort Worth	80%	40
Houston Northwest Medical Center	Houston	80%	228
Huguley Memorial Medical Center	Burleson	80%	142
Marshall Regional Medical Center	Marshall	80%	46
University of Texas Medical Branch Hospitals	Galveston	80%	74
West Houston Medical Center	Houston	80%	76
Methodist Hospital	Houston	79%	86
North Hills Hospital	N Richland Hills	79%	77
Christus Saint John Hospital	Houston	77%	82
Covenant Medical Center	Lubbock	77%	101
Harris Methodist Erath County	Stephenville	76%	29
Kings Daughters Hospital	Temple	76%	49
Christus Saint Elizabeth Hospital	Beaumont	75%	365
Doctors Hospital at Renaissance	Edinburg	74%	98
Wise Regional Health System	Decatur	74%	39
Brownwood Regional Medical Center	Brownwood	73%	64
Doctors Hospital	Dallas	71%	58
East Houston Regional Medical Center	Houston	71%	41
North Central Medical Center	McKinney	71%	48
Trinity Medical Center	Carrollton	71%	49
East Texas Medical Center-Tyler	Tyler	70%	60
Guadalupe Valley Hospital	Seguin	70%	69
Medical Center of Southeast Texas	Port Arthur	70%	83
Clear Lake Regional Medical Center	Webster	69%	101
San Angelo Community Medical Center	San Angelo	69%	103
Bayshore Medical Center	Pasadena	67%	94
Harris County Hospital District	Houston	63%	118
Nacogdoches Medical Center Hospital	Nacogdoches	59%	37
Presbyterian Hospital of Allen	Allen	59%	29
Methodist Sugar Land Hospital	Sugar Land	55%	31
Mainland Medical Center	Texas City	51%	67
Northeast Medical Center Hospital	Humble	50%	58
East Texas Medical Center-Athens	Athens	48%	52
Presbyterian Hospital of Greenville	Greenville	44%	108
Hopkins County Memorial Hospital	Sulphur Springs	25%	44

22. Prophylactic Antibiotic Stopped

Hospital Name	City	Rate	Cases
Austin Surgical Hospital	Austin	100%	67
Harris Methodist Southlake Ctr for Diag	Southlake	100%	28
Lubbock Heart Hospital	Lubbock	100%	29
Presbyterian Plano Ctr for Diag & Surgery	Plano	100%	42
Texsan Heart Hospital	San Antonio	100%	357
Baylor Medical Center-Ellis County	Waxahachie	98%	296
Central Texas Medical Center	San Marcos	97%	58
Henderson Memorial Hospital	Henderson	97%	37
Baylor Heart and Vascular Center	Dallas	96%	165
Fort Duncan Medical Center	Eagle Pass	95%	43
Texas Orthopedic Hospital	Houston	93%	683
Brownsville Surgical Hospital	Brownsville	92%	60
Cornerstone Regional Hospital	Edinburg	92%	51
Presbyterian Hospital of Dallas	Dallas	92%	261
Texoma Medical Center	Denison	92%	353
Wise Regional Health System	Decatur	92%	39
Baylor All Saints Med Ctr at Forth Worth	Fort Worth	90%	1323
El Paso Specialty Hospital	El Paso	90%	340
Baylor University Medical Center	Dallas	89%	3460
Heart Hospital of Austin	Austin	89%	107
Methodist Medical Center	Dallas	89%	191
Oakbend Medical Center	Richmond	89%	151
Saint Joseph Regional Health Center	Bryan	89%	1032
Baylor Regional Medical Center at Plano	Plano	88%	113
Hopkins County Memorial Hospital	Sulphur Springs	88%	130
Physicians Centre	Bryan	88%	57
Spine Hospital of South Texas	San Antonio	88%	80
Womans Hospital of Texas	Houston	88%	912
Baylor Medical Center at Irving	Irving	87%	719
College Station Medical Center	College Station	87%	268
Las Colinas Medical Center	Irving	87%	90
Seton Southwest Healthcare Center	Austin	86%	36
Baylor Medical Center at Garland	Garland	85%	699
Charlton Methodist Hospital	Dallas	85%	135
Denton Regional Medical Center	Denton	85%	211
Good Shepherd Medical Center	Longview	85%	68
Presbyterian Hospital of Greenville	Greenville	85%	249
Saint Joseph Medical Center	Houston	85%	713
South Texas Regional Medical Center	Jourdanton	85%	54
Walls Regional Hospital	Cleburne	85%	98
Pampa Regional Medical Center	Pampa	83%	103
Titus Regional Medical Center	Mount Pleasant	82%	40
Detar Hospital Navarro	Victoria	81%	444

NOTE: Hospital profiles are in alphabetical order by state, then city, then hospital within the city; Rankings are sorted by rate in descending order and exclude hospitals with less than 25 cases; (1) The number of cases is too small (n<25) for purposes of reliably predicting hospital performance; (2) Measure reflects the hospital's indication that its submission was based upon a sample of its relevant discharges; (3) Rate reflects fewer than the maximum possible quarters of data for the measure; (4) Inaccurate information submitted and suppressed for one or more quarters; (5) No data is available from the hospital for this measure; Please refer to the User's Guide for a full explanation of data

East Houston Regional Medical Center.	Houston	81%	93
Gulf Coast Medical Center	Wharton	81%	141
McKenna Memorial Hospital	New Braunfels	81%	113
Scott & White	Temple	81%	1719
Memorial Herman Katy Hospital.	Katy	80%	244
Mother Frances Hospital Jacksonville.	Jacksonville	80%	40
Saint Luke's Episcopal Hospital	Houston	80%	300
Baylor Regional Medical Center at Grapevine	Grapevine	79%	797
Brackenridge Hospital.	Austin	79%	135
Scenic Mountain Medical Center.	Big Spring	79%	34
Thomason General Hospital	El Paso	79%	162
University of Texas Health Center at Tyler.	Tyler	79%	80
Woodland Heights Medical Center	Lufkin	79%	396
Harris Methodist Continued Care Hospital.	Fort Worth	78%	234
Memorial Health System of East Texas-Lufkin	Lufkin	78%	94
Palo Pinto General Hospital	Mineral Wells	78%	92
Presbyterian Hospital of Denton	Denton	78%	437
Seton Medical Center.	Austin	78%	222
USMD Hospital at Arlington.	Arlington	78%	41
Harris Methodist HEB Hospital.	Bedford	77%	155
John Peter Smith Hospital	Fort Worth	77%	476
Ennis Regional Medical Center.	Ennis	76%	71
Harris Methodist Erath County.	Stephenville	76%	96
Midland Memorial Hospital.	Midland	76%	319
San Angelo Community Medical Center	San Angelo	76%	406
Cleveland Regional Medical Center.	Cleveland	75%	53
Del Sol Medical Center.	El Paso	75%	118
Mesquite Community Hospital.	Mesquite	75%	290
Odessa Regional Hospital.	Odessa	75%	137
Paris Regional Medical Center-South Campus.	Paris	75%	490
Christus Saint Catherine Hospital	Katy	73%	146
Hendrick Medical Center.	Abilene	73%	270
Medical City Dallas.	Dallas	73%	360
Methodist Hospital.	Houston	73%	415
Baylor Medical Center at Frisco.	Frisco	72%	58
South Austin Hospital.	Austin	72%	252
Baptist Medical Center.	San Antonio	71%	463
Doctors Hospital	Dallas	71%	223
Medical Center of Mesquite.	Mesquite	71%	158
Brownsville Medical Center.	Brownsville	70%	144
Tomball Regional Hospital.	Tomball	70%	50
Val Verde Regional Medical Center.	Del Rio	70%	97
Baptist-Saint Anthony's Health System	Amarillo	69%	296
Citizens Medical Center.	Victoria	69%	438
Conroe Regional Medical Center.	Conroe	69%	251
East Texas Medical Center-Athens	Athens	69%	120
East Texas Medical Center-Tyler.	Tyler	69%	150
Georgetown Healthcare System	Georgetown	69%	112
Methodist Hospital.	San Antonio	69%	456
University Medical Center.	Lubbock	69%	167
Memorial Hermann Healthcare System.	Houston	68%	2451
Memorial Hermann-Texas Medical Center.	Houston	68%	567
Mother Frances Hospital-Tyler.	Tyler	68%	253
University Hospital	San Antonio	68%	187
Doctors Hospital of Laredo	Laredo	67%	166
Harris County Hospital District	Houston	67%	289
Kings Daughters Hospital	Temple	67%	94
Matagorda County Hospital District	Bay City	67%	57
Richardson Medical Center.	Richardson	67%	178
Saint David's Rehabiltation Center.	Austin	67%	262
Las Palmas Medical Center.	El Paso	66%	209
Medical Center of Plano	Plano	66%	178
San Jacinto Methodist Hospital.	Baytown	66%	174
Trinity Medical Center.	Brenham	66%	70
Trinity Medical Center.	Carrollton	66%	184
Harris Methodist Southwest	Fort Worth	65%	100
Physicians Specialty Hospital of El Paso.	El Paso	65%	26
Presbyterian Hospital of Plano.	Plano	65%	174
Christus Spohn Hospital Kleberg	Kingsville	64%	64
Huguley Memorial Medical Center.	Burleson	64%	396
Longview Regional Medical Center	Longview	64%	367
North Austin Medical Center.	Austin	64%	214
Providence Memorial Hospital	El Paso	64%	323
Kingwood Medical Center.	Kingwood	63%	67
North Hills Hospital	N Richland Hills	63%	185
North Texas Medical Center	Gainesville	63%	75
Presbyterian Hospital of Allen.	Allen	63%	87
Twelve Oaks Hospital.	Houston	63%	35
University of Texas Medical Branch Hospitals.	Galveston	63%	345
Arlington Memorial Hospital.	Arlington	62%	169
Guadalupe Valley Hospital.	Seguin	62%	185
Harlingen Medical Center.	Harlingen	62%	255
Nacogdoches Memorial Hospital	Nacogdoches	61%	75
Navarro Regional Hospital	Corsicana	61%	114
Saint Luke's Community Med Ctr-The Woodlands	The Woodlands	61%	38

Valley Baptist Medical Center.	Harlingen	61%	190
Houston Northwest Medical Center.	Houston	60%	849
Nacogdoches Medical Center Hospital	Nacogdoches	60%	324
Abilene Regional Medical Center	Abilene	59%	584
Marshall Regional Medical Center.	Marshall	58%	162
Medical Center of Lewisville.	Lewisville	58%	135
North Central Medical Center	McKinney	58%	139
UT Southwestern Saint Paul Hospital	Dallas	58%	209
Wadley Regional Medical Center.	Texarkana	58%	294
Bayshore Medical Center.	Pasadena	57%	184
Centennial Medical Center.	Frisco	57%	127
Palestine Regional Medical Center.	Palestine	57%	258
Sid Peterson Memorial Hospital	Kerrville	57%	352
Sierra Medical Center.	El Paso	57%	312
Clear Lake Regional Medical Center.	Webster	56%	228
Methodist Willowbrook Hospital.	Houston	56%	39
Presbyterian Hospital of Kaufman.	Kaufman	56%	52
Lake Granbury Medical Center.	Granbury	55%	98
Shannon Medical Center.	San Angelo	55%	215
Memorial Hermann Baptist Beaumont	Beaumont	54%	101
Parkland Health & Hospital System.	Dallas	54%	136
Columbia Spring Branch Medical Center.	Houston	53%	155
Medical Center of Arlington.	Arlington	53%	177
Memorial Hermann Fort Bend Hospital.	Missouri City	53%	47
Uvalde Memorial Hospital.	Uvalde	53%	53
Brownwood Regional Medical Center.	Brownwood	52%	256
Christus Saint Elizabeth Hospital	Beaumont	52%	1312
Memorial Hermann Baptist Orange Hospital	Orange	52%	65
Methodist Sugar Land Hospital.	Sugar Land	52%	147
Northwest Texas Healthcare System	Amarillo	52%	961
RHD Memorial Medical Center.	Dallas	52%	100
Tops Surgical Specialty Hospital.	Houston	52%	25
Hill Country Memorial Hospital	Fredericksburg	51%	452
Lake Pointe Medical Center.	Rowlett	51%	138
Physicians Surgical Hospital at Quail Creek	Amarillo	51%	35
Rio Grande Regional Hospital.	McAllen	51%	121
Christus Jasper Memorial Hospital	Jasper	50%	44
Providence Health Center.	Waco	50%	189
Round Rock Medical Center.	Round Rock	50%	165
Brazosport Memorial Hospital	Lake Jackson	49%	92
Christus Santa Rosa Hospital-City Centre	San Antonio	48%	1164
Cypress Fairbanks Medical Center and Hospital	Houston	48%	106
Memorial Hermann Memorial City.	Houston	48%	770
Hillcrest Baptist Medical Center.	Waco	47%	204
Northeast Medical Center Hospital.	Humble	47%	217
Campbell Health System	Weatherford	46%	81
Christus Saint Michael Health System	Texarkana	46%	1223
Doctors Hospital at Renaissance	Edinburg	45%	346
Metroplex Hospital	Killeen	45%	211
Plaza Medical Center.	Fort Worth	45%	298
Valley Regional Medical Center.	Brownsville	45%	132
Zale-Lipshy University Hospital	Dallas	45%	65
Medical Center Hospital	Odessa	44%	447
Medical Center of Southeast Texas	Port Arthur	44%	255
Angleton-Danbury Medical Center	Angleton	43%	162
Covenant Medical Center.	Lubbock	43%	246
Permian General Hospital	Andrews	43%	67
Seton Northwest Hospital.	Austin	43%	110
Corpus Christi Medical Center-Bay Area	Corpus Christi	41%	282
Mainland Medical Center.	Texas City	41%	129
Nix Healthcare System	San Antonio	41%	157
Wilson N Jones Medical Center.	Sherman	40%	55
Christus Spohn Memorial Hospital	Corpus Christi	39%	1412
Park Plaza Hospital	Houston	36%	158
West Houston Medical Center.	Houston	35%	179
Laredo Medical Center.	Laredo	34%	367
Southwest General Hospital.	San Antonio	34%	184
Memorial Medical Center Livingston	Livingston	33%	30
Harris Methodist Northwest	Azle	31%	48
United Regional Healthcare System	Wichita Falls	30%	263
McAllen Medical Center.	McAllen	28%	238
Alliance Hospital	Odessa	27%	71
Mission Hospital.	Mission	26%	159
Christus Saint John Hospital	Houston	25%	335
Knapp Medical Center.	Weslaco	25%	170
Huntsville Memorial Hospital.	Huntsville	24%	143
Highland Community Hospital.	Lubbock	22%	79
The Hospital at Westlake Medical Center.	Austin	21%	29
Edinburg Regional Medical Center.	Edinburg	16%	55
Childress Regional Medical Center.	Childress	13%	46

NOTE: Hospital profiles are in alphabetical order by state, then city, then hospital within the city; Rankings are sorted by rate in descending order and exclude hospitals with less than 25 cases; (1) The number of cases is too small (n<25) for purposes of reliably predicting hospital performance; (2) Measure reflects the hospital's indication that its submission was based upon a sample of its relevant discharges; (3) Rate reflects fewer than the maximum possible quarters of data for the measure; (4) Inaccurate information submitted and suppressed for one or more quarters; (5) No data is available from the hospital for this measure; Please refer to the User's Guide for a full explanation of data

Pregnancy Care

23. Inpatient Neonatal Mortality

Hospital Name	City	Rate	Cases
Alice Regional Hospital	Alice	0.00%	580
Christus Spohn Hospital Kleberg	Kingsville	0.00%	345
East Texas Medical Center-Tyler	Tyler	0.00%	246
Kings Daughters Hospital	Temple	0.00%	769
Longview Regional Medical Center	Longview	0.00%	925
Matagorda County Hospital District	Bay City	0.00%	283
Memorial Health System of East Texas-Lufkin	Lufkin	0.00%	745
Tomball Regional Hospital	Tomball	0.00%	803
Metroplex Hospital	Killeen	0.08%	1313
Presbyterian Hospital of Allen	Allen	0.08%	1296
Citizens Medical Center	Victoria	0.10%	1039
West Houston Medical Center	Houston	0.14%	2170
Detar Hospital Navarro	Victoria	0.15%	1306
Saint Luke's Community Med Ctr-The Woodlands	The Woodlands	0.16%	1829
University Hospital	San Antonio	0.16%	607
Texoma Medical Center	Denison	0.17%	588
University of Texas Medical Branch Hospitals	Galveston	0.19%	1032
Corpus Christi Medical Center-Bay Area	Corpus Christi	0.20%	3506
McKenna Memorial Hospital	New Braunfels	0.20%	995
Charlton Methodist Hospital	Dallas	0.21%	2362
Round Rock Medical Center	Round Rock	0.22%	1782
Christus Spohn Hospital Beeville	Beeville	0.24%	412
Baptist Medical Center	San Antonio	0.26%	9512
Southwest General Hospital	San Antonio	0.28%	2169
Valley Regional Medical Center	Brownsville	0.28%	3174
Abilene Regional Medical Center	Abilene	0.34%	1464
Medical Center Hospital	Odessa	0.34%	1472
Medical Center of Arlington	Arlington	0.34%	3806
Huguley Memorial Medical Center	Burleson	0.35%	1143
Christus Spohn Memorial Hospital	Corpus Christi	0.39%	3588
Womans Hospital of Texas	Houston	0.41%	8798
Parkland Health & Hospital System	Dallas	0.45%	16281
Odessa Regional Hospital	Odessa	0.49%	2268
Memorial Medical Center Livingston	Livingston	0.70%	287
Methodist Medical Center	Dallas	0.76%	3839
Scott & White	Temple	1.21%	1077

24. Third or Fourth Degree Laceration

Hospital Name	City	Rate	Cases
Memorial Medical Center Livingston	Livingston	0.53%	188
Southwest General Hospital	San Antonio	0.65%	1376
Christus Spohn Hospital Kleberg	Kingsville	1.19%	168
Alice Regional Hospital	Alice	1.27%	393
Charlton Methodist Hospital	Dallas	1.31%	1681
Kings Daughters Hospital	Temple	1.55%	515
Texoma Medical Center	Denison	1.55%	386
Valley Regional Medical Center	Brownsville	1.57%	1652
Christus Spohn Hospital Beeville	Beeville	1.61%	249
West Houston Medical Center	Houston	1.70%	1415
Corpus Christi Medical Center-Bay Area	Corpus Christi	2.05%	2099
Memorial Health System of East Texas-Lufkin	Lufkin	2.07%	483
University of Texas Medical Branch Hospitals	Galveston	2.14%	5882
Medical Center of Arlington	Arlington	2.25%	2308
Methodist Medical Center	Dallas	2.26%	2612
Baptist Medical Center	San Antonio	2.40%	6040
Womans Hospital of Texas	Houston	2.63%	4638
Detar Hospital Navarro	Victoria	2.82%	710
Scott & White	Temple	3.13%	800
Citizens Medical Center	Victoria	3.27%	551
Saint Luke's Community Med Ctr-The Woodlands	The Woodlands	3.28%	1157
Christus Spohn Memorial Hospital	Corpus Christi	3.32%	2139
Metroplex Hospital	Killeen	3.33%	780
Tomball Regional Hospital	Tomball	3.52%	596
Medical Center Hospital	Odessa	4.01%	972
Round Rock Medical Center	Round Rock	4.11%	1169
University Hospital	San Antonio	4.31%	394
Presbyterian Hospital of Allen	Allen	4.54%	749
Longview Regional Medical Center	Longview	4.58%	589
Abilene Regional Medical Center	Abilene	4.72%	1038
Huguley Memorial Medical Center	Burleson	5.10%	824
Parkland Health & Hospital System	Dallas	5.13%	11763
Odessa Regional Hospital	Odessa	5.34%	1573
McKenna Memorial Hospital	New Braunfels	6.06%	693
East Texas Medical Center-Tyler	Tyler	6.21%	177
Matagorda County Hospital District	Bay City	6.76%	207

NOTE: Hospital profiles are in alphabetical order by state, then city, then hospital within the city; Rankings are sorted by rate in descending order and exclude hospitals with less than 25 cases; (1) The number of cases is too small (n<25) for purposes of reliably predicting hospital performance; (2) Measure reflects the hospital's indication that its submission was based upon a sample of its relevant discharges; (3) Rate reflects fewer than the maximum possible quarters of data for the measure; (4) Inaccurate information submitted and suppressed for one or more quarters; (5) No data is available from the hospital for this measure; Please refer to the User's Guide for a full explanation of data

Abilene Regional Medical Center

Alternate Name: Humana Hospital-Abilene
6250 Highway 83-84
Abilene, TX 79606
E-mail: debbie_mcclure@armc.net
URL: www.abileneregional.com
Ownership: Proprietary
Emergency Services: Yes

Phone: 915-695-9900
Fax: 325-428-1029

Accredited: Yes
Licensed Beds: 187

Key Personnel:
CEO/Administrator . . . . Michael Murphy
Chief Medical Staff . . . . Carl Turser, MD
Emergency Room . . . . Chrie Six, RN

Measure	Cases	This Hospital	State Average	U.S. Average	Top Hospital
Heart Attack Care					
ACE Inhibitor or ARB for LVSD	33	100%	85%	82%	100%
Aspirin at Arrival	66	100%	91%	92%	100%
Aspirin at Discharge	152	99%	90%	90%	100%
Beta Blocker at Arrival	58	100%	85%	87%	100%
Beta Blocker at Discharge	138	99%	86%	90%	100%
Fibrinolytic Medication Timing[1]	6	67%	30%	31%	100%
PCI Within 90 Minutes of Arrival	0	-	48%	54%	95%
Smoking Cessation Advice	57	100%	90%	88%	100%
Heart Failure Care					
ACE Inhibitor or ARB for LVSD	68	97%	82%	82%	100%
Discharge Instructions	136	100%	60%	61%	93%
Evaluation of LVS Function	166	100%	81%	83%	99%
Smoking Cessation Advice	49	100%	82%	82%	100%
Pneumonia Care					
Appropriate Initial Antibiotic	65	91%	79%	83%	94%
Blood Culture Timing	31	81%	89%	90%	100%
Influenza Vaccine[1]	22	82%	69%	70%	100%
Initial Antibiotic Timing	67	72%	78%	80%	93%
Oxygenation Assessment	87	100%	99%	99%	100%
Pneumococcal Vaccine	54	76%	68%	69%	94%
Smoking Cessation Advice	36	100%	83%	80%	100%
Surgical Infection Prevention					
Prophylactic Antibiotic Given	633	87%	67%	77%	95%
Prophylactic Antibiotic Selection	174	82%	86%	90%	100%
Prophylactic Antibiotic Stopped	584	59%	68%	72%	95%
Pregnancy Care					
Inpatient Neonatal Mortality	1,464	0.34%	-	-	-
Third or Fourth Degree Laceration	1,038	4.72%	3.23%	3.63%	3.27%

Hendrick Medical Center

1900 Pine Street
Abilene, TX 79601
URL: www.hendrickhealth.org
Ownership: Voluntary non-profit - Church
Emergency Services: Yes

Phone: 325-670-2000
Fax: 325-670-2293

Accredited: Yes
Licensed Beds: 525

Key Personnel:
Administrator/President . . . . Michael C Waters
Chief Medical Staff . . . . Jerry Strader, DDS
Cardiac Lab . . . . Steve Albrient
Catheterization Lab . . . . Steve Albrient
Emergency Room . . . . Connie Bowlin, RN
Infection Control . . . . Patty Bull
ICU . . . . Winnona Migliavacca, RN
Intensive/Coronary Care . . . . Steve Albright, RN
Director Medical/Surgical Nursing . . . . Winnona Migliavacca
OB/GYN Womens Health . . . . Sarah Mullkey
Respiratory/Cardiopulmonary . . . . Tim Riley

Measure	Cases	This Hospital	State Average	U.S. Average	Top Hospital
Heart Attack Care					
ACE Inhibitor or ARB for LVSD[2]	51	78%	85%	82%	100%
Aspirin at Arrival[2]	214	94%	91%	92%	100%
Aspirin at Discharge[2]	318	96%	90%	90%	100%
Beta Blocker at Arrival[2]	172	85%	85%	87%	100%
Beta Blocker at Discharge[2]	326	88%	86%	90%	100%
Fibrinolytic Medication Timing[1,2]	21	67%	30%	31%	100%
PCI Within 90 Minutes of Arrival[1,2]	9	33%	48%	54%	95%
Smoking Cessation Advice[2]	134	93%	90%	88%	100%

Measure	Cases	This Hospital	State Average	U.S. Average	Top Hospital
Heart Failure Care					
ACE Inhibitor or ARB for LVSD[2]	188	85%	82%	82%	100%
Discharge Instructions[2]	336	57%	60%	61%	93%
Evaluation of LVS Function[2]	411	96%	81%	83%	99%
Smoking Cessation Advice[2]	78	90%	82%	82%	100%
Pneumonia Care					
Appropriate Initial Antibiotic[2]	218	79%	79%	83%	94%
Blood Culture Timing[2]	175	87%	89%	90%	100%
Influenza Vaccine	70	89%	69%	70%	100%
Initial Antibiotic Timing[2]	259	73%	78%	80%	93%
Oxygenation Assessment[2]	317	100%	99%	99%	100%
Pneumococcal Vaccine[2]	179	87%	68%	69%	94%
Smoking Cessation Advice[2]	86	86%	83%	80%	100%
Surgical Infection Prevention					
Prophylactic Antibiotic Given[2]	276	88%	67%	77%	95%
Prophylactic Antibiotic Selection[2]	69	94%	86%	90%	100%
Prophylactic Antibiotic Stopped[2]	270	73%	68%	72%	95%
Pregnancy Care					
Inpatient Neonatal Mortality	-	-	-	-	-
Third or Fourth Degree Laceration	-	-	3.23%	3.63%	3.27%

Alice Regional Hospital

Alternate Name: CHRISTUS Spohn Hospital-Alice
2500 E Main
Alice, TX 78332
Ownership: Proprietary
Emergency Services: Yes

Phone: 361-664-4376
Fax: 361-883-6478
Accredited: Yes

Key Personnel:
President/CEO . . . . Leon Belila
Chief Medical Staff . . . . Judy Fenders
Cardiac Lab . . . . Jennifer Anbmendi
Emergency Room . . . . Stephen Dalrymple
Infection Control . . . . Traci Kreiszel
ICU . . . . Elvira DeTorres
OB/GYN Womens Health . . . . Patti Richard
Respiratory/Cardiopulmonary . . . . Cindi Bront

Measure	Cases	This Hospital	State Average	U.S. Average	Top Hospital
Heart Attack Care					
ACE Inhibitor or ARB for LVSD[1]	7	100%	85%	82%	100%
Aspirin at Arrival	76	97%	91%	92%	100%
Aspirin at Discharge	33	88%	90%	90%	100%
Beta Blocker at Arrival	60	97%	85%	87%	100%
Beta Blocker at Discharge	27	96%	86%	90%	100%
Fibrinolytic Medication Timing[3]	0	-	30%	31%	100%
PCI Within 90 Minutes of Arrival	0	-	48%	54%	95%
Smoking Cessation Advice[1,3]	2	100%	90%	88%	100%
Heart Failure Care					
ACE Inhibitor or ARB for LVSD	64	94%	82%	82%	100%
Discharge Instructions[3]	40	98%	60%	61%	93%
Evaluation of LVS Function	240	98%	81%	83%	99%
Smoking Cessation Advice[1,3]	10	100%	82%	82%	100%
Pneumonia Care					
Appropriate Initial Antibiotic[1,3]	22	91%	79%	83%	94%
Blood Culture Timing[3]	33	88%	89%	90%	100%
Influenza Vaccine[4,5]	-	-	69%	70%	100%
Initial Antibiotic Timing	213	83%	78%	80%	93%
Oxygenation Assessment	235	99%	99%	99%	100%
Pneumococcal Vaccine	137	92%	68%	69%	94%
Smoking Cessation Advice[1,3]	5	100%	83%	80%	100%
Surgical Infection Prevention					
Prophylactic Antibiotic Given[1,3]	16	94%	67%	77%	95%
Prophylactic Antibiotic Selection[5]	-	-	86%	90%	100%
Prophylactic Antibiotic Stopped[1,3]	15	53%	68%	72%	95%
Pregnancy Care					
Inpatient Neonatal Mortality	580	0.00%	-	-	-
Third or Fourth Degree Laceration	393	1.27%	3.23%	3.63%	3.27%

NOTE: Hospital profiles are in alphabetical order by state, then city, then hospital within the city; Rankings are sorted by rate in descending order and exclude hospitals with less than 25 cases; (1) The number of cases is too small (n<25) for purposes of reliably predicting hospital performance; (2) Measure reflects the hospital's indication that its submission was based upon a sample of its relevant discharges; (3) Rate reflects fewer than the maximum possible quarters of data for the measure; (4) Inaccurate information submitted and suppressed for one or more quarters; (5) No data is available from the hospital for this measure; Please refer to the User's Guide for a full explanation of data

Presbyterian Hospital of Allen

1105 Central Expressway North
Allen, TX 75013
Ownership: Government - Federal
Emergency Services: Yes

Phone: 972-747-1000

Accredited: Yes

Measure	Cases	This Hospital	State Average	U.S. Average	Top Hospital
Heart Attack Care					
ACE Inhibitor or ARB for LVSD[1]	1	100%	85%	82%	100%
Aspirin at Arrival[1]	7	100%	91%	92%	100%
Aspirin at Discharge[1]	4	100%	90%	90%	100%
Beta Blocker at Arrival[1]	7	100%	85%	87%	100%
Beta Blocker at Discharge[1]	5	100%	86%	90%	100%
Fibrinolytic Medication Timing	0	-	30%	31%	100%
PCI Within 90 Minutes of Arrival	0	-	48%	54%	95%
Smoking Cessation Advice[1]	2	100%	90%	88%	100%
Heart Failure Care					
ACE Inhibitor or ARB for LVSD[1]	20	85%	82%	82%	100%
Discharge Instructions	50	42%	60%	61%	93%
Evaluation of LVS Function	62	94%	81%	83%	99%
Smoking Cessation Advice[1]	15	100%	82%	82%	100%
Pneumonia Care					
Appropriate Initial Antibiotic	70	86%	79%	83%	94%
Blood Culture Timing	51	98%	89%	90%	100%
Influenza Vaccine[1]	17	88%	69%	70%	100%
Initial Antibiotic Timing	65	91%	78%	80%	93%
Oxygenation Assessment	87	100%	99%	99%	100%
Pneumococcal Vaccine	46	85%	68%	69%	94%
Smoking Cessation Advice	30	97%	83%	80%	100%
Surgical Infection Prevention					
Prophylactic Antibiotic Given[2,3]	93	48%	67%	77%	95%
Prophylactic Antibiotic Selection[2]	29	59%	86%	90%	100%
Prophylactic Antibiotic Stopped[2,3]	87	63%	68%	72%	95%
Pregnancy Care					
Inpatient Neonatal Mortality	1,296	0.08%	-	-	-
Third or Fourth Degree Laceration	749	4.54%	3.23%	3.63%	3.27%

Big Bend Regional Medical Center

2600 N Highway 118
Alpine, TX 79830
Ownership: Voluntary non-profit - Private
Emergency Services: Yes
Key Personnel:
President/CEO. . . . . Jimmy Stuart
Chief Medical Staff. . . . . David Sanchez, MD
Medical/Surgical Nursing Director . . . . Robin Byler
OB/GYN/Womens Health. . . . . Yolanda Morales
Chief of Radiology . . . . George Gonzales, MD
Respiratory Therapy Director . . . . Abe Miranda

Phone: 915-837-3447
Fax: 432-837-0255
Accredited: Yes
Licensed Beds: 40

Measure	Cases	This Hospital	State Average	U.S. Average	Top Hospital
Heart Attack Care					
ACE Inhibitor or ARB for LVSD	0	-	85%	82%	100%
Aspirin at Arrival[1]	8	100%	91%	92%	100%
Aspirin at Discharge[1]	5	100%	90%	90%	100%
Beta Blocker at Arrival[1]	9	100%	85%	87%	100%
Beta Blocker at Discharge[1]	5	80%	86%	90%	100%
Fibrinolytic Medication Timing	0	-	30%	31%	100%
PCI Within 90 Minutes of Arrival	0	-	48%	54%	95%
Smoking Cessation Advice[1]	1	0%	90%	88%	100%
Heart Failure Care					
ACE Inhibitor or ARB for LVSD[1]	14	71%	82%	82%	100%
Discharge Instructions	26	12%	60%	61%	93%
Evaluation of LVS Function	30	47%	81%	83%	99%
Smoking Cessation Advice[1]	4	75%	82%	82%	100%
Pneumonia Care					
Appropriate Initial Antibiotic	95	78%	79%	83%	94%
Blood Culture Timing	52	90%	89%	90%	100%
Influenza Vaccine	31	77%	69%	70%	100%
Initial Antibiotic Timing	113	91%	78%	80%	93%
Oxygenation Assessment	121	100%	99%	99%	100%
Pneumococcal Vaccine	79	91%	68%	69%	94%

Smoking Cessation Advice[1]	13	77%	83%	80%	100%
Surgical Infection Prevention					
Prophylactic Antibiotic Given[1,2,3]	3	0%	67%	77%	95%
Prophylactic Antibiotic Selection[1,2]	1	100%	86%	90%	100%
Prophylactic Antibiotic Stopped[1,2,3]	2	100%	68%	72%	95%
Pregnancy Care					
Inpatient Neonatal Mortality	-	-	-	-	-
Third or Fourth Degree Laceration	-	-	3.23%	3.63%	3.27%

Baptist-Saint Anthony's Health System

Alternate Name: BSA
1600 Wallace Boulevard
Amarillo, TX 79106
URL: www.bsahs.com
Ownership: Voluntary non-profit - Church
Emergency Services: Yes
Key Personnel:
Administrator/CEO. . . . . John Hicks
Chief Medical Staff. . . . . Kenneth Johnston, MD
Cardiac Lab . . . . Shay Christian
Catheterization Lab . . . . Terri Allen
Emergency Room . . . . Owen Grossman, MD
Infection Control. . . . . Charlotte Wheeler
ICU/Intensive Coronary Care . . . . Ronda Crow
Intensive Coronary. . . . . Kelly Fuller
Surgical Nursing. . . . . Susan Jones
OB/GYN Womens Health. . . . . Patty Mathies
Respiratory/Cardiopulmonary. . . . . Susan Young

Phone: 806-212-2000
Fax: 806-212-2853

Accredited: Yes
Licensed Beds: 451

Measure	Cases	This Hospital	State Average	U.S. Average	Top Hospital
Heart Attack Care					
ACE Inhibitor or ARB for LVSD[1]	23	83%	85%	82%	100%
Aspirin at Arrival	169	99%	91%	92%	100%
Aspirin at Discharge	257	95%	90%	90%	100%
Beta Blocker at Arrival	156	98%	85%	87%	100%
Beta Blocker at Discharge	262	98%	86%	90%	100%
Fibrinolytic Medication Timing[1]	2	50%	30%	31%	100%
PCI Within 90 Minutes of Arrival[1]	4	100%	48%	54%	95%
Smoking Cessation Advice	93	97%	90%	88%	100%
Heart Failure Care					
ACE Inhibitor or ARB for LVSD	72	75%	82%	82%	100%
Discharge Instructions	229	52%	60%	61%	93%
Evaluation of LVS Function	274	88%	81%	83%	99%
Smoking Cessation Advice	50	98%	82%	82%	100%
Pneumonia Care					
Appropriate Initial Antibiotic	97	78%	79%	83%	94%
Blood Culture Timing	70	86%	89%	90%	100%
Influenza Vaccine	27	41%	69%	70%	100%
Initial Antibiotic Timing	159	57%	78%	80%	93%
Oxygenation Assessment	175	100%	99%	99%	100%
Pneumococcal Vaccine	109	73%	68%	69%	94%
Smoking Cessation Advice	41	98%	83%	80%	100%
Surgical Infection Prevention					
Prophylactic Antibiotic Given	310	85%	67%	77%	95%
Prophylactic Antibiotic Selection	82	87%	86%	90%	100%
Prophylactic Antibiotic Stopped	296	69%	68%	72%	95%
Pregnancy Care					
Inpatient Neonatal Mortality	-	-	-	-	-
Third or Fourth Degree Laceration	-	-	3.23%	3.63%	3.27%

Northwest Texas Healthcare System

1501 Coulter Road
Amarillo, TX 79106
URL: www.nxtexashealthcare.com
Ownership: Proprietary
Emergency Services: Yes
CEO. . . . . Frank Lopez
CNO. . . . . Becky Hunter
Director Respiratory . . . . Randy Clarck

Phone: 806-354-1000
Fax: 806-354-1109

Accredited: Yes
Licensed Beds: 574

Measure	Cases	This Hospital	State Average	U.S. Average	Top Hospital
Heart Attack Care					

NOTE: Hospital profiles are in alphabetical order by state, then city, then hospital within the city; Rankings are sorted by rate in descending order and exclude hospitals with less than 25 cases; (1) The number of cases is too small (n<25) for purposes of reliably predicting hospital performance; (2) Measure reflects the hospital's indication that its submission was based upon a sample of its relevant discharges; (3) Rate reflects fewer than the maximum possible quarters of data for the measure; (4) Inaccurate information submitted and suppressed for one or more quarters; (5) No data is available from the hospital for this measure; Please refer to the User's Guide for a full explanation of data

ACE Inhibitor or ARB for LVSD	57	84%	85%	82%	100%
Aspirin at Arrival	205	96%	91%	92%	100%
Aspirin at Discharge	298	99%	90%	90%	100%
Beta Blocker at Arrival	180	96%	85%	87%	100%
Beta Blocker at Discharge	294	97%	86%	90%	100%
Fibrinolytic Medication Timing	0	-	30%	31%	100%
PCI Within 90 Minutes of Arrival[1]	12	33%	48%	54%	95%
Smoking Cessation Advice	157	97%	90%	88%	100%
Heart Failure Care					
ACE Inhibitor or ARB for LVSD	144	83%	82%	82%	100%
Discharge Instructions	264	83%	60%	61%	93%
Evaluation of LVS Function	326	88%	81%	83%	99%
Smoking Cessation Advice	94	94%	82%	82%	100%
Pneumonia Care					
Appropriate Initial Antibiotic	245	76%	79%	83%	94%
Blood Culture Timing	137	79%	89%	90%	100%
Influenza Vaccine	52	58%	69%	70%	100%
Initial Antibiotic Timing	229	69%	78%	80%	93%
Oxygenation Assessment	281	100%	99%	99%	100%
Pneumococcal Vaccine	123	64%	68%	69%	94%
Smoking Cessation Advice	103	89%	83%	80%	100%
Surgical Infection Prevention					
Prophylactic Antibiotic Given	979	81%	67%	77%	95%
Prophylactic Antibiotic Selection	211	81%	86%	90%	100%
Prophylactic Antibiotic Stopped	961	52%	68%	72%	95%
Pregnancy Care					
Inpatient Neonatal Mortality	-	-	-	-	-
Third or Fourth Degree Laceration	-	-	3.23%	3.63%	3.27%

Northwest Texas Surgery Center

3501 Soncy Rd Suite 118
Amarillo, TX 79109
Ownership: Proprietary
Emergency Services: Yes

Phone: 806-359-7999

Accredited: No

Measure	Cases	This Hospital	State Average	U.S. Average	Top Hospital
Heart Attack Care					
ACE Inhibitor or ARB for LVSD[5]	-	-	85%	82%	100%
Aspirin at Arrival[5]	-	-	91%	92%	100%
Aspirin at Discharge[5]	-	-	90%	90%	100%
Beta Blocker at Arrival[5]	-	-	85%	87%	100%
Beta Blocker at Discharge[5]	-	-	86%	90%	100%
Fibrinolytic Medication Timing[5]	-	-	30%	31%	100%
PCI Within 90 Minutes of Arrival[5]	-	-	48%	54%	95%
Smoking Cessation Advice[5]	-	-	90%	88%	100%
Heart Failure Care					
ACE Inhibitor or ARB for LVSD[5]	-	-	82%	82%	100%
Discharge Instructions[5]	-	-	60%	61%	93%
Evaluation of LVS Function[5]	-	-	81%	83%	99%
Smoking Cessation Advice[5]	-	-	82%	82%	100%
Pneumonia Care					
Appropriate Initial Antibiotic[5]	-	-	79%	83%	94%
Blood Culture Timing[5]	-	-	89%	90%	100%
Influenza Vaccine[5]	-	-	69%	70%	100%
Initial Antibiotic Timing[5]	-	-	78%	80%	93%
Oxygenation Assessment[5]	-	-	99%	99%	100%
Pneumococcal Vaccine[5]	-	-	68%	69%	94%
Smoking Cessation Advice[5]	-	-	83%	80%	100%
Surgical Infection Prevention					
Prophylactic Antibiotic Given[1,3]	1	0%	67%	77%	95%
Prophylactic Antibiotic Selection[5]	-	-	86%	90%	100%
Prophylactic Antibiotic Stopped[1,3]	1	100%	68%	72%	95%
Pregnancy Care					
Inpatient Neonatal Mortality	-	-	-	-	-
Third or Fourth Degree Laceration	-	-	3.23%	3.63%	3.27%

Physicians Surgical Hospital at Quail Creek

6819 Plum Creek
Amarillo, TX 79124
Ownership: Proprietary
Emergency Services: Yes

Phone: 806-354-6100

Accredited: No

Measure	Cases	This Hospital	State Average	U.S. Average	Top Hospital
Heart Attack Care					
ACE Inhibitor or ARB for LVSD[5]	-	-	85%	82%	100%
Aspirin at Arrival[5]	-	-	91%	92%	100%
Aspirin at Discharge[5]	-	-	90%	90%	100%
Beta Blocker at Arrival[5]	-	-	85%	87%	100%
Beta Blocker at Discharge[5]	-	-	86%	90%	100%
Fibrinolytic Medication Timing[5]	-	-	30%	31%	100%
PCI Within 90 Minutes of Arrival[5]	-	-	48%	54%	95%
Smoking Cessation Advice[5]	-	-	90%	88%	100%
Heart Failure Care					
ACE Inhibitor or ARB for LVSD[5]	-	-	82%	82%	100%
Discharge Instructions[5]	-	-	60%	61%	93%
Evaluation of LVS Function[5]	-	-	81%	83%	99%
Smoking Cessation Advice[5]	-	-	82%	82%	100%
Pneumonia Care					
Appropriate Initial Antibiotic[5]	-	-	79%	83%	94%
Blood Culture Timing[5]	-	-	89%	90%	100%
Influenza Vaccine[5]	-	-	69%	70%	100%
Initial Antibiotic Timing[5]	-	-	78%	80%	93%
Oxygenation Assessment[5]	-	-	99%	99%	100%
Pneumococcal Vaccine[5]	-	-	68%	69%	94%
Smoking Cessation Advice[5]	-	-	83%	80%	100%
Surgical Infection Prevention					
Prophylactic Antibiotic Given[3]	35	89%	67%	77%	95%
Prophylactic Antibiotic Selection[5]	-	-	86%	90%	100%
Prophylactic Antibiotic Stopped[3]	35	51%	68%	72%	95%
Pregnancy Care					
Inpatient Neonatal Mortality	-	-	-	-	-
Third or Fourth Degree Laceration	-	-	3.23%	3.63%	3.27%

Permian General Hospital

720 Hospital Drive
Andrews, TX 79714
E-mail: rrichards@permianregional.com
URL: www.permianregional.com
Ownership: Govt - Hospital District or Authority
Emergency Services: Yes

Phone: 423-523-2200
Fax: 423-464-2180

Accredited: Yes
Licensed Beds: 85

Key Personnel:
CEO. . . . . Randy Richards
Chief Medical Staff. Natver Jariwala, MD
Emergency Room Medical Director . . . . Paul Slaughter, MD
Director Infection/Disease Control . . . . Lynn Mock
Med/Surg Unit Director. . . . . Andrea Shaw, RN,BSN
OB/GYN Womens Health. . . . . Armand Wiltz
Director of Surgery. . . . . Tham Phan, RN
Director of Cardiopulmonary . . . . Dalton Jones, RRT

Measure	Cases	This Hospital	State Average	U.S. Average	Top Hospital
Heart Attack Care					
ACE Inhibitor or ARB for LVSD[3]	0	-	85%	82%	100%
Aspirin at Arrival[1,3]	1	100%	91%	92%	100%
Aspirin at Discharge[1,3]	1	100%	90%	90%	100%
Beta Blocker at Arrival[1,3]	1	100%	85%	87%	100%
Beta Blocker at Discharge[1,3]	1	100%	86%	90%	100%
Fibrinolytic Medication Timing[3]	0	-	30%	31%	100%
PCI Within 90 Minutes of Arrival[5]	-	-	48%	54%	95%
Smoking Cessation Advice[3]	0	-	90%	88%	100%
Heart Failure Care					
ACE Inhibitor or ARB for LVSD[1]	1	0%	82%	82%	100%
Discharge Instructions[1]	12	50%	60%	61%	93%
Evaluation of LVS Function[1]	10	10%	81%	83%	99%
Smoking Cessation Advice[1]	4	50%	82%	82%	100%
Pneumonia Care					
Appropriate Initial Antibiotic	25	88%	79%	83%	94%
Blood Culture Timing[1]	7	57%	89%	90%	100%
Influenza Vaccine[1]	8	100%	69%	70%	100%

NOTE: Hospital profiles are in alphabetical order by state, then city, then hospital within the city; Rankings are sorted by rate in descending order and exclude hospitals with less than 25 cases; (1) The number of cases is too small (n<25) for purposes of reliably predicting hospital performance; (2) Measure reflects the hospital's indication that its submission was based upon a sample of its relevant discharges; (3) Rate reflects fewer than the maximum possible quarters of data for the measure; (4) Inaccurate information submitted and suppressed for one or more quarters; (5) No data is available from the hospital for this measure; Please refer to the User's Guide for a full explanation of data

Measure	Cases	This Hospital	State Average	U.S. Average	Top Hospital
Initial Antibiotic Timing[1]	23	74%	78%	80%	93%
Oxygenation Assessment	34	94%	99%	99%	100%
Pneumococcal Vaccine[1]	15	53%	68%	69%	94%
Smoking Cessation Advice[1]	5	60%	83%	80%	100%
Surgical Infection Prevention					
Prophylactic Antibiotic Given	67	60%	67%	77%	95%
Prophylactic Antibiotic Selection	28	93%	86%	90%	100%
Prophylactic Antibiotic Stopped	67	43%	68%	72%	95%
Pregnancy Care					
Inpatient Neonatal Mortality	-	-	-	-	-
Third or Fourth Degree Laceration	-	-	3.23%	3.63%	3.27%

Angleton-Danbury Medical Center

Alternate Name: Angleton-Danbury General Hospital
132 Hospital Drive
Angleton, TX 77515
E-mail: hunte@admc.org
Ownership: Govt - Hospital District or Authority
Emergency Services: Yes

Phone: 979-849-7721
Fax: 979-849-0581

Accredited: Yes
Licensed Beds: 64

Key Personnel:
Administrator/CEO . . . . David Bleakney
Chief Medical Staff . . . . Marcia Filipp
Emergency Room . . . . Sheraz Pirali, MD
Director Infection/Disease Control . . . . Loretta Miles
Director Respiratory Therapy . . . . Mary Poole

Measure	Cases	This Hospital	State Average	U.S. Average	Top Hospital
Heart Attack Care					
ACE Inhibitor or ARB for LVSD[1]	4	0%	85%	82%	100%
Aspirin at Arrival[1]	11	91%	91%	92%	100%
Aspirin at Discharge[1]	8	88%	90%	90%	100%
Beta Blocker at Arrival[1]	11	100%	85%	87%	100%
Beta Blocker at Discharge[1]	8	75%	86%	90%	100%
Fibrinolytic Medication Timing[1]	1	0%	30%	31%	100%
PCI Within 90 Minutes of Arrival	0	-	48%	54%	95%
Smoking Cessation Advice[1]	1	100%	90%	88%	100%
Heart Failure Care					
ACE Inhibitor or ARB for LVSD[1]	20	60%	82%	82%	100%
Discharge Instructions	31	42%	60%	61%	93%
Evaluation of LVS Function	47	83%	81%	83%	99%
Smoking Cessation Advice[1]	7	86%	82%	82%	100%
Pneumonia Care					
Appropriate Initial Antibiotic	73	68%	79%	83%	94%
Blood Culture Timing	34	94%	89%	90%	100%
Influenza Vaccine[1]	14	36%	69%	70%	100%
Initial Antibiotic Timing	78	60%	78%	80%	93%
Oxygenation Assessment	99	98%	99%	99%	100%
Pneumococcal Vaccine	53	25%	68%	69%	94%
Smoking Cessation Advice[1]	24	92%	83%	80%	100%
Surgical Infection Prevention					
Prophylactic Antibiotic Given	170	53%	67%	77%	95%
Prophylactic Antibiotic Selection	37	86%	86%	90%	100%
Prophylactic Antibiotic Stopped	162	43%	68%	72%	95%
Pregnancy Care					
Inpatient Neonatal Mortality	-	-	-	-	-
Third or Fourth Degree Laceration	-	-	3.23%	3.63%	3.27%

Anson General Hospital

101 Avenue J
Anson, TX 79501
Ownership: Government - Local
Emergency Services: No

Phone: 915-823-3231
Fax: 325-823-3098
Accredited: No
Licensed Beds: 45

Key Personnel:
CEO . . . . Ted D Matthews
Chief Medical Staff . . . . G Kapla, MD
Director Infection/Disease Control . . . . Margaret Gates
Director Medical/Surgical Nursing . . . . Pat Cary, RN
Chief Radiology . . . . Herbert Sanders, DDS

Measure	Cases	This Hospital	State Average	U.S. Average	Top Hospital
Heart Attack Care					
ACE Inhibitor or ARB for LVSD[3]	0	-	85%	82%	100%

Measure	Cases	This Hospital	State Average	U.S. Average	Top Hospital
Aspirin at Arrival[1,3]	1	0%	91%	92%	100%
Aspirin at Discharge[3]	0	-	90%	90%	100%
Beta Blocker at Arrival[1,3]	1	0%	85%	87%	100%
Beta Blocker at Discharge[3]	0	-	86%	90%	100%
Fibrinolytic Medication Timing[3]	0	-	30%	31%	100%
PCI Within 90 Minutes of Arrival[5]	-	-	48%	54%	95%
Smoking Cessation Advice[3]	0	-	90%	88%	100%
Heart Failure Care					
ACE Inhibitor or ARB for LVSD[1]	3	100%	82%	82%	100%
Discharge Instructions[1]	13	15%	60%	61%	93%
Evaluation of LVS Function[1]	22	77%	81%	83%	99%
Smoking Cessation Advice[1]	3	67%	82%	82%	100%
Pneumonia Care					
Appropriate Initial Antibiotic	25	72%	79%	83%	94%
Blood Culture Timing[1]	9	100%	89%	90%	100%
Influenza Vaccine[1]	8	75%	69%	70%	100%
Initial Antibiotic Timing	29	100%	78%	80%	93%
Oxygenation Assessment	38	95%	99%	99%	100%
Pneumococcal Vaccine	27	70%	68%	69%	94%
Smoking Cessation Advice[1]	6	50%	83%	80%	100%
Surgical Infection Prevention					
Prophylactic Antibiotic Given[3]	0	-	67%	77%	95%
Prophylactic Antibiotic Selection[5]	-	-	86%	90%	100%
Prophylactic Antibiotic Stopped[3]	0	-	68%	72%	95%
Pregnancy Care					
Inpatient Neonatal Mortality	-	-	-	-	-
Third or Fourth Degree Laceration	-	-	3.23%	3.63%	3.27%

North Bay Hospital

1711 West Wheeler Avenue
Aransas Pass, TX 78336
URL: www.nbhtx.com
Ownership: Proprietary
Emergency Services: Yes

Phone: 361-758-8585
Fax: 361-758-3476

Accredited: No
Licensed Beds: 75

Key Personnel:
CEO . . . . Christopher W Dux

Measure	Cases	This Hospital	State Average	U.S. Average	Top Hospital
Heart Attack Care					
ACE Inhibitor or ARB for LVSD[3]	0	-	85%	82%	100%
Aspirin at Arrival[3]	0	-	91%	92%	100%
Aspirin at Discharge[3]	0	-	90%	90%	100%
Beta Blocker at Arrival[1,3]	1	100%	85%	87%	100%
Beta Blocker at Discharge[1,3]	1	0%	86%	90%	100%
Fibrinolytic Medication Timing[5]	-	-	30%	31%	100%
PCI Within 90 Minutes of Arrival[5]	-	-	48%	54%	95%
Smoking Cessation Advice[5]	-	-	90%	88%	100%
Heart Failure Care					
ACE Inhibitor or ARB for LVSD[1,3]	7	86%	82%	82%	100%
Discharge Instructions[1,3]	9	78%	60%	61%	93%
Evaluation of LVS Function[3]	27	74%	81%	83%	99%
Smoking Cessation Advice[1,3]	5	100%	82%	82%	100%
Pneumonia Care					
Appropriate Initial Antibiotic[1,3]	6	83%	79%	83%	94%
Blood Culture Timing[1,3]	6	83%	89%	90%	100%
Influenza Vaccine[5]	-	-	69%	70%	100%
Initial Antibiotic Timing[3]	30	77%	78%	80%	93%
Oxygenation Assessment[3]	36	94%	99%	99%	100%
Pneumococcal Vaccine[1,3]	18	83%	68%	69%	94%
Smoking Cessation Advice[1,3]	3	100%	83%	80%	100%
Surgical Infection Prevention					
Prophylactic Antibiotic Given[3]	0	-	67%	77%	95%
Prophylactic Antibiotic Selection[5]	-	-	86%	90%	100%
Prophylactic Antibiotic Stopped[3]	0	-	68%	72%	95%
Pregnancy Care					
Inpatient Neonatal Mortality	-	-	-	-	-
Third or Fourth Degree Laceration	-	-	3.23%	3.63%	3.27%

NOTE: Hospital profiles are in alphabetical order by state, then city, then hospital within the city; Rankings are sorted by rate in descending order and exclude hospitals with less than 25 cases; (1) The number of cases is too small (n<25) for purposes of reliably predicting hospital performance; (2) Measure reflects the hospital's indication that its submission was based upon a sample of its relevant discharges; (3) Rate reflects fewer than the maximum possible quarters of data for the measure; (4) Inaccurate information submitted and suppressed for one or more quarters; (5) No data is available from the hospital for this measure; Please refer to the User's Guide for a full explanation of data

Arlington Memorial Hospital

800 W Randol Mill Rd
Arlington, TX 76012   Phone: 817-548-6100
Ownership: Voluntary non-profit - Private   Accredited: Yes
Emergency Services: Yes

Measure	Cases	This Hospital	State Average	U.S. Average	Top Hospital
Heart Attack Care					
ACE Inhibitor or ARB for LVSD	65	82%	85%	82%	100%
Aspirin at Arrival	217	99%	91%	92%	100%
Aspirin at Discharge	210	98%	90%	90%	100%
Beta Blocker at Arrival	185	96%	85%	87%	100%
Beta Blocker at Discharge	200	97%	86%	90%	100%
Fibrinolytic Medication Timing[1]	6	83%	30%	31%	100%
PCI Within 90 Minutes of Arrival[1]	4	25%	48%	54%	95%
Smoking Cessation Advice	81	93%	90%	88%	100%
Heart Failure Care					
ACE Inhibitor or ARB for LVSD	197	81%	82%	82%	100%
Discharge Instructions	386	67%	60%	61%	93%
Evaluation of LVS Function	473	84%	81%	83%	99%
Smoking Cessation Advice	95	87%	82%	82%	100%
Pneumonia Care					
Appropriate Initial Antibiotic	244	87%	79%	83%	94%
Blood Culture Timing	264	91%	89%	90%	100%
Influenza Vaccine	62	81%	69%	70%	100%
Initial Antibiotic Timing	346	87%	78%	80%	93%
Oxygenation Assessment	396	100%	99%	99%	100%
Pneumococcal Vaccine	230	90%	68%	69%	94%
Smoking Cessation Advice	109	100%	83%	80%	100%
Surgical Infection Prevention					
Prophylactic Antibiotic Given[2,3]	180	84%	67%	77%	95%
Prophylactic Antibiotic Selection[2]	58	88%	86%	90%	100%
Prophylactic Antibiotic Stopped[2,3]	169	62%	68%	72%	95%
Pregnancy Care					
Inpatient Neonatal Mortality	-	-	-	-	-
Third or Fourth Degree Laceration	-	-	3.23%	3.63%	3.27%

Medical Center of Arlington

3301 Matlock Road   Phone: 817-465-3241
Arlington, TX 76015   Fax: 817-472-4878
URL: www.medicalcenterarlington.com
Ownership: Proprietary   Accredited: Yes
Emergency Services: Yes   Licensed Beds: 298
Key Personnel:
CEO. . . . . Patrick D Brilliant
Chief Medical Staff. . . . . Richard Wray, MD
Chief Catheterization Laboratory . . . . Charles Cramer, MD
Emergency Room . . . . Bill Crawley, RN
Infection Control. Carol Hill, RN
ICU Director . . . . Kathy Srokosz, RN
Medical/Surgical/Rehabilitation Director . . . . Rose Elam
OB/GYN Womens Health Director . . . . Leigh Wilson, RN
Respiratory Therapy Manager . . . . Pete Miholovich

Measure	Cases	This Hospital	State Average	U.S. Average	Top Hospital
Heart Attack Care					
ACE Inhibitor or ARB for LVSD	44	95%	85%	82%	100%
Aspirin at Arrival	240	100%	91%	92%	100%
Aspirin at Discharge	220	100%	90%	90%	100%
Beta Blocker at Arrival	167	99%	85%	87%	100%
Beta Blocker at Discharge	208	100%	86%	90%	100%
Fibrinolytic Medication Timing[1]	8	38%	30%	31%	100%
PCI Within 90 Minutes of Arrival[1]	13	31%	48%	54%	95%
Smoking Cessation Advice	96	99%	90%	88%	100%
Heart Failure Care					
ACE Inhibitor or ARB for LVSD	87	91%	82%	82%	100%
Discharge Instructions	234	74%	60%	61%	93%
Evaluation of LVS Function	282	96%	81%	83%	99%
Smoking Cessation Advice	48	96%	82%	82%	100%
Pneumonia Care					
Appropriate Initial Antibiotic	207	94%	79%	83%	94%
Blood Culture Timing	237	88%	89%	90%	100%
Influenza Vaccine	69	67%	69%	70%	100%

Measure	Cases	This Hospital	State Average	U.S. Average	Top Hospital
Initial Antibiotic Timing	298	91%	78%	80%	93%
Oxygenation Assessment	371	100%	99%	99%	100%
Pneumococcal Vaccine	195	56%	68%	69%	94%
Smoking Cessation Advice	76	100%	83%	80%	100%
Surgical Infection Prevention					
Prophylactic Antibiotic Given[2,3]	186	83%	67%	77%	95%
Prophylactic Antibiotic Selection[2]	87	91%	86%	90%	100%
Prophylactic Antibiotic Stopped[2,3]	177	53%	68%	72%	95%
Pregnancy Care					
Inpatient Neonatal Mortality	3,806	0.34%	-	-	-
Third or Fourth Degree Laceration	2,308	2.25%	3.23%	3.63%	3.27%

USMD Hospital at Arlington

Alternate Name: Arlington Memorial South Medical Center
801 West Interstate 20   Phone: 817-472-3400
Arlington, TX 76017   Fax: 817-472-3090
URL: www.usmdhospital.com
Ownership: Proprietary   Accredited: Yes
Emergency Services: Yes   Licensed Beds: 18
Key Personnel:
President . . . . Steven R Kamber

Measure	Cases	This Hospital	State Average	U.S. Average	Top Hospital
Heart Attack Care					
ACE Inhibitor or ARB for LVSD[5]	-	-	85%	82%	100%
Aspirin at Arrival[5]	-	-	91%	92%	100%
Aspirin at Discharge[5]	-	-	90%	90%	100%
Beta Blocker at Arrival[5]	-	-	85%	87%	100%
Beta Blocker at Discharge[5]	-	-	86%	90%	100%
Fibrinolytic Medication Timing[5]	-	-	30%	31%	100%
PCI Within 90 Minutes of Arrival[5]	-	-	48%	54%	95%
Smoking Cessation Advice[5]	-	-	90%	88%	100%
Heart Failure Care					
ACE Inhibitor or ARB for LVSD[5]	-	-	82%	82%	100%
Discharge Instructions[5]	-	-	60%	61%	93%
Evaluation of LVS Function[5]	-	-	81%	83%	99%
Smoking Cessation Advice[5]	-	-	82%	82%	100%
Pneumonia Care					
Appropriate Initial Antibiotic[5]	-	-	79%	83%	94%
Blood Culture Timing[5]	-	-	89%	90%	100%
Influenza Vaccine[5]	-	-	69%	70%	100%
Initial Antibiotic Timing[5]	-	-	78%	80%	93%
Oxygenation Assessment[5]	-	-	99%	99%	100%
Pneumococcal Vaccine[5]	-	-	68%	69%	94%
Smoking Cessation Advice[5]	-	-	83%	80%	100%
Surgical Infection Prevention					
Prophylactic Antibiotic Given[2,3]	46	70%	67%	77%	95%
Prophylactic Antibiotic Selection[5]	-	-	86%	90%	100%
Prophylactic Antibiotic Stopped[2,3]	41	78%	68%	72%	95%
Pregnancy Care					
Inpatient Neonatal Mortality	-	-	-	-	-
Third or Fourth Degree Laceration	-	-	3.23%	3.63%	3.27%

East Texas Medical Center-Athens

2000 S Palestine Street   Phone: 903-676-1000
Athens, TX 75751   Fax: 903-676-3153
E-mail: info@etmc.org
URL: www.etmc.org/athens
Ownership: Voluntary non-profit - Private   Accredited: Yes
Emergency Services: Yes   Licensed Beds: 117
Key Personnel:
President/CEO. . . . . Patrick Wallace

Measure	Cases	This Hospital	State Average	U.S. Average	Top Hospital
Heart Attack Care					
ACE Inhibitor or ARB for LVSD[1]	10	80%	85%	82%	100%
Aspirin at Arrival	86	98%	91%	92%	100%
Aspirin at Discharge	39	95%	90%	90%	100%
Beta Blocker at Arrival	85	93%	85%	87%	100%
Beta Blocker at Discharge	41	88%	86%	90%	100%
Fibrinolytic Medication Timing[1]	1	0%	30%	31%	100%
PCI Within 90 Minutes of Arrival	0	-	48%	54%	95%

NOTE: Hospital profiles are in alphabetical order by state, then city, then hospital within the city; Rankings are sorted by rate in descending order and exclude hospitals with less than 25 cases; (1) The number of cases is too small (n<25) for purposes of reliably predicting hospital performance; (2) Measure reflects the hospital's indication that its submission was based upon a sample of its relevant discharges; (3) Rate reflects fewer than the maximum possible quarters of data for the measure; (4) Inaccurate information submitted and suppressed for one or more quarters; (5) No data is available from the hospital for this measure; Please refer to the User's Guide for a full explanation of data

	Cases	This Hospital	State Average	U.S. Average	Top Hospital
Smoking Cessation Advice[1]	14	100%	90%	88%	100%
Heart Failure Care					
ACE Inhibitor or ARB for LVSD	68	79%	82%	82%	100%
Discharge Instructions	232	98%	60%	61%	93%
Evaluation of LVS Function	280	91%	81%	83%	99%
Smoking Cessation Advice	53	100%	82%	82%	100%
Pneumonia Care					
Appropriate Initial Antibiotic	130	86%	79%	83%	94%
Blood Culture Timing	79	95%	89%	90%	100%
Influenza Vaccine	33	73%	69%	70%	100%
Initial Antibiotic Timing	187	83%	78%	80%	93%
Oxygenation Assessment	208	99%	99%	99%	100%
Pneumococcal Vaccine	125	65%	68%	69%	94%
Smoking Cessation Advice	57	93%	83%	80%	100%
Surgical Infection Prevention					
Prophylactic Antibiotic Given[3]	124	79%	67%	77%	95%
Prophylactic Antibiotic Selection	52	48%	86%	90%	100%
Prophylactic Antibiotic Stopped[3]	120	69%	68%	72%	95%
Pregnancy Care					
Inpatient Neonatal Mortality	-	-	-	-	-
Third or Fourth Degree Laceration	-	-	3.23%	3.63%	3.27%

Atlanta Memorial Hospital

1077 South William Street
Atlanta, TX 75551
URL: www.atlanticmemorial.com
Ownership: Govt - Hospital District or Authority
Emergency Services: Yes

Phone: 903-799-3000
Fax: 903-799-3005

Accredited: No
Licensed Beds: 65

Key Personnel:
Administrator/CEO . . . . Tom Crow
Director Radiology . . . . Pam Purtle
Director Respiratory Therapy . . . . Karen Powell

Measure	Cases	This Hospital	State Average	U.S. Average	Top Hospital
Heart Attack Care					
ACE Inhibitor or ARB for LVSD[1]	2	100%	85%	82%	100%
Aspirin at Arrival[1]	8	75%	91%	92%	100%
Aspirin at Discharge[1]	6	100%	90%	90%	100%
Beta Blocker at Arrival[1]	5	40%	85%	87%	100%
Beta Blocker at Discharge[1]	6	67%	86%	90%	100%
Fibrinolytic Medication Timing	0	-	30%	31%	100%
PCI Within 90 Minutes of Arrival	0	-	48%	54%	95%
Smoking Cessation Advice	0	-	90%	88%	100%
Heart Failure Care					
ACE Inhibitor or ARB for LVSD	43	65%	82%	82%	100%
Discharge Instructions	97	42%	60%	61%	93%
Evaluation of LVS Function	112	79%	81%	83%	99%
Smoking Cessation Advice	25	36%	82%	82%	100%
Pneumonia Care					
Appropriate Initial Antibiotic	63	65%	79%	83%	94%
Blood Culture Timing[1]	7	100%	89%	90%	100%
Influenza Vaccine[4,5]	-	-	69%	70%	100%
Initial Antibiotic Timing	90	68%	78%	80%	93%
Oxygenation Assessment	107	93%	99%	99%	100%
Pneumococcal Vaccine	63	75%	68%	69%	94%
Smoking Cessation Advice	26	54%	83%	80%	100%
Surgical Infection Prevention					
Prophylactic Antibiotic Given[1,3]	9	100%	67%	77%	95%
Prophylactic Antibiotic Selection[5]	-	-	86%	90%	100%
Prophylactic Antibiotic Stopped[1,3]	9	44%	68%	72%	95%
Pregnancy Care					
Inpatient Neonatal Mortality	-	-	-	-	-
Third or Fourth Degree Laceration	-	-	3.23%	3.63%	3.27%

Austin Surgical Hospital

3003 Bee Caves Road
Austin, TX 78746
Ownership: Proprietary
Emergency Services: Yes

Phone: 512-347-9888

Accredited: Yes

Measure	Cases	This Hospital	State Average	U.S. Average	Top Hospital
Heart Attack Care					

	Cases	This Hospital	State Average	U.S. Average	Top Hospital
ACE Inhibitor or ARB for LVSD[5]	-	-	85%	82%	100%
Aspirin at Arrival[5]	-	-	91%	92%	100%
Aspirin at Discharge[5]	-	-	90%	90%	100%
Beta Blocker at Arrival[5]	-	-	85%	87%	100%
Beta Blocker at Discharge[5]	-	-	86%	90%	100%
Fibrinolytic Medication Timing[5]	-	-	30%	31%	100%
PCI Within 90 Minutes of Arrival[5]	-	-	48%	54%	95%
Smoking Cessation Advice[5]	-	-	90%	88%	100%
Heart Failure Care					
ACE Inhibitor or ARB for LVSD[5]	-	-	82%	82%	100%
Discharge Instructions[5]	-	-	60%	61%	93%
Evaluation of LVS Function[5]	-	-	81%	83%	99%
Smoking Cessation Advice[5]	-	-	82%	82%	100%
Pneumonia Care					
Appropriate Initial Antibiotic[5]	-	-	79%	83%	94%
Blood Culture Timing[5]	-	-	89%	90%	100%
Influenza Vaccine[5]	-	-	69%	70%	100%
Initial Antibiotic Timing[5]	-	-	78%	80%	93%
Oxygenation Assessment[5]	-	-	99%	99%	100%
Pneumococcal Vaccine[5]	-	-	68%	69%	94%
Smoking Cessation Advice[5]	-	-	83%	80%	100%
Surgical Infection Prevention					
Prophylactic Antibiotic Given[2,3]	67	99%	67%	77%	95%
Prophylactic Antibiotic Selection[5]	-	-	86%	90%	100%
Prophylactic Antibiotic Stopped[2,3]	67	100%	68%	72%	95%
Pregnancy Care					
Inpatient Neonatal Mortality	-	-	-	-	-
Third or Fourth Degree Laceration	-	-	3.23%	3.63%	3.27%

Brackenridge Hospital

601 E 15th Street
Austin, TX 78701
Ownership: Government - Local
Emergency Services: Yes

Phone: 512-324-7000

Accredited: Yes

Measure	Cases	This Hospital	State Average	U.S. Average	Top Hospital
Heart Attack Care					
ACE Inhibitor or ARB for LVSD[1]	11	100%	85%	82%	100%
Aspirin at Arrival	89	100%	91%	92%	100%
Aspirin at Discharge	90	100%	90%	90%	100%
Beta Blocker at Arrival	76	99%	85%	87%	100%
Beta Blocker at Discharge	86	99%	86%	90%	100%
Fibrinolytic Medication Timing[1]	2	0%	30%	31%	100%
PCI Within 90 Minutes of Arrival[1]	5	80%	48%	54%	95%
Smoking Cessation Advice	51	100%	90%	88%	100%
Heart Failure Care					
ACE Inhibitor or ARB for LVSD	108	99%	82%	82%	100%
Discharge Instructions	236	82%	60%	61%	93%
Evaluation of LVS Function	249	99%	81%	83%	99%
Smoking Cessation Advice	109	96%	82%	82%	100%
Pneumonia Care					
Appropriate Initial Antibiotic[2]	108	84%	79%	83%	94%
Blood Culture Timing[2]	86	85%	89%	90%	100%
Influenza Vaccine[1,2]	17	47%	69%	70%	100%
Initial Antibiotic Timing[2]	144	71%	78%	80%	93%
Oxygenation Assessment[2]	152	99%	99%	99%	100%
Pneumococcal Vaccine[2]	39	44%	68%	69%	94%
Smoking Cessation Advice[2]	56	70%	83%	80%	100%
Surgical Infection Prevention					
Prophylactic Antibiotic Given[2,3]	135	74%	67%	77%	95%
Prophylactic Antibiotic Selection[2]	40	92%	86%	90%	100%
Prophylactic Antibiotic Stopped[2,3]	135	79%	68%	72%	95%
Pregnancy Care					
Inpatient Neonatal Mortality	-	-	-	-	-
Third or Fourth Degree Laceration	-	-	3.23%	3.63%	3.27%

NOTE: Hospital profiles are in alphabetical order by state, then city, then hospital within the city; Rankings are sorted by rate in descending order and exclude hospitals with less than 25 cases; (1) The number of cases is too small (n<25) for purposes of reliably predicting hospital performance; (2) Measure reflects the hospital's indication that its submission was based upon a sample of its relevant discharges; (3) Rate reflects fewer than the maximum possible quarters of data for the measure; (4) Inaccurate information submitted and suppressed for one or more quarters; (5) No data is available from the hospital for this measure; Please refer to the User's Guide for a full explanation of data

Healthsouth Surgical Hospital of Austin

6818 Austin Center Blvd Suite 100   Phone: 512-346-1994
Austin, TX 78731
Ownership: Proprietary   Accredited: Yes
Emergency Services: No

Measure	Cases	This Hospital	State Average	U.S. Average	Top Hospital
Heart Attack Care					
ACE Inhibitor or ARB for LVSD[5]	-	-	85%	82%	100%
Aspirin at Arrival[5]	-	-	91%	92%	100%
Aspirin at Discharge[5]	-	-	90%	90%	100%
Beta Blocker at Arrival[5]	-	-	85%	87%	100%
Beta Blocker at Discharge[5]	-	-	86%	90%	100%
Fibrinolytic Medication Timing[5]	-	-	30%	31%	100%
PCI Within 90 Minutes of Arrival[5]	-	-	48%	54%	95%
Smoking Cessation Advice[5]	-	-	90%	88%	100%
Heart Failure Care					
ACE Inhibitor or ARB for LVSD[5]	-	-	82%	82%	100%
Discharge Instructions[5]	-	-	60%	61%	93%
Evaluation of LVS Function[5]	-	-	81%	83%	99%
Smoking Cessation Advice[5]	-	-	82%	82%	100%
Pneumonia Care					
Appropriate Initial Antibiotic[5]	-	-	79%	83%	94%
Blood Culture Timing[5]	-	-	89%	90%	100%
Influenza Vaccine[5]	-	-	69%	70%	100%
Initial Antibiotic Timing[5]	-	-	78%	80%	93%
Oxygenation Assessment[5]	-	-	99%	99%	100%
Pneumococcal Vaccine[5]	-	-	68%	69%	94%
Smoking Cessation Advice[5]	-	-	83%	80%	100%
Surgical Infection Prevention					
Prophylactic Antibiotic Given[1,2,3]	6	17%	67%	77%	95%
Prophylactic Antibiotic Selection[5]	-	-	86%	90%	100%
Prophylactic Antibiotic Stopped[1,2,3]	6	100%	68%	72%	95%
Pregnancy Care					
Inpatient Neonatal Mortality	-	-	-	-	-
Third or Fourth Degree Laceration	-	-	3.23%	3.63%	3.27%

Heart Hospital of Austin

3801 North Lamar Boulevard   Phone: 512-407-7000
Austin, TX 78756   Fax: 512-407-7525
URL: www.hearthospitalofaustin.com
Ownership: Proprietary   Accredited: Yes
Emergency Services: Yes   Licensed Beds: 58
Key Personnel:
President . . . . Roy C Vinson
Infection Control. . . . . Jack Bissett, MD

Measure	Cases	This Hospital	State Average	U.S. Average	Top Hospital
Heart Attack Care					
ACE Inhibitor or ARB for LVSD	105	89%	85%	82%	100%
Aspirin at Arrival	111	100%	91%	92%	100%
Aspirin at Discharge	454	99%	90%	90%	100%
Beta Blocker at Arrival	96	96%	85%	87%	100%
Beta Blocker at Discharge	426	96%	86%	90%	100%
Fibrinolytic Medication Timing	0	-	30%	31%	100%
PCI Within 90 Minutes of Arrival[1]	14	36%	48%	54%	95%
Smoking Cessation Advice	174	93%	90%	88%	100%
Heart Failure Care					
ACE Inhibitor or ARB for LVSD	232	85%	82%	82%	100%
Discharge Instructions	320	60%	60%	61%	93%
Evaluation of LVS Function	361	96%	81%	83%	99%
Smoking Cessation Advice	65	80%	82%	82%	100%
Pneumonia Care					
Appropriate Initial Antibiotic	25	56%	79%	83%	94%
Blood Culture Timing[1]	17	94%	89%	90%	100%
Influenza Vaccine[1]	7	57%	69%	70%	100%
Initial Antibiotic Timing	30	63%	78%	80%	93%
Oxygenation Assessment	35	97%	99%	99%	100%
Pneumococcal Vaccine[1]	23	61%	68%	69%	94%
Smoking Cessation Advice[1]	12	100%	83%	80%	100%
Surgical Infection Prevention					
Prophylactic Antibiotic Given[2,3]	106	82%	67%	77%	95%

Prophylactic Antibiotic Selection[2]	36	100%	86%	90%	100%
Prophylactic Antibiotic Stopped[2,3]	107	89%	68%	72%	95%
Pregnancy Care					
Inpatient Neonatal Mortality	-	-	-	-	-
Third or Fourth Degree Laceration	-	-	3.23%	3.63%	3.27%

North Austin Medical Center

12221 MoPac Expressway North   Phone: 512-901-1000
Austin, TX 78758   Fax: 512-901-1871
URL: www.northaustin.com
Ownership: Proprietary   Accredited: Yes
Emergency Services: Yes   Licensed Beds: 210
Key Personnel:
CEO. . . . . Donald H Wilkerson
Chief Medical Staff. . . . . Michael Romane
Emergency Room . . . . Robert Mills
Director Respiratory Therapy . . . . Michael Moore

Measure	Cases	This Hospital	State Average	U.S. Average	Top Hospital
Heart Attack Care					
ACE Inhibitor or ARB for LVSD	42	93%	85%	82%	100%
Aspirin at Arrival	159	96%	91%	92%	100%
Aspirin at Discharge	172	97%	90%	90%	100%
Beta Blocker at Arrival	81	91%	85%	87%	100%
Beta Blocker at Discharge	164	96%	86%	90%	100%
Fibrinolytic Medication Timing	0	-	30%	31%	100%
PCI Within 90 Minutes of Arrival[1]	13	69%	48%	54%	95%
Smoking Cessation Advice	81	96%	90%	88%	100%
Heart Failure Care					
ACE Inhibitor or ARB for LVSD	107	77%	82%	82%	100%
Discharge Instructions	237	64%	60%	61%	93%
Evaluation of LVS Function	277	96%	81%	83%	99%
Smoking Cessation Advice	72	93%	82%	82%	100%
Pneumonia Care					
Appropriate Initial Antibiotic	119	92%	79%	83%	94%
Blood Culture Timing	140	94%	89%	90%	100%
Influenza Vaccine	37	76%	69%	70%	100%
Initial Antibiotic Timing	177	71%	78%	80%	93%
Oxygenation Assessment	219	100%	99%	99%	100%
Pneumococcal Vaccine	129	77%	68%	69%	94%
Smoking Cessation Advice	48	94%	83%	80%	100%
Surgical Infection Prevention					
Prophylactic Antibiotic Given[2,3]	233	74%	67%	77%	95%
Prophylactic Antibiotic Selection[2]	111	93%	86%	90%	100%
Prophylactic Antibiotic Stopped[2,3]	214	64%	68%	72%	95%
Pregnancy Care					
Inpatient Neonatal Mortality	-	-	-	-	-
Third or Fourth Degree Laceration	-	-	3.23%	3.63%	3.27%

Saint David's Rehabiltation Center

1005 E 32nd Street   Phone: 512-476-7111
Austin, TX 78705   Fax: 512-867-5831
URL: stdavidsrehab.com
Ownership: Voluntary non-profit - Other   Accredited: Yes
Emergency Services: Yes   Licensed Beds: 107
Key Personnel:
CEO. . . . . Cole Eslyn
Chief Medical Staff. . . . . Cioo Race, MD

Measure	Cases	This Hospital	State Average	U.S. Average	Top Hospital
Heart Attack Care					
ACE Inhibitor or ARB for LVSD	34	82%	85%	82%	100%
Aspirin at Arrival	146	98%	91%	92%	100%
Aspirin at Discharge	166	98%	90%	90%	100%
Beta Blocker at Arrival	104	96%	85%	87%	100%
Beta Blocker at Discharge	172	97%	86%	90%	100%
Fibrinolytic Medication Timing[1]	1	0%	30%	31%	100%
PCI Within 90 Minutes of Arrival[1]	4	75%	48%	54%	95%
Smoking Cessation Advice	81	100%	90%	88%	100%
Heart Failure Care					
ACE Inhibitor or ARB for LVSD	175	88%	82%	82%	100%
Discharge Instructions	421	61%	60%	61%	93%

NOTE: Hospital profiles are in alphabetical order by state, then city, then hospital within the city; Rankings are sorted by rate in descending order and exclude hospitals with less than 25 cases; (1) The number of cases is too small (n<25) for purposes of reliably predicting hospital performance; (2) Measure reflects the hospital's indication that its submission was based upon a sample of its relevant discharges; (3) Rate reflects fewer than the maximum possible quarters of data for the measure; (4) Inaccurate information submitted and suppressed for one or more quarters; (5) No data is available from the hospital for this measure; Please refer to the User's Guide for a full explanation of data

Evaluation of LVS Function	492	98%	81%	83%	99%
Smoking Cessation Advice	110	99%	82%	82%	100%
Pneumonia Care					
Appropriate Initial Antibiotic	183	95%	79%	83%	94%
Blood Culture Timing	206	95%	89%	90%	100%
Influenza Vaccine	62	77%	69%	70%	100%
Initial Antibiotic Timing	276	82%	78%	80%	93%
Oxygenation Assessment	321	100%	99%	99%	100%
Pneumococcal Vaccine	188	76%	68%	69%	94%
Smoking Cessation Advice	87	97%	83%	80%	100%
Surgical Infection Prevention					
Prophylactic Antibiotic Given[2,3]	278	85%	67%	77%	95%
Prophylactic Antibiotic Selection[2]	135	93%	86%	90%	100%
Prophylactic Antibiotic Stopped[2,3]	262	67%	68%	72%	95%
Pregnancy Care					
Inpatient Neonatal Mortality	-	-	-	-	-
Third or Fourth Degree Laceration	-	-	3.23%	3.63%	3.27%

Seton Medical Center

1201 West 38th Street   Phone: 512-324-1000
Austin, TX 78705   Fax: 512-380-7527
URL: www.seton.net
Ownership: Voluntary non-profit - Church   Accredited: Yes
Emergency Services: Yes   Licensed Beds: 502
Key Personnel:
President/CEO . . . . John Brindley
Chief Medical Staff . . . . Phillip Church
Chief Cardiology . . . . Joseph Gallinger
Emergency Room . . . . Mark Vassallo
Director Respiratory Care . . . . Ron Boltonhouse

Measure	Cases	This Hospital	State Average	U.S. Average	Top Hospital
Heart Attack Care					
ACE Inhibitor or ARB for LVSD	56	98%	85%	82%	100%
Aspirin at Arrival	189	99%	91%	92%	100%
Aspirin at Discharge	326	99%	90%	90%	100%
Beta Blocker at Arrival	162	98%	85%	87%	100%
Beta Blocker at Discharge	293	98%	86%	90%	100%
Fibrinolytic Medication Timing[1]	1	0%	30%	31%	100%
PCI Within 90 Minutes of Arrival[1]	10	80%	48%	54%	95%
Smoking Cessation Advice	93	96%	90%	88%	100%
Heart Failure Care					
ACE Inhibitor or ARB for LVSD	244	98%	82%	82%	100%
Discharge Instructions	491	82%	60%	61%	93%
Evaluation of LVS Function	584	97%	81%	83%	99%
Smoking Cessation Advice	97	89%	82%	82%	100%
Pneumonia Care					
Appropriate Initial Antibiotic[2]	81	91%	79%	83%	94%
Blood Culture Timing[2]	66	92%	89%	90%	100%
Influenza Vaccine[1,2]	16	56%	69%	70%	100%
Initial Antibiotic Timing[2]	135	72%	78%	80%	93%
Oxygenation Assessment[2]	145	100%	99%	99%	100%
Pneumococcal Vaccine[2]	91	73%	68%	69%	94%
Smoking Cessation Advice[2]	28	71%	83%	80%	100%
Surgical Infection Prevention					
Prophylactic Antibiotic Given[2,3]	232	71%	67%	77%	95%
Prophylactic Antibiotic Selection[2]	81	96%	86%	90%	100%
Prophylactic Antibiotic Stopped[2,3]	222	78%	68%	72%	95%
Pregnancy Care					
Inpatient Neonatal Mortality	-	-	-	-	-
Third or Fourth Degree Laceration	-	-	3.23%	3.63%	3.27%

Seton Northwest Hospital

1113 Research Boulevard   Phone: 512-324-6000
Austin, TX 78759   Fax: 512-324-6924
URL: www.seton.net
Ownership: Voluntary non-profit - Church   Accredited: Yes
Emergency Services: Yes   Licensed Beds: 113
Key Personnel:
President/CEO . . . . Charles Barnett

Measure	Cases	This Hospital	State Average	U.S. Average	Top Hospital

Heart Attack Care

ACE Inhibitor or ARB for LVSD	0	-	85%	82%	100%
Aspirin at Arrival[1]	9	100%	91%	92%	100%
Aspirin at Discharge[1]	5	100%	90%	90%	100%
Beta Blocker at Arrival[1]	3	100%	85%	87%	100%
Beta Blocker at Discharge[1]	4	100%	86%	90%	100%
Fibrinolytic Medication Timing	0	-	30%	31%	100%
PCI Within 90 Minutes of Arrival	0	-	48%	54%	95%
Smoking Cessation Advice	0	-	90%	88%	100%
Heart Failure Care					
ACE Inhibitor or ARB for LVSD[1]	17	100%	82%	82%	100%
Discharge Instructions	39	62%	60%	61%	93%
Evaluation of LVS Function	45	100%	81%	83%	99%
Smoking Cessation Advice[1]	8	38%	82%	82%	100%
Pneumonia Care					
Appropriate Initial Antibiotic[2]	128	95%	79%	83%	94%
Blood Culture Timing[2]	96	82%	89%	90%	100%
Influenza Vaccine[4,5]	-	-	69%	70%	100%
Initial Antibiotic Timing[2]	152	77%	78%	80%	93%
Oxygenation Assessment[2]	168	99%	99%	99%	100%
Pneumococcal Vaccine[2]	82	84%	68%	69%	94%
Smoking Cessation Advice[2]	43	79%	83%	80%	100%
Surgical Infection Prevention					
Prophylactic Antibiotic Given[2,3]	113	66%	67%	77%	95%
Prophylactic Antibiotic Selection[2]	30	97%	86%	90%	100%
Prophylactic Antibiotic Stopped[2,3]	110	43%	68%	72%	95%
Pregnancy Care					
Inpatient Neonatal Mortality	-	-	-	-	-
Third or Fourth Degree Laceration	-	-	3.23%	3.63%	3.27%

Seton Southwest Healthcare Center

7900 FM 1826   Phone: 512-324-9000
Austin, TX 78737   Fax: 512-324-9040
URL: www.seton.net
Ownership: Voluntary non-profit - Church   Accredited: Yes
Emergency Services: Yes   Licensed Beds: 17
Key Personnel:
President/CEO . . . . Marry Farie

Measure	Cases	This Hospital	State Average	U.S. Average	Top Hospital
Heart Attack Care					
ACE Inhibitor or ARB for LVSD[5]	-	-	85%	82%	100%
Aspirin at Arrival[5]	-	-	91%	92%	100%
Aspirin at Discharge[5]	-	-	90%	90%	100%
Beta Blocker at Arrival[5]	-	-	85%	87%	100%
Beta Blocker at Discharge[5]	-	-	86%	90%	100%
Fibrinolytic Medication Timing[5]	-	-	30%	31%	100%
PCI Within 90 Minutes of Arrival[5]	-	-	48%	54%	95%
Smoking Cessation Advice[5]	-	-	90%	88%	100%
Heart Failure Care					
ACE Inhibitor or ARB for LVSD[3]	0	-	82%	82%	100%
Discharge Instructions[1,3]	2	0%	60%	61%	93%
Evaluation of LVS Function[1,3]	2	50%	81%	83%	99%
Smoking Cessation Advice[3]	0	-	82%	82%	100%
Pneumonia Care					
Appropriate Initial Antibiotic[1,3]	22	86%	79%	83%	94%
Blood Culture Timing[1,3]	14	100%	89%	90%	100%
Influenza Vaccine[5]	-	-	69%	70%	100%
Initial Antibiotic Timing[1,3]	24	92%	78%	80%	93%
Oxygenation Assessment[3]	26	100%	99%	99%	100%
Pneumococcal Vaccine[1,3]	10	80%	68%	69%	94%
Smoking Cessation Advice[1,3]	6	83%	83%	80%	100%
Surgical Infection Prevention					
Prophylactic Antibiotic Given[2,3]	37	70%	67%	77%	95%
Prophylactic Antibiotic Selection[1,2]	17	94%	86%	90%	100%
Prophylactic Antibiotic Stopped[2,3]	36	86%	68%	72%	95%
Pregnancy Care					
Inpatient Neonatal Mortality	-	-	-	-	-
Third or Fourth Degree Laceration	-	-	3.23%	3.63%	3.27%

South Austin Hospital

Alternate Name: HCA South Austin Medical Center

NOTE: Hospital profiles are in alphabetical order by state, then city, then hospital within the city; Rankings are sorted by rate in descending order and exclude hospitals with less than 25 cases; (1) The number of cases is too small (n<25) for purposes of reliably predicting hospital performance; (2) Measure reflects the hospital's indication that its submission was based upon a sample of its relevant discharges; (3) Rate reflects fewer than the maximum possible quarters of data for the measure; (4) Inaccurate information submitted and suppressed for one or more quarters; (5) No data is available from the hospital for this measure; Please refer to the User's Guide for a full explanation of data

901 W Ben White Boulevard
Austin, TX 78704
URL: www.southaustinhospital.com
Ownership: Proprietary
Emergency Services: Yes
Key Personnel:
CEO. . . . . Erol R Akdamar
Chief Medical Staff. . . . . Steve Berkowitz
Emergency Room . . . . Jerry Anderson

Phone: 512-447-2211
Fax: 512-416-6213

Accredited: Yes
Licensed Beds: 252

Measure	Cases	This Hospital	State Average	U.S. Average	Top Hospital
Heart Attack Care					
ACE Inhibitor or ARB for LVSD	100	84%	85%	82%	100%
Aspirin at Arrival	252	97%	91%	92%	100%
Aspirin at Discharge	232	97%	90%	90%	100%
Beta Blocker at Arrival	172	90%	85%	87%	100%
Beta Blocker at Discharge	204	98%	86%	90%	100%
Fibrinolytic Medication Timing[1]	1	0%	30%	31%	100%
PCI Within 90 Minutes of Arrival[1]	14	64%	48%	54%	95%
Smoking Cessation Advice	89	100%	90%	88%	100%
Heart Failure Care					
ACE Inhibitor or ARB for LVSD	199	85%	82%	82%	100%
Discharge Instructions	351	57%	60%	61%	93%
Evaluation of LVS Function	405	98%	81%	83%	99%
Smoking Cessation Advice	92	99%	82%	82%	100%
Pneumonia Care					
Appropriate Initial Antibiotic	183	87%	79%	83%	94%
Blood Culture Timing	179	94%	89%	90%	100%
Influenza Vaccine	57	79%	69%	70%	100%
Initial Antibiotic Timing	230	70%	78%	80%	93%
Oxygenation Assessment	303	100%	99%	99%	100%
Pneumococcal Vaccine	159	64%	68%	69%	94%
Smoking Cessation Advice	86	100%	83%	80%	100%
Surgical Infection Prevention					
Prophylactic Antibiotic Given[2,3]	262	74%	67%	77%	95%
Prophylactic Antibiotic Selection[2]	122	93%	86%	90%	100%
Prophylactic Antibiotic Stopped[2,3]	252	72%	68%	72%	95%
Pregnancy Care					
Inpatient Neonatal Mortality	-	-	-	-	-
Third or Fourth Degree Laceration	-	-	3.23%	3.63%	3.27%

The Hospital at Westlake Medical Center

5656 Bee Caves Road, Suite M-302
Austin, TX 78746
Ownership: Proprietary
Emergency Services: Yes

Phone: 512-327-0000

Accredited: No

Measure	Cases	This Hospital	State Average	U.S. Average	Top Hospital
Heart Attack Care					
ACE Inhibitor or ARB for LVSD[1,3]	3	100%	85%	82%	100%
Aspirin at Arrival[1,3]	9	100%	91%	92%	100%
Aspirin at Discharge[1,3]	16	100%	90%	90%	100%
Beta Blocker at Arrival[1,3]	6	100%	85%	87%	100%
Beta Blocker at Discharge[1,3]	14	100%	86%	90%	100%
Fibrinolytic Medication Timing[3]	0	-	30%	31%	100%
PCI Within 90 Minutes of Arrival[1]	1	100%	48%	54%	95%
Smoking Cessation Advice[1,3]	3	100%	90%	88%	100%
Heart Failure Care					
ACE Inhibitor or ARB for LVSD[1]	7	100%	82%	82%	100%
Discharge Instructions[1]	14	21%	60%	61%	93%
Evaluation of LVS Function[1]	16	100%	81%	83%	99%
Smoking Cessation Advice[1]	2	100%	82%	82%	100%
Pneumonia Care					
Appropriate Initial Antibiotic[1]	5	100%	79%	83%	94%
Blood Culture Timing[1]	4	100%	89%	90%	100%
Influenza Vaccine	0	-	69%	70%	100%
Initial Antibiotic Timing[1]	6	67%	78%	80%	93%
Oxygenation Assessment[1]	7	100%	99%	99%	100%
Pneumococcal Vaccine[1]	4	100%	68%	69%	94%
Smoking Cessation Advice[1]	1	100%	83%	80%	100%
Surgical Infection Prevention					
Prophylactic Antibiotic Given[3]	30	77%	67%	77%	95%

Prophylactic Antibiotic Selection	30	97%	86%	90%	100%
Prophylactic Antibiotic Stopped[3]	29	21%	68%	72%	95%
Pregnancy Care					
Inpatient Neonatal Mortality	-	-	-	-	-
Third or Fourth Degree Laceration	-	-	3.23%	3.63%	3.27%

Harris Methodist Northwest

108 Denver Trail
Azle, TX 76020
URL: www.hmhs.org
Ownership: Voluntary non-profit - Church
Emergency Services: Yes
Key Personnel:
President . . . . Brett McClung
Chief Medical Staff. . . . . Monica Goth
Director Infection/Disease Control . . . . Jean Earls

Phone: 817-444-8600
Fax: 817-882-2553

Accredited: Yes
Licensed Beds: 44

Measure	Cases	This Hospital	State Average	U.S. Average	Top Hospital
Heart Attack Care					
ACE Inhibitor or ARB for LVSD[1]	3	67%	85%	82%	100%
Aspirin at Arrival	30	93%	91%	92%	100%
Aspirin at Discharge[1]	9	100%	90%	90%	100%
Beta Blocker at Arrival[1]	21	95%	85%	87%	100%
Beta Blocker at Discharge[1]	9	89%	86%	90%	100%
Fibrinolytic Medication Timing[1]	5	100%	30%	31%	100%
PCI Within 90 Minutes of Arrival[1]	0	-	48%	54%	95%
Smoking Cessation Advice[1]	5	80%	90%	88%	100%
Heart Failure Care					
ACE Inhibitor or ARB for LVSD[1]	20	95%	82%	82%	100%
Discharge Instructions	73	92%	60%	61%	93%
Evaluation of LVS Function	91	93%	81%	83%	99%
Smoking Cessation Advice[1]	17	94%	82%	82%	100%
Pneumonia Care					
Appropriate Initial Antibiotic	139	86%	79%	83%	94%
Blood Culture Timing	114	93%	89%	90%	100%
Influenza Vaccine	44	84%	69%	70%	100%
Initial Antibiotic Timing	161	97%	78%	80%	93%
Oxygenation Assessment	210	100%	99%	99%	100%
Pneumococcal Vaccine	131	78%	68%	69%	94%
Smoking Cessation Advice	70	99%	83%	80%	100%
Surgical Infection Prevention					
Prophylactic Antibiotic Given[2,3]	52	52%	67%	77%	95%
Prophylactic Antibiotic Selection[1,2]	17	94%	86%	90%	100%
Prophylactic Antibiotic Stopped[2,3]	48	31%	68%	72%	95%
Pregnancy Care					
Inpatient Neonatal Mortality	-	-	-	-	-
Third or Fourth Degree Laceration	-	-	3.23%	3.63%	3.27%

Lakeside Hospital at Bastrop

3201 Hwy 71 East
Bastrop, TX 78602
Ownership: Proprietary
Emergency Services: Yes

Phone: 512-321-8234

Accredited: Yes

Measure	Cases	This Hospital	State Average	U.S. Average	Top Hospital
Heart Attack Care					
ACE Inhibitor or ARB for LVSD[5]	-	-	85%	82%	100%
Aspirin at Arrival[5]	-	-	91%	92%	100%
Aspirin at Discharge[5]	-	-	90%	90%	100%
Beta Blocker at Arrival[5]	-	-	85%	87%	100%
Beta Blocker at Discharge[5]	-	-	86%	90%	100%
Fibrinolytic Medication Timing[5]	-	-	30%	31%	100%
PCI Within 90 Minutes of Arrival[5]	-	-	48%	54%	95%
Smoking Cessation Advice[5]	-	-	90%	88%	100%
Heart Failure Care					
ACE Inhibitor or ARB for LVSD[1,3]	7	100%	82%	82%	100%
Discharge Instructions[1,3]	8	0%	60%	61%	93%
Evaluation of LVS Function[1,3]	14	50%	81%	83%	99%
Smoking Cessation Advice[1,3]	6	0%	82%	82%	100%
Pneumonia Care					
Appropriate Initial Antibiotic[1,3]	1	100%	79%	83%	94%
Blood Culture Timing[1,3]	3	100%	89%	90%	100%

NOTE: Hospital profiles are in alphabetical order by state, then city, then hospital within the city; Rankings are sorted by rate in descending order and exclude hospitals with less than 25 cases; (1) The number of cases is too small (n<25) for purposes of reliably predicting hospital performance; (2) Measure reflects the hospital's indication that its submission was based upon a sample of its relevant discharges; (3) Rate reflects fewer than the maximum possible quarters of data for the measure; (4) Inaccurate information submitted and suppressed for one or more quarters; (5) No data is available from the hospital for this measure; Please refer to the User's Guide for a full explanation of data

Measure	Cases	This Hospital	State Average	U.S. Average	Top Hospital
Influenza Vaccine[5]	-	-	69%	70%	100%
Initial Antibiotic Timing[1,3]	8	50%	78%	80%	93%
Oxygenation Assessment[1,3]	12	92%	99%	99%	100%
Pneumococcal Vaccine[1,3]	10	50%	68%	69%	94%
Smoking Cessation Advice[3]	0	-	83%	80%	100%
Surgical Infection Prevention					
Prophylactic Antibiotic Given[3]	0	-	67%	77%	95%
Prophylactic Antibiotic Selection[5]	-	-	86%	90%	100%
Prophylactic Antibiotic Stopped[3]	0	-	68%	72%	95%
Pregnancy Care					
Inpatient Neonatal Mortality	-	-	-	-	-
Third or Fourth Degree Laceration	-	-	3.23%	3.63%	3.27%

Matagorda County Hospital District

Alternate Name: Matagorda General Hospital
1115 Ave G
Bay City, TX 77414
Ownership: Govt - Hospital District or Authority
Emergency Services: Yes

Phone: 979-245-6383
Fax: 979-245-1525
Accredited: Yes
Licensed Beds: 100

Measure	Cases	This Hospital	State Average	U.S. Average	Top Hospital
Heart Attack Care					
ACE Inhibitor or ARB for LVSD[1]	4	75%	85%	82%	100%
Aspirin at Arrival	31	90%	91%	92%	100%
Aspirin at Discharge[1]	15	73%	90%	90%	100%
Beta Blocker at Arrival[1]	9	56%	85%	87%	100%
Beta Blocker at Discharge[1]	16	69%	86%	90%	100%
Fibrinolytic Medication Timing[1]	2	100%	30%	31%	100%
PCI Within 90 Minutes of Arrival	0	-	48%	54%	95%
Smoking Cessation Advice[1]	2	100%	90%	88%	100%
Heart Failure Care					
ACE Inhibitor or ARB for LVSD	28	79%	82%	82%	100%
Discharge Instructions	76	37%	60%	61%	93%
Evaluation of LVS Function	100	82%	81%	83%	99%
Smoking Cessation Advice[1]	20	90%	82%	82%	100%
Pneumonia Care					
Appropriate Initial Antibiotic	42	90%	79%	83%	94%
Blood Culture Timing	36	92%	89%	90%	100%
Influenza Vaccine[1]	12	83%	69%	70%	100%
Initial Antibiotic Timing	58	86%	78%	80%	93%
Oxygenation Assessment	83	98%	99%	99%	100%
Pneumococcal Vaccine	45	62%	68%	69%	94%
Smoking Cessation Advice[1]	10	90%	83%	80%	100%
Surgical Infection Prevention					
Prophylactic Antibiotic Given	63	94%	67%	77%	95%
Prophylactic Antibiotic Selection[1]	18	61%	86%	90%	100%
Prophylactic Antibiotic Stopped	57	67%	68%	72%	95%
Pregnancy Care					
Inpatient Neonatal Mortality	283	0.00%	-	-	-
Third or Fourth Degree Laceration	207	6.76%	3.23%	3.63%	3.27%

San Jacinto Methodist Hospital

4401 Garth Road
Baytown, TX 77521
URL: www.methodisthealth.com/sanjacinto
Ownership: Voluntary non-profit - Church
Emergency Services: Yes

Phone: 281-420-8600
Fax: 281-420-8852

Accredited: Yes
Licensed Beds: 335

Key Personnel:
President . . . . S Jeffrey Ackerman, MD
Director Infection/Disease Control . . . . Barbara Gils
Director Respiratory Therapy . . . . Gina Beard

Measure	Cases	This Hospital	State Average	U.S. Average	Top Hospital
Heart Attack Care					
ACE Inhibitor or ARB for LVSD[2]	47	87%	85%	82%	100%
Aspirin at Arrival[2]	217	99%	91%	92%	100%
Aspirin at Discharge[2]	152	89%	90%	90%	100%
Beta Blocker at Arrival[2]	198	96%	85%	87%	100%
Beta Blocker at Discharge[2]	166	94%	86%	90%	100%
Fibrinolytic Medication Timing[1,2]	14	21%	30%	31%	100%
PCI Within 90 Minutes of Arrival[1,2]	8	12%	48%	54%	95%
Smoking Cessation Advice[2]	52	100%	90%	88%	100%

Heart Failure Care

Measure	Cases	This Hospital	State Average	U.S. Average	Top Hospital
ACE Inhibitor or ARB for LVSD[2]	115	75%	82%	82%	100%
Discharge Instructions[2]	264	74%	60%	61%	93%
Evaluation of LVS Function[2]	314	90%	81%	83%	99%
Smoking Cessation Advice[2]	62	97%	82%	82%	100%
Pneumonia Care					
Appropriate Initial Antibiotic[2]	140	81%	79%	83%	94%
Blood Culture Timing[2]	88	90%	89%	90%	100%
Influenza Vaccine[2]	28	43%	69%	70%	100%
Initial Antibiotic Timing[2]	184	74%	78%	80%	93%
Oxygenation Assessment[2]	221	100%	99%	99%	100%
Pneumococcal Vaccine[2]	110	89%	68%	69%	94%
Smoking Cessation Advice[2]	59	97%	83%	80%	100%
Surgical Infection Prevention					
Prophylactic Antibiotic Given[2,3]	182	73%	67%	77%	95%
Prophylactic Antibiotic Selection[2]	37	86%	86%	90%	100%
Prophylactic Antibiotic Stopped[2,3]	174	66%	68%	72%	95%
Pregnancy Care					
Inpatient Neonatal Mortality	-	-	-	-	-
Third or Fourth Degree Laceration	-	-	3.23%	3.63%	3.27%

Beaumont Bone & Joint Institute

3650 Laurel Avenue
Beaumont, TX 77707
Ownership: Government - Federal
Emergency Services: No

Phone: 409-838-0346

Accredited: No

Measure	Cases	This Hospital	State Average	U.S. Average	Top Hospital
Heart Attack Care					
ACE Inhibitor or ARB for LVSD[5]	-	-	85%	82%	100%
Aspirin at Arrival[5]	-	-	91%	92%	100%
Aspirin at Discharge[5]	-	-	90%	90%	100%
Beta Blocker at Arrival[5]	-	-	85%	87%	100%
Beta Blocker at Discharge[5]	-	-	86%	90%	100%
Fibrinolytic Medication Timing[5]	-	-	30%	31%	100%
PCI Within 90 Minutes of Arrival[5]	-	-	48%	54%	95%
Smoking Cessation Advice[5]	-	-	90%	88%	100%
Heart Failure Care					
ACE Inhibitor or ARB for LVSD[5]	-	-	82%	82%	100%
Discharge Instructions[5]	-	-	60%	61%	93%
Evaluation of LVS Function[5]	-	-	81%	83%	99%
Smoking Cessation Advice[5]	-	-	82%	82%	100%
Pneumonia Care					
Appropriate Initial Antibiotic[5]	-	-	79%	83%	94%
Blood Culture Timing[5]	-	-	89%	90%	100%
Influenza Vaccine[5]	-	-	69%	70%	100%
Initial Antibiotic Timing[5]	-	-	78%	80%	93%
Oxygenation Assessment[5]	-	-	99%	99%	100%
Pneumococcal Vaccine[5]	-	-	68%	69%	94%
Smoking Cessation Advice[5]	-	-	83%	80%	100%
Surgical Infection Prevention					
Prophylactic Antibiotic Given[5]	-	-	67%	77%	95%
Prophylactic Antibiotic Selection[5]	-	-	86%	90%	100%
Prophylactic Antibiotic Stopped[5]	-	-	68%	72%	95%
Pregnancy Care					
Inpatient Neonatal Mortality	-	-	-	-	-
Third or Fourth Degree Laceration	-	-	3.23%	3.63%	3.27%

Christus Saint Elizabeth Hospital

Alternate Name: Saint Elizabeth Hospital
2830 Calder
Beaumont, TX 77702
E-mail: communications@christushealth.org
URL: www.christushealth.org
Ownership: Voluntary non-profit - Church
Emergency Services: Yes

Phone: 409-892-7171
Fax: 409-899-8191

Accredited: Yes
Licensed Beds: 461

Key Personnel:
Administrator . . . . Edward M Myers
Chief Medical Staff . . . . Herman William, MD
Director Infection/Disease Control . . . . Cindy Powell
Chief Radiology . . . . Elizabeth Blanchette
Director Respiratory Therapy . . . . Shelly Cooper

NOTE: Hospital profiles are in alphabetical order by state, then city, then hospital within the city; Rankings are sorted by rate in descending order and exclude hospitals with less than 25 cases; (1) The number of cases is too small (n<25) for purposes of reliably predicting hospital performance; (2) Measure reflects the hospital's indication that its submission was based upon a sample of its relevant discharges; (3) Rate reflects fewer than the maximum possible quarters of data for the measure; (4) Inaccurate information submitted and suppressed for one or more quarters; (5) No data is available from the hospital for this measure; Please refer to the User's Guide for a full explanation of data

Measure	Cases	This Hospital	State Average	U.S. Average	Top Hospital
Heart Attack Care					
ACE Inhibitor or ARB for LVSD	88	83%	85%	82%	100%
Aspirin at Arrival	352	95%	91%	92%	100%
Aspirin at Discharge	432	98%	90%	90%	100%
Beta Blocker at Arrival	301	89%	85%	87%	100%
Beta Blocker at Discharge	430	94%	86%	90%	100%
Fibrinolytic Medication Timing[1]	3	0%	30%	31%	100%
PCI Within 90 Minutes of Arrival[1]	21	71%	48%	54%	95%
Smoking Cessation Advice	188	99%	90%	88%	100%
Heart Failure Care					
ACE Inhibitor or ARB for LVSD	348	89%	82%	82%	100%
Discharge Instructions	812	90%	60%	61%	93%
Evaluation of LVS Function	928	93%	81%	83%	99%
Smoking Cessation Advice	236	96%	82%	82%	100%
Pneumonia Care					
Appropriate Initial Antibiotic	406	83%	79%	83%	94%
Blood Culture Timing	392	87%	89%	90%	100%
Influenza Vaccine	114	92%	69%	70%	100%
Initial Antibiotic Timing	564	81%	78%	80%	93%
Oxygenation Assessment	636	99%	99%	99%	100%
Pneumococcal Vaccine	339	87%	68%	69%	94%
Smoking Cessation Advice	179	89%	83%	80%	100%
Surgical Infection Prevention					
Prophylactic Antibiotic Given	1,358	64%	67%	77%	95%
Prophylactic Antibiotic Selection	365	75%	86%	90%	100%
Prophylactic Antibiotic Stopped	1,312	52%	68%	72%	95%
Pregnancy Care					
Inpatient Neonatal Mortality	-	-	-	-	-
Third or Fourth Degree Laceration	-	-	3.23%	3.63%	3.27%

Memorial Hermann Baptist Beaumont

3080 College Street
Beaumont, TX 77701   Phone: 409-212-5000
URL: www.mhbh.org   Fax: 409-212-6016
Ownership: Voluntary non-profit - Church   Accredited: Yes
Emergency Services: Yes   Licensed Beds: 352
Key Personnel:
President/CEO . . . . David Parmer
Chief Medical Staff . . . . Vicki Clark
Chief Catheterization Laboratory . . . . Bruce Hubbard
Director Respiratory Therapy . . . . Betty Wyble

Measure	Cases	This Hospital	State Average	U.S. Average	Top Hospital
Heart Attack Care					
ACE Inhibitor or ARB for LVSD	33	94%	85%	82%	100%
Aspirin at Arrival	130	94%	91%	92%	100%
Aspirin at Discharge	169	99%	90%	90%	100%
Beta Blocker at Arrival	101	90%	85%	87%	100%
Beta Blocker at Discharge	169	96%	86%	90%	100%
Fibrinolytic Medication Timing[3]	0	-	30%	31%	100%
PCI Within 90 Minutes of Arrival[1]	1	100%	48%	54%	95%
Smoking Cessation Advice[1,3]	11	100%	90%	88%	100%
Heart Failure Care					
ACE Inhibitor or ARB for LVSD	155	87%	82%	82%	100%
Discharge Instructions[3]	81	88%	60%	61%	93%
Evaluation of LVS Function	373	96%	81%	83%	99%
Smoking Cessation Advice[3]	28	96%	82%	82%	100%
Pneumonia Care					
Appropriate Initial Antibiotic[3]	29	83%	79%	83%	94%
Blood Culture Timing[3]	34	97%	89%	90%	100%
Influenza Vaccine[5]	-	-	69%	70%	100%
Initial Antibiotic Timing	250	82%	78%	80%	93%
Oxygenation Assessment	282	100%	99%	99%	100%
Pneumococcal Vaccine	149	72%	68%	69%	94%
Smoking Cessation Advice[1,3]	8	100%	83%	80%	100%
Surgical Infection Prevention					
Prophylactic Antibiotic Given	104	84%	67%	77%	95%
Prophylactic Antibiotic Selection[5]	-	-	86%	90%	100%
Prophylactic Antibiotic Stopped[3]	101	54%	68%	72%	95%
Pregnancy Care					
Inpatient Neonatal Mortality	-	-	-	-	-

Third or Fourth Degree Laceration	-	-	3.23%	3.63%	3.27%

Harris Methodist HEB Hospital

Alternate Name: HEB Hospital; Harris HEB
1600 Hospital Parkway   Phone: 817-685-4000
Bedford, TX 76022   Fax: 817-685-4890
URL: www.HarrisHospital.com
Ownership: Voluntary non-profit - Church   Accredited: Yes
Emergency Services: Yes   Licensed Beds: 287
Key Personnel:
President/CEO . . . . Douglas D Hawthorne
Chief Medical Staff . . . . Mary Brian, MD
Catheterization Lab . . . . Don Rogers
Emergency Room . . . . Grace Bosworth
Infection Control . . . . Rama Stevens
ICU . . . . Gary Wallace
Intensive Coronary . . . . Gary Wallace
Director Medical/Surgical Nursing . . . . Jerry Harrison, RN
OB/GYN/Women's Health . . . . Nanette Rix
Chief Radiology . . . . Stanley Cook, MD
Respiratory/Cardiopulmonary . . . . John Crowell

Measure	Cases	This Hospital	State Average	U.S. Average	Top Hospital
Heart Attack Care					
ACE Inhibitor or ARB for LVSD	25	96%	85%	82%	100%
Aspirin at Arrival	191	98%	91%	92%	100%
Aspirin at Discharge	185	100%	90%	90%	100%
Beta Blocker at Arrival	133	95%	85%	87%	100%
Beta Blocker at Discharge	186	97%	86%	90%	100%
Fibrinolytic Medication Timing	0	-	30%	31%	100%
PCI Within 90 Minutes of Arrival[1]	10	80%	48%	54%	95%
Smoking Cessation Advice	70	100%	90%	88%	100%
Heart Failure Care					
ACE Inhibitor or ARB for LVSD	93	98%	82%	82%	100%
Discharge Instructions	220	75%	60%	61%	93%
Evaluation of LVS Function	274	92%	81%	83%	99%
Smoking Cessation Advice	50	98%	82%	82%	100%
Pneumonia Care					
Appropriate Initial Antibiotic	194	85%	79%	83%	94%
Blood Culture Timing	212	92%	89%	90%	100%
Influenza Vaccine	71	89%	69%	70%	100%
Initial Antibiotic Timing	257	89%	78%	80%	93%
Oxygenation Assessment	327	100%	99%	99%	100%
Pneumococcal Vaccine	200	92%	68%	69%	94%
Smoking Cessation Advice	88	99%	83%	80%	100%
Surgical Infection Prevention					
Prophylactic Antibiotic Given[2,3]	180	74%	67%	77%	95%
Prophylactic Antibiotic Selection[2]	58	91%	86%	90%	100%
Prophylactic Antibiotic Stopped[2,3]	155	77%	68%	72%	95%
Pregnancy Care					
Inpatient Neonatal Mortality	-	-	-	-	-
Third or Fourth Degree Laceration	-	-	3.23%	3.63%	3.27%

Christus Spohn Hospital Beeville

Alternate Name: Spohn Bee County Hospital
1500 E Houston Street   Phone: 361-354-2000
Beeville, TX 78102   Fax: 361-358-9322
URL: www.christushealth.org
Ownership: Voluntary non-profit - Church   Accredited: Yes
Emergency Services: Yes   Licensed Beds: 69
Key Personnel:
President/CEO . . . . Kathy J McDonagh
Infection Control . . . . Michael G Bullen, MD

Measure	Cases	This Hospital	State Average	U.S. Average	Top Hospital
Heart Attack Care					
ACE Inhibitor or ARB for LVSD[1]	4	75%	85%	82%	100%
Aspirin at Arrival[1]	22	100%	91%	92%	100%
Aspirin at Discharge[1]	13	92%	90%	90%	100%
Beta Blocker at Arrival[1]	19	84%	85%	87%	100%
Beta Blocker at Discharge[1]	10	70%	86%	90%	100%
Fibrinolytic Medication Timing[3]	0	-	30%	31%	100%
PCI Within 90 Minutes of Arrival	0	-	48%	54%	95%

NOTE: Hospital profiles are in alphabetical order by state, then city, then hospital within the city; Rankings are sorted by rate in descending order and exclude hospitals with less than 25 cases; (1) The number of cases is too small (n<25) for purposes of reliably predicting hospital performance; (2) Measure reflects the hospital's indication that its submission was based upon a sample of its relevant discharges; (3) Rate reflects fewer than the maximum possible quarters of data for the measure; (4) Inaccurate information submitted and suppressed for one or more quarters; (5) No data is available from the hospital for this measure; Please refer to the User's Guide for a full explanation of data

Smoking Cessation Advice[1,3]	1	100%	90%	88%	100%
Heart Failure Care					
ACE Inhibitor or ARB for LVSD	49	98%	82%	82%	100%
Discharge Instructions[3]	38	82%	60%	61%	93%
Evaluation of LVS Function	222	95%	81%	83%	99%
Smoking Cessation Advice[1,3]	12	100%	82%	82%	100%
Pneumonia Care					
Appropriate Initial Antibiotic[1,3]	7	86%	79%	83%	94%
Blood Culture Timing[1,3]	9	100%	89%	90%	100%
Influenza Vaccine[5]	-	-	69%	70%	100%
Initial Antibiotic Timing	96	95%	78%	80%	93%
Oxygenation Assessment	115	99%	99%	99%	100%
Pneumococcal Vaccine	66	82%	68%	69%	94%
Smoking Cessation Advice[1,3]	6	100%	83%	80%	100%
Surgical Infection Prevention					
Prophylactic Antibiotic Given[1,3]	5	20%	67%	77%	95%
Prophylactic Antibiotic Selection[5]	-	-	86%	90%	100%
Prophylactic Antibiotic Stopped[1,3]	3	67%	68%	72%	95%
Pregnancy Care					
Inpatient Neonatal Mortality	412	0.24%	-	-	-
Third or Fourth Degree Laceration	249	1.61%	3.23%	3.63%	3.27%

Foundation Surgical Hospital

5410 West Loop South   Phone: 713-622-2262
Bellaire, TX 77401
Ownership: Proprietary   Accredited: No
Emergency Services: Yes

Measure	Cases	This Hospital	State Average	U.S. Average	Top Hospital
Heart Attack Care					
ACE Inhibitor or ARB for LVSD[5]	-	-	85%	82%	100%
Aspirin at Arrival[5]	-	-	91%	92%	100%
Aspirin at Discharge[5]	-	-	90%	90%	100%
Beta Blocker at Arrival[5]	-	-	85%	87%	100%
Beta Blocker at Discharge[5]	-	-	86%	90%	100%
Fibrinolytic Medication Timing[5]	-	-	30%	31%	100%
PCI Within 90 Minutes of Arrival[5]	-	-	48%	54%	95%
Smoking Cessation Advice[5]	-	-	90%	88%	100%
Heart Failure Care					
ACE Inhibitor or ARB for LVSD[5]	-	-	82%	82%	100%
Discharge Instructions[5]	-	-	60%	61%	93%
Evaluation of LVS Function[5]	-	-	81%	83%	99%
Smoking Cessation Advice[5]	-	-	82%	82%	100%
Pneumonia Care					
Appropriate Initial Antibiotic[5]	-	-	79%	83%	94%
Blood Culture Timing[5]	-	-	89%	90%	100%
Influenza Vaccine[5]	-	-	69%	70%	100%
Initial Antibiotic Timing[5]	-	-	78%	80%	93%
Oxygenation Assessment[5]	-	-	99%	99%	100%
Pneumococcal Vaccine[5]	-	-	68%	69%	94%
Smoking Cessation Advice[5]	-	-	83%	80%	100%
Surgical Infection Prevention					
Prophylactic Antibiotic Given[1,2,3]	19	63%	67%	77%	95%
Prophylactic Antibiotic Selection[5]	-	-	86%	90%	100%
Prophylactic Antibiotic Stopped[1,2,3]	19	95%	68%	72%	95%
Pregnancy Care					
Inpatient Neonatal Mortality	-	-	-	-	-
Third or Fourth Degree Laceration	-	-	3.23%	3.63%	3.27%

Bellville General Hospital

44 N Cummings Street   Phone: 979-865-3141
Bellville, TX 77418   Fax: 979-865-9631
URL: www.bellvillehospital.com
Ownership: Govt - Hospital District or Authority   Accredited: Yes
Emergency Services: Yes   Licensed Beds: 32
Key Personnel:
President . . . . Steve Lackey

Measure	Cases	This Hospital	State Average	U.S. Average	Top Hospital
Heart Attack Care					
ACE Inhibitor or ARB for LVSD[3]	0	-	85%	82%	100%
Aspirin at Arrival[1,3]	1	100%	91%	92%	100%

Aspirin at Discharge[3]	0	-	90%	90%	100%
Beta Blocker at Arrival[1,3]	1	100%	85%	87%	100%
Beta Blocker at Discharge[3]	0	-	86%	90%	100%
Fibrinolytic Medication Timing[3]	0	-	30%	31%	100%
PCI Within 90 Minutes of Arrival	0	-	48%	54%	95%
Smoking Cessation Advice[3]	0	-	90%	88%	100%
Heart Failure Care					
ACE Inhibitor or ARB for LVSD[1]	13	92%	82%	82%	100%
Discharge Instructions	29	100%	60%	61%	93%
Evaluation of LVS Function	36	83%	81%	83%	99%
Smoking Cessation Advice[1]	6	100%	82%	82%	100%
Pneumonia Care					
Appropriate Initial Antibiotic	29	48%	79%	83%	94%
Blood Culture Timing[1]	17	100%	89%	90%	100%
Influenza Vaccine[1]	12	58%	69%	70%	100%
Initial Antibiotic Timing	47	87%	78%	80%	93%
Oxygenation Assessment	56	91%	99%	99%	100%
Pneumococcal Vaccine	35	43%	68%	69%	94%
Smoking Cessation Advice[1]	12	100%	83%	80%	100%
Surgical Infection Prevention					
Prophylactic Antibiotic Given[1,3]	4	75%	67%	77%	95%
Prophylactic Antibiotic Selection[1]	2	50%	86%	90%	100%
Prophylactic Antibiotic Stopped[1,3]	4	100%	68%	72%	95%
Pregnancy Care					
Inpatient Neonatal Mortality	-	-	-	-	-
Third or Fourth Degree Laceration	-	-	3.23%	3.63%	3.27%

Scenic Mountain Medical Center

1601 W 11th Place   Phone: 432-263-1211
Big Spring, TX 79720   Fax: 432-268-4962
URL: www.smmccares.com
Ownership: Proprietary   Accredited: Yes
Emergency Services: Yes   Licensed Beds: 150
Key Personnel:
CEO. . . . . George N Parsley
Chief Medical Staff. . . . . James Huston, MD
Chief Radiology . . . . Vivian Gordon
Director Respiratory Therapy . . . . Robby Daniel

Measure	Cases	This Hospital	State Average	U.S. Average	Top Hospital
Heart Attack Care					
ACE Inhibitor or ARB for LVSD[1]	3	100%	85%	82%	100%
Aspirin at Arrival[1]	18	83%	91%	92%	100%
Aspirin at Discharge[1]	11	100%	90%	90%	100%
Beta Blocker at Arrival[1]	18	89%	85%	87%	100%
Beta Blocker at Discharge[1]	11	100%	86%	90%	100%
Fibrinolytic Medication Timing[1]	1	0%	30%	31%	100%
PCI Within 90 Minutes of Arrival	0	-	48%	54%	95%
Smoking Cessation Advice[1]	1	100%	90%	88%	100%
Heart Failure Care					
ACE Inhibitor or ARB for LVSD	26	81%	82%	82%	100%
Discharge Instructions	115	29%	60%	61%	93%
Evaluation of LVS Function	148	80%	81%	83%	99%
Smoking Cessation Advice	26	85%	82%	82%	100%
Pneumonia Care					
Appropriate Initial Antibiotic	64	58%	79%	83%	94%
Blood Culture Timing	35	86%	89%	90%	100%
Influenza Vaccine[1]	14	36%	69%	70%	100%
Initial Antibiotic Timing	68	87%	78%	80%	93%
Oxygenation Assessment	80	100%	99%	99%	100%
Pneumococcal Vaccine	39	56%	68%	69%	94%
Smoking Cessation Advice	29	79%	83%	80%	100%
Surgical Infection Prevention					
Prophylactic Antibiotic Given[2,3]	40	18%	67%	77%	95%
Prophylactic Antibiotic Selection[1,2]	13	85%	86%	90%	100%
Prophylactic Antibiotic Stopped[2,3]	34	79%	68%	72%	95%
Pregnancy Care					
Inpatient Neonatal Mortality	-	-	-	-	-
Third or Fourth Degree Laceration	-	-	3.23%	3.63%	3.27%

Northeast Medical Center

Alternate Name: Red River Regional Hospital

504 Lipscomb Boulevard
Bonham, TX 75418
Ownership: Proprietary
Emergency Services: No

Phone: 903-583-8585
Fax: 903-640-7601
Accredited: Yes
Licensed Beds: 75

Key Personnel:
CEO. . . . . Jay J Hodges
Chief Medical Staff. . . . . George George
Emergency Room . . . . Tina Elliotte

Measure	Cases	This Hospital	State Average	U.S. Average	Top Hospital
Heart Attack Care					
ACE Inhibitor or ARB for LVSD[1,3]	6	100%	85%	82%	100%
Aspirin at Arrival[3]	27	100%	91%	92%	100%
Aspirin at Discharge[1,3]	12	92%	90%	90%	100%
Beta Blocker at Arrival[3]	25	88%	85%	87%	100%
Beta Blocker at Discharge[1,3]	15	80%	86%	90%	100%
Fibrinolytic Medication Timing[1,3]	2	50%	30%	31%	100%
PCI Within 90 Minutes of Arrival	0	-	48%	54%	95%
Smoking Cessation Advice[1,3]	4	75%	90%	88%	100%
Heart Failure Care					
ACE Inhibitor or ARB for LVSD[1,3]	11	100%	82%	82%	100%
Discharge Instructions[3]	31	68%	60%	61%	93%
Evaluation of LVS Function[3]	63	67%	81%	83%	99%
Smoking Cessation Advice[1,3]	16	100%	82%	82%	100%
Pneumonia Care					
Appropriate Initial Antibiotic[3]	32	81%	79%	83%	94%
Blood Culture Timing	56	84%	89%	90%	100%
Influenza Vaccine	29	100%	69%	70%	100%
Initial Antibiotic Timing[3]	53	77%	78%	80%	93%
Oxygenation Assessment[3]	77	100%	99%	99%	100%
Pneumococcal Vaccine[3]	54	89%	68%	69%	94%
Smoking Cessation Advice[1,3]	16	100%	83%	80%	100%
Surgical Infection Prevention					
Prophylactic Antibiotic Given[3]	0	-	67%	77%	95%
Prophylactic Antibiotic Selection	0	-	86%	90%	100%
Prophylactic Antibiotic Stopped[3]	0	-	68%	72%	95%
Pregnancy Care					
Inpatient Neonatal Mortality	-	-	-	-	-
Third or Fourth Degree Laceration	-	-	3.23%	3.63%	3.27%

Bowie Memorial Hospital
705 East Greenwood Avenue
Bowie, TX 76230
Ownership: Govt - Hospital District or Authority
Emergency Services: Yes

Phone: 940-872-1126
Fax: 940-872-1561
Accredited: No
Licensed Beds: 49

Key Personnel:
President/CEO. . . . . Joyce Crumpler
Chief Medical Staff. . . . . Jay Turk
Emergency Room . . . . Marten Karlson
Infection Control. . . . . Peggy Raley, LVN
Medical/Surgical Nursing . . . . Anna Heller, RN
Director of Pulmonary . . . . Brenda Haile

Measure	Cases	This Hospital	State Average	U.S. Average	Top Hospital
Heart Attack Care					
ACE Inhibitor or ARB for LVSD[1]	2	100%	85%	82%	100%
Aspirin at Arrival[1]	16	94%	91%	92%	100%
Aspirin at Discharge[1]	13	100%	90%	90%	100%
Beta Blocker at Arrival[1]	14	100%	85%	87%	100%
Beta Blocker at Discharge[1]	12	100%	86%	90%	100%
Fibrinolytic Medication Timing	0	-	30%	31%	100%
PCI Within 90 Minutes of Arrival	0	-	48%	54%	95%
Smoking Cessation Advice[1]	3	100%	90%	88%	100%
Heart Failure Care					
ACE Inhibitor or ARB for LVSD[1]	18	100%	82%	82%	100%
Discharge Instructions	42	100%	60%	61%	93%
Evaluation of LVS Function	52	98%	81%	83%	99%
Smoking Cessation Advice[1]	3	100%	82%	82%	100%
Pneumonia Care					
Appropriate Initial Antibiotic	74	80%	79%	83%	94%
Blood Culture Timing[1]	22	91%	89%	90%	100%
Influenza Vaccine[4,5]	-	-	69%	70%	100%

Initial Antibiotic Timing	111	95%	78%	80%	93%
Oxygenation Assessment	134	100%	99%	99%	100%
Pneumococcal Vaccine	97	92%	68%	69%	94%
Smoking Cessation Advice	30	100%	83%	80%	100%
Surgical Infection Prevention					
Prophylactic Antibiotic Given[1,3]	4	25%	67%	77%	95%
Prophylactic Antibiotic Selection[1]	1	0%	86%	90%	100%
Prophylactic Antibiotic Stopped[1,3]	4	100%	68%	72%	95%
Pregnancy Care					
Inpatient Neonatal Mortality	-	-	-	-	-
Third or Fourth Degree Laceration	-	-	3.23%	3.63%	3.27%

Stephens Memorial Hospital
200 S Geneva Street
Breckenridge, TX 76424
Ownership: Government - Local
Emergency Services: Yes

Phone: 254-559-2241
Fax: 254-559-9000
Accredited: No
Licensed Beds: 40

Key Personnel:
CEO. . . . . Robbie Bewery
Chief Medical Staff. . . . . Connie Rankon, MD

Measure	Cases	This Hospital	State Average	U.S. Average	Top Hospital
Heart Attack Care					
ACE Inhibitor or ARB for LVSD[1]	1	100%	85%	82%	100%
Aspirin at Arrival[1]	4	75%	91%	92%	100%
Aspirin at Discharge[1]	5	100%	90%	90%	100%
Beta Blocker at Arrival[1]	4	75%	85%	87%	100%
Beta Blocker at Discharge[1]	3	100%	86%	90%	100%
Fibrinolytic Medication Timing[3]	0	-	30%	31%	100%
PCI Within 90 Minutes of Arrival	0	-	48%	54%	95%
Smoking Cessation Advice[3]	0	-	90%	88%	100%
Heart Failure Care					
ACE Inhibitor or ARB for LVSD[1]	16	81%	82%	82%	100%
Discharge Instructions[1,3]	7	100%	60%	61%	93%
Evaluation of LVS Function	68	84%	81%	83%	99%
Smoking Cessation Advice[1,3]	3	67%	82%	82%	100%
Pneumonia Care					
Appropriate Initial Antibiotic[1,3]	2	50%	79%	83%	94%
Blood Culture Timing[1,3]	3	100%	89%	90%	100%
Influenza Vaccine[4,5]	-	-	69%	70%	100%
Initial Antibiotic Timing	43	91%	78%	80%	93%
Oxygenation Assessment	57	100%	99%	99%	100%
Pneumococcal Vaccine	43	100%	68%	69%	94%
Smoking Cessation Advice[1,3]	1	100%	83%	80%	100%
Surgical Infection Prevention					
Prophylactic Antibiotic Given[3]	0	-	67%	77%	95%
Prophylactic Antibiotic Selection[5]	-	-	86%	90%	100%
Prophylactic Antibiotic Stopped[3]	0	-	68%	72%	95%
Pregnancy Care					
Inpatient Neonatal Mortality	-	-	-	-	-
Third or Fourth Degree Laceration	-	-	3.23%	3.63%	3.27%

Trinity Medical Center
700 Medical Parkway
Brenham, TX 77833
URL: www.trinitymed.com
Ownership: Voluntary non-profit - Church
Emergency Services: Yes

Phone: 979-836-6173
Fax: 979-830-2277

Accredited: Yes
Licensed Beds: 60

Key Personnel:
Administrator/CEO. . . . . John Simms
Chief Medical Staff. . . . . Bobby Marek, MD
Director of Cardiology/Cardiac Lab. . . . . Lynn Boeaer
Emergency Room . . . . D Opertriller
Respiratory Care . . . . Ken Banver

Measure	Cases	This Hospital	State Average	U.S. Average	Top Hospital
Heart Attack Care					
ACE Inhibitor or ARB for LVSD	0	-	85%	82%	100%
Aspirin at Arrival[1]	8	100%	91%	92%	100%
Aspirin at Discharge[1]	4	100%	90%	90%	100%
Beta Blocker at Arrival[1]	3	100%	85%	87%	100%
Beta Blocker at Discharge[1]	2	100%	86%	90%	100%

Fibrinolytic Medication Timing	0	-	30%	31%	100%
PCI Within 90 Minutes of Arrival	0	-	48%	54%	95%
Smoking Cessation Advice	0	-	90%	88%	100%
Heart Failure Care					
ACE Inhibitor or ARB for LVSD[1]	20	90%	82%	82%	100%
Discharge Instructions	35	80%	60%	61%	93%
Evaluation of LVS Function	54	67%	81%	83%	99%
Smoking Cessation Advice[1]	8	62%	82%	82%	100%
Pneumonia Care					
Appropriate Initial Antibiotic	32	75%	79%	83%	94%
Blood Culture Timing	33	82%	89%	90%	100%
Influenza Vaccine[1]	12	75%	69%	70%	100%
Initial Antibiotic Timing	48	83%	78%	80%	93%
Oxygenation Assessment	65	100%	99%	99%	100%
Pneumococcal Vaccine	32	69%	68%	69%	94%
Smoking Cessation Advice[1]	5	100%	83%	80%	100%
Surgical Infection Prevention					
Prophylactic Antibiotic Given[2,3]	78	77%	67%	77%	95%
Prophylactic Antibiotic Selection[1,2]	20	90%	86%	90%	100%
Prophylactic Antibiotic Stopped[2,3]	70	66%	68%	72%	95%
Pregnancy Care					
Inpatient Neonatal Mortality	-	-	-	-	-
Third or Fourth Degree Laceration	-	-	3.23%	3.63%	3.27%

Brownfield Regional Medical Center

705 E Felt
Brownfield, TX 79316
E-mail: webmaster@brownfield-rmc.org
URL: www.brownfield-rmc.org
Ownership: Govt - Hospital District or Authority
Emergency Services: Yes

Phone: 806-637-3551
Fax: 806-637-9083

Accredited: No
Licensed Beds: 71

Key Personnel:
CEO . . . . Mike Click, RN
Chief Medical Staff . . . . Paul Chebib, MD
Director Infection/Disease Control . . . . Michelle McElly, RN
Director Radiology . . . . David Cassarez
Director Respiratory Therapy . . . . Shannon Devine

Measure	Cases	This Hospital	State Average	U.S. Average	Top Hospital
Heart Attack Care					
ACE Inhibitor or ARB for LVSD[3]	0	-	85%	82%	100%
Aspirin at Arrival[1,3]	4	100%	91%	92%	100%
Aspirin at Discharge[1,3]	1	100%	90%	90%	100%
Beta Blocker at Arrival[1,3]	3	33%	85%	87%	100%
Beta Blocker at Discharge[1,3]	1	0%	86%	90%	100%
Fibrinolytic Medication Timing[3]	0	-	30%	31%	100%
PCI Within 90 Minutes of Arrival	0	-	48%	54%	95%
Smoking Cessation Advice[3]	0	-	90%	88%	100%
Heart Failure Care					
ACE Inhibitor or ARB for LVSD[1]	4	25%	82%	82%	100%
Discharge Instructions	36	0%	60%	61%	93%
Evaluation of LVS Function	40	42%	81%	83%	99%
Smoking Cessation Advice[1]	6	33%	82%	82%	100%
Pneumonia Care					
Appropriate Initial Antibiotic[1]	21	95%	79%	83%	94%
Blood Culture Timing[1]	3	100%	89%	90%	100%
Influenza Vaccine[4,5]	-	-	69%	70%	100%
Initial Antibiotic Timing	41	93%	78%	80%	93%
Oxygenation Assessment	45	100%	99%	99%	100%
Pneumococcal Vaccine	31	13%	68%	69%	94%
Smoking Cessation Advice[1]	3	33%	83%	80%	100%
Surgical Infection Prevention					
Prophylactic Antibiotic Given[5]	-	-	67%	77%	95%
Prophylactic Antibiotic Selection[5]	-	-	86%	90%	100%
Prophylactic Antibiotic Stopped[5]	-	-	68%	72%	95%
Pregnancy Care					
Inpatient Neonatal Mortality	-	-	-	-	-
Third or Fourth Degree Laceration	-	-	3.23%	3.63%	3.27%

Brownsville Medical Center

1040 W Jefferson Street
Brownsville, TX 78520
URL: www.brownsvillemedical.com
Ownership: Proprietary
Emergency Services: Yes

Phone: 956-544-1400
Fax: 956-698-5712

Accredited: Yes
Licensed Beds: 243

Key Personnel:
CEO . . . . Jim Wesson
Director Medical/Surgical Nursing . . . . Brenda Ivory, RN
OB/GYN Womens Health . . . . Rose Gonen, MD
Chief Radiology . . . . William McKinney, MD

Measure	Cases	This Hospital	State Average	U.S. Average	Top Hospital
Heart Attack Care					
ACE Inhibitor or ARB for LVSD	57	95%	85%	82%	100%
Aspirin at Arrival	205	97%	91%	92%	100%
Aspirin at Discharge	177	97%	90%	90%	100%
Beta Blocker at Arrival	174	99%	85%	87%	100%
Beta Blocker at Discharge	178	98%	86%	90%	100%
Fibrinolytic Medication Timing[1]	2	0%	30%	31%	100%
PCI Within 90 Minutes of Arrival[1]	4	0%	48%	54%	95%
Smoking Cessation Advice	31	97%	90%	88%	100%
Heart Failure Care					
ACE Inhibitor or ARB for LVSD	100	98%	82%	82%	100%
Discharge Instructions	263	94%	60%	61%	93%
Evaluation of LVS Function	253	96%	81%	83%	99%
Smoking Cessation Advice[1]	14	93%	82%	82%	100%
Pneumonia Care					
Appropriate Initial Antibiotic	107	75%	79%	83%	94%
Blood Culture Timing	89	81%	89%	90%	100%
Influenza Vaccine	47	30%	69%	70%	100%
Initial Antibiotic Timing	169	59%	78%	80%	93%
Oxygenation Assessment	198	97%	99%	99%	100%
Pneumococcal Vaccine	128	30%	68%	69%	94%
Smoking Cessation Advice[1]	20	95%	83%	80%	100%
Surgical Infection Prevention					
Prophylactic Antibiotic Given[3]	150	68%	67%	77%	95%
Prophylactic Antibiotic Selection	39	100%	86%	90%	100%
Prophylactic Antibiotic Stopped[3]	144	70%	68%	72%	95%
Pregnancy Care					
Inpatient Neonatal Mortality	-	-	-	-	-
Third or Fourth Degree Laceration	-	-	3.23%	3.63%	3.27%

Brownsville Surgical Hospital

4750 North Expressway
Brownsville, TX 78526
Ownership: Proprietary
Emergency Services: No

Phone: 956-554-2000

Accredited: Yes

Measure	Cases	This Hospital	State Average	U.S. Average	Top Hospital
Heart Attack Care					
ACE Inhibitor or ARB for LVSD[3]	0	-	85%	82%	100%
Aspirin at Arrival[1,3]	1	100%	91%	92%	100%
Aspirin at Discharge[1,3]	1	100%	90%	90%	100%
Beta Blocker at Arrival[1,3]	1	100%	85%	87%	100%
Beta Blocker at Discharge[1,3]	1	100%	86%	90%	100%
Fibrinolytic Medication Timing[1,3]	1	0%	30%	31%	100%
PCI Within 90 Minutes of Arrival[5]	-	-	48%	54%	95%
Smoking Cessation Advice[3]	0	-	90%	88%	100%
Heart Failure Care					
ACE Inhibitor or ARB for LVSD[3]	0	-	82%	82%	100%
Discharge Instructions[1,3]	1	100%	60%	61%	93%
Evaluation of LVS Function[1,3]	1	0%	81%	83%	99%
Smoking Cessation Advice[3]	0	-	82%	82%	100%
Pneumonia Care					
Appropriate Initial Antibiotic[1,3]	2	100%	79%	83%	94%
Blood Culture Timing[1]	1	100%	89%	90%	100%
Influenza Vaccine	0	-	69%	70%	100%
Initial Antibiotic Timing[1,3]	1	100%	78%	80%	93%
Oxygenation Assessment[1,3]	3	100%	99%	99%	100%
Pneumococcal Vaccine[1,3]	2	100%	68%	69%	94%
Smoking Cessation Advice[3]	0	-	83%	80%	100%

Surgical Infection Prevention					
Prophylactic Antibiotic Given	62	94%	67%	77%	95%
Prophylactic Antibiotic Selection[1]	20	100%	86%	90%	100%
Prophylactic Antibiotic Stopped	60	92%	68%	72%	95%
Pregnancy Care					
Inpatient Neonatal Mortality	-	-	-	-	-
Third or Fourth Degree Laceration	-	-	3.23%	3.63%	3.27%

Valley Regional Medical Center

100 A Alton Gloor
Brownsville, TX 78526
URL: www.valleyregionalmedicalcenter.com
Ownership: Proprietary
Emergency Services: Yes
Key Personnel:
CEO. . . . . David Handley

Phone: 956-350-7000
Fax: 956-350-7191

Accredited: Yes
Licensed Beds: 214

Measure	Cases	This Hospital	State Average	U.S. Average	Top Hospital
Heart Attack Care					
ACE Inhibitor or ARB for LVSD	46	85%	85%	82%	100%
Aspirin at Arrival	145	91%	91%	92%	100%
Aspirin at Discharge	133	87%	90%	90%	100%
Beta Blocker at Arrival	121	79%	85%	87%	100%
Beta Blocker at Discharge	134	86%	86%	90%	100%
Fibrinolytic Medication Timing[1]	5	20%	30%	31%	100%
PCI Within 90 Minutes of Arrival[1]	7	71%	48%	54%	95%
Smoking Cessation Advice	36	100%	90%	88%	100%
Heart Failure Care					
ACE Inhibitor or ARB for LVSD	70	81%	82%	82%	100%
Discharge Instructions	227	92%	60%	61%	93%
Evaluation of LVS Function	246	91%	81%	83%	99%
Smoking Cessation Advice	39	100%	82%	82%	100%
Pneumonia Care					
Appropriate Initial Antibiotic	135	92%	79%	83%	94%
Blood Culture Timing	113	93%	89%	90%	100%
Influenza Vaccine	43	23%	69%	70%	100%
Initial Antibiotic Timing	183	72%	78%	80%	93%
Oxygenation Assessment	206	98%	99%	99%	100%
Pneumococcal Vaccine	131	56%	68%	69%	94%
Smoking Cessation Advice	34	97%	83%	80%	100%
Surgical Infection Prevention					
Prophylactic Antibiotic Given[2,3]	137	86%	67%	77%	95%
Prophylactic Antibiotic Selection[2]	57	100%	86%	90%	100%
Prophylactic Antibiotic Stopped[2,3]	132	45%	68%	72%	95%
Pregnancy Care					
Inpatient Neonatal Mortality	3,174	0.28%	-	-	-
Third or Fourth Degree Laceration	1,652	1.57%	3.23%	3.63%	3.27%

Brownwood Regional Medical Center

1501 Burnet Drive
PO Box 760
Brownwood, TX 76801
URL: www.brmc-cares.com
Ownership: Proprietary
Emergency Services: Yes
Key Personnel:
CEO. . . . . Matt T Maxfield
Chief Medical Staff. . . . . David Morales, MD
Cardiac Lab . . . . Rick Jennings
Catheterization Lab . . . . Rick Jennings
Infection Control. . . . . Sandy Porter, RN
ICU . . . . Kasey Bonnema, RN
Intensive/Coronary Care . . . . Kasey Bonnema, RN
OB/GYN Women's Health . . . . Kyla Berry, RN
Respiratory/Cardiopulmonary. . . . . Kasey Bonnoma, RN

Phone: 325-646-8541
Fax: 325-649-3434

Accredited: Yes
Licensed Beds: 196

Measure	Cases	This Hospital	State Average	U.S. Average	Top Hospital
Heart Attack Care					
ACE Inhibitor or ARB for LVSD	0	-	85%	82%	100%
Aspirin at Arrival[1]	18	78%	91%	92%	100%
Aspirin at Discharge[1]	5	100%	90%	90%	100%
Beta Blocker at Arrival[1]	15	73%	85%	87%	100%
Beta Blocker at Discharge[1]	5	100%	86%	90%	100%

Fibrinolytic Medication Timing	0	-	30%	31%	100%
PCI Within 90 Minutes of Arrival	0	-	48%	54%	95%
Smoking Cessation Advice[1]	2	100%	90%	88%	100%
Heart Failure Care					
ACE Inhibitor or ARB for LVSD	50	94%	82%	82%	100%
Discharge Instructions	121	62%	60%	61%	93%
Evaluation of LVS Function	162	80%	81%	83%	99%
Smoking Cessation Advice	35	100%	82%	82%	100%
Pneumonia Care					
Appropriate Initial Antibiotic	130	72%	79%	83%	94%
Blood Culture Timing	135	92%	89%	90%	100%
Influenza Vaccine	70	87%	69%	70%	100%
Initial Antibiotic Timing	225	80%	78%	80%	93%
Oxygenation Assessment	272	100%	99%	99%	100%
Pneumococcal Vaccine	162	83%	68%	69%	94%
Smoking Cessation Advice	68	87%	83%	80%	100%
Surgical Infection Prevention					
Prophylactic Antibiotic Given	272	44%	67%	77%	95%
Prophylactic Antibiotic Selection	64	73%	86%	90%	100%
Prophylactic Antibiotic Stopped	256	52%	68%	72%	95%
Pregnancy Care					
Inpatient Neonatal Mortality	-	-	-	-	-
Third or Fourth Degree Laceration	-	-	3.23%	3.63%	3.27%

Physicians Centre

3131 University Drive East
Bryan, TX 77802
Ownership: Proprietary
Emergency Services: No

Phone: 979-731-3100

Accredited: Yes

Measure	Cases	This Hospital	State Average	U.S. Average	Top Hospital
Heart Attack Care					
ACE Inhibitor or ARB for LVSD[5]	-	-	85%	82%	100%
Aspirin at Arrival[5]	-	-	91%	92%	100%
Aspirin at Discharge[5]	-	-	90%	90%	100%
Beta Blocker at Arrival[5]	-	-	85%	87%	100%
Beta Blocker at Discharge[5]	-	-	86%	90%	100%
Fibrinolytic Medication Timing[5]	-	-	30%	31%	100%
PCI Within 90 Minutes of Arrival[5]	-	-	48%	54%	95%
Smoking Cessation Advice[5]	-	-	90%	88%	100%
Heart Failure Care					
ACE Inhibitor or ARB for LVSD[5]	-	-	82%	82%	100%
Discharge Instructions[5]	-	-	60%	61%	93%
Evaluation of LVS Function[5]	-	-	81%	83%	99%
Smoking Cessation Advice[5]	-	-	82%	82%	100%
Pneumonia Care					
Appropriate Initial Antibiotic[1,3]	1	0%	79%	83%	94%
Blood Culture Timing[3]	0	-	89%	90%	100%
Influenza Vaccine[5]	-	-	69%	70%	100%
Initial Antibiotic Timing[1,3]	5	100%	78%	80%	93%
Oxygenation Assessment[1,3]	5	100%	99%	99%	100%
Pneumococcal Vaccine[1,3]	2	0%	68%	69%	94%
Smoking Cessation Advice[3]	0	-	83%	80%	100%
Surgical Infection Prevention					
Prophylactic Antibiotic Given[2,3]	57	91%	67%	77%	95%
Prophylactic Antibiotic Selection[5]	-	-	86%	90%	100%
Prophylactic Antibiotic Stopped[2,3]	57	88%	68%	72%	95%
Pregnancy Care					
Inpatient Neonatal Mortality	-	-	-	-	-
Third or Fourth Degree Laceration	-	-	3.23%	3.63%	3.27%

Saint Joseph Regional Health Center

Alternate Name: Saint Joseph Hospital
2801 Franciscan Drive
Bryan, TX 77802
Ownership: Voluntary non-profit - Church
Emergency Services: Yes
Key Personnel:
CEO. . . . . Jack Buckley
Chief Medical Staff. Robert Emmick, MD
Emergency Room . . . . Bev Allen, RN
Infection Control. . . . . Jan Shay

Phone: 979-776-3777
Fax: 979-774-4590
Accredited: Yes
Licensed Beds: 205

NOTE: Hospital profiles are in alphabetical order by state, then city, then hospital within the city; Rankings are sorted by rate in descending order and exclude hospitals with less than 25 cases; (1) The number of cases is too small (n<25) for purposes of reliably predicting hospital performance; (2) Measure reflects the hospital's indication that its submission was based upon a sample of its relevant discharges; (3) Rate reflects fewer than the maximum possible quarters of data for the measure; (4) Inaccurate information submitted and suppressed for one or more quarters; (5) No data is available from the hospital for this measure; Please refer to the User's Guide for a full explanation of data

ICU . . . . Stephanie Cumpton

Measure	Cases	This Hospital	State Average	U.S. Average	Top Hospital
Heart Attack Care					
ACE Inhibitor or ARB for LVSD	71	86%	85%	82%	100%
Aspirin at Arrival	184	98%	91%	92%	100%
Aspirin at Discharge	247	98%	90%	90%	100%
Beta Blocker at Arrival	140	94%	85%	87%	100%
Beta Blocker at Discharge	235	95%	86%	90%	100%
Fibrinolytic Medication Timing	0	-	30%	31%	100%
PCI Within 90 Minutes of Arrival[1]	7	57%	48%	54%	95%
Smoking Cessation Advice	82	89%	90%	88%	100%
Heart Failure Care					
ACE Inhibitor or ARB for LVSD	336	80%	82%	82%	100%
Discharge Instructions	514	53%	60%	61%	93%
Evaluation of LVS Function	589	90%	81%	83%	99%
Smoking Cessation Advice	128	95%	82%	82%	100%
Pneumonia Care					
Appropriate Initial Antibiotic	172	85%	79%	83%	94%
Blood Culture Timing	169	85%	89%	90%	100%
Influenza Vaccine	66	44%	69%	70%	100%
Initial Antibiotic Timing	228	78%	78%	80%	93%
Oxygenation Assessment	315	97%	99%	99%	100%
Pneumococcal Vaccine	183	58%	68%	69%	94%
Smoking Cessation Advice	80	85%	83%	80%	100%
Surgical Infection Prevention					
Prophylactic Antibiotic Given	1,051	88%	67%	77%	95%
Prophylactic Antibiotic Selection	257	96%	86%	90%	100%
Prophylactic Antibiotic Stopped	1,032	89%	68%	72%	95%
Pregnancy Care					
Inpatient Neonatal Mortality	-	-	-	-	-
Third or Fourth Degree Laceration	-	-	3.23%	3.63%	3.27%

Seton Highland Lakes

Alternate Name: Shepperd Memorial Hospital
Highway 281 S
Burnet, TX 78611
URL: www.seton.net
Ownership: Voluntary non-profit - Church
Emergency Services: Yes
Phone: 512-715-3000
Fax: 512-756-6405
Accredited: Yes
Licensed Beds: 42

Key Personnel:
President/CEO . . . . Charles J Barnett
Chief Medical Staff . . . . Scott Liggett
Emergency Room . . . . Elizabeth Stevenson

Measure	Cases	This Hospital	State Average	U.S. Average	Top Hospital
Heart Attack Care					
ACE Inhibitor or ARB for LVSD	0	-	85%	82%	100%
Aspirin at Arrival[1]	10	80%	91%	92%	100%
Aspirin at Discharge[1]	9	67%	90%	90%	100%
Beta Blocker at Arrival[1]	6	67%	85%	87%	100%
Beta Blocker at Discharge[1]	8	38%	86%	90%	100%
Fibrinolytic Medication Timing	0	-	30%	31%	100%
PCI Within 90 Minutes of Arrival	0	-	48%	54%	95%
Smoking Cessation Advice	0	-	90%	88%	100%
Heart Failure Care					
ACE Inhibitor or ARB for LVSD[1]	5	60%	82%	82%	100%
Discharge Instructions	40	45%	60%	61%	93%
Evaluation of LVS Function	48	56%	81%	83%	99%
Smoking Cessation Advice[1]	3	67%	82%	82%	100%
Pneumonia Care					
Appropriate Initial Antibiotic	59	90%	79%	83%	94%
Blood Culture Timing	30	93%	89%	90%	100%
Influenza Vaccine[1]	10	90%	69%	70%	100%
Initial Antibiotic Timing	57	79%	78%	80%	93%
Oxygenation Assessment	73	100%	99%	99%	100%
Pneumococcal Vaccine	50	82%	68%	69%	94%
Smoking Cessation Advice[1]	13	77%	83%	80%	100%
Surgical Infection Prevention					
Prophylactic Antibiotic Given[5]	-	-	67%	77%	95%
Prophylactic Antibiotic Selection[5]	-	-	86%	90%	100%
Prophylactic Antibiotic Stopped[5]	-	-	68%	72%	95%

Measure	Cases	This Hospital	State Average	U.S. Average	Top Hospital
Pregnancy Care					
Inpatient Neonatal Mortality	-	-	-	-	-
Third or Fourth Degree Laceration	-	-	3.23%	3.63%	3.27%

Central Texas Hospital

806 N Crockett
Cameron, TX 76520
Ownership: Proprietary
Emergency Services: Yes
Phone: 254-697-6591
Accredited: No

Measure	Cases	This Hospital	State Average	U.S. Average	Top Hospital
Heart Attack Care					
ACE Inhibitor or ARB for LVSD[5]	-	-	85%	82%	100%
Aspirin at Arrival[5]	-	-	91%	92%	100%
Aspirin at Discharge[5]	-	-	90%	90%	100%
Beta Blocker at Arrival[5]	-	-	85%	87%	100%
Beta Blocker at Discharge[5]	-	-	86%	90%	100%
Fibrinolytic Medication Timing[5]	-	-	30%	31%	100%
PCI Within 90 Minutes of Arrival[5]	-	-	48%	54%	95%
Smoking Cessation Advice[5]	-	-	90%	88%	100%
Heart Failure Care					
ACE Inhibitor or ARB for LVSD[3]	0	-	82%	82%	100%
Discharge Instructions[1,3]	15	0%	60%	61%	93%
Evaluation of LVS Function[1,3]	24	25%	81%	83%	99%
Smoking Cessation Advice[1,3]	3	33%	82%	82%	100%
Pneumonia Care					
Appropriate Initial Antibiotic[1,3]	3	100%	79%	83%	94%
Blood Culture Timing[1,3]	3	100%	89%	90%	100%
Influenza Vaccine[5]	-	-	69%	70%	100%
Initial Antibiotic Timing[1,3]	5	80%	78%	80%	93%
Oxygenation Assessment[1,3]	7	100%	99%	99%	100%
Pneumococcal Vaccine[1,3]	8	0%	68%	69%	94%
Smoking Cessation Advice[1,3]	2	100%	83%	80%	100%
Surgical Infection Prevention					
Prophylactic Antibiotic Given[5]	-	-	67%	77%	95%
Prophylactic Antibiotic Selection[5]	-	-	86%	90%	100%
Prophylactic Antibiotic Stopped[5]	-	-	68%	72%	95%
Pregnancy Care					
Inpatient Neonatal Mortality	-	-	-	-	-
Third or Fourth Degree Laceration	-	-	3.23%	3.63%	3.27%

Hemphill County Hospital

1020 S 4th Street
Canadian, TX 79014
URL: www.hch.dst.ts.us
Ownership: Govt - Hospital District or Authority
Emergency Services: Yes
Phone: 806-323-6422
Fax: 806-323-8061
Accredited: No
Licensed Beds: 26

Key Personnel:
Administrator . . . . Robert Ezzell
Chief Medical Staff . . . . Valerie Verbi, MD
Emergency Room . . . . Valerie Verbi, MD
Director Infection/Disease Control . . . . Cary George

Measure	Cases	This Hospital	State Average	U.S. Average	Top Hospital
Heart Attack Care					
ACE Inhibitor or ARB for LVSD[5]	-	-	85%	82%	100%
Aspirin at Arrival[5]	-	-	91%	92%	100%
Aspirin at Discharge[5]	-	-	90%	90%	100%
Beta Blocker at Arrival[5]	-	-	85%	87%	100%
Beta Blocker at Discharge[5]	-	-	86%	90%	100%
Fibrinolytic Medication Timing[5]	-	-	30%	31%	100%
PCI Within 90 Minutes of Arrival[5]	-	-	48%	54%	95%
Smoking Cessation Advice[5]	-	-	90%	88%	100%
Heart Failure Care					
ACE Inhibitor or ARB for LVSD[1]	1	100%	82%	82%	100%
Discharge Instructions[3]	0	-	60%	61%	93%
Evaluation of LVS Function[1]	1	100%	81%	83%	99%
Smoking Cessation Advice[3]	0	-	82%	82%	100%
Pneumonia Care					
Appropriate Initial Antibiotic[1,3]	2	100%	79%	83%	94%
Blood Culture Timing[3]	0	-	89%	90%	100%
Influenza Vaccine[5]	-	-	69%	70%	100%

NOTE: Hospital profiles are in alphabetical order by state, then city, then hospital within the city; Rankings are sorted by rate in descending order and exclude hospitals with less than 25 cases; (1) The number of cases is too small (n<25) for purposes of reliably predicting hospital performance; (2) Measure reflects the hospital's indication that its submission was based upon a sample of its relevant discharges; (3) Rate reflects fewer than the maximum possible quarters of data for the measure; (4) Inaccurate information submitted and suppressed for one or more quarters; (5) No data is available from the hospital for this measure; Please refer to the User's Guide for a full explanation of data

Initial Antibiotic Timing[1]	22	95%	78%	80%	93%
Oxygenation Assessment[1]	23	100%	99%	99%	100%
Pneumococcal Vaccine[1]	16	81%	68%	69%	94%
Smoking Cessation Advice[1,3]	1	100%	83%	80%	100%
Surgical Infection Prevention					
Prophylactic Antibiotic Given[5]	-	-	67%	77%	95%
Prophylactic Antibiotic Selection[5]	-	-	86%	90%	100%
Prophylactic Antibiotic Stopped[5]	-	-	68%	72%	95%
Pregnancy Care					
Inpatient Neonatal Mortality	-	-	-	-	-
Third or Fourth Degree Laceration	-	-	3.23%	3.63%	3.27%

Dimmit County Memorial Hospital

704 Hospital Drive
Carrizo Springs, TX 78834
Ownership: Government - Local
Emergency Services: Yes

Phone: 830-876-2424
Fax: 830-876-2584
Accredited: No
Licensed Beds: 49

Key Personnel:
CEO . . . . Ernest Flores Jr
Chief of Medical Staff . . . . Carlos Salazer

Measure	Cases	This Hospital	State Average	U.S. Average	Top Hospital
Heart Attack Care					
ACE Inhibitor or ARB for LVSD[2,3]	0	-	85%	82%	100%
Aspirin at Arrival[1,2,3]	5	60%	91%	92%	100%
Aspirin at Discharge[1,2,3]	1	0%	90%	90%	100%
Beta Blocker at Arrival[1,2,3]	4	50%	85%	87%	100%
Beta Blocker at Discharge[1,2,3]	2	0%	86%	90%	100%
Fibrinolytic Medication Timing[2,3]	0	-	30%	31%	100%
PCI Within 90 Minutes of Arrival[2]	0	-	48%	54%	95%
Smoking Cessation Advice[2,3]	0	-	90%	88%	100%
Heart Failure Care					
ACE Inhibitor or ARB for LVSD[2]	0	-	82%	82%	100%
Discharge Instructions[1,2,3]	5	0%	60%	61%	93%
Evaluation of LVS Function[2]	40	0%	81%	83%	99%
Smoking Cessation Advice[2,3]	0	-	82%	82%	100%
Pneumonia Care					
Appropriate Initial Antibiotic[1,2,3]	3	100%	79%	83%	94%
Blood Culture Timing[1,2,3]	4	100%	89%	90%	100%
Influenza Vaccine[5]	-	-	69%	70%	100%
Initial Antibiotic Timing[2]	29	66%	78%	80%	93%
Oxygenation Assessment[2]	36	94%	99%	99%	100%
Pneumococcal Vaccine[1,2]	22	32%	68%	69%	94%
Smoking Cessation Advice[1,2,3]	2	0%	83%	80%	100%
Surgical Infection Prevention					
Prophylactic Antibiotic Given[2,3]	0	-	67%	77%	95%
Prophylactic Antibiotic Selection[5]	-	-	86%	90%	100%
Prophylactic Antibiotic Stopped[2,3]	0	-	68%	72%	95%
Pregnancy Care					
Inpatient Neonatal Mortality	-	-	-	-	-
Third or Fourth Degree Laceration	-	-	3.23%	3.63%	3.27%

Regency Hospital of North Dallas II

2225 Parker Road
Carrollton, TX 75010
Ownership: Proprietary
Emergency Services: Yes

Phone: 972-236-6800

Accredited: Yes

Measure	Cases	This Hospital	State Average	U.S. Average	Top Hospital
Heart Attack Care					
ACE Inhibitor or ARB for LVSD[5]	-	-	85%	82%	100%
Aspirin at Arrival[5]	-	-	91%	92%	100%
Aspirin at Discharge[5]	-	-	90%	90%	100%
Beta Blocker at Arrival[5]	-	-	85%	87%	100%
Beta Blocker at Discharge[5]	-	-	86%	90%	100%
Fibrinolytic Medication Timing[5]	-	-	30%	31%	100%
PCI Within 90 Minutes of Arrival[5]	-	-	48%	54%	95%
Smoking Cessation Advice[5]	-	-	90%	88%	100%
Heart Failure Care					
ACE Inhibitor or ARB for LVSD[5]	-	-	82%	82%	100%
Discharge Instructions[5]	-	-	60%	61%	93%
Evaluation of LVS Function[5]	-	-	81%	83%	99%

Smoking Cessation Advice[5]	-	-	82%	82%	100%
Pneumonia Care					
Appropriate Initial Antibiotic[3]	0	-	79%	83%	94%
Blood Culture Timing[3]	0	-	89%	90%	100%
Influenza Vaccine[5]	-	-	69%	70%	100%
Initial Antibiotic Timing[3]	0	-	78%	80%	93%
Oxygenation Assessment[3]	0	-	99%	99%	100%
Pneumococcal Vaccine[1,3]	1	0%	68%	69%	94%
Smoking Cessation Advice[3]	0	-	83%	80%	100%
Surgical Infection Prevention					
Prophylactic Antibiotic Given[5]	-	-	67%	77%	95%
Prophylactic Antibiotic Selection[5]	-	-	86%	90%	100%
Prophylactic Antibiotic Stopped[5]	-	-	68%	72%	95%
Pregnancy Care					
Inpatient Neonatal Mortality	-	-	-	-	-
Third or Fourth Degree Laceration	-	-	3.23%	3.63%	3.27%

Trinity Medical Center

4343 N Josey Lane
Carrollton, TX 75010
URL: www.trinitymedicalcenter.com
Ownership: Proprietary
Emergency Services: Yes

Phone: 972-492-1010
Fax: 972-394-4783

Accredited: Yes
Licensed Beds: 149

Key Personnel:
CEO . . . . Craig Sims
Chief Medical Staff . . . . Farrah Hamid
Emergency Room . . . . Sherry Armentor, RN
Coordinator Infection Control . . . . Denise Lavacak
CCU Spvg. Nurse . . . . Patty Jackson
Director Medical/Surgical Nursing . . . . Patty Jackson
OB/GYN Womens Health . . . . Brenda Axmann
Chief Radiology . . . . Laura Hanahan

Measure	Cases	This Hospital	State Average	U.S. Average	Top Hospital
Heart Attack Care					
ACE Inhibitor or ARB for LVSD[1]	3	33%	85%	82%	100%
Aspirin at Arrival	35	97%	91%	92%	100%
Aspirin at Discharge[1]	13	77%	90%	90%	100%
Beta Blocker at Arrival	35	89%	85%	87%	100%
Beta Blocker at Discharge[1]	15	80%	86%	90%	100%
Fibrinolytic Medication Timing	0	-	30%	31%	100%
PCI Within 90 Minutes of Arrival	0	-	48%	54%	95%
Smoking Cessation Advice[1]	4	75%	90%	88%	100%
Heart Failure Care					
ACE Inhibitor or ARB for LVSD	50	86%	82%	82%	100%
Discharge Instructions	111	57%	60%	61%	93%
Evaluation of LVS Function	143	93%	81%	83%	99%
Smoking Cessation Advice[1]	22	100%	82%	82%	100%
Pneumonia Care					
Appropriate Initial Antibiotic	167	84%	79%	83%	94%
Blood Culture Timing	130	95%	89%	90%	100%
Influenza Vaccine	46	96%	69%	70%	100%
Initial Antibiotic Timing	185	84%	78%	80%	93%
Oxygenation Assessment	228	99%	99%	99%	100%
Pneumococcal Vaccine	92	88%	68%	69%	94%
Smoking Cessation Advice	68	100%	83%	80%	100%
Surgical Infection Prevention					
Prophylactic Antibiotic Given[2]	183	69%	67%	77%	95%
Prophylactic Antibiotic Selection[2]	49	71%	86%	90%	100%
Prophylactic Antibiotic Stopped[2]	184	66%	68%	72%	95%
Pregnancy Care					
Inpatient Neonatal Mortality	-	-	-	-	-
Third or Fourth Degree Laceration	-	-	3.23%	3.63%	3.27%

East Texas Medical Center-Carthage

Alternate Name: Panola General Hospital

NOTE: Hospital profiles are in alphabetical order by state, then city, then hospital within the city; Rankings are sorted by rate in descending order and exclude hospitals with less than 25 cases; (1) The number of cases is too small (n<25) for purposes of reliably predicting hospital performance; (2) Measure reflects the hospital's indication that its submission was based upon a sample of its relevant discharges; (3) Rate reflects fewer than the maximum possible quarters of data for the measure; (4) Inaccurate information submitted and suppressed for one or more quarters; (5) No data is available from the hospital for this measure; Please refer to the User's Guide for a full explanation of data

409 Cottage Road
Carthage, TX 75633
E-mail: info@etmc.org
URL: www.etmc.org
Ownership: Government - Local
Emergency Services: Yes

Phone: 903-693-3841
Fax: 903-694-4625

Accredited: Yes
Licensed Beds: 49

Key Personnel:
Administrator . . . . Gary M Hudson
Chief Medical Staff. . . . . Linda Nagle
Emergency Room . . . . Gary Sweek, DO
Director Infection/Disease Control . . . . Royce Hill, MD
Chief Radiology . . . . John Crisp

Measure	Cases	This Hospital	State Average	U.S. Average	Top Hospital
Heart Attack Care					
ACE Inhibitor or ARB for LVSD[1]	1	100%	85%	82%	100%
Aspirin at Arrival[1]	7	100%	91%	92%	100%
Aspirin at Discharge[1]	4	100%	90%	90%	100%
Beta Blocker at Arrival[1]	5	40%	85%	87%	100%
Beta Blocker at Discharge[1]	5	80%	86%	90%	100%
Fibrinolytic Medication Timing	0	-	30%	31%	100%
PCI Within 90 Minutes of Arrival	0	-	48%	54%	95%
Smoking Cessation Advice	0	-	90%	88%	100%
Heart Failure Care					
ACE Inhibitor or ARB for LVSD[1]	16	81%	82%	82%	100%
Discharge Instructions	32	59%	60%	61%	93%
Evaluation of LVS Function	40	95%	81%	83%	99%
Smoking Cessation Advice[1]	7	57%	82%	82%	100%
Pneumonia Care					
Appropriate Initial Antibiotic	54	94%	79%	83%	94%
Blood Culture Timing	35	83%	89%	90%	100%
Influenza Vaccine[1]	13	69%	69%	70%	100%
Initial Antibiotic Timing	50	88%	78%	80%	93%
Oxygenation Assessment	69	100%	99%	99%	100%
Pneumococcal Vaccine	40	80%	68%	69%	94%
Smoking Cessation Advice[1]	17	65%	83%	80%	100%
Surgical Infection Prevention					
Prophylactic Antibiotic Given[1,3]	2	0%	67%	77%	95%
Prophylactic Antibiotic Selection[5]	-	-	86%	90%	100%
Prophylactic Antibiotic Stopped[1,3]	2	0%	68%	72%	95%
Pregnancy Care					
Inpatient Neonatal Mortality	-	-	-	-	-
Third or Fourth Degree Laceration	-	-	3.23%	3.63%	3.27%

Shelby Regional Medical Center

602 Hurst Street
Center, TX 75935
URL: www.shelbyregional.com
Ownership: Proprietary
Emergency Services: Yes

Phone: 936-598-2781
Fax: 936-598-4237

Accredited: Yes
Licensed Beds: 54

Key Personnel:
CEO. . . . . John Yeary
Chief Medical Staff. . . . . Charles Gutierrez
Emergency Room . . . . Steve Stuart
Director Respiratory Therapy . . . . Neasie Roberts

Measure	Cases	This Hospital	State Average	U.S. Average	Top Hospital
Heart Attack Care					
ACE Inhibitor or ARB for LVSD[3]	0	-	85%	82%	100%
Aspirin at Arrival[3]	0	-	91%	92%	100%
Aspirin at Discharge[3]	0	-	90%	90%	100%
Beta Blocker at Arrival[3]	0	-	85%	87%	100%
Beta Blocker at Discharge[3]	0	-	86%	90%	100%
Fibrinolytic Medication Timing[3]	0	-	30%	31%	100%
PCI Within 90 Minutes of Arrival	0	-	48%	54%	95%
Smoking Cessation Advice[3]	0	-	90%	88%	100%
Heart Failure Care					
ACE Inhibitor or ARB for LVSD[1]	12	83%	82%	82%	100%
Discharge Instructions	34	88%	60%	61%	93%
Evaluation of LVS Function	46	78%	81%	83%	99%
Smoking Cessation Advice[1]	7	100%	82%	82%	100%
Pneumonia Care					
Appropriate Initial Antibiotic	82	72%	79%	83%	94%

	48	90%	89%	90%	100%
Blood Culture Timing	48	90%	89%	90%	100%
Influenza Vaccine	25	64%	69%	70%	100%
Initial Antibiotic Timing	84	98%	78%	80%	93%
Oxygenation Assessment	105	99%	99%	99%	100%
Pneumococcal Vaccine	61	72%	68%	69%	94%
Smoking Cessation Advice	27	100%	83%	80%	100%
Surgical Infection Prevention					
Prophylactic Antibiotic Given[1,2]	9	89%	67%	77%	95%
Prophylactic Antibiotic Selection[2]	0	-	86%	90%	100%
Prophylactic Antibiotic Stopped[1,2]	8	62%	68%	72%	95%
Pregnancy Care					
Inpatient Neonatal Mortality	-	-	-	-	-
Third or Fourth Degree Laceration	-	-	3.23%	3.63%	3.27%

Childress Regional Medical Center

Highway 83 N
Childress, TX 79201
E-mail: crmc11@chipshot.net
URL: www.childresshospital.com
Ownership: Govt - Hospital District or Authority
Emergency Services: Yes

Phone: 940-937-6371
Fax: 940-937-9133

Accredited: No
Licensed Beds: 60

Key Personnel:
Administrator . . . . John Henderson
Chief Radiology . . . . Gary Swindell
Director Respiratory Therapy . . . . Sue Allen

Measure	Cases	This Hospital	State Average	U.S. Average	Top Hospital
Heart Attack Care					
ACE Inhibitor or ARB for LVSD[3]	0	-	85%	82%	100%
Aspirin at Arrival[1,3]	2	50%	91%	92%	100%
Aspirin at Discharge[1,3]	2	50%	90%	90%	100%
Beta Blocker at Arrival[1,3]	2	50%	85%	87%	100%
Beta Blocker at Discharge[1,3]	2	50%	86%	90%	100%
Fibrinolytic Medication Timing[3]	0	-	30%	31%	100%
PCI Within 90 Minutes of Arrival[5]	-	-	48%	54%	95%
Smoking Cessation Advice[1,3]	1	100%	90%	88%	100%
Heart Failure Care					
ACE Inhibitor or ARB for LVSD[1]	7	86%	82%	82%	100%
Discharge Instructions	26	38%	60%	61%	93%
Evaluation of LVS Function	31	84%	81%	83%	99%
Smoking Cessation Advice[1]	2	100%	82%	82%	100%
Pneumonia Care					
Appropriate Initial Antibiotic	32	94%	79%	83%	94%
Blood Culture Timing[1]	5	100%	89%	90%	100%
Influenza Vaccine[4,5]	-	-	69%	70%	100%
Initial Antibiotic Timing	55	82%	78%	80%	93%
Oxygenation Assessment	67	100%	99%	99%	100%
Pneumococcal Vaccine	41	83%	68%	69%	94%
Smoking Cessation Advice[1]	14	100%	83%	80%	100%
Surgical Infection Prevention					
Prophylactic Antibiotic Given[3]	46	87%	67%	77%	95%
Prophylactic Antibiotic Selection[1]	19	100%	86%	90%	100%
Prophylactic Antibiotic Stopped[3]	46	13%	68%	72%	95%
Pregnancy Care					
Inpatient Neonatal Mortality	-	-	-	-	-
Third or Fourth Degree Laceration	-	-	3.23%	3.63%	3.27%

East Texas Medical Center-Clarksville

Alternate Name: ETMC-Clarksville
3000 West Main Street
PO Drawer 1270
Clarksville, TX 75426
URL: www.etmc.org/hospital/page.php?pageID=297
Ownership: Voluntary non-profit - Other
Emergency Services: Yes

Phone: 903-427-6400
Fax: 903-427-2719

Accredited: Yes
Licensed Beds: 36

Key Personnel:
Chairman/CEO. . . . . Elmer Ellis
President . . . . Elmer Ellis
Administrator . . . . Stacy Holland
Emergency Room . . . . Linda Tabb, RN
Infection Control . . . . Amber Sims, RN
ICU . . . . Sharla McCulloch, RN
Intensive Coronary. . . . . Sharla McCulloch, RN

NOTE: Hospital profiles are in alphabetical order by state, then city, then hospital within the city; Rankings are sorted by rate in descending order and exclude hospitals with less than 25 cases; (1) The number of cases is too small (n<25) for purposes of reliably predicting hospital performance; (2) Measure reflects the hospital's indication that its submission was based upon a sample of its relevant discharges; (3) Rate reflects fewer than the maximum possible quarters of data for the measure; (4) Inaccurate information submitted and suppressed for one or more quarters; (5) No data is available from the hospital for this measure; Please refer to the User's Guide for a full explanation of data

Medical Surgical Nursing . . . . Carolyn Durham, RN
Surgical Services. . . . . Fonda Glover, RN
Respiratory/Cardiopulmonary. . . . . Gary Rodriguez, RCF

Measure	Cases	This Hospital	State Average	U.S. Average	Top Hospital
Heart Attack Care					
ACE Inhibitor or ARB for LVSD[1]	3	100%	85%	82%	100%
Aspirin at Arrival[1]	9	78%	91%	92%	100%
Aspirin at Discharge[1]	5	100%	90%	90%	100%
Beta Blocker at Arrival[1]	7	86%	85%	87%	100%
Beta Blocker at Discharge[1]	5	100%	86%	90%	100%
Fibrinolytic Medication Timing[3]	0	-	30%	31%	100%
PCI Within 90 Minutes of Arrival	0	-	48%	54%	95%
Smoking Cessation Advice[1,3]	1	100%	90%	88%	100%
Heart Failure Care					
ACE Inhibitor or ARB for LVSD	38	84%	82%	82%	100%
Discharge Instructions[3]	27	63%	60%	61%	93%
Evaluation of LVS Function	138	88%	81%	83%	99%
Smoking Cessation Advice[1,3]	9	67%	82%	82%	100%
Pneumonia Care					
Appropriate Initial Antibiotic[1,3]	8	100%	79%	83%	94%
Blood Culture Timing[1,3]	13	85%	89%	90%	100%
Influenza Vaccine[5]	-	-	69%	70%	100%
Initial Antibiotic Timing	116	87%	78%	80%	93%
Oxygenation Assessment	145	99%	99%	99%	100%
Pneumococcal Vaccine	91	62%	68%	69%	94%
Smoking Cessation Advice[1,3]	8	88%	83%	80%	100%
Surgical Infection Prevention					
Prophylactic Antibiotic Given[5]	-	-	67%	77%	95%
Prophylactic Antibiotic Selection[5]	-	-	86%	90%	100%
Prophylactic Antibiotic Stopped[5]	-	-	68%	72%	95%
Pregnancy Care					
Inpatient Neonatal Mortality	-	-	-	-	-
Third or Fourth Degree Laceration	-	-	3.23%	3.63%	3.27%

Walls Regional Hospital

201 Walls Drive
Cleburne, TX 76033
URL: www.texashealth.org
Ownership: Voluntary non-profit - Church
Emergency Services: Yes
Key Personnel:
President . . . . Brent D Magers
Chief Medical Staff. . . . . Barney Maddox, MD
Emergency Room . . . . Nettie Davis

Phone: 817-462-7900
Fax: 817-641-4346

Accredited: Yes
Licensed Beds: 137

Measure	Cases	This Hospital	State Average	U.S. Average	Top Hospital
Heart Attack Care					
ACE Inhibitor or ARB for LVSD[1]	7	100%	85%	82%	100%
Aspirin at Arrival	32	91%	91%	92%	100%
Aspirin at Discharge[1]	16	100%	90%	90%	100%
Beta Blocker at Arrival[1]	19	79%	85%	87%	100%
Beta Blocker at Discharge[1]	15	100%	86%	90%	100%
Fibrinolytic Medication Timing	0	-	30%	31%	100%
PCI Within 90 Minutes of Arrival	0	-	48%	54%	95%
Smoking Cessation Advice[1]	1	100%	90%	88%	100%
Heart Failure Care					
ACE Inhibitor or ARB for LVSD	61	100%	82%	82%	100%
Discharge Instructions	135	99%	60%	61%	93%
Evaluation of LVS Function	176	100%	81%	83%	99%
Smoking Cessation Advice	30	100%	82%	82%	100%
Pneumonia Care					
Appropriate Initial Antibiotic	156	90%	79%	83%	94%
Blood Culture Timing	124	99%	89%	90%	100%
Influenza Vaccine	44	89%	69%	70%	100%
Initial Antibiotic Timing	164	95%	78%	80%	93%
Oxygenation Assessment	216	100%	99%	99%	100%
Pneumococcal Vaccine	124	95%	68%	69%	94%
Smoking Cessation Advice	55	100%	83%	80%	100%
Surgical Infection Prevention					
Prophylactic Antibiotic Given[2,3]	108	90%	67%	77%	95%
Prophylactic Antibiotic Selection[2]	36	94%	86%	90%	100%

Prophylactic Antibiotic Stopped[2,3]	98	85%	68%	72%	95%
Pregnancy Care					
Inpatient Neonatal Mortality	-	-	-	-	-
Third or Fourth Degree Laceration	-	-	3.23%	3.63%	3.27%

Cleveland Regional Medical Center

300 East Crockett
Cleveland, TX 77327
Ownership: Proprietary
Emergency Services: Yes
Key Personnel:
Administrator . . . . Ron MacLaren

Phone: 281-593-1811
Fax: 281-432-4369
Accredited: Yes
Licensed Beds: 104

Measure	Cases	This Hospital	State Average	U.S. Average	Top Hospital
Heart Attack Care					
ACE Inhibitor or ARB for LVSD[1]	5	60%	85%	82%	100%
Aspirin at Arrival	29	97%	91%	92%	100%
Aspirin at Discharge[1]	12	67%	90%	90%	100%
Beta Blocker at Arrival[1]	24	83%	85%	87%	100%
Beta Blocker at Discharge[1]	15	73%	86%	90%	100%
Fibrinolytic Medication Timing[1]	1	0%	30%	31%	100%
PCI Within 90 Minutes of Arrival	0	-	48%	54%	95%
Smoking Cessation Advice[1]	1	100%	90%	88%	100%
Heart Failure Care					
ACE Inhibitor or ARB for LVSD	46	65%	82%	82%	100%
Discharge Instructions	112	6%	60%	61%	93%
Evaluation of LVS Function	141	83%	81%	83%	99%
Smoking Cessation Advice	38	79%	82%	82%	100%
Pneumonia Care					
Appropriate Initial Antibiotic	96	82%	79%	83%	94%
Blood Culture Timing	72	79%	89%	90%	100%
Influenza Vaccine[1]	23	52%	69%	70%	100%
Initial Antibiotic Timing	128	75%	78%	80%	93%
Oxygenation Assessment	144	98%	99%	99%	100%
Pneumococcal Vaccine	66	58%	68%	69%	94%
Smoking Cessation Advice	58	97%	83%	80%	100%
Surgical Infection Prevention					
Prophylactic Antibiotic Given[2,3]	54	30%	67%	77%	95%
Prophylactic Antibiotic Selection[2]	27	89%	86%	90%	100%
Prophylactic Antibiotic Stopped[2,3]	53	75%	68%	72%	95%
Pregnancy Care					
Inpatient Neonatal Mortality	-	-	-	-	-
Third or Fourth Degree Laceration	-	-	3.23%	3.63%	3.27%

Goodall-Witcher Healthcare Foundation

101 South Avenue T
Clifton, TX 76634
URL: www.gwhf.org
Ownership: Voluntary non-profit - Private
Emergency Services: Yes
Key Personnel:
President/CEO. . . . . Clarence Fields Jr, CHE
Infection Control. . . . . Pat Massingill, RN
Medical Surgical Nursing . . . . Anita Diebenow
Respiratory Therapy. . . . . Gina Wellborn, RRT

Phone: 254-675-8322
Fax: 254-675-2246

Accredited: No
Licensed Beds: 72

Measure	Cases	This Hospital	State Average	U.S. Average	Top Hospital
Heart Attack Care					
ACE Inhibitor or ARB for LVSD[1]	2	100%	85%	82%	100%
Aspirin at Arrival[1]	10	100%	91%	92%	100%
Aspirin at Discharge[1]	8	62%	90%	90%	100%
Beta Blocker at Arrival[1]	5	60%	85%	87%	100%
Beta Blocker at Discharge[1]	5	80%	86%	90%	100%
Fibrinolytic Medication Timing[1]	1	0%	30%	31%	100%
PCI Within 90 Minutes of Arrival	0	-	48%	54%	95%
Smoking Cessation Advice	0	-	90%	88%	100%
Heart Failure Care					
ACE Inhibitor or ARB for LVSD[1]	17	88%	82%	82%	100%
Discharge Instructions	39	97%	60%	61%	93%
Evaluation of LVS Function	65	77%	81%	83%	99%
Smoking Cessation Advice[1]	10	80%	82%	82%	100%
Pneumonia Care					

NOTE: Hospital profiles are in alphabetical order by state, then city, then hospital within the city; Rankings are sorted by rate in descending order and exclude hospitals with less than 25 cases; (1) The number of cases is too small (n<25) for purposes of reliably predicting hospital performance; (2) Measure reflects the hospital's indication that its submission was based upon a sample of its relevant discharges; (3) Rate reflects fewer than the maximum possible quarters of data for the measure; (4) Inaccurate information submitted and suppressed for one or more quarters; (5) No data is available from the hospital for this measure; Please refer to the User's Guide for a full explanation of data

Appropriate Initial Antibiotic	55	75%	79%	83%	94%
Blood Culture Timing	49	94%	89%	90%	100%
Influenza Vaccine	33	97%	69%	70%	100%
Initial Antibiotic Timing	83	86%	78%	80%	93%
Oxygenation Assessment	118	99%	99%	99%	100%
Pneumococcal Vaccine	92	85%	68%	69%	94%
Smoking Cessation Advice[1]	15	93%	83%	80%	100%
Surgical Infection Prevention					
Prophylactic Antibiotic Given[1,3]	6	50%	67%	77%	95%
Prophylactic Antibiotic Selection[5]	-	-	86%	90%	100%
Prophylactic Antibiotic Stopped[1,3]	6	33%	68%	72%	95%
Pregnancy Care					
Inpatient Neonatal Mortality	-	-	-	-	-
Third or Fourth Degree Laceration	-	-	3.23%	3.63%	3.27%

Coleman County Medical Center

Alternate Name: Ourall-Morris Memorial Hospital
310 S Pecos St
Coleman, TX 76834
Ownership: Govt - Hospital District or Authority
Emergency Services: No

Phone: 325-625-2135
Fax: 325-625-5730
Accredited: No
Licensed Beds: 46

Key Personnel:
President . . . . Mark Griffis
CEO . . . . Douglas Langley
Chief Medical Staff . . . . Michael Bailey, DO
Infection Control . . . . Lynn Corbelt
Respiratory Therapy . . . . Sam Bowden

Measure	Cases	This Hospital	State Average	U.S. Average	Top Hospital
Heart Attack Care					
ACE Inhibitor or ARB for LVSD[3]	0	-	85%	82%	100%
Aspirin at Arrival[1,3]	1	100%	91%	92%	100%
Aspirin at Discharge[1,3]	1	100%	90%	90%	100%
Beta Blocker at Arrival[1,3]	1	100%	85%	87%	100%
Beta Blocker at Discharge[3]	0	-	86%	90%	100%
Fibrinolytic Medication Timing[1,3]	1	100%	30%	31%	100%
PCI Within 90 Minutes of Arrival	0	-	48%	54%	95%
Smoking Cessation Advice[3]	0	-	90%	88%	100%
Heart Failure Care					
ACE Inhibitor or ARB for LVSD[1]	10	80%	82%	82%	100%
Discharge Instructions	26	54%	60%	61%	93%
Evaluation of LVS Function	36	67%	81%	83%	99%
Smoking Cessation Advice[1]	5	40%	82%	82%	100%
Pneumonia Care					
Appropriate Initial Antibiotic	52	71%	79%	83%	94%
Blood Culture Timing	43	100%	89%	90%	100%
Influenza Vaccine	29	100%	69%	70%	100%
Initial Antibiotic Timing	36	92%	78%	80%	93%
Oxygenation Assessment	96	100%	99%	99%	100%
Pneumococcal Vaccine	73	90%	68%	69%	94%
Smoking Cessation Advice[1]	15	60%	83%	80%	100%
Surgical Infection Prevention					
Prophylactic Antibiotic Given[5]	-	-	67%	77%	95%
Prophylactic Antibiotic Selection[5]	-	-	86%	90%	100%
Prophylactic Antibiotic Stopped[5]	-	-	68%	72%	95%
Pregnancy Care					
Inpatient Neonatal Mortality	-	-	-	-	-
Third or Fourth Degree Laceration	-	-	3.23%	3.63%	3.27%

College Station Medical Center

Alternate Name: Humana Hospital Brazos Valley
1604 Rock Prairie Road
College Station, TX 77842
URL: www.csmedcenter.com
Ownership: Proprietary
Emergency Services: Yes

Phone: 979-764-5100
Fax: 979-693-3294

Accredited: Yes
Licensed Beds: 119

Key Personnel:
CEO . . . . Thomas W Jackson
Chief Medical Staff . . . . Usha Venkatraj
Emergency Room . . . . Joe Jones, MD
Director Infection/Disease Control . . . . Yeojin Zee
OB/GYN Womens Health . . . . Ben Zivney
Chief Radiology . . . . Ron Rust, MD

Measure	Cases	This Hospital	State Average	U.S. Average	Top Hospital
Heart Attack Care					
ACE Inhibitor or ARB for LVSD[1]	18	94%	85%	82%	100%
Aspirin at Arrival	51	98%	91%	92%	100%
Aspirin at Discharge	61	98%	90%	90%	100%
Beta Blocker at Arrival	33	100%	85%	87%	100%
Beta Blocker at Discharge	61	100%	86%	90%	100%
Fibrinolytic Medication Timing	0	-	30%	31%	100%
PCI Within 90 Minutes of Arrival[1]	3	0%	48%	54%	95%
Smoking Cessation Advice[1]	20	100%	90%	88%	100%
Heart Failure Care					
ACE Inhibitor or ARB for LVSD	52	96%	82%	82%	100%
Discharge Instructions	93	69%	60%	61%	93%
Evaluation of LVS Function	103	99%	81%	83%	99%
Smoking Cessation Advice[1]	18	100%	82%	82%	100%
Pneumonia Care					
Appropriate Initial Antibiotic	54	94%	79%	83%	94%
Blood Culture Timing	43	95%	89%	90%	100%
Influenza Vaccine[1]	18	94%	69%	70%	100%
Initial Antibiotic Timing	60	90%	78%	80%	93%
Oxygenation Assessment	75	100%	99%	99%	100%
Pneumococcal Vaccine	44	91%	68%	69%	94%
Smoking Cessation Advice[1]	21	100%	83%	80%	100%
Surgical Infection Prevention					
Prophylactic Antibiotic Given	270	97%	67%	77%	95%
Prophylactic Antibiotic Selection	75	92%	86%	90%	100%
Prophylactic Antibiotic Stopped	268	87%	68%	72%	95%
Pregnancy Care					
Inpatient Neonatal Mortality	-	-	-	-	-
Third or Fourth Degree Laceration	-	-	3.23%	3.63%	3.27%

Mitchell County Hospital

1543 Chestnut Street
Colorado City, TX 79512
URL: www.mitchellcountyhospital.com
Ownership: Govt - Hospital District or Authority
Emergency Services: Yes

Phone: 325-728-3431
Fax: 325-728-8974

Accredited: No
Licensed Beds: 39

Key Personnel:
Chief Medical Staff . . . . Dee A Raach, MD
Director Radiology . . . . Mary Paul Proctor
Director Respiratory Therapy . . . . Gerald McGaha, RT

Measure	Cases	This Hospital	State Average	U.S. Average	Top Hospital
Heart Attack Care					
ACE Inhibitor or ARB for LVSD[3]	0	-	85%	82%	100%
Aspirin at Arrival[3]	0	-	91%	92%	100%
Aspirin at Discharge[3]	0	-	90%	90%	100%
Beta Blocker at Arrival[3]	0	-	85%	87%	100%
Beta Blocker at Discharge[3]	0	-	86%	90%	100%
Fibrinolytic Medication Timing[1,3]	4	50%	30%	31%	100%
PCI Within 90 Minutes of Arrival[5]	-	-	48%	54%	95%
Smoking Cessation Advice[3]	0	-	90%	88%	100%
Heart Failure Care					
ACE Inhibitor or ARB for LVSD[1]	4	50%	82%	82%	100%
Discharge Instructions[1]	12	17%	60%	61%	93%
Evaluation of LVS Function[1]	15	93%	81%	83%	99%
Smoking Cessation Advice[1]	1	0%	82%	82%	100%
Pneumonia Care					
Appropriate Initial Antibiotic	30	97%	79%	83%	94%
Blood Culture Timing[1]	11	100%	89%	90%	100%
Influenza Vaccine[1]	11	64%	69%	70%	100%
Initial Antibiotic Timing	50	92%	78%	80%	93%
Oxygenation Assessment	62	100%	99%	99%	100%
Pneumococcal Vaccine	35	71%	68%	69%	94%
Smoking Cessation Advice[1]	8	62%	83%	80%	100%
Surgical Infection Prevention					
Prophylactic Antibiotic Given[1]	4	25%	67%	77%	95%
Prophylactic Antibiotic Selection[1]	1	100%	86%	90%	100%
Prophylactic Antibiotic Stopped[1]	5	100%	68%	72%	95%
Pregnancy Care					
Inpatient Neonatal Mortality	-	-	-	-	-

NOTE: Hospital profiles are in alphabetical order by state, then city, then hospital within the city; Rankings are sorted by rate in descending order and exclude hospitals with less than 25 cases; (1) The number of cases is too small (n<25) for purposes of reliably predicting hospital performance; (2) Measure reflects the hospital's indication that its submission was based upon a sample of its relevant discharges; (3) Rate reflects fewer than the maximum possible quarters of data for the measure; (4) Inaccurate information submitted and suppressed for one or more quarters; (5) No data is available from the hospital for this measure; Please refer to the User's Guide for a full explanation of data

| Third or Fourth Degree Laceration | - | - | 3.23% | 3.63% | 3.27% |

Columbus Community Hospital

110 Shult Drive
PO Box 865
Columbus, TX 78934
URL: www.columbusch.com
Ownership: Voluntary non-profit - Private
Emergency Services: Yes

Phone: 979-732-2371
Fax: 979-732-9242

Accredited: No
Licensed Beds: 40

Key Personnel:
President/CEO. . . . . Rob Thomas
Chief Medical Staff. . . . . Troy Millican, MD
Emergency Services Director. . . . . Donna Campbell, MD
Emergency Room . . . . Jeno Hargrove, RN
Infection Control. . . . . Carol Rooks, RN
ICU . . . . Susie Janacek, RN
Respiratory/Cardiopulmonary. . . . . Bill Smith, RRT

Measure	Cases	This Hospital	State Average	U.S. Average	Top Hospital
Heart Attack Care					
ACE Inhibitor or ARB for LVSD	0	-	85%	82%	100%
Aspirin at Arrival[1]	2	100%	91%	92%	100%
Aspirin at Discharge[1]	2	100%	90%	90%	100%
Beta Blocker at Arrival[1]	3	100%	85%	87%	100%
Beta Blocker at Discharge[1]	3	100%	86%	90%	100%
Fibrinolytic Medication Timing[3]	0	-	30%	31%	100%
PCI Within 90 Minutes of Arrival	0	-	48%	54%	95%
Smoking Cessation Advice[3]	0	-	90%	88%	100%
Heart Failure Care					
ACE Inhibitor or ARB for LVSD[1]	12	75%	82%	82%	100%
Discharge Instructions[1,3]	3	100%	60%	61%	93%
Evaluation of LVS Function	34	91%	81%	83%	99%
Smoking Cessation Advice[3]	0	-	82%	82%	100%
Pneumonia Care					
Appropriate Initial Antibiotic[1,3]	3	67%	79%	83%	94%
Blood Culture Timing[1,3]	4	100%	89%	90%	100%
Influenza Vaccine[5]	-	-	69%	70%	100%
Initial Antibiotic Timing	37	89%	78%	80%	93%
Oxygenation Assessment	43	98%	99%	99%	100%
Pneumococcal Vaccine	30	90%	68%	69%	94%
Smoking Cessation Advice[3]	0	-	83%	80%	100%
Surgical Infection Prevention					
Prophylactic Antibiotic Given[1,3]	9	100%	67%	77%	95%
Prophylactic Antibiotic Selection[5]	-	-	86%	90%	100%
Prophylactic Antibiotic Stopped[1,3]	9	100%	68%	72%	95%
Pregnancy Care					
Inpatient Neonatal Mortality	-	-	-	-	-
Third or Fourth Degree Laceration	-	-	3.23%	3.63%	3.27%

Comanche County Medical Center

10201 Highway 16 North
PO Box 847
Comanche, TX 76442
URL: www.comanchecmc.org
Ownership: Govt - Hospital District or Authority
Emergency Services: Yes

Phone: 254-879-4900
Fax: 254-879-4990

Accredited: No
Licensed Beds: 25

Key Personnel:
Interim CEO. . . . . Kurt Meyer
Chief Medical Staff. S. Howard Dickey, DO
Infection Control. . . . . Sarah Anderson
Medical/Surgical Nursing . . . . Pana Surinale, RN
Surgical Services . . . . Carol Mahan, RN
Respiratory/Cardiopulmonary. . . . . Johnnie Robinson

Measure	Cases	This Hospital	State Average	U.S. Average	Top Hospital
Heart Attack Care					
ACE Inhibitor or ARB for LVSD[1]	4	100%	85%	82%	100%
Aspirin at Arrival[1]	13	77%	91%	92%	100%
Aspirin at Discharge[1]	8	88%	90%	90%	100%
Beta Blocker at Arrival[1]	10	80%	85%	87%	100%
Beta Blocker at Discharge[1]	3	100%	86%	90%	100%
Fibrinolytic Medication Timing	0	-	30%	31%	100%
PCI Within 90 Minutes of Arrival	0	-	48%	54%	95%

Smoking Cessation Advice	0	-	90%	88%	100%
Heart Failure Care					
ACE Inhibitor or ARB for LVSD[1]	13	92%	82%	82%	100%
Discharge Instructions	52	63%	60%	61%	93%
Evaluation of LVS Function	86	74%	81%	83%	99%
Smoking Cessation Advice[1]	11	82%	82%	82%	100%
Pneumonia Care					
Appropriate Initial Antibiotic	41	90%	79%	83%	94%
Blood Culture Timing[1]	22	95%	89%	90%	100%
Influenza Vaccine[1]	10	100%	69%	70%	100%
Initial Antibiotic Timing	49	78%	78%	80%	93%
Oxygenation Assessment	60	100%	99%	99%	100%
Pneumococcal Vaccine	40	90%	68%	69%	94%
Smoking Cessation Advice[1]	8	75%	83%	80%	100%
Surgical Infection Prevention					
Prophylactic Antibiotic Given[1]	18	72%	67%	77%	95%
Prophylactic Antibiotic Selection[1]	4	100%	86%	90%	100%
Prophylactic Antibiotic Stopped[1]	17	100%	68%	72%	95%
Pregnancy Care					
Inpatient Neonatal Mortality	-	-	-	-	-
Third or Fourth Degree Laceration	-	-	3.23%	3.63%	3.27%

Conroe Regional Medical Center

504 Medical Center Boulevard
Conroe, TX 77304

URL: www.conroeregional.com
Ownership: Proprietary
Emergency Services: Yes

Toll-Free: 888-633-2687
Phone: 936-539-1111
Fax: 936-539-7059

Accredited: Yes
Licensed Beds: 260

Key Personnel:
President/CEO. . . . . Jerry A Nash
Chief Medical Staff. Rochelle Evans, DO
Director Infection/Disease Control . . . . Elaine Whaley, RN
CCU Spvg. Nurse . . . . Sharla Shumaker, RN
OB/GYN Womens Health. . . . . Wayne Farley, DO
Director Respiratory Therapy . . . . Frank Bristow

Measure	Cases	This Hospital	State Average	U.S. Average	Top Hospital
Heart Attack Care					
ACE Inhibitor or ARB for LVSD	75	87%	85%	82%	100%
Aspirin at Arrival	225	100%	91%	92%	100%
Aspirin at Discharge	270	99%	90%	90%	100%
Beta Blocker at Arrival	149	95%	85%	87%	100%
Beta Blocker at Discharge	243	96%	86%	90%	100%
Fibrinolytic Medication Timing[1]	10	70%	30%	31%	100%
PCI Within 90 Minutes of Arrival[1]	16	81%	48%	54%	95%
Smoking Cessation Advice	138	99%	90%	88%	100%
Heart Failure Care					
ACE Inhibitor or ARB for LVSD	190	91%	82%	82%	100%
Discharge Instructions	498	62%	60%	61%	93%
Evaluation of LVS Function	482	96%	81%	83%	99%
Smoking Cessation Advice	154	97%	82%	82%	100%
Pneumonia Care					
Appropriate Initial Antibiotic	260	87%	79%	83%	94%
Blood Culture Timing	210	89%	89%	90%	100%
Influenza Vaccine	62	71%	69%	70%	100%
Initial Antibiotic Timing	337	77%	78%	80%	93%
Oxygenation Assessment	383	99%	99%	99%	100%
Pneumococcal Vaccine	216	77%	68%	69%	94%
Smoking Cessation Advice	130	97%	83%	80%	100%
Surgical Infection Prevention					
Prophylactic Antibiotic Given[2,3]	291	91%	67%	77%	95%
Prophylactic Antibiotic Selection[2]	168	88%	86%	90%	100%
Prophylactic Antibiotic Stopped[2,3]	251	69%	68%	72%	95%
Pregnancy Care					
Inpatient Neonatal Mortality	-	-	-	-	-
Third or Fourth Degree Laceration	-	-	3.23%	3.63%	3.27%

Christus Spohn Memorial Hospital

Alternate Name: Memorial Medical Center

NOTE: Hospital profiles are in alphabetical order by state, then city, then hospital within the city; Rankings are sorted by rate in descending order and exclude hospitals with less than 25 cases; (1) The number of cases is too small (n<25) for purposes of reliably predicting hospital performance; (2) Measure reflects the hospital's indication that its submission was based upon a sample of its relevant discharges; (3) Rate reflects fewer than the maximum possible quarters of data for the measure; (4) Inaccurate information submitted and suppressed for one or more quarters; (5) No data is available from the hospital for this measure; Please refer to the User's Guide for a full explanation of data

2606 Hospital Blvd
Corpus Christi, TX 78405
E-mail: Spohn@christushealth.org
URL: www.christusspohn.org
Ownership: Voluntary non-profit - Church
Emergency Services: Yes

Phone: 361-902-4000
Fax: 361-881-1427

Accredited: Yes
Licensed Beds: 397

Key Personnel:
CEO/President . . . . Peter Banko
Chief Medical Staff . . . . John McKeever
Director Infection/Disease Control . . . . Leona Kocinek
CCU Spvg. Nurse . . . . Brian Grant
Chief Radiology . . . . Dale Obermueller
Respiratory Care . . . . Liz Elivondo

Measure	Cases	This Hospital	State Average	U.S. Average	Top Hospital
Heart Attack Care					
ACE Inhibitor or ARB for LVSD	116	78%	85%	82%	100%
Aspirin at Arrival	402	96%	91%	92%	100%
Aspirin at Discharge	529	96%	90%	90%	100%
Beta Blocker at Arrival	369	94%	85%	87%	100%
Beta Blocker at Discharge	552	96%	86%	90%	100%
Fibrinolytic Medication Timing[1]	2	0%	30%	31%	100%
PCI Within 90 Minutes of Arrival[1]	6	67%	48%	54%	95%
Smoking Cessation Advice	175	100%	90%	88%	100%
Heart Failure Care					
ACE Inhibitor or ARB for LVSD	466	80%	82%	82%	100%
Discharge Instructions	1,028	74%	60%	61%	93%
Evaluation of LVS Function	1,190	96%	81%	83%	99%
Smoking Cessation Advice	192	99%	82%	82%	100%
Pneumonia Care					
Appropriate Initial Antibiotic	537	83%	79%	83%	94%
Blood Culture Timing	513	85%	89%	90%	100%
Influenza Vaccine[4,5]	-	-	69%	70%	100%
Initial Antibiotic Timing	801	72%	78%	80%	93%
Oxygenation Assessment	939	100%	99%	99%	100%
Pneumococcal Vaccine	533	78%	68%	69%	94%
Smoking Cessation Advice	208	98%	83%	80%	100%
Surgical Infection Prevention					
Prophylactic Antibiotic Given	1,444	77%	67%	77%	95%
Prophylactic Antibiotic Selection	533	93%	86%	90%	100%
Prophylactic Antibiotic Stopped	1,412	39%	68%	72%	95%
Pregnancy Care					
Inpatient Neonatal Mortality	3,588	0.39%	-	-	-
Third or Fourth Degree Laceration	2,139	3.32%	3.23%	3.63%	3.27%

Corpus Christi Medical Center-Bay Area

7101 S Padre Island Dr
Corpus Christi, TX 78412
URL: www.ccmedicalcenter.com
Ownership: Proprietary
Emergency Services: Yes

Phone: 361-761-1400
Fax: 361-761-3654

Accredited: Yes
Licensed Beds: 494

Key Personnel:
CEO . . . . Steve Woerner
Chief Medical Staff . . . . Sandy Diaz
Emergency Room . . . . Suzanne Low, DO
Director Infection/Disease Control . . . . Annette Enrriques

Measure	Cases	This Hospital	State Average	U.S. Average	Top Hospital
Heart Attack Care					
ACE Inhibitor or ARB for LVSD	31	87%	85%	82%	100%
Aspirin at Arrival	174	99%	91%	92%	100%
Aspirin at Discharge	242	95%	90%	90%	100%
Beta Blocker at Arrival	160	92%	85%	87%	100%
Beta Blocker at Discharge	248	92%	86%	90%	100%
Fibrinolytic Medication Timing[1]	1	0%	30%	31%	100%
PCI Within 90 Minutes of Arrival[1]	9	22%	48%	54%	95%
Smoking Cessation Advice	82	87%	90%	88%	100%
Heart Failure Care					
ACE Inhibitor or ARB for LVSD	153	79%	82%	82%	100%
Discharge Instructions	388	44%	60%	61%	93%
Evaluation of LVS Function	455	88%	81%	83%	99%
Smoking Cessation Advice	67	64%	82%	82%	100%
Pneumonia Care					

Measure	Cases	This Hospital	State Average	U.S. Average	Top Hospital
Appropriate Initial Antibiotic	204	72%	79%	83%	94%
Blood Culture Timing	185	89%	89%	90%	100%
Influenza Vaccine	79	58%	69%	70%	100%
Initial Antibiotic Timing	297	70%	78%	80%	93%
Oxygenation Assessment	377	99%	99%	99%	100%
Pneumococcal Vaccine	262	69%	68%	69%	94%
Smoking Cessation Advice	71	68%	83%	80%	100%
Surgical Infection Prevention					
Prophylactic Antibiotic Given[2,3]	291	69%	67%	77%	95%
Prophylactic Antibiotic Selection[2]	156	96%	86%	90%	100%
Prophylactic Antibiotic Stopped[2,3]	282	41%	68%	72%	95%
Pregnancy Care					
Inpatient Neonatal Mortality	3,506	0.20%	-	-	-
Third or Fourth Degree Laceration	2,099	2.05%	3.23%	3.63%	3.27%

Navarro Regional Hospital

3201 West Highway 22
Corsicana, TX 75110
URL: www.navarrohospital.com
Ownership: Proprietary
Emergency Services: Yes

Phone: 903-654-6800
Fax: 903-654-6964

Accredited: Yes
Licensed Beds: 162

Key Personnel:
CEO . . . . Nancy Byrnes
CNO . . . . Glenda Terry, RN

Measure	Cases	This Hospital	State Average	U.S. Average	Top Hospital
Heart Attack Care					
ACE Inhibitor or ARB for LVSD[1]	6	100%	85%	82%	100%
Aspirin at Arrival	35	83%	91%	92%	100%
Aspirin at Discharge[1]	16	75%	90%	90%	100%
Beta Blocker at Arrival	25	84%	85%	87%	100%
Beta Blocker at Discharge[1]	18	94%	86%	90%	100%
Fibrinolytic Medication Timing	0	-	30%	31%	100%
PCI Within 90 Minutes of Arrival	0	-	48%	54%	95%
Smoking Cessation Advice[1]	5	100%	90%	88%	100%
Heart Failure Care					
ACE Inhibitor or ARB for LVSD	56	91%	82%	82%	100%
Discharge Instructions	114	61%	60%	61%	93%
Evaluation of LVS Function	162	92%	81%	83%	99%
Smoking Cessation Advice[1]	24	100%	82%	82%	100%
Pneumonia Care					
Appropriate Initial Antibiotic	81	84%	79%	83%	94%
Blood Culture Timing	81	80%	89%	90%	100%
Influenza Vaccine	32	59%	69%	70%	100%
Initial Antibiotic Timing	136	75%	78%	80%	93%
Oxygenation Assessment	164	99%	99%	99%	100%
Pneumococcal Vaccine	101	81%	68%	69%	94%
Smoking Cessation Advice	34	97%	83%	80%	100%
Surgical Infection Prevention					
Prophylactic Antibiotic Given	120	88%	67%	77%	95%
Prophylactic Antibiotic Selection	28	93%	86%	90%	100%
Prophylactic Antibiotic Stopped	114	61%	68%	72%	95%
Pregnancy Care					
Inpatient Neonatal Mortality	-	-	-	-	-
Third or Fourth Degree Laceration	-	-	3.23%	3.63%	3.27%

East Texas Medical Center-Crockett

Alternate Name: Houston County Hospital
1100 Loop 304 E
Crockett, TX 75835
E-mail: info@etmc.org
URL: www.etmc.org/crockett
Ownership: Voluntary non-profit - Private
Emergency Services: Yes

Phone: 936-546-3862
Fax: 936-546-3892

Accredited: Yes
Licensed Beds: 93

Key Personnel:
CEO . . . . Nelda Welch
Chief Medical Staff . . . . Mike Cochran, MD
Emergency Room . . . . David Garner, RN

Measure	Cases	This Hospital	State Average	U.S. Average	Top Hospital
Heart Attack Care					
ACE Inhibitor or ARB for LVSD	0	-	85%	82%	100%

NOTE: Hospital profiles are in alphabetical order by state, then city, then hospital within the city; Rankings are sorted by rate in descending order and exclude hospitals with less than 25 cases; (1) The number of cases is too small (n<25) for purposes of reliably predicting hospital performance; (2) Measure reflects the hospital's indication that its submission was based upon a sample of its relevant discharges; (3) Rate reflects fewer than the maximum possible quarters of data for the measure; (4) Inaccurate information submitted and suppressed for one or more quarters; (5) No data is available from the hospital for this measure; Please refer to the User's Guide for a full explanation of data

Measure	Cases	This Hospital	State Average	U.S. Average	Top Hospital
Aspirin at Arrival[1]	22	77%	91%	92%	100%
Aspirin at Discharge[1]	15	67%	90%	90%	100%
Beta Blocker at Arrival[1]	17	82%	85%	87%	100%
Beta Blocker at Discharge[1]	13	77%	86%	90%	100%
Fibrinolytic Medication Timing	0	-	30%	31%	100%
PCI Within 90 Minutes of Arrival	0	-	48%	54%	95%
Smoking Cessation Advice[1]	1	100%	90%	88%	100%
Heart Failure Care					
ACE Inhibitor or ARB for LVSD[1]	22	95%	82%	82%	100%
Discharge Instructions	76	63%	60%	61%	93%
Evaluation of LVS Function	107	84%	81%	83%	99%
Smoking Cessation Advice	28	86%	82%	82%	100%
Pneumonia Care					
Appropriate Initial Antibiotic	48	67%	79%	83%	94%
Blood Culture Timing	25	96%	89%	90%	100%
Influenza Vaccine[4,5]	-	-	69%	70%	100%
Initial Antibiotic Timing	70	90%	78%	80%	93%
Oxygenation Assessment	87	98%	99%	99%	100%
Pneumococcal Vaccine	65	58%	68%	69%	94%
Smoking Cessation Advice[1]	12	83%	83%	80%	100%
Surgical Infection Prevention					
Prophylactic Antibiotic Given[1,3]	21	52%	67%	77%	95%
Prophylactic Antibiotic Selection[1]	6	100%	86%	90%	100%
Prophylactic Antibiotic Stopped[1,3]	20	95%	68%	72%	95%
Pregnancy Care					
Inpatient Neonatal Mortality	-	-	-	-	-
Third or Fourth Degree Laceration	-	-	3.23%	3.63%	3.27%

Cuero Community Hospital

2550 North Esplanade Street
Cuero, TX 77954
URL: www.cuerohosp.org
Ownership: Govt - Hospital District or Authority
Emergency Services: Yes

Phone: 361-275-6191
Fax: 361-275-3999

Accredited: No
Licensed Beds: 60

Key Personnel:
Administrator . . . . Darryl Stefka
Chief Medical Staff. . . . . Ramond Ruise
Emergency Room . . . . Patty Jetter
Director Infection/Disease Control . . . . Debbie Irving, RN
Director Medical/Surgical Nursing . . . . Melanie Guenther, RN
Chief Radiology . . . . James Newman, MD
Director Respiratory Therapy . . . . John Davis

Measure	Cases	This Hospital	State Average	U.S. Average	Top Hospital
Heart Attack Care					
ACE Inhibitor or ARB for LVSD[1]	1	100%	85%	82%	100%
Aspirin at Arrival[1]	14	93%	91%	92%	100%
Aspirin at Discharge[1]	6	83%	90%	90%	100%
Beta Blocker at Arrival[1]	14	86%	85%	87%	100%
Beta Blocker at Discharge[1]	7	86%	86%	90%	100%
Fibrinolytic Medication Timing[1]	1	0%	30%	31%	100%
PCI Within 90 Minutes of Arrival	0	-	48%	54%	95%
Smoking Cessation Advice[1]	1	100%	90%	88%	100%
Heart Failure Care					
ACE Inhibitor or ARB for LVSD[1]	20	95%	82%	82%	100%
Discharge Instructions	50	100%	60%	61%	93%
Evaluation of LVS Function	77	94%	81%	83%	99%
Smoking Cessation Advice[1]	8	75%	82%	82%	100%
Pneumonia Care					
Appropriate Initial Antibiotic	83	75%	79%	83%	94%
Blood Culture Timing	39	97%	89%	90%	100%
Influenza Vaccine[1]	18	100%	69%	70%	100%
Initial Antibiotic Timing	103	96%	78%	80%	93%
Oxygenation Assessment	119	100%	99%	99%	100%
Pneumococcal Vaccine	81	100%	68%	69%	94%
Smoking Cessation Advice[1]	11	100%	83%	80%	100%
Surgical Infection Prevention					
Prophylactic Antibiotic Given[1,3]	5	40%	67%	77%	95%
Prophylactic Antibiotic Selection[1]	1	100%	86%	90%	100%
Prophylactic Antibiotic Stopped[1,3]	4	100%	68%	72%	95%
Pregnancy Care					
Inpatient Neonatal Mortality	-	-	-	-	-
Third or Fourth Degree Laceration	-	-	3.23%	3.63%	3.27%

Coon Memorial Hospital

1411 Denver Avenue
Dalhart, TX 79022
URL: www.coonmemorial.org
Ownership: Govt - Hospital District or Authority
Emergency Services: Yes

Phone: 806-244-4571
Fax: 806-244-5013

Accredited: No
Licensed Beds: 23

Key Personnel:
CEO. . . . . Leroy Schaffner
President . . . . Sieto Mellema

Measure	Cases	This Hospital	State Average	U.S. Average	Top Hospital
Heart Attack Care					
ACE Inhibitor or ARB for LVSD[3]	0	-	85%	82%	100%
Aspirin at Arrival[1,3]	1	100%	91%	92%	100%
Aspirin at Discharge[1,3]	1	100%	90%	90%	100%
Beta Blocker at Arrival[1,3]	2	100%	85%	87%	100%
Beta Blocker at Discharge[1,3]	2	100%	86%	90%	100%
Fibrinolytic Medication Timing[3]	0	-	30%	31%	100%
PCI Within 90 Minutes of Arrival	0	-	48%	54%	95%
Smoking Cessation Advice[3]	0	-	90%	88%	100%
Heart Failure Care					
ACE Inhibitor or ARB for LVSD[1]	4	100%	82%	82%	100%
Discharge Instructions[1]	19	5%	60%	61%	93%
Evaluation of LVS Function	29	24%	81%	83%	99%
Smoking Cessation Advice[1]	3	0%	82%	82%	100%
Pneumonia Care					
Appropriate Initial Antibiotic[1]	20	45%	79%	83%	94%
Blood Culture Timing[1]	4	100%	89%	90%	100%
Influenza Vaccine[1]	9	67%	69%	70%	100%
Initial Antibiotic Timing	30	53%	78%	80%	93%
Oxygenation Assessment	36	100%	99%	99%	100%
Pneumococcal Vaccine[1]	23	70%	68%	69%	94%
Smoking Cessation Advice[1]	10	40%	83%	80%	100%
Surgical Infection Prevention					
Prophylactic Antibiotic Given[5]	-	-	67%	77%	95%
Prophylactic Antibiotic Selection[5]	-	-	86%	90%	100%
Prophylactic Antibiotic Stopped[5]	-	-	68%	72%	95%
Pregnancy Care					
Inpatient Neonatal Mortality	-	-	-	-	-
Third or Fourth Degree Laceration	-	-	3.23%	3.63%	3.27%

Baylor Heart and Vascular Center

621 North Hall Street Suite 150
Dallas, TX 75226
Ownership: Proprietary
Emergency Services: No

Phone: 214-820-0600

Accredited: Yes

Measure	Cases	This Hospital	State Average	U.S. Average	Top Hospital
Heart Attack Care					
ACE Inhibitor or ARB for LVSD[1]	23	100%	85%	82%	100%
Aspirin at Arrival[1]	12	100%	91%	92%	100%
Aspirin at Discharge	140	100%	90%	90%	100%
Beta Blocker at Arrival[1]	11	100%	85%	87%	100%
Beta Blocker at Discharge	136	99%	86%	90%	100%
Fibrinolytic Medication Timing	0	-	30%	31%	100%
PCI Within 90 Minutes of Arrival	0	-	48%	54%	95%
Smoking Cessation Advice	53	100%	90%	88%	100%
Heart Failure Care					
ACE Inhibitor or ARB for LVSD	234	100%	82%	82%	100%
Discharge Instructions	266	100%	60%	61%	93%
Evaluation of LVS Function	268	100%	81%	83%	99%
Smoking Cessation Advice	50	100%	82%	82%	100%
Pneumonia Care					
Appropriate Initial Antibiotic[5]	-	-	79%	83%	94%
Blood Culture Timing[5]	-	-	89%	90%	100%
Influenza Vaccine[5]	-	-	69%	70%	100%
Initial Antibiotic Timing[5]	-	-	78%	80%	93%
Oxygenation Assessment[5]	-	-	99%	99%	100%
Pneumococcal Vaccine[5]	-	-	68%	69%	94%
Smoking Cessation Advice[5]	-	-	83%	80%	100%
Surgical Infection Prevention					
Prophylactic Antibiotic Given	176	99%	67%	77%	95%

NOTE: Hospital profiles are in alphabetical order by state, then city, then hospital within the city; Rankings are sorted by rate in descending order and exclude hospitals with less than 25 cases; (1) The number of cases is too small (n<25) for purposes of reliably predicting hospital performance; (2) Measure reflects the hospital's indication that its submission was based upon a sample of its relevant discharges; (3) Rate reflects fewer than the maximum possible quarters of data for the measure; (4) Inaccurate information submitted and suppressed for one or more quarters; (5) No data is available from the hospital for this measure; Please refer to the User's Guide for a full explanation of data

Prophylactic Antibiotic Selection	48	100%	86%	90%	100%
Prophylactic Antibiotic Stopped	165	96%	68%	72%	95%

Pregnancy Care

Inpatient Neonatal Mortality	-	-	-	-	-
Third or Fourth Degree Laceration	-	-	3.23%	3.63%	3.27%

Baylor University Medical Center

Alternate Name: Irving Healthcare System
3500 Gaston Avenue
Dallas, TX 75246

Toll-Free: 800-4BA-YLOR
Phone: 214-820-0111
Fax: 214-820-7577

URL: www.baylorhealth.com
Ownership: Voluntary non-profit - Church
Emergency Services: Yes
Accredited: Yes
Licensed Beds: 998

Key Personnel:
President/CEO . . . . Joel Allison
Chief Medical Staff . . . . Michael Emmett, MD
Director Catheterization Laboratory . . . . John Hyland, MD
Emergency Room . . . . Leonard Riggs, MD
Director Infection/Disease Control . . . . William Sutker, MD
Director Medical/Surgical Nursing . . . . Remy Tolentino, RN
OB/GYN Womens Health . . . . C Allen Stringer, MD
Chief Radiology . . . . Michael Smerud, MD
Director Respiratory Therapy . . . . Charles Shuey, Jr, DM

Measure	Cases	This Hospital	State Average	U.S. Average	Top Hospital
Heart Attack Care					
ACE Inhibitor or ARB for LVSD	171	94%	85%	82%	100%
Aspirin at Arrival	313	98%	91%	92%	100%
Aspirin at Discharge	545	97%	90%	90%	100%
Beta Blocker at Arrival	227	97%	85%	87%	100%
Beta Blocker at Discharge	509	98%	86%	90%	100%
Fibrinolytic Medication Timing	0	-	30%	31%	100%
PCI Within 90 Minutes of Arrival[1]	10	90%	48%	54%	95%
Smoking Cessation Advice	236	100%	90%	88%	100%
Heart Failure Care					
ACE Inhibitor or ARB for LVSD	446	93%	82%	82%	100%
Discharge Instructions	805	88%	60%	61%	93%
Evaluation of LVS Function	944	99%	81%	83%	99%
Smoking Cessation Advice	249	100%	82%	82%	100%
Pneumonia Care					
Appropriate Initial Antibiotic	396	89%	79%	83%	94%
Blood Culture Timing	373	91%	89%	90%	100%
Influenza Vaccine	142	89%	69%	70%	100%
Initial Antibiotic Timing	573	79%	78%	80%	93%
Oxygenation Assessment	691	100%	99%	99%	100%
Pneumococcal Vaccine	367	86%	68%	69%	94%
Smoking Cessation Advice	170	99%	83%	80%	100%
Surgical Infection Prevention					
Prophylactic Antibiotic Given	3,530	94%	67%	77%	95%
Prophylactic Antibiotic Selection	877	88%	86%	90%	100%
Prophylactic Antibiotic Stopped	3,460	89%	68%	72%	95%
Pregnancy Care					
Inpatient Neonatal Mortality	-	-	-	-	-
Third or Fourth Degree Laceration	-	-	3.23%	3.63%	3.27%

Charlton Methodist Hospital

PO Box 225357
Dallas, TX 75222
Ownership: Voluntary non-profit - Private
Emergency Services: Yes
Phone: 214-947-7777
Fax: 214-947-7525
Accredited: Yes
Licensed Beds: 190

Key Personnel:
CEO/President . . . . Howard Chase
Emergency Room . . . . John Haupert

Measure	Cases	This Hospital	State Average	U.S. Average	Top Hospital
Heart Attack Care					
ACE Inhibitor or ARB for LVSD	44	98%	85%	82%	100%
Aspirin at Arrival	234	98%	91%	92%	100%
Aspirin at Discharge	194	99%	90%	90%	100%
Beta Blocker at Arrival	163	97%	85%	87%	100%
Beta Blocker at Discharge	228	100%	86%	90%	100%
Fibrinolytic Medication Timing[1]	1	100%	30%	31%	100%

PCI Within 90 Minutes of Arrival[1]	13	54%	48%	54%	95%
Smoking Cessation Advice	81	100%	90%	88%	100%
Heart Failure Care					
ACE Inhibitor or ARB for LVSD	250	96%	82%	82%	100%
Discharge Instructions	449	77%	60%	61%	93%
Evaluation of LVS Function	552	97%	81%	83%	99%
Smoking Cessation Advice	149	98%	82%	82%	100%
Pneumonia Care					
Appropriate Initial Antibiotic	169	80%	79%	83%	94%
Blood Culture Timing	156	90%	89%	90%	100%
Influenza Vaccine	50	88%	69%	70%	100%
Initial Antibiotic Timing	291	82%	78%	80%	93%
Oxygenation Assessment	312	100%	99%	99%	100%
Pneumococcal Vaccine	146	93%	68%	69%	94%
Smoking Cessation Advice	73	99%	83%	80%	100%
Surgical Infection Prevention					
Prophylactic Antibiotic Given[2,3]	139	98%	67%	77%	95%
Prophylactic Antibiotic Selection[2]	39	100%	86%	90%	100%
Prophylactic Antibiotic Stopped[2,3]	135	85%	68%	72%	95%
Pregnancy Care					
Inpatient Neonatal Mortality	2,362	0.21%	-	-	-
Third or Fourth Degree Laceration	1,681	1.31%	3.23%	3.63%	3.27%

Dallas Southwest Medical Center

Alternate Name: Dallas Family Hospital
2929 S Hampton Road
Dallas, TX 75224
Ownership: Proprietary
Emergency Services: Yes
Phone: 214-330-4611
Fax: 214-648-9835
Accredited: No
Licensed Beds: 107

Key Personnel:
President/CEO . . . . Jimmy Brown
Chief Medical Staff . . . . Richard Andrews
Emergency Room . . . . Tamra Albright, RN
Infection Control . . . . Rosemarie Onwunue
ICU . . . . Tania Albright
Medical/Surgical Nursing . . . . Marion Clark
OB/GYN Womens Health . . . . Susan Rushing, RN
Respiratory/Cardiopulmonary . . . . Robert Estrada

Measure	Cases	This Hospital	State Average	U.S. Average	Top Hospital
Heart Attack Care					
ACE Inhibitor or ARB for LVSD[3]	0	-	85%	82%	100%
Aspirin at Arrival[1,3]	4	100%	91%	92%	100%
Aspirin at Discharge[3]	0	-	90%	90%	100%
Beta Blocker at Arrival[1,3]	6	83%	85%	87%	100%
Beta Blocker at Discharge[3]	0	-	86%	90%	100%
Fibrinolytic Medication Timing[3]	0	-	30%	31%	100%
PCI Within 90 Minutes of Arrival	0	-	48%	54%	95%
Smoking Cessation Advice[3]	0	-	90%	88%	100%
Heart Failure Care					
ACE Inhibitor or ARB for LVSD[1,3]	6	83%	82%	82%	100%
Discharge Instructions[1,3]	14	0%	60%	61%	93%
Evaluation of LVS Function[3]	36	92%	81%	83%	99%
Smoking Cessation Advice[1,3]	5	20%	82%	82%	100%
Pneumonia Care					
Appropriate Initial Antibiotic[1,3]	4	50%	79%	83%	94%
Blood Culture Timing[1,3]	7	57%	89%	90%	100%
Influenza Vaccine[5]	-	-	69%	70%	100%
Initial Antibiotic Timing[1,3]	18	83%	78%	80%	93%
Oxygenation Assessment[1,3]	19	100%	99%	99%	100%
Pneumococcal Vaccine[1,3]	6	0%	68%	69%	94%
Smoking Cessation Advice[3]	0	-	83%	80%	100%
Surgical Infection Prevention					
Prophylactic Antibiotic Given[1,3]	18	44%	67%	77%	95%
Prophylactic Antibiotic Selection[5]	-	-	86%	90%	100%
Prophylactic Antibiotic Stopped[1,3]	18	100%	68%	72%	95%
Pregnancy Care					
Inpatient Neonatal Mortality	-	-	-	-	-
Third or Fourth Degree Laceration	-	-	3.23%	3.63%	3.27%

NOTE: Hospital profiles are in alphabetical order by state, then city, then hospital within the city; Rankings are sorted by rate in descending order and exclude hospitals with less than 25 cases; (1) The number of cases is too small (n<25) for purposes of reliably predicting hospital performance; (2) Measure reflects the hospital's indication that its submission was based upon a sample of its relevant discharges; (3) Rate reflects fewer than the maximum possible quarters of data for the measure; (4) Inaccurate information submitted and suppressed for one or more quarters; (5) No data is available from the hospital for this measure; Please refer to the User's Guide for a full explanation of data

Doctors Hospital

9330 Poppy Drive
#205 West
Dallas, TX 75218
URL: www.doctorshospitaldallas.com
Ownership: Proprietary
Emergency Services: Yes

Phone: 214-324-6100
Fax: 214-324-0612

Accredited: Yes
Licensed Beds: 228

Key Personnel:
CEO. . . . . Mitch Edgeworth
Chief Medical Staff. . . . . Leonard Comia, MD
OB/GYN Womens Health. . . . . Julie Pao, MD
Chief Radiology . . . . John Barnhill, MD
Director Respiratory Therapy . . . . Rick Plunk

Measure	Cases	This Hospital	State Average	U.S. Average	Top Hospital
Heart Attack Care					
ACE Inhibitor or ARB for LVSD	28	100%	85%	82%	100%
Aspirin at Arrival	141	99%	91%	92%	100%
Aspirin at Discharge	130	98%	90%	90%	100%
Beta Blocker at Arrival	119	99%	85%	87%	100%
Beta Blocker at Discharge	122	100%	86%	90%	100%
Fibrinolytic Medication Timing[1]	1	0%	30%	31%	100%
PCI Within 90 Minutes of Arrival[1]	3	67%	48%	54%	95%
Smoking Cessation Advice	45	98%	90%	88%	100%
Heart Failure Care					
ACE Inhibitor or ARB for LVSD	144	94%	82%	82%	100%
Discharge Instructions	292	90%	60%	61%	93%
Evaluation of LVS Function	365	98%	81%	83%	99%
Smoking Cessation Advice	75	93%	82%	82%	100%
Pneumonia Care					
Appropriate Initial Antibiotic	193	91%	79%	83%	94%
Blood Culture Timing	171	95%	89%	90%	100%
Influenza Vaccine	54	76%	69%	70%	100%
Initial Antibiotic Timing	225	77%	78%	80%	93%
Oxygenation Assessment	284	100%	99%	99%	100%
Pneumococcal Vaccine	172	74%	68%	69%	94%
Smoking Cessation Advice	68	84%	83%	80%	100%
Surgical Infection Prevention					
Prophylactic Antibiotic Given[2]	244	75%	67%	77%	95%
Prophylactic Antibiotic Selection[2]	58	71%	86%	90%	100%
Prophylactic Antibiotic Stopped[2]	223	71%	68%	72%	95%
Pregnancy Care					
Inpatient Neonatal Mortality	-	-	-	-	-
Third or Fourth Degree Laceration	-	-	3.23%	3.63%	3.27%

Healthsouth Medical Center

2124 Research Row
Dallas, TX 75235
Ownership: Proprietary
Emergency Services: No

Phone: 214-904-6100

Accredited: Yes

Key Personnel:
President, Diagnostic Division . . . . Greg Brophy
President, Inpatient Division. . . . . Mark J Tarr

Measure	Cases	This Hospital	State Average	U.S. Average	Top Hospital
Heart Attack Care					
ACE Inhibitor or ARB for LVSD[5]	-	-	85%	82%	100%
Aspirin at Arrival[5]	-	-	91%	92%	100%
Aspirin at Discharge[5]	-	-	90%	90%	100%
Beta Blocker at Arrival[5]	-	-	85%	87%	100%
Beta Blocker at Discharge[5]	-	-	86%	90%	100%
Fibrinolytic Medication Timing[5]	-	-	30%	31%	100%
PCI Within 90 Minutes of Arrival[5]	-	-	48%	54%	95%
Smoking Cessation Advice[5]	-	-	90%	88%	100%
Heart Failure Care					
ACE Inhibitor or ARB for LVSD[5]	-	-	82%	82%	100%
Discharge Instructions[5]	-	-	60%	61%	93%
Evaluation of LVS Function[5]	-	-	81%	83%	99%
Smoking Cessation Advice[5]	-	-	82%	82%	100%
Pneumonia Care					
Appropriate Initial Antibiotic[5]	-	-	79%	83%	94%
Blood Culture Timing[5]	-	-	89%	90%	100%
Influenza Vaccine[5]	-	-	69%	70%	100%

Measure	Cases	This Hospital	State Average	U.S. Average	Top Hospital
Initial Antibiotic Timing[5]	-	-	78%	80%	93%
Oxygenation Assessment[5]	-	-	99%	99%	100%
Pneumococcal Vaccine[5]	-	-	68%	69%	94%
Smoking Cessation Advice[5]	-	-	83%	80%	100%
Surgical Infection Prevention					
Prophylactic Antibiotic Given[5]	-	-	67%	77%	95%
Prophylactic Antibiotic Selection[5]	-	-	86%	90%	100%
Prophylactic Antibiotic Stopped[5]	-	-	68%	72%	95%
Pregnancy Care					
Inpatient Neonatal Mortality	-	-	-	-	-
Third or Fourth Degree Laceration	-	-	3.23%	3.63%	3.27%

Mary Shiels Hospital

3515 Howell Street
Dallas, TX 75204
URL: www.maryshiels.com
Ownership: Proprietary
Emergency Services: No

Phone: 214-443-3000
Fax: 214-443-3049

Accredited: Yes
Licensed Beds: 28

Key Personnel:
CEO. . . . . Suzanne Greever
Chief Medical Staff. Mark Armstrong, MD
Director Infection/Disease Control . . . . Kathy Dawson, RN

Measure	Cases	This Hospital	State Average	U.S. Average	Top Hospital
Heart Attack Care					
ACE Inhibitor or ARB for LVSD[5]	-	-	85%	82%	100%
Aspirin at Arrival[5]	-	-	91%	92%	100%
Aspirin at Discharge[5]	-	-	90%	90%	100%
Beta Blocker at Arrival[5]	-	-	85%	87%	100%
Beta Blocker at Discharge[5]	-	-	86%	90%	100%
Fibrinolytic Medication Timing[5]	-	-	30%	31%	100%
PCI Within 90 Minutes of Arrival[5]	-	-	48%	54%	95%
Smoking Cessation Advice[5]	-	-	90%	88%	100%
Heart Failure Care					
ACE Inhibitor or ARB for LVSD[5]	-	-	82%	82%	100%
Discharge Instructions[5]	-	-	60%	61%	93%
Evaluation of LVS Function[5]	-	-	81%	83%	99%
Smoking Cessation Advice[5]	-	-	82%	82%	100%
Pneumonia Care					
Appropriate Initial Antibiotic[5]	-	-	79%	83%	94%
Blood Culture Timing[5]	-	-	89%	90%	100%
Influenza Vaccine[5]	-	-	69%	70%	100%
Initial Antibiotic Timing[5]	-	-	78%	80%	93%
Oxygenation Assessment[5]	-	-	99%	99%	100%
Pneumococcal Vaccine[5]	-	-	68%	69%	94%
Smoking Cessation Advice[5]	-	-	83%	80%	100%
Surgical Infection Prevention					
Prophylactic Antibiotic Given[5]	-	-	67%	77%	95%
Prophylactic Antibiotic Selection[5]	-	-	86%	90%	100%
Prophylactic Antibiotic Stopped[5]	-	-	68%	72%	95%
Pregnancy Care					
Inpatient Neonatal Mortality	-	-	-	-	-
Third or Fourth Degree Laceration	-	-	3.23%	3.63%	3.27%

Medical City Dallas

Alternate Name: Humana Hospital-Medical City Dallas
7777 Forest Lane
Dallas, TX 75230
E-mail: medcity.main@hcahealthcare.com
URL: www.medicalcityhospital.com
Ownership: Proprietary
Emergency Services: Yes

Phone: 972-566-7000
Fax: 972-566-6248

Accredited: Yes
Licensed Beds: 598

Key Personnel:
President/CEO. . . . . Britt Berrett
Chief Medical Staff. Mitch Voelker, MD

Measure	Cases	This Hospital	State Average	U.S. Average	Top Hospital
Heart Attack Care					
ACE Inhibitor or ARB for LVSD[1]	24	88%	85%	82%	100%
Aspirin at Arrival	112	99%	91%	92%	100%
Aspirin at Discharge	136	96%	90%	90%	100%
Beta Blocker at Arrival	102	95%	85%	87%	100%

NOTE: Hospital profiles are in alphabetical order by state, then city, then hospital within the city; Rankings are sorted by rate in descending order and exclude hospitals with less than 25 cases; (1) The number of cases is too small (n<25) for purposes of reliably predicting hospital performance; (2) Measure reflects the hospital's indication that its submission was based upon a sample of its relevant discharges; (3) Rate reflects fewer than the maximum possible quarters of data for the measure; (4) Inaccurate information submitted and suppressed for one or more quarters; (5) No data is available from the hospital for this measure; Please refer to the User's Guide for a full explanation of data

Beta Blocker at Discharge	128	99%	86%	90%	100%
Fibrinolytic Medication Timing[1]	1	0%	30%	31%	100%
PCI Within 90 Minutes of Arrival[1]	8	25%	48%	54%	95%
Smoking Cessation Advice	52	96%	90%	88%	100%
Heart Failure Care					
ACE Inhibitor or ARB for LVSD	243	89%	82%	82%	100%
Discharge Instructions	412	47%	60%	61%	93%
Evaluation of LVS Function	479	94%	81%	83%	99%
Smoking Cessation Advice	86	95%	82%	82%	100%
Pneumonia Care					
Appropriate Initial Antibiotic	124	89%	79%	83%	94%
Blood Culture Timing	131	94%	89%	90%	100%
Influenza Vaccine	44	48%	69%	70%	100%
Initial Antibiotic Timing	189	79%	78%	80%	93%
Oxygenation Assessment	235	100%	99%	99%	100%
Pneumococcal Vaccine	138	57%	68%	69%	94%
Smoking Cessation Advice	46	78%	83%	80%	100%
Surgical Infection Prevention					
Prophylactic Antibiotic Given[2,3]	376	87%	67%	77%	95%
Prophylactic Antibiotic Selection[2]	173	90%	86%	90%	100%
Prophylactic Antibiotic Stopped[2,3]	360	73%	68%	72%	95%
Pregnancy Care					
Inpatient Neonatal Mortality	-	-	-	-	-
Third or Fourth Degree Laceration	-	-	3.23%	3.63%	3.27%

Methodist Medical Center

PO Box 655999
Dallas, TX 75265
URL: www.mhd.com
Ownership: Voluntary non-profit - Church
Emergency Services: Yes

Phone: 214-947-8181
Fax: 214-947-2519

Accredited: Yes
Licensed Beds: 478

Key Personnel:
President/CEO . . . . Stephen L Mansfield, FACHE
OB/GYN Womens Health . . . . Clare Edmon, MD
Chief Radiology . . . . James Camak, MD
Director Respiratory Therapy . . . . Pam Christian

Measure	Cases	This Hospital	State Average	U.S. Average	Top Hospital
Heart Attack Care					
ACE Inhibitor or ARB for LVSD	65	92%	85%	82%	100%
Aspirin at Arrival	173	99%	91%	92%	100%
Aspirin at Discharge	216	100%	90%	90%	100%
Beta Blocker at Arrival	146	99%	85%	87%	100%
Beta Blocker at Discharge	216	99%	86%	90%	100%
Fibrinolytic Medication Timing	0	-	30%	31%	100%
PCI Within 90 Minutes of Arrival[1]	16	69%	48%	54%	95%
Smoking Cessation Advice	93	100%	90%	88%	100%
Heart Failure Care					
ACE Inhibitor or ARB for LVSD	284	97%	82%	82%	100%
Discharge Instructions	508	97%	60%	61%	93%
Evaluation of LVS Function	529	98%	81%	83%	99%
Smoking Cessation Advice	131	100%	82%	82%	100%
Pneumonia Care					
Appropriate Initial Antibiotic	173	82%	79%	83%	94%
Blood Culture Timing	209	95%	89%	90%	100%
Influenza Vaccine	56	93%	69%	70%	100%
Initial Antibiotic Timing	266	80%	78%	80%	93%
Oxygenation Assessment	312	100%	99%	99%	100%
Pneumococcal Vaccine	143	97%	68%	69%	94%
Smoking Cessation Advice	98	100%	83%	80%	100%
Surgical Infection Prevention					
Prophylactic Antibiotic Given[2,3]	194	96%	67%	77%	95%
Prophylactic Antibiotic Selection[2]	65	94%	86%	90%	100%
Prophylactic Antibiotic Stopped[2,3]	191	89%	68%	72%	95%
Pregnancy Care					
Inpatient Neonatal Mortality	3,839	0.76%	-	-	-
Third or Fourth Degree Laceration	2,612	2.26%	3.23%	3.63%	3.27%

Parkland Health & Hospital System

5201 Harry Hines Boulevard
Dallas, TX 75235
URL: www.utsouthwestern.edu/parkland
Ownership: Govt - Hospital District or Authority
Emergency Services: Yes

Phone: 214-590-8000
Fax: 214-590-8096

Accredited: Yes
Licensed Beds: 997

Key Personnel:
President/CEO . . . . Ron J Anderson, MD
Interim COO/Chief Medical Officer . . . . Samuel Lee Ross, MD
Senior Vice President . . . . Annie Franklin
Senior Vice President . . . . Michael Korpiel
Director Emergency Room . . . . Randy Blanchard, RN
Emergency Room . . . . Gary Reed, MD
Director Infection/Disease Control . . . . Shirley Shores
Intensive Care/Coronary . . . . Annie Franklin
Medical Surgery . . . . Archie Drake, RN
OB/GYN Women's Health . . . . Kathleen Hanoldgham
Director Radiology . . . . Terry Napper

Measure	Cases	This Hospital	State Average	U.S. Average	Top Hospital
Heart Attack Care					
ACE Inhibitor or ARB for LVSD	65	85%	85%	82%	100%
Aspirin at Arrival	253	97%	91%	92%	100%
Aspirin at Discharge	207	98%	90%	90%	100%
Beta Blocker at Arrival	226	93%	85%	87%	100%
Beta Blocker at Discharge	227	99%	86%	90%	100%
Fibrinolytic Medication Timing[3]	0	-	30%	31%	100%
PCI Within 90 Minutes of Arrival[1]	12	33%	48%	54%	95%
Smoking Cessation Advice	98	94%	90%	88%	100%
Heart Failure Care					
ACE Inhibitor or ARB for LVSD	521	89%	82%	82%	100%
Discharge Instructions	790	61%	60%	61%	93%
Evaluation of LVS Function	820	100%	81%	83%	99%
Smoking Cessation Advice	366	96%	82%	82%	100%
Pneumonia Care					
Appropriate Initial Antibiotic	182	82%	79%	83%	94%
Blood Culture Timing	239	79%	89%	90%	100%
Influenza Vaccine	50	92%	69%	70%	100%
Initial Antibiotic Timing	315	39%	78%	80%	93%
Oxygenation Assessment	368	99%	99%	99%	100%
Pneumococcal Vaccine	70	80%	68%	69%	94%
Smoking Cessation Advice	180	84%	83%	80%	100%
Surgical Infection Prevention					
Prophylactic Antibiotic Given[2,3]	142	89%	67%	77%	95%
Prophylactic Antibiotic Selection[2]	144	98%	86%	90%	100%
Prophylactic Antibiotic Stopped[2,3]	136	54%	68%	72%	95%
Pregnancy Care					
Inpatient Neonatal Mortality	16,281	0.45%	-	-	-
Third or Fourth Degree Laceration	11,763	5.13%	3.23%	3.63%	3.27%

Pine Creek Medical Center

9032 Harry Hines Blvd
Dallas, TX 75235
Ownership: Government - Federal
Emergency Services: Yes

Phone: 214-231-2273

Accredited: Yes

Measure	Cases	This Hospital	State Average	U.S. Average	Top Hospital
Heart Attack Care					
ACE Inhibitor or ARB for LVSD[5]	-	-	85%	82%	100%
Aspirin at Arrival[5]	-	-	91%	92%	100%
Aspirin at Discharge[5]	-	-	90%	90%	100%
Beta Blocker at Arrival[5]	-	-	85%	87%	100%
Beta Blocker at Discharge[5]	-	-	86%	90%	100%
Fibrinolytic Medication Timing[5]	-	-	30%	31%	100%
PCI Within 90 Minutes of Arrival[5]	-	-	48%	54%	95%
Smoking Cessation Advice[5]	-	-	90%	88%	100%
Heart Failure Care					
ACE Inhibitor or ARB for LVSD[5]	-	-	82%	82%	100%
Discharge Instructions[5]	-	-	60%	61%	93%
Evaluation of LVS Function[5]	-	-	81%	83%	99%
Smoking Cessation Advice[5]	-	-	82%	82%	100%
Pneumonia Care					
Appropriate Initial Antibiotic[5]	-	-	79%	83%	94%

NOTE: Hospital profiles are in alphabetical order by state, then city, then hospital within the city; Rankings are sorted by rate in descending order and exclude hospitals with less than 25 cases; (1) The number of cases is too small (n<25) for purposes of reliably predicting hospital performance; (2) Measure reflects the hospital's indication that its submission was based upon a sample of its relevant discharges; (3) Rate reflects fewer than the maximum possible quarters of data for the measure; (4) Inaccurate information submitted and suppressed for one or more quarters; (5) No data is available from the hospital for this measure; Please refer to the User's Guide for a full explanation of data

Measure	Cases	This Hospital	State Average	U.S. Average	Top Hospital
Blood Culture Timing[5]	-	-	89%	90%	100%
Influenza Vaccine[5]	-	-	69%	70%	100%
Initial Antibiotic Timing[5]	-	-	78%	80%	93%
Oxygenation Assessment[5]	-	-	99%	99%	100%
Pneumococcal Vaccine[5]	-	-	68%	69%	94%
Smoking Cessation Advice[5]	-	-	83%	80%	100%
Surgical Infection Prevention					
Prophylactic Antibiotic Given[1,3]	3	100%	67%	77%	95%
Prophylactic Antibiotic Selection[5]	-	-	86%	90%	100%
Prophylactic Antibiotic Stopped[1,3]	3	100%	68%	72%	95%
Pregnancy Care					
Inpatient Neonatal Mortality	-	-	-	-	-
Third or Fourth Degree Laceration	-	-	3.23%	3.63%	3.27%

Presbyterian Hospital of Dallas

8200 Walnut Hill Lane
Dallas, TX 75231
URL: www.texashealth.org
Ownership: Voluntary non-profit - Private
Emergency Services: Yes

Phone: 214-345-6789
Fax: 214-345-6093

Accredited: Yes
Licensed Beds: 866

Key Personnel:
President . . . . Mark H Merrill
Chief Medical Staff. . . . . Bobby Abraham
Emergency Room . . . . A Compton Broders, MD
Director Respiratory Therapy . . . . Anne Jernigan

Measure	Cases	This Hospital	State Average	U.S. Average	Top Hospital
Heart Attack Care					
ACE Inhibitor or ARB for LVSD	49	86%	85%	82%	100%
Aspirin at Arrival	214	97%	91%	92%	100%
Aspirin at Discharge	290	99%	90%	90%	100%
Beta Blocker at Arrival	179	95%	85%	87%	100%
Beta Blocker at Discharge	287	97%	86%	90%	100%
Fibrinolytic Medication Timing	0	-	30%	31%	100%
PCI Within 90 Minutes of Arrival[1]	14	36%	48%	54%	95%
Smoking Cessation Advice	103	98%	90%	88%	100%
Heart Failure Care					
ACE Inhibitor or ARB for LVSD	300	84%	82%	82%	100%
Discharge Instructions	505	84%	60%	61%	93%
Evaluation of LVS Function	650	96%	81%	83%	99%
Smoking Cessation Advice	123	98%	82%	82%	100%
Pneumonia Care					
Appropriate Initial Antibiotic	249	89%	79%	83%	94%
Blood Culture Timing	260	95%	89%	90%	100%
Influenza Vaccine	83	95%	69%	70%	100%
Initial Antibiotic Timing	351	89%	78%	80%	93%
Oxygenation Assessment	412	100%	99%	99%	100%
Pneumococcal Vaccine	273	93%	68%	69%	94%
Smoking Cessation Advice	66	95%	83%	80%	100%
Surgical Infection Prevention					
Prophylactic Antibiotic Given[2,3]	263	90%	67%	77%	95%
Prophylactic Antibiotic Selection[2]	94	99%	86%	90%	100%
Prophylactic Antibiotic Stopped[2,3]	261	92%	68%	72%	95%
Pregnancy Care					
Inpatient Neonatal Mortality	-	-	-	-	-
Third or Fourth Degree Laceration	-	-	3.23%	3.63%	3.27%

RHD Memorial Medical Center

7 Medical Parkway
Dallas, TX 75234
URL: www.rhdmemorial.com
Ownership: Proprietary
Emergency Services: Yes

Phone: 972-247-1000
Fax: 972-888-7090

Accredited: Yes
Licensed Beds: 155

Key Personnel:
President/CEO. . . . . Travis Roderick
Chief Medical Staff. . . . . Eugene Wyszynski, DO
Chief Catheterization Laboratory . . . . James Rellas
Emergency Room . . . . Ralph Kelly, DO
Supervisor Infection Control . . . . Patti Grant, RN
Director Medical/Surgical Nursing . . . . Patsy Kidd
Chief Radiology . . . . Kevin McDonell, MD

Measure	Cases	This Hospital	State Average	U.S. Average	Top Hospital

Measure	Cases	This Hospital	State Average	U.S. Average	Top Hospital
Heart Attack Care					
ACE Inhibitor or ARB for LVSD[1]	23	70%	85%	82%	100%
Aspirin at Arrival	104	95%	91%	92%	100%
Aspirin at Discharge	87	79%	90%	90%	100%
Beta Blocker at Arrival	108	92%	85%	87%	100%
Beta Blocker at Discharge	95	83%	86%	90%	100%
Fibrinolytic Medication Timing[1]	4	25%	30%	31%	100%
PCI Within 90 Minutes of Arrival	0	-	48%	54%	95%
Smoking Cessation Advice	34	100%	90%	88%	100%
Heart Failure Care					
ACE Inhibitor or ARB for LVSD	55	71%	82%	82%	100%
Discharge Instructions	114	56%	60%	61%	93%
Evaluation of LVS Function	137	80%	81%	83%	99%
Smoking Cessation Advice	39	97%	82%	82%	100%
Pneumonia Care					
Appropriate Initial Antibiotic	97	79%	79%	83%	94%
Blood Culture Timing	126	94%	89%	90%	100%
Influenza Vaccine	43	88%	69%	70%	100%
Initial Antibiotic Timing	163	79%	78%	80%	93%
Oxygenation Assessment	212	100%	99%	99%	100%
Pneumococcal Vaccine	126	85%	68%	69%	94%
Smoking Cessation Advice	43	93%	83%	80%	100%
Surgical Infection Prevention					
Prophylactic Antibiotic Given[2]	105	69%	67%	77%	95%
Prophylactic Antibiotic Selection[1,2]	18	100%	86%	90%	100%
Prophylactic Antibiotic Stopped[2]	100	52%	68%	72%	95%
Pregnancy Care					
Inpatient Neonatal Mortality	-	-	-	-	-
Third or Fourth Degree Laceration	-	-	3.23%	3.63%	3.27%

Texas Inst for Surg at Presbyterian Hosp

7115 Greenville Avenue Suite 215
Dallas, TX 75231
Ownership: Proprietary
Emergency Services: Yes

Phone: 214-647-5300

Accredited: Yes

Measure	Cases	This Hospital	State Average	U.S. Average	Top Hospital
Heart Attack Care					
ACE Inhibitor or ARB for LVSD[5]	-	-	85%	82%	100%
Aspirin at Arrival[5]	-	-	91%	92%	100%
Aspirin at Discharge[5]	-	-	90%	90%	100%
Beta Blocker at Arrival[5]	-	-	85%	87%	100%
Beta Blocker at Discharge[5]	-	-	86%	90%	100%
Fibrinolytic Medication Timing[5]	-	-	30%	31%	100%
PCI Within 90 Minutes of Arrival[5]	-	-	48%	54%	95%
Smoking Cessation Advice[5]	-	-	90%	88%	100%
Heart Failure Care					
ACE Inhibitor or ARB for LVSD[5]	-	-	82%	82%	100%
Discharge Instructions[5]	-	-	60%	61%	93%
Evaluation of LVS Function[5]	-	-	81%	83%	99%
Smoking Cessation Advice[5]	-	-	82%	82%	100%
Pneumonia Care					
Appropriate Initial Antibiotic[5]	-	-	79%	83%	94%
Blood Culture Timing[5]	-	-	89%	90%	100%
Influenza Vaccine[5]	-	-	69%	70%	100%
Initial Antibiotic Timing[5]	-	-	78%	80%	93%
Oxygenation Assessment[5]	-	-	99%	99%	100%
Pneumococcal Vaccine[5]	-	-	68%	69%	94%
Smoking Cessation Advice[5]	-	-	83%	80%	100%
Surgical Infection Prevention					
Prophylactic Antibiotic Given[5]	-	-	67%	77%	95%
Prophylactic Antibiotic Selection[5]	-	-	86%	90%	100%
Prophylactic Antibiotic Stopped[5]	-	-	68%	72%	95%
Pregnancy Care					
Inpatient Neonatal Mortality	-	-	-	-	-
Third or Fourth Degree Laceration	-	-	3.23%	3.63%	3.27%

NOTE: Hospital profiles are in alphabetical order by state, then city, then hospital within the city; Rankings are sorted by rate in descending order and exclude hospitals with less than 25 cases; (1) The number of cases is too small (n<25) for purposes of reliably predicting hospital performance; (2) Measure reflects the hospital's indication that its submission was based upon a sample of its relevant discharges; (3) Rate reflects fewer than the maximum possible quarters of data for the measure; (4) Inaccurate information submitted and suppressed for one or more quarters; (5) No data is available from the hospital for this measure; Please refer to the User's Guide for a full explanation of data

UT Southwestern Saint Paul Hospital

5909 Harry Hines Blvd
Dallas, TX 75390
Ownership: Government - State
Emergency Services: Yes

Phone: 214-879-3758

Accredited: Yes

Measure	Cases	This Hospital	State Average	U.S. Average	Top Hospital
Heart Attack Care					
ACE Inhibitor or ARB for LVSD	36	75%	85%	82%	100%
Aspirin at Arrival	117	98%	91%	92%	100%
Aspirin at Discharge	118	97%	90%	90%	100%
Beta Blocker at Arrival	107	93%	85%	87%	100%
Beta Blocker at Discharge	115	96%	86%	90%	100%
Fibrinolytic Medication Timing	0	-	30%	31%	100%
PCI Within 90 Minutes of Arrival[1]	3	67%	48%	54%	95%
Smoking Cessation Advice	32	100%	90%	88%	100%
Heart Failure Care					
ACE Inhibitor or ARB for LVSD	210	84%	82%	82%	100%
Discharge Instructions	368	44%	60%	61%	93%
Evaluation of LVS Function	397	97%	81%	83%	99%
Smoking Cessation Advice	67	100%	82%	82%	100%
Pneumonia Care					
Appropriate Initial Antibiotic	99	77%	79%	83%	94%
Blood Culture Timing	113	89%	89%	90%	100%
Influenza Vaccine	35	51%	69%	70%	100%
Initial Antibiotic Timing	151	69%	78%	80%	93%
Oxygenation Assessment	231	99%	99%	99%	100%
Pneumococcal Vaccine	92	60%	68%	69%	94%
Smoking Cessation Advice	32	100%	83%	80%	100%
Surgical Infection Prevention					
Prophylactic Antibiotic Given[3]	235	70%	67%	77%	95%
Prophylactic Antibiotic Selection	73	93%	86%	90%	100%
Prophylactic Antibiotic Stopped[3]	209	58%	68%	72%	95%
Pregnancy Care					
Inpatient Neonatal Mortality	-	-	-	-	-
Third or Fourth Degree Laceration	-	-	3.23%	3.63%	3.27%

Zale-Lipshy University Hospital

5151 Harry Hines Boulevard
Dallas, TX 75235
URL: www.utsouthwestern.edu/utsw/home/pc/universityhospitals
Ownership: Government - State
Emergency Services: No
Key Personnel:
CEO . . . . Don Smithburg

Phone: 214-645-5555
Fax: 214-645-5663

Accredited: Yes
Licensed Beds: 151

Measure	Cases	This Hospital	State Average	U.S. Average	Top Hospital
Heart Attack Care					
ACE Inhibitor or ARB for LVSD[1,3]	1	100%	85%	82%	100%
Aspirin at Arrival[1,3]	2	100%	91%	92%	100%
Aspirin at Discharge[1,3]	6	100%	90%	90%	100%
Beta Blocker at Arrival[1,3]	2	50%	85%	87%	100%
Beta Blocker at Discharge[1,3]	7	100%	86%	90%	100%
Fibrinolytic Medication Timing[3]	0	-	30%	31%	100%
PCI Within 90 Minutes of Arrival[5]	-	-	48%	54%	95%
Smoking Cessation Advice[3]	0	-	90%	88%	100%
Heart Failure Care					
ACE Inhibitor or ARB for LVSD[1]	11	82%	82%	82%	100%
Discharge Instructions	29	52%	60%	61%	93%
Evaluation of LVS Function	29	90%	81%	83%	99%
Smoking Cessation Advice[1]	4	100%	82%	82%	100%
Pneumonia Care					
Appropriate Initial Antibiotic[1]	8	75%	79%	83%	94%
Blood Culture Timing[1]	2	100%	89%	90%	100%
Influenza Vaccine[1]	5	100%	69%	70%	100%
Initial Antibiotic Timing[1]	13	62%	78%	80%	93%
Oxygenation Assessment[1]	19	100%	99%	99%	100%
Pneumococcal Vaccine[1]	12	83%	68%	69%	94%
Smoking Cessation Advice[1]	3	100%	83%	80%	100%
Surgical Infection Prevention					
Prophylactic Antibiotic Given[3]	83	72%	67%	77%	95%
Prophylactic Antibiotic Selection	38	92%	86%	90%	100%

Prophylactic Antibiotic Stopped[3]	65	45%	68%	72%	95%
Pregnancy Care					
Inpatient Neonatal Mortality	-	-	-	-	-
Third or Fourth Degree Laceration	-	-	3.23%	3.63%	3.27%

Wise Regional Health System

609 Medical Center Drive
Decatur, TX 76234
Ownership: Govt - Hospital District or Authority   Accredited: Yes
Emergency Services: Yes

Phone: 940-627-5921

Measure	Cases	This Hospital	State Average	U.S. Average	Top Hospital
Heart Attack Care					
ACE Inhibitor or ARB for LVSD[1]	1	100%	85%	82%	100%
Aspirin at Arrival[1]	6	100%	91%	92%	100%
Aspirin at Discharge[1]	1	100%	90%	90%	100%
Beta Blocker at Arrival[1]	4	75%	85%	87%	100%
Beta Blocker at Discharge[1]	2	100%	86%	90%	100%
Fibrinolytic Medication Timing	0	-	30%	31%	100%
PCI Within 90 Minutes of Arrival	0	-	48%	54%	95%
Smoking Cessation Advice	0	-	90%	88%	100%
Heart Failure Care					
ACE Inhibitor or ARB for LVSD[1]	15	93%	82%	82%	100%
Discharge Instructions	52	85%	60%	61%	93%
Evaluation of LVS Function	58	95%	81%	83%	99%
Smoking Cessation Advice[1]	13	92%	82%	82%	100%
Pneumonia Care					
Appropriate Initial Antibiotic	49	90%	79%	83%	94%
Blood Culture Timing	53	94%	89%	90%	100%
Influenza Vaccine[1]	5	20%	69%	70%	100%
Initial Antibiotic Timing	61	80%	78%	80%	93%
Oxygenation Assessment	74	100%	99%	99%	100%
Pneumococcal Vaccine[1]	23	65%	68%	69%	94%
Smoking Cessation Advice[1]	21	100%	83%	80%	100%
Surgical Infection Prevention					
Prophylactic Antibiotic Given[2,3]	41	88%	67%	77%	95%
Prophylactic Antibiotic Selection[2]	39	74%	86%	90%	100%
Prophylactic Antibiotic Stopped[2,3]	39	92%	68%	72%	95%
Pregnancy Care					
Inpatient Neonatal Mortality	-	-	-	-	-
Third or Fourth Degree Laceration	-	-	3.23%	3.63%	3.27%

Val Verde Regional Medical Center

Alternate Name: Val Verde Memorial Hospital
801 Bedell Avenue
Del Rio, TX 78840
E-mail: info@vvrmc.org
URL: www.vvrmc.org
Ownership: Govt - Hospital District or Authority   Accredited: Yes
Emergency Services: Yes   Licensed Beds: 93
Key Personnel:
Administrator/CEO . . . . Mike Bowers
Emergency Department Manager . . . . Letty Ortiz, RN
Infection Control Director . . . . Charlie Linebaugh
Med/Surg Department Manager . . . . Tamara Rattay, RN
OB/GYN/Women's Health . . . . Michelle Hollingsworth
Surgery Manager . . . . Sheri Weathersbee
Respiratory Care Director . . . . Gayla Satterfield

Phone: 830-775-8566
Fax: 830-768-2630

Measure	Cases	This Hospital	State Average	U.S. Average	Top Hospital
Heart Attack Care					
ACE Inhibitor or ARB for LVSD[1]	5	60%	85%	82%	100%
Aspirin at Arrival	30	87%	91%	92%	100%
Aspirin at Discharge[1]	10	90%	90%	90%	100%
Beta Blocker at Arrival	26	92%	85%	87%	100%
Beta Blocker at Discharge[1]	12	92%	86%	90%	100%
Fibrinolytic Medication Timing	0	-	30%	31%	100%
PCI Within 90 Minutes of Arrival	0	-	48%	54%	95%
Smoking Cessation Advice[1]	2	100%	90%	88%	100%
Heart Failure Care					
ACE Inhibitor or ARB for LVSD	38	87%	82%	82%	100%
Discharge Instructions	105	77%	60%	61%	93%

NOTE: Hospital profiles are in alphabetical order by state, then city, then hospital within the city; Rankings are sorted by rate in descending order and exclude hospitals with less than 25 cases; (1) The number of cases is too small (n<25) for purposes of reliably predicting hospital performance; (2) Measure reflects the hospital's indication that its submission was based upon a sample of its relevant discharges; (3) Rate reflects fewer than the maximum possible quarters of data for the measure; (4) Inaccurate information submitted and suppressed for one or more quarters; (5) No data is available from the hospital for this measure; Please refer to the User's Guide for a full explanation of data

Evaluation of LVS Function	125	70%	81%	83%	99%
Smoking Cessation Advice[1]	13	69%	82%	82%	100%
Pneumonia Care					
Appropriate Initial Antibiotic	55	51%	79%	83%	94%
Blood Culture Timing	40	88%	89%	90%	100%
Influenza Vaccine[1]	20	40%	69%	70%	100%
Initial Antibiotic Timing	65	55%	78%	80%	93%
Oxygenation Assessment	81	98%	99%	99%	100%
Pneumococcal Vaccine	51	43%	68%	69%	94%
Smoking Cessation Advice[1]	11	64%	83%	80%	100%
Surgical Infection Prevention					
Prophylactic Antibiotic Given[2]	100	74%	67%	77%	95%
Prophylactic Antibiotic Selection[1,2]	20	75%	86%	90%	100%
Prophylactic Antibiotic Stopped[2]	97	70%	68%	72%	95%
Pregnancy Care					
Inpatient Neonatal Mortality	-	-	-	-	-
Third or Fourth Degree Laceration	-	-	3.23%	3.63%	3.27%

Texoma Medical Center

1000 Memorial Drive
Denison, TX 75020
E-mail: contactus@thcs.org
URL: www.thcs.org
Ownership: Voluntary non-profit - Private
Emergency Services: Yes

Phone: 903-416-4000
Fax: 903-416-4129

Accredited: Yes
Licensed Beds: 267

Key Personnel:
President/CEO . . . . W Mackey Watkins
Catheterization Lab . . . . Lisa Smith
Coordinator Infection Control . . . . Donna Glenn, RN
Nurse Manager OB/GYN Womens Health . . . . . Anna Hanley
Director Respiratory Therapy . . . . Lisa Smith

Measure	Cases	This Hospital	State Average	U.S. Average	Top Hospital
Heart Attack Care					
ACE Inhibitor or ARB for LVSD	39	92%	85%	82%	100%
Aspirin at Arrival	116	97%	91%	92%	100%
Aspirin at Discharge	130	98%	90%	90%	100%
Beta Blocker at Arrival	102	95%	85%	87%	100%
Beta Blocker at Discharge	138	96%	86%	90%	100%
Fibrinolytic Medication Timing	0	-	30%	31%	100%
PCI Within 90 Minutes of Arrival[1]	9	56%	48%	54%	95%
Smoking Cessation Advice	52	100%	90%	88%	100%
Heart Failure Care					
ACE Inhibitor or ARB for LVSD	88	94%	82%	82%	100%
Discharge Instructions	172	84%	60%	61%	93%
Evaluation of LVS Function	207	93%	81%	83%	99%
Smoking Cessation Advice	40	92%	82%	82%	100%
Pneumonia Care					
Appropriate Initial Antibiotic	169	93%	79%	83%	94%
Blood Culture Timing	133	97%	89%	90%	100%
Influenza Vaccine	43	100%	69%	70%	100%
Initial Antibiotic Timing	212	83%	78%	80%	93%
Oxygenation Assessment	236	100%	99%	99%	100%
Pneumococcal Vaccine	153	99%	68%	69%	94%
Smoking Cessation Advice	52	100%	83%	80%	100%
Surgical Infection Prevention					
Prophylactic Antibiotic Given[3]	374	89%	67%	77%	95%
Prophylactic Antibiotic Selection	124	97%	86%	90%	100%
Prophylactic Antibiotic Stopped[3]	353	92%	68%	72%	95%
Pregnancy Care					
Inpatient Neonatal Mortality	588	0.17%	-	-	-
Third or Fourth Degree Laceration	386	1.55%	3.23%	3.63%	3.27%

Denton Regional Medical Center

Alternate Name: Denton Regional Medical Center
3535 South Interstate 35
Denton, TX 76210
URL: www.dentonregional.com
Ownership: Proprietary
Emergency Services: Yes

Phone: 940-384-3535
Fax: 940-384-4702

Accredited: Yes
Licensed Beds: 288

Key Personnel:
CEO . . . . Jack Bovender
Chief Medical Staff . . . . Stephen Weinberg, MD

Emergency Room . . . . Susan Conn
Director Medical/Surgical Nursing . . . . Helene Kennedy, RN
OB/GYN Womens Health. . . . . Ron Wilson, MD
Chief Radiology . . . . Gregory Naugher, MD
Director Respiratory Therapy . . . . Jana Trevino

Measure	Cases	This Hospital	State Average	U.S. Average	Top Hospital
Heart Attack Care					
ACE Inhibitor or ARB for LVSD[1]	21	100%	85%	82%	100%
Aspirin at Arrival	128	99%	91%	92%	100%
Aspirin at Discharge	202	96%	90%	90%	100%
Beta Blocker at Arrival	114	98%	85%	87%	100%
Beta Blocker at Discharge	198	99%	86%	90%	100%
Fibrinolytic Medication Timing	0	-	30%	31%	100%
PCI Within 90 Minutes of Arrival[1]	5	80%	48%	54%	95%
Smoking Cessation Advice	77	96%	90%	88%	100%
Heart Failure Care					
ACE Inhibitor or ARB for LVSD	79	85%	82%	82%	100%
Discharge Instructions	220	93%	60%	61%	93%
Evaluation of LVS Function	272	92%	81%	83%	99%
Smoking Cessation Advice	52	100%	82%	82%	100%
Pneumonia Care					
Appropriate Initial Antibiotic	118	87%	79%	83%	94%
Blood Culture Timing	136	90%	89%	90%	100%
Influenza Vaccine	58	55%	69%	70%	100%
Initial Antibiotic Timing	200	81%	78%	80%	93%
Oxygenation Assessment	239	100%	99%	99%	100%
Pneumococcal Vaccine	141	62%	68%	69%	94%
Smoking Cessation Advice	55	96%	83%	80%	100%
Surgical Infection Prevention					
Prophylactic Antibiotic Given[2,3]	223	87%	67%	77%	95%
Prophylactic Antibiotic Selection[2]	109	98%	86%	90%	100%
Prophylactic Antibiotic Stopped[2,3]	211	85%	68%	72%	95%
Pregnancy Care					
Inpatient Neonatal Mortality	-	-	-	-	-
Third or Fourth Degree Laceration	-	-	3.23%	3.63%	3.27%

Mayhill Hospital

2809 Mayhill Road
Denton, TX 76208
Ownership: Proprietary
Emergency Services: Yes

Phone: 972-712-3394

Accredited: Yes

Key Personnel:
CEO . . . . Bill Brattvet

Measure	Cases	This Hospital	State Average	U.S. Average	Top Hospital
Heart Attack Care					
ACE Inhibitor or ARB for LVSD[5]	-	-	85%	82%	100%
Aspirin at Arrival[5]	-	-	91%	92%	100%
Aspirin at Discharge[5]	-	-	90%	90%	100%
Beta Blocker at Arrival[5]	-	-	85%	87%	100%
Beta Blocker at Discharge[5]	-	-	86%	90%	100%
Fibrinolytic Medication Timing[5]	-	-	30%	31%	100%
PCI Within 90 Minutes of Arrival[5]	-	-	48%	54%	95%
Smoking Cessation Advice[5]	-	-	90%	88%	100%
Heart Failure Care					
ACE Inhibitor or ARB for LVSD[5]	-	-	82%	82%	100%
Discharge Instructions[5]	-	-	60%	61%	93%
Evaluation of LVS Function[5]	-	-	81%	83%	99%
Smoking Cessation Advice[5]	-	-	82%	82%	100%
Pneumonia Care					
Appropriate Initial Antibiotic[5]	-	-	79%	83%	94%
Blood Culture Timing[5]	-	-	89%	90%	100%
Influenza Vaccine[5]	-	-	69%	70%	100%
Initial Antibiotic Timing[5]	-	-	78%	80%	93%
Oxygenation Assessment[5]	-	-	99%	99%	100%
Pneumococcal Vaccine[5]	-	-	68%	69%	94%
Smoking Cessation Advice[5]	-	-	83%	80%	100%
Surgical Infection Prevention					
Prophylactic Antibiotic Given[5]	-	-	67%	77%	95%
Prophylactic Antibiotic Selection[5]	-	-	86%	90%	100%
Prophylactic Antibiotic Stopped[5]	-	-	68%	72%	95%

NOTE: Hospital profiles are in alphabetical order by state, then city, then hospital within the city; Rankings are sorted by rate in descending order and exclude hospitals with less than 25 cases; (1) The number of cases is too small (n<25) for purposes of reliably predicting hospital performance; (2) Measure reflects the hospital's indication that its submission was based upon a sample of its relevant discharges; (3) Rate reflects fewer than the maximum possible quarters of data for the measure; (4) Inaccurate information submitted and suppressed for one or more quarters; (5) No data is available from the hospital for this measure; Please refer to the User's Guide for a full explanation of data

Pregnancy Care					
Inpatient Neonatal Mortality	-	-	-	-	-
Third or Fourth Degree Laceration	-	-	3.23%	3.63%	3.27%

North Texas Hospital

2801 South Mayhill Road
Denton, TX 76208
Ownership: Government - Federal
Emergency Services: Yes
Key Personnel:
Surgery . . . . Daryl Steward, MD

Phone: 940-220-0600

Accredited: No

Measure	Cases	This Hospital	State Average	U.S. Average	Top Hospital
Heart Attack Care					
ACE Inhibitor or ARB for LVSD[5]	-	-	85%	82%	100%
Aspirin at Arrival[5]	-	-	91%	92%	100%
Aspirin at Discharge[5]	-	-	90%	90%	100%
Beta Blocker at Arrival[5]	-	-	85%	87%	100%
Beta Blocker at Discharge[5]	-	-	86%	90%	100%
Fibrinolytic Medication Timing[5]	-	-	30%	31%	100%
PCI Within 90 Minutes of Arrival[5]	-	-	48%	54%	95%
Smoking Cessation Advice[5]	-	-	90%	88%	100%
Heart Failure Care					
ACE Inhibitor or ARB for LVSD[5]	-	-	82%	82%	100%
Discharge Instructions[5]	-	-	60%	61%	93%
Evaluation of LVS Function[5]	-	-	81%	83%	99%
Smoking Cessation Advice[5]	-	-	82%	82%	100%
Pneumonia Care					
Appropriate Initial Antibiotic[5]	-	-	79%	83%	94%
Blood Culture Timing[5]	-	-	89%	90%	100%
Influenza Vaccine[5]	-	-	69%	70%	100%
Initial Antibiotic Timing[5]	-	-	78%	80%	93%
Oxygenation Assessment[5]	-	-	99%	99%	100%
Pneumococcal Vaccine[5]	-	-	68%	69%	94%
Smoking Cessation Advice[5]	-	-	83%	80%	100%
Surgical Infection Prevention					
Prophylactic Antibiotic Given[3]	0	-	67%	77%	95%
Prophylactic Antibiotic Selection[5]	-	-	86%	90%	100%
Prophylactic Antibiotic Stopped[3]	0	-	68%	72%	95%
Pregnancy Care					
Inpatient Neonatal Mortality	-	-	-	-	-
Third or Fourth Degree Laceration	-	-	3.23%	3.63%	3.27%

Presbyterian Hospital of Denton

3000 N I-35
Denton, TX 76201
Ownership: Proprietary
Emergency Services: Yes
Key Personnel:
Cardiology . . . . Simon Allo, MD
OBGYN . . . . Frederick Cummings, MD
Pulmonary . . . . Jamal Mubarak, MD

Phone: 940-898-7000

Accredited: Yes

Measure	Cases	This Hospital	State Average	U.S. Average	Top Hospital
Heart Attack Care					
ACE Inhibitor or ARB for LVSD	33	91%	85%	82%	100%
Aspirin at Arrival	130	97%	91%	92%	100%
Aspirin at Discharge	158	94%	90%	90%	100%
Beta Blocker at Arrival	104	94%	85%	87%	100%
Beta Blocker at Discharge	161	96%	86%	90%	100%
Fibrinolytic Medication Timing[1]	1	0%	30%	31%	100%
PCI Within 90 Minutes of Arrival[1]	9	33%	48%	54%	95%
Smoking Cessation Advice	68	94%	90%	88%	100%
Heart Failure Care					
ACE Inhibitor or ARB for LVSD	73	75%	82%	82%	100%
Discharge Instructions	209	45%	60%	61%	93%
Evaluation of LVS Function	275	83%	81%	83%	99%
Smoking Cessation Advice	52	81%	82%	82%	100%
Pneumonia Care					
Appropriate Initial Antibiotic	130	76%	79%	83%	94%
Blood Culture Timing	119	96%	89%	90%	100%
Influenza Vaccine	57	60%	69%	70%	100%

Initial Antibiotic Timing	181	80%	78%	80%	93%
Oxygenation Assessment	253	100%	99%	99%	100%
Pneumococcal Vaccine	152	64%	68%	69%	94%
Smoking Cessation Advice	56	79%	83%	80%	100%
Surgical Infection Prevention					
Prophylactic Antibiotic Given	451	95%	67%	77%	95%
Prophylactic Antibiotic Selection	120	98%	86%	90%	100%
Prophylactic Antibiotic Stopped	437	78%	68%	72%	95%
Pregnancy Care					
Inpatient Neonatal Mortality	-	-	-	-	-
Third or Fourth Degree Laceration	-	-	3.23%	3.63%	3.27%

Community General Hospital

230 West Miller
Dilley, TX 78017
Ownership: Proprietary
Emergency Services: Yes

Phone: 830-965-2003

Accredited: Yes

Measure	Cases	This Hospital	State Average	U.S. Average	Top Hospital
Heart Attack Care					
ACE Inhibitor or ARB for LVSD[3]	0	-	85%	82%	100%
Aspirin at Arrival[1,3]	2	100%	91%	92%	100%
Aspirin at Discharge[3]	0	-	90%	90%	100%
Beta Blocker at Arrival[1,3]	2	100%	85%	87%	100%
Beta Blocker at Discharge[3]	0	-	86%	90%	100%
Fibrinolytic Medication Timing[5]	-	-	30%	31%	100%
PCI Within 90 Minutes of Arrival	0	-	48%	54%	95%
Smoking Cessation Advice[3]	0	-	90%	88%	100%
Heart Failure Care					
ACE Inhibitor or ARB for LVSD[3]	0	-	82%	82%	100%
Discharge Instructions[1,3]	3	100%	60%	61%	93%
Evaluation of LVS Function[1,3]	3	100%	81%	83%	99%
Smoking Cessation Advice[3]	0	-	82%	82%	100%
Pneumonia Care					
Appropriate Initial Antibiotic[1,3]	1	100%	79%	83%	94%
Blood Culture Timing[1,3]	1	100%	89%	90%	100%
Influenza Vaccine[5]	-	-	69%	70%	100%
Initial Antibiotic Timing[1,3]	2	100%	78%	80%	93%
Oxygenation Assessment[1,3]	2	100%	99%	99%	100%
Pneumococcal Vaccine[3]	0	-	68%	69%	94%
Smoking Cessation Advice[1,3]	1	100%	83%	80%	100%
Surgical Infection Prevention					
Prophylactic Antibiotic Given[5]	-	-	67%	77%	95%
Prophylactic Antibiotic Selection[5]	-	-	86%	90%	100%
Prophylactic Antibiotic Stopped[5]	-	-	68%	72%	95%
Pregnancy Care					
Inpatient Neonatal Mortality	-	-	-	-	-
Third or Fourth Degree Laceration	-	-	3.23%	3.63%	3.27%

Memorial Hospital

224 E 2nd Street
Dumas, TX 79029
Ownership: Govt - Hospital District or Authority
Emergency Services: Yes
Key Personnel:
CEO. . . . . Theron Park
CNO. . . . . Jackie Simpson
Emergency Room . . . . Bud Faris, DO
Director Infection/Disease Control . . . . Peggy Roberts, RN
Director Medical/Surgical Nursing . . . . Jackie Simpson, RN
OB/GYN Womens Health. . . . . Donald Maraist, MD
Chief Radiology . . . . Kristie Hajek, MD
Director Respiratory Therapy . . . . Sabrina Brown

Phone: 806-935-7171
Fax: 806-934-7842
Accredited: Yes
Licensed Beds: 60

Measure	Cases	This Hospital	State Average	U.S. Average	Top Hospital
Heart Attack Care					
ACE Inhibitor or ARB for LVSD[1,3]	1	100%	85%	82%	100%
Aspirin at Arrival[1,3]	6	67%	91%	92%	100%
Aspirin at Discharge[1,3]	3	100%	90%	90%	100%
Beta Blocker at Arrival[1,3]	6	67%	85%	87%	100%
Beta Blocker at Discharge[1,3]	3	67%	86%	90%	100%
Fibrinolytic Medication Timing[3]	0	-	30%	31%	100%

NOTE: Hospital profiles are in alphabetical order by state, then city, then hospital within the city; Rankings are sorted by rate in descending order and exclude hospitals with less than 25 cases; (1) The number of cases is too small (n<25) for purposes of reliably predicting hospital performance; (2) Measure reflects the hospital's indication that its submission was based upon a sample of its relevant discharges; (3) Rate reflects fewer than the maximum possible quarters of data for the measure; (4) Inaccurate information submitted and suppressed for one or more quarters; (5) No data is available from the hospital for this measure; Please refer to the User's Guide for a full explanation of data

PCI Within 90 Minutes of Arrival	0	-	48%	54%	95%
Smoking Cessation Advice[3]	0	-	90%	88%	100%
Heart Failure Care					
ACE Inhibitor or ARB for LVSD[1]	20	60%	82%	82%	100%
Discharge Instructions[1,3]	11	73%	60%	61%	93%
Evaluation of LVS Function	41	83%	81%	83%	99%
Smoking Cessation Advice[1,3]	6	100%	82%	82%	100%
Pneumonia Care					
Appropriate Initial Antibiotic[1,3]	6	50%	79%	83%	94%
Blood Culture Timing[1,3]	2	50%	89%	90%	100%
Influenza Vaccine[5]	-	-	69%	70%	100%
Initial Antibiotic Timing	50	86%	78%	80%	93%
Oxygenation Assessment	54	98%	99%	99%	100%
Pneumococcal Vaccine	26	62%	68%	69%	94%
Smoking Cessation Advice[1,3]	1	100%	83%	80%	100%
Surgical Infection Prevention					
Prophylactic Antibiotic Given[1,3]	6	33%	67%	77%	95%
Prophylactic Antibiotic Selection[5]	-	-	86%	90%	100%
Prophylactic Antibiotic Stopped[1,3]	6	83%	68%	72%	95%
Pregnancy Care					
Inpatient Neonatal Mortality	-	-	-	-	-
Third or Fourth Degree Laceration	-	-	3.23%	3.63%	3.27%

Fort Duncan Medical Center

Alternate Name: Maverick County Hospital District
350 S Adams Street   Phone: 830-773-5321
Eagle Pass, TX 78852   Fax: 830-758-4851
Ownership: Proprietary   Accredited: Yes
Emergency Services: Yes   Licensed Beds: 77
Key Personnel:
CEO. . . . . Elmo Lopez Jr
Chief Medical Staff. . . . . Carlos E Rodriguez, MD
Emergency Room . . . . Sebastian Padron, MD
Director Infection/Disease Control . . . . Trinidad Justo, RN
Director Medical/Surgical Nursing . . . . Jean Hardt, RN
Director Respiratory Therapy . . . . Samuel Garcia

Measure	Cases	This Hospital	State Average	U.S. Average	Top Hospital
Heart Attack Care					
ACE Inhibitor or ARB for LVSD[1]	4	100%	85%	82%	100%
Aspirin at Arrival	34	91%	91%	92%	100%
Aspirin at Discharge[1]	19	53%	90%	90%	100%
Beta Blocker at Arrival	28	61%	85%	87%	100%
Beta Blocker at Discharge[1]	19	47%	86%	90%	100%
Fibrinolytic Medication Timing	0	-	30%	31%	100%
PCI Within 90 Minutes of Arrival	0	-	48%	54%	95%
Smoking Cessation Advice[1]	3	100%	90%	88%	100%
Heart Failure Care					
ACE Inhibitor or ARB for LVSD	78	74%	82%	82%	100%
Discharge Instructions	217	68%	60%	61%	93%
Evaluation of LVS Function	220	39%	81%	83%	99%
Smoking Cessation Advice	39	79%	82%	82%	100%
Pneumonia Care					
Appropriate Initial Antibiotic	110	74%	79%	83%	94%
Blood Culture Timing	67	67%	89%	90%	100%
Influenza Vaccine[1]	20	35%	69%	70%	100%
Initial Antibiotic Timing	116	66%	78%	80%	93%
Oxygenation Assessment	126	96%	99%	99%	100%
Pneumococcal Vaccine	79	61%	68%	69%	94%
Smoking Cessation Advice[1]	14	79%	83%	80%	100%
Surgical Infection Prevention					
Prophylactic Antibiotic Given[3]	53	40%	67%	77%	95%
Prophylactic Antibiotic Selection[1]	19	89%	86%	90%	100%
Prophylactic Antibiotic Stopped[3]	43	95%	68%	72%	95%
Pregnancy Care					
Inpatient Neonatal Mortality	-	-	-	-	-
Third or Fourth Degree Laceration	-	-	3.23%	3.63%	3.27%

Eastland Memorial Hospital

304 S Daugherty Street   Phone: 254-629-2601
Eastland, TX 76448   Fax: 254-629-8929
E-mail: rrm@eastland-mh.com
URL: www.eastlandmemorial.com
Ownership: Govt - Hospital District or Authority   Accredited: No
Emergency Services: Yes   Licensed Beds: 83
Key Personnel:
President . . . . W H Hoffmann, JR
Administrator/CEO . . . . John Phillips

Measure	Cases	This Hospital	State Average	U.S. Average	Top Hospital
Heart Attack Care					
ACE Inhibitor or ARB for LVSD[3]	0	-	85%	82%	100%
Aspirin at Arrival[1,3]	1	100%	91%	92%	100%
Aspirin at Discharge[3]	0	-	90%	90%	100%
Beta Blocker at Arrival[1,3]	1	100%	85%	87%	100%
Beta Blocker at Discharge[3]	0	-	86%	90%	100%
Fibrinolytic Medication Timing[5]	-	-	30%	31%	100%
PCI Within 90 Minutes of Arrival[5]	-	-	48%	54%	95%
Smoking Cessation Advice[5]	-	-	90%	88%	100%
Heart Failure Care					
ACE Inhibitor or ARB for LVSD[1,2]	16	69%	82%	82%	100%
Discharge Instructions[1,2,3]	12	17%	60%	61%	93%
Evaluation of LVS Function[2]	71	52%	81%	83%	99%
Smoking Cessation Advice[1,2,3]	2	0%	82%	82%	100%
Pneumonia Care					
Appropriate Initial Antibiotic[1,3]	11	91%	79%	83%	94%
Blood Culture Timing[1,3]	17	88%	89%	90%	100%
Influenza Vaccine[5]	-	-	69%	70%	100%
Initial Antibiotic Timing	114	82%	78%	80%	93%
Oxygenation Assessment	121	83%	99%	99%	100%
Pneumococcal Vaccine	83	69%	68%	69%	94%
Smoking Cessation Advice[1,3]	3	100%	83%	80%	100%
Surgical Infection Prevention					
Prophylactic Antibiotic Given[1,3]	5	0%	67%	77%	95%
Prophylactic Antibiotic Selection[5]	-	-	86%	90%	100%
Prophylactic Antibiotic Stopped[1,3]	5	100%	68%	72%	95%
Pregnancy Care					
Inpatient Neonatal Mortality	-	-	-	-	-
Third or Fourth Degree Laceration	-	-	3.23%	3.63%	3.27%

Cornerstone Regional Hospital

2302 Cornerstone Boulevard   Phone: 956-618-4444
Edinburg, TX 78539
Ownership: Proprietary   Accredited: Yes
Emergency Services: Yes

Measure	Cases	This Hospital	State Average	U.S. Average	Top Hospital
Heart Attack Care					
ACE Inhibitor or ARB for LVSD[5]	-	-	85%	82%	100%
Aspirin at Arrival[5]	-	-	91%	92%	100%
Aspirin at Discharge[5]	-	-	90%	90%	100%
Beta Blocker at Arrival[5]	-	-	85%	87%	100%
Beta Blocker at Discharge[5]	-	-	86%	90%	100%
Fibrinolytic Medication Timing[5]	-	-	30%	31%	100%
PCI Within 90 Minutes of Arrival[5]	-	-	48%	54%	95%
Smoking Cessation Advice[5]	-	-	90%	88%	100%
Heart Failure Care					
ACE Inhibitor or ARB for LVSD[3]	0	-	82%	82%	100%
Discharge Instructions[3]	0	-	60%	61%	93%
Evaluation of LVS Function[3]	0	-	81%	83%	99%
Smoking Cessation Advice[3]	0	-	82%	82%	100%
Pneumonia Care					
Appropriate Initial Antibiotic[3]	0	-	79%	83%	94%
Blood Culture Timing[3]	0	-	89%	90%	100%
Influenza Vaccine[5]	-	-	69%	70%	100%
Initial Antibiotic Timing[1]	23	96%	78%	80%	93%
Oxygenation Assessment[1]	24	100%	99%	99%	100%
Pneumococcal Vaccine[1]	13	92%	68%	69%	94%
Smoking Cessation Advice[3]	0	-	83%	80%	100%
Surgical Infection Prevention					

NOTE: Hospital profiles are in alphabetical order by state, then city, then hospital within the city; Rankings are sorted by rate in descending order and exclude hospitals with less than 25 cases; (1) The number of cases is too small (n<25) for purposes of reliably predicting hospital performance; (2) Measure reflects the hospital's indication that its submission was based upon a sample of its relevant discharges; (3) Rate reflects fewer than the maximum possible quarters of data for the measure; (4) Inaccurate information submitted and suppressed for one or more quarters; (5) No data is available from the hospital for this measure; Please refer to the User's Guide for a full explanation of data

Prophylactic Antibiotic Given[3]	51	88%	67%	77%	95%
Prophylactic Antibiotic Selection[5]	-	-	86%	90%	100%
Prophylactic Antibiotic Stopped[3]	51	92%	68%	72%	95%
Pregnancy Care					
Inpatient Neonatal Mortality	-	-	-	-	-
Third or Fourth Degree Laceration	-	-	3.23%	3.63%	3.27%

Doctors Hospital at Renaissance

5501 South McColl Road
Edinburg, TX 78539
URL: www.dhr-rgv.com
Ownership: Voluntary non-profit - Other
Emergency Services: Yes

Phone: 956-661-7503
Fax: 956-661-7331

Accredited: Yes
Licensed Beds: 142

Key Personnel:
CEO. . . . . Joseph B Courtney

Measure	Cases	This Hospital	State Average	U.S. Average	Top Hospital
Heart Attack Care					
ACE Inhibitor or ARB for LVSD	51	69%	85%	82%	100%
Aspirin at Arrival	119	93%	91%	92%	100%
Aspirin at Discharge	203	88%	90%	90%	100%
Beta Blocker at Arrival	113	75%	85%	87%	100%
Beta Blocker at Discharge	212	81%	86%	90%	100%
Fibrinolytic Medication Timing[1]	1	0%	30%	31%	100%
PCI Within 90 Minutes of Arrival[1]	6	50%	48%	54%	95%
Smoking Cessation Advice	35	80%	90%	88%	100%
Heart Failure Care					
ACE Inhibitor or ARB for LVSD[2]	193	70%	82%	82%	100%
Discharge Instructions[2]	359	42%	60%	61%	93%
Evaluation of LVS Function[2]	425	90%	81%	83%	99%
Smoking Cessation Advice[2]	56	80%	82%	82%	100%
Pneumonia Care					
Appropriate Initial Antibiotic	85	80%	79%	83%	94%
Blood Culture Timing	65	92%	89%	90%	100%
Influenza Vaccine[1]	20	20%	69%	70%	100%
Initial Antibiotic Timing	112	46%	78%	80%	93%
Oxygenation Assessment	153	100%	99%	99%	100%
Pneumococcal Vaccine	102	18%	68%	69%	94%
Smoking Cessation Advice[1]	20	75%	83%	80%	100%
Surgical Infection Prevention					
Prophylactic Antibiotic Given[2]	372	76%	67%	77%	95%
Prophylactic Antibiotic Selection[2]	98	74%	86%	90%	100%
Prophylactic Antibiotic Stopped[2]	346	45%	68%	72%	95%
Pregnancy Care					
Inpatient Neonatal Mortality	-	-	-	-	-
Third or Fourth Degree Laceration	-	-	3.23%	3.63%	3.27%

Edinburg Regional Medical Center

Alternate Name: Edinburg Hospital
1102 W Trenton Road
Edinburg, TX 78539
URL: www.edinburgregional.com
Ownership: Proprietary
Emergency Services: Yes

Phone: 956-388-6000
Fax: 956-388-6020

Accredited: Yes
Licensed Beds: 250

Key Personnel:
CEO. . . . . James Christian Smolik

Measure	Cases	This Hospital	State Average	U.S. Average	Top Hospital
Heart Attack Care					
ACE Inhibitor or ARB for LVSD[1]	11	45%	85%	82%	100%
Aspirin at Arrival	46	87%	91%	92%	100%
Aspirin at Discharge	31	55%	90%	90%	100%
Beta Blocker at Arrival	35	77%	85%	87%	100%
Beta Blocker at Discharge	31	65%	86%	90%	100%
Fibrinolytic Medication Timing	0	-	30%	31%	100%
PCI Within 90 Minutes of Arrival	0	-	48%	54%	95%
Smoking Cessation Advice[1]	3	33%	90%	88%	100%
Heart Failure Care					
ACE Inhibitor or ARB for LVSD	43	44%	82%	82%	100%
Discharge Instructions	130	43%	60%	61%	93%
Evaluation of LVS Function	154	81%	81%	83%	99%
Smoking Cessation Advice[1]	17	65%	82%	82%	100%

Pneumonia Care					
Appropriate Initial Antibiotic[2]	78	83%	79%	83%	94%
Blood Culture Timing[2]	43	95%	89%	90%	100%
Influenza Vaccine[1,2]	15	73%	69%	70%	100%
Initial Antibiotic Timing[2]	90	56%	78%	80%	93%
Oxygenation Assessment[2]	120	99%	99%	99%	100%
Pneumococcal Vaccine[2]	73	55%	68%	69%	94%
Smoking Cessation Advice[2]	25	92%	83%	80%	100%
Surgical Infection Prevention					
Prophylactic Antibiotic Given[2]	55	36%	67%	77%	95%
Prophylactic Antibiotic Selection[1,2]	13	92%	86%	90%	100%
Prophylactic Antibiotic Stopped[2]	55	16%	68%	72%	95%
Pregnancy Care					
Inpatient Neonatal Mortality	-	-	-	-	-
Third or Fourth Degree Laceration	-	-	3.23%	3.63%	3.27%

El Campo Memorial Hospital

303 Sandy Corner Road
El Campo, TX 77437
E-mail: sgularte@ecmh.org
URL: www.ecmh.org
Ownership: Voluntary non-profit - Other
Emergency Services: Yes

Phone: 979-543-6251
Fax: 979-543-8420

Accredited: No
Licensed Beds: 49

Key Personnel:
Administrator/CEO. . . . . Steve Gularte
Chief Medical Staff. . . . . Ankus Sarkar, MD
Emergency Room . . . . Tom N Baccam, DO
Emergency Room . . . . Carlos Duqua, MD
Director Infection/Disease Control . . . . Sherrie Hardin, RN
ICU . . . . Sherrie Hardin, RN
Medical Surgical Nursing . . . . Jennifer Monroe, RN
CEO. . . . . Steven Gularte
Director Radiology . . . . Ron Price, RT
Respiratory/Cardiopulmonary. . . . . Jim Burger

Measure	Cases	This Hospital	State Average	U.S. Average	Top Hospital
Heart Attack Care					
ACE Inhibitor or ARB for LVSD	0	-	85%	82%	100%
Aspirin at Arrival[1]	17	71%	91%	92%	100%
Aspirin at Discharge[1]	4	100%	90%	90%	100%
Beta Blocker at Arrival[1]	14	64%	85%	87%	100%
Beta Blocker at Discharge[1]	5	60%	86%	90%	100%
Fibrinolytic Medication Timing	0	-	30%	31%	100%
PCI Within 90 Minutes of Arrival	0	-	48%	54%	95%
Smoking Cessation Advice	0	-	90%	88%	100%
Heart Failure Care					
ACE Inhibitor or ARB for LVSD[1]	5	60%	82%	82%	100%
Discharge Instructions	46	50%	60%	61%	93%
Evaluation of LVS Function	59	90%	81%	83%	99%
Smoking Cessation Advice[1]	6	0%	82%	82%	100%
Pneumonia Care					
Appropriate Initial Antibiotic	44	66%	79%	83%	94%
Blood Culture Timing	31	100%	89%	90%	100%
Influenza Vaccine[1]	11	82%	69%	70%	100%
Initial Antibiotic Timing	70	79%	78%	80%	93%
Oxygenation Assessment	77	100%	99%	99%	100%
Pneumococcal Vaccine	50	80%	68%	69%	94%
Smoking Cessation Advice[1]	10	20%	83%	80%	100%
Surgical Infection Prevention					
Prophylactic Antibiotic Given[1,3]	2	100%	67%	77%	95%
Prophylactic Antibiotic Selection[1]	2	0%	86%	90%	100%
Prophylactic Antibiotic Stopped[1,3]	2	100%	68%	72%	95%
Pregnancy Care					
Inpatient Neonatal Mortality	-	-	-	-	-
Third or Fourth Degree Laceration	-	-	3.23%	3.63%	3.27%

NOTE: Hospital profiles are in alphabetical order by state, then city, then hospital within the city; Rankings are sorted by rate in descending order and exclude hospitals with less than 25 cases; (1) The number of cases is too small (n<25) for purposes of reliably predicting hospital performance; (2) Measure reflects the hospital's indication that its submission was based upon a sample of its relevant discharges; (3) Rate reflects fewer than the maximum possible quarters of data for the measure; (4) Inaccurate information submitted and suppressed for one or more quarters; (5) No data is available from the hospital for this measure; Please refer to the User's Guide for a full explanation of data

Del Sol Medical Center

10301 Gateway West
El Paso, TX 79925
URL: www.delsolhealth.com
Ownership: Proprietary
Emergency Services: Yes

Phone: 915-595-9000
Fax: 915-594-5966

Accredited: Yes
Licensed Beds: 336

Key Personnel:
CEO . . . . Doug Matney
Emergency Room . . . . Jaime Moreno, MD
Director Infection/Disease Control . . . . Enid Seguinot
Chair OB/GYN . . . . Michiel Noe, MD
Director Radiology . . . . Carrie Gardy

Measure	Cases	This Hospital	State Average	U.S. Average	Top Hospital
Heart Attack Care					
ACE Inhibitor or ARB for LVSD	34	71%	85%	82%	100%
Aspirin at Arrival	207	98%	91%	92%	100%
Aspirin at Discharge	189	89%	90%	90%	100%
Beta Blocker at Arrival	139	91%	85%	87%	100%
Beta Blocker at Discharge	159	94%	86%	90%	100%
Fibrinolytic Medication Timing[1]	16	38%	30%	31%	100%
PCI Within 90 Minutes of Arrival[1]	8	50%	48%	54%	95%
Smoking Cessation Advice	67	96%	90%	88%	100%
Heart Failure Care					
ACE Inhibitor or ARB for LVSD	150	73%	82%	82%	100%
Discharge Instructions	378	84%	60%	61%	93%
Evaluation of LVS Function	429	81%	81%	83%	99%
Smoking Cessation Advice	76	95%	82%	82%	100%
Pneumonia Care					
Appropriate Initial Antibiotic	333	64%	79%	83%	94%
Blood Culture Timing	239	91%	89%	90%	100%
Influenza Vaccine	88	39%	69%	70%	100%
Initial Antibiotic Timing	451	67%	78%	80%	93%
Oxygenation Assessment	535	99%	99%	99%	100%
Pneumococcal Vaccine	315	33%	68%	69%	94%
Smoking Cessation Advice	123	93%	83%	80%	100%
Surgical Infection Prevention					
Prophylactic Antibiotic Given[2,3]	129	64%	67%	77%	95%
Prophylactic Antibiotic Selection[2]	49	84%	86%	90%	100%
Prophylactic Antibiotic Stopped[2,3]	118	75%	68%	72%	95%
Pregnancy Care					
Inpatient Neonatal Mortality	-	-	-	-	-
Third or Fourth Degree Laceration	-	-	3.23%	3.63%	3.27%

El Paso Specialty Hospital

1755 Curie Suite A
El Paso, TX 79902
Ownership: Proprietary
Emergency Services: Yes

Phone: 915-544-3636

Accredited: Yes

Measure	Cases	This Hospital	State Average	U.S. Average	Top Hospital
Heart Attack Care					
ACE Inhibitor or ARB for LVSD[5]	-	-	85%	82%	100%
Aspirin at Arrival[5]	-	-	91%	92%	100%
Aspirin at Discharge[5]	-	-	90%	90%	100%
Beta Blocker at Arrival[5]	-	-	85%	87%	100%
Beta Blocker at Discharge[5]	-	-	86%	90%	100%
Fibrinolytic Medication Timing[5]	-	-	30%	31%	100%
PCI Within 90 Minutes of Arrival[5]	-	-	48%	54%	95%
Smoking Cessation Advice[5]	-	-	90%	88%	100%
Heart Failure Care					
ACE Inhibitor or ARB for LVSD[5]	-	-	82%	82%	100%
Discharge Instructions[5]	-	-	60%	61%	93%
Evaluation of LVS Function[5]	-	-	81%	83%	99%
Smoking Cessation Advice[5]	-	-	82%	82%	100%
Pneumonia Care					
Appropriate Initial Antibiotic[5]	-	-	79%	83%	94%
Blood Culture Timing[5]	-	-	89%	90%	100%
Influenza Vaccine[5]	-	-	69%	70%	100%
Initial Antibiotic Timing[5]	-	-	78%	80%	93%
Oxygenation Assessment[5]	-	-	99%	99%	100%
Pneumococcal Vaccine[5]	-	-	68%	69%	94%

Measure	Cases	This Hospital	State Average	U.S. Average	Top Hospital
Smoking Cessation Advice[5]	-	-	83%	80%	100%
Surgical Infection Prevention					
Prophylactic Antibiotic Given[3]	341	88%	67%	77%	95%
Prophylactic Antibiotic Selection	109	100%	86%	90%	100%
Prophylactic Antibiotic Stopped[3]	340	90%	68%	72%	95%
Pregnancy Care					
Inpatient Neonatal Mortality	-	-	-	-	-
Third or Fourth Degree Laceration	-	-	3.23%	3.63%	3.27%

Las Palmas Medical Center

1801 N Oregon Street
El Paso, TX 79902
URL: www.laspalmashealth.com
Ownership: Proprietary
Emergency Services: Yes

Phone: 915-521-1200
Fax: 915-544-5203

Accredited: Yes
Licensed Beds: 317

Key Personnel:
CEO . . . . Hank Hernandez
Chief Medical Staff . . . . Emilio Gonzalez-Ayala, MD
Chief Catheterization Laboratory . . . . William Foote, MD
Emergency Room . . . . Mitchell Farrell, MD
Director Medical/Surgical Nursing . . . . Joann Owen
OB/GYN Womens Health . . . . Brion Gluck, MD
Chief Radiology . . . . Hugo Isuani, MD
Director Respiratory Therapy . . . . Danny Alvarel

Measure	Cases	This Hospital	State Average	U.S. Average	Top Hospital
Heart Attack Care					
ACE Inhibitor or ARB for LVSD[1]	13	77%	85%	82%	100%
Aspirin at Arrival	59	98%	91%	92%	100%
Aspirin at Discharge	71	93%	90%	90%	100%
Beta Blocker at Arrival	41	95%	85%	87%	100%
Beta Blocker at Discharge	58	95%	86%	90%	100%
Fibrinolytic Medication Timing[1]	3	67%	30%	31%	100%
PCI Within 90 Minutes of Arrival	0	-	48%	54%	95%
Smoking Cessation Advice	28	100%	90%	88%	100%
Heart Failure Care					
ACE Inhibitor or ARB for LVSD	65	77%	82%	82%	100%
Discharge Instructions	183	71%	60%	61%	93%
Evaluation of LVS Function	205	86%	81%	83%	99%
Smoking Cessation Advice	30	100%	82%	82%	100%
Pneumonia Care					
Appropriate Initial Antibiotic	81	72%	79%	83%	94%
Blood Culture Timing	87	87%	89%	90%	100%
Influenza Vaccine[4,5]	-	-	69%	70%	100%
Initial Antibiotic Timing	136	76%	78%	80%	93%
Oxygenation Assessment	178	98%	99%	99%	100%
Pneumococcal Vaccine	112	53%	68%	69%	94%
Smoking Cessation Advice	33	100%	83%	80%	100%
Surgical Infection Prevention					
Prophylactic Antibiotic Given[2,3]	211	92%	67%	77%	95%
Prophylactic Antibiotic Selection[2]	94	99%	86%	90%	100%
Prophylactic Antibiotic Stopped[2,3]	209	66%	68%	72%	95%
Pregnancy Care					
Inpatient Neonatal Mortality	-	-	-	-	-
Third or Fourth Degree Laceration	-	-	3.23%	3.63%	3.27%

Physicians Specialty Hospital of El Paso

1416 George Dieter
El Paso, TX 79936
Ownership: Proprietary
Emergency Services: Yes

Phone: 915-598-4240

Accredited: Yes

Measure	Cases	This Hospital	State Average	U.S. Average	Top Hospital
Heart Attack Care					
ACE Inhibitor or ARB for LVSD[1]	5	100%	85%	82%	100%
Aspirin at Arrival[1]	24	79%	91%	92%	100%
Aspirin at Discharge	28	82%	90%	90%	100%
Beta Blocker at Arrival[1]	24	75%	85%	87%	100%
Beta Blocker at Discharge	28	61%	86%	90%	100%
Fibrinolytic Medication Timing[3]	0	-	30%	31%	100%
PCI Within 90 Minutes of Arrival[1]	3	67%	48%	54%	95%
Smoking Cessation Advice[1,3]	3	67%	90%	88%	100%

NOTE: Hospital profiles are in alphabetical order by state, then city, then hospital within the city; Rankings are sorted by rate in descending order and exclude hospitals with less than 25 cases; (1) The number of cases is too small (n<25) for purposes of reliably predicting hospital performance; (2) Measure reflects the hospital's indication that its submission was based upon a sample of its relevant discharges; (3) Rate reflects fewer than the maximum possible quarters of data for the measure; (4) Inaccurate information submitted and suppressed for one or more quarters; (5) No data is available from the hospital for this measure; Please refer to the User's Guide for a full explanation of data

Heart Failure Care					
ACE Inhibitor or ARB for LVSD	40	70%	82%	82%	100%
Discharge Instructions[1,3]	18	0%	60%	61%	93%
Evaluation of LVS Function	81	84%	81%	83%	99%
Smoking Cessation Advice[1,3]	1	0%	82%	82%	100%
Pneumonia Care					
Appropriate Initial Antibiotic[1,3]	10	70%	79%	83%	94%
Blood Culture Timing[1,3]	4	25%	89%	90%	100%
Influenza Vaccine[5]	-	-	69%	70%	100%
Initial Antibiotic Timing	80	36%	78%	80%	93%
Oxygenation Assessment	109	100%	99%	99%	100%
Pneumococcal Vaccine	66	0%	68%	69%	94%
Smoking Cessation Advice[1,3]	2	100%	83%	80%	100%
Surgical Infection Prevention					
Prophylactic Antibiotic Given[3]	37	11%	67%	77%	95%
Prophylactic Antibiotic Selection[5]	-	-	86%	90%	100%
Prophylactic Antibiotic Stopped[3]	26	65%	68%	72%	95%
Pregnancy Care					
Inpatient Neonatal Mortality	-	-	-	-	-
Third or Fourth Degree Laceration	-	-	3.23%	3.63%	3.27%

Providence Memorial Hospital

2001 N Oregon Street
El Paso, TX 79902
URL: www.sphn.com
Ownership: Voluntary non-profit - Other
Emergency Services: Yes

Phone: 915-577-6011
Fax: 915-577-6109

Accredited: Yes
Licensed Beds: 508

Key Personnel:
CEO. . . . . Thomas E Casaday
Emergency Room . . . . Carl Templin
Director of Respiratory . . . . Vicente Carmone

Measure	Cases	This Hospital	State Average	U.S. Average	Top Hospital
Heart Attack Care					
ACE Inhibitor or ARB for LVSD	34	68%	85%	82%	100%
Aspirin at Arrival	136	100%	91%	92%	100%
Aspirin at Discharge	132	97%	90%	90%	100%
Beta Blocker at Arrival	106	93%	85%	87%	100%
Beta Blocker at Discharge	122	88%	86%	90%	100%
Fibrinolytic Medication Timing[1]	10	30%	30%	31%	100%
PCI Within 90 Minutes of Arrival[1]	6	0%	48%	54%	95%
Smoking Cessation Advice	32	97%	90%	88%	100%
Heart Failure Care					
ACE Inhibitor or ARB for LVSD	151	86%	82%	82%	100%
Discharge Instructions	377	69%	60%	61%	93%
Evaluation of LVS Function	406	89%	81%	83%	99%
Smoking Cessation Advice	28	93%	82%	82%	100%
Pneumonia Care					
Appropriate Initial Antibiotic	291	74%	79%	83%	94%
Blood Culture Timing	202	82%	89%	90%	100%
Influenza Vaccine[4,5]	-	-	69%	70%	100%
Initial Antibiotic Timing	361	70%	78%	80%	93%
Oxygenation Assessment	436	100%	99%	99%	100%
Pneumococcal Vaccine	274	91%	68%	69%	94%
Smoking Cessation Advice	39	62%	83%	80%	100%
Surgical Infection Prevention					
Prophylactic Antibiotic Given[2]	327	86%	67%	77%	95%
Prophylactic Antibiotic Selection[2]	78	96%	86%	90%	100%
Prophylactic Antibiotic Stopped[2]	323	64%	68%	72%	95%
Pregnancy Care					
Inpatient Neonatal Mortality	-	-	-	-	-
Third or Fourth Degree Laceration	-	-	3.23%	3.63%	3.27%

Sierra Medical Center

1625 Medical Center Drive
El Paso, TX 79902
URL: www.sphn.com
Ownership: Proprietary
Emergency Services: Yes

Phone: 915-747-4000
Fax: 915-747-2550

Accredited: Yes
Licensed Beds: 365

Key Personnel:
President/CEO. . . . . Thomas E Casaday

Measure	Cases	This Hospital	State Average	U.S. Average	Top Hospital
Heart Attack Care					
ACE Inhibitor or ARB for LVSD[1]	22	73%	85%	82%	100%
Aspirin at Arrival	127	99%	91%	92%	100%
Aspirin at Discharge	121	96%	90%	90%	100%
Beta Blocker at Arrival	87	89%	85%	87%	100%
Beta Blocker at Discharge	119	83%	86%	90%	100%
Fibrinolytic Medication Timing[1]	3	0%	30%	31%	100%
PCI Within 90 Minutes of Arrival[1]	4	0%	48%	54%	95%
Smoking Cessation Advice	30	93%	90%	88%	100%
Heart Failure Care					
ACE Inhibitor or ARB for LVSD	206	73%	82%	82%	100%
Discharge Instructions	425	35%	60%	61%	93%
Evaluation of LVS Function	490	90%	81%	83%	99%
Smoking Cessation Advice	60	82%	82%	82%	100%
Pneumonia Care					
Appropriate Initial Antibiotic	209	85%	79%	83%	94%
Blood Culture Timing	195	85%	89%	90%	100%
Influenza Vaccine	76	84%	69%	70%	100%
Initial Antibiotic Timing	303	67%	78%	80%	93%
Oxygenation Assessment	380	99%	99%	99%	100%
Pneumococcal Vaccine	268	86%	68%	69%	94%
Smoking Cessation Advice	63	76%	83%	80%	100%
Surgical Infection Prevention					
Prophylactic Antibiotic Given[2]	320	77%	67%	77%	95%
Prophylactic Antibiotic Selection[2]	81	98%	86%	90%	100%
Prophylactic Antibiotic Stopped[2]	312	57%	68%	72%	95%
Pregnancy Care					
Inpatient Neonatal Mortality	-	-	-	-	-
Third or Fourth Degree Laceration	-	-	3.23%	3.63%	3.27%

Southwestern General Hospital

Alternate Name: AMI Southwestern General Hospital
1221 N Cotton
El Paso, TX 79902
Ownership: Proprietary
Emergency Services: Yes

Phone: 915-496-9600
Fax: 915-496-9629
Accredited: Yes
Licensed Beds: 120

Key Personnel:
CEO. . . . . Joseph Wright
Chief Medical Staff. . . . . Irene Gomez
Emergency Room . . . . Jose Blanco, RN
Manager Radiology . . . . Joe Calderon
Manager Respiratory Therapy . . . . Melvin Bounds

Measure	Cases	This Hospital	State Average	U.S. Average	Top Hospital
Heart Attack Care					
ACE Inhibitor or ARB for LVSD[5]	-	-	85%	82%	100%
Aspirin at Arrival[5]	-	-	91%	92%	100%
Aspirin at Discharge[5]	-	-	90%	90%	100%
Beta Blocker at Arrival[5]	-	-	85%	87%	100%
Beta Blocker at Discharge[5]	-	-	86%	90%	100%
Fibrinolytic Medication Timing[5]	-	-	30%	31%	100%
PCI Within 90 Minutes of Arrival[5]	-	-	48%	54%	95%
Smoking Cessation Advice[5]	-	-	90%	88%	100%
Heart Failure Care					
ACE Inhibitor or ARB for LVSD[1]	2	100%	82%	82%	100%
Discharge Instructions[1,3]	9	100%	60%	61%	93%
Evaluation of LVS Function	31	48%	81%	83%	99%
Smoking Cessation Advice[1,3]	1	100%	82%	82%	100%
Pneumonia Care					
Appropriate Initial Antibiotic[1,3]	1	0%	79%	83%	94%
Blood Culture Timing[3]	0	-	89%	90%	100%
Influenza Vaccine[5]	-	-	69%	70%	100%
Initial Antibiotic Timing	32	59%	78%	80%	93%
Oxygenation Assessment	39	100%	99%	99%	100%
Pneumococcal Vaccine[1]	22	36%	68%	69%	94%
Smoking Cessation Advice[1,3]	1	100%	83%	80%	100%
Surgical infection Prevention					
Prophylactic Antibiotic Given[5]	-	-	67%	77%	95%
Prophylactic Antibiotic Selection[5]	-	-	86%	90%	100%
Prophylactic Antibiotic Stopped[5]	-	-	68%	72%	95%

NOTE: Hospital profiles are in alphabetical order by state, then city, then hospital within the city; Rankings are sorted by rate in descending order and exclude hospitals with less than 25 cases; (1) The number of cases is too small (n<25) for purposes of reliably predicting hospital performance; (2) Measure reflects the hospital's indication that its submission was based upon a sample of its relevant discharges; (3) Rate reflects fewer than the maximum possible quarters of data for the measure; (4) Inaccurate information submitted and suppressed for one or more quarters; (5) No data is available from the hospital for this measure; Please refer to the User's Guide for a full explanation of data

Pregnancy Care					
Inpatient Neonatal Mortality	-	-	-	-	-
Third or Fourth Degree Laceration	-	-	3.23%	3.63%	3.27%

Thomason General Hospital

4815 Alameda Avenue
El Paso, TX 79905
URL: www.thomasoncares.org
Ownership: Govt - Hospital District or Authority
Emergency Services: Yes

Phone: 915-544-1200
Fax: 915-521-7975

Accredited: Yes
Licensed Beds: 346

Key Personnel:
President/CEO........................ James N Valenti
Chief Medical Staff..................... Mathew J Walsh, MD
Director Medical/Surgical Nursing .... Dian Cassidy, RN
OB/GYN Womens Health................. Frederick E Harlass, MD
Director Respiratory Therapy.............. Robert Ontiveros

Measure	Cases	This Hospital	State Average	U.S. Average	Top Hospital
Heart Attack Care					
ACE Inhibitor or ARB for LVSD[1]	20	80%	85%	82%	100%
Aspirin at Arrival	86	100%	91%	92%	100%
Aspirin at Discharge	54	98%	90%	90%	100%
Beta Blocker at Arrival	81	96%	85%	87%	100%
Beta Blocker at Discharge	63	97%	86%	90%	100%
Fibrinolytic Medication Timing	0	-	30%	31%	100%
PCI Within 90 Minutes of Arrival	0	-	48%	54%	95%
Smoking Cessation Advice	25	100%	90%	88%	100%
Heart Failure Care					
ACE Inhibitor or ARB for LVSD	87	90%	82%	82%	100%
Discharge Instructions	183	83%	60%	61%	93%
Evaluation of LVS Function	185	97%	81%	83%	99%
Smoking Cessation Advice	92	100%	82%	82%	100%
Pneumonia Care					
Appropriate Initial Antibiotic[2]	125	91%	79%	83%	94%
Blood Culture Timing[2]	101	84%	89%	90%	100%
Influenza Vaccine[2]	29	83%	69%	70%	100%
Initial Antibiotic Timing[2]	145	63%	78%	80%	93%
Oxygenation Assessment[2]	156	100%	99%	99%	100%
Pneumococcal Vaccine[2]	62	76%	68%	69%	94%
Smoking Cessation Advice[2]	64	100%	83%	80%	100%
Surgical Infection Prevention					
Prophylactic Antibiotic Given[2]	173	77%	67%	77%	95%
Prophylactic Antibiotic Selection[2]	42	98%	86%	90%	100%
Prophylactic Antibiotic Stopped[2]	162	79%	68%	72%	95%
Pregnancy Care					
Inpatient Neonatal Mortality	-	-	-	-	-
Third or Fourth Degree Laceration	-	-	3.23%	3.63%	3.27%

Ennis Regional Medical Center

803 West Lampasas
Ennis, TX 75119
URL: www.ennisregional.com
Ownership: Proprietary
Emergency Services: Yes

Phone: 972-875-0900
Fax: 972-875-0537

Accredited: Yes
Licensed Beds: 45

Key Personnel:
CEO................................ Bernie Sweet

Measure	Cases	This Hospital	State Average	U.S. Average	Top Hospital
Heart Attack Care					
ACE Inhibitor or ARB for LVSD[3]	0	-	85%	82%	100%
Aspirin at Arrival[1,3]	4	100%	91%	92%	100%
Aspirin at Discharge[1,3]	2	50%	90%	90%	100%
Beta Blocker at Arrival[1,3]	4	100%	85%	87%	100%
Beta Blocker at Discharge[1,3]	2	100%	86%	90%	100%
Fibrinolytic Medication Timing[1,3]	1	0%	30%	31%	100%
PCI Within 90 Minutes of Arrival	0	-	48%	54%	95%
Smoking Cessation Advice[3]	0	-	90%	88%	100%
Heart Failure Care					
ACE Inhibitor or ARB for LVSD	30	93%	82%	82%	100%
Discharge Instructions	73	55%	60%	61%	93%
Evaluation of LVS Function	99	73%	81%	83%	99%
Smoking Cessation Advice[1]	23	83%	82%	82%	100%

Pneumonia Care					
Appropriate Initial Antibiotic	67	82%	79%	83%	94%
Blood Culture Timing	52	79%	89%	90%	100%
Influenza Vaccine	25	48%	69%	70%	100%
Initial Antibiotic Timing	96	77%	78%	80%	93%
Oxygenation Assessment	107	99%	99%	99%	100%
Pneumococcal Vaccine	68	46%	68%	69%	94%
Smoking Cessation Advice[1]	24	96%	83%	80%	100%
Surgical Infection Prevention					
Prophylactic Antibiotic Given[3]	72	43%	67%	77%	95%
Prophylactic Antibiotic Selection	26	100%	86%	90%	100%
Prophylactic Antibiotic Stopped[3]	71	76%	68%	72%	95%
Pregnancy Care					
Inpatient Neonatal Mortality	-	-	-	-	-
Third or Fourth Degree Laceration	-	-	3.23%	3.63%	3.27%

East Texas Medical Center-Fairfield

Alternate Name: Fairfield Memorial Hospital
125 Newman Street
Fairfield, TX 75840
URL: www.etmc.org
Ownership: Voluntary non-profit - Other
Emergency Services: Yes

Phone: 903-389-2121
Fax: 903-389-1601

Accredited: No
Licensed Beds: 48

Key Personnel:
Administrator .... Ruth Cook
Chief Medical Staff...................... Glenn Routhouska

Measure	Cases	This Hospital	State Average	U.S. Average	Top Hospital
Heart Attack Care					
ACE Inhibitor or ARB for LVSD[3]	0	-	85%	82%	100%
Aspirin at Arrival[1,3]	1	100%	91%	92%	100%
Aspirin at Discharge[3]	0	-	90%	90%	100%
Beta Blocker at Arrival[3]	0	-	85%	87%	100%
Beta Blocker at Discharge[1,3]	1	0%	86%	90%	100%
Fibrinolytic Medication Timing[3]	0	-	30%	31%	100%
PCI Within 90 Minutes of Arrival	0	-	48%	54%	95%
Smoking Cessation Advice[3]	0	-	90%	88%	100%
Heart Failure Care					
ACE Inhibitor or ARB for LVSD[1]	6	83%	82%	82%	100%
Discharge Instructions[1,3]	13	0%	60%	61%	93%
Evaluation of LVS Function	67	43%	81%	83%	99%
Smoking Cessation Advice[1,3]	2	50%	82%	82%	100%
Pneumonia Care					
Appropriate Initial Antibiotic[1,3]	10	80%	79%	83%	94%
Blood Culture Timing[1,3]	11	91%	89%	90%	100%
Influenza Vaccine[5]	-	-	69%	70%	100%
Initial Antibiotic Timing	34	71%	78%	80%	93%
Oxygenation Assessment	47	98%	99%	99%	100%
Pneumococcal Vaccine	30	43%	68%	69%	94%
Smoking Cessation Advice[1,3]	1	100%	83%	80%	100%
Surgical Infection Prevention					
Prophylactic Antibiotic Given[3]	0	-	67%	77%	95%
Prophylactic Antibiotic Selection[5]	-	-	86%	90%	100%
Prophylactic Antibiotic Stopped[3]	0	-	68%	72%	95%
Pregnancy Care					
Inpatient Neonatal Mortality	-	-	-	-	-
Third or Fourth Degree Laceration	-	-	3.23%	3.63%	3.27%

Connally Memorial Medical Center

499 10th Street
Floresville, TX 78114
Ownership: Government - Local
Emergency Services: No

Phone: 830-393-3122

Accredited: No

Measure	Cases	This Hospital	State Average	U.S. Average	Top Hospital
Heart Attack Care					
ACE Inhibitor or ARB for LVSD[1]	3	100%	85%	82%	100%
Aspirin at Arrival	34	82%	91%	92%	100%
Aspirin at Discharge[1]	23	78%	90%	90%	100%
Beta Blocker at Arrival	34	56%	85%	87%	100%
Beta Blocker at Discharge[1]	21	62%	86%	90%	100%
Fibrinolytic Medication Timing	0	-	30%	31%	100%

NOTE: Hospital profiles are in alphabetical order by state, then city, then hospital within the city; Rankings are sorted by rate in descending order and exclude hospitals with less than 25 cases; (1) The number of cases is too small (n<25) for purposes of reliably predicting hospital performance; (2) Measure reflects the hospital's indication that its submission was based upon a sample of its relevant discharges; (3) Rate reflects fewer than the maximum possible quarters of data for the measure; (4) Inaccurate information submitted and suppressed for one or more quarters; (5) No data is available from the hospital for this measure; Please refer to the User's Guide for a full explanation of data

PCI Within 90 Minutes of Arrival	0	-	48%	54%	95%
Smoking Cessation Advice[1]	2	100%	90%	88%	100%
Heart Failure Care					
ACE Inhibitor or ARB for LVSD[1,3]	5	60%	82%	82%	100%
Discharge Instructions[1,3]	9	22%	60%	61%	93%
Evaluation of LVS Function[1,3]	17	82%	81%	83%	99%
Smoking Cessation Advice[1,3]	1	100%	82%	82%	100%
Pneumonia Care					
Appropriate Initial Antibiotic[1]	24	42%	79%	83%	94%
Blood Culture Timing[1]	24	88%	89%	90%	100%
Influenza Vaccine[1]	11	100%	69%	70%	100%
Initial Antibiotic Timing	42	55%	78%	80%	93%
Oxygenation Assessment	52	100%	99%	99%	100%
Pneumococcal Vaccine	43	91%	68%	69%	94%
Smoking Cessation Advice[1]	9	100%	83%	80%	100%
Surgical Infection Prevention					
Prophylactic Antibiotic Given	25	48%	67%	77%	95%
Prophylactic Antibiotic Selection[1]	7	100%	86%	90%	100%
Prophylactic Antibiotic Stopped[1]	22	91%	68%	72%	95%
Pregnancy Care					
Inpatient Neonatal Mortality	-	-	-	-	-
Third or Fourth Degree Laceration	-	-	3.23%	3.63%	3.27%

Pecos County Memorial Hosptial

Sanderson Highway
Fort Stockton, TX 79735
Ownership: Voluntary non-profit - Other
Emergency Services: Yes

Phone: 432-336-2004
Fax: 432-336-4526
Accredited: No
Licensed Beds: 37

Key Personnel:
Administrator/CEO . . . . Nick Blythe
Chief Medical Staff . . . . Sandy Young
Emergency Room . . . . Cecil R George, MD
Director Infection/Disease Control . . . . Brenda Holiday, RN
Director Medical/Surgical Nursing . . . . Karen Romirea, RN
OB/GYN Womens Health. . . . . Cecil R George, MD
Director Respiratory Therapy . . . . Patty Reyna

Measure	Cases	This Hospital	State Average	U.S. Average	Top Hospital
Heart Attack Care					
ACE Inhibitor or ARB for LVSD[3]	0	-	85%	82%	100%
Aspirin at Arrival[1,3]	2	50%	91%	92%	100%
Aspirin at Discharge[1,3]	1	100%	90%	90%	100%
Beta Blocker at Arrival[1,3]	2	0%	85%	87%	100%
Beta Blocker at Discharge[1,3]	1	100%	86%	90%	100%
Fibrinolytic Medication Timing[3]	0	-	30%	31%	100%
PCI Within 90 Minutes of Arrival	0	-	48%	54%	95%
Smoking Cessation Advice[3]	0	-	90%	88%	100%
Heart Failure Care					
ACE Inhibitor or ARB for LVSD[1]	3	100%	82%	82%	100%
Discharge Instructions	33	18%	60%	61%	93%
Evaluation of LVS Function	38	16%	81%	83%	99%
Smoking Cessation Advice[1]	6	0%	82%	82%	100%
Pneumonia Care					
Appropriate Initial Antibiotic	54	61%	79%	83%	94%
Blood Culture Timing	27	93%	89%	90%	100%
Influenza Vaccine[4,5]	-	-	69%	70%	100%
Initial Antibiotic Timing	59	85%	78%	80%	93%
Oxygenation Assessment	76	100%	99%	99%	100%
Pneumococcal Vaccine	41	90%	68%	69%	94%
Smoking Cessation Advice[1]	7	43%	83%	80%	100%
Surgical Infection Prevention					
Prophylactic Antibiotic Given[1,3]	8	25%	67%	77%	95%
Prophylactic Antibiotic Selection[1]	3	100%	86%	90%	100%
Prophylactic Antibiotic Stopped[1,3]	7	86%	68%	72%	95%
Pregnancy Care					
Inpatient Neonatal Mortality	-	-	-	-	-
Third or Fourth Degree Laceration	-	-	3.23%	3.63%	3.27%

Baylor All Saints Med Ctr at Forth Worth

1400 8th Avenue
Fort Worth, TX 76104
URL: www.baylorhealth.com/locations/allsaints
Ownership: Voluntary non-profit - Private
Emergency Services: Yes

Phone: 817-926-2544
Fax: 817-922-1593

Accredited: Yes
Licensed Beds: 275

Key Personnel:
CEO . . . . Joel Allison
President . . . . Steven R Newton

Measure	Cases	This Hospital	State Average	U.S. Average	Top Hospital
Heart Attack Care					
ACE Inhibitor or ARB for LVSD	52	85%	85%	82%	100%
Aspirin at Arrival	175	95%	91%	92%	100%
Aspirin at Discharge	185	96%	90%	90%	100%
Beta Blocker at Arrival	150	95%	85%	87%	100%
Beta Blocker at Discharge	182	98%	86%	90%	100%
Fibrinolytic Medication Timing[1]	2	100%	30%	31%	100%
PCI Within 90 Minutes of Arrival[1]	9	100%	48%	54%	95%
Smoking Cessation Advice	58	100%	90%	88%	100%
Heart Failure Care					
ACE Inhibitor or ARB for LVSD	197	82%	82%	82%	100%
Discharge Instructions	387	79%	60%	61%	93%
Evaluation of LVS Function	459	95%	81%	83%	99%
Smoking Cessation Advice	91	91%	82%	82%	100%
Pneumonia Care					
Appropriate Initial Antibiotic	214	88%	79%	83%	94%
Blood Culture Timing	198	92%	89%	90%	100%
Influenza Vaccine	69	86%	69%	70%	100%
Initial Antibiotic Timing	257	91%	78%	80%	93%
Oxygenation Assessment	300	100%	99%	99%	100%
Pneumococcal Vaccine	172	92%	68%	69%	94%
Smoking Cessation Advice	65	92%	83%	80%	100%
Surgical Infection Prevention					
Prophylactic Antibiotic Given	1,383	97%	67%	77%	95%
Prophylactic Antibiotic Selection	329	97%	86%	90%	100%
Prophylactic Antibiotic Stopped	1,323	90%	68%	72%	95%
Pregnancy Care					
Inpatient Neonatal Mortality	-	-	-	-	-
Third or Fourth Degree Laceration	-	-	3.23%	3.63%	3.27%

Harris Methodist Continued Care Hospital

1301 Pennsylvania Avenue
Fort Worth, TX 76104
URL: www.texashealth.org
Ownership: Voluntary non-profit - Church
Emergency Services: Yes

Phone: 817-878-5500
Fax: 817-882-2865

Accredited: Yes
Licensed Beds: 628

Key Personnel:
President/CEO. . . . . Barclay Berdan
Chief Medical Staff. . . . . James Osborn, MD
Emergency Room . . . . John M Geesbreght, MD
Infection Control . . . . Carol Trickey
OB/GYN Womens Health. . . . . Iris Torvik
Respiratory/Cardiopulmonary. . . . . Gloria Whitcomb-Boyer

Measure	Cases	This Hospital	State Average	U.S. Average	Top Hospital
Heart Attack Care					
ACE Inhibitor or ARB for LVSD	108	79%	85%	82%	100%
Aspirin at Arrival	476	96%	91%	92%	100%
Aspirin at Discharge	620	99%	90%	90%	100%
Beta Blocker at Arrival	393	93%	85%	87%	100%
Beta Blocker at Discharge	640	98%	86%	90%	100%
Fibrinolytic Medication Timing[1]	4	0%	30%	31%	100%
PCI Within 90 Minutes of Arrival	33	70%	48%	54%	95%
Smoking Cessation Advice	288	94%	90%	88%	100%
Heart Failure Care					
ACE Inhibitor or ARB for LVSD	338	98%	82%	82%	100%
Discharge Instructions	686	72%	60%	61%	93%
Evaluation of LVS Function	849	92%	81%	83%	99%
Smoking Cessation Advice	143	85%	82%	82%	100%
Pneumonia Care					
Appropriate Initial Antibiotic	417	87%	79%	83%	94%
Blood Culture Timing	648	95%	89%	90%	100%

NOTE: Hospital profiles are in alphabetical order by state, then city, then hospital within the city; Rankings are sorted by rate in descending order and exclude hospitals with less than 25 cases; (1) The number of cases is too small (n<25) for purposes of reliably predicting hospital performance; (2) Measure reflects the hospital's indication that its submission was based upon a sample of its relevant discharges; (3) Rate reflects fewer than the maximum possible quarters of data for the measure; (4) Inaccurate information submitted and suppressed for one or more quarters; (5) No data is available from the hospital for this measure; Please refer to the User's Guide for a full explanation of data

Influenza Vaccine	180	85%	69%	70%	100%
Initial Antibiotic Timing	776	89%	78%	80%	93%
Oxygenation Assessment	903	100%	99%	99%	100%
Pneumococcal Vaccine	525	86%	68%	69%	94%
Smoking Cessation Advice	193	84%	83%	80%	100%
Surgical Infection Prevention					
Prophylactic Antibiotic Given[2,3]	248	89%	67%	77%	95%
Prophylactic Antibiotic Selection[2]	82	95%	86%	90%	100%
Prophylactic Antibiotic Stopped[2,3]	234	78%	68%	72%	95%
Pregnancy Care					
Inpatient Neonatal Mortality	-	-	-	-	-
Third or Fourth Degree Laceration	-	-	3.23%	3.63%	3.27%

Harris Methodist Southwest

6100 Harris Parkway
Fort Worth, TX 76132
URL: www.texahealth.org
Ownership: Voluntary non-profit - Private
Emergency Services: Yes

Phone: 817-433-5000
Fax: 817-433-6099

Accredited: Yes
Licensed Beds: 85

Key Personnel:
Administrator/President . . . . Stansel Harvey
Chief Medical Staff. . . . . Lynne R Tilkin, DO
Emergency Room . . . . Sharon Gibson
Director Infection/Disease Control . . . . Kim Strelczyk, RN
Director Medical/Surgical Nursing . . . . Jennifer Evans, RN
OB/GYN Womens Health. . . . . Cathy Johnson, RN
Chief Radiology . . . . Sanford Reitman, MD
Director Respiratory Therapy . . . . Marcy Graves

Measure	Cases	This Hospital	State Average	U.S. Average	Top Hospital
Heart Attack Care					
ACE Inhibitor or ARB for LVSD[1]	9	100%	85%	82%	100%
Aspirin at Arrival	87	98%	91%	92%	100%
Aspirin at Discharge	61	95%	90%	90%	100%
Beta Blocker at Arrival	78	100%	85%	87%	100%
Beta Blocker at Discharge	59	100%	86%	90%	100%
Fibrinolytic Medication Timing[1]	8	25%	30%	31%	100%
PCI Within 90 Minutes of Arrival	0	-	48%	54%	95%
Smoking Cessation Advice[1]	9	78%	90%	88%	100%
Heart Failure Care					
ACE Inhibitor or ARB for LVSD	57	100%	82%	82%	100%
Discharge Instructions	161	99%	60%	61%	93%
Evaluation of LVS Function	231	90%	81%	83%	99%
Smoking Cessation Advice	42	90%	82%	82%	100%
Pneumonia Care					
Appropriate Initial Antibiotic	165	81%	79%	83%	94%
Blood Culture Timing	187	90%	89%	90%	100%
Influenza Vaccine	63	84%	69%	70%	100%
Initial Antibiotic Timing	237	87%	78%	80%	93%
Oxygenation Assessment	292	100%	99%	99%	100%
Pneumococcal Vaccine	172	87%	68%	69%	94%
Smoking Cessation Advice	42	95%	83%	80%	100%
Surgical Infection Prevention					
Prophylactic Antibiotic Given[2,3]	110	85%	67%	77%	95%
Prophylactic Antibiotic Selection[2]	40	80%	86%	90%	100%
Prophylactic Antibiotic Stopped[2,3]	100	65%	68%	72%	95%
Pregnancy Care					
Inpatient Neonatal Mortality	-	-	-	-	-
Third or Fourth Degree Laceration	-	-	3.23%	3.63%	3.27%

Huguley Memorial Medical Center

11801 South Freeway (I-35W)
Burleson, TX 76028
URL: www.huguley.org
Ownership: Voluntary non-profit - Church
Emergency Services: Yes

Phone: 817-293-9110
Fax: 817-568-1296

Accredited: Yes
Licensed Beds: 213

Key Personnel:
President/CEO. . . . . Peter M Weber
Chief Medical Staff. . . . . Timothy Heath, MD
Emergency Room . . . . John K Griswell, MD
Director Infection/Disease Control . . . . Linda Stair, RN
Director Medical/Surgical Nursing . . . . Elizabeth Steger
OB/GYN Womens Health. . . . . Donna Duran, MD

Chief Radiology . . . . Tim Oltersdorf
Director Respiratory Therapy . . . . Joe Horn

Measure	Cases	This Hospital	State Average	U.S. Average	Top Hospital
Heart Attack Care					
ACE Inhibitor or ARB for LVSD[1]	24	92%	85%	82%	100%
Aspirin at Arrival	186	97%	91%	92%	100%
Aspirin at Discharge	167	97%	90%	90%	100%
Beta Blocker at Arrival	146	95%	85%	87%	100%
Beta Blocker at Discharge	179	98%	86%	90%	100%
Fibrinolytic Medication Timing[1]	3	0%	30%	31%	100%
PCI Within 90 Minutes of Arrival[1]	19	32%	48%	54%	95%
Smoking Cessation Advice	78	100%	90%	88%	100%
Heart Failure Care					
ACE Inhibitor or ARB for LVSD	75	95%	82%	82%	100%
Discharge Instructions	280	61%	60%	61%	93%
Evaluation of LVS Function	345	97%	81%	83%	99%
Smoking Cessation Advice	91	99%	82%	82%	100%
Pneumonia Care					
Appropriate Initial Antibiotic	226	80%	79%	83%	94%
Blood Culture Timing	193	83%	89%	90%	100%
Influenza Vaccine	73	73%	69%	70%	100%
Initial Antibiotic Timing	308	77%	78%	80%	93%
Oxygenation Assessment	371	98%	99%	99%	100%
Pneumococcal Vaccine	181	90%	68%	69%	94%
Smoking Cessation Advice	116	97%	83%	80%	100%
Surgical Infection Prevention					
Prophylactic Antibiotic Given[3]	407	86%	67%	77%	95%
Prophylactic Antibiotic Selection	142	80%	86%	90%	100%
Prophylactic Antibiotic Stopped[3]	396	64%	68%	72%	95%
Pregnancy Care					
Inpatient Neonatal Mortality	1,143	0.35%	-	-	-
Third or Fourth Degree Laceration	824	5.10%	3.23%	3.63%	3.27%

John Peter Smith Hospital

Alternate Name: JPS Health Network
1500 South Main Street
Fort Worth, TX 76104
URL: www.jpshealthnet.org
Ownership: Govt - Hospital District or Authority
Emergency Services: Yes

Phone: 817-924-3431
Fax: 817-927-1664

Accredited: Yes
Licensed Beds: 459

Key Personnel:
President/CEO. . . . . David M Cecero
Chief Medical Officer . . . . Jay Haynes, MD
Senior Director Cardiology Service Line . . . . Robert Bourassa
Manager Catheterization Lab . . . . Joe Elmore
Medical Director Emergency . . . . Jken Taub, MD
Coordinator Infection Control . . . . Jan Hawley
Administrative Director CCU . . . . Trudy Sander, RN
Director Medical/Surgical Nursing . . . . Audry Suggs
Director OB/GYN Womens Health . . . . Janet Figueroa
Director Surgical Services . . . . Pat Wright
Director Women/Infants/Children Svcs. . . . . Janet Figueroa
Director Respiratory Care. . . . . Joyce Gradel

Measure	Cases	This Hospital	State Average	U.S. Average	Top Hospital
Heart Attack Care					
ACE Inhibitor or ARB for LVSD	39	77%	85%	82%	100%
Aspirin at Arrival	199	91%	91%	92%	100%
Aspirin at Discharge	149	93%	90%	90%	100%
Beta Blocker at Arrival	185	86%	85%	87%	100%
Beta Blocker at Discharge	166	96%	86%	90%	100%
Fibrinolytic Medication Timing[1]	1	0%	30%	31%	100%
PCI Within 90 Minutes of Arrival[1]	11	27%	48%	54%	95%
Smoking Cessation Advice	103	70%	90%	88%	100%
Heart Failure Care					
ACE Inhibitor or ARB for LVSD	318	88%	82%	82%	100%
Discharge Instructions	485	14%	60%	61%	93%
Evaluation of LVS Function	505	99%	81%	83%	99%
Smoking Cessation Advice	214	70%	82%	82%	100%
Pneumonia Care					
Appropriate Initial Antibiotic	276	77%	79%	83%	94%
Blood Culture Timing	255	85%	89%	90%	100%

NOTE: Hospital profiles are in alphabetical order by state, then city, then hospital within the city; Rankings are sorted by rate in descending order and exclude hospitals with less than 25 cases; (1) The number of cases is too small (n<25) for purposes of reliably predicting hospital performance; (2) Measure reflects the hospital's indication that its submission was based upon a sample of its relevant discharges; (3) Rate reflects fewer than the maximum possible quarters of data for the measure; (4) Inaccurate information submitted and suppressed for one or more quarters; (5) No data is available from the hospital for this measure; Please refer to the User's Guide for a full explanation of data

Measure	Cases	This Hospital	State Average	U.S. Average	Top Hospital
Influenza Vaccine	58	2%	69%	70%	100%
Initial Antibiotic Timing	339	40%	78%	80%	93%
Oxygenation Assessment	389	100%	99%	99%	100%
Pneumococcal Vaccine	61	16%	68%	69%	94%
Smoking Cessation Advice	175	47%	83%	80%	100%
Surgical Infection Prevention					
Prophylactic Antibiotic Given	487	77%	67%	77%	95%
Prophylactic Antibiotic Selection	100	86%	86%	90%	100%
Prophylactic Antibiotic Stopped	476	77%	68%	72%	95%
Pregnancy Care					
Inpatient Neonatal Mortality	-	-	-	-	-
Third or Fourth Degree Laceration	-	-	3.23%	3.63%	3.27%

Medical Centre Surgical Hospital

750 13th Avenue
Fort Worth, TX 76104
Ownership: Voluntary non-profit - Private
Emergency Services: No

Phone: 817-334-5050

Accredited: Yes

Measure	Cases	This Hospital	State Average	U.S. Average	Top Hospital
Heart Attack Care					
ACE Inhibitor or ARB for LVSD[5]	-	-	85%	82%	100%
Aspirin at Arrival[5]	-	-	91%	92%	100%
Aspirin at Discharge[5]	-	-	90%	90%	100%
Beta Blocker at Arrival[5]	-	-	85%	87%	100%
Beta Blocker at Discharge[5]	-	-	86%	90%	100%
Fibrinolytic Medication Timing[5]	-	-	30%	31%	100%
PCI Within 90 Minutes of Arrival[5]	-	-	48%	54%	95%
Smoking Cessation Advice[5]	-	-	90%	88%	100%
Heart Failure Care					
ACE Inhibitor or ARB for LVSD[5]	-	-	82%	82%	100%
Discharge Instructions[5]	-	-	60%	61%	93%
Evaluation of LVS Function[5]	-	-	81%	83%	99%
Smoking Cessation Advice[5]	-	-	82%	82%	100%
Pneumonia Care					
Appropriate Initial Antibiotic[5]	-	-	79%	83%	94%
Blood Culture Timing[5]	-	-	89%	90%	100%
Influenza Vaccine[5]	-	-	69%	70%	100%
Initial Antibiotic Timing[5]	-	-	78%	80%	93%
Oxygenation Assessment[5]	-	-	99%	99%	100%
Pneumococcal Vaccine[5]	-	-	68%	69%	94%
Smoking Cessation Advice[5]	-	-	83%	80%	100%
Surgical Infection Prevention					
Prophylactic Antibiotic Given[1,2,3]	17	82%	67%	77%	95%
Prophylactic Antibiotic Selection[5]	-	-	86%	90%	100%
Prophylactic Antibiotic Stopped[1,2,3]	17	100%	68%	72%	95%
Pregnancy Care					
Inpatient Neonatal Mortality	-	-	-	-	-
Third or Fourth Degree Laceration	-	-	3.23%	3.63%	3.27%

Plaza Medical Center

Alternate Name: HCA Medical Plaza Hospital/Saint Joseph Hospital
900 8th Avenue
Fort Worth, TX 76104
URL: www.plazamedicalcenter.com
Ownership: Proprietary
Emergency Services: Yes
Key Personnel:
CEO . . . . Tony Villarreal
Chief Medical Staff . . . . MI Mughal
Emergency Room . . . . Daniela Wallace, RN
OB/GYN Womens Health . . . . Berkeley Merrill, MD

Phone: 817-336-2100
Fax: 817-347-5796

Accredited: Yes
Licensed Beds: 298

Measure	Cases	This Hospital	State Average	U.S. Average	Top Hospital
Heart Attack Care					
ACE Inhibitor or ARB for LVSD	58	97%	85%	82%	100%
Aspirin at Arrival	133	100%	91%	92%	100%
Aspirin at Discharge	335	99%	90%	90%	100%
Beta Blocker at Arrival	119	100%	85%	87%	100%
Beta Blocker at Discharge	352	99%	86%	90%	100%
Fibrinolytic Medication Timing	0	-	30%	31%	100%
PCI Within 90 Minutes of Arrival[1]	8	38%	48%	54%	95%

Measure	Cases	This Hospital	State Average	U.S. Average	Top Hospital
Smoking Cessation Advice	145	100%	90%	88%	100%
Heart Failure Care					
ACE Inhibitor or ARB for LVSD	172	90%	82%	82%	100%
Discharge Instructions	341	83%	60%	61%	93%
Evaluation of LVS Function	379	99%	81%	83%	99%
Smoking Cessation Advice	83	94%	82%	82%	100%
Pneumonia Care					
Appropriate Initial Antibiotic	133	75%	79%	83%	94%
Blood Culture Timing	137	91%	89%	90%	100%
Influenza Vaccine	51	57%	69%	70%	100%
Initial Antibiotic Timing	191	69%	78%	80%	93%
Oxygenation Assessment	241	99%	99%	99%	100%
Pneumococcal Vaccine	133	62%	68%	69%	94%
Smoking Cessation Advice	44	82%	83%	80%	100%
Surgical Infection Prevention					
Prophylactic Antibiotic Given[2,3]	304	88%	67%	77%	95%
Prophylactic Antibiotic Selection[2]	152	86%	86%	90%	100%
Prophylactic Antibiotic Stopped[2,3]	298	45%	68%	72%	95%
Pregnancy Care					
Inpatient Neonatal Mortality	-	-	-	-	-
Third or Fourth Degree Laceration	-	-	3.23%	3.63%	3.27%

Hill Country Memorial Hospital

1020 S State Highway 16
PO Box 835
Fredericksburg, TX 78624
E-mail: jyoung@hcmbs.org
URL: www.hcmbs.org
Ownership: Voluntary non-profit - Private
Emergency Services: Yes
Key Personnel:
CEO . . . . Jeff A Bourgeois
Chief Medical Staff . . . . Ottis Layne, MD
Chief Catheterization Laboratory . . . . Mell C Jackson, MD
Emergency Room . . . . Ottis Layne, MD
Director Infection/Disease Control . . . . Carl Evans, MD
Director Medical/Surgical Nursing . . . . Susan Ottmevs, RN
Manager Cardiopulmonary . . . . Cynthia Jacobson

Phone: 830-997-4353
Fax: 830-997-1348

Accredited: Yes
Licensed Beds: 84

Measure	Cases	This Hospital	State Average	U.S. Average	Top Hospital
Heart Attack Care					
ACE Inhibitor or ARB for LVSD[1]	2	100%	85%	82%	100%
Aspirin at Arrival[1]	15	60%	91%	92%	100%
Aspirin at Discharge[1]	10	70%	90%	90%	100%
Beta Blocker at Arrival[1]	12	92%	85%	87%	100%
Beta Blocker at Discharge[1]	12	92%	86%	90%	100%
Fibrinolytic Medication Timing	0	-	30%	31%	100%
PCI Within 90 Minutes of Arrival	0	-	48%	54%	95%
Smoking Cessation Advice[1]	1	100%	90%	88%	100%
Heart Failure Care					
ACE Inhibitor or ARB for LVSD[1]	20	85%	82%	82%	100%
Discharge Instructions	59	85%	60%	61%	93%
Evaluation of LVS Function	83	86%	81%	83%	99%
Smoking Cessation Advice[1]	5	100%	82%	82%	100%
Pneumonia Care					
Appropriate Initial Antibiotic	110	80%	79%	83%	94%
Blood Culture Timing	82	85%	89%	90%	100%
Influenza Vaccine	38	82%	69%	70%	100%
Initial Antibiotic Timing	160	79%	78%	80%	93%
Oxygenation Assessment	195	100%	99%	99%	100%
Pneumococcal Vaccine	149	87%	68%	69%	94%
Smoking Cessation Advice	26	73%	83%	80%	100%
Surgical Infection Prevention					
Prophylactic Antibiotic Given	459	85%	67%	77%	95%
Prophylactic Antibiotic Selection	108	96%	86%	90%	100%
Prophylactic Antibiotic Stopped	452	51%	68%	72%	95%
Pregnancy Care					
Inpatient Neonatal Mortality	-	-	-	-	-
Third or Fourth Degree Laceration	-	-	3.23%	3.63%	3.27%

NOTE: Hospital profiles are in alphabetical order by state, then city, then hospital within the city; Rankings are sorted by rate in descending order and exclude hospitals with less than 25 cases; (1) The number of cases is too small (n<25) for purposes of reliably predicting hospital performance; (2) Measure reflects the hospital's indication that its submission was based upon a sample of its relevant discharges; (3) Rate reflects fewer than the maximum possible quarters of data for the measure; (4) Inaccurate information submitted and suppressed for one or more quarters; (5) No data is available from the hospital for this measure; Please refer to the User's Guide for a full explanation of data

Baylor Medical Center at Frisco

5601 Warren Parkway
Frisco, TX 75034   Phone: 214-618-2000
Ownership: Proprietary   Accredited: Yes
Emergency Services: Yes

Key Personnel:
CEO . . . . William A Keaton
CNO . . . . Cheryl King, RN
Medical Staff Services . . . . Karen Murchison

Measure	Cases	This Hospital	State Average	U.S. Average	Top Hospital
Heart Attack Care					
ACE Inhibitor or ARB for LVSD[5]	-	-	85%	82%	100%
Aspirin at Arrival[5]	-	-	91%	92%	100%
Aspirin at Discharge[5]	-	-	90%	90%	100%
Beta Blocker at Arrival[5]	-	-	85%	87%	100%
Beta Blocker at Discharge[5]	-	-	86%	90%	100%
Fibrinolytic Medication Timing[5]	-	-	30%	31%	100%
PCI Within 90 Minutes of Arrival[5]	-	-	48%	54%	95%
Smoking Cessation Advice[5]	-	-	90%	88%	100%
Heart Failure Care					
ACE Inhibitor or ARB for LVSD[5]	-	-	82%	82%	100%
Discharge Instructions[5]	-	-	60%	61%	93%
Evaluation of LVS Function[5]	-	-	81%	83%	99%
Smoking Cessation Advice[5]	-	-	82%	82%	100%
Pneumonia Care					
Appropriate Initial Antibiotic[5]	-	-	79%	83%	94%
Blood Culture Timing[5]	-	-	89%	90%	100%
Influenza Vaccine[5]	-	-	69%	70%	100%
Initial Antibiotic Timing[5]	-	-	78%	80%	93%
Oxygenation Assessment[5]	-	-	99%	99%	100%
Pneumococcal Vaccine[5]	-	-	68%	69%	94%
Smoking Cessation Advice[5]	-	-	83%	80%	100%
Surgical Infection Prevention					
Prophylactic Antibiotic Given[3]	58	83%	67%	77%	95%
Prophylactic Antibiotic Selection	25	88%	86%	90%	100%
Prophylactic Antibiotic Stopped[3]	58	72%	68%	72%	95%
Pregnancy Care					
Inpatient Neonatal Mortality	-	-	-	-	-
Third or Fourth Degree Laceration	-	-	3.23%	3.63%	3.27%

Centennial Medical Center

12505 Lebanon Road
Frisco, TX 75035   Phone: 972-963-3333
URL: www.centennialmedcenter.com   Fax: 972-963-3624
Ownership: Proprietary   Accredited: Yes
Emergency Services: Yes   Licensed Beds: 118

Key Personnel:
CEO . . . . William C Henning

Measure	Cases	This Hospital	State Average	U.S. Average	Top Hospital
Heart Attack Care					
ACE Inhibitor or ARB for LVSD[1]	18	83%	85%	82%	100%
Aspirin at Arrival	62	98%	91%	92%	100%
Aspirin at Discharge	71	100%	90%	90%	100%
Beta Blocker at Arrival	59	97%	85%	87%	100%
Beta Blocker at Discharge	72	99%	86%	90%	100%
Fibrinolytic Medication Timing[1]	2	50%	30%	31%	100%
PCI Within 90 Minutes of Arrival[1]	7	71%	48%	54%	95%
Smoking Cessation Advice	31	90%	90%	88%	100%
Heart Failure Care					
ACE Inhibitor or ARB for LVSD	27	67%	82%	82%	100%
Discharge Instructions	60	30%	60%	61%	93%
Evaluation of LVS Function	81	88%	81%	83%	99%
Smoking Cessation Advice[1]	22	100%	82%	82%	100%
Pneumonia Care					
Appropriate Initial Antibiotic	66	79%	79%	83%	94%
Blood Culture Timing	56	96%	89%	90%	100%
Influenza Vaccine[1]	18	61%	69%	70%	100%
Initial Antibiotic Timing	68	94%	78%	80%	93%
Oxygenation Assessment	96	100%	99%	99%	100%
Pneumococcal Vaccine	48	71%	68%	69%	94%

Smoking Cessation Advice[1]	14	100%	83%	80%	100%
Surgical Infection Prevention					
Prophylactic Antibiotic Given[2]	142	92%	67%	77%	95%
Prophylactic Antibiotic Selection[2]	34	88%	86%	90%	100%
Prophylactic Antibiotic Stopped[2]	127	57%	68%	72%	95%
Pregnancy Care					
Inpatient Neonatal Mortality	-	-	-	-	-
Third or Fourth Degree Laceration	-	-	3.23%	3.63%	3.27%

North Texas Medical Center

1900 Hospital Blvd
Gainesville, TX 76240   Phone: 940-612-8600
Ownership: Govt - Hospital District or Authority   Accredited: No
Emergency Services: No

Key Personnel:
OBGYN . . . . Scott Brown, MD

Measure	Cases	This Hospital	State Average	U.S. Average	Top Hospital
Heart Attack Care					
ACE Inhibitor or ARB for LVSD[1]	4	100%	85%	82%	100%
Aspirin at Arrival[1]	24	75%	91%	92%	100%
Aspirin at Discharge[1]	12	83%	90%	90%	100%
Beta Blocker at Arrival[1]	21	71%	85%	87%	100%
Beta Blocker at Discharge[1]	14	71%	86%	90%	100%
Fibrinolytic Medication Timing[1]	2	50%	30%	31%	100%
PCI Within 90 Minutes of Arrival	0	-	48%	54%	95%
Smoking Cessation Advice[1]	5	40%	90%	88%	100%
Heart Failure Care					
ACE Inhibitor or ARB for LVSD[1]	13	54%	82%	82%	100%
Discharge Instructions	73	12%	60%	61%	93%
Evaluation of LVS Function	103	51%	81%	83%	99%
Smoking Cessation Advice[1]	22	59%	82%	82%	100%
Pneumonia Care					
Appropriate Initial Antibiotic	46	63%	79%	83%	94%
Blood Culture Timing	31	100%	89%	90%	100%
Influenza Vaccine[1]	17	59%	69%	70%	100%
Initial Antibiotic Timing	57	84%	78%	80%	93%
Oxygenation Assessment	70	99%	99%	99%	100%
Pneumococcal Vaccine	39	59%	68%	69%	94%
Smoking Cessation Advice[1]	14	71%	83%	80%	100%
Surgical Infection Prevention					
Prophylactic Antibiotic Given	81	65%	67%	77%	95%
Prophylactic Antibiotic Selection[1]	16	81%	86%	90%	100%
Prophylactic Antibiotic Stopped	75	63%	68%	72%	95%
Pregnancy Care					
Inpatient Neonatal Mortality	-	-	-	-	-
Third or Fourth Degree Laceration	-	-	3.23%	3.63%	3.27%

University of Texas Medical Branch Hospitals

301 University Boulevard
Galveston, TX 77555   Phone: 409-772-2618
E-mail: ccomer@utmb.edu, rgbrouil@utmb.edu   Fax: 409-772-6216
URL: www.utmb.edu
Ownership: Government - State   Accredited: Yes
Emergency Services: Yes   Licensed Beds: 804

Key Personnel:
President/CEO . . . . John D Stobo, MD
Chief Medical Staff . . . . Don Powell, MD
Chief Cardio-Thoracic Surgeon . . . . Vincent R Conti, MD
Chief Catheterization Laboratory . . . . Barry Uretsky, MD
Emergency Room . . . . Brian Zachariah, MD
Director Infection/Disease Control . . . . Norbert Roberts, MD
Director Medical/Surgical Nursing . . . . Dana Bjarnason
OB/GYN Womens Health . . . . Garland Anderson, MD
Chief Radiology . . . . Leonard E Swischuk, MD
Director Pulmonary Medicine . . . . Akhil Bidani, MD

Measure	Cases	This Hospital	State Average	U.S. Average	Top Hospital
Heart Attack Care					
ACE Inhibitor or ARB for LVSD[2]	98	80%	85%	82%	100%
Aspirin at Arrival[2]	214	97%	91%	92%	100%
Aspirin at Discharge[2]	271	98%	90%	90%	100%
Beta Blocker at Arrival[2]	182	98%	85%	87%	100%

NOTE: Hospital profiles are in alphabetical order by state, then city, then hospital within the city; Rankings are sorted by rate in descending order and exclude hospitals with less than 25 cases; (1) The number of cases is too small (n<25) for purposes of reliably predicting hospital performance; (2) Measure reflects the hospital's indication that its submission was based upon a sample of its relevant discharges; (3) Rate reflects fewer than the maximum possible quarters of data for the measure; (4) Inaccurate information submitted and suppressed for one or more quarters; (5) No data is available from the hospital for this measure; Please refer to the User's Guide for a full explanation of data

Measure	Cases	This Hospital	State Average	U.S. Average	Top Hospital
Beta Blocker at Discharge[2]	283	98%	86%	90%	100%
Fibrinolytic Medication Timing[2]	0	-	30%	31%	100%
PCI Within 90 Minutes of Arrival[1,2]	10	70%	48%	54%	95%
Smoking Cessation Advice[2]	119	97%	90%	88%	100%
Heart Failure Care					
ACE Inhibitor or ARB for LVSD[2]	243	77%	82%	82%	100%
Discharge Instructions[2]	311	45%	60%	61%	93%
Evaluation of LVS Function[2]	337	99%	81%	83%	99%
Smoking Cessation Advice[2]	100	88%	82%	82%	100%
Pneumonia Care					
Appropriate Initial Antibiotic[2]	100	83%	79%	83%	94%
Blood Culture Timing[2]	61	85%	89%	90%	100%
Influenza Vaccine[1,2]	20	20%	69%	70%	100%
Initial Antibiotic Timing[2]	143	41%	78%	80%	93%
Oxygenation Assessment[2]	177	98%	99%	99%	100%
Pneumococcal Vaccine[2]	80	36%	68%	69%	94%
Smoking Cessation Advice[2]	47	77%	83%	80%	100%
Surgical Infection Prevention					
Prophylactic Antibiotic Given[2,3]	348	49%	67%	77%	95%
Prophylactic Antibiotic Selection[2]	74	80%	86%	90%	100%
Prophylactic Antibiotic Stopped[2,3]	345	63%	68%	72%	95%
Pregnancy Care					
Inpatient Neonatal Mortality[2]	1,032	0.19%	-	-	-
Third or Fourth Degree Laceration	5,882	2.14%	3.23%	3.63%	3.27%

Baylor Medical Center at Garland

2300 Marie Curie
Garland, TX 75042
URL: www.baylorhealth.com/locations/garland
Ownership: Voluntary non-profit - Private
Emergency Services: Yes

Phone: 972-487-5000
Fax: 972-487-5005

Accredited: Yes
Licensed Beds: 220

Key Personnel:
CEO . . . . John McWhorter
Chief Medical Staff . . . . Michael Trombello, MD
Emergency Room . . . . Tom Button, RN
OB/GYN Womens Health . . . . Bernard Adami, MD
Chief Radiology . . . . Michael Trombello, MD
Director Respiratory Therapy . . . . Wayne Stewart

Measure	Cases	This Hospital	State Average	U.S. Average	Top Hospital
Heart Attack Care					
ACE Inhibitor or ARB for LVSD	36	100%	85%	82%	100%
Aspirin at Arrival	200	100%	91%	92%	100%
Aspirin at Discharge	189	98%	90%	90%	100%
Beta Blocker at Arrival	183	100%	85%	87%	100%
Beta Blocker at Discharge	190	99%	86%	90%	100%
Fibrinolytic Medication Timing[1]	3	0%	30%	31%	100%
PCI Within 90 Minutes of Arrival[1]	12	75%	48%	54%	95%
Smoking Cessation Advice	66	98%	90%	88%	100%
Heart Failure Care					
ACE Inhibitor or ARB for LVSD	122	93%	82%	82%	100%
Discharge Instructions	345	83%	60%	61%	93%
Evaluation of LVS Function	426	95%	81%	83%	99%
Smoking Cessation Advice	82	100%	82%	82%	100%
Pneumonia Care					
Appropriate Initial Antibiotic	179	89%	79%	83%	94%
Blood Culture Timing	172	96%	89%	90%	100%
Influenza Vaccine	50	52%	69%	70%	100%
Initial Antibiotic Timing	202	85%	78%	80%	93%
Oxygenation Assessment	281	100%	99%	99%	100%
Pneumococcal Vaccine	152	92%	68%	69%	94%
Smoking Cessation Advice	62	100%	83%	80%	100%
Surgical Infection Prevention					
Prophylactic Antibiotic Given	721	95%	67%	77%	95%
Prophylactic Antibiotic Selection	162	99%	86%	90%	100%
Prophylactic Antibiotic Stopped	699	85%	68%	72%	95%
Pregnancy Care					
Inpatient Neonatal Mortality	-	-	-	-	-
Third or Fourth Degree Laceration	-	-	3.23%	3.63%	3.27%

Vista Hospital of Dallas

2696 W Walnut St
Garland, TX 75042
URL: www.dynacq.com
Ownership: Proprietary
Emergency Services: Yes

Phone: 972-665-3000

Accredited: No
Licensed Beds: 113

Key Personnel:
CEO . . . . Gene Miller
Chief Medical Staff . . . . Wendy Curry
CCU Spvg. Nurse . . . . David Krumnow, RN
Director Medical/Surgical Nursing . . . . Paulette Murphy, RN
Chief Radiology . . . . Kendall Jones, MD
Director Respiratory Therapy . . . . Linda Semones

Measure	Cases	This Hospital	State Average	U.S. Average	Top Hospital
Heart Attack Care					
ACE Inhibitor or ARB for LVSD[5]	-	-	85%	82%	100%
Aspirin at Arrival[5]	-	-	91%	92%	100%
Aspirin at Discharge[5]	-	-	90%	90%	100%
Beta Blocker at Arrival[5]	-	-	85%	87%	100%
Beta Blocker at Discharge[5]	-	-	86%	90%	100%
Fibrinolytic Medication Timing[5]	-	-	30%	31%	100%
PCI Within 90 Minutes of Arrival[5]	-	-	48%	54%	95%
Smoking Cessation Advice[5]	-	-	90%	88%	100%
Heart Failure Care					
ACE Inhibitor or ARB for LVSD[5]	-	-	82%	82%	100%
Discharge Instructions[5]	-	-	60%	61%	93%
Evaluation of LVS Function[5]	-	-	81%	83%	99%
Smoking Cessation Advice[5]	-	-	82%	82%	100%
Pneumonia Care					
Appropriate Initial Antibiotic[5]	-	-	79%	83%	94%
Blood Culture Timing[5]	-	-	89%	90%	100%
Influenza Vaccine[5]	-	-	69%	70%	100%
Initial Antibiotic Timing[5]	-	-	78%	80%	93%
Oxygenation Assessment[5]	-	-	99%	99%	100%
Pneumococcal Vaccine[5]	-	-	68%	69%	94%
Smoking Cessation Advice[5]	-	-	83%	80%	100%
Surgical Infection Prevention					
Prophylactic Antibiotic Given[2,3]	0	-	67%	77%	95%
Prophylactic Antibiotic Selection[5]	-	-	86%	90%	100%
Prophylactic Antibiotic Stopped[2,3]	0	-	68%	72%	95%
Pregnancy Care					
Inpatient Neonatal Mortality	-	-	-	-	-
Third or Fourth Degree Laceration	-	-	3.23%	3.63%	3.27%

Coryell Memorial Hospital

1507 W Main
Gatesville, TX 76528
E-mail: adminsec@cmhos.org
URL: www.cmhos.org
Ownership: Govt - Hospital District or Authority
Emergency Services: Yes

Phone: 254-865-8251
Fax: 254-248-6306

Accredited: Yes
Licensed Beds: 55

Key Personnel:
President/CEO . . . . David K Byrom
Chief Medical Staff . . . . Regan Tipton
Respiratory/Cardiopulmonary . . . . Paul Rambue

Measure	Cases	This Hospital	State Average	U.S. Average	Top Hospital
Heart Attack Care					
ACE Inhibitor or ARB for LVSD[1]	3	100%	85%	82%	100%
Aspirin at Arrival[1]	11	91%	91%	92%	100%
Aspirin at Discharge[1]	7	100%	90%	90%	100%
Beta Blocker at Arrival[1]	13	85%	85%	87%	100%
Beta Blocker at Discharge[1]	9	78%	86%	90%	100%
Fibrinolytic Medication Timing[3]	0	-	30%	31%	100%
PCI Within 90 Minutes of Arrival	0	-	48%	54%	95%
Smoking Cessation Advice[3]	0	-	90%	88%	100%
Heart Failure Care					
ACE Inhibitor or ARB for LVSD[1]	2	50%	82%	82%	100%
Discharge Instructions[1,3]	4	100%	60%	61%	93%
Evaluation of LVS Function	34	41%	81%	83%	99%
Smoking Cessation Advice[1,3]	2	100%	82%	82%	100%
Pneumonia Care					

NOTE: Hospital profiles are in alphabetical order by state, then city, then hospital within the city; Rankings are sorted by rate in descending order and exclude hospitals with less than 25 cases; (1) The number of cases is too small (n<25) for purposes of reliably predicting hospital performance; (2) Measure reflects the hospital's indication that its submission was based upon a sample of its relevant discharges; (3) Rate reflects fewer than the maximum possible quarters of data for the measure; (4) Inaccurate information submitted and suppressed for one or more quarters; (5) No data is available from the hospital for this measure; Please refer to the User's Guide for a full explanation of data

Appropriate Initial Antibiotic[3]	0	-	79%	83%	94%
Blood Culture Timing[1,3]	4	75%	89%	90%	100%
Influenza Vaccine[5]	-	-	69%	70%	100%
Initial Antibiotic Timing	78	83%	78%	80%	93%
Oxygenation Assessment	98	100%	99%	99%	100%
Pneumococcal Vaccine	76	91%	68%	69%	94%
Smoking Cessation Advice[1,3]	1	100%	83%	80%	100%
Surgical Infection Prevention					
Prophylactic Antibiotic Given[1,3]	1	0%	67%	77%	95%
Prophylactic Antibiotic Selection[5]	-	-	86%	90%	100%
Prophylactic Antibiotic Stopped[1,3]	1	100%	68%	72%	95%
Pregnancy Care					
Inpatient Neonatal Mortality	-	-	-	-	-
Third or Fourth Degree Laceration	-	-	3.23%	3.63%	3.27%

Georgetown Healthcare System

Alternate Name: Georgetown Hospital
2000 Scenic Drive
Georgetown, TX 78626
E-mail: ghs@georgetownhealthcare.org
URL: www.georgetownhealthcare.org
Ownership: Govt - Hospital District or Authority
Emergency Services: Yes

Phone: 512-943-3000
Fax: 512-942-4477

Accredited: Yes
Licensed Beds: 104

Key Personnel:
President/CEO . . . . Kenneth W Poteete
Chief Medical Staff . . . . Stephen Garland
Emergency Room . . . . Porter Payne
Emergency Room . . . . Mark Shepherd, MD
Infection Control . . . . Crystal William
Director Respiratory Therapy . . . . Teresa Glenn

Measure	Cases	This Hospital	State Average	U.S. Average	Top Hospital
Heart Attack Care					
ACE Inhibitor or ARB for LVSD[1]	4	50%	85%	82%	100%
Aspirin at Arrival[1]	17	100%	91%	92%	100%
Aspirin at Discharge[1]	11	91%	90%	90%	100%
Beta Blocker at Arrival[1]	18	94%	85%	87%	100%
Beta Blocker at Discharge[1]	11	64%	86%	90%	100%
Fibrinolytic Medication Timing	0	-	30%	31%	100%
PCI Within 90 Minutes of Arrival	0	-	48%	54%	95%
Smoking Cessation Advice	0	-	90%	88%	100%
Heart Failure Care					
ACE Inhibitor or ARB for LVSD	27	74%	82%	82%	100%
Discharge Instructions	60	45%	60%	61%	93%
Evaluation of LVS Function	87	71%	81%	83%	99%
Smoking Cessation Advice[1]	8	75%	82%	82%	100%
Pneumonia Care					
Appropriate Initial Antibiotic	81	81%	79%	83%	94%
Blood Culture Timing	62	90%	89%	90%	100%
Influenza Vaccine[1]	23	43%	69%	70%	100%
Initial Antibiotic Timing	99	76%	78%	80%	93%
Oxygenation Assessment	140	99%	99%	99%	100%
Pneumococcal Vaccine	96	70%	68%	69%	94%
Smoking Cessation Advice[1]	18	56%	83%	80%	100%
Surgical Infection Prevention					
Prophylactic Antibiotic Given[3]	115	70%	67%	77%	95%
Prophylactic Antibiotic Selection	51	94%	86%	90%	100%
Prophylactic Antibiotic Stopped[3]	112	69%	68%	72%	95%
Pregnancy Care					
Inpatient Neonatal Mortality	-	-	-	-	-
Third or Fourth Degree Laceration	-	-	3.23%	3.63%	3.27%

East Texas Medical Center-Gilmer

712 North Wood
Gilmer, TX 75644
Ownership: Voluntary non-profit - Other
Emergency Services: Yes

Phone: 903-841-7100

Accredited: No

Measure	Cases	This Hospital	State Average	U.S. Average	Top Hospital
Heart Attack Care					
ACE Inhibitor or ARB for LVSD[3]	0	-	85%	82%	100%
Aspirin at Arrival[1,3]	5	40%	91%	92%	100%

Aspirin at Discharge[1,3]	3	67%	90%	90%	100%
Beta Blocker at Arrival[1,3]	4	100%	85%	87%	100%
Beta Blocker at Discharge[1,3]	4	75%	86%	90%	100%
Fibrinolytic Medication Timing[3]	0	-	30%	31%	100%
PCI Within 90 Minutes of Arrival	0	-	48%	54%	95%
Smoking Cessation Advice[3]	0	-	90%	88%	100%
Heart Failure Care					
ACE Inhibitor or ARB for LVSD[1]	21	90%	82%	82%	100%
Discharge Instructions[1,3]	24	17%	60%	61%	93%
Evaluation of LVS Function	88	70%	81%	83%	99%
Smoking Cessation Advice[1,3]	4	50%	82%	82%	100%
Pneumonia Care					
Appropriate Initial Antibiotic[1,3]	14	71%	79%	83%	94%
Blood Culture Timing[1,3]	7	86%	89%	90%	100%
Influenza Vaccine[5]	-	-	69%	70%	100%
Initial Antibiotic Timing	65	58%	78%	80%	93%
Oxygenation Assessment	93	100%	99%	99%	100%
Pneumococcal Vaccine	47	62%	68%	69%	94%
Smoking Cessation Advice[1,3]	1	100%	83%	80%	100%
Surgical Infection Prevention					
Prophylactic Antibiotic Given[5]	-	-	67%	77%	95%
Prophylactic Antibiotic Selection[5]	-	-	86%	90%	100%
Prophylactic Antibiotic Stopped[5]	-	-	68%	72%	95%
Pregnancy Care					
Inpatient Neonatal Mortality	-	-	-	-	-
Third or Fourth Degree Laceration	-	-	3.23%	3.63%	3.27%

Glen Rose Medical Center

1021 Holden Street
Glen Rose, TX 76043
Ownership: Govt - Hospital District or Authority
Emergency Services: Yes

Phone: 254-897-2215
Fax: 254-897-1427
Accredited: Yes
Licensed Beds: 16

Key Personnel:
President/CEO . . . . Gary Marks
Chief Medical Staff . . . . Aimee Coker, MD
Director Infection/Disease Control . . . . Jennifer Thrash
CNO . . . . Martha Nichols
Director Radiology . . . . Cherly Hatton
Director Respiratory Therapy . . . . Deborah Gray

Measure	Cases	This Hospital	State Average	U.S. Average	Top Hospital
Heart Attack Care					
ACE Inhibitor or ARB for LVSD[3]	0	-	85%	82%	100%
Aspirin at Arrival[1,3]	2	50%	91%	92%	100%
Aspirin at Discharge[1,3]	1	100%	90%	90%	100%
Beta Blocker at Arrival[1,3]	2	50%	85%	87%	100%
Beta Blocker at Discharge[3]	0	-	86%	90%	100%
Fibrinolytic Medication Timing[3]	0	-	30%	31%	100%
PCI Within 90 Minutes of Arrival	0	-	48%	54%	95%
Smoking Cessation Advice[3]	0	-	90%	88%	100%
Heart Failure Care					
ACE Inhibitor or ARB for LVSD[1]	15	100%	82%	82%	100%
Discharge Instructions[1,3]	3	67%	60%	61%	93%
Evaluation of LVS Function	34	91%	81%	83%	99%
Smoking Cessation Advice[3]	0	-	82%	82%	100%
Pneumonia Care					
Appropriate Initial Antibiotic[1,3]	8	62%	79%	83%	94%
Blood Culture Timing[1,3]	8	100%	89%	90%	100%
Influenza Vaccine[5]	-	-	69%	70%	100%
Initial Antibiotic Timing	94	93%	78%	80%	93%
Oxygenation Assessment	114	100%	99%	99%	100%
Pneumococcal Vaccine	65	95%	68%	69%	94%
Smoking Cessation Advice[1,3]	3	100%	83%	80%	100%
Surgical Infection Prevention					
Prophylactic Antibiotic Given[1,3]	9	89%	67%	77%	95%
Prophylactic Antibiotic Selection[5]	-	-	86%	90%	100%
Prophylactic Antibiotic Stopped[1,3]	9	100%	68%	72%	95%
Pregnancy Care					
Inpatient Neonatal Mortality	-	-	-	-	-
Third or Fourth Degree Laceration	-	-	3.23%	3.63%	3.27%

NOTE: Hospital profiles are in alphabetical order by state, then city, then hospital within the city; Rankings are sorted by rate in descending order and exclude hospitals with less than 25 cases; (1) The number of cases is too small (n<25) for purposes of reliably predicting hospital performance; (2) Measure reflects the hospital's indication that its submission was based upon a sample of its relevant discharges; (3) Rate reflects fewer than the maximum possible quarters of data for the measure; (4) Inaccurate information submitted and suppressed for one or more quarters; (5) No data is available from the hospital for this measure; Please refer to the User's Guide for a full explanation of data

Memorial Hospital

1110 N Sarah DeWitt Drive
Gonzales, TX 78629
Ownership: Voluntary non-profit - Other
Emergency Services: Yes

Phone: 830-672-7581
Fax: 830-672-2401
Accredited: No
Licensed Beds: 42

Key Personnel:

Administrator	Douglas Langley
Chief Medical Staff	Terry Eska, MD
Emergency Room	Robert Williamson, MD
Director Medical/Surgical Nursing	Rhea Lawlor
Director Respiratory Therapy	Barbara Langley

Measure	Cases	This Hospital	State Average	U.S. Average	Top Hospital
Heart Attack Care					
ACE Inhibitor or ARB for LVSD	0	-	85%	82%	100%
Aspirin at Arrival[1]	6	100%	91%	92%	100%
Aspirin at Discharge[1]	4	100%	90%	90%	100%
Beta Blocker at Arrival[1]	6	100%	85%	87%	100%
Beta Blocker at Discharge[1]	2	100%	86%	90%	100%
Fibrinolytic Medication Timing	0	-	30%	31%	100%
PCI Within 90 Minutes of Arrival	0	-	48%	54%	95%
Smoking Cessation Advice	0	-	90%	88%	100%
Heart Failure Care					
ACE Inhibitor or ARB for LVSD[1]	16	69%	82%	82%	100%
Discharge Instructions	38	0%	60%	61%	93%
Evaluation of LVS Function	51	69%	81%	83%	99%
Smoking Cessation Advice[1]	8	25%	82%	82%	100%
Pneumonia Care					
Appropriate Initial Antibiotic	33	82%	79%	83%	94%
Blood Culture Timing[1]	20	95%	89%	90%	100%
Influenza Vaccine[1]	22	23%	69%	70%	100%
Initial Antibiotic Timing	53	57%	78%	80%	93%
Oxygenation Assessment	56	100%	99%	99%	100%
Pneumococcal Vaccine	41	20%	68%	69%	94%
Smoking Cessation Advice[1]	7	14%	83%	80%	100%
Surgical Infection Prevention					
Prophylactic Antibiotic Given[1,3]	6	50%	67%	77%	95%
Prophylactic Antibiotic Selection[1]	2	100%	86%	90%	100%
Prophylactic Antibiotic Stopped[1,3]	5	100%	68%	72%	95%
Pregnancy Care					
Inpatient Neonatal Mortality	-	-	-	-	-
Third or Fourth Degree Laceration	-	-	3.23%	3.63%	3.27%

Graham Regional Medical Center

Alternate Name: Graham General Hospital
1301 Montgomery Road
Graham, TX 76450
URL: www.grahamrmc.com
Ownership: Government - Local
Emergency Services: Yes

Phone: 940-549-3400
Fax: 940-521-5158
Accredited: No
Licensed Beds: 37

Key Personnel:

Administrator	Blake Kretz
Chief Medical Staff	Pete Brown, MD
Emergency Room	Jadine Buckley, RN
Medical Surgical Nursing	Connie Beddingfield, RN
OB/GYN Women's Health	James Cawley, MD
Director Respiratory Therapy	Clint Grissom

Measure	Cases	This Hospital	State Average	U.S. Average	Top Hospital
Heart Attack Care					
ACE Inhibitor or ARB for LVSD[1]	1	100%	85%	82%	100%
Aspirin at Arrival[1]	5	80%	91%	92%	100%
Aspirin at Discharge[1]	2	100%	90%	90%	100%
Beta Blocker at Arrival[1]	3	100%	85%	87%	100%
Beta Blocker at Discharge[1]	1	100%	86%	90%	100%
Fibrinolytic Medication Timing	0	-	30%	31%	100%
PCI Within 90 Minutes of Arrival	0	-	48%	54%	95%
Smoking Cessation Advice	0	-	90%	88%	100%
Heart Failure Care					
ACE Inhibitor or ARB for LVSD[1]	18	100%	82%	82%	100%
Discharge Instructions	59	85%	60%	61%	93%
Evaluation of LVS Function	68	100%	81%	83%	99%
Smoking Cessation Advice[1]	20	100%	82%	82%	100%

Measure	Cases	This Hospital	State Average	U.S. Average	Top Hospital
Pneumonia Care					
Appropriate Initial Antibiotic	51	98%	79%	83%	94%
Blood Culture Timing	43	95%	89%	90%	100%
Influenza Vaccine[1]	17	94%	69%	70%	100%
Initial Antibiotic Timing	86	93%	78%	80%	93%
Oxygenation Assessment	101	100%	99%	99%	100%
Pneumococcal Vaccine	80	98%	68%	69%	94%
Smoking Cessation Advice[1]	23	100%	83%	80%	100%
Surgical Infection Prevention					
Prophylactic Antibiotic Given[1,3]	3	100%	67%	77%	95%
Prophylactic Antibiotic Selection[1]	3	100%	86%	90%	100%
Prophylactic Antibiotic Stopped[1,3]	3	100%	68%	72%	95%
Pregnancy Care					
Inpatient Neonatal Mortality	-	-	-	-	-
Third or Fourth Degree Laceration	-	-	3.23%	3.63%	3.27%

Lake Granbury Medical Center

Alternate Name: Hood General Hospital
1310 Paluxy Road
Granbury, TX 76048
URL: www.lakegranburymedicalcenter.com
Ownership: Proprietary
Emergency Services: Yes

Phone: 817-573-2683
Fax: 817-408-3038
Accredited: Yes
Licensed Beds: 56

Key Personnel:

CEO	Donnie L Romine
Director Emergency Services	Mark Kellar, RN
Emergency Room	Ken Filbeck, MD
Director Infection/Disease Control	Denise Pratz
CCU Spvg. Nurse	Gwen Aparicio
Chief Radiology	Rick Wright, DO
Director Respiratory Therapy	Connie Armstrong

Measure	Cases	This Hospital	State Average	U.S. Average	Top Hospital
Heart Attack Care					
ACE Inhibitor or ARB for LVSD[1]	1	100%	85%	82%	100%
Aspirin at Arrival[1]	10	100%	91%	92%	100%
Aspirin at Discharge[1]	6	100%	90%	90%	100%
Beta Blocker at Arrival[1]	10	100%	85%	87%	100%
Beta Blocker at Discharge[1]	5	100%	86%	90%	100%
Fibrinolytic Medication Timing	0	-	30%	31%	100%
PCI Within 90 Minutes of Arrival	0	-	48%	54%	95%
Smoking Cessation Advice[1]	2	50%	90%	88%	100%
Heart Failure Care					
ACE Inhibitor or ARB for LVSD[1]	22	82%	82%	82%	100%
Discharge Instructions	32	97%	60%	61%	93%
Evaluation of LVS Function	40	80%	81%	83%	99%
Smoking Cessation Advice[1]	9	100%	82%	82%	100%
Pneumonia Care					
Appropriate Initial Antibiotic	68	87%	79%	83%	94%
Blood Culture Timing	64	81%	89%	90%	100%
Influenza Vaccine[1]	22	73%	69%	70%	100%
Initial Antibiotic Timing	79	85%	78%	80%	93%
Oxygenation Assessment	108	100%	99%	99%	100%
Pneumococcal Vaccine	69	83%	68%	69%	94%
Smoking Cessation Advice	29	90%	83%	80%	100%
Surgical Infection Prevention					
Prophylactic Antibiotic Given[2,3]	103	89%	67%	77%	95%
Prophylactic Antibiotic Selection[2]	34	85%	86%	90%	100%
Prophylactic Antibiotic Stopped[2,3]	98	55%	68%	72%	95%
Pregnancy Care					
Inpatient Neonatal Mortality	-	-	-	-	-
Third or Fourth Degree Laceration	-	-	3.23%	3.63%	3.27%

Cozby-Germany Hospital

Alternate Name: East Texas Medical Center, Grande Saline Div.
707 N Waldrip Street
Grand Saline, TX 75140
E-mail: info@cozbygermanyhospital.com
URL: www.cozby-germanyhospital.com
Ownership: Voluntary non-profit - Private
Emergency Services: Yes

Phone: 903-962-4242
Fax: 903-962-3616
Accredited: No
Licensed Beds: 52

Key Personnel:

CEO	William Rowton

NOTE: Hospital profiles are in alphabetical order by state, then city, then hospital within the city; Rankings are sorted by rate in descending order and exclude hospitals with less than 25 cases; (1) The number of cases is too small (n<25) for purposes of reliably predicting hospital performance; (2) Measure reflects the hospital's indication that its submission was based upon a sample of its relevant discharges; (3) Rate reflects fewer than the maximum possible quarters of data for the measure; (4) Inaccurate information submitted and suppressed for one or more quarters; (5) No data is available from the hospital for this measure; Please refer to the User's Guide for a full explanation of data

Chief Medical Staff. . . . . Richard Ingrim, MD
Director Infection/Disease Control . . . . Nancy Carter
Director Medical/Surgical Nursing . . . . Margaret Smith
Chief Radiology . . . . Harold Smitson, MD
Director Respiratory Therapy . . . . Devin Rowe

Measure	Cases	This Hospital	State Average	U.S. Average	Top Hospital
Heart Attack Care					
ACE Inhibitor or ARB for LVSD[3]	0	-	85%	82%	100%
Aspirin at Arrival[1,3]	1	0%	91%	92%	100%
Aspirin at Discharge[1,3]	1	0%	90%	90%	100%
Beta Blocker at Arrival[1,3]	1	0%	85%	87%	100%
Beta Blocker at Discharge[1,3]	1	100%	86%	90%	100%
Fibrinolytic Medication Timing[3]	0	-	30%	31%	100%
PCI Within 90 Minutes of Arrival	0	-	48%	54%	95%
Smoking Cessation Advice[3]	0	-	90%	88%	100%
Heart Failure Care					
ACE Inhibitor or ARB for LVSD[1]	5	80%	82%	82%	100%
Discharge Instructions[1]	24	67%	60%	61%	93%
Evaluation of LVS Function	34	94%	81%	83%	99%
Smoking Cessation Advice[1]	9	89%	82%	82%	100%
Pneumonia Care					
Appropriate Initial Antibiotic	35	89%	79%	83%	94%
Blood Culture Timing	40	82%	89%	90%	100%
Influenza Vaccine[1]	16	44%	69%	70%	100%
Initial Antibiotic Timing	64	94%	78%	80%	93%
Oxygenation Assessment	74	100%	99%	99%	100%
Pneumococcal Vaccine	50	44%	68%	69%	94%
Smoking Cessation Advice[1]	13	69%	83%	80%	100%
Surgical Infection Prevention					
Prophylactic Antibiotic Given[5]	-	-	67%	77%	95%
Prophylactic Antibiotic Selection[5]	-	-	86%	90%	100%
Prophylactic Antibiotic Stopped[5]	-	-	68%	72%	95%
Pregnancy Care					
Inpatient Neonatal Mortality	-	-	-	-	-
Third or Fourth Degree Laceration	-	-	3.23%	3.63%	3.27%

Baylor Regional Medical Center at Grapevine

1650 West College
Grapevine, TX 76051
URL: www.baylorhealth.com
Ownership: Voluntary non-profit - Church
Emergency Services: Yes
Phone: 817-481-1588
Fax: 817-481-2962

Accredited: Yes
Licensed Beds: 104

Key Personnel:
CEO/President. . . . . Laura Lycan
Chief of Medical Staff. Stephen Lacey, MD
Director of Cardiology/Cardiac Lab. . . . . Phil Hecht, MD
Director Emergency Room. . . . . Kris Pawell
Director Infection/Disease Control . . . . Brady Allen
Director Medical/Surgical Nursing . . . . Lynn Curtis

Measure	Cases	This Hospital	State Average	U.S. Average	Top Hospital
Heart Attack Care					
ACE Inhibitor or ARB for LVSD[1]	22	95%	85%	82%	100%
Aspirin at Arrival	172	100%	91%	92%	100%
Aspirin at Discharge	162	98%	90%	90%	100%
Beta Blocker at Arrival	161	99%	85%	87%	100%
Beta Blocker at Discharge	150	96%	86%	90%	100%
Fibrinolytic Medication Timing[1]	1	100%	30%	31%	100%
PCI Within 90 Minutes of Arrival[1]	12	92%	48%	54%	95%
Smoking Cessation Advice	60	92%	90%	88%	100%
Heart Failure Care					
ACE Inhibitor or ARB for LVSD	46	96%	82%	82%	100%
Discharge Instructions	128	77%	60%	61%	93%
Evaluation of LVS Function	150	94%	81%	83%	99%
Smoking Cessation Advice[1]	23	100%	82%	82%	100%
Pneumonia Care					
Appropriate Initial Antibiotic	136	91%	79%	83%	94%
Blood Culture Timing	118	84%	89%	90%	100%
Influenza Vaccine	37	81%	69%	70%	100%
Initial Antibiotic Timing	159	86%	78%	80%	93%
Oxygenation Assessment	201	100%	99%	99%	100%

Pneumococcal Vaccine	105	86%	68%	69%	94%
Smoking Cessation Advice	51	96%	83%	80%	100%
Surgical Infection Prevention					
Prophylactic Antibiotic Given	805	96%	67%	77%	95%
Prophylactic Antibiotic Selection	184	92%	86%	90%	100%
Prophylactic Antibiotic Stopped	797	79%	68%	72%	95%
Pregnancy Care					
Inpatient Neonatal Mortality	-	-	-	-	-
Third or Fourth Degree Laceration	-	-	3.23%	3.63%	3.27%

Presbyterian Hospital of Greenville

Alternate Name: Presbyterian Hospital of Commerce
PO Drawer 1059
Greenville, TX 75401
E-mail: administration@hmhd.org
URL: www.hmhd.org
Ownership: Govt - Hospital District or Authority
Emergency Services: Yes
Phone: 903-886-3161
Fax: 903-408-1609

Accredited: Yes
Licensed Beds: 30

Key Personnel:
Administrator/CEO. . . . . Richard C Carter
Chief Medical Staff. . . . . Tom Selvaggi, MD
Emergency Room . . . . Rick Selveggi, MD
Director Respiratory Therapy . . . . Paul Loyd

Measure	Cases	This Hospital	State Average	U.S. Average	Top Hospital
Heart Attack Care					
ACE Inhibitor or ARB for LVSD[1]	9	44%	85%	82%	100%
Aspirin at Arrival	69	86%	91%	92%	100%
Aspirin at Discharge	32	72%	90%	90%	100%
Beta Blocker at Arrival	66	70%	85%	87%	100%
Beta Blocker at Discharge	32	81%	86%	90%	100%
Fibrinolytic Medication Timing[1]	1	0%	30%	31%	100%
PCI Within 90 Minutes of Arrival	0	-	48%	54%	95%
Smoking Cessation Advice[1]	7	100%	90%	88%	100%
Heart Failure Care					
ACE Inhibitor or ARB for LVSD	143	64%	82%	82%	100%
Discharge Instructions	267	1%	60%	61%	93%
Evaluation of LVS Function	338	93%	81%	83%	99%
Smoking Cessation Advice	62	89%	82%	82%	100%
Pneumonia Care					
Appropriate Initial Antibiotic	178	75%	79%	83%	94%
Blood Culture Timing	151	77%	89%	90%	100%
Influenza Vaccine	68	60%	69%	70%	100%
Initial Antibiotic Timing	221	69%	78%	80%	93%
Oxygenation Assessment	292	99%	99%	99%	100%
Pneumococcal Vaccine	162	58%	68%	69%	94%
Smoking Cessation Advice	88	85%	83%	80%	100%
Surgical Infection Prevention					
Prophylactic Antibiotic Given[3]	264	72%	67%	77%	95%
Prophylactic Antibiotic Selection	108	44%	86%	90%	100%
Prophylactic Antibiotic Stopped[3]	249	85%	68%	72%	95%
Pregnancy Care					
Inpatient Neonatal Mortality	-	-	-	-	-
Third or Fourth Degree Laceration	-	-	3.23%	3.63%	3.27%

Limestone Medical Center

701 McClintic Drive
Groesbeck, TX 76642
E-mail: swood@lmchospital.com
URL: lmchospital.com
Ownership: Govt - Hospital District or Authority
Emergency Services: Yes
Phone: 254-729-3281
Fax: 254-729-2689

Accredited: No
Licensed Beds: 20

Key Personnel:
President/CEO. . . . . Penny U Gray
Chief of Medical Staff. Larry Hughes
Emergency Room Director. . . . . Jude Wright
Respiratory/Cardiopulmonary. . . . . Joanie Isabell

Measure	Cases	This Hospital	State Average	U.S. Average	Top Hospital
Heart Attack Care					
ACE Inhibitor or ARB for LVSD[5]	-	-	85%	82%	100%
Aspirin at Arrival[5]	-	-	91%	92%	100%
Aspirin at Discharge[5]	-	-	90%	90%	100%

NOTE: Hospital profiles are in alphabetical order by state, then city, then hospital within the city; Rankings are sorted by rate in descending order and exclude hospitals with less than 25 cases; (1) The number of cases is too small (n<25) for purposes of reliably predicting hospital performance; (2) Measure reflects the hospital's indication that its submission was based upon a sample of its relevant discharges; (3) Rate reflects fewer than the maximum possible quarters of data for the measure; (4) Inaccurate information submitted and suppressed for one or more quarters; (5) No data is available from the hospital for this measure; Please refer to the User's Guide for a full explanation of data

			85%	87%	100%
Beta Blocker at Arrival[5]	-	-	85%	87%	100%
Beta Blocker at Discharge[5]	-	-	86%	90%	100%
Fibrinolytic Medication Timing[5]	-	-	30%	31%	100%
PCI Within 90 Minutes of Arrival[5]	-	-	48%	54%	95%
Smoking Cessation Advice[5]	-	-	90%	88%	100%
Heart Failure Care					
ACE Inhibitor or ARB for LVSD[2,3]	0	-	82%	82%	100%
Discharge Instructions[2,3]	0	-	60%	61%	93%
Evaluation of LVS Function[1,2,3]	2	100%	81%	83%	99%
Smoking Cessation Advice[2,3]	0	-	82%	82%	100%
Pneumonia Care					
Appropriate Initial Antibiotic[1,2,3]	13	77%	79%	83%	94%
Blood Culture Timing[1,2,3]	3	100%	89%	90%	100%
Influenza Vaccine[1,2]	5	100%	69%	70%	100%
Initial Antibiotic Timing[1,2,3]	3	100%	78%	80%	93%
Oxygenation Assessment[1,2,3]	17	100%	99%	99%	100%
Pneumococcal Vaccine[1,2,3]	14	93%	68%	69%	94%
Smoking Cessation Advice[1,2,3]	2	100%	83%	80%	100%
Surgical Infection Prevention					
Prophylactic Antibiotic Given[5]	-	-	67%	77%	95%
Prophylactic Antibiotic Selection[5]	-	-	86%	90%	100%
Prophylactic Antibiotic Stopped[5]	-	-	68%	72%	95%
Pregnancy Care					
Inpatient Neonatal Mortality	-	-	-	-	-
Third or Fourth Degree Laceration	-	-	3.23%	3.63%	3.27%

Renaissance Hospital-East Texas

5500 39th Street
Groves, TX 77619
URL: groves.renhealthcare.org
Ownership: Proprietary
Emergency Services: Yes

Phone: 409-962-5733
Fax: 409-963-5202

Accredited: Yes
Licensed Beds: 106

Key Personnel:
CEO . . . . David Cottey
Chief Medical Staff . . . . John Lee, Dr
Emergency Room . . . . Rhonda Smith

Measure	Cases	This Hospital	State Average	U.S. Average	Top Hospital
Heart Attack Care					
ACE Inhibitor or ARB for LVSD[1,3]	9	78%	85%	82%	100%
Aspirin at Arrival[3]	25	92%	91%	92%	100%
Aspirin at Discharge[3]	25	92%	90%	90%	100%
Beta Blocker at Arrival[3]	25	84%	85%	87%	100%
Beta Blocker at Discharge[3]	27	89%	86%	90%	100%
Fibrinolytic Medication Timing[1,3]	2	0%	30%	31%	100%
PCI Within 90 Minutes of Arrival	0	-	48%	54%	95%
Smoking Cessation Advice[1,3]	1	0%	90%	88%	100%
Heart Failure Care					
ACE Inhibitor or ARB for LVSD[1,2,3]	17	41%	82%	82%	100%
Discharge Instructions[1,2,3]	11	0%	60%	61%	93%
Evaluation of LVS Function[2,3]	71	58%	81%	83%	99%
Smoking Cessation Advice[1,2,3]	3	33%	82%	82%	100%
Pneumonia Care					
Appropriate Initial Antibiotic[1,2,3]	7	57%	79%	83%	94%
Blood Culture Timing[2,3]	0	-	89%	90%	100%
Influenza Vaccine[5]	-	-	69%	70%	100%
Initial Antibiotic Timing[2,3]	44	66%	78%	80%	93%
Oxygenation Assessment[2,3]	63	100%	99%	99%	100%
Pneumococcal Vaccine[2,3]	35	17%	68%	69%	94%
Smoking Cessation Advice[1,2,3]	4	50%	83%	80%	100%
Surgical Infection Prevention					
Prophylactic Antibiotic Given[1,3]	7	57%	67%	77%	95%
Prophylactic Antibiotic Selection[5]	-	-	86%	90%	100%
Prophylactic Antibiotic Stopped[1,3]	6	67%	68%	72%	95%
Pregnancy Care					
Inpatient Neonatal Mortality	-	-	-	-	-
Third or Fourth Degree Laceration	-	-	3.23%	3.63%	3.27%

Lavaca Medical Center

1400 N Texana Street
Hallettsville, TX 77964
Ownership: Government - Local
Emergency Services: No

Phone: 361-798-3671
Fax: 361-798-2682
Accredited: No
Licensed Beds: 43

Key Personnel:
CEO . . . . James E Vanek

Measure	Cases	This Hospital	State Average	U.S. Average	Top Hospital
Heart Attack Care					
ACE Inhibitor or ARB for LVSD[1]	2	100%	85%	82%	100%
Aspirin at Arrival[1]	8	100%	91%	92%	100%
Aspirin at Discharge[1]	4	100%	90%	90%	100%
Beta Blocker at Arrival[1]	8	75%	85%	87%	100%
Beta Blocker at Discharge[1]	4	100%	86%	90%	100%
Fibrinolytic Medication Timing	0	-	30%	31%	100%
PCI Within 90 Minutes of Arrival	0	-	48%	54%	95%
Smoking Cessation Advice	0	-	90%	88%	100%
Heart Failure Care					
ACE Inhibitor or ARB for LVSD[1]	8	100%	82%	82%	100%
Discharge Instructions[1]	21	71%	60%	61%	93%
Evaluation of LVS Function	44	61%	81%	83%	99%
Smoking Cessation Advice[1]	1	100%	82%	82%	100%
Pneumonia Care					
Appropriate Initial Antibiotic	39	77%	79%	83%	94%
Blood Culture Timing[1]	23	100%	89%	90%	100%
Influenza Vaccine[1]	14	86%	69%	70%	100%
Initial Antibiotic Timing	69	91%	78%	80%	93%
Oxygenation Assessment	82	100%	99%	99%	100%
Pneumococcal Vaccine	58	91%	68%	69%	94%
Smoking Cessation Advice[1]	7	86%	83%	80%	100%
Surgical Infection Prevention					
Prophylactic Antibiotic Given[5]	-	-	67%	77%	95%
Prophylactic Antibiotic Selection[5]	-	-	86%	90%	100%
Prophylactic Antibiotic Stopped[5]	-	-	68%	72%	95%
Pregnancy Care					
Inpatient Neonatal Mortality	-	-	-	-	-
Third or Fourth Degree Laceration	-	-	3.23%	3.63%	3.27%

Hamilton General Hospital

400 North Brown Street
Hamilton, TX 76531
URL: www.hamiltonhospital.org
Ownership: Govt - Hospital District or Authority   Accredited: No
Emergency Services: Yes

Phone: 254-386-1600
Fax: 254-386-5173

Key Personnel:
Administrator/CEO . . . . James Schafer
Chief of Medical Staff . . . . James R Lee, MD

Measure	Cases	This Hospital	State Average	U.S. Average	Top Hospital
Heart Attack Care					
ACE Inhibitor or ARB for LVSD[1]	2	100%	85%	82%	100%
Aspirin at Arrival[1]	14	100%	91%	92%	100%
Aspirin at Discharge[1]	9	78%	90%	90%	100%
Beta Blocker at Arrival[1]	15	80%	85%	87%	100%
Beta Blocker at Discharge[1]	8	75%	86%	90%	100%
Fibrinolytic Medication Timing	0	-	30%	31%	100%
PCI Within 90 Minutes of Arrival	0	-	48%	54%	95%
Smoking Cessation Advice	0	-	90%	88%	100%
Heart Failure Care					
ACE Inhibitor or ARB for LVSD[1]	18	89%	82%	82%	100%
Discharge Instructions	74	46%	60%	61%	93%
Evaluation of LVS Function	107	60%	81%	83%	99%
Smoking Cessation Advice[1]	7	57%	82%	82%	100%
Pneumonia Care					
Appropriate Initial Antibiotic	86	76%	79%	83%	94%
Blood Culture Timing[1]	18	89%	89%	90%	100%
Influenza Vaccine	36	56%	69%	70%	100%
Initial Antibiotic Timing	93	88%	78%	80%	93%
Oxygenation Assessment	128	96%	99%	99%	100%
Pneumococcal Vaccine	98	72%	68%	69%	94%
Smoking Cessation Advice[1]	11	82%	83%	80%	100%

NOTE: Hospital profiles are in alphabetical order by state, then city, then hospital within the city; Rankings are sorted by rate in descending order and exclude hospitals with less than 25 cases; (1) The number of cases is too small (n<25) for purposes of reliably predicting hospital performance; (2) Measure reflects the hospital's indication that its submission was based upon a sample of its relevant discharges; (3) Rate reflects fewer than the maximum possible quarters of data for the measure; (4) Inaccurate information submitted and suppressed for one or more quarters; (5) No data is available from the hospital for this measure; Please refer to the User's Guide for a full explanation of data

Surgical Infection Prevention					
Prophylactic Antibiotic Given[1,3]	3	33%	67%	77%	95%
Prophylactic Antibiotic Selection[1]	1	100%	86%	90%	100%
Prophylactic Antibiotic Stopped[1,3]	3	100%	68%	72%	95%
Pregnancy Care					
Inpatient Neonatal Mortality	-	-	-	-	-
Third or Fourth Degree Laceration	-	-	3.23%	3.63%	3.27%

Hamlin Memorial Hospital

632 Northwest Second Street
Hamlin, TX 79520
Ownership: Government - Local
Emergency Services: No
Key Personnel:
CEO. . . . . Jim Barnett

Phone: 325-576-3646
Fax: 325-576-2922
Accredited: No
Licensed Beds: 25

Measure	Cases	This Hospital	State Average	U.S. Average	Top Hospital
Heart Attack Care					
ACE Inhibitor or ARB for LVSD[3]	0	-	85%	82%	100%
Aspirin at Arrival[3]	0	-	91%	92%	100%
Aspirin at Discharge[3]	0	-	90%	90%	100%
Beta Blocker at Arrival[3]	0	-	85%	87%	100%
Beta Blocker at Discharge[3]	0	-	86%	90%	100%
Fibrinolytic Medication Timing[5]	-	-	30%	31%	100%
PCI Within 90 Minutes of Arrival[5]	-	-	48%	54%	95%
Smoking Cessation Advice[5]	-	-	90%	88%	100%
Heart Failure Care					
ACE Inhibitor or ARB for LVSD[1]	4	100%	82%	82%	100%
Discharge Instructions[1,3]	4	25%	60%	61%	93%
Evaluation of LVS Function[1]	17	53%	81%	83%	99%
Smoking Cessation Advice[1,3]	3	0%	82%	82%	100%
Pneumonia Care					
Appropriate Initial Antibiotic[1,3]	2	50%	79%	83%	94%
Blood Culture Timing[3]	0	-	89%	90%	100%
Influenza Vaccine[4,5]	-	-	69%	70%	100%
Initial Antibiotic Timing[1]	13	100%	78%	80%	93%
Oxygenation Assessment[1]	14	100%	99%	99%	100%
Pneumococcal Vaccine[1]	10	70%	68%	69%	94%
Smoking Cessation Advice[3]	0	-	83%	80%	100%
Surgical Infection Prevention					
Prophylactic Antibiotic Given[5]	-	-	67%	77%	95%
Prophylactic Antibiotic Selection[5]	-	-	86%	90%	100%
Prophylactic Antibiotic Stopped[5]	-	-	68%	72%	95%
Pregnancy Care					
Inpatient Neonatal Mortality	-	-	-	-	-
Third or Fourth Degree Laceration	-	-	3.23%	3.63%	3.27%

Harlingen Medical Center

5501 South Expressway 77
Harlingen, TX 78550
URL: www.harlingenmedicalcenter.com
Ownership: Proprietary
Emergency Services: Yes
Key Personnel:
President/CEO. . . . . Richard L Gamber
Chief Medical Staff. Ruby Byrd
Director Respiratory . . . . Alma Summers

Phone: 956-365-1000
Fax: 956-365-1875

Accredited: Yes
Licensed Beds: 80

Measure	Cases	This Hospital	State Average	U.S. Average	Top Hospital
Heart Attack Care					
ACE Inhibitor or ARB for LVSD[1]	17	100%	85%	82%	100%
Aspirin at Arrival	65	100%	91%	92%	100%
Aspirin at Discharge	72	100%	90%	90%	100%
Beta Blocker at Arrival	64	100%	85%	87%	100%
Beta Blocker at Discharge	67	100%	86%	90%	100%
Fibrinolytic Medication Timing	0	-	30%	31%	100%
PCI Within 90 Minutes of Arrival	0	-	48%	54%	95%
Smoking Cessation Advice[1]	13	100%	90%	88%	100%
Heart Failure Care					
ACE Inhibitor or ARB for LVSD	38	100%	82%	82%	100%
Discharge Instructions	146	96%	60%	61%	93%
Evaluation of LVS Function	168	97%	81%	83%	99%

Smoking Cessation Advice[1]	9	100%	82%	82%	100%
Pneumonia Care					
Appropriate Initial Antibiotic	101	88%	79%	83%	94%
Blood Culture Timing	99	92%	89%	90%	100%
Influenza Vaccine	42	62%	69%	70%	100%
Initial Antibiotic Timing	153	84%	78%	80%	93%
Oxygenation Assessment	165	100%	99%	99%	100%
Pneumococcal Vaccine	108	82%	68%	69%	94%
Smoking Cessation Advice[1]	17	100%	83%	80%	100%
Surgical Infection Prevention					
Prophylactic Antibiotic Given[3]	258	85%	67%	77%	95%
Prophylactic Antibiotic Selection	86	93%	86%	90%	100%
Prophylactic Antibiotic Stopped[3]	255	62%	68%	72%	95%
Pregnancy Care					
Inpatient Neonatal Mortality	-	-	-	-	-
Third or Fourth Degree Laceration	-	-	3.23%	3.63%	3.27%

Valley Baptist Medical Center

2101 Pease Street
Harlingen, TX 78550
URL: www.vbmc.org
Ownership: Voluntary non-profit - Church
Emergency Services: Yes
Key Personnel:
Administrator/President . . . . Ben McKibbens
Chief Medical Staff. Robert Minor, MD
Chief Catheterization Laboratory . . . . C Mild, MD
Emergency Room . . . . H Stephens, MD
Director Infection/Disease Control . . . . Pat Brattin, RN
CCU Spvg. Nurse . . . . Lucy Flores, RN
OB/GYN Womens Health. . . . . H Benavides, MD
Chief Radiology . . . . George Skye, MD
Director Respiratory Therapy . . . . Michelle Marantich

Phone: 956-389-1100
Fax: 956-389-1632

Accredited: Yes
Licensed Beds: 588

Measure	Cases	This Hospital	State Average	U.S. Average	Top Hospital
Heart Attack Care					
ACE Inhibitor or ARB for LVSD	65	100%	85%	82%	100%
Aspirin at Arrival	285	100%	91%	92%	100%
Aspirin at Discharge	256	100%	90%	90%	100%
Beta Blocker at Arrival	245	99%	85%	87%	100%
Beta Blocker at Discharge	251	99%	86%	90%	100%
Fibrinolytic Medication Timing	0	-	30%	31%	100%
PCI Within 90 Minutes of Arrival[1]	12	17%	48%	54%	95%
Smoking Cessation Advice	57	100%	90%	88%	100%
Heart Failure Care					
ACE Inhibitor or ARB for LVSD	228	100%	82%	82%	100%
Discharge Instructions	635	100%	60%	61%	93%
Evaluation of LVS Function	713	100%	81%	83%	99%
Smoking Cessation Advice	54	100%	82%	82%	100%
Pneumonia Care					
Appropriate Initial Antibiotic	332	85%	79%	83%	94%
Blood Culture Timing	251	89%	89%	90%	100%
Influenza Vaccine	86	42%	69%	70%	100%
Initial Antibiotic Timing	369	76%	78%	80%	93%
Oxygenation Assessment	440	100%	99%	99%	100%
Pneumococcal Vaccine	287	64%	68%	69%	94%
Smoking Cessation Advice	45	100%	83%	80%	100%
Surgical Infection Prevention					
Prophylactic Antibiotic Given[2,3]	197	79%	67%	77%	95%
Prophylactic Antibiotic Selection[2]	59	90%	86%	90%	100%
Prophylactic Antibiotic Stopped[2,3]	190	61%	68%	72%	95%
Pregnancy Care					
Inpatient Neonatal Mortality	-	-	-	-	-
Third or Fourth Degree Laceration	-	-	3.23%	3.63%	3.27%

NOTE: Hospital profiles are in alphabetical order by state, then city, then hospital within the city; Rankings are sorted by rate in descending order and exclude hospitals with less than 25 cases; (1) The number of cases is too small (n<25) for purposes of reliably predicting hospital performance; (2) Measure reflects the hospital's indication that its submission was based upon a sample of its relevant discharges; (3) Rate reflects fewer than the maximum possible quarters of data for the measure; (4) Inaccurate information submitted and suppressed for one or more quarters; (5) No data is available from the hospital for this measure; Please refer to the User's Guide for a full explanation of data

Henderson Memorial Hospital

300 Wilson
Henderson, TX 75652

Toll-Free: 800-329-7541
Phone: 903-657-7541
Fax: 903-655-3661

URL: www.hmhtx.org
Ownership: Voluntary non-profit - Other
Emergency Services: Yes

Accredited: Yes
Licensed Beds: 158

Key Personnel:

CEO................................... Mark Leitner
Chief Medical Staff...................... Yogesh Pai, MD
Emergency Room .... Tom Curtis, MD
Director Infection/Disease Control .... Tammy Koonce
CCU Spvg. Nurse .... Dorothy Boone, RN
Chief Radiology .... John Melvin, MD
Director Respiratory Therapy .... Marty Partida

Measure	Cases	This Hospital	State Average	U.S. Average	Top Hospital
Heart Attack Care					
ACE Inhibitor or ARB for LVSD[1]	3	100%	85%	82%	100%
Aspirin at Arrival[1]	16	100%	91%	92%	100%
Aspirin at Discharge[1]	10	100%	90%	90%	100%
Beta Blocker at Arrival[1]	14	93%	85%	87%	100%
Beta Blocker at Discharge[1]	9	89%	86%	90%	100%
Fibrinolytic Medication Timing	0	-	30%	31%	100%
PCI Within 90 Minutes of Arrival	0	-	48%	54%	95%
Smoking Cessation Advice[1]	2	50%	90%	88%	100%
Heart Failure Care					
ACE Inhibitor or ARB for LVSD	28	93%	82%	82%	100%
Discharge Instructions	96	67%	60%	61%	93%
Evaluation of LVS Function	125	75%	81%	83%	99%
Smoking Cessation Advice[1]	15	80%	82%	82%	100%
Pneumonia Care					
Appropriate Initial Antibiotic	80	81%	79%	83%	94%
Blood Culture Timing	56	86%	89%	90%	100%
Influenza Vaccine[1]	18	83%	69%	70%	100%
Initial Antibiotic Timing	108	85%	78%	80%	93%
Oxygenation Assessment	128	100%	99%	99%	100%
Pneumococcal Vaccine	76	72%	68%	69%	94%
Smoking Cessation Advice[1]	23	74%	83%	80%	100%
Surgical Infection Prevention					
Prophylactic Antibiotic Given[3]	40	70%	67%	77%	95%
Prophylactic Antibiotic Selection	39	85%	86%	90%	100%
Prophylactic Antibiotic Stopped[3]	37	97%	68%	72%	95%
Pregnancy Care					
Inpatient Neonatal Mortality	-	-	-	-	-
Third or Fourth Degree Laceration	-	-	3.23%	3.63%	3.27%

Hereford Regional Medical Center

Alternate Name: Deaf Smith General Hospital
801 E 3rd Street
Hereford, TX 79045

Phone: 806-364-2141
Fax: 806-349-9373

URL: www.herefordtx.org/DeafSmithCo/Healthcare.htm
Ownership: Govt - Hospital District or Authority
Emergency Services: No

Accredited: No
Licensed Beds: 40

Key Personnel:

CEO................................... James Taylor
Chief Medical Staff...................... Nadir Khuri, MD
Emergency Room .... Brinda Cozeby

Measure	Cases	This Hospital	State Average	U.S. Average	Top Hospital
Heart Attack Care					
ACE Inhibitor or ARB for LVSD[5]	-	-	85%	82%	100%
Aspirin at Arrival[5]	-	-	91%	92%	100%
Aspirin at Discharge[5]	-	-	90%	90%	100%
Beta Blocker at Arrival[5]	-	-	85%	87%	100%
Beta Blocker at Discharge[5]	-	-	86%	90%	100%
Fibrinolytic Medication Timing[5]	-	-	30%	31%	100%
PCI Within 90 Minutes of Arrival[5]	-	-	48%	54%	95%
Smoking Cessation Advice[5]	-	-	90%	88%	100%
Heart Failure Care					
ACE Inhibitor or ARB for LVSD[1]	5	60%	82%	82%	100%
Discharge Instructions[1,3]	5	0%	60%	61%	93%
Evaluation of LVS Function	31	35%	81%	83%	99%

	0	-	82%	82%	100%
Smoking Cessation Advice[3]					
Pneumonia Care					
Appropriate Initial Antibiotic[1,3]	3	100%	79%	83%	94%
Blood Culture Timing[1,3]	2	100%	89%	90%	100%
Influenza Vaccine[5]	-	-	69%	70%	100%
Initial Antibiotic Timing	44	80%	78%	80%	93%
Oxygenation Assessment	53	100%	99%	99%	100%
Pneumococcal Vaccine	34	18%	68%	69%	94%
Smoking Cessation Advice[1,3]	1	100%	83%	80%	100%
Surgical Infection Prevention					
Prophylactic Antibiotic Given[1,3]	2	0%	67%	77%	95%
Prophylactic Antibiotic Selection[5]	-	-	86%	90%	100%
Prophylactic Antibiotic Stopped[1,3]	1	0%	68%	72%	95%
Pregnancy Care					
Inpatient Neonatal Mortality	-	-	-	-	-
Third or Fourth Degree Laceration	-	-	3.23%	3.63%	3.27%

Hill Regional Hospital

101 Circle Drive
Hillsboro, TX 76645
Ownership: Proprietary
Emergency Services: Yes

Phone: 254-580-8500
Fax: 254-582-2144
Accredited: Yes
Licensed Beds: 92

Key Personnel:

CEO/President........................ Jan Mcclure
Chief Medical Staff.................... Paul Floy
Director Infection/Disease Control .... Patricia Perez
Head of Radiology .... Donna Rogers
Director Respiratory Therapy .... Kellie Harris

Measure	Cases	This Hospital	State Average	U.S. Average	Top Hospital
Heart Attack Care					
ACE Inhibitor or ARB for LVSD	0	-	85%	82%	100%
Aspirin at Arrival[1]	19	95%	91%	92%	100%
Aspirin at Discharge[1]	9	78%	90%	90%	100%
Beta Blocker at Arrival[1]	14	100%	85%	87%	100%
Beta Blocker at Discharge[1]	9	89%	86%	90%	100%
Fibrinolytic Medication Timing[1]	8	12%	30%	31%	100%
PCI Within 90 Minutes of Arrival	0	-	48%	54%	95%
Smoking Cessation Advice	0	-	90%	88%	100%
Heart Failure Care					
ACE Inhibitor or ARB for LVSD[1]	18	83%	82%	82%	100%
Discharge Instructions	86	56%	60%	61%	93%
Evaluation of LVS Function	122	79%	81%	83%	99%
Smoking Cessation Advice[1]	24	88%	82%	82%	100%
Pneumonia Care					
Appropriate Initial Antibiotic	69	88%	79%	83%	94%
Blood Culture Timing	37	89%	89%	90%	100%
Influenza Vaccine[1]	19	63%	69%	70%	100%
Initial Antibiotic Timing	86	97%	78%	80%	93%
Oxygenation Assessment	101	100%	99%	99%	100%
Pneumococcal Vaccine	67	82%	68%	69%	94%
Smoking Cessation Advice	25	80%	83%	80%	100%
Surgical Infection Prevention					
Prophylactic Antibiotic Given[1,2,3]	18	50%	67%	77%	95%
Prophylactic Antibiotic Selection[1,2]	11	91%	86%	90%	100%
Prophylactic Antibiotic Stopped[1,2,3]	16	69%	68%	72%	95%
Pregnancy Care					
Inpatient Neonatal Mortality	-	-	-	-	-
Third or Fourth Degree Laceration	-	-	3.23%	3.63%	3.27%

Columbia Spring Branch Medical Center

Alternate Name: Spring Branch Medical Center
8850 Long Point
Houston, TX 77055

Phone: 713-467-6555
Fax: 713-722-3785

URL: www.springbranchmedical.com
Ownership: Proprietary
Emergency Services: Yes

Accredited: Yes
Licensed Beds: 350

Key Personnel:

CEO................................... Scott Koenig
Chief Medical Staff.................... Caesar Bravo
Emergency Room .... Patty Torres
Director Infection/Disease Control .... Cathy Lamb
OB/GYN Womens Health................. Lucia Williams, MD

NOTE: Hospital profiles are in alphabetical order by state, then city, then hospital within the city; Rankings are sorted by rate in descending order and exclude hospitals with less than 25 cases; (1) The number of cases is too small (n<25) for purposes of reliably predicting hospital performance; (2) Measure reflects the hospital's indication that its submission was based upon a sample of its relevant discharges; (3) Rate reflects fewer than the maximum possible quarters of data for the measure; (4) Inaccurate information submitted and suppressed for one or more quarters; (5) No data is available from the hospital for this measure; Please refer to the User's Guide for a full explanation of data

Chief Radiology . . . . Julius Danziger
Director Respiratory Therapy . . . . Laura Williams

Measure	Cases	This Hospital	State Average	U.S. Average	Top Hospital
Heart Attack Care					
ACE Inhibitor or ARB for LVSD	35	83%	85%	82%	100%
Aspirin at Arrival	113	91%	91%	92%	100%
Aspirin at Discharge	114	84%	90%	90%	100%
Beta Blocker at Arrival	97	89%	85%	87%	100%
Beta Blocker at Discharge	121	90%	86%	90%	100%
Fibrinolytic Medication Timing[1]	1	100%	30%	31%	100%
PCI Within 90 Minutes of Arrival[1]	6	0%	48%	54%	95%
Smoking Cessation Advice	54	98%	90%	88%	100%
Heart Failure Care					
ACE Inhibitor or ARB for LVSD	119	81%	82%	82%	100%
Discharge Instructions	227	53%	60%	61%	93%
Evaluation of LVS Function	300	95%	81%	83%	99%
Smoking Cessation Advice	67	94%	82%	82%	100%
Pneumonia Care					
Appropriate Initial Antibiotic	127	74%	79%	83%	94%
Blood Culture Timing	149	93%	89%	90%	100%
Influenza Vaccine	42	79%	69%	70%	100%
Initial Antibiotic Timing	253	87%	78%	80%	93%
Oxygenation Assessment	266	98%	99%	99%	100%
Pneumococcal Vaccine	157	83%	68%	69%	94%
Smoking Cessation Advice	57	88%	83%	80%	100%
Surgical Infection Prevention					
Prophylactic Antibiotic Given[2,3]	158	66%	67%	77%	95%
Prophylactic Antibiotic Selection[2]	66	82%	86%	90%	100%
Prophylactic Antibiotic Stopped[2,3]	155	53%	68%	72%	95%
Pregnancy Care					
Inpatient Neonatal Mortality	-	-	-	-	-
Third or Fourth Degree Laceration	-	-	3.23%	3.63%	3.27%

Cypress Fairbanks Medical Center and Hospital
10655 Steepletop Drive   Phone: 281-890-4285
Houston, TX 77065   Fax: 281-890-0236
URL: www.cyfairhospital.com
Ownership: Proprietary   Accredited: Yes
Emergency Services: Yes   Licensed Beds: 140
Key Personnel:
President/CEO . . . . Bill Klier
Chief Medical Staff . . . . Colleen Hutson
Emergency Room . . . . Bob Shepherd, MD
Director Infection/Disease Control . . . . Cheryl Briggs, RN
CCU Spvg. Nurse . . . . Patti Bennett
Director Medical/Surgical Nursing . . . . Patti Bennett
Chief Radiology . . . . George Abdo, MD
Director Respiratory Therapy . . . . Jan Terry

Measure	Cases	This Hospital	State Average	U.S. Average	Top Hospital
Heart Attack Care					
ACE Inhibitor or ARB for LVSD[1]	5	100%	85%	82%	100%
Aspirin at Arrival	101	98%	91%	92%	100%
Aspirin at Discharge	78	100%	90%	90%	100%
Beta Blocker at Arrival	85	93%	85%	87%	100%
Beta Blocker at Discharge	70	96%	86%	90%	100%
Fibrinolytic Medication Timing[1]	3	33%	30%	31%	100%
PCI Within 90 Minutes of Arrival[1]	14	86%	48%	54%	95%
Smoking Cessation Advice	26	100%	90%	88%	100%
Heart Failure Care					
ACE Inhibitor or ARB for LVSD	81	84%	82%	82%	100%
Discharge Instructions	197	58%	60%	61%	93%
Evaluation of LVS Function	262	97%	81%	83%	99%
Smoking Cessation Advice	36	97%	82%	82%	100%
Pneumonia Care					
Appropriate Initial Antibiotic	202	92%	79%	83%	94%
Blood Culture Timing	219	88%	89%	90%	100%
Influenza Vaccine	76	87%	69%	70%	100%
Initial Antibiotic Timing	265	82%	78%	80%	93%
Oxygenation Assessment	379	100%	99%	99%	100%
Pneumococcal Vaccine	189	89%	68%	69%	94%

Measure	Cases	This Hospital	State Average	U.S. Average	Top Hospital
Smoking Cessation Advice	66	95%	83%	80%	100%
Surgical Infection Prevention					
Prophylactic Antibiotic Given[2]	119	85%	67%	77%	95%
Prophylactic Antibiotic Selection[2]	33	94%	86%	90%	100%
Prophylactic Antibiotic Stopped[2]	106	48%	68%	72%	95%
Pregnancy Care					
Inpatient Neonatal Mortality	-	-	-	-	-
Third or Fourth Degree Laceration	-	-	3.23%	3.63%	3.27%

Doctors Hospital Parkway+Tidwell
Alternate Name: Yale Clinic & Hospital
510 W Tidwell Road   Phone: 281-618-8500
Houston, TX 77091   Fax: 713-691-4790
URL: www.dhthcu.com
Ownership: Voluntary non-profit - Private   Accredited: Yes
Emergency Services: Yes   Licensed Beds: 263
Key Personnel:
President/CEO . . . . Max Ludeke
Chief Medical Staff . . . . Carlos Palacios, MD
Cardiac Lab . . . . Richard Barlow
Catheterization Lab . . . . Richard Barlow
Emergency Room . . . . Judith Reyers, RN
Infection Control . . . . Kathy Hudson
ICU . . . . Judith Reyes, RN
Intensive/Coronary Care . . . . Judith Reyer, RN
Medical/Surgical Nursing . . . . Allison Stasne, RN
OB/GYN Womens Health . . . . Jean Davis, RN
Respiratory/Cardiopulmonary . . . . Victor Yeldell

Measure	Cases	This Hospital	State Average	U.S. Average	Top Hospital
Heart Attack Care					
ACE Inhibitor or ARB for LVSD	27	81%	85%	82%	100%
Aspirin at Arrival	103	80%	91%	92%	100%
Aspirin at Discharge	100	66%	90%	90%	100%
Beta Blocker at Arrival	80	56%	85%	87%	100%
Beta Blocker at Discharge	97	65%	86%	90%	100%
Fibrinolytic Medication Timing[1,3]	1	0%	30%	31%	100%
PCI Within 90 Minutes of Arrival	0	-	48%	54%	95%
Smoking Cessation Advice[1,3]	14	79%	90%	88%	100%
Heart Failure Care					
ACE Inhibitor or ARB for LVSD	123	67%	82%	82%	100%
Discharge Instructions[3]	64	17%	60%	61%	93%
Evaluation of LVS Function	287	80%	81%	83%	99%
Smoking Cessation Advice[1,3]	22	45%	82%	82%	100%
Pneumonia Care					
Appropriate Initial Antibiotic[1,3]	9	78%	79%	83%	94%
Blood Culture Timing[1,3]	14	86%	89%	90%	100%
Influenza Vaccine[5]	-	-	69%	70%	100%
Initial Antibiotic Timing	126	60%	78%	80%	93%
Oxygenation Assessment	132	95%	99%	99%	100%
Pneumococcal Vaccine	58	10%	68%	69%	94%
Smoking Cessation Advice[1,3]	8	25%	83%	80%	100%
Surgical Infection Prevention					
Prophylactic Antibiotic Given[1,3]	24	29%	67%	77%	95%
Prophylactic Antibiotic Selection[5]	-	-	86%	90%	100%
Prophylactic Antibiotic Stopped[1,3]	24	17%	68%	72%	95%
Pregnancy Care					
Inpatient Neonatal Mortality	-	-	-	-	-
Third or Fourth Degree Laceration	-	-	3.23%	3.63%	3.27%

East Houston Regional Medical Center
13111 East Freeway   Phone: 713-393-2000
Houston, TX 77015
Ownership: Proprietary   Accredited: Yes
Emergency Services: Yes

Measure	Cases	This Hospital	State Average	U.S. Average	Top Hospital
Heart Attack Care					
ACE Inhibitor or ARB for LVSD	32	94%	85%	82%	100%
Aspirin at Arrival	156	94%	91%	92%	100%
Aspirin at Discharge	106	92%	90%	90%	100%
Beta Blocker at Arrival	130	88%	85%	87%	100%

Measure				
Beta Blocker at Discharge	106	92%	86%	90%	100%
Fibrinolytic Medication Timing[1]	15	27%	30%	31%	100%
PCI Within 90 Minutes of Arrival	0	-	48%	54%	95%
Smoking Cessation Advice	55	93%	90%	88%	100%
Heart Failure Care					
ACE Inhibitor or ARB for LVSD	149	87%	82%	82%	100%
Discharge Instructions	332	61%	60%	61%	93%
Evaluation of LVS Function	369	88%	81%	83%	99%
Smoking Cessation Advice	109	96%	82%	82%	100%
Pneumonia Care					
Appropriate Initial Antibiotic	170	79%	79%	83%	94%
Blood Culture Timing	139	94%	89%	90%	100%
Influenza Vaccine	40	52%	69%	70%	100%
Initial Antibiotic Timing	223	76%	78%	80%	93%
Oxygenation Assessment	245	98%	99%	99%	100%
Pneumococcal Vaccine	113	69%	68%	69%	94%
Smoking Cessation Advice	93	90%	83%	80%	100%
Surgical Infection Prevention					
Prophylactic Antibiotic Given[2,3]	105	70%	67%	77%	95%
Prophylactic Antibiotic Selection[2]	41	71%	86%	90%	100%
Prophylactic Antibiotic Stopped[2,3]	93	81%	68%	72%	95%
Pregnancy Care					
Inpatient Neonatal Mortality	-	-	-	-	-
Third or Fourth Degree Laceration	-	-	3.23%	3.63%	3.27%

Harris County Hospital District

2525 Holly Hall
Houston, TX 77054
Ownership: Govt - Hospital District or Authority   Accredited: Yes
Emergency Services: Yes
Phone: 713-566-6417

Measure	Cases	This Hospital	State Average	U.S. Average	Top Hospital
Heart Attack Care					
ACE Inhibitor or ARB for LVSD	68	93%	85%	82%	100%
Aspirin at Arrival	204	99%	91%	92%	100%
Aspirin at Discharge	228	97%	90%	90%	100%
Beta Blocker at Arrival	155	96%	85%	87%	100%
Beta Blocker at Discharge	229	95%	86%	90%	100%
Fibrinolytic Medication Timing[1]	7	0%	30%	31%	100%
PCI Within 90 Minutes of Arrival[1]	6	17%	48%	54%	95%
Smoking Cessation Advice	100	84%	90%	88%	100%
Heart Failure Care					
ACE Inhibitor or ARB for LVSD[2]	406	86%	82%	82%	100%
Discharge Instructions[2]	678	57%	60%	61%	93%
Evaluation of LVS Function[2]	697	97%	81%	83%	99%
Smoking Cessation Advice[2]	247	79%	82%	82%	100%
Pneumonia Care					
Appropriate Initial Antibiotic[2]	247	87%	79%	83%	94%
Blood Culture Timing[2]	237	82%	89%	90%	100%
Influenza Vaccine[4,5]	-	-	69%	70%	100%
Initial Antibiotic Timing[2]	332	48%	78%	80%	93%
Oxygenation Assessment[2]	371	98%	99%	99%	100%
Pneumococcal Vaccine[2]	96	36%	68%	69%	94%
Smoking Cessation Advice[2]	144	67%	83%	80%	100%
Surgical Infection Prevention					
Prophylactic Antibiotic Given[2,3]	296	72%	67%	77%	95%
Prophylactic Antibiotic Selection[2]	118	63%	86%	90%	100%
Prophylactic Antibiotic Stopped[2,3]	289	67%	68%	72%	95%
Pregnancy Care					
Inpatient Neonatal Mortality	-	-	-	-	-
Third or Fourth Degree Laceration	-	-	3.23%	3.63%	3.27%

Healthsouth Hospital for Specialized Surgery

5445 Labranch Street
Houston, TX 77004
Ownership: Proprietary
Emergency Services: Yes
Phone: 713-528-6800
Accredited: Yes

Measure	Cases	This Hospital	State Average	U.S. Average	Top Hospital
Heart Attack Care					
ACE Inhibitor or ARB for LVSD[5]	-	-	85%	82%	100%
Aspirin at Arrival[5]	-	-	91%	92%	100%

Measure				
Aspirin at Discharge[5]	-	-	90%	90%	100%
Beta Blocker at Arrival[5]	-	-	85%	87%	100%
Beta Blocker at Discharge[5]	-	-	86%	90%	100%
Fibrinolytic Medication Timing[5]	-	-	30%	31%	100%
PCI Within 90 Minutes of Arrival[5]	-	-	48%	54%	95%
Smoking Cessation Advice[5]	-	-	90%	88%	100%
Heart Failure Care					
ACE Inhibitor or ARB for LVSD[5]	-	-	82%	82%	100%
Discharge Instructions[5]	-	-	60%	61%	93%
Evaluation of LVS Function[5]	-	-	81%	83%	99%
Smoking Cessation Advice[5]	-	-	82%	82%	100%
Pneumonia Care					
Appropriate Initial Antibiotic[5]	-	-	79%	83%	94%
Blood Culture Timing[5]	-	-	89%	90%	100%
Influenza Vaccine[5]	-	-	69%	70%	100%
Initial Antibiotic Timing[5]	-	-	78%	80%	93%
Oxygenation Assessment[5]	-	-	99%	99%	100%
Pneumococcal Vaccine[5]	-	-	68%	69%	94%
Smoking Cessation Advice[5]	-	-	83%	80%	100%
Surgical Infection Prevention					
Prophylactic Antibiotic Given[2,3]	0	-	67%	77%	95%
Prophylactic Antibiotic Selection[5]	-	-	86%	90%	100%
Prophylactic Antibiotic Stopped[2,3]	0	-	68%	72%	95%
Pregnancy Care					
Inpatient Neonatal Mortality	-	-	-	-	-
Third or Fourth Degree Laceration	-	-	3.23%	3.63%	3.27%

Houston Northwest Medical Center

Alternate Name: HNMC
710 FM 1960 Road West
Houston, TX 77090
URL: www.hnmc.com
Ownership: Proprietary
Emergency Services: Yes
Phone: 281-440-1000
Fax: 281-440-2474
Accredited: Yes
Licensed Beds: 494

Key Personnel:
Interim CEO . . . . Drew Kahn
Chief Medical Staff . . . . Daniel Tuft
Emergency Room . . . . David Arai, MD
CCU Spvg. Nurse . . . . Grace Heffron, RN
Director Medical/Surgical Nursing . . . . Debby Drescher
OB/GYN Womens Health . . . . Patricia Laden
Chief Radiology . . . . David Boyd, MD
Director Respiratory Therapy . . . . John Hildreth

Measure	Cases	This Hospital	State Average	U.S. Average	Top Hospital
Heart Attack Care					
ACE Inhibitor or ARB for LVSD	91	92%	85%	82%	100%
Aspirin at Arrival	306	96%	91%	92%	100%
Aspirin at Discharge	333	96%	90%	90%	100%
Beta Blocker at Arrival	247	93%	85%	87%	100%
Beta Blocker at Discharge	321	97%	86%	90%	100%
Fibrinolytic Medication Timing[1]	3	33%	30%	31%	100%
PCI Within 90 Minutes of Arrival	25	92%	48%	54%	95%
Smoking Cessation Advice	145	99%	90%	88%	100%
Heart Failure Care					
ACE Inhibitor or ARB for LVSD	263	78%	82%	82%	100%
Discharge Instructions	487	56%	60%	61%	93%
Evaluation of LVS Function	568	90%	81%	83%	99%
Smoking Cessation Advice	119	99%	82%	82%	100%
Pneumonia Care					
Appropriate Initial Antibiotic	237	89%	79%	83%	94%
Blood Culture Timing	180	93%	89%	90%	100%
Influenza Vaccine	72	61%	69%	70%	100%
Initial Antibiotic Timing	353	64%	78%	80%	93%
Oxygenation Assessment	417	100%	99%	99%	100%
Pneumococcal Vaccine	199	70%	68%	69%	94%
Smoking Cessation Advice	94	93%	83%	80%	100%
Surgical Infection Prevention					
Prophylactic Antibiotic Given[2]	881	88%	67%	77%	95%
Prophylactic Antibiotic Selection[2]	228	80%	86%	90%	100%
Prophylactic Antibiotic Stopped[2]	849	60%	68%	72%	95%
Pregnancy Care					
Inpatient Neonatal Mortality	-	-	-	-	-

NOTE: Hospital profiles are in alphabetical order by state, then city, then hospital within the city; Rankings are sorted by rate in descending order and exclude hospitals with less than 25 cases; (1) The number of cases is too small (n<25) for purposes of reliably predicting hospital performance; (2) Measure reflects the hospital's indication that its submission was based upon a sample of its relevant discharges; (3) Rate reflects fewer than the maximum possible quarters of data for the measure; (4) Inaccurate information submitted and suppressed for one or more quarters; (5) No data is available from the hospital for this measure; Please refer to the User's Guide for a full explanation of data

Third or Fourth Degree Laceration	-	-	3.23%	3.63%	3.27%

Memorial Hermann Healthcare System

7737 Southwest Freeway Suite 200
Houston, TX 77074
Ownership: Voluntary non-profit - Other
Emergency Services: Yes

Phone: 713-776-6992

Accredited: Yes

Measure	Cases	This Hospital	State Average	U.S. Average	Top Hospital
Heart Attack Care					
ACE Inhibitor or ARB for LVSD	174	94%	85%	82%	100%
Aspirin at Arrival	752	98%	91%	92%	100%
Aspirin at Discharge	793	97%	90%	90%	100%
Beta Blocker at Arrival	629	97%	85%	87%	100%
Beta Blocker at Discharge	781	97%	86%	90%	100%
Fibrinolytic Medication Timing	39	23%	30%	31%	100%
PCI Within 90 Minutes of Arrival	25	44%	48%	54%	95%
Smoking Cessation Advice	244	99%	90%	88%	100%
Heart Failure Care					
ACE Inhibitor or ARB for LVSD	745	96%	82%	82%	100%
Discharge Instructions	1,575	55%	60%	61%	93%
Evaluation of LVS Function	1,905	99%	81%	83%	99%
Smoking Cessation Advice	395	97%	82%	82%	100%
Pneumonia Care					
Appropriate Initial Antibiotic	957	72%	79%	83%	94%
Blood Culture Timing	875	90%	89%	90%	100%
Influenza Vaccine[4,5]	-	-	69%	70%	100%
Initial Antibiotic Timing	1,245	78%	78%	80%	93%
Oxygenation Assessment	1,468	100%	99%	99%	100%
Pneumococcal Vaccine	820	83%	68%	69%	94%
Smoking Cessation Advice	320	95%	83%	80%	100%
Surgical Infection Prevention					
Prophylactic Antibiotic Given[2,3]	2,534	77%	67%	77%	95%
Prophylactic Antibiotic Selection[2]	815	93%	86%	90%	100%
Prophylactic Antibiotic Stopped[2,3]	2,451	68%	68%	72%	95%
Pregnancy Care					
Inpatient Neonatal Mortality	-	-	-	-	-
Third or Fourth Degree Laceration	-	-	3.23%	3.63%	3.27%

Memorial Hermann Memorial City

921 Gessner Road
Houston, TX 77024
URL: www.mhhs.org
Ownership: Voluntary non-profit - Private
Emergency Services: Yes
Key Personnel:

Phone: 713-242-3000
Fax: 713-827-4096

Accredited: Yes
Licensed Beds: 520

Administrator/CEO . . . . Wayne Voss
Chief Medical Staff . . . . BK Roy, MD
Director Infection/Disease Control . . . . Avis Thomas
CCU Spvg. Nurse . . . . Edith Woltman, RN
Director Medical/Surgical Nursing . . . . Marilyn Paine
OB/GYN Womens Health . . . . Rebecca Lueethcke, MD
Director Radiology . . . . Lonnie Cozad
Director Respiratory Therapy . . . . Kim Keilstrup

Measure	Cases	This Hospital	State Average	U.S. Average	Top Hospital
Heart Attack Care					
ACE Inhibitor or ARB for LVSD	64	92%	85%	82%	100%
Aspirin at Arrival	196	98%	91%	92%	100%
Aspirin at Discharge	281	96%	90%	90%	100%
Beta Blocker at Arrival	127	97%	85%	87%	100%
Beta Blocker at Discharge	284	97%	86%	90%	100%
Fibrinolytic Medication Timing[1]	4	25%	30%	31%	100%
PCI Within 90 Minutes of Arrival[1]	12	33%	48%	54%	95%
Smoking Cessation Advice	97	99%	90%	88%	100%
Heart Failure Care					
ACE Inhibitor or ARB for LVSD	206	91%	82%	82%	100%
Discharge Instructions	378	60%	60%	61%	93%
Evaluation of LVS Function	461	99%	81%	83%	99%
Smoking Cessation Advice	57	100%	82%	82%	100%
Pneumonia Care					
Appropriate Initial Antibiotic	162	83%	79%	83%	94%

Blood Culture Timing	157	95%	89%	90%	100%
Influenza Vaccine	53	81%	69%	70%	100%
Initial Antibiotic Timing	234	81%	78%	80%	93%
Oxygenation Assessment	286	100%	99%	99%	100%
Pneumococcal Vaccine	171	75%	68%	69%	94%
Smoking Cessation Advice	45	93%	83%	80%	100%
Surgical Infection Prevention					
Prophylactic Antibiotic Given[2,3]	792	53%	67%	77%	95%
Prophylactic Antibiotic Selection[2]	83	83%	86%	90%	100%
Prophylactic Antibiotic Stopped[2,3]	770	48%	68%	72%	95%
Pregnancy Care					
Inpatient Neonatal Mortality	-	-	-	-	-
Third or Fourth Degree Laceration	-	-	3.23%	3.63%	3.27%

Memorial Hermann-Texas Medical Center

Alternate Name: Hermann Hospital
6411 Fannin Street
Houston, TX 77030
URL: www.mhhs.org
Ownership: Voluntary non-profit - Private
Emergency Services: Yes
Key Personnel:

Phone: 713-704-4000
Fax: 713-448-5665

Accredited: Yes
Licensed Beds: 908

President/CEO . . . . James Eastham
Chief Medical Staff . . . . David Taylor, MD
Chief Catheterization Laboratory . . . . Richard Smalling, MD
OB/GYN Womens Health . . . . Larry Gilstrap, MD
Chief Radiology . . . . Stanford Goldman, MD
Director Respiratory Therapy . . . . Patti Roy

Measure	Cases	This Hospital	State Average	U.S. Average	Top Hospital
Heart Attack Care					
ACE Inhibitor or ARB for LVSD	85	94%	85%	82%	100%
Aspirin at Arrival	260	100%	91%	92%	100%
Aspirin at Discharge	472	95%	90%	90%	100%
Beta Blocker at Arrival	238	100%	85%	87%	100%
Beta Blocker at Discharge	454	95%	86%	90%	100%
Fibrinolytic Medication Timing[1]	9	67%	30%	31%	100%
PCI Within 90 Minutes of Arrival	26	96%	48%	54%	95%
Smoking Cessation Advice	290	98%	90%	88%	100%
Heart Failure Care					
ACE Inhibitor or ARB for LVSD	316	98%	82%	82%	100%
Discharge Instructions	518	86%	60%	61%	93%
Evaluation of LVS Function	562	99%	81%	83%	99%
Smoking Cessation Advice	180	100%	82%	82%	100%
Pneumonia Care					
Appropriate Initial Antibiotic	73	92%	79%	83%	94%
Blood Culture Timing	114	94%	89%	90%	100%
Influenza Vaccine	30	97%	69%	70%	100%
Initial Antibiotic Timing	135	76%	78%	80%	93%
Oxygenation Assessment	173	100%	99%	99%	100%
Pneumococcal Vaccine	60	87%	68%	69%	94%
Smoking Cessation Advice	58	97%	83%	80%	100%
Surgical Infection Prevention					
Prophylactic Antibiotic Given[2,3]	641	72%	67%	77%	95%
Prophylactic Antibiotic Selection[2]	186	91%	86%	90%	100%
Prophylactic Antibiotic Stopped[2,3]	567	68%	68%	72%	95%
Pregnancy Care					
Inpatient Neonatal Mortality	-	-	-	-	-
Third or Fourth Degree Laceration	-	-	3.23%	3.63%	3.27%

Methodist Hospital

6565 Fannin Street
Houston, TX 77030
URL: www.methodisthealth.com
Ownership: Voluntary non-profit - Church
Emergency Services: Yes
Key Personnel:

Phone: 713-790-3311
Fax: 713-790-2605

Accredited: Yes
Licensed Beds: 1,527

President/CEO . . . . Mark J Rappaport
Chief Medical Staff . . . . Catherine Williams, MD
Catheterization Lab . . . . Albert E Raizner, MD
Emergency Room . . . . Nicholas Hanno, RN
Emergency Room . . . . Robert Fromm, MD
Infection Control . . . . Fran Slater

NOTE: Hospital profiles are in alphabetical order by state, then city, then hospital within the city; Rankings are sorted by rate in descending order and exclude hospitals with less than 25 cases; (1) The number of cases is too small (n<25) for purposes of reliably predicting hospital performance; (2) Measure reflects the hospital's indication that its submission was based upon a sample of its relevant discharges; (3) Rate reflects fewer than the maximum possible quarters of data for the measure; (4) Inaccurate information submitted and suppressed for one or more quarters; (5) No data is available from the hospital for this measure; Please refer to the User's Guide for a full explanation of data

OB/GYN Womens Health. . . . . Joe Simpson
Chief Radiology . . . . James Harrell, MD

Measure	Cases	This Hospital	State Average	U.S. Average	Top Hospital
Heart Attack Care					
ACE Inhibitor or ARB for LVSD[2]	152	91%	85%	82%	100%
Aspirin at Arrival[2]	280	93%	91%	92%	100%
Aspirin at Discharge[2]	628	96%	90%	90%	100%
Beta Blocker at Arrival[2]	212	94%	85%	87%	100%
Beta Blocker at Discharge[2]	643	98%	86%	90%	100%
Fibrinolytic Medication Timing[1,2]	1	0%	30%	31%	100%
PCI Within 90 Minutes of Arrival[1,2]	9	44%	48%	54%	95%
Smoking Cessation Advice[2]	200	92%	90%	88%	100%
Heart Failure Care					
ACE Inhibitor or ARB for LVSD[2]	425	84%	82%	82%	100%
Discharge Instructions[2]	765	75%	60%	61%	93%
Evaluation of LVS Function[2]	842	98%	81%	83%	99%
Smoking Cessation Advice[2]	121	88%	82%	82%	100%
Pneumonia Care					
Appropriate Initial Antibiotic[2]	209	86%	79%	83%	94%
Blood Culture Timing[2]	277	94%	89%	90%	100%
Influenza Vaccine[2]	64	70%	69%	70%	100%
Initial Antibiotic Timing[2]	403	84%	78%	80%	93%
Oxygenation Assessment[2]	448	100%	99%	99%	100%
Pneumococcal Vaccine[2]	234	84%	68%	69%	94%
Smoking Cessation Advice[2]	73	90%	83%	80%	100%
Surgical Infection Prevention					
Prophylactic Antibiotic Given[2,3]	429	78%	67%	77%	95%
Prophylactic Antibiotic Selection[2]	86	79%	86%	90%	100%
Prophylactic Antibiotic Stopped[2,3]	415	73%	68%	72%	95%
Pregnancy Care					
Inpatient Neonatal Mortality	-	-	-	-	-
Third or Fourth Degree Laceration	-	-	3.23%	3.63%	3.27%

Methodist Willowbrook Hospital

18220 Tomball Parkway   Phone: 281-477-1000
Houston, TX 77070
Ownership: Voluntary non-profit - Church   Accredited: Yes
Emergency Services: Yes

Measure	Cases	This Hospital	State Average	U.S. Average	Top Hospital
Heart Attack Care					
ACE Inhibitor or ARB for LVSD[1]	11	73%	85%	82%	100%
Aspirin at Arrival	97	98%	91%	92%	100%
Aspirin at Discharge	68	87%	90%	90%	100%
Beta Blocker at Arrival	87	93%	85%	87%	100%
Beta Blocker at Discharge	75	92%	86%	90%	100%
Fibrinolytic Medication Timing[3]	0	-	30%	31%	100%
PCI Within 90 Minutes of Arrival[1]	1	0%	48%	54%	95%
Smoking Cessation Advice	25	96%	90%	88%	100%
Heart Failure Care					
ACE Inhibitor or ARB for LVSD	55	84%	82%	82%	100%
Discharge Instructions[3]	32	69%	60%	61%	93%
Evaluation of LVS Function	193	90%	81%	83%	99%
Smoking Cessation Advice[1,3]	13	100%	82%	82%	100%
Pneumonia Care					
Appropriate Initial Antibiotic[2]	120	88%	79%	83%	94%
Blood Culture Timing[2]	118	90%	89%	90%	100%
Influenza Vaccine[1,2]	23	83%	69%	70%	100%
Initial Antibiotic Timing[2]	140	85%	78%	80%	93%
Oxygenation Assessment[2]	189	99%	99%	99%	100%
Pneumococcal Vaccine[2]	100	91%	68%	69%	94%
Smoking Cessation Advice[1,2,3]	5	80%	83%	80%	100%
Surgical Infection Prevention					
Prophylactic Antibiotic Given[2,3]	196	85%	67%	77%	95%
Prophylactic Antibiotic Selection[5]	-	-	86%	90%	100%
Prophylactic Antibiotic Stopped[2,3]	39	56%	68%	72%	95%
Pregnancy Care					
Inpatient Neonatal Mortality	-	-	-	-	-
Third or Fourth Degree Laceration	-	-	3.23%	3.63%	3.27%

Park Plaza Hospital

1313 Hermann Drive   Phone: 713-527-5000
Houston, TX 77004   Fax: 713-524-6159
URL: www.parkplazahospital.com
Ownership: Proprietary   Accredited: Yes
Emergency Services: Yes   Licensed Beds: 468
Key Personnel:
CEO. . . . . Lex Guinn
Cardiac Lab . . . . Cathy Doughty
Director Emergency Room. . . . . Mike Davis
Director Infection Control . . . . Pam Diffenbach
ICU . . . . Mike Davis
Director Intensive/Coronary Care. . . . . Mike Davis
Director Medical/Surgical Nursing . . . . Mary Woodward
Director OB/GYN Womens Health . . . . Beth Garcia
Director Radiology . . . . Cathy Doughty
Director Respiratory/Cardiopulmonary . . . . Bill Dodds

Measure	Cases	This Hospital	State Average	U.S. Average	Top Hospital
Heart Attack Care					
ACE Inhibitor or ARB for LVSD[1]	11	73%	85%	82%	100%
Aspirin at Arrival	38	89%	91%	92%	100%
Aspirin at Discharge	27	96%	90%	90%	100%
Beta Blocker at Arrival	27	81%	85%	87%	100%
Beta Blocker at Discharge	28	96%	86%	90%	100%
Fibrinolytic Medication Timing[1]	1	0%	30%	31%	100%
PCI Within 90 Minutes of Arrival[1]	1	0%	48%	54%	95%
Smoking Cessation Advice[1]	12	100%	90%	88%	100%
Heart Failure Care					
ACE Inhibitor or ARB for LVSD	115	81%	82%	82%	100%
Discharge Instructions	295	76%	60%	61%	93%
Evaluation of LVS Function	339	92%	81%	83%	99%
Smoking Cessation Advice	75	100%	82%	82%	100%
Pneumonia Care					
Appropriate Initial Antibiotic	95	89%	79%	83%	94%
Blood Culture Timing	153	95%	89%	90%	100%
Influenza Vaccine[4,5]	-	-	69%	70%	100%
Initial Antibiotic Timing	210	74%	78%	80%	93%
Oxygenation Assessment	255	100%	99%	99%	100%
Pneumococcal Vaccine	142	71%	68%	69%	94%
Smoking Cessation Advice	40	100%	83%	80%	100%
Surgical Infection Prevention					
Prophylactic Antibiotic Given[2]	158	68%	67%	77%	95%
Prophylactic Antibiotic Selection[2]	42	90%	86%	90%	100%
Prophylactic Antibiotic Stopped[2]	158	36%	68%	72%	95%
Pregnancy Care					
Inpatient Neonatal Mortality	-	-	-	-	-
Third or Fourth Degree Laceration	-	-	3.23%	3.63%	3.27%

Renaissance Hospital Houston

2807 Little York Road   Phone: 713-697-7777
Houston, TX 77093   Fax: 713-696-4662
URL: www.renhealthcare.org/Default.aspx
Ownership: Proprietary   Accredited: No
Emergency Services: Yes   Licensed Beds: 39
Key Personnel:
CEO. . . . . Dan De La Garza
Chief Medical Staff. A Mauskar
Emergency Room . . . . Kevin Pallesen
Medical Surgical Nursing . . . . Diane Conner
Respiratory/Cardiopulmonary. . . . . K Peter

Measure	Cases	This Hospital	State Average	U.S. Average	Top Hospital
Heart Attack Care					
ACE Inhibitor or ARB for LVSD[3]	0	-	85%	82%	100%
Aspirin at Arrival[1,3]	4	75%	91%	92%	100%
Aspirin at Discharge[1,3]	1	100%	90%	90%	100%
Beta Blocker at Arrival[1,3]	4	50%	85%	87%	100%
Beta Blocker at Discharge[1,3]	1	100%	86%	90%	100%
Fibrinolytic Medication Timing[3]	0	-	30%	31%	100%
PCI Within 90 Minutes of Arrival	0	-	48%	54%	95%
Smoking Cessation Advice[3]	0	-	90%	88%	100%
Heart Failure Care					

NOTE: Hospital profiles are in alphabetical order by state, then city, then hospital within the city; Rankings are sorted by rate in descending order and exclude hospitals with less than 25 cases; (1) The number of cases is too small (n<25) for purposes of reliably predicting hospital performance; (2) Measure reflects the hospital's indication that its submission was based upon a sample of its relevant discharges; (3) Rate reflects fewer than the maximum possible quarters of data for the measure; (4) Inaccurate information submitted and suppressed for one or more quarters; (5) No data is available from the hospital for this measure; Please refer to the User's Guide for a full explanation of data

ACE Inhibitor or ARB for LVSD[1]	2	0%	82%	82%	100%
Discharge Instructions[1,3]	4	25%	60%	61%	93%
Evaluation of LVS Function	48	44%	81%	83%	99%
Smoking Cessation Advice[3]	0	-	82%	82%	100%
Pneumonia Care					
Appropriate Initial Antibiotic[1,3]	3	33%	79%	83%	94%
Blood Culture Timing[3]	0	-	89%	90%	100%
Influenza Vaccine[5]	-	-	69%	70%	100%
Initial Antibiotic Timing	29	83%	78%	80%	93%
Oxygenation Assessment	35	97%	99%	99%	100%
Pneumococcal Vaccine[1]	21	5%	68%	69%	94%
Smoking Cessation Advice[1,3]	2	0%	83%	80%	100%
Surgical Infection Prevention					
Prophylactic Antibiotic Given[1,3]	3	100%	67%	77%	95%
Prophylactic Antibiotic Selection[5]	-	-	86%	90%	100%
Prophylactic Antibiotic Stopped[1,3]	3	0%	68%	72%	95%
Pregnancy Care					
Inpatient Neonatal Mortality	-	-	-	-	-
Third or Fourth Degree Laceration	-	-	3.23%	3.63%	3.27%

Riverside General Hospital

3204 Ennis   Phone: 713-526-2441
Houston, TX 77004   Fax: 713-526-3554
URL: www.riversidegeneral.org
Ownership: Voluntary non-profit - Private   Accredited: Yes
Emergency Services: No   Licensed Beds: 98
Key Personnel:
Administrator . . . . Ernest Gibson
Chief Medical Staff. . . . . Edith Jones

Measure	Cases	This Hospital	State Average	U.S. Average	Top Hospital
Heart Attack Care					
ACE Inhibitor or ARB for LVSD[5]	-	-	85%	82%	100%
Aspirin at Arrival[5]	-	-	91%	92%	100%
Aspirin at Discharge[5]	-	-	90%	90%	100%
Beta Blocker at Arrival[5]	-	-	85%	87%	100%
Beta Blocker at Discharge[5]	-	-	86%	90%	100%
Fibrinolytic Medication Timing[5]	-	-	30%	31%	100%
PCI Within 90 Minutes of Arrival[5]	-	-	48%	54%	95%
Smoking Cessation Advice[5]	-	-	90%	88%	100%
Heart Failure Care					
ACE Inhibitor or ARB for LVSD[1,3]	1	100%	82%	82%	100%
Discharge Instructions[5]	-	-	60%	61%	93%
Evaluation of LVS Function[1,3]	2	50%	81%	83%	99%
Smoking Cessation Advice[5]	-	-	82%	82%	100%
Pneumonia Care					
Appropriate Initial Antibiotic[5]	-	-	79%	83%	94%
Blood Culture Timing[5]	-	-	89%	90%	100%
Influenza Vaccine[5]	-	-	69%	70%	100%
Initial Antibiotic Timing[5]	-	-	78%	80%	93%
Oxygenation Assessment[5]	-	-	99%	99%	100%
Pneumococcal Vaccine[5]	-	-	68%	69%	94%
Smoking Cessation Advice[5]	-	-	83%	80%	100%
Surgical Infection Prevention					
Prophylactic Antibiotic Given[5]	-	-	67%	77%	95%
Prophylactic Antibiotic Selection[5]	-	-	86%	90%	100%
Prophylactic Antibiotic Stopped[5]	-	-	68%	72%	95%
Pregnancy Care					
Inpatient Neonatal Mortality	-	-	-	-	-
Third or Fourth Degree Laceration	-	-	3.23%	3.63%	3.27%

Saint Joseph Medical Center

1401 Saint Joseph Parkway   Phone: 713-757-1000
Houston, TX 77002   Fax: 713-657-7123
E-mail: fritz.guthrie@hospitalpartners.com
URL: www.sjmctx.com
Ownership: Voluntary non-profit - Church   Accredited: Yes
Emergency Services: Yes   Licensed Beds: 792
Key Personnel:
Administrator/CEO. . . . . Phillip D Robinson
Director Emergency Department . . . . Dori Upton
Director Womens Health . . . . Janet Matthews

Measure	Cases	This Hospital	State Average	U.S. Average	Top Hospital
Heart Attack Care					
ACE Inhibitor or ARB for LVSD	38	100%	85%	82%	100%
Aspirin at Arrival	122	98%	91%	92%	100%
Aspirin at Discharge	119	97%	90%	90%	100%
Beta Blocker at Arrival	83	94%	85%	87%	100%
Beta Blocker at Discharge	100	97%	86%	90%	100%
Fibrinolytic Medication Timing[1]	5	0%	30%	31%	100%
PCI Within 90 Minutes of Arrival[1]	2	0%	48%	54%	95%
Smoking Cessation Advice	39	97%	90%	88%	100%
Heart Failure Care					
ACE Inhibitor or ARB for LVSD	171	95%	82%	82%	100%
Discharge Instructions	322	76%	60%	61%	93%
Evaluation of LVS Function	379	96%	81%	83%	99%
Smoking Cessation Advice	84	98%	82%	82%	100%
Pneumonia Care					
Appropriate Initial Antibiotic	179	93%	79%	83%	94%
Blood Culture Timing	167	98%	89%	90%	100%
Influenza Vaccine	44	86%	69%	70%	100%
Initial Antibiotic Timing	239	87%	78%	80%	93%
Oxygenation Assessment	258	99%	99%	99%	100%
Pneumococcal Vaccine	122	87%	68%	69%	94%
Smoking Cessation Advice	67	90%	83%	80%	100%
Surgical Infection Prevention					
Prophylactic Antibiotic Given	792	86%	67%	77%	95%
Prophylactic Antibiotic Selection	179	94%	86%	90%	100%
Prophylactic Antibiotic Stopped	713	85%	68%	72%	95%
Pregnancy Care					
Inpatient Neonatal Mortality	-	-	-	-	-
Third or Fourth Degree Laceration	-	-	3.23%	3.63%	3.27%

Saint Luke's Episcopal Hospital

6720 Bertner Avenue   Phone: 832-355-1000
Houston, TX 77030
URL: www.sleh.com
Ownership: Voluntary non-profit - Church   Accredited: Yes
Emergency Services: Yes   Licensed Beds: 946
Key Personnel:
CEO/President. . . . . David Pate, MD JD
Emergency Room Director. . . . . Jacklincs Lynch
OB/GYN Womens Health. . . . . Joe Leigh Simpson, MD
Chief Radiology . . . . P Milton Gray, MD

Measure	Cases	This Hospital	State Average	U.S. Average	Top Hospital
Heart Attack Care					
ACE Inhibitor or ARB for LVSD	120	91%	85%	82%	100%
Aspirin at Arrival	433	99%	91%	92%	100%
Aspirin at Discharge	648	97%	90%	90%	100%
Beta Blocker at Arrival	389	98%	85%	87%	100%
Beta Blocker at Discharge	670	97%	86%	90%	100%
Fibrinolytic Medication Timing[1]	6	17%	30%	31%	100%
PCI Within 90 Minutes of Arrival[1]	13	15%	48%	54%	95%
Smoking Cessation Advice	175	98%	90%	88%	100%
Heart Failure Care					
ACE Inhibitor or ARB for LVSD	754	67%	82%	82%	100%
Discharge Instructions	1,297	67%	60%	61%	93%
Evaluation of LVS Function	1,426	91%	81%	83%	99%
Smoking Cessation Advice	201	85%	82%	82%	100%
Pneumonia Care					
Appropriate Initial Antibiotic	255	85%	79%	83%	94%
Blood Culture Timing	265	88%	89%	90%	100%
Influenza Vaccine[4,5]	-	-	69%	70%	100%
Initial Antibiotic Timing	358	70%	78%	80%	93%
Oxygenation Assessment	470	100%	99%	99%	100%
Pneumococcal Vaccine	252	68%	68%	69%	94%
Smoking Cessation Advice	69	86%	83%	80%	100%
Surgical Infection Prevention					
Prophylactic Antibiotic Given[2,3]	310	53%	67%	77%	95%
Prophylactic Antibiotic Selection[2]	102	87%	86%	90%	100%
Prophylactic Antibiotic Stopped[2,3]	300	80%	68%	72%	95%
Pregnancy Care					

Inpatient Neonatal Mortality	-	-	-	-	-
Third or Fourth Degree Laceration	-	-	3.23%	3.63%	3.27%

Prophylactic Antibiotic Stopped[2,3]	25	52%	68%	72%	95%
Pregnancy Care					
Inpatient Neonatal Mortality	-	-	-	-	-
Third or Fourth Degree Laceration	-	-	3.23%	3.63%	3.27%

Texas Orthopedic Hospital

7401 South Main Street
Houston, TX 77030
Ownership: Proprietary
Emergency Services: Yes

Phone: 713-799-8600

Accredited: Yes

Measure	Cases	This Hospital	State Average	U.S. Average	Top Hospital
Heart Attack Care					
ACE Inhibitor or ARB for LVSD[5]	-	-	85%	82%	100%
Aspirin at Arrival[5]	-	-	91%	92%	100%
Aspirin at Discharge[5]	-	-	90%	90%	100%
Beta Blocker at Arrival[5]	-	-	85%	87%	100%
Beta Blocker at Discharge[5]	-	-	86%	90%	100%
Fibrinolytic Medication Timing[5]	-	-	30%	31%	100%
PCI Within 90 Minutes of Arrival[5]	-	-	48%	54%	95%
Smoking Cessation Advice[5]	-	-	90%	88%	100%
Heart Failure Care					
ACE Inhibitor or ARB for LVSD[5]	-	-	82%	82%	100%
Discharge Instructions[5]	-	-	60%	61%	93%
Evaluation of LVS Function[5]	-	-	81%	83%	99%
Smoking Cessation Advice[5]	-	-	82%	82%	100%
Pneumonia Care					
Appropriate Initial Antibiotic[5]	-	-	79%	83%	94%
Blood Culture Timing[5]	-	-	89%	90%	100%
Influenza Vaccine[5]	-	-	69%	70%	100%
Initial Antibiotic Timing[5]	-	-	78%	80%	93%
Oxygenation Assessment[5]	-	-	99%	99%	100%
Pneumococcal Vaccine[5]	-	-	68%	69%	94%
Smoking Cessation Advice[5]	-	-	83%	80%	100%
Surgical Infection Prevention					
Prophylactic Antibiotic Given[3]	690	97%	67%	77%	95%
Prophylactic Antibiotic Selection	223	100%	86%	90%	100%
Prophylactic Antibiotic Stopped[3]	683	93%	68%	72%	95%
Pregnancy Care					
Inpatient Neonatal Mortality	-	-	-	-	-
Third or Fourth Degree Laceration	-	-	3.23%	3.63%	3.27%

Tops Surgical Specialty Hospital

17080 Red Oak Drive
Houston, TX 77090
Ownership: Proprietary
Emergency Services: No

Phone: 281-539-2900

Accredited: Yes

Measure	Cases	This Hospital	State Average	U.S. Average	Top Hospital
Heart Attack Care					
ACE Inhibitor or ARB for LVSD[5]	-	-	85%	82%	100%
Aspirin at Arrival[5]	-	-	91%	92%	100%
Aspirin at Discharge[5]	-	-	90%	90%	100%
Beta Blocker at Arrival[5]	-	-	85%	87%	100%
Beta Blocker at Discharge[5]	-	-	86%	90%	100%
Fibrinolytic Medication Timing[5]	-	-	30%	31%	100%
PCI Within 90 Minutes of Arrival[5]	-	-	48%	54%	95%
Smoking Cessation Advice[5]	-	-	90%	88%	100%
Heart Failure Care					
ACE Inhibitor or ARB for LVSD[5]	-	-	82%	82%	100%
Discharge Instructions[5]	-	-	60%	61%	93%
Evaluation of LVS Function[5]	-	-	81%	83%	99%
Smoking Cessation Advice[5]	-	-	82%	82%	100%
Pneumonia Care					
Appropriate Initial Antibiotic[5]	-	-	79%	83%	94%
Blood Culture Timing[5]	-	-	89%	90%	100%
Influenza Vaccine[5]	-	-	69%	70%	100%
Initial Antibiotic Timing[5]	-	-	78%	80%	93%
Oxygenation Assessment[5]	-	-	99%	99%	100%
Pneumococcal Vaccine[5]	-	-	68%	69%	94%
Smoking Cessation Advice[5]	-	-	83%	80%	100%
Surgical Infection Prevention					
Prophylactic Antibiotic Given[2,3]	26	46%	67%	77%	95%
Prophylactic Antibiotic Selection[5]	-	-	86%	90%	100%

Twelve Oaks Hospital

Alternate Name: Sharpstown General Hospital
6700 Bellaire Boulevard at Tarnef
Houston, TX 77074
E-mail: info@twelveoaksmedicalcenter.com/
URL: www.twelveoaksmedicalcenter.com
Ownership: Proprietary
Emergency Services: Yes

Phone: 713-774-7611
Fax: 713-778-2666

Accredited: Yes
Licensed Beds: 190

Key Personnel:
CEO . . . . Kerry Teel
Emergency Room . . . . Elriede Salisbury, RN
OB/GYN Womens Health . . . . Ed Lord, MD
Director Respiratory Therapy . . . . Diane Blackmon

Measure	Cases	This Hospital	State Average	U.S. Average	Top Hospital
Heart Attack Care					
ACE Inhibitor or ARB for LVSD[1]	6	67%	85%	82%	100%
Aspirin at Arrival	31	94%	91%	92%	100%
Aspirin at Discharge	32	84%	90%	90%	100%
Beta Blocker at Arrival	32	72%	85%	87%	100%
Beta Blocker at Discharge	34	71%	86%	90%	100%
Fibrinolytic Medication Timing[3]	0	-	30%	31%	100%
PCI Within 90 Minutes of Arrival	0	-	48%	54%	95%
Smoking Cessation Advice[3]	0	-	90%	88%	100%
Heart Failure Care					
ACE Inhibitor or ARB for LVSD	85	75%	82%	82%	100%
Discharge Instructions[1,3]	24	50%	60%	61%	93%
Evaluation of LVS Function	179	81%	81%	83%	99%
Smoking Cessation Advice[1,3]	2	50%	82%	82%	100%
Pneumonia Care					
Appropriate Initial Antibiotic[1,3]	7	29%	79%	83%	94%
Blood Culture Timing[1,3]	5	100%	89%	90%	100%
Influenza Vaccine[5]	-	-	69%	70%	100%
Initial Antibiotic Timing	53	62%	78%	80%	93%
Oxygenation Assessment	70	100%	99%	99%	100%
Pneumococcal Vaccine	26	12%	68%	69%	94%
Smoking Cessation Advice[1,3]	4	50%	83%	80%	100%
Surgical Infection Prevention					
Prophylactic Antibiotic Given[3]	37	38%	67%	77%	95%
Prophylactic Antibiotic Selection[5]	-	-	86%	90%	100%
Prophylactic Antibiotic Stopped[3]	35	63%	68%	72%	95%
Pregnancy Care					
Inpatient Neonatal Mortality	-	-	-	-	-
Third or Fourth Degree Laceration	-	-	3.23%	3.63%	3.27%

University General Hospital

7501 Fannin
Houston, TX 77054
Ownership: Proprietary
Emergency Services: Yes

Phone: 713-652-3800

Accredited: Yes

Measure	Cases	This Hospital	State Average	U.S. Average	Top Hospital
Heart Attack Care					
ACE Inhibitor or ARB for LVSD[5]	-	-	85%	82%	100%
Aspirin at Arrival[5]	-	-	91%	92%	100%
Aspirin at Discharge[5]	-	-	90%	90%	100%
Beta Blocker at Arrival[5]	-	-	85%	87%	100%
Beta Blocker at Discharge[5]	-	-	86%	90%	100%
Fibrinolytic Medication Timing[5]	-	-	30%	31%	100%
PCI Within 90 Minutes of Arrival[5]	-	-	48%	54%	95%
Smoking Cessation Advice[5]	-	-	90%	88%	100%
Heart Failure Care					
ACE Inhibitor or ARB for LVSD[5]	-	-	82%	82%	100%
Discharge Instructions[5]	-	-	60%	61%	93%
Evaluation of LVS Function[5]	-	-	81%	83%	99%
Smoking Cessation Advice[5]	-	-	82%	82%	100%
Pneumonia Care					

NOTE: Hospital profiles are in alphabetical order by state, then city, then hospital within the city; Rankings are sorted by rate in descending order and exclude hospitals with less than 25 cases; (1) The number of cases is too small (n<25) for purposes of reliably predicting hospital performance; (2) Measure reflects the hospital's indication that its submission was based upon a sample of its relevant discharges; (3) Rate reflects fewer than the maximum possible quarters of data for the measure; (4) Inaccurate information submitted and suppressed for one or more quarters; (5) No data is available from the hospital for this measure; Please refer to the User's Guide for a full explanation of data

Measure			This Hospital	State Average	U.S. Average	Top Hospital
Appropriate Initial Antibiotic[5]	-	-	79%	83%	94%	
Blood Culture Timing[5]	-	-	89%	90%	100%	
Influenza Vaccine[5]	-	-	69%	70%	100%	
Initial Antibiotic Timing[5]	-	-	78%	80%	93%	
Oxygenation Assessment[5]	-	-	99%	99%	100%	
Pneumococcal Vaccine[5]	-	-	68%	69%	94%	
Smoking Cessation Advice[5]	-	-	83%	80%	100%	
Surgical Infection Prevention						
Prophylactic Antibiotic Given[5]	-	-	67%	77%	95%	
Prophylactic Antibiotic Selection[5]	-	-	86%	90%	100%	
Prophylactic Antibiotic Stopped[5]	-	-	68%	72%	95%	
Pregnancy Care						
Inpatient Neonatal Mortality	-	-	-	-	-	
Third or Fourth Degree Laceration	-	-	3.23%	3.63%	3.27%	

West Houston Medical Center

12141 Richmond Avenue
Houston, TX 77082
URL: www.westhoustonmedical.com
Ownership: Proprietary
Emergency Services: Yes

Phone: 281-558-3444
Fax: 281-558-7619

Accredited: Yes
Licensed Beds: 221

Key Personnel:
CEO. . . . . Jeffrey Holland
Chief Medical Staff. Waynens Alanis, MD
Emergency Room . . . . Lori Litzmger
Director Infection/Disease Control . . . . Kathy Lamb
OB/GYN Womens Health. . . . . Magdy W Rizk
Chief Radiology . . . . Stephanie Staten
Director Respiratory Therapy . . . . Debra Adams

Measure	Cases	This Hospital	State Average	U.S. Average	Top Hospital
Heart Attack Care					
ACE Inhibitor or ARB for LVSD	39	90%	85%	82%	100%
Aspirin at Arrival	156	94%	91%	92%	100%
Aspirin at Discharge	148	97%	90%	90%	100%
Beta Blocker at Arrival	99	92%	85%	87%	100%
Beta Blocker at Discharge	143	97%	86%	90%	100%
Fibrinolytic Medication Timing[1]	1	0%	30%	31%	100%
PCI Within 90 Minutes of Arrival[1]	6	33%	48%	54%	95%
Smoking Cessation Advice	67	99%	90%	88%	100%
Heart Failure Care					
ACE Inhibitor or ARB for LVSD	159	96%	82%	82%	100%
Discharge Instructions	311	56%	60%	61%	93%
Evaluation of LVS Function	383	98%	81%	83%	99%
Smoking Cessation Advice	93	98%	82%	82%	100%
Pneumonia Care					
Appropriate Initial Antibiotic	147	92%	79%	83%	94%
Blood Culture Timing	175	79%	89%	90%	100%
Influenza Vaccine	48	75%	69%	70%	100%
Initial Antibiotic Timing	236	63%	78%	80%	93%
Oxygenation Assessment	288	99%	99%	99%	100%
Pneumococcal Vaccine	173	83%	68%	69%	94%
Smoking Cessation Advice	65	95%	83%	80%	100%
Surgical Infection Prevention					
Prophylactic Antibiotic Given[2,3]	188	76%	67%	77%	95%
Prophylactic Antibiotic Selection[2]	76	80%	86%	90%	100%
Prophylactic Antibiotic Stopped[2,3]	179	35%	68%	72%	95%
Pregnancy Care					
Inpatient Neonatal Mortality	2,170	0.14%	-	-	-
Third or Fourth Degree Laceration	1,415	1.70%	3.23%	3.63%	3.27%

Womans Hospital of Texas

Alternate Name: Womens Hospital of Texas
7600 Fannin Street
Houston, TX 77054
URL: www.womenshospital.com
Ownership: Proprietary
Emergency Services: Yes

Phone: 713-790-1234
Fax: 713-790-0469

Accredited: Yes
Licensed Beds: 275

Key Personnel:
CEO. . . . . Linda Russell
Chief Medical Staff. Nicholas Sollene, MD
Director Infection/Disease Control . . . . Elena Zaccaria
Director Medical/Surgical Nursing . . . . Inez Williams

OB/GYN Womens Health. . . . . Ferdinand Plavidal, MD
Chief Radiology . . . . Ralph Sharman, MD
Director Respiratory Therapy . . . . Dale Camp

Measure	Cases	This Hospital	State Average	U.S. Average	Top Hospital
Heart Attack Care					
ACE Inhibitor or ARB for LVSD[5]	-	-	85%	82%	100%
Aspirin at Arrival[5]	-	-	91%	92%	100%
Aspirin at Discharge[5]	-	-	90%	90%	100%
Beta Blocker at Arrival[5]	-	-	85%	87%	100%
Beta Blocker at Discharge[5]	-	-	86%	90%	100%
Fibrinolytic Medication Timing[5]	-	-	30%	31%	100%
PCI Within 90 Minutes of Arrival[5]	-	-	48%	54%	95%
Smoking Cessation Advice[5]	-	-	90%	88%	100%
Heart Failure Care					
ACE Inhibitor or ARB for LVSD[5]	-	-	82%	82%	100%
Discharge Instructions[5]	-	-	60%	61%	93%
Evaluation of LVS Function[5]	-	-	81%	83%	99%
Smoking Cessation Advice[5]	-	-	82%	82%	100%
Pneumonia Care					
Appropriate Initial Antibiotic[1,3]	2	50%	79%	83%	94%
Blood Culture Timing[1,3]	1	100%	89%	90%	100%
Influenza Vaccine	0	-	69%	70%	100%
Initial Antibiotic Timing[1,3]	2	50%	78%	80%	93%
Oxygenation Assessment[1,3]	2	100%	99%	99%	100%
Pneumococcal Vaccine[1,3]	1	100%	68%	69%	94%
Smoking Cessation Advice[3]	0	-	83%	80%	100%
Surgical Infection Prevention					
Prophylactic Antibiotic Given[3]	943	92%	67%	77%	95%
Prophylactic Antibiotic Selection[3]	298	92%	86%	90%	100%
Prophylactic Antibiotic Stopped[3]	912	88%	68%	72%	95%
Pregnancy Care					
Inpatient Neonatal Mortality	8,798	0.41%	-	-	-
Third or Fourth Degree Laceration	4,638	2.63%	3.23%	3.63%	3.27%

Northeast Medical Center Hospital

18951 Memorial N
Humble, TX 77338
URL: www.nemch.org
Ownership: Govt - Hospital District or Authority
Emergency Services: Yes

Phone: 281-540-7700
Fax: 281-540-7846

Accredited: Yes
Licensed Beds: 237

Key Personnel:
President/CEO. . . . . Syble Missildine
Chief Medical Staff. Angel Munoz, MD
Catheterization Lab . . . . Ellen Pavela
Emergency Room . . . . Cas Luis
Emergency Room . . . . Dale Smith
Infection Control. . . . . Kathleen Bryne, RN
ICU . . . . Faye Helms, MD
Intensive/Coronary Care . . . . Faye Helms
Medical/Surgical Nursing . . . . Barbara Evans
OB/GYN Womens Health. . . . . Terry Buchalter
Respiratory/Cardiopulmonary. . . . . Ellen Pavela

Measure	Cases	This Hospital	State Average	U.S. Average	Top Hospital
Heart Attack Care					
ACE Inhibitor or ARB for LVSD[1]	15	53%	85%	82%	100%
Aspirin at Arrival	154	88%	91%	92%	100%
Aspirin at Discharge	61	85%	90%	90%	100%
Beta Blocker at Arrival	111	80%	85%	87%	100%
Beta Blocker at Discharge	53	87%	86%	90%	100%
Fibrinolytic Medication Timing[1]	12	8%	30%	31%	100%
PCI Within 90 Minutes of Arrival	0	-	48%	54%	95%
Smoking Cessation Advice[1]	8	100%	90%	88%	100%
Heart Failure Care					
ACE Inhibitor or ARB for LVSD	149	74%	82%	82%	100%
Discharge Instructions	416	37%	60%	61%	93%
Evaluation of LVS Function	503	86%	81%	83%	99%
Smoking Cessation Advice	88	99%	82%	82%	100%
Pneumonia Care					
Appropriate Initial Antibiotic	197	82%	79%	83%	94%
Blood Culture Timing	172	86%	89%	90%	100%
Influenza Vaccine	54	48%	69%	70%	100%

NOTE: Hospital profiles are in alphabetical order by state, then city, then hospital within the city; Rankings are sorted by rate in descending order and exclude hospitals with less than 25 cases; (1) The number of cases is too small (n<25) for purposes of reliably predicting hospital performance; (2) Measure reflects the hospital's indication that its submission was based upon a sample of its relevant discharges; (3) Rate reflects fewer than the maximum possible quarters of data for the measure; (4) Inaccurate information submitted and suppressed for one or more quarters; (5) No data is available from the hospital for this measure; Please refer to the User's Guide for a full explanation of data

Initial Antibiotic Timing	278	56%	78%	80%	93%
Oxygenation Assessment	324	99%	99%	99%	100%
Pneumococcal Vaccine	153	59%	68%	69%	94%
Smoking Cessation Advice	68	96%	83%	80%	100%
Surgical Infection Prevention					
Prophylactic Antibiotic Given[2,3]	230	73%	67%	77%	95%
Prophylactic Antibiotic Selection[2]	58	50%	86%	90%	100%
Prophylactic Antibiotic Stopped[2,3]	217	47%	68%	72%	95%
Pregnancy Care					
Inpatient Neonatal Mortality	-	-	-	-	-
Third or Fourth Degree Laceration	-	-	3.23%	3.63%	3.27%

Huntsville Memorial Hospital

110 Memorial Hospital Drive   Phone: 936-291-3411
Huntsville, TX 77340   Fax: 936-291-4241
E-mail: info@huntsvillememorial.com
URL: www.huntsvillememorial.com
Ownership: Voluntary non-profit - Private   Accredited: Yes
Emergency Services: Yes   Licensed Beds: 127
Key Personnel:
President/CEO . . . . Ralph Beaty
Emergency Room . . . . Jacquie Huff
Infection Control . . . . Deanna Hughes
ICU . . . . Debbie Grisham
Medical Surgical Nursing . . . . George Crippen
OB/GYN/Women's Health . . . . Ann Karr
Respiratory/Cardiopulmonary . . . . Doug Duncan

Measure	Cases	This Hospital	State Average	U.S. Average	Top Hospital
Heart Attack Care					
ACE Inhibitor or ARB for LVSD[1]	2	100%	85%	82%	100%
Aspirin at Arrival[1]	9	89%	91%	92%	100%
Aspirin at Discharge[1]	5	80%	90%	90%	100%
Beta Blocker at Arrival[1]	8	88%	85%	87%	100%
Beta Blocker at Discharge[1]	4	100%	86%	90%	100%
Fibrinolytic Medication Timing	0	-	30%	31%	100%
PCI Within 90 Minutes of Arrival	0	-	48%	54%	95%
Smoking Cessation Advice[1]	2	100%	90%	88%	100%
Heart Failure Care					
ACE Inhibitor or ARB for LVSD	37	89%	82%	82%	100%
Discharge Instructions	65	63%	60%	61%	93%
Evaluation of LVS Function	85	72%	81%	83%	99%
Smoking Cessation Advice[1]	18	61%	82%	82%	100%
Pneumonia Care					
Appropriate Initial Antibiotic	99	83%	79%	83%	94%
Blood Culture Timing	53	92%	89%	90%	100%
Influenza Vaccine[1]	16	69%	69%	70%	100%
Initial Antibiotic Timing	91	75%	78%	80%	93%
Oxygenation Assessment	103	97%	99%	99%	100%
Pneumococcal Vaccine	65	75%	68%	69%	94%
Smoking Cessation Advice[1]	14	71%	83%	80%	100%
Surgical Infection Prevention					
Prophylactic Antibiotic Given	166	94%	67%	77%	95%
Prophylactic Antibiotic Selection	33	91%	86%	90%	100%
Prophylactic Antibiotic Stopped	143	24%	68%	72%	95%
Pregnancy Care					
Inpatient Neonatal Mortality	-	-	-	-	-
Third or Fourth Degree Laceration	-	-	3.23%	3.63%	3.27%

Southwest Surgical Hospital

1612 Hurst Town Center Drive   Phone: 817-345-4100
Hurst, TX 76054
Ownership: Proprietary   Accredited: Yes
Emergency Services: Yes

Measure	Cases	This Hospital	State Average	U.S. Average	Top Hospital
Heart Attack Care					
ACE Inhibitor or ARB for LVSD[5]	-	-	85%	82%	100%
Aspirin at Arrival[5]	-	-	91%	92%	100%
Aspirin at Discharge[5]	-	-	90%	90%	100%
Beta Blocker at Arrival[5]	-	-	85%	87%	100%
Beta Blocker at Discharge[5]	-	-	86%	90%	100%

Fibrinolytic Medication Timing[5]	-	-	30%	31%	100%
PCI Within 90 Minutes of Arrival[5]	-	-	48%	54%	95%
Smoking Cessation Advice[5]	-	-	90%	88%	100%
Heart Failure Care					
ACE Inhibitor or ARB for LVSD[5]	-	-	82%	82%	100%
Discharge Instructions[5]	-	-	60%	61%	93%
Evaluation of LVS Function[5]	-	-	81%	83%	99%
Smoking Cessation Advice[5]	-	-	82%	82%	100%
Pneumonia Care					
Appropriate Initial Antibiotic[5]	-	-	79%	83%	94%
Blood Culture Timing[5]	-	-	89%	90%	100%
Influenza Vaccine[5]	-	-	69%	70%	100%
Initial Antibiotic Timing[5]	-	-	78%	80%	93%
Oxygenation Assessment[5]	-	-	99%	99%	100%
Pneumococcal Vaccine[5]	-	-	68%	69%	94%
Smoking Cessation Advice[5]	-	-	83%	80%	100%
Surgical Infection Prevention					
Prophylactic Antibiotic Given[1,3]	3	67%	67%	77%	95%
Prophylactic Antibiotic Selection[5]	-	-	86%	90%	100%
Prophylactic Antibiotic Stopped[1,3]	3	100%	68%	72%	95%
Pregnancy Care					
Inpatient Neonatal Mortality	-	-	-	-	-
Third or Fourth Degree Laceration	-	-	3.23%	3.63%	3.27%

Baylor Medical Center at Irving

1901 N Macarthur Blvd   Phone: 972-579-8100
Irving, TX 75061
Ownership: Voluntary non-profit - Private   Accredited: Yes
Emergency Services: Yes
Key Personnel:
OBGYN . . . . Barry Jacobs, MD
Pulmonary . . . . Mahendra Mahatma, MD
Cardiology . . . . Steven Shilling, MD

Measure	Cases	This Hospital	State Average	U.S. Average	Top Hospital
Heart Attack Care					
ACE Inhibitor or ARB for LVSD	36	97%	85%	82%	100%
Aspirin at Arrival	211	100%	91%	92%	100%
Aspirin at Discharge	198	97%	90%	90%	100%
Beta Blocker at Arrival	192	99%	85%	87%	100%
Beta Blocker at Discharge	183	99%	86%	90%	100%
Fibrinolytic Medication Timing	0	-	30%	31%	100%
PCI Within 90 Minutes of Arrival[1]	14	79%	48%	54%	95%
Smoking Cessation Advice	75	100%	90%	88%	100%
Heart Failure Care					
ACE Inhibitor or ARB for LVSD	136	96%	82%	82%	100%
Discharge Instructions	288	86%	60%	61%	93%
Evaluation of LVS Function	324	99%	81%	83%	99%
Smoking Cessation Advice	57	98%	82%	82%	100%
Pneumonia Care					
Appropriate Initial Antibiotic	173	94%	79%	83%	94%
Blood Culture Timing	194	88%	89%	90%	100%
Influenza Vaccine	64	75%	69%	70%	100%
Initial Antibiotic Timing	265	90%	78%	80%	93%
Oxygenation Assessment	299	100%	99%	99%	100%
Pneumococcal Vaccine	176	94%	68%	69%	94%
Smoking Cessation Advice	70	99%	83%	80%	100%
Surgical Infection Prevention					
Prophylactic Antibiotic Given	760	96%	67%	77%	95%
Prophylactic Antibiotic Selection	176	97%	86%	90%	100%
Prophylactic Antibiotic Stopped	719	87%	68%	72%	95%
Pregnancy Care					
Inpatient Neonatal Mortality	-	-	-	-	-
Third or Fourth Degree Laceration	-	-	3.23%	3.63%	3.27%

Irving Coppell Surgical Hospital

440 West Interstate 635   Phone: 972-868-4000
Irving, TX 75063
Ownership: Proprietary   Accredited: Yes
Emergency Services: Yes
Key Personnel:
Surgery . . . . Edward Clifford, MD

NOTE: Hospital profiles are in alphabetical order by state, then city, then hospital within the city; Rankings are sorted by rate in descending order and exclude hospitals with less than 25 cases; (1) The number of cases is too small (n<25) for purposes of reliably predicting hospital performance; (2) Measure reflects the hospital's indication that its submission was based upon a sample of its relevant discharges; (3) Rate reflects fewer than the maximum possible quarters of data for the measure; (4) Inaccurate information submitted and suppressed for one or more quarters; (5) No data is available from the hospital for this measure; Please refer to the User's Guide for a full explanation of data

Measure	Cases	This Hospital	State Average	U.S. Average	Top Hospital
Heart Attack Care					
ACE Inhibitor or ARB for LVSD[5]	-	-	85%	82%	100%
Aspirin at Arrival[5]	-	-	91%	92%	100%
Aspirin at Discharge[5]	-	-	90%	90%	100%
Beta Blocker at Arrival[5]	-	-	85%	87%	100%
Beta Blocker at Discharge[5]	-	-	86%	90%	100%
Fibrinolytic Medication Timing[5]	-	-	30%	31%	100%
PCI Within 90 Minutes of Arrival[5]	-	-	48%	54%	95%
Smoking Cessation Advice[5]	-	-	90%	88%	100%
Heart Failure Care					
ACE Inhibitor or ARB for LVSD[5]	-	-	82%	82%	100%
Discharge Instructions[5]	-	-	60%	61%	93%
Evaluation of LVS Function[5]	-	-	81%	83%	99%
Smoking Cessation Advice[5]	-	-	82%	82%	100%
Pneumonia Care					
Appropriate Initial Antibiotic[5]	-	-	79%	83%	94%
Blood Culture Timing[5]	-	-	89%	90%	100%
Influenza Vaccine[5]	-	-	69%	70%	100%
Initial Antibiotic Timing[1,3]	1	100%	78%	80%	93%
Oxygenation Assessment[1,3]	1	0%	99%	99%	100%
Pneumococcal Vaccine[3]	0	-	68%	69%	94%
Smoking Cessation Advice[5]	-	-	83%	80%	100%
Surgical Infection Prevention					
Prophylactic Antibiotic Given[1,3]	9	78%	67%	77%	95%
Prophylactic Antibiotic Selection[5]	-	-	86%	90%	100%
Prophylactic Antibiotic Stopped[1,3]	9	100%	68%	72%	95%
Pregnancy Care					
Inpatient Neonatal Mortality	-	-	-	-	-
Third or Fourth Degree Laceration	-	-	3.23%	3.63%	3.27%

Las Colinas Medical Center

6800 N MacArthur Boulevard
Irving, TX 75039
URL: www.lascolinas.com
Ownership: Voluntary non-profit - Private
Emergency Services: Yes

Phone: 972-969-2000
Fax: 972-969-2080

Accredited: Yes
Licensed Beds: 70

Key Personnel:
CEO . . . . Daniela Wallace
Emergency Room . . . . David Moikeha, MD

Measure	Cases	This Hospital	State Average	U.S. Average	Top Hospital
Heart Attack Care					
ACE Inhibitor or ARB for LVSD[1]	2	100%	85%	82%	100%
Aspirin at Arrival[1]	13	92%	91%	92%	100%
Aspirin at Discharge[1]	5	100%	90%	90%	100%
Beta Blocker at Arrival[1]	11	100%	85%	87%	100%
Beta Blocker at Discharge[1]	5	100%	86%	90%	100%
Fibrinolytic Medication Timing	0	-	30%	31%	100%
PCI Within 90 Minutes of Arrival	0	-	48%	54%	95%
Smoking Cessation Advice[1]	1	100%	90%	88%	100%
Heart Failure Care					
ACE Inhibitor or ARB for LVSD	33	88%	82%	82%	100%
Discharge Instructions	76	58%	60%	61%	93%
Evaluation of LVS Function	78	92%	81%	83%	99%
Smoking Cessation Advice[1]	8	100%	82%	82%	100%
Pneumonia Care					
Appropriate Initial Antibiotic	52	85%	79%	83%	94%
Blood Culture Timing	40	90%	89%	90%	100%
Influenza Vaccine[1]	14	79%	69%	70%	100%
Initial Antibiotic Timing	63	83%	78%	80%	93%
Oxygenation Assessment	65	100%	99%	99%	100%
Pneumococcal Vaccine	44	82%	68%	69%	94%
Smoking Cessation Advice[1]	12	58%	83%	80%	100%
Surgical Infection Prevention					
Prophylactic Antibiotic Given[2,3]	92	75%	67%	77%	95%
Prophylactic Antibiotic Selection[2]	43	91%	86%	90%	100%
Prophylactic Antibiotic Stopped[2,3]	90	87%	68%	72%	95%
Pregnancy Care					
Inpatient Neonatal Mortality	-	-	-	-	-
Third or Fourth Degree Laceration	-	-	3.23%	3.63%	3.27%

Faith Community Hospital

17 Magnolia Street
Jacksboro, TX 76458
E-mail: info@faithcommunityhospital.com
URL: www.faithcommunityhospital.com
Ownership: Govt - Hospital District or Authority
Emergency Services: Yes

Phone: 940-567-6633
Fax: 940-567-5714

Accredited: No
Licensed Beds: 41

Key Personnel:
Administrator/CEO . . . . Don Hopkins
Chief Medical Staff . . . . Syed Jamal, MD
Emergency Room . . . . Syed Jamal, MD
Medical Surgical Nursing . . . . Pete Peterson

Measure	Cases	This Hospital	State Average	U.S. Average	Top Hospital
Heart Attack Care					
ACE Inhibitor or ARB for LVSD[1]	1	100%	85%	82%	100%
Aspirin at Arrival[1]	7	71%	91%	92%	100%
Aspirin at Discharge[1]	4	75%	90%	90%	100%
Beta Blocker at Arrival[1]	8	25%	85%	87%	100%
Beta Blocker at Discharge[1]	7	71%	86%	90%	100%
Fibrinolytic Medication Timing	0	-	30%	31%	100%
PCI Within 90 Minutes of Arrival	0	-	48%	54%	95%
Smoking Cessation Advice[1]	2	50%	90%	88%	100%
Heart Failure Care					
ACE Inhibitor or ARB for LVSD[1]	9	78%	82%	82%	100%
Discharge Instructions[1]	12	67%	60%	61%	93%
Evaluation of LVS Function[1]	18	67%	81%	83%	99%
Smoking Cessation Advice[1]	3	100%	82%	82%	100%
Pneumonia Care					
Appropriate Initial Antibiotic[1]	12	83%	79%	83%	94%
Blood Culture Timing[1]	4	100%	89%	90%	100%
Influenza Vaccine[1]	7	86%	69%	70%	100%
Initial Antibiotic Timing[1]	17	94%	78%	80%	93%
Oxygenation Assessment[1]	20	100%	99%	99%	100%
Pneumococcal Vaccine[1]	11	100%	68%	69%	94%
Smoking Cessation Advice[1]	5	80%	83%	80%	100%
Surgical Infection Prevention					
Prophylactic Antibiotic Given[5]	-	-	67%	77%	95%
Prophylactic Antibiotic Selection[5]	-	-	86%	90%	100%
Prophylactic Antibiotic Stopped[5]	-	-	68%	72%	95%
Pregnancy Care					
Inpatient Neonatal Mortality	-	-	-	-	-
Third or Fourth Degree Laceration	-	-	3.23%	3.63%	3.27%

East Texas Medical Center-Jacksonville

Alternate Name: Nan Travis Memorial Hospital
501 S Ragsdale Street
Jacksonville, TX 75766
URL: www.etmc.org
Ownership: Voluntary non-profit - Private
Emergency Services: Yes

Phone: 903-541-5000
Fax: 903-541-5088

Accredited: Yes
Licensed Beds: 94

Key Personnel:
President . . . . Steve Bowen
Chief Medical Staff . . . . Larry Cunningham, MD
Emergency Room . . . . Donna Watson, RN
Infection Control . . . . Jana Batenar, RN
VP Medical Surgical Nursing . . . . Janet Blue
OB/GYN Womens Health . . . . Tammy Chastair, RN
Respiratory/Cardiopulmonary . . . . Hallie Peoples, RT

Measure	Cases	This Hospital	State Average	U.S. Average	Top Hospital
Heart Attack Care					
ACE Inhibitor or ARB for LVSD[3]	0	-	85%	82%	100%
Aspirin at Arrival[1,3]	10	80%	91%	92%	100%
Aspirin at Discharge[1,3]	7	86%	90%	90%	100%
Beta Blocker at Arrival[1,3]	8	75%	85%	87%	100%
Beta Blocker at Discharge[1,3]	7	100%	86%	90%	100%
Fibrinolytic Medication Timing[3]	0	-	30%	31%	100%
PCI Within 90 Minutes of Arrival	0	-	48%	54%	95%
Smoking Cessation Advice[1,3]	1	0%	90%	88%	100%
Heart Failure Care					
ACE Inhibitor or ARB for LVSD[1]	16	62%	82%	82%	100%
Discharge Instructions[1,3]	7	86%	60%	61%	93%

NOTE: Hospital profiles are in alphabetical order by state, then city, then hospital within the city; Rankings are sorted by rate in descending order and exclude hospitals with less than 25 cases; (1) The number of cases is too small (n<25) for purposes of reliably predicting hospital performance; (2) Measure reflects the hospital's indication that its submission was based upon a sample of its relevant discharges; (3) Rate reflects fewer than the maximum possible quarters of data for the measure; (4) Inaccurate information submitted and suppressed for one or more quarters; (5) No data is available from the hospital for this measure; Please refer to the User's Guide for a full explanation of data

Evaluation of LVS Function	64	94%	81%	83%	99%
Smoking Cessation Advice[1,3]	3	100%	82%	82%	100%
Pneumonia Care					
Appropriate Initial Antibiotic[1,3]	10	90%	79%	83%	94%
Blood Culture Timing[1,3]	11	100%	89%	90%	100%
Influenza Vaccine[5]	-	-	69%	70%	100%
Initial Antibiotic Timing	90	90%	78%	80%	93%
Oxygenation Assessment	106	100%	99%	99%	100%
Pneumococcal Vaccine	61	79%	68%	69%	94%
Smoking Cessation Advice[1,3]	4	100%	83%	80%	100%
Surgical Infection Prevention					
Prophylactic Antibiotic Given[1,3]	15	60%	67%	77%	95%
Prophylactic Antibiotic Selection[5]	-	-	86%	90%	100%
Prophylactic Antibiotic Stopped[1,3]	14	50%	68%	72%	95%
Pregnancy Care					
Inpatient Neonatal Mortality	-	-	-	-	-
Third or Fourth Degree Laceration	-	-	3.23%	3.63%	3.27%

Mother Frances Hospital Jacksonville

2026 S Jackson Street
Jacksonville, TX 75766   Phone: 903-541-4500
Ownership: Voluntary non-profit - Other   Accredited: Yes
Emergency Services: Yes

Measure	Cases	This Hospital	State Average	U.S. Average	Top Hospital
Heart Attack Care					
ACE Inhibitor or ARB for LVSD[3]	0	-	85%	82%	100%
Aspirin at Arrival[3]	0	-	91%	92%	100%
Aspirin at Discharge[3]	0	-	90%	90%	100%
Beta Blocker at Arrival[3]	0	-	85%	87%	100%
Beta Blocker at Discharge[3]	0	-	86%	90%	100%
Fibrinolytic Medication Timing[1,3]	1	0%	30%	31%	100%
PCI Within 90 Minutes of Arrival	0	-	48%	54%	95%
Smoking Cessation Advice[3]	0	-	90%	88%	100%
Heart Failure Care					
ACE Inhibitor or ARB for LVSD[1,3]	22	86%	82%	82%	100%
Discharge Instructions[1,3]	19	58%	60%	61%	93%
Evaluation of LVS Function[1,3]	24	96%	81%	83%	99%
Smoking Cessation Advice[1,3]	4	100%	82%	82%	100%
Pneumonia Care					
Appropriate Initial Antibiotic[3]	35	86%	79%	83%	94%
Blood Culture Timing[1,3]	37	89%	89%	90%	100%
Influenza Vaccine[1]	7	100%	69%	70%	100%
Initial Antibiotic Timing[3]	35	97%	78%	80%	93%
Oxygenation Assessment[3]	43	100%	99%	99%	100%
Pneumococcal Vaccine[1,3]	24	67%	68%	69%	94%
Smoking Cessation Advice[1,3]	8	62%	83%	80%	100%
Surgical Infection Prevention					
Prophylactic Antibiotic Given[3]	40	80%	67%	77%	95%
Prophylactic Antibiotic Selection[1]	19	95%	86%	90%	100%
Prophylactic Antibiotic Stopped[3]	40	80%	68%	72%	95%
Pregnancy Care					
Inpatient Neonatal Mortality	-	-	-	-	-
Third or Fourth Degree Laceration	-	-	3.23%	3.63%	3.27%

Christus Jasper Memorial Hospital

Alternate Name: Jasper Memorial Hospital
1275 Marvin Hancock Drive   Phone: 409-384-1872
Jasper, TX 75951   Fax: 409-384-4357
E-mail: deborah.wiegand@christushealth.org
URL: www.christusjasper.org
Ownership: Govt - Hospital District or Authority   Accredited: Yes
Emergency Services: Yes   Licensed Beds: 81
Key Personnel:
President/CEO . . . . George N Miller Jr
Chief Medical Staff . . . . Larry Brown

Measure	Cases	This Hospital	State Average	U.S. Average	Top Hospital
Heart Attack Care					
ACE Inhibitor or ARB for LVSD[1,3]	1	100%	85%	82%	100%
Aspirin at Arrival[1,3]	4	50%	91%	92%	100%
Aspirin at Discharge[1,3]	3	100%	90%	90%	100%

Beta Blocker at Arrival[1,3]	4	50%	85%	87%	100%
Beta Blocker at Discharge[1,3]	2	100%	86%	90%	100%
Fibrinolytic Medication Timing[3]	0	-	30%	31%	100%
PCI Within 90 Minutes of Arrival[5]	-	-	48%	54%	95%
Smoking Cessation Advice[3]	0	-	90%	88%	100%
Heart Failure Care					
ACE Inhibitor or ARB for LVSD[1]	22	82%	82%	82%	100%
Discharge Instructions	55	76%	60%	61%	93%
Evaluation of LVS Function	79	95%	81%	83%	99%
Smoking Cessation Advice[1]	17	100%	82%	82%	100%
Pneumonia Care					
Appropriate Initial Antibiotic	46	74%	79%	83%	94%
Blood Culture Timing	38	79%	89%	90%	100%
Influenza Vaccine[1]	22	55%	69%	70%	100%
Initial Antibiotic Timing	69	68%	78%	80%	93%
Oxygenation Assessment	78	100%	99%	99%	100%
Pneumococcal Vaccine	53	62%	68%	69%	94%
Smoking Cessation Advice[1]	16	94%	83%	80%	100%
Surgical Infection Prevention					
Prophylactic Antibiotic Given[3]	46	85%	67%	77%	95%
Prophylactic Antibiotic Selection[1]	16	88%	86%	90%	100%
Prophylactic Antibiotic Stopped[3]	44	50%	68%	72%	95%
Pregnancy Care					
Inpatient Neonatal Mortality	-	-	-	-	-
Third or Fourth Degree Laceration	-	-	3.23%	3.63%	3.27%

Dickerson Memorial Hospital

1001 Dickerson Drive   Phone: 409-489-0600
Jasper, TX 75951
Ownership: Voluntary non-profit - Private   Accredited: No
Emergency Services: Yes

Measure	Cases	This Hospital	State Average	U.S. Average	Top Hospital
Heart Attack Care					
ACE Inhibitor or ARB for LVSD	0	-	85%	82%	100%
Aspirin at Arrival[1]	5	80%	91%	92%	100%
Aspirin at Discharge[1]	2	0%	90%	90%	100%
Beta Blocker at Arrival[1]	5	60%	85%	87%	100%
Beta Blocker at Discharge[1]	3	33%	86%	90%	100%
Fibrinolytic Medication Timing[3]	0	-	30%	31%	100%
PCI Within 90 Minutes of Arrival	0	-	48%	54%	95%
Smoking Cessation Advice[1,3]	1	100%	90%	88%	100%
Heart Failure Care					
ACE Inhibitor or ARB for LVSD[3]	0	-	82%	82%	100%
Discharge Instructions[1,3]	8	0%	60%	61%	93%
Evaluation of LVS Function[1,3]	15	13%	81%	83%	99%
Smoking Cessation Advice[3]	0	-	82%	82%	100%
Pneumonia Care					
Appropriate Initial Antibiotic[1,3]	4	50%	79%	83%	94%
Blood Culture Timing[1,3]	1	0%	89%	90%	100%
Influenza Vaccine[5]	-	-	69%	70%	100%
Initial Antibiotic Timing[1]	7	86%	78%	80%	93%
Oxygenation Assessment[1]	22	100%	99%	99%	100%
Pneumococcal Vaccine[1,3]	3	0%	68%	69%	94%
Smoking Cessation Advice[1,3]	1	0%	83%	80%	100%
Surgical Infection Prevention					
Prophylactic Antibiotic Given[1,3]	2	0%	67%	77%	95%
Prophylactic Antibiotic Selection[5]	-	-	86%	90%	100%
Prophylactic Antibiotic Stopped[1,3]	2	50%	68%	72%	95%
Pregnancy Care					
Inpatient Neonatal Mortality	-	-	-	-	-
Third or Fourth Degree Laceration	-	-	3.23%	3.63%	3.27%

South Texas Regional Medical Center

Alternate Name: Tri City Community Hospital

NOTE: Hospital profiles are in alphabetical order by state, then city, then hospital within the city; Rankings are sorted by rate in descending order and exclude hospitals with less than 25 cases; (1) The number of cases is too small (n<25) for purposes of reliably predicting hospital performance; (2) Measure reflects the hospital's indication that its submission was based upon a sample of its relevant discharges; (3) Rate reflects fewer than the maximum possible quarters of data for the measure; (4) Inaccurate information submitted and suppressed for one or more quarters; (5) No data is available from the hospital for this measure; Please refer to the User's Guide for a full explanation of data

1905 Highway 97 E
PO Box 189
Jourdanton, TX 78026
URL: www.strmc.org
Ownership: Proprietary
Emergency Services: Yes

Toll-Free: 800-460-8224
Phone: 830-769-3515
Fax: 830-769-5264

Accredited: Yes
Licensed Beds: 47

Key Personnel:
CEO. . . . . Dennis Barts
Chief Medical Staff. . . . . Patricia Lovillarreal
Emergency Room . . . . R Castilleo
Director Respiratory Therapy . . . . Gayla Jones

Measure	Cases	This Hospital	State Average	U.S. Average	Top Hospital
Heart Attack Care					
ACE Inhibitor or ARB for LVSD[1]	2	100%	85%	82%	100%
Aspirin at Arrival	31	97%	91%	92%	100%
Aspirin at Discharge[1]	18	83%	90%	90%	100%
Beta Blocker at Arrival	28	71%	85%	87%	100%
Beta Blocker at Discharge[1]	23	70%	86%	90%	100%
Fibrinolytic Medication Timing	0	-	30%	31%	100%
PCI Within 90 Minutes of Arrival	0	-	48%	54%	95%
Smoking Cessation Advice[1]	1	100%	90%	88%	100%
Heart Failure Care					
ACE Inhibitor or ARB for LVSD	27	85%	82%	82%	100%
Discharge Instructions	141	75%	60%	61%	93%
Evaluation of LVS Function	165	87%	81%	83%	99%
Smoking Cessation Advice	27	93%	82%	82%	100%
Pneumonia Care					
Appropriate Initial Antibiotic	119	88%	79%	83%	94%
Blood Culture Timing	109	99%	89%	90%	100%
Influenza Vaccine	49	98%	69%	70%	100%
Initial Antibiotic Timing	162	79%	78%	80%	93%
Oxygenation Assessment	182	100%	99%	99%	100%
Pneumococcal Vaccine	100	96%	68%	69%	94%
Smoking Cessation Advice	41	90%	83%	80%	100%
Surgical Infection Prevention					
Prophylactic Antibiotic Given[2,3]	59	46%	67%	77%	95%
Prophylactic Antibiotic Selection[1,2]	15	93%	86%	90%	100%
Prophylactic Antibiotic Stopped[2,3]	54	85%	68%	72%	95%
Pregnancy Care					
Inpatient Neonatal Mortality	-	-	-	-	-
Third or Fourth Degree Laceration	-	-	3.23%	3.63%	3.27%

Christus Saint Catherine Hospital
701 South Fry Road
Katy, TX 77450
Ownership: Voluntary non-profit - Church
Emergency Services: Yes

Phone: 281-599-5700

Accredited: Yes

Measure	Cases	This Hospital	State Average	U.S. Average	Top Hospital
Heart Attack Care					
ACE Inhibitor or ARB for LVSD[1]	5	100%	85%	82%	100%
Aspirin at Arrival	47	96%	91%	92%	100%
Aspirin at Discharge[1]	22	91%	90%	90%	100%
Beta Blocker at Arrival	42	95%	85%	87%	100%
Beta Blocker at Discharge	27	96%	86%	90%	100%
Fibrinolytic Medication Timing[1]	3	0%	30%	31%	100%
PCI Within 90 Minutes of Arrival	0	-	48%	54%	95%
Smoking Cessation Advice[1]	6	100%	90%	88%	100%
Heart Failure Care					
ACE Inhibitor or ARB for LVSD	49	98%	82%	82%	100%
Discharge Instructions	130	85%	60%	61%	93%
Evaluation of LVS Function	155	100%	81%	83%	99%
Smoking Cessation Advice[1]	19	100%	82%	82%	100%
Pneumonia Care					
Appropriate Initial Antibiotic	151	90%	79%	83%	94%
Blood Culture Timing	78	92%	89%	90%	100%
Influenza Vaccine[1]	20	95%	69%	70%	100%
Initial Antibiotic Timing	143	89%	78%	80%	93%
Oxygenation Assessment	159	100%	99%	99%	100%
Pneumococcal Vaccine	86	93%	68%	69%	94%
Smoking Cessation Advice	28	100%	83%	80%	100%

Measure	Cases	This Hospital	State Average	U.S. Average	Top Hospital
Surgical Infection Prevention					
Prophylactic Antibiotic Given	155	68%	67%	77%	95%
Prophylactic Antibiotic Selection	31	94%	86%	90%	100%
Prophylactic Antibiotic Stopped	146	73%	68%	72%	95%
Pregnancy Care					
Inpatient Neonatal Mortality	-	-	-	-	-
Third or Fourth Degree Laceration	-	-	3.23%	3.63%	3.27%

Memorial Herman Katy Hospital
Alternate Name: Epic Health Care
5602 Medical Center Drive
Katy, TX 77494
Ownership: Voluntary non-profit - Private
Emergency Services: Yes

Phone: 281-392-1111
Fax: 281-644-7068
Accredited: Yes
Licensed Beds: 118

Key Personnel:
Administrator/CEO. . . . . Scott Barbe
Director Infection/Disease Control . . . . Phillis Godwin
OB/GYN Womens Health. . . . . Morris Gonik, MD

Measure	Cases	This Hospital	State Average	U.S. Average	Top Hospital
Heart Attack Care					
ACE Inhibitor or ARB for LVSD[1]	14	86%	85%	82%	100%
Aspirin at Arrival	75	100%	91%	92%	100%
Aspirin at Discharge	43	95%	90%	90%	100%
Beta Blocker at Arrival	68	100%	85%	87%	100%
Beta Blocker at Discharge	46	98%	86%	90%	100%
Fibrinolytic Medication Timing[1]	6	100%	30%	31%	100%
PCI Within 90 Minutes of Arrival	0	-	48%	54%	95%
Smoking Cessation Advice[1]	4	100%	90%	88%	100%
Heart Failure Care					
ACE Inhibitor or ARB for LVSD	63	98%	82%	82%	100%
Discharge Instructions	106	87%	60%	61%	93%
Evaluation of LVS Function	150	100%	81%	83%	99%
Smoking Cessation Advice[1]	10	100%	82%	82%	100%
Pneumonia Care					
Appropriate Initial Antibiotic	102	85%	79%	83%	94%
Blood Culture Timing	112	96%	89%	90%	100%
Influenza Vaccine[4,5]	-	-	69%	70%	100%
Initial Antibiotic Timing	145	92%	78%	80%	93%
Oxygenation Assessment	180	100%	99%	99%	100%
Pneumococcal Vaccine	103	98%	68%	69%	94%
Smoking Cessation Advice	39	100%	83%	80%	100%
Surgical Infection Prevention					
Prophylactic Antibiotic Given[2,3]	249	82%	67%	77%	95%
Prophylactic Antibiotic Selection[2]	92	88%	86%	90%	100%
Prophylactic Antibiotic Stopped[2,3]	244	80%	68%	72%	95%
Pregnancy Care					
Inpatient Neonatal Mortality	-	-	-	-	-
Third or Fourth Degree Laceration	-	-	3.23%	3.63%	3.27%

Presbyterian Hospital of Kaufman
850 Highway 243 W
PO Box 1108
Kaufman, TX 75142
URL: www.phscare.org/phk.htm
Ownership: Voluntary non-profit - Church
Emergency Services: Yes

Phone: 972-932-7200
Fax: 972-932-5425

Accredited: Yes
Licensed Beds: 91

Key Personnel:
Chief Medical Staff. . . . . Jeral Antone, MD
Emergency Room . . . . Michael Hueber, DO
Director Infection/Disease Control . . . . Janet Drummond
Director Medical/Surgical Nursing . . . . Stephanie Huckaby
Surgical Services . . . . Susan Stone
Director Respiratory Therapy . . . . Trisha Scarborough

Measure	Cases	This Hospital	State Average	U.S. Average	Top Hospital
Heart Attack Care					
ACE Inhibitor or ARB for LVSD[1]	3	67%	85%	82%	100%
Aspirin at Arrival[1]	22	95%	91%	92%	100%
Aspirin at Discharge[1]	13	77%	90%	90%	100%
Beta Blocker at Arrival[1]	11	82%	85%	87%	100%
Beta Blocker at Discharge[1]	11	82%	86%	90%	100%

NOTE: Hospital profiles are in alphabetical order by state, then city, then hospital within the city; Rankings are sorted by rate in descending order and exclude hospitals with less than 25 cases; (1) The number of cases is too small (n<25) for purposes of reliably predicting hospital performance; (2) Measure reflects the hospital's indication that its submission was based upon a sample of its relevant discharges; (3) Rate reflects fewer than the maximum possible quarters of data for the measure; (4) Inaccurate information submitted and suppressed for one or more quarters; (5) No data is available from the hospital for this measure; Please refer to the User's Guide for a full explanation of data

Measure		1	100%	30%	31%	100%
Fibrinolytic Medication Timing[1]		1	100%	30%	31%	100%
PCI Within 90 Minutes of Arrival		0	-	48%	54%	95%
Smoking Cessation Advice[1]		3	100%	90%	88%	100%
Heart Failure Care						
ACE Inhibitor or ARB for LVSD		33	91%	82%	82%	100%
Discharge Instructions		125	95%	60%	61%	93%
Evaluation of LVS Function		149	87%	81%	83%	99%
Smoking Cessation Advice		37	95%	82%	82%	100%
Pneumonia Care						
Appropriate Initial Antibiotic		76	80%	79%	83%	94%
Blood Culture Timing		64	95%	89%	90%	100%
Influenza Vaccine		33	97%	69%	70%	100%
Initial Antibiotic Timing		89	98%	78%	80%	93%
Oxygenation Assessment		116	100%	99%	99%	100%
Pneumococcal Vaccine		77	90%	68%	69%	94%
Smoking Cessation Advice		36	97%	83%	80%	100%
Surgical Infection Prevention						
Prophylactic Antibiotic Given[2,3]		55	78%	67%	77%	95%
Prophylactic Antibiotic Selection[1,2]		18	67%	86%	90%	100%
Prophylactic Antibiotic Stopped[2,3]		52	56%	68%	72%	95%
Pregnancy Care						
Inpatient Neonatal Mortality		-	-	-	-	-
Third or Fourth Degree Laceration		-	-	3.23%	3.63%	3.27%

Otto Kaiser Memorial Hospital

3349 S Highway 181
Kenedy, TX 78119
Phone: 830-583-3401
Ownership: Govt - Hospital District or Authority Accredited: No
Emergency Services: No

Measure	Cases	This Hospital	State Average	U.S. Average	Top Hospital
Heart Attack Care					
ACE Inhibitor or ARB for LVSD[3]	0	-	85%	82%	100%
Aspirin at Arrival[3]	0	-	91%	92%	100%
Aspirin at Discharge[3]	0	-	90%	90%	100%
Beta Blocker at Arrival[3]	0	-	85%	87%	100%
Beta Blocker at Discharge[3]	0	-	86%	90%	100%
Fibrinolytic Medication Timing[3]	0	-	30%	31%	100%
PCI Within 90 Minutes of Arrival[5]	-	-	48%	54%	95%
Smoking Cessation Advice[3]	0	-	90%	88%	100%
Heart Failure Care					
ACE Inhibitor or ARB for LVSD[1]	2	0%	82%	82%	100%
Discharge Instructions[1]	12	0%	60%	61%	93%
Evaluation of LVS Function	31	13%	81%	83%	99%
Smoking Cessation Advice[1]	1	100%	82%	82%	100%
Pneumonia Care					
Appropriate Initial Antibiotic[1,3]	17	88%	79%	83%	94%
Blood Culture Timing[1,3]	4	100%	89%	90%	100%
Influenza Vaccine[1]	8	50%	69%	70%	100%
Initial Antibiotic Timing[1,3]	19	74%	78%	80%	93%
Oxygenation Assessment[3]	25	100%	99%	99%	100%
Pneumococcal Vaccine[1,3]	18	56%	68%	69%	94%
Smoking Cessation Advice[1,3]	1	100%	83%	80%	100%
Surgical Infection Prevention					
Prophylactic Antibiotic Given[5]	-	-	67%	77%	95%
Prophylactic Antibiotic Selection[5]	-	-	86%	90%	100%
Prophylactic Antibiotic Stopped[5]	-	-	68%	72%	95%
Pregnancy Care					
Inpatient Neonatal Mortality	-	-	-	-	-
Third or Fourth Degree Laceration	-	-	3.23%	3.63%	3.27%

Sid Peterson Memorial Hospital

710 Water Street
Kerrville, TX 78028
URL: www.spmh.com
Ownership: Voluntary non-profit - Other
Emergency Services: Yes
Phone: 830-896-4200
Fax: 830-258-7381

Accredited: Yes
Licensed Beds: 148

Key Personnel:
Administrator . . . . James Patrick Murray
Chief Medical Staff . . . . D Barrington
ICU Supervising Nurse . . . . Katie Mosley-Clark

Measure	Cases	This Hospital	State Average	U.S. Average	Top Hospital
Heart Attack Care					
ACE Inhibitor or ARB for LVSD[1]	4	75%	85%	82%	100%
Aspirin at Arrival[1]	21	95%	91%	92%	100%
Aspirin at Discharge[1]	13	85%	90%	90%	100%
Beta Blocker at Arrival[1]	20	90%	85%	87%	100%
Beta Blocker at Discharge[1]	13	77%	86%	90%	100%
Fibrinolytic Medication Timing[1]	1	0%	30%	31%	100%
PCI Within 90 Minutes of Arrival	0	-	48%	54%	95%
Smoking Cessation Advice[1]	3	67%	90%	88%	100%
Heart Failure Care					
ACE Inhibitor or ARB for LVSD[1]	19	84%	82%	82%	100%
Discharge Instructions	107	66%	60%	61%	93%
Evaluation of LVS Function	117	80%	81%	83%	99%
Smoking Cessation Advice[1]	17	82%	82%	82%	100%
Pneumonia Care					
Appropriate Initial Antibiotic	142	80%	79%	83%	94%
Blood Culture Timing	105	89%	89%	90%	100%
Influenza Vaccine[4,5]	-	-	69%	70%	100%
Initial Antibiotic Timing	224	89%	78%	80%	93%
Oxygenation Assessment	269	100%	99%	99%	100%
Pneumococcal Vaccine	180	84%	68%	69%	94%
Smoking Cessation Advice	49	94%	83%	80%	100%
Surgical Infection Prevention					
Prophylactic Antibiotic Given[3]	363	88%	67%	77%	95%
Prophylactic Antibiotic Selection	131	95%	86%	90%	100%
Prophylactic Antibiotic Stopped[3]	352	57%	68%	72%	95%
Pregnancy Care					
Inpatient Neonatal Mortality	-	-	-	-	-
Third or Fourth Degree Laceration	-	-	3.23%	3.63%	3.27%

Laird Memorial Hospital

1612 S Henderson Boulevard
Kilgore, TX 75662
Ownership: Voluntary non-profit - Other
Emergency Services: Yes
Phone: 903-984-3505
Fax: 903-983-4354
Accredited: No
Licensed Beds: 60

Key Personnel:
President/CEO . . . . Bob S Ellzey
Chief Medical Staff . . . . Phil Denny, MD
Infection Control Coordinator . . . . Deborah Crager, RN
Director Respiratory Therapy . . . . Patti Fields

Measure	Cases	This Hospital	State Average	U.S. Average	Top Hospital
Heart Attack Care					
ACE Inhibitor or ARB for LVSD[3]	0	-	85%	82%	100%
Aspirin at Arrival[3]	0	-	91%	92%	100%
Aspirin at Discharge[3]	0	-	90%	90%	100%
Beta Blocker at Arrival[3]	0	-	85%	87%	100%
Beta Blocker at Discharge[3]	0	-	86%	90%	100%
Fibrinolytic Medication Timing[3]	0	-	30%	31%	100%
PCI Within 90 Minutes of Arrival[5]	-	-	48%	54%	95%
Smoking Cessation Advice[3]	0	-	90%	88%	100%
Heart Failure Care					
ACE Inhibitor or ARB for LVSD[1]	16	75%	82%	82%	100%
Discharge Instructions	55	58%	60%	61%	93%
Evaluation of LVS Function	74	73%	81%	83%	99%
Smoking Cessation Advice[1]	16	100%	82%	82%	100%
Pneumonia Care					
Appropriate Initial Antibiotic	62	58%	79%	83%	94%
Blood Culture Timing	44	80%	89%	90%	100%
Influenza Vaccine[1]	16	88%	69%	70%	100%
Initial Antibiotic Timing	86	92%	78%	80%	93%
Oxygenation Assessment	95	100%	99%	99%	100%
Pneumococcal Vaccine	57	72%	68%	69%	94%
Smoking Cessation Advice[1]	21	90%	83%	80%	100%
Surgical Infection Prevention					
Prophylactic Antibiotic Given[1,3]	23	48%	67%	77%	95%
Prophylactic Antibiotic Selection[1]	9	78%	86%	90%	100%
Prophylactic Antibiotic Stopped[1,3]	21	90%	68%	72%	95%
Pregnancy Care					
Inpatient Neonatal Mortality	-	-	-	-	-

NOTE: Hospital profiles are in alphabetical order by state, then city, then hospital within the city; Rankings are sorted by rate in descending order and exclude hospitals with less than 25 cases; (1) The number of cases is too small (n<25) for purposes of reliably predicting hospital performance; (2) Measure reflects the hospital's indication that its submission was based upon a sample of its relevant discharges; (3) Rate reflects fewer than the maximum possible quarters of data for the measure; (4) Inaccurate information submitted and suppressed for one or more quarters; (5) No data is available from the hospital for this measure; Please refer to the User's Guide for a full explanation of data

Third or Fourth Degree Laceration	-	-	3.23%	3.63%	3.27%

Metroplex Hospital

2201 S Clear Creek Road
Killeen, TX 76549
E-mail: dhewitt@ahcs.org
URL: www.mplex.org
Ownership: Voluntary non-profit - Church
Emergency Services: Yes

Phone: 254-526-7523
Fax: 254-526-3483

Accredited: Yes
Licensed Beds: 213

Measure	Cases	This Hospital	State Average	U.S. Average	Top Hospital
Heart Attack Care					
ACE Inhibitor or ARB for LVSD[1]	7	71%	85%	82%	100%
Aspirin at Arrival	42	93%	91%	92%	100%
Aspirin at Discharge	31	90%	90%	90%	100%
Beta Blocker at Arrival	39	95%	85%	87%	100%
Beta Blocker at Discharge	33	97%	86%	90%	100%
Fibrinolytic Medication Timing	0	-	30%	31%	100%
PCI Within 90 Minutes of Arrival	0	-	48%	54%	95%
Smoking Cessation Advice[1]	12	92%	90%	88%	100%
Heart Failure Care					
ACE Inhibitor or ARB for LVSD	83	75%	82%	82%	100%
Discharge Instructions	213	61%	60%	61%	93%
Evaluation of LVS Function	249	90%	81%	83%	99%
Smoking Cessation Advice	48	77%	82%	82%	100%
Pneumonia Care					
Appropriate Initial Antibiotic	61	80%	79%	83%	94%
Blood Culture Timing	51	90%	89%	90%	100%
Influenza Vaccine[1]	18	89%	69%	70%	100%
Initial Antibiotic Timing	84	61%	78%	80%	93%
Oxygenation Assessment	101	100%	99%	99%	100%
Pneumococcal Vaccine	51	76%	68%	69%	94%
Smoking Cessation Advice	34	82%	83%	80%	100%
Surgical Infection Prevention					
Prophylactic Antibiotic Given[3]	215	51%	67%	77%	95%
Prophylactic Antibiotic Selection	84	89%	86%	90%	100%
Prophylactic Antibiotic Stopped[3]	211	45%	68%	72%	95%
Pregnancy Care					
Inpatient Neonatal Mortality	1,313	0.08%	-	-	-
Third or Fourth Degree Laceration	780	3.33%	3.23%	3.63%	3.27%

Christus Spohn Hospital Kleberg

Alternate Name: Spohn-Kleberg Memorial Hospital
1311 E General Cavazos Boulevard
Kingsville, TX 78363
Ownership: Voluntary non-profit - Church
Emergency Services: Yes
Key Personnel:
President/CEO . . . . Kathy J McDonagh
OB/GYN . . . . Ronald Cole, MD

Phone: 361-595-1661
Fax: 361-595-5005
Accredited: Yes
Licensed Beds: 100

Measure	Cases	This Hospital	State Average	U.S. Average	Top Hospital
Heart Attack Care					
ACE Inhibitor or ARB for LVSD[1]	1	100%	85%	82%	100%
Aspirin at Arrival[1]	12	92%	91%	92%	100%
Aspirin at Discharge[1]	8	88%	90%	90%	100%
Beta Blocker at Arrival[1]	13	92%	85%	87%	100%
Beta Blocker at Discharge[1]	8	75%	86%	90%	100%
Fibrinolytic Medication Timing[1]	1	0%	30%	31%	100%
PCI Within 90 Minutes of Arrival	0	-	48%	54%	95%
Smoking Cessation Advice[1]	2	100%	90%	88%	100%
Heart Failure Care					
ACE Inhibitor or ARB for LVSD	50	64%	82%	82%	100%
Discharge Instructions	152	85%	60%	61%	93%
Evaluation of LVS Function	179	79%	81%	83%	99%
Smoking Cessation Advice	43	100%	82%	82%	100%
Pneumonia Care					
Appropriate Initial Antibiotic	167	89%	79%	83%	94%
Blood Culture Timing	63	94%	89%	90%	100%
Influenza Vaccine[4,5]	-	-	69%	70%	100%
Initial Antibiotic Timing	204	84%	78%	80%	93%
Oxygenation Assessment	226	97%	99%	99%	100%

Measure	Cases	This Hospital	State Average	U.S. Average	Top Hospital
Pneumococcal Vaccine	121	86%	68%	69%	94%
Smoking Cessation Advice	39	100%	83%	80%	100%
Surgical Infection Prevention					
Prophylactic Antibiotic Given	64	86%	67%	77%	95%
Prophylactic Antibiotic Selection[1]	14	93%	86%	90%	100%
Prophylactic Antibiotic Stopped	64	64%	68%	72%	95%
Pregnancy Care					
Inpatient Neonatal Mortality	345	0.00%	-	-	-
Third or Fourth Degree Laceration	168	1.19%	3.23%	3.63%	3.27%

Kingwood Medical Center

22999 US Highway 59
Kingwood, TX 77339
URL: www.kingwoodmedical.com
Ownership: Proprietary
Emergency Services: Yes
Key Personnel:
CEO . . . . Gay Nord

Phone: 281-348-8000
Fax: 281-348-8010

Accredited: Yes
Licensed Beds: 155

Measure	Cases	This Hospital	State Average	U.S. Average	Top Hospital
Heart Attack Care					
ACE Inhibitor or ARB for LVSD	27	100%	85%	82%	100%
Aspirin at Arrival	136	99%	91%	92%	100%
Aspirin at Discharge	83	99%	90%	90%	100%
Beta Blocker at Arrival	111	93%	85%	87%	100%
Beta Blocker at Discharge	83	99%	86%	90%	100%
Fibrinolytic Medication Timing[1]	20	60%	30%	31%	100%
PCI Within 90 Minutes of Arrival[1]	3	67%	48%	54%	95%
Smoking Cessation Advice	47	100%	90%	88%	100%
Heart Failure Care					
ACE Inhibitor or ARB for LVSD	96	90%	82%	82%	100%
Discharge Instructions	251	74%	60%	61%	93%
Evaluation of LVS Function	305	97%	81%	83%	99%
Smoking Cessation Advice	63	100%	82%	82%	100%
Pneumonia Care					
Appropriate Initial Antibiotic	181	90%	79%	83%	94%
Blood Culture Timing	158	84%	89%	90%	100%
Influenza Vaccine	61	90%	69%	70%	100%
Initial Antibiotic Timing	249	76%	78%	80%	93%
Oxygenation Assessment	300	98%	99%	99%	100%
Pneumococcal Vaccine	163	89%	68%	69%	94%
Smoking Cessation Advice	90	100%	83%	80%	100%
Surgical Infection Prevention					
Prophylactic Antibiotic Given[2,3]	70	49%	67%	77%	95%
Prophylactic Antibiotic Selection[1,2]	9	33%	86%	90%	100%
Prophylactic Antibiotic Stopped[2,3]	67	63%	68%	72%	95%
Pregnancy Care					
Inpatient Neonatal Mortality	-	-	-	-	-
Third or Fourth Degree Laceration	-	-	3.23%	3.63%	3.27%

Kingwood Specialty Hospital

300 Kingwood Medical Drive
Kingwood, TX 77339
Ownership: Proprietary
Emergency Services: No

Phone: 281-312-4000

Accredited: No

Measure	Cases	This Hospital	State Average	U.S. Average	Top Hospital
Heart Attack Care					
ACE Inhibitor or ARB for LVSD[5]	-	-	85%	82%	100%
Aspirin at Arrival[5]	-	-	91%	92%	100%
Aspirin at Discharge[5]	-	-	90%	90%	100%
Beta Blocker at Arrival[5]	-	-	85%	87%	100%
Beta Blocker at Discharge[5]	-	-	86%	90%	100%
Fibrinolytic Medication Timing[5]	-	-	30%	31%	100%
PCI Within 90 Minutes of Arrival[5]	-	-	48%	54%	95%
Smoking Cessation Advice[5]	-	-	90%	88%	100%
Heart Failure Care					
ACE Inhibitor or ARB for LVSD[5]	-	-	82%	82%	100%
Discharge Instructions[5]	-	-	60%	61%	93%
Evaluation of LVS Function[5]	-	-	81%	83%	99%
Smoking Cessation Advice[5]	-	-	82%	82%	100%
Pneumonia Care					

NOTE: Hospital profiles are in alphabetical order by state, then city, then hospital within the city; Rankings are sorted by rate in descending order and exclude hospitals with less than 25 cases; (1) The number of cases is too small (n<25) for purposes of reliably predicting hospital performance; (2) Measure reflects the hospital's indication that its submission was based upon a sample of its relevant discharges; (3) Rate reflects fewer than the maximum possible quarters of data for the measure; (4) Inaccurate information submitted and suppressed for one or more quarters; (5) No data is available from the hospital for this measure; Please refer to the User's Guide for a full explanation of data

Measure	Cases	This Hospital	State Average	U.S. Average	Top Hospital
Appropriate Initial Antibiotic[5]	-	-	79%	83%	94%
Blood Culture Timing[5]	-	-	89%	90%	100%
Influenza Vaccine[5]	-	-	69%	70%	100%
Initial Antibiotic Timing[5]	-	-	78%	80%	93%
Oxygenation Assessment[5]	-	-	99%	99%	100%
Pneumococcal Vaccine[5]	-	-	68%	69%	94%
Smoking Cessation Advice[5]	-	-	83%	80%	100%
Surgical Infection Prevention					
Prophylactic Antibiotic Given[1,2,3]	16	81%	67%	77%	95%
Prophylactic Antibiotic Selection[5]	-	-	86%	90%	100%
Prophylactic Antibiotic Stopped[1,2,3]	16	100%	68%	72%	95%
Pregnancy Care					
Inpatient Neonatal Mortality	-	-	-	-	-
Third or Fourth Degree Laceration	-	-	3.23%	3.63%	3.27%

Knox County Hospital

701 S 5th Street
PO Box 608
Knox City, TX 79529
E-mail: knoxhospital@srcaccess.net
URL: www.knoxcountytx.net
Ownership: Govt - Hospital District or Authority
Emergency Services: Yes

Phone: 940-657-3535
Fax: 940-657-3005

Accredited: No
Licensed Beds: 14

Key Personnel:
Administrator . . . . Stephan Kuehler
Chief Medical Staff. . . . . Shirley Barretto, MD
Emergency Room . . . . Dan Offutt
Director Infection/Disease Control . . . . Jan Rolston
Director Medical/Surgical Nursing . . . . Debbie Wilde, RN

Measure	Cases	This Hospital	State Average	U.S. Average	Top Hospital
Heart Attack Care					
ACE Inhibitor or ARB for LVSD[3]	0	-	85%	82%	100%
Aspirin at Arrival[1,3]	1	100%	91%	92%	100%
Aspirin at Discharge[1,3]	1	0%	90%	90%	100%
Beta Blocker at Arrival[1,3]	1	0%	85%	87%	100%
Beta Blocker at Discharge[1,3]	1	100%	86%	90%	100%
Fibrinolytic Medication Timing[5]	-	-	30%	31%	100%
PCI Within 90 Minutes of Arrival[5]	-	-	48%	54%	95%
Smoking Cessation Advice[5]	-	-	90%	88%	100%
Heart Failure Care					
ACE Inhibitor or ARB for LVSD[1,3]	2	50%	82%	82%	100%
Discharge Instructions[1,3]	1	100%	60%	61%	93%
Evaluation of LVS Function[1,3]	4	100%	81%	83%	99%
Smoking Cessation Advice[3]	0	-	82%	82%	100%
Pneumonia Care					
Appropriate Initial Antibiotic[1,3]	1	100%	79%	83%	94%
Blood Culture Timing[3]	0	-	89%	90%	100%
Influenza Vaccine[5]	-	-	69%	70%	100%
Initial Antibiotic Timing[1,3]	14	100%	78%	80%	93%
Oxygenation Assessment[1,3]	14	100%	99%	99%	100%
Pneumococcal Vaccine[1,3]	11	91%	68%	69%	94%
Smoking Cessation Advice[3]	0	-	83%	80%	100%
Surgical Infection Prevention					
Prophylactic Antibiotic Given[5]	-	-	67%	77%	95%
Prophylactic Antibiotic Selection[5]	-	-	86%	90%	100%
Prophylactic Antibiotic Stopped[5]	-	-	68%	72%	95%
Pregnancy Care					
Inpatient Neonatal Mortality	-	-	-	-	-
Third or Fourth Degree Laceration	-	-	3.23%	3.63%	3.27%

Saint Marks Medical Center

One Saint Mark's Place
La Grange, TX 78945
Ownership: Proprietary
Emergency Services: No

Phone: 979-242-2200

Accredited: No

Measure	Cases	This Hospital	State Average	U.S. Average	Top Hospital
Heart Attack Care					
ACE Inhibitor or ARB for LVSD[1]	2	50%	85%	82%	100%
Aspirin at Arrival[1]	7	86%	91%	92%	100%
Aspirin at Discharge[1]	5	100%	90%	90%	100%

Measure	Cases	This Hospital	State Average	U.S. Average	Top Hospital
Beta Blocker at Arrival[1]	10	70%	85%	87%	100%
Beta Blocker at Discharge[1]	6	83%	86%	90%	100%
Fibrinolytic Medication Timing[3]	0	-	30%	31%	100%
PCI Within 90 Minutes of Arrival	0	-	48%	54%	95%
Smoking Cessation Advice[3]	0	-	90%	88%	100%
Heart Failure Care					
ACE Inhibitor or ARB for LVSD[1]	17	94%	82%	82%	100%
Discharge Instructions[1,3]	12	42%	60%	61%	93%
Evaluation of LVS Function	77	65%	81%	83%	99%
Smoking Cessation Advice[1,3]	6	17%	82%	82%	100%
Pneumonia Care					
Appropriate Initial Antibiotic[1,3]	9	78%	79%	83%	94%
Blood Culture Timing[1,3]	18	94%	89%	90%	100%
Influenza Vaccine[5]	-	-	69%	70%	100%
Initial Antibiotic Timing	105	74%	78%	80%	93%
Oxygenation Assessment	118	98%	99%	99%	100%
Pneumococcal Vaccine	94	35%	68%	69%	94%
Smoking Cessation Advice[3]	0	-	83%	80%	100%
Surgical Infection Prevention					
Prophylactic Antibiotic Given[1,3]	9	33%	67%	77%	95%
Prophylactic Antibiotic Selection[5]	-	-	86%	90%	100%
Prophylactic Antibiotic Stopped[1,3]	8	25%	68%	72%	95%
Pregnancy Care					
Inpatient Neonatal Mortality	-	-	-	-	-
Third or Fourth Degree Laceration	-	-	3.23%	3.63%	3.27%

Brazosport Memorial Hospital

100 Medical Drive
Lake Jackson, TX 77566
URL: www.brazosportmemorial.com
Ownership: Voluntary non-profit - Private
Emergency Services: Yes

Phone: 979-297-4411
Fax: 979-299-2861

Accredited: Yes
Licensed Beds: 165

Key Personnel:
CEO. . . . . Daniel L Buche
Chief Medical Staff. . . . . LP Bui, MD
Emergency Room . . . . E Tow, DO
Infection Control Nurse. . . . . Kathy Jordan
CCU Spvg. Nurse . . . . Tina Mathews
Director Medical/Surgical Nursing . . . . Mary Gotcher
Chief Radiology . . . . J Fuchs, MD
Director Respiratory Therapy . . . . Ron Adams

Measure	Cases	This Hospital	State Average	U.S. Average	Top Hospital
Heart Attack Care					
ACE Inhibitor or ARB for LVSD[1]	4	50%	85%	82%	100%
Aspirin at Arrival	48	98%	91%	92%	100%
Aspirin at Discharge[1]	16	88%	90%	90%	100%
Beta Blocker at Arrival	51	86%	85%	87%	100%
Beta Blocker at Discharge[1]	22	82%	86%	90%	100%
Fibrinolytic Medication Timing[1]	15	73%	30%	31%	100%
PCI Within 90 Minutes of Arrival	0	-	48%	54%	95%
Smoking Cessation Advice[1]	2	50%	90%	88%	100%
Heart Failure Care					
ACE Inhibitor or ARB for LVSD	57	58%	82%	82%	100%
Discharge Instructions	117	74%	60%	61%	93%
Evaluation of LVS Function	142	97%	81%	83%	99%
Smoking Cessation Advice	28	54%	82%	82%	100%
Pneumonia Care					
Appropriate Initial Antibiotic	121	71%	79%	83%	94%
Blood Culture Timing	94	84%	89%	90%	100%
Influenza Vaccine	34	74%	69%	70%	100%
Initial Antibiotic Timing	160	83%	78%	80%	93%
Oxygenation Assessment	192	98%	99%	99%	100%
Pneumococcal Vaccine	111	83%	68%	69%	94%
Smoking Cessation Advice	44	73%	83%	80%	100%
Surgical Infection Prevention					
Prophylactic Antibiotic Given[3]	91	68%	67%	77%	95%
Prophylactic Antibiotic Selection	33	91%	86%	90%	100%
Prophylactic Antibiotic Stopped[3]	92	49%	68%	72%	95%
Pregnancy Care					
Inpatient Neonatal Mortality	-	-	-	-	-
Third or Fourth Degree Laceration	-	-	3.23%	3.63%	3.27%

NOTE: Hospital profiles are in alphabetical order by state, then city, then hospital within the city; Rankings are sorted by rate in descending order and exclude hospitals with less than 25 cases; (1) The number of cases is too small (n<25) for purposes of reliably predicting hospital performance; (2) Measure reflects the hospital's indication that its submission was based upon a sample of its relevant discharges; (3) Rate reflects fewer than the maximum possible quarters of data for the measure; (4) Inaccurate information submitted and suppressed for one or more quarters; (5) No data is available from the hospital for this measure; Please refer to the User's Guide for a full explanation of data

Medical Arts Hospital

1600 N Bryan Avenue
Lamesa, TX 79331
URL: www.medicalartshospital.org
Ownership: Government - Local
Emergency Services: Yes

Phone: 806-872-2183
Fax: 806-872-0823

Accredited: No
Licensed Beds: 44

Key Personnel:
CEO. . . . . Charles Butts
Chief Medical Staff. . . . . Dr Griengsak Chowpaknam
Manager ER. . . . . Jeana Amos
Manager/Infection Control . . . . Rebekah Parker
Manager/Surgical Services . . . . Rebekah Parker
CEO/Administrator. . . . . Charles N Butts

Measure	Cases	This Hospital	State Average	U.S. Average	Top Hospital
Heart Attack Care					
ACE Inhibitor or ARB for LVSD	0	-	85%	82%	100%
Aspirin at Arrival[1]	5	100%	91%	92%	100%
Aspirin at Discharge[1]	3	67%	90%	90%	100%
Beta Blocker at Arrival[1]	6	67%	85%	87%	100%
Beta Blocker at Discharge[1]	4	50%	86%	90%	100%
Fibrinolytic Medication Timing[3]	0	-	30%	31%	100%
PCI Within 90 Minutes of Arrival	0	-	48%	54%	95%
Smoking Cessation Advice[3]	0	-	90%	88%	100%
Heart Failure Care					
ACE Inhibitor or ARB for LVSD[1]	13	92%	82%	82%	100%
Discharge Instructions[1,3]	5	80%	60%	61%	93%
Evaluation of LVS Function	51	84%	81%	83%	99%
Smoking Cessation Advice[3]	0	-	82%	82%	100%
Pneumonia Care					
Appropriate Initial Antibiotic[1,3]	9	78%	79%	83%	94%
Blood Culture Timing[1,3]	4	75%	89%	90%	100%
Influenza Vaccine[5]	-	-	69%	70%	100%
Initial Antibiotic Timing	58	72%	78%	80%	93%
Oxygenation Assessment	69	100%	99%	99%	100%
Pneumococcal Vaccine	39	87%	68%	69%	94%
Smoking Cessation Advice[1,3]	2	100%	83%	80%	100%
Surgical Infection Prevention					
Prophylactic Antibiotic Given[5]	-	-	67%	77%	95%
Prophylactic Antibiotic Selection[5]	-	-	86%	90%	100%
Prophylactic Antibiotic Stopped[5]	-	-	68%	72%	95%
Pregnancy Care					
Inpatient Neonatal Mortality	-	-	-	-	-
Third or Fourth Degree Laceration	-	-	3.23%	3.63%	3.27%

Rollins Brook Community Hospital

608 N Key Avenue
Lampasas, TX 76550
Ownership: Voluntary non-profit - Church
Emergency Services: Yes

Phone: 512-556-3682
Fax: 512-556-8869
Accredited: Yes
Licensed Beds: 36

Key Personnel:
Administrator . . . . Larry Luce
Chief Radiology . . . . Lynn Bandas

Measure	Cases	This Hospital	State Average	U.S. Average	Top Hospital
Heart Attack Care					
ACE Inhibitor or ARB for LVSD	0	-	85%	82%	100%
Aspirin at Arrival[1]	3	100%	91%	92%	100%
Aspirin at Discharge[1]	3	100%	90%	90%	100%
Beta Blocker at Arrival[1]	2	100%	85%	87%	100%
Beta Blocker at Discharge[1]	2	100%	86%	90%	100%
Fibrinolytic Medication Timing	0	-	30%	31%	100%
PCI Within 90 Minutes of Arrival	0	-	48%	54%	95%
Smoking Cessation Advice	0	-	90%	88%	100%
Heart Failure Care					
ACE Inhibitor or ARB for LVSD[1]	5	80%	82%	82%	100%
Discharge Instructions	30	57%	60%	61%	93%
Evaluation of LVS Function	55	25%	81%	83%	99%
Smoking Cessation Advice[1]	2	0%	82%	82%	100%
Pneumonia Care					
Appropriate Initial Antibiotic	35	69%	79%	83%	94%
Blood Culture Timing[1]	18	100%	89%	90%	100%
Influenza Vaccine[1]	15	47%	69%	70%	100%

Medical Center at Lancaster

Alternate Name: Midway Park Medical Center
2600 W Pleasant Run Road
Lancaster, TX 75146
E-mail: laura.bogert@columbia.net
URL: www.mclancaster.com
Ownership: Proprietary
Emergency Services: Yes

Phone: 972-223-9600
Fax: 972-230-2966

Accredited: Yes
Licensed Beds: 90

Key Personnel:
CEO. . . . . Barry L Mousa

Measure	Cases	This Hospital	State Average	U.S. Average	Top Hospital
Heart Attack Care					
ACE Inhibitor or ARB for LVSD[1]	6	67%	85%	82%	100%
Aspirin at Arrival	41	90%	91%	92%	100%
Aspirin at Discharge[1]	20	85%	90%	90%	100%
Beta Blocker at Arrival	28	89%	85%	87%	100%
Beta Blocker at Discharge[1]	20	85%	86%	90%	100%
Fibrinolytic Medication Timing[1,3]	2	100%	30%	31%	100%
PCI Within 90 Minutes of Arrival	0	-	48%	54%	95%
Smoking Cessation Advice[1,3]	1	100%	90%	88%	100%
Heart Failure Care					
ACE Inhibitor or ARB for LVSD	57	65%	82%	82%	100%
Discharge Instructions[1,3]	12	0%	60%	61%	93%
Evaluation of LVS Function	176	73%	81%	83%	99%
Smoking Cessation Advice[1,3]	3	100%	82%	82%	100%
Pneumonia Care					
Appropriate Initial Antibiotic[1,3]	2	0%	79%	83%	94%
Blood Culture Timing[1,3]	8	100%	89%	90%	100%
Influenza Vaccine[5]	-	-	69%	70%	100%
Initial Antibiotic Timing	49	49%	78%	80%	93%
Oxygenation Assessment	75	100%	99%	99%	100%
Pneumococcal Vaccine	28	11%	68%	69%	94%
Smoking Cessation Advice[1,3]	3	100%	83%	80%	100%
Surgical Infection Prevention					
Prophylactic Antibiotic Given[1,3]	6	50%	67%	77%	95%
Prophylactic Antibiotic Selection[5]	-	-	86%	90%	100%
Prophylactic Antibiotic Stopped[1,3]	5	80%	68%	72%	95%
Pregnancy Care					
Inpatient Neonatal Mortality	-	-	-	-	-
Third or Fourth Degree Laceration	-	-	3.23%	3.63%	3.27%

Doctors Hospital of Laredo

10700 Mcpherson Road
Laredo, TX 78041
Ownership: Proprietary
Emergency Services: Yes

Phone: 956-523-2000

Accredited: Yes

Measure	Cases	This Hospital	State Average	U.S. Average	Top Hospital
Heart Attack Care					
ACE Inhibitor or ARB for LVSD[1]	9	100%	85%	82%	100%
Aspirin at Arrival	48	96%	91%	92%	100%
Aspirin at Discharge	29	90%	90%	90%	100%
Beta Blocker at Arrival	43	93%	85%	87%	100%
Beta Blocker at Discharge	28	86%	86%	90%	100%
Fibrinolytic Medication Timing[1]	10	50%	30%	31%	100%
PCI Within 90 Minutes of Arrival	0	-	48%	54%	95%
Smoking Cessation Advice[1]	9	89%	90%	88%	100%
Heart Failure Care					
ACE Inhibitor or ARB for LVSD	62	84%	82%	82%	100%

NOTE: Hospital profiles are in alphabetical order by state, then city, then hospital within the city; Rankings are sorted by rate in descending order and exclude hospitals with less than 25 cases; (1) The number of cases is too small (n<25) for purposes of reliably predicting hospital performance; (2) Measure reflects the hospital's indication that its submission was based upon a sample of its relevant discharges; (3) Rate reflects fewer than the maximum possible quarters of data for the measure; (4) Inaccurate information submitted and suppressed for one or more quarters; (5) No data is available from the hospital for this measure; Please refer to the User's Guide for a full explanation of data

Discharge Instructions	200	37%	60%	61%	93%
Evaluation of LVS Function	226	73%	81%	83%	99%
Smoking Cessation Advice	30	77%	82%	82%	100%
Pneumonia Care					
Appropriate Initial Antibiotic	64	75%	79%	83%	94%
Blood Culture Timing	67	64%	89%	90%	100%
Influenza Vaccine[1]	22	55%	69%	70%	100%
Initial Antibiotic Timing	121	65%	78%	80%	93%
Oxygenation Assessment	127	100%	99%	99%	100%
Pneumococcal Vaccine	78	51%	68%	69%	94%
Smoking Cessation Advice[1]	12	92%	83%	80%	100%
Surgical Infection Prevention					
Prophylactic Antibiotic Given	184	43%	67%	77%	95%
Prophylactic Antibiotic Selection	36	92%	86%	90%	100%
Prophylactic Antibiotic Stopped	166	67%	68%	72%	95%
Pregnancy Care					
Inpatient Neonatal Mortality	-	-	-	-	-
Third or Fourth Degree Laceration	-	-	3.23%	3.63%	3.27%

Laredo Medical Center

1700 E Saunders
Laredo, TX 78041
URL: www.mercylaredo.com
Ownership: Voluntary non-profit - Church
Emergency Services: Yes

Phone: 956-796-5000
Fax: 956-796-3221

Accredited: Yes
Licensed Beds: 325

Key Personnel:
President/CEO . . . . Abe Martinez
Associate CEO . . . . John Gallagher
OB/GYN Womens Health . . . . Doi Mariana
Chief Radiology . . . . Guillermo Salinas, MD
Director Respiratory Therapy . . . . Robert Gonzalez

Measure	Cases	This Hospital	State Average	U.S. Average	Top Hospital
Heart Attack Care					
ACE Inhibitor or ARB for LVSD	27	67%	85%	82%	100%
Aspirin at Arrival	146	90%	91%	92%	100%
Aspirin at Discharge	136	87%	90%	90%	100%
Beta Blocker at Arrival	57	72%	85%	87%	100%
Beta Blocker at Discharge	123	72%	86%	90%	100%
Fibrinolytic Medication Timing[1]	14	7%	30%	31%	100%
PCI Within 90 Minutes of Arrival[1]	6	33%	48%	54%	95%
Smoking Cessation Advice	51	67%	90%	88%	100%
Heart Failure Care					
ACE Inhibitor or ARB for LVSD[2]	113	58%	82%	82%	100%
Discharge Instructions[2]	265	51%	60%	61%	93%
Evaluation of LVS Function[2]	292	91%	81%	83%	99%
Smoking Cessation Advice[2]	33	76%	82%	82%	100%
Pneumonia Care					
Appropriate Initial Antibiotic[2]	111	75%	79%	83%	94%
Blood Culture Timing[2]	84	74%	89%	90%	100%
Influenza Vaccine[2]	27	52%	69%	70%	100%
Initial Antibiotic Timing[2]	140	72%	78%	80%	93%
Oxygenation Assessment[2]	154	100%	99%	99%	100%
Pneumococcal Vaccine[2]	88	49%	68%	69%	94%
Smoking Cessation Advice[1,2]	22	86%	83%	80%	100%
Surgical Infection Prevention					
Prophylactic Antibiotic Given[2,3]	384	58%	67%	77%	95%
Prophylactic Antibiotic Selection[2]	102	84%	86%	90%	100%
Prophylactic Antibiotic Stopped[2,3]	367	34%	68%	72%	95%
Pregnancy Care					
Inpatient Neonatal Mortality	-	-	-	-	-
Third or Fourth Degree Laceration	-	-	3.23%	3.63%	3.27%

Providence Hospital

230 Calle Del Norte
Laredo, TX 78041
Ownership: Proprietary
Emergency Services: Yes

Phone: 956-693-5000

Accredited: Yes

Measure	Cases	This Hospital	State Average	U.S. Average	Top Hospital
Heart Attack Care					
ACE Inhibitor or ARB for LVSD[5]	-	-	85%	82%	100%

Aspirin at Arrival[5]	-	-	91%	92%	100%
Aspirin at Discharge[5]	-	-	90%	90%	100%
Beta Blocker at Arrival[5]	-	-	85%	87%	100%
Beta Blocker at Discharge[5]	-	-	86%	90%	100%
Fibrinolytic Medication Timing[5]	-	-	30%	31%	100%
PCI Within 90 Minutes of Arrival[5]	-	-	48%	54%	95%
Smoking Cessation Advice[5]	-	-	90%	88%	100%
Heart Failure Care					
ACE Inhibitor or ARB for LVSD[5]	-	-	82%	82%	100%
Discharge Instructions[5]	-	-	60%	61%	93%
Evaluation of LVS Function[5]	-	-	81%	83%	99%
Smoking Cessation Advice[5]	-	-	82%	82%	100%
Pneumonia Care					
Appropriate Initial Antibiotic[1,3]	2	0%	79%	83%	94%
Blood Culture Timing[3]	0	-	89%	90%	100%
Influenza Vaccine[5]	-	-	69%	70%	100%
Initial Antibiotic Timing[1,3]	4	100%	78%	80%	93%
Oxygenation Assessment[1,3]	4	100%	99%	99%	100%
Pneumococcal Vaccine[1,3]	2	0%	68%	69%	94%
Smoking Cessation Advice[1,3]	2	0%	83%	80%	100%
Surgical Infection Prevention					
Prophylactic Antibiotic Given[1,3]	21	100%	67%	77%	95%
Prophylactic Antibiotic Selection[5]	-	-	86%	90%	100%
Prophylactic Antibiotic Stopped[1,3]	22	68%	68%	72%	95%
Pregnancy Care					
Inpatient Neonatal Mortality	-	-	-	-	-
Third or Fourth Degree Laceration	-	-	3.23%	3.63%	3.27%

Covenant Hospital Levelland

Alternate Name: Methodist Hospital Levelland
1900 College Avenue
Levelland, TX 79336
Ownership: Voluntary non-profit - Other
Emergency Services: Yes

Phone: 806-894-4963
Fax: 806-894-6461
Accredited: No
Licensed Beds: 78

Key Personnel:
Administrator . . . . Jerry Osburn
Chief Medical Staff . . . . Micheal Bailey
Emergency Room . . . . Harry Weaver
Director Infection/Disease Control . . . . Karen Seely
OB/GYN Womens Health . . . . Micheal Bailey, MD
Director Respiratory Therapy . . . . Vicky Bautista

Measure	Cases	This Hospital	State Average	U.S. Average	Top Hospital
Heart Attack Care					
ACE Inhibitor or ARB for LVSD[3]	0	-	85%	82%	100%
Aspirin at Arrival[1,3]	2	50%	91%	92%	100%
Aspirin at Discharge[3]	0	-	90%	90%	100%
Beta Blocker at Arrival[1,3]	3	0%	85%	87%	100%
Beta Blocker at Discharge[1,3]	1	0%	86%	90%	100%
Fibrinolytic Medication Timing[5]	-	-	30%	31%	100%
PCI Within 90 Minutes of Arrival[5]	-	-	48%	54%	95%
Smoking Cessation Advice[5]	-	-	90%	88%	100%
Heart Failure Care					
ACE Inhibitor or ARB for LVSD[1,3]	1	100%	82%	82%	100%
Discharge Instructions[1,3]	7	0%	60%	61%	93%
Evaluation of LVS Function[3]	25	4%	81%	83%	99%
Smoking Cessation Advice[1,3]	1	0%	82%	82%	100%
Pneumonia Care					
Appropriate Initial Antibiotic[1,3]	10	90%	79%	83%	94%
Blood Culture Timing[1,3]	1	100%	89%	90%	100%
Influenza Vaccine[5]	-	-	69%	70%	100%
Initial Antibiotic Timing	30	90%	78%	80%	93%
Oxygenation Assessment	43	95%	99%	99%	100%
Pneumococcal Vaccine[1]	21	24%	68%	69%	94%
Smoking Cessation Advice[1,3]	4	0%	83%	80%	100%
Surgical Infection Prevention					
Prophylactic Antibiotic Given[1,3]	6	17%	67%	77%	95%
Prophylactic Antibiotic Selection[5]	-	-	86%	90%	100%
Prophylactic Antibiotic Stopped[1,3]	1	100%	68%	72%	95%
Pregnancy Care					
Inpatient Neonatal Mortality	-	-	-	-	-
Third or Fourth Degree Laceration	-	-	3.23%	3.63%	3.27%

NOTE: Hospital profiles are in alphabetical order by state, then city, then hospital within the city; Rankings are sorted by rate in descending order and exclude hospitals with less than 25 cases; (1) The number of cases is too small (n<25) for purposes of reliably predicting hospital performance; (2) Measure reflects the hospital's indication that its submission was based upon a sample of its relevant discharges; (3) Rate reflects fewer than the maximum possible quarters of data for the measure; (4) Inaccurate information submitted and suppressed for one or more quarters; (5) No data is available from the hospital for this measure; Please refer to the User's Guide for a full explanation of data

Medical Center of Lewisville

Alternate Name: Lewisville Memorial Hospital
500 W Main Street
Lewisville, TX 75057
URL: www.lewisvillemedical.com
Ownership: Proprietary
Emergency Services: Yes
Phone: 972-420-1000
Fax: 972-420-1805

Accredited: Yes
Licensed Beds: 202

Key Personnel:
President/CEO . . . . Douglas Welch
Chief Medical Staff . . . . Barry Sanders
Director Infection/Disease Control . . . . P White
Director Medical/Surgical Nursing . . . . Cathy Riney, RN
OB/GYN Womens Health. . . . . Rebecca Collins
Chief Radiology . . . . Thomas Knight

Measure	Cases	This Hospital	State Average	U.S. Average	Top Hospital
Heart Attack Care					
ACE Inhibitor or ARB for LVSD[1]	5	60%	85%	82%	100%
Aspirin at Arrival	60	97%	91%	92%	100%
Aspirin at Discharge[1]	20	75%	90%	90%	100%
Beta Blocker at Arrival	52	92%	85%	87%	100%
Beta Blocker at Discharge[1]	19	84%	86%	90%	100%
Fibrinolytic Medication Timing	0	-	30%	31%	100%
PCI Within 90 Minutes of Arrival	0	-	48%	54%	95%
Smoking Cessation Advice[1]	2	100%	90%	88%	100%
Heart Failure Care					
ACE Inhibitor or ARB for LVSD	69	83%	82%	82%	100%
Discharge Instructions	203	53%	60%	61%	93%
Evaluation of LVS Function	223	96%	81%	83%	99%
Smoking Cessation Advice	42	86%	82%	82%	100%
Pneumonia Care					
Appropriate Initial Antibiotic	118	82%	79%	83%	94%
Blood Culture Timing	98	80%	89%	90%	100%
Influenza Vaccine	51	63%	69%	70%	100%
Initial Antibiotic Timing	192	64%	78%	80%	93%
Oxygenation Assessment	218	97%	99%	99%	100%
Pneumococcal Vaccine	122	58%	68%	69%	94%
Smoking Cessation Advice	52	85%	83%	80%	100%
Surgical Infection Prevention					
Prophylactic Antibiotic Given[2,3]	135	53%	67%	77%	95%
Prophylactic Antibiotic Selection[2]	63	81%	86%	90%	100%
Prophylactic Antibiotic Stopped[2,3]	135	58%	68%	72%	95%
Pregnancy Care					
Inpatient Neonatal Mortality	-	-	-	-	-
Third or Fourth Degree Laceration	-	-	3.23%	3.63%	3.27%

Good Shephard Medical Center-Linden

404 North Kaufman Street
Linden, TX 75563
Ownership: Govt - Hospital District or Authority
Emergency Services: Yes
Phone: 903-756-5561

Accredited: No

Measure	Cases	This Hospital	State Average	U.S. Average	Top Hospital
Heart Attack Care					
ACE Inhibitor or ARB for LVSD[1,3]	1	0%	85%	82%	100%
Aspirin at Arrival[1,3]	2	100%	91%	92%	100%
Aspirin at Discharge[1,3]	2	100%	90%	90%	100%
Beta Blocker at Arrival[1,3]	2	50%	85%	87%	100%
Beta Blocker at Discharge[1,3]	3	33%	86%	90%	100%
Fibrinolytic Medication Timing[3]	0	-	30%	31%	100%
PCI Within 90 Minutes of Arrival	0	-	48%	54%	95%
Smoking Cessation Advice[3]	0	-	90%	88%	100%
Heart Failure Care					
ACE Inhibitor or ARB for LVSD[1,3]	1	100%	82%	82%	100%
Discharge Instructions[1,3]	23	0%	60%	61%	93%
Evaluation of LVS Function[3]	28	21%	81%	83%	99%
Smoking Cessation Advice[1,3]	7	29%	82%	82%	100%
Pneumonia Care					
Appropriate Initial Antibiotic[1,3]	7	100%	79%	83%	94%
Blood Culture Timing[3]	0	-	89%	90%	100%
Influenza Vaccine[5]	-	-	69%	70%	100%
Initial Antibiotic Timing[1,3]	10	90%	78%	80%	93%

Measure	Cases	This Hospital	State Average	U.S. Average	Top Hospital
Oxygenation Assessment[1,3]	13	100%	99%	99%	100%
Pneumococcal Vaccine[1,3]	6	0%	68%	69%	94%
Smoking Cessation Advice[1,3]	2	0%	83%	80%	100%
Surgical Infection Prevention					
Prophylactic Antibiotic Given[1,3]	2	50%	67%	77%	95%
Prophylactic Antibiotic Selection	0	-	86%	90%	100%
Prophylactic Antibiotic Stopped[1,3]	1	100%	68%	72%	95%
Pregnancy Care					
Inpatient Neonatal Mortality	-	-	-	-	-
Third or Fourth Degree Laceration	-	-	3.23%	3.63%	3.27%

Lamb Healthcare Center

1500 S Sunset
Littlefield, TX 79339
Ownership: Voluntary non-profit - Other
Emergency Services: Yes
Phone: 806-385-6411
Fax: 806-385-3998
Accredited: No
Licensed Beds: 75

Key Personnel:
Chief Medical Staff . . . . Toni Hedges, MD
Emergency Room . . . . Enricke Rodriguez, MD

Measure	Cases	This Hospital	State Average	U.S. Average	Top Hospital
Heart Attack Care					
ACE Inhibitor or ARB for LVSD[3]	0	-	85%	82%	100%
Aspirin at Arrival[3]	0	-	91%	92%	100%
Aspirin at Discharge[3]	0	-	90%	90%	100%
Beta Blocker at Arrival[3]	0	-	85%	87%	100%
Beta Blocker at Discharge[3]	0	-	86%	90%	100%
Fibrinolytic Medication Timing[3]	0	-	30%	31%	100%
PCI Within 90 Minutes of Arrival	0	-	48%	54%	95%
Smoking Cessation Advice[3]	0	-	90%	88%	100%
Heart Failure Care					
ACE Inhibitor or ARB for LVSD[1]	4	25%	82%	82%	100%
Discharge Instructions[1]	21	19%	60%	61%	93%
Evaluation of LVS Function	37	35%	81%	83%	99%
Smoking Cessation Advice[1]	6	100%	82%	82%	100%
Pneumonia Care					
Appropriate Initial Antibiotic	38	42%	79%	83%	94%
Blood Culture Timing[1]	4	100%	89%	90%	100%
Influenza Vaccine[4,5]	-	-	69%	70%	100%
Initial Antibiotic Timing	44	82%	78%	80%	93%
Oxygenation Assessment	64	98%	99%	99%	100%
Pneumococcal Vaccine	44	25%	68%	69%	94%
Smoking Cessation Advice[1]	9	100%	83%	80%	100%
Surgical Infection Prevention					
Prophylactic Antibiotic Given[1,3]	4	25%	67%	77%	95%
Prophylactic Antibiotic Selection	0	-	86%	90%	100%
Prophylactic Antibiotic Stopped[1,3]	4	75%	68%	72%	95%
Pregnancy Care					
Inpatient Neonatal Mortality	-	-	-	-	-
Third or Fourth Degree Laceration	-	-	3.23%	3.63%	3.27%

Memorial Medical Center Livingston

Alternate Name: Polk County Memorial Hospital
602 E Church
Livingston, TX 77351
E-mail: sfranklin@memorialhealth.com
Ownership: Government - Local
Emergency Services: Yes
Phone: 936-327-4381
Fax: 936-329-8730

Accredited: Yes
Licensed Beds: 41

Measure	Cases	This Hospital	State Average	U.S. Average	Top Hospital
Heart Attack Care					
ACE Inhibitor or ARB for LVSD	0	-	85%	82%	100%
Aspirin at Arrival[1]	7	57%	91%	92%	100%
Aspirin at Discharge[1]	3	33%	90%	90%	100%
Beta Blocker at Arrival[1]	7	71%	85%	87%	100%
Beta Blocker at Discharge[1]	4	50%	86%	90%	100%
Fibrinolytic Medication Timing[3]	0	-	30%	31%	100%
PCI Within 90 Minutes of Arrival	0	-	48%	54%	95%
Smoking Cessation Advice[1,3]	2	100%	90%	88%	100%
Heart Failure Care					
ACE Inhibitor or ARB for LVSD	46	65%	82%	82%	100%
Discharge Instructions[1,3]	24	88%	60%	61%	93%

NOTE: Hospital profiles are in alphabetical order by state, then city, then hospital within the city; Rankings are sorted by rate in descending order and exclude hospitals with less than 25 cases; (1) The number of cases is too small (n<25) for purposes of reliably predicting hospital performance; (2) Measure reflects the hospital's indication that its submission was based upon a sample of its relevant discharges; (3) Rate reflects fewer than the maximum possible quarters of data for the measure; (4) Inaccurate information submitted and suppressed for one or more quarters; (5) No data is available from the hospital for this measure; Please refer to the User's Guide for a full explanation of data

Evaluation of LVS Function	107	77%	81%	83%	99%
Smoking Cessation Advice[1,3]	11	100%	82%	82%	100%
Pneumonia Care					
Appropriate Initial Antibiotic[1,3]	7	86%	79%	83%	94%
Blood Culture Timing[1,3]	6	100%	89%	90%	100%
Influenza Vaccine[5]	-	-	69%	70%	100%
Initial Antibiotic Timing	86	71%	78%	80%	93%
Oxygenation Assessment	87	95%	99%	99%	100%
Pneumococcal Vaccine	49	43%	68%	69%	94%
Smoking Cessation Advice[1,3]	7	100%	83%	80%	100%
Surgical Infection Prevention					
Prophylactic Antibiotic Given[3]	30	77%	67%	77%	95%
Prophylactic Antibiotic Selection[5]	-	-	86%	90%	100%
Prophylactic Antibiotic Stopped[3]	30	33%	68%	72%	95%
Pregnancy Care					
Inpatient Neonatal Mortality	287	0.70%	-	-	-
Third or Fourth Degree Laceration	188	0.53%	3.23%	3.63%	3.27%

Llano Memorial Hospital

200 W Ollie Street
Llano, TX 78643
Ownership: Govt - Hospital District or Authority
Emergency Services: Yes

Phone: 325-247-5040
Fax: 325-248-2108
Accredited: No
Licensed Beds: 30

Key Personnel:
CEO . . . . Ernie Parisi
Chief Medical Staff . . . . Tiffany Gainer
Director Medical/Surgical Nursing . . . . Terri Martin
Chief Radiology . . . . DD Stiles
Director Respiratory Therapy . . . . Clay Wagner

Measure	Cases	This Hospital	State Average	U.S. Average	Top Hospital
Heart Attack Care					
ACE Inhibitor or ARB for LVSD	0	-	85%	82%	100%
Aspirin at Arrival[1]	1	100%	91%	92%	100%
Aspirin at Discharge[1]	4	100%	90%	90%	100%
Beta Blocker at Arrival[1]	3	33%	85%	87%	100%
Beta Blocker at Discharge[1]	5	80%	86%	90%	100%
Fibrinolytic Medication Timing	0	-	30%	31%	100%
PCI Within 90 Minutes of Arrival	0	-	48%	54%	95%
Smoking Cessation Advice	0	-	90%	88%	100%
Heart Failure Care					
ACE Inhibitor or ARB for LVSD[1]	6	83%	82%	82%	100%
Discharge Instructions[1]	23	78%	60%	61%	93%
Evaluation of LVS Function	40	88%	81%	83%	99%
Smoking Cessation Advice[1]	5	100%	82%	82%	100%
Pneumonia Care					
Appropriate Initial Antibiotic[2]	66	95%	79%	83%	94%
Blood Culture Timing[2]	81	85%	89%	90%	100%
Influenza Vaccine	37	100%	69%	70%	100%
Initial Antibiotic Timing[2]	133	86%	78%	80%	93%
Oxygenation Assessment[2]	152	100%	99%	99%	100%
Pneumococcal Vaccine[2]	107	95%	68%	69%	94%
Smoking Cessation Advice[2]	27	85%	83%	80%	100%
Surgical Infection Prevention					
Prophylactic Antibiotic Given[1,2]	6	33%	67%	77%	95%
Prophylactic Antibiotic Selection[1,2]	2	100%	86%	90%	100%
Prophylactic Antibiotic Stopped[1,2]	6	83%	68%	72%	95%
Pregnancy Care					
Inpatient Neonatal Mortality	-	-	-	-	-
Third or Fourth Degree Laceration	-	-	3.23%	3.63%	3.27%

W J Mangold Memorial Hospital

Alternate Name: Lockney General Hospital
320 N Main Street
PO Box 37
Lockney, TX 79241
E-mail: mallen@mangold.lockney.isd.tenet.edu
URL: www.mangoldmemorial.org
Ownership: Govt - Hospital District or Authority
Emergency Services: Yes

Phone: 806-652-3373
Fax: 806-652-2172

Accredited: No
Licensed Beds: 27

Key Personnel:
Administrator . . . . Sharon Hunt
Chief Medical Staff . . . . Gary B Mangold, MD

Director Infection/Disease Control . . . . Trina Wilson, RN
OB/GYN Womens Health . . . . Gary B Mangold, MD
Director Respiratory Therapy . . . . Dimple Adams

Measure	Cases	This Hospital	State Average	U.S. Average	Top Hospital
Heart Attack Care					
ACE Inhibitor or ARB for LVSD[5]	-	-	85%	82%	100%
Aspirin at Arrival[5]	-	-	91%	92%	100%
Aspirin at Discharge[5]	-	-	90%	90%	100%
Beta Blocker at Arrival[5]	-	-	85%	87%	100%
Beta Blocker at Discharge[5]	-	-	86%	90%	100%
Fibrinolytic Medication Timing[5]	-	-	30%	31%	100%
PCI Within 90 Minutes of Arrival[5]	-	-	48%	54%	95%
Smoking Cessation Advice[5]	-	-	90%	88%	100%
Heart Failure Care					
ACE Inhibitor or ARB for LVSD[5]	-	-	82%	82%	100%
Discharge Instructions[5]	-	-	60%	61%	93%
Evaluation of LVS Function[5]	-	-	81%	83%	99%
Smoking Cessation Advice[5]	-	-	82%	82%	100%
Pneumonia Care					
Appropriate Initial Antibiotic[1,3]	3	100%	79%	83%	94%
Blood Culture Timing	28	100%	89%	90%	100%
Influenza Vaccine[1]	14	71%	69%	70%	100%
Initial Antibiotic Timing[3]	31	97%	78%	80%	93%
Oxygenation Assessment[3]	57	100%	99%	99%	100%
Pneumococcal Vaccine[3]	36	83%	68%	69%	94%
Smoking Cessation Advice[1,3]	11	91%	83%	80%	100%
Surgical Infection Prevention					
Prophylactic Antibiotic Given[5]	-	-	67%	77%	95%
Prophylactic Antibiotic Selection[5]	-	-	86%	90%	100%
Prophylactic Antibiotic Stopped[5]	-	-	68%	72%	95%
Pregnancy Care					
Inpatient Neonatal Mortality	-	-	-	-	-
Third or Fourth Degree Laceration	-	-	3.23%	3.63%	3.27%

Good Shepherd Medical Center

700 E Marshall Avenue
Longview, TX 75601
E-mail: webmaster@gsmc.org
URL: www.GoodShepherdHealth.org
Ownership: Voluntary non-profit - Private
Emergency Services: Yes

Phone: 903-315-2000
Fax: 903-315-2002

Accredited: Yes
Licensed Beds: 412

Key Personnel:
President/CEO . . . . Jerry D Adair
Medical Staff . . . . Edna York
OB/GYN Womens Health . . . . EA Clark, MD
Chief Radiology . . . . Kim Howard, MD

Measure	Cases	This Hospital	State Average	U.S. Average	Top Hospital
Heart Attack Care					
ACE Inhibitor or ARB for LVSD[2]	48	96%	85%	82%	100%
Aspirin at Arrival[2]	244	100%	91%	92%	100%
Aspirin at Discharge[2]	292	100%	90%	90%	100%
Beta Blocker at Arrival[2]	208	99%	85%	87%	100%
Beta Blocker at Discharge[2]	257	98%	86%	90%	100%
Fibrinolytic Medication Timing[2]	0	-	30%	31%	100%
PCI Within 90 Minutes of Arrival[2]	0	-	48%	54%	95%
Smoking Cessation Advice[2]	111	97%	90%	88%	100%
Heart Failure Care					
ACE Inhibitor or ARB for LVSD[2]	124	97%	82%	82%	100%
Discharge Instructions[2]	261	94%	60%	61%	93%
Evaluation of LVS Function[2]	318	91%	81%	83%	99%
Smoking Cessation Advice[2]	60	100%	82%	82%	100%
Pneumonia Care					
Appropriate Initial Antibiotic[2]	90	92%	79%	83%	94%
Blood Culture Timing[2]	91	86%	89%	90%	100%
Influenza Vaccine[2]	27	85%	69%	70%	100%
Initial Antibiotic Timing[2]	141	79%	78%	80%	93%
Oxygenation Assessment[2]	167	99%	99%	99%	100%
Pneumococcal Vaccine[2]	102	59%	68%	69%	94%
Smoking Cessation Advice[2]	51	90%	83%	80%	100%
Surgical Infection Prevention					

NOTE: Hospital profiles are in alphabetical order by state, then city, then hospital within the city; Rankings are sorted by rate in descending order and exclude hospitals with less than 25 cases; (1) The number of cases is too small (n<25) for purposes of reliably predicting hospital performance; (2) Measure reflects the hospital's indication that its submission was based upon a sample of its relevant discharges; (3) Rate reflects fewer than the maximum possible quarters of data for the measure; (4) Inaccurate information submitted and suppressed for one or more quarters; (5) No data is available from the hospital for this measure; Please refer to the User's Guide for a full explanation of data

Prophylactic Antibiotic Given[2,3]	70	64%	67%	77%	95%
Prophylactic Antibiotic Selection[2]	74	89%	86%	90%	100%
Prophylactic Antibiotic Stopped[2,3]	68	85%	68%	72%	95%
Pregnancy Care					
Inpatient Neonatal Mortality	-	-	-	-	-
Third or Fourth Degree Laceration	-	-	3.23%	3.63%	3.27%

Longview Regional Medical Center

Alternate Name: Longview Regional Hospital
2901 N 4th Street
Longview, TX 75605   Phone: 903-758-1818
URL: www.longviewregional.com   Fax: 903-758-5167
Ownership: Proprietary   Accredited: Yes
Emergency Services: Yes   Licensed Beds: 164
Key Personnel:
Interim CEO . . . . Allyn R Harris

Measure	Cases	This Hospital	State Average	U.S. Average	Top Hospital
Heart Attack Care					
ACE Inhibitor or ARB for LVSD[1]	14	93%	85%	82%	100%
Aspirin at Arrival	80	98%	91%	92%	100%
Aspirin at Discharge	82	98%	90%	90%	100%
Beta Blocker at Arrival	72	97%	85%	87%	100%
Beta Blocker at Discharge	83	96%	86%	90%	100%
Fibrinolytic Medication Timing	0	-	30%	31%	100%
PCI Within 90 Minutes of Arrival[1]	1	0%	48%	54%	95%
Smoking Cessation Advice	34	100%	90%	88%	100%
Heart Failure Care					
ACE Inhibitor or ARB for LVSD	59	86%	82%	82%	100%
Discharge Instructions	148	99%	60%	61%	93%
Evaluation of LVS Function	168	100%	81%	83%	99%
Smoking Cessation Advice	32	100%	82%	82%	100%
Pneumonia Care					
Appropriate Initial Antibiotic	131	89%	79%	83%	94%
Blood Culture Timing	126	92%	89%	90%	100%
Influenza Vaccine	34	97%	69%	70%	100%
Initial Antibiotic Timing	175	86%	78%	80%	93%
Oxygenation Assessment	197	99%	99%	99%	100%
Pneumococcal Vaccine	116	97%	68%	69%	94%
Smoking Cessation Advice	41	100%	83%	80%	100%
Surgical Infection Prevention					
Prophylactic Antibiotic Given	379	80%	67%	77%	95%
Prophylactic Antibiotic Selection	101	83%	86%	90%	100%
Prophylactic Antibiotic Stopped	367	64%	68%	72%	95%
Pregnancy Care					
Inpatient Neonatal Mortality	925	0.00%	-	-	-
Third or Fourth Degree Laceration	589	4.58%	3.23%	3.63%	3.27%

Covenant Medical Center

Alternate Name: Methodist Hospital
3615 19th Street
Lubbock, TX 79410   Phone: 806-725-1011
URL: www.covenanthealth.org   Fax: 806-723-6289
Ownership: Voluntary non-profit - Church
Emergency Services: Yes   Accredited: Yes
                                        Licensed Beds: 920
Key Personnel:
President/CEO . . . . Steven L Hunter
Emergency Room . . . . Karen Baggerly
Director Infection/Disease Control . . . . Clark Kerr
Director CCU . . . . Susan Sayari

Measure	Cases	This Hospital	State Average	U.S. Average	Top Hospital
Heart Attack Care					
ACE Inhibitor or ARB for LVSD	132	75%	85%	82%	100%
Aspirin at Arrival	225	95%	91%	92%	100%
Aspirin at Discharge	531	93%	90%	90%	100%
Beta Blocker at Arrival	189	83%	85%	87%	100%
Beta Blocker at Discharge	541	92%	86%	90%	100%
Fibrinolytic Medication Timing	0	-	30%	31%	100%
PCI Within 90 Minutes of Arrival[1]	17	41%	48%	54%	95%
Smoking Cessation Advice	214	100%	90%	88%	100%
Heart Failure Care					

Measure	Cases	This Hospital	State Average	U.S. Average	Top Hospital
ACE Inhibitor or ARB for LVSD[2]	314	66%	82%	82%	100%
Discharge Instructions[2]	665	33%	60%	61%	93%
Evaluation of LVS Function[2]	802	85%	81%	83%	99%
Smoking Cessation Advice[2]	127	98%	82%	82%	100%
Pneumonia Care					
Appropriate Initial Antibiotic[2]	329	78%	79%	83%	94%
Blood Culture Timing[2]	477	94%	89%	90%	100%
Influenza Vaccine	186	70%	69%	70%	100%
Initial Antibiotic Timing[2]	616	74%	78%	80%	93%
Oxygenation Assessment[2]	726	100%	99%	99%	100%
Pneumococcal Vaccine[2]	473	78%	68%	69%	94%
Smoking Cessation Advice[2]	158	97%	83%	80%	100%
Surgical Infection Prevention					
Prophylactic Antibiotic Given[2,3]	272	71%	67%	77%	95%
Prophylactic Antibiotic Selection[2]	101	77%	86%	90%	100%
Prophylactic Antibiotic Stopped[2,3]	246	43%	68%	72%	95%
Pregnancy Care					
Inpatient Neonatal Mortality	-	-	-	-	-
Third or Fourth Degree Laceration	-	-	3.23%	3.63%	3.27%

Highland Community Hospital

2412 50th Street   Phone: 806-788-4100
Lubbock, TX 79412   Fax: 806-788-4278
URL: www.highlandcommunityhospital.com
Ownership: Proprietary   Accredited: Yes
Emergency Services: Yes   Licensed Beds: 123
Key Personnel:
CEO . . . . Doak Enabnit
Chief Medical Staff . . . . Michael Chamales, MD
Catheterization Lab . . . . Ginny Ginithan
Emergency Room . . . . Rosemary Hernandez, RN
Intensive Coronary . . . . Rosemary Hernandez, RN
OB/GYN Women's Health . . . . Peggy Howell, RN
Respiratory/Cardiopulmonary . . . . Rieta Merrell

Measure	Cases	This Hospital	State Average	U.S. Average	Top Hospital
Heart Attack Care					
ACE Inhibitor or ARB for LVSD[3]	0	-	85%	82%	100%
Aspirin at Arrival[1,3]	3	100%	91%	92%	100%
Aspirin at Discharge[1,3]	2	100%	90%	90%	100%
Beta Blocker at Arrival[1,3]	1	100%	85%	87%	100%
Beta Blocker at Discharge[1,3]	1	100%	86%	90%	100%
Fibrinolytic Medication Timing[3]	0	-	30%	31%	100%
PCI Within 90 Minutes of Arrival	0	-	48%	54%	95%
Smoking Cessation Advice[3]	0	-	90%	88%	100%
Heart Failure Care					
ACE Inhibitor or ARB for LVSD[1]	4	100%	82%	82%	100%
Discharge Instructions[1]	13	54%	60%	61%	93%
Evaluation of LVS Function[1]	17	88%	81%	83%	99%
Smoking Cessation Advice[1]	5	80%	82%	82%	100%
Pneumonia Care					
Appropriate Initial Antibiotic	34	56%	79%	83%	94%
Blood Culture Timing[1]	20	80%	89%	90%	100%
Influenza Vaccine[1]	10	70%	69%	70%	100%
Initial Antibiotic Timing	34	79%	78%	80%	93%
Oxygenation Assessment	40	100%	99%	99%	100%
Pneumococcal Vaccine[1]	23	61%	68%	69%	94%
Smoking Cessation Advice[1]	12	83%	83%	80%	100%
Surgical Infection Prevention					
Prophylactic Antibiotic Given[3]	81	43%	67%	77%	95%
Prophylactic Antibiotic Selection	29	100%	86%	90%	100%
Prophylactic Antibiotic Stopped[3]	79	22%	68%	72%	95%
Pregnancy Care					
Inpatient Neonatal Mortality	-	-	-	-	-
Third or Fourth Degree Laceration	-	-	3.23%	3.63%	3.27%

NOTE: Hospital profiles are in alphabetical order by state, then city, then hospital within the city; Rankings are sorted by rate in descending order and exclude hospitals with less than 25 cases; (1) The number of cases is too small (n<25) for purposes of reliably predicting hospital performance; (2) Measure reflects the hospital's indication that its submission was based upon a sample of its relevant discharges; (3) Rate reflects fewer than the maximum possible quarters of data for the measure; (4) Inaccurate information submitted and suppressed for one or more quarters; (5) No data is available from the hospital for this measure; Please refer to the User's Guide for a full explanation of data

Lubbock Heart Hospital

4810 N Loop 289
Lubbock, TX 79416
URL: www.lubbockhearthospital.com
Ownership: Proprietary
Emergency Services: Yes

Phone: 806-687-7777
Fax: 806-687-7778

Accredited: No
Licensed Beds: 74

Key Personnel:
CEO. . . . . John McGreevy

Measure	Cases	This Hospital	State Average	U.S. Average	Top Hospital
Heart Attack Care					
ACE Inhibitor or ARB for LVSD[2]	29	66%	85%	82%	100%
Aspirin at Arrival[2]	78	96%	91%	92%	100%
Aspirin at Discharge[2]	180	97%	90%	90%	100%
Beta Blocker at Arrival[2]	66	76%	85%	87%	100%
Beta Blocker at Discharge[2]	158	79%	86%	90%	100%
Fibrinolytic Medication Timing[2,3]	0	-	30%	31%	100%
PCI Within 90 Minutes of Arrival[1,2]	2	0%	48%	54%	95%
Smoking Cessation Advice[1,2,3]	12	83%	90%	88%	100%
Heart Failure Care					
ACE Inhibitor or ARB for LVSD[2]	89	57%	82%	82%	100%
Discharge Instructions[2,3]	71	37%	60%	61%	93%
Evaluation of LVS Function[2]	275	87%	81%	83%	99%
Smoking Cessation Advice[1,2,3]	7	71%	82%	82%	100%
Pneumonia Care					
Appropriate Initial Antibiotic[1,3]	3	67%	79%	83%	94%
Blood Culture Timing[1,3]	2	50%	89%	90%	100%
Influenza Vaccine[5]	-	-	69%	70%	100%
Initial Antibiotic Timing[1]	16	50%	78%	80%	93%
Oxygenation Assessment[1]	18	100%	99%	99%	100%
Pneumococcal Vaccine[1]	18	94%	68%	69%	94%
Smoking Cessation Advice[1,3]	1	0%	83%	80%	100%
Surgical Infection Prevention					
Prophylactic Antibiotic Given[2,3]	32	59%	67%	77%	95%
Prophylactic Antibiotic Selection[5]	-	-	86%	90%	100%
Prophylactic Antibiotic Stopped[2,3]	29	100%	68%	72%	95%
Pregnancy Care					
Inpatient Neonatal Mortality	-	-	-	-	-
Third or Fourth Degree Laceration	-	-	3.23%	3.63%	3.27%

University Medical Center

602 Indiana Avenue
Lubbock, TX 79415
URL: www.teamumc.org
Ownership: Govt - Hospital District or Authority
Emergency Services: Yes

Phone: 806-775-8200
Fax: 806-775-9220

Accredited: Yes
Licensed Beds: 365

Key Personnel:
CEO. . . . . David G Allison
Chief Medical Staff. . . . . Sylvia Brito
Emergency Room . . . . Fred Hagedorn, MD
Director Infection/Disease Control . . . . Tim Howell
OB/GYN Womens Health. . . . . Daniel McGunegle
Chief Radiology . . . . Glenn Roberson, MD
Director Respiratory Therapy . . . . Vicki Higginbotham

Measure	Cases	This Hospital	State Average	U.S. Average	Top Hospital
Heart Attack Care					
ACE Inhibitor or ARB for LVSD	49	71%	85%	82%	100%
Aspirin at Arrival	233	94%	91%	92%	100%
Aspirin at Discharge	263	96%	90%	90%	100%
Beta Blocker at Arrival	161	92%	85%	87%	100%
Beta Blocker at Discharge	261	94%	86%	90%	100%
Fibrinolytic Medication Timing	0	-	30%	31%	100%
PCI Within 90 Minutes of Arrival[1]	6	67%	48%	54%	95%
Smoking Cessation Advice	117	89%	90%	88%	100%
Heart Failure Care					
ACE Inhibitor or ARB for LVSD[2]	125	84%	82%	82%	100%
Discharge Instructions[2]	239	49%	60%	61%	93%
Evaluation of LVS Function[2]	285	88%	81%	83%	99%
Smoking Cessation Advice[2]	74	68%	82%	82%	100%
Pneumonia Care					
Appropriate Initial Antibiotic[2]	88	76%	79%	83%	94%
Blood Culture Timing[2]	69	83%	89%	90%	100%

Memorial Health System of East Texas-Lufkin

Alternate Name: Memorial Medical Center of East Texas
1201 W Frank Avenue
Lufkin, TX 75904
URL: www.mymemorialhealth.org
Ownership: Voluntary non-profit - Private
Emergency Services: Yes

Phone: 936-634-8111
Fax: 936-639-7004

Accredited: Yes
Licensed Beds: 234

Key Personnel:
CEO. . . . . Gary L Whatley
Chief Medical Staff. . . . . Jerry Robbins, MD
Emergency Room . . . . Norma Sanford
Director Medical/Surgical Nursing . . . . Barbara Shadden
Chief Radiology . . . . Glenn Davis, MD
Director Respiratory Therapy . . . . David Henson

Measure	Cases	This Hospital	State Average	U.S. Average	Top Hospital
Heart Attack Care					
ACE Inhibitor or ARB for LVSD	39	72%	85%	82%	100%
Aspirin at Arrival	88	92%	91%	92%	100%
Aspirin at Discharge	131	85%	90%	90%	100%
Beta Blocker at Arrival	89	89%	85%	87%	100%
Beta Blocker at Discharge	128	88%	86%	90%	100%
Fibrinolytic Medication Timing[3]	0	-	30%	31%	100%
PCI Within 90 Minutes of Arrival[1]	1	0%	48%	54%	95%
Smoking Cessation Advice[1,3]	13	92%	90%	88%	100%
Heart Failure Care					
ACE Inhibitor or ARB for LVSD	107	76%	82%	82%	100%
Discharge Instructions[3]	35	69%	60%	61%	93%
Evaluation of LVS Function	274	78%	81%	83%	99%
Smoking Cessation Advice[1,3]	3	100%	82%	82%	100%
Pneumonia Care					
Appropriate Initial Antibiotic[1,3]	15	93%	79%	83%	94%
Blood Culture Timing[3]	35	100%	89%	90%	100%
Influenza Vaccine[5]	-	-	69%	70%	100%
Initial Antibiotic Timing	251	62%	78%	80%	93%
Oxygenation Assessment	272	97%	99%	99%	100%
Pneumococcal Vaccine	172	71%	68%	69%	94%
Smoking Cessation Advice[1,3]	8	100%	83%	80%	100%
Surgical Infection Prevention					
Prophylactic Antibiotic Given[3]	97	86%	67%	77%	95%
Prophylactic Antibiotic Selection[5]	-	-	86%	90%	100%
Prophylactic Antibiotic Stopped[3]	94	78%	68%	72%	95%
Pregnancy Care					
Inpatient Neonatal Mortality	745	0.00%	-	-	-
Third or Fourth Degree Laceration	483	2.07%	3.23%	3.63%	3.27%

Woodland Heights Medical Center

Alternate Name: Columbia Heights Medical Center
505 S John Redditt Drive
Lufkin, TX 75904
Ownership: Proprietary
Emergency Services: Yes

Phone: 936-634-8311
Fax: 936-637-8600

Accredited: Yes
Licensed Beds: 146

Key Personnel:
CEO. . . . . Lance Jones
Emergency Room . . . . Patrick Gummell
Director Infection/Disease Control . . . . Doris Weatherford, RN
Director Medical/Surgical Nursing . . . . Jeannine Stevens, RN
OB/GYN Womens Health. . . . . Cheryl Suiter, MD
Chief Radiology . . . . Cody DuVall, MD
Director Respiratory Therapy . . . . Sam Price

Influenza Vaccine and Surgical section for Lubbock Heart Hospital continued at top of right column:

Measure	Cases	This Hospital	State Average	U.S. Average	Top Hospital
Influenza Vaccine[1]	11	45%	69%	70%	100%
Initial Antibiotic Timing[2]	129	73%	78%	80%	93%
Oxygenation Assessment[2]	158	100%	99%	99%	100%
Pneumococcal Vaccine[2]	65	40%	68%	69%	94%
Smoking Cessation Advice[2]	32	62%	83%	80%	100%
Surgical Infection Prevention					
Prophylactic Antibiotic Given[3]	176	78%	67%	77%	95%
Prophylactic Antibiotic Selection	63	83%	86%	90%	100%
Prophylactic Antibiotic Stopped[3]	167	69%	68%	72%	95%
Pregnancy Care					
Inpatient Neonatal Mortality	-	-	-	-	-
Third or Fourth Degree Laceration	-	-	3.23%	3.63%	3.27%

NOTE: Hospital profiles are in alphabetical order by state, then city, then hospital within the city; Rankings are sorted by rate in descending order and exclude hospitals with less than 25 cases; (1) The number of cases is too small (n<25) for purposes of reliably predicting hospital performance; (2) Measure reflects the hospital's indication that its submission was based upon a sample of its relevant discharges; (3) Rate reflects fewer than the maximum possible quarters of data for the measure; (4) Inaccurate information submitted and suppressed for one or more quarters; (5) No data is available from the hospital for this measure; Please refer to the User's Guide for a full explanation of data

Measure	Cases	This Hospital	State Average	U.S. Average	Top Hospital
Heart Attack Care					
ACE Inhibitor or ARB for LVSD	38	89%	85%	82%	100%
Aspirin at Arrival	92	96%	91%	92%	100%
Aspirin at Discharge	122	94%	90%	90%	100%
Beta Blocker at Arrival	82	96%	85%	87%	100%
Beta Blocker at Discharge	114	96%	86%	90%	100%
Fibrinolytic Medication Timing[1]	2	0%	30%	31%	100%
PCI Within 90 Minutes of Arrival[1]	2	50%	48%	54%	95%
Smoking Cessation Advice	47	100%	90%	88%	100%
Heart Failure Care					
ACE Inhibitor or ARB for LVSD	119	95%	82%	82%	100%
Discharge Instructions	207	76%	60%	61%	93%
Evaluation of LVS Function	276	97%	81%	83%	99%
Smoking Cessation Advice	38	100%	82%	82%	100%
Pneumonia Care					
Appropriate Initial Antibiotic	122	71%	79%	83%	94%
Blood Culture Timing	73	90%	89%	90%	100%
Influenza Vaccine	37	92%	69%	70%	100%
Initial Antibiotic Timing	141	87%	78%	80%	93%
Oxygenation Assessment	169	100%	99%	99%	100%
Pneumococcal Vaccine	109	93%	68%	69%	94%
Smoking Cessation Advice	44	100%	83%	80%	100%
Surgical Infection Prevention					
Prophylactic Antibiotic Given	424	88%	67%	77%	95%
Prophylactic Antibiotic Selection	110	85%	86%	90%	100%
Prophylactic Antibiotic Stopped	396	79%	68%	72%	95%
Pregnancy Care					
Inpatient Neonatal Mortality	-	-	-	-	-
Third or Fourth Degree Laceration	-	-	3.23%	3.63%	3.27%

Seton Edgar B Davis Memorial Hospital

Alternate Name: Edgar B Davis Memorial Hospital
130 Hays Street   Toll-Free: 888-875-7000
Luling, TX 78648   Phone: 830-875-7000
                                     Fax: 830-875-7053
Ownership: Voluntary non-profit – Church   Accredited: No
Emergency Services: No   Licensed Beds: 30
Key Personnel:
President/CEO . . . . Carol A Hoke
Emergency Room . . . . Bertha Curtis

Measure	Cases	This Hospital	State Average	U.S. Average	Top Hospital
Heart Attack Care					
ACE Inhibitor or ARB for LVSD[3]	0	-	85%	82%	100%
Aspirin at Arrival[1,3]	1	0%	91%	92%	100%
Aspirin at Discharge[1,3]	1	100%	90%	90%	100%
Beta Blocker at Arrival[1,3]	1	0%	85%	87%	100%
Beta Blocker at Discharge[1,3]	1	100%	86%	90%	100%
Fibrinolytic Medication Timing[3]	0	-	30%	31%	100%
PCI Within 90 Minutes of Arrival	0	-	48%	54%	95%
Smoking Cessation Advice[3]	0	-	90%	88%	100%
Heart Failure Care					
ACE Inhibitor or ARB for LVSD[1,3]	12	92%	82%	82%	100%
Discharge Instructions[3]	25	32%	60%	61%	93%
Evaluation of LVS Function[3]	42	76%	81%	83%	99%
Smoking Cessation Advice[1,3]	10	90%	82%	82%	100%
Pneumonia Care					
Appropriate Initial Antibiotic[3]	34	88%	79%	83%	94%
Blood Culture Timing	38	92%	89%	90%	100%
Influenza Vaccine[1]	16	44%	69%	70%	100%
Initial Antibiotic Timing[3]	47	81%	78%	80%	93%
Oxygenation Assessment[3]	54	100%	99%	99%	100%
Pneumococcal Vaccine[3]	35	69%	68%	69%	94%
Smoking Cessation Advice[1,3]	6	100%	83%	80%	100%
Surgical Infection Prevention					
Prophylactic Antibiotic Given[5]	-	-	67%	77%	95%
Prophylactic Antibiotic Selection[5]	-	-	86%	90%	100%
Prophylactic Antibiotic Stopped[5]	-	-	68%	72%	95%
Pregnancy Care					
Inpatient Neonatal Mortality	-	-	-	-	-

Third or Fourth Degree Laceration	-	-	3.23%	3.63%	3.27%

Madison Saint Joseph Health Center

Alternate Name: Saint Francis Health Center
100 W Cross Street   Phone: 936-348-2631
Madisonville, TX 77864   Fax: 936-348-3404
URL: www.st.josephs.org
Ownership: Voluntary non-profit – Church   Accredited: Yes
Emergency Services: Yes   Licensed Beds: 45
Key Personnel:
Administrator . . . . Reed Edmundson
Chief of Medical Staff . . . . Anrew Eisenderg
Emergency Room . . . . Julia Jarrell
Emergency Room . . . . Anna McDonald
Director Medical/Surgical Nursing . . . . Carol Aufduncampe
Director of Pulmonary/Respiratory Care . . . . Michael Robinson

Measure	Cases	This Hospital	State Average	U.S. Average	Top Hospital
Heart Attack Care					
ACE Inhibitor or ARB for LVSD[3]	0	-	85%	82%	100%
Aspirin at Arrival[3]	0	-	91%	92%	100%
Aspirin at Discharge[1,3]	1	100%	90%	90%	100%
Beta Blocker at Arrival[3]	0	-	85%	87%	100%
Beta Blocker at Discharge[1,3]	1	100%	86%	90%	100%
Fibrinolytic Medication Timing[3]	0	-	30%	31%	100%
PCI Within 90 Minutes of Arrival	0	-	48%	54%	95%
Smoking Cessation Advice[3]	0	-	90%	88%	100%
Heart Failure Care					
ACE Inhibitor or ARB for LVSD[1,3]	7	86%	82%	82%	100%
Discharge Instructions[1,3]	5	60%	60%	61%	93%
Evaluation of LVS Function[1,3]	23	43%	81%	83%	99%
Smoking Cessation Advice[1,3]	3	67%	82%	82%	100%
Pneumonia Care					
Appropriate Initial Antibiotic[1,3]	22	95%	79%	83%	94%
Blood Culture Timing[1]	19	84%	89%	90%	100%
Influenza Vaccine[1]	5	100%	69%	70%	100%
Initial Antibiotic Timing[1,3]	21	90%	78%	80%	93%
Oxygenation Assessment[1,3]	24	100%	99%	99%	100%
Pneumococcal Vaccine[1,3]	16	100%	68%	69%	94%
Smoking Cessation Advice[1,3]	7	100%	83%	80%	100%
Surgical Infection Prevention					
Prophylactic Antibiotic Given[5]	-	-	67%	77%	95%
Prophylactic Antibiotic Selection[5]	-	-	86%	90%	100%
Prophylactic Antibiotic Stopped[5]	-	-	68%	72%	95%
Pregnancy Care					
Inpatient Neonatal Mortality	-	-	-	-	-
Third or Fourth Degree Laceration	-	-	3.23%	3.63%	3.27%

Falls Community Hospital

Alternate Name: Torbett-Hutchings-Smith Hospital
322 Coleman   Phone: 254-803-3561
PO Box 60   Fax: 254-883-6066
Marlin, TX 76661
E-mail: fallshosp@aol.com
URL: www.fallshospital.org
Ownership: Voluntary non-profit – Private   Accredited: No
Emergency Services: Yes   Licensed Beds: 44
Key Personnel:
Administrator . . . . Willis L Reese
Chief Medical Staff . . . . Dileep Bhateley, MD
Infection Control . . . . Betty Trotten, RN
Director Respiratory Therapy . . . . Melissa Aldermann

Measure	Cases	This Hospital	State Average	U.S. Average	Top Hospital
Heart Attack Care					
ACE Inhibitor or ARB for LVSD[1,3]	1	100%	85%	82%	100%
Aspirin at Arrival[1,3]	1	100%	91%	92%	100%
Aspirin at Discharge[1,3]	1	100%	90%	90%	100%
Beta Blocker at Arrival[1,3]	1	100%	85%	87%	100%
Beta Blocker at Discharge[1,3]	1	100%	86%	90%	100%
Fibrinolytic Medication Timing[3]	0	-	30%	31%	100%
PCI Within 90 Minutes of Arrival	0	-	48%	54%	95%
Smoking Cessation Advice[1,3]	1	100%	90%	88%	100%

NOTE: Hospital profiles are in alphabetical order by state, then city, then hospital within the city; Rankings are sorted by rate in descending order and exclude hospitals with less than 25 cases; (1) The number of cases is too small (n<25) for purposes of reliably predicting hospital performance; (2) Measure reflects the hospital's indication that its submission was based upon a sample of its relevant discharges; (3) Rate reflects fewer than the maximum possible quarters of data for the measure; (4) Inaccurate information submitted and suppressed for one or more quarters; (5) No data is available from the hospital for this measure; Please refer to the User's Guide for a full explanation of data

Heart Failure Care					
ACE Inhibitor or ARB for LVSD[1]	18	72%	82%	82%	100%
Discharge Instructions	85	85%	60%	61%	93%
Evaluation of LVS Function	105	96%	81%	83%	99%
Smoking Cessation Advice	25	100%	82%	82%	100%
Pneumonia Care					
Appropriate Initial Antibiotic	97	75%	79%	83%	94%
Blood Culture Timing	62	98%	89%	90%	100%
Influenza Vaccine[1]	24	96%	69%	70%	100%
Initial Antibiotic Timing	144	88%	78%	80%	93%
Oxygenation Assessment	165	100%	99%	99%	100%
Pneumococcal Vaccine	81	95%	68%	69%	94%
Smoking Cessation Advice	53	96%	83%	80%	100%
Surgical Infection Prevention					
Prophylactic Antibiotic Given[5]	-	-	67%	77%	95%
Prophylactic Antibiotic Selection[5]	-	-	86%	90%	100%
Prophylactic Antibiotic Stopped[5]	-	-	68%	72%	95%
Pregnancy Care					
Inpatient Neonatal Mortality	-	-	-	-	-
Third or Fourth Degree Laceration	-	-	3.23%	3.63%	3.27%

Marshall Regional Medical Center

Alternate Name: Marshall Memorial Hospital
811 S Washington Avenue
Marshall, TX 75670
URL: www.marshallregional.org
Ownership: Voluntary non-profit - Private
Emergency Services: Yes

Phone: 903-927-6000
Fax: 903-927-6101

Accredited: Yes
Licensed Beds: 139

Key Personnel:
CEO/CFO . . . . Russell J Collier
Chief Medical Staff. Bud Siebenlist, MD
Emergency Room . . . . Nick Zenarosa, MD
Director Infection/Disease Control . . . . Tena Tiller, RN
CCU Spvg. Nurse . . . . Sandy Sims
Director Medical/Surgical Nursing . . . . Linda Shaneman, RN
OB/GYN Womens Health. . . . . Eric McCathran, MD
Chief Radiology . . . . Bud R Siebenlist, MD
Director Respiratory Therapy . . . . Sandy Sims, RN

Measure	Cases	This Hospital	State Average	U.S. Average	Top Hospital
Heart Attack Care					
ACE Inhibitor or ARB for LVSD[1]	11	82%	85%	82%	100%
Aspirin at Arrival	39	95%	91%	92%	100%
Aspirin at Discharge[1]	22	91%	90%	90%	100%
Beta Blocker at Arrival	39	85%	85%	87%	100%
Beta Blocker at Discharge	25	88%	86%	90%	100%
Fibrinolytic Medication Timing	0	-	30%	31%	100%
PCI Within 90 Minutes of Arrival	0	-	48%	54%	95%
Smoking Cessation Advice[1]	3	100%	90%	88%	100%
Heart Failure Care					
ACE Inhibitor or ARB for LVSD	57	93%	82%	82%	100%
Discharge Instructions	102	88%	60%	61%	93%
Evaluation of LVS Function	124	97%	81%	83%	99%
Smoking Cessation Advice[1]	24	96%	82%	82%	100%
Pneumonia Care					
Appropriate Initial Antibiotic	129	72%	79%	83%	94%
Blood Culture Timing	60	93%	89%	90%	100%
Influenza Vaccine	25	96%	69%	70%	100%
Initial Antibiotic Timing	111	86%	78%	80%	93%
Oxygenation Assessment	133	99%	99%	99%	100%
Pneumococcal Vaccine	83	86%	68%	69%	94%
Smoking Cessation Advice	35	91%	83%	80%	100%
Surgical Infection Prevention					
Prophylactic Antibiotic Given[2,3]	161	54%	67%	77%	95%
Prophylactic Antibiotic Selection[2]	46	80%	86%	90%	100%
Prophylactic Antibiotic Stopped[2,3]	162	58%	68%	72%	95%
Pregnancy Care					
Inpatient Neonatal Mortality	-	-	-	-	-
Third or Fourth Degree Laceration	-	-	3.23%	3.63%	3.27%

McAllen Medical Center

301 W Expwy 83
McAllen, TX 78503
URL: www.mcallenmedicalcenter.com
Ownership: Proprietary
Emergency Services: Yes

Phone: 956-632-4000
Fax: 956-632-4010

Accredited: Yes
Licensed Beds: 552

Key Personnel:
CEO/Managing Director. . . . . Daniel P McLean
Chief Medical Staff. Terrance Posluszny, MD
Chief Catheterization Laboratory . . . . Jack Balmer
Emergency Room . . . . Oscar Tijerina, MD
Director Infection/Disease Control . . . . Michael Jelinek, MD
OB/GYN Womens Health. . . . . Hugo Zapata, MD
Chief Radiology . . . . Julio Astacio, MD
Director Respiratory Therapy . . . . Roger Luna

Measure	Cases	This Hospital	State Average	U.S. Average	Top Hospital
Heart Attack Care					
ACE Inhibitor or ARB for LVSD[2]	71	54%	85%	82%	100%
Aspirin at Arrival[2]	241	90%	91%	92%	100%
Aspirin at Discharge[2]	233	91%	90%	90%	100%
Beta Blocker at Arrival[2]	147	86%	85%	87%	100%
Beta Blocker at Discharge[2]	262	83%	86%	90%	100%
Fibrinolytic Medication Timing[2]	0	-	30%	31%	100%
PCI Within 90 Minutes of Arrival[1,2]	14	50%	48%	54%	95%
Smoking Cessation Advice[2]	69	84%	90%	88%	100%
Heart Failure Care					
ACE Inhibitor or ARB for LVSD[2]	135	64%	82%	82%	100%
Discharge Instructions[2]	271	59%	60%	61%	93%
Evaluation of LVS Function[2]	307	82%	81%	83%	99%
Smoking Cessation Advice[1,2]	22	64%	82%	82%	100%
Pneumonia Care					
Appropriate Initial Antibiotic[2]	87	83%	79%	83%	94%
Blood Culture Timing[2]	79	89%	89%	90%	100%
Influenza Vaccine[2]	25	60%	69%	70%	100%
Initial Antibiotic Timing[2]	133	54%	78%	80%	93%
Oxygenation Assessment[2]	156	97%	99%	99%	100%
Pneumococcal Vaccine[2]	85	72%	68%	69%	94%
Smoking Cessation Advice[1,2]	20	75%	83%	80%	100%
Surgical Infection Prevention					
Prophylactic Antibiotic Given[2]	251	58%	67%	77%	95%
Prophylactic Antibiotic Selection[2]	57	88%	86%	90%	100%
Prophylactic Antibiotic Stopped[2]	238	28%	68%	72%	95%
Pregnancy Care					
Inpatient Neonatal Mortality	-	-	-	-	-
Third or Fourth Degree Laceration	-	-	3.23%	3.63%	3.27%

Rio Grande Regional Hospital

101 E Ridge Road
McAllen, TX 78503
URL: www.riohealth.com
Ownership: Proprietary
Emergency Services: Yes

Phone: 956-632-6000
Fax: 956-632-6621

Accredited: Yes
Licensed Beds: 319

Key Personnel:
CEO. . . . . Stephen K Jones, JR
Chief Medical Staff. Michael Jelinek
Emergency Room . . . . Nanulea Sloref

Measure	Cases	This Hospital	State Average	U.S. Average	Top Hospital
Heart Attack Care					
ACE Inhibitor or ARB for LVSD	46	59%	85%	82%	100%
Aspirin at Arrival	166	93%	91%	92%	100%
Aspirin at Discharge	175	87%	90%	90%	100%
Beta Blocker at Arrival	104	82%	85%	87%	100%
Beta Blocker at Discharge	174	87%	86%	90%	100%
Fibrinolytic Medication Timing[1]	1	0%	30%	31%	100%
PCI Within 90 Minutes of Arrival[1]	6	50%	48%	54%	95%
Smoking Cessation Advice	33	94%	90%	88%	100%
Heart Failure Care					
ACE Inhibitor or ARB for LVSD	131	67%	82%	82%	100%
Discharge Instructions	369	67%	60%	61%	93%
Evaluation of LVS Function	417	76%	81%	83%	99%
Smoking Cessation Advice	54	91%	82%	82%	100%

Pneumonia Care					
Appropriate Initial Antibiotic	146	79%	79%	83%	94%
Blood Culture Timing	125	94%	89%	90%	100%
Influenza Vaccine	43	91%	69%	70%	100%
Initial Antibiotic Timing	238	71%	78%	80%	93%
Oxygenation Assessment	259	96%	99%	99%	100%
Pneumococcal Vaccine	168	75%	68%	69%	94%
Smoking Cessation Advice	28	82%	83%	80%	100%
Surgical Infection Prevention					
Prophylactic Antibiotic Given[2,3]	125	66%	67%	77%	95%
Prophylactic Antibiotic Selection[2]	49	94%	86%	90%	100%
Prophylactic Antibiotic Stopped[2,3]	121	51%	68%	72%	95%
Pregnancy Care					
Inpatient Neonatal Mortality	-	-	-	-	-
Third or Fourth Degree Laceration	-	-	3.23%	3.63%	3.27%

North Central Medical Center

Alternate Name: North Texas Medical Center-Westpark Campus
4500 Medical Center Drive
McKinney, TX 75069

Toll-Free: 972-569-8000
Phone: 972-547-8000
Fax: 972-547-8008

URL: www.ncentralmedical.com
Ownership: Proprietary
Emergency Services: Yes
Accredited: Yes
Licensed Beds: 270

Key Personnel:
CEO. . . . . George Miller
Chief Medical Staff. . . . . Dan Rex, MD
Emergency Room . . . . Tom Button

Measure	Cases	This Hospital	State Average	U.S. Average	Top Hospital
Heart Attack Care					
ACE Inhibitor or ARB for LVSD[1]	23	91%	85%	82%	100%
Aspirin at Arrival	142	99%	91%	92%	100%
Aspirin at Discharge	147	97%	90%	90%	100%
Beta Blocker at Arrival	116	95%	85%	87%	100%
Beta Blocker at Discharge	150	96%	86%	90%	100%
Fibrinolytic Medication Timing	0	-	30%	31%	100%
PCI Within 90 Minutes of Arrival[1]	9	56%	48%	54%	95%
Smoking Cessation Advice	60	100%	90%	88%	100%
Heart Failure Care					
ACE Inhibitor or ARB for LVSD	81	70%	82%	82%	100%
Discharge Instructions	188	65%	60%	61%	93%
Evaluation of LVS Function	256	93%	81%	83%	99%
Smoking Cessation Advice	46	100%	82%	82%	100%
Pneumonia Care					
Appropriate Initial Antibiotic	189	91%	79%	83%	94%
Blood Culture Timing	176	88%	89%	90%	100%
Influenza Vaccine	46	54%	69%	70%	100%
Initial Antibiotic Timing	263	93%	78%	80%	93%
Oxygenation Assessment	330	100%	99%	99%	100%
Pneumococcal Vaccine	199	59%	68%	69%	94%
Smoking Cessation Advice	59	97%	83%	80%	100%
Surgical Infection Prevention					
Prophylactic Antibiotic Given[2,3]	143	63%	67%	77%	95%
Prophylactic Antibiotic Selection[2]	48	71%	86%	90%	100%
Prophylactic Antibiotic Stopped[2,3]	139	58%	68%	72%	95%
Pregnancy Care					
Inpatient Neonatal Mortality	-	-	-	-	-
Third or Fourth Degree Laceration	-	-	3.23%	3.63%	3.27%

Medical Center of Mesquite

1011 N Galloway Avenue
Mesquite, TX 75149
URL: www.hma-corp.com
Ownership: Proprietary
Emergency Services: Yes

Phone: 214-320-7000
Fax: 972-289-9468

Accredited: Yes
Licensed Beds: 200

Key Personnel:
Emergency Room . . . . Penny Stillwell, RN
Director Infection Control . . . . Kim Salmon, RN
Director Radiology . . . . Tommy E Lanham
Director Respiratory Therapy . . . . Richard Hodgkins

Measure	Cases	This Hospital	State Average	U.S. Average	Top Hospital
Heart Attack Care					
ACE Inhibitor or ARB for LVSD	26	77%	85%	82%	100%
Aspirin at Arrival	164	88%	91%	92%	100%
Aspirin at Discharge	172	76%	90%	90%	100%
Beta Blocker at Arrival	169	87%	85%	87%	100%
Beta Blocker at Discharge	174	84%	86%	90%	100%
Fibrinolytic Medication Timing[1]	16	12%	30%	31%	100%
PCI Within 90 Minutes of Arrival[1]	13	31%	48%	54%	95%
Smoking Cessation Advice	72	62%	90%	88%	100%
Heart Failure Care					
ACE Inhibitor or ARB for LVSD	132	67%	82%	82%	100%
Discharge Instructions	346	62%	60%	61%	93%
Evaluation of LVS Function	394	67%	81%	83%	99%
Smoking Cessation Advice	102	80%	82%	82%	100%
Pneumonia Care					
Appropriate Initial Antibiotic	161	50%	79%	83%	94%
Blood Culture Timing	103	90%	89%	90%	100%
Influenza Vaccine	45	56%	69%	70%	100%
Initial Antibiotic Timing	192	62%	78%	80%	93%
Oxygenation Assessment	251	100%	99%	99%	100%
Pneumococcal Vaccine	136	44%	68%	69%	94%
Smoking Cessation Advice	59	92%	83%	80%	100%
Surgical Infection Prevention					
Prophylactic Antibiotic Given[2]	206	46%	67%	77%	95%
Prophylactic Antibiotic Selection[2]	48	83%	86%	90%	100%
Prophylactic Antibiotic Stopped[2]	158	71%	68%	72%	95%
Pregnancy Care					
Inpatient Neonatal Mortality	-	-	-	-	-
Third or Fourth Degree Laceration	-	-	3.23%	3.63%	3.27%

Mesquite Community Hospital

3500 Interstate 30
Motley Drive
Mesquite, TX 75150
URL: www.mchtx.com
Ownership: Proprietary
Emergency Services: Yes

Phone: 972-698-3000
Fax: 972-698-2465

Accredited: Yes
Licensed Beds: 172

Key Personnel:
CEO/Administrator . . . . Henry Hawthorne

Measure	Cases	This Hospital	State Average	U.S. Average	Top Hospital
Heart Attack Care					
ACE Inhibitor or ARB for LVSD[1]	8	50%	85%	82%	100%
Aspirin at Arrival	53	98%	91%	92%	100%
Aspirin at Discharge[1]	20	85%	90%	90%	100%
Beta Blocker at Arrival	52	90%	85%	87%	100%
Beta Blocker at Discharge[1]	23	96%	86%	90%	100%
Fibrinolytic Medication Timing[1]	5	100%	30%	31%	100%
PCI Within 90 Minutes of Arrival	0	-	48%	54%	95%
Smoking Cessation Advice[1]	11	100%	90%	88%	100%
Heart Failure Care					
ACE Inhibitor or ARB for LVSD	92	84%	82%	82%	100%
Discharge Instructions	202	59%	60%	61%	93%
Evaluation of LVS Function	248	90%	81%	83%	99%
Smoking Cessation Advice	78	100%	82%	82%	100%
Pneumonia Care					
Appropriate Initial Antibiotic	153	86%	79%	83%	94%
Blood Culture Timing	126	87%	89%	90%	100%
Influenza Vaccine	39	54%	69%	70%	100%
Initial Antibiotic Timing	175	81%	78%	80%	93%
Oxygenation Assessment	204	100%	99%	99%	100%
Pneumococcal Vaccine	77	77%	68%	69%	94%
Smoking Cessation Advice	80	98%	83%	80%	100%
Surgical Infection Prevention					
Prophylactic Antibiotic Given[2]	297	79%	67%	77%	95%
Prophylactic Antibiotic Selection[2]	69	81%	86%	90%	100%
Prophylactic Antibiotic Stopped[2]	290	75%	68%	72%	95%
Pregnancy Care					
Inpatient Neonatal Mortality	-	-	-	-	-
Third or Fourth Degree Laceration	-	-	3.23%	3.63%	3.27%

NOTE: Hospital profiles are in alphabetical order by state, then city, then hospital within the city; Rankings are sorted by rate in descending order and exclude hospitals with less than 25 cases; (1) The number of cases is too small (n<25) for purposes of reliably predicting hospital performance; (2) Measure reflects the hospital's indication that its submission was based upon a sample of its relevant discharges; (3) Rate reflects fewer than the maximum possible quarters of data for the measure; (4) Inaccurate information submitted and suppressed for one or more quarters; (5) No data is available from the hospital for this measure; Please refer to the User's Guide for a full explanation of data

Parkview Regional Hospital

Alternate Name: Harris Methodist-Mexia
600 S Bonham
Mexia, TX 76667
E-mail: timpadams@aol.com
URL: www.parkviewregional.com
Ownership: Proprietary
Emergency Services: Yes

Phone: 254-562-0408
Fax: 254-562-7532

Accredited: Yes
Licensed Beds: 59

Key Personnel:
Administrator . . . . Jimmy Stuart
Director of Pulmonary . . . . D Archer

Measure	Cases	This Hospital	State Average	U.S. Average	Top Hospital
Heart Attack Care					
ACE Inhibitor or ARB for LVSD	0	-	85%	82%	100%
Aspirin at Arrival[1]	10	90%	91%	92%	100%
Aspirin at Discharge[1]	7	71%	90%	90%	100%
Beta Blocker at Arrival[1]	4	75%	85%	87%	100%
Beta Blocker at Discharge[1]	9	67%	86%	90%	100%
Fibrinolytic Medication Timing	0	-	30%	31%	100%
PCI Within 90 Minutes of Arrival	0	-	48%	54%	95%
Smoking Cessation Advice[1]	2	100%	90%	88%	100%
Heart Failure Care					
ACE Inhibitor or ARB for LVSD[1]	16	94%	82%	82%	100%
Discharge Instructions	136	67%	60%	61%	93%
Evaluation of LVS Function	158	92%	81%	83%	99%
Smoking Cessation Advice[1]	21	90%	82%	82%	100%
Pneumonia Care					
Appropriate Initial Antibiotic	107	72%	79%	83%	94%
Blood Culture Timing	74	95%	89%	90%	100%
Influenza Vaccine[4,5]	-	-	69%	70%	100%
Initial Antibiotic Timing	151	88%	78%	80%	93%
Oxygenation Assessment	175	100%	99%	99%	100%
Pneumococcal Vaccine	94	73%	68%	69%	94%
Smoking Cessation Advice	45	96%	83%	80%	100%
Surgical Infection Prevention					
Prophylactic Antibiotic Given[1,3]	1	0%	67%	77%	95%
Prophylactic Antibiotic Selection[1]	1	0%	86%	90%	100%
Prophylactic Antibiotic Stopped[1,3]	1	100%	68%	72%	95%
Pregnancy Care					
Inpatient Neonatal Mortality	-	-	-	-	-
Third or Fourth Degree Laceration	-	-	3.23%	3.63%	3.27%

Midland Memorial Hospital

2200 W Illinois Avenue
Midland, TX 79701
E-mail: ljohnson@midland-memorial.com
URL: www.midland-memorial.com
Ownership: Govt - Hospital District or Authority
Emergency Services: Yes

Phone: 432-685-1111
Fax: 432-685-3488

Accredited: Yes
Licensed Beds: 321

Key Personnel:
President/CEO . . . . Russell Meyers
Chief Medical Staff . . . . Larry Oliver, MD
Emergency Room . . . . Ann Brewington, RN
Director Medical/Surgical Nursing . . . . Robyn Kedzie, RN
OB/GYN Womens Health . . . . James Welsh, MD
Chief Radiology . . . . Marlon Hughes, MD
Manager Respiratory Therapy . . . . Larry Harris

Measure	Cases	This Hospital	State Average	U.S. Average	Top Hospital
Heart Attack Care					
ACE Inhibitor or ARB for LVSD	44	95%	85%	82%	100%
Aspirin at Arrival	187	98%	91%	92%	100%
Aspirin at Discharge	202	90%	90%	90%	100%
Beta Blocker at Arrival	135	87%	85%	87%	100%
Beta Blocker at Discharge	215	87%	86%	90%	100%
Fibrinolytic Medication Timing	0	-	30%	31%	100%
PCI Within 90 Minutes of Arrival[1]	8	62%	48%	54%	95%
Smoking Cessation Advice	74	97%	90%	88%	100%
Heart Failure Care					
ACE Inhibitor or ARB for LVSD[2]	135	86%	82%	82%	100%
Discharge Instructions[2]	303	57%	60%	61%	93%
Evaluation of LVS Function[2]	333	80%	81%	83%	99%

Measure	Cases	This Hospital	State Average	U.S. Average	Top Hospital
Smoking Cessation Advice[2]	59	75%	82%	82%	100%
Pneumonia Care					
Appropriate Initial Antibiotic	200	65%	79%	83%	94%
Blood Culture Timing	102	88%	89%	90%	100%
Influenza Vaccine	47	68%	69%	70%	100%
Initial Antibiotic Timing	205	60%	78%	80%	93%
Oxygenation Assessment	257	100%	99%	99%	100%
Pneumococcal Vaccine	156	67%	68%	69%	94%
Smoking Cessation Advice	58	71%	83%	80%	100%
Surgical Infection Prevention					
Prophylactic Antibiotic Given[2,3]	320	85%	67%	77%	95%
Prophylactic Antibiotic Selection[2]	97	87%	86%	90%	100%
Prophylactic Antibiotic Stopped[2,3]	319	76%	68%	72%	95%
Pregnancy Care					
Inpatient Neonatal Mortality	-	-	-	-	-
Third or Fourth Degree Laceration	-	-	3.23%	3.63%	3.27%

West Texas Medical Center

25 Village Circle
Midland, TX 79701
Ownership: Voluntary non-profit - Private
Emergency Services: Yes

Phone: 432-571-7026

Accredited: No

Measure	Cases	This Hospital	State Average	U.S. Average	Top Hospital
Heart Attack Care					
ACE Inhibitor or ARB for LVSD[5]	-	-	85%	82%	100%
Aspirin at Arrival[5]	-	-	91%	92%	100%
Aspirin at Discharge[5]	-	-	90%	90%	100%
Beta Blocker at Arrival[5]	-	-	85%	87%	100%
Beta Blocker at Discharge[5]	-	-	86%	90%	100%
Fibrinolytic Medication Timing[5]	-	-	30%	31%	100%
PCI Within 90 Minutes of Arrival[5]	-	-	48%	54%	95%
Smoking Cessation Advice[5]	-	-	90%	88%	100%
Heart Failure Care					
ACE Inhibitor or ARB for LVSD[1,3]	8	75%	82%	82%	100%
Discharge Instructions[5]	-	-	60%	61%	93%
Evaluation of LVS Function[1,3]	9	100%	81%	83%	99%
Smoking Cessation Advice[5]	-	-	82%	82%	100%
Pneumonia Care					
Appropriate Initial Antibiotic[5]	-	-	79%	83%	94%
Blood Culture Timing[5]	-	-	89%	90%	100%
Influenza Vaccine[5]	-	-	69%	70%	100%
Initial Antibiotic Timing[1,3]	5	100%	78%	80%	93%
Oxygenation Assessment[1,3]	5	100%	99%	99%	100%
Pneumococcal Vaccine[1,3]	3	0%	68%	69%	94%
Smoking Cessation Advice[5]	-	-	83%	80%	100%
Surgical Infection Prevention					
Prophylactic Antibiotic Given[5]	-	-	67%	77%	95%
Prophylactic Antibiotic Selection[5]	-	-	86%	90%	100%
Prophylactic Antibiotic Stopped[5]	-	-	68%	72%	95%
Pregnancy Care					
Inpatient Neonatal Mortality	-	-	-	-	-
Third or Fourth Degree Laceration	-	-	3.23%	3.63%	3.27%

Palo Pinto General Hospital

400 SW 25th Avenue
Mineral Wells, TX 76067
E-mail: ppsl@txol.net
URL: www.ppgh.com
Ownership: Govt - Hospital District or Authority
Emergency Services: Yes

Phone: 940-325-7891
Fax: 940-325-7903

Accredited: Yes
Licensed Beds: 99

Key Personnel:
CEO . . . . Patricia J Dorris, RN
Chief Medical Staff . . . . John Jones, MD
Cardiac Lab . . . . Melony Hudson
Infection Control . . . . Sue Lamb, RN
ICU . . . . Robert Clark, RN
Medical/Surgical Unit . . . . Daniel T Valdez, RN
Women's Services . . . . Carolyn Holt, RN
Cardiopulmonary . . . . Sherry McAdory, RN

Measure	Cases	This Hospital	State Average	U.S. Average	Top Hospital

NOTE: Hospital profiles are in alphabetical order by state, then city, then hospital within the city; Rankings are sorted by rate in descending order and exclude hospitals with less than 25 cases; (1) The number of cases is too small (n<25) for purposes of reliably predicting hospital performance; (2) Measure reflects the hospital's indication that its submission was based upon a sample of its relevant discharges; (3) Rate reflects fewer than the maximum possible quarters of data for the measure; (4) Inaccurate information submitted and suppressed for one or more quarters; (5) No data is available from the hospital for this measure; Please refer to the User's Guide for a full explanation of data

Heart Attack Care					
ACE Inhibitor or ARB for LVSD	0	-	85%	82%	100%
Aspirin at Arrival[1]	20	70%	91%	92%	100%
Aspirin at Discharge[1]	6	67%	90%	90%	100%
Beta Blocker at Arrival[1]	21	67%	85%	87%	100%
Beta Blocker at Discharge[1]	7	43%	86%	90%	100%
Fibrinolytic Medication Timing	0	-	30%	31%	100%
PCI Within 90 Minutes of Arrival	0	-	48%	54%	95%
Smoking Cessation Advice[1]	3	33%	90%	88%	100%
Heart Failure Care					
ACE Inhibitor or ARB for LVSD	28	82%	82%	82%	100%
Discharge Instructions	90	100%	60%	61%	93%
Evaluation of LVS Function	105	60%	81%	83%	99%
Smoking Cessation Advice[1]	24	67%	82%	82%	100%
Pneumonia Care					
Appropriate Initial Antibiotic	101	72%	79%	83%	94%
Blood Culture Timing	27	85%	89%	90%	100%
Influenza Vaccine[1]	18	28%	69%	70%	100%
Initial Antibiotic Timing	103	70%	78%	80%	93%
Oxygenation Assessment	117	100%	99%	99%	100%
Pneumococcal Vaccine	70	69%	68%	69%	94%
Smoking Cessation Advice	42	67%	83%	80%	100%
Surgical Infection Prevention					
Prophylactic Antibiotic Given[3]	93	87%	67%	77%	95%
Prophylactic Antibiotic Selection	41	95%	86%	90%	100%
Prophylactic Antibiotic Stopped[3]	92	78%	68%	72%	95%
Pregnancy Care					
Inpatient Neonatal Mortality	-	-	-	-	-
Third or Fourth Degree Laceration	-	-	3.23%	3.63%	3.27%

Mission Hospital

900 S Bryan Road
Mission, TX 78572
E-mail: mgarza@missionmc.org
URL: www.missionhospital.org
Ownership: Government - Local
Emergency Services: No
Phone: 956-323-9000
Fax: 956-323-9102

Accredited: Yes
Licensed Beds: 138

Key Personnel:
CEO . . . . Javier Irruegas
Chief Medical Staff . . . . Daryl Stinch, MD
Emergency Department Manager . . . . Elijah Mydawbh
Emergency Room . . . . Andrew Robottom
Director Infection/Disease Control . . . . Gilbert Koschtial
Director Radiology . . . . Jim Johnson
Director Respiratory Therapy . . . . MaryLou Arguijo

Measure	Cases	This Hospital	State Average	U.S. Average	Top Hospital
Heart Attack Care					
ACE Inhibitor or ARB for LVSD[1]	23	70%	85%	82%	100%
Aspirin at Arrival	116	91%	91%	92%	100%
Aspirin at Discharge	99	79%	90%	90%	100%
Beta Blocker at Arrival	96	93%	85%	87%	100%
Beta Blocker at Discharge	85	86%	86%	90%	100%
Fibrinolytic Medication Timing[1]	1	0%	30%	31%	100%
PCI Within 90 Minutes of Arrival[1]	4	75%	48%	54%	95%
Smoking Cessation Advice	25	96%	90%	88%	100%
Heart Failure Care					
ACE Inhibitor or ARB for LVSD	60	75%	82%	82%	100%
Discharge Instructions	230	40%	60%	61%	93%
Evaluation of LVS Function	275	73%	81%	83%	99%
Smoking Cessation Advice	52	98%	82%	82%	100%
Pneumonia Care					
Appropriate Initial Antibiotic	177	75%	79%	83%	94%
Blood Culture Timing	115	89%	89%	90%	100%
Influenza Vaccine	58	29%	69%	70%	100%
Initial Antibiotic Timing	224	56%	78%	80%	93%
Oxygenation Assessment	243	98%	99%	99%	100%
Pneumococcal Vaccine	153	26%	68%	69%	94%
Smoking Cessation Advice	36	97%	83%	80%	100%
Surgical Infection Prevention					
Prophylactic Antibiotic Given[3]	172	40%	67%	77%	95%
Prophylactic Antibiotic Selection	56	88%	86%	90%	100%
Prophylactic Antibiotic Stopped[3]	159	26%	68%	72%	95%

Pregnancy Care					
Inpatient Neonatal Mortality	-	-	-	-	-
Third or Fourth Degree Laceration	-	-	3.23%	3.63%	3.27%

Memorial Hermann Fort Bend Hospital

Alternate Name: Fort Bend Medical Center
3803 FM 1092 Highway 6
Missouri City, TX 77459
URL: www.MHHS.org
Ownership: Voluntary non-profit - Private
Emergency Services: Yes
Phone: 281-499-4800
Fax: 281-725-5603

Accredited: Yes
Licensed Beds: 84

Key Personnel:
CEO . . . . Rod Brace
Chief Medical Staff . . . . Srinivas Nikam, MD
Director Emergency Room . . . . Allie Fonville
Director Infection/Disease Control . . . . Jeanne Wey
Director Medical/Surgical Nursing . . . . Bev Collings
OB/GYN Womens Health . . . . Michael Amaro, MD
Chief OB/GYN & Pediatrics . . . . Michael Amaro, MD
Chief Radiology . . . . Judson Snow, MD
Director Respiratory Therapy . . . . Linda McIntire

Measure	Cases	This Hospital	State Average	U.S. Average	Top Hospital
Heart Attack Care					
ACE Inhibitor or ARB for LVSD[1]	3	100%	85%	82%	100%
Aspirin at Arrival	29	93%	91%	92%	100%
Aspirin at Discharge[1]	10	90%	90%	90%	100%
Beta Blocker at Arrival[1]	22	100%	85%	87%	100%
Beta Blocker at Discharge[1]	10	100%	86%	90%	100%
Fibrinolytic Medication Timing	0	-	30%	31%	100%
PCI Within 90 Minutes of Arrival	0	-	48%	54%	95%
Smoking Cessation Advice[1]	2	100%	90%	88%	100%
Heart Failure Care					
ACE Inhibitor or ARB for LVSD	50	96%	82%	82%	100%
Discharge Instructions	114	96%	60%	61%	93%
Evaluation of LVS Function	131	98%	81%	83%	99%
Smoking Cessation Advice[1]	16	100%	82%	82%	100%
Pneumonia Care					
Appropriate Initial Antibiotic	81	88%	79%	83%	94%
Blood Culture Timing	73	100%	89%	90%	100%
Influenza Vaccine[4,5]	-	-	69%	70%	100%
Initial Antibiotic Timing	94	97%	78%	80%	93%
Oxygenation Assessment	116	100%	99%	99%	100%
Pneumococcal Vaccine	64	94%	68%	69%	94%
Smoking Cessation Advice	25	100%	83%	80%	100%
Surgical Infection Prevention					
Prophylactic Antibiotic Given[2,3]	50	84%	67%	77%	95%
Prophylactic Antibiotic Selection[1,2]	13	77%	86%	90%	100%
Prophylactic Antibiotic Stopped[2,3]	47	53%	68%	72%	95%
Pregnancy Care					
Inpatient Neonatal Mortality	-	-	-	-	-
Third or Fourth Degree Laceration	-	-	3.23%	3.63%	3.27%

Titus Regional Medical Center

Alternate Name: Titus County Memorial Hospital
2001 N Jefferson
Mount Pleasant, TX 75455
URL: www.titusregional.com
Ownership: Govt - Hospital District or Authority
Emergency Services: Yes
Phone: 903-577-6000
Fax: 903-577-6027

Accredited: Yes
Licensed Beds: 165

Key Personnel:
CEO . . . . Steve Jacobson
Emergency Room . . . . Peggy Helbert

Measure	Cases	This Hospital	State Average	U.S. Average	Top Hospital
Heart Attack Care					
ACE Inhibitor or ARB for LVSD[1]	3	100%	85%	82%	100%
Aspirin at Arrival[1]	12	75%	91%	92%	100%
Aspirin at Discharge[1]	7	57%	90%	90%	100%
Beta Blocker at Arrival[1]	6	67%	85%	87%	100%
Beta Blocker at Discharge[1]	6	67%	86%	90%	100%
Fibrinolytic Medication Timing[3]	0	-	30%	31%	100%
PCI Within 90 Minutes of Arrival	0	-	48%	54%	95%

NOTE: Hospital profiles are in alphabetical order by state, then city, then hospital within the city; Rankings are sorted by rate in descending order and exclude hospitals with less than 25 cases; (1) The number of cases is too small (n<25) for purposes of reliably predicting hospital performance; (2) Measure reflects the hospital's indication that its submission was based upon a sample of its relevant discharges; (3) Rate reflects fewer than the maximum possible quarters of data for the measure; (4) Inaccurate information submitted and suppressed for one or more quarters; (5) No data is available from the hospital for this measure; Please refer to the User's Guide for a full explanation of data

Smoking Cessation Advice[1,3]	1	0%	90%	88%	100%
Heart Failure Care					
ACE Inhibitor or ARB for LVSD	40	80%	82%	82%	100%
Discharge Instructions[3]	27	22%	60%	61%	93%
Evaluation of LVS Function	130	77%	81%	83%	99%
Smoking Cessation Advice[1,3]	3	33%	82%	82%	100%
Pneumonia Care					
Appropriate Initial Antibiotic[3]	27	67%	79%	83%	94%
Blood Culture Timing[1,3]	12	100%	89%	90%	100%
Influenza Vaccine[4,5]	-	-	69%	70%	100%
Initial Antibiotic Timing	221	53%	78%	80%	93%
Oxygenation Assessment	253	77%	99%	99%	100%
Pneumococcal Vaccine	136	20%	68%	69%	94%
Smoking Cessation Advice[1,3]	7	29%	83%	80%	100%
Surgical Infection Prevention					
Prophylactic Antibiotic Given[3]	51	47%	67%	77%	95%
Prophylactic Antibiotic Selection[5]	-	-	86%	90%	100%
Prophylactic Antibiotic Stopped[3]	40	82%	68%	72%	95%
Pregnancy Care					
Inpatient Neonatal Mortality	-	-	-	-	-
Third or Fourth Degree Laceration	-	-	3.23%	3.63%	3.27%

East Texas Medical Center-Mount Vernon

500 Highway 37 South   Phone: 903-537-4552
Mount Vernon, TX 75457   Fax: 903-537-8100
URL: www.etmc.org
Ownership: Voluntary non-profit - Private   Accredited: No
Emergency Services: Yes   Licensed Beds: 49
Key Personnel:
Administrator . . . . Stephen Pitts
Chief Medical Staff. . . . . Keith Gordan
Emergency Room . . . . Nancy Bolton
Director Infection/Disease Control . . . . Nilah Lahti
Chief Radiology . . . . Billy Parnell, MD

Measure	Cases	This Hospital	State Average	U.S. Average	Top Hospital
Heart Attack Care					
ACE Inhibitor or ARB for LVSD[3]	0	-	85%	82%	100%
Aspirin at Arrival[1,3]	2	0%	91%	92%	100%
Aspirin at Discharge[1,3]	3	67%	90%	90%	100%
Beta Blocker at Arrival[1,3]	3	67%	85%	87%	100%
Beta Blocker at Discharge[1,3]	3	67%	86%	90%	100%
Fibrinolytic Medication Timing[3]	0	-	30%	31%	100%
PCI Within 90 Minutes of Arrival[5]	-	-	48%	54%	95%
Smoking Cessation Advice[3]	0	-	90%	88%	100%
Heart Failure Care					
ACE Inhibitor or ARB for LVSD[1]	4	100%	82%	82%	100%
Discharge Instructions[1]	14	14%	60%	61%	93%
Evaluation of LVS Function	26	62%	81%	83%	99%
Smoking Cessation Advice[1]	3	67%	82%	82%	100%
Pneumonia Care					
Appropriate Initial Antibiotic[1]	15	87%	79%	83%	94%
Blood Culture Timing[1]	8	88%	89%	90%	100%
Influenza Vaccine[1]	1	100%	69%	70%	100%
Initial Antibiotic Timing[1]	15	93%	78%	80%	93%
Oxygenation Assessment[1]	19	100%	99%	99%	100%
Pneumococcal Vaccine[1]	13	85%	68%	69%	94%
Smoking Cessation Advice[1]	3	67%	83%	80%	100%
Surgical Infection Prevention					
Prophylactic Antibiotic Given[3]	0	-	67%	77%	95%
Prophylactic Antibiotic Selection	0	-	86%	90%	100%
Prophylactic Antibiotic Stopped[3]	0	-	68%	72%	95%
Pregnancy Care					
Inpatient Neonatal Mortality	-	-	-	-	-
Third or Fourth Degree Laceration	-	-	3.23%	3.63%	3.27%

Nacogdoches Medical Center Hospital
Alternate Name: AMI Nacogdoches Medical Center Hospital

4920 NE Stallings Drive   Phone: 936-569-9481
Nacogdoches, TX 75961   Fax: 936-568-3400
URL: www.nacmedicalcenter.com
Ownership: Proprietary
Emergency Services: Yes   Accredited: Yes
     Licensed Beds: 150

Measure	Cases	This Hospital	State Average	U.S. Average	Top Hospital
Heart Attack Care					
ACE Inhibitor or ARB for LVSD[1]	21	76%	85%	82%	100%
Aspirin at Arrival	81	86%	91%	92%	100%
Aspirin at Discharge	77	86%	90%	90%	100%
Beta Blocker at Arrival	69	80%	85%	87%	100%
Beta Blocker at Discharge	73	89%	86%	90%	100%
Fibrinolytic Medication Timing[1]	4	0%	30%	31%	100%
PCI Within 90 Minutes of Arrival[1]	1	0%	48%	54%	95%
Smoking Cessation Advice	29	97%	90%	88%	100%
Heart Failure Care					
ACE Inhibitor or ARB for LVSD	45	67%	82%	82%	100%
Discharge Instructions	112	47%	60%	61%	93%
Evaluation of LVS Function	134	82%	81%	83%	99%
Smoking Cessation Advice[1]	21	76%	82%	82%	100%
Pneumonia Care					
Appropriate Initial Antibiotic	93	69%	79%	83%	94%
Blood Culture Timing	89	97%	89%	90%	100%
Influenza Vaccine	33	82%	69%	70%	100%
Initial Antibiotic Timing	130	79%	78%	80%	93%
Oxygenation Assessment	162	100%	99%	99%	100%
Pneumococcal Vaccine	111	72%	68%	69%	94%
Smoking Cessation Advice	32	78%	83%	80%	100%
Surgical Infection Prevention					
Prophylactic Antibiotic Given[2]	346	70%	67%	77%	95%
Prophylactic Antibiotic Selection[2]	37	59%	86%	90%	100%
Prophylactic Antibiotic Stopped[2]	324	60%	68%	72%	95%
Pregnancy Care					
Inpatient Neonatal Mortality	-	-	-	-	-
Third or Fourth Degree Laceration	-	-	3.23%	3.63%	3.27%

Nacogdoches Memorial Hospital

1204 Mound Street   Phone: 936-564-4611
Nacogdoches, TX 75961   Fax: 936-568-3400
E-mail: info@nacmem.org
URL: www.nacmem.org
Ownership: Govt - Hospital District or Authority   Accredited: Yes
Emergency Services: Yes   Licensed Beds: 202
Key Personnel:
Director Infection/Disease Control . . . . Elenor Adams
Director Respiratory Therapy . . . . Richard McShan

Measure	Cases	This Hospital	State Average	U.S. Average	Top Hospital
Heart Attack Care					
ACE Inhibitor or ARB for LVSD[1]	13	85%	85%	82%	100%
Aspirin at Arrival	54	94%	91%	92%	100%
Aspirin at Discharge	72	83%	90%	90%	100%
Beta Blocker at Arrival	54	74%	85%	87%	100%
Beta Blocker at Discharge	75	80%	86%	90%	100%
Fibrinolytic Medication Timing[3]	0	-	30%	31%	100%
PCI Within 90 Minutes of Arrival[1]	3	33%	48%	54%	95%
Smoking Cessation Advice[1,3]	6	100%	90%	88%	100%
Heart Failure Care					
ACE Inhibitor or ARB for LVSD	114	81%	82%	82%	100%
Discharge Instructions[3]	50	34%	60%	61%	93%
Evaluation of LVS Function	281	80%	81%	83%	99%
Smoking Cessation Advice[1,3]	13	77%	82%	82%	100%
Pneumonia Care					
Appropriate Initial Antibiotic[1,3]	12	75%	79%	83%	94%
Blood Culture Timing[1,3]	12	100%	89%	90%	100%
Influenza Vaccine[5]	-	-	69%	70%	100%
Initial Antibiotic Timing	160	64%	78%	80%	93%
Oxygenation Assessment	185	98%	99%	99%	100%
Pneumococcal Vaccine	117	52%	68%	69%	94%
Smoking Cessation Advice[1,3]	4	50%	83%	80%	100%
Surgical Infection Prevention					

NOTE: Hospital profiles are in alphabetical order by state, then city, then hospital within the city; Rankings are sorted by rate in descending order and exclude hospitals with less than 25 cases; (1) The number of cases is too small (n<25) for purposes of reliably predicting hospital performance; (2) Measure reflects the hospital's indication that its submission was based upon a sample of its relevant discharges; (3) Rate reflects fewer than the maximum possible quarters of data for the measure; (4) Inaccurate information submitted and suppressed for one or more quarters; (5) No data is available from the hospital for this measure; Please refer to the User's Guide for a full explanation of data

Prophylactic Antibiotic Given[3]	75	81%	67%	77%	95%
Prophylactic Antibiotic Selection[5]	-	-	86%	90%	100%
Prophylactic Antibiotic Stopped[3]	75	61%	68%	72%	95%
Pregnancy Care					
Inpatient Neonatal Mortality	-	-	-	-	-
Third or Fourth Degree Laceration	-	-	3.23%	3.63%	3.27%

Christus Saint John Hospital

Alternate Name: Saint John Hospital
18300 Saint John Drive
Houston, TX 77058
URL: www.christushealth.org
Ownership: Voluntary non-profit - Private
Emergency Services: Yes

Phone: 281-333-5503
Fax: 281-333-8891

Accredited: Yes
Licensed Beds: 135

Key Personnel:
CEO . . . . Tom Permetti
Chief Medical Staff . . . . Daniel Casso, MD
Director Catheterization Lab . . . . Lisa Mizell
Director Emergency Room . . . . Steve Deacon
Infection Control . . . . Eileen Haag

Measure	Cases	This Hospital	State Average	U.S. Average	Top Hospital
Heart Attack Care					
ACE Inhibitor or ARB for LVSD	31	100%	85%	82%	100%
Aspirin at Arrival	119	99%	91%	92%	100%
Aspirin at Discharge	101	98%	90%	90%	100%
Beta Blocker at Arrival	121	98%	85%	87%	100%
Beta Blocker at Discharge	100	98%	86%	90%	100%
Fibrinolytic Medication Timing[1]	1	100%	30%	31%	100%
PCI Within 90 Minutes of Arrival[1]	8	25%	48%	54%	95%
Smoking Cessation Advice	50	98%	90%	88%	100%
Heart Failure Care					
ACE Inhibitor or ARB for LVSD	87	100%	82%	82%	100%
Discharge Instructions	177	73%	60%	61%	93%
Evaluation of LVS Function	210	100%	81%	83%	99%
Smoking Cessation Advice	36	100%	82%	82%	100%
Pneumonia Care					
Appropriate Initial Antibiotic	160	84%	79%	83%	94%
Blood Culture Timing	135	99%	89%	90%	100%
Influenza Vaccine	35	100%	69%	70%	100%
Initial Antibiotic Timing	165	92%	78%	80%	93%
Oxygenation Assessment	191	100%	99%	99%	100%
Pneumococcal Vaccine	119	95%	68%	69%	94%
Smoking Cessation Advice	34	100%	83%	80%	100%
Surgical Infection Prevention					
Prophylactic Antibiotic Given	348	78%	67%	77%	95%
Prophylactic Antibiotic Selection	82	77%	86%	90%	100%
Prophylactic Antibiotic Stopped	335	25%	68%	72%	95%
Pregnancy Care					
Inpatient Neonatal Mortality	-	-	-	-	-
Third or Fourth Degree Laceration	-	-	3.23%	3.63%	3.27%

Grimes-Saint Joseph's Health Center

Alternate Name: Navasota Regional Hospital
210 S Judson
Navasota, TX 77868
Ownership: Voluntary non-profit - Church
Emergency Services: Yes

Phone: 936-825-6585
Fax: 936-825-6007
Accredited: Yes
Licensed Beds: 47

Key Personnel:
Administrator . . . . Molly Hurst

Measure	Cases	This Hospital	State Average	U.S. Average	Top Hospital
Heart Attack Care					
ACE Inhibitor or ARB for LVSD[5]	-	-	85%	82%	100%
Aspirin at Arrival[5]	-	-	91%	92%	100%
Aspirin at Discharge[5]	-	-	90%	90%	100%
Beta Blocker at Arrival[5]	-	-	85%	87%	100%
Beta Blocker at Discharge[5]	-	-	86%	90%	100%
Fibrinolytic Medication Timing[5]	-	-	30%	31%	100%
PCI Within 90 Minutes of Arrival[5]	-	-	48%	54%	95%
Smoking Cessation Advice[5]	-	-	90%	88%	100%
Heart Failure Care					

Measure	Cases	This Hospital	State Average	U.S. Average	Top Hospital
ACE Inhibitor or ARB for LVSD[1,3]	1	100%	82%	82%	100%
Discharge Instructions[3]	0	-	60%	61%	93%
Evaluation of LVS Function[1,3]	1	100%	81%	83%	99%
Smoking Cessation Advice[3]	0	-	82%	82%	100%
Pneumonia Care					
Appropriate Initial Antibiotic[1,3]	4	75%	79%	83%	94%
Blood Culture Timing[5]	-	-	89%	90%	100%
Influenza Vaccine[5]	-	-	69%	70%	100%
Initial Antibiotic Timing[1,3]	3	67%	78%	80%	93%
Oxygenation Assessment[1,3]	4	100%	99%	99%	100%
Pneumococcal Vaccine[1,3]	2	100%	68%	69%	94%
Smoking Cessation Advice[3]	0	-	83%	80%	100%
Surgical Infection Prevention					
Prophylactic Antibiotic Given[5]	-	-	67%	77%	95%
Prophylactic Antibiotic Selection[5]	-	-	86%	90%	100%
Prophylactic Antibiotic Stopped[5]	-	-	68%	72%	95%
Pregnancy Care					
Inpatient Neonatal Mortality	-	-	-	-	-
Third or Fourth Degree Laceration	-	-	3.23%	3.63%	3.27%

McKenna Memorial Hospital

600 North Union Avenue
New Braunfels, TX 78130
URL: www.mckenna.org
Ownership: Proprietary
Emergency Services: Yes

Phone: 830-606-9111
Fax: 830-620-0796

Accredited: Yes
Licensed Beds: 132

Key Personnel:
CEO . . . . Tim Brierty
Emergency Room . . . . Joann Polledo
ICU . . . . Patty Toney
OB/GYN . . . . Pat Toney
Director Respiratory Therapy . . . . Jim Little

Measure	Cases	This Hospital	State Average	U.S. Average	Top Hospital
Heart Attack Care					
ACE Inhibitor or ARB for LVSD[1]	8	75%	85%	82%	100%
Aspirin at Arrival	39	97%	91%	92%	100%
Aspirin at Discharge	26	92%	90%	90%	100%
Beta Blocker at Arrival	40	98%	85%	87%	100%
Beta Blocker at Discharge	26	96%	86%	90%	100%
Fibrinolytic Medication Timing[1]	1	0%	30%	31%	100%
PCI Within 90 Minutes of Arrival	0	-	48%	54%	95%
Smoking Cessation Advice[1]	4	25%	90%	88%	100%
Heart Failure Care					
ACE Inhibitor or ARB for LVSD	36	81%	82%	82%	100%
Discharge Instructions	123	67%	60%	61%	93%
Evaluation of LVS Function	165	73%	81%	83%	99%
Smoking Cessation Advice[1]	23	74%	82%	82%	100%
Pneumonia Care					
Appropriate Initial Antibiotic	135	76%	79%	83%	94%
Blood Culture Timing	90	90%	89%	90%	100%
Influenza Vaccine	40	58%	69%	70%	100%
Initial Antibiotic Timing	164	76%	78%	80%	93%
Oxygenation Assessment	196	100%	99%	99%	100%
Pneumococcal Vaccine	125	54%	68%	69%	94%
Smoking Cessation Advice	37	81%	83%	80%	100%
Surgical Infection Prevention					
Prophylactic Antibiotic Given[3]	121	79%	67%	77%	95%
Prophylactic Antibiotic Selection	118	89%	86%	90%	100%
Prophylactic Antibiotic Stopped[3]	113	81%	68%	72%	95%
Pregnancy Care					
Inpatient Neonatal Mortality	995	0.20%	-	-	-
Third or Fourth Degree Laceration	693	6.06%	3.23%	3.63%	3.27%

Nocona General Hospital

100 Park Road
Nocona, TX 76255
Ownership: Govt - Hospital District or Authority
Emergency Services: Yes

Phone: 940-825-3235
Fax: 940-825-3604
Accredited: No
Licensed Beds: 38

Key Personnel:
Administrator . . . . Michael Graham
Chief Medical Staff . . . . Barbara Perry
Emergency Room . . . . Len Dingler, MD

NOTE: Hospital profiles are in alphabetical order by state, then city, then hospital within the city; Rankings are sorted by rate in descending order and exclude hospitals with less than 25 cases; (1) The number of cases is too small (n<25) for purposes of reliably predicting hospital performance; (2) Measure reflects the hospital's indication that its submission was based upon a sample of its relevant discharges; (3) Rate reflects fewer than the maximum possible quarters of data for the measure; (4) Inaccurate information submitted and suppressed for one or more quarters; (5) No data is available from the hospital for this measure; Please refer to the User's Guide for a full explanation of data

Respiratory . . . . Shelly Parker

Measure	Cases	This Hospital	State Average	U.S. Average	Top Hospital
Heart Attack Care					
ACE Inhibitor or ARB for LVSD[3]	0	-	85%	82%	100%
Aspirin at Arrival[1,3]	5	60%	91%	92%	100%
Aspirin at Discharge[1,3]	1	100%	90%	90%	100%
Beta Blocker at Arrival[1,3]	5	60%	85%	87%	100%
Beta Blocker at Discharge[1,3]	1	100%	86%	90%	100%
Fibrinolytic Medication Timing[1,3]	1	0%	30%	31%	100%
PCI Within 90 Minutes of Arrival	0	-	48%	54%	95%
Smoking Cessation Advice[3]	0	-	90%	88%	100%
Heart Failure Care					
ACE Inhibitor or ARB for LVSD[1]	4	50%	82%	82%	100%
Discharge Instructions[1,3]	7	57%	60%	61%	93%
Evaluation of LVS Function[1]	23	35%	81%	83%	99%
Smoking Cessation Advice[1,3]	3	67%	82%	82%	100%
Pneumonia Care					
Appropriate Initial Antibiotic[1,3]	1	100%	79%	83%	94%
Blood Culture Timing[3]	0	-	89%	90%	100%
Influenza Vaccine[5]	-	-	69%	70%	100%
Initial Antibiotic Timing	44	89%	78%	80%	93%
Oxygenation Assessment	45	96%	99%	99%	100%
Pneumococcal Vaccine	33	88%	68%	69%	94%
Smoking Cessation Advice[1,3]	1	100%	83%	80%	100%
Surgical Infection Prevention					
Prophylactic Antibiotic Given[1,3]	1	0%	67%	77%	95%
Prophylactic Antibiotic Selection[5]	-	-	86%	90%	100%
Prophylactic Antibiotic Stopped[1,3]	1	100%	68%	72%	95%
Pregnancy Care					
Inpatient Neonatal Mortality	-	-	-	-	-
Third or Fourth Degree Laceration	-	-	3.23%	3.63%	3.27%

North Hills Hospital

Alternate Name: North Hills Hospital
4401 Booth Calloway Road
N Richland Hills, TX 76180
URL: www.northhillshospital.com
Ownership: Proprietary
Emergency Services: Yes

Phone: 817-255-1000
Fax: 817-255-1991

Accredited: Yes
Licensed Beds: 144

Key Personnel:
CEO. . . . . Randolph Moresi
Chief Medical Staff. . . . . David Haefeli, MD
Emergency Room . . . . Deborah Morris

Measure	Cases	This Hospital	State Average	U.S. Average	Top Hospital
Heart Attack Care					
ACE Inhibitor or ARB for LVSD	25	96%	85%	82%	100%
Aspirin at Arrival	162	98%	91%	92%	100%
Aspirin at Discharge	137	100%	90%	90%	100%
Beta Blocker at Arrival	131	100%	85%	87%	100%
Beta Blocker at Discharge	138	100%	86%	90%	100%
Fibrinolytic Medication Timing	0	-	30%	31%	100%
PCI Within 90 Minutes of Arrival[1]	9	78%	48%	54%	95%
Smoking Cessation Advice	53	100%	90%	88%	100%
Heart Failure Care					
ACE Inhibitor or ARB for LVSD	83	100%	82%	82%	100%
Discharge Instructions	197	55%	60%	61%	93%
Evaluation of LVS Function	266	99%	81%	83%	99%
Smoking Cessation Advice	50	98%	82%	82%	100%
Pneumonia Care					
Appropriate Initial Antibiotic	180	91%	79%	83%	94%
Blood Culture Timing	216	93%	89%	90%	100%
Influenza Vaccine	59	63%	69%	70%	100%
Initial Antibiotic Timing	240	82%	78%	80%	93%
Oxygenation Assessment	299	100%	99%	99%	100%
Pneumococcal Vaccine	177	85%	68%	69%	94%
Smoking Cessation Advice	81	94%	83%	80%	100%
Surgical Infection Prevention					
Prophylactic Antibiotic Given[2,3]	197	52%	67%	77%	95%
Prophylactic Antibiotic Selection[2]	77	79%	86%	90%	100%
Prophylactic Antibiotic Stopped[2,3]	185	63%	68%	72%	95%

Pregnancy Care					
Inpatient Neonatal Mortality	-	-	-	-	-
Third or Fourth Degree Laceration	-	-	3.23%	3.63%	3.27%

Alliance Hospital

515 North Adams
Odessa, TX 79761
URL: www.alliancehospital.com
Ownership: Proprietary
Emergency Services: Yes

Toll-Free: 888-550-1904
Phone: 432-550-1000

Accredited: No
Licensed Beds: 70

Key Personnel:
CEO. . . . . Timothy Parker

Measure	Cases	This Hospital	State Average	U.S. Average	Top Hospital
Heart Attack Care					
ACE Inhibitor or ARB for LVSD[1]	19	68%	85%	82%	100%
Aspirin at Arrival	33	82%	91%	92%	100%
Aspirin at Discharge	106	92%	90%	90%	100%
Beta Blocker at Arrival	32	62%	85%	87%	100%
Beta Blocker at Discharge	105	83%	86%	90%	100%
Fibrinolytic Medication Timing[3]	0	-	30%	31%	100%
PCI Within 90 Minutes of Arrival	0	-	48%	54%	95%
Smoking Cessation Advice[1,3]	12	75%	90%	88%	100%
Heart Failure Care					
ACE Inhibitor or ARB for LVSD	70	76%	82%	82%	100%
Discharge Instructions[3]	46	41%	60%	61%	93%
Evaluation of LVS Function	223	70%	81%	83%	99%
Smoking Cessation Advice[1,3]	9	67%	82%	82%	100%
Pneumonia Care					
Appropriate Initial Antibiotic[1,3]	11	55%	79%	83%	94%
Blood Culture Timing[1,3]	7	86%	89%	90%	100%
Influenza Vaccine[5]	-	-	69%	70%	100%
Initial Antibiotic Timing	56	68%	78%	80%	93%
Oxygenation Assessment	71	100%	99%	99%	100%
Pneumococcal Vaccine	48	33%	68%	69%	94%
Smoking Cessation Advice[1,3]	4	75%	83%	80%	100%
Surgical Infection Prevention					
Prophylactic Antibiotic Given[3]	71	80%	67%	77%	95%
Prophylactic Antibiotic Selection[5]	-	-	86%	90%	100%
Prophylactic Antibiotic Stopped[3]	71	27%	68%	72%	95%
Pregnancy Care					
Inpatient Neonatal Mortality	-	-	-	-	-
Third or Fourth Degree Laceration	-	-	3.23%	3.63%	3.27%

Medical Center Hospital

500 W 4th Street
Odessa, TX 79761
URL: www.mchodessa.com
Ownership: Govt - Hospital District or Authority
Emergency Services: Yes

Phone: 432-640-4000
Fax: 432-640-2349

Accredited: Yes
Licensed Beds: 382

Key Personnel:
CEO. . . . . William W Webster
Chief Medical Officer . . . . Dr. Bruce Becker
Cardiac Lab . . . . Ervin Miller
Emergency Room . . . . Cece Wilmes
Director Surgery. . . . . Kelly Stanley
Director Respiratory/Cardiopulmonary . . . . Terry Calloway

Measure	Cases	This Hospital	State Average	U.S. Average	Top Hospital
Heart Attack Care					
ACE Inhibitor or ARB for LVSD	124	81%	85%	82%	100%
Aspirin at Arrival	276	95%	91%	92%	100%
Aspirin at Discharge	380	94%	90%	90%	100%
Beta Blocker at Arrival	222	88%	85%	87%	100%
Beta Blocker at Discharge	354	91%	86%	90%	100%
Fibrinolytic Medication Timing	0	-	30%	31%	100%
PCI Within 90 Minutes of Arrival[1]	12	50%	48%	54%	95%
Smoking Cessation Advice	143	87%	90%	88%	100%
Heart Failure Care					
ACE Inhibitor or ARB for LVSD	188	85%	82%	82%	100%
Discharge Instructions	341	66%	60%	61%	93%
Evaluation of LVS Function	362	90%	81%	83%	99%

NOTE: Hospital profiles are in alphabetical order by state, then city, then hospital within the city; Rankings are sorted by rate in descending order and exclude hospitals with less than 25 cases; (1) The number of cases is too small (n<25) for purposes of reliably predicting hospital performance; (2) Measure reflects the hospital's indication that its submission was based upon a sample of its relevant discharges; (3) Rate reflects fewer than the maximum possible quarters of data for the measure; (4) Inaccurate information submitted and suppressed for one or more quarters; (5) No data is available from the hospital for this measure; Please refer to the User's Guide for a full explanation of data

Smoking Cessation Advice	94	80%	82%	82%	100%
Pneumonia Care					
Appropriate Initial Antibiotic	181	80%	79%	83%	94%
Blood Culture Timing	114	85%	89%	90%	100%
Influenza Vaccine	58	43%	69%	70%	100%
Initial Antibiotic Timing	188	74%	78%	80%	93%
Oxygenation Assessment	240	100%	99%	99%	100%
Pneumococcal Vaccine	139	42%	68%	69%	94%
Smoking Cessation Advice	76	39%	83%	80%	100%
Surgical Infection Prevention					
Prophylactic Antibiotic Given[3]	483	67%	67%	77%	95%
Prophylactic Antibiotic Selection	140	86%	86%	90%	100%
Prophylactic Antibiotic Stopped[3]	447	44%	68%	72%	95%
Pregnancy Care					
Inpatient Neonatal Mortality	1,472	0.34%	-	-	-
Third or Fourth Degree Laceration	972	4.01%	3.23%	3.63%	3.27%

Odessa Regional Hospital

520 E 6th Street
Odessa, TX 79761

Toll-Free: 800-288-9203
Phone: 432-582-8200
Fax: 432-582-8913

E-mail: achurchill@iasishealthcare.com
URL: www.odessaregionalhospital.com
Ownership: Proprietary
Emergency Services: Yes

Accredited: Yes
Licensed Beds: 146

Key Personnel:
CEO . . . . R Craig Preston
Chief Medical Staff . . . . Anne Acreman, MD
Director Infection/Disease Control . . . . Micki Barnett
Director Respiratory Therapy . . . . Darlene Spencer

Measure	Cases	This Hospital	State Average	U.S. Average	Top Hospital
Heart Attack Care					
ACE Inhibitor or ARB for LVSD[3]	0	-	85%	82%	100%
Aspirin at Arrival[1,3]	5	60%	91%	92%	100%
Aspirin at Discharge[1,3]	1	100%	90%	90%	100%
Beta Blocker at Arrival[1,3]	5	80%	85%	87%	100%
Beta Blocker at Discharge[1,3]	1	0%	86%	90%	100%
Fibrinolytic Medication Timing[3]	0	-	30%	31%	100%
PCI Within 90 Minutes of Arrival	0	-	48%	54%	95%
Smoking Cessation Advice[3]	0	-	90%	88%	100%
Heart Failure Care					
ACE Inhibitor or ARB for LVSD[1]	4	100%	82%	82%	100%
Discharge Instructions	25	64%	60%	61%	93%
Evaluation of LVS Function	26	77%	81%	83%	99%
Smoking Cessation Advice[1]	3	100%	82%	82%	100%
Pneumonia Care					
Appropriate Initial Antibiotic	47	72%	79%	83%	94%
Blood Culture Timing	30	73%	89%	90%	100%
Influenza Vaccine[1]	13	38%	69%	70%	100%
Initial Antibiotic Timing	44	73%	78%	80%	93%
Oxygenation Assessment	52	100%	99%	99%	100%
Pneumococcal Vaccine[1]	21	67%	68%	69%	94%
Smoking Cessation Advice[1]	21	81%	83%	80%	100%
Surgical Infection Prevention					
Prophylactic Antibiotic Given[3]	140	69%	67%	77%	95%
Prophylactic Antibiotic Selection	54	87%	86%	90%	100%
Prophylactic Antibiotic Stopped[3]	137	75%	68%	72%	95%
Pregnancy Care					
Inpatient Neonatal Mortality	2,268	0.49%	-	-	-
Third or Fourth Degree Laceration	1,573	5.34%	3.23%	3.63%	3.27%

Memorial Herman Baptist Orange Hospital

Alternate Name: Baptist Hospital-Orange
608 Strickland Drive
Orange, TX 77630
URL: www.mhbh.org
Ownership: Voluntary non-profit - Church
Emergency Services: Yes

Phone: 409-883-9361
Fax: 409-883-1223

Accredited: Yes
Licensed Beds: 199

Key Personnel:
CEO . . . . Rossane Atkin
Chief Medical Staff . . . . Steve Mazzola, MD
Emergency Room . . . . Carolyn Knight, RN

Cardiology . . . . Miguel Casttllanos
Director Medical/Surgical Nursing . . . . Jeanie David
OB/GYN Womens Health . . . . Louis McIntyre, MD
Chief Radiology . . . . Charles Day, MD
Director Respiratory Therapy . . . . Jaen Jackson

Measure	Cases	This Hospital	State Average	U.S. Average	Top Hospital
Heart Attack Care					
ACE Inhibitor or ARB for LVSD[1]	2	100%	85%	82%	100%
Aspirin at Arrival	39	100%	91%	92%	100%
Aspirin at Discharge[1]	15	100%	90%	90%	100%
Beta Blocker at Arrival	38	97%	85%	87%	100%
Beta Blocker at Discharge[1]	14	100%	86%	90%	100%
Fibrinolytic Medication Timing[1]	2	0%	30%	31%	100%
PCI Within 90 Minutes of Arrival	0	-	48%	54%	95%
Smoking Cessation Advice[1]	7	100%	90%	88%	100%
Heart Failure Care					
ACE Inhibitor or ARB for LVSD	54	96%	82%	82%	100%
Discharge Instructions	108	97%	60%	61%	93%
Evaluation of LVS Function	141	98%	81%	83%	99%
Smoking Cessation Advice	32	100%	82%	82%	100%
Pneumonia Care					
Appropriate Initial Antibiotic	96	78%	79%	83%	94%
Blood Culture Timing	62	84%	89%	90%	100%
Influenza Vaccine[1]	24	67%	69%	70%	100%
Initial Antibiotic Timing	107	68%	78%	80%	93%
Oxygenation Assessment	121	100%	99%	99%	100%
Pneumococcal Vaccine	57	79%	68%	69%	94%
Smoking Cessation Advice	38	100%	83%	80%	100%
Surgical Infection Prevention					
Prophylactic Antibiotic Given[3]	65	35%	67%	77%	95%
Prophylactic Antibiotic Selection[1]	21	90%	86%	90%	100%
Prophylactic Antibiotic Stopped[3]	65	52%	68%	72%	95%
Pregnancy Care					
Inpatient Neonatal Mortality	-	-	-	-	-
Third or Fourth Degree Laceration	-	-	3.23%	3.63%	3.27%

Palestine Regional Medical Center

Alternate Name: Trinity Valley Medical Center
2900 South Loop 256
Palestine, TX 75801
E-mail: dprice@prhc.net
URL: www.palestineregional.com
Ownership: Proprietary
Emergency Services: Yes

Phone: 903-731-1000
Fax: 903-731-2217

Accredited: Yes
Licensed Beds: 258

Key Personnel:
CEO . . . . Randall L Hoover
Director Infection/Disease Control . . . . Sandra Knight
CCU Spvg. Nurse . . . . Leah Vintila
Director Medical/Surgical Nursing . . . . Debbie Stayffer
Director Respiratory Therapy . . . . Brandy Statham

Measure	Cases	This Hospital	State Average	U.S. Average	Top Hospital
Heart Attack Care					
ACE Inhibitor or ARB for LVSD[1]	12	92%	85%	82%	100%
Aspirin at Arrival	51	96%	91%	92%	100%
Aspirin at Discharge	27	89%	90%	90%	100%
Beta Blocker at Arrival	47	98%	85%	87%	100%
Beta Blocker at Discharge	33	91%	86%	90%	100%
Fibrinolytic Medication Timing[1]	4	25%	30%	31%	100%
PCI Within 90 Minutes of Arrival	0	-	48%	54%	95%
Smoking Cessation Advice[1]	7	86%	90%	88%	100%
Heart Failure Care					
ACE Inhibitor or ARB for LVSD	51	96%	82%	82%	100%
Discharge Instructions	115	85%	60%	61%	93%
Evaluation of LVS Function	153	89%	81%	83%	99%
Smoking Cessation Advice[1]	20	95%	82%	82%	100%
Pneumonia Care					
Appropriate Initial Antibiotic	80	88%	79%	83%	94%
Blood Culture Timing	86	88%	89%	90%	100%
Influenza Vaccine	25	88%	69%	70%	100%
Initial Antibiotic Timing	130	82%	78%	80%	93%

NOTE: Hospital profiles are in alphabetical order by state, then city, then hospital within the city; Rankings are sorted by rate in descending order and exclude hospitals with less than 25 cases; (1) The number of cases is too small (n<25) for purposes of reliably predicting hospital performance; (2) Measure reflects the hospital's indication that its submission was based upon a sample of its relevant discharges; (3) Rate reflects fewer than the maximum possible quarters of data for the measure; (4) Inaccurate information submitted and suppressed for one or more quarters; (5) No data is available from the hospital for this measure; Please refer to the User's Guide for a full explanation of data

Oxygenation Assessment	165	100%	99%	99%	100%
Pneumococcal Vaccine	98	96%	68%	69%	94%
Smoking Cessation Advice	29	90%	83%	80%	100%
Surgical Infection Prevention					
Prophylactic Antibiotic Given[3]	270	42%	67%	77%	95%
Prophylactic Antibiotic Selection	90	91%	86%	90%	100%
Prophylactic Antibiotic Stopped[3]	258	57%	68%	72%	95%
Pregnancy Care					
Inpatient Neonatal Mortality	-	-	-	-	-
Third or Fourth Degree Laceration	-	-	3.23%	3.63%	3.27%

Pampa Regional Medical Center

Alternate Name: Columbia Panhandle Regional Medical Center
1 Medical Plaza
Pampa, TX 79065
Ownership: Proprietary
Emergency Services: Yes

Phone: 806-665-3721
Fax: 806-665-5222
Accredited: Yes
Licensed Beds: 115

Key Personnel:
CEO. . . . . Alan N King
Chief Medical Staff. Laxman Bhatia, MD
Emergency Room . . . . Brenda Carter, RN

Measure	Cases	This Hospital	State Average	U.S. Average	Top Hospital
Heart Attack Care					
ACE Inhibitor or ARB for LVSD[1]	3	67%	85%	82%	100%
Aspirin at Arrival[1]	15	87%	91%	92%	100%
Aspirin at Discharge[1]	14	79%	90%	90%	100%
Beta Blocker at Arrival[1]	8	100%	85%	87%	100%
Beta Blocker at Discharge[1]	14	86%	86%	90%	100%
Fibrinolytic Medication Timing[1]	3	67%	30%	31%	100%
PCI Within 90 Minutes of Arrival	0	-	48%	54%	95%
Smoking Cessation Advice[1]	4	50%	90%	88%	100%
Heart Failure Care					
ACE Inhibitor or ARB for LVSD	42	98%	82%	82%	100%
Discharge Instructions	73	42%	60%	61%	93%
Evaluation of LVS Function	107	73%	81%	83%	99%
Smoking Cessation Advice[1]	13	46%	82%	82%	100%
Pneumonia Care					
Appropriate Initial Antibiotic	74	88%	79%	83%	94%
Blood Culture Timing	40	95%	89%	90%	100%
Influenza Vaccine	29	62%	69%	70%	100%
Initial Antibiotic Timing	103	88%	78%	80%	93%
Oxygenation Assessment	119	99%	99%	99%	100%
Pneumococcal Vaccine	73	59%	68%	69%	94%
Smoking Cessation Advice	27	70%	83%	80%	100%
Surgical Infection Prevention					
Prophylactic Antibiotic Given	107	79%	67%	77%	95%
Prophylactic Antibiotic Selection	25	96%	86%	90%	100%
Prophylactic Antibiotic Stopped	103	83%	68%	72%	95%
Pregnancy Care					
Inpatient Neonatal Mortality	-	-	-	-	-
Third or Fourth Degree Laceration	-	-	3.23%	3.63%	3.27%

Paris Regional Medical Center-South Campus

820 Clarksville Street
PO Box 9070
Paris, TX 75460
URL: www.parisrmc.com
Ownership: Proprietary
Emergency Services: Yes

Phone: 903-785-4521
Fax: 903-737-3848

Accredited: Yes
Licensed Beds: 405

Key Personnel:
President/CEO. . . . . Monty McLaurin
Chief Medical Staff. Arthur Tijerina, MD
Cardiac Lab . . . . JR Lindsey
Catheterization Lab . . . . JR Lindsey
Emergency Room . . . . Mark Mallory
Infection Control. . . . . Caren Jones
ICU . . . . Paula Ashford
Medical Surgical Nursing . . . . Rhonda Ground
OB/GYN/Women's Health . . . . Sue Moyer
Respiratory/Cardiopulmonary. . . . . JR Lindsey

Measure	Cases	This Hospital	State Average	U.S. Average	Top Hospital

Measure	Cases	This Hospital	State Average	U.S. Average	Top Hospital
Heart Attack Care					
ACE Inhibitor or ARB for LVSD	54	96%	85%	82%	100%
Aspirin at Arrival	119	97%	91%	92%	100%
Aspirin at Discharge	163	98%	90%	90%	100%
Beta Blocker at Arrival	105	96%	85%	87%	100%
Beta Blocker at Discharge	155	99%	86%	90%	100%
Fibrinolytic Medication Timing[1]	1	0%	30%	31%	100%
PCI Within 90 Minutes of Arrival[1]	7	43%	48%	54%	95%
Smoking Cessation Advice	65	97%	90%	88%	100%
Heart Failure Care					
ACE Inhibitor or ARB for LVSD	121	85%	82%	82%	100%
Discharge Instructions	217	46%	60%	61%	93%
Evaluation of LVS Function	292	95%	81%	83%	99%
Smoking Cessation Advice	55	82%	82%	82%	100%
Pneumonia Care					
Appropriate Initial Antibiotic	182	89%	79%	83%	94%
Blood Culture Timing	153	94%	89%	90%	100%
Influenza Vaccine	82	72%	69%	70%	100%
Initial Antibiotic Timing	272	76%	78%	80%	93%
Oxygenation Assessment	348	99%	99%	99%	100%
Pneumococcal Vaccine	207	69%	68%	69%	94%
Smoking Cessation Advice	98	80%	83%	80%	100%
Surgical Infection Prevention					
Prophylactic Antibiotic Given[2,3]	508	91%	67%	77%	95%
Prophylactic Antibiotic Selection[2]	157	88%	86%	90%	100%
Prophylactic Antibiotic Stopped[2,3]	490	75%	68%	72%	95%
Pregnancy Care					
Inpatient Neonatal Mortality	-	-	-	-	-
Third or Fourth Degree Laceration	-	-	3.23%	3.63%	3.27%

Bayshore Medical Center

Alternate Name: Columbia Bayshore Medical Center
4000 Spencer Highway
Pasadena, TX 77504
URL: www.bayshoremedical.com
Ownership: Proprietary
Emergency Services: Yes

Phone: 713-359-2000
Fax: 713-359-1958

Accredited: Yes
Licensed Beds: 373

Key Personnel:
President/CEO. . . . . Jeff Holland
Chief Medical Staff. D Patel
Chief Catheterization Laboratory . . . . J Mullins, MD
Director Infection/Disease Control . . . . Janet Dougherty
Director Medical/Surgical Nursing . . . . C Wormuth
OB/GYN Womens Health. . . . . H Sarria, MD
Surgical Services . . . . Mary Sartor

Measure	Cases	This Hospital	State Average	U.S. Average	Top Hospital
Heart Attack Care					
ACE Inhibitor or ARB for LVSD	35	74%	85%	82%	100%
Aspirin at Arrival	212	90%	91%	92%	100%
Aspirin at Discharge	194	88%	90%	90%	100%
Beta Blocker at Arrival	162	86%	85%	87%	100%
Beta Blocker at Discharge	188	87%	86%	90%	100%
Fibrinolytic Medication Timing[1]	4	0%	30%	31%	100%
PCI Within 90 Minutes of Arrival[1]	10	10%	48%	54%	95%
Smoking Cessation Advice	87	99%	90%	88%	100%
Heart Failure Care					
ACE Inhibitor or ARB for LVSD	149	67%	82%	82%	100%
Discharge Instructions	432	30%	60%	61%	93%
Evaluation of LVS Function	592	87%	81%	83%	99%
Smoking Cessation Advice	138	96%	82%	82%	100%
Pneumonia Care					
Appropriate Initial Antibiotic	262	73%	79%	83%	94%
Blood Culture Timing	231	85%	89%	90%	100%
Influenza Vaccine	72	85%	69%	70%	100%
Initial Antibiotic Timing	369	69%	78%	80%	93%
Oxygenation Assessment	445	97%	99%	99%	100%
Pneumococcal Vaccine	241	83%	68%	69%	94%
Smoking Cessation Advice	130	96%	83%	80%	100%
Surgical Infection Prevention					
Prophylactic Antibiotic Given[2,3]	202	39%	67%	77%	95%
Prophylactic Antibiotic Selection[2]	94	67%	86%	90%	100%

NOTE: Hospital profiles are in alphabetical order by state, then city, then hospital within the city; Rankings are sorted by rate in descending order and exclude hospitals with less than 25 cases; (1) The number of cases is too small (n<25) for purposes of reliably predicting hospital performance; (2) Measure reflects the hospital's indication that its submission was based upon a sample of its relevant discharges; (3) Rate reflects fewer than the maximum possible quarters of data for the measure; (4) Inaccurate information submitted and suppressed for one or more quarters; (5) No data is available from the hospital for this measure; Please refer to the User's Guide for a full explanation of data

Prophylactic Antibiotic Stopped[2,3]	184	57%	68%	72%	95%
Pregnancy Care					
Inpatient Neonatal Mortality	-	-	-	-	-
Third or Fourth Degree Laceration	-	-	3.23%	3.63%	3.27%

Vista Medical Center Hospital

4301 B Vista
Pasadena, TX 77504 Phone: 713-378-3000
Ownership: Proprietary Accredited: No
Emergency Services: Yes

Measure	Cases	This Hospital	State Average	U.S. Average	Top Hospital
Heart Attack Care					
ACE Inhibitor or ARB for LVSD[5]	-	-	85%	82%	100%
Aspirin at Arrival[5]	-	-	91%	92%	100%
Aspirin at Discharge[5]	-	-	90%	90%	100%
Beta Blocker at Arrival[5]	-	-	85%	87%	100%
Beta Blocker at Discharge[5]	-	-	86%	90%	100%
Fibrinolytic Medication Timing[5]	-	-	30%	31%	100%
PCI Within 90 Minutes of Arrival[5]	-	-	48%	54%	95%
Smoking Cessation Advice[5]	-	-	90%	88%	100%
Heart Failure Care					
ACE Inhibitor or ARB for LVSD[5]	-	-	82%	82%	100%
Discharge Instructions[5]	-	-	60%	61%	93%
Evaluation of LVS Function[5]	-	-	81%	83%	99%
Smoking Cessation Advice[5]	-	-	82%	82%	100%
Pneumonia Care					
Appropriate Initial Antibiotic[5]	-	-	79%	83%	94%
Blood Culture Timing[5]	-	-	89%	90%	100%
Influenza Vaccine[5]	-	-	69%	70%	100%
Initial Antibiotic Timing[5]	-	-	78%	80%	93%
Oxygenation Assessment[5]	-	-	99%	99%	100%
Pneumococcal Vaccine[5]	-	-	68%	69%	94%
Smoking Cessation Advice[5]	-	-	83%	80%	100%
Surgical Infection Prevention					
Prophylactic Antibiotic Given[2,3]	0	-	67%	77%	95%
Prophylactic Antibiotic Selection[5]	-	-	86%	90%	100%
Prophylactic Antibiotic Stopped[2,3]	0	-	68%	72%	95%
Pregnancy Care					
Inpatient Neonatal Mortality	-	-	-	-	-
Third or Fourth Degree Laceration	-	-	3.23%	3.63%	3.27%

Frio Hospital

200 IH 35 South
Pearsall, TX 78061 Phone: 830-334-3617
E-mail: fhosp@vsta.net Fax: 830-334-9812
URL: www.frioregionalhospital.com
Ownership: Proprietary Accredited: No
Emergency Services: No Licensed Beds: 22
Key Personnel:
CEO. . . . . Alan Holnds
Chief Medical Staff. Ostar Garza
Emergency Room . . . . Becky Waldrum

Measure	Cases	This Hospital	State Average	U.S. Average	Top Hospital
Heart Attack Care					
ACE Inhibitor or ARB for LVSD[3]	0	-	85%	82%	100%
Aspirin at Arrival[1,3]	2	100%	91%	92%	100%
Aspirin at Discharge[3]	0	-	90%	90%	100%
Beta Blocker at Arrival[1,3]	2	100%	85%	87%	100%
Beta Blocker at Discharge[1,3]	1	100%	86%	90%	100%
Fibrinolytic Medication Timing[3]	0	-	30%	31%	100%
PCI Within 90 Minutes of Arrival	0	-	48%	54%	95%
Smoking Cessation Advice[3]	0	-	90%	88%	100%
Heart Failure Care					
ACE Inhibitor or ARB for LVSD[1]	11	100%	82%	82%	100%
Discharge Instructions	34	91%	60%	61%	93%
Evaluation of LVS Function	29	93%	81%	83%	99%
Smoking Cessation Advice[1]	3	100%	82%	82%	100%
Pneumonia Care					
Appropriate Initial Antibiotic	31	90%	79%	83%	94%
Blood Culture Timing	25	80%	89%	90%	100%

Influenza Vaccine[1]	14	100%	69%	70%	100%
Initial Antibiotic Timing	36	94%	78%	80%	93%
Oxygenation Assessment	44	100%	99%	99%	100%
Pneumococcal Vaccine[1]	18	100%	68%	69%	94%
Smoking Cessation Advice[1]	14	93%	83%	80%	100%
Surgical Infection Prevention					
Prophylactic Antibiotic Given	0	-	67%	77%	95%
Prophylactic Antibiotic Selection	0	-	86%	90%	100%
Prophylactic Antibiotic Stopped[3]	0	-	68%	72%	95%
Pregnancy Care					
Inpatient Neonatal Mortality	-	-	-	-	-
Third or Fourth Degree Laceration	-	-	3.23%	3.63%	3.27%

Reeves County Hospital

2323 Texas Street
Pecos, TX 79772 Phone: 432-447-3551
E-mail: nsmith@trhta.net Fax: 432-447-5434
URL: www.reevescountyhospital.com
Ownership: Proprietary Accredited: No
Emergency Services: Yes Licensed Beds: 49
Key Personnel:
President/CEO. . . . . Al LaRochelle
Chief Medical Staff. WJ Bang, MD
Infection Control. Faye Lease
Medical/Surgical Nursing . . . . Carla Winsor-Rivas, RN
Respiratory/Cardiopulmonary. . . . . Frank Vasquez

Measure	Cases	This Hospital	State Average	U.S. Average	Top Hospital
Heart Attack Care					
ACE Inhibitor or ARB for LVSD[3]	0	-	85%	82%	100%
Aspirin at Arrival[3]	0	-	91%	92%	100%
Aspirin at Discharge[3]	0	-	90%	90%	100%
Beta Blocker at Arrival[3]	0	-	85%	87%	100%
Beta Blocker at Discharge[3]	0	-	86%	90%	100%
Fibrinolytic Medication Timing[5]	-	-	30%	31%	100%
PCI Within 90 Minutes of Arrival[5]	-	-	48%	54%	95%
Smoking Cessation Advice[5]	-	-	90%	88%	100%
Heart Failure Care					
ACE Inhibitor or ARB for LVSD	0	-	82%	82%	100%
Discharge Instructions[1,3]	6	17%	60%	61%	93%
Evaluation of LVS Function[1]	24	8%	81%	83%	99%
Smoking Cessation Advice[1,3]	4	100%	82%	82%	100%
Pneumonia Care					
Appropriate Initial Antibiotic[1,3]	5	100%	79%	83%	94%
Blood Culture Timing[1,3]	3	67%	89%	90%	100%
Influenza Vaccine[4,5]	-	-	69%	70%	100%
Initial Antibiotic Timing	36	83%	78%	80%	93%
Oxygenation Assessment	40	100%	99%	99%	100%
Pneumococcal Vaccine	26	27%	68%	69%	94%
Smoking Cessation Advice[1,3]	4	75%	83%	80%	100%
Surgical Infection Prevention					
Prophylactic Antibiotic Given[3]	0	-	67%	77%	95%
Prophylactic Antibiotic Selection[5]	-	-	86%	90%	100%
Prophylactic Antibiotic Stopped[3]	0	-	68%	72%	95%
Pregnancy Care					
Inpatient Neonatal Mortality	-	-	-	-	-
Third or Fourth Degree Laceration	-	-	3.23%	3.63%	3.27%

East Texas Medical Center-Pittsburg

Alternate Name: ETMC Pittsburgh
414 Quitman Street Phone: 903-856-6663
Pittsburg, TX 75686 Fax: 903-856-4598
URL: www.etmc.org
Ownership: Voluntary non-profit - Private Accredited: No
Emergency Services: No Licensed Beds: 49
Key Personnel:
Administrator . . . . W Perry Henderson
Chief Medical Staff. Blair MacBeath, MD
Emergency Room . . . . Ann Henderson
Infection Control. Clarice Hampton, RN
Surgery Manager . . . . Paulia Hays, RN
Respiratory/Cardiopulmonary. . . . . Sharissa Barrett

NOTE: Hospital profiles are in alphabetical order by state, then city, then hospital within the city; Rankings are sorted by rate in descending order and exclude hospitals with less than 25 cases; (1) The number of cases is too small (n<25) for purposes of reliably predicting hospital performance; (2) Measure reflects the hospital's indication that its submission was based upon a sample of its relevant discharges; (3) Rate reflects fewer than the maximum possible quarters of data for the measure; (4) Inaccurate information submitted and suppressed for one or more quarters; (5) No data is available from the hospital for this measure; Please refer to the User's Guide for a full explanation of data

Measure	Cases	This Hospital	State Average	U.S. Average	Top Hospital
Heart Attack Care					
ACE Inhibitor or ARB for LVSD[3]	0	-	85%	82%	100%
Aspirin at Arrival[3]	0	-	91%	92%	100%
Aspirin at Discharge[3]	0	-	90%	90%	100%
Beta Blocker at Arrival[3]	0	-	85%	87%	100%
Beta Blocker at Discharge[3]	0	-	86%	90%	100%
Fibrinolytic Medication Timing[3]	0	-	30%	31%	100%
PCI Within 90 Minutes of Arrival	0	-	48%	54%	95%
Smoking Cessation Advice[3]	0	-	90%	88%	100%
Heart Failure Care					
ACE Inhibitor or ARB for LVSD[1,3]	14	79%	82%	82%	100%
Discharge Instructions[3]	54	54%	60%	61%	93%
Evaluation of LVS Function[3]	79	49%	81%	83%	99%
Smoking Cessation Advice[1,3]	21	71%	82%	82%	100%
Pneumonia Care					
Appropriate Initial Antibiotic[3]	27	81%	79%	83%	94%
Blood Culture Timing[1]	12	100%	89%	90%	100%
Influenza Vaccine[4,5]	-	-	69%	70%	100%
Initial Antibiotic Timing[3]	32	78%	78%	80%	93%
Oxygenation Assessment[3]	40	100%	99%	99%	100%
Pneumococcal Vaccine[1,3]	22	77%	68%	69%	94%
Smoking Cessation Advice[1,3]	9	100%	83%	80%	100%
Surgical Infection Prevention					
Prophylactic Antibiotic Given[1,3]	3	67%	67%	77%	95%
Prophylactic Antibiotic Selection[1]	1	100%	86%	90%	100%
Prophylactic Antibiotic Stopped[1,3]	3	100%	68%	72%	95%
Pregnancy Care					
Inpatient Neonatal Mortality	-	-	-	-	-
Third or Fourth Degree Laceration	-	-	3.23%	3.63%	3.27%

Covenant Hospital Plainview

Alternate Name: Methodist Hospital Plainview
2601 Dimmitt Road
Plainview, TX 79072
E-mail: info@covenantplainview.org
URL: www.covenantplainview.org
Ownership: Voluntary non-profit - Church
Emergency Services: No

Phone: 806-296-5531
Fax: 806-293-1885

Accredited: Yes
Licensed Beds: 100

Key Personnel:
President/CEO . . . . Steve Hunter
Chief Medical Staff . . . . Ponnie Vering

Measure	Cases	This Hospital	State Average	U.S. Average	Top Hospital
Heart Attack Care					
ACE Inhibitor or ARB for LVSD[3]	0	-	85%	82%	100%
Aspirin at Arrival[1,3]	1	100%	91%	92%	100%
Aspirin at Discharge[1,3]	1	100%	90%	90%	100%
Beta Blocker at Arrival[1,3]	1	100%	85%	87%	100%
Beta Blocker at Discharge[1,3]	1	0%	86%	90%	100%
Fibrinolytic Medication Timing[3]	0	-	30%	31%	100%
PCI Within 90 Minutes of Arrival	0	-	48%	54%	95%
Smoking Cessation Advice[3]	0	-	90%	88%	100%
Heart Failure Care					
ACE Inhibitor or ARB for LVSD[1]	15	80%	82%	82%	100%
Discharge Instructions[1,3]	14	36%	60%	61%	93%
Evaluation of LVS Function	60	40%	81%	83%	99%
Smoking Cessation Advice[1,3]	1	0%	82%	82%	100%
Pneumonia Care					
Appropriate Initial Antibiotic[1,3]	7	71%	79%	83%	94%
Blood Culture Timing[1,3]	4	100%	89%	90%	100%
Influenza Vaccine[5]	-	-	69%	70%	100%
Initial Antibiotic Timing	49	71%	78%	80%	93%
Oxygenation Assessment	63	100%	99%	99%	100%
Pneumococcal Vaccine	42	57%	68%	69%	94%
Smoking Cessation Advice[1,3]	2	50%	83%	80%	100%
Surgical Infection Prevention					
Prophylactic Antibiotic Given[1,3]	15	20%	67%	77%	95%
Prophylactic Antibiotic Selection[5]	-	-	86%	90%	100%
Prophylactic Antibiotic Stopped[1,3]	13	100%	68%	72%	95%
Pregnancy Care					
Inpatient Neonatal Mortality	-	-	-	-	-

			3.23%	3.63%	3.27%
Third or Fourth Degree Laceration	-	-	3.23%	3.63%	3.27%

Baylor Regional Medical Center at Plano

4700 Alliance Boulevard   Phone: 469-814-2000
Plano, TX 75093
Ownership: Govt - Hospital District or Authority   Accredited: Yes
Emergency Services: No

Measure	Cases	This Hospital	State Average	U.S. Average	Top Hospital
Heart Attack Care					
ACE Inhibitor or ARB for LVSD	35	100%	85%	82%	100%
Aspirin at Arrival	87	100%	91%	92%	100%
Aspirin at Discharge	122	100%	90%	90%	100%
Beta Blocker at Arrival	77	100%	85%	87%	100%
Beta Blocker at Discharge	122	98%	86%	90%	100%
Fibrinolytic Medication Timing[3]	0	-	30%	31%	100%
PCI Within 90 Minutes of Arrival[1]	3	100%	48%	54%	95%
Smoking Cessation Advice[1,3]	17	100%	90%	88%	100%
Heart Failure Care					
ACE Inhibitor or ARB for LVSD	177	95%	82%	82%	100%
Discharge Instructions[3]	65	95%	60%	61%	93%
Evaluation of LVS Function	266	99%	81%	83%	99%
Smoking Cessation Advice[1,3]	9	100%	82%	82%	100%
Pneumonia Care					
Appropriate Initial Antibiotic[1,3]	10	100%	79%	83%	94%
Blood Culture Timing[1,3]	17	94%	89%	90%	100%
Influenza Vaccine[5]	-	-	69%	70%	100%
Initial Antibiotic Timing	75	92%	78%	80%	93%
Oxygenation Assessment	106	100%	99%	99%	100%
Pneumococcal Vaccine	58	86%	68%	69%	94%
Smoking Cessation Advice[1,3]	2	100%	83%	80%	100%
Surgical Infection Prevention					
Prophylactic Antibiotic Given[3]	124	98%	67%	77%	95%
Prophylactic Antibiotic Selection[5]	-	-	86%	90%	100%
Prophylactic Antibiotic Stopped[3]	113	88%	68%	72%	95%
Pregnancy Care					
Inpatient Neonatal Mortality	-	-	-	-	-
Third or Fourth Degree Laceration	-	-	3.23%	3.63%	3.27%

Medical Center of Plano

3901 West 15th Street   Toll-Free: 800-783-6941
Plano, TX 75075   Phone: 972-596-6800
                                         Fax: 972-519-1423
URL: www.medicalcenterofplano.com
Ownership: Proprietary   Accredited: Yes
Emergency Services: Yes   Licensed Beds: 427
Key Personnel:
President/CEO . . . . Harvey Fishero

Measure	Cases	This Hospital	State Average	U.S. Average	Top Hospital
Heart Attack Care					
ACE Inhibitor or ARB for LVSD	34	91%	85%	82%	100%
Aspirin at Arrival	139	99%	91%	92%	100%
Aspirin at Discharge	132	96%	90%	90%	100%
Beta Blocker at Arrival	109	99%	85%	87%	100%
Beta Blocker at Discharge	154	95%	86%	90%	100%
Fibrinolytic Medication Timing	0	-	30%	31%	100%
PCI Within 90 Minutes of Arrival[1]	11	82%	48%	54%	95%
Smoking Cessation Advice	45	98%	90%	88%	100%
Heart Failure Care					
ACE Inhibitor or ARB for LVSD	131	80%	82%	82%	100%
Discharge Instructions	260	52%	60%	61%	93%
Evaluation of LVS Function	356	94%	81%	83%	99%
Smoking Cessation Advice	57	96%	82%	82%	100%
Pneumonia Care					
Appropriate Initial Antibiotic[2]	136	90%	79%	83%	94%
Blood Culture Timing[2]	148	96%	89%	90%	100%
Influenza Vaccine	58	0%	69%	70%	100%
Initial Antibiotic Timing[2]	211	83%	78%	80%	93%
Oxygenation Assessment[2]	259	100%	99%	99%	100%
Pneumococcal Vaccine[2]	167	83%	68%	69%	94%
Smoking Cessation Advice[2]	49	94%	83%	80%	100%

NOTE: Hospital profiles are in alphabetical order by state, then city, then hospital within the city; Rankings are sorted by rate in descending order and exclude hospitals with less than 25 cases; (1) The number of cases is too small (n<25) for purposes of reliably predicting hospital performance; (2) Measure reflects the hospital's indication that its submission was based upon a sample of its relevant discharges; (3) Rate reflects fewer than the maximum possible quarters of data for the measure; (4) Inaccurate information submitted and suppressed for one or more quarters; (5) No data is available from the hospital for this measure; Please refer to the User's Guide for a full explanation of data

Surgical Infection Prevention					
Prophylactic Antibiotic Given[2,3]	194	83%	67%	77%	95%
Prophylactic Antibiotic Selection[2]	93	89%	86%	90%	100%
Prophylactic Antibiotic Stopped[2,3]	178	66%	68%	72%	95%
Pregnancy Care					
Inpatient Neonatal Mortality	-	-	-	-	-
Third or Fourth Degree Laceration	-	-	3.23%	3.63%	3.27%

Presbyterian Hospital of Plano

6200 W Parker Boulevard
Plano, TX 75093
URL: www.texashealth.org
Ownership: Voluntary non-profit - Private
Emergency Services: Yes

Phone: 972-981-8000
Fax: 972-981-3010

Accredited: Yes
Licensed Beds: 231

Key Personnel:
President . . . . Philip M Wentworth

Measure	Cases	This Hospital	State Average	U.S. Average	Top Hospital
Heart Attack Care					
ACE Inhibitor or ARB for LVSD	28	89%	85%	82%	100%
Aspirin at Arrival	133	100%	91%	92%	100%
Aspirin at Discharge	178	92%	90%	90%	100%
Beta Blocker at Arrival	108	98%	85%	87%	100%
Beta Blocker at Discharge	170	96%	86%	90%	100%
Fibrinolytic Medication Timing	0	-	30%	31%	100%
PCI Within 90 Minutes of Arrival[1]	10	40%	48%	54%	95%
Smoking Cessation Advice	57	98%	90%	88%	100%
Heart Failure Care					
ACE Inhibitor or ARB for LVSD	46	89%	82%	82%	100%
Discharge Instructions	146	88%	60%	61%	93%
Evaluation of LVS Function	172	98%	81%	83%	99%
Smoking Cessation Advice	36	97%	82%	82%	100%
Pneumonia Care					
Appropriate Initial Antibiotic	115	79%	79%	83%	94%
Blood Culture Timing	93	98%	89%	90%	100%
Influenza Vaccine	27	56%	69%	70%	100%
Initial Antibiotic Timing	120	82%	78%	80%	93%
Oxygenation Assessment	150	100%	99%	99%	100%
Pneumococcal Vaccine	66	86%	68%	69%	94%
Smoking Cessation Advice	37	100%	83%	80%	100%
Surgical Infection Prevention					
Prophylactic Antibiotic Given[2,3]	180	74%	67%	77%	95%
Prophylactic Antibiotic Selection[2]	55	95%	86%	90%	100%
Prophylactic Antibiotic Stopped[2,3]	174	65%	68%	72%	95%
Pregnancy Care					
Inpatient Neonatal Mortality	-	-	-	-	-
Third or Fourth Degree Laceration	-	-	3.23%	3.63%	3.27%

Presbyterian Plano Ctr for Diag & Surgery

6020 W Parker Road
Plano, TX 75093
Ownership: Proprietary
Emergency Services: Yes

Phone: 972-403-2700

Accredited: Yes

Measure	Cases	This Hospital	State Average	U.S. Average	Top Hospital
Heart Attack Care					
ACE Inhibitor or ARB for LVSD[5]	-	-	85%	82%	100%
Aspirin at Arrival[5]	-	-	91%	92%	100%
Aspirin at Discharge[5]	-	-	90%	90%	100%
Beta Blocker at Arrival[5]	-	-	85%	87%	100%
Beta Blocker at Discharge[5]	-	-	86%	90%	100%
Fibrinolytic Medication Timing[5]	-	-	30%	31%	100%
PCI Within 90 Minutes of Arrival[5]	-	-	48%	54%	95%
Smoking Cessation Advice[5]	-	-	90%	88%	100%
Heart Failure Care					
ACE Inhibitor or ARB for LVSD[5]	-	-	82%	82%	100%
Discharge Instructions[5]	-	-	60%	61%	93%
Evaluation of LVS Function[5]	-	-	81%	83%	99%
Smoking Cessation Advice[5]	-	-	82%	82%	100%
Pneumonia Care					
Appropriate Initial Antibiotic[5]	-	-	79%	83%	94%
Blood Culture Timing[5]	-	-	89%	90%	100%

Influenza Vaccine[5]	-	-	69%	70%	100%
Initial Antibiotic Timing[5]	-	-	78%	80%	93%
Oxygenation Assessment[5]	-	-	99%	99%	100%
Pneumococcal Vaccine[5]	-	-	68%	69%	94%
Smoking Cessation Advice[5]	-	-	83%	80%	100%
Surgical Infection Prevention					
Prophylactic Antibiotic Given[3]	42	88%	67%	77%	95%
Prophylactic Antibiotic Selection[5]	-	-	86%	90%	100%
Prophylactic Antibiotic Stopped[3]	42	100%	68%	72%	95%
Pregnancy Care					
Inpatient Neonatal Mortality	-	-	-	-	-
Third or Fourth Degree Laceration	-	-	3.23%	3.63%	3.27%

Medical Center of Southeast Texas

2555 Jimmy Johnson Boulevard
Port Arthur, TX 76640
URL: www.medicalcentertexas.com
Ownership: Proprietary
Emergency Services: No

Phone: 409-724-7389
Fax: 409-853-5182

Accredited: Yes
Licensed Beds: 224

Key Personnel:
CEO. . . . . Craig Desmond

Measure	Cases	This Hospital	State Average	U.S. Average	Top Hospital
Heart Attack Care					
ACE Inhibitor or ARB for LVSD	27	78%	85%	82%	100%
Aspirin at Arrival	101	92%	91%	92%	100%
Aspirin at Discharge	107	94%	90%	90%	100%
Beta Blocker at Arrival	92	83%	85%	87%	100%
Beta Blocker at Discharge	106	94%	86%	90%	100%
Fibrinolytic Medication Timing[1]	1	0%	30%	31%	100%
PCI Within 90 Minutes of Arrival[1]	9	33%	48%	54%	95%
Smoking Cessation Advice	32	100%	90%	88%	100%
Heart Failure Care					
ACE Inhibitor or ARB for LVSD	97	84%	82%	82%	100%
Discharge Instructions	236	67%	60%	61%	93%
Evaluation of LVS Function	283	92%	81%	83%	99%
Smoking Cessation Advice	52	100%	82%	82%	100%
Pneumonia Care					
Appropriate Initial Antibiotic	135	63%	79%	83%	94%
Blood Culture Timing	52	75%	89%	90%	100%
Influenza Vaccine	26	31%	69%	70%	100%
Initial Antibiotic Timing	134	54%	78%	80%	93%
Oxygenation Assessment	165	98%	99%	99%	100%
Pneumococcal Vaccine	97	41%	68%	69%	94%
Smoking Cessation Advice	35	100%	83%	80%	100%
Surgical Infection Prevention					
Prophylactic Antibiotic Given[3]	259	63%	67%	77%	95%
Prophylactic Antibiotic Selection	83	70%	86%	90%	100%
Prophylactic Antibiotic Stopped[3]	255	44%	68%	72%	95%
Pregnancy Care					
Inpatient Neonatal Mortality	-	-	-	-	-
Third or Fourth Degree Laceration	-	-	3.23%	3.63%	3.27%

Memorial Medical Center

Alternate Name: Champ Traylor Memorial
815 N Virginia
Port Lavaca, TX 77979
URL: www.mmcportlavaca.com
Ownership: Proprietary
Emergency Services: No

Phone: 361-552-6713
Fax: 361-552-0312

Accredited: No
Licensed Beds: 49

Key Personnel:
CEO. . . . . Eowod Corrier Jr
Chief Medical Staff. . . . . Richard Aroyo, MD
Director of Cardiology/Cardiac Lab. . . . . Mau Shoun Lin
Emergency Room . . . . Richerd Lorenz
Emergency Room . . . . Paul Bunnell
Director Infection/Disease Control . . . . Nadine Arnold, RN
Intensive Coronary Care . . . . Darleen Tripp, RN
Medical Surgical Nursing . . . . Pat Delgodo
OB/GYN Womens Health. . . . . GA William, MD
Director Respiratory Therapy . . . . Art Mabray

Measure	Cases	This Hospital	State Average	U.S. Average	Top Hospital

NOTE: Hospital profiles are in alphabetical order by state, then city, then hospital within the city; Rankings are sorted by rate in descending order and exclude hospitals with less than 25 cases; (1) The number of cases is too small (n<25) for purposes of reliably predicting hospital performance; (2) Measure reflects the hospital's indication that its submission was based upon a sample of its relevant discharges; (3) Rate reflects fewer than the maximum possible quarters of data for the measure; (4) Inaccurate information submitted and suppressed for one or more quarters; (5) No data is available from the hospital for this measure; Please refer to the User's Guide for a full explanation of data

	Heart Attack Care				
ACE Inhibitor or ARB for LVSD[1]	5	100%	85%	82%	100%
Aspirin at Arrival[1]	9	100%	91%	92%	100%
Aspirin at Discharge[1]	6	100%	90%	90%	100%
Beta Blocker at Arrival[1]	9	89%	85%	87%	100%
Beta Blocker at Discharge[1]	6	83%	86%	90%	100%
Fibrinolytic Medication Timing[1]	1	100%	30%	31%	100%
PCI Within 90 Minutes of Arrival	0	-	48%	54%	95%
Smoking Cessation Advice[1]	1	0%	90%	88%	100%
Heart Failure Care					
ACE Inhibitor or ARB for LVSD[1]	15	40%	82%	82%	100%
Discharge Instructions	43	70%	60%	61%	93%
Evaluation of LVS Function	51	45%	81%	83%	99%
Smoking Cessation Advice[1]	9	67%	82%	82%	100%
Pneumonia Care					
Appropriate Initial Antibiotic	64	52%	79%	83%	94%
Blood Culture Timing[1]	10	90%	89%	90%	100%
Influenza Vaccine[1]	13	46%	69%	70%	100%
Initial Antibiotic Timing	48	73%	78%	80%	93%
Oxygenation Assessment	65	98%	99%	99%	100%
Pneumococcal Vaccine	36	58%	68%	69%	94%
Smoking Cessation Advice[1]	14	86%	83%	80%	100%
Surgical Infection Prevention					
Prophylactic Antibiotic Given[1,3]	8	38%	67%	77%	95%
Prophylactic Antibiotic Selection[1]	1	100%	86%	90%	100%
Prophylactic Antibiotic Stopped[1,3]	8	62%	68%	72%	95%
Pregnancy Care					
Inpatient Neonatal Mortality	-	-	-	-	-
Third or Fourth Degree Laceration	-	-	3.23%	3.63%	3.27%

East Texas Medical Center-Quitman

Alternate Name: Wood County Central Hospital District
117 Winnsboro Street   Phone: 903-763-6300
Quitman, TX 75783   Fax: 903-763-6120
URL: www.etmc.org
Ownership: Voluntary non-profit - Private   Accredited: Yes
Emergency Services: Yes   Licensed Beds: 30
Key Personnel:
Administrator/CEO . . . . Ernest R Parisi

Measure	Cases	This Hospital	State Average	U.S. Average	Top Hospital
Heart Attack Care					
ACE Inhibitor or ARB for LVSD	0	-	85%	82%	100%
Aspirin at Arrival[1]	8	88%	91%	92%	100%
Aspirin at Discharge[1]	6	83%	90%	90%	100%
Beta Blocker at Arrival[1]	7	71%	85%	87%	100%
Beta Blocker at Discharge[1]	6	83%	86%	90%	100%
Fibrinolytic Medication Timing	0	-	30%	31%	100%
PCI Within 90 Minutes of Arrival	0	-	48%	54%	95%
Smoking Cessation Advice[1]	1	100%	90%	88%	100%
Heart Failure Care					
ACE Inhibitor or ARB for LVSD[1]	12	100%	82%	82%	100%
Discharge Instructions	55	58%	60%	61%	93%
Evaluation of LVS Function	80	74%	81%	83%	99%
Smoking Cessation Advice[1]	8	75%	82%	82%	100%
Pneumonia Care					
Appropriate Initial Antibiotic	43	86%	79%	83%	94%
Blood Culture Timing	37	81%	89%	90%	100%
Influenza Vaccine[1]	17	76%	69%	70%	100%
Initial Antibiotic Timing	57	91%	78%	80%	93%
Oxygenation Assessment	75	100%	99%	99%	100%
Pneumococcal Vaccine	51	94%	68%	69%	94%
Smoking Cessation Advice[1]	16	81%	83%	80%	100%
Surgical Infection Prevention					
Prophylactic Antibiotic Given[1,3]	13	62%	67%	77%	95%
Prophylactic Antibiotic Selection[1]	6	100%	86%	90%	100%
Prophylactic Antibiotic Stopped[1,3]	13	23%	68%	72%	95%
Pregnancy Care					
Inpatient Neonatal Mortality	-	-	-	-	-
Third or Fourth Degree Laceration	-	-	3.23%	3.63%	3.27%

Richardson Medical Center

401 W Campbell Road   Phone: 972-498-4000
Richardson, TX 75080   Fax: 972-498-7660
E-mail: webmaster@richardsonhealth.com
URL: www.richardsonregional.com
Ownership: Govt - Hospital District or Authority   Accredited: Yes
Emergency Services: Yes   Licensed Beds: 205
Key Personnel:
CEO. . . . . Ronald L Boring
Chief Medical Staff. . . . . Miriam Siblay, MD
Chief Medical Staff. . . . . Steve Hebert, MD
Manager Cardiac Lab. . . . . Ian Chenevert
Manager Catheterization Lab. . . . . Ian Chenevert
Manager ER. . . . . Melissa Oliver
Emergency Room . . . . Bryan Scott, MD
Director Infection Control . . . . Nancy Viamonte
ICU . . . . Dawn Partner
Manager Intensive Coronary . . . . Dawn Parten
Manager Surgical. . . . . Marlene Spadini
Director OB/GYN/Women's Health. . . . . TM Snyder
Director Radiology . . . . Greg Cooper
Director Respiratory/Cardiopulmonary . . . . Suzanne Grayson

Measure	Cases	This Hospital	State Average	U.S. Average	Top Hospital
Heart Attack Care					
ACE Inhibitor or ARB for LVSD	35	100%	85%	82%	100%
Aspirin at Arrival	104	99%	91%	92%	100%
Aspirin at Discharge	93	98%	90%	90%	100%
Beta Blocker at Arrival	84	100%	85%	87%	100%
Beta Blocker at Discharge	85	98%	86%	90%	100%
Fibrinolytic Medication Timing[1]	1	100%	30%	31%	100%
PCI Within 90 Minutes of Arrival[1]	6	83%	48%	54%	95%
Smoking Cessation Advice[1]	23	100%	90%	88%	100%
Heart Failure Care					
ACE Inhibitor or ARB for LVSD	59	98%	82%	82%	100%
Discharge Instructions	105	67%	60%	61%	93%
Evaluation of LVS Function	147	95%	81%	83%	99%
Smoking Cessation Advice[1]	14	100%	82%	82%	100%
Pneumonia Care					
Appropriate Initial Antibiotic	109	83%	79%	83%	94%
Blood Culture Timing	103	95%	89%	90%	100%
Influenza Vaccine	27	44%	69%	70%	100%
Initial Antibiotic Timing	159	91%	78%	80%	93%
Oxygenation Assessment	192	100%	99%	99%	100%
Pneumococcal Vaccine	114	73%	68%	69%	94%
Smoking Cessation Advice	34	97%	83%	80%	100%
Surgical Infection Prevention					
Prophylactic Antibiotic Given[2,3]	182	64%	67%	77%	95%
Prophylactic Antibiotic Selection[2]	53	87%	86%	90%	100%
Prophylactic Antibiotic Stopped[2,3]	178	67%	68%	72%	95%
Pregnancy Care					
Inpatient Neonatal Mortality	-	-	-	-	-
Third or Fourth Degree Laceration	-	-	3.23%	3.63%	3.27%

Oakbend Medical Center

1705 Jackson Street   Phone: 281-341-3000
Richmond, TX 77469   Fax: 281-341-2883
URL: www.oakbendmedcenter.org
Ownership: Govt - Hospital District or Authority   Accredited: Yes
Emergency Services: Yes   Licensed Beds: 185
Key Personnel:
CEO. . . . . David B Rowe

Measure	Cases	This Hospital	State Average	U.S. Average	Top Hospital
Heart Attack Care					
ACE Inhibitor or ARB for LVSD[1]	9	56%	85%	82%	100%
Aspirin at Arrival	36	97%	91%	92%	100%
Aspirin at Discharge[1]	18	67%	90%	90%	100%
Beta Blocker at Arrival	35	97%	85%	87%	100%
Beta Blocker at Discharge[1]	18	67%	86%	90%	100%
Fibrinolytic Medication Timing[1]	4	0%	30%	31%	100%
PCI Within 90 Minutes of Arrival	0	-	48%	54%	95%
Smoking Cessation Advice[1]	2	100%	90%	88%	100%

NOTE: Hospital profiles are in alphabetical order by state, then city, then hospital within the city; Rankings are sorted by rate in descending order and exclude hospitals with less than 25 cases; (1) The number of cases is too small (n<25) for purposes of reliably predicting hospital performance; (2) Measure reflects the hospital's indication that its submission was based upon a sample of its relevant discharges; (3) Rate reflects fewer than the maximum possible quarters of data for the measure; (4) Inaccurate information submitted and suppressed for one or more quarters; (5) No data is available from the hospital for this measure; Please refer to the User's Guide for a full explanation of data

Heart Failure Care				
ACE Inhibitor or ARB for LVSD	70	71%	82%	82%	100%
Discharge Instructions	144	91%	60%	61%	93%
Evaluation of LVS Function	180	81%	81%	83%	99%
Smoking Cessation Advice[1]	24	92%	82%	82%	100%
Pneumonia Care					
Appropriate Initial Antibiotic	156	74%	79%	83%	94%
Blood Culture Timing	138	95%	89%	90%	100%
Influenza Vaccine[4,5]	-	-	69%	70%	100%
Initial Antibiotic Timing	221	84%	78%	80%	93%
Oxygenation Assessment	257	97%	99%	99%	100%
Pneumococcal Vaccine	150	59%	68%	69%	94%
Smoking Cessation Advice	40	88%	83%	80%	100%
Surgical Infection Prevention					
Prophylactic Antibiotic Given[3]	166	67%	67%	77%	95%
Prophylactic Antibiotic Selection	63	89%	86%	90%	100%
Prophylactic Antibiotic Stopped[3]	151	89%	68%	72%	95%
Pregnancy Care					
Inpatient Neonatal Mortality	-	-	-	-	-
Third or Fourth Degree Laceration	-	-	3.23%	3.63%	3.27%

Starr County Memorial Hospital

PO Box 78
Rio Grande City, TX 78582
E-mail: contact@starrcountyhospital.com
URL: www.starrcountyhospital.com
Ownership: Govt - Hospital District or Authority
Emergency Services: No

Phone: 956-487-5561
Fax: 956-487-0332

Accredited: No
Licensed Beds: 49

Key Personnel:
President/CEO........................ Thalia H Munoz
Chief Medical Staff.................... Porfirio Rodriguez, MD
Emergency Room .... Mario Segura, RN
Director Infection/Disease Control .... Mario Segura, RN
Director Medical/Surgical Nursing .... Mario Segura, RN

Measure	Cases	This Hospital	State Average	U.S. Average	Top Hospital
Heart Attack Care					
ACE Inhibitor or ARB for LVSD[1]	5	40%	85%	82%	100%
Aspirin at Arrival	35	97%	91%	92%	100%
Aspirin at Discharge	25	100%	90%	90%	100%
Beta Blocker at Arrival	34	91%	85%	87%	100%
Beta Blocker at Discharge	25	88%	86%	90%	100%
Fibrinolytic Medication Timing[3]	0	-	30%	31%	100%
PCI Within 90 Minutes of Arrival	0	-	48%	54%	95%
Smoking Cessation Advice[3]	0	-	90%	88%	100%
Heart Failure Care					
ACE Inhibitor or ARB for LVSD[1]	14	93%	82%	82%	100%
Discharge Instructions[1,3]	14	0%	60%	61%	93%
Evaluation of LVS Function	69	59%	81%	83%	99%
Smoking Cessation Advice[1,3]	2	0%	82%	82%	100%
Pneumonia Care					
Appropriate Initial Antibiotic[1,3]	8	62%	79%	83%	94%
Blood Culture Timing[1,3]	6	100%	89%	90%	100%
Influenza Vaccine[5]	-	-	69%	70%	100%
Initial Antibiotic Timing	46	59%	78%	80%	93%
Oxygenation Assessment	61	98%	99%	99%	100%
Pneumococcal Vaccine	42	10%	68%	69%	94%
Smoking Cessation Advice[1,3]	1	0%	83%	80%	100%
Surgical Infection Prevention					
Prophylactic Antibiotic Given[5]	-	-	67%	77%	95%
Prophylactic Antibiotic Selection[5]	-	-	86%	90%	100%
Prophylactic Antibiotic Stopped[5]	-	-	68%	72%	95%
Pregnancy Care					
Inpatient Neonatal Mortality	-	-	-	-	-
Third or Fourth Degree Laceration	-	-	3.23%	3.63%	3.27%

Round Rock Medical Center

2400 Round Rock Avenue
Round Rock, TX 78681
URL: www.roundrockmedicalcenter.com
Ownership: Proprietary
Emergency Services: Yes

Phone: 512-341-1000
Fax: 512-341-5216

Accredited: Yes
Licensed Beds: 107

Key Personnel:
CEO................................ Deborah Ryle
Chief Medical Staff.................. Dr. John Costanz
Director Emergency Department .... Camille Compton, RN
Emergency Room .... Arthur Boone, MD
Director Medical Surgical Nursing .... Donna Trickey
Director Womens Services................ Darlene McQueen
Director Surgical Services .... Tom Williamson

Measure	Cases	This Hospital	State Average	U.S. Average	Top Hospital
Heart Attack Care					
ACE Inhibitor or ARB for LVSD[1]	24	96%	85%	82%	100%
Aspirin at Arrival	125	99%	91%	92%	100%
Aspirin at Discharge	126	93%	90%	90%	100%
Beta Blocker at Arrival	105	97%	85%	87%	100%
Beta Blocker at Discharge	117	93%	86%	90%	100%
Fibrinolytic Medication Timing	0	-	30%	31%	100%
PCI Within 90 Minutes of Arrival[1]	12	67%	48%	54%	95%
Smoking Cessation Advice	52	98%	90%	88%	100%
Heart Failure Care					
ACE Inhibitor or ARB for LVSD	50	86%	82%	82%	100%
Discharge Instructions	114	54%	60%	61%	93%
Evaluation of LVS Function	145	94%	81%	83%	99%
Smoking Cessation Advice[1]	19	100%	82%	82%	100%
Pneumonia Care					
Appropriate Initial Antibiotic	172	87%	79%	83%	94%
Blood Culture Timing	136	95%	89%	90%	100%
Influenza Vaccine	36	78%	69%	70%	100%
Initial Antibiotic Timing	206	77%	78%	80%	93%
Oxygenation Assessment	222	100%	99%	99%	100%
Pneumococcal Vaccine	121	78%	68%	69%	94%
Smoking Cessation Advice	61	97%	83%	80%	100%
Surgical Infection Prevention					
Prophylactic Antibiotic Given[2,3]	172	78%	67%	77%	95%
Prophylactic Antibiotic Selection[2]	79	96%	86%	90%	100%
Prophylactic Antibiotic Stopped[2,3]	165	50%	68%	72%	95%
Pregnancy Care					
Inpatient Neonatal Mortality	1,782	0.22%	-	-	-
Third or Fourth Degree Laceration	1,169	4.11%	3.23%	3.63%	3.27%

Lake Pointe Medical Center

6800 Scenic Drive
Rowlett, TX 75088
URL: www.lakepointemedical.com
Ownership: Proprietary
Emergency Services: Yes

Phone: 972-412-2273
Fax: 972-475-8345

Accredited: Yes
Licensed Beds: 99

Key Personnel:
CEO................................ John Harris
Chief Medical Staff.................. David Lensch, MD
Emergency Room .... John MacKenzie, DO
Director Infection/Disease Control .... Maria Sparks, RN
CCU Spvg. Nurse .... Patricia Batseli, RN
Director Medical/Surgical Nursing .... Jan Jones, RN
OB/GYN Womens Health................ Tom Sudela
Chief Radiology .... Joel Carp, MD
Director Respiratory Therapy .... Allen Blunt, RRT

Measure	Cases	This Hospital	State Average	U.S. Average	Top Hospital
Heart Attack Care					
ACE Inhibitor or ARB for LVSD[1]	8	100%	85%	82%	100%
Aspirin at Arrival	52	100%	91%	92%	100%
Aspirin at Discharge[1]	22	100%	90%	90%	100%
Beta Blocker at Arrival	50	98%	85%	87%	100%
Beta Blocker at Discharge[1]	24	100%	86%	90%	100%
Fibrinolytic Medication Timing	0	-	30%	31%	100%
PCI Within 90 Minutes of Arrival	0	-	48%	54%	95%
Smoking Cessation Advice[1]	2	100%	90%	88%	100%

NOTE: Hospital profiles are in alphabetical order by state, then city, then hospital within the city; Rankings are sorted by rate in descending order and exclude hospitals with less than 25 cases; (1) The number of cases is too small (n<25) for purposes of reliably predicting hospital performance; (2) Measure reflects the hospital's indication that its submission was based upon a sample of its relevant discharges; (3) Rate reflects fewer than the maximum possible quarters of data for the measure; (4) Inaccurate information submitted and suppressed for one or more quarters; (5) No data is available from the hospital for this measure; Please refer to the User's Guide for a full explanation of data

Heart Failure Care					
ACE Inhibitor or ARB for LVSD	43	100%	82%	82%	100%
Discharge Instructions	97	93%	60%	61%	93%
Evaluation of LVS Function	147	100%	81%	83%	99%
Smoking Cessation Advice[1]	20	100%	82%	82%	100%
Pneumonia Care					
Appropriate Initial Antibiotic	100	89%	79%	83%	94%
Blood Culture Timing	166	97%	89%	90%	100%
Influenza Vaccine[4,5]	-	-	69%	70%	100%
Initial Antibiotic Timing	207	93%	78%	80%	93%
Oxygenation Assessment	290	100%	99%	99%	100%
Pneumococcal Vaccine	170	99%	68%	69%	94%
Smoking Cessation Advice	64	100%	83%	80%	100%
Surgical Infection Prevention					
Prophylactic Antibiotic Given[2]	164	73%	67%	77%	95%
Prophylactic Antibiotic Selection[2]	41	88%	86%	90%	100%
Prophylactic Antibiotic Stopped[2]	138	51%	68%	72%	95%
Pregnancy Care					
Inpatient Neonatal Mortality	-	-	-	-	-
Third or Fourth Degree Laceration	-	-	3.23%	3.63%	3.27%

San Angelo Community Medical Center

Alternate Name: Columbia Medical Center of San Angelo
3501 Knickerbocker Road
San Angelo, TX 76904
Phone: 915-947-6436
Fax: 325-947-6523
URL: www.sacmc.com
Ownership: Proprietary
Emergency Services: Yes
Accredited: Yes
Licensed Beds: 168

Key Personnel:
CEO . . . . Samuel G Feazell
OB/GYN Womens Health . . . . Brenda Spence

Measure	Cases	This Hospital	State Average	U.S. Average	Top Hospital
Heart Attack Care					
ACE Inhibitor or ARB for LVSD[1]	12	100%	85%	82%	100%
Aspirin at Arrival	76	99%	91%	92%	100%
Aspirin at Discharge	84	100%	90%	90%	100%
Beta Blocker at Arrival	64	98%	85%	87%	100%
Beta Blocker at Discharge	82	100%	86%	90%	100%
Fibrinolytic Medication Timing[1]	9	44%	30%	31%	100%
PCI Within 90 Minutes of Arrival	0	-	48%	54%	95%
Smoking Cessation Advice	28	100%	90%	88%	100%
Heart Failure Care					
ACE Inhibitor or ARB for LVSD[1]	23	100%	82%	82%	100%
Discharge Instructions	105	76%	60%	61%	93%
Evaluation of LVS Function	149	97%	81%	83%	99%
Smoking Cessation Advice	26	96%	82%	82%	100%
Pneumonia Care					
Appropriate Initial Antibiotic	123	84%	79%	83%	94%
Blood Culture Timing	129	96%	89%	90%	100%
Influenza Vaccine	57	60%	69%	70%	100%
Initial Antibiotic Timing	190	78%	78%	80%	93%
Oxygenation Assessment	224	100%	99%	99%	100%
Pneumococcal Vaccine	156	83%	68%	69%	94%
Smoking Cessation Advice	32	100%	83%	80%	100%
Surgical Infection Prevention					
Prophylactic Antibiotic Given	432	85%	67%	77%	95%
Prophylactic Antibiotic Selection	103	69%	86%	90%	100%
Prophylactic Antibiotic Stopped	406	76%	68%	72%	95%
Pregnancy Care					
Inpatient Neonatal Mortality	-	-	-	-	-
Third or Fourth Degree Laceration	-	-	3.23%	3.63%	3.27%

Shannon Medical Center

Alternate Name: Shannon West Texas Memorial Hospital
120 E Harris Street
San Angelo, TX 76903
Phone: 325-653-6741
Fax: 325-657-5706
E-mail: hr@shannonhealth.org
URL: www.shannonhealth.com
Ownership: Voluntary non-profit - Other
Emergency Services: Yes
Accredited: Yes
Licensed Beds: 400

Key Personnel:
President/CEO . . . . Bryan Horner

Director Medical/Surgical Nursing . . . . Becky Ellis
Director Respiratory Therapy . . . . W Longoria

Measure	Cases	This Hospital	State Average	U.S. Average	Top Hospital
Heart Attack Care					
ACE Inhibitor or ARB for LVSD	63	84%	85%	82%	100%
Aspirin at Arrival	125	98%	91%	92%	100%
Aspirin at Discharge	121	96%	90%	90%	100%
Beta Blocker at Arrival	105	92%	85%	87%	100%
Beta Blocker at Discharge	146	99%	86%	90%	100%
Fibrinolytic Medication Timing[1,3]	3	33%	30%	31%	100%
PCI Within 90 Minutes of Arrival[1]	6	0%	48%	54%	95%
Smoking Cessation Advice[1,3]	10	100%	90%	88%	100%
Heart Failure Care					
ACE Inhibitor or ARB for LVSD	92	90%	82%	82%	100%
Discharge Instructions[3]	33	64%	60%	61%	93%
Evaluation of LVS Function	220	88%	81%	83%	99%
Smoking Cessation Advice[1,3]	11	100%	82%	82%	100%
Pneumonia Care					
Appropriate Initial Antibiotic[3]	29	72%	79%	83%	94%
Blood Culture Timing[3]	28	96%	89%	90%	100%
Influenza Vaccine[5]	-	-	69%	70%	100%
Initial Antibiotic Timing	255	74%	78%	80%	93%
Oxygenation Assessment	308	100%	99%	99%	100%
Pneumococcal Vaccine	222	86%	68%	69%	94%
Smoking Cessation Advice[1,3]	15	100%	83%	80%	100%
Surgical Infection Prevention					
Prophylactic Antibiotic Given[3]	218	89%	67%	77%	95%
Prophylactic Antibiotic Selection[5]	-	-	86%	90%	100%
Prophylactic Antibiotic Stopped[3]	215	55%	68%	72%	95%
Pregnancy Care					
Inpatient Neonatal Mortality	-	-	-	-	-
Third or Fourth Degree Laceration	-	-	3.23%	3.63%	3.27%

Baptist Medical Center

111 Dallas Street
San Antonio, TX 78205
Phone: 210-297-7000
Fax: 210-297-0700
URL: www.baptisthealthsystem.org
Ownership: Proprietary
Emergency Services: Yes
Accredited: No
Licensed Beds: 375

Key Personnel:
President/CEO . . . . Kent H Wallace
President Medical Staff . . . . Harry Hernandez
VP/Assistant Admin. Catheterization Lab. . . . . . Lea Martinez
Director Emergency Room . . . . Nathan Cobburn
Director Infection Control . . . . Claudia Doss
Intensive Coronary Care Unit . . . . Dot Brosig
Director Med/Surg . . . . Karen Ricks
Director OB/GYN/Women's Health . . . . Christi Garfield
Director Respiratory Therapy . . . . Raul Bocanggrai

Measure	Cases	This Hospital	State Average	U.S. Average	Top Hospital
Heart Attack Care					
ACE Inhibitor or ARB for LVSD[2]	50	66%	85%	82%	100%
Aspirin at Arrival[2]	239	95%	91%	92%	100%
Aspirin at Discharge[2]	262	91%	90%	90%	100%
Beta Blocker at Arrival[2]	154	95%	85%	87%	100%
Beta Blocker at Discharge[2]	273	94%	86%	90%	100%
Fibrinolytic Medication Timing[2]	0	-	30%	31%	100%
PCI Within 90 Minutes of Arrival[1,2]	8	38%	48%	54%	95%
Smoking Cessation Advice[2]	84	98%	90%	88%	100%
Heart Failure Care					
ACE Inhibitor or ARB for LVSD[2]	113	68%	82%	82%	100%
Discharge Instructions[2]	344	78%	60%	61%	93%
Evaluation of LVS Function[2]	431	88%	81%	83%	99%
Smoking Cessation Advice[2]	71	94%	82%	82%	100%
Pneumonia Care					
Appropriate Initial Antibiotic[2]	166	88%	79%	83%	94%
Blood Culture Timing[2]	260	93%	89%	90%	100%
Influenza Vaccine[2]	100	77%	69%	70%	100%
Initial Antibiotic Timing[2]	376	80%	78%	80%	93%
Oxygenation Assessment[2]	441	100%	99%	99%	100%

NOTE: Hospital profiles are in alphabetical order by state, then city, then hospital within the city; Rankings are sorted by rate in descending order and exclude hospitals with less than 25 cases; (1) The number of cases is too small (n<25) for purposes of reliably predicting hospital performance; (2) Measure reflects the hospital's indication that its submission was based upon a sample of its relevant discharges; (3) Rate reflects fewer than the maximum possible quarters of data for the measure; (4) Inaccurate information submitted and suppressed for one or more quarters; (5) No data is available from the hospital for this measure; Please refer to the User's Guide for a full explanation of data

Pneumococcal Vaccine[2]	289	71%	68%	69%	94%
Smoking Cessation Advice[2]	83	90%	83%	80%	100%
Surgical Infection Prevention					
Prophylactic Antibiotic Given[2]	498	87%	67%	77%	95%
Prophylactic Antibiotic Selection[2]	117	96%	86%	90%	100%
Prophylactic Antibiotic Stopped[2]	463	71%	68%	72%	95%
Pregnancy Care					
Inpatient Neonatal Mortality	9,512	0.26%	-	-	-
Third or Fourth Degree Laceration	6,040	2.40%	3.23%	3.63%	3.27%

Christus Santa Rosa Hospital-City Centre

Alternate Name: Santa Rosa Health Care
333 North Santa Rosa Street
San Antonio, TX 78207
URL: www.christussantarosa.org
Ownership: Voluntary non-profit - Church
Emergency Services: Yes

Phone: 210-704-2011
Fax: 210-704-3632

Accredited: Yes
Licensed Beds: 1,034

Key Personnel:
President/CEO . . . . Don A Beeler
Chief Medical Staff . . . . Richard Wayne
Emergency Room . . . . Prentis Vaughn, MD
Director Infection/Disease Control . . . . Nancy Mendicino
Chief Radiology . . . . Joaquin Mira, MD

Measure	Cases	This Hospital	State Average	U.S. Average	Top Hospital
Heart Attack Care					
ACE Inhibitor or ARB for LVSD	28	96%	85%	82%	100%
Aspirin at Arrival	161	100%	91%	92%	100%
Aspirin at Discharge	160	98%	90%	90%	100%
Beta Blocker at Arrival	143	98%	85%	87%	100%
Beta Blocker at Discharge	164	98%	86%	90%	100%
Fibrinolytic Medication Timing[1]	2	0%	30%	31%	100%
PCI Within 90 Minutes of Arrival[1]	6	33%	48%	54%	95%
Smoking Cessation Advice	49	98%	90%	88%	100%
Heart Failure Care					
ACE Inhibitor or ARB for LVSD	129	95%	82%	82%	100%
Discharge Instructions	554	96%	60%	61%	93%
Evaluation of LVS Function	602	99%	81%	83%	99%
Smoking Cessation Advice	90	100%	82%	82%	100%
Pneumonia Care					
Appropriate Initial Antibiotic	192	86%	79%	83%	94%
Blood Culture Timing	167	95%	89%	90%	100%
Influenza Vaccine[4,5]	-	-	69%	70%	100%
Initial Antibiotic Timing	257	80%	78%	80%	93%
Oxygenation Assessment	281	100%	99%	99%	100%
Pneumococcal Vaccine	143	96%	68%	69%	94%
Smoking Cessation Advice	54	100%	83%	80%	100%
Surgical Infection Prevention					
Prophylactic Antibiotic Given	1,183	83%	67%	77%	95%
Prophylactic Antibiotic Selection	335	94%	86%	90%	100%
Prophylactic Antibiotic Stopped	1,164	48%	68%	72%	95%
Pregnancy Care					
Inpatient Neonatal Mortality	-	-	-	-	-
Third or Fourth Degree Laceration	-	-	3.23%	3.63%	3.27%

Methodist Ambulatory Surgery Hospital NW

9150 Huebner Rd Suite 100
San Antonio, TX 78240
Ownership: Proprietary
Emergency Services: Yes

Phone: 210-691-8000

Accredited: Yes

Measure	Cases	This Hospital	State Average	U.S. Average	Top Hospital
Heart Attack Care					
ACE Inhibitor or ARB for LVSD[5]	-	-	85%	82%	100%
Aspirin at Arrival[5]	-	-	91%	92%	100%
Aspirin at Discharge[5]	-	-	90%	90%	100%
Beta Blocker at Arrival[5]	-	-	85%	87%	100%
Beta Blocker at Discharge[5]	-	-	86%	90%	100%
Fibrinolytic Medication Timing[5]	-	-	30%	31%	100%
PCI Within 90 Minutes of Arrival[5]	-	-	48%	54%	95%
Smoking Cessation Advice[5]	-	-	90%	88%	100%
Heart Failure Care					

Measure	Cases	This Hospital	State Average	U.S. Average	Top Hospital
ACE Inhibitor or ARB for LVSD[5]	-	-	82%	82%	100%
Discharge Instructions[5]	-	-	60%	61%	93%
Evaluation of LVS Function[5]	-	-	81%	83%	99%
Smoking Cessation Advice[5]	-	-	82%	82%	100%
Pneumonia Care					
Appropriate Initial Antibiotic[5]	-	-	79%	83%	94%
Blood Culture Timing[5]	-	-	89%	90%	100%
Influenza Vaccine[5]	-	-	69%	70%	100%
Initial Antibiotic Timing[5]	-	-	78%	80%	93%
Oxygenation Assessment[5]	-	-	99%	99%	100%
Pneumococcal Vaccine[5]	-	-	68%	69%	94%
Smoking Cessation Advice[5]	-	-	83%	80%	100%
Surgical Infection Prevention					
Prophylactic Antibiotic Given[1,2,3]	17	82%	67%	77%	95%
Prophylactic Antibiotic Selection[1,2]	8	100%	86%	90%	100%
Prophylactic Antibiotic Stopped[1,2,3]	17	100%	68%	72%	95%
Pregnancy Care					
Inpatient Neonatal Mortality	-	-	-	-	-
Third or Fourth Degree Laceration	-	-	3.23%	3.63%	3.27%

Methodist Hospital

Alternate Name: San Antonio Regional Hospital
7700 Floyd Curl Drive
San Antonio, TX 78229
URL: www.sahealth.com
Ownership: Proprietary
Emergency Services: Yes

Phone: 210-575-4000
Fax: 210-575-0246

Accredited: Yes
Licensed Beds: 672

Key Personnel:
CEO . . . . John E Hornbeak
Director Infection/Disease Control . . . . Cecil Robinson
CCU Spvg. Nurse . . . . J Pitcock
Director Respiratory Therapy . . . . Juan Vasquez

Measure	Cases	This Hospital	State Average	U.S. Average	Top Hospital
Heart Attack Care					
ACE Inhibitor or ARB for LVSD	116	75%	85%	82%	100%
Aspirin at Arrival	558	94%	91%	92%	100%
Aspirin at Discharge	614	94%	90%	90%	100%
Beta Blocker at Arrival	412	89%	85%	87%	100%
Beta Blocker at Discharge	657	95%	86%	90%	100%
Fibrinolytic Medication Timing	0	-	30%	31%	100%
PCI Within 90 Minutes of Arrival	25	24%	48%	54%	95%
Smoking Cessation Advice	239	97%	90%	88%	100%
Heart Failure Care					
ACE Inhibitor or ARB for LVSD	546	76%	82%	82%	100%
Discharge Instructions	1,224	54%	60%	61%	93%
Evaluation of LVS Function	1,525	87%	81%	83%	99%
Smoking Cessation Advice	232	92%	82%	82%	100%
Pneumonia Care					
Appropriate Initial Antibiotic	575	83%	79%	83%	94%
Blood Culture Timing	615	83%	89%	90%	100%
Influenza Vaccine	231	55%	69%	70%	100%
Initial Antibiotic Timing	955	67%	78%	80%	93%
Oxygenation Assessment	1,147	99%	99%	99%	100%
Pneumococcal Vaccine	646	48%	68%	69%	94%
Smoking Cessation Advice	235	83%	83%	80%	100%
Surgical Infection Prevention					
Prophylactic Antibiotic Given[2,3]	460	62%	67%	77%	95%
Prophylactic Antibiotic Selection[2]	219	92%	86%	90%	100%
Prophylactic Antibiotic Stopped[2,3]	456	69%	68%	72%	95%
Pregnancy Care					
Inpatient Neonatal Mortality	-	-	-	-	-
Third or Fourth Degree Laceration	-	-	3.23%	3.63%	3.27%

Nix Healthcare System

Alternate Name: Nix Medical Center

NOTE: Hospital profiles are in alphabetical order by state, then city, then hospital within the city; Rankings are sorted by rate in descending order and exclude hospitals with less than 25 cases; (1) The number of cases is too small (n<25) for purposes of reliably predicting hospital performance; (2) Measure reflects the hospital's indication that its submission was based upon a sample of its relevant discharges; (3) Rate reflects fewer than the maximum possible quarters of data for the measure; (4) Inaccurate information submitted and suppressed for one or more quarters; (5) No data is available from the hospital for this measure; Please refer to the User's Guide for a full explanation of data

414 Navarro Street
San Antonio, TX 78205
E-mail: nmc@NixHealth.com
URL: www.nixhealth.com
Ownership: Proprietary
Emergency Services: No
Key Personnel:
CEO. . . . . John Strieby

Phone: 210-271-1800
Fax: 210-271-2023

Accredited: Yes
Licensed Beds: 244

Measure	Cases	This Hospital	State Average	U.S. Average	Top Hospital
Heart Attack Care					
ACE Inhibitor or ARB for LVSD[1]	7	86%	85%	82%	100%
Aspirin at Arrival	39	100%	91%	92%	100%
Aspirin at Discharge	43	100%	90%	90%	100%
Beta Blocker at Arrival	37	97%	85%	87%	100%
Beta Blocker at Discharge	42	100%	86%	90%	100%
Fibrinolytic Medication Timing	0	-	30%	31%	100%
PCI Within 90 Minutes of Arrival	0	-	48%	54%	95%
Smoking Cessation Advice[1]	10	100%	90%	88%	100%
Heart Failure Care					
ACE Inhibitor or ARB for LVSD[1]	17	82%	82%	82%	100%
Discharge Instructions	64	98%	60%	61%	93%
Evaluation of LVS Function	83	96%	81%	83%	99%
Smoking Cessation Advice[1]	3	100%	82%	82%	100%
Pneumonia Care					
Appropriate Initial Antibiotic	68	79%	79%	83%	94%
Blood Culture Timing	25	100%	89%	90%	100%
Influenza Vaccine[1]	23	100%	69%	70%	100%
Initial Antibiotic Timing	58	95%	78%	80%	93%
Oxygenation Assessment	93	100%	99%	99%	100%
Pneumococcal Vaccine	68	100%	68%	69%	94%
Smoking Cessation Advice[1]	14	100%	83%	80%	100%
Surgical Infection Prevention					
Prophylactic Antibiotic Given[3]	164	55%	67%	77%	95%
Prophylactic Antibiotic Selection	43	86%	86%	90%	100%
Prophylactic Antibiotic Stopped[3]	157	41%	68%	72%	95%
Pregnancy Care					
Inpatient Neonatal Mortality	-	-	-	-	-
Third or Fourth Degree Laceration	-	-	3.23%	3.63%	3.27%

Southwest General Hospital
7400 Barlite Boulevard
San Antonio, TX 78224
E-mail: swgh_hr@iasishealthcare.com
URL: www.swgeneralhospital.com
Ownership: Proprietary
Emergency Services: Yes
Key Personnel:
CEO. . . . . Richard D Gonzalez
Chief Medical Staff. . . . . Damaso Oliva

Phone: 210-921-2000
Fax: 210-921-3508

Accredited: Yes
Licensed Beds: 319

Measure	Cases	This Hospital	State Average	U.S. Average	Top Hospital
Heart Attack Care					
ACE Inhibitor or ARB for LVSD[1]	1	100%	85%	82%	100%
Aspirin at Arrival	45	93%	91%	92%	100%
Aspirin at Discharge[1]	14	64%	90%	90%	100%
Beta Blocker at Arrival	34	82%	85%	87%	100%
Beta Blocker at Discharge[1]	13	77%	86%	90%	100%
Fibrinolytic Medication Timing[1]	3	67%	30%	31%	100%
PCI Within 90 Minutes of Arrival	0	-	48%	54%	95%
Smoking Cessation Advice[1]	5	100%	90%	88%	100%
Heart Failure Care					
ACE Inhibitor or ARB for LVSD	52	73%	82%	82%	100%
Discharge Instructions	243	25%	60%	61%	93%
Evaluation of LVS Function	293	95%	81%	83%	99%
Smoking Cessation Advice	72	100%	82%	82%	100%
Pneumonia Care					
Appropriate Initial Antibiotic	114	78%	79%	83%	94%
Blood Culture Timing	117	84%	89%	90%	100%
Influenza Vaccine[4,5]	-	-	69%	70%	100%
Initial Antibiotic Timing	152	81%	78%	80%	93%
Oxygenation Assessment	182	99%	99%	99%	100%
Pneumococcal Vaccine	90	67%	68%	69%	94%

Measure	Cases	This Hospital	State Average	U.S. Average	Top Hospital
Smoking Cessation Advice	48	96%	83%	80%	100%
Surgical Infection Prevention					
Prophylactic Antibiotic Given[3]	190	23%	67%	77%	95%
Prophylactic Antibiotic Selection	51	88%	86%	90%	100%
Prophylactic Antibiotic Stopped[3]	184	34%	68%	72%	95%
Pregnancy Care					
Inpatient Neonatal Mortality	2,169	0.28%	-	-	-
Third or Fourth Degree Laceration	1,376	0.65%	3.23%	3.63%	3.27%

Spine Hospital of South Texas
18600 North Hardy Oak
San Antonio, TX 78258
Ownership: Voluntary non-profit - Private
Emergency Services: Yes

Phone: 210-404-0800

Accredited: Yes

Measure	Cases	This Hospital	State Average	U.S. Average	Top Hospital
Heart Attack Care					
ACE Inhibitor or ARB for LVSD[5]	-	-	85%	82%	100%
Aspirin at Arrival[5]	-	-	91%	92%	100%
Aspirin at Discharge[5]	-	-	90%	90%	100%
Beta Blocker at Arrival[5]	-	-	85%	87%	100%
Beta Blocker at Discharge[5]	-	-	86%	90%	100%
Fibrinolytic Medication Timing[5]	-	-	30%	31%	100%
PCI Within 90 Minutes of Arrival[5]	-	-	48%	54%	95%
Smoking Cessation Advice[5]	-	-	90%	88%	100%
Heart Failure Care					
ACE Inhibitor or ARB for LVSD[5]	-	-	82%	82%	100%
Discharge Instructions[5]	-	-	60%	61%	93%
Evaluation of LVS Function[5]	-	-	81%	83%	99%
Smoking Cessation Advice[5]	-	-	82%	82%	100%
Pneumonia Care					
Appropriate Initial Antibiotic[5]	-	-	79%	83%	94%
Blood Culture Timing[5]	-	-	89%	90%	100%
Influenza Vaccine[5]	-	-	69%	70%	100%
Initial Antibiotic Timing[5]	-	-	78%	80%	93%
Oxygenation Assessment[5]	-	-	99%	99%	100%
Pneumococcal Vaccine[5]	-	-	68%	69%	94%
Smoking Cessation Advice[5]	-	-	83%	80%	100%
Surgical Infection Prevention					
Prophylactic Antibiotic Given[3]	81	68%	67%	77%	95%
Prophylactic Antibiotic Selection[5]	-	-	86%	90%	100%
Prophylactic Antibiotic Stopped[3]	80	88%	68%	72%	95%
Pregnancy Care					
Inpatient Neonatal Mortality	-	-	-	-	-
Third or Fourth Degree Laceration	-	-	3.23%	3.63%	3.27%

Texsan Heart Hospital
6700 IH-10 West
San Antonio, TX 78201
URL: www.texsanhearthospital.com
Ownership: Proprietary
Emergency Services: Yes
Key Personnel:
CEO/President. . . . . Craig Desmond
Surgery Team Leader . . . . Mitsy Pubrak
Respiratory Therapy Team Leader. . . . . Kirk Bellinger

Phone: 210-736-6700
Fax: 210-736-8400

Accredited: Yes
Licensed Beds: 60

Measure	Cases	This Hospital	State Average	U.S. Average	Top Hospital
Heart Attack Care					
ACE Inhibitor or ARB for LVSD	48	88%	85%	82%	100%
Aspirin at Arrival	75	100%	91%	92%	100%
Aspirin at Discharge	321	98%	90%	90%	100%
Beta Blocker at Arrival	64	97%	85%	87%	100%
Beta Blocker at Discharge	306	95%	86%	90%	100%
Fibrinolytic Medication Timing	0	-	30%	31%	100%
PCI Within 90 Minutes of Arrival[1]	1	0%	48%	54%	95%
Smoking Cessation Advice	95	97%	90%	88%	100%
Heart Failure Care					
ACE Inhibitor or ARB for LVSD	119	83%	82%	82%	100%
Discharge Instructions	156	62%	60%	61%	93%
Evaluation of LVS Function	172	100%	81%	83%	99%
Smoking Cessation Advice[1]	23	91%	82%	82%	100%

NOTE: Hospital profiles are in alphabetical order by state, then city, then hospital within the city; Rankings are sorted by rate in descending order and exclude hospitals with less than 25 cases; (1) The number of cases is too small (n<25) for purposes of reliably predicting hospital performance; (2) Measure reflects the hospital's indication that its submission was based upon a sample of its relevant discharges; (3) Rate reflects fewer than the maximum possible quarters of data for the measure; (4) Inaccurate information submitted and suppressed for one or more quarters; (5) No data is available from the hospital for this measure; Please refer to the User's Guide for a full explanation of data

Pneumonia Care					
Appropriate Initial Antibiotic[1]	12	33%	79%	83%	94%
Blood Culture Timing[1]	13	77%	89%	90%	100%
Influenza Vaccine[1]	7	43%	69%	70%	100%
Initial Antibiotic Timing[1]	16	81%	78%	80%	93%
Oxygenation Assessment[1]	18	100%	99%	99%	100%
Pneumococcal Vaccine[1]	15	67%	68%	69%	94%
Smoking Cessation Advice[1]	6	67%	83%	80%	100%
Surgical Infection Prevention					
Prophylactic Antibiotic Given[3]	361	89%	67%	77%	95%
Prophylactic Antibiotic Selection	143	100%	86%	90%	100%
Prophylactic Antibiotic Stopped[3]	357	100%	68%	72%	95%
Pregnancy Care					
Inpatient Neonatal Mortality	-	-	-	-	-
Third or Fourth Degree Laceration	-	-	3.23%	3.63%	3.27%

University Hospital

4502 Medical Drive
San Antonio, TX 78229
URL: www.universityhealthsystem.com
Ownership: Govt - Hospital District or Authority
Emergency Services: No

Phone: 210-358-4000
Fax: 210-358-4090

Accredited: Yes
Licensed Beds: 604

Key Personnel:
Administrator . . . . Greg Rufe
President/CEO. . . . . George B Hernandez Jr
Chief Medical Staff. Charles Bauer
Head of Emergency Room. . . . . Marilyn McFarlane
Director Infection/Disease Control . . . . Becky Sanchez
OB/GYN Womens Health. . . . . Marlene Upright
Chief Radiology . . . . Stewart R Reuter, MD
Director Respiratory Therapy . . . . Donnie Holman

Measure	Cases	This Hospital	State Average	U.S. Average	Top Hospital
Heart Attack Care					
ACE Inhibitor or ARB for LVSD	46	74%	85%	82%	100%
Aspirin at Arrival	122	99%	91%	92%	100%
Aspirin at Discharge	151	98%	90%	90%	100%
Beta Blocker at Arrival	91	87%	85%	87%	100%
Beta Blocker at Discharge	141	98%	86%	90%	100%
Fibrinolytic Medication Timing	0	-	30%	31%	100%
PCI Within 90 Minutes of Arrival[1]	7	14%	48%	54%	95%
Smoking Cessation Advice	65	42%	90%	88%	100%
Heart Failure Care					
ACE Inhibitor or ARB for LVSD	191	87%	82%	82%	100%
Discharge Instructions	296	5%	60%	61%	93%
Evaluation of LVS Function	309	96%	81%	83%	99%
Smoking Cessation Advice	106	35%	82%	82%	100%
Pneumonia Care					
Appropriate Initial Antibiotic	88	83%	79%	83%	94%
Blood Culture Timing	67	78%	89%	90%	100%
Influenza Vaccine[1]	14	21%	69%	70%	100%
Initial Antibiotic Timing	109	47%	78%	80%	93%
Oxygenation Assessment	137	100%	99%	99%	100%
Pneumococcal Vaccine	29	31%	68%	69%	94%
Smoking Cessation Advice	42	29%	83%	80%	100%
Surgical Infection Prevention					
Prophylactic Antibiotic Given	204	71%	67%	77%	95%
Prophylactic Antibiotic Selection	43	93%	86%	90%	100%
Prophylactic Antibiotic Stopped	187	68%	68%	72%	95%
Pregnancy Care					
Inpatient Neonatal Mortality[2]	607	0.16%	-	-	-
Third or Fourth Degree Laceration[2]	394	4.31%	3.23%	3.63%	3.27%

Dolly Vinsant Memorial Hospital

400 E US Highway 77
San Benito, TX 78586
Ownership: Proprietary
Emergency Services: Yes

Phone: 956-365-5236
Fax: 956-365-5233

Accredited: Yes
Licensed Beds: 81

Key Personnel:
CEO. . . . . Igor Kozlik
Chief Medical Staff. Fred Perez
Emergency Room . . . . Rafael Lopez, MD

Director Infection/Disease Control . . . . Candi Constantine
Director Medical/Surgical Nursing . . . . Della Anderson, DO
Chief Radiology . . . . CM Sokolosky, MD
Director Respiratory Therapy . . . . Edna Canales

Measure	Cases	This Hospital	State Average	U.S. Average	Top Hospital
Heart Attack Care					
ACE Inhibitor or ARB for LVSD[3]	0	-	85%	82%	100%
Aspirin at Arrival[1,3]	1	0%	91%	92%	100%
Aspirin at Discharge[3]	0	-	90%	90%	100%
Beta Blocker at Arrival[1,3]	1	0%	85%	87%	100%
Beta Blocker at Discharge[3]	0	-	86%	90%	100%
Fibrinolytic Medication Timing[3]	0	-	30%	31%	100%
PCI Within 90 Minutes of Arrival[5]	-	-	48%	54%	95%
Smoking Cessation Advice[3]	0	-	90%	88%	100%
Heart Failure Care					
ACE Inhibitor or ARB for LVSD[2]	0	-	82%	82%	100%
Discharge Instructions[1,2]	17	82%	60%	61%	93%
Evaluation of LVS Function[1,2]	14	100%	81%	83%	99%
Smoking Cessation Advice[1,2]	1	100%	82%	82%	100%
Pneumonia Care					
Appropriate Initial Antibiotic[2]	29	41%	79%	83%	94%
Blood Culture Timing[1,2]	5	100%	89%	90%	100%
Influenza Vaccine[1]	4	50%	69%	70%	100%
Initial Antibiotic Timing[2]	34	71%	78%	80%	93%
Oxygenation Assessment[2]	40	100%	99%	99%	100%
Pneumococcal Vaccine[1,2]	15	53%	68%	69%	94%
Smoking Cessation Advice[1,2]	9	89%	83%	80%	100%
Surgical Infection Prevention					
Prophylactic Antibiotic Given[2,3]	0	-	67%	77%	95%
Prophylactic Antibiotic Selection[2]	0	-	86%	90%	100%
Prophylactic Antibiotic Stopped[2,3]	0	-	68%	72%	95%
Pregnancy Care					
Inpatient Neonatal Mortality	-	-	-	-	-
Third or Fourth Degree Laceration	-	-	3.23%	3.63%	3.27%

Central Texas Medical Center

1301 Wonder World Drive
San Marcos, TX 78666
E-mail: webmasterctmc@ahss.org
URL: www.ctmc.org
Ownership: Voluntary non-profit - Church
Emergency Services: Yes

Phone: 512-353-8979
Fax: 512-753-3598

Accredited: Yes
Licensed Beds: 113

Key Personnel:
President/CEO. . . . . Gary L Jepson
Chief Staff . . . . Charles Matthis, MD
Catheterization Laboratory Director . . . . Karen Morris
Emergency Room . . . . Lana Cameron, RN
Infection Control. . . . . Faye Wright
ICU/CCU . . . . Lana Cameron, RN
OB/GYN. . . . . Terri Balogac, RN
Surgical Services/OR. . . . . Madelyn Smith, RN
Respiratory Therapy/Occupational Therapy . . . . Karen Morris

Measure	Cases	This Hospital	State Average	U.S. Average	Top Hospital
Heart Attack Care					
ACE Inhibitor or ARB for LVSD[1]	9	89%	85%	82%	100%
Aspirin at Arrival	47	98%	91%	92%	100%
Aspirin at Discharge	25	92%	90%	90%	100%
Beta Blocker at Arrival	43	95%	85%	87%	100%
Beta Blocker at Discharge	26	88%	86%	90%	100%
Fibrinolytic Medication Timing[1,3]	1	100%	30%	31%	100%
PCI Within 90 Minutes of Arrival	0	-	48%	54%	95%
Smoking Cessation Advice[3]	0	-	90%	88%	100%
Heart Failure Care					
ACE Inhibitor or ARB for LVSD	52	77%	82%	82%	100%
Discharge Instructions[3]	28	61%	60%	61%	93%
Evaluation of LVS Function	132	92%	81%	83%	99%
Smoking Cessation Advice[1,3]	3	100%	82%	82%	100%
Pneumonia Care					
Appropriate Initial Antibiotic[1,3]	14	57%	79%	83%	94%
Blood Culture Timing[1,3]	17	71%	89%	90%	100%
Influenza Vaccine[5]	-	-	69%	70%	100%

NOTE: Hospital profiles are in alphabetical order by state, then city, then hospital within the city; Rankings are sorted by rate in descending order and exclude hospitals with less than 25 cases; (1) The number of cases is too small (n<25) for purposes of reliably predicting hospital performance; (2) Measure reflects the hospital's indication that its submission was based upon a sample of its relevant discharges; (3) Rate reflects fewer than the maximum possible quarters of data for the measure; (4) Inaccurate information submitted and suppressed for one or more quarters; (5) No data is available from the hospital for this measure; Please refer to the User's Guide for a full explanation of data

Measure				
Initial Antibiotic Timing	123	78%	78%	80%	93%
Oxygenation Assessment	158	99%	99%	99%	100%
Pneumococcal Vaccine	92	83%	68%	69%	94%
Smoking Cessation Advice[1,3]	3	67%	83%	80%	100%
Surgical Infection Prevention					
Prophylactic Antibiotic Given[3]	59	90%	67%	77%	95%
Prophylactic Antibiotic Selection[5]	-	-	86%	90%	100%
Prophylactic Antibiotic Stopped[3]	58	97%	68%	72%	95%
Pregnancy Care					
Inpatient Neonatal Mortality	-	-	-	-	-
Third or Fourth Degree Laceration	-	-	3.23%	3.63%	3.27%

Guadalupe Valley Hospital

1215 E Court Street
Seguin, TX 78155

Toll-Free: 800-506-6394
Phone: 830-379-2411
Fax: 830-372-1582

E-mail: fbennett@gvh.com
URL: www.gvh.com
Ownership: Government - Local
Emergency Services: Yes

Accredited: Yes
Licensed Beds: 117

Key Personnel:
Administrator . . . . Don L Richie
Chief of Medical Staff. . . . . Steven White, MD
Director of Cardiology/Cardiac Lab. . . . . Steven Sokolyk, MD
Emergency Room . . . . Debra Baumler
Emergency Room . . . . Wendy Deleon
Infection Control. . . . . Barbara Haas
ICU . . . . Julia Abrameit
Medical Surgical Nursing . . . . Juanita Hathaway
Director Respiratory/Cardiology . . . . Tommy Aguirre

Measure	Cases	This Hospital	State Average	U.S. Average	Top Hospital
Heart Attack Care					
ACE Inhibitor or ARB for LVSD[1]	3	100%	85%	82%	100%
Aspirin at Arrival	29	83%	91%	92%	100%
Aspirin at Discharge[1]	12	92%	90%	90%	100%
Beta Blocker at Arrival[1]	23	83%	85%	87%	100%
Beta Blocker at Discharge[1]	12	83%	86%	90%	100%
Fibrinolytic Medication Timing	0	-	30%	31%	100%
PCI Within 90 Minutes of Arrival	0	-	48%	54%	95%
Smoking Cessation Advice[1]	2	100%	90%	88%	100%
Heart Failure Care					
ACE Inhibitor or ARB for LVSD	50	76%	82%	82%	100%
Discharge Instructions	121	71%	60%	61%	93%
Evaluation of LVS Function	193	67%	81%	83%	99%
Smoking Cessation Advice[1]	18	67%	82%	82%	100%
Pneumonia Care					
Appropriate Initial Antibiotic	47	87%	79%	83%	94%
Blood Culture Timing	56	93%	89%	90%	100%
Influenza Vaccine	25	8%	69%	70%	100%
Initial Antibiotic Timing	91	78%	78%	80%	93%
Oxygenation Assessment	103	100%	99%	99%	100%
Pneumococcal Vaccine	72	36%	68%	69%	94%
Smoking Cessation Advice[1]	12	67%	83%	80%	100%
Surgical Infection Prevention					
Prophylactic Antibiotic Given[3]	200	61%	67%	77%	95%
Prophylactic Antibiotic Selection	69	70%	86%	90%	100%
Prophylactic Antibiotic Stopped[3]	185	62%	68%	72%	95%
Pregnancy Care					
Inpatient Neonatal Mortality	-	-	-	-	-
Third or Fourth Degree Laceration	-	-	3.23%	3.63%	3.27%

Seymour Hospital

200 Stadium Drive
Seymour, TX 76380
Ownership: Govt - Hospital District or Authority
Emergency Services: Yes

Phone: 940-889-5572
Fax: 940-889-3337
Accredited: No
Licensed Beds: 49

Key Personnel:
CEO. . . . . Leslie Hardin
Chief Medical Staff. Richard Niles, MD
Director Pulmonary Therapy . . . . Julie Samstrala

Measure	Cases	This Hospital	State Average	U.S. Average	Top Hospital

Measure	Cases	This Hospital	State Average	U.S. Average	Top Hospital
Heart Attack Care					
ACE Inhibitor or ARB for LVSD[3]	0	-	85%	82%	100%
Aspirin at Arrival[1,3]	2	50%	91%	92%	100%
Aspirin at Discharge[3]	0	-	90%	90%	100%
Beta Blocker at Arrival[1,3]	2	50%	85%	87%	100%
Beta Blocker at Discharge[3]	0	-	86%	90%	100%
Fibrinolytic Medication Timing[3]	0	-	30%	31%	100%
PCI Within 90 Minutes of Arrival[5]	-	-	48%	54%	95%
Smoking Cessation Advice[3]	0	-	90%	88%	100%
Heart Failure Care					
ACE Inhibitor or ARB for LVSD[1]	3	67%	82%	82%	100%
Discharge Instructions[1]	15	27%	60%	61%	93%
Evaluation of LVS Function[1]	23	52%	81%	83%	99%
Smoking Cessation Advice[1]	7	29%	82%	82%	100%
Pneumonia Care					
Appropriate Initial Antibiotic[1]	15	100%	79%	83%	94%
Blood Culture Timing[1]	1	100%	89%	90%	100%
Influenza Vaccine[1]	6	100%	69%	70%	100%
Initial Antibiotic Timing[1]	24	83%	78%	80%	93%
Oxygenation Assessment	32	100%	99%	99%	100%
Pneumococcal Vaccine	25	84%	68%	69%	94%
Smoking Cessation Advice[1]	4	50%	83%	80%	100%
Surgical Infection Prevention					
Prophylactic Antibiotic Given[5]	-	-	67%	77%	95%
Prophylactic Antibiotic Selection[5]	-	-	86%	90%	100%
Prophylactic Antibiotic Stopped[5]	-	-	68%	72%	95%
Pregnancy Care					
Inpatient Neonatal Mortality	-	-	-	-	-
Third or Fourth Degree Laceration	-	-	3.23%	3.63%	3.27%

Willson N Jones

Alternate Name: Community Specialty Hospital
1111 Gallagher Drive
Sherman, TX 75090
Ownership: Voluntary non-profit - Private
Emergency Services: Yes

Phone: 903-870-4611
Fax: 903-870-4378
Accredited: Yes
Licensed Beds: 160

Key Personnel:
CEO. . . . . Steve Rowly

Measure	Cases	This Hospital	State Average	U.S. Average	Top Hospital
Heart Attack Care					
ACE Inhibitor or ARB for LVSD[5]	-	-	85%	82%	100%
Aspirin at Arrival[5]	-	-	91%	92%	100%
Aspirin at Discharge[5]	-	-	90%	90%	100%
Beta Blocker at Arrival[5]	-	-	85%	87%	100%
Beta Blocker at Discharge[5]	-	-	86%	90%	100%
Fibrinolytic Medication Timing[5]	-	-	30%	31%	100%
PCI Within 90 Minutes of Arrival[5]	-	-	48%	54%	95%
Smoking Cessation Advice[5]	-	-	90%	88%	100%
Heart Failure Care					
ACE Inhibitor or ARB for LVSD[5]	-	-	82%	82%	100%
Discharge Instructions[5]	-	-	60%	61%	93%
Evaluation of LVS Function[5]	-	-	81%	83%	99%
Smoking Cessation Advice[5]	-	-	82%	82%	100%
Pneumonia Care					
Appropriate Initial Antibiotic[5]	-	-	79%	83%	94%
Blood Culture Timing[5]	-	-	89%	90%	100%
Influenza Vaccine[5]	-	-	69%	70%	100%
Initial Antibiotic Timing[5]	-	-	78%	80%	93%
Oxygenation Assessment[5]	-	-	99%	99%	100%
Pneumococcal Vaccine[5]	-	-	68%	69%	94%
Smoking Cessation Advice[5]	-	-	83%	80%	100%
Surgical Infection Prevention					
Prophylactic Antibiotic Given[5]	-	-	67%	77%	95%
Prophylactic Antibiotic Selection[5]	-	-	86%	90%	100%
Prophylactic Antibiotic Stopped[5]	-	-	68%	72%	95%
Pregnancy Care					
Inpatient Neonatal Mortality	-	-	-	-	-
Third or Fourth Degree Laceration	-	-	3.23%	3.63%	3.27%

Wilson N Jones Medical Center

Alternate Name: Wilson N Jones Memorial Hospital

NOTE: Hospital profiles are in alphabetical order by state, then city, then hospital within the city; Rankings are sorted by rate in descending order and exclude hospitals with less than 25 cases; (1) The number of cases is too small (n<25) for purposes of reliably predicting hospital performance; (2) Measure reflects the hospital's indication that its submission was based upon a sample of its relevant discharges; (3) Rate reflects fewer than the maximum possible quarters of data for the measure; (4) Inaccurate information submitted and suppressed for one or more quarters; (5) No data is available from the hospital for this measure; Please refer to the User's Guide for a full explanation of data

500 N Highland
Sherman, TX 75092
URL: www.wnj.org
Ownership: Voluntary non-profit - Private
Emergency Services: Yes

Phone: 903-870-4611
Fax: 903-870-4378

Accredited: Yes
Licensed Beds: 404

Key Personnel:
President/CEO. . . . . K Steven Rowley
Chief Medical Staff. . . . . John Sciortino, DO
Cardiac Lab . . . . Robert Bums
Emergency Room . . . . Judy Kelley
Medical Director Emergency Room . . . . Jerry L Gray, MD
Infection Control. . . . . JoAnn Smith
ICU . . . . Ken Johnson
Director Medical/Surgical Nursing . . . . Kathy Wyatt, RN
Director Respiratory/Neurology . . . . Cheyrl Wood

Measure	Cases	This Hospital	State Average	U.S. Average	Top Hospital
Heart Attack Care					
ACE Inhibitor or ARB for LVSD	52	79%	85%	82%	100%
Aspirin at Arrival	172	95%	91%	92%	100%
Aspirin at Discharge	160	91%	90%	90%	100%
Beta Blocker at Arrival	153	86%	85%	87%	100%
Beta Blocker at Discharge	165	87%	86%	90%	100%
Fibrinolytic Medication Timing[3]	0	-	30%	31%	100%
PCI Within 90 Minutes of Arrival[1]	10	100%	48%	54%	95%
Smoking Cessation Advice[1,3]	16	100%	90%	88%	100%
Heart Failure Care					
ACE Inhibitor or ARB for LVSD	147	86%	82%	82%	100%
Discharge Instructions[3]	65	82%	60%	61%	93%
Evaluation of LVS Function	403	85%	81%	83%	99%
Smoking Cessation Advice[1,3]	19	95%	82%	82%	100%
Pneumonia Care					
Appropriate Initial Antibiotic[3]	25	80%	79%	83%	94%
Blood Culture Timing[3]	37	76%	89%	90%	100%
Influenza Vaccine[4,5]	-	-	69%	70%	100%
Initial Antibiotic Timing	248	83%	78%	80%	93%
Oxygenation Assessment	288	99%	99%	99%	100%
Pneumococcal Vaccine	184	66%	68%	69%	94%
Smoking Cessation Advice[1,3]	13	85%	83%	80%	100%
Surgical Infection Prevention					
Prophylactic Antibiotic Given[2,3]	56	46%	67%	77%	95%
Prophylactic Antibiotic Selection[5]	-	-	86%	90%	100%
Prophylactic Antibiotic Stopped[2,3]	55	40%	68%	72%	95%
Pregnancy Care					
Inpatient Neonatal Mortality	-	-	-	-	-
Third or Fourth Degree Laceration	-	-	3.23%	3.63%	3.27%

Smithville Regional Hospital
800 East Highway 71
Smithville, TX 78957
Ownership: Govt - Hospital District or Authority
Emergency Services: No

Phone: 512-237-3214

Accredited: No

Measure	Cases	This Hospital	State Average	U.S. Average	Top Hospital
Heart Attack Care					
ACE Inhibitor or ARB for LVSD[3]	0	-	85%	82%	100%
Aspirin at Arrival[1,3]	4	75%	91%	92%	100%
Aspirin at Discharge[1,3]	2	100%	90%	90%	100%
Beta Blocker at Arrival[1,3]	4	50%	85%	87%	100%
Beta Blocker at Discharge[1,3]	2	50%	86%	90%	100%
Fibrinolytic Medication Timing[3]	0	-	30%	31%	100%
PCI Within 90 Minutes of Arrival[5]	-	-	48%	54%	95%
Smoking Cessation Advice[3]	0	-	90%	88%	100%
Heart Failure Care					
ACE Inhibitor or ARB for LVSD[1]	22	73%	82%	82%	100%
Discharge Instructions	51	55%	60%	61%	93%
Evaluation of LVS Function	80	69%	81%	83%	99%
Smoking Cessation Advice[1]	17	71%	82%	82%	100%
Pneumonia Care					
Appropriate Initial Antibiotic	83	86%	79%	83%	94%
Blood Culture Timing	62	84%	89%	90%	100%
Influenza Vaccine	28	39%	69%	70%	100%
Initial Antibiotic Timing	129	88%	78%	80%	93%

Oxygenation Assessment	148	100%	99%	99%	100%
Pneumococcal Vaccine	93	41%	68%	69%	94%
Smoking Cessation Advice	28	71%	83%	80%	100%
Surgical Infection Prevention					
Prophylactic Antibiotic Given[1,3]	22	32%	67%	77%	95%
Prophylactic Antibiotic Selection[1]	12	100%	86%	90%	100%
Prophylactic Antibiotic Stopped[1,3]	22	100%	68%	72%	95%
Pregnancy Care					
Inpatient Neonatal Mortality	-	-	-	-	-
Third or Fourth Degree Laceration	-	-	3.23%	3.63%	3.27%

D M Cogdell Memorial Hospital
1700 Cogdell Boulevard
Snyder, TX 79549
E-mail: cbrown@snydertex.com
URL: www.cogdellhospital.com
Ownership: Government - Local
Emergency Services: Yes

Phone: 325-573-6374
Fax: 325-574-7433

Accredited: No
Licensed Beds: 99

Key Personnel:
CEO. . . . . Carol H Hanes
Chief Medical Staff. . . . . Christy Brown
Emergency Room . . . . Marcia Odal, MD
Director Infection/Disease Control . . . . Leslie Leucke, RN
CCU Spvg. Nurse . . . . Cheryl Chance, RN
Director Medical/Surgical Nursing . . . . Leslie Luecke, RN
Chief Radiology . . . . Brian Moffett
Director Respiratory Therapy . . . . Carl Burleson

Measure	Cases	This Hospital	State Average	U.S. Average	Top Hospital
Heart Attack Care					
ACE Inhibitor or ARB for LVSD[1]	1	100%	85%	82%	100%
Aspirin at Arrival[1]	1	100%	91%	92%	100%
Aspirin at Discharge[1]	1	100%	90%	90%	100%
Beta Blocker at Arrival	0	-	85%	87%	100%
Beta Blocker at Discharge[1]	1	100%	86%	90%	100%
Fibrinolytic Medication Timing[3]	0	-	30%	31%	100%
PCI Within 90 Minutes of Arrival	0	-	48%	54%	95%
Smoking Cessation Advice[3]	0	-	90%	88%	100%
Heart Failure Care					
ACE Inhibitor or ARB for LVSD	0	-	82%	82%	100%
Discharge Instructions[1,3]	6	0%	60%	61%	93%
Evaluation of LVS Function	40	18%	81%	83%	99%
Smoking Cessation Advice[1,3]	1	100%	82%	82%	100%
Pneumonia Care					
Appropriate Initial Antibiotic[1,3]	5	100%	79%	83%	94%
Blood Culture Timing[1,3]	6	83%	89%	90%	100%
Influenza Vaccine[5]	-	-	69%	70%	100%
Initial Antibiotic Timing	39	72%	78%	80%	93%
Oxygenation Assessment	54	83%	99%	99%	100%
Pneumococcal Vaccine[1]	20	20%	68%	69%	94%
Smoking Cessation Advice[1,3]	5	100%	83%	80%	100%
Surgical Infection Prevention					
Prophylactic Antibiotic Given[5]	-	-	67%	77%	95%
Prophylactic Antibiotic Selection[5]	-	-	86%	90%	100%
Prophylactic Antibiotic Stopped[5]	-	-	68%	72%	95%
Pregnancy Care					
Inpatient Neonatal Mortality	-	-	-	-	-
Third or Fourth Degree Laceration	-	-	3.23%	3.63%	3.27%

Harris Methodist Southlake Ctr for Diag
1545 E Southlake Blvd
Southlake, TX 76092
Ownership: Proprietary
Emergency Services: Yes

Phone: 817-748-8700

Accredited: No

Measure	Cases	This Hospital	State Average	U.S. Average	Top Hospital
Heart Attack Care					
ACE Inhibitor or ARB for LVSD[5]	-	-	85%	82%	100%
Aspirin at Arrival[5]	-	-	91%	92%	100%
Aspirin at Discharge[5]	-	-	90%	90%	100%
Beta Blocker at Arrival[5]	-	-	85%	87%	100%
Beta Blocker at Discharge[5]	-	-	86%	90%	100%

NOTE: Hospital profiles are in alphabetical order by state, then city, then hospital within the city; Rankings are sorted by rate in descending order and exclude hospitals with less than 25 cases; (1) The number of cases is too small (n<25) for purposes of reliably predicting hospital performance; (2) Measure reflects the hospital's indication that its submission was based upon a sample of its relevant discharges; (3) Rate reflects fewer than the maximum possible quarters of data for the measure; (4) Inaccurate information submitted and suppressed for one or more quarters; (5) No data is available from the hospital for this measure; Please refer to the User's Guide for a full explanation of data

Measure	Cases	This Hospital	State Average	U.S. Average	Top Hospital
Fibrinolytic Medication Timing[5]	-	-	30%	31%	100%
PCI Within 90 Minutes of Arrival[5]	-	-	48%	54%	95%
Smoking Cessation Advice[5]	-	-	90%	88%	100%
Heart Failure Care					
ACE Inhibitor or ARB for LVSD[5]	-	-	82%	82%	100%
Discharge Instructions[5]	-	-	60%	61%	93%
Evaluation of LVS Function[5]	-	-	81%	83%	99%
Smoking Cessation Advice[5]	-	-	82%	82%	100%
Pneumonia Care					
Appropriate Initial Antibiotic[5]	-	-	79%	83%	94%
Blood Culture Timing[5]	-	-	89%	90%	100%
Influenza Vaccine[5]	-	-	69%	70%	100%
Initial Antibiotic Timing[5]	-	-	78%	80%	93%
Oxygenation Assessment[5]	-	-	99%	99%	100%
Pneumococcal Vaccine[5]	-	-	68%	69%	94%
Smoking Cessation Advice[5]	-	-	83%	80%	100%
Surgical Infection Prevention					
Prophylactic Antibiotic Given[3]	31	71%	67%	77%	95%
Prophylactic Antibiotic Selection[5]	-	-	86%	90%	100%
Prophylactic Antibiotic Stopped[3]	28	100%	68%	72%	95%
Pregnancy Care					
Inpatient Neonatal Mortality	-	-	-	-	-
Third or Fourth Degree Laceration	-	-	3.23%	3.63%	3.27%

Stamford Memorial Hospital

E Highway 6
Stamford, TX 79553
Ownership: Govt - Hospital District or Authority
Emergency Services: Yes

Phone: 915-773-2725
Fax: 915-773-3781
Accredited: No
Licensed Beds: 34

Key Personnel:
CEO . . . . Jim Robertson

Measure	Cases	This Hospital	State Average	U.S. Average	Top Hospital
Heart Attack Care					
ACE Inhibitor or ARB for LVSD[3]	0	-	85%	82%	100%
Aspirin at Arrival[3]	0	-	91%	92%	100%
Aspirin at Discharge[3]	0	-	90%	90%	100%
Beta Blocker at Arrival[3]	0	-	85%	87%	100%
Beta Blocker at Discharge[3]	0	-	86%	90%	100%
Fibrinolytic Medication Timing[5]	-	-	30%	31%	100%
PCI Within 90 Minutes of Arrival[5]	-	-	48%	54%	95%
Smoking Cessation Advice[5]	-	-	90%	88%	100%
Heart Failure Care					
ACE Inhibitor or ARB for LVSD[1]	3	100%	82%	82%	100%
Discharge Instructions[1,3]	2	100%	60%	61%	93%
Evaluation of LVS Function[1]	18	100%	81%	83%	99%
Smoking Cessation Advice[3]	0	-	82%	82%	100%
Pneumonia Care					
Appropriate Initial Antibiotic[1,3]	3	67%	79%	83%	94%
Blood Culture Timing[3]	0	-	89%	90%	100%
Influenza Vaccine[5]	-	-	69%	70%	100%
Initial Antibiotic Timing[1]	19	100%	78%	80%	93%
Oxygenation Assessment[1]	23	100%	99%	99%	100%
Pneumococcal Vaccine[1]	16	94%	68%	69%	94%
Smoking Cessation Advice[3]	0	-	83%	80%	100%
Surgical Infection Prevention					
Prophylactic Antibiotic Given[5]	-	-	67%	77%	95%
Prophylactic Antibiotic Selection[5]	-	-	86%	90%	100%
Prophylactic Antibiotic Stopped[5]	-	-	68%	72%	95%
Pregnancy Care					
Inpatient Neonatal Mortality	-	-	-	-	-
Third or Fourth Degree Laceration	-	-	3.23%	3.63%	3.27%

Harris Methodist Erath County

Alternate Name: Harris Methodist Stephenville

411 N Belknap
Stephenville, TX 76401
E-mail: barbaramcmahan@hmhs.com
URL: www.texashealth.org/hospitals
Ownership: Voluntary non-profit - Private
Emergency Services: Yes

Phone: 254-965-1500
Fax: 254-965-1561

Accredited: Yes
Licensed Beds: 98

Key Personnel:
President . . . . Deborah Paganelli
Chief Medical Staff . . . . Karen Burroughs, MD
Emergency Room . . . . Jimmy Harris, MD
Infection Control . . . . Laura Parker, RN
Medical Surgical Nursing . . . . Julie Thomas, RN
OB/GYN/Women's Health . . . . Devra Lefevre, RN

Measure	Cases	This Hospital	State Average	U.S. Average	Top Hospital
Heart Attack Care					
ACE Inhibitor or ARB for LVSD[1]	4	75%	85%	82%	100%
Aspirin at Arrival	42	98%	91%	92%	100%
Aspirin at Discharge[1]	22	95%	90%	90%	100%
Beta Blocker at Arrival	34	91%	85%	87%	100%
Beta Blocker at Discharge[1]	22	95%	86%	90%	100%
Fibrinolytic Medication Timing[1]	7	71%	30%	31%	100%
PCI Within 90 Minutes of Arrival	0	-	48%	54%	95%
Smoking Cessation Advice[1]	4	100%	90%	88%	100%
Heart Failure Care					
ACE Inhibitor or ARB for LVSD[1]	15	100%	82%	82%	100%
Discharge Instructions	62	94%	60%	61%	93%
Evaluation of LVS Function	71	93%	81%	83%	99%
Smoking Cessation Advice[1]	6	100%	82%	82%	100%
Pneumonia Care					
Appropriate Initial Antibiotic	83	58%	79%	83%	94%
Blood Culture Timing	91	95%	89%	90%	100%
Influenza Vaccine	42	83%	69%	70%	100%
Initial Antibiotic Timing	122	89%	78%	80%	93%
Oxygenation Assessment	160	99%	99%	99%	100%
Pneumococcal Vaccine	92	87%	68%	69%	94%
Smoking Cessation Advice	40	100%	83%	80%	100%
Surgical Infection Prevention					
Prophylactic Antibiotic Given[2,3]	99	94%	67%	77%	95%
Prophylactic Antibiotic Selection[2]	29	76%	86%	90%	100%
Prophylactic Antibiotic Stopped[2,3]	96	76%	68%	72%	95%
Pregnancy Care					
Inpatient Neonatal Mortality	-	-	-	-	-
Third or Fourth Degree Laceration	-	-	3.23%	3.63%	3.27%

Methodist Sugar Land Hospital

16655 Southwest Freeway
Sugar Land, TX 77479
URL: www.methodisthealth.com
Ownership: Voluntary non-profit - Church
Emergency Services: Yes

Phone: 281-274-7000
Fax: 281-274-8361

Accredited: Yes
Licensed Beds: 54

Key Personnel:
President/CEO . . . . James F Heitzenrater
Emergency Room . . . . Dennise Davis
Director Respiratory Therapy . . . . Sally Shan

Measure	Cases	This Hospital	State Average	U.S. Average	Top Hospital
Heart Attack Care					
ACE Inhibitor or ARB for LVSD[1]	3	100%	85%	82%	100%
Aspirin at Arrival	30	97%	91%	92%	100%
Aspirin at Discharge[1]	12	92%	90%	90%	100%
Beta Blocker at Arrival[1]	22	86%	85%	87%	100%
Beta Blocker at Discharge[1]	10	70%	86%	90%	100%
Fibrinolytic Medication Timing[1]	1	0%	30%	31%	100%
PCI Within 90 Minutes of Arrival	0	-	48%	54%	95%
Smoking Cessation Advice[1]	3	67%	90%	88%	100%
Heart Failure Care					
ACE Inhibitor or ARB for LVSD[1]	21	90%	82%	82%	100%
Discharge Instructions	69	70%	60%	61%	93%
Evaluation of LVS Function	87	94%	81%	83%	99%
Smoking Cessation Advice[1]	9	89%	82%	82%	100%
Pneumonia Care					
Appropriate Initial Antibiotic[2]	73	60%	79%	83%	94%

NOTE: Hospital profiles are in alphabetical order by state, then city, then hospital within the city; Rankings are sorted by rate in descending order and exclude hospitals with less than 25 cases; (1) The number of cases is too small (n<25) for purposes of reliably predicting hospital performance; (2) Measure reflects the hospital's indication that its submission was based upon a sample of its relevant discharges; (3) Rate reflects fewer than the maximum possible quarters of data for the measure; (4) Inaccurate information submitted and suppressed for one or more quarters; (5) No data is available from the hospital for this measure; Please refer to the User's Guide for a full explanation of data

Measure					
Blood Culture Timing[2]	81	91%	89%	90%	100%
Influenza Vaccine[1,2]	19	95%	69%	70%	100%
Initial Antibiotic Timing[2]	111	84%	78%	80%	93%
Oxygenation Assessment[2]	140	100%	99%	99%	100%
Pneumococcal Vaccine[2]	90	87%	68%	69%	94%
Smoking Cessation Advice[1,2]	17	88%	83%	80%	100%
Surgical Infection Prevention					
Prophylactic Antibiotic Given[2,3]	148	61%	67%	77%	95%
Prophylactic Antibiotic Selection[2]	31	55%	86%	90%	100%
Prophylactic Antibiotic Stopped[2,3]	147	52%	68%	72%	95%
Pregnancy Care					
Inpatient Neonatal Mortality	-	-	-	-	-
Third or Fourth Degree Laceration	-	-	3.23%	3.63%	3.27%

Surgical Specialty Hospital of Sugar Land

1211 Highway 6, Suite 70　　　　Phone: 281-243-1000
Sugar Land, TX 77478
Ownership: Proprietary　　　　Accredited: Yes
Emergency Services: No

Measure	Cases	This Hospital	State Average	U.S. Average	Top Hospital
Heart Attack Care					
ACE Inhibitor or ARB for LVSD[5]	-	-	85%	82%	100%
Aspirin at Arrival[5]	-	-	91%	92%	100%
Aspirin at Discharge[5]	-	-	90%	90%	100%
Beta Blocker at Arrival[5]	-	-	85%	87%	100%
Beta Blocker at Discharge[5]	-	-	86%	90%	100%
Fibrinolytic Medication Timing[5]	-	-	30%	31%	100%
PCI Within 90 Minutes of Arrival[5]	-	-	48%	54%	95%
Smoking Cessation Advice[5]	-	-	90%	88%	100%
Heart Failure Care					
ACE Inhibitor or ARB for LVSD[5]	-	-	82%	82%	100%
Discharge Instructions[5]	-	-	60%	61%	93%
Evaluation of LVS Function[5]	-	-	81%	83%	99%
Smoking Cessation Advice[5]	-	-	82%	82%	100%
Pneumonia Care					
Appropriate Initial Antibiotic[5]	-	-	79%	83%	94%
Blood Culture Timing[5]	-	-	89%	90%	100%
Influenza Vaccine[5]	-	-	69%	70%	100%
Initial Antibiotic Timing[5]	-	-	78%	80%	93%
Oxygenation Assessment[5]	-	-	99%	99%	100%
Pneumococcal Vaccine[5]	-	-	68%	69%	94%
Smoking Cessation Advice[5]	-	-	83%	80%	100%
Surgical Infection Prevention					
Prophylactic Antibiotic Given[1,2,3]	12	83%	67%	77%	95%
Prophylactic Antibiotic Selection[5]	-	-	86%	90%	100%
Prophylactic Antibiotic Stopped[1,2,3]	12	0%	68%	72%	95%
Pregnancy Care					
Inpatient Neonatal Mortality	-	-	-	-	-
Third or Fourth Degree Laceration	-	-	3.23%	3.63%	3.27%

Hopkins County Memorial Hospital

115 Airport Rd　　　　Phone: 903-885-7671
Sulphur Springs, TX 75482
Ownership: Govt - Hospital District or Authority　Accredited: Yes
Emergency Services: Yes

Measure	Cases	This Hospital	State Average	U.S. Average	Top Hospital
Heart Attack Care					
ACE Inhibitor or ARB for LVSD[1]	7	100%	85%	82%	100%
Aspirin at Arrival	31	84%	91%	92%	100%
Aspirin at Discharge[1]	22	77%	90%	90%	100%
Beta Blocker at Arrival	27	81%	85%	87%	100%
Beta Blocker at Discharge[1]	23	83%	86%	90%	100%
Fibrinolytic Medication Timing	0	-	30%	31%	100%
PCI Within 90 Minutes of Arrival	0	-	48%	54%	95%
Smoking Cessation Advice[1]	7	71%	90%	88%	100%
Heart Failure Care					
ACE Inhibitor or ARB for LVSD	46	96%	82%	82%	100%
Discharge Instructions	110	86%	60%	61%	93%
Evaluation of LVS Function	143	77%	81%	83%	99%
Smoking Cessation Advice	29	83%	82%	82%	100%

Measure					
Pneumonia Care					
Appropriate Initial Antibiotic	139	69%	79%	83%	94%
Blood Culture Timing	66	85%	89%	90%	100%
Influenza Vaccine	37	70%	69%	70%	100%
Initial Antibiotic Timing	164	73%	78%	80%	93%
Oxygenation Assessment	209	100%	99%	99%	100%
Pneumococcal Vaccine	139	66%	68%	69%	94%
Smoking Cessation Advice	54	85%	83%	80%	100%
Surgical Infection Prevention					
Prophylactic Antibiotic Given[3]	153	47%	67%	77%	95%
Prophylactic Antibiotic Selection	44	25%	86%	90%	100%
Prophylactic Antibiotic Stopped[3]	130	88%	68%	72%	95%
Pregnancy Care					
Inpatient Neonatal Mortality	-	-	-	-	-
Third or Fourth Degree Laceration	-	-	3.23%	3.63%	3.27%

Rolling Plains Memorial Hospital

200 E Arizona　　　　Phone: 325-235-1701
Sweetwater, TX 79556　　　　Fax: 325-235-8705
Ownership: Govt - Hospital District or Authority　Accredited: Yes
Emergency Services: Yes　　　　Licensed Beds: 85
Key Personnel:
Administrator . . . . Tom Kennedy
Chief Medical Staff . . . . Mickey Williams, RN
Director Infection/Disease Control . . . . Dody Barnes, RN
CCU Spvg. Nurse . . . . Kevin Herm, RN
Director Medical/Surgical Nursing . . . . Sally Flores, RN
Chief Radiology . . . . Randy Lehrmann, ART
Director Respiratory Therapy . . . . Carla Lehrmann, LVN

Measure	Cases	This Hospital	State Average	U.S. Average	Top Hospital
Heart Attack Care					
ACE Inhibitor or ARB for LVSD	0	-	85%	82%	100%
Aspirin at Arrival[1]	5	80%	91%	92%	100%
Aspirin at Discharge[1]	1	100%	90%	90%	100%
Beta Blocker at Arrival[1]	2	0%	85%	87%	100%
Beta Blocker at Discharge[1]	1	0%	86%	90%	100%
Fibrinolytic Medication Timing	0	-	30%	31%	100%
PCI Within 90 Minutes of Arrival	0	-	48%	54%	95%
Smoking Cessation Advice	0	-	90%	88%	100%
Heart Failure Care					
ACE Inhibitor or ARB for LVSD[1]	15	93%	82%	82%	100%
Discharge Instructions	42	98%	60%	61%	93%
Evaluation of LVS Function	57	96%	81%	83%	99%
Smoking Cessation Advice[1]	10	100%	82%	82%	100%
Pneumonia Care					
Appropriate Initial Antibiotic	77	71%	79%	83%	94%
Blood Culture Timing	40	85%	89%	90%	100%
Influenza Vaccine[1]	18	94%	69%	70%	100%
Initial Antibiotic Timing	102	73%	78%	80%	93%
Oxygenation Assessment	111	100%	99%	99%	100%
Pneumococcal Vaccine	74	93%	68%	69%	94%
Smoking Cessation Advice[1]	21	100%	83%	80%	100%
Surgical Infection Prevention					
Prophylactic Antibiotic Given[1,3]	9	44%	67%	77%	95%
Prophylactic Antibiotic Selection[1]	1	100%	86%	90%	100%
Prophylactic Antibiotic Stopped[1,3]	8	75%	68%	72%	95%
Pregnancy Care					
Inpatient Neonatal Mortality	-	-	-	-	-
Third or Fourth Degree Laceration	-	-	3.23%	3.63%	3.27%

Kings Daughters Hospital

1901 SW H K Dodgen Loop　　　　Phone: 254-771-8600
Temple, TX 76502　　　　Fax: 254-771-8665
E-mail: contact@kdhosp.org
URL: www.kdhosp.org
Ownership: Voluntary non-profit - Other　Accredited: Yes
Emergency Services: Yes　　　　Licensed Beds: 150
Key Personnel:
President/CEO . . . . Tucker Bonner
VP . . . . Eric Lashbrook
Chief of Staff . . . . Gopal Guttikonda, MD
Infection Control . . . . Jennifer Middleton

NOTE: Hospital profiles are in alphabetical order by state, then city, then hospital within the city; Rankings are sorted by rate in descending order and exclude hospitals with less than 25 cases; (1) The number of cases is too small (n<25) for purposes of reliably predicting hospital performance; (2) Measure reflects the hospital's indication that its submission was based upon a sample of its relevant discharges; (3) Rate reflects fewer than the maximum possible quarters of data for the measure; (4) Inaccurate information submitted and suppressed for one or more quarters; (5) No data is available from the hospital for this measure; Please refer to the User's Guide for a full explanation of data

Intensive/Coronary Care . . . . Kathy Kabobel, RN
Medical/Surgical Nursing . . . . Nancy Urbantke, RN
OB/GYN Womens Health. . . . . Peggy Luna, RN
Respiratory/Cardiopulmonary. . . . . Mitzi Bane

Measure	Cases	This Hospital	State Average	U.S. Average	Top Hospital
Heart Attack Care					
ACE Inhibitor or ARB for LVSD[1]	3	67%	85%	82%	100%
Aspirin at Arrival[1]	23	100%	91%	92%	100%
Aspirin at Discharge[1]	15	100%	90%	90%	100%
Beta Blocker at Arrival	25	96%	85%	87%	100%
Beta Blocker at Discharge[1]	13	100%	86%	90%	100%
Fibrinolytic Medication Timing	0	-	30%	31%	100%
PCI Within 90 Minutes of Arrival	0	-	48%	54%	95%
Smoking Cessation Advice[1]	2	100%	90%	88%	100%
Heart Failure Care					
ACE Inhibitor or ARB for LVSD[1]	12	75%	82%	82%	100%
Discharge Instructions	35	86%	60%	61%	93%
Evaluation of LVS Function	39	100%	81%	83%	99%
Smoking Cessation Advice[1]	11	82%	82%	82%	100%
Pneumonia Care					
Appropriate Initial Antibiotic	49	92%	79%	83%	94%
Blood Culture Timing	35	80%	89%	90%	100%
Influenza Vaccine[1]	13	62%	69%	70%	100%
Initial Antibiotic Timing	59	85%	78%	80%	93%
Oxygenation Assessment	62	100%	99%	99%	100%
Pneumococcal Vaccine	44	91%	68%	69%	94%
Smoking Cessation Advice[1]	24	92%	83%	80%	100%
Surgical Infection Prevention					
Prophylactic Antibiotic Given[3]	93	82%	67%	77%	95%
Prophylactic Antibiotic Selection	49	76%	86%	90%	100%
Prophylactic Antibiotic Stopped[3]	94	67%	68%	72%	95%
Pregnancy Care					
Inpatient Neonatal Mortality	769	0.00%	-	-	-
Third or Fourth Degree Laceration	515	1.55%	3.23%	3.63%	3.27%

Scott & White

2401 S 31st Street
Temple, TX 76508

Toll-Free: 800-324-7947
Phone: 254-724-2111
Fax: 254-724-5579

E-mail: swhpques@swmail.sw.org
URL: www.sw.org
Ownership: Voluntary non-profit - Private
Emergency Services: Yes

Accredited: Yes
Licensed Beds: 625

Key Personnel:
President/CEO. . . . . Alfred B Knight, MD
Chief Medical Staff. . . . . Virginia Hunt

Measure	Cases	This Hospital	State Average	U.S. Average	Top Hospital
Heart Attack Care					
ACE Inhibitor or ARB for LVSD	91	96%	85%	82%	100%
Aspirin at Arrival	339	100%	91%	92%	100%
Aspirin at Discharge	571	100%	90%	90%	100%
Beta Blocker at Arrival	311	99%	85%	87%	100%
Beta Blocker at Discharge	567	100%	86%	90%	100%
Fibrinolytic Medication Timing	0	-	30%	31%	100%
PCI Within 90 Minutes of Arrival[1]	10	80%	48%	54%	95%
Smoking Cessation Advice	208	100%	90%	88%	100%
Heart Failure Care					
ACE Inhibitor or ARB for LVSD	267	96%	82%	82%	100%
Discharge Instructions	442	64%	60%	61%	93%
Evaluation of LVS Function	566	95%	81%	83%	99%
Smoking Cessation Advice	104	98%	82%	82%	100%
Pneumonia Care					
Appropriate Initial Antibiotic	183	85%	79%	83%	94%
Blood Culture Timing	229	93%	89%	90%	100%
Influenza Vaccine[4,5]	-	-	69%	70%	100%
Initial Antibiotic Timing	317	80%	78%	80%	93%
Oxygenation Assessment	416	100%	99%	99%	100%
Pneumococcal Vaccine	293	82%	68%	69%	94%
Smoking Cessation Advice	91	93%	83%	80%	100%
Surgical Infection Prevention					

Measure	Cases	This Hospital	State Average	U.S. Average	Top Hospital
Prophylactic Antibiotic Given	1,772	83%	67%	77%	95%
Prophylactic Antibiotic Selection	436	88%	86%	90%	100%
Prophylactic Antibiotic Stopped	1,719	81%	68%	72%	95%
Pregnancy Care					
Inpatient Neonatal Mortality[2]	1,077	1.21%	-	-	-
Third or Fourth Degree Laceration[2]	800	3.13%	3.23%	3.63%	3.27%

Medical Center at Terrell

Alternate Name: Terrell Community Hospital
1551 Highway 34 S
Terrell, TX 75160
Ownership: Proprietary
Emergency Services: Yes

Phone: 972-563-7611
Fax: 972-551-6808
Accredited: Yes
Licensed Beds: 130

Key Personnel:
Administrator/CEO. . . . . Ronald J Ensor
Chief Medical Staff. . . . . Steven Altshuler, MD
Director Respiratory Therapy . . . . Charles Blackshear
Director Surgical Services . . . . Sharon Zajic, RN
Director Infection/Disease Control . . . . DeLinda Garrett, RN
Director ICU/CCU . . . . Sharon Zajic, RN
Director Medical/Surgical Nursing . . . . Gay Nelle Gaskey, RN
Coordinator Women's Clinical Services . . . . Beverly Foulkrod, RN
Director Radiology . . . . Rhonda Bowling

Measure	Cases	This Hospital	State Average	U.S. Average	Top Hospital
Heart Attack Care					
ACE Inhibitor or ARB for LVSD[1]	5	80%	85%	82%	100%
Aspirin at Arrival	54	94%	91%	92%	100%
Aspirin at Discharge	32	97%	90%	90%	100%
Beta Blocker at Arrival	48	85%	85%	87%	100%
Beta Blocker at Discharge	31	97%	86%	90%	100%
Fibrinolytic Medication Timing[1]	3	0%	30%	31%	100%
PCI Within 90 Minutes of Arrival	0	-	48%	54%	95%
Smoking Cessation Advice[1]	5	80%	90%	88%	100%
Heart Failure Care					
ACE Inhibitor or ARB for LVSD	36	72%	82%	82%	100%
Discharge Instructions	88	61%	60%	61%	93%
Evaluation of LVS Function	118	53%	81%	83%	99%
Smoking Cessation Advice[1]	24	96%	82%	82%	100%
Pneumonia Care					
Appropriate Initial Antibiotic	80	79%	79%	83%	94%
Blood Culture Timing	71	87%	89%	90%	100%
Influenza Vaccine[1]	19	79%	69%	70%	100%
Initial Antibiotic Timing	112	80%	78%	80%	93%
Oxygenation Assessment	137	100%	99%	99%	100%
Pneumococcal Vaccine	83	77%	68%	69%	94%
Smoking Cessation Advice	31	84%	83%	80%	100%
Surgical Infection Prevention					
Prophylactic Antibiotic Given[1,3]	1	100%	67%	77%	95%
Prophylactic Antibiotic Selection[1]	2	100%	86%	90%	100%
Prophylactic Antibiotic Stopped[3]	0	-	68%	72%	95%
Pregnancy Care					
Inpatient Neonatal Mortality	-	-	-	-	-
Third or Fourth Degree Laceration	-	-	3.23%	3.63%	3.27%

Christus Saint Michael Health System

2600 Saint Michael Drive
Texarkana, TX 75503
URL: www.christusstmichael.org
Ownership: Voluntary non-profit - Church
Emergency Services: Yes

Phone: 903-614-1000
Fax: 903-614-2588

Accredited: Yes
Licensed Beds: 278

Key Personnel:
CEO. . . . . Chris Karan
Chief Medical Staff. . . . . Mike Finley
Emergency Room . . . . Claire Donohua
Director Radiology . . . . Wayne East
Director of Pulmonary . . . . Kevin Houck

Measure	Cases	This Hospital	State Average	U.S. Average	Top Hospital
Heart Attack Care					
ACE Inhibitor or ARB for LVSD	125	91%	85%	82%	100%
Aspirin at Arrival	321	99%	91%	92%	100%

NOTE: Hospital profiles are in alphabetical order by state, then city, then hospital within the city; Rankings are sorted by rate in descending order and exclude hospitals with less than 25 cases; (1) The number of cases is too small (n<25) for purposes of reliably predicting hospital performance; (2) Measure reflects the hospital's indication that its submission was based upon a sample of its relevant discharges; (3) Rate reflects fewer than the maximum possible quarters of data for the measure; (4) Inaccurate information submitted and suppressed for one or more quarters; (5) No data is available from the hospital for this measure; Please refer to the User's Guide for a full explanation of data

Aspirin at Discharge	363	97%	90%	90%	100%
Beta Blocker at Arrival	257	95%	85%	87%	100%
Beta Blocker at Discharge	356	97%	86%	90%	100%
Fibrinolytic Medication Timing[1]	3	67%	30%	31%	100%
PCI Within 90 Minutes of Arrival[1]	9	0%	48%	54%	95%
Smoking Cessation Advice	150	100%	90%	88%	100%
Heart Failure Care					
ACE Inhibitor or ARB for LVSD	324	90%	82%	82%	100%
Discharge Instructions	515	80%	60%	61%	93%
Evaluation of LVS Function	660	97%	81%	83%	99%
Smoking Cessation Advice	96	100%	82%	82%	100%
Pneumonia Care					
Appropriate Initial Antibiotic	253	88%	79%	83%	94%
Blood Culture Timing	227	95%	89%	90%	100%
Influenza Vaccine	66	89%	69%	70%	100%
Initial Antibiotic Timing	358	82%	78%	80%	93%
Oxygenation Assessment	413	100%	99%	99%	100%
Pneumococcal Vaccine	252	87%	68%	69%	94%
Smoking Cessation Advice	125	100%	83%	80%	100%
Surgical Infection Prevention					
Prophylactic Antibiotic Given	1,260	92%	67%	77%	95%
Prophylactic Antibiotic Selection	296	90%	86%	90%	100%
Prophylactic Antibiotic Stopped	1,223	46%	68%	72%	95%
Pregnancy Care					
Inpatient Neonatal Mortality	-	-	-	-	-
Third or Fourth Degree Laceration	-	-	3.23%	3.63%	3.27%

Wadley Regional Medical Center

1000 Pine Street   Phone: 903-798-8000
Texarkana, TX 75501   Fax: 903-798-8030
URL: www.wadleyhealth.com
Ownership: Voluntary non-profit - Private   Accredited: Yes
Emergency Services: Yes   Licensed Beds: 407
Key Personnel:
President/CEO . . . . James Summersett
Chief Medical Staff . . . . Stanley Knowles
Director Infection/Disease Control . . . . Barbara Clingan
Director Medical/Surgical Services . . . . Kristi Ragland
Director Surgical Services . . . . Sandra Morris
Director Radiology . . . . Bill Saling
Director Cardiopulmonary . . . . Cindy Biggar

Measure	Cases	This Hospital	State Average	U.S. Average	Top Hospital
Heart Attack Care					
ACE Inhibitor or ARB for LVSD	47	91%	85%	82%	100%
Aspirin at Arrival	164	98%	91%	92%	100%
Aspirin at Discharge	171	93%	90%	90%	100%
Beta Blocker at Arrival	148	94%	85%	87%	100%
Beta Blocker at Discharge	172	94%	86%	90%	100%
Fibrinolytic Medication Timing[1]	4	0%	30%	31%	100%
PCI Within 90 Minutes of Arrival[1]	4	0%	48%	54%	95%
Smoking Cessation Advice	64	97%	90%	88%	100%
Heart Failure Care					
ACE Inhibitor or ARB for LVSD	177	86%	82%	82%	100%
Discharge Instructions	317	72%	60%	61%	93%
Evaluation of LVS Function	423	90%	81%	83%	99%
Smoking Cessation Advice	71	87%	82%	82%	100%
Pneumonia Care					
Appropriate Initial Antibiotic	123	89%	79%	83%	94%
Blood Culture Timing	121	79%	89%	90%	100%
Influenza Vaccine	49	76%	69%	70%	100%
Initial Antibiotic Timing	207	78%	78%	80%	93%
Oxygenation Assessment	227	100%	99%	99%	100%
Pneumococcal Vaccine	146	79%	68%	69%	94%
Smoking Cessation Advice	67	85%	83%	80%	100%
Surgical Infection Prevention					
Prophylactic Antibiotic Given[3]	311	61%	67%	77%	95%
Prophylactic Antibiotic Selection	124	94%	86%	90%	100%
Prophylactic Antibiotic Stopped[3]	294	58%	68%	72%	95%
Pregnancy Care					
Inpatient Neonatal Mortality	-	-	-	-	-
Third or Fourth Degree Laceration	-	-	3.23%	3.63%	3.27%

Mainland Medical Center

Alternate Name: Mainland Center Hospital
6801 Emmett F Lowry Expwy   Phone: 409-938-5000
Texas City, TX 77591   Fax: 409-938-5001
URL: www.mainlandmedical.com
Ownership: Proprietary   Accredited: Yes
Emergency Services: Yes   Licensed Beds: 226
Key Personnel:
CEO . . . . Maura Walsh
Chief Medical Staff . . . . William Bondurant, MD
Emergency Room . . . . Donna Dollimont
Infection Control . . . . Donna Robertson, RN
ICU . . . . Richard Hart, RN
Intensive/Coronary Care . . . . Richard Hart, RN
OB/GYN Womens Health . . . . Sylvia Godinich
Respiratory/Cardiopulmonary . . . . Mary Salenger

Measure	Cases	This Hospital	State Average	U.S. Average	Top Hospital
Heart Attack Care					
ACE Inhibitor or ARB for LVSD[1]	21	90%	85%	82%	100%
Aspirin at Arrival	110	96%	91%	92%	100%
Aspirin at Discharge	60	93%	90%	90%	100%
Beta Blocker at Arrival	113	88%	85%	87%	100%
Beta Blocker at Discharge	69	91%	86%	90%	100%
Fibrinolytic Medication Timing[1]	6	67%	30%	31%	100%
PCI Within 90 Minutes of Arrival[1]	4	75%	48%	54%	95%
Smoking Cessation Advice[1]	13	100%	90%	88%	100%
Heart Failure Care					
ACE Inhibitor or ARB for LVSD[2]	143	90%	82%	82%	100%
Discharge Instructions[2]	301	54%	60%	61%	93%
Evaluation of LVS Function[2]	359	96%	81%	83%	99%
Smoking Cessation Advice[2]	66	97%	82%	82%	100%
Pneumonia Care					
Appropriate Initial Antibiotic	140	84%	79%	83%	94%
Blood Culture Timing	128	98%	89%	90%	100%
Influenza Vaccine	42	81%	69%	70%	100%
Initial Antibiotic Timing	192	88%	78%	80%	93%
Oxygenation Assessment	227	99%	99%	99%	100%
Pneumococcal Vaccine	129	78%	68%	69%	94%
Smoking Cessation Advice	62	90%	83%	80%	100%
Surgical Infection Prevention					
Prophylactic Antibiotic Given[2,3]	132	72%	67%	77%	95%
Prophylactic Antibiotic Selection[2]	67	51%	86%	90%	100%
Prophylactic Antibiotic Stopped[2,3]	129	41%	68%	72%	95%
Pregnancy Care					
Inpatient Neonatal Mortality	-	-	-	-	-
Third or Fourth Degree Laceration	-	-	3.23%	3.63%	3.27%

Saint Luke's Community Med Ctr-The Woodlands

17200 Saint Luke's Way   Phone: 936-266-4050
The Woodlands, TX 77384   Fax: 936-266-4001
URL: www.stlukeswoodlands.com
Ownership: Voluntary non-profit - Church   Accredited: Yes
Emergency Services: Yes   Licensed Beds: 76
Key Personnel:
President/CEO . . . . David Fine

Measure	Cases	This Hospital	State Average	U.S. Average	Top Hospital
Heart Attack Care					
ACE Inhibitor or ARB for LVSD[1]	15	80%	85%	82%	100%
Aspirin at Arrival	89	94%	91%	92%	100%
Aspirin at Discharge	83	86%	90%	90%	100%
Beta Blocker at Arrival	89	78%	85%	87%	100%
Beta Blocker at Discharge	77	84%	86%	90%	100%
Fibrinolytic Medication Timing[1,3]	1	0%	30%	31%	100%
PCI Within 90 Minutes of Arrival[1]	7	0%	48%	54%	95%
Smoking Cessation Advice[1,3]	8	100%	90%	88%	100%
Heart Failure Care					
ACE Inhibitor or ARB for LVSD	48	75%	82%	82%	100%
Discharge Instructions[1,3]	16	88%	60%	61%	93%
Evaluation of LVS Function	107	86%	81%	83%	99%
Smoking Cessation Advice[1,3]	5	100%	82%	82%	100%
Pneumonia Care					

NOTE: Hospital profiles are in alphabetical order by state, then city, then hospital within the city; Rankings are sorted by rate in descending order and exclude hospitals with less than 25 cases; (1) The number of cases is too small (n<25) for purposes of reliably predicting hospital performance; (2) Measure reflects the hospital's indication that its submission was based upon a sample of its relevant discharges; (3) Rate reflects fewer than the maximum possible quarters of data for the measure; (4) Inaccurate information submitted and suppressed for one or more quarters; (5) No data is available from the hospital for this measure; Please refer to the User's Guide for a full explanation of data

	Cases	This Hospital	State Average	U.S. Average	Top Hospital
Appropriate Initial Antibiotic[1,3]	16	69%	79%	83%	94%
Blood Culture Timing[1,3]	20	80%	89%	90%	100%
Influenza Vaccine[5]	-	-	69%	70%	100%
Initial Antibiotic Timing	105	64%	78%	80%	93%
Oxygenation Assessment	145	99%	99%	99%	100%
Pneumococcal Vaccine	71	63%	68%	69%	94%
Smoking Cessation Advice[1,3]	8	75%	83%	80%	100%
Surgical Infection Prevention					
Prophylactic Antibiotic Given[2,3]	38	53%	67%	77%	95%
Prophylactic Antibiotic Selection[5]	-	-	86%	90%	100%
Prophylactic Antibiotic Stopped[2,3]	38	61%	68%	72%	95%
Pregnancy Care					
Inpatient Neonatal Mortality	1,829	0.16%	-	-	-
Third or Fourth Degree Laceration	1,157	3.28%	3.23%	3.63%	3.27%

Tomball Regional Hospital

605 Holderrieth
Tomball, TX 77375
URL: www.tomballhospital.org
Ownership: Govt - Hospital District or Authority
Emergency Services: Yes

Phone: 281-401-7500
Fax: 281-351-4904

Accredited: Yes
Licensed Beds: 205

Key Personnel:
President/CEO . . . . Lynn LeBouef
Chief Medical Staff. Cotton Feray
Director Infection/Disease Control . . . . Lisa Shaklovitz
Director Respiratory Therapy . . . . Kathy LeBouef

Measure	Cases	This Hospital	State Average	U.S. Average	Top Hospital
Heart Attack Care					
ACE Inhibitor or ARB for LVSD	36	81%	85%	82%	100%
Aspirin at Arrival	168	93%	91%	92%	100%
Aspirin at Discharge	161	96%	90%	90%	100%
Beta Blocker at Arrival	149	79%	85%	87%	100%
Beta Blocker at Discharge	155	92%	86%	90%	100%
Fibrinolytic Medication Timing[3]	0	-	30%	31%	100%
PCI Within 90 Minutes of Arrival[1]	9	11%	48%	54%	95%
Smoking Cessation Advice[1,3]	10	100%	90%	88%	100%
Heart Failure Care					
ACE Inhibitor or ARB for LVSD	127	89%	82%	82%	100%
Discharge Instructions[3]	84	100%	60%	61%	93%
Evaluation of LVS Function	413	97%	81%	83%	99%
Smoking Cessation Advice[1,3]	10	100%	82%	82%	100%
Pneumonia Care					
Appropriate Initial Antibiotic[3]	41	73%	79%	83%	94%
Blood Culture Timing[3]	34	74%	89%	90%	100%
Influenza Vaccine[5]	-	-	69%	70%	100%
Initial Antibiotic Timing	249	71%	78%	80%	93%
Oxygenation Assessment	310	100%	99%	99%	100%
Pneumococcal Vaccine	156	72%	68%	69%	94%
Smoking Cessation Advice[1,3]	17	100%	83%	80%	100%
Surgical Infection Prevention					
Prophylactic Antibiotic Given[2,3]	55	87%	67%	77%	95%
Prophylactic Antibiotic Selection[5]	-	-	86%	90%	100%
Prophylactic Antibiotic Stopped[2,3]	50	70%	68%	72%	95%
Pregnancy Care					
Inpatient Neonatal Mortality	803	0.00%	-	-	-
Third or Fourth Degree Laceration	596	3.52%	3.23%	3.63%	3.27%

East Texas Medical Center-Trinity

Alternate Name: Trinity Memorial Hospital
317 Prospect Drive
Trinity, TX 75862
URL: www.etmc.org
Ownership: Voluntary non-profit - Other
Emergency Services: Yes

Phone: 936-594-3541
Fax: 936-744-1182

Accredited: No
Licensed Beds: 30

Key Personnel:
Administrator/COO. . . . . Terry Cutler

Measure	Cases	This Hospital	State Average	U.S. Average	Top Hospital
Heart Attack Care					
ACE Inhibitor or ARB for LVSD[1]	1	100%	85%	82%	100%
Aspirin at Arrival[1]	4	75%	91%	92%	100%

	Cases	This Hospital	State Average	U.S. Average	Top Hospital
Aspirin at Discharge[1]	2	100%	90%	90%	100%
Beta Blocker at Arrival[1]	4	100%	85%	87%	100%
Beta Blocker at Discharge[1]	2	50%	86%	90%	100%
Fibrinolytic Medication Timing[3]	0	-	30%	31%	100%
PCI Within 90 Minutes of Arrival	0	-	48%	54%	95%
Smoking Cessation Advice[3]	0	-	90%	88%	100%
Heart Failure Care					
ACE Inhibitor or ARB for LVSD[1]	11	73%	82%	82%	100%
Discharge Instructions[1,3]	3	67%	60%	61%	93%
Evaluation of LVS Function	48	52%	81%	83%	99%
Smoking Cessation Advice[1,3]	1	100%	82%	82%	100%
Pneumonia Care					
Appropriate Initial Antibiotic[1,3]	3	67%	79%	83%	94%
Blood Culture Timing[3]	0	-	89%	90%	100%
Influenza Vaccine[5]	-	-	69%	70%	100%
Initial Antibiotic Timing	41	46%	78%	80%	93%
Oxygenation Assessment	51	100%	99%	99%	100%
Pneumococcal Vaccine	31	32%	68%	69%	94%
Smoking Cessation Advice[1,3]	2	100%	83%	80%	100%
Surgical Infection Prevention					
Prophylactic Antibiotic Given[5]	-	-	67%	77%	95%
Prophylactic Antibiotic Selection[5]	-	-	86%	90%	100%
Prophylactic Antibiotic Stopped[5]	-	-	68%	72%	95%
Pregnancy Care					
Inpatient Neonatal Mortality	-	-	-	-	-
Third or Fourth Degree Laceration	-	-	3.23%	3.63%	3.27%

Trophy Club Medical Center

2850 South Highway 114e
Trophy Club, TX 76262
Ownership: Proprietary
Emergency Services: Yes

Phone: 817-837-4600

Accredited: Yes

Measure	Cases	This Hospital	State Average	U.S. Average	Top Hospital
Heart Attack Care					
ACE Inhibitor or ARB for LVSD[5]	-	-	85%	82%	100%
Aspirin at Arrival[5]	-	-	91%	92%	100%
Aspirin at Discharge[5]	-	-	90%	90%	100%
Beta Blocker at Arrival[5]	-	-	85%	87%	100%
Beta Blocker at Discharge[5]	-	-	86%	90%	100%
Fibrinolytic Medication Timing[5]	-	-	30%	31%	100%
PCI Within 90 Minutes of Arrival[5]	-	-	48%	54%	95%
Smoking Cessation Advice[5]	-	-	90%	88%	100%
Heart Failure Care					
ACE Inhibitor or ARB for LVSD[5]	-	-	82%	82%	100%
Discharge Instructions[5]	-	-	60%	61%	93%
Evaluation of LVS Function[5]	-	-	81%	83%	99%
Smoking Cessation Advice[5]	-	-	82%	82%	100%
Pneumonia Care					
Appropriate Initial Antibiotic[5]	-	-	79%	83%	94%
Blood Culture Timing[5]	-	-	89%	90%	100%
Influenza Vaccine[5]	-	-	69%	70%	100%
Initial Antibiotic Timing[5]	-	-	78%	80%	93%
Oxygenation Assessment[5]	-	-	99%	99%	100%
Pneumococcal Vaccine[5]	-	-	68%	69%	94%
Smoking Cessation Advice[5]	-	-	83%	80%	100%
Surgical Infection Prevention					
Prophylactic Antibiotic Given[1,3]	6	83%	67%	77%	95%
Prophylactic Antibiotic Selection[5]	-	-	86%	90%	100%
Prophylactic Antibiotic Stopped[1,3]	6	50%	68%	72%	95%
Pregnancy Care					
Inpatient Neonatal Mortality	-	-	-	-	-
Third or Fourth Degree Laceration	-	-	3.23%	3.63%	3.27%

East Texas Medical Center-Tyler

Alternate Name: Medical Center Hospital

NOTE: Hospital profiles are in alphabetical order by state, then city, then hospital within the city; Rankings are sorted by rate in descending order and exclude hospitals with less than 25 cases; (1) The number of cases is too small (n<25) for purposes of reliably predicting hospital performance; (2) Measure reflects the hospital's indication that its submission was based upon a sample of its relevant discharges; (3) Rate reflects fewer than the maximum possible quarters of data for the measure; (4) Inaccurate information submitted and suppressed for one or more quarters; (5) No data is available from the hospital for this measure; Please refer to the User's Guide for a full explanation of data

1000 South Beckham
PO Box 6400
Tyler, TX 75701
URL: www.etmc.org
Ownership: Voluntary non-profit - Private
Emergency Services: Yes

Phone: 903-597-0351
Fax: 903-535-6334

Accredited: Yes
Licensed Beds: 454

Key Personnel:
President/CEO...........................Elmer Ellis
Administrator/CEO.......................Robert B Evans
Chief Medical Staff.....................Bill Moore, MD
Day Surgery............................Chesley Walters
VP Cardiac Services ....John Stewart
Catheterization Lab ....Mike Fountain
Emergency Room ....Robert Creath, MD
Infection Control ....Annette Moore
Respiratory/Cardiopulmonary.............Robert Jackson

Measure	Cases	This Hospital	State Average	U.S. Average	Top Hospital
Heart Attack Care					
ACE Inhibitor or ARB for LVSD	66	82%	85%	82%	100%
Aspirin at Arrival	106	95%	91%	92%	100%
Aspirin at Discharge	275	97%	90%	90%	100%
Beta Blocker at Arrival	93	92%	85%	87%	100%
Beta Blocker at Discharge	276	93%	86%	90%	100%
Fibrinolytic Medication Timing[1]	2	0%	30%	31%	100%
PCI Within 90 Minutes of Arrival[1]	4	50%	48%	54%	95%
Smoking Cessation Advice	110	79%	90%	88%	100%
Heart Failure Care					
ACE Inhibitor or ARB for LVSD	188	71%	82%	82%	100%
Discharge Instructions	293	25%	60%	61%	93%
Evaluation of LVS Function	383	88%	81%	83%	99%
Smoking Cessation Advice	77	60%	82%	82%	100%
Pneumonia Care					
Appropriate Initial Antibiotic	52	73%	79%	83%	94%
Blood Culture Timing	37	81%	89%	90%	100%
Influenza Vaccine[1]	16	31%	69%	70%	100%
Initial Antibiotic Timing	81	57%	78%	80%	93%
Oxygenation Assessment	101	100%	99%	99%	100%
Pneumococcal Vaccine	68	34%	68%	69%	94%
Smoking Cessation Advice	38	47%	83%	80%	100%
Surgical Infection Prevention					
Prophylactic Antibiotic Given[3]	159	36%	67%	77%	95%
Prophylactic Antibiotic Selection	60	70%	86%	90%	100%
Prophylactic Antibiotic Stopped[3]	150	69%	68%	72%	95%
Pregnancy Care					
Inpatient Neonatal Mortality[2]	246	0.00%	-	-	-
Third or Fourth Degree Laceration[2]	177	6.21%	3.23%	3.63%	3.27%

Mother Frances Hospital-Tyler
800 E Dawson
Tyler, TX 75701
E-mail: lukerr@trimofran.org
URL: www.tmfhs.org
Ownership: Voluntary non-profit - Other
Emergency Services: Yes

Phone: 903-593-8441
Fax: 903-531-4067

Accredited: Yes
Licensed Beds: 358

Key Personnel:
President/CEO...........................J Linsey Bradley, Jr
Chief Medical Staff.....................Dr. Ed McClusky
Clinical Director/Cardiac................Linda Bowles
Director Cardiac Catheterization Lab ....Anne Nugent
Emergency Room ....John Montalto
Director Infection/Disease Control ....Sylvia Radcliffe, RN
ICU ....Melanie Schulte
Intensive Coronary.....................Linda Bowles
Medical Surgical Nursing ....Melanie Schulte
Clinical Director/Women Services ....Jeanine Henegan
Director Respiratory Therapy ....Marty Partida

Measure	Cases	This Hospital	State Average	U.S. Average	Top Hospital
Heart Attack Care					
ACE Inhibitor or ARB for LVSD	111	86%	85%	82%	100%
Aspirin at Arrival	323	98%	91%	92%	100%
Aspirin at Discharge	501	95%	90%	90%	100%

Measure	Cases	This Hospital	State Average	U.S. Average	Top Hospital
Beta Blocker at Arrival	210	98%	85%	87%	100%
Beta Blocker at Discharge	290	96%	86%	90%	100%
Fibrinolytic Medication Timing[1]	1	0%	30%	31%	100%
PCI Within 90 Minutes of Arrival[1]	22	64%	48%	54%	95%
Smoking Cessation Advice	216	100%	90%	88%	100%
Heart Failure Care					
ACE Inhibitor or ARB for LVSD	238	95%	82%	82%	100%
Discharge Instructions	511	94%	60%	61%	93%
Evaluation of LVS Function	641	98%	81%	83%	99%
Smoking Cessation Advice	110	99%	82%	82%	100%
Pneumonia Care					
Appropriate Initial Antibiotic	268	84%	79%	83%	94%
Blood Culture Timing	242	88%	89%	90%	100%
Influenza Vaccine	109	70%	69%	70%	100%
Initial Antibiotic Timing	328	74%	78%	80%	93%
Oxygenation Assessment	448	100%	99%	99%	100%
Pneumococcal Vaccine	289	60%	68%	69%	94%
Smoking Cessation Advice	101	100%	83%	80%	100%
Surgical Infection Prevention					
Prophylactic Antibiotic Given[2,3]	255	65%	67%	77%	95%
Prophylactic Antibiotic Selection[2]	82	85%	86%	90%	100%
Prophylactic Antibiotic Stopped[2,3]	253	68%	68%	72%	95%
Pregnancy Care					
Inpatient Neonatal Mortality	-	-	-	-	-
Third or Fourth Degree Laceration	-	-	3.23%	3.63%	3.27%

Texas Spine and Joint Hospital
1814 Roseland Boulevard
Tyler, TX 75701
Ownership: Proprietary
Emergency Services: Yes

Phone: 903-525-3488

Accredited: No

Measure	Cases	This Hospital	State Average	U.S. Average	Top Hospital
Heart Attack Care					
ACE Inhibitor or ARB for LVSD[5]	-	-	85%	82%	100%
Aspirin at Arrival[5]	-	-	91%	92%	100%
Aspirin at Discharge[5]	-	-	90%	90%	100%
Beta Blocker at Arrival[5]	-	-	85%	87%	100%
Beta Blocker at Discharge[5]	-	-	86%	90%	100%
Fibrinolytic Medication Timing[5]	-	-	30%	31%	100%
PCI Within 90 Minutes of Arrival[5]	-	-	48%	54%	95%
Smoking Cessation Advice[5]	-	-	90%	88%	100%
Heart Failure Care					
ACE Inhibitor or ARB for LVSD[5]	-	-	82%	82%	100%
Discharge Instructions[5]	-	-	60%	61%	93%
Evaluation of LVS Function[5]	-	-	81%	83%	99%
Smoking Cessation Advice[5]	-	-	82%	82%	100%
Pneumonia Care					
Appropriate Initial Antibiotic[5]	-	-	79%	83%	94%
Blood Culture Timing[5]	-	-	89%	90%	100%
Influenza Vaccine[5]	-	-	69%	70%	100%
Initial Antibiotic Timing[5]	-	-	78%	80%	93%
Oxygenation Assessment[5]	-	-	99%	99%	100%
Pneumococcal Vaccine[5]	-	-	68%	69%	94%
Smoking Cessation Advice[5]	-	-	83%	80%	100%
Surgical Infection Prevention					
Prophylactic Antibiotic Given[1,2,3]	23	70%	67%	77%	95%
Prophylactic Antibiotic Selection[1,2]	23	96%	86%	90%	100%
Prophylactic Antibiotic Stopped[1,2,3]	22	77%	68%	72%	95%
Pregnancy Care					
Inpatient Neonatal Mortality	-	-	-	-	-
Third or Fourth Degree Laceration	-	-	3.23%	3.63%	3.27%

University of Texas Health Center at Tyler
11937 US Highway 271
Tyler, TX 75708
E-mail: sally.stuart@uthct.edu
URL: www.uthct.edu
Ownership: Government - State
Emergency Services: Yes

Phone: 903-877-3451
Fax: 903-877-5725

Accredited: Yes
Licensed Beds: 204

Key Personnel:
President ....Kirk A Calhoun

NOTE: Hospital profiles are in alphabetical order by state, then city, then hospital within the city; Rankings are sorted by rate in descending order and exclude hospitals with less than 25 cases; (1) The number of cases is too small (n<25) for purposes of reliably predicting hospital performance; (2) Measure reflects the hospital's indication that its submission was based upon a sample of its relevant discharges; (3) Rate reflects fewer than the maximum possible quarters of data for the measure; (4) Inaccurate information submitted and suppressed for one or more quarters; (5) No data is available from the hospital for this measure; Please refer to the User's Guide for a full explanation of data

Chief Medical Officer . . . . Steven Brown, MD
Emergency Room . . . . Gary Kempt, RN
Infection Control. . . . . Doris Jarvis, RN
ICU . . . . Gary Kempt, RN
Medical/Surgical Nursing . . . . Teresa Serratt, RN
OB/GYN/Women's Health . . . . Dr Kenna Stephenson
Director Respiratory Therapy . . . . Willie Blevins

Measure	Cases	This Hospital	State Average	U.S. Average	Top Hospital
Heart Attack Care					
ACE Inhibitor or ARB for LVSD[1]	11	91%	85%	82%	100%
Aspirin at Arrival	47	94%	91%	92%	100%
Aspirin at Discharge	51	92%	90%	90%	100%
Beta Blocker at Arrival	32	94%	85%	87%	100%
Beta Blocker at Discharge	58	93%	86%	90%	100%
Fibrinolytic Medication Timing[1]	1	0%	30%	31%	100%
PCI Within 90 Minutes of Arrival[1]	1	0%	48%	54%	95%
Smoking Cessation Advice	28	86%	90%	88%	100%
Heart Failure Care					
ACE Inhibitor or ARB for LVSD	82	95%	82%	82%	100%
Discharge Instructions	161	19%	60%	61%	93%
Evaluation of LVS Function	186	88%	81%	83%	99%
Smoking Cessation Advice	47	89%	82%	82%	100%
Pneumonia Care					
Appropriate Initial Antibiotic	110	85%	79%	83%	94%
Blood Culture Timing	78	95%	89%	90%	100%
Influenza Vaccine	35	83%	69%	70%	100%
Initial Antibiotic Timing	199	61%	78%	80%	93%
Oxygenation Assessment	225	100%	99%	99%	100%
Pneumococcal Vaccine	122	84%	68%	69%	94%
Smoking Cessation Advice	68	90%	83%	80%	100%
Surgical Infection Prevention					
Prophylactic Antibiotic Given[3]	87	71%	67%	77%	95%
Prophylactic Antibiotic Selection[1]	22	77%	86%	90%	100%
Prophylactic Antibiotic Stopped[3]	80	79%	68%	72%	95%
Pregnancy Care					
Inpatient Neonatal Mortality	-	-	-	-	-
Third or Fourth Degree Laceration	-	-	3.23%	3.63%	3.27%

Uvalde Memorial Hospital

1025 Garner Field Road   Phone: 830-278-6251
Uvalde, TX 78801   Fax: 830-278-8529
URL: www.umhtx.org
Ownership: Govt - Hospital District or Authority   Accredited: Yes
Emergency Services: Yes   Licensed Beds: 52
Key Personnel:
Administrator . . . . Jim Buckner
Chief Medical Staff. . . . . Dr Carl Utterback
Cardiac Lab . . . . Linda Griffin
Infection Control. . . . . Jacqueline Gillette
ICU . . . . Linda Griffin
Medical Surgical Nursing . . . . Suzanne Rue
OB/GYN/Women's Health . . . . Pauline Garcia
Respiratory/Cardiopulmonary. . . . . George Gear

Measure	Cases	This Hospital	State Average	U.S. Average	Top Hospital
Heart Attack Care					
ACE Inhibitor or ARB for LVSD[1]	11	100%	85%	82%	100%
Aspirin at Arrival[1]	23	100%	91%	92%	100%
Aspirin at Discharge[1]	16	94%	90%	90%	100%
Beta Blocker at Arrival[1]	21	76%	85%	87%	100%
Beta Blocker at Discharge[1]	19	84%	86%	90%	100%
Fibrinolytic Medication Timing	0	-	30%	31%	100%
PCI Within 90 Minutes of Arrival	0	-	48%	54%	95%
Smoking Cessation Advice[1]	2	100%	90%	88%	100%
Heart Failure Care					
ACE Inhibitor or ARB for LVSD	44	95%	82%	82%	100%
Discharge Instructions	79	81%	60%	61%	93%
Evaluation of LVS Function	99	96%	81%	83%	99%
Smoking Cessation Advice[1]	9	78%	82%	82%	100%
Pneumonia Care					
Appropriate Initial Antibiotic	51	71%	79%	83%	94%
Blood Culture Timing	44	91%	89%	90%	100%

Measure	Cases	This Hospital	State Average	U.S. Average	Top Hospital
Influenza Vaccine[1]	21	95%	69%	70%	100%
Initial Antibiotic Timing	73	79%	78%	80%	93%
Oxygenation Assessment	87	100%	99%	99%	100%
Pneumococcal Vaccine	52	92%	68%	69%	94%
Smoking Cessation Advice[1]	10	60%	83%	80%	100%
Surgical Infection Prevention					
Prophylactic Antibiotic Given[3]	59	53%	67%	77%	95%
Prophylactic Antibiotic Selection[1]	13	38%	86%	90%	100%
Prophylactic Antibiotic Stopped[3]	53	53%	68%	72%	95%
Pregnancy Care					
Inpatient Neonatal Mortality	-	-	-	-	-
Third or Fourth Degree Laceration	-	-	3.23%	3.63%	3.27%

Wilbarger General Hospital

920 Hillcrest Drive   Phone: 940-552-9351
Vernon, TX 76384   Fax: 940-553-2981
Ownership: Govt - Hospital District or Authority   Accredited: No
Emergency Services: Yes   Licensed Beds: 47
Key Personnel:
President/CEO. . . . . Jonathan Vocikel
Chief Medical Staff. . . . . Joe Mendoza Jr, MD
Infection Control. . . . . Joe Richie, RN
Administrator . . . . Larry Parsons
Medical Surgical Nursing . . . . Joe Richie
Operating Room/Surgical Services . . . . Tami Ferguson, RN
Respiratory/Cardiopulmonary. . . . . Lance Jameson

Measure	Cases	This Hospital	State Average	U.S. Average	Top Hospital
Heart Attack Care					
ACE Inhibitor or ARB for LVSD[1,3]	1	0%	85%	82%	100%
Aspirin at Arrival[1,3]	6	83%	91%	92%	100%
Aspirin at Discharge[1,3]	6	50%	90%	90%	100%
Beta Blocker at Arrival[1,3]	4	75%	85%	87%	100%
Beta Blocker at Discharge[1,3]	6	83%	86%	90%	100%
Fibrinolytic Medication Timing[3]	0	-	30%	31%	100%
PCI Within 90 Minutes of Arrival	0	-	48%	54%	95%
Smoking Cessation Advice[3]	0	-	90%	88%	100%
Heart Failure Care					
ACE Inhibitor or ARB for LVSD[1]	18	89%	82%	82%	100%
Discharge Instructions	43	91%	60%	61%	93%
Evaluation of LVS Function	51	94%	81%	83%	99%
Smoking Cessation Advice[1]	18	94%	82%	82%	100%
Pneumonia Care					
Appropriate Initial Antibiotic	37	73%	79%	83%	94%
Blood Culture Timing[1]	13	100%	89%	90%	100%
Influenza Vaccine[1]	7	57%	69%	70%	100%
Initial Antibiotic Timing	38	68%	78%	80%	93%
Oxygenation Assessment	47	100%	99%	99%	100%
Pneumococcal Vaccine	28	100%	68%	69%	94%
Smoking Cessation Advice[1]	13	92%	83%	80%	100%
Surgical Infection Prevention					
Prophylactic Antibiotic Given[1,3]	1	0%	67%	77%	95%
Prophylactic Antibiotic Selection[1]	2	100%	86%	90%	100%
Prophylactic Antibiotic Stopped[1,3]	1	100%	68%	72%	95%
Pregnancy Care					
Inpatient Neonatal Mortality	-	-	-	-	-
Third or Fourth Degree Laceration	-	-	3.23%	3.63%	3.27%

Citizens Medical Center

2701 Hospital Drive   Phone: 361-573-9181
Victoria, TX 77901   Fax: 361-573-0611
E-mail: info@citizensmedicalcenter.org
URL: www.citizensmedicalcenter.org
Ownership: Government - Local   Accredited: Yes
Emergency Services: Yes   Licensed Beds: 344
Key Personnel:
Chief Medical Staff. . . . . Kurtis Krueger
Chief Radiology . . . . Steven Schnicker, MD

Measure	Cases	This Hospital	State Average	U.S. Average	Top Hospital
Heart Attack Care					
ACE Inhibitor or ARB for LVSD[1]	22	100%	85%	82%	100%

NOTE: Hospital profiles are in alphabetical order by state, then city, then hospital within the city; Rankings are sorted by rate in descending order and exclude hospitals with less than 25 cases; (1) The number of cases is too small (n<25) for purposes of reliably predicting hospital performance; (2) Measure reflects the hospital's indication that its submission was based upon a sample of its relevant discharges; (3) Rate reflects fewer than the maximum possible quarters of data for the measure; (4) Inaccurate information submitted and suppressed for one or more quarters; (5) No data is available from the hospital for this measure; Please refer to the User's Guide for a full explanation of data

	133	100%	91%	92%	100%
Aspirin at Arrival	133	100%	91%	92%	100%
Aspirin at Discharge	157	100%	90%	90%	100%
Beta Blocker at Arrival	112	100%	85%	87%	100%
Beta Blocker at Discharge	147	100%	86%	90%	100%
Fibrinolytic Medication Timing[1]	6	67%	30%	31%	100%
PCI Within 90 Minutes of Arrival[1]	1	100%	48%	54%	95%
Smoking Cessation Advice	44	100%	90%	88%	100%
Heart Failure Care					
ACE Inhibitor or ARB for LVSD	88	100%	82%	82%	100%
Discharge Instructions	247	100%	60%	61%	93%
Evaluation of LVS Function	296	100%	81%	83%	99%
Smoking Cessation Advice	33	97%	82%	82%	100%
Pneumonia Care					
Appropriate Initial Antibiotic	94	89%	79%	83%	94%
Blood Culture Timing	79	96%	89%	90%	100%
Influenza Vaccine	50	38%	69%	70%	100%
Initial Antibiotic Timing	150	84%	78%	80%	93%
Oxygenation Assessment	175	100%	99%	99%	100%
Pneumococcal Vaccine	111	81%	68%	69%	94%
Smoking Cessation Advice	33	85%	83%	80%	100%
Surgical Infection Prevention					
Prophylactic Antibiotic Given[3]	447	89%	67%	77%	95%
Prophylactic Antibiotic Selection	172	94%	86%	90%	100%
Prophylactic Antibiotic Stopped[3]	438	69%	68%	72%	95%
Pregnancy Care					
Inpatient Neonatal Mortality	1,039	0.10%	-	-	-
Third or Fourth Degree Laceration	551	3.27%	3.23%	3.63%	3.27%

Detar Hospital Navarro

506 E San Antonio St
Victoria, TX 77901
URL: www.detar.com
Ownership: Proprietary
Emergency Services: Yes

Phone: 361-575-7441
Fax: 361-788-6114

Accredited: Yes
Licensed Beds: 234

Key Personnel:
CEO . . . . William R Blanchard
Director Medical/Surgical Nursing . . . . Sammie Knebel, RN
Director Respiratory Therapy . . . . Mack Dorton

Measure	Cases	This Hospital	State Average	U.S. Average	Top Hospital
Heart Attack Care					
ACE Inhibitor or ARB for LVSD	35	100%	85%	82%	100%
Aspirin at Arrival	82	98%	91%	92%	100%
Aspirin at Discharge	159	100%	90%	90%	100%
Beta Blocker at Arrival	62	97%	85%	87%	100%
Beta Blocker at Discharge	173	99%	86%	90%	100%
Fibrinolytic Medication Timing[1]	4	25%	30%	31%	100%
PCI Within 90 Minutes of Arrival[1]	2	50%	48%	54%	95%
Smoking Cessation Advice	62	100%	90%	88%	100%
Heart Failure Care					
ACE Inhibitor or ARB for LVSD	72	99%	82%	82%	100%
Discharge Instructions	197	100%	60%	61%	93%
Evaluation of LVS Function	296	98%	81%	83%	99%
Smoking Cessation Advice	47	100%	82%	82%	100%
Pneumonia Care					
Appropriate Initial Antibiotic	93	88%	79%	83%	94%
Blood Culture Timing	88	99%	89%	90%	100%
Influenza Vaccine	36	83%	69%	70%	100%
Initial Antibiotic Timing	118	83%	78%	80%	93%
Oxygenation Assessment	152	100%	99%	99%	100%
Pneumococcal Vaccine	107	97%	68%	69%	94%
Smoking Cessation Advice	44	100%	83%	80%	100%
Surgical Infection Prevention					
Prophylactic Antibiotic Given	450	94%	67%	77%	95%
Prophylactic Antibiotic Selection	113	96%	86%	90%	100%
Prophylactic Antibiotic Stopped	444	81%	68%	72%	95%
Pregnancy Care					
Inpatient Neonatal Mortality	1,306	0.15%	-	-	-
Third or Fourth Degree Laceration	710	2.82%	3.23%	3.63%	3.27%

Hillcrest Baptist Medical Center

3000 Herring Avenue
Waco, TX 76708
E-mail: info@hillcrest.net
URL: www.hillcrest.net
Ownership: Voluntary non-profit - Church
Emergency Services: Yes

Phone: 254-202-2000
Fax: 254-202-9420

Accredited: Yes
Licensed Beds: 393

Key Personnel:
President/CEO . . . . Arthur L Hohenberger, FACHE
Chief Medical Staff . . . . David G Hoffman, MD
Cardiac Lab Manager . . . . Lisa Perry
Catheterization Lab Manager . . . . Mike Heussner
Emergency Room Director . . . . Tammy Owens
OB/GYN Womens Health . . . . Sherry Baker, RN
Technical Director Respiratory Therapy . . . . Dan Bollier

Measure	Cases	This Hospital	State Average	U.S. Average	Top Hospital
Heart Attack Care					
ACE Inhibitor or ARB for LVSD	32	81%	85%	82%	100%
Aspirin at Arrival	169	97%	91%	92%	100%
Aspirin at Discharge	199	93%	90%	90%	100%
Beta Blocker at Arrival	150	99%	85%	87%	100%
Beta Blocker at Discharge	192	97%	86%	90%	100%
Fibrinolytic Medication Timing[1]	2	0%	30%	31%	100%
PCI Within 90 Minutes of Arrival[1]	4	50%	48%	54%	95%
Smoking Cessation Advice	87	94%	90%	88%	100%
Heart Failure Care					
ACE Inhibitor or ARB for LVSD	102	67%	82%	82%	100%
Discharge Instructions	210	53%	60%	61%	93%
Evaluation of LVS Function	283	87%	81%	83%	99%
Smoking Cessation Advice	68	75%	82%	82%	100%
Pneumonia Care					
Appropriate Initial Antibiotic	99	76%	79%	83%	94%
Blood Culture Timing	87	92%	89%	90%	100%
Influenza Vaccine[4,5]	-	-	69%	70%	100%
Initial Antibiotic Timing	136	76%	78%	80%	93%
Oxygenation Assessment	188	100%	99%	99%	100%
Pneumococcal Vaccine	96	44%	68%	69%	94%
Smoking Cessation Advice	68	79%	83%	80%	100%
Surgical Infection Prevention					
Prophylactic Antibiotic Given[3]	222	65%	67%	77%	95%
Prophylactic Antibiotic Selection	78	92%	86%	90%	100%
Prophylactic Antibiotic Stopped[3]	204	47%	68%	72%	95%
Pregnancy Care					
Inpatient Neonatal Mortality	-	-	-	-	-
Third or Fourth Degree Laceration	-	-	3.23%	3.63%	3.27%

Providence Health Center

6901 Medical Parkway
Waco, TX 76712
URL: www.providence.net
Ownership: Voluntary non-profit - Church
Emergency Services: Yes

Phone: 254-751-4000
Fax: 254-751-4769

Accredited: Yes
Licensed Beds: 426

Key Personnel:
Administrator/CEO . . . . Kent A Keahey
Chief Medical Staff . . . . Joe Cunningham, MD
Cardiac Lab . . . . Debbie Kucera
Catheterization Lab . . . . Debbie Kucera
Emergency Room . . . . Brenda Davis, RN
Medical Director Emergency Room . . . . John Hamilton, MD
ICU . . . . Brenda Davis, RN
Director Respiratory Therapy . . . . Jerry Balzen

Measure	Cases	This Hospital	State Average	U.S. Average	Top Hospital
Heart Attack Care					
ACE Inhibitor or ARB for LVSD	49	76%	85%	82%	100%
Aspirin at Arrival	251	93%	91%	92%	100%
Aspirin at Discharge	312	89%	90%	90%	100%
Beta Blocker at Arrival	199	88%	85%	87%	100%
Beta Blocker at Discharge	305	91%	86%	90%	100%
Fibrinolytic Medication Timing[1]	5	60%	30%	31%	100%
PCI Within 90 Minutes of Arrival[1]	10	40%	48%	54%	95%

NOTE: Hospital profiles are in alphabetical order by state, then city, then hospital within the city; Rankings are sorted by rate in descending order and exclude hospitals with less than 25 cases; (1) The number of cases is too small (n<25) for purposes of reliably predicting hospital performance; (2) Measure reflects the hospital's indication that its submission was based upon a sample of its relevant discharges; (3) Rate reflects fewer than the maximum possible quarters of data for the measure; (4) Inaccurate information submitted and suppressed for one or more quarters; (5) No data is available from the hospital for this measure; Please refer to the User's Guide for a full explanation of data

	113	96%	90%	88%	100%
Smoking Cessation Advice	113	96%	90%	88%	100%
Heart Failure Care					
ACE Inhibitor or ARB for LVSD	166	78%	82%	82%	100%
Discharge Instructions	378	61%	60%	61%	93%
Evaluation of LVS Function	483	88%	81%	83%	99%
Smoking Cessation Advice	77	90%	82%	82%	100%
Pneumonia Care					
Appropriate Initial Antibiotic	217	87%	79%	83%	94%
Blood Culture Timing	182	86%	89%	90%	100%
Influenza Vaccine	69	26%	69%	70%	100%
Initial Antibiotic Timing	261	77%	78%	80%	93%
Oxygenation Assessment	322	100%	99%	99%	100%
Pneumococcal Vaccine	213	28%	68%	69%	94%
Smoking Cessation Advice	71	96%	83%	80%	100%
Surgical Infection Prevention					
Prophylactic Antibiotic Given[2,3]	196	68%	67%	77%	95%
Prophylactic Antibiotic Selection[2]	72	92%	86%	90%	100%
Prophylactic Antibiotic Stopped[2,3]	189	50%	68%	72%	95%
Pregnancy Care					
Inpatient Neonatal Mortality	-	-	-	-	-
Third or Fourth Degree Laceration	-	-	3.23%	3.63%	3.27%

Baylor Medical Center-Ellis County

Alternate Name: Baylor Medical Center-Waxahachie

1405 W Jefferson Street
Waxahachie, TX 75165
URL: www.bhcs.com/locations/waxahachie
Ownership: Voluntary non-profit - Church
Emergency Services: Yes

Phone: 972-923-9095
Fax: 972-937-5948

Accredited: Yes
Licensed Beds: 69

Key Personnel:
Chief Medical Staff . . . . Janet Fain
Emergency Room . . . . William O'Malley, MD
Director Infection/Disease Control . . . . Iris Wilson
Coord. CCU . . . . Brenda Dodge
Director Medical/Surgical Nursing . . . . Brenda Dodge
OB/GYN Womens Health . . . . Annette Garcia
Chief Radiology . . . . Ronny Rose
Director Respiratory Therapy . . . . A Sue Simmons

Measure	Cases	This Hospital	State Average	U.S. Average	Top Hospital
Heart Attack Care					
ACE Inhibitor or ARB for LVSD[1]	3	100%	85%	82%	100%
Aspirin at Arrival[1]	12	100%	91%	92%	100%
Aspirin at Discharge[1]	9	100%	90%	90%	100%
Beta Blocker at Arrival[1]	12	92%	85%	87%	100%
Beta Blocker at Discharge[1]	9	100%	86%	90%	100%
Fibrinolytic Medication Timing[1]	1	100%	30%	31%	100%
PCI Within 90 Minutes of Arrival	0	-	48%	54%	95%
Smoking Cessation Advice	0	-	90%	88%	100%
Heart Failure Care					
ACE Inhibitor or ARB for LVSD	25	100%	82%	82%	100%
Discharge Instructions	66	83%	60%	61%	93%
Evaluation of LVS Function	88	95%	81%	83%	99%
Smoking Cessation Advice[1]	18	89%	82%	82%	100%
Pneumonia Care					
Appropriate Initial Antibiotic	106	91%	79%	83%	94%
Blood Culture Timing	96	93%	89%	90%	100%
Influenza Vaccine	29	93%	69%	70%	100%
Initial Antibiotic Timing	139	91%	78%	80%	93%
Oxygenation Assessment	167	100%	99%	99%	100%
Pneumococcal Vaccine	83	90%	68%	69%	94%
Smoking Cessation Advice	36	81%	83%	80%	100%
Surgical Infection Prevention					
Prophylactic Antibiotic Given	306	97%	67%	77%	95%
Prophylactic Antibiotic Selection	76	96%	86%	90%	100%
Prophylactic Antibiotic Stopped	296	98%	68%	72%	95%
Pregnancy Care					
Inpatient Neonatal Mortality	-	-	-	-	-
Third or Fourth Degree Laceration	-	-	3.23%	3.63%	3.27%

Campbell Health System

Alternate Name: Campbell Memorial Hospital

713 E Anderson Street
Weatherford, TX 76086
URL: www.campbellhealth.com
Ownership: Govt - Hospital District or Authority
Emergency Services: Yes

Phone: 817-596-8751
Fax: 817-598-0326

Accredited: Yes
Licensed Beds: 99

Key Personnel:
CEO . . . . Scott M Landrum
Chief Medical Staff . . . . James B Newton, MD
Emergency Room . . . . Donna Ivey, MD
Director Infection/Disease Control . . . . Debbie Weaber
CCU Spvg. Nurse . . . . Geri Lindsey
OB/GYN Womens Health . . . . William C Martin, MD
Director Radiology . . . . Sheryl Barnes

Measure	Cases	This Hospital	State Average	U.S. Average	Top Hospital
Heart Attack Care					
ACE Inhibitor or ARB for LVSD[1]	2	50%	85%	82%	100%
Aspirin at Arrival	27	89%	91%	92%	100%
Aspirin at Discharge[1]	10	70%	90%	90%	100%
Beta Blocker at Arrival	31	84%	85%	87%	100%
Beta Blocker at Discharge[1]	11	82%	86%	90%	100%
Fibrinolytic Medication Timing[3]	0	-	30%	31%	100%
PCI Within 90 Minutes of Arrival	0	-	48%	54%	95%
Smoking Cessation Advice[1,3]	1	100%	90%	88%	100%
Heart Failure Care					
ACE Inhibitor or ARB for LVSD	26	54%	82%	82%	100%
Discharge Instructions[3]	25	88%	60%	61%	93%
Evaluation of LVS Function	130	65%	81%	83%	99%
Smoking Cessation Advice[1,3]	3	100%	82%	82%	100%
Pneumonia Care					
Appropriate Initial Antibiotic[1,3]	21	81%	79%	83%	94%
Blood Culture Timing[1,3]	23	91%	89%	90%	100%
Influenza Vaccine[5]	-	-	69%	70%	100%
Initial Antibiotic Timing	158	93%	78%	80%	93%
Oxygenation Assessment	214	100%	99%	99%	100%
Pneumococcal Vaccine	128	19%	68%	69%	94%
Smoking Cessation Advice[1,3]	9	78%	83%	80%	100%
Surgical Infection Prevention					
Prophylactic Antibiotic Given[3]	90	52%	67%	77%	95%
Prophylactic Antibiotic Selection[5]	-	-	86%	90%	100%
Prophylactic Antibiotic Stopped[3]	81	46%	68%	72%	95%
Pregnancy Care					
Inpatient Neonatal Mortality	-	-	-	-	-
Third or Fourth Degree Laceration	-	-	3.23%	3.63%	3.27%

Clear Lake Regional Medical Center

500 Medical Center Boulevard
Webster, TX 77598
URL: www.clearlakermc.com
Ownership: Proprietary
Emergency Services: Yes

Phone: 281-332-2511
Fax: 281-338-3352

Accredited: Yes
Licensed Beds: 434

Key Personnel:
President/CEO . . . . Donald Shaffett
Chief Medical Staff . . . . James Searcy, MD
Catheterization Lab . . . . Lois Hershey
Emergency Room . . . . Maureen Fuhrmann
Infection Control . . . . Donna Outlaw
ICU/Intensive Coronary Care . . . . Ramona Taylor
OB/GYN Womens Health . . . . Carol Forsberg
Respiratory/Cardiopulmonary . . . . Dedra Walker

Measure	Cases	This Hospital	State Average	U.S. Average	Top Hospital
Heart Attack Care					
ACE Inhibitor or ARB for LVSD	97	95%	85%	82%	100%
Aspirin at Arrival	372	98%	91%	92%	100%
Aspirin at Discharge	409	97%	90%	90%	100%
Beta Blocker at Arrival	315	95%	85%	87%	100%
Beta Blocker at Discharge	390	97%	86%	90%	100%
Fibrinolytic Medication Timing[1]	2	100%	30%	31%	100%
PCI Within 90 Minutes of Arrival[1]	20	95%	48%	54%	95%
Smoking Cessation Advice	168	98%	90%	88%	100%
Heart Failure Care					
ACE Inhibitor or ARB for LVSD	219	84%	82%	82%	100%

NOTE: Hospital profiles are in alphabetical order by state, then city, then hospital within the city; Rankings are sorted by rate in descending order and exclude hospitals with less than 25 cases; (1) The number of cases is too small (n<25) for purposes of reliably predicting hospital performance; (2) Measure reflects the hospital's indication that its submission was based upon a sample of its relevant discharges; (3) Rate reflects fewer than the maximum possible quarters of data for the measure; (4) Inaccurate information submitted and suppressed for one or more quarters; (5) No data is available from the hospital for this measure; Please refer to the User's Guide for a full explanation of data

Measure	Cases	This Hospital	State Average	U.S. Average	Top Hospital
Discharge Instructions	386	44%	60%	61%	93%
Evaluation of LVS Function	526	100%	81%	83%	99%
Smoking Cessation Advice	74	89%	82%	82%	100%
Pneumonia Care					
Appropriate Initial Antibiotic	178	86%	79%	83%	94%
Blood Culture Timing	213	96%	89%	90%	100%
Influenza Vaccine	72	90%	69%	70%	100%
Initial Antibiotic Timing	267	79%	78%	80%	93%
Oxygenation Assessment	338	99%	99%	99%	100%
Pneumococcal Vaccine	197	90%	68%	69%	94%
Smoking Cessation Advice	100	94%	83%	80%	100%
Surgical Infection Prevention					
Prophylactic Antibiotic Given[2,3]	238	76%	67%	77%	95%
Prophylactic Antibiotic Selection[2]	101	69%	86%	90%	100%
Prophylactic Antibiotic Stopped[2,3]	228	56%	68%	72%	95%
Pregnancy Care					
Inpatient Neonatal Mortality	-	-	-	-	-
Third or Fourth Degree Laceration	-	-	3.23%	3.63%	3.27%

Houston Physicians' Hospital

333 N Texas Avenue
Webster, TX 77598
Ownership: Proprietary
Emergency Services: Yes

Phone: 281-335-1700

Accredited: No

Measure	Cases	This Hospital	State Average	U.S. Average	Top Hospital
Heart Attack Care					
ACE Inhibitor or ARB for LVSD[5]	-	-	85%	82%	100%
Aspirin at Arrival[5]	-	-	91%	92%	100%
Aspirin at Discharge[5]	-	-	90%	90%	100%
Beta Blocker at Arrival[5]	-	-	85%	87%	100%
Beta Blocker at Discharge[5]	-	-	86%	90%	100%
Fibrinolytic Medication Timing[5]	-	-	30%	31%	100%
PCI Within 90 Minutes of Arrival[5]	-	-	48%	54%	95%
Smoking Cessation Advice[5]	-	-	90%	88%	100%
Heart Failure Care					
ACE Inhibitor or ARB for LVSD[5]	-	-	82%	82%	100%
Discharge Instructions[5]	-	-	60%	61%	93%
Evaluation of LVS Function[5]	-	-	81%	83%	99%
Smoking Cessation Advice[5]	-	-	82%	82%	100%
Pneumonia Care					
Appropriate Initial Antibiotic[5]	-	-	79%	83%	94%
Blood Culture Timing[5]	-	-	89%	90%	100%
Influenza Vaccine[5]	-	-	69%	70%	100%
Initial Antibiotic Timing[5]	-	-	78%	80%	93%
Oxygenation Assessment[5]	-	-	99%	99%	100%
Pneumococcal Vaccine[5]	-	-	68%	69%	94%
Smoking Cessation Advice[5]	-	-	83%	80%	100%
Surgical Infection Prevention					
Prophylactic Antibiotic Given[1,2,3]	5	20%	67%	77%	95%
Prophylactic Antibiotic Selection[5]	-	-	86%	90%	100%
Prophylactic Antibiotic Stopped[1,2,3]	5	0%	68%	72%	95%
Pregnancy Care					
Inpatient Neonatal Mortality	-	-	-	-	-
Third or Fourth Degree Laceration	-	-	3.23%	3.63%	3.27%

Colorado Fayette Medical Center

400 Youens Drive
Weimar, TX 78962
E-mail: info@cfmc-online.com
URL: www.cfmc-online.com
Ownership: Proprietary
Emergency Services: Yes
Key Personnel:
CEO . . . . James M Robinson Sr

Phone: 979-725-9531
Fax: 979-725-8132

Accredited: No
Licensed Beds: 38

Measure	Cases	This Hospital	State Average	U.S. Average	Top Hospital
Heart Attack Care					
ACE Inhibitor or ARB for LVSD	0	-	85%	82%	100%
Aspirin at Arrival[1]	9	89%	91%	92%	100%
Aspirin at Discharge[1]	5	100%	90%	90%	100%
Beta Blocker at Arrival[1]	7	86%	85%	87%	100%

Measure	Cases	This Hospital	State Average	U.S. Average	Top Hospital
Beta Blocker at Discharge[1]	6	100%	86%	90%	100%
Fibrinolytic Medication Timing[3]	0	-	30%	31%	100%
PCI Within 90 Minutes of Arrival	0	-	48%	54%	95%
Smoking Cessation Advice[3]	0	-	90%	88%	100%
Heart Failure Care					
ACE Inhibitor or ARB for LVSD[1]	1	0%	82%	82%	100%
Discharge Instructions[1,3]	5	0%	60%	61%	93%
Evaluation of LVS Function	46	15%	81%	83%	99%
Smoking Cessation Advice[1,3]	1	0%	82%	82%	100%
Pneumonia Care					
Appropriate Initial Antibiotic[1,3]	5	100%	79%	83%	94%
Blood Culture Timing[1,3]	2	100%	89%	90%	100%
Influenza Vaccine[5]	-	-	69%	70%	100%
Initial Antibiotic Timing	48	79%	78%	80%	93%
Oxygenation Assessment	57	100%	99%	99%	100%
Pneumococcal Vaccine	40	58%	68%	69%	94%
Smoking Cessation Advice[1,3]	2	0%	83%	80%	100%
Surgical Infection Prevention					
Prophylactic Antibiotic Given[1,3]	4	25%	67%	77%	95%
Prophylactic Antibiotic Selection[5]	-	-	86%	90%	100%
Prophylactic Antibiotic Stopped[1,3]	3	100%	68%	72%	95%
Pregnancy Care					
Inpatient Neonatal Mortality	-	-	-	-	-
Third or Fourth Degree Laceration	-	-	3.23%	3.63%	3.27%

Knapp Medical Center

1401 E 8th Street
Weslaco, TX 78599
E-mail: JVasquez@Knappmed.org
URL: www.knappmed.org
Ownership: Voluntary non-profit - Private
Emergency Services: Yes
Key Personnel:
President/CEO . . . . Robert W Vanderveer
Emergency Room . . . . Ramiro Falas

Phone: 956-968-8567
Fax: 956-969-5132

Accredited: Yes
Licensed Beds: 200

Measure	Cases	This Hospital	State Average	U.S. Average	Top Hospital
Heart Attack Care					
ACE Inhibitor or ARB for LVSD[1]	6	33%	85%	82%	100%
Aspirin at Arrival	73	92%	91%	92%	100%
Aspirin at Discharge	27	89%	90%	90%	100%
Beta Blocker at Arrival	43	81%	85%	87%	100%
Beta Blocker at Discharge	31	90%	86%	90%	100%
Fibrinolytic Medication Timing[1]	1	0%	30%	31%	100%
PCI Within 90 Minutes of Arrival	0	-	48%	54%	95%
Smoking Cessation Advice[1]	2	0%	90%	88%	100%
Heart Failure Care					
ACE Inhibitor or ARB for LVSD	104	68%	82%	82%	100%
Discharge Instructions	295	58%	60%	61%	93%
Evaluation of LVS Function	337	90%	81%	83%	99%
Smoking Cessation Advice	32	66%	82%	82%	100%
Pneumonia Care					
Appropriate Initial Antibiotic	189	77%	79%	83%	94%
Blood Culture Timing	151	91%	89%	90%	100%
Influenza Vaccine[4,5]	-	-	69%	70%	100%
Initial Antibiotic Timing	278	63%	78%	80%	93%
Oxygenation Assessment	309	96%	99%	99%	100%
Pneumococcal Vaccine	213	59%	68%	69%	94%
Smoking Cessation Advice	30	70%	83%	80%	100%
Surgical Infection Prevention					
Prophylactic Antibiotic Given[3]	174	73%	67%	77%	95%
Prophylactic Antibiotic Selection	73	97%	86%	90%	100%
Prophylactic Antibiotic Stopped[3]	170	25%	68%	72%	95%
Pregnancy Care					
Inpatient Neonatal Mortality	-	-	-	-	-
Third or Fourth Degree Laceration	-	-	3.23%	3.63%	3.27%

NOTE: Hospital profiles are in alphabetical order by state, then city, then hospital within the city; Rankings are sorted by rate in descending order and exclude hospitals with less than 25 cases; (1) The number of cases is too small (n<25) for purposes of reliably predicting hospital performance; (2) Measure reflects the hospital's indication that its submission was based upon a sample of its relevant discharges; (3) Rate reflects fewer than the maximum possible quarters of data for the measure; (4) Inaccurate information submitted and suppressed for one or more quarters; (5) No data is available from the hospital for this measure; Please refer to the User's Guide for a full explanation of data

Gulf Coast Medical Center

1400 Highway 59
Wharton, TX 77488
URL: www.gulfcoastmedical.com
Ownership: Proprietary
Emergency Services: Yes

Phone: 979-532-2500
Fax: 979-282-6844

Accredited: Yes
Licensed Beds: 161

Key Personnel:
CEO. . . . . Donnie Frederic

Measure	Cases	This Hospital	State Average	U.S. Average	Top Hospital
Heart Attack Care					
ACE Inhibitor or ARB for LVSD[1]	3	100%	85%	82%	100%
Aspirin at Arrival	25	92%	91%	92%	100%
Aspirin at Discharge[1]	11	91%	90%	90%	100%
Beta Blocker at Arrival[1]	13	85%	85%	87%	100%
Beta Blocker at Discharge[1]	12	92%	86%	90%	100%
Fibrinolytic Medication Timing[1]	6	0%	30%	31%	100%
PCI Within 90 Minutes of Arrival	0	-	48%	54%	95%
Smoking Cessation Advice[1]	3	67%	90%	88%	100%
Heart Failure Care					
ACE Inhibitor or ARB for LVSD	31	94%	82%	82%	100%
Discharge Instructions	75	36%	60%	61%	93%
Evaluation of LVS Function	88	92%	81%	83%	99%
Smoking Cessation Advice[1]	17	59%	82%	82%	100%
Pneumonia Care					
Appropriate Initial Antibiotic	50	88%	79%	83%	94%
Blood Culture Timing	38	92%	89%	90%	100%
Influenza Vaccine[1]	10	40%	69%	70%	100%
Initial Antibiotic Timing	71	85%	78%	80%	93%
Oxygenation Assessment	80	95%	99%	99%	100%
Pneumococcal Vaccine	47	89%	68%	69%	94%
Smoking Cessation Advice[1]	17	82%	83%	80%	100%
Surgical Infection Prevention					
Prophylactic Antibiotic Given	145	88%	67%	77%	95%
Prophylactic Antibiotic Selection	35	91%	86%	90%	100%
Prophylactic Antibiotic Stopped	141	81%	68%	72%	95%
Pregnancy Care					
Inpatient Neonatal Mortality	-	-	-	-	-
Third or Fourth Degree Laceration	-	-	3.23%	3.63%	3.27%

Parkview Hospital

901 S. Sweetwater
Wheeler, TX 79096
Ownership: Govt - Hospital District or Authority
Emergency Services: No

Phone: 806-826-5581

Accredited: No

Measure	Cases	This Hospital	State Average	U.S. Average	Top Hospital
Heart Attack Care					
ACE Inhibitor or ARB for LVSD[5]	-	-	85%	82%	100%
Aspirin at Arrival[5]	-	-	91%	92%	100%
Aspirin at Discharge[5]	-	-	90%	90%	100%
Beta Blocker at Arrival[5]	-	-	85%	87%	100%
Beta Blocker at Discharge[5]	-	-	86%	90%	100%
Fibrinolytic Medication Timing[5]	-	-	30%	31%	100%
PCI Within 90 Minutes of Arrival[5]	-	-	48%	54%	95%
Smoking Cessation Advice[5]	-	-	90%	88%	100%
Heart Failure Care					
ACE Inhibitor or ARB for LVSD[3]	0	-	82%	82%	100%
Discharge Instructions[1,3]	2	100%	60%	61%	93%
Evaluation of LVS Function[1,3]	2	50%	81%	83%	99%
Smoking Cessation Advice[3]	0	-	82%	82%	100%
Pneumonia Care					
Appropriate Initial Antibiotic[1,3]	21	62%	79%	83%	94%
Blood Culture Timing[1,3]	3	67%	89%	90%	100%
Influenza Vaccine[1]	2	100%	69%	70%	100%
Initial Antibiotic Timing[1,3]	16	81%	78%	80%	93%
Oxygenation Assessment[1,3]	22	100%	99%	99%	100%
Pneumococcal Vaccine[1,3]	17	41%	68%	69%	94%
Smoking Cessation Advice[1,3]	8	75%	83%	80%	100%
Surgical Infection Prevention					
Prophylactic Antibiotic Given[5]	-	-	67%	77%	95%
Prophylactic Antibiotic Selection[5]	-	-	86%	90%	100%

Prophylactic Antibiotic Stopped[5]	-	-	68%	72%	95%
Pregnancy Care					
Inpatient Neonatal Mortality	-	-	-	-	-
Third or Fourth Degree Laceration	-	-	3.23%	3.63%	3.27%

Lake Whitney Medical Center

200 N San Jacinto Street
PO Box 458
Whitney, TX 76692
Ownership: Voluntary non-profit - Private
Emergency Services: Yes

Phone: 254-694-3165
Fax: 254-694-3299

Accredited: No
Licensed Beds: 49

Key Personnel:
Administrator . . . . Ted Howard
Chief Medical Staff . . . . Clayton Pickering, DO
Emergency Room . . . . Elaine Morrow, DON

Measure	Cases	This Hospital	State Average	U.S. Average	Top Hospital
Heart Attack Care					
ACE Inhibitor or ARB for LVSD[3]	0	-	85%	82%	100%
Aspirin at Arrival[1,3]	3	67%	91%	92%	100%
Aspirin at Discharge[1,3]	4	25%	90%	90%	100%
Beta Blocker at Arrival[1,3]	2	100%	85%	87%	100%
Beta Blocker at Discharge[1,3]	3	67%	86%	90%	100%
Fibrinolytic Medication Timing[3]	0	-	30%	31%	100%
PCI Within 90 Minutes of Arrival	0	-	48%	54%	95%
Smoking Cessation Advice[1,3]	1	0%	90%	88%	100%
Heart Failure Care					
ACE Inhibitor or ARB for LVSD[1,3]	2	50%	82%	82%	100%
Discharge Instructions[1,3]	3	0%	60%	61%	93%
Evaluation of LVS Function[1,3]	6	33%	81%	83%	99%
Smoking Cessation Advice[1,3]	1	0%	82%	82%	100%
Pneumonia Care					
Appropriate Initial Antibiotic[1,3]	4	100%	79%	83%	94%
Blood Culture Timing[1,3]	2	100%	89%	90%	100%
Influenza Vaccine[5]	-	-	69%	70%	100%
Initial Antibiotic Timing[1,3]	7	71%	78%	80%	93%
Oxygenation Assessment[1,3]	14	100%	99%	99%	100%
Pneumococcal Vaccine[1,3]	11	18%	68%	69%	94%
Smoking Cessation Advice[1,3]	1	0%	83%	80%	100%
Surgical Infection Prevention					
Prophylactic Antibiotic Given[5]	-	-	67%	77%	95%
Prophylactic Antibiotic Selection[5]	-	-	86%	90%	100%
Prophylactic Antibiotic Stopped[5]	-	-	68%	72%	95%
Pregnancy Care					
Inpatient Neonatal Mortality	-	-	-	-	-
Third or Fourth Degree Laceration	-	-	3.23%	3.63%	3.27%

Kell West Regional Hospital

5402 Kell West Boulevard
Wichita Falls, TX 76310
E-mail: info@kellwest.com
URL: www.kellwest.com
Ownership: Proprietary
Emergency Services: Yes

Phone: 940-692-5888
Fax: 940-692-0915

Accredited: Yes
Licensed Beds: 41

Measure	Cases	This Hospital	State Average	U.S. Average	Top Hospital
Heart Attack Care					
ACE Inhibitor or ARB for LVSD[3]	0	-	85%	82%	100%
Aspirin at Arrival[3]	0	-	91%	92%	100%
Aspirin at Discharge[3]	0	-	90%	90%	100%
Beta Blocker at Arrival[3]	0	-	85%	87%	100%
Beta Blocker at Discharge[3]	0	-	86%	90%	100%
Fibrinolytic Medication Timing[3]	0	-	30%	31%	100%
PCI Within 90 Minutes of Arrival	0	-	48%	54%	95%
Smoking Cessation Advice[3]	0	-	90%	88%	100%
Heart Failure Care					
ACE Inhibitor or ARB for LVSD[1]	4	100%	82%	82%	100%
Discharge Instructions[1,3]	1	100%	60%	61%	93%
Evaluation of LVS Function[1]	9	78%	81%	83%	99%
Smoking Cessation Advice[3]	0	-	82%	82%	100%
Pneumonia Care					
Appropriate Initial Antibiotic[1,3]	2	100%	79%	83%	94%

NOTE: Hospital profiles are in alphabetical order by state, then city, then hospital within the city; Rankings are sorted by rate in descending order and exclude hospitals with less than 25 cases; (1) The number of cases is too small (n<25) for purposes of reliably predicting hospital performance; (2) Measure reflects the hospital's indication that its submission was based upon a sample of its relevant discharges; (3) Rate reflects fewer than the maximum possible quarters of data for the measure; (4) Inaccurate information submitted and suppressed for one or more quarters; (5) No data is available from the hospital for this measure; Please refer to the User's Guide for a full explanation of data

Measure	Cases	This Hospital	State Average	U.S. Average	Top Hospital
Blood Culture Timing[1,3]	1	100%	89%	90%	100%
Influenza Vaccine[5]	-	-	69%	70%	100%
Initial Antibiotic Timing	34	79%	78%	80%	93%
Oxygenation Assessment	39	100%	99%	99%	100%
Pneumococcal Vaccine[1]	23	65%	68%	69%	94%
Smoking Cessation Advice[1,3]	1	100%	83%	80%	100%
Surgical Infection Prevention					
Prophylactic Antibiotic Given[3]	0	-	67%	77%	95%
Prophylactic Antibiotic Selection[5]	-	-	86%	90%	100%
Prophylactic Antibiotic Stopped[3]	0	-	68%	72%	95%
Pregnancy Care					
Inpatient Neonatal Mortality	-	-	-	-	-
Third or Fourth Degree Laceration	-	-	3.23%	3.63%	3.27%

United Regional Healthcare System

Alternate Name: Bethania Regional Health Care Center
1600 11th Street
Wichita Falls, TX 76301
URL: www.urhcs.org
Ownership: Voluntary non-profit - Church
Emergency Services: Yes

Phone: 940-764-7000
Fax: 940-764-3996

Accredited: Yes
Licensed Beds: 541

Key Personnel:
President/CEO......................... Ms. Phyllis Cowling
Chief Medical Staff....................... Ashwin Patel, MD
Director Cardiology .... Ms. Lisa Green
Emergency Room .... Kim Felder, RN
Medical Director Emergency Room .... Rodrigo Menechaca, MD
Infection Control........................ Charlene Mossman, RN
ICU .... Pam Bradshaw, RN
Intensive Coronary Care .... Pam Bradshaw, RN
Director OB/GYN/Women's Health........... Charla Hoff, RN
Surgical Services/Anes. Director .... Mr. Wayne Cure
Director Respiratory Therapy .... Ms. Shelley Moser

Measure	Cases	This Hospital	State Average	U.S. Average	Top Hospital
Heart Attack Care					
ACE Inhibitor or ARB for LVSD	64	91%	85%	82%	100%
Aspirin at Arrival	199	97%	91%	92%	100%
Aspirin at Discharge	301	93%	90%	90%	100%
Beta Blocker at Arrival	185	95%	85%	87%	100%
Beta Blocker at Discharge	291	95%	86%	90%	100%
Fibrinolytic Medication Timing[1]	6	50%	30%	31%	100%
PCI Within 90 Minutes of Arrival[1]	16	88%	48%	54%	95%
Smoking Cessation Advice	119	92%	90%	88%	100%
Heart Failure Care					
ACE Inhibitor or ARB for LVSD	116	83%	82%	82%	100%
Discharge Instructions	262	42%	60%	61%	93%
Evaluation of LVS Function	323	90%	81%	83%	99%
Smoking Cessation Advice	62	77%	82%	82%	100%
Pneumonia Care					
Appropriate Initial Antibiotic	166	81%	79%	83%	94%
Blood Culture Timing	138	82%	89%	90%	100%
Influenza Vaccine	44	59%	69%	70%	100%
Initial Antibiotic Timing	222	76%	78%	80%	93%
Oxygenation Assessment	272	100%	99%	99%	100%
Pneumococcal Vaccine	156	72%	68%	69%	94%
Smoking Cessation Advice	88	84%	83%	80%	100%
Surgical Infection Prevention					
Prophylactic Antibiotic Given[3]	276	32%	67%	77%	95%
Prophylactic Antibiotic Selection	87	92%	86%	90%	100%
Prophylactic Antibiotic Stopped[3]	263	30%	68%	72%	95%
Pregnancy Care					
Inpatient Neonatal Mortality	-	-	-	-	-
Third or Fourth Degree Laceration	-	-	3.23%	3.63%	3.27%

Presbyterian Hospital of Winnsboro

719 W Coke Road
Winnsboro, TX 75494
URL: www.texashealth.org
Ownership: Voluntary non-profit - Private
Emergency Services: Yes

Phone: 903-342-5227
Fax: 903-342-3952

Accredited: Yes
Licensed Beds: 50

Key Personnel:
President .... Matthew Troup

Measure	Cases	This Hospital	State Average	U.S. Average	Top Hospital
Heart Attack Care					
ACE Inhibitor or ARB for LVSD[3]	0	-	85%	82%	100%
Aspirin at Arrival[1,3]	3	100%	91%	92%	100%
Aspirin at Discharge[1,3]	1	100%	90%	90%	100%
Beta Blocker at Arrival[1,3]	1	100%	85%	87%	100%
Beta Blocker at Discharge[3]	0	-	86%	90%	100%
Fibrinolytic Medication Timing[3]	0	-	30%	31%	100%
PCI Within 90 Minutes of Arrival	0	-	48%	54%	95%
Smoking Cessation Advice[3]	0	-	90%	88%	100%
Heart Failure Care					
ACE Inhibitor or ARB for LVSD[1]	9	89%	82%	82%	100%
Discharge Instructions	32	91%	60%	61%	93%
Evaluation of LVS Function	45	93%	81%	83%	99%
Smoking Cessation Advice[1]	11	91%	82%	82%	100%
Pneumonia Care					
Appropriate Initial Antibiotic[1]	23	91%	79%	83%	94%
Blood Culture Timing	30	97%	89%	90%	100%
Influenza Vaccine[1]	14	100%	69%	70%	100%
Initial Antibiotic Timing	35	91%	78%	80%	93%
Oxygenation Assessment	51	100%	99%	99%	100%
Pneumococcal Vaccine	41	98%	68%	69%	94%
Smoking Cessation Advice[1]	6	100%	83%	80%	100%
Surgical Infection Prevention					
Prophylactic Antibiotic Given[1,3]	10	60%	67%	77%	95%
Prophylactic Antibiotic Selection[1]	2	100%	86%	90%	100%
Prophylactic Antibiotic Stopped[1,3]	9	89%	68%	72%	95%
Pregnancy Care					
Inpatient Neonatal Mortality	-	-	-	-	-
Third or Fourth Degree Laceration	-	-	3.23%	3.63%	3.27%

North Runnels Hospital

East Highway 53
Winters, TX 79567
E-mail: viper@camalott.com
Ownership: Govt - Hospital District or Authority
Emergency Services: Yes

Phone: 325-754-4553
Fax: 325-754-5097

Accredited: No
Licensed Beds: 25

Key Personnel:
Administrator .... Roland K Rickard

Measure	Cases	This Hospital	State Average	U.S. Average	Top Hospital
Heart Attack Care					
ACE Inhibitor or ARB for LVSD[5]	-	-	85%	82%	100%
Aspirin at Arrival[5]	-	-	91%	92%	100%
Aspirin at Discharge[5]	-	-	90%	90%	100%
Beta Blocker at Arrival[5]	-	-	85%	87%	100%
Beta Blocker at Discharge[5]	-	-	86%	90%	100%
Fibrinolytic Medication Timing[5]	-	-	30%	31%	100%
PCI Within 90 Minutes of Arrival[5]	-	-	48%	54%	95%
Smoking Cessation Advice[5]	-	-	90%	88%	100%
Heart Failure Care					
ACE Inhibitor or ARB for LVSD[5]	-	-	82%	82%	100%
Discharge Instructions[5]	-	-	60%	61%	93%
Evaluation of LVS Function[5]	-	-	81%	83%	99%
Smoking Cessation Advice[5]	-	-	82%	82%	100%
Pneumonia Care					
Appropriate Initial Antibiotic[5]	-	-	79%	83%	94%
Blood Culture Timing[5]	-	-	89%	90%	100%
Influenza Vaccine[5]	-	-	69%	70%	100%
Initial Antibiotic Timing[5]	-	-	78%	80%	93%
Oxygenation Assessment[5]	-	-	99%	99%	100%
Pneumococcal Vaccine[5]	-	-	68%	69%	94%
Smoking Cessation Advice[5]	-	-	83%	80%	100%
Surgical Infection Prevention					
Prophylactic Antibiotic Given[5]	-	-	67%	77%	95%
Prophylactic Antibiotic Selection[5]	-	-	86%	90%	100%
Prophylactic Antibiotic Stopped[5]	-	-	68%	72%	95%
Pregnancy Care					
Inpatient Neonatal Mortality	-	-	-	-	-
Third or Fourth Degree Laceration	-	-	3.23%	3.63%	3.27%

NOTE: Hospital profiles are in alphabetical order by state, then city, then hospital within the city; Rankings are sorted by rate in descending order and exclude hospitals with less than 25 cases; (1) The number of cases is too small (n<25) for purposes of reliably predicting hospital performance; (2) Measure reflects the hospital's indication that its submission was based upon a sample of its relevant discharges; (3) Rate reflects fewer than the maximum possible quarters of data for the measure; (4) Inaccurate information submitted and suppressed for one or more quarters; (5) No data is available from the hospital for this measure; Please refer to the User's Guide for a full explanation of data

Tyler County Hospital

PO Drawer 549
Woodville, TX 75979
E-mail: vphillips@tchospital.us
URL: www.tchospital.us
Ownership: Govt - Hospital District or Authority
Emergency Services: Yes

Phone: 409-283-6192
Fax: 409-283-7424

Accredited: No
Licensed Beds: 49

Key Personnel:
President/CEO . . . . Sandra Smith Jackson, RN EdD
Chief Medical Staff . . . . Paula Schuttz, MD
Emergency Room . . . . Curtisad Garner, MD
Infection Control . . . . Sondra Wilson, RN
Respiratory Therapy Director . . . . Janay James, CRT

Measure	Cases	This Hospital	State Average	U.S. Average	Top Hospital
Heart Attack Care					
ACE Inhibitor or ARB for LVSD[1]	1	100%	85%	82%	100%
Aspirin at Arrival[1]	7	100%	91%	92%	100%
Aspirin at Discharge[1]	1	100%	90%	90%	100%
Beta Blocker at Arrival[1]	7	86%	85%	87%	100%
Beta Blocker at Discharge[1]	2	50%	86%	90%	100%
Fibrinolytic Medication Timing[3]	0	-	30%	31%	100%
PCI Within 90 Minutes of Arrival	0	-	48%	54%	95%
Smoking Cessation Advice[3]	0	-	90%	88%	100%
Heart Failure Care					
ACE Inhibitor or ARB for LVSD[1]	6	100%	82%	82%	100%
Discharge Instructions[1,3]	6	33%	60%	61%	93%
Evaluation of LVS Function	54	70%	81%	83%	99%
Smoking Cessation Advice[1,3]	2	100%	82%	82%	100%
Pneumonia Care					
Appropriate Initial Antibiotic[1,3]	6	83%	79%	83%	94%
Blood Culture Timing[1,3]	8	75%	89%	90%	100%
Influenza Vaccine[5]	-	-	69%	70%	100%
Initial Antibiotic Timing	63	86%	78%	80%	93%
Oxygenation Assessment	70	100%	99%	99%	100%
Pneumococcal Vaccine	45	53%	68%	69%	94%
Smoking Cessation Advice[1,3]	1	100%	83%	80%	100%
Surgical Infection Prevention					
Prophylactic Antibiotic Given[5]	-	-	67%	77%	95%
Prophylactic Antibiotic Selection[5]	-	-	86%	90%	100%
Prophylactic Antibiotic Stopped[5]	-	-	68%	72%	95%
Pregnancy Care					
Inpatient Neonatal Mortality	-	-	-	-	-
Third or Fourth Degree Laceration	-	-	3.23%	3.63%	3.27%

Yoakum Community Hospital

1200 Carl Ramert Drive
Yoakum, TX 77995
URL: www.yoakumhospital.com
Ownership: Govt - Hospital District or Authority
Emergency Services: Yes

Phone: 361-293-2321
Fax: 361-293-6172

Accredited: No
Licensed Beds: 25

Key Personnel:
CEO . . . . Wayne Ogburn
Chief Medical Staff . . . . Marshall C Bishop, MD
Emergency Room . . . . Pat Bembow
Infection Control . . . . Kim Mraz, RN
Medical/Surgical Nursing . . . . Patricia Benbow, RN

Measure	Cases	This Hospital	State Average	U.S. Average	Top Hospital
Heart Attack Care					
ACE Inhibitor or ARB for LVSD	0	-	85%	82%	100%
Aspirin at Arrival[1]	9	89%	91%	92%	100%
Aspirin at Discharge[1]	5	80%	90%	90%	100%
Beta Blocker at Arrival[1]	9	56%	85%	87%	100%
Beta Blocker at Discharge[1]	5	40%	86%	90%	100%
Fibrinolytic Medication Timing[3]	0	-	30%	31%	100%
PCI Within 90 Minutes of Arrival[5]	-	-	48%	54%	95%
Smoking Cessation Advice	0	-	90%	88%	100%
Heart Failure Care					
ACE Inhibitor or ARB for LVSD[1]	21	86%	82%	82%	100%
Discharge Instructions	42	31%	60%	61%	93%
Evaluation of LVS Function	60	82%	81%	83%	99%

Measure	Cases	This Hospital	State Average	U.S. Average	Top Hospital
Smoking Cessation Advice[1]	7	71%	82%	82%	100%
Pneumonia Care					
Appropriate Initial Antibiotic[1]	19	74%	79%	83%	94%
Blood Culture Timing[1]	9	67%	89%	90%	100%
Influenza Vaccine[1]	9	89%	69%	70%	100%
Initial Antibiotic Timing	30	83%	78%	80%	93%
Oxygenation Assessment	34	100%	99%	99%	100%
Pneumococcal Vaccine[1]	24	67%	68%	69%	94%
Smoking Cessation Advice[1]	7	29%	83%	80%	100%
Surgical Infection Prevention					
Prophylactic Antibiotic Given[5]	-	-	67%	77%	95%
Prophylactic Antibiotic Selection[5]	-	-	86%	90%	100%
Prophylactic Antibiotic Stopped[5]	-	-	68%	72%	95%
Pregnancy Care					
Inpatient Neonatal Mortality	-	-	-	-	-
Third or Fourth Degree Laceration	-	-	3.23%	3.63%	3.27%

NOTE: Hospital profiles are in alphabetical order by state, then city, then hospital within the city; Rankings are sorted by rate in descending order and exclude hospitals with less than 25 cases; (1) The number of cases is too small (n<25) for purposes of reliably predicting hospital performance; (2) Measure reflects the hospital's indication that its submission was based upon a sample of its relevant discharges; (3) Rate reflects fewer than the maximum possible quarters of data for the measure; (4) Inaccurate information submitted and suppressed for one or more quarters; (5) No data is available from the hospital for this measure; Please refer to the User's Guide for a full explanation of data

ALABAMA

Hospital	Heart Attack Care 1	2	3	4	5	6	7	8	Heart Failure Care 9	10	11	12	13	14	Pneumonia Care 15	16	17	18	Surgical Infection Prevention 19	20	21	22	Pregnancy Care 23	24
Andalusia Regional Hospital, Andalusia, AL	-	50 2	67 3	100 3	100 4	- 0	- 0	- 0	59 0	86 149	80 183	100 22	76 95	81 52	45 31	85 106	100 134	51 73	84 38	73 118	94 51	52 118	-	-
Athens-Limestone Hospital, Athens, AL	33 3	92 13	100 4	69 16	100 4	- 0	- 0	- 0	90 51	16 115	86 154	92 25	79 167	88 85	- 8	64 171	96 211	62 95	80 56	38 183	100 38	65 179	-	-
Atmore Community Hospital, Atmore, AL	100 1	71 7	67 3	0	100 2	-	-	100 1	81 26	69 59	89 70	95 21	78 32	94 18	62 8	89 37	98 46	79 33	90 10	-	-	-	-	-
Baptist Medical Center, Montgomery, AL	78 64	95 106	98 220	95 86	97 251	0	20 5	100 113	80 145	84 268	89 291	100 81	73 73	84 81	62 16	70 116	99 153	68 72	100 50	77 208	81 69	69 196	1.32 303	0.63 158
Baptist Medical Center East, Montgomery, AL	67 3	97 29	88 16	100 32	95 21	-	-	100 5	77 57	58 186	92 200	83 24	81 106	80 80	74 27	80 130	99 162	78 96	94 32	80 87	94 31	80 83	0.63 638	3.86 2148
Bibb Medical Center, Centreville, AL	-	-	-	-	-	-	-	-	100 3	7 14	19 16	67 3	94 36	75 8	27 11	99 36	100 49	57 28	71 7	-	-	-	-	-
Brookwood Medical Center, Birmingham, AL	94 50	97 146	96 182	97 138	99 184	-	71 14	98 65	84 182	72 355	92 424	94 94	82 292	87 212	69 11	91 337	100 426	87 250	93 70	88 1059	94 145	69 1001	-	-
Bryan W Whitfield Memorial Hospital, Demopolis, AL	100 1	56 18	92 12	47 19	58 12	-	-	0	100 7	93 1	37 105	22 18	53 58	86 7	0 13	65 80	97 97	16 43	50 22	61 23	88 8	83 23	-	-
Bullock County Hospital, Union Springs, AL	-	-	-	0	100 1	-	-	100 1	100 1	1 12	13 38	50 2	83 12	86 7	25 8	83 18	100 20	44 9	0 2	-	-	-	-	-
Callahan Eye Foundation Hospital, Birmingham, AL	-	-	-	-	-	-	-	-	-	-	-	-	-	-	-	-	-	-	-	-	-	-	-	-
Cherokee Medical Center, Centre, AL	50 2	43 7	100 2	67 3	100 2	50 2	-	-	77 31	49 43	79 67	83 12	82 44	75 28	45 11	86 58	100 66	61 38	75 16	0	0	0	-	-
Chilton Medical Center, Clanton, AL	-	0	0	0	0	-	-	100 1	67 1	58 12	93 15	0	78 36	74 19	71 7	80 44	100 46	67 24	100 7	-	0	0	-	-
Citizens Baptist Medical Center, Talladega, AL	100 4	88 24	94 16	64 11	94 16	-	-	100 1	73 49	44 110	87 126	78 27	80 86	92 61	50 24	90 99	97 117	55 55	82 33	68 77	85 26	90 72	-	-
Clay County Hospital, Ashland, AL	-	75 4	75 4	33 3	40 5	-	-	-	64 11	1 67	37 83	58 12	83 59	89 18	60 15	79 71	97 86	38 47	63 19	-	-	-	-	-
Community Hospital, Tallassee, AL	0	86 7	67 6	100 7	83 6	-	-	-	93 43	52 73	100 87	53 19	85 52	94 34	75 12	60 100	99 100	74 34	82 17	83 12	100 3	92 12	-	-
Cooper Green Mercy Hospital, Birmingham, AL	100 4	100 25	100 21	100 24	100 23	-	-	85 20	100 62	71 107	93 108	82 61	77 70	60 43	33 9	46 94	99 100	70 10	64 59	40 65	66 29	62 50	-	-
Coosa Valley Baptist Medical Center, Sylacauga, AL	67 6	97 32	93 14	89 27	93 15	-	-	67 3	79 57	51 84	80 112	86 21	89 101	92 74	60 20	89 104	97 122	44 61	82 33	72 87	100 27	24 83	-	-
Crenshaw Baptist Hospital, Luverne, AL	100 1	75 4	100 3	75 4	100 3	-	-	100 1	55 11	26 56	56 32	17 6	79 38	100 21	62 8	42 55	95 62	29 38	13 15	0	0	0	-	-
Crestwood Medical Center, Huntsville, AL	87 15	90 84	94 79	86 70	91 77	0	100 4	87 31	89 87	68 189	86 234	83 12	78 155	95 101	74 31	64 173	99 197	72 109	81 32	83 797	89 106	69 764	-	-
Cullman Regional Medical Center, Cullman, AL	86 7	97 62	87 31	90 49	88 32	0	-	100 7	92 89	87 172	87 193	92 37	81 171	93 122	78 45	85 193	100 238	84 156	68 37	98 440	95 132	82 423	-	-
D W McMillan Memorial Hospital, Brewton, AL	100 1	100 3	50 2	90 10	50 2	100 2	-	0	63 19	42 74	95 78	84 19	90 50	96 50	92 12	97 64	100 80	77 44	91 22	81 26	93 14	85 26	-	-
Dale Medical Center, Ozark, AL	0	84 19	80 5	79 14	67 6	100 1	-	100 1	89 9	21 56	86 63	69 16	61 74	85 53	100 8	84 80	100 106	44 57	78 32	27 11	100 8	73 11	-	-
DCH Regional Medical Center, Tuscaloosa, AL	77 60	98 161	98 258	86 126	96 252	0	78 9	100 119	83 116	73 245	86 288	100 45	78 199	85 155	88 59	69 301	99 385	82 196	90 90	86 262	86 69	71 241	-	-
Decatur General Hospital, Decatur, AL	86 44	99 142	97 149	94 131	95 153	67	100 3	94 54	87 143	85 304	91 364	70	81 171	95 136	91 35	83 235	99 279	94 146	86 95	97 246	95 132	89 236	-	-
DeKalb Regional Medical Center, Fort Payne, AL	80 5	92 24	83 12	95 19	92 12	24 17	50 10	60 5	83 60	78 95	96 119	100 20	81 104	88 65	69 36	78 127	99 153	62 85	37 26	56 171	93 14	55 164	-	-
East Alabama Medical Center, Opelika, AL	91 80	97 233	96 310	90 156	97 305	75	75 8	99 144	97 304	79 583	99 648	100 143	91 108	82 74	96 27	83 148	99 178	94 96	100 51	96 1021	97 253	91 961	0.12 1658	2.02 1140
Elba General Hospital & Nursing Home, Elba, AL	-	100 2	100 2	100 2	100 2	-	-	-	100 1	100 16	100 17	100 2	94 47	100 26	-	96 48	100 70	100 42	100 12	-	-	-	-	-
Eliza Coffee Memorial Hospital, Florence, AL	92 87	99 213	99 336	96 191	93 330	0	82 22	97 160	81 138	65 346	92 409	93 61	90 316	93 135	57 94	92 458	100 470	79 285	94 89	89 678	97 196	85 650	-	-
Elmore Community Hospital, Wetumpka, AL	-	-	-	0	0	-	-	-	50 4	0 6	48 23	0	67 3	100 5	-	85 109	100 94	0 11	33 3	0	0	0	-	-
Fayette Medical Center, Fayette, AL	0	67 12	67 6	64 11	80 5	-	-	-	58 19	44 55	86 28	80 10	81 85	95 62	69 26	83 119	94 119	71 72	85 33	93 29	100 9	31 29	-	-
Florala Memorial Hospital, Florala, AL	-	100 2	-	0	-	-	-	-	100 1	100 3	0	0	80 10	100 2	-	86 63	100 87	98 56	100 3	-	-	-	-	-
Flowers Hospital, Dothan, AL	98 56	99 158	100 274	100 121	100 282	0	78 9	100 123	100 109	94 274	100 304	100 50	89 194	86 206	94 49	91 170	100 230	97 153	58 100	100 1133	99 285	99 1097	0.00 1190	6.51 676
Gadsden Regional Medical Center, Gadsden, AL	72 39	86 120	92 146	78 98	88 157	24	50 10	100 77	79 131	44 260	97 348	97 60	77 70	94 50	89 65	72 318	100 390	85 220	95 102	94 758	94 206	48 726	-	-
George H Lanier Memorial Hospital, Valley, AL	33 3	84 25	78 9	91 23	70 10	1	-	0	93 87	38 178	96 187	89 47	84 193	70 94	63 19	78 83	98 95	82 51	77 26	65 104	0	77 98	-	-
Georgiana Hospital, Georgiana, AL	100 1	97 18	71 14	50 18	60 15	4	-	0	31 16	92 52	54 35	12	74 19	100	75 8	87 38	98 46	67 24	100 10	-	-	-	-	-
Greene County Hospital, Eutaw, AL	-	100	-	0	0	-	-	-	100 1	22 9	38 47	0	100 2	100 1	-	44 9	100 15	0 6	-	0	-	-	-	-
Grove Hill Memorial Hospital, Grove Hill, AL	0 1	62 8	100 2	57 7	100 2	-	-	-	64 11	24 54	71 56	20 5	83 41	91 11	56 9	83 29	100 48	55 22	0 7	0	0	0	-	-
Hale County Hospital, Greensboro, AL	-	-	-	0	0	-	-	-	92 13	92 13	39 23	100 3	100 5	100 2	-	80 5	100 14	0 8	-	0	-	-	-	-
Hartselle Medical Center, Hartselle, AL	-	-	-	100 1	100 1	-	-	-	50 2	70 10	70 100	8	95 70	56 37	15	96 75	100 86	91 58	100 18	60 5	100 4	20 5	-	-
HealthSouth Medical Center, Birmingham, AL	-	-	-	-	-	-	-	-	-	-	-	-	100	-	-	-	100 10	40 5	1	78 27	100 23	26	-	-
Helen Keller Memorial Hospital, Sheffield, AL	50 6	91 34	84 19	85 26	79 19	-	83 64	86	83 64	70 181	85 215	45	90 90	92 75	100 20	86 125	100 147	87 94	39	91 121	40 117	77 119	-	-
Highlands Medical Center, Scottsboro, AL	50 2	68 19	60 15	52 21	53 15	-	-	67 3	63 19	50 125	48 157	85 34	84 193	90 92	50 38	82 232	100 272	56 156	95 61	1 73	91 23	88 72	-	-
Hill Hospital of Sumter County, York, AL	-	-	-	-	-	-	-	-	100	-	-	-	100 1	100 1	-	75 4	100 5	40 5	0 1	60	5 100	4 20	-	-
Huntsville Hospital, Huntsville, AL	88 260	98 557	97 985	95 468	97 946	25 4	88 33	98 415	84 591	75 1126	93 1301	96 254	81 525	81 458	77 159	63 784	100 934	83 474	83 240	89 836	87 192	78 830	0.71 983	4.65 581
Infirmary West, Mobile, AL	50 2	85 20	88 8	80 15	89 9	-	-	100 2	89 44	31 59	92 63	80	88 57	63 88	57 14	73 61	92 92	48 33	36	80 98	69 16	75 99	-	-
J Paul Jones Hospital, Camden, AL	-	80 5	100 4	75 4	100 3	-	-	0	63 3	50	0 12	0	69	100	26	85 27	100 33	65	-	-	0	-	-	-
Jackson Hospital and Clinic, Montgomery, AL	62 52	86 173	92 235	76 124	87 239	0	33 9	81 95	78 114	58 311	85 353	89 85	69 91	87 89	69 26	55 164	95 190	65 113	90 40	93 359	94 103	84 357	-	-

NOTE: The first number in each column (boldface) is the rate in percent, the second number is the number of patients; Please refer to the main entry for footnotes; **Heart Attack Care:** 1. ACE Inhibitor or ARB for LVSD; 2. Aspirin at Arrival; 3. Aspirin at Discharge; 4. Beta Blocker at Arrival; 5. Beta Blocker at Discharge; 6. Fibrinolytic Medication Timing; 7. PCI Within 90 Minutes of Arrival; 8. Smoking Cessation Advice; **Heart Failure Care:** 9. ACE Inhibitor or ARB for LVSD; 10. Discharge Instructions; 11. Evaluation of LVS Function; 12. Smoking Cessation Advice; 13. Appropriate Initial Antibiotic; 14. Blood Culture Timing; 15. Influenza Vaccine; 16. Initial Antibiotic Timing; 17. Oxygenation Assessment; 18. Pneumococcal Vaccine; 19. Smoking Cessation Advice; **Surgical Infection Prevention:** 20. Prophylactic Antibiotic Given; 21. Prophylactic Antibiotic Selection; 22. Prophylactic Antibiotic Stopped; **Pregnancy Care:** 23. Inpatient Neonatal Mortality; 24. Third or Fourth Degree Laceration.

Hospital	Heart Attack Care 1	2	3	4	5	6	7	8	Heart Failure Care 9	10	11	12	13	14	Pneumonia Care 15	16	17	18	Surgical Infection Prevention 19	20	21	22	Pregnancy Care 23	24
Jackson Medical Center, Jackson, AL	·	0 100	·	·	·	·	·	·	60 5	6 47	60 52	43 7	89 76	94 16	47 17	85 78	84	61 33	47 19	80 107	68 19	90 104	·	·
Jacksonville Medical Center, Jacksonville, AL	100	1 100	8 100	2	6 75	4	·	0	100	9 76	94 53	100	76 80	88 50	90 10	74 82	93	84 55	100 23	85 33	92 12	85 33	0.00 242	0.50 202
L V Stabler Memorial Hospital, Greenville, AL	0	82 11	86 7	82 11	86 7	·	·	0	78 36	90 79	92 92	95	70 69	93 14	93 84	74 83	89	89 45	88 16	·	·	·	·	·
Lake Martin Community Hospital, Dadeville, AL	0	2 60	10 25	8 80	10 57	7	·	0	1 18	33 43	49 22	9	77 26	93 14	57 7	74 38	100	24 29	32 19	·	·	33	·	·
Lakeland Community Hospital, Haleyville, AL	·	91 11	100 7	85 13	100 8	·	·	0 100	87 15	91 68	88 90	94	91 58	58	3 71	85 346	96 114	39 75	97 102	25 4	4 100	1 25	·	4
Lakeview Community Hospital, Eufaula, AL	·	0 100	4 50	2 50	2 50	0	·	0	74 23	65 63	58 89	93	80 76	78 51	53 19	85 88	96 114	39 75	90 42	67 6	0 2	50 4	·	·
Lawrence Medical Center, Moulton, AL	80 5	89 37	71 28	71 34	67 30	·	·	0 100	91 11	98 42	76 45	89	83 106	85 39	78 27	89 91	100 127	54 48	98 43	67	2	·	·	·
Marion Regional Wellness Center, Hamilton, AL	100	100 3	100 2	83 6	100 3	·	·	0 100	82 17	76 46	90 50	100	79 94	89 64	97 32	93 123	100 153	98 101	91 33	100	2 100	2	·	·
Marshall Medical Center North, Guntersville, AL	·	75 4	100 1	83 6	100 3	·	·	0	95 21	66 71	95 94	100	83 132	89 114	89 38	90 178	100 219	82 124	94 50	89 151	91 54	91 152	0.25 403	9.44 286
Marshall Medical Center South, Boaz, AL	62 8	60 30	82 11	44 25	70 10	·	·	0 100	79 66	81 116	98 168	85	73 172	92 136	77 26	84 221	100 263	90 126	84 69	91 148	80 41	85 142	·	·
Medical Center Blount, Oneonta, AL	0	86 7	80 5	100 7	100 5	0	2	0	76 17	35 40	85 66	71	78 79	83 58	47 19	88 121	99 134	58 76	68 28	62 8	100 7	1 100	·	7
Medical Center East, Birmingham, AL	92 90	97 274	95 298	95 249	95 315	100	84	19 100	88 136	85 271	98 316	98	82 297	79 135	48 58	74 288	100 376	39 221	89	88 1249	96 318	57 1222	·	·
Medical Center Enterprise, Enterprise, AL	100	90 10	71 7	71 7	83 6	0	·	0 100	94 32	76 89	97 103	100	93 118	95 97	92 42	92 160	100 192	97 114	100 42	96 341	100 84	98 328	·	·
Mizell Memorial Hospital, Opp, AL	100	100 5	100 4	100 4	100 6	50	·	0 100	100 29	19 77	88 92	83	74 87	82 33	7 15	58 85	95 128	75 80	83 24	73 11	80 5	90 10	·	·
Mobile Infirmary Medical Center, Mobile, AL	74 61	98 168	97 231	96 116	96 246	0	50	10 95	65 130	57 262	90 309	87	74 77	86 78	64 28	67 147	100 174	78 81	76 41	93 361	95 93	65 343	·	·
Monroe County Hospital, Monroeville, AL	100	100 10	83 6	100 11	100 7	·	·	0	89 9	90 119	85 132	100	79 102	93 54	65 17	82 102	100 134	66 73	100 55	94 51	100 9	92 50	·	·
North Baldwin Infirmary, Bay Minette, AL	·	0 100	2 100	100 1	100 1	0	·	0	89 9	40 87	62 8	80	·	·	40 5	76 58	100 63	34 38	55 11	74 39	92 12	69 35	·	·
Northeast Alabama Regional Medical Center, Anniston, AL	82 50	97 177	94 180	90 108	89 184	0	91	11 100	78 226	71 430	88 502	99	85 169	95 167	·	69 286	100 345	56 189	98 88	77 415	91 125	62 382	·	·
Northport Medical Center, Northport, AL	100	100 5	100 3	100 6	100 5	0	11	100	75 28	89 70	78 79	100	90 68	90 62	·	75 100	99 123	52 54	88 42	94 468	96 110	85 445	·	·
Northwest Medical Center, Winfield, AL	100	88 8	100 4	92 12	88 8	0	·	100	89 28	47 76	83 103	86	91 114	96 50	48 25	89 130	100 151	76 80	83 24	94 111	88 26	62 110	·	·
Parkway Medical Center Hospital, Decatur, AL	100 2	79 14	75 4	82 17	80 5	·	50	10 95	93 30	30 100	97 127	100	78 93	86 78	21	96 106	100 119	78 81	76 32	55 143	88 40	97 134	·	2 100
Physicians Medical Center Carraway, Birmingham, AL	88 32	100 105	95 137	98 99	98 143	50	68	78 100	88 64	88 191	93 224	97	83 140	73 105	49 61	75 212	98 246	64 144	92 75	53 167	90 49	56 121	·	·
Pickens County Medical Center, Carrollton, AL	100 2	43 7	100 4	29 7	67 3	·	4	0 100	94 17	27 48	55 0	0	86 87	89 37	50 24	79 104	94 108	60 68	29 28	77 13	100 2	100 13	·	·
Prattville Baptist Hospital, Prattville, AL	50 2	82 17	80 5	87 15	83 6	33	15	29 100	91 33	81 88	104 95	100	78 120	90 122	29	88 145	99 177	89 93	100 49	85 13	71 7	80 15	·	1
Princeton Baptist Medical Center, Birmingham, AL	87 131	97 299	97 409	96 239	100 381	33	33	6 99	81 238	67 383	97 443	100	89 212	92 167	44 70	88 281	100 341	44 186	98 102	95 319	89 82	51 335	·	·
Providence Hospital, Mobile, AL	79 38	97 181	95 207	87 107	94 217	0	54	13 98	91 149	65 477	99 527	100	83 270	94 152	43 83	72 297	97 353	57 214	94 78	77 235	96 78	66 230	·	·
Randolph Health Systems Medical Center, Roanoke, AL	·	0 100	2	·	0	·	·	0	81 26	8 37	87 55	25	100 17	80 10	0 4	67 21	100 29	7 15	14 7	94 111	62	100 2	·	·
Red Bay Hospital, Red Bay, AL	·	·	·	·	·	·	·	·	·	8	20 5	0	67 3	100 1	·	67 3	60 5	67 3	0 1	·	·	100 1	·	·
Riverview Regional Medical Center, Gadsden, AL	67 52	90 171	92 171	87 130	88 175	50	40	5 100	79 130	47 277	82 366	100	85 229	78 134	47 53	73 246	99 315	57 183	100 72	90 360	71 68	42 336	·	·
Russell Medical Center, Alexander City, AL	75 12	98 52	91 46	98 52	98 46	0	25	4 74	79 28	56 62	92 92	66	68 53	83 62	53 19	73 206	100 281	53 70	58 54	84 231	90 50	79 223	·	·
Russellville Hospital, Russellville, AL	100	100 1	86 14	88 17	93 14	·	·	0 100	89 19	97 65	95 80	94	83 109	89 37	23	87 143	98 176	81 95	100 34	86 86	83 24	69 85	·	·
Saint Clair Regional Hospital, Pell City, AL	0	86 7	67 3	43 7	33 3	33	·	0 100	61 28	69 89	70 98	35	78 130	88 50	24	82 116	99 146	58 72	47 38	0 1	100	100 1	·	·
Saint Vincent's Hospital, Birmingham, AL	72 60	99 224	99 227	98 174	92 225	3	75	8 97	77 195	66 422	87 468	96	78 395	75 231	63 79	76 404	100 508	52 307	94 82	81 358	89 82	54 546	1.93 831	·
Shelby Baptist Medical Center, Alabaster, AL	80 61	91 171	93 180	78 128	94 170	0	43	14 78	62 121	32 271	93 305	66	82 176	89 96	50 54	73 231	100 298	58 168	59 95	76 401	79 139	69 384	·	·
Shoals Hospital, Muscle Shoals, AL	100	83 12	100 3	100 3	100 4	0	·	0 50	86 14	81 59	96 68	78	81 88	96 57	·	78 98	97 115	77 77	62 16	91 44	100 8	77 43	·	·
South Baldwin Regional Medical Center, Foley, AL	83 6	100 54	96 26	88 42	96 28	·	60	5 100	78 67	72 192	96 225	98	77 108	84 75	88 34	68 137	99 153	76 95	100 34	15 151	48 40	38 147	·	·
Southeast Alabama Medical Center, Dothan, AL	90 148	96 284	98 511	93 233	97 505	·	15	99 218	87 319	78 696	94 773	94	88 209	89 116	77 48	75 195	99 270	72 169	92 88	94 212	100 70	75 203	·	·
Springhill Medical Center, Mobile, AL	94 32	92 116	95 111	88 60	98 125	·	33	0 93	97 177	45 455	98 496	86	82 121	71 45	59 29	80 156	98 195	49 112	79 43	64 659	92 283	70 798	·	·
Stringfellow Memorial Hospital, Anniston, AL	88 8	97 59	96 53	70 40	79 56	0	17	6 100	81 101	51 208	95 232	100	83 156	94 97	37	78 163	99 216	87 110	100 77	65 75	58 12	55 66	·	·
Summit Hospital, Phenix City, AL	·	50 2	2 100	100 1	100 1	·	·	0 100	·	6 17	82 0	0	73 103	94 67	·	67 3	100 3	0 1	50 2	100 1	100	100 1	·	·
Thomas Hospital, Fairhope, AL	90 59	1 75	8 100	89 134	97 242	·	75	16 96	76 97	71 201	92 240	92	73 103	94 67	74 27	91 35	100 116	68 95	78 27	79 471	93 72	76 457	·	·
Thomasville Infirmary, Thomasville, AL	100 1	75	·	50 2	6 100	2	·	0 100	82 18	6 17	0 5	0	100 3	100 3	·	100	43 91	22	91 12	·	100	12 17	·	·
Trinity Medical Center, Birmingham, AL	92 114	98 208	100 418	97 190	99 416	50	67	94 172	99 146	78 308	95 372	77	88 133	78 135	·	78 206	100 281	71 165	78 64	83 760	99 255	72 738	·	·
Troy Regional Medical Center, Troy, AL	100 2	73 11	75 8	75 8	71 7	·	0	2 100	59 17	35 48	80 64	80	63 52	94 31	62 21	81 75	96 83	61 46	78 18	41 41	85 20	76 41	·	·
UAB Hospital, Birmingham, AL	81 88	98 177	99 325	94 156	95 316	·	71	87 127	83 320	41 516	95 549	63	84 88	74 139	19	64 180	100 243	28 110	48 64	72 556	73 85	54 546	1.93 831	2.52 2774
UAB Medical West, Bessemer, AL	94 16	96 56	90 39	86 59	93 43	0	·	100	96 75	55 186	99 200	100	86 172	91 158	33 46	81 302	99 336	65 177	100 78	87 349	89 91	58 329	·	·
University of South Alabama Medical Center, Mobile, AL	94 31	99 68	95 97	98 55	92 95	·	67	3 100	92 140	80 232	94 232	100	79 72	84 70	50 8	78 101	100 106	23 13	100 52	82 182	91 44	50 173	·	·
Vaughan Evergreen Medical Center, Evergreen, AL	·	0 100	5 100	2	83 6	100	·	0 81	42	81 42	42 144	72	81 74	47	81 74	67 42	99 57	47 30	90 10	·	·	·	·	·

NOTE: The first number in each column (boldface) is the rate in percent, the second number is the number of patients; Please refer to the main entry for footnotes; Heart Attack Care: 1. ACE Inhibitor or ARB for LVSD; 2. Aspirin at Discharge; 3. Aspirin at Arrival; 4. Beta Blocker at Arrival; 5. Beta Blocker at Discharge; 6. Fibrinolytic Medication Timing; 7. PCI Within 90 Minutes of Arrival; 8. Smoking Cessation Advice; Heart Failure Care: 9. ACE Inhibitor or ARB for LVSD; 10. Discharge Instructions; 11. Evaluation of LVS Function; 12. Smoking Cessation Advice; Pneumonia Care: 13. Appropriate Initial Antibiotic; 14. Blood Culture; 15. Influenza Vaccine; 16. Initial Antibiotic Timing; 17. Oxygenation Assessment; 18. Pneumococcal Vaccine; Surgical Infection Prevention: 19. Smoking Cessation Advice; 20. Prophylactic Antibiotic Given; 21. Prophylactic Antibiotic Selection; 22. Prophylactic Antibiotic Stopped; Pregnancy Care: 23. Inpatient Neonatal Mortality; 24. Third or Fourth Degree Laceration.

Hospital	Heart Attack Care								Heart Failure Care						Pneumonia Care					Surgical Infection Prevention			Pregnancy Care	
	1	2	3	4	5	6	7	8	9	10	11	12	13	14	15	16	17	18	19	20	21	22	23	24
Vaughan Regional Med Ctr-Parkway Campus, Selma, AL	74/27	84/97	93/56	86/87	90/59	43/7	0/–	100/8	80/192	31/364	87/412	89/75	70/117	87/68	48/23	60/139	100/164	53/89	90/29	28/157	68/40	62/115	–	–
Walker Baptist Medical Center, Jasper, AL	100/9	98/57	100/43	100/47	100/37	40/5	–	100/26	99/91	99/165	100/205	100/0	95/269	97/287	78/51	90/393	100/459	90/242	100/163	96/275	100/90	81/258	–	–
Washington County Hospital, Chatom, AL	–	–	–	–	–	0/1	–	–	33/3	0/10	38/13	0/2	100/8	100/2	0/–	100/10	100/11	20/5	100/0	–	–	–	–	–
Wedowee Hospital, Wedowee, AL	100/1	–	0/–	0/–	0/–	0/–	–	0/–	80/10	4/55	49/59	9/22	81/21	100/3	0/7	82/22	88/24	14/14	50/2	–	–	–	–	–
Wiregrass Medical Center, Geneva, AL	–	100/9	60/5	56/9	80/5	–	–	0/–	22/9	87/67	46/76	100/21	55/131	98/40	50/32	86/120	97/159	67/83	100/42	47/15	14/7	27/15	–	–
Woodland Medical Center, Cullman, AL	75/4	81/16	44/9	78/18	82/11	–	–	100/3	72/40	82/87	85/140	92/25	87/98	96/75	71/17	85/124	100/145	76/87	81/81	75/59	83/18	69/58	–	–
ARKANSAS																								
Arkansas Heart Hospital, Little Rock, AR	75/126	99/87	91/435	88/80	89/414	–	0/–	99/195	69/327	77/461	88/512	99/75	41/29	80/15	0/4	86/29	100/35	31/26	91/11	91/605	100/186	81/595	–	–
Arkansas Methodist Medical Center, Paragould, AR	100/6	92/98	91/82	89/76	91/78	–	0/–	100/29	96/49	89/146	94/214	93/41	78/232	88/161	–	82/272	100/320	83/168	96/112	92/117	90/29	94/113	–	–
Arkansas Surgical Hospital, North Little Rock, AR	–	–	–	–	–	–	–	–	–	–	–	–	–	–	–	–	–	83/18	100/9	80/586	100/185	72/584	–	–
Ashley County Medical Center, Crossett, AR	0/–	69/13	25/4	60/15	50/2	0/1	–	0/–	50/8	75/32	59/39	100/3	88/16	100/9	60/5	90/29	100/31	83/18	100/14	–	–	–	–	–
Baptist Health Medical Center, Heber Springs, AR	100/1	–	0/–	0/–	0/–	–	–	0/–	100/2	79/19	100/26	100/6	63/23	94/34	94/16	85/72	100/88	90/56	100/14	100/15	100/15	67/15	–	–
Baptist Health Medical Center, Arkadelphia, AR	–	50/2	50/2	100/2	100/2	–	–	0/–	50/8	85/33	78/46	100/3	83/23	100/19	100/11	92/53	98/59	90/40	86/7	100/85	88/158	80/475	–	–
Baptist Health Medical Center, Little Rock, AR	90/88	99/163	98/327	99/131	98/340	0/–	31/13	97/153	89/362	65/649	96/762	99/110	73/251	90/192	75/56	60/345	100/413	76/229	96/76	85/486	88/158	80/475	**0.60**/2853	**2.96**/1553
Baptist Health Med Ctr-North Little Rock, North Little Rock, AR	74/43	98/171	95/213	90/126	97/211	0/–	44/9	99/99	83/133	54/247	98/285	98/59	79/118	95/60	76/21	82/173	100/193	88/113	95/39	92/747	99/192	86/720	–	–
Baptist Memorial Hospital-Forrest City, Forrest City, AR	50/2	70/10	86/7	100/7	88/8	–	–	100/0	100/34	100/88	96/98	100/23	84/62	92/65	96/24	83/89	100/108	97/61	100/28	93/55	94/17	76/54	–	–
Baxter Regional Medical Center, Mountain Home, AR	84/88	94/270	89/300	93/256	94/297	–	32/19	100/109	68/169	71/279	94/357	96/52	79/207	93/172	51/75	91/291	100/341	91/229	99/96	78/713	86/170	70/681	–	–
Booneville Community Hospital, Booneville, AR	0/–	50/2	100/1	0/–	100/1	–	–	0/–	60/5	63/19	65/34	83/6	70/37	100/5	30/10	93/45	100/60	55/38	69/16	51/37	–	89/27	–	–
Bradley County Medical Center, Warren, AR	100/1	94/18	56/16	62/8	60/15	–	–	0/–	67/3	77/53	13/62	100/4	88/48	90/10	36/14	91/79	100/66	21/39	50/55	50/8	38/8	88/8	–	–
Chambers Memorial Hospital, Danville, AR	0/–	50/6	50/2	100/5	50/2	–	–	0/–	57/7	12/141	6/140	53/34	85/61	100/14	24/56	83/65	97/71	68/40	88/16	80/15	100/3	100/15	–	–
Chicot Memorial Hospital, Lake Village, AR	73/37	96/123	87/140	82/119	80/141	67/3	56/32	89/55	66/73	75/134	69/156	97/32	81/160	97/106	32/38	85/189	100/238	47/142	93/54	76/617	81/146	67/601	–	–
Conway Regional Medical Center, Conway, AR	75/4	100/20	100/10	100/19	82/11	–	4/–	100/3	94/72	95/209	91/236	80/5	74/72	93/61	61/23	78/88	93/105	52/46	100/24	60/83	93/30	70/84	**1.00**/799	**1.05**/569
Crittenden Memorial Hospital, West Memphis, AR	–	100/1	100/1	0/–	100/1	–	–	100/3	73/15	67/36	82/50	80/5	89/18	100/12	95/10	89/92	100/102	85/79	87/15	–	–	–	–	–
CrossRidge Community Hospital, Wynne, AR	–	–	–	–	–	–	–	–	47/15	53/15	69/36	25/4	73/26	88/16	50/10	55/20	100/29	65/20	12/8	93/214	94/34	28/191	–	–
De Queen Regional Medical Center, De Queen, AR	–	100/1	100/1	0/1	100/1	–	–	0/–	0/1	100/19	15/26	100/1	73/26	100/3	8/6	94/31	94/34	11/11	67/3	26/19	67/6	78/18	–	–
De Witt Hospital & Nursing Home, De Witt, AR	–	0/–	2/100	100/1	100/1	–	–	0/–	0/100	59/3	67/21	80/5	79/28	94/16	5/–	77/31	100/37	67/15	86/7	71/14	100/4	93/15	–	–
Delta Memorial Hospital, Dumas, AR	–	0/–	0/–	0/–	0/–	–	–	0/100	73/15	57/42	75/52	94/17	74/70	100/22	62/16	75/85	108/52	35/52	100/30	62/13	100/7	85/13	–	–
Drew Memorial Hospital, Monticello, AR	100/1	74/31	82/17	73/30	88/17	–	–	100/6	73/30	48/62	87/87	83/30	85/54	91/33	36/8	72/68	96/80	27/33	89/18	27/49	11/11	68/47	–	–
Great River Medical Center, Blytheville, AR	100/4	91/11	11/100	100/5	100/5	75/8	–	100/1	90/67	82/22	53/127	62/13	83/92	92/36	6/15	83/104	100/107	81/54	88/33	30/73	80/20	52/64	**0.00**/–	**0.00**/0
Harris Hospital and Clinic, Newport, AR	–	–	–	–	–	–	–	100/–	100/1	57/7	100/0	100/2	87/63	100/19	50/6	83/18	100/21	63/19	0/–	93/214	94/34	28/191	–	–
Healthpark Hospital, Hot Springs, AR	100/1	78/9	67/6	73/11	60/5	0/1	–	67/3	67/61	58/167	76/254	93/55	69/108	90/62	33/33	91/151	99/161	59/95	88/41	26/19	67/6	78/18	–	–
Helena Regional Medical Center, Helena, AR	100/1	89/9	80/5	50/6	86/7	–	–	67/3	67/36	33/111	71/135	65/23	87/109	93/76	–	93/176	98/180	50/98	82/49	71/14	100/4	93/15	–	–
Hot Springs County Medical Center, Malvern, AR	0/100	0/100	4/100	2/75	50/2	–	–	0/97	67/9	22/18	68/25	83/6	85/20	96/27	10/–	84/45	100/49	89/35	80/5	88/8	0/1	12/8	–	–
Howard Memorial Hospital, Nashville, AR	0/–	0/–	0/–	0/–	0/–	–	–	0/100	73/15	59/3	67/21	80/5	79/28	94/16	17/–	77/31	100/37	67/15	86/7	100/–	–	12/8	–	–
Levi Hospital, Hot Springs Natl Pk, AR	100/1	92/13	75/1	4/100	93/232	22/9	–	95/98	78/232	62/343	97/440	92/107	82/197	85/134	16/52	75/267	98/298	66/155	79/73	74/933	91/237	77/892	–	–
Magnolia Hospital, Magnolia, AR	0/–	33/3	3/67	33/3	3/67	–	–	0/100	73/6	22/53	53/30	30/100	85/54	91/31	33/15	84/49	100/59	62/34	100/0	27/49	11/11	68/47	–	–
McGehee-Desha County Hospital, McGehee, AR	100/5	89/27	91/23	90/30	29/100	75/2	–	100/1	81/16	55/128	99/173	100/10	92/66	92/51	28/6	86/143	100/107	81/99	88/3	30/73	80/20	52/64	–	–
Medical Center of South Arkansas, El Dorado, AR	100/2	95/20	100/12	90/100	100/10	8/–	–	100/1	90/42	94/66	99/173	100/29	80/70	92/51	28/6	92/132	100/157	81/101	100/38	83/23	100/5	70/23	–	–
Medical Park Hospital, Hope, AR	100/2	100/0	89/9	33/6	100/8	–	–	100/1	43/14	53/59	62/74	100/9	76/101	81/34	33/9	79/81	95/95	49/67	77/22	80/30	82/11	93/27	–	–
Mena Medical Center, Mena, AR	57/14	98/59	92/60	88/52	89/54	–	–	97/–	88/43	52/196	95/106	94/16	76/101	95/81	68/19	88/129	100/144	78/78	93/58	88/213	90/42	86/200	–	–
National Park Medical Center, Hot Springs, AR	95/20	97/92	92/173	90/68	89/141	57/–	75/–	99/78	93/102	82/196	98/222	100/–	84/141	96/93	44/–	88/174	100/212	94/131	65/–	97/379	99/105	71/375	–	–
NEA Medical Center, Jonesboro, AR	75/12	97/33	100/100	21/79	94/18	–	–	100/1	74/38	68/109	97/142	84/25	80/191	93/130	28/–	89/218	100/285	79/192	89/61	96/185	97/35	89/174	–	–
North Arkansas Regional Medical Center, Harrison, AR	77/35	98/165	199/8	81/127	92/207	–	80/–	95/100	88/92	75/152	92/198	97/30	80/110	91/94	64/28	67/158	100/189	68/116	81/52	81/420	97/118	56/409	**0.38**/3661	**3.31**/2511
Northwest Medical Center, Springdale, AR	94/51	99/143	97/126	94/104	98/133	0/2	5/–	95/57	82/38	80/75	90/93	88/24	82/71	78/72	86/35	81/100	100/127	90/94	76/27	82/254	94/62	50/242	–	–
NW Medical Center Benton County, Bentonville, AR																								

NOTE: The first number in each column (boldface) is the rate in percent, the second number is the number of patients; Please refer to the main entry for footnotes; **Heart Attack Care:** 1. ACE Inhibitor or ARB for LVSD; 2. Aspirin at Arrival; 3. Aspirin at Discharge; 4. Beta Blocker at Arrival; 5. Beta Blocker at Discharge; 6. Fibrinolytic Medication Timing; 7. PCI Within 90 Minutes of Arrival; 8. Smoking Cessation Advice; **Heart Failure Care:** 9. ACE Inhibitor or ARB for LVSD; 10. Discharge Instructions; 11. Evaluation of LVS Function; 12. Smoking Cessation Advice; **Pneumonia Care:** 13. Appropriate Initial Antibiotic; 14. Blood Culture Timing; 15. Influenza Vaccine; 16. Initial Antibiotic Timing; 17. Oxygenation Assessment; 18. Pneumococcal Vaccine; 19. Smoking Cessation Advice; **Surgical Infection Prevention:** 20. Prophylactic Antibiotic Selection; 21. Prophylactic Antibiotic Given; 22. Prophylactic Antibiotic Stopped; **Pregnancy Care:** 23. Inpatient Neonatal Mortality; 24. Third or Fourth Degree Laceration

Hospital	Heart Attack Care								Heart Failure Care				Pneumonia Care							Surgical Infection Prevention			Pregnancy Care	
	1	2	3	4	5	6	7	8	9	10	11	12	13	14	15	16	17	18	19	20	21	22	23	24
Ouachita Medical Center, Camden, AR	**75** 4	**83** 23	**90** 10	**91** 23	**86** 14	**75** 4	- 0	**100** 1	**96** 28	**62** 87	**67** 105	**89** 19	**84** 91	**84** 73	**76** 33	**86** 142	**99** 167	**59** 104	**100** 24	**20** 15	**100** 16	**84** 62	- -	- -
Ozark Health Medical Center, Clinton, AR	- -	- -	- -	- -	- -	- -	- -	- -	- -	**65** 26	**67** 46	- -	**96** 73	**98** 64	**100** 14	**88** 98	**100** 119	**86** 80	**71** 28	- -	- -	- -	- -	- -
Piggott Community Hospital, Piggott, AR	**80** 5	**100** 11	**80** 10	**80** 10	**50** 8	- 0	- 0	**100** 3	**80** 15	**94** 16	**97** 39	**80** 5	**92** 24	- -	**100** 13	**94** 36	**100** 45	**100** 35	**100** 8	- -	- -	- -	- -	- -
Pike County Memorial Hospital, Murfreesboro, AR	- 0	**100** 3	**100** 1	**20** 5	**50** 2	**12** 8	- 0	- 0	- 0	**64** 14	**7** 14	**75** 4	**92** 12	- 0	- 0	**94** 16	**100** 22	**30** 10	**60** 5	- -	- -	- -	- -	- -
Randolph County Medical Center, Pocahontas, AR	**100** 1	**83** 6	**75** 4	**83** 6	**67** 3	- 0	- -	- 0	**88** 8	**20** 25	**54** 39	**100** 6	**80** 65	**100** 30	**41** 22	**87** 69	**100** 85	**62** 61	**100** 12	**62** 40	**95** 22	**44** 32	- -	- -
Rebsamen Medical Center, Jacksonville, AR	**50** 6	**97** 30	**64** 14	**89** 27	**81** 16	- 0	- 0	**100** 2	**72** 29	**13** 15	**90** 91	**67** 3	**83** 18	**89** 18	- -	**84** 116	**100** 149	**44** 95	**67** 6	**89** 36	- -	**93** 29	**0.00** 466	**1.57** 318
Saint Anthony's Healthcare Center, Morrilton, AR	- 0	**100** 2	**100** 2	**100** 4	**100** 3	- 0	- 0	- 0	**89** 18	**71** 24	**97** 38	**88** 8	**76** 50	**94** 18	**100** 9	**78** 45	**100** 72	**73** 48	**80** 20	- -	- -	- -	- -	- -
Saint Bernard's Medical Center, Jonesboro, AR	**90** 100	**97** 215	**96** 368	**89** 140	**95** 368	- 0	**100** 7	**99** 192	**85** 317	**59** 506	**99** 613	**99** 151	**88** 266	**93** 210	**75** 76	**76** 372	**99** 448	**81** 262	**94** 172	**94** 728	**97** 144	**87** 698	**0.07** 1412	**4.00** 925
Saint Edward Mercy Medical Center, Fort Smith, AR	**90** 91	**96** 157	**97** 253	**97** 118	**97** 257	**11** 9	**40** 5	**100** 137	**84** 103	**60** 229	**99** 286	**97** 59	**82** 101	**90** 92	**100** 26	**66** 140	**100** 178	**81** 95	**92** 49	**89** 227	**95** 65	**76** 221	- -	- -
Saint John's Hospital-Berryville, Berryville, AR	**100** 2	**85** 13	**92** 12	**75** 16	**100** 10	- 0	- 0	**100** 3	**100** 6	**29** 41	**55** 49	**43** 7	**88** 95	**91** 44	**73** 22	**92** 97	**100** 122	**73** 79	**61** 23	- -	- -	- -	- -	- -
Saint Joseph's Mercy Health Center, Hot Springs Natl Pk, AR	**83** 53	**99** 181	**100** 209	**91** 145	**94** 156	**60** 20	**50** 2	**100** 93	**96** 135	**80** 282	**97** 345	**98** 87	**85** 253	**93** 233	**89** 72	**84** 344	**100** 433	**92** 282	**96** 118	**95** 587	**97** 58	**79** 540	- -	- -
Saint Mary's Regional Medical Center, Russellville, AR	**88** 8	**95** 41	**94** 17	**94** 32	**93** 15	**56** 9	- 0	**100** 2	**79** 53	**72** 116	**92** 153	**86** 29	**88** 178	**87** 129	**88** 42	**91** 195	**100** 253	**88** 135	**83** 65	**93** 376	**97** 101	**71** 369	- -	- -
Saint Mary-Rogers Memorial Hospital, Rogers, AR	**92** 26	**99** 120	**100** 132	**98** 93	**99** 142	- 0	**100** 7	**96** 53	**96** 78	**74** 165	**100** 211	**96** 25	**88** 154	**99** 133	**94** 51	**92** 200	**100** 251	**88** 170	**95** 61	**79** 224	**95** 62	**90** 212	- -	- -
Saint Vincent Infirmary Medical Center, Little Rock, AR	**68** 63	**96** 145	**96** 244	**91** 104	**95** 243	- 0	**20** 5	**100** 111	**86** 228	**44** 423	**91** 508	**99** 100	**81** 187	**92** 166	**71** 72	**80** 264	**100** 317	**72** 191	**98** 93	**83** 221	**99** 74	**77** 216	**0.54** 2042	**5.88** 1446
Saint Vincent Medical Center North, Sherwood, AR	**50** 2	**94** 18	**100** 8	**83** 18	**100** 8	- 0	- 0	**100** 1	**85** 20	**60** 53	**87** 68	**100** 15	**75** 71	**97** 30	**71** 17	**67** 81	**100** 87	**49** 49	**100** 20	**58** 89	**93** 14	**99** 84	- -	- -
Saline Memorial Hospital, Benton, AR	**50** 4	**93** 43	**54** 13	**73** 33	**83** 12	**57** 7	- 0	**75** 4	**50** 52	**42** 90	**92** 116	**93** 15	**81** 117	**95** 106	**38** 39	**86** 169	**100** 211	**39** 111	**63** 38	**60** 224	**88** 51	**36** 225	**0.00** 492	**4.68** 342
Siloam Springs Memorial Hospital, Siloam Springs, AR	**0** 1	**91** 11	**100** 6	**67** 12	**86** 7	- 0	- 0	**0** 1	**93** 14	**25** 71	**67** 85	**56** 18	**81** 91	**100** 53	**62** 24	**82** 127	**99** 147	**51** 75	**69** 35	**30** 23	**83** 6	**69** 16	- -	- -
South Mississippi County Regional Med Ctr, Osceola, AR	- 0	**50** 2	**0** 1	**100** 2	**100** 1	- 0	- 0	**0** 1	**14** 7	**75** 48	**82** 65	**80** 15	**82** 34	**100** 14	**83** 12	**63** 51	**97** 65	**86** 35	**62** 16	- -	- -	- -	- -	- -
Southwest Regional Medical Centre, Little Rock, AR	**89** 9	**93** 15	**100** 16	**88** 17	**88** 17	- 0	- 0	- 0	**80** 15	**67** 3	**71** 31	**0** 1	**75** 4	**75** 8	- -	**75** 48	**100** 61	**39** 28	**0** 1	**73** 89	- -	**57** 83	- -	- -
Sparks Regional Medical Center, Fort Smith, AR	**78** 46	**93** 188	**94** 220	**94** 186	**95** 224	**21** 24	**14** 7	**84** 85	**79** 151	**69** 323	**89** 430	**65** 60	**82** 212	**95** 194	**75** 60	**67** 317	**99** 390	**66** 212	**79** 86	**66** 299	**96** 98	**76** 287	**0.00** 1135	**3.84** 730
Stone County Medical Center, Mountain View, AR	**100** 2	**100** 3	**100** 2	**100** 2	**100** 1	- 0	- 0	- 0	**100** 13	**64** 22	**91** 33	**33** 3	**84** 98	**92** 52	**76** 25	**88** 82	**100** 116	**75** 76	**83** 18	- -	- -	- -	- -	- -
Stuttgart Regional Medical Center, Stuttgart, AR	- 0	**88** 8	**100** 4	**88** 8	**100** 5	- 0	- 0	- 0	**88** 32	**67** 96	**95** 127	**93** 15	**89** 53	**94** 49	**95** 19	**89** 91	**99** 103	**84** 61	**89** 28	**100** 22	**100** 2	**95** 20	- -	- -
Summit Medical Center, Van Buren, AR	**67** 3	**90** 29	**64** 14	**86** 28	**93** 14	**0** 2	- 0	**100** 1	**81** 26	**54** 80	**82** 122	**79** 14	**74** 117	**91** 87	**94** 31	**85** 131	**99** 154	**95** 77	**72** 60	**80** 82	**100** 26	**27** 82	- -	- -
Surgical Hospital of Jonesboro, Jonesboro, AR	- -	- -	- -	- -	- -	- -	- -	- -	- -	- -	- -	- -	- -	- -	- -	- -	- -	- -	- -	**74** 192	**100** 19	**92** 190	- -	- -
UAMS Medical Center, Little Rock, AR	**82** 33	**96** 97	**95** 88	**85** 67	**96** 102	**0** 1	**50** 4	**100** 57	**79** 192	**71** 263	**97** 288	**100** 98	**87** 119	**86** 176	**49** 51	**55** 228	**100** 335	**36** 118	**99** 106	**74** 303	**56** 73	**88** 292	**1.97** 2029	**6.37** 1224
Washington Regional Medical Center, Fayetteville, AR	**88** 64	**94** 183	**97** 267	**88** 161	**90** 267	- 0	**67** 6	**86** 101	**85** 148	**91** 258	**97** 292	**99** 67	**79** 103	**94** 72	**58** 26	**64** 138	**100** 169	**64** 98	**80** 45	**31** 80	**94** 79	**64** 189	- -	- -
White County Medical Center, Searcy, AR	**75** 36	**94** 102	**97** 99	**83** 88	**95** 110	**50** 6	**36** 11	**98** 51	**77** 91	**76** 202	**93** 254	**91** 35	**89** 141	**93** 138	- -	**86** 195	**94** 236	**70** 163	**93** 54	**78** 331	**99** 149	**90** 300	- -	- -
White River Medical Center, Batesville, AR	**96** 54	**99** 136	**96** 132	**100** 119	**96** 144	**50** 12	**75** 4	**98** 52	**95** 125	**82** 253	**100** 333	**93** 54	**91** 132	**93** 132	**98** 59	**77** 184	**100** 229	**85** 144	**84** 50	**94** 354	**94** 132	**82** 342	- -	- -
FLORIDA																								
Aventura Hospital and Medical Center, Aventura, FL	**97** 79	**98** 284	**99** 277	**97** 204	**98** 314	**50** 2	**50** 4	**100** 70	**92** 173	**92** 425	**99** 552	**100** 42	**81** 225	**86** 290	**40** 73	**48** 370	**97** 464	**71** 307	**100** 62	**81** 234	**97** 67	**70** 213	- -	- -
Baptist Hospital, Pensacola, FL	**81** 54	**96** 145	**96** 206	**91** 116	**97** 204	- 0	**60** 5	**96** 93	**82** 136	**56** 351	**86** 400	**93** 108	**89** 238	**82** 217	**71** 73	**74** 318	**100** 350	**69** 194	**100** 98	**77** 741	**90** 157	**63** 699	- -	- -
Baptist Hospital, Miami, FL	**94** 127	**98** 439	**99** 490	**95** 343	**100** 510	**50** 2	**100** 14	**100** 168	**92** 319	**82** 660	**99** 760	**99** 85	**95** 421	**91** 459	**85** 120	**62** 535	**100** 695	**89** 388	**100** 117	**96** 296	**100** 73	**93** 286	- -	- -
Baptist Medical Center, Jacksonville, FL	**86** 63	**96** 152	**98** 402	**94** 147	**97** 404	**33** 3	**14** 7	**99** 170	**82** 251	**36** 502	**97** 622	**81** 149	**80** 301	**85** 324	**59** 99	**61** 468	**98** 576	**64** 252	**77** 151	**76** 1325	**74** 78	**73** 1224	- -	- -
Baptist Medical Center Beaches, Jacksonville Bch, FL	**75** 12	**98** 105	**92** 49	**98** 95	**89** 56	- 0	- 0	**71** 7	**82** 85	**75** 162	**92** 222	**89** 27	**84** 202	**92** 170	**51** 55	**70** 261	**100** 284	**77** 169	**94** 50	**89** 356	**97** 33	**49** 333	**0.13** 791	**4.60** 695
Baptist Medical Center Nassau, Fernandina Bch, FL	- 0	**88** 8	**60** 5	**88** 8	**80** 5	- 0	- 0	- 0	**63** 27	**8** 65	**99** 76	**70** 10	**89** 97	**92** 105	**72** 25	**79** 125	**97** 143	**77** 73	**73** 33	**86** 109	**86** 21	**90** 105	**0.38** 261	**0.44** 228
Bartow Regional Medical Center, Bartow, FL	**100** 2	**62** 13	**50** 4	**83** 12	**71** 7	- 0	- 0	- 0	**86** 37	**25** 139	**69** 159	**77** 35	**58** 108	**85** 73	**25** 24	**73** 122	**100** 152	**24** 82	**75** 40	**44** 36	**40** 5	**75** 36	- -	- -
Bascom Palmer Eye Institute, Miami, FL	- -	- -	- -	- -	- -	- -	- -	- -	- -	- -	- -	- -	- -	- -	- -	- -	- -	- -	- -	- -	- -	- -	- -	- -
Bay Medical Center, Panama City, FL	**74** 126	**97** 312	**94** 359	**93** 290	**94** 367	**0** 4	**43** 14	**97** 145	**81** 376	**48** 876	**86** 1003	**91** 238	**81** 344	**78** 294	- -	**71** 475	**100** 571	**65** 344	**98** 163	**95** 799	**95** 203	**80** 769	- -	- -
Bayfront Medical Center, Saint Petersburg, FL	**77** 26	**98** 143	**91** 168	**87** 124	**88** 168	**0** 2	**36** 14	**99** 69	**90** 134	**57** 247	**98** 291	**94** 94	**95** 166	**86** 162	**78** 23	**89** 218	**100** 244	**77** 115	**94** 63	**69** 586	**94** 64	**66** 559	- -	- -
Bert Fish Medical Center, New Smyrna Beach, FL	**82** 28	**95** 146	**78** 65	**95** 133	**95** 65	**62** 32	- 0	**100** 10	**76** 70	**34** 156	**82** 181	**80** 15	**80** 127	**80** 86	**68** 34	**86** 170	**100** 193	**78** 125	**74** 43	**77** 173	**98** 48	**76** 162	- -	- -
Bethesda Memorial Hospital, Boynton Beach, FL	**89** 18	**90** 125	**93** 69	**79** 77	**96** 92	- 0	- 0	**100** 11	**77** 78	**63** 204	**95** 263	**100** 21	**88** 139	**87** 134	**85** 41	**82** 237	**100** 263	**86** 162	**98** 48	**97** 206	**98** 41	**62** 193	**0.26** 766	**2.57** 544
Blake Medical Center, Bradenton, FL	**85** 67	**95** 312	**97** 282	**93** 228	**97** 249	**33** 3	**50** 4	**97** 73	**84** 130	**71** 408	**91** 514	**98** 47	**87** 217	**90** 159	**56** 75	**64** 272	**100** 322	**60** 231	**96** 45	**86** 895	**95** 96	**39** 878	- -	- -
Boca Raton Community Hospital, Boca Raton, FL	**82** 17	**90** 126	**86** 42	**87** 127	**94** 53	**0** 2	- 0	**62** 8	**72** 206	**88** 460	**87** 614	**85** 26	**88** 289	**86** 239	**41** 85	**79** 304	**98** 421	**53** 309	**80** 35	**82** 1075	**78** 210	**71** 1036	**0.00** 413	**4.20** 1144
Brandon Regional Hospital, Brandon, FL	**70** 107	**95** 361	**87** 350	**87** 230	**95** 434	- 0	**60** 20	**98** 180	**60** 179	**34** 350	**95** 445	**93** 71	**80** 319	**78** 161	**44** 61	**49** 388	**99** 466	**44** 264	**98** 116	**77** 299	**82** 99	**63** 283	- -	- -
Brooksville Regional Hospital, Brooksville, FL	**73** 22	**87** 164	**76** 59	**89** 157	**91** 75	**69** 13	- 0	**100** 17	**82** 141	**32** 336	**92** 396	**99** 86	**85** 227	**93** 185	**79** 66	**77** 284	**100** 347	**84** 191	**100** 92	**89** 387	**93** 55	**69** 372	- -	- -
Broward General Medical Center, Fort Lauderdale, FL	**78** 81	**94** 155	**93** 208	**97** 112	**93** 215	**0** 1	**50** 8	**98** 96	**90** 177	**95** 263	**97** 282	**99** 76	**88** 113	**89** 133	**14** 22	**69** 183	**100** 210	**19** 67	**98** 62	**77** 245	**79** 66	**56** 233	**0.65** 3524	**2.00** 2101
Campbellton Graceville Hospital, Graceville, FL	- -	- -	- -	- -	- -	- -	- -	- -	**25** 4	**0** 4	**50** 8	- 0	**100** 2	- 0	- -	**100** 3	**100** 3	**0** 3	- 0	- -	- -	- -	- -	- -
Cape Canaveral Hospital, Cocoa Beach, FL	**100** 14	**97** 90	**91** 56	**95** 100	**97** 71	**0** 1	- 0	**100** 11	**89** 95	**92** 197	**96** 239	**98** 45	**89** 192	**95** 203	**96** 57	**79** 247	**100** 286	**92** 192	**96** 56	**96** 437	**92** 95	**86** 414	- -	- -

NOTE: The first number in each column (boldface) is the rate in percent, the second number is the number of patients; Please refer to the main entry for footnotes; ***Heart Attack Care:*** *1. ACE Inhibitor or ARB for LVSD; 2. Aspirin at Arrival; 3. Aspirin at Discharge; 4. Beta Blocker at Arrival; 5. Beta Blocker at Discharge; 6. Fibrinolytic Medication Timing; 7. PCI Within 90 Minutes of Arrival; 8. Smoking Cessation Advice;* ***Heart Failure Care:*** *9. ACE Inhibitor or ARB for LVSD; 10. Discharge Instructions; 11. Evaluation of LVS Function; 12. Smoking Cessation Advice;* ***Pneumonia Care:*** *13. Appropriate Initial Antibiotic; 14. Blood Culture Timing; 15. Influenza Vaccine; 16. Initial Antibiotic Timing; 17. Oxygenation Assessment; 18. Pneumococcal Vaccine; 19. Smoking Cessation Advice;* ***Surgical Infection Prevention:*** *20. Prophylactic Antibiotic Given; 21. Prophylactic Antibiotic Selection; 22. Prophylactic Antibiotic Stopped;* ***Pregnancy Care:*** *23. Inpatient Neonatal Mortality; 24. Third or Fourth Degree Laceration*

Hospital	Heart Attack Care								Heart Failure Care				Pneumonia Care							Surgical Infection Prevention			Pregnancy Care	
	1	2	3	4	5	6	7	8	9	10	11	12	13	14	15	16	17	18	19	20	21	22	23	24
Cape Coral Hospital, Cape Coral, FL	80 15	94 93	96 49	89 73	95 62	- 0	- 0	89 9	84 49	44 117	90 143	96 23	83 92	90 97	71 21	83 121	100 140	81 95	93 30	90 105	90 41	71 100	- -	- -
Capital Regional Medical Center, Tallahassee, FL	79 39	88 89	88 86	86 69	83 95	- 0	50 4	97 33	70 158	17 307	96 395	86 73	80 86	84 86	50 22	68 139	100 152	68 77	90 40	87 321	73 26	61 312	0.41 972	3.24 617
Cedars Medical Center, Miami, FL	66 118	90 242	80 286	82 239	79 299	18 28	- 0	80 94	65 371	37 663	92 777	85 199	82 170	75 195	25 59	54 314	98 343	33 203	85 67	96 468	89 101	62 462	- -	- -
Central Florida Regional Hospital, Sanford, FL	77 48	96 160	96 224	89 113	94 240	33 3	17 6	97 89	75 118	66 283	91 356	92 97	87 149	80 104	49 45	56 217	98 244	47 124	87 68	83 390	92 100	75 364	- -	- -
Charlotte Regional Medical Center, Punta Gorda, FL	80 85	99 151	95 311	93 146	89 332	0 1	77 13	96 103	81 253	67 407	93 464	99 70	85 127	95 137	58 48	77 177	99 232	67 164	98 52	65 464	94 70	78 450	- -	- -
Citrus Memorial Hospital, Inverness, FL	73 55	96 282	96 272	85 260	93 278	100 1	62 13	94 103	74 112	54 241	86 297	90 41	83 139	90 123	- -	75 178	100 231	81 167	94 36	86 529	97 150	89 483	- -	- -
Cleveland Clinic Florida, Weston, FL	100 41	100 87	100 140	100 86	100 142	- 0	83 12	100 44	100 97	93 207	100 220	100 20	95 83	96 90	96 28	86 84	100 120	96 71	100 8	97 320	97 76	67 312	- -	- -
Columbia Hospital, West Palm Beach, FL	0 6	80 65	88 32	72 47	69 32	100 2	- 0	71 7	63 67	53 186	75 275	71 42	82 62	95 80	19 16	83 103	100 132	47 66	71 17	73 219	98 47	54 213	- -	- -
Columbia Memorial Hospital of Jacksonville, Jacksonville, FL	85 65	92 245	95 335	88 184	94 349	50 4	31 13	99 177	77 239	43 498	93 615	97 128	88 301	90 346	43 74	75 416	99 530	42 294	96 147	83 314	88 137	60 290	- -	- -
Community Hospital, New Port Richey, FL	76 38	94 219	82 89	89 122	86 127	50 14	- 0	100 28	78 156	63 346	84 494	99 72	90 167	80 117	33 61	76 245	99 296	84 193	100 87	88 273	87 79	66 265	- -	- -
Coral Gables Hospital, Miami, FL	83 12	97 119	81 59	99 108	95 64	50 8	- 0	100 6	90 90	94 223	96 295	100 27	87 223	92 197	- -	82 251	98 283	80 203	96 27	95 145	100 31	37 145	- -	- -
Coral Springs Medical Center, Coral Springs, FL	82 11	96 93	69 36	94 67	86 36	38 8	- 0	100 5	79 72	93 175	89 195	100 20	83 116	89 115	80 25	71 133	100 174	83 86	96 46	69 170	82 40	44 164	- -	- -
Delray Medical Center, Delray Beach, FL	99 118	100 506	100 548	99 474	99 541	14 21	95 19	100 73	97 178	100 497	99 688	100 21	93 257	100 211	- -	95 257	100 305	93 216	100 22	96 1176	96 252	81 1134	- -	- -
DeSoto Memorial Hospital, Arcadia, FL	0 1	89 28	43 7	75 24	86 7	- 0	- 0	0 2	59 22	18 78	56 89	22 9	92 61	91 45	67 15	70 63	99 67	47 38	21 14	100 3	0 1	33 3	- -	- -
Doctors Hospital of Sarasota, Sarasota, FL	75 8	89 65	91 35	79 29	94 34	0 2	- 0	100 4	85 65	66 129	96 194	96 25	87 122	87 103	70 53	76 193	100 229	67 171	90 59	92 226	97 72	73 219	- -	- -
Doctors Memorial Hospital, Perry, FL	100 1	94 16	83 12	94 16	75 12	- -	- -	- -	68 28	23 22	66 74	88 8	50 18	100 6	- -	79 58	97 75	51 37	100 6	100 7	- -	0 7	- -	- -
Doctors Memorial Hospital, Bonifay, FL	- -	- -	- -	- -	- -	- -	- -	- -	38 8	90 48	22 74	94 17	67 60	86 7	87 15	79 61	88 82	79 39	89 19	- -	- -	- -	- -	- -
Edward White Hospital, Saint Petersburg, FL	100 5	97 30	94 17	81 21	94 18	0 1	- 0	80 5	82 33	23 93	86 148	90 21	88 92	91 112	47 38	92 154	99 182	53 115	84 45	89 126	94 33	69 118	- -	- -
Englewood Community Hospital, Englewood, FL	79 24	93 116	78 63	80 118	78 76	0 6	- 0	91 11	76 59	76 131	80 169	77 13	71 92	83 58	56 27	74 104	100 116	48 79	94 18	88 168	90 51	86 161	- -	- -
Fawcett Memorial Hospital, Port Charlotte, FL	78 23	82 85	82 50	81 75	90 61	- 0	- 0	92 13	76 103	77 246	84 312	97 38	80 121	91 105	53 38	80 173	100 220	72 160	93 44	91 425	95 87	61 409	- -	- -
Fishermen's Hospital, Marathon, FL	- 0	100 3	- 0	100 3	100 1	- 0	- 0	- 0	100 9	25 20	82 22	100 4	79 28	93 14	88 8	79 29	100 36	70 23	90 10	78 69	87 15	16 68	- -	- -
Flagler Hospital, Saint Augustine, FL	74 27	89 289	91 257	80 224	86 245	0 1	25 12	94 78	82 144	35 366	98 458	86 78	81 160	86 115	- -	67 216	100 265	65 142	92 71	59 259	87 75	44 254	- -	- -
Florida Hospital DeLand, Deland, FL	85 26	96 138	97 72	90 112	96 77	37 19	- 0	100 18	78 120	38 242	98 351	100 59	92 225	95 251	- -	87 342	99 387	64 228	100 87	91 410	98 90	89 398	- -	- -
Florida Hospital Fish Memorial, Orange City, FL	71 31	92 206	87 112	90 145	96 109	24 25	100 1	95 19	76 123	41 342	92 437	93 58	88 262	89 228	53 77	58 349	100 372	52 226	91 80	87 432	82 118	76 415	- -	- -
Florida Hospital Flagler, Palm Coast, FL	75 24	92 177	86 86	91 165	91 79	45 11	- 0	100 15	83 69	25 191	90 241	97 36	74 92	84 85	83 24	86 113	99 145	69 77	100 37	75 371	91 96	65 365	- -	- -
Florida Hospital Heartland Medical Center, Sebring, FL	90 31	87 119	92 59	86 90	99 77	0 2	- 0	77 13	71 206	58 382	94 476	91 87	90 193	87 137	74 57	69 257	100 287	78 210	88 50	88 434	97 94	71 418	0.94 1069	1.24 726
Florida Hospital Orlando, Orlando, FL	87 253	96 598	94 982	88 520	95 1021	0 1	67 15	100 355	84 776	75 1762	94 2113	99 342	90 929	85 951	- -	76 1482	100 1744	90 894	99 405	86 1434	94 363	75 1383	- -	- -
Florida Hospital Waterman, Tavares, FL	82 28	89 158	86 86	83 145	92 89	- 0	- 0	80 20	76 234	75 403	94 485	87 67	77 180	88 206	79 66	77 255	100 323	77 205	91 64	72 579	90 134	64 541	- -	- -
Florida Hospital Wauchula, Wauchula, FL	- 0	- 0	- 0	- 0	- 0	- 0	- -	- 0	- 0	100 4	75 4	- 0	90 21	90 21	50 8	83 30	100 35	59 17	100 5	- -	- -	- -	- -	- -
Florida Hospital Zephyrhills, Zephyrhills, FL	69 55	92 226	92 185	85 206	89 184	14 14	67 3	75 56	82 110	53 294	85 349	49 53	86 176	79 101	29 59	75 174	96 233	47 143	75 57	79 328	88 67	78 308	0.14 705	1.54 456
Florida Hospital-Ormond Memorial, Ormond Beach, FL	73 96	95 280	94 413	83 232	89 419	50 4	43 7	98 133	72 211	70 372	94 503	97 77	90 154	91 138	- -	76 218	98 259	76 171	87 71	79 866	93 195	58 845	- -	- -
Florida Medical Center, Lauderdale Lakes, FL	89 127	97 323	94 420	94 325	95 434	33 3	56 18	100 101	76 203	57 393	87 528	100 35	83 90	91 89	73 30	83 125	100 147	80 103	100 25	89 460	94 82	53 454	- -	- -
Fort Walton Beach Medical Center, Fort Walton Beach, FL	100 54	99 164	99 282	100 130	99 262	- 0	42 12	99 110	100 74	95 219	97 283	100 55	79 156	89 132	65 40	69 218	100 245	67 138	95 76	87 246	91 110	53 230	- -	- -
Glades General Hospital, Belle Glade, FL	- 0	100 8	100 2	100 6	100 2	- 0	- 0	0 1	88 51	89 122	99 128	96 26	82 50	85 55	- -	82 55	100 66	85 26	83 12	96 24	100 8	91 23	- -	- -
Good Samaritan Medical Center, West Palm Beach, FL	75 8	96 51	96 23	98 46	100 30	0 1	- 0	100 3	86 77	67 206	95 263	100 27	89 217	95 221	98 63	84 298	100 349	94 210	100 61	70 227	97 62	78 219	- -	- -
Gulf Breeze Hospital, Gulf Breeze, FL	80 5	97 29	100 20	88 25	95 19	- 0	- 0	100 9	88 25	57 92	88 110	93 15	92 114	91 76	73 22	81 127	100 153	76 95	100 35	76 419	97 93	60 394	- -	- -
Gulf Coast Hospital, Fort Meyers, FL	- 0	79 14	50 4	77 13	83 6	- 0	- 0	- 0	86 7	4 23	60 25	100 1	73 59	90 49	67 15	68 79	100 92	52 54	100 20	83 354	98 85	81 351	- -	- -
Gulf Coast Medical Center, Panama City, FL	67 3	94 16	60 5	100 13	100 8	- 0	- 0	100 1	74 43	40 98	84 132	100 17	78 181	73 83	55 44	66 269	99 304	45 179	97 69	70 416	66 82	65 395	- -	- -
Halifax Medical Center, Daytona Beach, FL	93 68	97 367	99 364	98 301	97 378	12 8	25 4	100 160	94 311	96 641	99 786	100 201	90 381	68 285	- -	88 471	100 576	86 286	99 144	91 794	91 385	77 779	- -	- -
Health Central, Ocoee, FL	82 11	85 94	88 48	76 96	91 53	- 0	- 0	91 11	78 110	39 200	93 268	85 53	82 114	84 101	64 22	53 187	100 202	69 108	88 40	84 170	91 44	80 167	- -	- -
Healthmark Regional Medical Center, Defuniak Springs, FL	- 0	80 5	0 1	60 5	0 1	- 0	- 0	- 0	67 3	38 8	33 30	67 3	43 14	- 0	- -	60 40	90 48	56 32	38 8	- 0	- -	- 0	- -	- -
HealthSouth Doctors' Hospital, Miami, FL	100 3	97 62	100 10	98 57	100 17	100 3	- 0	100 1	96 45	87 153	100 177	100 15	87 167	90 165	96 57	89 174	100 250	94 161	100 51	99 546	96 137	94 525	- -	- -
Heart of Florida Regional Medical Center, Davenport, FL	68 19	79 106	69 54	68 102	73 59	- 0	- 0	83 12	81 160	20 398	82 439	84 56	85 173	84 105	66 47	59 211	100 231	56 131	90 59	89 748	85 72	61 740	- -	- -
Helen Ellis Memorial Hospital, Tarpon Springs, FL	87 31	92 134	68 87	90 126	88 96	- 0	100 6	82 28	79 122	12 235	91 308	63 43	84 108	89 73	48 23	73 139	99 155	35 97	64 39	91 47	81 47	55 47	- -	- -
Hendry Regional Medical Center, Clewiston, FL	100 1	100 5	50 2	100 3	100 1	100 1	- 0	100 2	50 8	97 29	70 30	100 6	92 12	92 13	0 1	56 9	100 15	86 7	100 7	100 3	- -	100 3	- -	- -
Hialeah Hospital, Miami, FL	91 35	97 216	95 87	93 170	94 94	87 15	- 0	100 11	96 163	99 368	100 446	100 66	84 279	94 281	95 77	86 390	100 438	92 299	100 53	95 123	89 28	67 96	- -	- -
Highlands Regional Medical Center, Sebring, FL	40 5	91 44	71 21	95 39	75 24	0 2	- 0	100 4	66 58	29 160	83 208	95 21	71 150	93 123	46 56	60 183	100 206	64 149	79 28	53 135	96 23	62 126	- -	- -
Holmes Regional Medical Center, Melbourne, FL	85 298	94 426	98 744	92 383	95 762	25 4	35 20	97 256	74 412	73 661	89 818	93 132	85 388	93 403	57 96	86 517	100 602	62 377	88 121	91 947	94 241	65 920	- -	- -

NOTE: The first number in each column (boldface) is the rate in percent, the second number is the number of patients; Please refer to the main entry for footnotes; ***Heart Attack Care:*** *1. ACE Inhibitor or ARB for LVSD; 2. Aspirin at Arrival; 3. Aspirin at Discharge; 4. Beta Blocker at Arrival; 5. Beta Blocker at Discharge; 6. Fibrinolytic Medication Timing; 7. PCI Within 90 Minutes of Arrival; 8. Smoking Cessation Advice;* ***Heart Failure Care:*** *9. ACE Inhibitor or ARB for LVSD; 10. Discharge Instructions; 11. Evaluation of LVS Function; 12. Smoking Cessation Advice;* ***Pneumonia Care:*** *13. Appropriate Initial Antibiotic; 14. Blood Culture Timing; 15. Influenza Vaccine; 16. Initial Antibiotic Timing; 17. Oxygenation Assessment; 18. Pneumococcal Vaccine; 19. Smoking Cessation Advice;* ***Surgical Infection Prevention:*** *20. Prophylactic Antibiotic Given; 21. Prophylactic Antibiotic Selection; 22. Prophylactic Antibiotic Stopped;* ***Pregnancy Care:*** *23. Inpatient Neonatal Mortality; 24. Third or Fourth Degree Laceration*

Hospital	Heart Attack Care								Heart Failure Care				Pneumonia Care							Surgical Infection Prevention			Pregnancy Care	
	1	2	3	4	5	6	7	8	9	10	11	12	13	14	15	16	17	18	19	20	21	22	23	24
Holy Cross Hospital, Fort Lauderdale, FL	98 45	100 188	99 266	99 172	99 271	20 5	25 4	100 71	99 191	100 446	100 544	100 57	85 172	87 182	100 55	81 211	100 266	100 170	100 29	74 292	94 77	61 279	- -	- -
Homestead Hospital, Homestead, FL	100 8	100 88	100 18	100 77	100 20	0 2	- 0	100 5	98 126	94 291	100 323	100 84	98 241	95 249	83 52	80 298	100 344	95 160	100 103	86 73	95 20	87 62	- -	- -
Imperial Point Medical Center, Fort Lauderdale, FL	67 3	79 33	82 11	85 20	82 11	100 1	- 0	100 3	82 50	71 119	86 139	100 38	85 94	86 97	- -	86 125	100 135	54 72	100 35	75 138	97 33	26 131	- -	- -
Indian River Memorial Hospital, Vero Beach, FL	79 19	96 134	89 62	90 144	90 72	40 5	- 0	100 2	76 142	65 63	80 458	100 15	79 42	87 38	- -	72 270	100 350	37 247	89 9	92 59	- -	60 58	- -	- -
Jackson Hospital, Marianna, FL	90 10	97 30	100 16	86 29	95 19	- 0	- 0	100 5	92 50	24 125	87 167	94 31	74 91	86 56	32 25	78 101	100 128	26 70	97 36	87 86	100 29	86 84	- -	- -
Jackson Memorial Hospital, Miami, FL	91 66	96 223	96 212	94 180	96 231	33 18	0 4	95 96	84 275	41 509	97 569	73 137	94 200	68 182	41 46	51 326	99 352	45 139	70 86	60 298	82 60	68 280	- -	- -
Jay Hospital, Jay, FL	100 1	86 7	75 4	83 6	100 2	100 1	- 0	100 1	89 18	96 46	90 58	57 7	61 49	96 28	44 9	82 50	96 73	70 37	60 20	- -	- -	- -	- -	- -
JFK Medical Center, Atlantis, FL	87 245	96 729	95 944	93 517	95 946	100 1	47 34	99 272	85 493	82 1037	93 1223	99 170	80 351	78 379	65 129	56 547	100 668	64 434	97 118	87 905	97 274	60 881	- -	- -
Jupiter Medical Center, Jupiter, FL	75 8	86 70	87 30	89 72	91 32	50 2	- 0	100 1	72 81	52 178	90 219	71 14	85 116	87 103	42 31	77 155	100 192	52 129	76 25	70 178	96 45	67 174	- -	- -
Kendall Medical Center, Miami, FL	63 180	94 455	93 409	83 322	90 494	14 7	60 20	99 139	65 342	72 679	97 777	100 65	91 464	94 424	41 116	76 619	100 660	52 444	93 86	86 330	97 134	75 310	- -	- -
Lake City Medical Center, Lake City, FL	70 10	79 48	53 19	89 47	65 20	0 2	- 0	100 5	54 56	46 160	91 214	94 32	69 177	92 80	56 52	62 227	98 256	58 170	96 52	26 19	0 5	100 10	- -	- -
Lake Wales Medical Center, Lake Wales, FL	67 6	78 23	50 12	76 17	71 14	- 0	- 0	75 4	74 68	22 180	88 214	23 35	82 94	97 77	30 20	74 137	100 151	64 86	36 33	50 52	92 12	96 50	- -	- -
Lakeland Regional Medical Center, Lakeland, FL	82 67	97 284	97 309	92 261	95 303	0 3	38 8	100 115	84 157	84 280	91 322	86 49	88 163	97 169	68 41	72 240	100 291	64 170	87 91	83 534	97 127	72 510	0.67 896	2.13 657
Lakewood Ranch Medical Center, Bradenton, FL	86 7	83 46	74 23	79 47	83 23	33 3	- 0	33 3	79 19	62 66	91 78	100 6	84 93	85 82	69 16	81 100	100 127	70 77	65 23	81 155	88 26	61 145	- -	- -
Largo Medical Center, Largo, FL	90 48	97 267	96 255	94 170	96 278	33 3	25 12	98 98	91 110	41 332	97 429	100 59	82 211	88 171	61 82	71 303	100 333	63 226	100 75	95 279	97 103	89 241	- -	- -
Larkin Community Hospital, South Miami, FL	100 3	97 31	92 13	93 27	93 15	0 1	- 0	100 9	100 12	98 41	89 73	100 8	75 65	90 83	76 29	75 120	100 135	86 77	100 49	100 24	100 3	100 9	- -	- -
Lawnwood Regional Med Ctr & Heart Inst, Fort Pierce, FL	99 115	99 189	98 369	97 163	98 398	38 8	12 8	100 147	95 261	90 493	98 586	99 135	90 219	94 288	95 80	81 356	99 411	92 240	97 106	86 428	91 119	75 415	- -	- -
Lee Memorial Health System, Fort Myers, FL	80 59	93 161	96 199	92 119	98 220	0 1	33 12	99 87	81 100	46 195	91 238	95 42	82 105	93 116	81 31	73 155	100 193	77 118	90 39	88 339	91 86	80 328	- -	- -
Leesburg Regional Medical Center, Leesburg, FL	82 114	97 262	97 355	90 170	97 401	- 0	30 20	98 114	89 178	69 343	99 426	99 73	89 210	84 251	- -	64 344	100 362	75 233	92 61	94 467	99 124	93 460	- -	- -
Lehigh Regional Medical Center, Lehigh Acres, FL	70 10	87 52	57 21	75 48	65 20	- 0	- 0	33 3	88 66	28 164	95 174	48 33	80 172	92 74	- -	75 171	100 202	57 119	47 57	54 140	93 29	67 133	- -	- -
Lower Keys Medical Center, Key West, FL	100 2	91 22	86 7	89 18	100 7	0 1	- 0	50 2	81 31	83 90	94 104	100 21	50 98	91 93	52 25	70 105	100 140	52 77	97 35	57 120	58 31	48 94	- -	- -
Manatee Memorial Hospital, Bradenton, FL	75 93	95 414	91 410	89 364	87 422	45 11	64 14	95 154	83 233	84 475	94 630	94 144	85 215	85 153	64 50	70 264	99 312	79 181	90 77	80 468	90 126	62 452	- -	- -
Mariners Hospital, Tavernier, FL	67 3	100 32	100 7	94 16	100 6	- 0	- 0	100 3	93 27	100 39	100 46	100 11	90 60	94 47	82 11	93 60	100 73	93 44	100 18	92 13	100 5	62 13	- -	- -
Martin Memorial Medical Center, Stuart, FL	78 36	95 149	91 91	90 106	90 109	30 10	40 5	100 16	84 101	42 208	94 270	100 34	87 82	85 105	- -	78 153	100 179	57 127	100 29	91 241	94 71	72 221	- -	- -
Mease Hospital-Countryside, Safety Harbor, FL	89 19	97 158	88 57	88 75	97 88	- 0	- 0	100 9	91 150	68 337	93 434	98 47	85 265	95 286	74 91	78 281	100 445	75 296	98 85	73 168	93 61	78 145	- -	- -
Mease Hospital-Dunedin, Dunedin, FL	100 15	95 60	88 25	94 32	98 46	- 0	- 0	100 10	87 90	70 159	91 199	100 25	85 107	95 109	52 42	88 115	100 208	57 137	100 48	81 103	97 30	84 87	- -	- -
Memorial Hospital Miramar, Miramar, FL	100 3	100 39	100 7	92 39	100 10	- 0	- 0	100 1	96 24	88 122	98 133	89 9	89 134	98 125	100 26	93 150	100 174	100 92	100 26	89 213	95 21	86 210	- -	- -
Memorial Hospital of Tampa, Tampa, FL	100 3	91 22	88 8	94 18	100 8	- 0	- 0	100 3	98 44	94 107	99 144	100 17	88 139	94 144	75 32	79 203	100 208	68 120	100 39	81 129	89 36	64 127	- -	- -
Memorial Hospital Pembroke, Pembroke Pines, FL	100 3	98 103	94 32	99 85	100 32	- 0	- 0	100 6	100 73	96 237	100 270	100 46	90 263	98 286	96 73	92 266	100 376	97 196	100 68	97 169	97 39	96 155	- -	- -
Memorial Hospital West, Pembroke Pines, FL	94 36	97 264	95 160	98 167	99 171	- 0	89 19	100 56	90 178	84 463	100 523	100 52	95 320	91 341	94 81	87 436	100 502	98 264	100 80	91 583	95 41	83 553	- -	- -
Memorial Regional Hospital, Hollywood, FL	92 150	99 412	99 652	97 357	98 652	- 0	87 30	99 222	93 486	85 869	99 992	100 208	97 305	95 359	95 65	85 403	100 506	96 236	100 118	93 1000	95 63	85 971	- -	- -
Mercy Hospital, Miami, FL	94 79	99 251	99 355	99 250	97 374	0 1	75 4	100 64	95 298	96 496	99 551	100 75	95 202	94 234	- -	89 295	100 354	84 261	100 44	96 1252	97 316	84 1229	- -	- -
Miami Jewish Home & Hosp for the Aged, Miami, FL	- 0	50 2	50 2	50 2	100 2	- 0	- 0	- 0	- 0	0 5	75 16	- 0	40 5	100 14	58 12	80 46	100 64	46 52	0 1	- 0	- 0	- 0	- -	- -
Morton Plant Hospital, Clearwater, FL	96 155	97 415	98 601	94 245	99 695	- 0	- 0	97 232	90 240	67 523	93 701	100 93	90 262	95 239	73 89	65 289	100 463	72 312	91 102	75 224	87 67	92 200	- -	- -
Mount Sinai Medical Center, Miami, FL	81 99	96 184	86 313	91 163	89 339	0 1	56 9	91 97	80 173	50 305	94 373	91 35	90 128	85 153	40 25	65 193	95 219	53 138	94 32	79 547	84 316	74 538	0.19 2158	1.70 1115
Munroe Regional Medical Center, Ocala, FL	82 170	94 319	95 345	86 213	96 397	- 0	50 10	93 143	84 229	43 364	91 454	82 73	86 176	89 135	84 55	59 245	100 306	82 225	89 90	90 673	94 173	81 628	- -	- -
Nature Coast Regional Hospital, Williston, FL	- 0	- 0	- 0	- 0	- 0	- 0	- 0	- 0	87 15	0 1	78 41	0 1	100 10	100 4	- -	71 41	100 49	14 21	50 2	- -	- -	- -	- -	- -
NCH Downtown Naples Hospital, Naples, FL	91 120	100 577	99 700	98 507	98 666	- 0	40 20	99 158	80 456	45 887	89 1121	97 122	88 496	85 384	28 143	72 527	100 654	44 482	76 124	88 2605	94 593	80 2452	- -	- -
North Bay Medical Center, New Port Richey, FL	89 9	93 73	86 28	91 33	83 36	33 3	- 0	100 8	89 71	53 152	91 196	93 30	81 99	92 92	40 25	78 103	100 157	62 80	95 43	68 111	97 34	74 89	- -	- -
North Broward Medical Center, Deerfield Beach, FL	88 33	91 164	94 64	91 112	93 91	40 5	- 0	100 10	83 115	82 214	89 257	100 45	86 123	90 96	- -	73 152	100 175	55 78	88 40	69 186	96 47	33 180	- -	- -
North Florida Regional Medical Center, Gainesville, FL	62 98	98 194	97 314	87 143	90 316	- 0	58 12	98 115	64 220	44 470	88 573	98 82	91 204	76 203	64 76	73 309	97 384	51 241	98 90	86 315	90 136	65 313	- -	- -
North Okaloosa Medical Center, Crestview, FL	88 8	89 46	71 28	89 45	73 26	- 0	- 0	100 5	73 52	31 135	95 165	89 35	86 110	70 64	40 20	72 142	100 158	58 96	86 44	65 227	82 40	77 221	- -	- -
North Ridge Medical Center, Fort Lauderdale, FL	96 54	95 148	99 251	95 142	97 260	0 2	40 15	100 68	90 94	97 176	90 221	100 24	90 50	91 44	73 11	90 71	99 81	67 61	92 12	93 580	96 150	62 570	- -	- -
North Shore Medical Center, Miami, FL	76 41	84 171	88 82	88 145	96 101	50 8	- 0	100 16	85 271	92 494	97 571	100 124	94 187	84 211	86 36	63 262	100 314	75 145	100 54	95 79	100 19	91 76	- -	- -
Northside Hospital, Saint Petersburg, FL	95 37	95 210	97 257	93 150	96 270	100 1	62 16	97 120	83 98	54 252	98 321	97 60	81 275	94 222	41 73	65 373	100 411	41 253	92 105	85 228	95 74	59 211	- -	- -
Northwest Florida Community Hospital, Chipley, FL	- 0	- 0	- 0	- 0	- 0	- 0	- -	- 0	100 13	26 35	60 40	100 7	85 33	95 20	100 7	80 41	100 46	62 16	79 14	- -	- -	- -	- -	- -
Northwest Medical Center, Margate, FL	89 27	88 165	90 72	89 102	99 93	25 8	- 0	90 10	87 95	88 260	93 333	100 37	88 194	90 156	70 53	70 225	100 274	73 175	96 52	86 318	82 110	79 312	- -	- -
Oak Hill Hospital, Brooksville, FL	87 39	87 223	73 158	83 189	85 176	100 3	60 10	98 48	71 108	25 357	80 418	93 61	79 237	86 149	43 68	63 321	98 360	49 249	97 72	87 435	96 126	57 414	- -	- -

NOTE: The first number in each column (boldface) is the rate in percent, the second number is the number of patients; Please refer to the main entry for footnotes; ***Heart Attack Care:*** *1. ACE Inhibitor or ARB for LVSD; 2. Aspirin at Arrival; 3. Aspirin at Discharge; 4. Beta Blocker at Arrival; 5. Beta Blocker at Discharge; 6. Fibrinolytic Medication Timing; 7. PCI Within 90 Minutes of Arrival; 8. Smoking Cessation Advice;* ***Heart Failure Care:*** *9. ACE Inhibitor or ARB for LVSD; 10. Discharge Instructions; 11. Evaluation of LVS Function; 12. Smoking Cessation Advice;* ***Pneumonia Care:*** *13. Appropriate Initial Antibiotic; 14. Blood Culture Timing; 15. Influenza Vaccine; 16. Initial Antibiotic Timing; 17. Oxygenation Assessment; 18. Pneumococcal Vaccine; 19. Smoking Cessation Advice;* ***Surgical Infection Prevention:*** *20. Prophylactic Antibiotic Given; 21. Prophylactic Antibiotic Selection; 22. Prophylactic Antibiotic Stopped;* ***Pregnancy Care:*** *23. Inpatient Neonatal Mortality; 24. Third or Fourth Degree Laceration*

Hospital	Heart Attack Care								Heart Failure Care				Pneumonia Care							Surgical Infection Prevention			Pregnancy Care	
	1	2	3	4	5	6	7	8	9	10	11	12	13	14	15	16	17	18	19	20	21	22	23	24
Ocala Regional Medical Center, Ocala, FL	86 106	94 220	95 219	79 112	97 260	- 0	82 11	99 90	80 204	49 343	93 440	93 85	90 294	82 211	84 92	69 401	100 482	80 296	93 144	93 983	94 242	92 902	- -	- -
Orange Park Medical Center, Orange Park, FL	89 9	93 84	97 33	94 65	100 46	17 6	- 0	93 14	86 122	67 257	98 371	93 75	90 303	92 447	59 118	75 501	100 669	70 409	87 134	90 519	89 120	84 498	- -	- -
Orlando Regional Healthcare, Orlando, FL	89 196	93 388	95 607	86 266	96 671	- 0	57 23	96 246	84 743	37 1408	99 1651	92 334	89 664	85 564	75 224	65 956	100 1188	76 581	89 330	93 3356	96 847	86 3065	- -	- -
Osceola Regional Medical Center, Kissimmee, FL	82 66	91 221	83 245	80 196	81 254	- 0	31 13	99 81	73 211	95 401	98 458	100 44	79 298	80 202	49 79	53 342	100 396	34 243	96 56	80 528	94 144	83 484	- -	- -
Palm Beach Grdns Medical Center, Palm Beach Grdns, FL	64 198	95 364	92 782	91 333	93 815	0 2	74 19	100 219	75 351	85 567	91 672	99 90	87 143	90 126	78 40	77 166	99 203	70 132	96 28	95 599	98 129	42 566	- -	- -
Palm Springs General Hospital, Miami, FL	83 23	97 139	83 46	89 123	87 52	40 15	- 0	- 0	78 160	80 316	91 380	85 26	67 247	95 189	- -	73 292	96 341	53 248	100 26	75 123	80 41	73 121	- -	- -
Palmetto General Hospital, Hialeah, FL	88 16	97 189	90 40	99 177	92 51	0 3	- 0	100 12	80 177	81 395	95 462	100 71	87 244	77 213	65 40	75 263	100 311	73 174	100 46	88 179	93 44	63 180	- -	- -
Palms of Pasadena Hospital, Saint Petersburg, FL	100 4	100 44	100 20	98 44	100 19	- 0	- 0	100 2	93 42	70 132	86 176	78 23	87 136	69 150	- -	73 199	98 247	63 188	77 39	92 336	91 80	42 313	- -	- -
Palms West Hospital, Loxahatchee, FL	56 9	83 52	57 28	95 22	76 25	- 0	- 0	100 9	65 83	47 215	93 245	82 34	81 137	82 80	62 32	46 140	99 165	69 89	91 34	74 307	92 79	54 298	- -	- -
Pan American Hospital, Miami, FL	83 18	97 116	93 44	89 119	87 46	- 0	- 0	100 4	80 127	95 240	96 323	96 28	65 223	96 162	89 44	84 207	100 236	97 155	100 25	83 242	87 75	89 240	- -	- -
Parrish Medical Center, Titusville, FL	97 38	94 143	80 60	96 118	96 76	100 1	- 0	100 25	93 104	92 182	94 234	100 39	87 130	90 132	57 42	74 194	100 243	74 133	100 49	90 231	92 59	80 225	- -	- -
Pasco Regional Medical Center, Dade City, FL	100 4	98 44	100 14	97 34	95 19	50 16	- 0	83 6	97 70	54 166	96 205	95 37	76 131	94 125	85 55	81 141	100 204	87 135	89 55	83 280	98 51	63 252	- -	- -
Peace River Regional Medical Center, Port Charlotte, FL	100 3	98 54	96 28	86 37	100 33	- 0	- 0	100 8	97 66	45 175	99 222	100 17	79 160	91 129	90 41	67 214	99 266	94 168	97 68	82 401	88 68	76 377	- -	- -
Physicians Regional Medical Center, Naples, FL	100 2	95 20	100 10	100 22	100 11	- 0	- 0	- 0	100 19	27 11	98 60	50 2	89 9	86 7	- -	84 49	100 63	71 35	100 2	74 77	- -	95 77	0.00 0	0.00 0
Plantation General Hospital, Plantation, FL	100 3	90 20	80 10	71 21	75 12	- 0	- 0	0 1	71 76	64 131	86 153	89 37	86 84	83 102	10 20	68 148	99 162	47 43	93 45	94 146	96 46	77 146	0.63 3780	2.43 2060
Putnam Community Medical Center, Palatka, FL	100 9	92 86	94 33	94 78	100 43	43 7	- 0	100 11	96 77	81 236	100 275	100 66	90 185	94 141	92 60	79 275	99 302	92 182	100 77	72 141	92 40	48 135	- -	- -
Raulerson Hospital, Okeechobee, FL	100 6	88 49	94 16	89 44	94 18	0 4	- 0	100 4	89 54	79 234	67 258	100 58	72 149	88 102	73 49	79 189	100 226	69 143	100 53	82 67	92 25	52 67	- -	- -
Regional Medical Center Bayonet Point, Hudson, FL	85 163	92 344	94 625	85 324	94 640	30 10	33 3	95 208	80 304	51 549	94 674	91 115	86 125	68 84	51 47	62 185	100 233	54 158	95 43	62 566	95 155	60 542	- -	- -
Sacred Heart Health System, Pensacola, FL	97 74	98 226	96 312	98 221	96 310	50 4	22 9	95 128	95 188	80 342	98 389	98 102	64 219	94 131	66 41	58 228	100 299	62 176	75 60	54 349	93 86	57 336	0.43 691	1.34 373
Sacred Heart Hospital on the Emerald Coast, Destin, FL	100 1	100 15	100 5	88 8	80 5	- 0	- 0	100 2	90 29	74 74	96 90	86 7	80 55	87 38	70 23	94 48	100 93	86 63	91 23	80 183	90 51	73 177	- -	- -
Saint Anthony's Hospital, Saint Petersburg, FL	94 17	93 104	93 73	93 85	92 75	- 0	- 0	100 30	89 98	83 217	87 281	100 69	88 188	92 200	62 58	75 219	100 372	64 183	98 112	84 149	84 49	57 136	- -	- -
Saint Cloud Regional Medical Center, Saint Cloud, FL	100 1	90 21	71 7	60 20	86 7	- 0	- 0	- 0	88 25	11 19	88 80	75 4	79 14	100 12	- -	71 84	100 102	70 61	100 8	44 32	- -	16 31	- -	- -
Saint Joseph's Hospital, Tampa, FL	93 178	99 494	96 517	99 379	95 529	- 0	0 1	100 197	91 422	62 811	95 975	100 171	87 252	70 290	76 95	77 391	100 648	73 274	97 162	80 225	96 69	86 198	- -	- -
Saint Lucie Medical Center, Port Saint Lucie, FL	85 26	92 200	82 68	90 185	87 79	42 33	- 0	100 6	84 185	86 369	91 503	99 68	86 243	89 206	55 53	66 307	100 383	63 241	98 58	90 472	71 100	45 464	- -	- -
Saint Luke's Hospital, Jacksonville, FL	94 32	100 146	97 143	97 118	95 181	100 1	78 9	100 59	90 115	59 245	96 306	100 42	90 87	87 106	77 26	84 147	99 209	85 153	100 39	78 282	92 75	77 278	- -	- -
Saint Mary's Medical Center, West Palm Beach, FL	67 3	96 46	79 19	98 45	86 22	0 2	- 0	100 4	86 81	92 168	95 209	96 46	93 165	95 207	92 40	78 287	100 301	90 94	100 95	84 192	89 37	74 185	- -	- -
Saint Petersburg General Hospital, Saint Petersburg, FL	75 4	88 60	90 21	97 33	100 24	- 0	- 0	100 5	77 39	42 85	94 134	86 28	84 136	83 149	40 45	77 228	99 278	39 162	89 66	91 225	93 67	71 221	0.06 1587	1.87 1125
Saint Vincent's Medical Center, Jacksonville, FL	87 69	97 140	95 283	96 139	95 293	0 1	0 3	86 104	83 125	79 244	94 310	100 42	79 117	90 117	58 33	57 175	100 241	60 139	97 29	62 321	83 83	91 316	- -	- -
Santa Rosa Medical Center, Milton, FL	71 7	96 52	54 24	90 50	76 29	0 1	- 0	100 7	89 45	66 122	91 142	94 48	77 137	97 131	85 46	78 151	100 193	82 98	99 67	88 156	89 35	80 153	- -	- -
Sarasota Memorial Health Care Systems, Sarasota, FL	87 141	96 420	97 528	95 389	94 548	0 1	29 7	91 142	84 233	35 423	93 580	94 68	82 221	87 222	67 57	79 320	100 421	86 282	82 78	83 771	96 192	73 754	- -	- -
Sebastian River Medical Center, Sebastian, FL	91 11	98 63	96 25	95 59	100 24	0 2	- 0	67 3	92 96	62 175	47 153	91 32	77 187	79 121	75 60	73 188	99 239	78 198	86 57	94 204	93 46	93 195	- -	- -
Seven Rivers Regional Medical Center, Crystal River, FL	100 24	98 112	96 45	100 113	96 50	- 0	- 0	100 12	100 126	99 216	95 280	100 53	82 154	100 115	69 42	74 149	100 202	84 142	74 39	93 497	100 57	78 469	- -	- -
Shands at Lake Shore, Lake City, FL	56 9	86 81	71 51	82 82	75 53	- 0	- 0	58 12	52 33	11 141	88 166	74 35	70 97	89 47	45 22	61 102	99 118	39 56	66 38	57 101	100 18	32 91	0.84 238	1.70 176
Shands at Starke, Starke, FL	- 0	67 3	100 1	0 3	100 1	100 1	- 0	- 0	90 21	93 43	93 58	92 13	82 39	78 23	100 6	83 52	100 64	83 30	75 8	100 1	0 1	100 1	- -	- -
Shands at the University of Florida, Gainesville, FL	82 128	97 280	97 401	90 246	96 403	0 1	62 8	96 161	86 324	32 548	96 617	87 122	81 160	87 166	34 50	55 238	100 319	42 146	96 99	86 589	95 133	72 570	1.66 1807	2.03 1032
Shands Jacksonville, Jacksonville, FL	95 65	99 208	97 276	97 181	97 271	100 1	67 6	96 144	91 176	68 257	97 298	96 83	79 96	71 113	- -	52 162	99 201	49 78	95 57	93 270	91 70	79 263	1.09 733	2.19 548
Shands Live Oak, Live Oak, FL	- 0	100 3	- 0	67 3	- 0	- 0	- 0	- 0	56 16	62 47	59 61	100 9	87 39	85 26	60 10	80 59	100 60	87 31	94 16	- -	- -	- -	- -	- -
South Bay Hospital, Sun City Center, FL	54 13	84 95	79 42	71 62	92 53	- 0	- 0	100 3	59 102	49 253	93 338	95 41	79 174	91 170	60 70	73 238	98 286	47 206	100 60	87 227	92 66	61 219	- -	- -
South Florida Baptist Hospital, Plant City, FL	100 9	100 33	100 14	100 33	100 19	- 0	- 0	100 4	94 63	71 119	99 146	100 43	86 132	94 178	62 45	84 166	100 261	83 148	98 66	81 114	97 30	73 92	- -	- -
South Lake Hospital, Clermont, FL	56 9	92 71	85 20	84 43	90 30	- 0	- 0	75 4	76 75	82 208	94 240	94 34	91 92	87 92	- -	82 110	100 144	84 89	62 32	90 329	97 73	92 326	- -	- -
South Miami Hospital, Miami, FL	100 84	100 185	99 277	97 146	99 297	100 1	78 9	99 100	98 144	87 311	100 360	98 41	94 288	98 341	100 106	90 372	100 475	99 310	100 63	93 245	95 62	95 237	- -	- -
Southwest Florida Regional Medical Center, Fort Myers, FL	72 86	96 226	96 274	91 207	97 286	0 1	42 12	99 89	83 219	52 460	87 531	97 87	88 262	86 285	51 110	73 437	100 509	54 336	92 102	77 345	94 234	62 341	- -	- -
Sun Coast Hospital, Largo, FL	55 11	97 39	92 25	93 42	93 30	- 0	- 0	33 6	91 54	21 111	91 150	84 19	85 116	86 118	- -	85 156	100 210	56 109	56 55	86 198	94 51	58 188	- -	- -
Tallahassee Memorial Health Care Foundation, Tallahassee, FL	91 121	96 314	99 399	96 229	97 436	0 1	76 17	98 168	82 209	84 355	97 432	100 88	87 173	84 152	80 46	62 226	100 270	92 149	97 66	92 713	94 180	75 690	- -	- -
Tampa General Healthcare, Tampa, FL	79 102	94 252	97 329	89 198	94 339	- 0	50 18	96 137	85 336	71 556	93 605	99 154	86 145	89 181	60 55	48 255	99 328	65 110	96 101	81 1985	89 517	72 1823	0.65 5567	3.43 3699
Town and Country Hospital, Tampa, FL	83 6	94 33	81 16	86 37	83 23	100 1	- 0	50 4	90 39	32 112	94 154	75 24	80 112	70 88	- -	70 145	99 160	73 84	85 27	92 136	86 28	66 128	- -	- -
Trinity Community Hospital, Jasper, FL	- 0	- 0	- 0	- 0	- 0	0 1	- 0	- 0	- 0	26 43	30 44	0 4	80 5	- 0	0 1	43 7	100 7	17 6	100 1	- -	- -	- -	- -	- -
Twin Cities Hospital, Niceville, FL	- 0	100 7	100 1	86 7	100 1	- 0	- 0	100 1	92 24	74 46	98 53	100 8	81 58	91 34	93 14	74 85	100 108	79 66	100 21	92 99	68 40	85 99	- -	- -

NOTE: The first number in each column (boldface) is the rate in percent, the second number is the number of patients; Please refer to the main entry for footnotes; ***Heart Attack Care:*** *1. ACE Inhibitor or ARB for LVSD; 2. Aspirin at Arrival; 3. Aspirin at Discharge; 4. Beta Blocker at Arrival; 5. Beta Blocker at Discharge; 6. Fibrinolytic Medication Timing; 7. PCI Within 90 Minutes of Arrival; 8. Smoking Cessation Advice;* ***Heart Failure Care:*** *9. ACE Inhibitor or ARB for LVSD; 10. Discharge Instructions; 11. Evaluation of LVS Function; 12. Smoking Cessation Advice;* ***Pneumonia Care:*** *13. Appropriate Initial Antibiotic; 14. Blood Culture Timing; 15. Influenza Vaccine; 16. Initial Antibiotic Timing; 17. Oxygenation Assessment; 18. Pneumococcal Vaccine; 19. Smoking Cessation Advice;* ***Surgical Infection Prevention:*** *20. Prophylactic Antibiotic Given; 21. Prophylactic Antibiotic Selection; 22. Prophylactic Antibiotic Stopped;* ***Pregnancy Care:*** *23. Inpatient Neonatal Mortality; 24. Third or Fourth Degree Laceration*

Hospital	Heart Attack Care								Heart Failure Care				Pneumonia Care							Surgical Infection Prevention			Pregnancy Care	
	1	2	3	4	5	6	7	8	9	10	11	12	13	14	15	16	17	18	19	20	21	22	23	24
University Community Hospital, Tampa, FL	**69** 77	**95** 287	**95** 372	**92** 245	**96** 394	**-** 0	**65** 20	**98** 138	**78** 176	**51** 351	**94** 461	**100** 68	**86** 180	**84** 150	**36** 25	**61** 236	**99** 296	**42** 160	**88** 56	**69** 323	**74** 90	**76** 312	**-** -	**-** -
University Community Hospital of Carrollwood, Tampa, FL	**60** 5	**95** 19	**67** 9	**68** 22	**100** 9	**0** 1	**-** 0	**-** 0	**64** 42	**70** 97	**87** 120	**100** 21	**89** 146	**79** 99	**33** 12	**67** 172	**99** 193	**42** 95	**100** 40	**82** 76	**89** 37	**54** 72	**-** -	**-** -
University Hospital & Medical Center, Tamarac, FL	**80** 15	**87** 109	**84** 32	**86** 66	**86** 50	**25** 4	**-** 0	**83** 6	**72** 97	**70** 244	**89** 318	**96** 26	**89** 143	**86** 137	**70** 50	**76** 202	**97** 226	**62** 162	**100** 35	**90** 178	**90** 50	**71** 167	**-** -	**-** -
Venice Regional Medical Center, Venice, FL	**100** 74	**100** 311	**100** 260	**99** 269	**100** 320	**0** 1	**83** 6	**100** 81	**100** 140	**93** 254	**100** 323	**100** 43	**91** 164	**93** 176	**84** 75	**91** 263	**100** 306	**87** 241	**100** 47	**95** 449	**89** 93	**87** 433	**-** -	**-** -
Villages Regional Hospital, The Villages, FL	**67** 6	**94** 64	**78** 18	**84** 64	**86** 21	**-** 0	**-** 0	**100** 3	**75** 93	**63** 247	**88** 279	**86** 35	**88** 202	**84** 180	**79** 71	**71** 235	**99** 303	**74** 223	**90** 41	**80** 123	**100** 32	**69** 118	**-** -	**-** -
Wellington Regional Medical Center, Wellington, FL	**55** 11	**96** 51	**88** 24	**85** 40	**84** 25	**-** 0	**-** 0	**75** 4	**82** 62	**56** 208	**81** 200	**85** 33	**90** 124	**87** 143	**62** 37	**83** 163	**100** 205	**56** 126	**96** 46	**79** 547	**97** 137	**66** 542	**0.04** 2652	**3.78** 1665
West Boca Medical Center, Boca Raton, FL	**92** 12	**97** 119	**95** 57	**98** 118	**93** 61	**75** 4	**-** 0	**100** 2	**96** 52	**81** 168	**93** 223	**100** 14	**88** 192	**92** 171	**80** 44	**90** 234	**99** 268	**78** 160	**100** 32	**90** 163	**88** 42	**70** 162	**-** -	**-** -
West Florida Regional Medical Center, Pensacola, FL	**87** 46	**95** 146	**99** 201	**85** 98	**96** 210	**-** 0	**73** 11	**99** 101	**76** 127	**46** 240	**96** 272	**96** 54	**84** 146	**97** 139	**78** 46	**65** 202	**100** 247	**76** 155	**98** 45	**64** 288	**94** 114	**51** 281	**-** -	**-** -
Westchester General Hospital, Miami, FL	**50** 4	**93** 14	**64** 11	**86** 14	**100** 11	**0** 1	**-** 0	**100** 2	**50** 12	**30** 27	**72** 47	**80** 5	**82** 65	**71** 41	**38** 13	**62** 71	**97** 74	**67** 54	**56** 9	**84** 45	**93** 14	**89** 44	**-** -	**-** -
Westside Regional Medical Center, Plantation, FL	**99** 68	**99** 328	**99** 333	**98** 307	**99** 334	**-** 0	**60** 15	**95** 64	**90** 117	**71** 325	**99** 394	**98** 48	**83** 186	**90** 166	**67** 49	**78** 249	**99** 264	**66** 146	**100** 45	**96** 540	**94** 133	**79** 526	**-** -	**-** -
Winter Haven Hospital, Winter Haven, FL	**80** 85	**97** 299	**92** 324	**89** 265	**94** 328	**-** 0	**67** 12	**99** 108	**93** 300	**89** 436	**96** 532	**97** 72	**86** 367	**93** 379	**79** 141	**77** 532	**99** 605	**78** 386	**90** 114	**92** 738	**97** 198	**87** 693	**-** -	**-** -
Wuesthoff Health Systems, Rockledge, FL	**100** 68	**98** 205	**99** 223	**95** 154	**98** 255	**0** 1	**54** 13	**100** 115	**99** 180	**83** 413	**98** 486	**100** 108	**84** 185	**92** 189	**94** 52	**71** 241	**100** 294	**81** 171	**99** 91	**95** 664	**90** 151	**74** 635	**-** -	**-** -
Wuesthoff Medical Center-Melbourne, Melbourne, FL	**100** 7	**90** 30	**100** 14	**87** 15	**100** 18	**-** 0	**-** 0	**100** 2	**77** 71	**60** 121	**93** 149	**100** 25	**74** 85	**93** 58	**73** 22	**66** 91	**100** 115	**76** 70	**100** 23	**93** 290	**88** 76	**67** 283	**-** -	**-** -
GEORGIA																								
Appling Hospital, Baxley, GA	**100** 1	**89** 9	**100** 1	**100** 8	**100** 2	**-** 0	**-** 0	**100** 1	**86** 7	**81** 42	**82** 44	**100** 10	**78** 73	**86** 22	**38** 21	**75** 113	**100** 138	**66** 82	**96** 28	**20** 15	**40** 5	**100** 12	**0.77** 261	**2.41** 166
Athens Regional Medical Center, Athens, GA	**85** 110	**97** 253	**98** 345	**90** 164	**96** 332	**58** 12	**62** 8	**100** 171	**89** 94	**68** 260	**98** 281	**97** 62	**86** 107	**83** 89	**62** 26	**85** 124	**100** 170	**60** 83	**98** 46	**57** 163	**88** 83	**68** 159	**-** -	**-** -
Atlanta Medical Center, Atlanta, GA	**100** 25	**98** 65	**99** 67	**98** 51	**98** 65	**-** 0	**25** 4	**92** 24	**99** 150	**96** 232	**98** 258	**96** 77	**81** 47	**90** 60	**25** 20	**70** 96	**100** 119	**44** 41	**86** 36	**50** 238	**86** 65	**66** 232	**-** -	**-** -
Bacon County Hospital System, Alma, GA	**100** 1	**50** 2	**-** 0	**50** 2	**100** 1	**-** 0	**-** 0	**-** 0	**43** 7	**69** 32	**82** 39	**89** 9	**83** 35	**94** 18	**70** 10	**97** 39	**100** 54	**71** 35	**100** 10	**-** -	**-** -	**-** -	**-** -	**-** -
Barrow Regional Medical Center, Winder, GA	**50** 2	**58** 12	**33** 6	**70** 10	**33** 6	**-** 0	**-** 0	**-** 0	**56** 16	**6** 65	**47** 51	**89** 19	**52** 82	**74** 39	**-** -	**68** 76	**100** 103	**38** 52	**83** 35	**44** 39	**89** 9	**94** 36	**-** -	**-** -
Berrien County Hospital, Nashville, GA	**100** 1	**100** 1	**100** 1	**100** 1	**100** 1	**-** 0	**-** 0	**-** 0	**100** 1	**19** 16	**13** 23	**20** 5	**58** 36	**100** 9	**57** 7	**85** 40	**96** 57	**36** 33	**57** 14	**-** -	**-** -	**-** -	**-** -	**-** -
BJC Medical Center, Commerce, GA	**75** 8	**89** 27	**67** 15	**79** 28	**80** 15	**0** 2	**-** 0	**100** 4	**61** 18	**24** 59	**63** 75	**82** 11	**59** 32	**93** 15	**33** 9	**39** 57	**100** 71	**34** 41	**71** 7	**44** 32	**100** 5	**90** 31	**-** -	**-** -
Bleckley Memorial Hospital, Cochran, GA	**-** -	**-** -	**-** -	**-** -	**-** -	**-** -	**-** -	**-** -	**100** 5	**82** 34	**32** 37	**88** 8	**80** 20	**100** 4	**75** 4	**81** 16	**100** 23	**64** 11	**100** 6	**-** -	**-** -	**-** -	**-** -	**-** -
Brooks County Hospital, Quitman, GA	**-** -	**-** -	**-** -	**-** -	**-** -	**-** -	**-** -	**-** -	**100** 3	**100** 13	**84** 19	**100** 5	**100** 14	**100** 9	**80** 5	**71** 21	**100** 26	**85** 13	**100** 7	**-** -	**-** -	**-** -	**-** -	**-** -
Burke Medical Center, Waynesboro, GA	**0** 1	**73** 11	**71** 7	**73** 11	**100** 9	**-** 0	**-** 0	**-** 0	**89** 9	**46** 80	**29** 86	**45** 11	**74** 65	**87** 23	**25** 12	**90** 93	**95** 110	**22** 65	**59** 22	**100** 3	**100** 3	**100** 3	**0.00** 318	**0.45** 221
Candler County Hospital, Metter, GA	**-** 0	**100** 1	**100** 1	**100** 1	**100** 1	**-** 0	**-** 0	**-** 0	**100** 4	**41** 46	**15** 68	**77** 13	**71** 34	**100** 19	**75** 8	**75** 56	**100** 63	**48** 25	**92** 12	**-** -	**-** -	**-** -	**-** -	**-** -
Candler Hospital, Savannah, GA	**100** 7	**97** 30	**100** 18	**100** 19	**100** 21	**-** 0	**-** 0	**100** 4	**100** 126	**72** 366	**98** 425	**100** 59	**89** 217	**93** 224	**73** 71	**77** 328	**100** 423	**81** 244	**99** 101	**65** 74	**73** 22	**66** 74	**0.27** 2972	**3.54** 1693
Charlton Memorial Hospital, Folkston, GA	**-** -	**-** -	**-** -	**-** -	**-** -	**-** -	**-** -	**-** -	**-** -	**-** -	**-** -	**-** -	**-** 0	**-** 0	**-** 0	**-** 0	**100** 1	**-** 0	**0** 1	**-** -	**-** -	**-** -	**-** -	**-** -
Chatuge Regional Hospital & Nursing Home, Hiawassee, GA	**-** 0	**100** 2	**100** 2	**100** 2	**100** 2	**-** 0	**-** 0	**0** 1	**71** 7	**60** 20	**97** 33	**60** 5	**100** 34	**97** 36	**100** 11	**87** 47	**100** 55	**100** 40	**88** 16	**-** -	**-** -	**-** -	**-** -	**-** -
Chestatee Regional Hospital, Dahlonega, GA	**50** 2	**100** 6	**50** 2	**100** 7	**100** 3	**0** 1	**-** 0	**-** 0	**100** 11	**28** 29	**74** 43	**73** 11	**87** 70	**91** 22	**67** 15	**72** 69	**99** 102	**52** 62	**93** 29	**82** 28	**96** 28	**69** 26	**0.74** 135	**5.56** 90
Clinch Memorial Hospital, Homerville, GA	**-** -	**-** -	**-** -	**-** -	**-** -	**-** -	**-** -	**-** -	**50** 2	**0** 16	**69** 16	**67** 3	**95** 20	**100** 3	**43** 7	**81** 16	**96** 28	**38** 13	**0** 2	**-** -	**-** -	**-** -	**-** -	**-** -
Cobb Memorial Hospital, Royston, GA	**67** 3	**75** 12	**67** 6	**88** 8	**100** 5	**33** 3	**-** 0	**-** 0	**92** 13	**59** 41	**96** 55	**94** 16	**87** 52	**94** 54	**54** 13	**90** 88	**99** 106	**67** 67	**80** 25	**78** 32	**100** 13	**66** 32	**-** -	**-** -
Coffee Regional Medical Center, Douglas, GA	**-** 0	**81** 21	**60** 5	**95** 22	**100** 4	**100** 2	**-** 0	**-** 0	**88** 78	**64** 232	**69** 254	**89** 53	**80** 128	**94** 32	**73** 26	**86** 168	**99** 169	**58** 71	**88** 33	**33** 9	**89** 9	**56** 9	**-** -	**-** -
Coliseum Medical Center, Macon, GA	**55** 49	**90** 73	**93** 123	**87** 71	**86** 133	**50** 2	**33** 3	**98** 44	**69** 94	**49** 229	**82** 253	**100** 58	**85** 131	**87** 109	**73** 44	**72** 195	**98** 214	**80** 123	**100** 60	**76** 230	**93** 101	**68** 215	**-** -	**-** -
Colquitt Regional Medical Center, Moultrie, GA	**100** 2	**100** 39	**100** 17	**100** 36	**94** 17	**25** 4	**-** 0	**100** 3	**79** 52	**73** 125	**92** 153	**100** 35	**79** 67	**92** 38	**82** 11	**89** 9	**97** 109	**83** 54	**97** 34	**38** 45	**100** 4	**83** 42	**-** -	**-** -
Columbus Medical Center, Columbus, GA	**88** 8	**85** 75	**97** 39	**84** 63	**95** 40	**33** 6	**-** 0	**89** 19	**87** 106	**72** 314	**94** 353	**96** 130	**79** 151	**73** 110	**28** 25	**69** 197	**100** 240	**56** 79	**91** 89	**85** 260	**98** 58	**60** 247	**-** -	**-** -
Crisp Regional Hospital, Cordele, GA	**67** 3	**76** 34	**55** 20	**66** 35	**86** 21	**100** 1	**-** 0	**67** 3	**82** 55	**50** 162	**86** 184	**89** 35	**81** 102	**95** 108	**61** 31	**54** 155	**94** 216	**83** 131	**82** 38	**60** 5	**80** 5	**60** 5	**-** -	**-** -
DeKalb Medical Center, Decatur, GA	**87** 39	**98** 171	**94** 117	**96** 156	**97** 109	**36** 11	**-** 0	**100** 36	**86** 302	**70** 500	**94** 580	**96** 118	**84** 227	**87** 273	**78** 85	**61** 410	**100** 504	**62** 237	**96** 113	**87** 304	**88** 67	**59** 290	**-** -	**-** -
Dekalb Medical Center at Hillandale, Lithonia, GA	**86** 7	**94** 36	**69** 16	**91** 34	**65** 17	**17** 6	**-** 0	**100** 2	**86** 70	**48** 136	**93** 139	**100** 39	**80** 71	**75** 64	**11** 9	**63** 82	**100** 95	**30** 40	**100** 25	**64** 97	**81** 26	**57** 93	**-** -	**-** -
Doctors Hospital, Columbus, GA	**80** 5	**90** 31	**93** 15	**100** 24	**89** 18	**-** 0	**-** 0	**100** 2	**84** 91	**46** 203	**92** 223	**100** 45	**81** 143	**77** 117	**63** 35	**76** 177	**100** 211	**72** 103	**100** 48	**78** 176	**92** 127	**72** 177	**-** -	**-** -
Doctors Hospital, Augusta, GA	**83** 6	**92** 39	**95** 21	**88** 25	**94** 18	**-** 0	**-** 0	**100** 8	**64** 73	**30** 210	**81** 232	**95** 42	**95** 129	**94** 94	**62** 45	**64** 190	**100** 234	**59** 131	**96** 52	**87** 207	**91** 95	**76** 199	**-** -	**-** -
Dodge County Hospital, Eastman, GA	**0** 1	**87** 15	**57** 7	**67** 15	**44** 9	**50** 4	**-** 0	**0** 3	**56** 9	**89** 54	**21** 72	**54** 24	**67** 67	**83** 35	**-** -	**84** 95	**97** 111	**20** 60	**19** 21	**67** 3	**100** 3	**100** 3	**-** -	**-** -
Donalsonville Hospital, Donalsonville, GA	**-** 0	**50** 4	**67** 3	**25** 4	**33** 3	**-** 0	**-** 0	**0** 1	**50** 2	**12** 26	**45** 33	**80** 5	**67** 101	**100** 3	**48** 21	**83** 99	**91** 114	**37** 49	**73** 30	**45** 40	**80** 10	**57** 35	**0.34** 290	**3.19** 188
Dorminy Medical Center, Fitzgerald, GA	**-** 0	**75** 16	**80** 5	**60** 15	**83** 6	**0** 2	**-** 0	**100** 2	**68** 19	**61** 33	**66** 77	**100** 5	**79** 19	**92** 13	**-** -	**78** 64	**99** 68	**51** 37	**100** 11	**0** 2	**100** 1	**100** 1	**0.00** 200	**1.00** 100
Early Memorial Hospital, Blakely, GA	**-** -	**-** -	**-** -	**-** -	**-** -	**-** -	**-** -	**-** -	**50** 2	**91** 11	**80** 15	**100** 1	**92** 12	**83** 6	**67** 3	**62** 13	**100** 18	**27** 11	**100** 3	**-** -	**-** -	**-** -	**-** -	**-** -
East Georgia Regional Medical Center, Statesboro, GA	**78** 9	**86** 37	**85** 26	**80** 41	**81** 27	**0** 3	**-** 0	**86** 7	**72** 61	**17** 180	**69** 204	**95** 41	**70** 155	**92** 74	**-** -	**70** 159	**98** 196	**13** 84	**91** 55	**78** 274	**86** 43	**44** 259	**-** -	**-** -
Effingham Hospital, Springfield, GA	**-** -	**-** -	**-** -	**-** -	**-** -	**-** -	**-** -	**-** -	**-** 0	**0** 8	**38** 8	**100** 1	**-** -	**-** -	**-** -	**-** -	**-** -	**-** -	**-** -	**-** -	**-** -	**-** -	**-** -	**-** -
Elbert Memorial Hospital, Elberton, GA	**-** 0	**89** 19	**93** 15	**86** 14	**91** 11	**-** 0	**-** 0	**100** 2	**91** 23	**83** 72	**86** 98	**89** 19	**71** 73	**97** 39	**-** -	**70** 81	**99** 111	**65** 63	**96** 24	**64** 11	**100** 5	**82** 11	**-** -	**-** -
Emanuel Medical Center, Swainsboro, GA	**100** 1	**100** 3	**100** 1	**60** 5	**50** 2	**-** 0	**-** 0	**-** 0	**62** 40	**64** 151	**88** 164	**73** 33	**83** 71	**69** 39	**-** -	**89** 95	**100** 119	**65** 60	**85** 40	**88** 60	**100** 18	**57** 58	**0.00** 204	**1.41** 142

NOTE: The first number in each column (boldface) is the rate in percent, the second number is the number of patients; Please refer to the main entry for footnotes; ***Heart Attack Care:*** *1. ACE Inhibitor or ARB for LVSD; 2. Aspirin at Arrival; 3. Aspirin at Discharge; 4. Beta Blocker at Arrival; 5. Beta Blocker at Discharge; 6. Fibrinolytic Medication Timing; 7. PCI Within 90 Minutes of Arrival; 8. Smoking Cessation Advice;* ***Heart Failure Care:*** *9. ACE Inhibitor or ARB for LVSD; 10. Discharge Instructions; 11. Evaluation of LVS Function; 12. Smoking Cessation Advice;* ***Pneumonia Care:*** *13. Appropriate Initial Antibiotic; 14. Blood Culture Timing; 15. Influenza Vaccine; 16. Initial Antibiotic Timing; 17. Oxygenation Assessment; 18. Pneumococcal Vaccine; 19. Smoking Cessation Advice;* ***Surgical Infection Prevention:*** *20. Prophylactic Antibiotic Given; 21. Prophylactic Antibiotic Selection; 22. Prophylactic Antibiotic Stopped;* ***Pregnancy Care:*** *23. Inpatient Neonatal Mortality; 24. Third or Fourth Degree Laceration*

Hospital	Heart Attack Care								Heart Failure Care				Pneumonia Care							Surgical Infection Prevention			Pregnancy Care	
	1	2	3	4	5	6	7	8	9	10	11	12	13	14	15	16	17	18	19	20	21	22	23	24
Emory Cartersville Medical Center, Cartersville, GA	78 9	94 52	100 21	89 38	96 25	- 0	- 0	88 8	82 56	21 167	93 187	88 43	92 199	90 184	63 38	87 264	100 304	44 162	91 111	64 143	97 68	63 134	- -	- -
Emory Crawford Long Hospital, Atlanta, GA	72 98	97 100	95 296	95 92	94 315	- 0	44 9	98 132	78 259	46 325	92 342	96 73	86 104	73 113	38 32	63 208	100 224	39 107	98 54	84 551	79 89	80 539	- -	- -
Emory Dunwoody Medical Center, Atlanta, GA	75 4	100 14	90 10	100 10	100 9	100 1	- 0	100 2	84 38	58 88	91 80	90 21	84 44	97 37	58 12	76 49	100 58	64 28	75 16	62 52	90 21	47 47	- -	- -
Emory Eastside Medical Center, Snellville, GA	91 11	93 86	87 31	95 80	100 33	52 21	- 0	80 5	81 83	86 269	99 303	100 41	92 246	90 241	86 77	84 301	100 394	96 243	94 69	93 211	95 119	81 201	- -	- -
Emory Northlake Regional Medical Center, Tucker, GA	60 5	100 24	83 12	95 19	92 12	0 1	- 0	50 2	74 46	85 112	87 129	72 32	73 78	78 73	40 20	67 104	98 118	37 54	64 33	26 76	93 28	86 72	- -	- -
Emory University Hospital, Atlanta, GA	86 72	94 112	99 244	95 93	95 284	0 1	25 4	98 115	92 218	71 307	100 337	100 53	89 55	89 83	74 23	59 125	100 149	78 73	100 24	89 575	87 84	85 556	- -	- -
Emory-Adventist Hospital, Smyrna, GA	100 1	86 7	100 3	100 6	100 4	- 0	- 0	- 0	88 24	38 90	98 99	41 32	74 66	96 67	69 32	78 74	97 101	60 53	40 30	34 44	55 11	69 42	- -	- -
Evans Memorial Hospital, Claxton, GA	50 2	100 2	67 3	75 4	100 1	- 0	- 0	100 2	93 14	100 66	78 59	100 8	75 64	95 21	70 20	71 96	100 118	76 74	100 21	50 2	100 2	100 2	- -	- -
Fairview Park Hospital, Dublin, GA	82 17	94 79	87 55	96 76	95 59	60 15	75 4	100 21	74 97	46 224	82 251	100 54	68 125	97 67	8 48	57 199	97 225	40 123	97 35	78 92	85 40	78 91	- -	- -
Fannin Regional Hospital, Blue Ridge, GA	- 0	100 9	67 3	100 9	67 3	- 0	- 0	- 0	91 23	69 58	86 74	100 12	86 77	98 80	88 26	90 124	100 151	91 97	100 37	85 158	82 33	64 153	- -	- -
Flint River Community Hospital, Montezuma, GA	- 0	50 2	0 1	0 1	0 1	- 0	- 0	0 1	80 15	36 44	70 56	54 13	74 34	88 17	29 14	74 53	99 69	14 28	73 11	75 16	100 1	7 15	- -	- -
Floyd Medical Center, Rome, GA	86 7	98 61	78 18	89 28	92 24	- 0	- 0	91 11	68 122	12 211	92 246	95 62	82 195	91 235	75 72	77 332	100 420	74 219	94 118	73 498	94 127	83 494	0.30 2014	7.12 1461
Gordon Hospital, Calhoun, GA	64 11	91 64	90 29	90 63	87 31	33 3	- 0	78 9	67 39	51 106	90 129	85 26	80 167	93 99	71 52	85 171	100 219	64 140	82 67	86 133	100 28	86 131	- -	- -
Grady General Hospital, Cairo, GA	50 2	86 14	71 7	79 14	100 9	- 0	- 0	0 1	67 6	47 15	85 20	100 3	86 42	67 15	71 7	85 40	96 55	62 32	67 9	33 15	100 3	83 12	- -	- -
Grady Memorial Hospital, Atlanta, GA	91 103	93 260	99 231	92 173	98 207	33 3	- 0	44 124	89 206	1 338	93 348	25 161	83 115	65 106	24 21	32 214	99 231	33 48	19 97	69 184	88 50	73 183	0.36 833	2.37 2485
Habersham County Medical Center, Demorest, GA	- 0	83 6	100 2	100 6	100 2	- 0	- 0	- 0	79 19	59 44	92 53	80 5	86 79	74 69	93 14	92 78	100 111	81 72	86 29	94 36	97 36	74 35	- -	- -
Hamilton Medical Center, Dalton, GA	67 15	94 97	86 43	95 73	93 54	38 26	50 8	100 17	78 125	42 327	97 390	96 75	84 208	91 163	84 67	67 301	98 389	78 217	94 121	91 239	98 40	84 228	- -	- -
Hamilton Medical Center, Chatsworth, GA	- 0	100 5	- 0	75 4	50 2	0 1	- 0	- 0	93 14	87 63	59 69	100 18	76 78	85 61	9 32	86 98	100 114	34 58	95 44	100 1	0 1	100 1	- -	- -
Hart County Hospital, Hartwell, GA	67 3	77 22	65 17	61 18	80 15	0 1	- 0	100 3	67 12	61 66	69 94	67 15	80 45	83 29	- -	85 65	97 77	54 56	50 16	50 6	83 6	0 6	- -	- -
Henry Medical Center, Stockbridge, GA	70 20	98 164	86 71	97 146	92 73	62 45	- 0	96 25	88 130	83 266	88 303	98 42	87 139	74 96	37 30	65 164	98 200	51 94	95 44	81 149	88 50	38 149	0.48 414	6.32 570
Higgins General Hospital, Bremen, GA	- -	- -	- -	- -	- -	- -	- -	- -	94 16	75 28	94 36	67 9	93 56	61 33	95 21	84 77	100 95	92 48	85 26	- -	- -	- -	- -	- -
Houston Medical Center, Warner Robins, GA	100 2	94 36	83 12	84 32	78 9	25 8	- 0	50 2	84 86	53 195	79 211	90 72	87 92	94 62	48 29	61 133	100 175	83 89	78 51	74 174	83 48	48 173	- -	- -
Hughston Orthopedic Hospital, Columbus, GA	- -	- -	- -	- -	- -	- -	- -	- -	- 0	- 0	0 1	- 0	- 0	- 0	- -	- 0	- 0	- 0	- 0	74 1491	100 419	65 1475	- -	- -
Hutcheson Medical Center, Fort Oglethrope, GA	47 19	88 78	60 65	69 68	54 59	12 17	- 0	48 25	66 50	60 222	71 250	57 58	60 210	89 211	18 93	74 352	99 474	13 229	40 183	62 112	93 54	100 110	- -	- -
Irwin County Hospital, Ocilla, GA	- -	- -	- -	- -	- -	- -	- -	- -	100 5	54 13	63 19	100 1	82 22	80 5	0 1	55 22	96 27	38 13	40 10	90 10	100 11	100 10	0.21 478	5.45 275
Jasper Mem Hosp & Retreat Nursing Home, Monticello, GA	- -	- -	- -	- -	- -	- -	- -	- -	- -	- -	- -	- -	- -	- -	- -	- -	- -	- -	- -	- -	- -	- -	- -	- -
Jefferson Hospital, Louisville, GA	- 0	- 0	- 0	- 0	- 0	0 1	- 0	- 0	100 16	75 64	62 78	43 7	79 47	82 33	33 12	78 77	94 86	44 48	59 17	- -	- -	- -	- -	- -
John D Archbold Memorial Hospital, Thomasville, GA	96 28	100 122	100 106	99 106	98 100	14 14	50 4	100 40	97 118	80 282	98 320	100 86	91 132	90 101	88 34	85 177	100 225	90 122	100 60	85 470	93 56	74 423	- -	- -
Legacy Medical Center of Atlanta, Atlanta, GA	- -	- -	- -	- -	- -	- -	- -	- -	- 0	- 0	- 0	- 0	- -	- -	- -	- -	- -	- -	- -	- -	- -	- -	- -	- -
Liberty Regional Medical Center, Hinesville, GA	- 0	- 0	- 0	- 0	- 0	- 0	- 0	- 0	67 6	61 36	55 44	91 11	92 52	87 30	42 12	45 80	100 91	34 38	82 17	68 57	100 19	98 50	- -	- -
Macon Northside Hospital, Macon, GA	100 2	89 9	100 4	100 4	83 6	0 1	- 0	100 1	74 47	72 109	82 128	100 34	86 51	93 58	62 26	73 86	100 107	76 68	100 32	50 74	92 26	80 81	- -	- -
McDuffie Regional Medical Center, Thomson, GA	100 1	80 5	100 3	40 5	50 4	- 0	- 0	- 0	83 12	55 33	81 31	100 2	58 77	95 66	70 20	85 138	99 144	71 90	71 21	0 12	93 14	10 10	- -	- -
Meadows Regional Medical Center, Vidalia, GA	82 11	90 40	86 37	81 37	84 37	30 10	- 0	100 18	93 45	68 136	80 177	94 47	80 79	84 49	32 31	82 118	100 156	27 75	92 38	34 85	96 26	79 86	0.58 520	2.84 388
Medical Center of Central Georgia, Macon, GA	58 84	97 121	90 236	93 88	94 265	0 1	57 7	98 92	78 157	50 241	93 284	90 50	86 80	90 106	44 25	64 150	100 174	55 86	92 51	71 266	79 117	47 255	- -	- -
Medical College of Georgia Hospital & Clinics, Augusta, GA	92 59	97 116	97 159	97 77	100 130	- 0	0 2	98 102	86 222	45 303	99 325	81 127	86 69	85 106	29 31	61 168	100 190	45 87	67 49	75 257	80 54	60 240	0.91 110	6.03 315
Memorial Hospital & Manor, Bainbridge, GA	60 5	93 15	70 10	77 13	80 10	50 2	- 0	- 0	84 31	59 76	71 78	79 14	74 57	61 28	46 13	74 70	99 79	34 35	65 17	58 33	97 29	100 29	- -	- -
Memorial Hospital of Adel, Adel, GA	100 1	88 8	100 5	89 9	100 6	- 0	- 0	- 0	83 12	93 14	71 59	100 5	50 6	100 1	- -	65 48	100 59	58 31	100 4	50 8	- -	75 8	- -	- -
Memorial Medical Center, Savannah, GA	92 91	98 233	99 386	98 199	99 409	- 0	50 18	99 169	92 252	85 556	94 606	86 161	85 226	98 207	69 48	79 281	100 344	83 136	90 91	89 215	97 75	75 204	1.59 3203	1.67 1732
Mitchell County Hospital, Camilla, GA	- -	- -	- -	- -	- -	- -	- -	- -	100 2	50 8	70 10	50 4	91 22	69 13	100 5	67 18	100 29	47 17	60 5	- -	- -	- -	- -	- -
Monroe County Hospital, Forsyth, GA	- -	- -	- -	- -	- -	- -	- -	- -	- -	- -	- -	- -	84 37	80 15	6 16	68 40	98 46	3 38	0 6	- -	- -	- -	- -	- -
Newton Medical, Covington, GA	86 7	96 84	83 48	96 78	92 49	57 7	- 0	100 14	91 105	74 236	97 268	76 51	90 153	88 112	60 53	80 231	100 248	68 143	83 60	52 48	77 47	73 48	0.00 712	3.23 527
North Fulton Regional Hospital, Roswell, GA	75 8	98 64	96 25	98 58	92 25	0 2	- 0	50 2	88 59	70 184	99 206	96 27	82 243	97 240	90 58	91 302	100 370	92 214	89 61	89 233	90 70	84 221	- -	- -
North Georgia Medical Center, Ellijay, GA	0 1	60 5	100 4	20 5	0 3	- 0	- 0	- 0	50 12	71 42	67 67	43 7	70 46	83 18	33 9	67 55	99 69	54 39	35 17	40 10	100 9	78 9	- -	- -
Northeast Georgia Medical Center, Gainesville, GA	89 123	99 387	99 560	94 327	99 558	0 1	76 17	100 227	75 217	52 474	87 570	98 84	86 280	88 185	65 92	90 343	100 412	75 244	96 96	54 79	- -	94 68	0.23 3520	2.33 2531
Northside Hospital, Atlanta, GA	75 8	96 49	89 18	98 43	100 26	100 1	- 0	100 3	88 86	66 185	99 211	93 30	95 181	99 164	92 61	92 228	100 312	94 154	100 52	96 114	95 114	62 110	0.37 18311	4.59 11482
Northside Hospital, Cumming, GA	67 3	94 81	96 25	83 66	83 24	100 6	- 0	100 7	61 66	68 207	91 230	100 44	90 239	97 256	93 58	90 306	100 397	94 246	97 91	86 63	93 61	59 59	- -	- -
Northside Hospital-Cherokee, Canton, GA	75 4	100 27	100 8	100 24	100 8	0 1	- 0	100 2	80 44	64 96	94 125	87 23	94 170	97 184	80 41	84 246	100 303	85 169	93 82	92 38	79 38	61 38	0.00 1101	1.47 816
Oconee Regional Medical Center, Milledgeville, GA	71 7	97 34	70 10	86 29	64 11	0 1	- 0	100 2	85 107	67 184	92 198	83 42	84 126	86 146	34 32	71 211	100 236	40 106	77 56	82 40	88 40	80 40	0.00 533	1.86 431

NOTE: The first number in each column (boldface) is the rate in percent, the second number is the number of patients; Please refer to the main entry for footnotes; ***Heart Attack Care:*** *1. ACE Inhibitor or ARB for LVSD; 2. Aspirin at Arrival; 3. Aspirin at Discharge; 4. Beta Blocker at Arrival; 5. Beta Blocker at Discharge; 6. Fibrinolytic Medication Timing; 7. PCI Within 90 Minutes of Arrival; 8. Smoking Cessation Advice;* ***Heart Failure Care:*** *9. ACE Inhibitor or ARB for LVSD; 10. Discharge Instructions; 11. Evaluation of LVS Function; 12. Smoking Cessation Advice;* ***Pneumonia Care:*** *13. Appropriate Initial Antibiotic; 14. Blood Culture Timing; 15. Influenza Vaccine; 16. Initial Antibiotic Timing; 17. Oxygenation Assessment; 18. Pneumococcal Vaccine; 19. Smoking Cessation Advice;* ***Surgical Infection Prevention:*** *20. Prophylactic Antibiotic Given; 21. Prophylactic Antibiotic Selection; 22. Prophylactic Antibiotic Stopped;* ***Pregnancy Care:*** *23. Inpatient Neonatal Mortality; 24. Third or Fourth Degree Laceration*

Hospital	Heart Attack Care								Heart Failure Care				Pneumonia Care							Surgical Infection Prevention			Pregnancy Care	
	1	2	3	4	5	6	7	8	9	10	11	12	13	14	15	16	17	18	19	20	21	22	23	24
Palmyra Medical Centers, Albany, GA	- 0	100 12	100 1	64 11	100 2	- 0	- 0	- 0	74 58	82 106	93 123	100 24	81 69	97 36	67 18	57 102	100 130	47 60	100 32	55 388	79 95	49 376	- -	- -
Peach Regional Medical Center, Fort Valley, GA	- -	- -	- -	- -	- -	- -	- -	- -	89 27	52 67	84 76	69 13	79 39	92 36	75 4	82 39	100 44	79 14	73 15	- -	- -	- -	- -	- -
Perry Hospital, Perry, GA	- 0	89 18	100 6	71 14	60 5	- 0	- 0	- 0	91 11	71 38	79 53	100 5	91 75	98 46	70 23	85 97	98 129	87 75	84 19	63 30	100 12	59 27	- -	- -
Phoebe Putney Memorial Hospital, Albany, GA	73 128	94 176	98 455	88 162	93 423	60 5	32 22	97 207	82 182	40 381	90 414	76 99	84 135	86 97	46 35	60 220	100 240	43 127	60 65	36 72	55 74	61 72	1.30 3150	2.85 1998
Piedmont Fayette Hospital, Fayetteville, GA	67 12	94 82	91 35	91 69	92 37	- 0	- 0	100 2	74 88	87 53	88 243	80 10	87 31	90 41	- -	77 234	100 266	84 140	100 6	91 87	- -	76 87	- -	- -
Piedmont Hospital, Atlanta, GA	94 103	91 95	98 365	88 81	97 350	- 0	43 7	96 139	77 234	78 376	98 403	97 75	89 201	84 209	72 64	68 311	100 363	62 181	92 73	94 436	90 102	88 425	- -	- -
Piedmont Mountainside Hospital, Jasper, GA	100 2	100 10	86 7	100 12	100 8	- 0	- 0	100 1	86 14	44 87	87 102	79 28	77 149	92 75	48 44	66 145	99 187	51 118	92 40	79 126	80 30	62 120	- -	- -
Polk Medical Center, Cedartown, GA	- -	- -	- -	- -	- -	- -	- -	- -	- 0	22 18	14 29	100 4	53 36	91 32	44 16	90 58	99 68	59 39	80 10	- -	- -	- -	- -	- -
Promina Gwinnett Health System, Lawrenceville, GA	76 25	92 225	94 81	94 199	97 91	64 47	- 0	92 13	93 159	75 370	99 435	99 76	96 283	86 289	89 62	78 377	100 450	91 241	100 107	90 68	71 68	88 67	- -	- -
Putnam General Hospital, Eatonton, GA	- -	- -	- -	- -	- -	- -	- -	- -	- -	- -	- -	- -	88 43	88 33	56 16	86 57	99 83	50 56	80 10	- -	- -	- -	- -	- -
Redmond Regional Medical Center, Rome, GA	86 140	99 336	99 568	95 242	97 584	- 0	83 18	100 284	86 314	51 574	97 636	99 139	86 276	87 270	69 81	72 332	100 424	81 285	92 108	94 330	98 138	69 319	- -	- -
Rockdale Hospital, Conyers, GA	100 10	100 125	100 58	100 123	100 57	- 0	- 0	100 9	100 84	97 306	95 346	100 42	88 172	92 158	80 59	87 246	100 292	61 154	100 56	96 300	92 65	96 295	- -	- -
Saint Francis Hospital, Columbus, GA	92 123	96 285	98 361	97 253	97 342	40 5	56 18	99 132	82 217	55 482	88 560	89 123	89 255	94 247	- -	80 342	100 409	63 245	90 86	87 331	97 65	46 324	- -	- -
Saint Joseph Candler Hospital, Savannah, GA	100 55	97 124	99 380	96 91	99 401	50 2	45 11	99 178	100 92	71 307	97 338	100 56	80 107	95 105	69 42	76 160	100 215	77 142	98 56	87 113	96 51	60 104	- -	- -
Saint Joseph's Hospital, Atlanta, GA	77 324	98 317	98 1323	97 260	98 1275	0 1	79 19	100 466	63 420	66 634	99 700	97 87	85 256	94 211	65 57	74 318	100 397	59 278	92 59	77 262	84 89	64 261	- -	- -
Saint Mary's Hospital, Athens, GA	89 18	93 54	83 35	92 40	89 47	8 13	- 0	89 19	93 105	50 220	97 242	80 66	82 85	96 72	58 24	74 107	100 129	60 70	85 34	64 72	87 70	96 68	- -	- -
Satilla Regional Medical Center, Waycross, GA	71 7	91 74	58 31	92 64	86 28	50 2	- 0	89 9	73 111	67 252	86 308	98 41	84 166	97 141	79 61	80 219	100 270	80 154	89 56	59 63	- -	32 59	0.25 799	2.61 574
Smith Northview Hospital, Valdosta, GA	60 5	100 19	100 17	96 23	89 19	0 2	- 0	50 2	91 34	32 79	78 88	20 10	78 54	88 17	17 12	65 51	96 67	20 30	75 16	32 59	86 22	63 57	- -	- -
South Fulton Medical Center, East Point, GA	83 18	92 118	85 52	99 84	98 52	33 12	- 0	89 19	92 128	58 310	92 350	97 98	84 182	80 167	31 52	64 263	100 309	48 131	81 77	76 221	95 56	68 213	- -	- -
South Georgia Medical Center, Valdosta, GA	78 23	100 156	98 208	97 117	96 211	55 11	25 4	95 85	80 126	47 318	85 359	96 75	87 141	94 53	66 29	64 199	99 240	55 130	88 50	75 64	86 66	73 62	- -	- -
Southeast Georgia Health Sys, Brunswick, GA	73 11	93 89	92 36	86 77	91 43	28 18	0 1	77 13	71 115	77 299	97 346	85 73	79 169	96 109	55 42	65 182	98 230	45 132	57 51	64 463	98 116	55 446	- -	- -
Southeast Georgia Health Sys-Camden Campus, St Marys, GA	100 1	75 4	50 2	100 4	100 3	- 0	- 0	- 0	64 22	66 59	77 69	90 10	68 59	87 31	47 17	84 55	97 67	38 34	93 15	91 79	94 16	84 74	- -	- -
Southern Regional Medical Center, Riverdale, GA	85 26	95 178	81 91	90 144	88 94	58 36	14 7	100 30	83 289	72 623	83 694	100 166	85 254	82 219	55 60	68 314	99 357	72 160	89 100	82 530	86 76	73 506	- -	- -
Spalding Regional Medical Center, Griffin, GA	87 15	98 112	95 44	96 107	88 43	57 14	- 0	100 19	85 146	93 354	95 408	97 111	91 224	94 188	- -	84 323	100 367	84 201	95 95	94 468	94 126	80 444	- -	- -
Stephens County Hospital, Toccoa, GA	- 0	84 19	62 8	56 18	56 9	- 0	- 0	33 3	48 31	41 138	49 162	36 28	60 124	97 93	71 34	74 166	99 190	61 106	35 43	48 31	87 31	42 31	- -	- -
Sumter Regional Hospital, Americus, GA	50 2	88 17	80 10	75 16	78 9	0 1	- 0	100 3	81 27	65 92	82 107	93 15	66 64	84 69	80 15	71 104	99 127	71 72	92 25	74 140	89 35	59 130	- -	- -
Sylvan Grove Hospital, Jackson, GA	- -	- -	- -	- -	- -	- -	- -	- -	- 0	83 6	50 10	100 3	100 18	100 12	50 2	100 17	100 25	91 11	100 5	- -	- -	- -	- -	- -
Tailor Telfair Regional Hospital, McRae, GA	- -	- -	- -	- -	- -	- -	- -	- -	100 1	38 26	26 39	67 9	31 29	100 6	100 5	78 18	97 34	55 20	75 4	- -	- -	- -	- -	- -
Tanner Medical Center, Villa Rica, GA	100 4	97 29	90 10	86 28	89 9	67 3	- 0	100 5	94 47	78 100	96 106	100 16	89 104	86 57	95 20	87 106	100 121	94 54	86 42	86 21	100 9	90 20	- -	- -
Tanner Medical Center, Carrollton, GA	58 19	96 135	89 62	94 111	94 63	73 15	- 0	92 26	60 111	43 224	89 272	89 57	87 211	78 113	58 55	72 218	100 292	65 172	79 62	70 401	96 83	93 393	- -	- -
Taylor Regional Hospital, Hawkinsville, GA	0 2	90 21	100 7	86 14	100 6	25 4	- 0	- 0	85 27	66 64	97 76	57 14	69 52	94 32	55 22	70 92	100 100	36 56	52 21	94 108	100 32	86 107	- -	- -
Tift Regional Medical Hospital, Tifton, GA	95 19	93 60	85 54	96 53	89 53	- 0	100 2	95 20	89 147	84 255	98 279	97 62	86 138	94 66	62 21	65 138	100 160	98 96	100 33	51 136	92 40	81 125	0.07 1436	2.16 925
Trinity Hospital of Augusta, Augusta, GA	- 0	100 3	100 3	100 3	33 3	- 0	- 0	- 0	72 25	83 77	88 96	79 14	82 79	88 77	56 27	79 113	100 138	65 82	60 25	86 125	98 43	77 123	- -	- -
Turning Point Hospital, Moultrie, GA	- -	- -	- -	- -	- -	- -	- -	- -	- -	- -	- -	- -	- -	- -	- -	- -	- -	- -	- -	- -	- -	- -	- -	- -
Union General Hospital, Blairsville, GA	- 0	73 11	100 5	53 17	100 6	- 0	- 0	- 0	83 23	49 61	84 75	100 8	83 84	91 65	50 24	81 104	100 125	64 81	89 28	77 64	94 18	87 61	- -	- -
University Hospital, Augusta, GA	91 113	97 360	98 506	96 252	98 447	0 4	38 13	100 186	98 288	91 613	99 683	100 108	90 300	95 400	83 120	82 524	100 660	87 399	94 128	92 1934	92 439	46 1927	- -	- -
Upson Regional Medical Center, Thomaston, GA	100 4	87 46	70 20	82 39	95 22	45 11	- 0	86 7	89 71	70 145	80 171	91 46	98 91	87 75	48 29	87 138	100 171	54 90	80 46	63 35	94 34	17 35	- -	- -
Walton Regional Medical Center, Monroe, GA	50 2	100 17	100 6	73 15	62 8	- 0	- 0	0 1	69 51	52 153	84 172	79 24	83 135	85 79	56 55	77 198	100 226	74 150	81 52	65 80	100 11	70 80	- -	- -
Washington County Regional Medical Center, Sandersville, GA	- 0	57 7	100 2	80 5	100 2	- 0	- 0	- 0	75 16	84 50	75 59	100 11	74 171	91 100	80 35	77 221	100 256	80 128	96 51	12 8	12 8	50 8	- -	- -
Wayne Memorial Hospital, Jesup, GA	100 2	95 22	78 9	86 21	78 9	- 0	- 0	100 1	93 54	98 103	86 124	100 25	90 40	97 34	86 7	95 55	100 65	82 33	100 18	97 29	94 31	100 28	- -	- -
WellStar Cobb Hospital, Austell, GA	89 18	89 113	90 58	96 94	90 58	60 5	100 1	90 21	82 192	33 458	94 510	99 126	86 244	84 218	82 71	59 336	100 417	63 218	95 111	87 110	92 113	65 110	- -	- -
WellStar Douglas Hospital, Douglasville, GA	100 4	97 65	100 19	85 54	90 21	0 5	- 0	80 5	79 99	21 224	91 255	98 61	88 174	90 142	55 33	72 214	100 255	62 117	96 80	83 29	97 29	57 28	- -	- -
WellStar Kennestone Hospital, Marietta, GA	84 159	97 494	96 607	95 382	97 605	- 0	64 25	96 207	80 332	50 698	98 770	97 174	81 354	89 367	57 97	63 503	100 624	54 333	91 145	87 181	91 184	78 178	- -	- -
WellStar Paulding Hospital, Dallas, GA	100 4	92 13	100 7	90 10	100 7	- 0	- 0	100 1	82 17	28 39	89 44	100 10	92 78	92 59	75 16	80 88	100 107	65 57	96 25	67 6	100 6	83 6	- -	- -
Wesley Woods Geriatric Hospital, Atlanta, GA	- 0	100 2	100 3	0 2	100 3	- 0	- -	- 0	100 5	60 20	100 38	100 1	55 11	- 0	73 11	53 15	100 17	64 39	67 9	- 0	- 0	- 0	- -	- -
West Georgia Medical Center, La Grange, GA	96 24	100 140	100 63	98 110	100 68	44 18	0 1	100 36	77 150	81 253	93 285	100 55	90 181	86 142	78 49	86 259	100 288	68 153	99 67	90 86	88 74	82 84	- -	- -
LOUISIANA																								
Abbeville General Hospital, Abbeville, LA	50 2	80 10	50 6	60 5	17 6	- 0	- 0	100 2	72 25	94 87	82 134	88 25	73 49	91 44	94 18	85 82	97 97	97 66	100 13	77 83	73 26	100 75	- -	- -

*NOTE: The first number in each column (boldface) is the rate in percent, the second number is the number of patients; Please refer to the main entry for footnotes; **Heart Attack Care:** 1. ACE Inhibitor or ARB for LVSD; 2. Aspirin at Arrival; 3. Aspirin at Discharge; 4. Beta Blocker at Arrival; 5. Beta Blocker at Discharge; 6. Fibrinolytic Medication Timing; 7. PCI Within 90 Minutes of Arrival; 8. Smoking Cessation Advice; **Heart Failure Care:** 9. ACE Inhibitor or ARB for LVSD; 10. Discharge Instructions; 11. Evaluation of LVS Function; 12. Smoking Cessation Advice; **Pneumonia Care:** 13. Appropriate Initial Antibiotic; 14. Blood Culture Timing; 15. Influenza Vaccine; 16. Initial Antibiotic Timing; 17. Oxygenation Assessment; 18. Pneumococcal Vaccine; 19. Smoking Cessation Advice; **Surgical Infection Prevention:** 20. Prophylactic Antibiotic Given; 21. Prophylactic Antibiotic Selection; 22. Prophylactic Antibiotic Stopped; **Pregnancy Care:** 23. Inpatient Neonatal Mortality; 24. Third or Fourth Degree Laceration*

Hospital	Heart Attack Care									Heart Failure Care					Pneumonia Care					Surgical Infection Prevention			Pregnancy Care	
	1	2	3	4	5	6	7	8	9	10	11	12	13	14	15	16	17	18	19	20	21	22	23	24
Abrom Kaplan Memorial Hospital, Kaplan, LA	-	0	0	0	0 1	0	0	-	0	27 11	53 19	100 1	83 12	86 14	67 3	74 23	100 28	53 19	40 5	11 9	100 2	62 8	-	-
Acadian Medical Center, Eunice, LA	100 1	100 1	100 1	100 2	100 2	75 4	0	-	0	96 95	80 98	100 24	75 32	85 33	93 14	87 69	100 87	93 43	19 22	80 30	77 13	83 29	-	-
Allen Parish Hospital, Kinder, LA	0	100 1	100 1	100 1	100 1	-	0	-	100 1	0 2	50 22	0	100 1	100 3	38 24	68 25	94 36	0 23	0	80 22	13	-	-
American Legion Hospital, Crowley, LA	100 5	100 5	100 4	80 5	100 4	-	0	100 1	100 1	38 76	57 102	81 27	84 107	86 57	38 24	71 163	96 192	72 104	73 45	25 144	96 45	37 139	-	-
Assumption Community Hospital, Napoleonville, LA	-	50 2	100 2	-	-	-	-	-	-	80 74	89 112	81 26	91 46	94 68	57 21	93 94	100 121	68 79	74 19	100 100	-	0 2	-	-
Avoyelles Hospital, Marksville, LA	74 113	95 328	87 361	93 287	94 359	40 5	10	97 32	88 24	89 151	84 851	85 48	85 39	85 61	-	66 512	99 637	68 320	72 29	92 327	62 320	-	-	-
Baton Rouge General Medical Center, Baton Rouge, LA	100 5	98 44	80 25	91 33	88 25	27 11	0	86 7	90 41	60 70	85 101	88 17	49 104	92 51	-	87 126	99 164	62 95	100 36	81 100	26 35	16 98	-	-
Beauregard Memorial Hospital, DeRidder, LA	-	-	-	-	-	-	-	-	-	-	-	-	0	-	-	0 100	100 1	0	-	60 10	-	67 9	-	-
Bossier Specialty Hospital, Bossier City, LA	5	88 25	82 11	92 26	86 14	38 8	-	100 1	100 5	47 145	86 166	96 54	84 134	90 83	62 42	83 196	100 235	72 116	100 69	40 87	83 29	36 66	-	-
Byrd Regional Hospital, Leesville, LA	0	0 1	0	0 100	0	-	0	-	88 8	23 13	31 61	25 4	25 8	0	-	93 43	71 48	38 24	40 5	60 10	-	-	-	-
Caldwell Memorial Hospital, Columbia, LA	100 44	98 128	100 215	97 115	99 237	0 1	60 10	97 116	98 242	87 468	99 533	98 87	75 174	91 176	95 62	68 241	99 318	93 189	67	77 1292	90 302	56 1255	0.09 1135	4.55 549
Christus Saint Frances Cabrini Hospital, Alexandria, LA	100 80	100 177	100 302	100 159	100 288	100 1	85 13	100 131	99 197	92 358	100 400	95 80	83 196	94 210	100 51	91 256	100 309	100 184	70	76 438	61 122	59 418	-	-
CHRISTUS Saint Patrick Hospital, Lake Charles, LA	79 33	96 109	96 149	95 94	96 135	0 3	33	96 57	86 194	91 396	98 484	90	89 158	98 169	-	87 277	100 342	93 223	91 76	85 279	91 70	45 267	-	-
Christus Schumpert Health System, Shreveport, LA	0 100	-	0 1	0	0	-	-	-	-	20 5	66 29	0	67 3	4	-	68 40	98 54	50 32	0	0	-	0	-	-
Citizens Medical Center, Columbia, LA	87 15	91 66	89 57	80 51	84 56	8	50	93 28	64 110	45 190	85 209	84 61	75 60	94 50	50 20	78 81	99 92	40 53	30	64 58	87 23	40 57	-	-
Community Specialty Hosp of N Louisiana, Minden, LA	100 2	50 8	0 5	67 6	50 4	0 1	-	0 1	86 22	7 44	65 68	14 14	67 48	81 16	-	55 42	98 56	54 35	22 9	58	45 13	11 61	-	-
Dauterive Hospital, New Iberia, LA	50 2	100 6	100 6	100 6	83 6	0	0	0	75 20	98 41	0 65	100	73 30	80 15	12 8	45 45	98 61	49 41	100	54 63	46 13	44 78	-	-
DeSoto Regional Health System, Mansfield, LA	100 6	100 39	97 29	97 35	97 33	-	0	94 17	90 51	81 139	86 172	94 35	63 68	79 42	-	70 90	100 106	91 53	81 31	88 82	94 36	71 17	-	-
Doctors Hospital, Shreveport, LA	-	100 1	-	0	0 1	-	-	0	50 6	20 5	66 29	0 3	100 1	100 4	-	100 1	100 2	50	0 1	76 17	-	17 17	-	-
Doctors Hospital of Opelousas, Opelousas, LA	10 10	94 84	100 44	96 67	100 46	50 10	4	85 34	98 126	65 192	97 195	82 61	91 102	92 53	29 17	73 108	95 119	83 12	63	95 250	99 80	88 240	0.85 1062	3.87 750
Doctors' Hospital of Slidell, Slidell, LA	20 20	95 77	90 67	95 65	98 64	57 7	0	75 40	95 100	60 149	91 156	80 81	73 60	79 67	18 11	54 91	99 98	11 9	46	83 167	71 45	85 137	0.09 1113	3.90 616
E A Conway Medical Center, Monroe, LA	0	0	0	0	0	-	-	0	0	0 10	0 65	25	100 3	0	-	94 33	100 35	0 14	0	12 8	-	0 8	-	-
Earl K Long Medical Center, Baton Rouge, LA	48 77	92 264	92 254	96 240	93 262	0 2	28	18 18	79 106	51 234	88 284	91 44	76 100	92	30	68 144	96 178	40 113	41 78	78 215	81 74	42 203	-	-
East Carroll Parish Hospital, Lake Providence, LA	-	-	-	-	0	-	-	-	14 7	0 25	45 33	100	85 20	75	7	65 20	96 26	65 74	5	75 12	-	50 10	-	-
East Jefferson General Hospital, Metairie, LA	0	65 17	67 9	69 16	79 14	-	0	0 1	88 8	36 14	49 61	0	100	60 5	-	86 90	95 108	65 74	0	14 7	-	71 7	-	-
Fairway Medical Center, Covington, LA	72 57	96 137	97 184	87 94	93 201	0	0	84 91	65 133	46 286	93 369	70	77 98	88 64	26	74 168	99 174	72 123	43	83 188	61 70	48 182	0.09 1113	3.90 616
Franklin Medical Center, Winnsboro, LA	-	-	-	-	-	-	-	-	0	0 3	49 61	0 3	100 1	60 1	-	88 152	99 161	77 115	80 5	12 8	-	46 35	-	-
Glenwood Regional Medical Center, West Monroe, LA	100 2	-	-	0 100	-	-	-	0	0	0 2	80 5	5	92 38	0	-	-	100 2	0 2	0	58 59	-	0 8	-	-
Greater Baton Rouge Surgical Hospital, Baton Rouge, LA	100 1	-	0	-	80 5	-	-	0	0 3	0	80 5	33 100	93 18	56	-	100 1	100 1	80 54	15	-	73 56	-	-
Green Clinic Surgical Hospital, Ruston, LA	-	83 12	75	4 100	100 4	-	0 2	98	14 7	22 25	135 100	9	93 11	18	-	67 3	100 3	48	21	58	0 1	79 58	-	-
Hardtner Medical Center, Olla, LA	31 100	44 100	200 100	100 4	100 43	-	14	7 100	98 64	22 100	45 33	100	85	20 75	-	72 57	96 67	64 39	3	88 59	-	100 1	-	-
Heart Hospital of Lafayette, Lafayette, LA	3 94	16 86	86 7	90	100 10	40 5	0	33	100 4	12 17	66 56	9	18 11	86 7	6	72 57	100 67	64 67	20	89 106	90 41	80 102	1.11 181	2.78 108
Homer Memorial Hospital, Homer, LA	3 100	100 14	90 10	92 13	89 9	100 1	0	100 7	94 48	90 58	98 62	32 100	88 25	97 30	5	67 43	100 50	67 6	40 95	93 192	84 69	65 189	-	-
Huey P Long Medical Center, Pineville, LA	92 24	94 111	94 80	77 75	96 85	-	44	89 46	86 63	85 164	90 184	90 39	80 88	79 96	31	85 142	99 184	89 113	14	93 192	84 69	65 189	-	-
Iberia Medical Center, New Iberia, LA	-	-	-	-	-	-	-	-	80 15	67 54	90 81	83	82 60	95 19	10	92 63	94 67	36 44	14	83 36	-	46 35	-	-
Jackson Parish Hospital, Jonesboro, LA	100 2	97 33	93 14	96 27	100 19	-	50	0 100	100 24	97 30	92 153	86 7	89 18	93 29	-	88 152	100 161	77 115	5	83 36	-	46 35	-	-
Jennings American Legion Hospital, Jennings, LA	97 29	75 108	56	60 5	97 115	0	50 4	84 100	90 124	92 220	99 240	100 61	75 158	90 121	-	73 243	99 262	87 156	57	89 275	83 159	82 253	1.26 1748	2.94 1054
Kenner Regional Medical Center, Kenner, LA	25 69	93 69	75 89	55 91	78	1	50	2 95	67 89	73 194	88 236	86 42	83 83	65 65	29	66 157	99 190	72 128	47	55 202	86 99	51 192	-	-
La Salle General Hospital, Jena, LA	100 1	100 2	0	100 4	100 1	-	-	100	82 22	87 38	90 41	95 19	67 24	15	0 5	44 25	100 29	40 10	13	84 67	95 21	85 61	-	-
Lady of the Sea General Hospital, Cut Off, LA	-	-	-	-	-	-	-	-	70 56	65 172	92 230	82 66	84 129	88 166	60 65	83 242	100 319	95 165	90	87 69	84 19	20 66	-	-
Lane Regional Memorial Hospital, Zachary, LA	100 1	91	33 87	15 86	21 79	50 2	-	86 7	70	65														

NOTE: The first number in each column (boldface) is the rate in percent; the second number is the number of patients; Please refer to the main entry for footnotes; **Heart Attack Care:** 1. ACE Inhibitor or ARB for LVSD; 2. Aspirin at Arrival; 3. Aspirin at Discharge; 4. Beta Blocker at Arrival; 5. Beta Blocker at Discharge; 6. Fibrinolytic Medication Timing; 7. PCI Within 90 Minutes of Arrival; 8. Smoking Cessation Advice; **Heart Failure Care:** 9. ACE Inhibitor or ARB for LVSD; 10. Discharge Instructions; 11. Evaluation of LVS Function; 12. Smoking Cessation Advice; **Pneumonia Care:** 13. Blocker at Discharge; 14. Blood Culture Timing; 15. Influenza Vaccine; 16. Initial Antibiotic Timing; 17. Oxygenation Assessment; 18. Pneumococcal Vaccine; 19. Smoking Cessation Advice; **Surgical Infection Prevention:** 20. Prophylactic Antibiotic Given; 21. Prophylactic Antibiotic Selection; 22. Prophylactic Antibiotic Stopped; **Pregnancy Care:** 23. Inpatient Neonatal Mortality; 24. Third or Fourth Degree Laceration

Hospital	Heart Attack Care 1	2	3	4	5	6	7	8	Heart Failure Care 9	10	11	12	13	14	Pneumonia Care 15	16	17	18	19	Surgical Infection Prevention 20	21	22	Pregnancy Care 23	24
Leonard J Chabert Medical Center, Houma, LA	83 12	100 56	94 36	100 46	98 44	0 1	·	92 24	91 106	55 152	97 152	95 78	93 45	96 54	53 15	56 62	100 78	64 11	66 32	77 245	87 75	83 230	0.43 470	2.72 294
Lincoln General Hospital, Ruston, LA	100 5	98 58	97 38	96 55	95 37	100 1	·	100 1	66 61	67 42	92 263	100 11	89 18	72 18	·	89 133	98 145	80 83	100 6	74 31	·	86 29	·	·
Lindy Boggs Medical Center, New Orleans, LA	100 20	100 64	100 134	98 57	99 136	·	80 5	100 71	96 107	100 251	98 267	100 43	85 26	85 20	·	88 25	100 35	89 19	92 12	88 223	96 82	57 219	·	·
Louisiana Heart Hospital, Lacombe, LA	98 43	98 117	98 174	96 101	99 174	·	0 5	86 22	94 215	73 62	99 324	89 19	71 14	88 17	·	44 126	94 152	26 31	75 12	68 53	·	51 51	·	·
Louisiana State Univ Hosp-Shreveport, Shreveport, LA	86 7	82 22	75 16	79 14	91 22	0 1	·	0 1	79 73	63 141	83 160	96 45	84 124	94 72	43 14	73 122	99 143	59 51	100 56	65 65	81 27	67 57	2.02 397	4.47 1163
LSU-Bogalusa Medical Center, Bogalusa, LA	86 7	82 22	75 16	79 14	91 22	0 1	·	0 1	79 73	63 141	83 160	96 45	84 124	94 72	·	·	·	·	·	·	·	·	·	·
Meadowcrest Hospital, Gretna, LA	·	·	·	·	·	·	·	·	·	·	·	·	·	·	·	·	·	·	·	43 7	5	57 7	·	·
Medical Center of Louisiana at New Orleans, New Orleans, LA	·	·	·	·	·	·	·	·	·	·	·	·	·	·	·	·	·	·	·	·	·	·	·	·
Methodist Hospital, New Orleans, LA	·	·	·	·	·	·	·	·	·	·	·	·	·	·	·	·	·	·	·	·	·	·	·	·
Minden Medical Center, Minden, LA	100 6	96 27	100 21	95 20	100 19	0 1	·	100 1	87 63	99 137	94 180	100 32	83 63	95 66	93 27	80 137	100 177	89 100	100 39	47 172	41 32	56 167	·	·
Monroe Surgical Hospital, Monroe, LA	·	·	·	·	·	·	·	·	·	0 100	0 1	·	·	·	25 4	0 16	100 6	33 3	0 1	90 31	41 32	68 31	·	·
Morehouse General Hospital, Bastrop, LA	67 3	75 20	62 8	65 17	75 8	75 4	·	0 1	71 28	70 61	55 96	80 15	53 55	0 20	0 16	67 115	78 129	58 72	67 21	45 112	75 4	79 110	·	·
Natchitoches Regional Medical Center, Natchitoches, LA	33 3	95 21	33 3	85 20	100 4	43 7	·	0 1	59 51	66 101	89 123	68 25	80 152	92 103	51 35	80 230	99 282	52 180	60 42	61 76	56 16	44 68	·	·
Neuromedical Center Hospital, Baton Rouge, LA	·	·	·	·	·	·	·	·	·	·	·	·	·	·	·	·	·	·	·	14 14	·	43 14	·	·
North Oaks Medical System, Hammond, LA	84 55	96 191	94 172	91 129	97 206	0 1	44 9	100 95	85 369	68 688	95 816	94 177	87 213	97 121	84 63	79 334	100 407	89 214	94 108	93 428	88 60	89 407	·	·
Northshore Regional Medical Center, Slidell, LA	95 22	98 97	95 100	98 92	100 103	25 4	100 2	100 44	96 114	89 249	100 277	99 76	80 193	99 196	100 62	90 240	99 303	99 181	98 88	90 343	90 103	67 328	0.19 522	2.97 404
Oakdale Community Hospital, Oakdale, LA	·	0 100	·	0 100	0 3	·	·	·	0 100	100 1	0 1	100 1	0 85	0 11	75 ·	89 152	100 182	76 107	90 41	80 5	100 2	0 5	·	·
Ochsner Baptist Medical Center, New Orleans, LA	·	·	·	·	·	·	·	·	·	·	·	·	·	·	·	·	0 100	0 1	·	42 12	·	57 7	·	·
Ochsner Clinic Foundation, New Orleans, LA	93 81	97 220	97 215	99 168	99 262	0 1	100 10	98 83	92 168	46 270	100 288	93 57	83 115	86 94	84 ·	66 131	100 173	88 112	72 36	52 623	97 156	59 616	·	·
Ochsner Medical Center-Baton Rouge, Baton Rouge, LA	90 77	99 134	96 120	95 110	93 119	1 ·	30 23	69 51	90 130	51 210	93 211	46 39	70 122	88 113	62 ·	70 182	99 207	13 114	71 52	62 278	81 80	99 272	·	·
Opelousas General Hospital, Opelousas, LA	64 11	97 79	96 70	85 80	95 76	0 ·	33 6	100 36	76 105	72 284	86 332	93 88	71 122	80 133	51 45	68 228	98 269	59 150	87 70	45 270	96 75	57 236	·	·
Ouachita Community Hospital, West Monroe, LA	·	·	·	·	·	·	·	·	·	·	·	·	·	·	·	·	·	·	·	14 14	43 14	43 14	·	·
Our Lady of Lourdes Regional Medical Center, Lafayette, LA	90 20	94 124	85 138	84 100	89 149	2 ·	0 5	100 51	73 141	74 327	89 394	100 68	74 152	94 121	82 45	60 194	99 253	92 144	100 58	84 156	91 53	64 154	·	·
Our Lady of the Lake Regional Medical Center, Baton Rouge, LA	93 88	99 239	97 349	95 216	97 338	4 ·	73 15	100 36	86 347	83 166	94 873	99 27	85 46	87 52	75 40	79 312	100 378	79 219	100 19	83 175	90 103	76 168	·	·
P & S Surgical Hospital, Monroe, LA	·	·	·	·	·	·	·	·	·	·	·	·	·	·	·	·	0 100	0 1	·	77 226	·	75 225	·	·
Park Place Surgical Hospital, Lafayette, LA	·	·	·	·	·	·	·	·	·	·	·	·	·	·	·	·	·	0 1	·	42 12	57 7	57 7	·	·
Physicians Surgical Specialty Hospital, Houma, LA	·	·	·	·	·	·	·	·	·	·	·	·	·	·	·	·	·	·	·	44 27	92 26	92 26	·	·
Rapides Regional Medical Center, Alexandria, LA	80 60	91 194	95 194	86 88	94 212	0 ·	12 8	97 97	76 224	57 421	90 502	94 102	80 131	96 180	96 55	77 282	100 316	91 201	88 60	44 234	67 107	42 227	·	·
Richardson Medical Center, Rayville, LA	·	100 7	67 3	71 7	100 3	·	·	100 1	50 4	0 6	35 46	0 1	25 4	100 4	·	69 58	83 69	46 35	·	33 3	·	100 2	·	·
River Parishes Hospital, La Place, LA	83 6	97 30	87 23	83 24	82 22	33 ·	0 ·	100 7	86 72	87 179	93 196	100 54	82 49	97 34	45 11	77 62	97 74	54 39	93 28	58 83	82 34	81 97	·	·
River West Medical Center, Plaquemine, LA	88 8	100 30	95 22	86 28	91 23	0 ·	0 ·	100 7	82 62	44 105	90 121	78 23	87 75	92 85	53 17	71 116	99 153	13 61	77 30	38 55	70 20	96 47	·	·
Sabine Medical Center, Many, LA	100 2	71 24	75 16	57 14	93 14	0 ·	0 ·	67 3	79 14	82 67	49 101	25 ·	50 38	91 22	91 11	89 63	78 ·	84 55	91 11	50 6	0 1	100 5	·	·
Saint Anne General Medical Center, Raceland, LA	100 3	100 5	100 5	80 5	40 5	0 1	·	0 ·	63 19	59 61	88 66	89 27	81 27	93 14	90 10	86 35	95 38	72 25	67 9	87 54	0 16	70 53	0.00 208	9.88 81
Saint Charles Parish Hospital, Luling, LA	100 5	86 21	100 14	80 20	81 16	·	55 ·	0 ·	100 51	80 15	99 114	56 9	56 9	75 8	·	78 63	100 71	31 42	100 3	100 3	·	50 2	·	·
Saint Elizabeth Hospital, Gonzales, LA	67 6	91 23	83 12	90 21	91 11	1 100	0 ·	0 ·	77 110	91 33	95 167	6 ·	90 21	96 23	·	75 128	99 155	86 95	91 11	91 11	·	0 11	·	·
Saint Francis Medical Center, Monroe, LA	66 59	95 130	94 217	84 128	84 247	100 ·	17 ·	100 6	83 169	45 422	84 519	76 ·	83 152	95 160	70 46	65 209	100 263	73 167	48 ·	69 213	80 210	76 209	·	·
Saint Tammany Parish Hospital, Covington, LA	100 38	99 102	99 115	100 100	100 131	0 ·	6 ·	100 5	100 153	78 362	100 401	74 ·	92 173	92 166	92 53	90 215	100 266	79 161	82 ·	84 615	89 200	55 603	·	·
Savoy Medical Center, Mamou, LA	100 2	89 9	80 5	88 8	75 4	1 ·	100 ·	90 ·	61 44	86 86	71 112	93 29	82 45	100 76	52 21	90 109	98 132	66 79	92 37	79 66	86 21	47 64	0.28 359	0.52 194
Slidell Memorial Hospital, Slidell, LA	73 33	98 120	95 111	94 111	94 116	1 ·	73 ·	58 ·	81 117	54 297	82 317	61 59	85 208	88 121	49 67	66 242	98 307	48 166	70 96	70 265	82 71	57 258	·	·
Southpark Community Hospital, Slidell, LA	·	·	·	·	·	·	·	·	·	·	·	·	·	·	·	·	·	·	0 ·	100 30	0 ·	43 30	·	·
Southwest Community Hospital, Lafayette, LA	·	·	·	·	·	·	·	·	·	0 9	19 16	0 1	0 1	100 2	·	0 100	100 4	0 3	·	44 27	0 ·	92 26	·	·
Southwest Medical Center, Lafayette, LA	88 17	90 73	88 85	85 70	86 88	1 ·	5 ·	98 ·	81 74	55 170	88 192	29 ·	79 102	91 45	58 31	72 110	99 123	47 68	77 43	86 144	92 66	55 134	·	·
Springhill Medical Center, Springhill, LA	0 1	89 9	80 5	50 8	60 5	0 ·	0 ·	0 ·	75 16	47 17	79 96	80 5	86 7	86 7	·	89 64	100 79	52 52	100 3	100 2	66 ·	50 2	·	·
Surgical Specialty Hospital, Baton Rouge, LA	·	·	·	·	·	·	·	·	·	·	·	·	·	·	·	·	0 100	0 ·	3 100	3 100	·	·	·	·
Teche Regional Medical Center, Morgan City, LA	100 8	100 22	100 11	100 24	87 15	0 100	0 100	100 2	85 46	90 139	70 155	59 34	73 55	92 50	63 19	91 77	99 90	44 54	52 21	77 43	67 15	74 42	·	·
Terrebonne General Medical Center, Houma, LA	85 52	94 200	94 214	95 180	95 232	20 ·	55 ·	95 110	77 158	78 339	90 385	88 ·	70 150	91 126	64 45	66 213	99 237	67 141	50 ·	86 458	84 57	62 440	0.23 2190	3.61 1245
Thibodaux Regional Medical Center, Thibodaux, LA	97 31	100 118	98 188	97 96	99 177	4 100	75 ·	100 ·	95 86	88 235	95 279	98 42	81 113	89 94	90 39	88 165	99 198	80 122	95 43	46 214	65 102	56 190	0.16 625	7.85 293
Touro Infirmary, New Orleans, LA	67 24	95 83	91 76	84 79	85 81	14 ·	7 ·	72 ·	81 261	46 347	91 462	61 80	80 98	94 124	26 38	80 147	95 187	29 91	43 35	81 410	89 157	75 403	·	·

NOTE: The first number in each column (boldface) is the rate in percent; the second number is the number of patients; Please refer to the main entry for footnotes; **Heart Attack Care**: 1. ACE Inhibitor or ARB for LVSD; 2. Aspirin at Arrival; 3. Aspirin at Discharge; 4. Beta Blocker at Arrival; 5. Beta Blocker at Discharge; 6. Fibrinolytic Medication Timing; 7. PCI Within 90 Minutes of Arrival; 8. Smoking Cessation Advice; **Heart Failure Care**: 9. ACE Inhibitor or ARB for LVSD; 10. Discharge Instructions; 11. Evaluation of LVS Function; 12. Smoking Cessation Advice; **Pneumonia Care**: 13. Appropriate Initial Antibiotic; 14. Blood Culture Timing; 15. Influenza Vaccine; 16. Initial Antibiotic Timing; 17. Oxygenation Assessment; 18. Pneumococcal Vaccine; 19. Smoking Cessation Advice; **Surgical Infection Prevention**: 20. Prophylactic Antibiotic Given; 21. Prophylactic Antibiotic Selection; 22. Prophylactic Antibiotic Stopped; **Pregnancy Care**: 23. Inpatient Neonatal Mortality; 24. Third or Fourth Degree Laceration.

Hospital	Heart Attack Care 1	2	3	4	5	6	7	8	Heart Failure Care 9	10	11	12	13	14	Pneumonia Care 15	16	17	18	19	Surgical Infection Prevention 20	21	22	Pregnancy Care 23	24
Tri-Ward Rural Health Clinic, Bernice, LA	-	0 100	2 100	-	-	0	-	-	-	-	-	-	-	-	-	-	-	-	-	-	-	-	-	-
Tulane University Hospital & Clinic, New Orleans, LA	94 17	100 50	98 55	97 34	100 52	0	10	84 31	92 106	78 175	96 176	76 62	93 27	79 24	40 5	59 27	100 34	50 6	53 17	78 261	92 51	87 260	-	-
University Medical Center, Lafayette, LA	91 11	100 45	98 50	97 33	96 52	12 8	0 1	88 33	92 91	23 151	95 152	75 69	78 69	59 46	10 10	64 81	99 90	14 7	73 49	64 200	72 64	78 185	1.29 466	3.23 310
Villa Feliciana Medical Complex, Jackson, LA	-	-	-	-	-	-	-	-	-	-	-	-	-	-	-	100	100	100	-	-	-	-	-	-
Ville Platte Medical Center, Ville Platte, LA	100 1	94 18	64 11	92 12	89 9	0 5	-	50 2	73 77	40 142	89 185	82 40	80 97	85 82	85 41	83 163	99 175	70 101	89 56	27 11	60 5	82 11	-	-
Vista Surgical Hospital of Baton Rouge, Baton Rouge, LA	-	100 1	-	100 1	-	-	-	-	-	-	-	-	100 1	-	0 2	14 100	16	0 1	25 4	83 89	100 25	56 87	-	-
W O Moss Regional Medical Center, Lake Charles, LA	-	100 1	-	100 1	-	-	-	-	89 18	48 31	100 31	64 11	100 15	50 8	0 2	93 14	100 16	0 1	25 4	83 89	100 25	56 87	-	-
West Calcasieu-Cameron Hospital, Sulphur, LA	89 18	96 56	94 47	94 48	96 53	0 3	0	91 23	73 48	90 68	98 117	100 17	86 46	83 41	79 14	83 72	97 88	67 51	90 20	80 150	91 46	36 150	0.00 271	1.68 179
West Carroll Memorial Hospital, Oak Grove, LA	-	-	-	-	-	-	-	-	-	-	-	3	86 7	7 2	-	63 111	100 127	52 89	-	80 99	46	46 96	-	-
West Jefferson Medical Center, Marrero, LA	76 80	96 279	94 260	96 243	97 265	0 1	17	95 112	72 335	35 578	91 675	85 193	80 169	123	42 31	55 191	98 230	29 93	82 79	57 328	74 158	57 304	-	-
Willis Knighton Bossier Health Center, Bossier City, LA	48 33	94 100	88 99	86 76	78 113	0	33 3	100	46 87	29 38	83 184	100 11	81 16	83 12	0	78 172	99 201	61 114	100 8	68 57	57	57 49	-	-
Willis Knighton Medical Center, Shreveport, LA	68 131	98 231	94 338	86 169	92 377	0	18 11	100 53	67 344	33 106	88 700	100 22	83 29	90 42	-	80 381	100 456	51 280	94 17	80 99	91	46 96	-	-
Winn Parish Medical Center, Winnfield, LA	0	50 2	0	0 1	-	0 1	0	-	89 28	88 50	89 91	94 16	86 50	98 48	100 17	93 91	100 110	100 58	27	50 2	100 1	0 1	-	-
Woman's Hospital Foundation, Baton Rouge, LA	-	-	-	-	-	-	-	-	-	-	-	-	-	-	-	-	-	-	-	96 55	74 158	87 53	1.00 8762	3.63 5154
Women and Children's Hospital, Lake Charles, LA	-	100 1	100 1	100 1	100 1	-	-	-	83	14	100 14	100 4	100 4	100 12	0 6	83 30	97 33	83 12	92 12	87 326	91 104	86 322	0.66 1818	2.50 1082
Women and Children's Hospital, Lafayette, LA	-	100 1	100 1	100 2	100 2	-	-	2 100	-	-	-	-	50	100 2	0 6	0 1	100 2	0	50 2	93 262	86 85	86 260	0.84 3551	2.89 2041
MISSISSIPPI																								
Alliance Health Center, Meridian, MS	-	-	-	-	-	-	-	-	-	-	-	-	-	-	-	-	-	-	-	-	-	-	-	-
Alliance Healthcare System, Holly Springs, MS	-	0 1	-	-	0 1	-	-	0 1	83 6	0 9	57 47	0 1	100 1	50 2	-	68 34	98 43	50 22	0 1	0 1	100 1	-	-	-
Baptist Memorial Hospital Desoto, Southaven, MS	92 52	97 269	95 279	84 202	90 290	50 4	36	99 130	90 156	82 460	96 538	97 130	84 234	50 173	90 51	59 237	100 279	86 140	108	90 455	98 58	75 428	-	-
Baptist Memorial Hospital-Booneville, Booneville, MS	100 2	83 6	100 4	67 6	113	44 9	50	97 35	86 63	75 142	92 164	94 31	81 142	89 120	91 22	69 158	99 194	74 93	96 51	89 516	85 156	78 495	-	-
Baptist Memorial Hospital-Golden Triangle, Columbus, MS	76 21	93 91	93 93	86 75	87 86	9	50	97 35	86 63	75 142	92 164	94 31	81 142	89 120	91 22	69 158	99 194	74 93	96 51	89 516	85 156	78 495	-	-
Baptist Memorial Hospital-North Mississippi, Oxford, MS	85 20	96 119	97 148	92 101	93 147	8	-	100 67	76 127	82 233	97 273	64 108	82 131	94 109	83 52	86 161	100 216	87 134	97 60	88 442	61	72 401	-	-
Baptist Memorial Hospital-Union County, New Albany, MS	75 4	100 13	90 10	90 10	83 6	0	17	100	97 30	100 84	98 105	93 15	74 80	91 47	94 17	86 83	100 90	88 51	95 22	94 126	94 34	68 116	0.29 1049	1.46 751
Beacham Memorial Hospital, Magnolia, MS	-	80 5	75 4	40 5	50 4	-	-	-	67 15	50 10	71 76	0 2	67 3	0	-	85 80	89 104	25 64	0	68 37	37	-	-	-
Biloxi Regional Medical Center, Biloxi, MS	80 5	85 13	100 4	20 5	100 8	0	0	0	76 147	42 259	92 288	90	54 111	88	55 29	69 138	99 169	72 85	86 76	84 206	78 36	67 188	-	-
Bolivar Medical Center, Cleveland, MS	67 12	90 51	64 22	70 47	67 24	60	5	100	76 157	75 288	87 371	95	87 89	86 64	56 16	75 110	100 133	53 64	97 35	84 100	94 32	48 96	-	-
Calhoun Health Services, Calhoun City, MS	-	83 6	67 6	100 6	83 6	0	-	98 53	82 11	80 44	80 51	88 17	88 16	92 13	100 3	95 19	100 26	92 13	100	90 26	-	-	-	-
Central Mississippi Medical Center, Jackson, MS	64 33	93 124	88 115	79 108	85 123	88	67	98	71 128	51 206	91 249	97	73 111	85 86	88 32	62 157	98 187	79 89	50	90 432	97 63	66 419	-	-
Choctaw Health Center, Philadelphia, MS	-	-	-	-	-	-	-	0 1	0 1	-	-	-	-	-	-	0	4 100	5 100	0	2	-	-	-	-
Claiborne County Hospital, Port Gibson, MS	-	-	-	-	-	-	-	-	-	-	80 5	5	0	0	-	0	100 4	100 5	0	0	-	-	-	-
Clay County Medical Center, West Point, MS	100	100 3	-	100 4	100 3	0	0	0	91 57	73 26	74 129	100 5	92 12	83 12	-	92 78	97 91	67 60	100 2	68	78 33	79	0.19 517	0.90 332
Covington County Hospital, Collins, MS	-	0 1	-	0 1	-	0	-	100	69 16	25 12	89 18	3	67	89 9	0 6	56 34	98 43	5 21	14 7	37	36	67	-	-
Delta Regional Medical Center, Greenville, MS	100 16	98 105	87 124	86 71	82 113	25 8	8	92 48	95 44	90 144	97 154	93 26	90 98	87 127	90 50	75 142	98 167	83 94	91 35	93 129	94 64	84 116	0.13 746	1.89 529
Field Memorial Community Hospital, Centreville, MS	67 3	82 17	70 10	100 10	90 10	0 1	-	100	67 24	37 60	52 73	27	100 17	100 5	88 8	91 22	100 32	27 22	9	9	-	-	-	-
Forrest County General Hospital, Hattiesburg, MS	96 71	98 315	97 497	96 183	97 514	0	67	100 225	91 224	72 505	95 572	100 108	88 236	91 246	66 67	73 329	97 432	77 207	100 117	82 320	76 130	55 313	-	-
Franklin County Memorial Hospital, Meadville, MS	-	100 2	-	100 2	100 1	2	67	100	57 14	44 9	88 41	0 35	29 7	0	8	91 33	100 41	91 22	100	89 140	81	39 135	-	-
Garden Park Medical Center, Gulfport, MS	100 2	88 24	100 4	64 14	67 3	0 2	-	100	88 32	75 115	90 121	0	77 64	86 28	15	65 81	100 84	73 33	20	89 176	88 43	67 3	-	-
George County Hospital, Lucedale, MS	100	93 15	100 6	67 12	83 6	5	-	0	81 21	44 9	86 87	0	71 7	7	-	86 63	98 85	17 53	2	75 4	81	67 3	-	-
Gilmore Memorial Hospital, Amory, MS	100	92 13	100 4	91 11	100 6	0	1	0	75 16	61 67	81 101	93	87 90	95 66	59 17	87 98	100 120	75 67	33	80 176	88 43	81 175	-	-
Greenwood LeFlore Hospital, Greenwood, MS	67 9	88 52	73 26	86 49	82 28	12	8	100	68 99	20 244	78 279	59	84 73	88 52	44 18	85 108	100 128	45 65	91	53 193	94 62	45 185	0.44 226	2.88 416
Grenada Lake Medical Center, Grenada, MS	67 6	81 31	75 12	79 28	62 16	25 4	4	83	77 73	30 135	93 169	79	78 76	89 63	46 13	81 107	100 121	90 49	57 28	89 141	28	93 129	-	-
Gulf Coast Medical Center/Gulf Oaks Hospital, Biloxi, MS	0 1	90 10	100 3	62 13	100 5	4	-	100	64 11	58 40	90 50	83 6	83 48	86 21	13	96 49	100 100	62 29	73 11	95 99	91 35	81 99	-	-
H C Watkins Memorial Hospital, Quitman, MS	-	-	-	-	-	-	-	100	100 1	4	30 10	10 100	27	11 100	-	38 8	94 17	25 12	2	9	-	-	-	-
Hancock Medical Center, Bay Saint Louis, MS	-	-	-	-	-	-	-	-	65 23	55 51	88 59	100	76 63	84 38	81 31	88 59	98 66	82 28	29	4	25 4	50 4	-	-
Hancock Medical Center, Bay Saint Louis, MS	-	100 22	100 4	96 26	100 14	0	-	0	100 14	77 13	44	100	87 23	86	-	73 169	100 209	30 102	8	100 2	81 35	-	-	-
Highland Community Hospital, Picayune, GF	-	-	-	-	-	-	-	0 1	-	-	-	-	0 1	-	-	100 2	100 4	33 3	0	100	91	100 2	-	-
Jasper General Hospital, Bay Springs, MS	-	-	-	-	-	-	-	-	-	-	-	-	-	-	-	-	-	-	-	-	-	-	-	-

NOTE: The first number in each column (boldface) is the rate in percent, the second number is the number of patients; Please refer to the main entry for footnotes; **Heart Attack Care:** 1. ACE Inhibitor or ARB for LVSD; 2. Aspirin at Arrival; 3. Aspirin at Discharge; 4. Beta Blocker at Arrival; 5. Beta Blocker at Discharge; 6. Fibrinolytic Medication Timing; 7. PCI Within 90 Minutes of Arrival; 8. Smoking Cessation Advice; **Heart Failure Care:** 9. ACE Inhibitor or ARB for LVSD; 10. Discharge Instructions; 11. Evaluation of LVS Function; 12. Smoking Cessation Advice; **Pneumonia Care:** 13. Appropriate Initial Antibiotic; 14. Blood Culture Timing; 15. Influenza Vaccine; 16. Initial Antibiotic Timing; 17. Oxygenation Assessment; 18. Pneumococcal Vaccine; 19. Smoking Cessation Advice; **Surgical Infection Prevention:** 20. Prophylactic Antibiotic Given; 21. Prophylactic Antibiotic Selection; 22. Prophylactic Antibiotic Stopped; **Pregnancy Care:** 23. Inpatient Neonatal Mortality; 24. Third or Fourth Degree Laceration

Hospital	Heart Attack Care								Heart Failure Care				Pneumonia Care							Surgical Infection Prevention			Pregnancy Care	
	1	2	3	4	5	6	7	8	9	10	11	12	13	14	15	16	17	18	19	20	21	22	23	24
Jeff Anderson Regional Medical Center, Meridian, MS	100 36	99 109	99 153	99 102	99 172	- 0	0 2	97 65	99 102	54 311	99 368	96 52	70 172	90 88	- -	67 287	98 352	57 221	93 60	73 377	92 142	70 361	- -	- -
Jefferson County Hospital, Fayette, MS	- -	- -	- -	- -	- -	- -	- -	- -	- 0	100 2	0 19	100 1	0 2	- 0	- -	67 3	81 16	0 6	- 0	- -	- -	- -	- -	- -
Jefferson Davis Community Hospital, Prentiss, MS	- -	- -	- -	- -	- -	- -	- -	- -	100 7	35 17	56 16	75 8	93 14	75 8	80 5	80 20	100 22	79 14	57 7	- -	- -	- -	- -	- -
Kilmichael Hospital, Kilmichael, MS	- -	- -	- -	- -	- -	- -	- -	- -	- 0	50 6	0 20	0 1	- 0	- 0	- -	100 11	100 20	6 16	- 0	- -	- -	- -	- -	- -
King's Daughters Medical Center, Brookhaven, MS	100 2	100 13	80 5	80 10	88 8	- 0	- 0	- 0	96 55	70 135	94 155	100 24	93 68	91 55	81 27	82 94	100 125	73 70	96 26	85 86	93 27	80 84	- -	- -
Lackey Memorial Hospital, Forest, MS	- 0	- 0	- 0	- 0	- 0	- 0	- -	- 0	100 4	0 12	67 18	- 0	78 54	88 8	71 14	83 60	91 68	59 29	13 23	- -	- -	- -	- -	- -
Laird Hospital, Union, MS	0 1	80 5	75 4	60 5	100 4	- 0	- 0	- 0	75 4	33 21	34 41	0 6	95 20	67 3	71 7	100 12	82 51	65 23	36 11	- -	- -	- -	- -	- -
Madison County Medical Center, Canton, MS	100 2	71 34	71 17	69 32	71 17	- 0	- 0	67 3	63 27	2 84	63 95	70 20	83 18	78 9	33 6	73 30	88 33	23 13	50 6	18 39	50 10	56 36	- -	- -
Magee General Hospital, Magee, MS	100 1	75 8	100 3	75 8	100 4	- 0	- 0	- 0	90 29	56 63	98 83	95 20	95 112	97 88	94 35	97 173	99 191	94 121	94 35	- -	- -	- -	- -	- -
Magnolia Regional Health Center, Corinth, MS	80 30	93 112	93 108	82 94	86 112	57 23	100 1	74 39	68 148	52 225	95 272	89 55	77 182	89 114	59 46	78 208	99 242	71 118	76 58	83 288	94 80	16 284	- -	- -
Marion General Hospital, Columbia, MS	- 0	81 16	80 10	82 11	90 10	0 3	- 0	67 3	79 42	79 71	87 87	85 20	97 72	100 44	46 13	90 91	100 99	90 51	90 29	- 0	- 0	- 0	- -	- -
Memorial Hospital at Gulfport, Gulfport, MS	87 99	94 177	99 298	81 134	92 329	50 4	40 10	96 159	77 275	42 616	90 703	93 180	87 171	97 150	56 48	45 271	98 336	64 174	82 109	70 449	92 145	76 443	- -	- -
Mississippi Baptist Health Systems, Jackson, MS	84 101	98 200	96 382	89 172	94 400	- 0	14 14	98 154	96 329	83 675	97 760	97 134	81 77	96 51	74 23	70 123	99 150	68 90	68 28	77 305	90 73	79 295	- -	- -
Mississippi Methodist Rehab Center, Jackson, MS	- -	- -	- -	- -	- -	- -	- -	- -	- -	- -	- -	- -	- -	- -	- -	- 0	100 1	- 0	- -	- -	- -	- -	- -	- -
Montfort Jones Memorial Hospital, Kosciusko, MS	100 2	100 16	100 2	72 18	100 3	- 0	- 0	0 1	70 23	8 65	62 74	33 9	73 63	84 19	86 21	70 64	100 87	90 49	39 18	50 4	0 1	33 3	- -	- -
Natchez Community Hospital, Natchez, MS	0 1	79 29	62 16	59 22	76 17	0 1	- 0	57 7	87 76	37 177	92 200	80 41	58 130	92 95	46 24	72 168	98 190	48 96	81 47	86 94	75 24	72 87	- -	- -
Natchez Regional Medical Center, Natchez, MS	33 9	98 52	78 45	98 47	84 50	0 5	50 2	71 21	82 51	21 159	76 187	50 26	66 68	84 55	60 15	76 111	98 129	51 85	42 33	87 164	92 49	78 160	0.00 247	0.71 425
Neshoba County General Hospital, Philadelphia, MS	- 0	67 3	67 3	0 2	0 2	- 0	- 0	- 0	71 21	64 59	87 68	87 15	89 36	90 30	72 18	98 40	100 47	88 26	100 11	100 1	- 0	100 1	- -	- -
Newton Regional Hospital, Newton, MS	- 0	100 4	100 1	50 2	100 1	- 0	- 0	- 0	57 14	92 12	67 54	100 2	100 1	- 0	- -	80 20	100 24	60 15	100 1	- -	- -	- -	- -	- -
North Mississippi Medical Center, Tupelo, MS	92 208	99 360	100 781	97 310	99 722	33 6	45 22	99 347	90 430	97 645	95 725	100 210	84 206	88 158	59 88	76 251	100 370	91 251	98 112	92 951	84 255	72 903	1.04 483	6.35 315
North Mississippi Medical Center-Eupora, Eupora, MS	100 1	100 2	- 0	100 2	100 1	- 0	- 0	- 0	87 30	60 20	88 81	83 6	63 19	100 12	- -	94 128	98 181	70 106	43 7	- 0	- -	- 0	- -	- -
North Mississippi Medical Center-Iuka, Iuka, MS	100 1	50 8	67 6	62 8	57 7	- 0	- 0	- 0	88 8	74 23	81 120	100 5	83 6	100 2	- -	78 51	97 65	61 28	100 3	- -	- -	- -	- -	- -
North Oak Regional Medical Center, Senatobia, MS	- 0	50 2	100 1	25 4	33 3	- 0	- 0	- 0	40 5	83 18	79 80	100 1	100 1	100 1	- -	80 41	96 47	83 24	- 0	67 6	- -	67 6	- -	- -
North Sunflower County Hospital, Ruleville, MS	- -	- -	- -	- -	- -	- -	- -	- -	89 9	23 13	81 27	100 2	80 20	83 18	60 10	78 49	100 59	71 38	100 6	- -	- -	- -	- -	- -
Northwest Mississippi Regional Medical Center, Clarksdale, MS	70 27	85 68	88 49	66 70	92 51	14 7	- 0	100 18	77 183	61 318	91 343	99 84	45 55	95 21	0 4	58 55	100 70	18 28	100 23	78 129	95 40	57 126	- -	- -
Oktibbeha County Hospital, Starkville, MS	100 1	100 3	100 3	67 3	100 2	- 0	- -	- 0	80 20	33 54	73 60	29 7	70 86	90 67	76 17	79 103	91 121	74 66	78 18	56 305	68 88	80 296	- -	- -
Pearl River County Hospital and Nursing Home, Poplarville, MS	- -	- -	- -	- -	- -	- -	- -	- -	- 0	- -	75 4	- -	- 0	100 1	- -	80 10	100 13	80 5	- 0	- -	- -	- -	- -	- -
Rankin Medical Center, Brandon, MS	100 1	94 17	71 7	94 16	86 7	- 0	- 0	50 2	84 70	62 145	93 194	92 50	93 99	92 60	- -	90 109	100 134	97 63	94 51	86 69	74 19	75 65	- -	- -
Regency Hospital of Jackson, Jackson, MS	- -	- -	- -	- -	- -	- -	- -	- -	- -	- -	- -	- -	- 0	- 0	- -	- 0	- 0	- 0	- 0	- -	- -	- -	- -	- -
Riley Memorial Hospital, Meridian, MS	100 7	95 20	100 15	90 21	93 15	- 0	- 0	100 4	92 53	95 125	93 150	94 34	56 70	94 62	80 15	70 89	98 118	84 58	92 25	67 114	78 23	75 107	- -	- -
River Oaks Hospital, Jackson, MS	100 1	89 19	78 9	93 15	71 7	0 4	- 0	33 3	55 20	30 104	79 122	70 20	73 115	95 56	35 26	72 118	100 160	49 68	63 43	60 823	80 69	76 814	- -	- -
River Region Health System, Vicksburg, MS	83 35	96 130	95 141	87 83	92 142	58 19	29 7	97 66	91 162	63 395	97 466	100 98	78 181	95 147	93 58	89 221	99 275	96 135	95 86	80 406	91 99	64 386	- -	- -
Rush Foundation Hospital, Meridian, MS	97 32	97 79	100 116	99 68	98 107	- 0	80 5	93 55	93 89	86 186	97 208	90 50	82 76	96 46	94 16	86 63	97 91	75 44	89 28	73 174	78 60	64 165	- -	- -
Saint Dominic Jackson Memorial Hospital, Jackson, MS	90 69	99 153	97 272	91 134	96 270	0 2	40 5	100 84	86 145	81 284	89 312	98 42	86 90	87 84	- -	79 110	100 145	71 79	96 24	72 268	90 69	66 254	- -	- -
Scott Regioanl Hospital, Morton, MS	- 0	50 2	0 1	0 2	0 1	- 0	- 0	- 0	0 1	62 26	47 38	78 9	90 99	100 2	45 31	83 132	100 136	92 49	93 46	- -	- -	- -	- -	- -
Sharkey Issaquena Community Hospital, Rolling Fork, MS	- -	- -	- -	- -	- -	- -	- -	- -	0 1	0 2	7 14	- 0	- 0	- 0	- -	83 6	100 6	0 5	- 0	- -	- -	- -	- -	- -
Simpson General Hospital, Mendenhall, MS	- -	- -	- -	- -	- -	- -	- -	- -	67 6	47 15	74 27	82 11	20 15	75 4	0 8	64 11	79 19	13 15	60 5	- -	- -	- -	- -	- -
Singing River Hospital, Pascagoula, MS	93 67	97 263	96 258	95 217	93 243	- 0	50 10	100 109	91 259	95 494	95 532	100 129	84 245	86 183	81 68	91 293	100 352	80 183	100 93	86 175	89 175	76 172	- -	- -
South Central Regional Medical Center, Laurel, MS	75 16	90 112	85 53	80 105	82 55	70 10	- 0	92 12	69 75	45 149	81 177	97 34	87 156	86 92	47 34	90 191	96 210	44 116	98 49	78 490	92 117	26 485	- -	- -
South Sunflower County Hospital, Indianola, MS	50 4	57 21	53 17	53 17	71 17	- 0	- 0	100 1	62 34	0 19	86 79	50 6	86 7	- 0	- -	71 63	83 87	67 52	0 2	100 8	- -	88 8	0.24 413	2.68 261
Southwest Mississippi Regional Medical Center, McComb, MS	70 27	81 79	94 94	69 54	92 104	0 1	25 4	97 36	70 113	64 255	72 297	100 53	71 139	90 92	11 35	78 181	99 225	58 128	94 48	89 475	95 98	80 467	- -	- -
Tippah County Hospital, Ripley, MS	- 0	100 2	100 2	0 1	0 2	- -	- -	- -	73 15	44 9	71 42	33 3	100 1	86 7	- -	84 64	98 91	59 58	- 0	- 0	- -	- 0	- -	- -
Trace Regional Hospital, Houston, MS	100 1	92 13	100 10	88 8	89 9	- 0	- 0	- 0	86 7	38 8	84 50	- 0	100 2	67 3	- -	92 74	100 86	67 54	50 2	- -	- -	- -	- -	- -
Tri-Lakes Medical Center, Batesville, MS	- 0	100 6	100 1	33 3	100 1	- 0	- 0	- 0	57 14	48 23	63 110	60 5	91 11	71 7	- -	81 64	98 80	15 34	20 5	33 3	- -	100 3	- -	- -
University of Mississippi Medical Center, Jackson, MS	85 40	98 121	98 135	95 97	98 150	- 0	50 8	98 107	86 242	46 304	97 310	88 114	83 59	84 69	6 18	59 106	99 137	5 37	79 53	88 326	94 206	76 320	2.32 3925	1.70 2349
Walthall County General Hospital, Tylertown, MS	- 0	50 2	100 2	100 2	67 3	- 0	- 0	- 0	67 3	30 40	43 63	29 7	75 44	100 6	17 12	89 46	79 63	3 32	23 13	- -	- -	- -	- -	- -
Wayne General Hospital, Waynesboro, MS	100 1	67 9	60 5	56 9	40 5	- 0	- 0	- 0	81 53	63 19	89 73	0 1	86 7	83 6	- -	92 62	100 79	79 39	100 3	0 4	- -	33 3	- -	- -
Wesley Medical Center, Hattiesburg, MS	96 27	97 94	99 132	97 74	100 122	0 3	100 2	100 47	99 121	86 220	100 261	98 64	87 131	96 113	97 32	86 138	100 190	98 104	100 52	92 1007	91 250	83 995	- -	- -

NOTE: The first number in each column (boldface) is the rate in percent, the second number is the number of patients; Please refer to the main entry for footnotes; ***Heart Attack Care:*** *1. ACE Inhibitor or ARB for LVSD; 2. Aspirin at Arrival; 3. Aspirin at Discharge; 4. Beta Blocker at Arrival; 5. Beta Blocker at Discharge; 6. Fibrinolytic Medication Timing; 7. PCI Within 90 Minutes of Arrival; 8. Smoking Cessation Advice;* ***Heart Failure Care:*** *9. ACE Inhibitor or ARB for LVSD; 10. Discharge Instructions; 11. Evaluation of LVS Function; 12. Smoking Cessation Advice;* ***Pneumonia Care:*** *13. Appropriate Initial Antibiotic; 14. Blood Culture Timing; 15. Influenza Vaccine; 16. Initial Antibiotic Timing; 17. Oxygenation Assessment; 18. Pneumococcal Vaccine; 19. Smoking Cessation Advice;* ***Surgical Infection Prevention:*** *20. Prophylactic Antibiotic Given; 21. Prophylactic Antibiotic Selection; 22. Prophylactic Antibiotic Stopped;* ***Pregnancy Care:*** *23. Inpatient Neonatal Mortality; 24. Third or Fourth Degree Laceration*

Column groups: **Heart Attack Care** (1–8) · **Heart Failure Care** (9–12) · **Pneumonia Care** (13–19) · **Surgical Infection Prevention** (20–22) · **Pregnancy Care** (23–24)

Hospital	1	2	3	4	5	6	7	8	9	10	11	12	13	14	15	16	17	18	19	20	21	22	23	24
Whitfield Medical Surgical Hospital, Whitfield, MS	-	0 100	1 100	1 100	1 0	-	-	-	- 100	2	- 100	2	-	0	0	- 100	18 100	86 7	0	-	-	-	-	-
Winston Medical Center, Louisville, MS	-	0 100	1 0	1 100	1 0	-	-	-	0 75	8 97	29 93	41 78	9	83 29	93 14	85 33	100 44	87 23	88 8	-	-	-	-	-
Woman's Hospital at River Oaks, Jackson, MS	0 1	0 1	0 1	0 1	0 1	0 5	0 1	-	-	-	-	-	-	-	-	-	-	-	-	86 339	78 18	84 337	0.33 1530	4.03 769
Yalobusha General Hospital, Water Valley, MS	-	-	-	-	-	-	-	-	50 4	14 7	48 33	0 100	3	0 100	3	96 25	83 29	27 22	100 3	76 748	97 307	99 742	-	-
PUERTO RICO																								
Admin de Servicios Medicos Puerto Rico, San Juan, PR	-	-	-	-	-	-	-	-	-	-	-	-	-	-	-	-	-	-	-	-	-	-	-	-
Ashford Presbyterian Community Hospital, San Juan, PR	100 10	93 45	71 24	89 46	91 23	-	0	100	4 100	33 100	69 93	91 68	79 85	66 71	45 45	248 81	268 49	144 71	7	72 368	97 108	24 328	0.00	7.04 1222
Auxilio Mutuo Hospital, San Juan, PR	73 33	85 132	85 138	73 105	81 150	0	0 2	81 16	64 86	35 302	82 304	91 137	61 213	71 66	9 47	45 248	81 268	49 144	42 12	77 171	99 89	100 158	-	0
Bella Vista Hospital, Mayaguez, PR	80 15	74 54	72 39	53 51	60 47	60	5	50 4	75 36	82 140	65 142	67 121	79 112	66 3	35 43	148 100	165 5	96 89	9	56 313	96 51	6 303	-	-
Cardiovascular Center of Puerto Rico, Rio Piedras, PR	90 77	97 69	99 259	97 70	96 226	-	-	89 55	97 239	94 373	87 373	83 18	0	-	-	96 25	83 29	27 22	100 3	76 748	97 307	99 742	0.33 1530	4.03 769
Castaner General Hospital, Castaner, PR	-	-	-	-	-	-	-	-	0 2	0 2	2 0	-	-	-	-	-	-	-	-	-	-	-	-	-
Clinica Espanola, Mayaguez, PR	0	0 100	100 1	0 100	1	-	-	100	1 100	20 100	25 80	100 67	12	50 8	100 3	91 11	79 14	100 11	100 2	62 332	97 88	24 328	-	-
Doctor I Gonzalez Martinez Oncologic Hospital, San Juan, PR	-	-	100	-	-	-	-	-	100	-	100 1	100	-	100 1	-	- 100	3	100	3	-	-	-	-	-
Doctors Center Hospital, Manati, PR	100 3	100 12	100 5	73 11	80 5	0	33	0	1 100	13 100	35 89	100 79	19 38	16	28 100	21 28	100 28	-	3	45 29	35 17	24 29	-	-
Hima Humacao, Humacao, PR	100 13	96 55	100 48	96 51	100 48	0	1	100	10 100	31 93	122 100	91 141	88 89	80 34	35 63	151 99	155 34	91 100	23	26 43	0 100	36	-	-
Hima-San Pablo Fajardo, Fajardo, PR	86 7	86 21	92 12	82 17	100 11	0	1	0 100	89 65	95 107	85 110	91 75	48 75	78 36	0 54	78 93	83 10	48 100	6	74 27	100 2	100 36	-	-
Hospital Comunitario Buen Samaritano, Aguadilla, PR	50 42	79 136	42 118	75 134	52 118	0	2	72 18	44 63	259 62	260 65	222 77	113 84	85 39	16 30	115 97	118 6	64 85	12	64 52	88 75	52 193	-	-
Hospital Damas, Ponce, PR	100 42	95 132	96 124	92 125	97 139	47	19	93 15	99 73	100 211	89 373	100 70	71 87	60 26	64 20	5 92	124 10	73 70	10	64 195	88 75	52 193	-	-
Hospital De La Concepcion, San German, PR	98 43	93 111	96 124	91 104	95 110	-	-	100	99 16	100 178	96 175	93 70	40 5	-	83	20 5	92 124	10 73	70	14 63	- 100	20	-	-
Hospital Del Maestro, San Juan, PR	67 3	77 13	67 15	60 15	56 16	0	-	100	7 100	15 57	106 58	93 76	55 76	72	35 62	76 99	83 24	45 92	12	29 14	100 27	79 70	-	-
Hospital Doctor Cayetano Coll Y Toste, Arecibo, PR	68 37	92 77	90 80	68 74	79 80	33	24	100	82 27	82 160	86 152	100 73	62 73	78 64	22 42	81 81	87 71	52 100	26	47 78	-	45 78	-	-
Hospital Doctor Dominguez, Humacao, PR	100 8	81 16	100 21	75 16	95 20	33	12	80	5 100	49 41	62 26	100 83	59 79	75 8	5 10	58 92	79 14	49 100	12	-	-	-	-	-
Hospital Doctor Pila, Ponce, PR	-	71 167	-	-	-	24	33	-	85	111 85	103	-	60 111	61 59	-	63 150	93 47	79	3	57 88	85 27	95 88	-	-
Hospital Doctor Susoni, Arecibo, PR	56 18	96 53	80 46	81 42	59 39	36	14	0 100	4 91	23 28	65 46	100 67	64 71	38 5	19 41	66 77	69 10	42 100	6	44 50	100 6	100 33	-	-
Hospital Episcopal Cristo Redentor, Guayama, PR	88 8	77 53	72 18	66 58	80 20	0	2	100	82 28	69 88	72 88	94 55	42 82	11 14	40 47	90 49	36 25	75	4	14 63	95 21	52 63	-	-
Hospital Hermanos Melendez, Bayamon, PR	-	91 270	70 283	94 71	72 261	33	6	93 108	73 55	18 228	99 226	90 64	119 92	65 100	8 26	12 145	87 154	25 84	93 34	30 98	118 100	88 172	-	-
Hospital Interamericano de Medicina, Caguas, PR	-	-	-	94	11	-	-	100	94 81	99 112	89 112	100	0 100	2 0	100 2	100 2	100 2	0 1	100 6	73 30	-	88 32	-	-
Hospital Matilde Brenes, Bayamon, PR	67 3	100 10	71 14	88 8	75 12	0	-	0 98	55 11	60 95	204 52	50 71	14 73	52 60	204 46	54 90	59 59	2 0	1	29 14	98 17	88 32	-	-
Hospital Menonita De Cayey, Cayey, PR	100 2	96 49	80 30	80 51	83 41	0	5	0 100	93 60	41 224	65 222	97 32	67 64	73 8	54 13	34 68	96 73	39 94	17	60 55	97 31	89 54	-	-
Hospital Metropolitano, San German, PR	94 17	97 31	100 33	97 31	91 35	0	0	0 100	100 19	100 52	100 52	100 70	10 94	33	13 100	7 34	100 35	100 100	19 6	88 8	- 100	8	-	-
Hospital Metropolitano Doctor Tito Mattei, Yauco, PR	67 43	94 36	85 34	100 18	72 4	0	-	93 29	85 20	18 79	59 80	90 81	75 45	42 16	8 29	68 92	154 58	14 100	5 29	36 55	80 20	20 100	20	-
Hospital Oncologico Andres Grillasca, Ponce, PR	-	-	50	-	25 4	-	-	0 100	70 10	9 11	100 0	66 32	0	100 2	100 0	100 2	100 0	21 0	1	29 14	33 3	100 16	-	-
Hospital Pavia Hato Rey, Hato Rey, PR	71 21	79 150	93 205	91 11	95 77	-	-	0 61	31 60	15 84	134 54	134 78	51 80	27 73	15 80	47 19	82 33	0 21	17	40 20	-	100 135	-	-
Hospital Pavia Santurce, Fernandez Juncos, PR	78 89	75 238	-	-	-	50	2	0 98	75 185	60 215	-	100 97	37 59	185 46	13 55	285 98	291 17	202 88	53	84 603	89 151	70	-	-
Hospital Perea, Mayaguez, PR	100 1	89 9	100 3	100 10	100 9	-	-	5 77	13 70	40 70	29 100	100 33	5 77	13	- 100	20 18	94 46	13 100	3	50 4	100 1	50 4	-	-
Hospital San Carlos Borromeo, Moca, PR	60 5	81 16	61 18	68 19	75 20	0	3	0 93	68 32	25 64	60 222	97 8	10 60	154	29 21	14 64	73 39	20 10	100 6	0	97 31	100 2	-	-
Hospital San Cristobal, Coto Laurel, PR	94 31	85 67	100	99 69	95 73	50	-	0 100	50 8	69 42	52 100	33 94	42 18	-	100 4	67 27	100 100	89 18	14	88 8	- 100	8	0 100	55
Hospital San Francisco, San Juan, PR	100 5	94 36	94 17	85 34	100 18	0	4	93 9	85 20	18 69	88 226	90 100	81 75	28 81	8 100	52 29	92 91	14 58	29	36 55	80 20	20 100	20	-
Hospital San Gerardo, Rio Piedras, PR	0	71 7	50 4	29 7	25 4	0	-	100	4 85	20 70	10 9	11 66	32	0 32	24 47	19 82	33 0	21 0	1	29 14	33 3	100 16	-	-
Hospital San Juan Bautista Medical Center, Caguas, PR	-	-	-	91 11	-	-	-	0 98	60 1	84 100	134 54	78 51	80 15	31 100	2 100	46 54	90 59	88 17	89 27	73 30	89 151	100 135	-	-
Hospital Santa Rosa, Guayama, PR	100 1	89 9	100 3	100 10	100 9	0	-	100	5 100	29 100	29 100	100 5	77 13	-	- 100	18	94 291	17 202	98 53	50 4	100 1	50 4	-	-
Hospital Universitario Doctor Ramon Ruiz Arnau, Bayamon, PR	75 12	98 41	50 22	90 41	52 21	29	7	0 100	9 100	21 100	58 59	100 11	57 127	64 18	29 67	51 150	100 155	56 89	50 28	0	2 100	2	-	-
Hospital Wilma N Vazquez, Vega Baja, PR	100 4	100 33	100 23	96 23	100 18	-	50	0 100	1 100	4 100	46 100	100 4	44 18	-	100 4	67 27	76 29	89 18	100 2	- 100	-	100 8	-	-
Lafayette Hospital, Arroyo, PR	100 6	91 23	75 12	80 15	78 9	0	4	2 100	85 9	79 17	41 100	100 57	28 81	16 4	100 52	29 92	97 83	24 100	7	30 20	80 20	100 20	0 100	7
Manati Medical Center Doctor Otero Lopez, Manati, PR	100 32	99 195	100 91	95 162	95 77	0	-	100	60 15	35 100	493 100	78 493	57 100	394 92	56 92	393 100	100 394	40 232	135 100	84 603	91 22	95 22	-	-
Mennonite General Hospital, Aibonito, PR	100 1	95 20	60 5	70 20	40 5	-	-	0 100	73 11	63 57	63 134	100 97	80 30	75 28	0 1	41 27	97 33	35 20	100 9	-	91 70	50 4	-	-
Metropolitan Hospital, San Juan, PR	-	100 22	-	100 22	-	-	-	0 100	100 10	100 232	100 58	98 58	88 119	-	-	-	98 47	-	-	-	-	100 6	-	-

NOTE: The first number in each column (boldface) is the rate in percent, the second number is the number of patients; Please refer to the main entry for footnotes; **Heart Attack Care**: 1. ACE Inhibitor or ARB for LVSD; 2. Aspirin at Arrival; 3. Aspirin at Discharge; 4. Beta Blocker at Arrival; 5. Beta Blocker at Discharge; 6. Fibrinolytic Medication Timing; 7. PCI Within 90 Minutes of Arrival; 8. Smoking Cessation Advice; **Heart Failure Care**: 9. ACE Inhibitor or ARB for LVSD; 10. Discharge Instructions; 11. Evaluation of LVS Function; 12. Smoking Cessation Advice; **Pneumonia Care**: 13. Appropriate Initial Antibiotic; 14. Blood Culture Timing; 15. Influenza Vaccine; 16. Initial Antibiotic Timing; 17. Oxygenation Assessment; 18. Pneumococcal Vaccine; 19. Smoking Cessation Advice; **Surgical Infection Prevention**: 20. Prophylactic Antibiotic Given; 21. Prophylactic Antibiotic Selection; 22. Prophylactic Antibiotic Stopped; **Pregnancy Care**: 23. Inpatient Neonatal Mortality; 24. Third or Fourth Degree Laceration

Hospital	Heart Attack Care								Heart Failure Care				Pneumonia Care							Surgical Infection Prevention			Pregnancy Care	
	1	2	3	4	5	6	7	8	9	10	11	12	13	14	15	16	17	18	19	20	21	22	23	24
Professional Hospital, Manati, PR	- -	- -	- -	- -	- -	- -	- -	- -	- -	- -	- -	- -	- -	- -	- -	- -	- -	- -	- -	38 13	- -	8 13	- -	- -
Ramon E Betances Hospital, Mayaguez, PR	66 50	95 78	80 110	80 79	78 113	- 0	0 1	96 25	66 65	77 146	84 146	100 21	62 48	79 29	36 11	- -	97 74	41 34	100 10	- -	- -	- -	- -	- -
Ryder Memorial Hospital, Humacao, PR	100 4	96 27	86 22	89 27	87 23	100 1	- 0	- -	86 7	- -	81 48	- -	- -	97 29	- -	27 26	100 29	24 25	- -	- -	100 10	100 15	- -	- -
San Juan Municipal Hospital, Rio Piedras, PR	75 8	91 22	68 22	68 25	81 26	- -	- -	100 13	93 14	95 43	59 41	100 17	- -	- -	- -	78 37	97 58	5 20	100 32	- -	- -	100 28	- -	- -
San Luke's Memorial Hospital, Ponce, PR	87 30	94 187	88 105	62 190	85 110	10 10	- 0	100 16	92 65	71 171	74 170	100 22	79 121	75 64	- -	51 123	100 124	88 67	100 19	68 137	97 34	65 137	- -	- -
University District Hospital, Rio Piedras, PR	0 1	100 1	100 1	100 1	100 1	- 0	- 0	0 1	67 3	0 6	83 6	75 4	29 7	0 1	- 0	33 9	89 9	0 1	33 3	73 237	84 67	69 231	- -	- -
UPR Carolina, Carolina, PR	88 142	93 238	86 175	88 190	90 173	38 21	- 0	90 40	93 101	27 318	100 319	82 38	57 292	69 84	11 46	39 372	97 409	9 206	80 80	77 112	100 27	73 101	- -	- -
SOUTH CAROLINA																								
Abbeville County Memorial Hospital, Abbeville, SC	100 1	89 9	100 1	100 7	100 1	- 0	- 0	- 0	75 4	81 16	94 17	60 5	90 10	86 7	- -	93 14	100 17	75 8	25 4	- -	- -	- -	- -	- -
Aiken Regional Medical Centers, Aiken, SC	100 36	99 126	100 134	95 85	100 125	- 0	56 9	95 60	99 138	47 226	99 276	98 42	88 104	92 116	85 34	94 164	100 197	97 120	100 39	91 574	98 128	81 538	- -	- -
Allen Bennett Memorial Hospital, Greer, SC	- 0	100 1	- 0	100 1	- 0	- 0	- -	- 0	86 36	78 76	94 104	94 18	93 123	99 74	88 34	92 148	100 187	87 119	96 55	82 94	94 32	90 89	- -	- -
Anderson Area Medical Center, Anderson, SC	100 54	100 322	100 326	100 272	100 309	- 0	96 23	100 138	89 212	75 448	96 567	100 124	92 443	98 567	77 156	78 715	99 868	91 558	100 219	90 582	86 64	85 531	- -	- -
Bamberg County Memorial Hospital, Bamberg, SC	- 0	100 3	- 0	100 3	100 2	- 0	- 0	- 0	75 12	67 46	77 53	14 7	64 45	84 32	79 14	82 57	99 83	65 49	70 20	- -	- -	- -	0.00 60	1.59 63
Barnwell County Hospital, Barnwell, SC	- 0	92 13	88 8	100 7	89 9	- 0	- 0	100 1	92 12	40 5	78 46	50 2	67 6	83 12	- -	82 93	98 118	29 63	0 2	0 1	- -	100 1	- -	- -
Beaufort Memorial Hospital, Beaufort, SC	100 14	93 72	92 38	99 68	95 37	- 0	- 0	100 10	86 118	73 243	83 264	91 46	84 92	77 48	50 14	67 87	98 106	47 57	91 34	88 542	97 155	79 535	- -	- -
Bon Secours Saint Francis Hospital, Charleston, SC	0 1	91 22	100 6	76 21	100 5	- 0	- 0	100 1	89 45	81 137	95 167	85 26	92 138	92 131	90 48	86 181	100 219	84 138	82 51	97 497	99 99	90 487	0.12 1707	3.28 1159
Cannon Memorial Hospital, Pickens, SC	100 1	77 13	80 5	83 12	100 6	20 5	- 0	100 1	100 11	87 31	78 37	100 5	86 81	92 91	100 24	81 100	100 140	88 86	88 34	79 24	100 10	92 24	- -	- -
Carolina Pines Regional Medical Center, Hartsville, SC	50 2	86 37	81 16	81 32	78 18	75 4	- 0	100 4	76 109	60 226	98 252	84 62	87 196	95 175	57 49	90 292	100 336	69 169	90 101	90 150	91 34	70 145	- -	- -
Carolinas Hospital System-Florence, Florence, SC	73 49	95 144	94 192	93 109	98 205	- 0	67 3	97 73	87 210	64 394	97 477	99 98	77 190	97 172	73 45	79 277	98 336	81 187	100 87	89 674	95 167	79 658	- -	- -
Carolinas Hospital System-Lake City, Lake City, SC	100 1	100 4	- 0	20 5	50 2	- 0	- 0	- 0	67 27	91 55	92 64	72 25	97 64	90 42	100 8	87 70	100 73	86 35	85 13	50 2	- 0	100 2	- -	- -
Charleston Memorial Hospital, Charleston, SC	- -	- -	- -	- -	- -	- -	- -	- -	- -	- -	- -	- -	- -	- -	- -	- -	- -	- -	- -	- -	- -	- -	- -	- -
Chester Regional Medical Center, Chester, SC	20 5	71 17	67 6	76 17	86 7	0 1	- 0	- 0	64 39	54 123	89 146	70 44	64 94	89 37	29 17	65 101	98 109	53 60	78 37	68 28	89 9	18 28	- -	- -
Chesterfield General Hospital, Cheraw, SC	- 0	100 6	100 5	100 5	100 5	- 0	- 0	- 0	97 39	66 87	91 101	64 14	81 98	86 86	61 31	94 132	99 154	74 93	76 46	45 22	100 6	100 15	- -	- -
Clarendon Memorial Hospital, Manning, SC	0 1	70 10	40 5	50 6	60 5	- 0	- 0	- 0	83 35	84 103	83 112	92 24	81 132	90 87	- -	83 156	99 193	71 95	97 36	49 86	89 28	88 84	- -	- -
Coastal Carolina Medical Center, Hardeeville, SC	- 0	50 4	100 1	100 3	100 1	- 0	- 0	0 1	100 6	62 39	63 41	83 6	83 30	96 24	86 7	67 18	97 38	71 21	33 3	54 13	100 5	58 12	- -	- -
Colleton Medical Center, Walterboro, SC	75 4	67 12	88 8	71 7	100 6	0 1	- 0	100 1	78 83	42 265	94 287	95 56	67 83	97 59	79 24	88 127	99 150	69 78	75 28	83 167	98 41	69 154	- -	- -
Conway Medical Center, Conway, SC	100 8	100 85	87 39	96 75	95 37	80 10	- 0	100 5	91 86	90 49	92 260	100 12	82 17	91 33	- -	88 248	100 294	71 145	100 15	93 41	- -	76 38	- -	- -
East Cooper Regional Medical Center, Mount Pleasant, SC	100 1	100 4	67 3	100 6	100 5	- 0	- 0	- 0	85 26	88 75	82 94	100 7	89 103	87 97	76 34	85 139	100 169	94 111	100 16	82 222	83 48	93 224	- -	- -
Edgefield County Hospital, Edgefield, SC	100 1	100 2	67 3	67 3	67 3	- 0	- 0	100 1	85 13	67 45	68 59	73 15	75 40	100 24	89 18	100 47	100 60	91 46	44 9	- -	- -	- -	- -	- -
Fairfield Memorial Hospital, Winnsboro, SC	- 0	100 2	0 1	100 1	100 1	- 0	- -	- 0	83 6	18 34	63 41	50 2	76 38	85 20	43 7	93 43	100 49	44 32	42 12	- -	- -	- -	- -	- -
Georgetown Memorial Hospital, Georgetown, SC	86 14	95 81	90 60	92 74	90 60	- 0	- 0	100 30	83 102	77 209	97 237	96 50	90 84	94 118	37 30	87 162	100 188	85 109	95 43	90 328	94 77	34 319	- -	- -
Grand Strand Regional Medical Center, Myrtle Beach, SC	89 106	100 322	98 416	98 273	99 413	67 3	83 29	99 167	89 181	99 479	99 534	100 97	88 182	84 197	64 74	85 277	100 349	81 242	98 116	93 363	97 224	67 354	- -	- -
Greenville Memorial Medical Campus, Greenville, SC	88 220	97 492	98 658	94 383	97 744	100 1	68 34	100 404	94 395	70 694	98 800	96 195	93 294	95 268	83 98	67 456	100 552	82 301	94 174	93 253	94 88	90 239	- -	- -
Hampton Regional Medical Center, Varnville, SC	100 1	75 4	67 3	67 3	100 3	0 1	- 0	- 0	50 6	0 25	48 25	0 3	90 29	100 7	86 7	92 12	100 32	58 26	43 7	0 1	100 2	100 1	- -	- -
Hillcrest Hospital, Simpsonville, SC	75 4	88 17	100 5	78 9	91 11	- 0	- 0	100 1	84 19	71 41	94 54	100 9	94 85	100 48	83 18	85 109	99 129	89 81	100 32	87 69	100 20	78 69	- -	- -
Hilton Head Regional Medical Center, Hilton Head Isl, SC	79 14	100 80	99 93	96 54	98 92	- 0	20 5	93 29	79 78	58 155	94 199	86 21	96 98	90 92	74 27	94 108	100 167	78 125	96 23	84 238	97 37	86 232	- -	- -
Kershaw County Medical Center, Camden, SC	60 5	78 41	71 17	82 38	79 19	40 5	- 0	50 4	77 90	56 200	96 252	89 62	89 161	85 114	62 48	73 230	100 293	64 183	73 66	90 209	100 50	54 205	- -	- -
Laurens County Hospital, Clinton, SC	67 3	90 31	75 12	77 30	69 13	0 3	- 0	67 3	90 31	62 66	78 112	67 24	82 122	85 86	73 30	82 131	100 181	71 105	50 38	73 172	88 40	71 168	- -	- -
Lexington Medical Center, West Columbia, SC	68 28	95 183	95 91	87 131	97 92	- 0	- 0	79 24	76 105	59 217	99 268	93 58	82 122	92 98	92 26	76 138	100 184	95 94	83 47	88 205	83 48	59 201	- -	- -
Loris Community Hospital, Loris, SC	83 6	98 56	94 34	98 52	94 35	- 0	- 0	88 8	88 59	89 165	93 175	89 45	77 82	95 59	79 28	81 93	100 140	74 92	96 48	94 195	89 38	84 191	- -	- -
Marion County Medical Center, Marion, SC	90 10	93 54	94 35	96 48	92 38	0 1	- 0	100 3	89 100	66 221	94 248	93 69	74 57	84 58	74 19	73 85	100 112	74 50	98 44	86 153	100 24	37 145	- -	- -
Marlboro Park Hospital, Bennettsville, SC	100 2	100 7	100 1	86 7	100 3	0 2	- 0	100 1	97 31	58 73	81 79	85 26	77 70	90 50	65 17	77 75	99 91	47 49	86 28	47 17	80 5	91 11	- -	- -
Mary Black Memorial Hospital, Spartanburg, SC	100 5	98 42	85 20	93 45	89 19	0 1	- 0	100 2	90 63	57 141	98 174	95 43	87 107	86 122	81 42	84 152	100 205	92 130	97 65	87 635	96 171	78 616	- -	- -
McLeod Medical Center Dillon, Dillon, SC	80 5	90 21	80 15	93 14	94 18	0 1	- 0	100 1	78 46	75 36	76 178	100 4	67 12	82 11	- -	85 93	100 133	34 56	100 5	100 14	- -	62 13	- -	- -
McLeod Regional Medical Center-Pee Dee, Florence, SC	87 188	98 323	98 503	95 253	99 609	67 3	79 14	100 270	88 355	82 679	93 747	99 174	86 235	96 244	90 63	79 319	99 421	85 227	99 129	96 255	95 66	80 245	- -	- -
Medical University of S Carolina Med Ctr, Charleston, SC	85 60	99 122	100 266	99 114	99 276	- 0	55 11	98 112	87 290	86 449	99 475	94 131	88 107	99 145	84 32	76 210	100 249	71 87	81 81	95 693	74 169	85 665	2.52 634	3.29 1643
Newberry County Memorial Hospital, Newberry, SC	100 3	92 13	57 7	100 9	100 9	- 0	- 0	- 0	74 42	83 119	77 144	93 27	75 64	84 50	83 18	92 88	100 92	71 58	91 22	80 83	84 19	65 83	- -	- -
Oconee Memorial Hospital, Seneca, SC	90 10	93 44	95 21	89 28	83 23	45 29	- 0	100 11	72 71	57 162	82 203	100 28	89 248	91 127	72 90	90 349	100 488	73 291	100 137	88 186	100 33	77 175	- -	- -

NOTE: The first number in each column (boldface) is the rate in percent, the second number is the number of patients; Please refer to the main entry for footnotes; ***Heart Attack Care:*** *1. ACE Inhibitor or ARB for LVSD; 2. Aspirin at Arrival; 3. Aspirin at Discharge; 4. Beta Blocker at Arrival; 5. Beta Blocker at Discharge; 6. Fibrinolytic Medication Timing; 7. PCI Within 90 Minutes of Arrival; 8. Smoking Cessation Advice;* ***Heart Failure Care:*** *9. ACE Inhibitor or ARB for LVSD; 10. Discharge Instructions; 11. Evaluation of LVS Function; 12. Smoking Cessation Advice;* ***Pneumonia Care:*** *13. Appropriate Initial Antibiotic; 14. Blood Culture Timing; 15. Influenza Vaccine; 16. Initial Antibiotic Timing; 17. Oxygenation Assessment; 18. Pneumococcal Vaccine; 19. Smoking Cessation Advice;* ***Surgical Infection Prevention:*** *20. Prophylactic Antibiotic Given; 21. Prophylactic Antibiotic Selection; 22. Prophylactic Antibiotic Stopped;* ***Pregnancy Care:*** *23. Inpatient Neonatal Mortality; 24. Third or Fourth Degree Laceration*

Hospital	Heart Attack Care 1	2	3	4	5	6	7	8	Heart Failure Care 9	10	11	12	13	14	Pneumonia Care 15	16	17	18	19	Surgical Infection Prevention 20	21	22	Pregnancy Care 23	24
Palmetto Baptist Medical Center Easley, Easley, SC	100 12	93 68	92 40	93 46	95 44	40 5	0	88 16	98 48	85 117	95 147	100 34	91 127	94 125	100 25	77 201	100 233	99 144	92 59	95 259	90 70	86 246		
Palmetto Health Baptist Columbia, Columbia, SC	100 5	98 60	97 33	100 43	100 34	0	0	80 5	93 87	86 198	98 232	95 63	81 172	94 175	73 52	81 222	100 274	85 144	88 83	92 1182	95 302	91 1154	0.20 3946	3.47 2364
Palmetto Health Richland Hospital, Columbia, SC	91 85	94 185	98 363	92 131	96 344	0	8 25	100 191	87 279	74 472	99 530	99 176	88 130	93 121	83 30	70 195	100 249	84 112	100 88	95 1725	93 478	84 1671		
Piedmont Medical Center, Rock Hill, SC	89 92	99 298	98 347	93 280	97 338	0	63 19	99 151	84 160	75 293	99 355	100 85	83 336	79 291	90 102	77 511	100 584	88 315	99 151	93 796	93 81	86 785		
Providence Hosp/Providence Heart Inst, Columbia, SC	92 59	96 171	98 302	94 162	95 292	0	25	100 124	90 181	96 277	99 326	100 67	83 150	100 20	92 51	64 164	100 221	84 142	100 59	89 268	93	69 261		
Regional Med Ctr of Orangeburg & Calhoun, Orangeburg, SC	81 16	96 114	91 57	93 82	96 67	55 11		94 16	82 119	53 373	89 412	98 98	78 184	94 204	58 48	87 303	100 360	68 174	98 88	86 194	92 59	87 182		
Roper Hospital, Charleston, SC	86 51	97 147	97 297	97 129	95 270		60 15	86 104	93 297	75 602	98 705	84 128	85 155	97 139	87 75	84 248	100 309	77 226	65 83	94 365	96 85	90 353	0.00 666	3.15 444
Saint Francis Hospital, Greenville, SC	97 37	100 139	99 171	100 102	99 193	100 2		100 65	99 193	66 325	100 372	100 97	92 225	96 232	87 73	79 274	99 345	86 292	100 99	96 812	99 85	93 310		
Self Regional Healthcare Center, Greenwood, SC	100 53	99 175	98 180	98 132	98 186	40 5	8 13	99 74	88 286	90 333	97 380	100 85	84 187	95 346	89 82	82 499	100 604	78 210	99 86	95 1545	88 310	81 1478		
Spartanburg Regional Health Care System, Spartanburg, SC	86 160	97 406	99 557	98 315	99 603	67 3	68 25	100 307	86 286	90 631	100 737	99 184	92 325	95 346	89 82	82 499	100 604	95 356	100 173	95 1545	88 310	81 1478		
Springs Memorial Hospital, Lancaster, SC	76 21	90 123	81 75	86 105	84 77	50 10		97 31	72 103	81 189	95 256	100 57	71 148	84 89	40	87 187	99 200	88 108	63	68 121	66 38	52 112		
Trident Medical Center, Charleston, SC	82 76	96 205	95 326	85 186	92 317		59 17	96 135	77 248	38 591	87 671	93 121	90 277	83 208	91	54 402	100 527	54 297	92 140	75 517	86 351	68 496	0.03 3533	1.91 2511
Tuomey Regional Medical Center, Sumter, SC	100 17	81 53	77 30	85 33	91 45			90 10	87 206	51 472	85 571	92 135	79 162	85 117	76 34	66 241	100 292	77 145	92 75	78 426	99 117	81 417		
Upstate Carolina Medical Center, Gaffney, SC	100 1	84 32	92 12	62 29	92 12	5	25 4	25 4	69 36	54 110	84 141	68 37	66 109	96 113		82 164	99 218	83 124	80 66	92 110	93 27	84 102		
Waccamaw Community Hospital, Murrells Inlet, SC	83 6	93 59	84 31	91 54	100 32	3		100 10	96 54	69 153	92 178	94 35	83 103	90 94	83 36	93 166	100 198	93 128	100 44	95 295	76 67	79 290		
Wallace Thomson Hospital, Union, SC		71 21	67 9	80 15	78 9	10		0	77 30	46 145	67 163	52 29	61 82	85 47	68 22	77 111	99 140	70 79	42 36	31 29	85 13	96 27		
Williamsburg Regional Hospital, Kingstree, SC	100 1	80 5	5 100	3 20	33 3			0	86 14	17 29	65 31	50 4	56 32	93 44		79 38	93 93	15 27	40 5	0 1		0		
Wilson Medical Center, Darlington, SC	100 1	100 1	0	0	100 1	1		0	93 27	17 6	49 100	100 1	100 1	93 15		72 29	100 33	90 21	100 1	0 1				
TEXAS																								
Abilene Regional Medical Center, Abilene, TX	100 33	100 66	99 152	100 58	99 138	67 6	38 8	100 57	97 68	100 136	100 166	100 49	91 65	81 31	82 22	72 67	100 87	76 54	100 36	87 633	82 174	59 584	0.34 1464	4.72 1038
Alice Regional Hospital, Alice, TX	100 7	97 76	88 33	97 60	96 27		100 2	100 2	94 64	98 40	98 240	100 10	91 22	88 33		83 213	99 235	92 137	100 5	94 16		53 15	0.00 580	1.27 393
Alliance Hospital, Odessa, TX	68 19	82 33	92 106	62 32	83 105	1	75 12	75 12	76 70	41 46	70 223	67 9	55 11	86 7		68 56	100 71	33 48	75 4	80 71	86 37	27 71		
Angleton-Danbury Medical Center, Angleton, TX	0 4	91 11	88 8	100 11	75 8		1	100 1	60 20	42 31	83 47	86 7	68 73	94 34	36 14	60 78	98 99	25 53	92 24	53 170	86 37	43 162		
Anson General Hospital, Anson, TX		0 1	0	0 1	0			0	100 3	15 13	77 22	67 3	72 25	100 9	75 8	100 29	95 38	70 27	50 6	0		0		
Arlington Memorial Hospital, Arlington, TX	82 65	99 217	98 210	96 185	97 200	83 6	25	93 81	81 197	67 386	84 473	87	87 244	91 264	81 62	87 346	100 396	90 230	100 109	84 180	88 58	62 169		
Atlanta Memorial Hospital, Atlanta, TX	100 2	75 8	100 8	40 5	67 6			0	65 43	42 97	79 112	36	65 63	100 7		68 90	93 107	75 63	54 26	100 9	44 9			
Austin Surgical Hospital, Austin, TX																				99 67		100 67		
Baptist Medical Center, San Antonio, TX	66 50	95 239	91 262	95 154	94 273		38 8	98 84	68 113	78 344	88 431	94 71	88 166	93 260	77 100	80 376	100 441	71 289	90 83	87 498	96 117	71 463	0.26 9512	2.40 6040
Baptist-Saint Anthony's Health System, Amarillo, TX	83 23	99 169	95 257	98 156	98 262	50	100 2	97 93	75 72	52 229	88 274	98 10	78 97	86 70	41 27	57 159	99 235	73 109	98 41	85 310	87 82	69 296		
Baylor All Saints Med Ctr at Forth Worth, Fort Worth, TX	85 52	95 175	96 185	95 150	98 182	100	100 2	82 58	82 197	79 387	95 459	91 91	88 214	92 198	66 69	91 257	100 300	92 172	92 65	97 1383	97 329	90 1323		
Baylor Heart and Vascular Center, Dallas, TX	100 23	100 12	100 140	100 140	99 136		100 9	100 53	100 234	100 266	100 268	100 50	100 100	100		92 75	100 106	86 58	100 2	99 176	83 58	88 165		
Baylor Medical Center at Frisco, Frisco, TX																				83 58	72 58			
Baylor Medical Center at Garland, Garland, TX	100 36	100 200	98 189	100 183	99 190	0	75 12	98 66	93 122	83 345	95 426	100 82	89 179	96 172	52 50	85 202	100 281	92 152	100 62	95 721	99 162	85 699		
Baylor Medical Center at Irving, Irving, TX	97 36	100 211	97 198	99 192	99 183		79 14	100 75	96 136	86 288	99 324	98 57	94 173	88 194	75 64	90 265	100 299	94 176	99 70	96 760	97 176	87 719		
Baylor Medical Center-Ellis County, Waxahachie, TX	100 3	100 12	100 9	92 12	100 9	100 1		0	96 25	83 66	95 88	89 18	91 106	93 96	93 29	91 139	100 167	90 83	81 36	97 306	96 76	98 296		
Baylor Regional Medical Center at Grapevine, Grapevine, TX	95 22	100 172	98 162	99 161	96 150	100 1	92 12	92 60	96 46	77 128	94 150	100 23	91 136	84 118	81 37	86 159	100 201	86 105	96 51	96 805	92 184	79 797		
Baylor Regional Medical Center at Plano, Plano, TX	100 35	100 87	100 122	100 77	98 122		100 3	100 17	95 177	95 65	99 266	100 9	100 10	94 17	37	92 75	100 106	86 58	100 2	98 124		88 113		
Baylor University Medical Center, Dallas, TX	94 171	98 313	97 545	97 227	98 509		90	100 236	93 446	88 805	99 944	100 249	89 396	91 373	89 142	79 573	100 691	86 367	99 170	94 3530	88 877	89 3460		
Bayshore Medical Center, Pasadena, TX	74 35	90 212	88 194	86 162	87 188	73 15		99 87	67 149	30 432	87 592	96 138	73 262	85 231	85 72	69 369	100 445	83 241	96 130	39 202	67 94	57 184		
Beaumont Bone & Joint Institute, Beaumont, TX																								
Bellville General Hospital, Bellville, TX		0 100		0 100				0 100	92	29 100	83	100 6	48	100	58 12	87 47	91 56	43 35	100 12	75 4	50 2	100 4		
Big Bend Regional Medical Center, Alpine, TX	0 100	8 100	8 100	9 100	80 5			0	71 14	12 26	47 30	75 4	78 50	86	77 31	91 113	100 121	91 79	77 13	79	87	69		
Bowie Memorial Hospital, Bowie, TX	100 2	94 16	100 13	100 14	98 12			100 3	47	26	52 100	100 3	80 74	91	31	95 111	100 134	92	30	25 4	0 1	100 4		
Brackenridge Hospital, Austin, TX	100 11	100 89	100 90	99 99	99 86	0	80	100 51	99 108	82 236	99 249	96 109	84 108	85 86	47 17	71 144	99 152	44 39	70 56	74 135	40 79	79 135		
Brazosport Memorial Hospital, Lake Jackson, TX	50 4	98 48	88 16	86 51	82 22	73 15		50 2	58 57	74 117	97 142	54 28	71 121	84 94	74 34	83 160	98 192	83 111	73 44	68 91	91	49 92		
Brownfield Regional Medical Center, Brownfield, TX	0 100	100 4	100	100 1	0 1	0		25 4	4 0	0 36	42 40	33 6	95 21	100	30 47	93 41	100 45	13 31	33 3	39 202	67	57		
Brownsville Medical Center, Brownsville, TX	95 57	97 205	97 177	99 174	98 178	2	4	97 31	98 100	94 263	96 253	93 14	75 107	81 89	30	59 169	97 198	30 128	95 20	68 150	100 39	70 144		
Brownsville Surgical Hospital, Brownsville, TX		0 100	100 1	100 1	100 1	1		100 1	100	0 100	0 1	100 1	100	100 1	47	0 100	100 3	100 2		94 62	100 20	92 60		

NOTE: The first number in each column (boldface) is the rate in percent; the second number is the number of patients; Please refer to the main entry for footnotes; **Heart Attack Care:** 1. ACE Inhibitor or ARB for LVSD; 2. Aspirin at Arrival; 3. Aspirin at Discharge; 4. Beta Blocker at Arrival; 5. Beta Blocker at Discharge; 6. Fibrinolytic Medication Timing; 7. PCI Within 90 Minutes of Arrival; 8. Smoking Cessation Advice; **Heart Failure Care:** 9. ACE Inhibitor or ARB for LVSD; 10. Discharge Instructions; 11. Evaluation of LVS Function; 12. Smoking Cessation Advice; **Pneumonia Care:** 13. Appropriate Initial Antibiotic; 14. Blood Culture Timing; 15. Influenza Vaccine; 16. Initial Antibiotic Timing; 17. Oxygenation Assessment; 18. Pneumococcal Vaccine; 19. Smoking Cessation Advice; **Surgical Infection Prevention:** 20. Prophylactic Antibiotic Given; 21. Prophylactic Antibiotic Selection; 22. Prophylactic Antibiotic Stopped; **Pregnancy Care:** 23. Inpatient Neonatal Mortality; 24. Third or Fourth Degree Laceration

Hospital	Heart Attack Care								Heart Failure Care				Pneumonia Care							Surgical Infection Prevention			Pregnancy Care	
	1	2	3	4	5	6	7	8	9	10	11	12	13	14	15	16	17	18	19	20	21	22	23	24
Brownwood Regional Medical Center, Brownwood, TX	- 0	78 18	100 5	73 15	100 5	- 0	- 0	100 2	94 50	62 121	80 162	100 35	72 130	92 135	87 70	80 225	100 272	83 162	87 68	44 272	73 64	52 256	- -	- -
Campbell Health System, Weatherford, TX	50 2	89 27	70 10	84 31	82 11	- 0	- 0	100 1	54 26	88 25	65 130	100 3	81 21	91 23	- -	93 158	100 214	19 128	78 9	52 90	- -	46 81	- -	- -
Centennial Medical Center, Frisco, TX	83 18	98 62	100 71	97 59	99 72	50 2	71 7	90 31	67 27	30 60	88 81	100 22	79 66	96 56	61 18	94 68	100 96	71 48	100 14	92 142	88 34	57 127	- -	- -
Central Texas Hospital, Cameron, TX	- -	- -	- -	- -	- -	- -	- -	- -	- 0	0 15	25 24	33 3	100 3	100 3	- -	80 5	100 7	0 8	100 2	- -	- -	- -	- -	- -
Central Texas Medical Center, San Marcos, TX	89 9	98 47	92 25	95 43	88 26	100 1	- 0	- 0	77 52	61 28	92 132	100 3	57 14	71 17	- -	78 123	99 158	83 92	67 3	90 59	- -	97 58	- -	- -
Charlton Methodist Hospital, Dallas, TX	98 44	98 234	99 194	97 163	100 228	100 1	54 13	100 81	96 250	77 449	97 552	98 149	80 169	90 156	88 50	82 291	100 312	93 146	99 73	98 139	100 39	85 135	0.21 2362	1.31 1681
Childress Regional Medical Center, Childress, TX	- 0	50 2	50 2	50 2	50 2	- 0	- -	100 1	86 7	38 26	84 31	100 2	94 32	100 5	- -	82 55	100 67	83 41	100 14	87 46	100 19	13 46	- -	- -
Christus Jasper Memorial Hospital, Jasper, TX	100 1	50 4	100 3	50 4	100 2	- 0	- -	- 0	82 22	76 55	95 79	100 17	74 46	79 38	55 22	68 69	100 78	62 53	94 16	85 46	88 16	50 44	- -	- -
Christus Saint Catherine Hospital, Katy, TX	100 5	96 47	91 22	95 42	96 27	0 3	- 0	100 6	98 49	85 130	100 155	100 19	90 151	92 78	95 20	89 143	100 159	93 86	100 28	68 155	94 31	73 146	- -	- -
Christus Saint Elizabeth Hospital, Beaumont, TX	83 88	95 352	98 432	89 301	94 430	0 3	71 21	99 188	89 348	90 812	93 928	96 236	83 406	87 392	92 114	81 564	99 636	87 339	89 179	64 1358	75 365	52 1312	- -	- -
Christus Saint John Hospital, Houston, TX	100 31	99 119	98 101	98 121	98 100	100 1	25 8	98 50	100 87	73 177	100 210	100 36	84 160	99 135	100 35	92 165	100 191	95 119	100 34	78 348	77 82	25 335	- -	- -
Christus Saint Michael Health System, Texarkana, TX	91 125	99 321	97 363	95 257	97 356	67 3	0 9	100 150	90 324	80 515	97 660	100 96	88 253	95 227	89 66	82 358	100 413	87 252	100 125	92 1260	90 296	46 1223	- -	- -
Christus Santa Rosa Hospital-City Centre, San Antonio, TX	96 28	100 161	98 160	98 143	98 164	0 2	33 6	98 49	95 129	96 554	99 602	100 90	86 192	95 167	- -	80 257	100 281	96 143	100 54	83 1183	94 335	48 1164	- -	- -
Christus Spohn Hospital Beeville, Beeville, TX	75 4	100 22	92 13	84 19	70 10	- 0	- 0	100 1	98 49	82 38	95 222	100 12	86 7	100 9	- -	95 96	99 115	82 66	100 6	20 5	- -	67 3	0.24 412	1.61 249
Christus Spohn Hospital Kleberg, Kingsville, TX	100 1	92 12	88 8	92 13	75 8	0 1	- 0	100 2	64 50	85 152	79 179	100 43	89 167	94 63	- -	84 204	97 226	86 121	100 39	86 64	93 14	64 64	0.00 345	1.19 168
Christus Spohn Memorial Hospital, Corpus Christi, TX	78 116	96 402	96 529	94 369	96 552	0 2	67 6	100 175	80 466	74 1028	96 1190	99 192	83 537	85 513	- -	72 801	100 939	78 533	98 208	77 1444	93 533	39 1412	0.39 3588	3.32 2139
Citizens Medical Center, Victoria, TX	100 22	100 133	100 157	100 112	100 147	67 6	100 1	100 44	100 88	100 247	100 296	97 33	89 94	96 79	38 50	84 150	100 175	81 111	85 33	89 447	94 172	69 438	0.10 1039	3.27 551
Clear Lake Regional Medical Center, Webster, TX	95 97	98 372	97 409	95 315	97 390	100 2	95 20	98 168	84 219	44 386	100 526	89 74	86 178	96 213	90 72	79 267	99 338	90 197	94 100	76 238	69 101	56 228	- -	- -
Cleveland Regional Medical Center, Cleveland, TX	60 5	97 29	67 12	83 24	73 15	0 1	- 0	100 1	65 46	6 112	83 141	79 38	82 96	79 72	52 23	75 128	98 144	58 66	97 58	30 54	89 27	75 53	- -	- -
Coleman County Medical Center, Coleman, TX	- 0	100 1	100 1	100 1	- 0	100 1	- 0	- 0	80 10	54 26	67 36	40 5	71 52	100 43	100 29	92 36	100 96	90 73	60 15	- -	- -	- -	- -	- -
College Station Medical Center, College Station, TX	94 18	98 51	98 61	100 33	100 61	- 0	0 3	100 20	96 52	69 93	99 103	100 18	94 54	95 43	94 18	90 60	100 75	91 44	100 21	97 270	92 75	87 268	- -	- -
Colorado Fayette Medical Center, Weimar, TX	- 0	89 9	100 5	86 7	100 6	- 0	- 0	- 0	0 1	0 5	15 46	0 1	100 5	100 2	- -	79 48	100 57	58 40	0 2	25 4	- -	100 3	- -	- -
Columbia Spring Branch Medical Center, Houston, TX	83 35	91 113	84 114	89 97	90 121	100 1	0 6	98 54	81 119	53 227	95 300	94 67	74 127	93 149	79 42	87 253	98 266	83 157	88 57	66 158	82 66	53 155	- -	- -
Columbus Community Hospital, Columbus, TX	- 0	100 2	100 2	100 3	100 3	- 0	- 0	- 0	75 12	100 3	91 34	- 0	67 3	100 4	- -	89 37	98 43	90 30	- 0	100 9	- -	100 9	- -	- -
Comanche County Medical Center, Comanche, TX	100 4	77 13	88 8	80 10	100 3	- 0	- 0	- 0	92 13	63 52	74 86	82 11	90 41	95 22	100 10	78 49	100 60	90 40	75 8	72 18	100 4	100 17	- -	- -
Community General Hospital, Dilley, TX	- 0	100 2	- 0	100 2	- 0	- 0	- 0	- 0	- 0	100 3	100 3	- 0	100 1	100 1	- -	100 2	100 2	- 0	100 1	- -	- -	- -	- -	- -
Connally Memorial Medical Center, Floresville, TX	100 3	82 34	78 23	56 34	62 21	- 0	- 0	100 2	60 5	22 9	82 17	100 1	42 24	88 24	100 11	55 42	100 52	91 43	100 9	48 25	100 7	91 22	- -	- -
Conroe Regional Medical Center, Conroe, TX	87 75	100 225	99 270	95 149	96 243	70 10	81 16	99 138	91 190	62 498	96 482	97 154	87 260	89 210	71 62	77 337	99 383	77 216	97 130	91 291	88 168	69 251	- -	- -
Coon Memorial Hospital, Dalhart, TX	- 0	100 1	100 1	100 2	100 2	- 0	- 0	- 0	100 4	5 19	24 29	0 3	45 20	100 4	67 9	53 30	100 36	70 23	40 10	- -	- -	- -	- -	- -
Cornerstone Regional Hospital, Edinburg, TX	- -	- -	- -	- -	- -	- -	- -	- -	- 0	- 0	- 0	- 0	- 0	- 0	- -	96 23	100 24	92 13	- 0	88 51	- -	92 51	- -	- -
Corpus Christi Medical Center-Bay Area, Corpus Christi, TX	87 31	99 174	95 242	92 160	92 248	0 1	22 9	87 82	79 153	44 388	88 455	64 67	72 204	89 185	58 79	70 297	99 377	69 262	68 71	69 291	96 156	41 282	0.20 3506	2.05 2099
Coryell Memorial Hospital, Gatesville, TX	100 3	91 11	100 7	85 13	78 9	- 0	- 0	- 0	50 2	100 4	41 34	100 2	- 0	75 4	- -	83 78	100 98	91 76	100 1	0 1	- -	100 1	- -	- -
Covenant Hospital Levelland, Levelland, TX	- 0	50 2	- 0	0 3	0 1	- -	- -	- -	100 1	0 7	4 25	0 1	90 10	100 1	- -	90 30	95 43	24 21	0 4	17 6	- -	100 1	- -	- -
Covenant Hospital Plainview, Plainview, TX	- 0	100 1	100 1	100 1	0 1	- 0	- 0	- 0	80 15	36 14	40 60	0 1	71 7	100 4	- -	71 49	100 63	57 42	50 2	20 15	- -	100 13	- -	- -
Covenant Medical Center, Lubbock, TX	75 132	95 225	93 531	83 189	92 541	- 0	41 17	100 214	66 314	33 665	85 802	98 127	78 329	94 477	70 186	74 616	100 726	78 473	97 158	71 272	77 101	43 246	- -	- -
Cozby-Germany Hospital, Grand Saline, TX	- 0	0 1	0 1	0 1	100 1	- 0	- 0	- 0	80 5	67 24	94 34	89 9	89 35	82 40	44 16	94 64	100 74	44 50	69 13	- -	- -	- -	- -	- -
Cuero Community Hospital, Cuero, TX	100 1	93 14	83 6	86 14	86 7	0 1	- 0	100 1	95 20	100 50	94 77	75 8	75 83	97 39	100 18	96 103	100 119	100 81	100 11	40 5	100 1	100 4	- -	- -
Cypress Fairbanks Medical Center and Hospital, Houston, TX	100 5	98 101	100 78	93 85	96 70	33 3	86 14	100 26	84 81	58 197	97 262	97 36	92 202	88 219	87 76	82 265	100 379	89 189	95 66	85 119	94 33	48 106	- -	- -
D M Cogdell Memorial Hospital, Snyder, TX	100 1	100 1	100 1	- 0	100 1	- 0	- 0	- 0	- 0	0 6	18 40	100 1	100 5	83 6	- -	72 39	83 54	20 20	100 5	- -	- -	- -	- -	- -
Dallas Southwest Medical Center, Dallas, TX	- 0	100 4	- 0	83 6	- 0	- 0	- 0	- 0	83 6	0 14	92 36	20 5	50 4	57 7	- -	83 18	100 19	0 6	- 0	44 18	- -	100 18	- -	- -
Del Sol Medical Center, El Paso, TX	71 34	98 207	89 189	91 139	94 159	38 16	50 8	96 67	73 150	84 378	81 429	95 76	64 333	91 239	39 88	67 451	99 535	33 315	93 123	64 129	84 49	75 118	- -	- -
Denton Regional Medical Center, Denton, TX	100 21	99 128	96 202	98 114	99 198	- 0	80 5	96 77	85 79	93 220	92 272	100 52	87 118	90 136	55 58	81 200	100 239	62 141	96 55	87 223	98 109	85 211	- -	- -
Detar Hospital Navarro, Victoria, TX	100 35	98 82	100 159	97 62	99 173	25 4	50 2	100 62	99 72	100 197	98 296	100 47	88 93	99 88	83 36	83 118	100 152	97 107	100 44	94 450	96 113	81 444	0.15 1306	2.82 710
Dickerson Memorial Hospital, Jasper, TX	- 0	80 5	0 2	60 5	33 3	- 0	- -	100 1	- 0	0 8	13 15	- 0	50 4	0 1	- -	86 7	100 22	0 3	0 1	0 2	- -	50 2	- -	- -
Dimmit County Memorial Hospital, Carrizo Springs, TX	- 0	60 5	0 1	50 4	0 2	- 0	- 0	- 0	- 0	0 5	0 40	- 0	100 3	100 4	- -	66 29	94 36	32 22	0 2	- 0	- -	- 0	- -	- -
Doctors Hospital, Dallas, TX	100 28	99 141	98 130	99 119	100 122	0 1	67 3	98 45	94 144	90 292	98 365	93 75	91 193	95 171	76 54	77 225	100 284	74 172	84 68	75 244	71 58	71 223	- -	- -
Doctors Hospital at Renaissance, Edinburg, TX	69 51	93 119	88 203	75 113	81 212	0 1	50 6	80 35	70 193	42 359	90 425	80 56	80 85	92 65	20 20	46 112	100 153	18 102	75 20	76 372	74 98	45 346	- -	- -
Doctors Hospital of Laredo, Laredo, TX	100 9	96 48	90 29	93 43	86 28	50 10	- 0	89 9	84 62	37 200	73 226	77 30	75 64	64 67	55 22	65 121	100 127	51 78	92 12	43 184	92 36	67 166	- -	- -

NOTE: The first number in each column (boldface) is the rate in percent, the second number is the number of patients; Please refer to the main entry for footnotes; ***Heart Attack Care:*** *1. ACE Inhibitor or ARB for LVSD; 2. Aspirin at Arrival; 3. Aspirin at Discharge; 4. Beta Blocker at Arrival; 5. Beta Blocker at Discharge; 6. Fibrinolytic Medication Timing; 7. PCI Within 90 Minutes of Arrival; 8. Smoking Cessation Advice;* ***Heart Failure Care:*** *9. ACE Inhibitor or ARB for LVSD; 10. Discharge Instructions; 11. Evaluation of LVS Function; 12. Smoking Cessation Advice;* ***Pneumonia Care:*** *13. Appropriate Initial Antibiotic; 14. Blood Culture Timing; 15. Influenza Vaccine; 16. Initial Antibiotic Timing; 17. Oxygenation Assessment; 18. Pneumococcal Vaccine; 19. Smoking Cessation Advice;* ***Surgical Infection Prevention:*** *20. Prophylactic Antibiotic Given; 21. Prophylactic Antibiotic Selection; 22. Prophylactic Antibiotic Stopped;* ***Pregnancy Care:*** *23. Inpatient Neonatal Mortality; 24. Third or Fourth Degree Laceration*

Hospital	Heart Attack Care								Heart Failure Care				Pneumonia Care							Surgical Infection Prevention			Pregnancy Care	
	1	2	3	4	5	6	7	8	9	10	11	12	13	14	15	16	17	18	19	20	21	22	23	24
Doctors Hospital Parkway+Tidwell, Houston, TX	**81** 27	**80** 103	**66** 100	**56** 80	**65** 97	**0** 1	- 0	**79** 14	**67** 123	**17** 64	**80** 287	**45** 22	**78** 9	**86** 14	- -	**60** 126	**95** 132	**10** 58	**25** 8	**29** 24	- -	**17** 24	- -	- -
Dolly Vinsant Memorial Hospital, San Benito, TX	- 0	**0** 1	- 0	**0** 1	- 0	- 0	- -	- 0	- 0	**82** 17	**100** 14	**100** 1	**41** 29	**100** 5	**50** 4	**71** 34	**100** 40	**53** 15	**89** 9	- 0	- 0	- 0	- -	- -
East Houston Regional Medical Center, Houston, TX	**94** 32	**94** 156	**92** 106	**88** 130	**92** 106	**27** 15	- 0	**93** 55	**87** 149	**61** 332	**88** 369	**96** 109	**79** 170	**94** 139	**52** 40	**76** 223	**98** 245	**69** 113	**90** 93	**70** 105	**71** 41	**81** 93	- -	- -
East Texas Medical Center-Athens, Athens, TX	**80** 10	**98** 86	**95** 39	**93** 85	**88** 41	**0** 1	- 0	**100** 14	**79** 68	**98** 232	**91** 280	**100** 53	**86** 130	**95** 79	**73** 33	**83** 187	**99** 208	**65** 125	**93** 57	**79** 124	**48** 52	**69** 120	- -	- -
East Texas Medical Center-Carthage, Carthage, TX	**100** 1	**100** 7	**100** 4	**40** 5	**80** 5	- 0	- 0	- 0	**81** 16	**59** 32	**95** 40	**57** 7	**94** 54	**83** 35	**69** 13	**88** 50	**100** 69	**80** 40	**65** 17	**0** 2	- -	**0** 2	- -	- -
East Texas Medical Center-Clarksville, Clarksville, TX	**100** 3	**78** 9	**100** 5	**86** 7	**100** 5	- 0	- 0	**100** 1	**84** 38	**63** 27	**88** 138	**67** 9	**100** 8	**85** 13	- -	**87** 116	**99** 145	**62** 91	**88** 8	- -	- -	- -	- -	- -
East Texas Medical Center-Crockett, Crockett, TX	- 0	**77** 22	**67** 15	**82** 17	**77** 13	- 0	- 0	**100** 1	**95** 22	**63** 76	**84** 107	**86** 28	**67** 48	**96** 25	- -	**90** 70	**98** 87	**58** 65	**83** 12	**52** 21	**100** 6	**95** 20	- -	- -
East Texas Medical Center-Fairfield, Fairfield, TX	- 0	**100** 1	- 0	- 0	**0** 1	- 0	- 0	- 0	**83** 6	**0** 13	**43** 67	**50** 2	**80** 10	**91** 11	- -	**71** 34	**98** 47	**43** 30	**100** 1	- 0	- -	- 0	- -	- -
East Texas Medical Center-Gilmer, Gilmer, TX	- 0	**40** 5	**67** 3	**100** 4	**75** 4	- 0	- 0	- 0	**90** 21	**17** 24	**70** 88	**50** 4	**71** 14	**86** 7	- -	**58** 65	**100** 93	**62** 47	**100** 1	- -	- -	- -	- -	- -
East Texas Medical Center-Jacksonville, Jacksonville, TX	- 0	**80** 10	**86** 7	**75** 8	**100** 7	- 0	- 0	**0** 1	**62** 16	**86** 7	**94** 64	**100** 3	**90** 10	**100** 11	- -	**90** 90	**100** 106	**79** 61	**100** 4	**60** 15	- -	**50** 14	- -	- -
East Texas Medical Center-Mount Vernon, Mount Vernon, TX	- 0	**0** 2	**67** 3	**67** 3	**67** 3	- 0	- -	- 0	**100** 4	**14** 14	**62** 26	**67** 3	**87** 15	**88** 8	**100** 1	**93** 15	**100** 19	**85** 13	**67** 3	- 0	- 0	- 0	- -	- -
East Texas Medical Center-Pittsburg, Pittsburg, TX	- 0	- 0	- 0	- 0	- 0	- 0	- 0	- 0	**79** 14	**54** 54	**49** 79	**71** 21	**81** 27	**100** 12	- -	**78** 32	**100** 40	**77** 22	**100** 9	**67** 3	**100** 1	**100** 3	- -	- -
East Texas Medical Center-Quitman, Quitman, TX	- 0	**88** 8	**83** 6	**71** 7	**83** 6	- 0	- 0	**100** 1	**100** 12	**58** 55	**74** 80	**75** 8	**86** 43	**81** 37	**76** 17	**91** 57	**100** 75	**94** 51	**81** 16	**62** 13	**100** 6	**23** 13	- -	- -
East Texas Medical Center-Trinity, Trinity, TX	**100** 1	**75** 4	**100** 2	**100** 4	**50** 2	- 0	- 0	- 0	**73** 11	**67** 3	**52** 48	**100** 1	**67** 3	- 0	- -	**46** 41	**100** 51	**32** 31	**100** 2	- -	- -	- -	- -	- -
East Texas Medical Center-Tyler, Tyler, TX	**82** 66	**95** 106	**97** 275	**92** 93	**93** 276	**0** 2	**50** 4	**79** 110	**71** 188	**25** 293	**88** 383	**60** 77	**73** 52	**81** 37	**31** 16	**57** 81	**100** 101	**34** 68	**47** 38	**36** 159	**70** 60	**69** 150	**0.00** 246	**6.21** 177
Eastland Memorial Hospital, Eastland, TX	- 0	**100** 1	- 0	**100** 1	- 0	- -	- -	- -	**69** 16	**17** 12	**52** 71	**0** 2	**91** 11	**88** 17	- -	**82** 114	**83** 121	**69** 83	**100** 3	**0** 5	- -	**100** 5	- -	- -
Edinburg Regional Medical Center, Edinburg, TX	**45** 11	**87** 46	**55** 31	**77** 35	**65** 31	- 0	- 0	**33** 3	**44** 43	**43** 130	**81** 154	**65** 17	**83** 78	**95** 43	**73** 15	**56** 90	**99** 120	**55** 73	**92** 25	**36** 55	**92** 13	**16** 55	- -	- -
El Campo Memorial Hospital, El Campo, TX	- 0	**71** 17	**100** 4	**64** 14	**60** 5	- 0	- 0	- 0	**60** 5	**50** 46	**90** 59	**0** 6	**66** 44	**100** 31	**82** 11	**79** 70	**100** 77	**80** 50	**20** 10	**100** 2	**0** 2	**100** 2	- -	- -
El Paso Specialty Hospital, El Paso, TX	- -	- -	- -	- -	- -	- -	- -	- -	- -	- -	- -	- -	- -	- -	- -	- -	- -	- -	- -	**88** 341	**100** 109	**90** 340	- -	- -
Ennis Regional Medical Center, Ennis, TX	- 0	**100** 4	**50** 2	**100** 4	**100** 2	**0** 1	- 0	- 0	**93** 30	**55** 73	**73** 99	**83** 23	**82** 67	**79** 52	**48** 25	**77** 96	**99** 107	**46** 68	**96** 24	**43** 72	**100** 26	**76** 71	- -	- -
Faith Community Hospital, Jacksboro, TX	**100** 1	**71** 7	**75** 4	**25** 8	**71** 7	- 0	- 0	**50** 2	**78** 9	**67** 12	**67** 18	**100** 3	**83** 12	**100** 4	**86** 7	**94** 17	**100** 20	**100** 11	**80** 5	- -	- -	- -	- -	- -
Falls Community Hospital, Marlin, TX	**100** 1	**100** 1	**100** 1	**100** 1	**100** 1	- 0	- 0	**100** 1	**72** 18	**85** 85	**96** 105	**100** 25	**75** 97	**98** 62	**96** 24	**88** 144	**100** 165	**95** 81	**96** 53	- -	- -	- -	- -	- -
Fort Duncan Medical Center, Eagle Pass, TX	**100** 4	**91** 34	**53** 19	**61** 28	**47** 19	- 0	- 0	**100** 3	**74** 78	**68** 217	**39** 220	**79** 39	**74** 110	**67** 67	**35** 20	**66** 116	**96** 126	**61** 79	**79** 14	**40** 53	**89** 19	**95** 43	- -	- -
Foundation Surgical Hospital, Bellaire, TX	- -	- -	- -	- -	- -	- -	- -	- -	- -	- -	- -	- -	- -	- -	- -	- -	- -	- -	- -	**63** 19	- -	**95** 19	- -	- -
Frio Hospital, Pearsall, TX	- 0	**100** 2	- 0	**100** 2	**100** 1	- 0	- 0	- 0	**100** 11	**91** 34	**93** 29	**100** 3	**90** 31	**80** 25	**100** 14	**94** 36	**100** 44	**100** 18	**93** 14	- 0	- 0	- 0	- -	- -
Georgetown Healthcare System, Georgetown, TX	**50** 4	**100** 17	**91** 11	**94** 18	**64** 11	- 0	- 0	- 0	**74** 27	**45** 60	**71** 87	**75** 8	**81** 81	**90** 62	**43** 23	**76** 99	**99** 140	**70** 96	**56** 18	**70** 115	**94** 51	**69** 112	- -	- -
Glen Rose Medical Center, Glen Rose, TX	- 0	**50** 2	**100** 1	**50** 2	- 0	- 0	- 0	- 0	**100** 15	**67** 3	**91** 34	- 0	**62** 8	**100** 8	- -	**93** 94	**100** 114	**95** 65	**100** 3	**89** 9	- -	**100** 9	- -	- -
Good Shephard Medical Center-Linden, Linden, TX	**0** 1	**100** 2	**100** 2	**50** 2	**33** 3	- 0	- 0	- 0	**100** 1	**0** 23	**21** 28	**29** 7	**100** 7	- 0	- -	**90** 10	**100** 13	**0** 6	**0** 2	**50** 2	- 0	**100** 1	- -	- -
Good Shepherd Medical Center, Longview, TX	**96** 48	**100** 244	**100** 292	**99** 208	**98** 257	- 0	- 0	**97** 111	**97** 124	**94** 261	**91** 318	**100** 60	**92** 90	**86** 91	**85** 27	**79** 141	**99** 167	**59** 102	**90** 51	**64** 70	**89** 74	**85** 68	- -	- -
Goodall-Witcher Healthcare Foundation, Clifton, TX	**100** 2	**100** 10	**62** 8	**60** 5	**80** 5	**0** 1	- 0	- 0	**88** 17	**97** 39	**77** 65	**80** 10	**75** 55	**94** 49	**97** 33	**86** 83	**99** 118	**85** 92	**93** 15	**50** 6	- -	**33** 6	- -	- -
Graham Regional Medical Center, Graham, TX	**100** 1	**80** 5	**100** 2	**100** 3	**100** 1	- 0	- 0	- 0	**100** 18	**85** 59	**100** 68	**100** 20	**98** 51	**95** 43	**94** 17	**93** 86	**100** 101	**98** 80	**100** 23	**100** 3	**100** 3	**100** 3	- -	- -
Grimes-Saint Joseph's Health Center, Navasota, TX	- -	- -	- -	- -	- -	- -	- -	- -	**100** 1	- 0	**100** 1	- 0	**75** 4	- -	- -	**67** 3	**100** 4	**100** 2	- 0	- -	- -	- -	- -	- -
Guadalupe Valley Hospital, Seguin, TX	**100** 3	**83** 29	**92** 12	**83** 23	**83** 12	- 0	- 0	**100** 2	**76** 50	**71** 121	**67** 193	**67** 18	**87** 47	**93** 56	**8** 25	**78** 91	**100** 103	**36** 72	**67** 12	**61** 200	**70** 69	**62** 185	- -	- -
Gulf Coast Medical Center, Wharton, TX	**100** 3	**92** 25	**91** 11	**85** 13	**92** 12	**0** 6	- 0	**67** 3	**94** 31	**36** 75	**92** 88	**59** 17	**88** 50	**92** 38	**40** 10	**85** 71	**95** 80	**89** 47	**82** 17	**88** 145	**91** 35	**81** 141	- -	- -
Hamilton General Hospital, Hamilton, TX	**100** 2	**100** 14	**78** 9	**80** 15	**75** 8	- 0	- 0	- 0	**89** 18	**46** 74	**60** 107	**57** 7	**76** 86	**89** 18	**56** 36	**88** 93	**96** 128	**72** 98	**82** 11	**33** 3	**100** 1	**100** 3	- -	- -
Hamlin Memorial Hospital, Hamlin, TX	- 0	- 0	- 0	- 0	- 0	- -	- -	- -	**100** 4	**25** 4	**53** 17	**0** 3	**50** 2	- 0	- -	**100** 13	**100** 14	**70** 10	- 0	- -	- -	- -	- -	- -
Harlingen Medical Center, Harlingen, TX	**100** 17	**100** 65	**100** 72	**100** 64	**100** 67	- 0	- 0	**100** 13	**100** 38	**96** 146	**97** 168	**100** 9	**88** 101	**92** 99	**62** 42	**84** 153	**100** 165	**82** 108	**100** 17	**85** 258	**93** 86	**62** 255	- -	- -
Harris County Hospital District, Houston, TX	**93** 68	**99** 204	**97** 228	**96** 155	**95** 229	**0** 7	**17** 6	**84** 100	**86** 406	**57** 678	**97** 697	**79** 247	**87** 247	**82** 237	- -	**48** 332	**98** 371	**36** 96	**67** 144	**72** 296	**63** 118	**67** 289	- -	- -
Harris Methodist Continued Care Hospital, Fort Worth, TX	**79** 108	**96** 476	**99** 620	**93** 393	**98** 640	**0** 4	**70** 33	**94** 288	**98** 338	**72** 686	**92** 849	**85** 143	**87** 417	**95** 648	**85** 180	**89** 776	**100** 903	**86** 525	**84** 193	**89** 248	**95** 82	**78** 234	- -	- -
Harris Methodist Erath County, Stephenville, TX	**75** 4	**98** 42	**95** 22	**91** 34	**95** 22	**71** 7	- 0	**100** 4	**100** 15	**94** 62	**93** 71	**100** 6	**58** 83	**95** 91	**83** 42	**89** 122	**99** 160	**87** 92	**100** 40	**94** 99	**76** 29	**76** 96	- -	- -
Harris Methodist HEB Hospital, Bedford, TX	**96** 25	**98** 191	**100** 185	**95** 133	**97** 186	- 0	**80** 10	**100** 70	**98** 93	**75** 220	**92** 274	**98** 50	**85** 194	**92** 212	**89** 71	**89** 257	**100** 327	**92** 200	**99** 88	**74** 180	**91** 58	**77** 155	- -	- -
Harris Methodist Northwest, Azle, TX	**67** 3	**93** 30	**100** 9	**95** 21	**89** 9	**100** 5	- 0	**80** 5	**95** 20	**92** 73	**93** 91	**94** 17	**86** 139	**93** 114	**84** 44	**97** 161	**100** 210	**78** 131	**99** 70	**52** 52	**94** 17	**31** 48	- -	- -
Harris Methodist Southlake Ctr for Diag, Southlake, TX	- -	- -	- -	- -	- -	- -	- -	- -	- -	- -	- -	- -	- -	- -	- -	- -	- -	- -	- -	**71** 31	- -	**100** 28	- -	- -
Harris Methodist Southwest, Fort Worth, TX	**100** 9	**98** 87	**95** 61	**100** 78	**100** 59	**25** 8	- 0	**78** 9	**100** 57	**99** 161	**90** 231	**90** 42	**81** 165	**90** 187	**84** 63	**87** 237	**100** 292	**87** 172	**95** 42	**85** 110	**80** 40	**65** 100	- -	- -
Healthsouth Hospital For Specialized Surgery, Houston, TX	- -	- -	- -	- -	- -	- -	- -	- -	- -	- -	- -	- -	- -	- -	- -	- -	- -	- -	- -	- 0	- -	- 0	- -	- -
Healthsouth Medical Center, Dallas, TX	- -	- -	- -	- -	- -	- -	- -	- -	- -	- -	- -	- -	- -	- -	- -	- -	- -	- -	- -	- -	- -	- -	- -	- -
Healthsouth Surgical Hospital of Austin, Austin, TX	- -	- -	- -	- -	- -	- -	- -	- -	- -	- -	- -	- -	- -	- -	- -	- -	- -	- -	- -	**17** 6	- -	**100** 6	- -	- -
Heart Hospital of Austin, Austin, TX	**89** 105	**100** 111	**99** 454	**96** 96	**96** 426	- 0	**36** 14	**93** 174	**85** 232	**60** 320	**96** 361	**80** 65	**56** 25	**94** 17	**57** 7	**63** 30	**97** 35	**61** 23	**100** 12	**82** 106	**100** 36	**89** 107	- -	- -

NOTE: The first number in each column (boldface) is the rate in percent, the second number is the number of patients; Please refer to the main entry for footnotes; ***Heart Attack Care:*** *1. ACE Inhibitor or ARB for LVSD; 2. Aspirin at Arrival; 3. Aspirin at Discharge; 4. Beta Blocker at Arrival; 5. Beta Blocker at Discharge; 6. Fibrinolytic Medication Timing; 7. PCI Within 90 Minutes of Arrival; 8. Smoking Cessation Advice;* ***Heart Failure Care:*** *9. ACE Inhibitor or ARB for LVSD; 10. Discharge Instructions; 11. Evaluation of LVS Function; 12. Smoking Cessation Advice;* ***Pneumonia Care:*** *13. Appropriate Initial Antibiotic; 14. Blood Culture Timing; 15. Influenza Vaccine; 16. Initial Antibiotic Timing; 17. Oxygenation Assessment; 18. Pneumococcal Vaccine; 19. Smoking Cessation Advice;* ***Surgical Infection Prevention:*** *20. Prophylactic Antibiotic Given; 21. Prophylactic Antibiotic Selection; 22. Prophylactic Antibiotic Stopped;* ***Pregnancy Care:*** *23. Inpatient Neonatal Mortality; 24. Third or Fourth Degree Laceration*

Each cell below shows the rate in percent (first, boldface number) and the number of patients (second number).

Hospital	Heart Attack Care 1	2	3	4	5	6	7	8	Heart Failure Care 9	10	11	12	13	14	Pneumonia Care 15	16	17	18	19	Surgical Infection Prevention 20	21	22	Pregnancy Care 23	24
Hemphill County Hospital, Canadian, TX	100 3								100 1		100 0	80 0	100 0	0		95 22	100 23	81 16	100 1					
Henderson Memorial Hospital, Henderson, TX		16 100		93 14	89 9	0		50 2	93 28	67 96	75 125	80 15	81 80	86 56	83 18	85 108	100 128	72 76	74 23	70 40	85 39	97 37		
Hendrick Medical Center, Abilene, TX	78 51	94 214	96 318	85 172	88 326	67 21	33 9	93 134	60 188	57 336	96 411	90 78	79 218	87 175	89 70	73 259	100 317	87 179	86 86	88 276	94 69	73 270		
Hereford Regional Medical Center, Hereford, TX			100 10	100 6	100 1				100 4	5	35 31	90 5	100 3	100 2	10	44 100	100 40	34 100	34 12	81 12	100 0	0 2	0 1	
Highland Community Hospital, Lubbock, TX		100 3	100 2	100 1					100 0	54 13	88 17	80 5	56 34	100 3	70 10	79 44	100 40	18 34	83 12	43 81	100 29	22 79		0 1
Hill Country Memorial Hospital, Fredericksburg, TX	100 2	60 15	70 10	92 12	92 12			100 1	85 20	85 59	86 83	100 5	80 110	85 82	82 38	79 160	100 195	87 149	73 26	85 459	96 108	51 452		
Hill Regional Hospital, Hillsboro, TX		95 19	78 9	100 14	89 9	12 8			83 18	56 86	79 122	88 24	88 69	89 37	63 19	97 86	100 101	82 67	80 25	50 18	91 11	69 16		
Hillcrest Baptist Medical Center, Waco, TX	81 32	97 169	93 199	99 150	97 192	0 2	50 4	94 87	67 102	53 210	87 283	75 68	76 99	92 87		76 136	100 188	44 96	79 68	65 222	92 78	47 204		
Hopkins County Memorial Hospital, Sulphur Springs, TX	100 7	84 31	77 22	81 27	83 23	0	0	71 7	96 46	86 110	77 143	83 29	69 139	85 66	70 37	73 164	100 209	66 139	85 54	47 153	25 44	88 130		
Houston Northwest Medical Center, Houston, TX	92 91	96 306	96 333	93 247	97 321	33 3	92 25	99 145	78 263	56 487	90 568	99 119	89 237	93 180	61 72	64 353	100 417	70 199	93 94	88 881	80 228	60 849		
Houston Physicians' Hospital, Webster, TX																100 0	0 1	0		20 5	0 5			
Huguley Memorial Medical Center, Burleson, TX	92 24	97 186	97 167	95 146	98 179	0 3	32	19 100	95 75	61 280	97 345	99 91	80 226	83 193	73 73	77 308	98 371	90 181	97 116	86 407	80 142	64 396	0.35 1143	5.10 824
Huntsville Memorial Hospital, Huntsville, TX	100 2	89 9	80 5	88 8	100 4			100 2	89 37	63 65	72 85	61 18	83 99	92 53	69 16	75 91	97 103	75 65	71 14	94 166	91 33	24 143		
Irving Coppell Surgical Hospital, Irving, TX																100 0	0 1	0		78 9	100	9		
John Peter Smith Hospital, Fort Worth, TX	77 39	93 199	93 149	86 185	96 166	0 1	27 11	70 103	88 318	14 485	99 505	70 214	77 276	85 255	2 58	40 339	100 389	59 213	47 175	77 487	86 100	77 476		
Kell West Regional Hospital, Wichita Falls, TX		0	0	0 1	100 1				100 4	100 1	78 9	100 2	100 1	100	58	34 39	39	65 23	100	9		25 170		
Kings Daughters Hospital, Temple, TX	67 3	100 23	100 15	96 25	100 13	0	0	100 2	75 12	86 35	80 39	82 11	92 49	80 35	62 13	89 59	100 62	91 44	92 24	82 93	76 49	67 94	0.00 769	1.55 515
Kingwood Medical Center, Kingwood, TX	100 27	99 136	99 83	93 111	99 83	60 20	67	3 100	90 96	74 251	97 305	100 63	90 181	84 158	90 61	76 249	98 300	89 163	100 90	49 70	63 33	63 67		
Kingwood Specialty Hospital, Kingwood, TX											100 0	0 1	100 0	0 1	100 0	100 3	0 1	0	0	81 16	100	16		
Knapp Medical Center, Weslaco, TX	33 6	92 73	89 27	81 43	90 31	0 1		0	68 104	58 295	90 337	66 32	77 189	91 151	2 58	63 278	96 309	59 213	70 30	73 174	97 73	25 170		
Knox County Hospital, Knox City, TX		0 100	0 1	0 1	100 1				50 2	100 1	100 4	0	100 2	100 1		100 14	100 14	91 11	0		0	4		
Laird Memorial Hospital, Kilgore, TX	67 27	87 136	72 57	72 57	72 123	7	33	67 51	75 113	58 113	73 74	76 33	58 62	80 44	88 16	92 86	100 95	72 57	90 21	48 23	78 9	90 21		
Lake Granbury Medical Center, Granbury, TX	100 2	92 13	100 6	100 11	100 5			100 1	82 22	97 32	80 40	64 4	87 68	81 64	73 22	85 79	100 108	83 69	90 29	89 103	85 34	55 98	0.00 925	4.58 589
Las Colinas Medical Center, Irving, TX	77 13	98 59	93 71	95 41	95 58	67	75	80 28	77 65	71 65	86 205	30 100	89 100	97 166	79 14	93 207	100 290	99 170	64 100	73 164	88 41	51 138		0 1
Lake Pointe Medical Center, Rowlett, TX	100 2	100 8	4 100	75 4	8 100			0	50 2	0 3	61 44	0 1	100 4	100 2	86 14	71 7	100 82	18 11	100 7	81 16	100	100 16		0 1
Lake Whitney Medical Center, Whitney, TX		67 3	25 4		67 3				100 7	0	33 6	6 100	100 1	100 3	100 5	50 8	100 17	93 14	0 2	78 9	91	100 16		
Lakeside Hospital at Bastrop, Bastrop, TX									100	0	50 14	0	42 38	100 4	37	82 44	92 12	50 10	0	25 4	0	0		
Lamb Healthcare Center, Littlefield, TX	0	0 100	0 1	33 3	80 5			0	25 4	19 21	35 37	42 38	75 111	81 100	52 27	72 140	98 64	44 25	9 22	58 384	84 102	83 6		
Laredo Medical Center, Laredo, TX	14 98	80 98	82 97	97 72	96 83		1 100	100 34	86 59	99 148	100 168	90 100	89 131	92 126	34	86 175	99 197	97 116	86 41	80 379	83 101	64 367	0.00 283	6.76 207
Las Palmas Medical Center, El Paso, TX	29 66	96 78	97 180	76 66	79 158		2 83		57 89	37 71	87 275	71 74	67 3	50 2	40	50 16	100 18	94 18	0 1	59 32	32	100 29		
Lavaca Medical Center, Hallettsville, TX	0	0 100	67 3	67 6	100 1			0 100	86 7	60 5	43 23	67 3	95 22	84 19	100 5	90 21	100 24	100 16	100 7	50 6		80 5		
Limestone Medical Center, Groesbeck, TX	67 6	90 41	85 20	89 28	85 20	6	75	4 100	90 143	54 301	96 359	97 66	84 140	98 128	81 42	88 192	99 227	78 129	90 62	72 132	51 67	41 129		0 1
Llano Memorial Hospital, Llano, TX	80 5	94 54	97 32	85 48	97 31			80 5	72 36	61 88	53 118	96 24	79 80	87 71	79 19	80 112	100 137	77 83	31 100	54 161	67 46	58 162		
Longview Regional Medical Center, Longview, TX	81 124	95 276	94 380	88 222	91 354		50 12	87 143	85 188	66 341	90 362	80 94	80 181	85 114	43 58	74 188	100 240	86 83	39 76	67 483	86 140	44 447	0.34 1472	4.01 972
Lubbock Heart Hospital, Lubbock, TX																								
Madison Saint Joseph Health Center, Madisonville, TX																								
Mainland Medical Center, Texas City, TX	90 21	96 110	93 60	88 113	91 69	6		4 100	90 143	54 301	96 359	97 66								72 132				
Marshall Regional Medical Center, Marshall, TX	82 11	95 39	91 22	85 39	88 25			0 100	93 57	88 102	97 124	96 24	72 129	93 60	25	86 111	99 133	86 83	91 35	54 161	46	58 162		
Mary Shiels Hospital, Dallas, TX																								
Matagorda County Hospital District, Bay City, TX	93 14	98 80	73 15	33 3	80 5			0	83 6	78 23	88 40	90	95 66	85 81	83 12	86 133	100 152	95 107	85 27	33 6	2	83 6		
Mayhill Hospital, Denton, TX																								
McAllen Medical Center, McAllen, TX	54 71	90 241	91 233	86 147	83 262	14	50	84 69	64 135	59 271	82 307	64 20	83 87	89 79	60 25	54 133	97 156	72 85	75 20	58 251	88 57	28 238		
McKenna Memorial Hospital, New Braunfels, TX	75 8	97 39	92 26	98 40	96 26	1		25 4	81 36	67 123	73 165	74	76 135	90 90	58 40	76 164	100 196	54 125	37 81	79 121	89 118	81 113	0.20 995	6.06 693
Medical Arts Hospital, Lamesa, TX		0 100	67 3	67 6	50 4			0 100	92 13	80 5	84 51	0 78	78 9	75 4	100 5	72 58	100 69	87 39	100 7	50 6		0		
Medical Center at Lancaster, Lancaster, TX	67 6	90 41	85 20	89 28	85 20	6	75	0 100	65 57	0 12	73 176	100 3	0	8 100	79 19	49 49	100 75	11 28	3 100	50 6		80 5		
Medical Center at Terrell, Terrell, TX	80 5	94 54	97 32	85 48	97 31			80 5	72 36	61 88	53 118	96 24	79 80	87 71	79 19	80 112	100 137	77 83	31 84	67 132	51 67	41 129		0 1
Medical Center Hospital, Odessa, TX	81 124	95 276	94 380	88 222	91 354	8	50 12	87 143	85 188	66 341	90 362	80 94	80 181	85 114	43 58	74 188	100 240	42 139	39 76	67 483	86 140	44 447	0.34 1472	4.01 972
Medical Center of Arlington, Arlington, TX	95 44	100 240	100 220	99 167	100 208	38	8 31	13 99	91 87	74 234	96 282	96 48	94 207	88 237	67	96 298	100 371	56 195	100 76	83 186	91 87	53 177	0.34 3806	2.25 2308

NOTE: The first number in each column (boldface) is the rate in percent, the second number is the number of patients; Please refer to the main entry for footnotes; *Heart Attack Care*: 1. ACE Inhibitor or ARB for LVSD; 2. Aspirin at Arrival; 3. Aspirin at Discharge; 4. Beta Blocker at Arrival; 5. Beta Blocker at Discharge; 6. Fibrinolytic Medication Timing; 7. PCI Within 90 Minutes of Arrival; 8. Smoking Cessation Advice; *Heart Failure Care*: 9. ACE Inhibitor or ARB for LVSD; 10. Discharge Instructions; 11. Evaluation of LVS Function; 12. Smoking Cessation Advice; *Pneumonia Care*: 13. Appropriate Initial Antibiotic; 14. Blood Culture Timing; 15. Influenza Vaccine; 16. Initial Antibiotic Timing; 17. Oxygenation Assessment; 18. Pneumococcal Vaccine; 19. Smoking Cessation Advice; *Surgical Infection Prevention*: 20. Prophylactic Antibiotic Given; 21. Prophylactic Antibiotic Selection; 22. Prophylactic Antibiotic Stopped; *Pregnancy Care*: 23. Inpatient Neonatal Mortality; 24. Third or Fourth Degree Laceration

Each cell shows the rate in percent (boldface) followed by the number of patients.

Hospital	1	2	3	4	5	6	7	8	9	10	11	12	13	14	15	16	17	18	19	20	21	22	23	24
Medical Center of Lewisville, Lewisville, TX	60 5	97 60	75 20	92 52	84 19			0 100	83 69	53 203	96 223	86 42	82 118	80 98	63 51	64 192	97 218	58 122	85 52	53 135	81 63	58 135		
Medical Center of Mesquite, Mesquite, TX	77 26	88 164	76 172	87 169	84 174	12 16	31 13	62 72	67 132	62 346	67 394	80 102	50 161	90 103	56 45	62 192	100 251	44 136	92 59	46 206	83 48	71 158		
Medical Center of Plano, Plano, TX	91 34	99 139	96 132	99 109	95 154	0	82 11	98 45	80 131	52 260	94 356	96 57	90 136	96 148	0 58	83 211	100 259	83 167	94 49	83 194	89 93	66 178		
Medical Center of Southeast Texas, Port Arthur, TX	78 27	92 101	94 107	83 92	94 106	0 1	33	100 9	84 97	67 236	92 283	100 52	63 135	75 52	31 26	54 134	98 165	41 97	100 35	63 259	70 83	44 255		
Medical Centre Surgical Hospital, Fort Worth, TX	88 24	99 112	96 136	95 102	99 128		25 8	96 52												82 17		100 17		
Medical City Dallas, Dallas, TX	72 39	92 88	85 131	89 89	88 128	0	0 1	92 13	76 107	69 35	78 274	100 3	93 15	100 35	48 44	62 251	97 272	71 172	78 46	87 376	90 173	73 360		
Memorial Health System of East Texas-Lufkin, Lufkin, TX	100 174	88 752	85 793	89 629	97 781	0 2	44 25	99 244	96 745	35	78 141	32 395	78 957	94 875	67 24	68 107	100 121	79 57	100 8	35 65	90 21	94 97	0.00 745	2.07 483
Memorial Hermann Baptist Orange Hospital, Orange, TX	86 14	100 75	95 43	97 38	100 14	0 2	33	100 7	96 54	69 108	100 100	100 57	78 96	84 157	24	68 100	100 100	79 100	100 39	35 65	90 21	52 65		
Memorial Hermann Katy Hospital, Katy, TX	94 33	94 130	95 169	100 101	96 169	100	96 46	0 100	87 155	87 106	96 373	96 28	83 102	97 112		92 145	100 180	72 103	100 8	84 104	88 92	80 244		
Memorial Hermann Baptist Beaumont, Beaumont, TX	100 3	93 29	90 10	100 22	100 10	0	100	100 2	96 50	88 81	96 131	100 16	88 81	100 73		82 250	100 282	72 149	100 8	84 104		54 101		
Memorial Hermann Fort Bend Hospital, Missouri City, TX	94 174	98 752	97 793	97 629	97 781	23 39	44	99 244	96 745	55 1575	99 1905	97 395	72 957	90 875		78 1245	100 1468	94 64	64 100	84 50	77 13	53 47		
Memorial Hermann Healthcare System, Houston, TX	92 64	98 196	96 281	97 127	97 284	25 4	33 12	99 97	91 206	60 378	99 461	57 100	83 162	95 157	53	81 234	100 286	75 171	95 93	53 792	83 83	68 2451		
Memorial Hermann Memorial City, Houston, TX	94 85	100 260	95 472	100 238	95 454	67 9	96	98 290	98 316	86 518	99 562	100 180	92 73	94 114	30	76 135	100 173	87 60	97 58	72 641	91 186	48 770	0.70 287	0.53 188
Memorial Hermann-Texas Medical Center, Houston, TX	100 1	67	100 3	67	67 3	0			60 20	73 11	83 41	100 6	50 6	50 2		86 50	98 54	62 26	100 1	33 6		68 567		
Memorial Hospital, Dumas, TX		100 6	100 4	100 6	100 2		100	0 100	69 16	0 38	69 51	25	82 33	95 20	23 22	57 53	100 56	20 41	14	50 6	2 100	83 6		
Memorial Hospital, Gonzales, TX	100 5	100 9	100 6	100 9	83 6	100	0	100 2	40 15	70 43	45 51	67	52 64	90 10	13	73 48	98 65	58 36	86	38 8	100 2	62 8		
Memorial Medical Center, Port Lavaca, TX	50 8	57 7	33 3	71 7	50 4	100		100 11	65 46	88 24	77 107	100	86 7	94 6		71 86	100 95	43 49	100 7	77 30		33 30	0.70 287	30 287
Memorial Medical Center Livingston, Livingston, TX		98 53	85 20	90 52	96 23	5	78	100 100	84 92	59 202	90 248	100	86 153	87 126	39	81 175	100 204	77 77	80	79 297	81 69	75 290		
Mesquite Community Hospital, Mesquite, TX	91 152	93 280	96 628	94 212	98 643	0	44 9	92 200	84 425	75 765	98 842	88 121	86 209	94 277	64	84 403	100 448	84 234	90 73	78 429	79 86	73 415		
Methodist Ambulatory Surgery Hospital NW, San Antonio, TX																				82 17	100 8			
Methodist Hospital, Houston, TX	75 116	94 558	94 614	94 412	95 657	0	24 25	97 239	76 546	54 1224	87 1525	92 232	83 575	83 615	55 231	67 955	99 1147	48 646	83 235	62 460	92 219	69 456	0.76 3839	2.26 2612
Methodist Hospital, San Antonio, TX	92 65	99 173	100 216	99 146	99 216	16	69	100 93	97 284	97 508	98 529	100 131	82 173	95 209	56	80 266	100 312	97 143	100 98	96 194	94 65	89 191		
Methodist Medical Center, Dallas, TX	100 3	97 30	95 501	98 210	96 290	0 1	64 22	100 216	90 21	70 69	94 87	89 110	60 73	91 81	19	84 111	100 140	87 90	88 17	61 148	55 31	52 147		
Methodist Sugar Land Hospital, Sugar Land, TX	73 11	98 81	87 68	80 93	70 10	1	0	67 3	90 55	69 32	90 193	76 21	69 93	90 118	23	85 140	99 189	91 100	80 5	85 196	56 39	60 324		
Methodist Willowbrook Hospital, Houston, TX	71 7	93 42	90 31	95 39	92 75	4	33	3 100	67 83	61 213	90 249	77 13	80 61	90 51	18	61 84	100 101	76 51	82 34	51 215	89 84	45 211	0.08 1313	3.33 780
Metroplex Hospital, Killeen, TX	95 44	98 187	90 202	87 135	87 215	62 8	75	92 74	86 135	57 303	80 333	75 24	65 200	88 102	47	60 205	100 257	67 156	71 58	85 320	87 97	76 319		
Midland Memorial Hospital, Midland, TX	70 23	91 116	79 99	93 96	86 85	1	75 4	96 25	75 60	40 230	73 275	98 52	75 177	89 115	58	56 224	98 243	26 153	97 36	40 172	88 56	26 159		
Mission Hospital, Mission, TX		0	0	0	0			0	50 4	17 12	93 15	0 1	97 30	100 11	11	92 45	100 62	71 35	62 8	25 4	100 5			
Mitchell County Hospital, Colorado City, TX		60 5	100 1	60 5	100 1	50 4	4	40 5	86 22	58 107	96	67	86 35	89 37	100	89 44	100 100	88 33	8	4 100	19	40		
Mother Frances Hospital Jacksonville, Jacksonville, TX		96 159	97 172	91 81	96 164	0 1	69 81	96	77 107	64 237	96 277	93 72	92 119	94 140	76 37	71 177	100 219	77 129	94 48	74 233	93 111	64 214		
Mother Frances Hospital-Tyler, Tyler, TX		0	0	100 1	0 1	12	86 7	75 4	86 7	78 9	74 27	100 5	83 6	83 6	29	77 30	94 36	83 18	100 3	0	0	0		
Nacogdoches Medical Center Hospital, Nacogdoches, TX	86 111	98 323	95 501	98 210	96 290	0 1	64 22	97 29	70 81	65 188	93 256	99 88	91 189	88 176	54 46	93 263	100 330	59 199	97 59	63 143	59 37	58 139		
Nacogdoches Memorial Hospital, Nacogdoches, TX	76 21	86 81	86 77	80 111	95 116	4	0	100 60	81 114	34 50	80 281	77 13	80 81	93 216	52	64 160	99 164	85 177	94 81	52 197	79 77	63 185		
Navarro Regional Hospital, Corsicana, TX	100 6	83 35	75 16	84 25	86 85	0	78	3 100	91 56	61 114	92 162	100 24	84 81	80 81	59	75 136	99 164	81 101	100 97	88 120	93 28	61 114		
Nix Healthcare System, San Antonio, TX	86 7	100 39	100 43	97 37	94 42	1	75	0 100	82 17	98 64	96 83	3 100	79 68	89 68	100 23	95 58	93 100	26 153	97 36	40 172	88 56	41 157		
Nocona General Hospital, Nocona, TX		60 5	100 1	60 5	100 1	50 4	4	40 5	50 4	57 7	35 23	67	97 30	11 100	100	89 44	100 62	88 33	100	25 4	100 5	100 1		
North Austin Medical Center, Austin, TX	93 42	96 159	97 172	91 81	96 164	13	69 81	96	77 107	64 237	96 277	93 72	92 119	94 140	76 37	71 177	100 219	77 129	94 48	74 233	93 111	64 214		
North Bay Hospital, Aransas Pass, TX	96	0	0	100 1	0 1	12	86 7	75	86 7	78 9	74 27	100 5	83 6	83 6	29	77 30	94 36	83 18	100 3	0	0	0		
North Central Medical Center, McKinney, TX	91 23	99 142	97 147	95 116	96 150	4	56	9 100	70 81	65 188	93 256	46	91 189	88 176	54 46	93 263	100 330	59 199	97 59	63 143	71 48	58 139		
North Hills Hospital, N Richland Hills, TX	96 25	98 162	100 137	100 131	100 138	0	78	9 100	83 100	55 197	88 266	50	91 180	93 216	59	82 240	100 299	85 177	94 81	52 197	79 77	63 185		
North Runnels Hospital, Winters, TX																				0	0	100 1		
North Texas Hospital, Denton, TX	56 9	97 36	67 18	97 35	67 18	4		0 100	71 70	91 144	81 180	92 24	74 156	95 138		84 221	97 257	59 150	88 40	67 166	89 63	89 151		
North Texas Medical Center, Gainesville, TX	100 4	75 24	83 12	71 21	71 14	50	0	40 5	54 13	12 73	51 103	59 22	63 46	100 31	59 17	84 57	99 70	59 39	71 14	65 81	81 16	63 75		
Northeast Medical Center, Bonham, TX	100 6	100 27	92 12	88 25	80 15	50 2	13	75	100 11	68 31	67 63	100 16	81 32	84 56	100 29	77 53	100 77	89 54	80 16	80	0	0		
Northeast Medical Center Hospital, Humble, TX	53 15	88 154	85 61	80 111	87 53	8 12	56	9 100	74 149	37 416	86 503	88	91 197	86 172	54	56 278	99 324	99 153	96	73 230	50 58	47 217		
Northwest Texas Healthcare System, Amarillo, TX	84 57	96 205	99 298	96 180	97 294	0	78	12 97	83 144	83 264	88 326	94 94	76 245	79 137	58	69 229	100 281	64 123	89 103	52 197	81 211	52 961		
Northwest Texas Surgery Center, Amarillo, TX																				0	0	100 1		
Oakbend Medical Center, Richmond, TX	56 9	97 36	67 18	97 35	67 18	4		0 100	71 70	91 144	81 180	92 24	74 156	95 138		84 221	97 257	59 150	88 40	67 166	89 63	89 151		

NOTE: The first number in each column (boldface) is the rate in percent; the second number is the number of patients; Please refer to the main entry for footnotes; **Heart Attack Care:** 1. ACE Inhibitor or ARB for LVSD; 2. Aspirin at Arrival; 3. Aspirin at Discharge; 4. Beta Blocker at Arrival; 5. Beta Blocker at Discharge; 6. Fibrinolytic Medication Timing; 7. PCI Within 90 Minutes of Arrival; 8. Smoking Cessation Advice; **Heart Failure Care:** 9. ACE Inhibitor or ARB for LVSD; 10. Discharge Instructions; 11. Evaluation of LVS Function; 12. Smoking Cessation Advice; **Pneumonia Care:** 13. Appropriate Initial Antibiotic; 14. Blood Culture Timing; 15. Influenza Vaccine; 16. Initial Antibiotic Timing; 17. Oxygenation Assessment; 18. Pneumococcal Vaccine; 19. Smoking Cessation Advice; **Surgical Infection Prevention:** 20. Prophylactic Antibiotic Given; 21. Prophylactic Antibiotic Selection; 22. Prophylactic Antibiotic Stopped; **Pregnancy Care:** 23. Inpatient Neonatal Mortality; 24. Third or Fourth Degree Laceration

Hospital	Heart Attack Care 1	2	3	4	5	6	7	8	Heart Failure Care 9	10	11	12	13	14	Pneumonia Care 15	16	17	18	19	Surgical Infection Prevention 20	21	22	Pregnancy Care 23	24
Odessa Regional Hospital, Odessa, TX	–	60 5	100 1	80 5	0 1	– 0	– 0	– 0	0 4	64 25	77 26	100 3	72 47	73 30	38 13	73 44	52 100	67 21	81 21	69 140	87 54	75 137	0.49 2268	5.34 1573
Otto Kaiser Memorial Hospital, Kenedy, TX	–	– 0	– 0	– 0	– 0	– 0	– 0	– 0	0 2	0 12	13 31	100 1	88 17	100 4	50 8	74 19	100 25	56 18	100 1	42 270	91 90	57 258	–	–
Palestine Regional Medical Center, Palestine, TX	92 12	96 51	89 27	98 47	91 33	25 4	– 0	86 7	96 51	85 115	89 153	95 20	88 80	88 86	88 25	82 130	100 165	96 98	90 29	87 93	95 41	83 103	–	–
Palo Pinto General Hospital, Mineral Wells, TX	0	70 20	67 6	67 21	43 7	–	0	33 3	82 28	100 90	60 105	67 24	72 101	85 27	28 18	70 103	100 117	69 70	67 42	79 107	96 25	41 78	–	92
Pampa Regional Medical Center, Pampa, TX	67 3	87 15	79 14	100 8	86 14	67	43	65	85 121	73 217	73 107	46 13	88 74	95 40	62 29	88 103	99 119	59 207	80 27	79 508	83 157	25 83	–	103
Paris Regional Medical Center-South Campus, Paris, TX	96 54	97 119	96 105	96 163	99 155	0	0	7 97	85 121	76 295	95 292	82 55	89 95	95 153	72 82	76 272	99 348	59 207	80 80	68 158	90 157	75 490	–	–
Park Plaza Hospital, Houston, TX	73 11	89 38	96 27	81 27	96 28	0	0	1 100	81 115	76 295	92 339	100 75	89 95	95 153	50 2	74 210	100 255	71 142	100 40	68 158	90 42	36 158	–	–
Parkland Health & Hospital System, Dallas, TX	85 65	97 253	98 207	93 226	99 227	0	33 12	98	89 521	61 790	100 820	96 366	82 182	79 239	92 50	39 315	99 368	80 70	84 180	89 142	98 144	54 136	0.45 16281	5.13 11763
Parkview Hospital, Wheeler, TX	–	0	–	–	–	–	–	–	0 100	100 2	50 2	–	62 21	67 3	100 2	81 16	100 22	41 17	75 8	0 1	0 1	100 1	–	–
Parkview Regional Hospital, Mexia, TX	0	90 10	71 7	75 4	67 9	–	–	100	94 16	67 136	92 158	90 21	72 107	95 74	2	88 151	100 175	73 94	96 45	25 8	3 86	88 57	1	–
Pecos County Memorial Hospital, Fort Stockton, TX	–	50 2	100	0	100 1	–	–	0	100 3	18 33	16 38	0	61 54	93 27	6	85 59	100 76	90 41	43 7	60 67	100 3	51 35	7	–
Permian General Hospital, Andrews, TX	0	100 1	100	100 1	100 1	–	–	0	50 12	50 10	10 10	50 4	88 25	57 7	100 8	74 23	94 34	53 15	60 5	60 67	28 43	67	–
Physicians Centre, Bryan, TX	100	0 100	0	0	0	0	0	0	0 1	0 2	0 2	0	0 1	0	100 5	100 5	100 5	0 2	0	91 57	88 57	57	–
Physicians Specialty Hospital of El Paso, El Paso, TX	100 5	79 24	82 28	75 24	61 28	0	67	3 67	70 40	0 18	84 81	0 1	70 10	25 4	36	80 100	100 109	0 66	100 2	11 37	65 26	–	–
Physicians Surgical Hospital at Quail Creek, Amarillo, TX	–	–	–	–	–	–	–	–	–	–	–	–	–	–	–	–	–	–	–	89 35	51 35	35	–
Pine Creek Medical Center, Dallas, TX	–	–	–	–	–	–	–	–	0 100	2	50 2	12	–	3	100 3	–	–	–	–	100 3	100 3	–	–
Plaza Medical Center, Fort Worth, TX	97 49	100 133	99 335	100 119	99 352	0	38 8	100 145	90 172	83 341	99 379	94 83	75 133	91 137	57 51	69 191	99 241	62 133	82 44	68 196	86 152	45 298	–	–
Presbyterian Hospital of Allen, Allen, TX	100 1	100 7	100	100 4	100 5	0	0	0 100 2	85 20	42 50	94 62	100 15	86 70	98 51	88 17	91 65	100 87	85 46	97 30	100 21	59 29	63 87	0.08 1296	4.54 749
Presbyterian Hospital of Dallas, Dallas, TX	86 49	97 214	99 290	95 179	97 287	0	36 14	98 103	84 300	84 505	96 650	98 123	89 249	95 260	95 83	89 351	100 412	93 273	95 66	86 327	94 94	92 261	–	–
Presbyterian Hospital of Denton, Denton, TX	91 33	97 130	94 158	94 104	96 161	0	33 9	94 68	75 73	45 209	83 275	81 52	76 130	96 119	60 57	80 181	100 253	64 152	79 56	90 263	99 94	78 437	–	–
Presbyterian Hospital of Greenville, Greenville, TX	44 9	86 69	72 32	70 66	81 32	0	0	100 7	64 143	1 267	93 338	89 62	75 178	77 151	60 68	69 221	99 292	58 162	85 88	95 451	98 120	85 249	–	–
Presbyterian Hospital of Kaufman, Kaufman, TX	67 3	95 22	77 13	82 11	82 11	100	40	0	91 33	95 125	87 149	95 37	80 76	95 64	97 33	98 89	100 116	90 77	97 36	72 264	44 108	56 52	0 3	–
Presbyterian Hospital of Plano, Plano, TX	89 28	100 133	92 178	98 108	96 170	1	10 98	89 46	88 146	98 172	91 11	79 115	98 93	56 27	82 120	100 150	86 66	100 37	78 55	67 18	65 174	67 6	–
Presbyterian Hospital of Winnsboro, Winnsboro, TX	–	0 100	3 100	100 1	1	0	0	0	89	91 32	93 45	91 11	91 23	97 30	100 14	91 35	51	41 100	6	74 180	95 55	89 9	–	–
Presbyterian Plano Ctr for Diag & Surgery, Plano, TX	76 49	93 251	89 312	88 199	91 305	60	40 10	96 113	78 166	61 378	88 483	90 77	87 217	86 182	26 69	77 261	100 322	28 213	96 71	60 10	2 89	100 42	–	–
Providence Health Center, Waco, TX	–	100 3	100	2 100	2 100	5	40	10	93 15	98 42	96 57	100	0 2	0	100	100 4	4	0 2	0	88 42	50 189	–	–
Providence Hospital, Laredo, TX	34 100	100 136	97 132	93 106	88 122	30	0 6	97 32	86 151	69 377	89 406	93 28	74 291	82 202	70	83 361	100 436	91 274	62 39	86 327	78 96	64 323	–	–
Providence Memorial Hospital, El Paso, TX	68 34	100 136	97 132	70 10	83 6	10	0	6 97	84 300	6	8 24	100 4	100	67 3	–	100 40	100	27 26	75 4	100 21	68 22	0	–
Reeves County Hospital, Pecos, TX	0	0	0	0	0	0	0	0	17 6	8	24 100	–	100	67	36 100	75	0 1	75	100	86 327	96 78	0	–
Regency Hospital of North Dallas II, Carrollton, TX	–	0 75	4 100	1 50	4 100	1	0	0	0	25 4	44 48	3	33 3	0	43	29 97	0	5 21	0 2	100 3	0 3	–	–
Renaissance Hospital Houston, Houston, TX	78 9	92 25	92 25	84 25	89 27	0 2	0	0	41 17	0 11	58 71	33	57 7	0	100	44 100	63	17 35	50 4	57 7	67 6	100	–
Renaissance Hospital-East Texas, Groves, TX	70 23	95 104	79 87	92 108	83 95	25	4	100 34	71 55	56 114	80 137	97	79 97	94 126	88 43	79 163	100 212	85 126	93 43	69 105	100 18	52 100	0 3	–
RHD Memorial Medical Center, Dallas, TX	100 35	99 104	98 93	100 84	98 85	100	83	6 100	98 59	67 105	95 147	100	83 109	95 103	44 27	91 159	100 192	73 114	97 34	64 182	87 53	67 178	67 6	–
Richardson Medical Center, Richardson, TX	59 46	93 166	87 175	82 104	87 174	1	50	94 33	67 131	67 369	76 417	91	79 146	94 125	91 43	71 238	96 259	75 168	82 28	66 125	94 49	51 121	–	–
Rio Grande Regional Hospital, McAllen, TX	86 71	98 184	98 247	94 140	95 235	0	57	7 89	100 1	53 514	50 589	95 128	85 172	85 169	44 66	66 228	97 315	58 183	85 80	88 1051	96 257	89 1032	–	–
Riverside General Hospital, Houston, TX	–	–	–	–	–	–	–	–	100 1	–	50 2	–	–	–	–	–	–	–	–	–	–	–	–	–
Rolling Plains Memorial Hospital, Sweetwater, TX	80 15	80 5	86 8	78 89	84 77	0 1	0	7 100	93 15	98 16	86 107	100	71 77	85 40	94 18	73 102	100 111	93 74	75	44	9 100	61 38	0.16	8
Rollins Brook Community Hospital, Lampasas, TX	0 100	3 100	3 100	3 100	2 100	6	15	13	80 5	57 30	25 55	0	69 35	100 18	47 15	88 50	100 70	71 59	100 7	57	1 100	75 8	1829	–
Round Rock Medical Center, Round Rock, TX	96 24	99 125	93 126	97 105	93 117	0	67	12 98	86 50	54 114	94 145	100	87 172	95 136	78 36	77 206	100 222	78 121	61	78 172	96 79	50 165	0.22 1782	4.11 1169
Saint David's Rehabilitation Center, Austin, TX	82 34	98 146	98 166	96 104	97 172	1	75	4 100	88 175	61 421	98 492	99 110	95 183	95 206	77 62	82 276	100 321	76 188	87	86 278	93 135	67 262	–	–
Saint Joseph Medical Center, Houston, TX	100 38	98 122	97 119	98 83	97 100	0	0	2 97	95 171	76 322	86 379	98 84	93 179	98 167	86 44	87 239	99 258	87 122	90 67	86 792	94 179	76 713	–	–
Saint Joseph Regional Health Center, Bryan, TX	86 71	98 184	98 247	94 140	95 235	0	57	7 89	80 336	53 514	95 589	95 128	85 172	85 169	44 66	66 228	97 315	58 183	85 80	88 1051	96 257	89 1032	–	–
Saint Luke's Community Med Ctr-The Woodlands, The Woodlands, TX	–	–	–	–	–	–	–	–	100 1	–	50 2	–	–	–	–	–	–	–	–	–	–	–	3.28 1157	–
Saint Luke's Episcopal Hospital, Houston, TX	91 120	99 433	97 648	98 389	97 670	17	6	175	67 754	67 1297	91 1426	85 201	85 255	88 265	94 18	70 358	100 470	68 252	69	53 310	93 102	80 300	–	–
Saint Marks Medical Center, La Grange, TX	50 2	86 7	100	5 70	83 6	0 1	15	13 98	94 17	42 12	65 77	17	78 9	94 18	47 15	74 105	98 118	35 94	7	33 9	25 8	25 8	–	–
San Angelo Community Medical Center, San Angelo, TX	100 12	96 76	100 84	98 64	100 82	44	0	100 28	100	76 105	97 149	96	84 123	96 129	60 57	78 190	100 224	83 156	100 32	85 432	69 103	76 406	–	–
San Jacinto Methodist Hospital, Baytown, TX	87 47	99 217	89 152	96 198	94 166	21	14	12 100	75 115	74 264	90 314	97 62	81 140	90 20	44 28	74 184	100 221	89 110	97 59	73 682	96 257	66 174	–	–

NOTE: The first number in each column (boldface) is the rate in percent, the second number is the number of patients; Please refer to the main entry for footnotes; **Heart Attack Care:** 1. ACE Inhibitor or ARB for LVSD; 2. Aspirin at Arrival; 3. Aspirin at Discharge; 4. Beta Blocker at Arrival; 5. Beta Blocker at Discharge; 6. Fibrinolytic Medication Timing; 7. PCI Within 90 Minutes of Arrival; 8. Smoking Cessation Advice; **Heart Failure Care:** 9. ACE Inhibitor or ARB for LVSD; 10. Discharge Instructions; 11. Evaluation of LVS Function; 12. Smoking Cessation Advice; **Pneumonia Care:** 13. Appropriate Initial Antibiotic; 14. Blood Culture Timing; 15. Influenza Vaccine; 16. Initial Antibiotic Timing; 17. Oxygenation Assessment; 18. Pneumococcal Vaccine; 19. Smoking Cessation Advice; **Surgical Infection Prevention:** 20. Prophylactic Antibiotic Given; 21. Prophylactic Antibiotic Selection; 22. Prophylactic Antibiotic Stopped; **Pregnancy Care:** 23. Inpatient Neonatal Mortality; 24. Third or Fourth Degree Laceration

Column groups: **Heart Attack Care** = columns 1–8; **Heart Failure Care** = columns 9–12; **Pneumonia Care** = columns 13–19; **Surgical Infection Prevention** = columns 20–22; **Pregnancy Care** = columns 23–24. In each cell the first (boldface) number is the rate in percent and the second number is the number of patients.

Hospital	1	2	3	4	5	6	7	8	9	10	11	12	13	14	15	16	17	18	19	20	21	22	23	24
Scenic Mountain Medical Center, Big Spring, TX	100 3	83 18	100 11	89 18	100 11	0 1	-	100 1	81 26	29 115	80 148	85 26	58 64	86 35	36 14	87 68	100 80	56 39	79 29	18 40	85 13	79 34	-	-
Scott & White, Temple, TX	96 91	100 339	100 571	99 311	100 567	80 10	10 100	100 208	96 267	64 442	95 566	98 104	85 183	93 229	-	80 317	100 416	82 293	93 91	83 1772	88 436	81 1719	1.21 1077	3.13 800
Seton Edgar B Davis Memorial Hospital, Luling, TX	-	0 0	100 1	0 0	100 1	-	-	0 0	92 12	32 25	76 42	90 10	88 34	92 38	44 16	81 47	100 54	69 35	100 6	-	-	-	-	-
Seton Highland Lakes, Burnet, TX	-	80 10	67 9	67 6	38 8	-	-	-	60 5	45 40	56 48	90 10	90 59	93 30	90 10	79 57	100 73	82 50	77 13	-	-	-	-	-
Seton Medical Center, Austin, TX	98 56	99 189	99 326	98 162	98 293	0 1	80 10	96 93	98 244	82 491	97 584	89 97	91 81	92 66	56 16	72 135	100 145	73 91	71 28	71 232	96 81	78 222	-	-
Seton Northwest Hospital, Austin, TX	-	100 9	100 5	100 3	100 4	-	-	-	100 17	62 39	100 45	38 8	95 128	82 96	-	77 152	99 168	84 82	79 43	66 113	97 30	43 110	-	-
Seton Southwest Healthcare Center, Austin, TX	0 0	50 2	0 0	50 2	0 0	-	-	0 0	0 0	2 50	50 2	29 7	86 22	100 14	-	92 24	100 32	80 10	83 6	70 37	94 17	86 36	-	-
Seymour Hospital, Seymour, TX	84 63	0 0	0 0	0 0	0 0	-	-	0 0	67 3	27 15	52 23	29 7	100 15	100 1	6	92 24	100 32	84 25	50 4	89 218	0 9	55 215	-	-
Shannon Medical Center, San Angelo, TX	84 63	98 125	96 121	92 105	99 146	33 3	0 6	100 10	90 92	64 33	88 220	100 11	72 29	90 48	64 25	74 255	100 306	86 222	100 15	89 218	0 9	55 215	-	-
Shelby Regional Medical Center, Center, TX	-	0 0	0 0	-	0 0	-	-	-	83 12	88 34	78 46	100 7	72 82	90 48	28	98 84	99 105	72 61	100 27	89 9	0	62 8	-	-
Sid Peterson Memorial Hospital, Kerrville, TX	75 4	95 21	85 13	90 20	77 13	0 1	-	67 3	84 19	66 107	80 117	82 17	80 142	89 105	-	89 224	100 269	84 180	94 49	88 363	95 131	57 352	-	-
Sierra Medical Center, El Paso, TX	73 22	99 127	96 121	89 87	83 119	0 3	0 4	93 30	73 206	35 425	90 490	82 60	85 209	85 195	84 76	67 303	99 380	86 268	76 63	77 320	98 81	57 312	-	-
Smithville Regional Hospital, Smithville, TX	-	75 4	100 2	50 4	50 2	-	-	-	73 22	55 51	69 80	71 17	86 83	84 62	39 28	88 129	100 148	41 93	100 28	32 22	100 12	100 22	-	-
South Austin Hospital, Austin, TX	84 100	97 252	97 232	90 172	98 204	0	14 100	100 89	85 199	57 351	98 405	99 92	87 183	94 179	79 57	70 230	100 303	64 159	90 86	74 262	93 122	72 252	-	-
South Texas Regional Medical Center, Jourdanton, TX	100 2	93 45	83 18	71 28	70 23	0	0	100 1	85 27	75 141	87 165	93 27	88 119	99 109	98 49	79 162	100 182	96 100	90 41	46 59	93 15	85 54	-	-
Southwest General Hospital, San Antonio, TX	100 1	93 45	64 14	82 34	77 13	67 3	-	100 5	73 52	25 243	95 293	100 72	78 114	84 117	-	81 152	99 182	67 90	96 48	23 190	88 51	34 184	0.28 2169	0.65 1376
Southwest Surgical Hospital, Hurst, TX	-	-	-	-	-	-	-	-	-	-	-	-	-	-	-	-	-	-	-	67 3	-	100 3	-	-
Southwestern General Hospital, El Paso, TX	-	-	-	-	-	-	-	-	100 2	2 100	48 31	100 1	0 1	0	-	59 32	100 39	36 22	22 100	68 81	-	88 80	-	-
Spine Hospital of South Texas, San Antonio, TX	-	-	-	-	-	-	-	-	-	-	-	-	-	-	-	-	-	-	-	-	-	-	-	-
Stamford Memorial Hospital, Stamford, TX	-	-	-	-	0 0	-	-	-	100 3	100 2	100 18	0 2	67 3	0	-	100 19	100 23	94 16	0	68 81	-	88 80	-	-
Starr County Memorial Hospital, Rio Grande City, TX	40 5	97 35	100 25	91 34	88 25	-	-	0 0	93 14	14 59	59 69	0 2	62 8	8 100	29	59 46	98 61	10 40	64 7	77 30	30 97	79 162	-	-
Stephens Memorial Hospital, Breckenridge, TX	100 1	75 4	100 5	75 4	100 3	-	-	100 1	81 16	100 7	84 68	67 3	50 2	100 3	-	91 43	100 57	100 43	100 1	47 51	98 42	82 40	-	-
Surgical Specialty Hospital of Sugar Land, Sugar Land, TX	-	-	-	-	-	-	-	-	-	-	-	-	-	-	-	-	-	-	0	83 12	100 12	0 12	-	-
Texas Inst for Surg at Presbyterian Hosp, Dallas, TX	-	-	-	-	-	-	-	-	-	-	-	-	-	-	-	-	-	-	-	-	-	-	-	-
Texas Orthopedic Hospital, Houston, TX	-	-	-	-	-	-	-	-	-	-	-	-	-	-	-	-	-	-	12	46 26	100 223	52 25	-	-
Texas Spine and Joint Hospital, Tyler, TX	-	-	-	-	-	-	-	-	-	-	-	-	-	-	-	-	-	-	-	70 23	96 23	77 22	-	-
Texoma Medical Center, Denison, TX	92 39	97 116	98 130	95 102	96 138	9 56	14 65	9 100	94 88	84 172	93 207	92 40	93 169	97 133	21 14	83 212	100 236	99 153	52 42	89 374	97 124	92 353	0.16 607	4.31 394
Texsan Heart Hospital, San Antonio, TX	88 48	100 75	98 321	97 64	95 306	0 1	0 1	1 97	83 119	62 156	100 172	91 23	33 12	77 13	45 11	16 18	100 18	67 15	6	89 361	100 143	100 357	-	-
The Hospital at Westlake Medical Center, Austin, TX	100 3	100 9	100 16	100 6	100 6	1 100	100 1	3 100	100 7	21 14	100 16	100 2	100 5	100 4	0	67 6	100 7	100 4	100	77 30	100 97	82 79	-	-
Thomason General Hospital, El Paso, TX	80 20	97 214	98 271	98 182	98 283	0	70 10	97 119	77 243	45 311	99 337	88 100	83 100	85 177	20 20	41 143	98 177	36 80	77 47	49 348	80 74	63 345	0.19 1032	2.14 882
Titus Regional Medical Center, Mount Pleasant, TX	100 3	75 12	57 7	67 6	67 6	-	-	-	80 40	22 27	77 130	33 3	67 27	27 100	51 5	53 221	77 253	20 156	29 7	47 55	98 51	82 40	-	-
Tomball Regional Hospital, Tomball, TX	81 36	93 168	96 161	79 149	92 155	50 6	11 88	92 119	89 127	42 262	90 323	77 62	81 166	82 138	59 44	71 249	100 310	72 156	84 88	87 55	92 87	70 50	0.00 803	3.52 596
Tops Surgical Specialty Hospital, Houston, TX	-	-	-	-	-	-	-	-	-	-	-	-	-	-	-	-	-	-	-	46 26	100 223	52 25	-	-
Trinity Medical Center, Brenham, TX	-	0 0	100 8	100 4	100 2	-	-	-	90 20	80 35	67 54	62 8	75 32	82 33	75 12	83 48	100 65	69 32	100 5	77 78	90 20	66 70	-	-
Trinity Medical Center, Carrollton, TX	71 49	94 233	96 263	92 161	94 261	6 33	6 89	0	84 125	49 239	88 285	68 74	76 88	83 69	45 11	84 185	99 228	88 92	68	69 183	71 49	66 184	-	-
Trophy Club Medical Center, Trophy Club, TX	33 3	97 35	77 13	89 35	80 15	0	1 86	75	86 28	57 111	93 143	100 22	84 167	95 130	46	61 199	100 225	84 122	100 90	83 6	100 6	50 6	-	-
Twelve Oaks Hospital, Houston, TX	67 6	94 31	84 32	72 32	71 34	0	0	0	75 85	50 24	81 179	50 2	29 7	100 5	21	62 53	100 70	12 26	50 4	38 37	30 37	63 35	-	-
Tyler County Hospital, Woodville, TX	100 1	100 7	100 1	86 7	50 2	0	0	0	100 6	33 6	70 54	83 6	83 6	75 8	35	86 63	100 70	53 45	100 1	70 46	-	-	-	-
United Regional Healthcare System, Wichita Falls, TX	91 64	97 199	93 301	95 185	95 291	50	11	92	83 116	42 262	90 323	77 62	81 166	82 138	44	76 222	100 272	72 156	84 88	32 276	92 87	70 50	-	-
University General Hospital, Houston, TX	74 46	99 122	98 151	87 91	98 141	0	7 42	7 14	87 191	5 296	96 309	35 106	83 88	78 67	21 14	47 109	100 137	31 29	29 42	71 204	93 43	68 187	-	-
University Hospital, San Antonio, TX	71 49	94 233	96 263	92 161	94 261	6	67 6	89 117	84 125	49 239	88 285	68 74	76 88	83 69	45 11	73 129	100 158	40 65	62 32	78 176	83 63	69 167	0.17 588	1.55 386
University Medical Center, Lubbock, TX	91 11	94 47	92 51	94 32	93 58	1 86	67	1 86	95 82	19 161	93 143	89 22	85 110	95 78	83 35	61 199	100 225	84 122	90 68	69 183	77 49	79 80	-	-
University of Texas Health Center at Tyler, Tyler, TX	91 11	94 47	92 51	94 32	93 58	0	0	10 97	77 243	45 311	99 337	88 100	83 100	61 44	20 20	41 143	98 177	36 80	77 47	80 74	80 74	79 80	-	-
University of Texas Medical Branch Hospitals, Galveston, TX	80 98	97 214	98 271	98 182	98 283	0	10 97	119	77 243	45 311	99 337	69 13	51 55	88 40	40 20	41 143	98 177	43 51	64 11	49 348	80 74	63 345	0.19 1032	2.14 882
USMD Hospital at Arlington, Arlington, TX	-	-	-	-	-	-	-	-	-	-	-	-	-	-	-	-	-	-	-	70 46	-	78 41	-	-
UT Southwestern Saint Paul Hospital, Dallas, TX	75 36	98 117	97 118	93 107	96 115	0	3 100	92 119	84 210	44 368	97 397	99 67	77 99	89 113	51 35	69 151	99 231	60 92	29 32	70 235	93 73	58 209	-	-
Uvalde Memorial Hospital, Uvalde, TX	100 11	100 23	94 16	76 21	84 19	0	0	0	95 44	81 79	96 99	78 9	71 51	91 44	95 21	79 73	100 87	92 52	60 10	53 59	38 13	53 53	-	-
Val Verde Regional Medical Center, Del Rio, TX	60 5	87 30	90 10	92 26	92 12	0	0	100 2	87 38	77 105	70 125	69 13	51 55	88 40	40 20	55 65	98 81	43 51	64 11	74 100	75 20	70 97	-	-

NOTE: The first number in each column (boldface) is the rate in percent, the second number is the number of patients; Please refer to the main entry for footnotes; Heart Attack Care: 1. ACE Inhibitor or ARB for LVSD; 2. Aspirin at Arrival; 3. Aspirin at Discharge; 4. Beta Blocker at Arrival; 5. Beta Blocker at Discharge; 6. Fibrinolytic Medication Timing; 7. PCI Within 90 Minutes of Arrival; 8. Smoking Cessation Advice; Heart Failure Care: 9. ACE Inhibitor or ARB for LVSD; 10. Discharge Instructions; 11. Evaluation of LVS Function; 12. Smoking Cessation Advice; Pneumonia Care: 13. Appropriate Initial Antibiotic; 14. Blood Culture Timing; 15. Influenza Vaccine; 16. Initial Antibiotic Timing; 17. Oxygenation Assessment; 18. Pneumococcal Vaccine; 19. Smoking Cessation Advice; Surgical Infection Prevention: 20. Prophylactic Antibiotic Given; 21. Prophylactic Antibiotic Selection; 22. Prophylactic Antibiotic Stopped; Pregnancy Care: 23. Inpatient Neonatal Mortality; 24. Third or Fourth Degree Laceration

Hospital	Heart Attack Care								Heart Failure Care						Pneumonia Care					Surgical Infection Prevention			Pregnancy Care	
	1	2	3	4	5	6	7	8	9	10	11	12	13	14	15	16	17	18	19	20	21	22	23	24
Valley Baptist Medical Center, Harlingen, TX	**100** 65	**100** 285	**100** 256	**99** 245	**99** 251	**0**	**17**	**12** 100	**100** 228	**100** 635	**100** 713	**100** 54	**85** 332	**89** 251	**42** 86	**76** 369	**100** 440	**64** 287	**100** 45	**79** 197	**90** 59	**61** 190	·	·
Valley Regional Medical Center, Brownsville, TX	**85** 46	**91** 145	**87** 133	**79** 121	**86** 134	**20** 5	**71** 7	**100** 36	**81** 70	**92** 227	**91** 246	**100** 39	**92** 135	**93** 113	**23** 43	**72** 183	**98** 206	**56** 131	**97** 34	**86** 137	**100** 57	**45** 132	**0.28** 3174	**1.57** 1652
Vista Hospital of Dallas, Garland, TX	·	·	·	·	·	·	·	·	·	·	·	·	·	·	·	·	·	·	·	**0**	·	·	·	**0**
Vista Medical Center Hospital, Pasadena, TX	·	·	·	·	·	·	·	·	·	·	·	·	·	·	·	·	·	·	·	**0**	·	·	·	**0**
W J Mangold Memorial Hospital, Lockney, TX	·	·	·	·	·	·	·	·	·	·	·	·	**100** 3	**100** 28	**71** 14	**97** 31	**100** 57	**83** 36	**91** 11	·	·	·	·	·
Wadley Regional Medical Center, Texarkana, TX	**91** 47	**98** 164	**93** 171	**94** 148	**94** 172	**0** 4	**0** 4	**97** 64	**86** 177	**72** 317	**90** 423	**87** 71	**89** 123	**79** 121	**76** 49	**78** 207	**100** 227	**79** 146	**85** 67	**61** 311	**94** 124	**58** 294	·	·
Walls Regional Hospital, Cleburne, TX	**100** 7	**91** 32	**100** 16	**79** 19	**100** 15	·	**0**	**100**	**100** 61	**99** 135	**100** 176	**100** 30	**90** 156	**99** 124	**89** 44	**95** 164	**100** 216	**95** 124	**100** 55	**90** 108	**94** 36	**85** 98	·	·
West Houston Medical Center, Houston, TX	**90** 39	**94** 156	**97** 148	**92** 99	**97** 143	**0** 1	**33** 6	**99** 67	**96** 159	**56** 311	**98** 383	**98** 93	**92** 147	**79** 175	**75** 48	**63** 236	**99** 288	**83** 173	**95** 65	**76** 188	**80** 76	**35** 179	**0.14** 2170	**1.70** 1415
West Texas Medical Center, Midland, TX	**0** 1	**83** 6	**50** 6	**75** 4	**83** 6	·	·	·	**75** 8	·	**100** 9	·	·	·	·	**100** 5	**100** 5	**0** 3	·	**0**	·	·	·	·
Wilbarger General Hospital, Vernon, TX	·	·	·	·	·	·	·	·	**89** 18	**91** 43	**94** 51	**94** 18	**73** 37	**100** 13	**57** 7	**68** 38	**47** 100	**100** 28	**92** 13	**0**	**100** 1	**100** 2	·	·
Wilson N Jones, Sherman, TX	·	·	·	·	·	·	·	·	·	·	·	·	·	·	·	·	·	·	·	·	·	·	·	·
Wilson N Jones Medical Center, Sherman, TX	**79** 52	**95** 172	**91** 160	**86** 153	**87** 165	**0**	**100** 10	**100** 16	**86** 147	**82** 65	**85** 403	**95** 19	**80** 25	**76** 37	**20** 5	**83** 248	**99** 288	**66** 184	**85** 13	**46** 56	·	**40** 55	·	·
Wise Regional Health System, Decatur, TX	**100** 1	**100** 6	**100** 1	**75** 4	**100** 2	·	·	·	**93** 15	**85** 52	**95** 58	**92** 13	**90** 49	**94** 53	**5** 80	**80** 61	**100** 74	**65** 23	**100** 21	**88** 41	**74** 39	**92** 39	·	·
Womans Hospital of Texas, Houston, TX	·	·	·	·	·	·	·	·	·	·	·	·	**50** 2	**100** 2	· 0	**50** 2	**100** 2	**100** 1	· 0	**92** 943	**92** 298	**88** 912	**0.41** 8798	**2.63** 4638
Woodland Heights Medical Center, Lufkin, TX	**89** 38	**96** 92	**94** 122	**96** 82	**96** 114	**0** 2	**50** 2	**100** 47	**95** 119	**76** 207	**97** 276	**100** 38	**71** 122	**90** 73	**92** 37	**87** 141	**100** 169	**93** 109	**100** 44	**88** 424	**85** 110	**79** 396	·	·
Yoakum Community Hospital, Yoakum, TX	**0**	**89** 9	**80** 5	**56** 9	**40** 5	·	·	·	**86** 21	**31** 42	**82** 60	**71** 7	**74** 19	**67** 9	**89** 9	**83** 30	**100** 34	**67** 24	**29** 7	·	·	·	·	·
Zale-Lipshy University Hospital, Dallas, TX	**100** 1	**100** 2	**100** 6	**50** 2	**100** 7	·	·	·	**82** 11	**52** 29	**90** 29	**100** 4	**75** 8	**100** 2	**5**	**62** 13	**100** 19	**83** 12	**100** 3	**72** 83	**92** 38	**45** 65	·	·

NOTE: The first number in each column (boldface) is the rate in percent, the second number is the number of patients; Please refer to the main entry for footnotes; **Heart Attack Care:** 1. ACE Inhibitor or ARB for LVSD; 2. Aspirin at Arrival; 3. Aspirin at Discharge; 4. Beta Blocker at Discharge; 5. Beta Blocker at Arrival; 6. Fibrinolytic Medication Timing; 7. PCI Within 90 Minutes of Arrival; 8. Smoking Cessation Advice; **Heart Failure Care:** 9. ACE Inhibitor or ARB for LVSD; 10. Discharge Instructions; 11. Evaluation of LVS Function; 12. Smoking Cessation Advice; **Pneumonia Care:** 13. Appropriate Initial Antibiotic; 14. Blood Culture Timing; 15. Influenza Vaccine; 16. Initial Antibiotic Timing; 17. Oxygenation Assessment; 18. Pneumococcal Vaccine; 19. Smoking Cessation Advice; **Surgical Infection Prevention:** 20. Prophylactic Antibiotic Given; 21. Prophylactic Antibiotic Selection; 22. Prophylactic Antibiotic Stopped; **Pregnancy Care:** 23. Inpatient Neonatal Mortality; 24. Third or Fourth Degree Laceration

Hospitals whose Mortality Rate is Better than the U.S. National Rate

Heart Attack

Hospital	City	State	Phone	Web Site
Abbott-Northwestern Hospital	Minneapolis	Minnesota	612-863-4000	www.abbottnorthwestern.com
Advocate Lutheran General Hospital	Park Ridge	Illinois	847-723-2210	www.advocatehealth.com
Aurora Saint Lukes Medical Center	Milwaukee	Wisconsin	414-649-6000	www.aurorahealthcare.org
Avera Heart Hospital of South Dakota	Sioux Falls	South Dakota	605-977-7000	www.southdakotaheart.com
Barnes Jewish Hospital	Saint Louis	Missouri	314-747-3000	www.barnesjewish.org
Cape Cod Hospital	Hyannis	Massachusetts	508-771-1800	www.capecodhealth.org/
Evergreen Hospital Medical Center	Kirkland	Washington	425-899-1000	www.evergreenhealthcare.org
Hartford Hospital	Hartford	Connecticut	860-545-5000	www.harthosp.org
Hillcrest Hospital	Mayfield Heights	Ohio	440-312-4500	www.hillcresthospital.org
Maimonides Medical Center	Brooklyn	New York	718-283-6000	www.maimonidesmed.org
Maine Medical Center	Portland	Maine	207-871-0111	www.mmc.org
New York-Presbyterian Hospital	New York	New York	212-746-5454	www.nyp.org
Rex Hospital	Raleigh	North Carolina	919-784-3100	www.rexhealth.com
Saint Vincent Heart Center of Indiana	Indianapolis	Indiana	317-583-5000	www.theheartcenter.com
Saint Vincent's Medical Center	Bridgeport	Connecticut	203-576-6000	www.stvincents.org
Suburban Hospital Association	Bethesda	Maryland	301-896-3100	www.suburbanhospital.org
Trumbull Memorial Hospital	Warren	Ohio	330-841-9011	www.trumhosp.org

Note: Table shows hospitals whose 30-day risk-adjusted death (mortality) rate from heart attack is lower than the U.S. national rate of 16%

Heart Failure

Hospital	City	State	Phone	Web Site
Aventura Hospital & Medical Center	Aventura	Florida	305-682-7000	www.aventurahospital.com
Bay Medical Center	Panama City	Florida	850-769-1511	www.baymedical.org
Bayonne Medical Center	Bayonne	New Jersey	201-858-5000	www.bayonnemedicalcenter.org
Beth Israel Deaconess Medical Center	Boston	Massachusetts	617-667-7000	www.bidmc.harvard.edu
Beth Israel Medical Center	New York	New York	212-420-2000	www.bethisraelny.com
Brigham and Women's Hosptial	Boston	Massachusetts	617-732-5500	www.brighamandwomens.org
Christiana Hospital	Newark	Delaware	302-733-1000	www.christianacare.org
Community Hospital	Munster	Indiana	219-836-1600	www.comhs.org/community
Genesys Regional Medical Center	Grand Blanc	Michigan	810-606-5000	www.genesys.org
Glendale Memorial Hospital & Health Center	Glendale	California	818-502-1900	www.glendalememorial.com
Good Samaritan Hospital	Baltimore	Maryland	410-532-8000	www.goodsam-md.org
Hackensack University Medical Center	Hackensack	New Jersey	201-996-3760	www.humed.com
Harper University Hospital	Detroit	Michigan	313-745-8040	www.harperhospital.org
Healtheast Saint John's Hospital	Maplewood	Minnesota	651-232-7000	www.stjohnshospital-mn.org
Hillcrest Hospital	Mayfield Heights	Ohio	440-312-4500	www.hillcresthospital.org
Liberty Hospital	Liberty	Missouri	816-781-7200	www.libertyhospital.org
Loyola University Medical Center	Maywood	Illinois	708-216-9000	www.luhs.org
Maimonides Medical Center	Brooklyn	New York	718-283-6000	www.maimonidesmed.org
Marymount Hospital	Garfield Heights	Ohio	216-581-0500	www.marymount.org
Mclaren Regional Medical Center	Flint	Michigan	810-342-2000	www.mclaren.org
Memorial Hermann Healthcare System	Houston	Texas	281-929-6100	www.mhhs.org
Mercy Hospital	Miami	Florida	305-854-4400	www.mercymiami.com
Methodist Hospitals	Gary	Indiana	219-886-4000	www.methodisthospital.org
Miami Valley Hospital	Dayton	Ohio	937-208-8000	www.miamivalleyhospital.com
Mount Sinai Medical Center	Miami Beach	Florida	305-674-2121	www.msmc.com
New York-Presbyterian Hospital	New York	New York	212-746-5454	www.nyp.org
Northwestern Memorial Hospital	Chicago	Illinois	312-926-2000	www.nmh.org
Olympia Medical Center	Los Angeles	California	310-657-5900	www.olympiamedicalcenter.com
Providence Hospital	Southfield	Michigan	248-849-3000	www.stjohn.org/Providence/
Saint Agnes Hospital	Baltimore	Maryland	410-368-6000	www.stagnes.org
Sinai-Grace Hospital	Detroit	Michigan	313-966-3300	www.sinaigrace.org
Southcoast Hospital Group	Fall River	Massachusetts	508-679-3131	www.southcoast.org/charlton/
Southwest General Health Center	Middleburg Heights	Ohio	440-816-8000	www.swgeneral.com
Saint Catherine Hospital	East Chicago	Indiana	219-392-1700	www.comhs.org/stcatherine/
Western Pennsylvania Hospital Forbes Reg Campus	Monroeville	Pennsylvania	412-858-2000	www.wpahs.org
White Plains Hospital Center	White Plains	New York	914-681-0600	www.wphospital.org
William Beaumont Hospital	Royal Oak	Michigan	248-898-5000	www.beaumonthospitals.com
Willis Knighton Medical Center	Shreveport	Louisiana	318-212-4000	www.wkmc.com

Note: Table shows hospitals whose 30-day risk-adjusted death (mortality) rate from heart failure is lower than the U.S. national rate of 11%

Hospitals whose Mortality Rate is Worse than the U.S. National Rate

Heart Attack

Hospital	City	State	Phone	Web Site
Christus Saint Michael Health System	Texarkana	Texas	903-614-1000	www.christusstmichael.org/
Danville Regional Medical Center	Danville	Virginia	434-799-2100	www.danvilleregional.org
Kingman Regional Medical Center	Kingman	Arizona	928-757-2101	www.azkrmc.com
Southern Ohio Medical Center	Portsmouth	Ohio	740-356-5000	www.somc.org
Sparks Regional Medical Center	Fort Smith	Arkansas	479-441-4000	www.sparks.org
SVCMC-Catholic Medical Center of Brooklyn Queens	Jamaica	New York		
Yuma Regional Medical Center	Yuma	Arizona	928-344-2000	www.yumaregional.org

Note: Table shows hospitals whose 30-day risk-adjusted death (mortality) rate from heart attack is lower than the U.S. national rate of 16%

Heart Failure

Hospital	City	State	Phone	Web Site
Advocate Christ Hospital & Medical Center	Oak Lawn	Illinois	708-684-8000	www.advocatehealth.com
Athens Regional Medical Center	Athens	Tennessee	423-745-1411	www.athensrmc.com
Banner Thunderbird Medical Center	Glendale	Arizona	602-865-5555	www.bannerhealth.com
Baptist Memorial Hospital	Memphis	Tennessee	901-226-5000	www.baptistonline.org
Baylor All Saints Medical Center at Fort Worth	Fort Worth	Texas	817-926-2544	www.baylorhealth.com/locations/allsaints
Bromenn Healthcare	Normal	Illinois	309-454-1400	www.bromenn.org
Christus Saint Francis Cabrini Hospital	Alexandria	Louisiana	318-448-6760	www.cabrini.org
Claremore Regional Hospital	Claremore	Oklahoma	918-341-2556	www.claremorereghospital.com
Conway Regional Medical Center	Conway	Arkansas	501-329-3831	www.conwayregional.org
Corona Regional Medical Center	Corona	California	951-737-4343	www.coronaregional.com
Danville Regional Medical Center	Danville	Virginia	434-799-2100	www.danvilleregional.org
Faith Regional Health Services	Norfolk	Nebraska	402-371-3402	www.frhs.org
Forrest General Hospital	Hattiesburg	Mississippi	601-288-7000	www.forrestgeneral.com
Gnaden Huetten Memorial Hospital	Lehighton	Pennsylvania	610-377-1300	www.bluemountainhealthsystem.org
Hardin Medical Center	Savannah	Tennessee	731-926-8000	www.hardinmedicacenter.org
Hendrick Medical Center	Abilene	Texas	325-670-2000	www.hendrickhealth.org
Huguley Health System	Fort Worth	Texas	817-293-9110	www.huguley.org
Jackson Hospital & Clinic	Montgomery	Alabama	334-293-8000	www.jackson.org
Kenmore Mercy Hospital	Kenmore	New York	716-447-6100	www.chsbuffalo.org
Lodi Memorial Hospital	Lodi	California	209-334-3411	www.lodihealth.org
Manatee Memorial Hospital	Bradenton	Florida	941-745-6862	www.manateememorial.com
Massena Memorial Hospital	Massena	New York	315-769-4233	www.massenahospital.org
Medical Center of Central Georgia	Macon	Georgia	478-633-1000	www.mccg.org
Mercy Medical Center	Redding	California	530-225-6000	www.redding.mercy.org
Olympic Medical Center	Port Angeles	Washington	360-417-7000	www.olympicmedical.org
Plainview Hospital	Plainview	New York	516-719-3000	www.northshorelij.com
Port Huron Hospital	Port Huron	Michigan	810-987-5000	www.porthuronhospital.org
Providence Hospital	Mobile	Alabama	251-633-1000	www.providencehospital.org
Providence Saint Vincent Medical Center	Portland	Oregon	503-216-1234	www.providence.org
Sacred Heart Medical Center	Eugene	Oregon	541-686-7300	www.peacehealth.org
Samaritan Hospital	Troy	New York	518-271-3300	www.nehealth.com
Saint Josephs Medical Center of Stockton	Stockton	California	209-943-2000	www.stjospehscares.org
Saint Marys Hospital Medical Center	Green Bay	Wisconsin	920-498-4200	www.stmgb.org
Sutter General Hospital	Sacramento	California	916-454-2222	www.suttermedicalcenter.org
Tri-City Medical Center	Oceanside	California	760-940-5780	www.tricitymed.org

Note: Table shows hospitals whose 30-day risk-adjusted death (mortality) rate from heart failure is lower than the U.S. national rate of 11%

Hospital Mortality from Heart Attack and Heart Failure: State Summary

State	Number of Hospitals					
	Heart Attack			Heart Failure		
	Better than U.S. National Rate[1]	No Different than U.S. National Rate[2]	Worse than U.S. National Rate[3]	Better than U.S. National Rate[4]	No Different than U.S. National Rate[5]	Worse than U.S. National Rate[6]
Alabama	0	93	0	0	99	2
Alaska	0	13	0	0	20	0
Arizona	0	62	2	0	71	1
Arkansas	0	81	1	0	82	1
California	0	316	0	2	323	6
Colorado	0	61	0	0	68	0
Connecticut	2	29	0	0	32	0
Delaware	0	5	0	1	4	0
District of Columbia	0	7	0	0	7	0
Florida	0	182	0	4	180	1
Georgia	0	134	0	0	141	1
Guam	0	1	0	0	1	0
Hawaii	0	15	0	0	18	0
Idaho	0	33	0	0	37	0
Illinois	1	184	0	2	184	2
Indiana	1	117	0	3	119	0
Iowa	0	112	0	0	125	0
Kansas	0	114	0	0	132	0
Kentucky	0	100	0	0	103	0
Louisiana	0	108	0	1	117	1
Maine	1	37	0	0	39	0
Maryland	1	44	0	2	43	0
Massachusetts	1	63	0	3	62	0
Michigan	0	132	0	6	131	1
Minnesota	1	131	0	1	137	0
Mississippi	0	80	0	0	98	1
Missouri	1	117	0	1	123	0
Montana	0	41	0	0	60	0
N. Mariana Islands	0	1	0	0	1	0
Nebraska	0	74	0	0	87	1
Nevada	0	28	0	0	31	0
New Hampshire	0	26	0	0	26	0
New Jersey	0	75	0	2	73	0
New Mexico	0	38	0	0	42	0
New York	2	185	1	4	187	4
North Carolina	1	108	0	0	114	0
North Dakota	0	33	0	0	43	0
Ohio	2	155	1	4	159	0
Oklahoma	0	100	0	0	115	1
Oregon	0	57	0	0	56	2
Pennsylvania	0	170	0	1	170	1
Puerto Rico	0	47	0	0	49	0
Rhode Island	0	10	0	0	11	0
South Carolina	0	57	0	0	58	0
South Dakota	1	44	0	0	54	0
Tennessee	0	116	0	0	116	3
Texas	0	320	1	1	357	3
Utah	0	31	0	0	39	0
Vermont	0	15	0	0	16	0
Virgin Islands	0	2	0	0	2	0
Virginia	0	79	1	0	83	1
Washington	1	75	0	0	85	1
West Virginia	0	53	0	0	53	0
Wisconsin	1	118	0	0	124	1
Wyoming	0	23	0	0	26	0
U.S. and Territories	17	4453	7	38	4734	35

Note: (1) 30-day risk-adjusted death rate is lower than U.S. rate of 16%; (2) 30-day risk-adjusted death rate is about the same as U.S. rate of 16% or difference is uncertain; (3) 30-day risk-adjusted death rate is higher than U.S. rate of 16%; (4) 30-day risk-adjusted death rate is lower than U.S. rate of 11%; (2) 30-day risk-adjusted death rate is about the same as U.S. rate of 11% or difference is uncertain; (3) 30-day risk-adjusted death rate is higher than U.S. rate of 11%

What Do These Mortality Categories Show?

These categories show how hospitals' risk-adjusted 30-Day Death (mortality) rates compare to the rate across the U.S., after making adjustments for how sick patients were before they were admitted to the hospital and taking into account differences in death rates that might be due to chance.

Hospitals are shown to be Better or Worse Than U.S. National Rate only if we can be 95% certain that the difference between their risk-adjusted death (mortality) rates and the U.S. National rate is not due to chance. All others are shown in the No Different Than U.S. National Rate category.

Better than U.S. National Rate. Hospitals in the Better Than U.S. National Rate category have risk-adjusted 30-day death (mortality) rates that are lower than the U.S. National rate, and we can be 95% certain that this difference is not due to chance.

No Different than U.S. National Rate. Many hospitals in the No Different Than U.S. National Rate category have risk-adjusted 30-day death (mortality) rates that are about the same as the U.S. National rate. Other hospitals in this category have rates that are higher or lower than the U.S. National rate, but we cannot be 95% certain that these differences are not due to chance. One cannot be certain about differences when a hospital has very few relevant patients.

Worse than U.S. National Rate. Hospitals in the Worse Than U.S. National Rate category have risk-adjusted 30-day death (mortality) rates that are higher than the U.S. National rate, and we can be 95% certain that this difference is not due to chance.

Why are Death Rates for Individual Hospitals Not Shown?

Comparisons based on estimated death (mortality) rates alone can be misleading. Risk-adjusted death (mortality) rates are estimated for individual hospitals based on information taken from a particular time period (in this case, July 1, 2005 - June 30, 2006). If a slightly different time period had been chosen, chances are that each hospital's results would have been somewhat different.

Researchers almost always report a range ("confidence interval" or in this case an "interval estimate") around their estimates, to show how much variation might be due to this kind of chance. A confidence interval or interval estimate tells us we can be reasonably "confident" (in this case, 95% confident) that a hospital's death (mortality) rate fell somewhere within this specified range. The smaller the range, the more precise the estimate.

When hospitals treat a very large number of patients, chance differences will not have much effect on the overall rates. The range will be small, and the estimated death (mortality) rates will be more precise. In hospitals that treat smaller numbers of patients, however, even small chance differences could have a big impact on death (mortality) rates. The 95% confidence interval, or range, will be large, and the estimated death (mortality) rates will be much less precise.

Because the number of patients treated at U.S. hospitals varies widely, the precision of hospitals' estimated death (mortality) rates also varies.

Calculation of 30-Day Risk-Adjusted Mortality Rates

CMS calculates 30-day death (mortality) rates for heart attack and heart failure. The rates are "risk-adjusted" using Medicare claims and enrollment data in a complex statistical model. The model predicts how many patients will die within 30 days of being admitted to each hospital for heart attack or heart failure. It includes deaths whether the patients die in the hospital or after leaving, and whether or not they die for heart attack/heart failure or something else. By "risk-adjusted", we mean that the model calculates a death (mortality) rate that adjusts for the kinds of patients who go to that hospital so that hospitals that take care of sicker patients won't have a worse rate just because their patients were sicker before they arrived at the hospital.

For each hospital's rate, the model also calculates an "interval estimate" (which is like a confidence interval), which describes how much uncertainty there is around the rate-how much bigger or smaller

the rate might really be. A hospital with many relevant patients will have a rate that is more precise or certain; that is, the "interval estimate" will be relatively narrow. A hospital with few relevant patients will have a rate that is less precise or certain; that is, will have a wide "interval estimate." The "risk-adjusted" hospital rate with its "interval estimate" can be compared to the U.S. National death (mortality) rate (the "national crude mortality rate"). If the interval estimate includes (overlaps with) the national crude mortality rate, the hospital's performance is considered to be "no different than U.S. National rate" and so is placed in that category. If the entire interval estimate is below the national crude mortality rate, then the hospital's performance is "worse than U.S. National rate." If the entire interval estimate is above the national crude mortality rate, the hospital's performance is "better than U.S. National rate."

Data Collection Methods

Cases Included in the Model. All Medicare beneficiaries aged 65 or older who were enrolled in Original Medicare (traditional fee-for-service Medicare) for the entire 12 months prior to their hospital admission for heart attack or heart failure, and for whom complete administrative data for that 12-month period are available, are included in the model. The model identifies (1) all short-stay acute-care hospital discharges for heart attack or heart failure in the reference year based on a principal discharge diagnosis on the Medicare beneficiary's inpatient claim, and (2) all deaths (for all causes) within 30 days of admission. Hospital stays that lasted one day or less are excluded, provided the patient was discharged alive and not against medical advice. (For the initial publication of the rates in June 2007, the reference year used for calculating mortality rates is July 2005 through June 2006. Subsequent updates to the rates are expected to use the same July/June reference year.)

Hospital mortality rates for heart attack are calculated based on all admissions for heart attack, even if an individual Medicare beneficiary was hospitalized more than once for this condition during the 12-month period. However, for purposes of calculating heart failure mortality rates, if a beneficiary had multiple admissions during the 12-month period, one admission is chosen randomly for inclusion in the model.

Use of a 30-Day Period to Assess Mortality

The model tracks deaths that occur within 30 days of a hospital admission, rather than inpatient mortality only, or mortality over some other post-discharge period. Thirty-day mortality was chosen over inpatient mortality because variability across hospitals in lengths of stay can make differences in inpatient mortality hard to interpret. For example, a heart attack patient hospitalized for 12 days may have a higher chance of dying during the hospital stay than a patient hospitalized for only 7 days, merely because the first patient's outcome is tracked for 5 days longer than the second patient's. Thirty-day mortality was chosen over longer windows (such as 90 days or one year), because mortality over longer periods may have less to do with the care received in the hospital and more to do with other complicating illnesses, patients' own behavior, or the care they received after discharge.

Use of Administrative Claims Data

Administrative claims data, rather than medical records data, are used to predict 30-day mortality. These data are widely available for Original Medicare (traditional fee-for-service) beneficiaries, are relatively inexpensive to acquire, and are timely. Using administrative data makes it possible to calculate mortality without having to do chart reviews or requiring hospitals to report additional data. Research conducted when the measures were being developed demonstrated that the administrative claims-based models perform well in predicting mortality compared with models based on chart reviews.

Risk-Adjustment and Covariates Included in the Model

Risk-Adjustment. The model adjusts for differences in patients' risks unrelated to their hospital care (risk-adjustment). The characteristics that Medicare patients bring with them when they arrive at a hospital with a heart attack or heart failure are not under the control of the hospital. However, some patient characteristics may make death more likely (increase the "risk" of death), no matter where the patient is treated or how good the care is. Moreover, some hospitals may treat people with a history of more severe disease. Therefore, when mortality rates are calculated for each hospital for a 12-month period, they are adjusted based on the unique mix of patients that hospital treated during that period. Factors included in the risk-adjustment model include age, gender, past medical history, and other diseases or conditions (comorbidities) that patients had when they arrived at the hospital that are known to increase their risk.

Past medical history and comorbidities are included in the model using CMS's hierarchical condition categories (HCCs) and a history of certain procedures. Medicare patients are assigned to one or more HCCs based on diagnoses (ICD-9 codes) obtained from the patient's discharge claim, and from the hospital inpatient, hospital outpatient, and physician Medicare claims submitted for the patient one year prior to the admission. Secondary diagnoses from the patient's hospital discharge claim that might represent complications that occurred while the patient was in the hospital, rather than conditions that were present on admission, are not included in assigning the patient's HCC. Research has shown that coding differences among providers affect HCCs only slightly. Diagnoses from unreliable sources (such as laboratory or other claims that were not based on face-to-face encounters) are not included when assigning the HCCs in the model.

To "risk-adjust" mortality rates for patient characteristics, the statistical model estimates the independent effects of age, gender, comorbidities, and a hospital-specific component of quality on mortality of patients within 30 days of hospital admission (the dependent variable). Using these estimates, the model calculates an adjusted mortality rate for each hospital that can be compared with those of other hospitals with different case mixes.

Covariates in 30-Day Mortality Risk-Adjustment Models	
Heart Attack	Heart Failure
Age-65	Age-65
Gender (male)	Gender (male)
History of PTCA	History of PTCA
History of CABG	History of CABG
History of heart failure	History of heart failure
History of MI	History of MI
AMI location (Group 1): anterior, anterolateral	
AMI location (Group 2): inferolateral, inferoposterior, inferior, other lateral, and true posterior	
Unstable angina	Unstable angina
Chronic atherosclerosis	Chronic atherosclerosis
Cardiopulmonary-respiratory failure and shock	Cardiopulmonary-respiratory failure and shock
Valvular heart disease	Valvular heart disease
Hypertension	Hypertension
Stroke	Stroke
Cerebrovascular disease	
Renal failure	Renal failure
COPD	COPD
Pneumonia	Pneumonia
Diabetes	Diabetes
Protein-calorie malnutrition	Protein-calorie malnutrition
Dementia	Dementia
Functional disability	Functional disability
Peripheral vascular disease	Peripheral vascular disease
Metastatic cancer	Metastatic cancer
Trauma in last year	Trauma in last year
Major psych disorder	Major psych disorder
Chronic liver disease	Chronic liver disease

Statistical Methods Used to Calculate Mortality Rates

Hierarchical Regression Model. The statistical model for computing 30-day risk-adjusted mortality rate measures is a "hierarchical regression model." This type of model is based on the assumption that any heart attack or heart failure patients treated at a particular hospital will experience a level of quality of care that applies to all patients treated for the same condition in that hospital. In other words, the expected risk of death for two similar heart attack or heart failure patients treated in the same hospital would be more alike than the risk of death for the same two patients treated in two different hospitals.

The likelihood that an individual patient will die is therefore a combination of (1) his or her individual risk characteristics (for example, gender, comorbidities, and past medical history) and 2) the hospital's unique quality of care for all patients treated for that condition in that hospital. The model estimates the effects of both of these components on mortality.

Calculating Mortality Rates. Each hospital's "30-day risk-adjusted mortality rate" (also called the "Risk Standardized Mortality Rate" or RSMR) is computed in several steps. First, the predicted 30-day mortality for a particular hospital obtained from the hierarchical regression model is divided by the expected mortality for that hospital, which is also obtained from the regression model. Predicted mortality is the rate of deaths from heart attack or heart failure that would be anticipated in the particular hospital during the 12-month period, given the patient case mix and the hospital's unique quality of care effect on mortality. Expected mortality is the rate of deaths from heart attack or heart failure that would be expected if the same patients with the same characteristics had instead been treated at an "average" hospital, given the "average" hospital's quality of care effect on mortality for patients with that condition. This ratio is then multiplied by the national unadjusted mortality rate for the condition for all hospitals to compute a "risk-adjusted mortality rate" for the hospital. So, the higher a hospital's predicted 30-day mortality rate, relative to expected mortality for the hospital's particular case mix of patients, the higher its adjusted mortality rate will be. Hospitals with better quality will have lower rates.

(Predicted 30-day mortality/Expected mortality) * U.S. National mortality rate = RSMR

For example, suppose the model predicts that 10 percent of Hospital A's heart attack patients would die within 30 days of admission in a given year, based on their ages, gender mix, and pre-existing health conditions, and based on the estimate of the hospital's specific quality of care. Then, suppose that the expected rate of 30-day deaths for those same patients were higher – say, 15 percent – if they had instead been treated at an "average" U.S. hospital. If the actual mortality rate for the 12-month period for all heart attack patients in all hospitals in the U.S. is 12 percent, then the hospital's risk-adjusted 30-day mortality rate would be 8 percent.

(10%/15%)* 12% = RSMR for Hospital A 8%

If, instead, 9 percent of these patients would be expected to have died if treated at the average hospital, then the hospital's mortality rate would be 13.3 percent.

(10%/9%)* 12% = RSMR for Hospital A 13.3%

In the first case, the hospital performed better than the average hospital and had a relatively low risk-adjusted mortality rate (8 percent); in the second case it performed worse and had a relatively high rate (13.3 percent).

Hospitals with relatively low-risk patients whose predicted mortality rate is the same as the expected mortality rate for the average hospital for the same group of low-risk patients would have an adjusted mortality rate equal to the national rate (12 percent in this example). Similarly, hospitals with high-risk patients whose predicted mortality rate is the same as the expected mortality rate for the average hospital for the same group of high-risk patients would also have an adjusted mortality rate equal to the national rate of 12 percent. Thus, each hospital's case mix should not affect the adjusted mortality rates used to compare hospitals.

Adjusting for Small Hospitals or a Small Number of Cases. The hierarchical regression model also adjusts mortality rates results for small hospitals or hospitals with few heart attack or heart failure cases in a given year. This reduces the chance that such hospitals' performance will fluctuate wildly from year to year or that they will be wrongly classified as either a worse or better performer. For these hospitals, the model not only considers deaths among patients treated for the condition in the small sample size of cases, but pools together patients from all hospitals treated for the given condition, to make the result more reliable. In essence, the predicted mortality rate for a hospital with a small number of cases is moved toward the overall U.S. National mortality rate for all hospitals. The estimates of mortality for hospitals with few patients will rely considerably on the pooled data for all hospitals, making it less likely that small hospitals will fall into either of the outlier categories. This pooling affords a "borrowing of statistical strength" that provides more confidence in the results.

Significance Testing, Interval Estimates, and Comparing Rates Among Hospitals

Significance Testing and Interval Estimates. The model also calculates how precise the estimates of the adjusted mortality rate are, and determines upper and lower bounds (Interval Estimates) for each hospital's risk-adjusted rate. Interval estimates, which are like confidence intervals, describe how much uncertainty there is around the rate—how much bigger or smaller the rate might really be. Larger hospitals typically have more precise estimates and smaller interval estimates, since more data are available to estimate mortality. The smaller the sample size, the greater the difference in mortality rates between a hospital and the national rate must be in order for that difference to be statistically meaningful.

Comparing Mortality Rates Among Hospitals. The risk-adjusted hospital rate with its interval estimate can be compared to the U.S. National crude mortality rate. If the interval estimate includes (overlaps with) the national crude mortality rate, the hospital's performance is in the "no different than U.S. National rate" category. If the entire interval estimate is below the national crude mortality rate, then the hospital is performing "worse than U.S. National rate." If the entire interval estimate is above the national crude mortality rate, it is "better than U.S. National rate."

Glossary of Terms

Accreditation
An evaluative process in which a healthcare organization undergoes an examination of its policies, procedures and performance by an external private sector organization ("accrediting body") to ensure that it is meeting predetermined criteria. It usually involves both on- and off-site surveys. Also see the terms AOA, The Joint Commission, and Medicare-Certified Hospitals.

Acute Care Hospital
A hospital that provides inpatient medical care and other related services for surgery, acute medical conditions or injuries (usually for a short term illness or condition).

Acute Myocardial Infarction (AMI)
A condition (also called a heart attack) that occurs when the arteries leading to the heart become blocked and the blood supply is slowed or stopped. When the heart muscle can't get the oxygen and nutrients it needs, the part of the heart tissue that is affected may die.

Additional Measures
Measures included in the Hospital Quality Alliance measure set, reflecting care for discharges occurring on or after April 1, 2004 (Collection period varies by measure).

Acute Myocardial Infarction
- Fibrinolytic agent received within 30 minutes of hospital arrival
- Percutaneous Coronary Intervention (PCI) received within 90 minutes of hospital arrival (previously PCI received within 120 minutes of hospital arrival, as well as, Percutaneous Transluminal Coronary Angioplasty (PTCA) received within 90 minutes of hospital arrival)
- Smoking cessation advice/counseling
- 30-Day Risk Adjusted Heart Attack Mortality

Heart Failure
- Discharge instructions
- Smoking cessation advice/counseling
- 30-Day Risk Adjusted Heart Failure Mortality

Pneumonia
- Blood culture performed in the emergency department prior to initial antibiotic received in hospital (previously Blood culture performed prior to first antibiotic received in hospital)
- Smoking cessation advice/counseling
- Appropriate initial antibiotic selection
- Influenza vaccination status

Surgical Care Improvement/Surgical Infection Prevention
- Prophylactic antibiotic received within 1 hour prior to surgical incision
- Prophylactic antibiotic selection
- Prophylactic antibiotic discontinued within 24 hours after surgery end time

American Hospital Association (AHA)
The national organization that represents and serves all types of hospitals, health care networks, and their patients and communities. AHA takes part in national health policy development, legislative and regulatory debates, and legal matters. AHA provides education for health care leaders and is a source of information on health care issues and trends.

American Osteopathic Association (AOA)
A member association representing approximately 52,000 osteopathic physicians (D.O.s). The AOA serves as the primary certifying body for D.O.s, and is the accrediting agency for all osteopathic medical colleges and health care facilities.

The AOA writes a performance report on each hospital that it checks. You can call or write to AOA to find out a hospital's level of accreditation.

Angioplasty
In angioplasty, a catheter is used to insert a balloon that is inflated to open a blocked blood vessel. Percutaneous transluminal coronary angioplasty (PTCA) is one of several procedures used to open a blocked blood vessel, known collectively as a percutaneous coronary intervention or PCI.

Angiotensin Converting Enzyme (ACE) Inhibitor
A medicine used to treat heart attacks, heart failure, or a decreased function of the left heart. They stop production of a hormone that can narrow blood vessels. This helps reduce the pressure in the heart and lower blood pressure.

Angiotensin Receptor Blocker (ARB)
A medicine used to treat patients with heart failure and a decreased function of the left heart. ARBs block the action of a hormone that can narrow blood vessels. This helps reduce the pressure in the heart and lower blood pressure.

Antibiotic
Medicine used to fight bacteria in the body.

Atherectomy
A procedure where a blade or laser on a catheter cuts through and removes blockages in blood vessels. It is one of several procedures used to open a blocked blood vessel (known as a Percutaneous Coronary Intervention or PCI).

Beta Blocker
A type of medicine that is used to lower blood pressure, treat chest pain (angina) and heart failure, and to help prevent a heart attack. Beta blockers relieve the stress on the heart by slowing the heart rate and reducing the force with which the heart muscles contract to pump blood. They also help keep blood vessels from constricting in the heart, brain, and body.

Blood Culture
A blood test that shows if there are bacteria in the blood, and what type of bacteria it is. It helps your doctor decide which antibiotic to use to treat a bacterial infection.

Centers for Medicare & Medicaid Services (CMS)
The federal agency that runs the Medicare program for the elderly aged and disabled. In addition, CMS works with the states to run the Medicaid program for low-income individuals. CMS works to make sure that the people in these programs are able to get high quality health care. Also see the term DHHS.

Certification (Medicare-Certified)
State government agencies inspect health care providers, including hospitals, nursing homes, dialysis facilities and home health agencies, as well as other health care providers. These providers are certified if they pass inspection. Being certified is not the same as being accredited. Medicare or Medicaid only pays for care provided by certified or accredited providers.

Critical Access Hospital (CAH)
A small, generally geographically remote facility that provides outpatient and inpatient hospital services to people in rural areas. The designation was established by law, for special payments under the Medicare program. To be designated as a CAH, a hospital must be located in a rural area, provide 24-hour emergency services; have an average length-of-stay for its patients of 96 hours or less; be located more than 35 miles (or more than 15 miles in areas with mountainous terrain) from the nearest hospital or be designated by its State as a "necessary provider". Hospitals may have no more than 25 beds.

Department of Health and Human Services (DHHS)
A division of the U.S. government that administers many of the social programs at the Federal level dealing with the health and welfare of the citizens of the United States. CMS is an agency within DHHS.

Diastolic Pressure
The lowest pressure in the artery when the heart is filling with blood. In a blood pressure reading, the diastolic pressure is the second number recorded.

Do hospitals that treat sicker patients have worse death rates? (Risk-adjustment)
Hospitals that treat sicker patients do not necessarily have worse death rates. The hospital-specific 30-day death (mortality) rates used in this report have been adjusted to account for differences in patients' health before their hospital admission.

Sicker patients or patients with more health-related risks may be more likely to die than healthier patients. Moreover, patients who are sicker may be more likely to be treated at particular hospitals while patients who are healthier may be more likely to be treated at other hospitals.

To compare hospitals fairly (and to avoid penalizing those that treat sicker patients) it is therefore important to consider differences in patients' health before they were admitted to the hospital. The statistical process of accounting for differences in patients' sickness before they were admitted to the hospital is called risk-adjustment. This statistical process aims to 'level the playing field' by accounting for health risks that patients have before they enter the hospital.

Fibrinolysis, Fibrinolytic Drugs
Fibrinolytic drugs are "clot-busting" medicines that can help dissolve blood clots in blood vessels and improve blood flow to your heart. They are important for treating heart attacks. If you have a heart attack, your doctor may give you a fibrinolytic drug, perform a percutaneous coronary intervention (PCI), or both.

Hospital Quality Alliance (HQA): Improving Care Through Information
In December 2002, the American Hospital Association (AHA), Federation of American Hospitals (FAH), and Association of American Medical Colleges (AAMC) launched the Hospital Quality Alliance (HQA), a national public-private collaboration to encourage hospitals to voluntarily collect and report hospital quality performance information. This effort is intended to make important information about hospital performance accessible to the public and to inform and invigorate efforts to improve quality. CMS and the Joint Commission participate in the HQA, along with the AHA, the FAH, the AAMC, the American Medical Association, the American Nurses Association, the National Association of Children's Hospitals and Related Organizations, American Association of Retired People, American Federation of Labor and Council of Industrial Organizations, the Consumer-Purchaser Disclosure Project, the Agency for Healthcare Research and Quality, the National Quality Forum, the Blue Cross and Blue Shield Association, the National Business Coalition on Health, General Electric, and the U.S. Chamber of Commerce.

Influenza
Influenza is a serious and sometimes deadly lung infection that can spread quickly in a community. Symptoms include fever-often a high temperature of more than 102° Fahrenheit (38.9° Celsius), headache, muscle aches and pains, chills, cough and chest pain when you take a breath ("pleuritic chest pain"). Although most people recover from the illness, the Centers for Disease Control and Prevention (the CDC) estimates that in the United States more than 200,000 people are hospitalized and about 36,000 people die from the flu and its complications every year.

Influenza Vaccination ("Flu Shot")
The main way to keep from getting flu is to get a yearly flu vaccination. Scientists make a different vaccine every year because the strains of flu viruses change from year to year. Nine to 10 months before the flu season begins, they prepare a new vaccine made from inactivated (killed) flu viruses. Because the viruses have been killed, they cannot cause infection. The vaccine preparation is based on the strains of the flu viruses that are in circulation at the time.

Hospitals should check to make sure that pneumonia patients get a flu shot during flu season to protect them from another lung infection and to help prevent the spread of influenza in the community. You can also get the vaccine at your doctor's office or a local clinic, and in many communities at workplaces, supermarkets, and drugstores. You must get the vaccine every year because it changes.

Inpatient Hospital Services
Services provided to patients admitted to a hospital that include bed and board, nursing services, diagnostic or therapeutic services, and medical or surgical services.

Left Ventricular Function Assessment
A test to check how well the heart is pumping.

Long-term Care Hospital
A facility, like a nursing home, that provides a variety of services that help people with health or personal needs and activities of daily living (like walking, eating, and going to the bathroom) over a period of time. Most long-term care is custodial care, for which Medicare does not pay.

Measurement
The process of collecting data to assess performance conducted at a single point in time or repeated over time.

Medicaid
A joint federal and state program that helps with medical costs for some people with low incomes and limited resources. Medicaid programs vary from state to state, but most health care costs are covered if you qualify for both Medicare and Medicaid.

Medicare-Certified Hospital
In order to receive any payment from either the Medicare or Medicaid programs, a hospital must meet a set of basic standards for quality of care, called "conditions of participation". Medicare-certified hospitals are reviewed periodically (every three years) to assure that they are continuing to provide services of acceptable quality.

Medicare also considers or "deems" hospitals as Medicare-certified that meet the accreditation requirements of the The Joint Commission or the American Osteopathic Association. Most short-term acute care hospitals in the United States choose to be Medicare-certified, either directly or through accreditation.

Medicare Provider Number
Medicare identifies the hospitals with which it works using a unique number. These numbers were used to identify the facilities that reported data for Hospital Compare. If hospitals share a Medicare Provider Number (for example, they bill Medicare for services as a single legal entity), the performance data for those hospitals are, in effect, combined into an aggregate rate representing all of the hospitals represented by the Medicare Provider Number. If you are interested in a hospital that is part of a system or network, you may not be able to find your specific hospital.

Medigap Policy
A Medicare supplement insurance policy sold by private insurance companies to fill "gaps" in Original Medicare Plan coverage. Except in Massachusetts, Minnesota and Wisconsin, there are 10 standardized plans labeled Plan A through Plan J. Medigap policies only work with the Original Medicare Plan.

Original Medicare Plan
A pay-per-visit health plan that lets you go to any doctor, hospital, or other health care supplier who accepts Medicare and is accepting new Medicare patients. You must pay the deductible. Medicare pays its share of the Medicare-approved amount, and you pay your share (coinsurance). In some cases you may be charged more than the Medicare-approved amount. The Original Medicare Plan has two parts: Part A (Hospital Insurance) and Part B (Medical Insurance).

Osteopathic Doctor
A licensed physician who can do surgery and prescribe drugs who has training in manipulative therapy. Also called a Doctor of Osteopathy or DO.

Outcome Measures
Measures designed to reflect the results of care, rather than how frequently a specific treatment or intervention was performed.

Oxygenation Assessment
Test that measures the amount of oxygen in your blood to see if you need oxygen therapy.

Percutaneous Coronary Interventions (PCI)
The procedures called Percutaneous Coronary Interventions (PCI), such as angioplasty and atherectomy are among those that are the most effective for opening blocked blood vessels that cause heart attacks. Doctors may perform a PCI, or give medicine to open the blockage, and in some cases, may do both.

Plan of Care
A written plan of care created with your physician and hospital staff. It tells what services you will get to reach and keep your best physical, mental, and social well being. The hospital staff keeps your doctor up-to-date on how you are doing and updates your care plan as needed.

Pneumonia
An inflammation of the lungs caused by a viral or bacterial infection. This fills your lungs with mucus and lowers the oxygen level in your blood. Symptoms can include fever, fatigue, difficulty breathing, chills, a "wet" cough, and chest pain.

Pneumonia (pneumococcal) Vaccination
Vaccine given to prevent pneumonia, estimated to protect against 80% of bacteria causing pneumonia.

Process of Care Measures
Measures that show, in percentage form or as a rate, how often a health care provider gives recommended care; that is, the treatment known to give the best results for most patients with a particular condition.

Provider
A doctor, hospital, health care professional, or health care facility.

Psychiatric Hospital
A facility that provides inpatient psychiatric services for the diagnosis and treatment of mental illness on a 24-hour basis, by or under the supervision of a physician.

Quality
Quality health care is how well a doctor, hospital, health plan, or other provider of health care, keeps its members healthy or treats them when they are sick. Good quality health care means doing the right thing at the right time, in the right way, for the right person and getting the best possible results.

Quality Assurance
The process of looking at how well a medical service is provided. The process may include formally reviewing health care given to a person, or group of persons, locating the problem, correcting the problem, and then checking to see if what you did worked.

Quality Improvement Organizations (QIOs)
Groups of practicing doctors and other health care experts who are paid by the federal government to check and improve the care given to Medicare patients. They must review your complaints about the quality of care given by: inpatient hospitals, hospital outpatient departments, hospital emergency rooms, skilled nursing facilities, home health agencies, Private Fee-for-Service plans, and ambulatory surgical centers.

Rehabilitation Hospital
A hospital that specializes in improving or restoring a patient's functional ability through therapies. Sometimes called a post-acute hospital.

Risk-Adjusted 30-Day Death (Mortality) Rates
The 30-day Risk-Adjusted Death (Mortality) Rates are produced using a complex statistical model, that relies on Medicare claims and enrollment information. The model predicts patient deaths for any cause within 30 days of hospital admission for heart attack or heart failure, whether the patients die while still in the hospital or after

discharge. Thirty-day mortality is used because this is the time period when deaths are most likely to be related to the care patients received in the hospital. Deaths that occur outside the hospital within 30 days are included along with deaths that occur in the hospital, because some hospitals discharge patients sooner than others.

"Starter Set" Measures

Heart Attack
- Aspirin at arrival
- Aspirin at discharge
- ACE Inhibitor or ARB for Left Ventricular Systolic Dysfunction*
- Beta Blocker at arrival
- Beta Blocker at discharge

Heart Failure
- Evaluation of Left Ventricular Systolic (LVS) Function**
- ACE Inhibitor or ARB for Left Ventricular Systolic Dysfunction*

Pneumonia
- Oxygenation Assessment
- Initial Antibiotic Timing
- Pneumococcal Vaccination Status

*Modified, effective 1Q2005 discharges. For more information, see http://www.cms.hhs.gov/HospitalQualityInits/downloads/HospitalSummaryOfMeeting1.pdf.

**Modified, effective 1Q2006 discharges.

Stent
A small wire tube inserted in a blood vessel by a catheter to hold open a blocked blood vessel. One of several procedures to open a blocked blood vessel called a percutaneous coronary intervention (PCI).

The Joint Commission
An organization that evaluates and accredits health care organizations and programs in the United States. The Joint Commission is an independent, not-for-profit organization. The Joint Commission looks at how well a hospital treats patients and how good a hospital's staff and equipment are. A hospital is accredited by The Joint Commission if it meets certain quality standards. These checks are done at least every 3 years. Most hospitals take part in these accreditations.

The Joint Commission writes a "performance report" on each hospital that it checks. You can order these reports free of charge.

Thirty-Day Mortality Model Information
See Krumholtz, H., et al. "An Administrative Claims Model Suitable for Profiling Hospital Performance Based on 30-Day Mortality Rates Among Patients with an Acute Myocardial Infarction." Circulation. Vol. 113: 1683-1692, 2006, for details on the development of the AMI model. An accompanying article in the same volume discusses the heart failure model.

Treatment
Something done to help with a health problem. For example, medicine and surgery are treatments.

Treatment Options
The choices you have when there is more than one way to treat your health problem.

Abbeville County Memorial Hospital Abbeville, SC, 290
Abbeville General Hospital Abbeville, LA, 200
Abilene Regional Medical Center Abilene, TX, 332
Abrom Kaplan Memorial Hospital Kaplan, LA, 211
Acadian Medical Center Eunice, LA, 207
Admin de Servicios Medicos Puerto Rico San Juan, PR, 280
Advanced Cardiology Center (alternate name) Mayaguez, PR, 277
Aiken Regional Medical Centers Aiken, SC, 290
Alice Regional Hospital Alice, TX, 332
Allen Bennett Memorial Hospital Greer, SC, 299
Allen Parish Hospital Kinder, LA, 212
Alliance Health Center Meridian, MS, 254
Alliance Healthcare System Holly Springs, MS, 247
Alliance Hospital Odessa, TX, 405
American Legion Hospital Crowley, LA, 206
AMI East Cooper Community Hospital (alternate name) Mount Pleasant, SC, 302
AMI Nacogdoches Medical Center Hospital (alternate name) Nacogdoches, TX, 403
AMI National Park Medical Center (alternate name) Hot Springs, AR, 54
AMI Southwestern General Hospital (alternate name) El Paso, TX, 365
AMI Town and Country Medical Center (alternate name) Tampa, FL, 135
Andalusia Regional Hospital Andalusia, AL, 9
Anderson Area Medical Center Anderson, SC, 290
Angleton-Danbury General Hospital (alternate name) Angleton, TX, 335
Angleton-Danbury Medical Center Angleton, TX, 335
Anmed Health (alternate name) Anderson, SC, 290
Anson General Hospital Anson, TX, 335
Appling Hospital Baxley, GA, 159
Arkansas Heart Hospital Little Rock, AR, 56
Arkansas Methodist Hospital Paragould, AR, 62
Arkansas Surgical Hospital North Little Rock, AR, 61
Arlington Memorial Hospital Arlington, TX, 336
Arlington Memorial South Medical Center (alternate name) Arlington, TX, 336
Ashford Presbyterian Community Hospital San Juan, PR, 281
Ashley County Medical Center Crossett, AR, 49
Ashley Memorial Hospital (alternate name) Crossett, AR, 49
Assumption Community Hospital Napoleonville, LA, 222
Assumption General Hospital (alternate name) Napoleonville, LA, 222
Athens Regional Medical Center Athens, GA, 153
Athens-Limestone Hospital Athens, AL, 10
Atlanta Medical Center Atlanta, GA, 154
Atlanta Memorial Hospital Atlanta, TX, 337
Atmore Community Hospital Atmore, AL, 11
Austin Surgical Hospital Austin, TX, 337
Auxilio Mutuo Hospital San Juan, PR, 274
Aventura Hospital and Medical Center Aventura, FL, 86
Avoyelles Hospital Marksville, LA, 219
Bacon County Hospital System Alma, GA, 152
Bamberg County Memorial Hospital Bamberg, SC, 291
Baptist Health Med Ctr-North Little Rock North Little Rock, AR, 61
Baptist Health Medical Center Arkadelphia, AR, 46
Baptist Health Medical Center Heber Springs, AR, 52
Baptist Health Medical Center Little Rock, AR, 56
Baptist Hospital of Gadsden (alternate name) Gadsden, AL, 23
Baptist Hospital of Miami (alternate name) Miami, FL, 112
Baptist Hospital-Orange (alternate name) Orange, TX, 406
Baptist Hospital Miami, FL, 112
Baptist Hospital Pensacola, FL, 123
Baptist Medical Center Beaches Jacksonville Bch, FL, 105
Baptist Medical Center East Montgomery, AL, 30
Baptist Medical Center Nassau Fernandina Bch, FL, 96
Baptist Medical Center-Easley (alternate name) Easley, SC, 296
Baptist Medical Center (alternate name) Little Rock, AR, 56
Baptist Medical Center Jacksonville, FL, 103
Baptist Medical Center Montgomery, AL, 30
Baptist Medical Center San Antonio, TX, 413
Baptist Memorial Hospital Desoto Southaven, MS, 261
Baptist Memorial Hospital-Booneville Booneville, MS, 241
Baptist Memorial Hospital-Forrest City Forrest City, AR, 51
Baptist Memorial Hospital-Golden Triangle Columbus, MS, 244
Baptist Memorial Hospital-North Mississippi Oxford, MS, 257
Baptist Memorial Hospital-Union County New Albany, MS, 256
Baptist North Hospital (alternate name) Cumming, GA, 166
Baptist-Saint Anthony's Health System Amarillo, TX, 333
Barnwell County Hospital Barnwell, SC, 291
Barrow Regional Medical Center Winder, GA, 191
Bartow Regional Medical Center Bartow, FL, 87
Bascom Palmer Eye Institute Miami, FL, 112
Baton Rouge General Medical Center Baton Rouge, LA, 201

Baxter Regional Medical Center Mountain Home, AR, 59
Bay Medical Center Panama City, FL, 122
Bayfront Medical Center Saint Petersburg, FL, 128
Baylor All Saints Med Ctr at Forth Worth Fort Worth, TX, 367
Baylor Heart and Vascular Center Dallas, TX, 354
Baylor Medical Center at Frisco Frisco, TX, 370
Baylor Medical Center at Garland Garland, TX, 371
Baylor Medical Center at Irving Irving, TX, 385
Baylor Medical Center-Ellis County Waxahachie, TX, 427
Baylor Medical Center-Waxahachie (alternate name) Waxahachie, TX, 427
Baylor Regional Medical Center at Grapevine Grapevine, TX, 374
Baylor Regional Medical Center at Plano Plano, TX, 409
Baylor University Medical Center Dallas, TX, 355
Bayshore Medical Center Pasadena, TX, 407
Beacham Memorial Hospital Magnolia, MS, 253
Beaufort Memorial Hospital Beaufort, SC, 291
Beaumont Bone & Joint Institute Beaumont, TX, 341
Beauregard Memorial Hospital DeRidder, LA, 207
Bella Vista Hospital Mayaguez, PR, 276
Bellville General Hospital Bellville, TX, 343
Berrien County Hospital Nashville, GA, 181
Bert Fish Medical Center New Smyrna Beach, FL, 117
Bethania Regional Health Care Center (alternate name) Wichita Falls, TX, 430
Bethesda Memorial Hospital Boynton Beach, FL, 88
Bibb Medical Center Centreville, AL, 16
Bienville Medical Center Arcadia, LA, 200
Big Bend Regional Medical Center Alpine, TX, 333
Biloxi Regional Medical Center Biloxi, MS, 240
BJC Medical Center Commerce, GA, 165
Blake Medical Center Bradenton, FL, 88
Bleckley Memorial Hospital Cochran, GA, 163
Blount Memorial Hospital (alternate name) Oneonta, AL, 32
Boaz-Albertville Medical Center (alternate name) Boaz, AL, 15
Boca Raton Community Hospital Boca Raton, FL, 87
Bolivar Medical Center Cleveland, MS, 243
Bon Secours Saint Francis Hospital Charleston, SC, 292
Booneville Community Hospital Booneville, AR, 47
Bossier Specialty Hospital Bossier City, LA, 204
Bowie Memorial Hospital Bowie, TX, 344
Brackenridge Hospital Austin, TX, 337
Bradford Hospital (alternate name) Starke, FL, 132
Bradley County Medical Center Warren, AR, 66
Brandon Regional Hospital Brandon, FL, 89
Brazosport Memorial Hospital Lake Jackson, TX, 391
Brooks County Hospital Quitman, GA, 182
Brooksville Regional Hospital Brooksville, FL, 90
Brookwood Medical Center Birmingham, AL, 12
Broward General Medical Center Fort Lauderdale, FL, 97
Brownfield Regional Medical Center Brownfield, TX, 345
Brownsville Medical Center Brownsville, TX, 345
Brownsville Surgical Hospital Brownsville, TX, 345
Brownwood Regional Medical Center Brownwood, TX, 346
Bryan W Whitfield Memorial Hospital Demopolis, AL, 19
BSA (alternate name) Amarillo, TX, 333
Bullock County Hospital Union Springs, AL, 38
Burke Medical Center Waynesboro, GA, 191
Byerly Hospital (alternate name) Hartsville, SC, 300
Byrd Regional Hospital Leesville, LA, 217
Caldwell Memorial Hospital Columbia, LA, 205
Calhoun Health Services Calhoun City, MS, 242
Callahan Eye Foundation Hospital Birmingham, AL, 12
Campbell Health System Weatherford, TX, 427
Campbell Memorial Hospital (alternate name) Weatherford, TX, 427
Campbellton Graceville Hospital Graceville, FL, 100
Candler County Hospital Metter, GA, 179
Candler Hospital Savannah, GA, 184
Cannon Memorial Hospital Pickens, SC, 304
Cape Canaveral Hospital (alternate name) Cocoa Beach, FL, 92
Cape Canaveral Hospital Cocoa Beach, FL, 92
Cape Coral Hospital Cape Coral, FL, 90
Capital Regional Medical Center Tallahassee, FL, 133
Cardiovascular Center of Puerto Rico Rio Piedras, PR, 279
Carolina Pines Regional Medical Center Hartsville, SC, 300
Carolinas Hospital System-Florence Florence, SC, 297
Carolinas Hospital System-Lake City Lake City, SC, 301
Cartersville Medical Center (alternate name) Cartersville, GA, 162
Castaner General Hospital Castaner, PR, 272
Cedars Medical Center Miami, FL, 112
Central Alabama Medical Center (alternate name) Wetumpka, AL, 39
Central Florida Regional Hospital Sanford, FL, 129
Central Mississippi Medical Center Jackson, MS, 249
Central Texas Hospital Cameron, TX, 347
Central Texas Medical Center San Marcos, TX, 416

Centurion Hospital of Carrollwood (alternate name) Tampa, FL, 135
Chambers Memorial Hospital Danville, AR, 49
Champ Traylor Memorial (alternate name) Port Lavaca, TX, 410
Charleston Memorial Hospital Charleston, SC, 292
Charlotte Regional Medical Center Punta Gorda, FL, 126
Charlton Memorial Hospital Folkston, GA, 171
Charlton Methodist Hospital Dallas, TX, 355
Chatuge Regional Hospital & Nursing Home Hiawassee, GA, 174
Cherokee Medical Center Centre, AL, 16
Chestatee Hospital (alternate name) Dahlonega, GA, 166
Chestatee Regional Hospital Dahlonega, GA, 166
Chester Regional Medical Center Chester, SC, 294
Chesterfield General Hospital Cheraw, SC, 294
Chicot Memorial Hospital Lake Village, AR, 56
Childress Regional Medical Center Childress, TX, 349
Chilton Medical Center Clanton, AL, 17
Choctaw Health Center Philadelphia, MS, 257
Christus Jasper Memorial Hospital Jasper, TX, 387
Christus Saint Catherine Hospital Katy, TX, 388
Christus Saint Elizabeth Hospital Beaumont, TX, 341
Christus Saint Frances Cabrini Hospital Alexandria, LA, 200
Christus Saint John Hospital Houston, TX, 404
Christus Saint Michael Health System Texarkana, TX, 421
CHRISTUS Saint Patrick Hospital Lake Charles, LA, 215
Christus Santa Rosa Hospital-City Centre San Antonio, TX, 414
Christus Schumpert Health System Shreveport, LA, 228
Christus Spohn Hospital Beeville Beeville, TX, 342
Christus Spohn Hospital Kleberg Kingsville, TX, 390
CHRISTUS Spohn Hospital-Alice (alternate name) Alice, TX, 332
Christus Spohn Memorial Hospital Corpus Christi, TX, 352
Citizens Baptist Medical Center Talladega, AL, 36
Citizens Hospital (alternate name) Talladega, AL, 36
Citizens Medical Center Columbia, LA, 205
Citizens Medical Center Victoria, TX, 425
Citrus Memorial Hospital Inverness, FL, 103
Claiborne County Hospital Port Gibson, MS, 259
Clarendon Memorial Hospital Manning, SC, 302
Clay County Hospital & Nursing Home (alternate name) Ashland, AL, 10
Clay County Hospital Ashland, AL, 10
Clay County Medical Center West Point, MS, 263
Clear Lake Regional Medical Center Webster, TX, 427
Cleveland Clinic Florida Weston, FL, 139
Cleveland Regional Medical Center Cleveland, TX, 350
Clinch Memorial Hospital Homerville, GA, 175
Clinica Espanola Mayaguez, PR, 276
Coastal Carolina Medical Center Hardeeville, SC, 300
Cobb Memorial Hospital Royston, GA, 183
Coffee Regional Hospital (alternate name) Douglas, GA, 168
Coffee Regional Medical Center Douglas, GA, 168
Coleman County Medical Center Coleman, TX, 351
Coliseum Medical Center Macon, GA, 177
Coliseum Northside Hospital (alternate name) Macon, GA, 177
College Station Medical Center College Station, TX, 351
Colleton Medical Center Walterboro, SC, 307
Colorado Fayette Medical Center Weimar, TX, 428
Colquitt Regional Medical Center Moultrie, GA, 180
Columbia Aventura Hospital and Medical Center (alternate name) Aventura, FL, 86
Columbia Bartow Memorial Hospital (alternate name) Bartow, FL, 87
Columbia Bayshore Medical Center (alternate name) Pasadena, TX, 407
Columbia De Queen Regional Medical Center (alternate name) De Queen, AR, 50
Columbia Heights Medical Center (alternate name) Lufkin, TX, 397
Columbia Hospital West Palm Beach, FL, 138
Columbia Medical Center of San Angelo (alternate name) San Angelo, TX, 413
Columbia Medical Center Sanford (alternate name) Sanford, FL, 129
Columbia Memorial Hospital of Jacksonville Jacksonville, FL, 103
Columbia Panhandle Regional Medical Center (alternate name) Pampa, TX, 407
Columbia Saint Petersburg Medical Center (alternate name) Saint Petersburg, FL, 129
Columbia Spring Branch Medical Center Houston, TX, 377
Columbus Community Hospital Columbus, TX, 352
Columbus Medical Center Columbus, GA, 163
Comanche County Medical Center Comanche, TX, 352
Community General Hospital Dilley, TX, 361
Community Hospital of Andalusia (alternate name) Andalusia, AL, 9
Community Hospital New Port Richey, FL, 117

Community Hospital Tallassee, AL, 36
Community Specialty Hosp of N Louisiana Minden, LA, 220
Community Specialty Hospital (alternate name) Sherman, TX, 417
Connally Memorial Medical Center Floresville, TX, 366
Conroe Regional Medical Center Conroe, TX, 352
Conway Medical Center Conway, SC, 295
Conway Regional Medical Center Conway, AR, 49
Coon Memorial Hospital Dalhart, TX, 354
Cooper Green Mercy Hospital Birmingham, AL, 12
Coosa Valley Baptist Medical Center Sylacauga, AL, 36
Coosa Valley Medical Center (alternate name) Sylacauga, AL, 36
Coral Gables Hospital Miami, FL, 92
Coral Springs Medical Center Coral Springs, FL, 93
Cornerstone Regional Hospital Edinburg, TX, 362
Corpus Christi Medical Center-Bay Area Corpus Christi, TX, 353
Coryell Memorial Hospital Gatesville, TX, 371
Covenant Hospital Levelland Levelland, TX, 393
Covenant Hospital Plainview Plainview, TX, 409
Covenant Medical Center Lubbock, TX, 396
Covington County Hospital Collins, MS, 243
Cozby-Germany Hospital Grand Saline, TX, 373
Crenshaw Baptist Hospital Luverne, AL, 28
Crestwood Medical Center Huntsville, AL, 26
Crisp Regional Hospital Cordele, GA, 165
Crittenden Memorial Hospital West Memphis, AR, 66
CrossRidge Community Hospital Wynne, AR, 67
Cuero Community Hospital Cuero, TX, 354
Cullman Regional Medical Center Cullman, AL, 17
Cypress Fairbanks Medical Center and Hospital Houston, TX, 378
D M Cogdell Memorial Hospital Snyder, TX, 418
D W McMillan Memorial Hospital Brewton, AL, 15
Dale County Hospital (alternate name) Ozark, AL, 33
Dale Medical Center Ozark, AL, 33
Dallas Family Hospital (alternate name) Dallas, TX, 355
Dallas Southwest Medical Center Dallas, TX, 355
Dauterive Hospital New Iberia, LA, 222
DCH Regional Medical Center Tuscaloosa, AL, 37
De Queen Regional Medical Center De Queen, AR, 50
De Soto General Hospital (alternate name) Mansfield, LA, 218
De Witt Hospital & Nursing Home De Witt, AR, 50
Deaf Smith General Hospital (alternate name) Hereford, TX, 377
Decatur General Hospital Decatur, AL, 18
Dekalb Medical Center at Hillandale Lithonia, GA, 176
DeKalb Medical Center Decatur, GA, 167
DeKalb Regional Medical Center Fort Payne, AL, 23
Del Sol Medical Center El Paso, TX, 364
Delray Community Hospital (alternate name) Delray Beach, FL, 95
Delray Medical Center Delray Beach, FL, 95
Delta Memorial Hospital Dumas, AR, 50
Delta Regional Medical Center Greenville, MS, 245
Denton Regional Medical Center (alternate name) Denton, TX, 360
Denton Regional Medical Center Denton, TX, 360
DeSoto Memorial Hospital Arcadia, FL, 86
DeSoto Regional Health System Mansfield, LA, 218
Detar Hospital Navarro Victoria, TX, 426
Dickerson Memorial Hospital Jasper, TX, 387
Dimmit County Memorial Hospital Carrizo Springs, TX, 348
Doctor I Gonzalez Martinez Oncologic Hospital San Juan, PR, 281
Doctor's Hospital (alternate name) Sarasota, FL, 130
Doctors Center Hospital Manati, PR, 275
Doctors Hospital at Renaissance Edinburg, TX, 363
Doctors Hospital of Augusta (alternate name) Augusta, GA, 157
Doctors Hospital of Laredo Laredo, TX, 392
Doctors Hospital of Opelousas Opelousas, LA, 226
Doctors Hospital of Sarasota Sarasota, FL, 130
Doctors Hospital Parkway+Tidwell Houston, TX, 378
Doctors Hospital Augusta, GA, 157
Doctors Hospital Columbus, GA, 164
Doctors Hospital Dallas, TX, 356
Doctors Hospital Shreveport, LA, 229
Doctors Memorial Hospital Bonifay, FL, 88
Doctors Memorial Hospital Perry, FL, 124
Doctors' Hospital of Slidell Slidell, LA, 229
Dodge County Hospital Eastman, GA, 170
Dolly Vinsant Memorial Hospital San Benito, TX, 416
Donalsonville Hospital Donalsonville, GA, 168
Dorminy Medical Center Fitzgerald, GA, 171
Drew Memorial Hospital Monticello, AR, 59
E A Conway Medical Center Monroe, LA, 220
Earl K Long Medical Center Baton Rouge, LA, 201
Early Memorial Hospital Blakely, GA, 159

East Alabama Medical Center Opelika, AL, 32
East Carroll Parish Hospital Lake Providence, LA, 217
East Cooper Regional Medical Center Mount Pleasant, SC, 302
East Georgia Regional Medical Center Statesboro, GA, 186
East Houston Regional Medical Center Houston, TX, 378
East Jefferson General Hospital Metairie, LA, 219
East Texas Medical Center, Grande Saline Div. (alternate name) Grand Saline, TX, 373
East Texas Medical Center-Athens Athens, TX, 336
East Texas Medical Center-Carthage Carthage, TX, 348
East Texas Medical Center-Clarksville Clarksville, TX, 349
East Texas Medical Center-Crockett Crockett, TX, 353
East Texas Medical Center-Fairfield Fairfield, TX, 366
East Texas Medical Center-Gilmer Gilmer, TX, 372
East Texas Medical Center-Jacksonville Jacksonville, TX, 386
East Texas Medical Center-Mount Vernon Mount Vernon, TX, 403
East Texas Medical Center-Pittsburg Pittsburg, TX, 408
East Texas Medical Center-Quitman Quitman, TX, 411
East Texas Medical Center-Trinity Trinity, TX, 423
East Texas Medical Center-Tyler Tyler, TX, 423
Eastland Memorial Hospital Eastland, TX, 362
Edgar B Davis Memorial Hospital (alternate name) Luling, TX, 398
Edgefield County Hospital Edgefield, SC, 297
Edinburg Hospital (alternate name) Edinburg, TX, 363
Edinburg Regional Medical Center Edinburg, TX, 363
Edward White Hospital Saint Petersburg, FL, 128
Effingham County Hospital & Extended Care Facility (alternate name) Springfield, GA, 186
Effingham Hospital Springfield, GA, 186
El Campo Memorial Hospital El Campo, TX, 363
El Paso Specialty Hospital El Paso, TX, 364
Elba General Hospital & Nursing Home Elba, AL, 19
Elbert Memorial Hospital Elberton, GA, 170
Eliza Coffee Memorial Hospital Florence, AL, 22
Elliott White Springs Memorial Hospital (alternate name) Lancaster, SC, 301
Elmore Community Hospital Wetumpka, AL, 39
Emanuel County Hospital (alternate name) Swainsboro, GA, 187
Emanuel Medical Center Swainsboro, GA, 187
Emory Cartersville Medical Center Cartersville, GA, 162
Emory Crawford Long Hospital Atlanta, GA, 154
Emory Dunwoody Medical Center Atlanta, GA, 154
Emory Eastside Medical Center Snellville, GA, 185
Emory Northlake Regional Medical Center Tucker, GA, 188
Emory University Hospital Atlanta, GA, 155
Emory-Adventist Hospital Smyrna, GA, 185
Englewood Community Hospital Englewood, FL, 96
Ennis Regional Medical Center Ennis, TX, 366
Epic Health Care (alternate name) Katy, TX, 388
ETMC Pittsburgh (alternate name) Pittsburg, TX, 408
ETMC-Clarksville (alternate name) Clarksville, TX, 349
Evans Memorial Hospital Claxton, GA, 163
Evergreen Medical Center (alternate name) Evergreen, AL, 21
Fairfield Memorial Hospital (alternate name) Fairfield, TX, 366
Fairfield Memorial Hospital Winnsboro, SC, 308
Fairview Park Hospital Dublin, GA, 169
Fairway Medical Center Covington, LA, 205
Faith Community Hospital Jacksboro, TX, 386
Falls Community Hospital Marlin, TX, 398
Fannin Regional Hospital Blue Ridge, GA, 159
Fawcett Memorial Hospital Port Charlotte, FL, 125
Fayette Medical Center Fayette, AL, 21
Field Memorial Community Hospital Centreville, MS, 242
Fish Memorial Hospital (alternate name) New Smyrna Beach, FL, 117
Fishermen's Hospital Marathon, FL, 110
Flagler Hospital Saint Augustine, FL, 127
Flint River Community Hospital Montezuma, GA, 179
Florala Memorial Hospital Florala, AL, 22
Florence General Hospital (alternate name) Florence, SC, 297
Florida Hospital DeLand Deland, FL, 95
Florida Hospital Fish Memorial Orange City, FL, 119
Florida Hospital Flagler Palm Coast, FL, 121
Florida Hospital Heartland Medical Center Sebring, FL, 131
Florida Hospital Orlando Orlando, FL, 120
Florida Hospital Waterman Tavares, FL, 136
Florida Hospital Wauchula Wauchula, FL, 138
Florida Hospital Zephyrhills Zephyrhills, FL, 140
Florida Hospital-Ormond Memorial Ormond Beach, FL, 120
Florida Medical Center Lauderdale Lakes, FL, 109
Flowers Hospital Dothan, AL, 19
Floyd Medical Center Rome, GA, 182
Forrest County General Hospital Hattiesburg, MS, 247
Forrest General Hospital (alternate name) Hattiesburg, MS, 247
Fort Bend Medical Center (alternate name) Missouri City, TX, 402

Fort Duncan Medical Center Eagle Pass, TX, 362
Fort Walton Beach Medical Center Fort Walton Beach, FL, 99
Foundation Surgical Hospital Bellaire, TX, 343
Franklin County Memorial Hospital Meadville, MS, 253
Franklin Medical Center Winnsboro, LA, 233
Franklin Parish Hospital (alternate name) Winnsboro, LA, 233
Frio Hospital Pearsall, TX, 408
Gadsden Regional Medical Center Gadsden, AL, 23
Garden Park Medical Center Gulfport, MS, 246
George County Hospital Lucedale, MS, 252
George H Lanier Memorial Hospital Valley, AL, 38
Georgetown Healthcare System Georgetown, TX, 372
Georgetown Hospital (alternate name) Georgetown, TX, 372
Georgetown Memorial Hospital Georgetown, SC, 298
Georgia Baptist Health Care System (alternate name) Atlanta, GA, 154
Georgiana Doctors Community Hospital (alternate name) Georgiana, AL, 24
Georgiana Hospital Georgiana, AL, 24
Gilmore Memorial Hospital Amory, MS, 239
Glades General Hospital Belle Glade, FL, 87
Glen Rose Medical Center Glen Rose, TX, 372
Glenwood Regional Medical Center West Monroe, LA, 232
Golden Triangle Regional Medical Center (alternate name) Columbus, MS, 244
Good Samaritan Medical Center (alternate name) West Palm Beach, FL, 139
Good Samaritan Medical Center West Palm Beach, FL, 139
Good Shephard Medical Center-Linden Linden, TX, 394
Good Shepherd Medical Center Longview, TX, 395
Goodall-Witcher Healthcare Foundation Clifton, TX, 350
Gordon Hospital Calhoun, GA, 161
Grady General Hospital Cairo, GA, 160
Grady Memorial Hospital Atlanta, GA, 155
Graham General Hospital (alternate name) Graham, TX, 373
Graham Regional Medical Center Graham, TX, 373
Grand Strand Regional Medical Center (alternate name) Myrtle Beach, SC, 303
Grand Strand Regional Medical Center Myrtle Beach, SC, 303
Great River Medical Center Blytheville, AR, 47
Greater Baton Rouge Surgical Hospital Baton Rouge, LA, 202
Green Clinic Surgical Hospital Ruston, LA, 228
Greene County Hospital Eutaw, AL, 20
Greenlawn Hospital (alternate name) Atmore, AL, 11
Greenville Memorial Hospital (alternate name) Greenville, SC, 298
Greenville Memorial Medical Campus Greenville, SC, 298
Greenwood LeFlore Hospital Greenwood, MS, 246
Grenada Lake Medical Center Grenada, MS, 246
Grimes-Saint Joseph's Health Center Navasota, TX, 404
GRMC Glenwood Hospital (alternate name) West Monroe, LA, 232
Grove Hill Memorial Hospital Grove Hill, AL, 25
Guadalupe Valley Hospital Seguin, TX, 417
Gulf Breeze Hospital Gulf Breeze, FL, 101
Gulf Coast Hospital (alternate name) Panama City, FL, 122
Gulf Coast Hospital Fort Meyers, FL, 98
Gulf Coast Medical Center/Gulf Oaks Hospital Biloxi, MS, 240
Gulf Coast Medical Center Panama City, FL, 122
Gulf Coast Medical Center Wharton, TX, 429
Guntersville-Arab Medical Center (alternate name) Guntersville, AL, 25
Gwinnett Medical Center (alternate name) Lawrenceville, GA, 176
H C Watkins Memorial Hospital Quitman, MS, 259
Habersham County Medical Center Demorest, GA, 168
Hale County Hospital Greensboro, AL, 24
Halifax Medical Center Daytona Beach, FL, 94
Hamilton General Hospital Hamilton, TX, 375
Hamilton Medical Center Chatsworth, GA, 163
Hamilton Medical Center Dalton, GA, 167
Hamilton Memorial Hospital (alternate name) Jasper, FL, 105
Hamlin Memorial Hospital Hamlin, TX, 376
Hampton General Hospital (alternate name) Varnville, SC, 307
Hampton Regional Medical Center Varnville, SC, 307
Hancock Medical Center Bay Saint Louis, MS, 239
Hardtner Medical Center Olla, LA, 225
Harlingen Medical Center Harlingen, TX, 376
Harris County Hospital District Houston, TX, 379
Harris Hospital and Clinic Newport, AR, 61
Harris Methodist Continued Care Hospital Fort Worth, TX, 367
Harris Methodist Erath County Stephenville, TX, 419
Harris Methodist HEB Hospital Bedford, TX, 342
Harris Methodist Northwest Azle, TX, 340
Harris Methodist Southlake Ctr for Diag Southlake, TX, 418
Harris Methodist Southwest Fort Worth, TX, 368
Harris Methodist Stephenville (alternate name) Stephenville, TX, 419
Harris Methodist-Mexia (alternate name) Mexia, TX, 401
Hart County Hospital Hartwell, GA, 173

Hartselle Medical Center Hartselle, AL, 26
HCA Aiken Regional Medical Center (alternate name) Aiken, SC, 290
HCA Bayonet/Hudson Point Medical Center (alternate name) Hudson, FL, 102
HCA Medical Plaza Hospital/Saint Joseph Hospital (alternate name) Fort Worth, TX, 369
HCA Newport Richey Hospital (alternate name) New Port Richey, FL, 117
HCA Palmyra Medical Center (alternate name) Albany, GA, 152
HCA South Austin Medical Center (alternate name) Austin, TX, 339
HCA, Cedars Medical Center (alternate name) Miami, FL, 112
Health Central Ocoee, FL, 118
Healthmark Regional Medical Center Defuniak Springs, FL, 95
Healthpark Hospital Hot Springs, AR, 53
HealthSouth Doctors' Hospital Miami, FL, 92
Healthsouth Hospital for Specialized Surgery Houston, TX, 379
HealthSouth Medical Center Birmingham, AL, 13
Healthsouth Medical Center Dallas, TX, 356
Healthsouth Surgical Hospital of Austin Austin, TX, 338
Heart Hospital of Austin Austin, TX, 338
Heart Hospital of Lafayette Lafayette, LA, 212
Heart of Florida Regional Medical Center Davenport, FL, 94
HEB Hospital
        Harris HEB (alternate name) Bedford, TX, 342
Helen Ellis Memorial Hospital Tarpon Springs, FL, 136
Helen Keller Memorial Hospital Sheffield, AL, 35
Helena Regional Medical Center Helena, AR, 53
Hemphill County Hospital Canadian, TX, 347
Henderson Memorial Hospital Henderson, TX, 377
Hendrick Medical Center Abilene, TX, 332
Hendry General Hospital (alternate name) Clewiston, FL, 91
Hendry Regional Medical Center Clewiston, FL, 91
Henry Medical Center Stockbridge, GA, 186
Hereford Regional Medical Center Hereford, TX, 377
Hermann Hospital (alternate name) Houston, TX, 380
Hialeah Hospital Miami, FL, 101
Higgins General Hospital Bremen, GA, 160
Highland Community Hospital Lubbock, TX, 396
Highland Community Hospital Picayune, GF, 258
Highlands Medical Center Scottsboro, AL, 35
Highlands Regional Medical Center Sebring, FL, 131
Hill Country Memorial Hospital Fredericksburg, TX, 369
Hill Hospital of Sumter County York, AL, 39
Hill Hospital of York (alternate name) York, AL, 39
Hill Regional Hospital Hillsboro, TX, 377
Hillcrest Baptist Medical Center Waco, TX, 426
Hillcrest Hospital Simpsonville, SC, 305
Hilton Head Regional Medical Center Hilton Head Isl, SC, 300
Hima Humacao Humacao, PR, 274
Hima-San Pablo Fajardo Fajardo, PR, 273
HNMC (alternate name) Houston, TX, 379
Holmes Regional Medical Center Melbourne, FL, 111
Holy Cross Hospital Fort Lauderdale, FL, 97
Holy Name of Jesus Medical Center (alternate name) Gadsden, AL, 23
Homer Memorial Hospital Homer, LA, 208
Homestead Hospital Homestead, FL, 102
Hood General Hospital (alternate name) Granbury, TX, 373
Hopkins County Memorial Hospital Sulphur Springs, TX, 420
Hospital Comunitario Buen Samaritano Aguadilla, PR, 269
Hospital Damas Ponce, PR, 278
Hospital De Area Doctor Buitrago (alternate name) Guayama, PR, 273
Hospital De La Concepcion San German, PR, 280
Hospital Del Maestro San Juan, PR, 281
Hospital Doctor Cayetano Coll Y Toste Arecibo, PR, 269
Hospital Doctor Dominguez Humacao, PR, 275
Hospital Doctor Pila Ponce, PR, 278
Hospital Doctor Susoni Arecibo, PR, 269
Hospital Episcopal Cristo Redentor Guayama, PR, 273
Hospital Hermanos Melendez Bayamon, PR, 270
Hospital Interamericano de Medicina Caguas, PR, 271
Hospital Matilde Brenes Bayamon, PR, 270
Hospital Menonita De Cayey Cayey, PR, 272
Hospital Metropolitano Doctor Tito Mattei Yauco, PR, 283
Hospital Metropolitano San German, PR, 280
Hospital Oncologico Andres Grillasca Ponce, PR, 278
Hospital Pavia Hato Rey Hato Rey, PR, 274
Hospital Pavia Santurce Fernandez Juncos, PR, 273
Hospital Perea Mayaguez, PR, 277
Hospital San Carlos Borromeo Moca, PR, 277
Hospital San Cristobal Coto Laurel, PR, 272
Hospital San Francisco San Juan, PR, 282
Hospital San Gerardo Rio Piedras, PR, 279
Hospital San Juan Bautista Medical Center Caguas, PR, 271
Hospital San Pablo Bayamon, PR, 271
Hospital Santa Rosa Guayama, PR, 274

Hospital Universitario Doctor Ramon Ruiz Arnau Bayamon, PR, 271
Hospital Wilma N Vazquez Vega Baja, PR, 282
Hot Springs County Medical Center Malvern, AR, 58
Houston Community Hospital (alternate name) Houston, MS, 248
Houston County Hospital (alternate name) Crockett, TX, 353
Houston Medical Center Warner Robins, GA, 190
Houston Northwest Medical Center Houston, TX, 379
Houston Physicians' Hospital Webster, TX, 428
Howard Memorial Hospital Nashville, AR, 60
Huey P Long Medical Center Pineville, LA, 226
Hughston Orthopedic Hospital Columbus, GA, 164
Huguley Memorial Medical Center Burleson, TX, 368
Humana Hospital Brazos Valley (alternate name) College Station, TX, 351
Humana Hospital Orange Park (alternate name) Orange Park, FL, 119
Humana Hospital Pasco (alternate name) Dade City, FL, 93
Humana Hospital-Abilene (alternate name) Abilene, TX, 332
Humana Hospital-Brandon (alternate name) Brandon, FL, 89
Humana Hospital-Fort Walton Beach (alternate name) Fort Walton Beach, FL, 99
Humana Hospital-Gwinnett (alternate name) Snellville, GA, 185
Humana Hospital-Medical City Dallas (alternate name) Dallas, TX, 356
Humana Hospital-Oakdale (alternate name) Oakdale, LA, 225
Humana Hospital-Winn Parish (alternate name) Winnfield, LA, 232
Huntsville Hospital Huntsville, AL, 27
Huntsville Memorial Hospital Huntsville, TX, 385
Hutcheson Medical Center Fort Oglethorpe, GA, 172
Iberia General Hospital & Medical Center (alternate name) New Iberia, LA, 223
Iberia Medical Center New Iberia, LA, 223
Imperial Point Medical Center Fort Lauderdale, FL, 97
Indian River Memorial Hospital Vero Beach, FL, 137
Infirmary West Mobile, AL, 28
Irving Coppell Surgical Hospital Irving, TX, 385
Irving Healthcare System (alternate name) Dallas, TX, 355
Irwin County Hospital Ocilla, GA, 181
J Paul Jones Hospital Camden, AL, 15
Jackson Hospital and Clinic Montgomery, AL, 31
Jackson Hospital Marianna, FL, 111
Jackson Medical Center Jackson, AL, 27
Jackson Memorial Hospital Miami, FL, 113
Jackson Parish Hospital Jonesboro, LA, 211
Jacksonville Medical Center Jacksonville, AL, 27
Jasper General Hospital Bay Springs, MS, 240
Jasper Mem Hosp & Retreat Nursing Home Monticello, GA, 180
Jasper Memorial Hospital (alternate name) Jasper, TX, 387
Jay Hospital Jay, FL, 105
Jeff Anderson Regional Medical Center Meridian, MS, 254
Jefferson County Hospital Fayette, MS, 245
Jefferson Davis Community Hospital Prentiss, MS, 259
Jefferson Davis Memorial Hospital (alternate name) Natchez, MS, 256
Jefferson Hospital Louisville, GA, 177
Jefferson Regional Medical Center Pine Bluff, AR, 62
Jennings American Legion Hospital Jennings, LA, 211
JFK Medical Center Atlantis, FL, 86
John D Archbold Memorial Hospital Thomasville, GA, 187
John M Meadows Memorial Hospital (alternate name) Vidalia, GA, 189
John Peter Smith Hospital Fort Worth, TX, 368
Johnson County Regional Hospital (alternate name) Clarksville, AR, 48
Johnson Regional Medical Center Clarksville, AR, 48
Jones County Community Hospital (alternate name) Laurel, MS, 251
JPS Health Network (alternate name) Fort Worth, TX, 368
Jupiter Medical Center Jupiter, FL, 106
Kell West Regional Hospital Wichita Falls, TX, 429
Kendall Medical Center Miami, FL, 113
Kenner Regional Medical Center Kenner, LA, 211
Kershaw County Medical Center Camden, SC, 292
Kershaw County Memorial Hospital (alternate name) Camden, SC, 292
Kilmichael Hospital Kilmichael, MS, 251
King's Daughters Medical Center Brookhaven, MS, 241
Kings Daughters Hospital Temple, TX, 420
Kingwood Medical Center Kingwood, TX, 390
Kingwood Specialty Hospital Kingwood, TX, 390
Knapp Medical Center Weslaco, TX, 428
Knox County Hospital Knox City, TX, 391
L V Stabler Memorial Hospital Greenville, AL, 24
La Salle General Hospital Jena, LA, 210
Lackey Memorial Hospital Forest, MS, 245
Lady of the Sea General Hospital Cut Off, LA, 207

Lafayette General Medical Center Lafayette, LA, 213
Lafayette General Surgical Hospital Lafayette, LA, 213
Lafayette Hospital Arroyo, PR, 270
Lafayette Surgical Specialty Hospital Lafayette, LA, 213
Laird Hospital Union, MS, 262
Laird Memorial Hospital Kilgore, TX, 389
Lake Area Medical Center (alternate name) Lake Charles, LA, 216
Lake Charles Memorial Hospital Lake Charles, LA, 216
Lake City Community Hospital (alternate name) Lake City, SC, 301
Lake City Medical Center Lake City, FL, 107
Lake Granbury Medical Center Granbury, TX, 373
Lake Martin Community Hospital Dadeville, AL, 18
Lake Pointe Medical Center Rowlett, TX, 412
Lake Shore Hospital (alternate name) Lake City, FL, 107
Lake Wales Medical Center Lake Wales, FL, 107
Lake Whitney Medical Center Whitney, TX, 429
Lakeland Community Hospital Haleyville, AL, 25
Lakeland Regional Medical Center Lakeland, FL, 108
Lakeside Hospital at Bastrop Bastrop, TX, 340
Lakeview Community Hospital Eufaula, AL, 20
Lakeview Regional Medical Center Covington, LA, 206
Lakewood Medical Center (alternate name) Morgan City, LA, 221
Lakewood Ranch Medical Center Bradenton, FL, 89
Lallie Kemp/Regional Medical Center Independence, LA, 210
Lamb Healthcare Center Littlefield, TX, 394
Lane Regional Memorial Hospital Zachary, LA, 233
Laredo Medical Center Laredo, TX, 393
Largo Medical Center Largo, FL, 108
Larkin Community Hospital South Miami, FL, 131
Las Colinas Medical Center Irving, TX, 386
Las Palmas Medical Center El Paso, TX, 364
Laurens County Hospital Clinton, SC, 294
Lavaca Medical Center Hallettsville, TX, 375
Lawnwood Regional Med Ctr & Heart Inst Fort Pierce, FL, 99
Lawrence County Hospital (alternate name) Moulton, AL, 31
Lawrence Medical Center Moulton, AL, 31
Lawrence Memorial Hospital Walnut Ridge, AR, 66
Lee Memorial Health System Fort Myers, FL, 98
Leesburg Regional Medical Center Leesburg, FL, 109
Legacy Medical Center of Atlanta Atlanta, GA, 155
Lehigh Regional Medical Center Lehigh Acres, FL, 109
Leonard J Chabert Medical Center Houma, LA, 209
Levi Hospital Hot Springs Natl Pk, AR, 54
Lewisville Memorial Hospital (alternate name) Lewisville, TX, 394
Lexington Medical Center West Columbia, SC, 307
Liberty Memorial Hospital (alternate name) Hinesville, GA, 174
Liberty Regional Medical Center Hinesville, GA, 174
Limestone Medical Center Groesbeck, TX, 374
Lincoln General Hospital Ruston, LA, 228
Lindy Boggs Medical Center New Orleans, LA, 223
Llano Memorial Hospital Llano, TX, 395
Lockney General Hospital (alternate name) Lockney, TX, 395
Longview Regional Hospital (alternate name) Longview, TX, 396
Longview Regional Medical Center Longview, TX, 396
Loris Community Hospital Loris, SC, 302
Louisiana Heart Hospital Lacombe, LA, 212
Louisiana State Univ Hosp-Shreveport Shreveport, LA, 229
Lower Florida Keys Health System (alternate name) Key West, FL, 106
Lower Keys Medical Center Key West, FL, 106
LRMC (alternate name) Leesburg, FL, 109
LSU-Bogalusa Medical Center Bogalusa, LA, 204
Lubbock Heart Hospital Lubbock, TX, 397
Macon Northside Hospital Macon, GA, 177
Madison County Medical Center Canton, MS, 242
Madison General Hospital (alternate name) Canton, MS, 242
Madison Saint Joseph Health Center Madisonville, TX, 398
Magee General Hospital Magee, MS, 252
Magnolia Hospital (alternate name) Corinth, MS, 244
Magnolia Hospital Magnolia, AR, 57
Magnolia Regional Health Center Corinth, MS, 244
Mainland Center Hospital (alternate name) Texas City, TX, 422
Mainland Medical Center Texas City, TX, 422
Manatee Memorial Hospital Bradenton, FL, 89
Manati Medical Center Doctor Otero Lopez Manati, PR, 276
Mariners Hospital Tavernier, FL, 136
Marion Community Hospital (alternate name) Ocala, FL, 118
Marion County Medical Center Marion, SC, 302
Marion General Hospital Columbia, MS, 244
Marion Regional Wellness Center Hamilton, AL, 26
Marlboro Park Hospital Bennettsville, SC, 291
Marshall Medical Center North Guntersville, AL, 25
Marshall Medical Center South Boaz, AL, 15
Marshall Memorial Hospital (alternate name) Marshall, TX, 399
Marshall Regional Medical Center Marshall, TX, 399

Martin Memorial Hospital (alternate name) Stuart, FL, 132
Martin Memorial Medical Center Stuart, FL, 132
Martinez Oncologic Hospital, I. G. (alternate name) San Juan, PR, 281
Mary Black Memorial Hospital Spartanburg, SC, 305
Mary Shiels Hospital Dallas, TX, 356
Matagorda County Hospital District Bay City, TX, 341
Matagorda General Hospital (alternate name) Bay City, TX, 341
Maverick County Hospital District (alternate name) Eagle Pass, TX, 362
Mayhill Hospital Denton, TX, 360
McAllen Medical Center McAllen, TX, 399
McDuffie Regional Medical Center Thomson, GA, 187
MCG Health System (alternate name) Augusta, GA, 157
McGehee-Desha County Hospital McGehee, AR, 58
McKenna Memorial Hospital New Braunfels, TX, 404
McLeod Medical Center Dillon Dillon, SC, 296
Mcleod Medical Center-Darlington (alternate name) Darlington, SC, 296
McLeod Regional Medical Center-Pee Dee Florence, SC, 297
Meadowcrest Hospital Gretna, LA, 208
Meadows Regional Medical Center Vidalia, GA, 189
Mease Hospital-Countryside Safety Harbor, FL, 127
Mease Hospital-Dunedin Dunedin, FL, 96
Medical Arts Hospital Lamesa, TX, 392
Medical Center at Lancaster Lancaster, TX, 392
Medical Center at Terrell Terrell, TX, 421
Medical Center Blount Oneonta, AL, 32
Medical Center East Birmingham, AL, 13
Medical Center Enterprise Enterprise, AL, 20
Medical Center Hospital (alternate name) Punta Gorda, FL, 126
Medical Center Hospital (alternate name) Tyler, TX, 423
Medical Center Hospital Odessa, TX, 405
Medical Center of Arlington Arlington, TX, 336
Medical Center of Central Georgia Macon, GA, 178
Medical Center of Lewisville Lewisville, TX, 394
Medical Center of Louisiana at New Orleans New Orleans, LA, 223
Medical Center of Mesquite Mesquite, TX, 400
Medical Center of Plano Plano, TX, 409
Medical Center of South Arkansas El Dorado, AR, 50
Medical Center of Southeast Texas Port Arthur, TX, 410
Medical Center Shoals (alternate name) Muscle Shoals, AL, 31
Medical Centre Surgical Hospital Fort Worth, TX, 369
Medical City Dallas Dallas, TX, 356
Medical College of Georgia Hospital & Clinics Augusta, GA, 157
Medical Park Hospital (alternate name) Hope, AR, 53
Medical Park Hospital Hope, AR, 53
Medical University Hospital (alternate name) Charleston, SC, 293
Medical University of S Carolina Med Ctr Charleston, SC, 293
Memorial Health System of East Texas-Lufkin Lufkin, TX, 397
Memorial Health University Medical Center (alternate name) Savannah, GA, 184
Memorial Herman Baptist Orange Hospital Orange, TX, 406
Memorial Herman Katy Hospital Katy, TX, 388
Memorial Hermann Baptist Beaumont Beaumont, TX, 342
Memorial Hermann Fort Bend Hospital Missouri City, TX, 402
Memorial Hermann Healthcare System Houston, TX, 380
Memorial Hermann Memorial City Houston, TX, 380
Memorial Hermann-Texas Medical Center Houston, TX, 380
Memorial Hospital & Manor Bainbridge, GA, 158
Memorial Hospital at Gulfport Gulfport, MS, 246
Memorial Hospital Holly Springs (alternate name) Holly Springs, MS, 247
Memorial Hospital Miramar Miramar, FL, 116
Memorial Hospital of Adel Adel, GA, 152
Memorial Hospital of Tampa Tampa, FL, 134
Memorial Hospital of Washington County (alternate name) Sandersville, GA, 184
Memorial Hospital Pembroke Pembroke Pines, FL, 122
Memorial Hospital West Pembroke Pines, FL, 123
Memorial Hospital (alternate name) Bainbridge, GA, 158
Memorial Hospital (alternate name) Siloam Springs, AR, 64
Memorial Hospital Dumas, TX, 361
Memorial Hospital Gonzales, TX, 373
Memorial Medical Center Livingston Livingston, TX, 394
Memorial Medical Center of East Texas (alternate name) Lufkin, TX, 397
Memorial Medical Center of Jacksonville (alternate name) Jacksonville, FL, 103
Memorial Medical Center (alternate name) Corpus Christi, TX, 352
Memorial Medical Center Port Lavaca, TX, 410
Memorial Medical Center Savannah, GA, 184
Memorial Regional Hospital Hollywood, FL, 102
Mena Medical Center Mena, AR, 58
Mennonite General Hospital Aibonito, PR, 269
Mercy Hospital Miami, FL, 113

Mesquite Community Hospital Mesquite, TX, 400
Methodist Ambulatory Surgery Hospital NW San Antonio, TX, 414
Methodist Hospital Levelland (alternate name) Levelland, TX, 393
Methodist Hospital Plainview (alternate name) Plainview, TX, 409
Methodist Hospital (alternate name) Lubbock, TX, 396
Methodist Hospital Houston, TX, 380
Methodist Hospital New Orleans, LA, 223
Methodist Hospital San Antonio, TX, 414
Methodist Medical Center Dallas, TX, 357
Methodist Sugar Land Hospital Sugar Land, TX, 419
Methodist Willowbrook Hospital Houston, TX, 381
Metroplex Hospital Killeen, TX, 390
Metropolitan Hospital San Juan, PR, 282
Miami Jewish Home & Hosp for the Aged Miami, FL, 114
Midland Memorial Hospital Midland, TX, 401
Midway Park Medical Center (alternate name) Lancaster, TX, 392
Minden Medical Center Minden, LA, 220
Mission Hospital Mission, TX, 402
Mississippi Baptist Health Systems Jackson, MS, 249
Mississippi Methodist Rehab Center Jackson, MS, 249
Mitchell County Hospital Camilla, GA, 161
Mitchell County Hospital Colorado City, TX, 351
Mizell Memorial Hospital Opp, AL, 33
Mobile Infirmary Medical Center Mobile, AL, 28
Monroe County Hospital Forsyth, GA, 172
Monroe County Hospital Monroeville, AL, 30
Monroe Surgical Hospital Monroe, LA, 221
Montfort Jones Memorial Hospital Kosciusko, MS, 251
Morehouse General Hospital Bastrop, LA, 201
Morrow Memorial Hospital (alternate name) Winter Haven, FL, 140
Morton Plant Hospital Clearwater, FL, 91
Morton Plant North Bay Hospital (alternate name) New Port Richey, FL, 117
Mother Frances Hospital Jacksonville Jacksonville, TX, 387
Mother Frances Hospital-Tyler Tyler, TX, 424
Mount Sinai Medical Center Miami, FL, 115
Munroe Regional Medical Center Ocala, FL, 118
Murray Medical Center (alternate name) Chatsworth, GA, 163
Nacogdoches Medical Center Hospital Nacogdoches, TX, 403
Nacogdoches Memorial Hospital Nacogdoches, TX, 403
Nan Travis Memorial Hospital (alternate name) Jacksonville, TX, 386
Naples Community Hospital (alternate name) Naples, FL, 116
Natchez Community Hospital Natchez, MS, 256
Natchez Regional Medical Center Natchez, MS, 256
Natchitoches Regional Medical Center Natchitoches, LA, 222
National Park Medical Center Hot Springs, AR, 54
Nature Coast Regional Hospital Williston, FL, 139
Navarro Regional Hospital Corsicana, TX, 353
Navasota Regional Hospital (alternate name) Navasota, TX, 404
NCH Downtown Naples Hospital Naples, FL, 116
NEA Medical Center Jonesboro, AR, 55
Neshoba County General Hospital Philadelphia, MS, 258
Neuromedical Center Hospital Baton Rouge, LA, 202
Newberry County Memorial Hospital Newberry, SC, 303
Newton Medical Covington, GA, 166
Newton Regional Hospital Newton, MS, 256
Nix Healthcare System San Antonio, TX, 414
Nix Medical Center (alternate name) San Antonio, TX, 414
NMMC-Hamilton (alternate name) Hamilton, AL, 26
Nocona General Hospital Nocona, TX, 404
North Arkansas Regional Medical Center Harrison, AR, 52
North Austin Medical Center Austin, TX, 338
North Baldwin Infirmary Bay Minette, AL, 11
North Bay Hospital Aransas Pass, TX, 335
North Bay Medical Center New Port Richey, FL, 117
North Beach Community Hospital (alternate name) Weston, FL, 139
North Broward Medical Center Deerfield Beach, FL, 94
North Central Medical Center McKinney, TX, 400
North Florida Regional Medical Center Gainesville, FL, 100
North Fulton Regional Hospital Roswell, GA, 183
North Georgia Medical Center Ellijay, GA, 170
North Hills Hospital (alternate name) N Richland Hills, TX, 405
North Hills Hospital N Richland Hills, TX, 405
North Mississippi Medical Center-Eupora Eupora, MS, 244
North Mississippi Medical Center-Iuka Iuka, MS, 248
North Mississippi Medical Center Tupelo, MS, 261
North Oak Regional Medical Center Senatobia, MS, 260
North Oaks Medical System Hammond, LA, 208
North Okaloosa Medical Center Crestview, FL, 93
North Ridge Medical Center Fort Lauderdale, FL, 98
North Runnels Hospital Winters, TX, 430
North Shore Medical Center Miami, FL, 114

North Sunflower County Hospital Ruleville, MS, 260
North Texas Hospital Denton, TX, 361
North Texas Medical Center-Westpark Campus (alternate name) McKinney, TX, 400
North Texas Medical Center Gainesville, TX, 370
Northeast Alabama Regional Medical Center Anniston, AL, 9
Northeast Georgia Medical Center Gainesville, GA, 173
Northeast Medical Center Hospital Humble, TX, 384
Northeast Medical Center Bonham, TX, 343
Northlake Regional Medical Center (alternate name) Tucker, GA, 188
Northport Hospital-DCH (alternate name) Northport, AL, 32
Northport Medical Center Northport, AL, 32
Northridge Medical Center (alternate name) Prattville, AL, 34
Northshore Regional Medical Center Slidell, LA, 230
Northside Hospital-Cherokee Canton, GA, 161
Northside Hospital Atlanta, GA, 155
Northside Hospital Cumming, GA, 166
Northside Hospital Saint Petersburg, FL, 128
Northwest Florida Community Hospital Chipley, FL, 90
Northwest Medical Center Margate, FL, 110
Northwest Medical Center Springdale, AR, 65
Northwest Medical Center Winfield, AL, 39
Northwest Mississippi Regional Medical Center Clarksdale, MS, 243
Northwest Texas Healthcare System Amarillo, TX, 333
Northwest Texas Surgery Center Amarillo, TX, 334
NW Medical Center Benton County Bentonville, AR, 46
Oak Hill Hospital Brooksville, FL, 90
Oakbend Medical Center Richmond, TX, 411
Oakdale Community Hospital Oakdale, LA, 225
Ocala Regional Medical Center Ocala, FL, 118
Ochsner Baptist Medical Center New Orleans, LA, 224
Ochsner Clinic Foundation New Orleans, LA, 224
Ochsner Medical Center-Baton Rouge Baton Rouge, LA, 202
Ochsner Medical Center-Kenner (alternate name) Kenner, LA, 211
Ochsner Medical Center (alternate name) Gretna, LA, 208
Oconee Memorial Hospital Seneca, SC, 305
Oconee Regional Medical Center Milledgeville, GA, 179
Odessa Regional Hospital Odessa, TX, 406
Oktibbeha County Hospital Starkville, MS, 261
Opelousas General Hospital Opelousas, LA, 226
Orange Park Medical Center Orange Park, FL, 119
Orlando Regional Healthcare Orlando, FL, 120
Osceola Regional Medical Center Kissimmee, FL, 106
Otto Kaiser Memorial Hospital Kenedy, TX, 389
Ouachita Community Hospital West Monroe, LA, 232
Ouachita Medical Center Camden, AR, 48
Our Lady of Lourdes Regional Medical Center Lafayette, LA, 214
Our Lady of the Lake Regional Medical Center Baton Rouge, LA, 203
Ourall-Morris Memorial Hospital (alternate name) Coleman, TX, 351
Ozark Health Medical Center Clinton, AR, 48
P & S Surgical Hospital Monroe, LA, 221
Palestine Regional Medical Center Palestine, TX, 406
Palm Beach Grdns Medical Center Palm Beach Grdns, FL, 121
Palm Springs General Hospital Miami, FL, 101
Palmetto Baptist Medical Center Easley Easley, SC, 296
Palmetto General Hospital Hialeah, FL, 101
Palmetto Health Baptist Columbia Columbia, SC, 295
Palmetto Health Richland Hospital Columbia, SC, 295
Palms of Pasadena Hospital Saint Petersburg, FL, 129
Palms West Hospital (alternate name) Loxahatchee, FL, 110
Palms West Hospital Loxahatchee, FL, 110
Palmyra Medical Centers Albany, GA, 152
Palo Pinto General Hospital Mineral Wells, TX, 401
Pampa Regional Medical Center Pampa, TX, 407
Pan American Hospital Miami, FL, 114
Panola General Hospital (alternate name) Carthage, TX, 348
Paris Regional Medical Center-South Campus Paris, TX, 407
Park Place Surgical Hospital Lafayette, LA, 214
Park Plaza Hospital Houston, TX, 381
Parkland Health & Hospital System Dallas, TX, 357
Parkview Hospital Wheeler, TX, 429
Parkview Regional Hospital Mexia, TX, 401
Parkway Medical Center Hospital Decatur, AL, 18
Parrish Medical Center Titusville, FL, 137
Pasco Regional Medical Center Dade City, FL, 93
Peace River Regional Medical Center Port Charlotte, FL, 125
Peach County Hospital (alternate name) Fort Valley, GA, 172
Peach Regional Medical Center Fort Valley, GA, 172
Pearl River County Hospital and Nursing Home Poplarville, MS, 258
Pearl River Medical Complex (alternate name) Poplarville, MS, 258
Pecos County Memorial Hosptial Fort Stockton, TX, 367

Pembroke Pines General Hospital (alternate name) Pembroke Pines, FL, 122
Permian General Hospital Andrews, TX, 334
Perry Hospital Perry, GA, 181
PGH (alternate name) Plantation, FL, 124
Phoebe Putney Memorial Hospital Albany, GA, 152
Physicians Centre Bryan, TX, 346
Physicians Medical Center Carraway Birmingham, AL, 13
Physicians Regional Medical Center Naples, FL, 116
Physicians Specialty Hospital of El Paso El Paso, TX, 364
Physicians Surgical Hospital at Quail Creek Amarillo, TX, 334
Physicians Surgical Specialty Hospital Houma, LA, 209
Pickens County Medical Center Carrollton, AL, 16
Pickens General Hospital (alternate name) Jasper, GA, 175
Piedmont Fayette Hospital Fayetteville, GA, 171
Piedmont Hospital Atlanta, GA, 156
Piedmont Medical Center Rock Hill, SC, 304
Piedmont Mountainside Hospital Jasper, GA, 175
Piggott Community Hospital Piggott, AR, 62
Pike County Memorial Hospital Murfreesboro, AR, 60
Pilas Hospital, Dr. (alternate name) Ponce, PR, 278
Pine Creek Medical Center Dallas, TX, 357
Plantation General Hospital Plantation, FL, 124
Plaza Medical Center Fort Worth, TX, 369
Polk County Memorial Hospital (alternate name) Livingston, TX, 394
Polk Medical Center Cedartown, GA, 162
Prattville Baptist Hospital Prattville, AL, 34
Presbyterian Community Hospital (alternate name) San Juan, PR, 281
Presbyterian Hospital of Allen Allen, TX, 333
Presbyterian Hospital of Commerce (alternate name) Greenville, TX, 374
Presbyterian Hospital of Dallas Dallas, TX, 358
Presbyterian Hospital of Denton Denton, TX, 361
Presbyterian Hospital of Greenville Greenville, TX, 374
Presbyterian Hospital of Kaufman Kaufman, TX, 388
Presbyterian Hospital of Plano Plano, TX, 410
Presbyterian Hospital of Winnsboro Winnsboro, TX, 430
Presbyterian Plano Ctr for Diag & Surgery Plano, TX, 410
Princeton Baptist Medical Center Birmingham, AL, 14
Professional Hospital Manati, PR, 276
Promina Cobb Hospital (alternate name) Austell, GA, 158
Promina Gwinnett Health System Lawrenceville, GA, 176
Providence Health Center Waco, TX, 426
Providence Hosp/Providence Heart Inst Columbia, SC, 295
Providence Hospital Laredo, TX, 393
Providence Hospital Mobile, AL, 29
Providence Memorial Hospital El Paso, TX, 365
Putnam Community Hospital (alternate name) Palatka, FL, 121
Putnam Community Medical Center Palatka, FL, 121
Putnam General Hospital Eatonton, GA, 170
Ramon E Betances Hospital Mayaguez, PR, 277
Randolph County Medical Center Pocahontas, AR, 63
Randolph Health Systems Medical Center Roanoke, AL, 34
Rankin Medical Center Brandon, MS, 241
Rapides Regional Medical Center Alexandria, LA, 200
Raulerson Hospital Okeechobee, FL, 119
Rebsamen Medical Center Jacksonville, AR, 54
Red Bay Hospital Red Bay, AL, 34
Red River Regional Hospital (alternate name) Bonham, TX, 343
Redmond Park Hospital (alternate name) Rome, GA, 183
Redmond Regional Medical Center Rome, GA, 183
Reeves County Hospital Pecos, TX, 408
Regency Hospital of Jackson Jackson, MS, 249
Regency Hospital of North Dallas II Carrollton, TX, 348
Regional Med Ctr of Orangeburg & Calhoun Orangeburg, SC, 304
Regional Medical Center Bayonet Point Hudson, FL, 102
Renaissance Hospital Houston Houston, TX, 381
Renaissance Hospital-East Texas Groves, TX, 375
RHD Memorial Medical Center Dallas, TX, 358
Richardson Medical Center Rayville, LA, 227
Richardson Medical Center Richardson, TX, 411
Richland Parish Hospital Service District (alternate name) Rayville, LA, 227
Riley Memorial Hospital Meridian, MS, 255
Rio Grande Regional Hospital McAllen, TX, 399
River Oaks Hospital Jackson, MS, 250
River Parishes Hospital La Place, LA, 217
River Parishes Medical Center (alternate name) La Place, LA, 217
River Region Health System Vicksburg, MS, 262
River West Medical Center Plaquemine, LA, 227
Riverside General Hospital Houston, TX, 382
Riverview Regional Medical Center Gadsden, AL, 23
Rockdale Hospital Conyers, GA, 165
Rolling Plains Memorial Hospital Sweetwater, TX, 420
Rollins Brook Community Hospital Lampasas, TX, 392
Roper Hospital Charleston, SC, 293

Round Rock Medical Center Round Rock, TX, 412
Rush Foundation Hospital Meridian, MS, 255
Rush Hospital-Newton (alternate name) Newton, MS, 256
Russell Hospital (alternate name) Alexander City, AL, 9
Russell Medical Center Alexander City, AL, 9
Russellville Hospital Russellville, AL, 35
Ryder Memorial Hospital Humacao, PR, 275
Sabine Medical Center Many, LA, 218
Sacred Heart Health System Pensacola, FL, 123
Sacred Heart Hospital on the Emerald Coast Destin, FL, 96
Saint Anne General Hospital Raceland, LA, 227
Saint Anthony's Healthcare Center Morrilton, AR, 59
Saint Anthony's Hospital (alternate name) Morrilton, AR, 59
Saint Anthony's Hospital Saint Petersburg, FL, 129
Saint Bernard's Medical Center Jonesboro, AR, 55
Saint Charles Parish Hospital Luling, LA, 218
Saint Clair Regional Hospital Pell City, AL, 33
Saint Cloud Regional Medical Center Saint Cloud, FL, 127
Saint David's Rehabilitation Center Austin, TX, 338
Saint Dominic Jackson Memorial Hospital Jackson, MS, 250
Saint Edward Mercy Medical Center Fort Smith, AR, 51
Saint Elizabeth Hospital (alternate name) Beaumont, TX, 341
Saint Elizabeth Hospital Gonzales, LA, 208
Saint Eugene Community Hospital (alternate name) Dillon, SC, 296
Saint Francis Health Center (alternate name) Madisonville, TX, 398
Saint Francis Health System (alternate name) Greenville, SC, 299
Saint Francis Hospital Columbus, GA, 164
Saint Francis Hospital Greenville, SC, 299
Saint Francis Medical Center Monroe, LA, 221
Saint John Hospital (alternate name) Houston, TX, 404
Saint John's Hospital-Berryville Berryville, AR, 47
Saint Joseph Candler Hospital Savannah, GA, 185
Saint Joseph Hospital (alternate name) Bryan, TX, 346
Saint Joseph Hospital (alternate name) Port Charlotte, FL, 125
Saint Joseph Medical Center Houston, TX, 382
Saint Joseph Regional Health Center Bryan, TX, 346
Saint Joseph's Hospital Atlanta, GA, 156
Saint Joseph's Hospital Tampa, FL, 134
Saint Joseph's Mercy Health Center Hot Springs Natl Pk, AR, 54
Saint Joseph's/ Saint Anthony's Health System (alternate name) Saint Petersburg, FL, 129
Saint Lucie Medical Center Port Saint Lucie, FL, 126
Saint Luke's Community Med Ctr-The Woodlands The Woodlands, TX, 422
Saint Luke's Episcopal Hospital Houston, TX, 382
Saint Luke's Hospital Jacksonville, FL, 104
Saint Marks Medical Center La Grange, TX, 391
Saint Mary's Hospital Athens, GA, 153
Saint Mary's Medical Center West Palm Beach, FL, 139
Saint Mary's Regional Medical Center Russellville, AR, 63
Saint Mary-Rogers Memorial Hospital Rogers, AR, 63
Saint Petersburg General Hospital Saint Petersburg, FL, 129
Saint Tammany Parish Hospital Covington, LA, 206
Saint Vincent Infirmary Medical Center Little Rock, AR, 57
Saint Vincent Medical Center North Sherwood, AR, 64
Saint Vincent's Hospital Birmingham, AL, 14
Saint Vincent's Medical Center Jacksonville, FL, 104
Saline Memorial Hospital Benton, AR, 46
San Angelo Community Medical Center San Angelo, TX, 413
San Antonio Regional Hospital (alternate name) San Antonio, TX, 414
San German Area Hospital (alternate name) San German, PR, 280
San Jacinto Methodist Hospital Baytown, TX, 341
San Juan Municipal Hospital Rio Piedras, PR, 279
San Luke's Memorial Hospital Ponce, PR, 279
Santa Rosa Clinic (alternate name) Guayama, PR, 274
Santa Rosa Health Care (alternate name) San Antonio, TX, 414
Santa Rosa Medical Center Milton, FL, 115
Sarasota Memorial Health Care Systems Sarasota, FL, 130
Sarasota Memorial Hospital (alternate name) Sarasota, FL, 130
Satilla Regional Medical Center Waycross, GA, 190
Savoy Medical Center Mamou, LA, 218
Scenic Mountain Medical Center Big Spring, TX, 343
Schumpert Medical Center (alternate name) Shreveport, LA, 228
Scott & White Temple, TX, 421
Scott Regioanl Hospital Morton, MS, 255
Sebastian River Medical Center Sebastian, FL, 130
Self Memorial Hospital (alternate name) Greenwood, SC, 299
Self Regional Healthcare Center Greenwood, SC, 299
Senatobia Community Hospital (alternate name) Senatobia, MS, 260
Seton Edgar B Davis Memorial Hospital Luling, TX, 398
Seton Highland Lakes Burnet, TX, 347
Seton Medical Center Austin, TX, 339

Seton Northwest Hospital Austin, TX, 339
Seton Southwest Healthcare Center Austin, TX, 339
Seven Rivers Regional Medical Center Crystal River, FL, 93
Seventh Ward General Hospital (alternate name) Hammond, LA, 208
Seymour Hospital Seymour, TX, 417
Shallowford Community Hospital (alternate name) Atlanta, GA, 154
Shands at Lake Shore Lake City, FL, 107
Shands at Starke Starke, FL, 132
Shands at the University of Florida Gainesville, FL, 100
Shands Hospital at the University of Florida (alternate name) Gainesville, FL, 100
Shands Jacksonville Jacksonville, FL, 104
Shands Live Oak Live Oak, FL, 109
Shannon Medical Center San Angelo, TX, 413
Shannon West Texas Memorial Hospital (alternate name) San Angelo, TX, 413
Sharkey Issaquena Community Hospital Rolling Fork, MS, 260
Sharpstown General Hospital (alternate name) Houston, TX, 383
Shelby Baptist Medical Center Alabaster, AL, 9
Shelby Regional Medical Center Center, TX, 349
Shepperd Memorial Hospital (alternate name) Burnet, TX, 347
Shoals Hospital Muscle Shoals, AL, 31
Sid Peterson Memorial Hospital Kerrville, TX, 389
Sierra Medical Center El Paso, TX, 365
Siloam Springs Memorial Hospital Siloam Springs, AR, 64
Simpson General Hospital Mendenhall, MS, 254
Singing River Hospital Pascagoula, MS, 257
Slidell Memorial Hospital Slidell, LA, 230
SMC Regional Medical Center (alternate name) Osceola, AR, 61
Smith Northview Hospital Valdosta, GA, 189
Smithville Regional Hospital Smithville, TX, 418
Smyrna Hospital (alternate name) Smyrna, GA, 185
South Austin Hospital Austin, TX, 339
South Baldwin Hospital (alternate name) Foley, AL, 22
South Baldwin Regional Medical Center Foley, AL, 22
South Bay Hospital Sun City Center, FL, 132
South Central Regional Medical Center Laurel, MS, 251
South Florida Baptist Hospital Plant City, FL, 124
South Fulton Medical Center East Point, GA, 169
South Georgia Medical Center Valdosta, GA, 189
South Lake Hospital Clermont, FL, 91
South Louisiana Medical Center (alternate name) Houma, LA, 209
South Miami Hospital Miami, FL, 114
South Mississippi County Regional Med Ctr Osceola, AR, 61
South Sunflower County Hospital Indianola, MS, 248
South Texas Regional Medical Center Jourdanton, TX, 387
Southeast Alabama Medical Center Dothan, AL, 19
Southeast Georgia Health System-Camden Campus Saint Marys, GA, 184
Southeast Georgia Health System Brunswick, GA, 160
Southern Regional Medical Center Riverdale, GA, 182
Southern Surgical Hospital Slidell, LA, 230
Southpark Community Hospital Lafayette, LA, 214
Southwest Florida Regional Medical Center Fort Myers, FL, 99
Southwest General Hospital San Antonio, TX, 415
Southwest Medical Center Lafayette, LA, 214
Southwest Mississippi Regional Medical Center McComb, MS, 253
Southwest Regional Medical Centre Little Rock, AR, 57
Southwest Surgical Hospital Hurst, TX, 385
Southwestern General Hospital El Paso, TX, 365
Spalding Regional Medical Center Griffin, GA, 173
Sparks Regional Medical Center Fort Smith, AR, 52
Spartanburg Regional Health Care System Spartanburg, SC, 306
Spine Hospital of South Texas San Antonio, TX, 415
Spohn Bee County Hospital (alternate name) Beeville, TX, 342
Spohn-Kleberg Memorial Hospital (alternate name) Kingsville, TX, 390
Spring Branch Medical Center (alternate name) Houston, TX, 377
Springdale Memorial Hospital (alternate name) Springdale, AR, 65
Springhill Medical Center Mobile, AL, 29
Springhill Medical Center Springhill, LA, 231
Springhill Memorial Hospital (alternate name) Mobile, AL, 29
Springs Memorial Hospital Lancaster, SC, 301
Stamford Memorial Hospital Stamford, TX, 419
Starr County Memorial Hospital Rio Grande City, TX, 412
Stephens County Hospital Toccoa, GA, 188
Stephens Memorial Hospital Breckenridge, TX, 344
Stone County Medical Center Mountain View, AR, 60
Stringfellow Memorial Hospital Anniston, AL, 10
Stuttgart Regional Medical Center Stuttgart, AR, 65
Summit Hospital Phenix City, AL, 33

Summit Medical Center Van Buren, AR, 65
Sumter Regional Hospital Americus, GA, 153
Sun Coast Hospital Largo, FL, 108
Surgical Hospital of Jonesboro Jonesboro, AR, 55
Surgical Specialty Hospital of Sugar Land Sugar Land, TX, 420
Surgical Specialty Hospital Baton Rouge, LA, 203
Suwannee County Hospital (alternate name) Live Oak, FL, 109
Sylvan Grove Hospital Jackson, GA, 175
Tailor Telfair Regional Hospital McRae, GA, 178
Tallahassee Memorial Health Care Foundation Tallahassee, FL, 133
Tampa General Care (alternate name) Tampa, FL, 134
Tampa General Healthcare Tampa, FL, 134
Tanner Medical Center Carrollton, GA, 162
Tanner Medical Center Villa Rica, GA, 190
Taylor Regional Hospital Hawkinsville, GA, 174
Teche Regional Medical Center Morgan City, LA, 221
Terrebonne General Medical Center Houma, LA, 209
Terrell Community Hospital (alternate name) Terrell, TX, 421
Texas Inst for Surg at Presbyterian Hosp Dallas, TX, 358
Texas Orthopedic Hospital Houston, TX, 383
Texas Spine and Joint Hospital Tyler, TX, 424
Texoma Medical Center Denison, TX, 360
Texsan Heart Hospital San Antonio, TX, 415
The Hospital at Westlake Medical Center Austin, TX, 340
Thibodaux Regional Medical Center Thibodaux, LA, 231
Thomas Hospital Fairhope, AL, 21
Thomason General Hospital El Paso, TX, 366
Thomasville Infirmary Thomasville, AL, 37
Three Rivers Hospital and Medical Center (alternate name) McRae, GA, 178
Tift Regional Medical Hospital Tifton, GA, 188
Tippah County Hospital Ripley, MS, 260
Titus County Memorial Hospital (alternate name) Mount Pleasant, TX, 402
Titus Regional Medical Center Mount Pleasant, TX, 402
Tomball Regional Hospital Tomball, TX, 423
Tops Surgical Specialty Hospital Houston, TX, 383
Torbett-Hutchings-Smith Hospital (alternate name) Marlin, TX, 398
Touro Infirmary New Orleans, LA, 224
Town and Country Hospital Tampa, FL, 135
Trace Regional Hospital Houston, MS, 248
Tri City Community Hospital (alternate name) Jourdanton, TX, 387
Trident Medical Center Charleston, SC, 293
Tri-Lakes Medical Center Batesville, MS, 239
Trinity Community Hospital Jasper, FL, 105
Trinity Hospital of Augusta Augusta, GA, 157
Trinity Medical Center Birmingham, AL, 14
Trinity Medical Center Brenham, TX, 344
Trinity Medical Center Carrollton, TX, 348
Trinity Memorial Hospital (alternate name) Trinity, TX, 423
Trinity Valley Medical Center (alternate name) Palestine, TX, 406
Tri-Ward Rural Health Clinic Bernice, LA, 204
Trophy Club Medical Center Trophy Club, TX, 423
Troy Regional Medical Center Troy, AL, 37
Tulane University Hospital & Clinic New Orleans, LA, 225
Tuomey Regional Medical Center Sumter, SC, 306
Turning Point Hospital Moultrie, GA, 180
Twelve Oaks Hospital Houston, TX, 383
Twin Cities Hospital Niceville, FL, 118
Tyler County Hospital Woodville, TX, 431
UAB Hospital Birmingham, AL, 14
UAB Medical West Bessemer, AL, 11
UAMS Medical Center Little Rock, AR, 57
UCH (alternate name) Tampa, FL, 135
Union General Hospital Blairsville, GA, 159
United Regional Healthcare System Wichita Falls, TX, 430
University Community Hospital of Carrollwood Tampa, FL, 135
University Community Hospital Tampa, FL, 135
University District Hospital Rio Piedras, PR, 280
University General Hospital Houston, TX, 383
University Hospital & Medical Center Tamarac, FL, 133
University Hospital (alternate name) Tamarac, FL, 133
University Hospital Augusta, GA, 158
University Hospital San Antonio, TX, 416
University Medical Center (alternate name) Jacksonville, FL, 104
University Medical Center Lafayette, LA, 215
University Medical Center Lubbock, TX, 397
University of Alabama Hospital (alternate name) Birmingham, AL, 14
University of Mississippi Medical Center Jackson, MS, 250
University of South Alabama Medical Center Mobile, AL, 29
University of Texas Health Center at Tyler Tyler, TX, 424

University of Texas Medical Branch Hospitals Galveston, TX, 370
UPR Carolina Carolina, PR, 272
Upson County Hospital (alternate name) Thomaston, GA, 187
Upson Regional Medical Center Thomaston, GA, 187
Upstate Carolina Medical Center Gaffney, SC, 298
Upstate Carolina Memorial Center (alternate name) Gaffney, SC, 298
USMD Hospital at Arlington Arlington, TX, 336
UT Southwestern Saint Paul Hospital Dallas, TX, 359
Uvalde Memorial Hospital Uvalde, TX, 425
Val Verde Memorial Hospital (alternate name) Del Rio, TX, 359
Val Verde Regional Medical Center Del Rio, TX, 359
Valley Baptist Medical Center Harlingen, TX, 376
Valley Regional Medical Center Brownsville, TX, 346
Van Buren County Memorial Hospital (alternate name) Clinton, AR, 48
Vaughan Evergreen Medical Center Evergreen, AL, 21
Vaughan Jackson Medical Center (alternate name) Jackson, AL, 27
Vaughan Regional Med Ctr-Parkway Campus Selma, AL, 35
Venice Regional Medical Center Venice, FL, 137
Villa Feliciana Medical Complex Jackson, LA, 210
Villages Regional Hospital The Villages, FL, 137
Ville Platte Medical Center Ville Platte, LA, 232
Vista Hospital of Dallas Garland, TX, 371
Vista Medical Center Hospital Pasadena, TX, 408
Vista Surgical Hospital of Baton Rouge Baton Rouge, LA, 203
W J Mangold Memorial Hospital Lockney, TX, 395
W O Moss Regional Medical Center Lake Charles, LA, 216
Waccamaw Community Hospital Murrells Inlet, SC, 303
Wadley Regional Medical Center Texarkana, TX, 422
Walker Baptist Medical Center Jasper, AL, 28
Walker Memorial Medical Center/Wauchula (alternate name) Wauchula, FL, 138
Wallace Thomson Hospital Union, SC, 306
Walls Regional Hospital Cleburne, TX, 350
Walter Olin Moss Regional Hospital (alternate name) Lake Charles, LA, 216
Walthall County General Hospital Tylertown, MS, 262
Walton Regional Medical Center Monroe, GA, 179
Washington County Hospital & Nursing Home (alternate name) Chatom, AL, 16
Washington County Hospital Chatom, AL, 16
Washington County Regional Medical Center Sandersville, GA, 184
Washington Regional Medical Center Fayetteville, AR, 51
Wayne General Hospital Waynesboro, MS, 263
Wayne Memorial Hospital Jesup, GA, 176
Wedowee Hospital Wedowee, AL, 38
Wellington Regional Medical Center Wellington, FL, 138
WellStar Cobb Hospital Austell, GA, 158
WellStar Douglas Hospital Douglasville, GA, 169
WellStar Kennestone Hospital Marietta, GA, 178
WellStar Paulding Hospital Dallas, GA, 167
Wesley Medical Center Hattiesburg, MS, 247
Wesley Woods Geriatric Hospital Atlanta, GA, 156
West Boca Medical Center Boca Raton, FL, 87
West Calcasieu-Cameron Hospital Sulphur, LA, 231
West Carroll Memorial Hospital Oak Grove, LA, 225
West Florida Hospital (alternate name) Pensacola, FL, 124
West Florida Regional Medical Center Pensacola, FL, 124
West Georgia Medical Center La Grange, GA, 176
West Houston Medical Center Houston, TX, 384
West Jefferson Medical Center Marrero, LA, 219
West Orange Hospital (alternate name) Ocoee, FL, 118
West Texas Medical Center Midland, TX, 401
Westchester General Hospital Miami, FL, 115
Westside Regional Medical Center (alternate name) Plantation, FL, 125
Westside Regional Medical Center Plantation, FL, 125
White County Medical Center Searcy, AR, 64
White River Medical Center Batesville, AR, 46
Whitfield Medical Surgical Hospital Whitfield, MS, 263
Wilbarger General Hospital Vernon, TX, 425
Williamsburg County Memorial Hospital (alternate name) Kingstree, SC, 300
Williamsburg Regional Hospital Kingstree, SC, 300
Willis Knighton Bossier Health Center Bossier City, LA, 205
Willis Knighton Medical Center Shreveport, LA, 229
Williston Memorial Hospital (alternate name) Williston, FL, 139
Wilson N Jones Sherman, TX, 417
Wilson Medical Center Darlington, SC, 296
Wilson N Jones Medical Center Sherman, TX, 417
Wilson N Jones Memorial Hospital (alternate name) Sherman, TX, 417
Winfield Carraway Hospital (alternate name) Winfield, AL, 39
Winn Parish Medical Center Winnfield, LA, 232
Winston Medical Center Louisville, MS, 252
Winter Haven Hospital Winter Haven, FL, 140

Wiregrass Medical Center Geneva, AL, 24
Wise Regional Health System Decatur, TX, 359
Woman's Hospital at River Oaks Jackson, MS, 251
Woman's Hospital Foundation Baton Rouge, LA, 203
Woman's Hospital (alternate name) Jackson, MS, 251
Womans Hospital of Texas Houston, TX, 384
Women and Children's Hospital Lake Charles, LA, 216
Women's and Children's Hospital Lafayette, LA, 215
Womens Hospital of Acadiana (alternate name) Lafayette, LA, 215
Womens Hospital of Texas (alternate name) Houston, TX, 384
Wood County Central Hospital District (alternate name) Quitman, TX, 411
Woodland Community Hospital (alternate name) Cullman, AL, 17
Woodland Heights Medical Center Lufkin, TX, 397
Woodland Medical Center Cullman, AL, 17
Wuesthoff Health Systems Rockledge, FL, 126
Wuesthoff Medical Center-Melbourne Melbourne, FL, 111
Yale Clinic & Hospital (alternate name) Houston, TX, 378
Yalobusha General Hospital Water Valley, MS, 262
Yoakum Community Hospital Yoakum, TX, 431
Zale-Lipshy University Hospital Dallas, TX, 359

Sedgwick Press
Hospital & Health Plan Directories

The Directory of Hospital Personnel, 2007

The Directory of Hospital Personnel is the best resource you can have at your fingertips when researching or marketing a product or service to the hospital market. A "Who's Who" of the hospital universe, this directory puts you in touch with over 150,000 key decision-makers. With 100% verification of data you can rest assured that you will reach the right person with just one call. Every hospital in the U.S. is profiled, listed alphabetically by city within state. Plus, three easy-to-use, cross-referenced indexes put the facts at your fingertips faster and more easily than any other directory: Hospital Name Index, Bed Size Index and Personnel Index. *The Directory of Hospital Personnel* is the only complete source for key hospital decision-makers by name. Whether you want to define or restructure sales territories… locate hospitals with the purchasing power to accept your proposals… keep track of important contacts or colleagues… or find information on which insurance plans are accepted, *The Directory of Hospital Personnel* gives you the information you need – easily, efficiently, effectively and accurately.

"Recommended for college, university and medical libraries." –ARBA

1,500 pages; Softcover ISBN 1-59237-178-7 $325.00 ◆ Online Database $545.00 ◆ Online Database & Directory Combo, $650.00

The Directory of Health Care Group Purchasing Organizations, 2006

This comprehensive directory provides the important data you need to get in touch with over 800 Group Purchasing Organizations. By providing in-depth information on this growing market and its members, *The Directory of Health Care Group Purchasing Organizations* fills a major need for the most accurate and comprehensive information on over 800 GPOs – Mailing Address, Phone & Fax Numbers, E-mail Addresses, Key Contacts, Purchasing Agents, Group Descriptions, Membership Categorization, Standard Vendor Proposal Requirements, Membership Fees & Terms, Expanded Services, Total Member Beds & Outpatient Visits represented and more. Five indexes provide a number of ways to locate the right GPO: Alphabetical Index, Expanded Services Index, Organization Type Index, Geographic Index and Member Institution Index. With its comprehensive and detailed information on each purchasing organization, *The Directory of Health Care Group Purchasing Organizations* is the go-to source for anyone looking to target this market.

"The information is clearly arranged and easy to access…recommended for those needing this very specialized information." –ARBA

1,000 pages; Softcover ISBN 1-59237-0091-8, $325.00 ◆ Online Database, $650.00 ◆ Online Database & Directory Combo, $750.00

The HMO/PPO Directory, 2007

The HMO/PPO Directory is a comprehensive source that provides detailed information about Health Maintenance Organizations and Preferred Provider Organizations nationwide. This comprehensive directory details more information about more managed health care organizations than ever before. Over 1,100 HMOs, PPOs, Medicare Advantage Plans and affiliated companies are listed, arranged alphabetically by state. Detailed listings include Key Contact Information, Prescription Drug Benefits, Enrollment, Geographical Areas Served, Affiliated Physicians & Hospitals, Federal Qualifications, Status, Year Founded, Managed Care Partners, Employer References, Fees & Payment Information and more. Plus, five years of historical information is included related to Revenues, Net Income, Medical Loss Ratios, Membership Enrollment and Number of Patient Complaints. Five easy-to-use, cross-referenced indexes will put this vast array of information at your fingertips immediately: HMO Index, PPO Index, Other Providers Index, Personnel Index and Enrollment Index. *The HMO/PPO Directory* provides the most comprehensive data on the most companies available on the market place today.

"Helpful to individuals requesting certain HMO/PPO issues such as co-payment costs, subscription costs and patient complaints. Individuals concerned (or those with questions) about their insurance may find this text to be of use to them." –ARBA

600 pages; Softcover ISBN 1-59237-158-2, $325.00 ◆ Online Database, $495.00 ◆ Online Database & Directory Combo, $600.00

To preview any of our Directories Risk-Free for 30 days, call (800) 562-2139 or fax to (518) 789-0556

Medical Device Register, 2007

The only one-stop resource of every medical supplier licensed to sell products in the US. This award-winning directory offers immediate access to over 13,000 companies - and more than 65,000 products – in two information-packed volumes. This comprehensive resource saves hours of time and trouble when searching for medical equipment and supplies and the manufacturers who provide them. Volume I: The Product Directory, provides essential information for purchasing or specifying medical supplies for every medical device, supply, and diagnostic available in the US. Listings provide FDA codes & Federal Procurement Eligibility, Contact information for every manufacturer of the product along with Prices and Product Specifications. Volume 2 - Supplier Profiles, offers the most complete and important data about Suppliers, Manufacturers and Distributors. Company Profiles detail the number of employees, ownership, method of distribution, sales volume, net income, key executives detailed contact information medical products the company supplies, plus the medical specialties they cover. Four indexes provide immediate access to this wealth of information: Keyword Index, Trade Name Index, Supplier Geographical Index and OEM (Original Equipment Manufacturer) Index. Medical Device Register, 2007 is the only one-stop source for locating suppliers and products; looking for new manufacturers or hard-to-find medical devices; comparing products and companies; know who's selling what and who to buy from cost effectively. This directory has become the standard in its field and will be a welcome addition to the reference collection of any medical library, large public library, university library along with the collections that serve the medical community.

"A wealth of information on medical devices, medical device companies… and key personnel in the industry is provide in this comprehensive reference work... A valuable reference work, one of the best hardcopy compilations available." -Doody Publishing

3,000 pages Two Volumes; Hardcover ISBN 1-59237-181-7; $325.00

The Directory of Independent Ambulatory Care Centers

This first edition of *The Directory of Independent Ambulatory Care Centers* provides access to detailed information that, before now, could only be found scattered in hundreds of different sources. This comprehensive and up-to-date directory pulls together a vast array of contact information for over 7,200 Ambulatory Surgery Centers, Ambulatory General and Urgent Care Clinics, and Diagnostic Imaging Centers that are not affiliated with a hospital or major medical center. Detailed listings include Mailing Address, Phone & Fax Numbers, E-mail and Web Site addresses, Contact Name and Phone Numbers of the Medical Director and other Key Executives and Purchasing Agents, Specialties & Services Offered, Year Founded, Numbers of Employees and Surgeons, Number of Operating Rooms, Number of Cases seen per year, Overnight Options, Contracted Services and much more. Listings are arranged by State, by Center Category and then alphabetically by Organization Name. Two indexes provide quick and easy access to this wealth of information: Entry Name Index and Specialty/Service Index. *The Directory of Independent Ambulatory Care Centers* is a must-have resource for anyone marketing a product or service to this important industry and will be an invaluable tool for those searching for a local care center that will meet their specific needs.

"Among the numerous hospital directories, no other provides information on independent ambulatory centers. A handy, well-organized resource that would be useful in medical center libraries and public libraries." –Choice

986 pages; Softcover ISBN 1-930956-90-8, $185.00 ◆ Online Database, $365.00 ◆ Online Database & Directory Combo, $450.00

To preview any of our Directories Risk-Free for 30 days, call (800) 562-2139 or fax to (518) 789-0556

Sedgwick Press
Health Directories

The Complete Directory for People with Disabilities, 2007

wealth of information, now in one comprehensive sourcebook. Completely updated, this edition contains more information than ever before, including thousands of new entries and enhancements to existing entries and thousands of additional web sites and e-mail addresses. This up-to-date directory is the most comprehensive resource available for people with disabilities, detailing Independent Living Centers, Rehabilitation Facilities, State & Federal Agencies, Associations, Support Groups, Periodicals & Books, Assistive Devices, Employment & Education Programs, Camps and Travel Groups. Each year, more libraries, schools, colleges, hospitals, rehabilitation centers and individuals add *The Complete Directory for People with Disabilities* to their collections, making sure that this information is readily available to the families, individuals and professionals who can benefit most from the amazing wealth of resources cataloged here.

"No other reference tool exists to meet the special needs of the disabled in one convenient resource for information." –Library Journal

1200 pages; Softcover ISBN 1-59237-147-7, $165.00 ◆ Online Database $215.00 ◆ Online Database & Directory Combo $300.00

The Complete Directory for People with Chronic Illness, 2007/08

Thousands of hours of research have gone into this completely updated 2005/06 edition – several new chapters have been added along with thousands of new entries and enhancements to existing entries. Plus, each chronic illness chapter has been reviewed by an medical expert in the field. This widely-hailed directory is structured around the 90 most prevalent chronic illnesses – from Asthma to Cancer to Wilson's Disease – and provides a comprehensive overview of the support services and information resources available for people diagnosed with a chronic illness. Each chronic illness has its own chapter and contains a brief description in layman's language, followed by important resources for National & Local Organizations, State Agencies, Newsletters, Books & Periodicals, Libraries & Research Centers, Support Groups & Hotlines, Web Sites and much more. This directory is an important resource for health care professionals, the collections of hospital and health care libraries, as well as an invaluable tool for people with a chronic illness and their support network.

"A must purchase for all hospital and health care libraries and is strongly recommended for all public library reference departments." –ARBA

1200 pages; Softcover ISBN 1-59237-183-3, $165.00 ◆ Online Database $215.00 ◆ Online Database & Directory Combo $300.00

The Complete Learning Disabilities Directory, 2007

The Complete Learning Disabilities Directory is the most comprehensive database of Programs, Services, Curriculum Materials, Professional Meetings & Resources, Camps, Newsletters and Support Groups for teachers, students and families concerned with learning disabilities. This information-packed directory includes information about Associations & Organizations, Schools, Colleges & Testing Materials, Government Agencies, Legal Resources and much more. For quick, easy access to information, this directory contains four indexes: Entry Name Index, Subject Index and Geographic Index. With every passing year, the field of learning disabilities attracts more attention and the network of caring, committed and knowledgeable professionals grows every day. This directory is an invaluable research tool for these parents, students and professionals.

"Due to its wealth and depth of coverage, parents, teachers and others... should find this an invaluable resource." –Booklist

900 pages; Softcover ISBN 1-59237-122-1, $145.00 ◆ Online Database $195.00 ◆ Online Database & Directory Combo $280.00

The Complete Mental Health Directory, 2006/07

This is the most comprehensive resource covering the field of behavioral health, with critical information for both the layman and the mental health professional. For the layman, this directory offers understandable descriptions of 25 Mental Health Disorders as well as detailed information on Associations, Media, Support Groups and Mental Health Facilities. For the professional, *The Complete Mental Health Directory* offers critical and comprehensive information on Managed Care Organizations, Information Systems, Government Agencies and Provider Organizations. This comprehensive volume of needed information will be widely used in any reference collection.

"... the strength of this directory is that it consolidates widely dispersed information into a single volume." –Booklist

800 pages; Softcover ISBN 1-59237-124-8, $165.00 ◆ Online Database $215.00 ◆ Online & Directory Combo $300.00

To preview any of our Directories Risk-Free for 30 days, call (800) 562-2139 or fax to (518) 789-0556

Older Americans Information Directory, 2006/07

Completely updated for 2006/07, this sixth edition has been completely revised and now contains 1,000 new listings, over 8,000 updates to existing listings and over 3,000 brand new e-mail addresses and web sites. You'll find important resources for Older Americans including National, Regional, State & Local Organizations, Government Agencies, Research Centers, Libraries & Information Centers, Legal Resources, Discount Travel Information, Continuing Education Programs, Disability Aids & Assistive Devices, Health, Print Media and Electronic Media. Three indexes: Entry Index, Subject Index and Geographic Index make it easy to find just the right source of information. This comprehensive guide to resources for Older Americans will be a welcome addition to any reference collection.

"Highly recommended for academic, public, health science and consumer libraries…" –Choic

1,200 pages; Softcover ISBN 1-59237-136-1, $165.00 ◆ Online Database $215.00 ◆ Online Database & Directory Combo $300.00

The Complete Directory for Pediatric Disorders, 2007

This important directory provides parents and caregivers with information about Pediatric Conditions, Disorders, Diseases and Disabilities, including Blood Disorders, Bone & Spinal Disorders, Brain Defects & Abnormalities, Chromosomal Disorders, Congenital Heart Defects, Movement Disorders, Neuromuscular Disorders and Pediatric Tumors & Cancers. This carefully written directory offers: understandable Descriptions of 15 major bodily systems; Descriptions of more than 200 Disorders and a Resources Section, detailing National Agencies & Associations, State Associations, Online Services, Libraries & Resource Centers, Research Centers, Support Groups & Hotlines, Camps, Books and Periodicals. This resource will provide immediate access to information crucial to families and caregivers when coping with children's illnesses.

"Recommended for public and consumer health libraries." –Library Journe

1,200 pages; Softcover ISBN 1-59237-150-7 $165.00 ◆ Online Database $215.00 ◆ Online Database & Directory Combo $300.00

The Directory of Drug & Alcohol Residential Rehabilitation Facilities

This brand new directory is the first-ever resource to bring together, all in one place, data on the thousands of drug and alcohol residential rehabilitation facilities in the United States. *The Directory of Drug & Alcohol Residential Rehabilitation Facilities* covers over 1,000 facilities, with detailed contact information for each one, including mailing address, phone and fax numbers, email addresses and web sites, mission statement, type of treatment programs, cost, average length of stay, numbers of residents and counselors, accreditation, insurance plans accepted, type of environment, religious affiliation, education components and much more. It also contains a helpful chapter on General Resources that provides contact information for Associations, Print & Electronic Media, Support Groups and Conferences. Multiple indexes allow the user to pinpoint the facilities that meet very specific criteria. This time-saving tool is what so many counselors, parents and medical professionals have been asking for. *The Directory of Drug & Alcohol Residential Rehabilitation Facilities* will be a helpful tool in locating the right source for treatment for a wide range of individuals. This comprehensive directory will be an important acquisition for all reference collections: public and academic libraries, case managers, social workers, state agencies and many more.

"This is an excellent, much needed directory that fills an important gap…" –Bookli

300 pages; Softcover ISBN 1-59237-031-4, $135.00

To preview any of our Directories Risk-Free for 30 days, call (800) 562-2139 or fax to (518) 789-0556

Sedgwick Press
Education Directories

The Comparative Guide to American Elementary & Secondary Schools, 2007

The only guide of its kind, this award winning compilation offers a snapshot profile of every public school district in the United States serving 1,500 or more students – more than 5,900 districts are covered. Organized alphabetically by district within state, each chapter begins with a Statistical Overview of the state. Each district listing includes contact information (name, address, phone number and web site) plus Grades Served, the Numbers of Students and Teachers and the Number of Regular, Special Education, Alternative and vocational Schools in the district along with statistics on Student/Classroom Teacher Ratios, Drop Out Rates, Ethnicity, the Numbers of Librarians and Guidance Counselors and District Expenditures per student. As an added bonus, *The Comparative Guide to American Elementary and Secondary Schools* provides important ranking tables, both by state and nationally, for each data element. For easy navigation through this wealth of information, this handbook contains a useful City Index that lists all districts that operate schools within a city. These important comparative statistics are necessary for anyone considering relocation or doing comparative research on their own district and would be a perfect acquisition for any public library or school district library.

"This straightforward guide is an easy way to find general information. Valuable for academic and large public library collections." –ARBA

1,400 pages; Softcover ISBN 1-59237-223-6, $125.00

Educators Resource Directory, 2007/08

Educators Resource Directory is a comprehensive resource that provides the educational professional with thousands of resources and statistical data for professional development. This directory saves hours of research time by providing immediate access to Associations & Organizations, Conferences & Trade Shows, Educational Research Centers, Employment Opportunities & Teaching Abroad, School Library Services, Scholarships, Financial Resources, Professional Consultants, Computer Software & Testing Resources and much more. Plus, this comprehensive directory also includes a section on Statistics and Rankings with over 100 tables, including statistics on Average Teacher Salaries, SAT/ACT scores, Revenues & Expenditures and more. These important statistics will allow the user to see how their school rates among others, make relocation decisions and so much more. For quick access to information, this directory contains four indexes: Entry & Publisher Index, Geographic Index, a Subject & Grade Index and Web Sites Index. *Educators Resource Directory* will be a well-used addition to the reference collection of any school district, education department or public library.

"Recommended for all collections that serve elementary and secondary school professionals." –Choice

1,000 pages; Softcover ISBN 1-59237-179-5, $145.00 ✦ Online Database $195.00 ✦ Online Database & Directory Combo $280.00

To preview any of our Directories Risk-Free for 30 days, call (800) 562-2139 or fax to (518) 789-0556

Grey House Publishing
Business Directories

The Directory of Business Information Resources, 2007

With 100% verification, over 1,000 new listings and more than 12,000 updates, this 2007 edition of *The Directory of Business Information Resources* is the most up-to-date source for contacts in over 98 business areas – from advertising and agriculture to utilities and wholesalers. This carefully researched volume details: the Associations representing each industry; the Newsletters that keep members current; the Magazines and Journals - with their "Special Issues" - that are important to the trade, the Conventions that are "must attends," Databases, Directories and Industry Web Sites that provide access to must-have marketing resources. Includes contact names, phone & fax numbers, web sites and e-mail addresses. This one-volume resource is a gold mine of information and would be a welcome addition to any reference collection.

"This is a most useful and easy-to-use addition to any researcher's library." –The Information Professionals Institute

2,500 pages; Softcover ISBN 1-59237-146-9, $195.00 ♦ Online Database $495.00

Nations of the World, 2007/08 A Political, Economic and Business Handbook

This completely revised edition covers all the nations of the world in an easy-to-use, single volume. Each nation is profiled in a single chapter that includes Key Facts, Political & Economic Issues, a Country Profile and Business Information. In this fast-changing world, it is extremely important to make sure that the most up-to-date information is included in your reference collection. This edition is just the answer. Each of the 200+ country chapters have been carefully reviewed by a political expert to make sure that the text reflects the most current information on Politics, Travel Advisories, Economics and more. You'll find such vital information as a Country Map, Population Characteristics, Inflation, Agricultural Production, Foreign Debt, Political History, Foreign Policy, Regional Insecurity, Economics, Trade & Tourism, Historical Profile, Political Systems, Ethnicity, Languages, Media, Climate, Hotels, Chambers of Commerce, Banking, Travel Information and more. Five Regional Chapters follow the main text and include a Regional Map, an Introductory Article, Key Indicators and Currencies for the Region. As an added bonus, an all-inclusive CD-ROM is available as a companion to the printed text. Noted for its sophisticated, up-to-date and reliable compilation of political, economic and business information, this brand new edition will be an important acquisition to any public, academic or special library reference collection.

"A useful addition to both general reference collections and business collections." –RUSQ

1,700 pages; Print Version Only Softcover ISBN 1-59237-177-9, $155.00

The Directory of Venture Capital & Private Equity Firms, 2007

This edition has been extensively updated and broadly expanded to offer direct access to over 2,800 Domestic and International Venture Capital Firms, including address, phone & fax numbers, e-mail addresses and web sites for both primary and branch locations. Entries include details on the firm's Mission Statement, Industry Group Preferences, Geographic Preferences, Average and Minimum Investments and Investment Criteria. You'll also find details that are available nowhere else, including the Firm's Portfolio Companies and extensive information on each of the firm's Managing Partners, such as Education, Professional Background and Directorships held, along with the Partner's E-mail Address. *The Directory of Venture Capital & Private Equity Firms* offers five important indexes: Geographic Index, Executive Name Index, Portfolio Company Index, Industry Preference Index and College & University Index. With its comprehensive coverage and detailed, extensive information on each company, *The Directory of Venture Capital & Private Equity Firms* is an important addition to any finance collection.

"The sheer number of listings, the descriptive information provided and the outstanding indexing make this directory a better value than its principal competitor, Pratt's Guide to Venture Capital Sources. Recommended for business collections in large public, academic and business libraries." –Choice

1,300 pages; Softcover ISBN 1-59237-176-0, $565.00/$450.00 Library ♦ Online Database (includes a free copy of the directory) $889.00

To preview any of our Directories Risk-Free for 30 days, call (800) 562-2139 or fax to (518) 789-0556

The Directory of Mail Order Catalogs, 2007

Published since 1981, the *Directory of Mail Order Catalogs* is the premier source of information on the mail order catalog industry. It is the source that business professionals and librarians have come to rely on for the thousands of catalog companies in the US. New for 2007, The Directory of Mail Order Catalogs has been combined with its companion volume, *The Directory of Business to Business Catalogs*, to offer all 13,000 catalog companies in one easy-to-use volume. Section I: Consumer Catalogs, covers over 9,000 consumer catalog companies in 44 different product chapters from Animals to Toys & Games. Section II: Business to Business Catalogs, details 5,000 business catalogs, everything from computers to laboratory supplies, building construction and much more. Listings contain detailed contact information including mailing address, phone & fax numbers, web sites, e-mail addresses and key contacts along with important business details such as product descriptions, employee size, years in business, sales volume, catalog size, number of catalogs mailed and more. Three indexes are included for easy access to information: Catalog & Company Name Index, Geographic Index and Product Index. *The Directory of Mail Order Catalogs*, now with its expanded business to business catalogs, is the largest and most comprehensive source covering this billion-dollar industry. It is the standard in its field. This important resource is a useful tool for entrepreneurs searching for catalogs to pick up their product, vendors looking to expand their customer base in the catalog industry, market researchers, small businesses investigating new supply vendors, along with the library patron who is exploring the available catalogs in their areas of interest.

"This is a godsend for those looking for information." –Reference Book Review

1,700 pages; Softcover ISBN 1-59237-156-6 $350.00/$250.00 Library ◆ Online Database (includes a free copy of the directory) $495.00

Sports Market Place Directory, 2007

For over 20 years, this comprehensive, up-to-date directory has offered direct access to the Who, What, When & Where of the Sports Industry. With over 20,000 updates and enhancements, the *Sports Market Place Directory* is the most detailed, comprehensive and current sports business reference source available. In 1,800 information-packed pages, *Sports Market Place Directory* profiles contact information and key executives for: Single Sport Organizations, Professional Leagues, Multi-Sport Organizations, Disabled Sports, High School & Youth Sports, Military Sports, Olympic Organizations, Media, Sponsors, Sponsorship & Marketing Event Agencies, Event & Meeting Calendars, Professional Services, College Sports, Manufacturers & Retailers, Facilities and much more. *The Sports Market Place Directory* provides organization's contact information with detailed descriptions including: Key Contacts, physical, mailing, email and web addresses plus phone and fax numbers. Plus, nine important indexes make sure that you can find the information you're looking for quickly and easily: Entry Index, Single Sport Index, Media Index, Sponsor Index, Agency Index, Manufacturers Index, Brand Name Index, Facilities Index and Executive/Geographic Index. For over twenty years, *The Sports Market Place Directory* has assisted thousands of individuals in their pursuit of a career in the sports industry. Why not use "THE SOURCE" that top recruiters, headhunters and career placement centers use to find information on or about sports organizations and key hiring contacts.

1,800 pages; Softcover ISBN 1-59237-189-2, $225.00 ◆ Online Database $479.00

Food and Beverage Market Place, 2007

Food and Beverage Market Place is bigger and better than ever with thousands of new companies, thousands of updates to existing companies and two revised and enhanced product category indexes. This comprehensive directory profiles over 18,000 Food & Beverage Manufacturers, 12,000 Equipment & Supply Companies, 2,200 Transportation & Warehouse Companies, 2,000 Brokers & Wholesalers, 8,000 Importers & Exporters, 900 Industry Resources and hundreds of Mail Order Catalogs. Listings include detailed contact Information, Sales Volumes, Key Contacts, Brand & Product Information, Packaging Details and much more. *Thomas Food and Beverage Market Place* is available as a three-volume printed set, a subscription-based Online Database via the Internet, on CD-ROM, as well as mailing lists and a licensable database.

"An essential purchase for those in the food industry but will also be useful in public libraries where needed. Much of the information will be difficult and time consuming to locate without this handy three-volume ready-reference source." –ARBA

8,500 pages, 3 Volume Set; Softcover ISBN 1-59237-152-3, $595.00 ◆ Online Database $795.00 ◆ Online Database & 3 Volume Set Combo, $995.00

To preview any of our Directories Risk-Free for 30 days, call (800) 562-2139 or fax to (518) 789-0556

The Grey House Homeland Security Directory, 2007

This updated edition features the latest contact information for government and private organizations involved with Homeland Security along with the latest product information and provides detailed profiles of nearly 1,000 Federal & State Organizations & Agencies and over 3,000 Officials and Key Executives involved with Homeland Security. These listings are incredibly detailed and include Mailing Address, Phone & Fax Numbers, Email Addresses & Web Sites, a complete Description of the Agency and a complete list of the Officials and Key Executives associated with the Agency. Next, *The Grey House Homeland Security Directory* provides the go-to source for Homeland Security Products & Services. This section features over 2,000 Companies that provide Consulting, Products or Services. With this Buyer's Guide at their fingertips, users can locate suppliers of everything from Training Materials to Access Controls, from Perimeter Security to BioTerrorism Countermeasures and everything in between – complete with contact information and product descriptions. A handy Product Locator Index is provided to quickly and easily locate suppliers of a particular product. Lastly, an Information Resources Section provides immediate access to contact information for hundreds of Associations, Newsletters, Magazines, Trade Shows, Databases and Directories that focus on Homeland Security. This comprehensive, information-packed resource will be a welcome tool for any company or agency that is in need of Homeland Security information and will be a necessary acquisition for the reference collection of all public libraries and large school districts.

"Compiles this information in one place and is discerning in content. A useful purchase for public and academic libraries." –Booklis

800 pages; Softcover ISBN 1-59237-151-5, $195.00 ◆ Online Database (includes a free copy of the directory) $385.00

The Grey House Transportation Security Directory & Handbook

This brand new title is the only reference of its kind that brings together current data on Transportation Security. With information on everything from Regulatory Authorities to Security Equipment, this top-flight database brings together the relevant information necessary for creating and maintaining a security plan for a wide range of transportation facilities. With this current, comprehensive directory at the ready you'll have immediate access to: Regulatory Authorities & Legislation; Information Resources; Sample Security Plans & Checklists; Contact Data for Major Airports, Seaports, Railroads, Trucking Companies and Oil Pipelines; Security Service Providers; Recommended Equipment & Product Information and more. Using the *Grey House Transportation Security Directory & Handbook*, managers will be able to quickly and easily assess their current security plans; develop contacts to create and maintain new security procedures; and source the products and services necessary to adequately maintain a secure environment. This valuable resource is a must for all Security Managers at Airports, Seaports, Railroads, Trucking Companies and Oil Pipelines.

800 pages; Softcover ISBN 1-59237-075-6, $195

The Grey House Safety & Security Directory, 2007

The Grey House Safety & Security Directory is the most comprehensive reference tool and buyer's guide for the safety and security industry. Arranged by safety topic, each chapter begins with OSHA regulations for the topic, followed by Training Articles written by top professionals in the field and Self-Inspection Checklists. Next, each topic contains Buyer's Guide sections that feature related products and services. Topics include Administration, Insurance, Loss Control & Consulting, Protective Equipment & Apparel, Noise & Vibration, Facilities Monitoring & Maintenance, Employee Health Maintenance & Ergonomics, Retail Food Services, Machine Guards, Process Guidelines & Tool Handling, Ordinary Materials Handling, Hazardous Materials Handling, Workplace Preparation & Maintenance, Electrical Lighting & Safety, Fire & Rescue and Security. The Buyer's Guide sections are carefully indexed within each topic area to ensure that you can find the supplies needed to meet OSHA's regulations. Six important indexes make finding information and product manufacturers quick and easy: Geographical Index of Manufacturers and Distributors, Company Profile Index, Brand Name Index, Product Index, Index of Web Sites and Index of Advertisers. This comprehensive, up-to-date reference will provide every tool necessary to make sure a business is in compliance with OSHA regulations and locate the products and services needed to meet those regulations.

"Presents industrial safety information for engineers, plant managers, risk managers, and construction site supervisors…" –Choi

1,500 pages, 2 Volume Set; Softcover ISBN 1-59237-160-4, $225.00

The Grey House Biometric Information Directory

The Biometric Information Directory is the only comprehensive source for current biometric industry information. This 2006 edition is the first published by Grey House. With 100% updated information, this latest edition offers a complete, current look, in both print and online form, of biometric companies and products – one of the fastest growing industries in today's economy. Detailed profiles of manufacturers of the latest biometric technology, including Finger, Voice, Face, Hand, Signature, Iris, Vein and Palm Identification systems. Data on the companies include key executives, company size and a detailed, indexed description of their product line. Plus, the Directory also includes valuable business resources, and current editorial make this edition the easiest way for the business community and consumers alike to access the largest, most current compilation of biometric industry information available on the market today. The new edition boasts increased numbers of companies, contact names and company data, with over 700 manufacturers and service providers. Information in the directory includes: Editorial on Advancements in Biometrics; Profiles of 700+ companies listed with contact information; Organizations, Trade & Educational Associations, Publications, Conferences, Trade Shows and Expositions Worldwide; Web Site Index; Biometric & Vendors Services Index by Types of Biometrics; and a Glossary of Biometric Terms. This resource will be an important source for anyone who is considering the use of a biometric product, investing in the development of biometric technology, support existing marketing and sales efforts and will be an important acquisition for the business reference collection for large public and business libraries.

00 pages; Softcover ISBN 1-59237-121-3, $225

The Rauch Guide to the US Adhesives & Sealants, Cosmetics & Toiletries, Ink, Paint, Plastics, Pulp & Paper and Rubber Industries

The Rauch Guides are known worldwide for their comprehensive marketing information. Acquired by Grey House Publishing in 2005, new updated and revised editions will be published throughout 2005 and 2006. Each Guide provides market facts and figures in a highly organized format, ideal for today's busy personnel, serving as ready-references for top executives as well as the industry newcomer. *The Rauch Guides* save time and money by organizing widely scattered information and providing estimates for important business decisions, some of which are available nowhere else. Each Guide is organized into several information-packed chapters. After a brief introduction, the ECONOMICS section provides data on industry shipments; long-term growth and forecasts; prices; company performance; employment, expenditures, and productivity; transportation and geographical patterns; packaging; foreign trade; and government regulations. Next, TECHNOLOGY & RAW MATERIALS provide market, technical, and raw material information for chemicals, equipment and related materials, including market size and leading suppliers, prices, end uses, and trends. PRODUCTS & MARKETS provide information for each major industry product, including market size and historical trends, leading suppliers, five-year forecasts, industry structure, and major end uses. For easy access, each *Guide* contains a chapter on INDUSTRY ACTIVITIES, ORGANIZATIONS & SOURCES OF INFORMATION with detailed information on meetings, exhibits, and trade shows, sources of statistical information, trade associations, technical and professional societies, and trade and technical periodicals. Next, the COMPANY DIRECTORY profiles major industry companies, both public and private. Generally several hundred companies are analyzed. Information includes complete contact information, web address, estimated total and domestic sales, product description, and recent mergers and acquisitions. Each Guide also contains several APPENDICES that provide a cross-reference of suppliers, subsidiaries and divisions. The Rauch Guides will prove to be an invaluable source of market information, company data, trends and forecasts that anyone in these fast-paced industries.

The Rauch Guide to the U.S. Paint Industry Softcover ISBN 1-59237-127-2 $595 ◆ The Rauch Guide to the U.S. Plastics Industry Softcover ISBN 1-59237-128-0 $595 ◆ The Rauch Guide to the U.S. Adhesives and Sealants Industry Softcover ISBN 1-59237-129-9 $595 ◆ The Rauch Guide to the U.S. Ink Industry Softcover ISBN 1-59237-126-4 $595 ◆ The Rauch Guide to the U.S. Rubber Industry Softcover ISBN 1-59237-130-2 $595 ◆ The Rauch Guide to the U.S. Pulp and Paper Industry Softcover ISBN 1-59237-131-0 $595 ◆ The Rauch Guide to the U.S. Cosmetic and Toiletries Industry Softcover ISBN 1-59237-132-9 $895

The Grey House Performing Arts Directory, 2007

The Grey House Performing Arts Directory is the most comprehensive resource covering the Performing Arts. This important directory provides current information on over 8,500 Dance Companies, Instrumental Music Programs, Opera Companies, Choral Groups, Theater Companies, Performing Arts Series and Performing Arts Facilities. Plus, this edition now contains a brand new section on Artist Management Groups. In addition to mailing address, phone & fax numbers, e-mail addresses and web sites, dozens of other fields of available information include mission statement, key contacts, facilities, seating capacity, season, attendance and more. This directory also provides an important Information Resources section that covers hundreds of Performing Arts Associations, Magazines, Newsletters, Trade Shows, Directories, Databases and Industry Web Sites. Five indexes provide immediate access to this wealth of information: Entry Name, Executive Name, Performance Facilities, Geographic and Information Resources. *The Grey House Performing Arts Directory* pulls together thousands of Performing Arts Organizations, Facilities and Information Resources into an easy-to-use source – this kind of comprehensiveness and extensive detail is not available in any resource on the market place today.

"Immensely useful and user-friendly ... recommended for public, academic and certain special library reference collections." –Booklist

500 pages; Softcover ISBN 1-59237-138-8, $185.00 ◆ Online Database $335.00

To preview any of our Directories Risk-Free for 30 days, call (800) 562-2139 or fax to (518) 789-0556

New York State Directory, 2007/08

The New York State Directory, published annually since 1983, is a comprehensive and easy-to-use guide to accessing public officials and private sector organizations and individuals who influence public policy in the state of New York. *The New York State Directory* include important information on all New York state legislators and congressional representatives, including biographies and key committee assignments. It also includes staff rosters for all branches of New York state government and for federal agencies and departments that impact the state policy process. Following the state government section are 25 chapters covering policy areas from agriculture through veterans' affairs. Each chapter identifies the state, local and federal agencies and officials that formulate or implement policy. In addition, each chapter contains a roster of private sector experts and advocates who influence the policy process. The directory also offers appendices that include statewide party officials; chambers of commerce; lobbying organizations; public and private universities and colleges; television, radio and print media; and local government agencies and officials.

New York State Directory - 800 pages; Softcover ISBN 1-59237-190-6; $145.00
New York State Directory with Profiles of New York – 2 volumes; 1,600 pages; Softcover ISBN 1-59237-191-4; $225

Profiles of New York ✦ Profiles of Florida ✦ Profiles of Texas ✦ Profiles of Illinois ✦ Profiles of Michigan ✦ Profiles of Ohio ✦ Profiles of New Jersey ✦ Profiles of Massachusetts ✦ Profiles of Pennsylvania ✦ Profiles of Wisconsin ✦ Profiles of Connecticut ✦ Profiles of Indiana ✦ Profiles of North Carolina ✦ Profiles of Virginia ✦ Profiles of California

Packed with over 50 pieces of data that make up a complete, user-friendly profile of each state, these directories go even further by then pulling selected data and providing it in ranking list form for even easier comparisons between the 100 largest towns and cities! The careful layout gives the user an easy-to-read snapshot of every single place and county in the state, from the biggest metropolis to the smallest unincorporated hamlet. The richness of each place or county profile is astounding in its depth, from history to weather, all packed in an easy-to-navigate, compact format. No need for piles of multiple sources with this volume on your desk. Here is a look at just a few of the data sets you'll find in each profile: History, Geography, Climate, Population, Vital Statistics, Economy, Income, Taxes Education, Housing, Health & Environment, Public Safety, Newspapers, Transportation, Presidential Election Results, Information Contacts and Chambers of Commerce. As an added bonus, there is a section on Selected Statistics, where data from the 100 largest towns and cities is arranged into easy-to-use charts. Each of 22 different data points has its own two-page spread with the cities listed in alpha order so researchers can easily compare and rank cities. A remarkable compilation that offers overviews and insights into each corner of the state, *Profiles of New York, Profiles of Florida* and *Profiles of Texas* go beyond Census statistics, beyond metro area coverage, beyond the 100 best places to live. Drawn from official census information, other government statistics and original research, you will have at your fingertips data that's available nowhere else in one single source. Data will be published on additional states in 2006 and 2007.

Each Profiles of... title ranges from 400-800 pages, priced at $149.00 each

Research Services Directory: Commercial & Corporate Research Centers

This Ninth Edition provides access to well over 8,000 independent Commercial Research Firms, Corporate Research Centers and Laboratories offering contract services for hands-on, basic or applied research. *Research Services Directory* covers the thousands of types of research companies, including Biotechnology & Pharmaceutical Developers, Consumer Product Research, Defense Contractors, Electronics & Software Engineers, Think Tanks, Forensic Investigators, Independent Commercial Laboratories, Information Brokers, Market & Survey Research Companies, Medical Diagnostic Facilities, Product Research & Development Firms and more. Each entry provides the company's name, mailing address, phone & fax numbers, key contacts, web site, e-mail address, as well as a company description and research and technical fields served. Four indexes provide immediate access to this wealth of information: Research Firms Index, Geographic Index, Personnel Name Index and Subject Index.

"An important source for organizations in need of information about laboratories, individuals and other facilities." –ARB

1,400 pages; Softcover ISBN 1-59237-003-9, $395.00 ✦ Online Database (includes a free copy of the directory) $850.00

International Business and Trade Directories

Completely updated, the Third Edition of *International Business and Trade Directories* now contains more than 10,000 entries, over 2,000 more than the last edition, making this directory the most comprehensive resource of the worlds business and trade directories. Entrie include content descriptions, price, publisher's name and address, web site and e-mail addresses, phone and fax numbers and editorial staff. Organized by industry group, and then by region, this resource puts over 10,000 industry-specific business and trade directories at the reader's fingertips. Three indexes are included for quick access to information: Geographic Index, Publisher Index and Title Index. Public, college and corporate libraries, as well as individuals and corporations seeking critical market information will want to add this directory to their marketing collection.

"Reasonably priced for a work of this type, this directory should appeal to larger academi public and corporate libraries with an international focus." –Library Journ

1,800 pages; Softcover ISBN 1-930956-63-0, $225.00 ✦ Online Database (includes a free copy of the directory) $450.00

To preview any of our Directories Risk-Free for 30 days, call (800) 562-2139 or fax to (518) 789-0556

Grey House Publishing Canada
Canadian Information Resources

Canadian Almanac & Directory, 2007

The Canadian Almanac & Directory contains ten directories in one – giving you all the facts and figures you will ever need about Canada. No other single source provides users with the quality and depth of up-to-date information for all types of research. This national directory and guide gives you access to statistics, images and over 45,000 names and addresses for everything from Airlines to zoos - updated every year. It's Ten Directories in One! Each section is a directory in itself, providing robust information on business and finance, communications, government, associations, arts and culture (museums, zoos, libraries, etc.), health, transportation, law, education, and more. Government information includes federal, provincial and territorial - and includes an easy-to-use quick index to find key information. A separate municipal government section includes every municipality in Canada, with full profiles of Canada's largest urban centers. A complete legal directory lists judges and judicial officials, court locations and law firms across the country. A wealth of general information, the Canadian Almanac & Directory also includes national statistics on population, employment, imports and exports, and more. National awards and honors are presented, along with forms of address, Commonwealth information and full color photos of Canadian symbols. Postal information, weights, measures, distances and other useful charts are also incorporated. Complete almanac information includes perpetual calendars, five-year holiday planners and astronomical information. Published continuously for 160 years, The Canadian Almanac & Directory is the best single reference source for business executives, managers and assistants; government and public affairs executives; lawyers; marketing, sales and advertising executives; researchers, editors and journalists.

Hardcover ISBN 978-1-89502-149-3; 1,600 pages; $315.00

Associations Canada, 2007

The Most Powerful Fact-Finder to Business, Trade, Professional and Consumer Organizations
Associations Canada covers Canadian organizations and international groups including industry, commercial and professional associations, registered charities, special interest and common interest organizations. This annually revised compendium provides detailed listings and abstracts for nearly 20,000 regional, national and international organizations. This popular volume provides the most comprehensive picture of Canada's non-profit sector. Detailed listings enable users to identify an organization's budget, founding date, scope of activity, licensing body, sources of funding, executive information, full address and complete contact information, just to name a few. Powerful indexes help researchers find information quickly and easily. The following indexes are included: subject, acronym, geographic, budget, executive name, conferences & conventions, mailing list, defunct and unreachable associations and registered charitable organizations. In addition to annual spending of over $1 billion on transportation and conventions alone, Canadian associations account for many millions more in pursuit of membership interests. Associations Canada provides complete access to this highly lucrative market. Associations Canada is a strong source of prospects for sales and marketing executives, tourism and convention officials, researchers, government officials - anyone who wants to locate non-profit interest groups and trade associations.

Hardcover ISBN 978-1-59237-219-5; 1,600 pages; $315.00

Financial Services Canada, 2007/08

Financial Services Canada is the only master file of current contacts and information that serves the needs of the entire financial services industry in Canada. With over 18,000 organizations and hard-to-find business information, Financial Services Canada is the most up-to-date source for names and contact numbers of industry professionals, senior executives, portfolio managers, financial advisors, agency bureaucrats and elected representatives. Financial Services Canada incorporates the latest changes in the industry to provide you with the most current details on each company, including: name, title, organization, telephone and fax numbers, e-mail and web addresses. Financial Services Canada also includes private company listings never before compiled, government agencies, association and consultant services - to ensure that you'll never miss a client or a contact. Current listings include: banks and branches, non-depository institutions, stock exchanges and brokers, investment management firms, insurance companies, major accounting and law firms, government agencies and financial associations. Powerful indexes assist researchers with locating the vital financial information they need. The following indexes are included: alphabetic, geographic, executive name, corporate web site/e-mail, government quick reference and subject. Financial Services Canada is a valuable resource for financial executives, bankers, financial planners, sales and marketing professionals, lawyers and chartered accountants, government officials, investment dealers, journalists, librarians and reference specialists.

00 pages; Hardcover ISBN 978-1-59237-221-8 $315.00

To preview any of our Directories Risk-Free for 30 days, call (800) 562-2139 or fax to (518) 789-0556

Directory of Libraries in Canada, 2007/08

The Directory of Libraries in Canada brings together almost 7,000 listings including libraries and their branches, information resource centers, archives and library associations and learning centers. The directory offers complete and comprehensive information on Canadian libraries, resource centers, business information centers, professional associations, regional library systems, archives, library schools and library technical programs. The Directory of Libraries in Canada includes important features of each library and service, including library information; personnel details, including contact names and e-mail addresses; collection information; services available to users; acquisitions budgets; and computers and automated systems. Useful information on each library's electronic access is also included, such as Internet browser, connectivity and public Internet/CD-ROM/subscription database access. The directory also provides powerful indexes for subject, location, personal name and Web site/e-mail to assist researchers with locating the crucial information they need. The Directory of Libraries in Canada is a vital reference tool for publishers, advocacy groups, students, research institutions, computer hardware suppliers, and other diverse groups that provide products and services to this unique market.

850 pages; Hardcover ISBN 978-1-59237-222-5; $315.00

Canadian Environmental Directory, 2007/08

The Canadian Environmental Directory is Canada's most complete and only national listing of environmental associations and organizations, government regulators and purchasing groups, product and service companies, special libraries, and more! The extensive Products and Services section provides detailed listings enabling users to identify the company name, address, phone, fax, e-mail, Web address, firm type, contact names (and titles), product and service information, affiliations, trade information, branch and affiliate data. The Government section gives you all the contact information you need at every government level – federal, provincial and municipal. We also include descriptions of current environmental initiatives, programs and agreements, names of environment-related acts administered by each ministry or department PLUS information and tips on who to contact and how to sell to governments in Canada. The Associations section provides complete contact information and a brief description of activities. Included are Canadian environmental organizations and international groups including industry, commercial and professional associations, registered charities, special interest and common interest organizations. All the Information you need about the Canadian environmental industry directory of products and services, special libraries and resource, conferences, seminars and tradeshows, chronology of environmental events, law firms and major Canadian companies, The Canadian Environmental Directory is ideal for business, government, engineers and anyone conducting research on the environment.

Hardcover ISBN 978-1-59237-218-8; 900 pages; $315.00

Grey House Publishing
General Reference Titles

he Value of a Dollar 1600-1859, The Colonial Era to The Civil War

llowing the format of the widely acclaimed, T*he Value of a Dollar, 1860-2004, The Value of a Dollar 1600-1859, The Colonial Era to The il War* records the actual prices of thousands of items that consumers purchased from the Colonial Era to the Civil War. Our torial department had been flooded with requests from users of our Value of a Dollar for the same type of information, just from an lier time period. This new volume is just the answer – with pricing data from 1600 to 1859. Arranged into five-year chapters, each ear chapter includes a Historical Snapshot, Consumer Expenditures, Investments, Selected Income, Income/Standard Jobs, Food sket, Standard Prices and Miscellany. There is also a section on Trends. This informative section charts the change in price over e and provides added detail on the reasons prices changed within the time period, including industry developments, changes in sumer attitudes and important historical facts. This fascinating survey will serve a wide range of research needs and will be useful in high school, public and academic library reference collections.

 pages; Hardcover ISBN 1-59237-094-2, $135.00

he Value of a Dollar 1860-2004, Third Edition

guide to practical economy, *The Value of a Dollar* records the actual prices of thousands of items that consumers purchased from the il War to the present, along with facts about investment options and income opportunities. This brand new Third Edition boasts a nd new addition to each five-year chapter, a section on Trends. This informative section charts the change in price over time and ovides added detail on the reasons prices changed within the time period, including industry developments, changes in consumer itudes and important historical facts. Plus, a brand new chapter for 2000-2004 has been added. Each 5-year chapter includes a storical Snapshot, Consumer Expenditures, Investments, Selected Income, Income/Standard Jobs, Food Basket, Standard Prices and scellany. This interesting and useful publication will be widely used in any reference collection.

"Recommended for high school, college and public libraries." –ARBA

 pages; Hardcover ISBN 1-59237-074-8, $135.00

orking Americans 1880-1999
lume I: The Working Class, Volume II: The Middle Class, Volume III: The Upper Class

ch of the volumes in the *Working Americans 1880-1999* series focuses on a particular class of Americans, The Working Class, The ddle Class and The Upper Class over the last 120 years. Chapters in each volume focus on one decade and profile three to five nilies. Family Profiles include real data on Income & Job Descriptions, Selected Prices of the Times, Annual Income, Annual dgets, Family Finances, Life at Work, Life at Home, Life in the Community, Working Conditions, Cost of Living, Amusements and ch more. Each chapter also contains an Economic Profile with Average Wages of other Professions, a selection of Typical Pricing, y Events & Inventions, News Profiles, Articles from Local Media and Illustrations. The *Working Americans* series captures the estyles of each of the classes from the last twelve decades, covers a vast array of occupations and ethnic backgrounds and travels the tire nation. These interesting and useful compilations of portraits of the American Working, Middle and Upper Classes during the t 120 years will be an important addition to any high school, public or academic library reference collection.

"These interesting, unique compilations of economic and social facts, figures and graphs will support multiple research needs. They will engage and enlighten patrons in high school, public and academic library collections." –Booklist

lume I: The Working Class ◆ 558 pages; Hardcover ISBN 1-891482-81-5, $145.00 ◆ Volume II: The Middle Class ◆ 591 pages; rdcover ISBN 1-891482-72-6; $145.00 ◆ Volume III: The Upper Class ◆ 567 pages; Hardcover ISBN 1-930956-38-X, $145.00

orking Americans 1880-1999 Volume IV: Their Children

is Fourth Volume in the highly successful *Working Americans 1880-1999* series focuses on American children, decade by decade from 80 to 1999. This interesting and useful volume introduces the reader to three children in each decade, one from each of the Working, iddle and Upper classes. Like the first three volumes in the series, the individual profiles are created from interviews, diaries, atistical studies, biographies and news reports. Profiles cover a broad range of ethnic backgrounds, geographic area and lifestyles – erything from an orphan in Memphis in 1882, following the Yellow Fever epidemic of 1878 to an eleven-year-old nephew of a beer ron and owner of the New York Yankees in New York City in 1921. Chapters also contain important supplementary materials cluding News Features as well as information on everything from Schools to Parks, Infectious Diseases to Childhood Fears along th Entertainment, Family Life and much more to provide an informative overview of the lifestyles of children from each decade. is interesting account of what life was like for Children in the Working, Middle and Upper Classes will be a welcome addition to the ference collection of any high school, public or academic library.

0 pages; Hardcover ISBN 1-930956-35-5, $145.00

To preview any of our Directories Risk-Free for 30 days, call (800) 562-2139 or fax to (518) 789-0556

Working Americans 1880-2003 Volume V: Americans At War

Working Americans 1880-2003 Volume V: Americans At War is divided into 11 chapters, each covering a decade from 1880-2003 and examines the lives of Americans during the time of war, including declared conflicts, one-time military actions, protests, and preparations for war. Each decade includes several personal profiles, whether on the battlefield or on the homefront, that tell the storie of civilians, soldiers, and officers during the decade. The profiles examine: Life at Home; Life at Work; and Life in the Community. Each decade also includes an Economic Profile with statistical comparisons, a Historical Snapshot, News Profiles, local News Articles, and Illustrations that provide a solid historical background to the decade being examined. Profiles range widely not only geographically, but also emotionally, from that of a girl whose leg was torn off in a blast during WWI, to the boredom of being stationed in the Dakotas as the Indian Wars were drawing to a close. As in previous volumes of the *Working Americans* series, information is presented in narrative form, but hard facts and real-life situations back up each story. The basis of the profiles come from diaries, private print books, personal interviews, family histories, estate documents and magazine articles. For easy reference, *Working Americans 1880-2003 Volume V: Americans At War* includes an in-depth Subject Index. The *Working Americans* series has become an important reference for public libraries, academic libraries and high school libraries. This fifth volume will be a welcome addition to all of these types of reference collections.

600 pages; Hardcover ISBN 1-59237-024-1; $145.00
Five Volume Set (Volumes I-V), Hardcover ISBN 1-59237-034-9, $675.00

Working Americans 1880-2005 Volume VI: Women at Work

Unlike any other volume in the *Working Americans* series, this Sixth Volume, is the first to focus on a particular gender of Americans. *Volume VI: Women at Work*, traces what life was like for working women from the 1860's to the present time. Beginning with the life of a maid in 1890 and a store clerk in 1900 and ending with the life and times of the modern working women, this text captures the struggle, strengths and changing perception of the American woman at work. Each chapter focuses on one decade and profiles three to five women with real data on Income & Job Descriptions, Selected Prices of the Times, Annual Income, Annual Budgets, Family Finances, Life at Work, Life at Home, Life in the Community, Working Conditions, Cost of Living, Amusements and much more. For even broader access to the events, economics and attitude towards women throughout the past 130 years, each chapter is supplemented with News Profiles, Articles from Local Media, Illustrations, Economic Profiles, Typical Pricing, Key Events, Inventions and more. This important volume illustrates what life was like for working women over time and allows the reader to develop an understanding of the changing role of women at work. These interesting and useful compilations of portraits of women at work will be an important addition to any high school public or academic library reference collection.

600 pages; Hardcover ISBN 1-59237-063-2; $145.00

Working Americans 1880-2005 Volume VII: Social Movements

The newest addition to the widely-successful *Working Americans* series, *Volume VII: Social Movements* explores how Americans sought and fought for change from the 1880s to the present time. Following the format of previous volumes in the Working Americans series, the tex examines the lives of 34 individuals who have worked — often behind the scenes — to bring about change. Issues include topics as diverse as the Anti-smoking movement of 1901 to efforts by Native Americans to reassert their long lost rights. Along the way, the book will profile individuals brave enough to demand suffrage for Kansas women in 1912 or demand an end to lynching during a March on Washington in 1923. Each profile is enriched with real data on Income & Job Descriptions, Selected Prices of the Times, Annual Incomes & Budgets, Life at Work, Life at Home, Life in the Community, along with News Features, Key Events, and Illustrations. The depth of information contained in each profile allow the user to explore the private, financial and public lives of these subjects, deepening our understanding of how calls for change took place in our society. A must-purchase for the reference collections of high school libraries, public libraries and academic libraries.

600 pages; Hardcover ISBN 1-59237-101-9; $145.00
Seven Volume Set (Volumes I-VII), Hardcover ISBN 1-59237-133-7, $945.00

The Encyclopedia of Warrior Peoples & Fighting Groups

Many military groups throughout the world have excelled in their craft either by fortuitous circumstances, outstanding leadership, or intense training. This new second edition of The Encyclopedia of Warrior Peoples and Fighting Groups explores the origins and leadership of these outstanding combat forces, chronicles their conquests and accomplishments, examines the circumstances surrounding their decline or disbanding, and assesses their influence on the groups and methods of warfare that followed. This edition has been completely updated with information through 2005 and contains over 20 new entries. Readers will encounter ferocious tribes charismatic leaders, and daring militias, from ancient times to the present, including Amazons, Buffalo Soldiers, Green Berets, Iron Brigade, Kamikazes, Peoples of the Sea, Polish Winged Hussars, Sacred Band of Thebes, Teutonic Knights, and Texas Rangers. With over 100 alphabetical entries, numerous cross-references and illustrations, a comprehensive bibliography, and index, the Encyclopedia of Warrior Peoples and Fighting Groups is a valuable resource for readers seeking insight into the bold history of distinguished fighting forces.

"This work is especially useful for high school students, undergraduates, and gener.
readers with an interest in military history." –Library Journ

Pub. Date: May 2006; Hardcover ISBN 1-59237-116-7; $135.00

To preview any of our Directories Risk-Free for 30 days, call (800) 562-2139 or fax to (518) 789-0556

The Encyclopedia of Invasions & Conquests, From the Ancient Times to the Present

Throughout history, invasions and conquests have played a remarkable role in shaping our world and defining our boundaries, both physically and culturally. This second edition of the popular Encyclopedia of Invasions & Conquests, a comprehensive guide to over [?] invasions, conquests, battles and occupations from ancient times to the present, takes readers on a journey that includes the Roman conquest of Britain, the Portuguese colonization of Brazil, and the Iraqi invasion of Kuwait, to name a few. New articles will explore the late 20th and 21st centuries, with a specific focus on recent conflicts in Afghanistan, Kuwait, Iraq, Yugoslavia, Grenada and Chechnya. Categories of entries include countries, invasions and conquests, and individuals. In addition to covering the military aspects of invasions and conquests, entries cover some of the political, economic, and cultural aspects, for example, the effects of a conquest on the invade country's political and monetary system and in its language and religion. The entries on leaders – among them Sargon, Alexander the Great, William the Conqueror, and Adolf Hitler – deal with the people who sought to gain control, expand power, or exert religious or political influence over others through military means. Revised and updated for this second edition, entries are arranged alphabetically within historical periods. Each chapter provides a map to help readers locate key areas and geographical features, and bibliographical references appear at the end of each entry. Other useful features include cross-references, a cumulative bibliography and a comprehensive subject index. This authoritative, well-organized, lucidly written volume will prove invaluable for a variety of readers, including high school students, military historians, members of the armed forces, history buffs and hobbyists.

> *"Engaging writing, sensible organization, nice illustrations, interesting and obscure facts, and useful maps make this book a pleasure to read." –ARBA*

Pub. Date: March 2006; Hardcover ISBN 1-59237-114-0; $135.00

Encyclopedia of Prisoners of War & Internment

This authoritative second edition provides a valuable overview of the history of prisoners of war and interned civilians, from earliest times to the present. Written by an international team of experts in the field of POW studies, this fascinating and thought-provoking volume includes entries on a wide range of subjects including the Crusades, Plains Indian Warfare, concentration camps, the two world wars, and famous POWs throughout history, as well as atrocities, escapes, and much more. Written in a clear and easily understandable style, this informative reference details over 350 entries, 30% larger than the first edition, that survey the history of prisoners of war and interned civilians from the earliest times to the present, with emphasis on the 19th and 20th centuries. Medical conditions, international law, exchanges of prisoners, organizations working on behalf of POWs, and trials associated with the treatment of captives are just some of the themes explored. Entries range from the Ardeatine Caves Massacre to Kurt Vonnegut. Entries are arranged alphabetically, plus illustrations and maps are provided for easy reference. The text also includes an introduction, bibliography, appendix of selected documents, and end-of-entry reading suggestions. This one-of-a-kind reference will be a helpful addition to the reference collections of all public libraries, high schools, and university libraries and will prove invaluable to historians and military enthusiasts.

> *"Thorough and detailed yet accessible to the lay reader. Of special interest to subject specialists and historians; recommended for public and academic libraries." - Library Journal*

Pub. Date: March 2006; Hardcover ISBN 1-59237-120-5; $135.00

The Religious Right, A Reference Handbook

Timely and unbiased, this third edition updates and expands its examination of the religious right and its influence on our government, citizens, society, and politics. From the fight to outlaw the teaching of Darwin's theory of evolution to the struggle to outlaw abortion, the religious right is continually exerting an influence on public policy. This text explores the influence of religion on legislation and society, while examining the alignment of the religious right with the political right. A historical survey of the movement highlights the shift to "hands-on" approach to politics and the struggle to present a unified front. The coverage offers a critical historical survey of the religious right movement, focusing on its increased involvement in the political arena, attempts to forge coalitions, and notable successes and failures. The text offers complete coverage of biographies of the men and women who have advanced the cause and an up to date chronology illuminate the movement's goals, including their accomplishments and failures. This edition offers an extensive update to all sections along with several brand new entries. Two new sections complement this third edition, a chapter on legal issues and court decisions and a chapter on demographic statistics and electoral patterns. To aid in further research, The Religious Right, offers an entire section of annotated listings of print and non-print resources, as well as of organizations affiliated with the religious right, and those opposing it. Comprehensive in its scope, this work offers easy-to-read, pertinent information for those seeking to understand the religious right and its evolving role in American society. A must for libraries of all sizes, university religion departments, activists, high schools and for those interested in the evolving role of the religious right.

> *" Recommended for all public and academic libraries." - Library Journal*

Pub. Date: November 2006; Hardcover ISBN 1-59237-113-2; $135.00

To preview any of our Directories Risk-Free for 30 days, call (800) 562-2139 or fax to (518) 789-0556

From Suffrage to the Senate, America's Political Women

From Suffrage to the Senate is a comprehensive and valuable compendium of biographies of leading women in U.S. politics, past and present, and an examination of the wide range of women's movements. Up to date through 2006, this dynamically illustrated reference work explores American women's path to political power and social equality from the struggle for the right to vote and the abolition of slavery to the first African American woman in the U.S. Senate and beyond. This new edition includes over 150 new entries and a brand new section on trends and demographics of women in politics. The in-depth coverage also traces the political heritage of the abolition, labor, suffrage, temperance, and reproductive rights movements. The alphabetically arranged entries include biographies of every woman from across the political spectrum who has served in the U.S. House and Senate, along with women in the Judiciary and the U.S. Cabinet and, new to this edition, biographies of activists and political consultants. Bibliographical references follow each entry. For easy reference, a handy chronology is provided detailing 150 years of women's history. This up-to-date reference will be a must-purchase for women's studies departments, high schools and public libraries and will be a handy resource for those researching the key players in women's politics, past and present.

"An engaging tool that would be useful in high school, public, and academic libraries looking for an overview of the political history of women in the US." –Booklist

Pub. Date: October 2006; Two Volume Set; Hardcover ISBN 1-59237-117-5; $195.00

An African Biographical Dictionary

This landmark second edition is the only biographical dictionary to bring together, in one volume, cultural, social and political leaders – both historical and contemporary – of the sub-Saharan region. Over 800 biographical sketches of prominent Africans, as well as foreigners who have affected the continent's history, are featured, 150 more than the previous edition. The wide spectrum of leaders includes religious figures, writers, politicians, scientists, entertainers, sports personalities and more. Access to these fascinating individuals is provided in a user-friendly format. The biographies are arranged alphabetically, cross-referenced and indexed. Entries include the country or countries in which the person was significant and the commonly accepted dates of birth and death. Each biographical sketch is chronologically written; entries for cultural personalities add an evaluation of their work. This information is followed by a selection of references often found in university and public libraries, including autobiographies and principal biographical works. Appendixes list each individual by country and by field of accomplishment – rulers, musicians, explorers, missionaries, businessmen, physicists – nearly thirty categories in all. Another convenient appendix lists heads of state since independence by country. Up-to-date and representative of African societies as a whole, An African Biographical Dictionary provides a wealth of vital information for students of African culture and is an indispensable reference guide for anyone interested in African affairs.

"An unquestionable convenience to have these concise, informative biographies gathered into one source, indexed, and analyzed by appendixes listing entrants by nation and occupational field." –Wilson Library Bulletin

Pub. Date: July 2006; Hardcover ISBN 1-59237-112-4; $125.00

American Environmental Leaders, From Colonial Times to the Present

A comprehensive and diverse award winning collection of biographies of the most important figures in American environmentalism. Few subjects arouse the passions the way the environment does. How will we feed an ever-increasing population and how can that food be made safe for consumption? Who decides how land is developed? How can environmental policies be made fair for everyone, including multiethnic groups, women, children, and the poor? American Environmental Leaders presents more than 350 biographies of men and women who have devoted their lives to studying, debating, and organizing these and other controversial issues over the last 200 years. In addition to the scientists who have analyzed how human actions affect nature, we are introduced to poets, landscape architects, presidents, painters, activists, even sanitation engineers, and others who have forever altered how we think about the environment. The easy to use A–Z format provides instant access to these fascinating individuals, and frequent cross references indicate others with whom individuals worked (and sometimes clashed). End of entry references provide users with a starting point for further research.

"Highly recommended for high school, academic, and public libraries needing environmental biographical information." –Library Journal/Starred Review

Two Volume Set; Hardcover ISBN 1-57607-385-8 $175.00

World Cultural Leaders of the Twentieth Century

An expansive two volume set that covers 450 worldwide cultural icons, World Cultural Leaders of the Twentieth Century includes each person's works, achievements, and professional careers in a thorough essay. Who was the originator of the term "documentary"? Which poet married the daughter of the famed novelist Thomas Mann in order to help her escape Nazi Germany? Which British writer served as an agent in Russia against the Bolsheviks before the 1917 revolution? These and many more questions are answered in this illuminating text. A handy two volume set that makes it easy to look up 450 worldwide cultural icons: novelists, poets, playwrights, painters, sculptors, architects, dancers, choreographers, actors, directors, filmmakers, singers, composers, and musicians. World Cultural Leaders of the Twentieth Century provides entries (many of them illustrated) covering the person's works, achievements, and professional career in a thorough essay and offers interesting facts and statistics. Entries are fully cross-referenced so that readers can learn how various individuals influenced others. A thorough general index completes the coverage.

"Fills a need for handy, concise information on a wide array of international cultural figures." –ARBA

Two Volume Set; Hardcover ISBN 1-57607-038-7 $175.00

To preview any of our Directories Risk-Free for 30 days, call (800) 562-2139 or fax to (518) 789-0556

Universal Reference Publications
Statistical & Demographic Reference Books

America's Top-Rated Cities, 2007

America's Top-Rated Cities provides current, comprehensive statistical information and other essential data in one easy-to-use source on the 100 "top" cities that have been cited as the best for business and living in the U.S. This handbook allows readers to see, at a glance, a concise social, business, economic, demographic and environmental profile of each city, including brief evaluative comments. In addition to detailed data on Cost of Living, Finances, Real Estate, Education, Major Employers, Media, Crime and Climate, city reports now include Housing Vacancies, Tax Audits, Bankruptcy, Presidential Election Results and more. This outstanding source of information will be widely used in any reference collection.

"The only source of its kind that brings together all of this information into one easy-to-use source. It will be beneficial to many business and public libraries." –ARBA

00 pages, 4 Volume Set; Softcover ISBN 1-59237-184-1, $195.00

America's Top-Rated Smaller Cities, 2006/07

A perfect companion to *America's Top-Rated Cities*, *America's Top-Rated Smaller Cities* provides current, comprehensive business and living profiles of smaller cities (population 25,000-99,999) that have been cited as the best for business and living in the United States. Sixty cities make up this 2004 edition of *America's Top-Rated Smaller Cities*, all are top-ranked by Population Growth, Median Income, Unemployment Rate and Crime Rate. City reports reflect the most current data available on a wide-range of statistics, including Employment & Earnings, Household Income, Unemployment Rate, Population Characteristics, Taxes, Cost of Living, Education, Health Care, Public Safety, Recreation, Media, Air & Water Quality and much more. Plus, each city report contains a Background of the City, and an Overview of the State Finances. *America's Top-Rated Smaller Cities* offers a reliable, one-stop source for statistical data that, before now, could only be found scattered in hundreds of sources. This volume is designed for a wide range of readers: individuals considering relocating a residence or business; professionals considering expanding their business or changing careers; general and market researchers; real estate consultants; human resource personnel; urban planners and investors.

"Provides current, comprehensive statistical information in one easy-to-use source... Recommended for public and academic libraries and specialized collections." –Library Journal

00 pages; Softcover ISBN 1-59237-135-3, $160.00

Profiles of America: Facts, Figures & Statistics for Every Populated Place in the United States

Profiles of America is the only source that pulls together, in one place, statistical, historical and descriptive information about every place in the United States in an easy-to-use format. This award winning reference set, now in its second edition, compiles statistics and data from over 20 different sources – the latest census information has been included along with more than nine brand new statistical topics. This Four-Volume Set details over 40,000 places, from the biggest metropolis to the smallest unincorporated hamlet, and provides statistical details and information on over 50 different topics including Geography, Climate, Population, Vital Statistics, Economy, Income, Taxes, Education, Housing, Health & Environment, Public Safety, Newspapers, Transportation, Presidential Election Results and Information Contacts or Chambers of Commerce. Profiles are arranged, for ease-of-use, by state and then by county. Each county begins with a County-Wide Overview and is followed by information for each Community in that particular county. The Community profiles within the county are arranged alphabetically. *Profiles of America* is a virtual snapshot of America at your fingertips and a unique compilation of information that will be widely used in any reference collection.

A Library Journal Best Reference Book "An outstanding compilation." –Library Journal

,000 pages; Four Volume Set; Softcover ISBN 1-891482-80-7, $595.00

The Comparative Guide to American Suburbs, 2007

The Comparative Guide to American Suburbs is a one-stop source for Statistics on the 2,000+ suburban communities surrounding the 50 largest metropolitan areas – their population characteristics, income levels, economy, school system and important data on how they compare to one another. Organized into 50 Metropolitan Area chapters, each chapter contains an overview of the Metropolitan Area, a detailed Map followed by a comprehensive Statistical Profile of each Suburban Community, including Contact Information, Physical Characteristics, Population Characteristics, Income, Economy, Unemployment Rate, Cost of Living, Education, Chambers of Commerce and more. Next, statistical data is sorted into Ranking Tables that rank the suburbs by twenty different criteria, including Population, Per Capita Income, Unemployment Rate, Crime Rate, Cost of Living and more. *The Comparative Guide to American Suburbs* is the best source for locating data on suburbs. Those looking to relocate, as well as those doing preliminary market research, will find this an invaluable timesaving resource.

"Public and academic libraries will find this compilation useful...The work draws together figures from many sources and will be especially helpful for job relocation decisions." – Booklist

700 pages; Softcover ISBN 1-59237-180-9, $130.00

To preview any of our Directories Risk-Free for 30 days, call (800) 562-2139 or fax to (518) 789-0556

The Asian Databook: Statistics for all US Counties & Cities with Over 10,000 Population

This is the first-ever resource that compiles statistics and rankings on the US Asian population. *The Asian Databook* presents over 20 statistical data points for each city and county, arranged alphabetically by state, then alphabetically by place name. Data reported for each place includes Population, Languages Spoken at Home, Foreign-Born, Educational Attainment, Income Figures, Poverty Status, Homeownership, Home Values & Rent, and more. Next, in the Rankings Section, the top 75 places are listed for each data element. These easy-to-access ranking tables allow the user to quickly determine trends and population characteristics. This kind of comparative data can not be found elsewhere, in print or on the web, in a format that's as easy-to-use or more concise. A useful resource for those searching for demographics data, career search and relocation information and also for market research. With data ranging from Ancestry to Education, *The Asian Databook* presents a useful compilation of information that will be a much-needed resource in the reference collection of any public or academic library along with the marketing collection of any company whose primary focus in on the Asian population.

1,000 pages; Softcover ISBN 1-59237-044-6 $150.00

The Hispanic Databook: Statistics for all US Counties & Cities with Over 10,000 Population

Previously published by Toucan Valley Publications, this second edition has been completely updated with figures from the latest census and has been broadly expanded to include dozens of new data elements and a brand new Rankings section. The Hispanic population in the United States has increased over 42% in the last 10 years and accounts for 12.5% of the total US population. For ease-of-use, *The Hispanic Databook* presents over 20 statistical data points for each city and county, arranged alphabetically by state, then alphabetically by place name. Data reported for each place includes Population, Languages Spoken at Home, Foreign-Born, Educational Attainment, Income Figures, Poverty Status, Homeownership, Home Values & Rent, and more. Next, in the Rankings Section, the top 75 places are listed for each data element. These easy-to-access ranking tables allow the user to quickly determine trends and population characteristics. This kind of comparative data can not be found elsewhere, in print or on the web, in a format that's as easy-to-use or more concise. A useful resource for those searching for demographics data, career search and relocation information and also for market research. With data ranging from Ancestry to Education, *The Hispanic Databook* presents a useful compilation of information that will be a much-needed resource in the reference collection of any public or academic library along with the marketing collection of any company whose primary focus in on the Hispanic population.

*"This accurate, clearly presented volume of selected Hispanic demographics i
recommended for large public libraries and research collections."-Library Journal*

1,000 pages; Softcover ISBN 1-59237-008-X, $150.00

Ancestry in America: A Comparative Guide to Over 200 Ethnic Backgrounds

This brand new reference work pulls together thousands of comparative statistics on the Ethnic Backgrounds of all populated places in the United States with populations over 10,000. Never before has this kind of information been reported in a single volume. Section One, Statistics by Place, is made up of a list of over 200 ancestry and race categories arranged alphabetically by each of the 5,000 different places with populations over 10,000. The population number of the ancestry group in that city or town is provided along with the percent that group represents of the total population. This informative city-by-city section allows the user to quickly and easily explore the ethnic makeup of all major population bases in the United States. Section Two, Comparative Rankings, contains three table for each ethnicity and race. In the first table, the top 150 populated places are ranked by population number for that particular ancestry group, regardless of population. In the second table, the top 150 populated places are ranked by the percent of the total population for that ancestry group. In the third table, those top 150 populated places with 10,000 population are ranked by population number for each ancestry group. These easy-to-navigate tables allow users to see ancestry population patterns and make city-by-city comparisons as well. Plus, as an added bonus with the purchase of *Ancestry in America*, a free companion CD-ROM is available that lists statistics and rankings for all of the 35,000 populated places in the United States. This brand new, information-packed resource will serve a wide-range or research requests for demographics, population characteristics, relocation information and much more. *Ancestry in America: A Comparative Guide to Over 200 Ethnic Backgrounds* will be an important acquisition to all reference collections.

*"This compilation will serve a wide range of research requests for population characteristi
... it offers much more detail than other sources." —Bookli*

1,500 pages; Softcover ISBN 1-59237-029-2, $225.00

To preview any of our Directories Risk-Free for 30 days, call (800) 562-2139 or fax to (518) 789-0556

he American Tally: Statistics & Comparative Rankings for U.S. Cities with Populations over 10,000

his important statistical handbook compiles, all in one place, comparative statistics on all U.S. cities and towns with a 10,000+ pulation. *The American Tally* provides statistical details on over 4,000 cities and towns and profiles how they compare with one other in Population Characteristics, Education, Language & Immigration, Income & Employment and Housing. Each section begins th an alphabetical listing of cities by state, allowing for quick access to both the statistics and relative rankings of any city. Next, the ghest and lowest cities are listed in each statistic. These important, informative lists provide quick reference to which cities are at th extremes of the spectrum for each statistic. Unlike any other reference, *The American Tally* provides quick, easy access to mparative statistics – a must-have for any reference collection.

"A solid library reference." -Bookwatch

0 pages; Softcover ISBN 1-930956-29-0, $125.00

he Environmental Resource Handbook, 2007/08

e *Environmental Resource Handbook* is the most up-to-date and comprehensive source for Environmental Resources and Statistics. ction I: Resources provides detailed contact information for thousands of information sources, including Associations & ganizations, Awards & Honors, Conferences, Foundations & Grants, Environmental Health, Government Agencies, National Parks Wildlife Refuges, Publications, Research Centers, Educational Programs, Green Product Catalogs, Consultants and much more. ction II: Statistics, provides statistics and rankings on hundreds of important topics, including Children's Environmental Index, unicipal Finances, Toxic Chemicals, Recycling, Climate, Air & Water Quality and more. This kind of up-to-date environmental data, in one place, is not available anywhere else on the market place today. This vast compilation of resources and statistics is a must-ve for all public and academic libraries as well as any organization with a primary focus on the environment.

"…the intrinsic value of the information make it worth consideration by libraries with environmental collections and environmentally concerned users." –Booklist

00 pages; Softcover ISBN 1-59237-195-7, $155.00 ◆ Online Database $300.00

eather America, A Thirty-Year Summary of Statistical Weather Data and Rankings

is valuable resource provides extensive climatological data for over 4,000 National and Cooperative Weather Stations throughout e United States. *Weather America* begins with a new Major Storms section that details major storm events of the nation and a tional Rankings section that details rankings for several data elements, such as Maximum Temperature and Precipitation. The main dy of *Weather America* is organized into 50 state sections. Each section provides a Data Table on each Weather Station, organized phabetically, that provides statistics on Maximum and Minimum Temperatures, Precipitation, Snowfall, Extreme Temperatures, ggy Days, Humidity and more. State sections contain two brand new features in this edition – a City Index and a narrative escription of the climatic conditions of the state. Each section also includes a revised Map of the State that includes not only weather tions, but cities and towns.

"Best Reference Book of the Year." –Library Journal

013 pages; Softcover ISBN 1-891482-29-7, $175.00

rime in America's Top-Rated Cities

is volume includes over 20 years of crime statistics in all major crime categories: violent crimes, property crimes and total crime. *ime in America's Top-Rated Cities* is conveniently arranged by city and covers 76 top-rated cities. *Crime in America's Top-Rated Cities* fers details that compare the number of crimes and crime rates for the city, suburbs and metro area along with national crime trends r violent, property and total crimes. Also, this handbook contains important information and statistics on Anti-Crime Programs, ime Risk, Hate Crimes, Illegal Drugs, Law Enforcement, Correctional Facilities, Death Penalty Laws and much more. A much-eded resource for people who are relocating, business professionals, general researchers, the press, law enforcement officials and udents of criminal justice.

"Data is easy to access and will save hours of searching." –Global Enforcement Review

2 pages; Softcover ISBN 1-891482-84-X, $155.00

To preview any of our Directories Risk-Free for 30 days, call (800) 562-2139 or fax to (518) 789-0556